Diseases of the Nervous System

Arthur K. Asbury is Van Meter Professor Emeritus of
Neurology, Hospital of the University of Pennsylvania,
Philadelphia, USA

Guy M. McKhann is Professor of Neurology, The Zanvyl
Krieger Mind and Brain Institute, Johns Hopkins
University, Baltimore, Maryland, USA

W. Ian McDonald is Professor Emeritus, Institute of
Neurology, The National Hospital for Neurology and
Neurosurgery, Queen Square, London, UK

Peter J. Goadsby is Professor of Neurology, Institute of
Neurology, The National Hospital for Neurology and
Neurosurgery, Queen Square, London, UK

Justin C. McArthur is Professor of Neurology and
Epidemiology, Johns Hopkins University School of
Medicine, Baltimore, Maryland, USA

The third edition of a neurology classic, this two-volume
text is the most comprehensive neurology reference available. It encompasses epidemiology, pathology, pathophysiology, and clinical features of the full range of neurological
disorders. The basic principles of neurological dysfunction
are covered at cellular and molecular level by leading
experts in the field. Disease mechanisms are reviewed
comprehensively, with particular relevance to the principles of therapy.

Sections cover the general principles of neurological
disease, disorders of higher function, motor control,
special senses, spine and spinal cord, bodily function,
headache and pain, neuromuscular disorders, epilepsy,
cerebrovascular disorders, neoplastic disorders, autoimmune disorders, disorders of myelin, infections, trauma
and toxic disorders, degenerative disorders, and neurological manifestations of systemic conditions. Each section,
under the direction of one of the distinguished editors, is a
text-within-a-text, offering the most reliable account of its
topic currently available.

Contributors to this work include the leading clinicians
and clinical neuroscientists internationally. Current, comprehensive and authoritative, this is the definitive reference for neurologists, neurosurgeons, neuropsychiatrists,
indeed everyone with a professional or research interest in
the neurosciences.

From reviews of previous editions:

'A scholarly, well-crafted and attractive book . . . *Diseases of the
Nervous System* deserves a place in the library of every medical
school, neurology department, and neuroscience department'
New England Journal of Medicine

'All clinical neurologists and trainees in neurology will find it
invaluable as a reference and a way into the latest scientific
literature' *British Medical Journal*

'This is a superb book'
Journal of Neurology, Neurosurgery and Psychiatry

Diseases of the Nervous System

Clinical Neuroscience and Therapeutic Principles

Third Edition

VOLUME 1

Edited by

Arthur K. Asbury, MD
University of Pennsylvania School of Medicine
Philadelphia, USA

Guy M. McKhann, MD
The Zanvyl Krieger Mind and Brain Institute
Johns Hopkins University, Baltimore, MD, USA

W. Ian McDonald, MB, ChB, PhD
Institute of Neurology
The National Hospital for Neurology and Neurosurgery, London, UK

Peter J. Goadsby, MD, PhD
Institute of Neurology
The National Hospital for Neurology and Neurosurgery, London, UK

Justin C. McArthur, MB BS, MPH
Departments of Neurology and Epidemiology
Johns Hopkins University School of Medicine, Baltimore, MD, USA

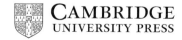

CAMBRIDGE
UNIVERSITY PRESS

PUBLISHED BY THE PRESS SYNDICATE OF THE UNIVERSITY OF CAMBRIDGE
The Pitt Building, Trumpington Street, Cambridge, United Kingdom

CAMBRIDGE UNIVERSITY PRESS
The Edinburgh Building, Cambridge CB2 2RU, UK
40 West 20th Street, New York, NY 10011-4211, USA
477 Williamstown Road, Port Melbourne, VIC 3207, Australia
Ruiz de Alarcón 13, 28014 Madrid, Spain
Dock House, The Waterfront, Cape Town 8001, South Africa

http://www. cambridge.org

Third edition © Cambridge University Press, 2002

First and second editions published by W.B. Saunders 1986, 1992

Third edition published by Cambridge University Press 2002

Printed in the United Kingdom at the University Press, Cambridge

Typeface Utopia 8.5/12pt.   *System* QuarkXPress™ [SE]

A catalogue record for this book is available from the British Library

Library of Congress Cataloguing in Publication data

Diseases of the nervous system / edited by Arthur K. Asbury . . . [et al.]. – 3rd ed.
    p. ;   cm.
Includes bibliographical references and indexes.
ISBN 0 521 79351 3 (hardback)
1. Nervous system – Diseases. I. Asbury, Arthur K., 1928–
[DNLM: 1. Nervous System Diseases. WL 140 D611 2001]
RC346 .M33 2001
616.8 – dc21   2001043713

ISBN 0 521 79351 3 hardback in two volumes

This text is dedicated to our many friends and colleagues who wrote the chapters, for their diligence, for their intellectual rigour, and for their belief in the vision of scientific and clinical excellence on which these volumes are predicated.

Contents

Contributors

EDITORS

Arthur K. Asbury
Department of Neurology
Hospital of the University of Pennsylvania
3400 Spruce Street
Philadelphia
PA 19104-4283
USA

Guy M. McKhann
The Zanvyl Krieger Mind and Brain Institute
Johns Hopkins University
338 Krieger Hall
3400 N. Charles Street
Baltimore
MD 21218-2689
USA

W. Ian McDonald
The National Hospital for Neurology and Neurosurgery
Queen Square
London WC1N 3BG, UK

Peter J. Goadsby
Institute of Neurology
National Hospital for Neurology and Neurosurgery
Queen Square
London WC1N 3BG
UK

Justin C. McArthur
Departments of Neurology and Epidemiology
Johns Hopkins University School of Medicine
600 N. Wolfe Street
Baltimore
MD 21287-7609
USA

CONTRIBUTORS

Ted Abel
Department of Biology
University of Pennsylvania
319 Leidy Laboratories
Philadelphia
PA 19104
USA

Gary M. Abrams
Department of Neurology
UCSF Mount Zion Medical Center
1600 Divisadero Street
San Francisco
CA 94115
USA

Paul D. Acton
Department of Radiology
University of Pennsylvania School of Medicine
Room 305
3700 Market Street
Philadelphia
PA 19104-3147
USA

Marilyn S. Albert
Department of Geriatrics
– Massachusetts General Hospital East
Department of Psychiatry and Neurology
Harvard Medical School
149 13th Street
Charlestown
MA 02129
USA

Jeffrey R. Alger
Department of Radiology
University of California at Los Angeles
Los Angeles, CA
USA

Douglas Arnold
Department of Neurology
Montreal Neurological Institute
Canada

Arthur K. Asbury
Department of Neurology
Hospital of the University of Pennsylvania
3400 Spruce Street
Philadelphia
PA 19104-4283
USA

James Ashe
Brain Sciences Center, VAMC
Department of Neurology and Neuroscience
University of Minnesota
One Veterans Drive
Minneapolis
MN 55417
USA

Mohammed BenDebba
Department of Neurosurgery
Johns Hopkins Medical Institute
Meyer 7-109
600 N. Wolfe Street
Baltimore
MD 21287
USA

James L. Bernat
Neurology Section
Dartmouth-Hitchcock Medical Ctr.
1 Medical Center Drive
Lebanon
NH 03756
USA

Kailash P. Bhatia
National Hospital for Neurology and Neurosurgery
Institute of Neurology
Queen Square
London WC1N 3BG
UK

Shawn J. Bird
Department of Neurology
Hospital of the University of Pennsylvania
3 W Gates
3400 Spruce Street
Philadelphia
PA 19104-4283
USA

Thomas P. Bleck
Department of Neurology, 394
University of Virginia Health Sciences Center
McKim Hall 2025
Charlottesville
VA 22908-0001
USA

Peter C. Blumbergs
Department of Neuropathology
Institute of Medical and Veterinary Science
University of Adelaide
Adelaide 5000
South Australia

Nikolai Bogduk
Newcastle Bone and Joint Institute
University of Newcastle
Royal Newcastle Hospital
PO Box 664J
Newcastle
NSW 2300
Australia

Charles F. Bolton
University Western Ontario
London Health Sciences Centre
375 South Street
London
Ontario N5A 4G5
Canada

David R. Borchelt
Department of Pathology
Johns Hopkins University School of Medicine
558 Ross Research Building
720 Rutland Avenue
Baltimore
MD 21205-2196
USA

Michael Brada
Department of Clinical Oncology
The Institute of Cancer Research
The Royal Marsden NHS Trust
Downs Road
Sutton
Surrey SM2 5PT
UK

Thomas Brandt
Department of Neurology
Klinikum Grosshadern
University of Munich
Marchioninistr. 15
Munich 81377
Germany

Henry Brem
Department of Neurosurgery
Johns Hopkins Medical Institutions
466 Carnegie
Baltimore
MD 21287
USA

Steven M. Bromley
Neurological Institute of New York
Columbia-Presbyterian Medical Center
New York
NY 10032
USA

Peter Brown
Sobell Department of Motor Neuroscience
Institute of Neurology
Queen Square
London WC2N 3BG
UK

John C.M. Brust
College of Physicians & Surgeons of Columbia University
Harlem Hospital Center
506 Lenox Avenue
New York
NY 10037
USA

Silvia A. Bunge
Department of Psychology
Stanford University School of Medicine
Stanford
CA 94305
USA

Huaibin Cai
Department of Pathology
Johns Hopkins University School of Medicine
558 Ross Research Building
720 Rutland Avenue
Baltimore
MD 21205-2196
USA

Stephen C. Cannon
Department of Neurobiology
Harvard Medical School
Department of Neurology
Massachusetts General Hospital
55 Fruit Street
Boston
MA 02114
USA

Louis R. Caplan
Harvard Medical School and Department of Neurology
Beth Israel Deaconess Medical Center
330 Brookline Avenue
Boston
MA 02215
USA

Juan Ricardo Carhuapoma
Division of Critical Care Neurology
Neurological Institute
New York Presbyterian Hospital
Columbia University College of Physicians and Surgeons
New York
NY
USA

Lucinda J. Carr
Consultant Pediatric Neurologist
Great Ormond Street Hospital for Children
NHS Trust
Great Ormond Street
London WC1N 3JN
UK

Borka Ceranic
Neuro-otology Department
The National Hospital for Neurology and Neurosurgery
Queen Square
London WC2N 3BG
UK

Richard E. Chaisson
Johns Hopkins Medical Institutions
455 1830 East Monument Street
Baltimore
MD 21205
USA

Vinay Chaudhry
Department of Neurology
Johns Hopkins School of Medicine
600 N. Wolfe Street
Meyer 6-119
Baltimore
MD 21287
USA

Dennis W. Choi
Department of Neurosciences
Merck Research Laboratories
Merck & Co. Inc., 770 Sumneytown Pike
West Point, PA 19486, USA

Hannah Cock
Institute of Neurology
Queen Square
London WC1N 3BG
UK

Alastair Compston
University of Cambridge Clinical School
Addenbrooke's Hospital
Hills Road
Cambridge CB2 2QQ
UK

Patricia K. Coyle
Department of Neurology
SUNY at Stony Brook
HSC T12/020
Stony Brook
NY 11794-8121
USA

Charles A. Dackis
Treatment and Research Center
Department of Psychiatry
University of Pennsylvania
3900 Chesnut Street
Philadelphia
PA 19104-6178
USA

Antonio R. Damasio
Department of Neurology
University of Iowa
College of Medicine
200 Hawkins Drive
Iowa City
IA 52242-1053
USA

Larry E. Davis
Neurology Service
VA Hospital
2100 Ridgecrest Drive S.E.
Albuquerque
NM 87108
USA

Mahlon R. DeLong
Department of Neurology
Emory University School of Medicine
Woodruff Memorial Building
Suite 600
1639 Pierce Drive
Atlanta
GA 30322
USA

Martha Bridge Denckla
Kennedy–Krieger Institute
707 North Broadway
Suite 516
Baltimore
MD 21205
USA

J. Raymond DePaulo
Department of Psychiatry
Johns Hopkins University School of Medicine
600 N. Wolfe Street
Baltimore
MD 21287
USA

John A. Detre
Department of Neurology
Hospital of the University of Pennsylvania
3400 Spruce Street
Philadelphia
PA 19104-4283
USA

Ivan F. Diamond
Ernest Gallo Clinic and Research Center
University of California, San Francisco
5858 Horton Street
Suite 200
Emoryville
CA 94608
USA

Martin Dichgans
Department of Neurology
Kliniken Grosshadern
Mardiounivistrasse 15
Munchen, D-81377
Germany

Salvatore DiMauro
Department of Neurology
Columbia University
College of Physicians and Surgeons
630 West 168th Street
New York
NY 10032
USA

Richard L. Doty
Smell and Taste Center
Hospital of the University of Pennsylvania
5 Ravdin Building
3400 Spruce Street
Philadelphia
PA 19104-4283
USA

Patrick M. Dougherty
Department of Anesthesiology
M.D. Anderson Hospital
Houston
TX
USA

David A. Drachman
Department of Neurology
University of Massachusetts Medical School
55 Lake Avenue North
Worcester
MA 06155
USA

Daniel B. Drachman
Neurology/Neuromuscular Unit
Johns Hopkins School of Medicine
6-119 Meyer Building
600 N. Wolfe Street
Baltimore
MD 21287-0001
USA

John S. Duncan
Institute of Neurology
Queen Square
London WC1N 4BG
UK

Benjamin H. Eidelman
Department of Neurology
Mayo Clinic, Jacksonville
4500 San Pablo Road
Jacksonville
FL 32224-1865
USA

Marian L. Evatt
Department of Neurology
Emory University School of Medicine
Woodruff Building
Suite 600
139 Pierce Drive
Atlanta
GA 30322
USA

Simon F. Farmer
National Hospital for Neurology and Neurosurgery
Queen Square
London WC1N 3BG
UK

Thomas E. Feasby
Department of Clinical Neurosciences
University of Calgary
Foothills Hospital
1403 29th Street NW
Calgary
AB T2N 2T9
Canada

Robert A. Felberg
Department of Neurology
Ochsner Clinic Foundation
1514 Jefferson Highway
New Orleans
LA 70121
USA

Michael D. Ferrari
Department of Neurology
Leiden University Medical Centre
PO Box 9600
2300 RC Leiden
The Netherlands

Kenneth H. Fischbeck
Neurogenetics Branch
National Institute of Neurological Disorders and Stroke
National Institutes of Health
Building 10, Room 3B-14
10 Center Drive
Bethesda
MD 20892-1250
USA

Robert S. Fisher
Department of Neurology
Stanford University School of Medicine
Room H3160
300 Pasteur Drive
Stanford
CA 94305-5235
USA

Clare J. Fowler
Institute of Neurology
Queen Square
London WC1N 3BG
UK

Hans-Joachim Freund
Medizinische Einrichtungen
Universitat Dusseldorf
Neurologische Klinik
Moorenstrasse 5
Dusseldorf 40225
Germany

John D.E. Gabrieli
Department of Psychology
Stanford University
Stanford
CA 94305
USA

Romergryko G. Geocadin
Departments of Neurology and Anesthesiology Critical
   Care Medicine
Johns Hopkins University Hospital
400 N. Wolfe Street
Baltimore
MD 21287
USA

Alfred L. George, Jr
Departments of Medicine and Pharmacology
Vanderbilt University Medical Center
451 Preston Building
Nashville
TN 37232-6304
USA

Apostolos P. Georgopoulos
Veterans Administration Medical Center
Department of Neurology
Neuroscience and Psychiatry
University of Minnesota
One Veterans Drive
Minneapolis
MN 55417
USA

Gavin Giovannoni
Institute of Neurology
Queen Square
London WC1N 3BG
UK

Jonathan D. Glass
Department of Neurology
Emory University School of Medicine
Whitehead Biomedical Research Building
615 Michael Street
WWB 600
Atlanta GA 30322
USA

Peter J. Goadsby
Institute of Neurology
The National Hospital for Neurology and Neurosurgery
Queen Square
London WC1N 3BG
UK

Susanne Goldstein
Human Motor Control Section
National Institute of Neurological Disorders and Stroke
National Institutes of Health
Bldg 10, Room 5N226
10 Center Drive, MSC 1428
Bethesda
MD 20892-1428
USA

Estrella Gómez-Tortosa
Servicio de Neurología
Fundación Jiménez Díaz
Avda. Reyes Católicos 2
Madrid 28040
Spain

Barry Gordon
Division of Cognitive Neurology
The Johns Hopkins University School of Medicine
222 Meyer, 600 N. Wolfe St.
Baltimore
MD 21287-7222
USA

M. Sean Grady
Department of Neurosurgery
Hospital of the University of Pennsylvania
5th floor, Silverstein Pavilion
3400 Spruce Street
Philadelphia
PA 19104-4283
USA

Steven B. Graff-Radford
Cedars–Sinai Medical Center
444 South San Vicente, Suite 1101
Los Angeles
CA 90048
USA

Joel D. Greenspan
Department of OCB5
Dental School
University of Maryland
Baltimore, MD, USA

Michael D. Greicius
Department of Psychiatry and Behavioral Sciences
Stanford University
416 Quarry Road
CA 94305
USA

Diane E. Griffin
Department of Molecular Microbiology and Immunology
Johns Hopkins University Bloomberg School of Public
    Health
615 N. Wolfe Street
Baltimore
MD 21205
USA

Robert C. Griggs
Department of Neurology
University of Rochester School of Medicine and Dentistry
601 Elmwood Avenue
Rochester
NY 14642
USA

James C. Grotta
Department of Neurology
University of Texas Houston
Medical School Bldg. MSB 7-044
6431 Fannin Street
Houston
TX 77030
USA

Michael A. Grotzer
Division of Oncology/Hematology
University Children's Hospital
Steinwiesstrasse 75
CH-8032
Zurich
Switzerland

John H. Growdon
Department of Neurology
Harvard Medical School Memory Disorders Unit
Neurology Service
Massachusetts General Hospital
WACC 830
Boston
MA 02115
USA

Renzo Guerrini
Neurosciences Unit
Institute of Child Health and Great Ormond Street
    Hospital
University College
The Wolfson Centre
Mecklenburgh Square
London WC1N 2AP, UK

Dakshin Gullapalli
Department of Neurology
University of Virginia School of Medicine
Charlottesville
VA 22908
USA

Joost Haan
Department of Neurology
Leiden University Medical Centre
PO Box 9600
2300 RC Leiden
The Netherlands

Ronald G. Haller
Neuromuscular Center
Institute for Exercise and Environmental Medicine
Presbyterian Hospital
7232 Greenville
Dallas
TX 75231
USA

Mark Hallett
NINDS
National Institutes of Health
Building 10, Room 5N 226
10 Center Drive, MSC 1428
Bethesda
MD 20892-1428
USA

Shaheen Hamdy
Department of GI Science
Clinical Sciences Building
Hope Hospital
Eccles Old Road
Salford
Manchester M6 8HD
UK

Daniel F. Hanley
Department of Neurology
Johns Hopkins Hospital
600 N. Wolfe Street
Meyer 6-113
Baltimore
MD 21287
USA

Paul J. Harrison
University Departments of Psychiatry and Clinical
   Neurology (Neuropathology)
Warneford Hospital
Neurosciences Building
Oxford OX3 7JX
UK

John Hart, Jr
Donald W. Reynolds Center on Aging
University of Arkansas Medical School
4301 W. Markham St.
Little Rock
AR 72205, USA

Hans-Peter Hartung
Department of Neurology
Heinrich-Heine-University
Duesseldorf
Moorenstr. 5
D-40225 Duesseldorf
Germany

Kenneth M. Heilman
Department of Neurology
University of Florida College of Medicine
Box 100238
Gainesville
Fl 32610
USA

Hans-Joachen Heinze
Klin. Neurophysiologie
Otto-von-Guericke
Universitat Magdeburg
Leipziger Street
Magdeburg 44,3910
Germany

David B. Hellmann
Department of Medicine
Johns Hopkins Bayview Medical Center
Johns Hopkins University School of Medicine
4940 Eastern Avenue
Baltimore
MD 21224
USA

Michael D. Hill
Department of Clinical Neurosciences
University of Calgary
6020 Dalcastle Crescent N.W.
Calgary
AB T3A 1S4
Canada

Jeremy Hobart
Department of Neurology
The Peninsula Medical School
Derriford Hospital
Plymouth, Devon, UK

Reinhard Hohlfeld
Institute for Clinical Neuroimmunology and Department
   of Neurology
Ludwig-Maximillians University
Klinikum Grosshaden
Marchioninistrasse 15
D-81366 Munich
Germany

Alexander H. Hoon, Jr
Department of Pediatrics
Johns Hopkins University School of Medicine
Kennedy–Krieger Institute
707 N. Broadway
Baltimore
MD 21205
USA

Fay B. Horak
Neurological Sciences Institute
Department of Pharmacology and Physiology
Oregon Health Sciences University
Portland
OR 97201
USA

Jyh-Gong Hou
Parkinson's Disease Center and Movement Disorders
    Clinic
Department of Neurology
Baylor College of Medicine
6550 Fannin, Suite 1801
Houston
TX 77030
USA

Matthew A. Howard III
Division of Neurosurgery
University of Iowa Hospitals and Clinics
200 Hawkins Drive
Iowa City
IA 52242
USA

Orest Hurko
Department of Investigational Medicine
GlaxoSmithKline Pharmaceuticals
Neurology Centre for Excellence in Drug Discovery
New Frontiers Science Park North H17 2-233
Third Avenue
Harlow
Essex CM19 5AW
UK

Bradley T. Hyman
Department of Neurology
Massachusetts General Hospital East
149 13th Street
Charlestown
MA 02129
USA

David N. Irani
Department of Molecular Biology and Immunology
Bloomberg School of Public Health
Johns Hopkins University
615 N. Wolfe Street
Baltimore
MD 21205
USA

Michael C. Irizarry
Department of Neurology
Massachusetts General Hospital East
149 13th Street
Charlestown
MA 02129
 USA

Joseph Jankovic
Parkinson's Disease Center and Movement Disorders
    Clinic
Department of Neurology
Baylor College of Medicine
6550 Fannin, Suite 1801
Houston
TX 77030
USA

James L. Januzzi, Jr
Cardiology Division and Department of Medicine
Massachusetts General Hospital
Harvard Medical School
55 Fruit Street
Boston MA 02114
USA

Cheryl A. Jay
UCSF Department of Neurology
Neurology Service, 4M62
San Francisco General Hospital
1001 Potrero Avenue
San Francisco
CA 94110
USA

David C. Jimerson
Department of Psychiatry
Beth Israel Deaconess Medical Center and Harvard
    Medical School
330 Brookline Avenue
Boston
MA 02215
USA

Michael V. Johnston
Kennedy–Krieger Institute
Departments of Neurology and Pediatrics
Johns Hopkins University School of Medicine
Suite 610
707 North Broadway
Baltimore
MD 21205
USA

Ricardo E. Jorge
Department of Psychiatry
University of Iowa College of Medicine
200 Hawkins Drive
Iowa City
IA 52242
USA

Peter W. Kaplan
Department of Neurology
Johns Hopkins Medical Center at Bayview
4940 Eastern Avenue
Baltimore
MD 21224-2780
USA

Barbara Illowsky Karp
Office of the Clinical Director and Human Motor Control
    Section NINDS
National Institutes of Health
Building 10, Room 5N 226
10 Center Drive, MSC 1428
Bethesda
MD 20892-1428
USA

Raymond J. Kelleher, III
Massachusetts Institute of Technology
77 Massachusetts Avenue
Bldg. E25-435
Cambridge
MA 02139-4307
USA

Christopher Kennard
Division of Neurosciences and Psychological Medicine
Imperial College School of Medicine
Charing Cross Hospital
St Dunstan's Road
London W6 8RP
UK

Bernd C. Kieseier
Department of Neurology
Heinrich-Heine-University
Moorenstrasse 5
D-40225 Düsseldorf
Germany

John Laterra
Department of Neurology
Johns Hopkins Medical Institutions
Carnegie Room 490
600 N. Wolfe Street
Baltimore
MD 21287-7709
USA

Jin-Moo Lee
Department of Neurology Box 8111
Washington University School of Medicine
660 South Euclid Avenue
St. Louis
MO 63105
USA

R. John Leigh
Department of Neurology
University Hospitals of Cleveland
11100 Euclid Avenue
Cleveland
OH 44106
USA

Ramon C. Leiguarda
Raúl Carrea Institute of Neurological Research
FLENI
Montanueses 2325
Buenos Aires
1428 1112
Argentina

Frederick A. Lenz
Department of Neurosurgery
Johns Hopkins Hospital
7-113 Meyer
600 N. Wolfe Street
Baltimore
MD 21287
USA

Andrew P. Lieberman
Neurogenetics Branch
National Institute of Neurological Disorders and Stroke
National Institutes of Health
Building 10, Room 3B-14
10 Center Drive
Bethesda
MD 20892-1250
USA

Richard B. Lipton
Department of Neurology, Epidemiology and Social
    Medicine
Albert Einstein College of Medicine
New York
USA
and Innovative Medical Research
1200 High Ridge Road
Stamford, CT 06905, USA

xxiv   List of contributors

Donlin M. Long
Department of Neurosurgery
Johns Hopkins Hospital
600 N. Wolfe Street
Meyer 7-109
Baltimore
MD 21287
USA

Linda M. Luxon
Neuro-otology Department
The National Hospital for Neurology and Neurosurgery
Queen Square
London WC2N 3BG
UK

Dean F. MacKinnon
Department of Psychiatry
Johns Hopkins University School of Medicine
600 N. Wolfe Street
Baltimore
MD 21287
USA

Yukari C. Manabe
Department of Medicine
Johns Hopkins Medical Institutions
455 1830 East Monument Street
Baltimore
MD 21205
USA

Richard J. Mannion
Neural Plasticity Research Group
Department of Anesthesia and Critical Care
Massachusetts General Hospital East and Harvard
    Medical School
149 13th Street
Charlestown
MA 02129
USA

Russell L. Margolis
Department of Psychiatry and Behavioral Sciences
Johns Hopkins University
600 N. Wolfe Street
Baltimore
MD 21205
USA

Christopher J. Mathias
Imperial College School of Medicine
Neurovascular Medicine Unit
St. Mary's Hospital
Praed Street
London W2 1NY
UK

Justin C. McArthur
Departments of Neurology and Epidemiology
Johns Hopkins University
600 N. Wolfe Street
Baltimore
MD 21287-7609
USA

W. Ian McDonald
Institute of Neurology
The National Hospital for Neurology and Neurosurgery
Queen Square
London WC1N 3BG, UK

John W. McDonald, III
Department of Neurology and Neurological Surgery
Center for the Study of Nervous System Injury
McMillan Bldg.
Washington University School of Medicine
Campus Box 8111, Room 204
660 South Euclid Avenue
St. Louis
MO 63110-1010
USA

Steven L. McIntire
Department of Neurology, UCSF
Suite 200
5858 Horton Street
Emoryville
CA 94608
USA

Tracy K. McIntosh
Department of Neurosurgery
Hospital of the University of Pennsylvania
5th floor, Silverstein Pavilion
Philadelphia
PA 19104-4283
USA

Guy M. McKhann
The Zanvyl Krieger Mind & Brain Institute
Johns Hopkins University
338 Krieger Hall
3400 N. Charles Street
Baltimore
MD 21218-2689
USA

Guy M. McKhann, II
Department of Neurological Surgery
Columbia University
Neurological Institute Room 428
710 168th Street
New York
NY 10032
USA

Pamela J. McLean
Department of Neurology
Massachusetts General Hospital East
149 13th Street
Charlestown
MA 02129
USA

Gillian E. Mead
Department of Clinical and Surgical Sciences (Geriatric
    Medicine)
University of Edinburgh
21 Chalmers Street
Edinburgh EH3 9EW
UK

Donna Mergler
CINBOISE
University of Quebec at Montreal
CP 8888 succ Centre-ville
Montreal
Quebec H3C 3P8
Canada

Bruce L. Miller
Department of Neurology
UCSF School of Medicine
Parnassus Avenue
San Francisco CA 94143
USA

David H. Miller
University Department of Clinical Neurology
Institute of Neurology
Queen Square
London WC2N 3BG
UK

Ganeshwaran H. Mochida
Department of Neurology
Beth Israel Deaconess Medical Center
Harvard Institutes of Medicine, Room 816
77 Avenue Louis Pasteur
Boston
MA 02115
USA

Robert Y. Moore
Department of Neurology
University of Pittsburgh
Liliane S. Kaufmann Building
3471 5th Avenue, Suite 811
Pittsburgh
PA 15213
USA

Antony Morland
Department of Psychology
Royal Holloway College
Egham
Surrey TW20 0EX
UK

Hugo W. Moser
Departments of Neurology and Pediatrics
Johns Hopkins University
Kennedy–Krieger Institute
707 N. Broadway
Room 503
Baltimore
MD 21205
USA

Eric A. Nofzinger
Department of Psychiatry and Neuroscience
University of Pittsburgh School of Medicine
3811 O'Hara Street
Pittsburgh
PA 15213
USA

John G. Nutt
Department of Neurology L226
Oregon Health Sciences University
3181 SW Sam Jackson Park Road
Portland
OR 97201
USA

Charles P. O'Brien
Treatment and Research Center
University of Pennsylvania Department of Psychiatry
3900 Chesnut Street
Philadelphia
PA 19104-6178
USA

Puneet Opal
Institute for Molecular Genetics
Department of Pediatrics
Baylor College of Medicine
One Baylor Plaza
Houston
TX 77030
USA

Richard W. Orrell
Department of Clinical Neurosciences
Royal Free and University College Medical School
Royal Free Campus
Rowland Hill Street
London NW3 2PF
UK

Mitsuhiro Osame
The Third Dept. of Internal Medicine
Faculty of Medicine
Kagoshima University Hospital
Sakuragaoka 8 35-1
Kagoshima 890-8520
Japan

Lucio Parmeggiani
Institute of Child Health and Great Ormond Street
    Hospital for Children
University College London
The Wolfson Centre
Mecklenburgh Square
London WC1N 2AP
UK

Roy A. Patchell
Department of Neurosurgery and Neurology
University of Kentucky Medical Center
800 Rose Street
Lexington
KY 40536
USA

Emilio Perucca
Clinical Pharmacology Unit
Department of Internal Medicine and Therapeutics
University of Pavia
Piazza Botta 10
27100 Pavia
Italy

Ognen A.C. Petroff
Department of Neurology
Yale University Medical School
333 Cedar Street
New Haven, CT 06510
USA

Peter C. Phillips
Department of Neurology
Children's Hospital of Philadelphia
34th & Civic Center Blvd.
4th Floor Wood Bldg.
Philadelphia
PA 19104-4399
USA

David E. Pleasure
Departments of Neurology and Pediatrics
Children's Hospital of Philadelphia
Room 516H Abramson Research Building
3517 Civic Center Boulevard
Philadelphia
PA 19104
USA

Samuel J. Pleasure
Department of Neurology
University of California, San Francisco
Room S-256C
513 Parnassus Avenue
San Francisco
CA 94143
USA

John D. Pollard
Institute of Clinical Neurosciences
Royal Prince Alfred Hospital
University of Sydney
Camperdown
Sydney NSW 2050
Australia

Russell K. Portenoy
Department of Pain Medicine and Palliative Care
Beth Israel Medical Center
First Avenue at 16th Street
New York
NY 10003
USA

Jerome B. Posner
Department of Neurology
Memorial Sloan-Kettering Cancer Center
1275 York Avenue
New York
NY 10021
USA

Donald L. Price
Division of Neuropathology
Departments of Neurology, Pathology and Neuroscience
Johns Hopkins Medical Institutions
558 Ross Research Bldg.
720 Rutland Avenue
Baltimore
MD 21205
USA

James W. Prichard
Department of Neurology Box 60
Yale Medical School
West Tisbury
MA 02575
USA

Stanley B. Prusiner
Institute for Neurodegenerative Diseases
Departments of Neurology and of Biochemistry and
  Biophysics
Box 0518, Parnassus Avenue
University of California, San Francisco
San Francisco
CA 94143-0518
USA

Scott L. Rauch
Department of Psychiatry, Harvard Medical School
Massachusetts General Hospital East
149 13th Street
Boston
MA 02129
USA

Gerald V. Raymond
Department of Neurology
Johns Hopkins University School of Medicine
Kennedy–Krieger Institute
707 N. Broadway
Baltimore
MD 21205
USA

Jeremy H. Rees
National Hospital for Neurology and Neurosurgery
Queen Square
London WC1N 3BG
UK

Michael J. Regan
Division of Rheumatology
Johns Hopkins University School of Medicine
1830 East Monument Street
Suite 7500
Baltimore
MD 21205
USA

Louis Reik, Jr.
Department of Neurology
University of Connecticut Health Center
263 Farmington Avenue
Farmington
CT 06030
USA

Mary Reilly
Department of Clinical Neurology
The National Hospital for Neurology and Neurosurgery
Queen Square
London WC2N 3BG
UK

E. Steve Roach
Department of Neurology
University of Texas
Southwestern Medical Center
5323 Harry Hines Blvd.
Dallas
TX 75235
USA

Robert G. Robinson
Department of Psychiatry
University of Iowa College of Medicine
200 Hawkins Drive
Iowa City
IA 52242
USA

Maria A. Ron
Institute of Neurology
Queen Square
London WC1N 3BG
UK

Howard J. Rosen
Department of Neurology
UCSF School of Medicine
1600 Divisadero Street
San Francisco CA 94115
USA

Christopher A. Ross
Departments of Psychiatry and Neuroscience
Johns Hopkins University School of Medicine
720 Rutland Avenue
Baltimore
MD 21205
USA

Douglas L. Rothman
Department of Diagnostic Radiology
Yale University Medical School
333 Cedar Street
New Haven, CT 06510
USA

Roberto Salvatori
Division of Endocrinology and Metabolism
Department of Medicine
Johns Hopkins University School of Medicine
Suite 333
1830 E. Monument Street
Baltimore
MD 21287
USA

Martin A. Samuels
Department of Neurology
Brigham and Women's Hospital
75 Francis Street
Boston
MA 02115
USA

Jennifer B. Sass
Program in Human Health and the Environment
University of Maryland School of Medicine
9–34 MSTF
10 South Pine Street
Baltimore
MD 21201-1596
USA

Anthony H.V. Schapira
University Department of Clinical Neurosciences
Royal Free & UCH Medical School
Rowland Hill Street
London NW3 2PF
UK

Ola A. Selnes
Department of Neurology
School of Medicine
Department of Cognitive Science
Krieger Mind/Brain Institute
Johns Hopkins University
600 N. Wolfe Street
Baltimore
MD 21287-7222
USA

Michael E. Selzer
Department of Neurology
Hospital of the University of Pennsylvania
3 W. Gates
3400 Spruce Street
Philadelphia
PA 19104-4283
USA

Sudha Seshadri
Framingham Heart Study
Department of Neurology
Boston University School of Medicine
Framingham
Boston
MA 01702
USA

Pamela J. Shaw
Department of Neurology
E Floor
Medical School University of Sheffield
Beech Hill Road
Sheffield S10 2RX
UK

Simon Shorvon
Institute of Neurology
Queen Square
London WC1N 3BG
UK

Ellen K. Silbergeld
Department of Environmental Health Sciences
Bloomberg School of Public Health
Johns Hopkins University
615 North Wolfe Street
Baltimore
MD 21205
USA

Stephen D. Silberstein
Jefferson Headache Center
Department of Neurology
Thomas Jefferson University Hospital
111 South 11 Street
Suite 8130
Philadelphia
PA 19107
USA

Harvey S. Singer
Department of Neurology
Johns Hopkins University
600 N. Wolfe Street
Harvey 811
Baltimore
MD 21287
USA

Julio Sotelo
National Institute of Neurology of Mexico
Insurgentes Sur 3877
Mexico City 14269
Mexico

Judith M. Spies
Institute of Clinical Neuroscience
University of Sydney
Royal Prince Alfred Hospital
Missenden Road
Camperdown NSW 2050
Australia

Dan J. Stein
MRC Anxiety Disorders Unit
Department of Psychiatry
University of Stellenbosch
Cape Town
South Africa

Donna J. Stephenson
Department of Neurology
Johns Hopkins University
600 N. Wolfe Street
Harvey 811
Baltimore
MD 21287
USA

John H. Stone
Johns Hopkins Vasculitis Center
Johns Hopkins School of Medicine
1830 East Monument Street
Suite 7500
Baltimore
MD 21205
USA

Marcus A. Stoodley
University of New South Wales
Institute of Neurological Science
Prince of Wales Hospital
Randwick
NSW 1031
Australia

Kunihiko Suzuki
Neuroscience Center-CB 7250
University of North Carolina
Chapel Hill
NC 27599-7250
USA

J. Paul Taylor
Neurogenetics Branch
National Institute of Neurological Disorders and Stroke
National Institutes of Health
Building 10, Room 3B-14
10 Center Drive
Bethesda
MD 20892-1250
USA

Peter K. Thomas
Department of Clinical Neurology
Institute of Neurology
Queen Square
London WC2N 3BG
UK

Pierre Thomas
Service de Neurologie and Consultation d'Epileptologie
CHU de NICE
France

Alan J. Thompson
Neurological Outcome Measurement Unit
Institute of Neurology
Queen Square
London WC2N 3BG
UK

Philip D. Thompson
Department of Neurology
Royal Adelaide Hospital
University Department of Medicine
University of Adelaide
Adelaide 5000
South Australia

Klaus V. Toyka
Department of Neurology
Julius-Maximilians-University
Josef-Schneider-Strasse 11
97080 Würzburg
Germany

Jerrold L. Vitek
Department of Neurology
Emory University School of Medicine
PO Box Drawer V
Suite 600
1639 Pierce Drive
Atlanta
GA 30322
USA

Bavanisha Vythilingum
MRC Anxiety Disorders
Department of Psychiatry
University of Stellenbosch
Cape Town
South Africa

Christopher A. Walsh
Department of Neurology
Beth Israel Deaconess Medical Center
Harvard Medical School
77 Avenue Louis Pasteur
Boston
MA 02115
USA

Gary S. Wand
Department of Medicine
The Johns Hopkins University School of Medicine
Suite 333
1830 E. Monument Street
Baltimore
MD 21205
USA

Charles P. Warlow
Department of Clinical Neurosciences
The University of Edinburgh
Edinburgh
UK

Bryce K.A. Weir
Section of Neurosurgery, Department of Surgery
University of Chicago Pritzker School of Medicine
5841 S. Maryland Avenue
Chicago
IL 60637
USA

Richard P. White
Institute of Neurology
National Hospital for Neurology and Neurosurgery
Queen Square
London WC1N 3BG
UK

Eelco F.M. Wijdicks
Department of Neurology
Mayo Clinic and Mayo Foundation
200 First Street, S.W.
Rochester
MN 55905
USA

Robert G. Will
National CJD Surveillance Unit
Western General Hospital
University of Edinburgh
UK

Michael A. Williams
Department of Neurology
Johns Hopkins University School of Medicine
600 N. Wolfe Street
Baltimore
MD 21287
USA

Kaethe Willms
Department of Microbiology
Faculty of Medicine
National University of Mexico
Insurgentes Sur 3877 C.P.
Mexico City 14269
Mexico

Oliver J. Wiseman
The National Hospital for Neurology and Neurosurgery
Queen Square
London WC1N 3BG
UK

Barbara E. Wolfe
Department of Psychiatry
Beth Israel Deaconess Medical Center
Harvard Medical School
330 Brookline Avenue
Boston
MA 02215
USA

Philip C. Wong
Division of Neuropathology
Department of Pathology
Johns Hopkins University School of Medicine
558 Ross Research Building
720 Rutland Avenue
Baltimore
MD 21205-2196
USA

Clifford J. Woolf
Neural Plasticity Research Group
Department of Anesthesia and Critical Care
Massachusetts General Hospital East and Harvard
    Medical School
149 13th Street
Charlestown
MA 02129
USA

Jie Wu
Department of Neurology
Barrow Neurological Institute
St. Joseph Hospital and Medical Center
350 W. Thomas Road
Phoenix
AZ 85013-4496
USA

G. Bryan Young
Clinical Neurological Sciences
University Western Ontario
London Health Sciences Centre
375 South Street
London
Ontario N5A 4G5
Canada

John Zajicek
Department of Neurology
Level 10, Derriford Hospital
Derriford Road
Plymouth
Devon PL6 8DH
UK

David S. Zee
Department of Neurology
Johns Hopkins Hospital
600 N. Wolfe Street
Baltimore
MD 21287
USA

Huda V. Zoghbi
Department of Molecular and Human Genetics
Howard Hughes Medical Institute
Baylor College of Medicine, T807
One Baylor Plaza
Mail Stop 225
Houston
TX 77030
USA

Preface

In the 10 years since the second edition of *Diseases of the Nervous System* appeared, extraordinary change has taken place in the field of neurosciences, both basic and clinical. In accordance with what is happening in the neurosciences, major changes have occurred with this third edition. Organization of subject matter and ordering of topics has changed substantially, in some cases dramatically. Of the contributors, a number of the authors for the previous two editions have written again in their special fields of expertise, but overall, more than three-quarters of the contributors are new to these pages. Two new editors have been added, Peter J. Goadsby and Justin C. McArthur; Cambridge University Press is the new publisher; and a new subtitle, *Clinical Neuroscience and Therapeutic Principles* has supplanted the previous one.

Despite these changes, the purpose of these reference volumes remains the same, namely to summarize what the scientific method, as applied to problems of neurological dysfunction, has taught us about the pathophysiology of neurological disorders. To say it differently, our purpose is not to focus on incidence, natural history, phenomenology and semeiology of neurological disorders, although these aspects are touched upon, but rather to focus on the mechanisms of neurological disease and the principles that form the basis for management and therapeutics. In addition to the emphasis on pathophysiology and principles of therapy, three other axioms guided the planning of this edition, just as they did for the previous editions. First, contributors were chosen who brought clinical expertise to bear as well as scientific authoritativeness. Second, we tried to assure that the depth with which each topic covered was relatively uniform from one chapter to the next. There is a corollary to this principle of uniformity. Given that these volumes are a general reference covering the entire field of neurological disorders, each chapter is, by necessity, a relatively brief summary of where matters stand in that particular disorder or area of interest. This level of detail will be insufficient for some readers. When this is the case, readers are urged to consult the primary literature listed in the references.

The third point has to do with the intended readership. It is assumed that the reader will have a grasp of the terminology of everyday neurology and of the neurological examination, and will have a working knowledge of the basic concepts of nervous system anatomy and physiology. With this proviso, these volumes are designed to be of use to medical students, physicians in training, physicians trained in fields other than the nervous system, and of course to those trained or training in the fields of neurology, psychiatry, neurosurgery and related specialties. Neuroscientists of any background or level of training should have no difficulty using these volumes, and indeed it is this readership whom we particularly have in mind.

A project of this size requires many hands. The editors owe a debt of gratitude to the many who worked so diligently to make these volumes a reality. Particular thanks go to Ms Barbara C. Williams, the overall coordinator, Ms Theresa Daly at the School of Medicine, University of Pennsylvania, Ms Nancy Rosenberg at Johns Hopkins Hospital, Ms Olga Shapeero and Ms Sophie Ryan at the Institute of Neurology Queen Square, and Ms Susan Soohoo at the Krieger Mind-Brain Institute, Johns Hopkins University. Ms Mary Sanders performed the copy editing thoroughly and skilfully. Dr Richard Barling, director of medical and professional publishing at the Cambridge University Press, provided excellent guidance and support. But it is the chapter authors to whom we most deeply indebted, and to whom these volumes are dedicated. The publisher provided the loom, the editors made the design, but it was the 213 contributors who wove the fabric.

Arthur K. Asbury
Guy M. McKhann
W. Ian McDonald
Peter J. Goadsby
Justin C. McArthur

Part I

Introduction and general principles

Pathophysiology of nervous system diseases

Justin C. McArthur[1], Guy M. McKhann[2], W. Ian McDonald[3], Peter J. Goadsby[4] and Arthur K. Asbury[5]

[1] Departments of Neurology and Epidemiology, Johns Hopkins University Baltimore, MD, USA
[2] The Zanvyl Krieger Mind and Brain Institute, Johns Hopkins University School of Medicine, Baltimore, MD, USA
[3] Institute of Neurology, University College London, Royal College of Physicians, London, UK
[4] Institute of Neurology, The National Hospital for Neurology and Neurosurgery, London, UK
[5] University of Pennsylvania School of Medicine, Philadelphia, PA, USA

Since the last edition of this textbook, the field of Neurology and the Neurosciences has witnessed remarkable advances in the technologies available for the study of the brain and our concepts about the nervous system and its diseases. There has been progress in our ability to modify, prevent or treat these disease processes and to evaluate clinical outcomes, and in the resources available to handle and disperse data. There is, however, always a competition between the advancement of knowledge and the challenges of disease. We face challenges that demand that we put these advances to good use.

This introduction provides a brief, and necessarily incomplete, overview of some of the advances, and the many remaining challenges, for the study and treatment of diseases of the nervous system. A number of new therapeutic strategies have already been developed, and are already impacting on the quality of life of those with neurological disease. Many new treatments, both symptomatic and disease-modifying, are in the developmental pipeline. With the delineation of the human genome in 2001, a particular problem has emerged: the need to delineate protein production (proteomics) and protein modifications on a cellular basis. 'The emerging challenge in understanding the pathogenesis of the neurodegenerative disorders will be to characterize and elucidate aberrant protein interactions in the affected cells' (Martin, 1999). Future efforts will be focused on determining the tertiary structure of proteins which is currently determined using X-ray crystallography and nuclear magnetic resonance. Because of their relatively low through-put, complexity and high cost, these techniques have not generally been used for therapeutic targeting in drug discovery programmes. Recent technological advances, coupled with the information from human genome sequencing, are beginning to enable construction of a database to predict protein

structure from sequence, and may be relevant for up to one-third of all gene targets (Christendat et al., 2000).

Global challenges in the developed and developing world

The world's aging population is increasingly affected by both acute and chronic neurological diseases. These include cerebrovascular disease, Alzheimer's disease and other dementias and Parkinson's disease. In the USA, the number of the very old (older than 85) is expected to increase sevenfold, from 2 million in 1990 to 14 million in 2040 and is increasingly vulnerable to chronic neurodegenerative disorders.

Since the original descriptions in the 1870s that microbes caused infections, specifically the discovery by Koch that *Bacillus anthracis* caused anthrax, major neurological complications of systemic infections continue to affect millions annually, particularly in developing nations. These infections include malaria, HIV-1 infection, tuberculosis, and leprosy, as well as 'new' infections that have emerged in previously unaffected areas. Malaria remains a major scourge across the world, with approximately 1.5 million deaths annually, many from cerebral involvement. Until recently, research efforts have been scattered and underfunded, with little coordinated effort for the development of a vaccine. In sub-Saharan Africa, the AIDS epidemic has produced an enormous sociopolitical crisis because it has literally decimated a generation, with seroprevalence rates exceeding 25% of the population, and an estimated 13.2 million 'AIDS orphans' (UNAIDS, 2000). Despite the availability of effective treatment, leprosy remains the commonest cause of peripheral neuropathy worldwide. Increasingly, developed and developing countries are linked by diseases which have spread because of the ease and speed of global travel. As one recently developing example of 'emerging' infections, the appearance of West Nile encephalitis in the eastern USA in the past few years is thought to reflect the introduction of infected *Anopheles* mosquitoes from increased air travel (Lanciotti et al., 1999).

One of the major challenges facing our society will be how to equitably distribute therapeutic advances, many of which may be both costly and complex, particularly to underserved populations. The AIDS epidemic provides a stark warning of how an inadequate global response can fail to deliver currently available and effective treatments to millions. It serves as an example to avoid as improved pathogenesis-based treatments for neurological diseases such as Alzheimer's are developed (Steinbrook & Drazen, 2001).

The impact of imaging on neurosciences

No technology has changed the practice of the clinical neurosciences more than cranial imaging. Within the past two decades we have witnessed the development first of structural imaging (CT and MRI), then functional imaging (PET and fMRI), and now refined morphological and physiological imaging (diffusion-weighted and perfusion-weighted imaging), and biochemical characterization with magnetic resonance spectroscopy (MRS). Advances in imaging techniques during the past two decades have literally revolutionized our ability to localize pathology within the nervous system, establish diagnoses, and guide therapies. Rather than devalue the role of neuropathology in the clinical neurosciences, the improvements in imaging have facilitated an even closer integration of clinical neurology with pathology. We can now see the brain, ask what part is involved in neural and cognitive processing, evaluate the extent and distribution of injury, and characterize mechanisms of plasticity and recovery.

Of all of the various imaging modalities: computerized tomography, positron emission tomography, angiography, arguably magnetic resonance imaging (MRI) has become the most widely used modality because of its sensitivity, and lack of radiation risk. The field of MRI has now taken on two new functions: (i) magnetic resonance spectroscopy, identifying the biochemical profile of the living brain through the identification of specific chemical spectra and (ii) the development of functional MRI using changes in deoxyhemoglobin to detect regional brain activation. Both of these techniques are non-invasive, repeatable, and involve no radiation risk. Specialized MR techniques such as diffusion-weighted imaging and perfusion-imaging have pushed forward our understanding of cerebrovascular pathophysiology. They allow for the identification of

Table 1.1. Physiologic processes accessible in humans by functional and metabolic imaging

Physiologic processes	Methods
Glucose metabolism	FDG-PET[a]
Blood flow or volume	[^{15}O]H$_2$O-PET, perfusion MRI
Tissue oxygenation	nitroimidazole-PET, fMRI
Tissue pH	^{31}P-MRS
Protein synthesis	Amino acid-PET
Cell proliferation (mitotic rate)	Thymidine-PET
Receptor concentration or occupancy	PET
Enzyme kinetics	PET
Endogenous metabolite concentration	MRS(I)[a]
Water diffusion	DWI
Tissue anisotropy	DTI
Drug pharmacokinetics/dynamics	PET, MRS
Vascular permeability	Dynamic MR

Notes:
DTI, diffuse tensor imaging; DWI, diffusion-weighted MR imaging; FDG, [^{18}F]fluorodeoxyglucose; fMRI, functional magnetic resonance imaging; MR, magnetic resonance; MRS(I), magnetic resonance spectroscopy–spectroscopic imaging; PET, positron emission tomography. [a] Technique used routinely in clinical practice for oncology.
Source: From Pomper, M.G. (2000). Table 27.3–1, p. 680. Reproduced with permission from the publisher.

'vulnerable' brain tissue within the first few hours after onset of stroke. The identification of diffusion–perfusion 'mismatch' can now lead directly to treatment with thrombolytic therapies or induced hypertension.

These remarkable advances are incomplete. We are still not 'online' with the timing of the brain's processing of information. The dependence of current methods of functional imaging, both PET and fMRI, on changes in blood oxygenation and blood flow associated with neural activity remains a limiting factor. Other imaging techniques based on electrophysiological or magnetophysiological principles may provide further advances. Nonetheless, current physiological imaging as detailed in Table 1.1 can now permit the detection of a variety of metabolic alterations within the living brain, including blood flow, metabolism and perturbations in neurotransmitters (Fig. 1.1, see colour plate section). The recent development of the National Institute of Biomedical Imaging and Bioengineering (NIBIB) at the National Institutes of Health will probably further facilitate and accelerate the progress of imaging research.

Neuropsychiatric disorders have been extensively studied using both structural and functional neuroimaging. Mood disorders have a neurochemical origin, but may also be associated with regionally selective alterations in brain structure. For example, a 40% reduction has been found in grey matter volume in prefrontal cortex in patients with bipolar disorders or familiar recurrent unipolar depression (Drevets et al., 1997). As an example of an investigative approach which combines genetic studies, neuropsychological testing and functional imaging, a specific gene variant in the dopamine-degrading enzyme, catechol-o-methyltransferase, is more common in schizophrenics and the prefrontal cortex appears to be metabolically more active (Egan et al., 2001). Positron emission tomography scans during reading tasks showed reduced activity in the left hemisphere in dyslexics from three different countries, suggesting that there is a universal neurocognitive basis for dyslexia (Paulesu et al., 2001). Multidisciplinary studies such as these will become more common and will undoubtedly facilitate an improved understanding of how genetic variation may influence brain behaviour in health and disease.

The genetics of neurological diseases

Over 50% of genetic disorders affect the nervous system and are detailed in the online textbook *Online Mendelian Inheritance in Man (OMIM)*. This database is a catalogue of human genes and genetic disorders authored and edited by Dr Victor A. McKusick and his colleagues at Johns Hopkins and elsewhere, and developed for the World Wide Web by NCBI, the National Center for Biotechnology Information. OMIM contains 12 749 genetic disorders and 9365 established gene locations.

The elucidation of the genetic mechanisms of disease using molecular techniques has advanced rapidly, in large part because most neurogenetic disorders are inherited in a simple Mendelian fashion. Linkage analysis, positional cloning and searches for mutations in candidate genes have led to the identification of mutant genes in more than 50 disorders. The elucidation of the human genome through the Human Genome Project and the surprising observation that the number of identifiable human genes (26 000) is only a few thousand more than the number identified for a much smaller organism, the round worm, sets the stage for a detailed exploration of genes and proteins associated with specific neurological diseases.

Extraordinary progress has been made in identifying specific genes that pose risk factors for many common neurodegenerative disorders and the ways in which pro-

teins coded by these genes are associated with loss of function or gain of adverse properties (Price et al., 1998a; Hardy & Gwinn-Hardy, 1998; Price et al., 1998b). Even before the Human Genome Project was completed in 2001, the mapping and cloning of genes involved in inherited neurological disorders had been performed. It is now anticipated that the genomes of given individuals will be highly variable, as compared to the reference human sequence. Thus, it should be possible to analyse disease genes from studies of a single individual, rather than large kindreds, as has been required up to now. For a number of disorders long considered 'sporadic', the findings from genetics have changed our ways of thinking. Advances in Alzheimer's disease (AD) are illustrative, but we could equally have chosen Parkinson's disease (PD), frontotemporal dementia, or amyotrophic lateral sclerosis. It has been known for some time that rare families existed with an early onset of Alzheimer's disease (under age 60) and an apparently dominant pattern of inheritance. Evaluation of these families has yielded four genetic loci with numerous mutations, all involved in the processing of the protein beta amyloid. These findings not only strengthened the amyloid hypothesis as the underlying mechanism of Alzheimer's disease, but provided information leading to the development of transgenic mouse models. Allelic variation in apo-E appears to act as a time dependent susceptibility gene (Price et al., 1998a).

In an example of a multidisciplinary approach to improve the sensitivity of preventive treatment trials for AD, genetic testing has been combined with functional imaging in an innovative approach to more efficiently test preventive treatments. Positron emission tomography is used in cognitively normal apolipoprotein E4 heterozygotes to identify those with decreased glucose metabolism in several brain regions typically affected in AD. Those with PET abnormalities are considered to be at greatest risk for the development of AD and participate in the clinical trial (Reiman et al., 2001).

Alzheimer's disease also provides an example of the identification of genes associated with an increased risk of disease, rather than disease mechanisms. The first such genotype, Apo-E4, is associated with a fourfold increased risk of late-onset AD and appears to act as a time-dependent susceptibility gene (Price et al., 1998a). Two other genetic loci, A2M and LRPAP1 have also recently been reported as risk-associated genes (Sanchez et al., 2001; Nicosia et al., 2001), and perhaps only operate in selected populations. The concept of risk factor genes has been proposed for some time, but finally there is specific evidence for such a phenomenon. Manipulation of transgenic mice models has suggested therapeutic strategies for the much larger group of patients with late-onset Alzheimer's disease through manipulation of the secretases involved in processing amyloid, or vaccines aimed against possibly toxic fragments of amyloid. As outlined in Chapter 115, similar strategies have been used to explore the role of the protein alpha synuclein in Parkinson's disease, and the protein tau in frontotemporal dementia.

The mechanisms of cellular injury for most neurogenetic disorders remain uncertain, even when a gene product can be identified. Another genetic abnormality, the triplet repeat mechanism for diseases such as Huntington's disease, fragile X syndrome, and various spinocerebellar ataxias, has focused attention on how proteins determine abnormal cellular function and ultimately cell death. There has been a shift away from thinking about enzymatic abnormalities to abnormalities of protein structure and function. This consideration of proteins as mechanisms of disease applies not only to the triplet repeat diseases, but also to other diseases involving proteins such as prion diseases and neurodegenerative diseases.

Common mechanisms may exist for a number of neurodegenerative diseases, including Alzheimer's disease and Parkinson's disease. Most neurodegenerative diseases have been linked to abnormal protein aggregates interfering with neuronal function and viability. Genetic errors and mutations may produce misfolded proteins which tend to accumulate within neurons and may impair the function of proteasomes, which is normally critical in the ubiquitin proteasome system for breaking down proteins. Further accumulation, over a prolonged period, may lead to additional accumulation and even more proteasomal dysfunction (Bence et al., 2001). In Huntington's disease, polyglutamine expansions in the huntingtin and atrophin-1 proteins can be identified, and have been proposed to lead to neuronal toxicity by interference with gene transcription (Fig. 1.2) (Nucifora, Jr. et al., 2001). Mitochondrial disorders can affect almost every tissue and organ system, typically with maternal transmission. Mitochondrial genetics have become increasingly important since the first descriptions of mutations in mitochondrial DNA in 1988 (Holt et al., 1988). A wide range of systemic and neurological diseases have now been linked to specific mutations, including chronic progressive external ophthalmoplegia (CPEO), Leber's optic atrophy, MELAS and MERRF. In addition, mutations in mtDNA may contribute to aging and neurodegenerative diseases.

The accurate diagnosis of many neurogenetic disorders is now possible; and both antenatal and presymptomatic disease diagnosis is also feasible. Genotypic diagnosis by DNA testing allows for precision in diagnosis, and facilitates genetic counselling and predictive testing. It can also identify patients with specific genetic disorders for natural history studies, and ultimately, for therapeutic interventions. These technological advances bring their own set of ethical concerns, however, including the potential misuse of genetic testing to screen 'at risk' individuals for employment or health insurance.

The field of gene therapy was introduced with tremendous fanfare over a decade ago, and had the potential to introduce functional genes into a diseased cell. There have been persistent technical challenges with the delivery systems used to deliver the genes, and the entire field suffered a major setback following an unanticipated patient death in one gene therapy trial. Nonetheless, the recent demonstration of a non-viral gene-transfer therapy for hemophilia A has generated renewed excitement at the potential to cure selected genetic diseases (Roth et al., 2001).

Ion channels and neurotransmitters in neurological disease

The study of ion channels and their distribution in muscle and nerve has expanded tremendously in the past decade, and has led to an improved understanding of the molecular basis for a collection of disorders termed 'channelopathies', including the familial myotonias and periodic paralyses. In epilepsy, different types of rare seizure disorders are now known to be inherited in either an autosomal dominant or autosomal recessive pattern. Mutations have recently been identified in a widely distributed sodium channel, SCN1A in an inherited form of epilepsy, Generalized Epilepsy with Febrile Seizures Plus type 2 (Escayg et al., 2000). The underlying mechanisms have now been clarified for febrile seizures inherited in an autosomal dominant pattern and have been linked to a point mutation in the beta subunit of voltage-gated sodium channel (Wallace et al., 1998). Identification of the mutant genes underlying rare forms of human epilepsy could facilitate recognition of molecular targets and the development of new treatments, for example, drugs acting on potassium channels to enhance potassium current and inhibit seizures. In other areas, the study of genetically determined dysfunction in ion channels has been productive. Several channelopathies with know genetic alterations have been identified in diseases as phenotypically diverse as familial hemiplegic migraine, episodic ataxia, benign neonatal epilepsy type I, and congenital myotonia. These can affect calcium, potassium or chloride channels, with molecular alterations ranging from point mutations, to prematurely truncated proteins, to pathological expansion of terminal sequences (Nappi et al., 2000).

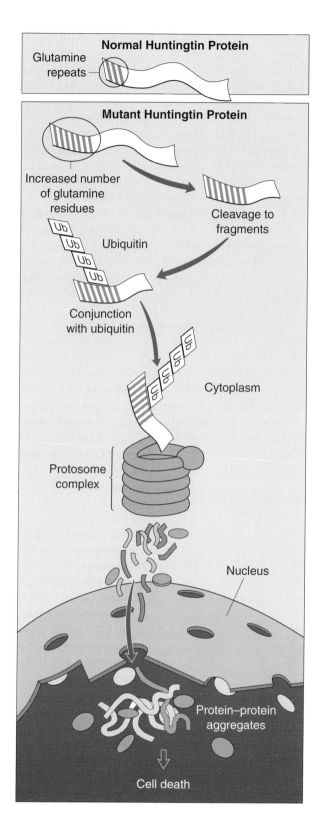

Normal Huntingtin Protein

Glutamine repeats

Mutant Huntingtin Protein

Increased number of glutamine residues

Cleavage to fragments

Ubiquitin

Conjunction with ubiquitin

Cytoplasm

Protosome complex

Nucleus

Protein–protein aggregates

Cell death

Fig. 1.2. Proposed mechanism of huntingtin-induced death of neuronal cells. The mutant huntingtin protein produced by an increase in the number of CAG repeats in the DH gene is cleaved to fragments that retain the increased number of glutamine residues. These fragments are conjugated with ubiquitin and carried to the proteasome complex. Subsequent cleavage is incomplete, and components of both huntingtin and the proteasome are translocated to the nucleus, where aggregates form, resulting in intranuclear inclusions. Over time, this process leads to cell death. (From Martin, 1999.)

With the description of the neurotoxicity of glutamate in 1957, there has been an explosion in our understanding of the biology of neurotransmitters in the CNS. Much of this work has focused on glutamate, the principal excitatory neurotransmitter, and its inhibitory counterpart gamma-amino butyric acid (GABA). To date, five high-affinity glutamate transporters have been cloned, with differential cellular and anatomical localization. In addition to its neurotoxicity, glutamate plays important roles in synaptic plasticity, learning, and development (Maragakis & Rothstein, 2001).

The molecular pathways underlying learning, memory and drug addiction have begun to converge with the recognition that drugs of abuse can cause long-lasting neural changes in the brain (Nestler, 2001).

The impact of stem cells for neurological diseases

Most of us were brought up with the concept that individuals are born with all of the neurons that they are ever going to have, and that neurons are gradually lost with aging. This concept has now been clearly proven wrong, at least for specific areas of brain such as the hippocampus. The adult brain and spinal cord contain neural stem cells that have the capacity to form neurons, astrocytes, and oligodendrocytes from cells in the ependyma and subventricular zone. Although widely viewed as a 'new' observation, in fact progenitor cells were identified in the periventricular zones in the 1950s. What functional significance this neurogenesis has in later life for the processing of memories or in response to injury remains to be determined. In addition, marrow stroma cells transplanted to the brain are able to generate astrocytes (Kopen et al., 1999). Cell lines developed from pluripotent human fetal or embryonic stem cells have now been developed (Shihabuddin et al., 1999), and successful transplantation has been achieved in animal models of Parkinson's disease, motor neuron disease, and spinal cord injury. The long-term efficacy of such treatments, particularly in Parkinson's disease, is a particularly active area of investigation. Stem cells are usually derived from aborted fetuses or embryos, and in the USA, ethical concerns have effectively halted the public funding of stem cell research using these embryonic stem cells. The field of stem cell transplant has achieved even greater promise, both scientifically and politically, through the recognition that pluripotential embryonic stems cells can develop into a wide range of differentiated tissues, including neurons and muscle cells. Although embryonic stem cells appear to proliferate much more efficiently than adult stem cells, these cells are being actively developed and may avoid some of the ethical issues of the use of embryonic tissue. There are many questions still to be answered regarding the relative potential of embryonic stem cells and adult-derived progenitor cells. The exciting possibility exists, however, that these cells could be used as therapeutic agents, either as cell transplants, as sources of trophic factors or gene products to modify neurodegenerative processes in the brain or spinal cord. Functional recovery has been achieved in damaged spinal cords with some restoration of neurological function after injury (Kocsis, 1999) and early human trials have been completed in stroke with positive results.

The development of animal models

Animal models have, of course, been available for the study of neurological diseases for many years. These models usually occurred spontaneously and were utilized when an astute observer realized their implications for neuroscience research. The development of molecular biological techniques has allowed the insertion and removal of genes at the will of the investigator, particularly in easily manipulated species like the mouse and the fruit fly. This has permitted the development of reproducible animal models of common neurological diseases. Transgenic animals engineered to express human genes linked to Alzheimer's disease, amyotrophic lateral sclerosis and Huntington's disease have produced critically valuable advances in our understanding of the pathophysiological mechanisms. Although the exact pathophysiological mechanisms of Alzheimer's disease remain unclear, several transgenic animal models have already been used to delineate discrete pathways of injury. The application of transgenic technology should allow us to modify tumour-suppressor genes and to test pharmacological, biological, or genetic manipulations to prevent progression or even reverse the neurological disease. Small animal models will also allow

for the efficient testing of new therapies for PD and other chronic neurodegenerative disorders. For example, in Parkinson's disease, animal models have been developed in the fly and mouse, which duplicate many of the cardinal features of Parkinson's disease (Fig. 1.3) (Dawson, 2000). Transgenic mice or flies over-expressing alpha synuclein develop pathology within dopamine neurons and age-dependent motor deficits (Masliah et al., 2000; Feany & Bender, 2000). Shimura et al. (2001) showed that the products of two genes, Parkin and alpha-synuclein, functionally interact and may lead to Parkinsonian degeneration.

A genetic model of Tauopathies has been developed by expressing human wild type and mutant Tau in the nervous system of the fruit fly. Transgenic flies die early after developing progressive neurodegeneration, but, at least in this model, show no signs of the large filamentous aggregates of Tau that compose neurofibrillary tangles (Wittmann et al., 2001).

Even more complex functions and neurological disorders can now be evaluated in large animal models. These have traditionally been used for physiological experiments, but are now being developed for the study of neuro-psychiatric disorders such as schizophrenia. For example, by disrupting the development of fetal pigs brains chemically with a toxin that impedes cell division, pathological changes can be induced that mimic the abnormalities evident in the brains of some schizophrenics (Anon, 2001).

Mechanisms of cellular injury

Work since the last edition of this book has delineated more clearly how neurons and astrocytes may be injured during neurological diseases. The role of excitotoxic substances including glutamate has been studied extensively and the 'traditional' dichotomous model of two forms of cell death (necrotic or apoptotic) has been challenged. Substantial advances have been made in understanding the pathophysiological mechanisms underlying neuronal cell death in diverse neurological disorders. Great efforts have been made both in dissecting the cellular mechanisms mediating neuronal death, and in developing therapeutic strategies to prevent this, broadly defined as 'neuroprotection'. The two basic mechanisms of neuronal death, necrosis and apoptosis (or programmed cell death), have been extensively researched. In excitotoxic cell death, exposure to exogenous toxic substances, including glutamate, leads to an energy-independent cell destruction. Glutamate exposure can trigger neuronal death within the brain and has been implicated in the pathogenesis of numerous CNS diseases, including ischemic brain injury,

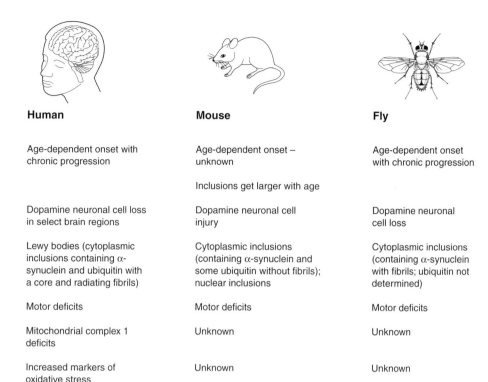

Human	Mouse	Fly
Age-dependent onset with chronic progression	Age-dependent onset – unknown	Age-dependent onset with chronic progression
	Inclusions get larger with age	
Dopamine neuronal cell loss in select brain regions	Dopamine neuronal cell injury	Dopamine neuronal cell loss
Lewy bodies (cytoplasmic inclusions containing α-synuclein and ubiquitin with a core and radiating fibrils)	Cytoplasmic inclusions (containing α-synuclein and some ubiquitin without fibrils); nuclear inclusions	Cytoplasmic inclusions (containing α-synuclein with fibrils; ubiquitin not determined)
Motor deficits	Motor deficits	Motor deficits
Mitochondrial complex 1 deficits	Unknown	Unknown
Increased markers of oxidative stress	Unknown	Unknown

Fig. 1.3. A comparison of animal models of PD. Recent molecular advances have enabled the engineering of mice and flies that carry wild-type or mutant versions of the protein α-synuclein, which is implicated in PD. A comparison of the features of the fly and mouse animal models of PD and how they correlate with the characteristics of the disease in human patients is shown. (From Dawson, 2000.)

amyotrophic lateral sclerosis, trauma, and seizures (Choi, 1988). NMDA receptors appear to be critical in acute glutamate neurotoxicity, for example, in ischemic brain injury. Hypoxic–ischemic brain injury may lead not only to excitotoxic cell death, but also to apoptosis or programmed cell death wherein cells die with negligible inflammation. Lee and Choi (Lee et al., 1999) have proposed that ischemic brain injury most likely represents an 'admixture' of morphologic features of both excitotoxicity and apoptosis. In apoptosis, caspase activation results in cell death through the destruction of critical molecules and the activation of others which mediate an energy-dependent 'suicide programme'. Mediators of apoptosis have been defined and several genes identified, including a family of 'cell death' sustained proteases, the caspases. Activation of caspase1 occurs in diverse models including cerebral ischemia, cerebral trauma, and neurodegenerative diseases such as ALS and Huntington's disease (Hara et al., 1997; Ona et al., 1999). Caspase inhibition may therefore be yet another avenue for targeted therapies, both for acute and chronic neurological disorders. Caspase activation also occurs in cerebral trauma, amyotrophic lateral sclerosis and Huntington's disease. Caspase pathways are

activated in territories subjected to moderate hypoxia and lead to apoptotic cell death over a more prolonged period than that occurring with necrotic cell death. The importance of this is that apoptosis can be aborted either by timely reperfusion of the brain or by caspase inhibition (Friedlander, 2000). Despite the clear effectiveness of NMDA antagonists in experimental models of stroke, numerous clinical trials have unfortunately failed to show any clinical efficacy. Rather than being the result of faulty trial design or poor outcome measures, it seems more likely that other forms of cellular injury may play critical roles in ischemic brain injury. These may include AMPA/kainate receptor-mediated toxicity and extracellular zinc.

An important new concept in pathology is the description of the role of inflammation in diseases previously thought not to involve an inflammatory component. For example, in Alzheimer's disease there are now clear descriptions of local microglial activation, cytokine release, reactive astrocytosis and a multiprotein inflammatory response (McGeer & McGeer, 1995; Eikelenboom et al., 1994). Whether these responses are critical, or simply reflect an epiphenomenon, remains to be determined, but already clinical trials of anti-inflammatory agents are in progress, and their results eagerly awaited.

Multiple sclerosis has traditionally been referred to as an inflammatory demyelinating disease and most of us were taught in medical school that it 'spared CNS axons'. Though degeneration of axons in multiple sclerosis lesions was first recognized by Charcot in 1877, recent elegant work has reinforced the frequency with which axonal transection and both neuronal and axonal loss occurs in multiple sclerosis. Axonal pathology has been identified as a determinant of irreversible disability (Matthews et al., 1998; Davie et al., 1995). This has led directly to change in treatment philosophy, ie, to begin treatment early before there is irreversible axonal injury. Refinement of non-invasive MR-based techniques to quantify underlying pathological lesions in MS will be relevant to the rational development of new treatments.

Plasticity in adult brains

In the past three decades, there has been an increased understanding of the synaptic and molecular basis of plasticity within the adult human brain. Current research indicates that experience-dependent plasticity may not decrease dramatically with age, as had previously been thought. This research may produce effective remediation for neurological impairments following trauma, stroke, or surgery. Functional magnetic resonance imaging has been widely used to examine the neural mechanisms underlying the acquisition of skilled behaviours. In epilepsy, the development of circuitry with recurrent excitatory synapses has emerged as common to numerous experimental models of epilepsy and could potentially occur within the sclerotic hippocampus of humans (McNamara, 1999).

Dendrites may have the capacity to synthesize proteins, thus could modulate the strength of connections between neurons, ultimately influencing neural activities including learning and memory. Protein synthesis occurs in intact dendrites, and this local protein synthesis could facilitate the ability of synapses to make synapse-specific changes (Aakalu et al., 2001).

Information processing and computational neuroscience

The ability to store, integrate and rapidly analyse large amounts of data has been a crucial advance in facilitating the progress in areas such as genomics and imaging. Data management, data handling, and statistics have all

advanced to a point where more than adequate computational power is available on the average laptop computer. In addition, the Internet has revolutionized how most neuroscientists access, publish and disperse information, making use of large publicly available databases. One exciting application is the potential for the Internet to enhance remote or long-distance collaborations, without the need for travel or telephone communications. Systems are now in place which can permit the control of experimental equipment remotely in real time. For example, the Great Lakes Regional Center for AIDS Research facilitates telemicroscopy, distance learning, and video conferencing with real-time document and image sharing (Teasley & Wolinsky, 2001).

The objectives of computational neuroscience span the development of alternative test systems to model biological processes to the working of physiological systems, such as explaining how the brain might process information. This field has obviously been advanced by the revolution in affordable computers, which can be applied to produce neural networks and artificial intelligence, or systems which 'learn' how to address a neurobiological problem. The concept of neural networks has increasingly focused on attempts to understand complex human behaviour. For example, complex human memory is likely mediated by assemblies of interconnected neural networks with different components contributing towards memory function and dysfunction. At the same time, our patients and non-scientists have become our partners because they have the potential to tap into the same information sources as clinicians and scientists. In this new era, there is increasing need for clinicians and investigators to be sources of understandable, accurate and unbiased information.

Advances in neuroepidemiology and clinical trials

Here, neurological clinical trials research has advanced on several different fronts. At a national level in the USA, programmes and resources sponsored by the NIH to train and develop well-trained clinical researchers have been expanded. One example of this is the NIH-funded K23 programme, which is designed to foster the career development of clinician–investigators in patient-oriented research. The widespread application of evidence-based neurology in the past two decades has greatly improved clinical practice, the quality of patient-oriented neurology publications and the education of neurologists. Many neurological therapies and interventions have been submitted to rigorous and systematic analyses and meta-analyses to examine both the efficacy and effectiveness of therapies. Detailed literature reviews and practice guidelines have been developed for most neurological disorders and their treatments through mechanisms such as the *Cochrane Review* and the *American Academy of Neurology*.

The design of clinical trials has improved markedly with the more accurate modelling of sample size calculations to ensure that clinical trials are adequately powered to show statistically significant differences, where they exist. The interactions of neuroscientists and statisticians have led to new strategies to more efficiently test new therapies in controlled clinical trials. As an example, it is now recognized by clinical trialists that even small overestimates in the efficacy of an intervention can lead to a significant reduction in the statistical power of a trial. Cost-effectiveness modelling techniques can be used to better define minimum clinically important differences (Samsa & Matchar, 2001). Finally, new outcome measures have been developed and refined both for the study of central and peripheral nervous system disorders in clinical trials. For example, in multiple sclerosis, clinical trials now routinely incorporate magnetic resonance imaging as one of the important outcome measures. In the study of painful peripheral neuropathies, skin biopsy, a technique originally developed in the 1960s has now been 'rediscovered' and is now being used as an outcome measure in trials of regenerative agents for sensory neuropathies.

Some of the great successes in clinical neurosciences have actually been in prevention with the development of effective vaccines. Thus, we rarely encounter poliomyelitis, postrubella mental retardation, or postinfectious demyelination after measles (at least in the developed world). Recognition of risk factors and changes in life style have led to a significant decline in cardiovascular and cerebrovascular diseases, but strategies for preventing or delaying neurodegenerative diseases are still lacking. Possible protective effects of estrogens, antioxidants, and non-steroidal anti-inflammatory agents for neurodegenerative diseases are promising, but firm recommendations can still not be made.

The ultimate value of deciphering pathophysiological processes at a molecular level will arise in the development of targeted therapies. These should both reduce toxicity and permit a direct attack on disease process. Examples include the development of Herceptin, a 'monoclonal antibody', which has been proved useful for treatment of metastatic breast cancer which has been linked to the over-expression of the HER-2 allele. More recently, a targeted treatment for CML has been approved which blocks the expression of AB-1, a 'tumour promoting gene' (Druker et al., 2001). Gene and cell-based therapies are being devel-

oped for stroke, anoxic brain injury and other neurological disorders. In global ischemia models in gerbils, it appears that new neurons are produced within the hippocampus, raising the possibility that recovery after brain ischemia may, in part, reflect neurogenesis (Frank R. Sharp, University of Cincinnati, personal communication 2001). Fetal stem cells have been implanted in rodent models and continue dividing for several weeks. Cell lines in a marmocet model of stroke have restored some functional recovery (Svendsen & Smith, 1999; Ostenfeld et al., 2000).

At the same time, clinical research has come under closer scrutiny. Potential conflicts of interest by investigators, adequacy of informed consent procedures and the adequacy of monitoring of ongoing studies are subjects of concern, not only among investigators, but among the general public as well. As we proceed into the intervention phase of neurologic disease research and care, it is essential that investigators maintain their credibility for accurate, unbiased clinical research trial design, implementation and interpretation.

Therapeutic impact of translational neurosciences research

The concept of translational research, the delivery of laboratory discoveries to patient-oriented applications has many examples in neurological diseases. One increasingly important aspect of translational research is the development of new therapies, focused on pathogenic mechanisms. There are now FDA-approved agents for neurological diseases for which, until recently, we had no therapeutic options. These include Alzheimer's disease, amyotrophic lateral sclerosis, and multiple sclerosis, with agents that, at least for ALS and MS, are truly 'disease modifying', rather than symptomatic. One intervention which has changed clinical practice substantially is the introduction of TPA in appropriately selected patients with acute ischemic stroke. Acute ischemic strokes are now considered, like myocardial infarction, as 'brain attacks' requiring urgent evaluation and consideration for specific treatment. In stroke, the concept of neuroprotection has been tested successfully in ischemic animal models, but has failed to translate successfully to human trials. In fact, the last 15 years have seen a series of failures for a variety of treatments for ischemic stroke. Some of these failures may have been due to underpowered trials, or incorrect estimates of treatment effect (Samsa & Matchar, 2001) In Alzheimer's disease, transgenic models have been used to probe possible effectiveness of disease-modifying therapies, including inhibitors of beta secretase, the enzyme critical for A-production, vaccination strategies directed against A-beta, neuroprotective strategies with antioxidants or estrogens to protect neurons from the downstream effects of A-beta accumulation, and other strategies. In other neurodegenerative diseases, such as Parkinson's disease, strategies to replace critical neurotransmitters have been attempted. Disappointingly, fetal neuronal grafts into the basal ganglia have as yet produced only modest effect on symptoms of Parkinson's disease with the added concern that dyskinesias developed in a proportion of patients (Freed et al., 2001)

In the tremendous potential of the basic and clinical neurosciences to permit an ever finer dissection of disease processes, we must never lose sight that these same processes affect a person, a family, a mind.

Ask not what disease the person has, rather what person the disease has.   *William Osler, 1889*

References

Anon. (2001). Creating the schizophrenic pig. *Science*, **292**, 2247.

Aakalu, G., Smith, W.B., Nguyen, N., Jiang, C. & Schuman, E.M. (2001). Dynamic visualization of local protein synthesis in hippocampal neurons. *Neuron*, **30**, 489–502.

Bence, N.F., Sampat, R.M. & Kopito, R.R. (2001). Impairment of the ubiquitin–proteasome system by protein aggregation. *Science*, **292**, 1552–5.

Choi, D.W. (1988). Calcium-mediated neurotoxicity: relationship to specific channel types and role in ischemic damage. *Trends Neurosci.*, **11**, 465–9.

Christendat, D., Yee, A., Dharamsi, A. et al. (2000). Structural proteomics of an archaeon. *Nat. Struct. Biol.*, **7**, 903–9.

Davie, C.A., Barker, G.J., Webb, S. et al. (1995). Persistent functional deficit in multiple sclerosis and autosomal dominant cerebellar ataxia is associated with axon loss. *Brain*, **118** (6), 1583–92.

Dawson, V.L. (2000). Neurobiology. Of flies and mice. *Science*, **288**, 631–2.

Drevets, W.C., Price, J.L., Simpson, J.R., Jr. et al. (1997). Subgenual prefrontal cortex abnormalities in mood disorders. *Nature*, **386**, 824–7.

Druker, B.J., Talpaz, M., Resta, D.J. et al. (2001). Efficacy and safety of a specific inhibitor of the BCR-ABL tyrosine kinase in chronic myeloid leukemia. *N. Engl. J. Med.*, **344**, 1031–7.

Egan, M.F., Goldberg, T.E., Kolachana, B.S. et al. (2001). Effect of COMT Val108/158 Met genotype on frontal lobe function and risk for schizophrenia. *Proc. Natl Acad. Sci. USA*, **98**, 6917–22.

Eikelenboom, P., Zhan, S.S., van Gool, W.A. & Allsop, D. (1994). Inflammatory mechanisms in Alzheimer's disease. *Trends Pharmacol. Sci.*, **15**, 447–50.

Escayg, A., MacDonald, B.T., Meisler, M.H. et al. (2000). Mutations of SCN1A, encoding a neuronal sodium channel, in two families with GEFS+2. *Nat. Genet.*, **24**, 343–5.

Feany, M.B. and Bender, W.W. (2000). A Drosophila model of Parkinson's disease. *Nature*, **404**, 394–8.

Freed, C.R., Greene, P.E., Breeze, R.E. et al. (2001). Transplantation of embryonic dopamine neurons for severe Parkinson's disease. *N. Engl. J. Med.*, **344**, 710–19.

Friedlander, R.M. (2000). Role of caspase 1 in neurologic disease. *Arch. Neurol.*, **57**, 1273–6.

Hara, H., Friedlander, R.M., Gagliardini, V. et al. (1997). Inhibition of interleukin 1 beta converting enzyme family proteases reduces ischemic and excitotoxic neuronal damage. *Proc. Natl Acad. Sci. USA*, **94**, 2007–12.

Hardy, J. & Gwinn-Hardy, K. (1998). Genetic classification of primary neurodegenerative disease. *Science*, **282**, 1075–9.

Holt, I.J., Harding, A.E. & Morgan-Hughes, J.A. (1988). Deletions of muscle mitochondrial DNA in patients with mitochondrial myopathies. *Nature*, **331**, 717–19.

Kocsis, J.D. (1999). Restoration of function by glial cell transplantation into demyelinated spinal cord. *J. Neurotrauma*, **16**, 695–703.

Kopen, G.C., Prockop, D.J. & Phinney, D.G. (1999). Marrow stromal cells migrate throughout forebrain and cerebellum, and they differentiate into astrocytes after injection into neonatal mouse brains. *Proc. Natl Acad. Sci. USA*, **96**, 10711–16.

Kraut, M.A., Kremen, S., Segal, J.B., Calhoun, V. & Moo, L. (2001). Object activation from features in the semantic system. *J. Cognit. Neurosci.*, in press.

Lanciotti, R.S., Roehrig, J.T., Deubel, V. et al. (1999). Origin of the West Nile virus responsible for an outbreak of encephalitis in the northeastern United States. *Science*, **286**, 2333–7.

Lee, J.M., Zipfel, G.J. & Choi, D.W. (1999). The changing landscape of ischaemic brain injury mechanisms. *Nature*, **399**, A7–A14.

Maragakis, N.J. & Rothstein, J.D. (2001). Glutamate transporters in neurologic disease. *Arch. Neurol.*, **58**, 365–70.

Martin, J.B. (1999). Molecular basis of the neurodegenerative disorders. *N. Engl. J. Med.*, **340**, 1970–80.

Masliah, E., Rockenstein, E., Veinbergs, I. et al. (2000). Dopaminergic loss and inclusion body formation in alpha-synuclein mice: implications for neurodegenerative disorders. *Science*, **287**, 1265–9.

Matthews, P.M., De Stefano, N., Narayanan, S. et al. (1998). Putting magnetic resonance spectroscopy studies in context: axonal damage and disability in multiple sclerosis. *Semin. Neurol.*, **18**, 327–36.

McGeer, P.L. & McGeer, E.G. (1995). The inflammatory response system of brain: implications for therapy of Alzheimer and other neurodegenerative diseases. *Brain Res. Brain Res. Rev.*, **21**, 195–218.

McNamara, J.O. (1999). Emerging insights into the genesis of epilepsy. *Nature*, **399**, A15–A22.

Nappi, G., Costa, A., Tassorelli, C. & Santorelli, F.M. (2000). Migraine as a complex disease: heterogeneity, comorbidity and genotype–phenotype interactions. *Funct. Neurol.*, **15**, 87–93.

Nestler, E.J. (2001). Neurobiology. Total recall – the memory of addiction. *Science*, **292**, 2266–7.

Nicosia, F., Alberici, A., Benussi, L. et al. (2001). Analysis of alpha-2-macroglobulin-2 allele as a risk factor in alzheimer's disease. *Dement. Geriatr. Cogn. Disord.*, **12**, 305–8.

Nucifora, F.C., Jr., Sasaki, M., Peters, M.F. et al. (2001). Interference by huntingtin and atrophin-1 with cbp-mediated transcription leading to cellular toxicity. *Science*, **291**, 2423–8.

Ona, V.O., Li, M., Vonsattel, J.P. et al. (1999). Inhibition of caspase-1 slows disease progression in a mouse model of Huntington's disease. *Nature*, **399**, 263–7.

Ostenfeld, T., Caldwell, M.A., Prowse, K.R., Linskens, M.H., Jauniaux, E. & Svendsen, C.N. (2000). Human neural precursor cells express low levels of telomerase in vitro and show diminishing cell proliferation with extensive axonal outgrowth following transplantation. *Exp. Neurol.*, **164**, 215–26.

Paulesu, E., Demonet, J.F., Fazio, F. et al. (2001). Dyslexia: cultural diversity and biological unity. *Science*, **291**, 2165–7.

Pomper, M.G. (2000). Functional and metabolic imaging. In *Cancer: Principles and Practice of Oncology*, ed. V. DeVita, S. Hellman & S.A. Rosenberg, pp. 679–89. Philadelphia: Lippincott, Williams & Wilkins.

Price, D.L., Sisodia, S.S. & Borchelt, D.R. (1998b). Genetic neurodegenerative diseases: the human illness and transgenic models. *Science*, **282**, 1079–83.

Price, D.L., Tanzi, R.E., Borchelt, D.R. & Sisodia, S.S. (1998a). Alzheimer's disease: genetic studies and transgenic models. *Annu. Rev. Genet.*, **32**, 461–93.

Reiman, E.M., Caselli, R.J., Chen, K., Alexander, G.E., Bandy, D. & Frost, J. (2001). Declining brain activity in cognitively normal apolipoprotein E varepsilon 4 heterozygotes: a foundation for using positron emission tomography to efficiently test treatments to prevent Alzheimer's disease. *Proc. Natl Acad. Sci. USA*, **98**, 3334–9.

Roth, D.A., Tawa, N.E., Jr., O'Brien, J.M., Treco, D.A. & Selden, R.F. (2001). Nonviral transfer of the gene encoding coagulation factor VIII in patients with severe hemophilia A . *N. Engl. J. Med.*, **344**, 1735–42.

Samsa, G.P. & Matchar, D.B. (2001). Have randomized controlled trials of neuroprotective drugs been underpowered? An illustration of three statistical principles. *Stroke*, **32**, 669–74.

Sanchez, L., Alvarez, V., Gonzalez, P., Gonzalez, I., Alvarez, R. & Coto, E. (2001). Variation in the LRP-associated protein gene (LRPAP1) is associated with late-onset Alzheimer disease. *Am. J. Med. Genet.*, **105**, 76–8.

Shihabuddin, L.S., Palmer, T.D. & Gage, F.H. (1999). The search for neural progenitor cells: prospects for the therapy of neurodegenerative disease. *Mol. Med. Today*, **5**, 474–80.

Shimura, H., Schlossmacher, M.G., Hattori, N. et al. (2001). Ubiquitination of a new form of alpha-synuclein by parkin from human brain: implications for Parkinson's disease. *Science*, **293**, 263–9.

Steinbrook, R. & Drazen, J.M. (2001). AIDS—will the next 20 years be different? *N. Engl. J. Med.*, **344**, 1781–2.

Svendsen, C.N. & Smith, A.G. (1999). New prospects for human stem-cell therapy in the nervous system. *Trends Neurosci.*, **22**, 357–64.

Teasley, S. & Wolinsky, S. (2001). Communication. Scientific collaborations at a distance. *Science*, **292**, 2254–5.

UNAIDS (2000). AIDS Epidemic: Update December 2000. (Geneva: Joint United Nations Programme on HIV/AIDS).

Wallace, R.H., Wang, D.W., Singh, R. et al. (1998). Febrile seizures and generalized epilepsy associated with a mutation in the Na$^+$-channel beta1 subunit gene SCN1B. *Nat. Genet.*, **19**, 366–70.

Wittmann, C.W., Wszolek, M.F., Shulman, J.M. et al. (2001). Tauopathy in drosophilia: neurodegeneration without neurofibrillary tangles. *Science*, **293**, 711–14.

2

Genetics of common neurological disorders

Orest Hurko

Department of Investigational Medicine, GlaxoSmithKline Pharamaceuticals,
Neurology Centre for Excellence in Drug Discovery, Harlow, Essex, UK

There is growing appreciation of the influence of genetic constitution on predisposition to disease, even that not usually considered 'genetic'. Approximately 40% of the estimated 30 000 human genes are expressed in the nervous system, the majority of these exclusively (Hurko, 1997; International Human Genome Sequencing Consortium, 2001; Sutcliffe, 1988; Venter et al., 2001). Neurological and psychiatric health might thus be especially susceptible to genetic influence. Furthermore, the nervous system can be uniquely vulnerable to mutations in genes expressed ubiquitously, as with huntingtin (Trottier et al., 1995), and to primary metabolic derangements in non-neural tissue, as with hepatic porphyrias (Strand et al., 1970) or diabetes mellitus. A disproportionate number of single gene disorders manifest as neurological or psychiatric dysfunction (Hurko, 2001).

Many of the successes of human molecular genetics have come from study of neurological disease. Neurological patients suffering from monogenic disorders have thus far only benefited from improved diagnosis. Identification of pathogenic genes has provided powerful reagents, transgenic animals, lessons from homologues in lower organisms and other insights into pathophysiology. These will hasten the development of effective therapies. However, most of these benefits, both realized and anticipated, have been confined to monogenic disorders. Such single gene, or Mendelian, disorders are rare.

Complexity in single gene disorders

Furthermore, even in monogenic disorders the relationship to clinical phenotype is not always straightforward (Estivill 1996). A given phenotype can result from mutation of any of a number of genes. Genetic heterogeneity exists in early-onset Alzheimer's disease (Dartigues & Letenneur,

2000), autosomal dominant spinocerebellar atrophies (Durr & Brice, 2000), limb-girdle muscular dystrophies (Beckmann, 1999; Bushby, 1999; Kissel & Mendell, 1999) and X-linked mental retardation (Toniolo & D'Adamo, 2000), among others.

Allelic heterogeneity

Different mutations within a single gene also contribute complexity. Frame-shift mutations abolish activity of dystrophin, causing Duchenne muscular dystrophy (DMD); mutations that do not shift reading frame compromise function only partially, resulting in milder Becker dystrophy or just subclinical elevation of serum creatine kinase (England et al., 1990; Matsuo et al., 1990). Similarly, variations in the length of triplet repeat expansions underlying Huntington disease (Reddy et al.,1999; Trottier et al., 1994), several of the spinocerebellar atrophies (Cummings & Zoghbi, 2000; Stevanin et al., 2000), fragile-X mental retardation, (Jin & Warren, 2000; Kooy et al., 2000), and myotonic dystrophy (Lieberman & Fischbeck, 2000) determine the severity of the neurological disorder. Allelic differences can be qualitative as well as quantitative. For example, some mutations of the ryanodine receptor result in central core myopathy (Zhang et al., 1993); others confer susceptibility to malignant hyperthermia without clinically evident myopathy (Gillard et al., 1992; McCarthy et al., 2000).

Mosaicism, the presence or expression of more than one genotype in an individual, results either from lyonization in X-linked disorders (Lupski et al., 1991), heteroplasmy in mitochondrial disorders (Hurko, 2001), or somatic mutations, as in tumours. In mosaics, clinical phenotype depends not only on which gene is mutant, but also on distribution and frequency. Parental imprinting adds further complexity. Inheritance of a certain mutation from father results in the Prader–Willi syndrome, whereas inheritance of a similar mutation from mother causes the very different Angelman syndrome (Fridman & Koiffmann, 2000; Greenstein, 1990; Hulten et al., 1991).

Further complexity results from interaction of a pathogenic gene with the environment and with other genes. Mutation of the ryanodine receptor gene may be inapparent until exposure to halothane; mutations underlying hepatic porphyria inapparent until exposure to barbiturates. No gene is expressed in isolation. 'Monogenic' disorders can be modified by epistatic interactions with other genes (Maestri & Beaty 1992).

Genetically complex disorders

Even more complicated genetic and environmental interactions determine susceptibility to many common neurological and psychiatric disorders. Because of this complexity, delineation of genetic factors for common diseases has lagged behind those of rare Mendelian traits (Risch & Botstein, 1996). Analyses suitable for monogenic disorders are often suboptimal for complex traits. However, recent technical and analytical advances promise identification of susceptibility genes for several common neurological and psychiatric disorders.

Is a disease genetic?

Before turning to specific examples, it is useful to consider the meaning of genetic disorder. All biological phenomena result from complex interactions of thousands of genes and innumerable environmental factors. Diseases are no exception. In a given setting, some factors are more important than others. As a start, it is useful to estimate the relative contribution of genetic and environmental factors.

For many genetic diseases familial grouping is inapparent, particularly given the small size of modern nuclear families. These days, most cases of autosomal recessive disorders, such as metabolic disorders and progressive neurodegenerations of infancy like Tay–Sachs disease, occur as singletons in families with no previous history. Even if 1/100 healthy individuals carry a single copy of recessive mutation, there is only 1/10000 chance that two such heterozygotes will marry, and only 1/4 of their offspring will fall ill because of homozygosity for the mutant gene. With a typical family size of two children, the overwhelming likelihood is that there will not be additional cases in siblings or in other generations. Only systematic analyses of large populations or consideration of biological data will reveal the genetic nature of such disorders. Similar considerations apply to new autosomal dominant

mutations (Rudnik-Schoneborn et al., 1994), mitochondrial disorders like Kearns–Sayre syndrome (Butler & Gadoth, 1976), and chromosomal anomalies like Down's syndrome (Antonarakis, 1993).

Furthermore, not all diseases that 'run in families' are genetic. Members of a family share environmental factors: diet, socioeconomic class, as well as exposure to infectious, physical and chemical pathogens. A classic method for estimating the relative contributions of genetic and environmental factors has been the adoption study. Significantly higher similarity to biological rather than adoptive parents was the seminal indicator of the importance of genetics in schizophrenia (Heston, 1996) and alcoholism (Goodwin et al., 1974). However, the adoption method is limited. It will not detect recessive disorders or new mutations, and it also suffers from selective placement of adopted children into environments similar to those into which they were born. Adoption studies have not been used extensively in the study of neurological diseases.

A useful alternative is the comparison of concordance rates in monozygotic (MZ) and dizygotic (DZ) twins (Hawkes, 1997; Maher & Reik, 2000; Martin et al., 1997). MZ twins share all their genes, whereas DZ twins share only half. Therefore, a higher concordance rate in MZ than DZ twins is evidence of a genetic contribution. The higher the ratio of MZ concordance to DZ concordance, the higher the estimate of heritability. In the simplest case of a genetically determined disease, one would expect that all MZ twins would be perfectly concordant. For complex disorders this is usually not the case, for reasons only partially understood. There may be genetic heterogeneity: some twin pairs may have a highly heritable form of the disease, whereas others have a nonheritable phenocopy. In part, discordance may be an artefact of disease definition: MZ concordance for an expanded definition that includes schizoids is an almost perfect 1.0, twice that for classic schizophrenia. Furthermore, twin discordance has been seen even in well-defined single gene disorders. In X-linked DMD, dramatic discordance between MZ twin carriers is the rule rather than the exception, because of asymmetries in X-inactivation (Lupski et al., 1991). Not only environmental but also other developmental factors such as gene imprinting, may contribute to twin discordance, as has been shown for the Beckwith–Wiedemann tumour and mental retardation syndrome (Maher & Reik, 2000). In theory, the twin method is subject to the possible criticism that MZ twins share more environmental factors both prenatally and postnatally than do DZ twins. However, many of these concerns have proven more apparent than real (Kendler, 1993).

Although not perfect, twin studies have provided useful initial evidence of genetic factors in neurological and

Table 2.1. Comparative heritabilities

Disorder	λ	MZ	DZ	Heritability (%)
Autism	84–210	73%	7%	93
Schizophrenia	11	46%	14%	89
Anorexia nervosa	41			80
Multiple sclerosis	30	25.9%	2.3	
Febrile seizures	6–12	39%	12	
Alzheimer's disease	5			
ADHD	2–4	58%	31%	79
Lacunar stroke volume	2.5	61%	38%	73
Obsessive compulsive disorder				47–68
Bipolar depression	7	62%	8%	59
Migraine		34%	21%	52
Panic disorder	2.4–4.75			35–46
Unipolar depression		40%	17%	21–45
Sciatica		18%	12%	21
Pressure pain threshhold		57%	51%	10

psychiatric diseases, among them, multiple sclerosis (Ebers et al., 1986, 1995; James, 1996), autism (Bailey et al., 1995; Folstein & Rutter, 1977), schizophrenia (Gottesman, 1994), and attention deficit hyperactivity disorder (ADHD) (Sherman et al., 1997; Sutcliffe, 1988).

Other types of segregation analysis consider the relative risk among first-, second- and third-degree relatives of affected probands. The ratio of the risk to each class of relative is compared to the general population risk, expressed as the statistic λ_x. For example, λ_1 of 10 indicates that a first-degree relative of an affected individual has a tenfold higher risk of developing the disorder than does an unrelated individual in the same population. The more heritable the disorder the higher the value of λ_1. The more common the disorder in the general population, the lower is λ_1. This statistic serves as a rough guide to the tractability of a complex disorder for genetic analysis. Modest successes have now been achieved for complex human disorders such as schizophrenia, with λ_1 of about 10 (Table 2.1).

Genetic models

Further evidence of a genetic contribution can be provided by a distinctive pattern of transmission. For example, transmission of DMD from unaffected mothers to half of their sons strongly implicated the X chromosome, long before the dystrophin gene, or, for that matter, anything about DNA or the physical structure of any gene, were known. Identification of genetic patterns of transmission

requires an explicit model against which to test data. There are two fundamentally different types of genetic model (Murphy & Chase, 1975). Neurologists are most familiar with the qualitative Mendelian model. An alternative Galtonian model has been used to describe quantitative traits, largely by agricultural and behavioural geneticists. Both models are simplifications, but are demonstrably useful in certain circumstances. Analysis of complex neurological and psychiatric diseases may require a synthesis of the two.

The Mendelian model posits that each phenotype is dichotomous. Either a bean is wrinkled or smooth, green or yellow. In Mendelian disorders, an individual either has the disease or is well. The Mendelian model further posits that each trait is determined exclusively by a single gene represented by two alleles, which can be either identical (homozygous) or different (heterozygous) in a given individual. Each allele is either recessive or dominant with respect to expression of a given trait. Segregation of a mendelian dominant disorder such as Huntington disease can be be modelled by a single coin toss representing the allele a child receives from her affected parent, heads for the wild-type allele, tails for the mutation (Murphy & Chase, 1975). If one scores 1 for heads, there are only two possible outcomes: a score of 1 and she will be healthy, a score of 0 and she will get Huntington disease.

The Galtonian genetic model has been used for metric rather than dichotomous traits. For example, the weight of livestock is more accurately described as a continuum rather than as a simple dichotomy of heavy or light. Genetic transmission of many metric traits behaves as if there were a large number of genes contributing to the phenotype (Falconer, 1960). An appropriate analogy is a coin tossing game with a hundred equally weighted coins, again scoring 1 for heads and 0 for tails (Murphy & Chase, 1975). In this game there are a large variety of possible outcomes ranging from 0 to 100. The distribution of expected winnings will approximate a normal distribution with a mean of 50. From the score, one is able to tell how many times one flipped heads, but one wouldn't be able to tell which particular coins did so. The agricultural geneticist studying the weight of livestock will be able to estimate the aggregate number of heavy alleles inherited by a given animal, but will be unable to determine in which genes these heavy alleles reside. Some disease states, such as hypertension, are more accurately modelled as a continuum rather than as dichotomous states. Even when diseases can be considered dichotomous, such as stroke, the severity, age of onset and susceptibility may be modelled along a continuum.

For many complex traits, reality is somewhere in between the extreme Mendelian and Galtonian models. Even though multiple genes affect susceptibility, they are unlikely to be of equal effect. A single gene of dominant effect, as occurs in a Mendelian disorder, would be represented by a silver dollar, ten genes of low effect modifying the course of the illness would each be represented by a penny. Possible winnings would be represented by two nonoverlapping normal distributions with means of 5 cents and $1.05. If disease threshold were 50 cents, only the toss of the silver dollar would determine if the person became ill. Furthermore, even though refined measurements might provide an estimate of the total number of modifying genes mutant in an individual, only the presence or absence of mutation in the single gene of major effect could be determined unequivocally.

It is likely that many complex genetic disorders result from alterations of a small number of genes with different degrees of influence. An appropriate analogy is a coin tossing game with pennies, nickels, dimes and quarters. The total score could be determined, but the outcome of any particular toss may be indeterminate. Similarly, mutation of a given susceptibility gene could be present in an unaffected individual or absent in someone affected by virtue of the remainder of the genome. Furthermore, the relative importance of a given gene may vary according to the environment. A gene affecting lipid metabolism may be an importantant determinant of stroke in those consuming a lot of animal fat, but have only negligible significance for vegetarians.

Gene identification

Gene identification in single gene disorders

Definitive proof of monogenic determination requires identification of a gene mutant in affected individuals and normal in those that are healthy. Pathogenic mutations have been identified by one of two general methods: one beginning with biology, the other with genetics. In certain disorders, biochemical definition of abnormal patterns of metabolites or storage products in diseased individuals led to identification of a defective enzyme and subsequent analysis of the encoding gene. This method has been most successful in the delineation of autosomal recessive neurological disorders occurring in infants and children (Online Mendelian Inheritance in Man, 2001).

Many neurological disorders occuring later in life do not leave leave a sufficiently clear biological signature for unambiguous identification of a mutant protein. This calls for an alternative strategy based on identification of the chromosomal location of the mutant gene. This approach of 'reverse genetics' was appropriately renamed 'positional cloning' (Collins, 1990). The favoured method has been linkage analysis in large families segregating the disorder in a Mendelian pattern (Ott, 1985). Naturally occuring variants in the DNA sequence are used as markers. Originally, these markers were polymorphisms of surface antigens or electrophoretic patterns of proteins, then restriction fragment length polymorphisms (RFLPs) (Botstein et al., 1980) and later more ubiquitous microsatellites or short tandem repeats (Bently & Durham, 1995). The chromosomal locations of these markers had previously been determined and assembled into maps. One by one the segregation of these markers is compared to the segregation of the disease phenotype in large families. Unlinked markers are transmitted from affected parent to affected offspring at random, on average, 50% of the time. Those markers in the immediate vicinity of the disease gene are transmitted to affected offspring more often than expected by chance, and are thereby linked.

The observed frequency of recombination, separation of the marker and the disease in offspring, is an estimate of the genetic distance between the two loci. This value is expressed as θ. Because estimates of genetic distance are subject to sampling error, the accuracy of the estimate is given as a likelihood, expressed as a lod score, logarithm of odds. For example, a family study reporting a maximum lod score of 3 for $\theta = 0.04$ to a marker means that it is 1000 times more likely that the true genetic distance between that marker and the pathogenic mutation is 4 centiMorgans (cM), than is the null hypothesis that the two are unlinked. The larger the number of informative family members observed, the more accurate the estimate.

With current technology, most genome-wide scans are undertaken with about 300 markers, spaced roughly every 10 cM (Brzustowicz et al., 2000; Kehoe et al., 1999b; Morissette et al., 1999; Weeks et al., 2000). Areas of the genome that give positive signals are then re-examined with a denser array of markers confined to that region. In theory, it should be possible to resolve any genetic distance given a sufficient number of observed transmissions and informative meioses. However, there are practical limitations. Accuracy improves by a square of the number of informative meioses sampled. Precise definition of a disease-causing mutation by strictly genetic methods requires analysis of hundreds of thousands of meioses. In actual practice, the accuracy of human linkage studies is limited to about 2–3 cM, roughly 2–3 million base pairs. Current estimates of the total number of human genes have converged on about 30000 (International Human Genome Sequencing Consortium, 2001; Venter et al., 2001), having previously ranged from 35000 to 140000 (Aparicio, 2000; Liang et al., 2000), distributed over the 3300 cM of the human genome. Therefore linkage analysis on practicable human sample sizes can only resolve down to the 20 to 30 genes within that region. Each of these genes becomes a 'positional candidate'. Sometimes this number can be whittled down further by identification of deletions or translocations, overlaps of which define a narrower critical region. In the absence of such physical rearrangements, biological clues such as tissue distribution and predicted gene function guide a series of guesses until a gene mutant only in affected individuals is found. The majority of monogenic disorders have been resolved by a combination of genetic and biological information.

When large families are unavailable, multiple smaller kinships are analysed under the assumption that the gene responsible for the disorder is the same in each family. This assumption proved valid for many neurological disorders, a tribute to the diagnostic precision afforded by clinical neurology. However, for many others, the assumption does not hold. Notably, the demyelinating forms of Charcot Marie Tooth disease, the limb–girdle muscular dystrophies, the adult-onset spinocerebellar degenerations as well as many other Mendelian neurological disorders proved to be genetically heterogeneous (Online Mendelian Inheritance in Man, 2001). Results from linkage data from several small families each segregating a phenotypically indistinguishable but genetically distinct spinocerebellar atrophy would cancel each other out. Ideally, this problem is avoided by the use of a single large family. However, if only small families are available, allowances for heterogeneity can be made, but only by increasing sample size (Lander & Botstein, 1986). Allowances also have to be made for age-dependent penetrance, with care taken not to score individuals as unaffected if below likely age of onset. These considerations, and others, also apply to complex disorders.

Gene identification in complex disorders

Linkage approaches similar to those for monogenic disorders have also been applied to genetically complex diseases, chiefly diabetes, asthma and psychiatric disorders (Brzustowicz et al., 2000; Morissette et al., 1999). However, despite many successes with monogenics, linkage analysis of complex traits has proven much more difficult. Even with strict diagnostic criteria and large samples, most of these linkage analyses have yielded only weak and irreproducible findings (Risch & Botstein, 1996). This failure could mean that even highly heritable common disorders are influenced by a very large number of genes, each of small effect, approaching a Galtonian model. If so, then their identification would be impossible by any feasible linkage study. However, the failures may simply be methodological.

If most of the susceptibility for a given disease results from a small number of genes with large or moderate effect, modifications of the linkage approach may prove successful. One such modification is a non-parametric technique, not requiring specification of a pattern of inheritance (Kruglyak et al., 1996). In the standard parametric linkage analyses used for monogenic disorders, one must specify whether the disease mutation segregates as a dominant or a recessive. In many complex disorders, this is not known. Furthermore, many gene effects are semidominant, a heterozygote is phenotypically distinguishable from either homozygote, unlike the classic Mendelian model (Falconer, 1960). One nonparametric linkage approach is the method of affected sibling pairs. Regardless of mode of inheritance, any marker shared by affected siblings more often than expected by chance must be linked to a susceptibility gene. The closer the marker to the disease gene, the more frequently will it be shared by affected individuals in a given family. The utility of this approach depends not only on the distance between the marker and the disease gene but also on the frequency of the disease allele in the population and the magnitude of its effect on disease susceptibility. In a favourable situation, for example, if individuals with a copy of a susceptibility allele were at four-fold or greater risk of developing the disorder than were those without that allele, then several hundred sibling pairs are sufficient to establish linkage in a genome-wide search (Risch & Merikangas, 1996).

However, if the disease allele confers less susceptibility or is unusually rare or frequent in the population, linkage can only be established by analysis of tens or hundreds of thousands of sibling pairs. For this reason, alternatives to linkage analysis have to be considered.

The major alternative to linkage analysis in families is allelic association in populations: the presence of a marker allele more frequently in affected individuals than in matched controls from the same population. In properly designed studies, allelic association is more powerful than linkage analysis, detecting associations with genes of only modest effect (genotype relative risk of 1.5) in samples of only a few hundred individuals. In an association study, the goal is to find linkage disequilibrium (not to be confused with linkage analysis) between a marker and a disease-susceptibility gene. Linkage disequilibrium is based on the assumption that a significant proportion of disease susceptibility attributable to a given gene results from an ancestral mutation in a single individual (Jorde, 1995; Kruglyak, 1997). Markers are usually nucleotide polymorphisms in the immediate vicinity of an ancestral mutation, rather than the pathogenic mutation itself. Such markers are transmitted together with the disease allele until separated by recombination. Unless the marker happens to be a unique disease susceptibility mutation, the correlation between it and disease would not be perfect in present-day populations.

In present-day populations, some unaffected individuals with the marker will be descendants of the diseased ancestor, but will have had the marker and disease allele separated by recombination. Such an event can be recognised by the use of multiple markers arranged in a haplotype that brackets the disease susceptibility locus. Other unaffected individuals will have inherited the marker not from the diseased ancestor but from her unaffected sibling. Some affected individuals may not have the marker, either because of recombination or by virtue of having inherited a disease allele from another ancestor with a different background set of markers. For these reasons, the success of association studies depends not only on the proximity of the markers to the actual disease susceptibility locus, but also on the history of the population.

There are two major limitations to association studies, population stratification and the inability to survey beyond the immediate vicinity of the marker. Spurious associations can arise if the ethnicity of affected and control individuals is not matched carefully. For example, both sickle cell anemia and G6PD deficiency are more common in individuals of African and Mediterranean descent than they are in Northern Europeans. In a sample that included both Europeans and Africans, a G6PD marker would show a strong association with sickle cell disease even though the genes are on separate chromosomes. In such a case, allelic association is not an indication of linkage disquilbrium. An identical association study in sub-Saharan Africa would show no association.

A number of methods have been suggested to guard against spurious associations from population stratification (Pritchard & Rosenberg, 1999). However, their utility in population-based case control studies of allelic association of complex disorders resulting from genes of small to modest effect is still untested. An alternative to case-controlled population-based allelic association studies is the transmission/disequilibrium test (TDT) (Spielman et al., 1993), which is immune to errors of population stratification. In this test, nonrandom distribution of a marker from heterozygous parents to an affected offspring provides robust evidence of linkage disequilibrium to a disease susceptibility gene. A thousand trios of affected offspring with both parents should be sufficient in a genome-wide scan to identify markers in linkage disequilibrium with genes of modest effect (Risch & Merikangas, 1996).

The remaining limitation of TDT, as of all association studies, is that in most populations, linkage disequilibrium only extends for very short distances, tens of thousands of bases. Linkage analysis can be undertaken with markers separated by tens of centiMorgans, tens of millions of base pairs, from the disease locus, because the experiment only requires detection of cross-overs in a few generations. A complete linkage scan can therefore be accomplished with 300 markers. In contrast, association studies for linkage disequilibrium depend on the absence of recombination between marker and disease loci in the many generations that separate the study population from the ancestral mutation (Kruglyak, 1997). Thus, even a marker within the same gene but 100 kilobases distant from a pathogenic mutation may fail to show an association. A complete survey of the human genome by association might require testing of as many as 1 000 000 markers (Risch & Merikangas, 1996). The technology to accomplish this will likely require the use of a different type of marker, the single nucleotide polymorphism [SNP], detection of which is amenable to automation. A consortium to develop the necessary SNP markers is already under way (Gray et al., 2000). The technical and statistical problems posed by this number of assays on hundreds of individuals are formidable, but soluble. Pooling of DNA from affected and unaffected individuals in case control studies followed by quantitation of allele frequencies in each of the two pools requires that an assay need only be done twice, rather than separately for each of hundreds of individuals (Germer et al., 2000; Shaw et al., 1998) Genotyping using dense oligonucleotide arrays on solid supports or other technologies will significantly increase throughput and reduce costs (Fan et al., 2000).

Presently, association studies are limited to analysis of a few candidate genes, selected because of a biological rationale. Many association studies will be mentioned in the sections on specific neurological diseases, but most of them have used single markers and a case-control rather than TDT design. Both negative and positive studies are thus suspect. Ideally, association studies should use TDT with a dense array of multiple markers spanning the gene of interest, something not yet done in most neurological studies. An excellent example of the candidate gene TDT approach has been the robust demonstration of association of ADHD with polymorphisms in the dopamine D4 gene (Muglia et al., 2000; Smalley et al., 1998; Tahir et al., 2000). The recent completion of a first rough draft of the human genome (Bentley, 2000; Butler & Smaglik, 2000; International Human Genome Sequencing Consortium, 2001; Venter et al., 2001) and increased understanding of pathophysiology of neurological diseases will aid in the selection of candidates for allelic association studies as will reference to tissue- or disease-specific patterns of gene expression made possible by high-density nucleotide arrays (Gaasterland & Bekiranov, 2000; Lee et al., 2000).

In addition to the top-down allelic association methods used in case-controlled population studies and TDT, the bottom-up approach of cladistic analysis may prove useful (Haviland et al., 1997; Templeton et al., 1987). In this approach, haplotypes constructed for a randomly selected population sample are used to construct trees, where each branchpoint represents an alteration of one marker. Comparisons of disease frequency are then made on either side of each branchpoint. A significant difference implies that the individuals on either side of the branchpoint must differ by the presence of a mutation affecting susceptibility. Although this method is mathematically more powerful than conventional association studies, it has not been used widely, in part because of the difficulties with accurate estimation of haplotypes and the use of population-based samples in which only a minority of individuals have a clinical phenotype of interest. However, cladistics may prove useful in very common neurological disorders such as stroke or migraine.

Neurological disorders with complex inheritance

In contrast to psychiatric and autoimmune disorders, the emphasis on neurological genetics has been on monogenic disorders. In the last two decades, in excess of 650 monogenic neurological disorders have been mapped. Of these, the responsible gene has been identified for over 460 (Hurko, 2001; Online Mendelian Inheritance in Man, 2001). Over two-thirds of these mapped disorders present in childhood, many of them autosomal recessive disorders such as Tay–Sachs disease for which biochemical analysis revealed an a enzymatic deficiency that was subsequently confirmed by sequencing of a mapped gene in affected individuals. Since homozygosity for many of these mutations precludes reproduction, the mutant alleles survive in the gene pool in the much larger reservoir of asymptomatic heterozygous carriers. Although the total burden of heritable neurological disease in children is low compared to that of adults, the number of discrete diagnoses is considerably higher (Childs, 1998).

In both single-gene and complex disorders, deleterious alleles can survive in the gene pool as dominants if serious disease only becomes manifest after child-bearing years. In contrast to the many rare, single-gene, autosomal recessive neurological diseases in childhood, the number of neurological diagnoses are in adults are fewer even though the total burden of neurological disease is higher. The genetic propensity for most of these diseases is complex. Some neurological diseases are grouped under the same diagnosis, such as Alzheimer's disease, even though they may result from any of a number of distinct genetic abnormalities.

As a general rule, genetic diseases of chidhood are rare, many and monogenic, those of adults are common, few and polygenic (Childs, 1998).

Adult-onset dementias

Some of the heterogeneity of adult-onset dementia is readily apparent clinically, as with multi-infarct dementia, vitamin B12 deficiency, hypothyroidism, Creutzfeld–Jacob disease or late syphilis. More careful clinical and pathological analysis further subdivides late-onset dementia into frontotemporal dementia, Lewy body dementia, Alzheimer's disease, and multiple rarer disorders. The genetic contribution to each of these disorders ranges from negligible to major. As shown in Table 2.2 several of these segregate as single-gene disorders. Allelic heterogeneity has been demonstrated for the amyloid precursor protein and tau genes, mutations of which can cause a variety of clinical phenotypes (Table 2.2).

Table 2.2. Single-gene adult-onset dementias

Disorder	MIM	Location	Gene product
(Early-onset) Alzheimer's disease 1, APP related	104300	21q21.3–q22.05	amyloid beta 4 precursor
Dementia, presenile, and cerebroarterial amyloidosis	104760 0.0005	21q21.3–q22.05	amyloid beta A4 precursor
Amyloid angiopathy (Dutch)	104760	21q21.3–q22.05	amyloid beta A4 precursor
(Early-onset) Alzheimer's disease 3	104311	14q24.3	presenilin-1, seven transmembrane domain protein
Alzheimer's disease, familial, with spastic paraparesis and unusual plaques	104311 0.0017	14q24.3	presenilin-1, seven transmembrane domain protein
(Early-onset) Alzheimer's disease 4	600759	1q31–q42	presenilin-2, seven transmembrane domain protein
Alzheimer's disease, familial, Type 5	602096	12p11.23–q13.12	association with transcription factor CP2; TFCP2 (189889)
Alzheimer's disease without neurofibrillary tangles	604154	3	
Hereditary frontotemporal dementia (FTD)	601630	17q21–q22	microtubule-associated protein tau; MAPT (157140)
Disinhibition–dementia–Parkinsonism–amyotrophy complex (DDPAC)	600274	17q21–q22	tau
Progressive subcortical gliosis (PSG) of Neumann	221820	17q21–q22	?
Parkinsonism-dementia with pallido-ponto-nigral degeneration (PPND)	168610	17q21–q22	tau
Multiple system tauopathy with presenile dementia	601875	17q21	tau
Familial British dementia; presenile dementia with spastic ataxia cerebral amyloid angiopathy, British type	176500	13q14	BRI 603904, integral membrane protein 2B; ITM2B
Creutzfeld–Jakob disease	123400	20pter–p12	prion protein (176640)
Cerebral autosomal dominant angiopathy with subcortical infarctions and leukoariosis [CADASIL]	125310	19q12	Homologue 3 of Drosophila NOTCH (600276)
Dementia, familial nonspecific	600795	3p11.1–q11.2	
Atherosclerosis, premature, with deafness, nephropathy, diabetes mellitus, photomyoclonus, and degenerative neurologic disease	209010		
Lewy body dysphasic dementia	127750		associated with allele of debrisoquine 4-hydroxylase (CYP2D6B)
ALS-Parkinson–Dementia complex	105500		
Ceroid lipofuscinosis, adult type (Kufs disease) (CLN4)	204300		

Autosomal dominant Alzheimer's disease is rare, accounting for only 0.3% of cases (Campion et al., 1999). Mutations of any of three genes account for the majority of these autosomal dominant cases (Table 2.2). All of these lead to early onset, by age 60 (Dartigues & Letenneur, 2000). The prevalence of early-onset Alzheimer's disease has been estimated to be 41.2/100 000

of which only 12.9% were autosomal dominant. In the same population survey, 56% of these autosomal dominant families were found to have a mutation of presenilin-1, and another 15% to have a mutation in amyloid precursor protein APP. Although the vast majority of Alzheimer cases have not been associated with mutations in either presenilins-1, -2 or APP, these rare families have had great heuristic value in supporting a primary role for amyloid pathology.

In contrast, no simple inheritance pattern is evident in the more common late-onset Alzheimer's disease (AD). That notwithstanding, genetic factors play a major role in predisposition to AD, which has a λ_1 of 5. The only major susceptibility gene unequivocally identified to date is apolipoprotein E, with the presence of the E4 allele increasing the relative risk for AD by a factor of 4.5 in the heterozygous state (Scott et al., 1999). Although this was discovered in the course of linkage analysis, the positive marker was in linkage disequilibrium with apoE, and might not have been detected had a slightly more distant marker been used (Martin et al., 2000; Risch & Merikangas, 1997). However, the E4 allele is neither necessary nor sufficient for Alzheimer's disease: most apoE4 carriers do not dement and about one-half of Alzheimer's disease is not associated with apoE4 (Myers et al., 1996).

Furthermore, the effect of apoE is not specific for Alzheimer's disease, associations with ApoE 4 having been observed for susceptibility to Creutzfeld–Jakob disease (Amouyel et al., 1994), age of onset and susceptibility to Pick's disease (Farrer et al., 1995), susceptibility to schizophrenia (Harrington et al., 1995), age of onset of Huntington's disease in males (Kehoe et al., 1999a) though not disease susceptibility (Kalman et al., 2000), as well as poor outcomes after head trauma and intracerebral hemorrhage (Friedman et al., 1999; Horsburgh et al., 2000).

Although the total λ_1 for AD is 5, the gene-specific λ_1 for apoE is only 2, implying that a substantial part the genetic risk for AD results from other genes. It appears likely that there may be as many as 4 additional susceptibility genes for late-onset AD with effect comparable or greater than that of apoE (Martinez et al., 1998; Warwick Daw et al., 2000). Candidates include an alpha-2-macroglublin in 12p13.3–p12.3, supported in some studies (Blacker et al., 1998; Liao et al., 1998), but not others (Shibata et al., 2000); a perhaps unrelated gene in 12p11.23–q13.12 (Scott et al., 2000); very low density lipoprotein receptor encoded on 9p24 (Okuizumi et al., 1995); bleomycin hydrolase on 17q11.2 (Papassotiropoulos et al., 2000); interleukin 1α (Du et al., 2000); and certain variations of the mitochondrial genome (Hutchin & Cortopassi, 1995). Genetic studies with these candidates have either given mixed results or await confirmation.

Multiple sclerosis

Unlike the adult-onset dementias, no monogenic forms of multiple sclerosis have been reported. Although there may be initial diagnostic confusion presented by the clinical features of adult-onset spinocerebellar atrophies and hereditary spastic paraplegias (Durr & Brice, 2000) or with the radiographic appearance of CADASIL or some of the leukodystrophies, routine clinical evaluation easily distinguishes these Mendelian disorders from multiple sclerosis (Hutchin & Cortopassi, 1995).

Neverthess, this disorder is highly heritable, with a λ_1 of 30, five times that of late-onset Alzheimer's disease. Six per cent of MS probands have an affected first-degree relative, considerably in excess of that predicted by a population frequency of 3/10000. Monozygotic twins have a concordance rate of 25.9% compared to a 2.3% concordance rate in dizygotic twins, suggesting polygenic inheritance. The number of concordant twins in these studies is low, however, and the twin data need to be viewed with some circumspection (Ebers et al., 1995). Despite this apparently high heritability, three recently completed genome-wide linkage scans have failed to identify a susceptibility locus unequivocally (Ebers et al., 1995; Multiple Sclerosis Genetics Group, 1996; Sawcer et al., 1996). The strongest signals from these linkage studies clustered around the HLA region on chromosome 6p21. Even though the HLA locus contributes little to overall susceptibility, it has been clearly identified in a number of case-controlled and TDT studies that have demonstrated an association with HLA-DR2 alleles (Haines et al., 1998).

Weaker positive associations have been observed with interferon gamma in patients at low risk because of their HLA status (Goris et al., 1999; Vandenbroeck et al., 1998) and the I-cell adhesion molecule (Mycko et al., 1998). Severity of but not susceptibility to MS (Reboul et al., 2000) has been reported to be associated with a certain combination of interleukin-1beta and interleukin-1 receptor antagonist genes. An association has been reported with TNF-α, independent of the association with the nearby HLA region (Fernandez-Arquero et al., 1999) as has an association with the immunogobulin heavy chain region (Walter et al., 1991). Association studies with myelin basic protein (Wood et al., 1994) and complement factors 6 and 7 (Chataway et al., 1999) have been negative. Both the negative and positive associations deserve to be re-examined and other regions of the genome examined in larger populations with denser marker arrays. However, at present, there is no strong evidence to support the existence of any susceptibility genes of moderate or major effect other than HLA.

Parkinson's disease

Although there is little evidence for substantial genetic contribution to typical late-onset Parkinson's disease, some early-onset disease is attributable to either mono-genic or polygenic disorders. A rare autosomal dominant form of parkinsonism associated with dysautonomia and dementia has been associated with mutations of the alpha-synuclein gene (Polymeropoulos et al., 1996). An autoso-mal recessive juvenile-onset parkinsonian syndrome with atypical clinical features has been associated with muta-tions in the parkin gene (Kitada et al., 1998). Parkinsonian features can sometimes be seen in several other Mendelian disorders, including some of the dominantly inherited spinocerebellar atrophies associated with triplet repeat expansions (Durr & Brice, 2000); the X-linked Segawa syn-drome resulting from mutations in GTP cyclohydrolase (Ischinose et al., 1994; Nygaard & Duvoisin, 1986); Filipino dystonia syndrome (Muller et al., 1990); as part of the phe-notype of a single infant with tyrosine hydroxylase defi-ciency (Ludecke et al., 1996); in several of the syndromes associated with mutations in the microtubule tau gene (Lynch et al., 1994; Wijker et al., 1996); and in the X-linked Waisman syndrome of early-onset parkinsonism, mega-encephaly and seizures (Gregg et al., 1991).

However, these rare Mendelian disorders can be distin-guished readily from classic Parkinson's disease, a common disorder of late adult life with incidence of about 1/10 000 (Bower et al., 1999; Tanner et al., 1999). A large twin study demonstrated no difference in concordance for monozygotic or dizygotic twins with late-onset Parkinson's disease (Tanner et al., 1999). The same study demonstrated a sixfold higher monozygotic concordance rate in those twins for whom disease onset was before age 50. These data imply that there is a significant genetic risk for early-onset disease, but none for typical late-onset Parkinson's disease. Segregation analysis has ruled out Mendelian inheritance as an explanation for occasional familial clus-tering of Parkinson's disease (Zareparsi et al., 1998). Biochemical and cell fusion studies have suggested that a non-Mendelian susceptibility factor might be mitochon-drial DNA (Swerdlow et al., 1996), a plausible hypothesis for which the evidence remains inconclusive.

Epilepsy

Although described by Hippocrates as a familial disease, epilepsy is present in siblings in only a minority of families (Baraitser, 1982). Heritability differs by seizure type and age of onset. For idiopathic grand mal epilepsy beginning before age 35, the concordance rate for MZ twins is 0.30 and for DZ twins it is only 0.13 (Miller et al., 1999) whereas for late-onset cases there is no significant difference. Overall, the frequency in close relatives ranges from 3 to 6%, compared to a general population risk of 0.5%

(Alstrom, 1950). Febrile seizures have a recurrence rate of 0.39 in MZ twins and 0.12 in DZ twins, indicating signifi-cant heritability. The frequency of febrile seizures in sib-lings is 20% (Frantzen et al., 1970), compared to a general population risk of 3% (Baraitser, 1982). Other studies suggest common genetic factors for febrile convulsions, temporal lobe epilepsy and early status epilepticus (Baraitser, 1982).

Some of this familial clustering results from rare mono-genic disorders that segregate as simple Mendelian traits (Table 2.3). However, a larger number of cases appear to result from multigenic inheritance. Susceptibility loci have been mapped, but genes not yet identified. (Table 2.4). In some types of epilepsy, there are a few genes of major effect, none of which is either necessary or sufficient to cause the disorder. In nocturnal frontal lobe epilepsy the effects of two single genes were so strong that they were located with a modified Mendelian model, with allowances for low penetrance (Phillips et al., 1995) (Table 2.3). In con-trast juvenile myoclonic epilepsy proved more difficult to map using a Mendelian model, but more tractable using a complex genetic model (Elmslie et al., 1997; Greenberg et al., 2000) using which, two susceptibility loci have been identified. Reduced penetrance in a Mendelian model and complex genetics can simply be different ways of model-ling the same reality.

Migraine

The genetics of migraine has proven difficult in part because of the high prevalence of this disorder, with a life-time incidence of 33% in women and 13.3% in men (Launer et al., 1999). Studies in monozygotic and dizygotic twins raised either together or apart, have yielded herit-ability estimates of 52% (Ziegler et al., 1998). Twin studies of migraine with aura show a concordance rate of 34% in MZ twins and only 21% in DZ twins, similar to that of non-twin siblings (Ulrich et al., 2000). In migraine without aura, the concordance ratios were similar: 28% in MZ and 18% in DZ twin pairs (Gervil et al., 1999). Although many MZ twin migraineurs are concordant for the presence or absence of aura, a significant proportion are not (Kallela et al., 1999). Rare severe forms of migraine with aura, familial hemi-plegic migraine, have been shown to be monogenic disor-ders. Fifty per cent of these families have mutations of the CACNL1A4 gene on chromosome 19p13 (Ophoff et al., 1996). The same locus appears to contribute to some cases of non-hemiplegic migraine, either with or without aura. There are at least two other monogenic forms of hemi-plegic migraine, one of which has been mapped to chromosome 1q31 (Gardner et al., 1997). There is evidence

Table 2.3. 'Monogenic' epilepsy syndromes

Disorder	OMIM	Locus	Gene
Benign adult familial myoclonus epilepsy (BAFME; FAME) (autosomal dominant)	601068	8q23.3–q24.11	
Benign neonatal convulsions, type I (BFNC1) (autosomal dominant)	121200	20q13.3	potassium channel, voltage-gated, subfamily Q, member 2; KCNQ2 (602235)
Benign neonatal convulsions, type II (EBN2; BFNC2) (autosomal dominant)	121201	8q24	potassium channel, voltage-gated, subfamily Q, member 3 KCNQ3 gene (602232
Idiopathic generalized epilepsy (EGI)	600669	8q24	? allelic to EBN2
Benign familial infantile convulsions BFIC (autosomal dominant)	601764	19q	
Benign Rolandic epilepsy; Centrotemporal epilepsy	117100		(mouse gene found on 9)
Childhood Absence Epilepsy 1 (ECA1)	600131	8q24	
Childhood Absence Epilepsy 2 (ECA2)	600131	5q31.1–q33.1	gamma-aminobutyric acid receptor, gamma-2 (GABRG2) (137164)
Febrile convulsions, familial, 1 FEB1 (autosomal dominant, penetrance 60%)	602476	8q13–q21	
Febrile convulsions, familial, 2 FEB2 (autosomal dominant)	602477	19p13.3	
Febrile convulsions, familial, 3 FEB3 (autosomal dominant)	604403	2q23–q24	
Generalized epilepsy with febrile seizures plus; GEFS+, TYPE 1 (autosomal dominant)	604236	19q13	voltage-gated sodium channel beta-1 subunit gene (SCN1B) (600235)
Generalized epilepsy with febrile seizures plus, type 2; GEFS+, TYPE 2 (GEFSP2)(autosomal dominant)	604233	2q21–q33	alpha-subunit voltage-gated sodium channels (SCN1A)(182389)
Generalized epilepsy with febrile seizures plus, type 3; GEFS+, TYPE 3 (GEFSP3)	614233	5q31.1–q33.1	gamma-aminobutyric acid receptor, gamma-2 (GABRG2) (137164)
Nocturnal frontal lobe epilepsy ENFL 1 (autosomal dominant, low penetrance)	600513	20q13.2	neuronal nicotinic acetylcholine receptor, alpha polypeptide 4 (CHRNA4) (118504)
Nocturnal frontal lobe epilepsy ENFL 2 (autosomal dominant, low penetrance)	603204	15q24	close to the CHRNA3 (118503)/CHRNA5 (118505)/CHRNB4 (118509) cluster.
Nocturnal frontal lobe epilepsy ENFL 3 (autosomal dominant, low penetrance)	605375	1p21	Acetylcholine receptor, neuronal nicotinic, beta-2 subunit (CHRNB2) (118507)
Partial epilepsy (autosomal dominant)	600512	10q23.3–q24.1	
Reading epilepsy	132300		
Rolandic epilepsy and speech dyspraxia	601085		

Table 2.4. Susceptibility loci for epilepsy

Disorder	Susceptibility locus
Febrile convulsions, familial, 4 (FEB4)	5q14–q15
Idiopathic generalized epilepsy EGI	8q24
Idiopathic generalized epilepsy EGI	2q22–q23
Juvenile myoclonic epilepsy EJM1, Janz syndrome	6p
Juvenile myoclonic epilepsy EJM2	15q14

Table 2.5. Heritability of stroke

Aneurysm/SAH	$\lambda = 4.2$	(2.2–8.0)
Intraparenchymal hemorrhage	$\lambda = 2.39$	
Dissection	$\lambda = 6.3$	(2.2–18.3)
All ischemic	$\lambda = 1.4$	(1.1–2.0)
Large artery	$\lambda = 1.85$	
Lacunar	$\lambda = 2.53$	
heritability	= 73%	
twin concordance	= 61% MZ, 38% DZ	

for susceptibility loci on the X chromosome and elsewhere for non-hemiplegic migraine (Nyholt et al., 1998)

Genetic analyses have been undertaken not only for susceptibility but also for specific characteristics of the migraine syndrome. For example, preliminary observations suggest that predisposition to aura in migraineurs may be influenced by a locus on chromosome 6p (Gardner et al., 1997), predisposition to migraine-related strokes by variations in the mitochondrial genome (Nyholt et al., 1998), and the frequency of migraine attacks by a gene in the vicinity of angiotensin-converting enzyme (Martelletti et al., 1999).

Stroke

Although individually rare, there are a large number of Mendelian disorders associated with stroke, which have been reviewed extensively (Hassan & Markus, 2000; Natowicz & Kelley, 1987). Of particular interest is CADASIL, resulting from mutations of the notch3 gene (Viitanen & Kalimo, 2000) and homocystinuria, which can result from deficiency of any of several enzymes (Mudd et al., 1998). Although homozygotes for classic homocystinuria are very rare, heterozygotes are relatively common. An elevated plasma level of homocystine is a significant risk factor for stroke in the general population (Giles et al., 1998) but the relationship to specific genes has not yet been established (Kiely et al., 1993).

Except for these rare Mendelian disorders it is difficult to demonstrate a significant degree of heritability for stroke, in large part because of the high incidence in the general population. The sex-averaged relative risk of having a stroke by virtue of having an affected parent is only 1.9 (Kiely et al., 1993). Population studies demonstrate ethnic differences, which could either be genetic or environmental (Kiely et al., 1993; Reed, 1993). Although a twin concordance study has suggested an influence of genetic factors, generalizations from this small sample must be made with caution (Howard et al., 1994).

However, if stroke is subdivided by type, certain groupings appear to have a higher heritability than others (Table 2.5). A large number of association studies have been undertaken in an effort to identify susceptibility genes underlying ischemic stroke in the general population. Of these, studies with the fibrinogen gene have been positive, showing a modest but consistent effect, whereas studies with genes encoding other clotting factors have been either negative or irreproducible (Hassan & Markus, 2000). Complex genetic analyses of the stroke-prone spontaneously hypertensive rat have identified three distinct quantitative trait loci that account for most of the variance in incidence and severity of stroke (Jeffs et al., 1997; Rubattu et al., 1996) in these laboratory strains. The genes underlying such susceptibility remain to be identified, as does its relevance to human disease (Rubattu et al., 1999).

Myasthenia gravis

About 4% of myasthenics have an affected relative, higher than would be expected from a population prevalence of 2 to 4/100 000. There is a sharp dichotomy in heritability between early- and late-onset forms (Online Mendelian Inheritance in Man, 2001). Forty-two per cent of familial cases have onset before 2 years of age, and perhaps are more appropriately described as myasthenic syndromes. Some of this familial clustering is not genetic, but results from maternal transmission of antibody, whereas others result from rare mutations affecting end-plate acetylcholinesterase or the alpha, beta or gamma subunit of nicotinic receptor. Infantile cases only account for 1% of all myasthenics.

Genetic susceptibility to the more common adult-onset form is complex. Some of this genetic susceptibility resides in the HLA region, particularly HLA-DR3 and -B8 (Janer et al., 1999), especially for females. The predisposing haplotypes are the same as for juvenile-onset diabetes mellitus, systemic lupus erythematosus and susceptibility to HIV

(Price et al., 1999). Other HLA associations have been reported for polymyositis and dermatomyositis (Rider et al., 1998). An association with myasthenia gravis has also been reported for the beta-adrenergic receptor (Xu et al., 2000). Although there has been no association independent of HLA between TNFβ and myasthenia (Manz et al., 1998), differences in this site may discriminate myasthenics with thymic hyperplasia from those with thymomas (Zelano et al., 1998). Similarly, there may be an allelic association between interleukin-10 and levels of circulating antinicotinic receptor antibodies in myasthenics but no association with disease susceptibility (Huang et al., 1999).

Pain

Weak associations with the HLA locus have been demonstrated for susceptibility to reflex sympathetic dystrophy (Huang et al., 1999) now renamed the complex regional pain syndrome. Rare instances of monogenic congenital insensitivity to pain have been mapped (Online Mendelian Inheritance in Man, 2001), and, in one instance, the mutant gene identified (Kemler et al., 1999).

However, the heritability of overall pain sensitivity in the general population is a low 10%, with MZ and DZ concordances almost identical. Genetic studies with inbred rodents tested for specific pain mechanisms have shown much higher heritability, attributable in most instances to a small number of genes of major effect (Mogil et al., 1999). Susceptibility to one type of painful stimulus can be either positively or negatively correlated with responses to other stimuli. Genetic analysis of mechanism-based pain susceptibility has yet to be undertaken in humans.

Sleep disorders

Several types of sleep disorder have been described, of which narcolepsy is the best understood. Strong association with the HLA region on chromosome 6 p21.3 has long been known (Mignot et al., 1997). The segregation pattern is complex. Mutations of orexin receptor 2, encoded by a gene on human chromosome 6p21, give rise to a monogenic narcolepsy in dogs (Lin et al., 1999). To date, mutations in the orexin receptor 2 gene have not been reported in humans with narcolepsy although low CSF levels of orexin are common (Nishino et al., 2000). It appears that the proximity of the two genes is fortuitous, and orexin deficiency in most cases of narcolepsy may be the result of immune attack on the hypothalamus. A mutation in the preproorexin gene has been reported in a single case of atypical narcolepsy (Peyron et al., 2000), but this mutation appears exceptional.

Other types of sleep disorder have been shown to segregate as simple Mendelians traits: rare instances of fatal familial insomnia, an autosomal dominant disease resulting from mutations of the prion protein gene (Harder et al., 1999) and a circadian rhythm disturbance (Toh et al., 2000). Genetic definition of other sleep disorders will depend in part on a better definition of phenotype.

References

Alstrom, C.H. (1950). A study of epilepsy in its clinical, social and genetic aspects. *Acta Psychiat. Neurol. Scand. Suppl*, **63**, 1–284.

Amouyel, P., Vidal, O., Launay, J.M. & Laplanch, J.L. (1994). The apolipoprotein E alleles as major susceptibility factors for Creutzfeldt–Jakob disease. The French Research Group on Epidemiology of Human Spongiform Encephalopathies. *Lancet*, **344**, 1315–18.

Antonarakis, S.E. (1993). Human chromosome 21: genome mapping and exploration circa. *Trends Genet.*, **9**, 142–8.

Aparicio, S.A. (2000). How to count . . . human genes. *Nat. Genet.*, **25**, 129–30.

Bailey, A., LeCouteur, A., Gottesman, I. I. et al. (1995). Autism as a strong genetic disorder: evidence from a British twin study. *Psychol. Med.*, **25**, 63–77.

Baraitser, M. (1982). *The Genetics of Neurological Disorders.* Oxford: Oxford University Press.

Beckmann, J.S. (1999). Disease taxonomy – monogenic muscular dystrophy. *Br. Med. Bull.*, **55**, 340–57.

Bentley, D.R. (2000). The Human Genome Project – an overview. *Med. Res. Rev.*, **20**, 189–96.

Bently, D.R. & Dunham, I. (1995). Mapping human chromosomes. *Curr. Opin. Genet. Dev.*, **5**, 328–34.

Blacker, D., Wilcox, M.A., Laird, N.M. et al. (1998). Alpha-2 macroglobulin is genetically associated with Alzheimer's disease. *Nat. Genet.*, **19**, 357–60.

Botstein, D., White, R.L., Skolnick, M. & Davis, R.W. (1980). Construction of a genetic linkage map in man using restriction fragment length polymorphisms. *Am. J. Hum. Genet.*, **32**, 314–31.

Bower, J.H., Maraganore, D.M., McDonnell, S.K. & Rocca, W.A. (1999). Incidence and distribution of parkinsonism in Olmstead County, Minnesota. *Neurology*, **12** (52), 1214–20.

Brzustowicz, L.M., Hodgkinson, K.A., Chow, E.W., & Honer, W.G. (2000). Location of a major susceptibility locus for familial schizophrenia on chromosome 1q21–q22. *Science*, **288**, 678–82.

Bushby, K M. (1999). The limb–girdle muscular dystrophies: diagnostic guidelines. *Europ. J. Paediatr. Neurol.*, **3**, 53–8.

Butler, I.J. & Gadoth, N. (1976). Kearns–Sayre syndrome: a review of a multisystem disorder of children and young adults. *Arch. Intern. Med.*, **136**, 1290–3.

Butler, D. & Smaglik, P. (2000). Draft data leave geneticists with a mountain still to climb. *Nature*, **405**, 984–5.

Campion, D., Dumanchin, C., Hannequin, D. et al. (1999).

Early-onset autosomal dominant Alzheimer's disease: prevalence, genetic heterogeneity, and mutation spectrum. *Am. J. Hum. Genet.*, **65**, 664–70.

Chataway, J., Sawcer, S., Sherman, D et al. (1999). No evidence for association of multiple sclerosis with the complement factors C6 and C7. *J. Neuroimmunol.*, **99**, 150–6.

Childs, B. (1998). A logic of disease. In *The Metabolic and Molecular Bases of Inherited Disease*, ed. C.R. Scriver, A.L. Beaudet, S. Sly & D. Valle, 7th edn, pp. 229–58, New York: McGraw-Hill, Inc.

Collins, F.S. (1990). Identifying human disease genes by positional cloning. *Harvey Lect.*, **91** (86), 149–64.

Cummings, C.J. & Zoghbi, H.Y. (2000). Fourteen and counting: unraveling trinucleotide repeat diseases. *Hum. Mol. Genet.*, **9**, 909–16.

Dartigues, J.F. & Letenneur, L. (2000). Genetic epidemiology of Alzheimer's disease. *Curr. Opin. Neurol.*, **13**, 385–9.

Du, Y., Dodel, R.C., Eastwood, B.J. et al. (2000). Association of an interleukin 1 alpha polymorphism with Alzheimer's disease. *Neurology*, **22** (55), 480–3.

Durr, A. & Brice, A. (2000). Clinical and genetic aspects of spinocerebellar degeneration. *Curr. Opin. Neurol.*, **13**, 407–13.

Ebers, G.C., Bulman, D.E., Sadovnick, A.D. et al. (1986). A population-based study of multiple sclerosis in twins. *New Engl. J. Med.*, **315**, 1638–42.

Ebers, G.C., Sadovnick, A.D. & Risch, N.J. (1995). A genetic basis for familial aggregation in multiple sclerosis. Canadian Collaborative Study Group. *Nature*, **14** (377), 150–1.

Ebers, G.C., Kukay, K., Bulman, D.E. et al. (1990). A full genome search in multiple sclerosis. *Nat. Genet.*, **13**, 472–6.

Elmslie, F.V., Rees, M., Williamson, M.P. et al. (1997). Genetic mapping of a major susceptibility locus for juvenile myoclonic epilepsy on chromosome 15q. *Hum. Mol. Genet.*, **6**, 1329–34.

England, S.B., Nicholson, L.V.B., Johnson, M.A. et al. (1990). Very mild muscular dystrophy associated with the deletion of 46% of dystrophin. *Nature*, **343**, 180–2.

Estivill, X. (1996). Complexity in a monogenic disease. *Nat. Genet.*, **12**, 348–50.

Falconer, D.S. (1960). *Introduction to Quantitative Genetics*. New York: Ronald Press.

Fan, J-B., Chen, X., Halushka, M.K. et al. (2000). Parallel genotyping of human SNPs using generic high-density oligonucleotide tag arrays. *Genome Res.*, **10**, 853–60.

Farrer, L.A., Abraham, C.R., Volicer, L. et al. (1995). Allele epsilon 4 of apolipoprotein E shows a dose effect on age at onset of Pick disease. *Exp. Neurol.*, **136**, 162–70.

Fernandez-Arquero, M., Arroyo, R., Rubio, A. et al. (1999). Primary association of a TNF gene polymorphism with susceptibility to multiple sclerosis. *Neurology*, **53**, 1361–3.

Folstein, S. & Rutter, M. (1977). Infantile autism: a genetic study of 21 twin pairs. *J. Child Psychol. Psychiat.*, **18**, 297–321.

Frantzen, E., Lennox-Buchthal, M., Nygaard, A. & Stene, J.A. (1970). A genetic study of febrile convulsions. *Neurology*, **20**, 909–17.

Fridman, C. & Koiffmann, C.P. (2000). Origin of uniparental disomy 15 in patients with Prader-Willi or Angelman syndrome, *Am. J. Med. Genet.*, **94**, 249–53.

Friedman, G., Froom, P., Sazbon, L. et al. (1999). Apolipoprotein E-epsilon-4 genotype predicts a poor outcome in survivors of traumatic brain injury. *Neurology*, **52**, 244–8.

Gaasterland, T. & Bekiranov, S. (2000). Making the most of microarray data. *Nat. Genet.*, **24**, 204–6.

Gardner, K., Barmada, M.M., Ptacek, L.J. & Hoffman, E.P. (1997). A new locus for hemiplegic migraine maps to chromosome 1q31. *Neurology*, **49**, 1231–8.

Germer, S., Holland, M.J. & Higuchi, R. (2000). High-throughput SNP allele-frequency determination in pooled DNA samples by kinetic PCR. *Genome Res.*, **10**, 258–66.

Gervil, M., Ulrich, V., Kyvik, K O., Olesen, J. & Russell, M.B. (1999). Migraine without aura: a population-based twin study. *Ann. Neurol.*, **1999**, (46), 606–11.

Giles, W.H., Croft, J.B., Greenlund, K.J., Ford, E.S. & Kittner, S.J. (1998). Total homocyst(e)ine concentration and the likelihood of nonfatal stroke: results from the Third National Health and Nutrition Examination Survey. *Stroke*, **29**, 2473–7.

Gillard, E.F., Otsu, K., Fujii, J. et al. (1992). Polymorphisms and deduced amino acid substitutions in the coding sequence of the ryanodine receptor (RYR1) gene in individuals with malignant hyperthermia. *Genomics*, **13**, 1247–54.

Goodwin, D.W., Schulsinger, F., Moller, N., Hermansen, L., Winokur, G. & Guze, S.B. (1974). Drinking problems in adopted and nonadopted sons of alcoholics. *Arch. Gen. Psychiat.*, **31**, 164–9.

Goris, A., Epplen, C., Fiten, P. et al. (1999). Analysis of an IFN-gamma gene (IFNG) polymorphism in multiple sclerosis in Europe: effect of population structure on association with disease. *J. Interferon Cytokine Res.*, **19**, 1037–46.

Gottesman, I.I. (1994). Schizophrenia epigenesis: past, present, and future. *Acta Psychiatr. Scand. Suppl.*, **384**, 26–33.

Gray, I.C., Campbell, D.A. & Spurr, N.K. (2000). Single nucleotide polymorphisms as tools in human genetics. *Hum. Mol. Genet.*, **9**, 2403–8.

Greenberg, D.A., Durner, M., Keddache, M. et al. (2000). Reproducibility and complications in gene searches: linkage on chromosome 6, heterogeneity, association, and maternal inheritance in juvenile myoclonic epilepsy. *Am. J. Hum. Genet.*, **66** (508), 516.

Greenstein, M.A. (1990). Prader–Willi and Angelman syndromes in one kindred with expression consistent with genetic imprinting. *Am. J. Hum. Genet.*, **47**, A59.

Gregg, R.G., Metzenberg, A.B., Hogan, K., Sekhon, G. & Laxova, R. (1991). Waisman syndrome, a human X-linked recessive basal ganglia disorder with mental retardation: localization to Xq27.3-dter. *Genomics*, **9**, 701–6.

Haines, J.L., Terwedow, H.A., Burgess, K. et al. (1998). Linkage of the MHC to familial multiple sclerosis suggests genetic heterogeneity. *Hum. Mol. Genet.*, **7**, 1229–34.

Harder, A., Jendroska, K., Kreuz, F. et al. (1999). Novel twelve-generation kindred of fatal familial insomnia form Germany representing the entire spectrum of disease expression. *Am. J. Med. Genet.*, **87**, 311–16.

Harrington, C.R., Roth, M., Xuereb, J.H., McKenna, P.J. & Wischik,

C.M. (1995). Apolipoprotein E type epsilon-4 allele frequency is increased in patients with schizophrenia. *Neurosci. Lett.*, **202**, 101–4.

Hassan, A. & Markus, H.S. (2000). Genetics and ischaemic stroke. *Brain*, **123**, 1784–812.

Haviland, M.B., Ferrell, R.E. & Sing, C.F. (1997). Association between common alleles of the low-density lipoprotein gene region and interindividuals variation in plasma lipids and alpoliprotein levels in a population based sample from Rochester, Minnesota. *Hum. Genet.*, **99**, 108–14.

Hawkes, C.H. (1997). Twin studies in medicine – what do they tell us?. *Q. J. Med.*, **90**, 311–21.

Heston, L.L. (1996). Psychiatric disorders in foster-home reared children of schizophrenic mothers. *Br. J. Psychiat.*, **112**, 819–25.

Horsburgh, K., McCarron, M.O., White, F. & Nicoll, J.A. (2000). The role of apolipoprotein E in Alzheimer's disease, acute brain injury and cerebrovascular disease: evidence of common mechanisms and utility of animal models. *Neurobiol. Aging*, **21**, 245–55.

Howard, G., Anderson, R., Sorlie, P., Andrews, V., Backlund, E. & Burke, G.L. (1994). Ethnic differences in stroke mortality between non-Hispanic whites, Hispanic whites, and blacks. The National Longitudinal Mortality Study. *Stroke*, **25**, 2120–5.

Huang, D.R., Zhou, Y.H., Xia, S.Q., Liu, L., Pirskanen, R. & Lefvert, A.K. (1999). Markers in the promoter region of interleukin-10 (IL-10) gene in myasthenia gravis: implications of diverse effects of IL-10 in the pathogenesis of the disease. *J. Neuroimmunol.*, **1**, (94), 82–7.

Hulten, M., Armstrong, S., Challinor, P. (1991). Genomic imprinting in an Angelman and Prader-Willi translocation family. *Lancet*, **338**, 638–9.

Hurko, O. (1997). The explosion of neurogenetics. *Curr. Opin. Neurol.*, **10**, 77–83.

Hurko, O. (2001). Genetics and genomics in neuropharmacology: the impact on drug discovery and development. *Europ. Neuropsychopharmacol.*, **11**, 491–9.

Hurko, O., Johns, D.R., Rutledge, S.L. et al. (1990). Heteroplasmy in chronic external ophthalmoplegia: clinical and molecular observations. *Pediatr. Res.*, **19** (28), 542–8.

Hutchin, T. & Cortopassi, G.A. (1995). A mitochondrial DNA clone is associated with increased risk for Alzheimer's disease. *Proc. Nat. Acad. Sci. USA*, **92**, 6892–5.

International Human Genome Sequencing Consortium (2001). Initial sequencing and analysis of the human genome. *Nature*, **409**, 860–921.

Ischinose, H., Ohye, T., Takahashi, E. et al. (1994). Hereditary progressive dystonia with marked diurnal fluctuation caused by mutations in the GTP cyclohydrolase I gene. *Nat. Genet.*, **8**, 236–42.

James, W.H. (1996). Review of the contribution of twin studies in the search for non-genetic causes of multiple sclerosis. *Neuroepidemiology*, **15**, 132–41.

Janer, M., Cowland, A., Picard, J. et al. (1999). A susceptibility region for myasthenia gravis extending into the HLA-class I sector telomeric to HLA-C. *Hum. Immunol.*, **60**, 909–17.

Jeffs, B., Clark, J.S., Anderson, N.H. et al. (1997). Sensitivity to cerebral ischemic insult in a rat model of stroke is determined by a single genetic locus. *Nat. Genet.*, **16**, 364–7.

Jin, P. & Warren, S.T. (2000). Understanding the molecular basis of fragile X syndrome. *Hum. Mol. Genet.*, **9**, 901–8.

Jorde, L.B. (1995). Linkage disequilibrium as a gene-mapping tool. *Am. J. Hum. Genet.*, **56**, 11–14.

Kallela, M., Wessman, M., Fakkila, M., Palotie, A., Koskenvuo, M.L. & Kaprio, J. (1999). Clinical characteristics of migraine concordant monozygotic twin pairs. *Acta Neurol. Scand.*, **100**, 254–9.

Kalman, J., Juhasz, A., Majtenyi, K. et al. (2000). Apolipoprotein E polymorphism in Pick's disease and in Huntington's disease. *Neurobiol. Aging*, **21**, 555–8.

Kehoe, P., Krawczak, M., Harper, P.S., Owen, M.J. & Jones, A.L. (1999a). Age of onset in Huntington disease: sex specific influence of apolipoprotein E genotype and normal CAG repeat length. *J. Med. Genet.*, **36**, 108–11.

Kehoe, P., Wavrant-De Vrieze, F., Crook, R. et al. (1999b). Full genome scan for late onset Alzheimer's disease. *Hum. Mol. Genet.*, **8**, 237–45.

Kemler, M.A., van de Vusse, A.C., van den Berg-Loonen, E.M., Barendse, G.A., van Kleef, M. & Weber, W.E.J. (1999). HLA-DQ1 associated with reflex sympathetic dystrophy, *Neurology*, **53**, 1350–1.

Kendler, K. (1993). A test of the equal-environment assumption in twin studies of psychiatric illness. *Behav. Genet.*, **23**, 21–7.

Kiely, D.K., Wolf, P.A., Cupples, L.A., Beiser, A.S. & Myers, R.H. (1993). Familial aggregation of stroke. The Framingham Study. *Stroke*, **24**, 1366–71.

Kissel, J.T. & Mendell, J.R. (1999). Muscular dystrophy: historical overview and classification in the genetic era. *Semin. Neurol.*, **19**, 5–7.

Kitada, T., Asakawa, S., Hattori, N. et al. (1998). Mutations in the parkin gene cause autosomal recessive juvenile parkinsonism. *Nature*, **392**, 605–8.

Kooy, R.F., Willemsen, R., & Oostra, B.A. (2000). Fragile X syndrome at the turn of the century. *Mol. Med. Today*, **6**, 193–8.

Kruglyak, L. (1997). What is significant in whole-genome linkage disequilibrium studies? *Am. J. Hum. Genet.*, **61**, 810–12.

Kruglyak, L., Daly, M.J., Reeve-Daly, M.P. & Lander, E.S. (1996). Parametric and nonparametric linkage analysis: a unified multipoint approach. *American Journal of Human Genetics*, **58**, 1347–63.

Lander, E.S. & Botstein, D. (1986). Strategies for studying heterogeneous genetic traits in humans by using a linkage map of restriction fragment length polymorphisms. *Proc. Nat. Acad. Sci. USA*, **83**, 7353–7.

Launer, L.J., Terwindt, G.M. & Ferrari, M.D. (1999). The prevalence and characteristics of migraine in a population-based cohort: the GEM study. *Neurology*, **11** (53), 537–42.

Lee, C.K., Weindruch, R. & Prolla, T.A. (2000). Gene-expression profile of the ageing brain in mice. *Nat. Genet.*, **25**, 294–7.

Liang, F., Holt, I., Pertea, G., Karamycheva, S., Salzberg, S.L. & Quackenbush, J. (2000). Gene index analysis of the human genome estimates approximately 120, 000 genes. *Nat. Genet.*, **25**, 239–40.

Liao, A., Nitsch, R.M., Greenberg, S.M. et al. (1998). Genetic association of an alpha2-macroglobulin polymorphism and Alzheimer's disease. *Hum. Molec. Genet.*, **7**, 1953–6.

Lieberman, A.P. & Fischbeck, K.H. (2000). Triplet repeat expansion in neuromuscular disease. *Muscle Nerve*, **23**, 843–50.

Lin, L., Faraco, J., Li, R. et al. (1999). The sleep disorder canine narcolepsy is caused by a mutation in the hypocretin (orexin) receptor 2 gene, *Cell*, **98**, 365–76.

Ludecke, B., Knappskog, P.M., Clayton, P.T. et al. (1996). Recessively inherited L-DOPA-responsive parkinsonism in infancy caused by a point mutation (L205P) in the tyrosine hydroxylase gene. *Hum. Molec. Genet.*, **5**, 1023–8.

Lupski, J.R., Garcia, C.A., Zoghbi, H.Y., Hoffman, E.P. & Fenwick, R.G. (1991). Discordance of muscular dystrophy in monozygotic female twins: evidence supporting asymmetric splitting of the inner cell mass in a manifesting carrier of Duchenne dystrophy. *Am. J. Med. Genet.*, **40**, 354–64.

Lynch, T., Sano, M., Marder, K.S. et al. (1994). Clinical characteristics of a family with chromosome 17-linked disinhibition-dementia-parkinsonism-amyotrophy complex. *Neurology*, **44**, 1878–84.

McCarthy, T.V., Quane, K.A. & Lynch, P.J. (2000). Ryanodine receptor mutations in malignant hyperthermia and central core disease. *Hum. Mutat*, **15**, 410–17.

Maestri, N.E. & Beaty, T.H. (1992). Predictions of a 2-locus model for disease heterogeneity: application to adrenoleukodystrophy. *Am. J. Med. Genet.*, **44**, 576–82.

Maher, E.R. & Reik, W. (2000). Beckwith–Wiedemann syndrome: imprinting in clusters revisited. *J. Clin. Invest.*, **105**, 247–52.

Manz, M.G., Melms, A., Sommer, N. & Muller, C.A. (1998). Myasthenia gravis and tumor necrosis factor beta polymorphisms: linkage disequilibrium but no association beyond HLA-B8. *J. Neuroimmunol.*, **90**, 187–91.

Martelletti, P., Lulli, P., Morellini, M. et al. (1999). Chromosome 6p-encoded HLA-DR2 determination discriminates migraine without aura from migraine with aura. *Hum. Immunol.*, **60**, 69–74.

Martin, E.R., Lai, E.H., Gilbert, J.R. et al. (2000). SNPing away at complex diseases: analysis of single-nucleotide polymorphisms around APOE in Alzheimer's disease. *Am. J. Hum. Genet.*, **67**, 383–94.

Martin, N., Boomsma, D. & Machin, G. (1997). A twin-pronged attack on complex traits. *Nat. Genet.*, **17**, 387–92.

Martinez, M., Campion, D., Brice, A. et al. (1998). Apolipoprotein E epsilon4 allele and familial aggregation of Alzheimer's disease. *Arch. Neurol.*, **55**, 810–16.

Matsuo, M., Masumura, T., Nakajima, T. et al. (1990). A very small frame-shifting deletion within exon 19 of the Duchenne muscular dystrophy gene. *Biochem. Biophys. Res. Commun.*, **170**, 963–7.

Mendelian Inheritance in Man OMIM (TM) [Online]. World Wide Web URL http: //www.ncbi.nlm.nih.gov/omim/ (2001). McKusick–Nathans Institute for Genetic Medicine, Ref Type: Electronic Citation.

Mignot, E., Hayduk, R., Black, J., Grumet, F.C. & Guilleminault, C. (1997). HLA DQB1*0602 is associated with cataplexy in 509 narcoleptic patients. *Sleep*, **20**, 1012–20.

Miller, L.L., Pellock, J.M., Boggs, J.G., DeLorenzo, R.J., Meyer, J.M. & Corey, L.A. (1999). Epilepsy and seizure occurence in a population-based sample of Virginian twins and their families. *Epilepsy Res.*, **34**, 135–43.

Mogil, J.S., Wilson, S.G., Bon, K. et al. (1999). Heritability of nociception I: responses of 11 inbred mouse strains on 12 measures of nociception. *Pain*, **80**, 67–82.

Morissette, J., Villeneuve, A., Bordeleau, L. et al. (1999). Genome-wide search for linkage of bipolar affective disorders in a very large pedigree derived from a homogeneous population in Quebec points to a locus of major effect on chromosome 12q23–q24. 4. *Am. J. Med. Genet.*, **88**, 567–87.

Mudd, S.H., Levy, H.L. & Skovby, F. (1998). Disorders of transsulfuration. In *The Metabolic and Molecular Bases of Inherited Disease*, 7th Edn., ed. C.R. Scriver., A.L. Beaudet, S. Sly & D. Valley. no. 1279, p. 1327. New York: McGraw-Hill Inc.

Muglia, P., Jain, U., Macciardi, F. & Kennedy, J.L. (2000). Adult attention deficit hyperactivity disorder and the dopamine D4 receptor gene. *Am. J. Med. Genet.*, **96**, 273–7.

Muller, U., Lee, L.V., Viterbo, G. et al. (1990). The phenotype of X-linked torsion dystonia (XLTD). *Am. J. Hum. Genet.*, **47**, A69.

Multiple Sclerosis Genetics Group (1996). A complete genomic screen for multiple sclerosis underscores a role for the major histocompatability (sic) complex. *Nat. Genet.*, vol. 13, pp. 472–6.

Murphy, E.A. & Chase, G.A. (1975). *Principles of Genetic Counseling.* Chicago: Year Book Medical Publishers, Inc.

Mycko, M.P., Kwinkowski, M., Tronczynska, E., Szymanska, B. & Selmaj, K W. (1998). Multiple sclerosis: the increased frequency of the ICAM-1 exon 6 gene point mutation genetic type K469. *Ann. Neurol.*, **44**, 70–5.

Myers, R.H., Schaefer, E.J., Wilson, P.W.F. et al. (1996). Apolipoprotein E epsilon-4 associated with dementia in a population-based study: the Framingham study. *Neurology*, **46**, 673–7.

Natowicz, M. & Kelley, R.I. (1987). Mendelian etiologies of stroke. *Ann. Neurol.*, **22**, 175–92.

Nishino, S., Ripley, B., Overeem, S., Lammers, G.J. & Mignot, E. (2000). Hypocretin (orexin) deficiency in human narcolepsy. *Lancet*, **355**, 39–40.

Nygaard, T.G. & Duvoisin, R.C. (1986). Hereditary dystonia-parkinsonism syndrome of juvenile onset. *Neurology*, **36**, 1424–8.

Nyholt, D.R., Lea, R.A., Goadsby, P.J. & Brimage, P.J. (1998). Familial typical migraine: linkage to chromosome 19p13 and evidence for genetic heterogeneity. *Neurology*, **50**, 1428–30.

Okuizumi, K., Onodera, O., Namba, Y. et al. (1995). Genetic association of the very low density lipoprotein (VLDL) receptor gene with sporadic Alzheimer's disease. *Nat. Genet.*, **11**, 207–9.

Ophoff, R.A., Terwindt, G.M., Vergouwe, M.N. et al. (1996). Familial hemiplegic migraine and episodic ataxia type-2 are caused by mutations in the Ca^{2+} channel gene CACNL1A4. *Cell*, **87**, 543–52.

Ott, J. (1985). *Analysis of Human Genetic Linkage.* Baltimore: The Johns Hopkins University Press.

Papassotiropoulos, A., Bagli, M., Jessen, F. et al. (2000). Confirmation of the association between bleomycin hydrolase genotype and Alzheimer's disease. *Molec. Psychiat.*, **5**, 213–15.

Peyron, C., Faraco, J., Rogers, W. et al. (2000). A mutation in a case of early onset narcolepsy and a generalized absence of hypocretin peptides in human narcoleptic brains. *Nat. Med.*, **6**, 991–7.

Phillips, H.A., Scheffer, I.E., Berkovic, S.F., Hollway, G.E., Sutherland, G R. & Mulley, J.C. (1995). Localization of a gene for autosomal dominant nocturnal frontal lobe epilepsy to chromosome 20q13.2. *Nat. Genet.*, **10**, 117–18.

Polymeropoulos, M.H., Higgins, J.J., Golbe, L.I. et al. (1996). Mapping of a gene for Parkinson's disease to chromosome 4q21–q23. *Science*, **274**, 1197–8.

Price, P., Witt, C., Allcock, R. et al. (1999). The genetic basis for the association of the 8.1 ancestral haplotype (A1, B8, DR3) with multiple immunopathological diseases. *Immunol. Rev.*, **167**, 257–74.

Pritchard, J.K. & Rosenberg, N.A. (1999). Use of unlinked genetic markers to detect population stratification in associated studies. *Am. J. Hum. Genet.*, **65**, 220–8.

Reboul, J., Mertens, C., Levillayer, F. et al. (2000). Cytokines in genetic susceptibility to multiple sclerosis: a candidate gene approach. French Multiple Sclerosis Genetics Group. *J. Neuroimmunol.*, **102**, 107–12.

Reddy, P., Williams, M. & Tagle, D. (1999). Recent advances in understanding the pathogenesis of Huntington's disease. *Trends Neurosci.*, **22**, 248–55.

Reed, D.M. (1993). The paradox of high risk of stroke in populations with low risk of coronary heart disease. *Am. J Epidemiol.*, **131**, 579–88.

Rider, L.G., Gurley, R.C., Pandey, J.P. et al. (1998). Clinical, serologic, and immunogenetic features of familial idiopathic inflammatory myopathy. *Arthritis Rheum.*, **41**, 710–19.

Risch, N. & Botstein, D.A. (1996). A manic depressive history, *Nat. Genet.*, **12**, 351–3.

Risch, N. & Merikangas, K. (1996). The future of genetic studies of complex human diseases. *Science*, **273**, 1516–17.

Risch, N. & Merikangas, K. (1997). Genetic analysis of complex diseases. *Science*, **275**, 1329–30.

Rubattu, S., Ridker, P., Stampfer, M.J., Volpe, M., Hennekens, C.H. & Lindpainter, K. (1999). The gene encoding atrial natriuretic peptide and the risk of human stroke. *Circulation*, **19** (100), 1722–6.

Rubattu, S., Volpe, M., Kreutz, R., Ganten, U., Ganten, D. & Lindpaintner, K. (1996). Chromosomal mapping of quantitative trait loci contributing to stroke in a rat model of complex human disease. *Nat. Genet.*, **13**, 429–34.

Rudnik-Schoneborn, S., Wirth, B. & Zerres, K. (1994). Evidence of autosomal dominant mutations in childhood-onset proximal spinal muscular atrophy. *Am. J. Hum. Genet.*, **55**, 112–19.

Sawcer, S., Jones, H.B., Feakes, R. et al. (1996). A genome screen in multiple sclerosis reveals susceptibility loci on chromosome 6p21 and 17q22. *Nat. Genet.*, **13**, 464–8.

Schrijver, H.M., Crusius, J.B., Uitdehaag, B.M. et al. (1999). Association of interleukin-1beta and interleukin-1 receptor antagonist genes with disease severity in MS. *Neurology*, **52**, 595–9.

Scott, W.K., Pericak-Vance, M.A. & Haines, J.L. (1999). Genetic analysis of complex diseases. *Science*, **275**, 1327.

Scott, W.K., Grubber, J.M., Conneally, P. M. et al. (2000). Fine mapping of the chromosome 12 late-onset Alzheimer's disease locus: potential genetic and phenotypic heterogeneity. *Am. J. Hum. Genet.*, **66**, 922–32.

Shaw, S.H., Carrasquillo, M.M., Kashuk, C., Puffenberger, E.G. & Chakravarti, A. (1998). Allele frequency distributions in pooled DNA samples: applications to mapping complex disease genes. *Genome Res.*, **8**, 111–23.

Sherman, D.K., McGue, M.K. & Iacono, W.G. (1997). Twin concordance for attention deficit hyperactivity disorder: a comparison of teachers' and mother's reports. *Am. J. Psychiat.*, **154**, 532–5.

Shibata, N., Ohnuma, T., Takahashi, T. et al. (2000). No genetic association between alpha-2 macroglobulin I1000V polymorphism and Japanese sporadic Alzheimer's disease. *Neurosci. Lett.*, **290**, 154–6.

Smalley, S.L., Bailey, J.N., Palmer, C.G. et al. (1998). Evidence for the dopamine D4 receptor in a susceptibility gene in attention deficit hyperactivity disorder. *Molec. Psychiat.*, **3**, 427–30.

Spielman, R.S., McGinnis, R.E. & Ewens, W.J. (1993). Transmission test for linkage disequilibrium: the insulin gene region and insulin-dependent diabetes mellitus (IDDM). *Am. J. Hum. Genet.*, **52**, 502–16.

Stevanin, G., Durr, A. & Brice, A. (2000). Clinical and molecular advances in autosomal dominant cerebellar ataxias: from genotype to phenotype and physiopathology. *Eur. J. Hum. Genet.*, **8**, 4–18.

Strand, L.J., Felsher, B.F., Redeker, A.G. & Marver, H.S. (1970). Heme biosynthesis in intermittent acute porphyria: decreased hepatic conversion of porphobilinogen to porphyrins and increased delta aminolevulinic acid synthetase activity. *Proc. Natl. Acad. Sci. USA*, **67**, 1315–20.

Sutcliffe, J.G. (1988). mRNA in the mammalian central nervous system. *Ann. Rev. Neurosci.*, **11**, 157–98.

Swerdlow, R.H., Parks, J.K., Miller, S.W. et al. (1996). Origin and functional consequences of the complex I defect in Parkinson's disease. *Ann. Neurol.*, **40**, 663–71.

Tahir, E., Yazgan, Y., Cirakoglu, B., Ozbay, F., Waldman, I. & Asherson, P.J. (2000). Association and linkage of DRD4 and DRD5 with attention deficit hyperactivity disorder (ADHD) in a sample of Turkish children. *Mol. Psychiat.*, **5**, 396–404.

Tanner, C.M., Ottman, R., Goldman, S.M. et al. (1999). Parkinson disease in twins: an etiologic study. *J. Am. Med. Ass.*, **27** (281), 341–6.

Templeton, A.R., Boerwinkle, E. & Sing, C.F. (1987). A cladistic analysis of phenotypic associations with haplotypes inferred from restriction endonuclease mapping. I. Basic theory and an analysis of alcohol dehydrogenase activity in *Drosophila*. *Genetics*, **117**, 343–51.

Toh, K.I., Jones, C.R., He, Y. et al. (2000). An hPer2 phosphorylation site mutation in familial advanced sleep phase syndrome. *Science*, **291**, 1040–3.

Toniolo, D. & D'Adamo, P. (2000). X-linked non-specific mental retardation. *Curr. Opin. Genet. Dev.*, **10**, 280–5.

Trottier, Y., Biancalana, V. & Mandel, J-L. (1994). Instability of CAG repeats in Huntington's disease: relation to parental transmission and age of onset. *J. Med. Genet.*, **31**, 377–82.

Trottier, Y., Devys, D., Imbert, G. et al. (1995). Cellular localization of the Huntington's disease protein and discrimination of the normal and mutated form. *Nat. Genet.*, **10**, 104–10.

Ulrich, V., Gervil, M., Kyvik, K. O., Olesen, J. & Russell, M.B. (2000). The significance of genetic and environmental factors for migraine with aura. A genetic epidemiologic study of Danish twins. *Ugeskr. Laeger.*, **10** (162), 167–70.

Vandenbroeck, K., Opdenakker, G., Goris, A., Murru, R., Billiau, A. & Marrosu, M.G. (1998). Interferon-gamma gene polymorphism-associated risk for multiple sclerosis in Sardinia. *Ann Neurol*, **44**, 841–2.

Venter, J.C., Adams, M.D., Myers, E.W. et al. (2001). The sequence of the human genome. *Science*, **291**, 1304–51.

Viitanen, M. & Kalimo, H. (2000). CADASIL: hereditary arteriopathy leading to multiple brain infarcts and dementia. *Ann. NY. Acad. Sci.*, **903**, 273–84.

Walter, M.A., Gibson, W.T., Ebers, G.C. & Cox, D.W. (1991). Susceptibility to multiple sclerosis is associated with the proximal immunoglobulin heavy chain variable region. *J. Clin. Invest.*, **87**, 1266–73.

Warwick Daw, E., Payami, H., Nemens, E.J. et al. (2000). The number of trait loci in human late-onset Alzheimer's disease. *Am. J. Hum. Genet.*, **66**, 196–204.

Weeks, D.E., Conley, Y.P., Mah, T.S. et al. (2000). A full genome scan for age-related maculopathy. *Science*, **288**, 678–82.

Wijker, M., Wszolek, Z.K., Wolters, E.C.H. et al. (1996). Localization of the gene for rapidly progressive autosomal dominant parkinsonism and dementia with pallido-ponto-nigral degeneration to chromosome 17q21. *Hum. Mol. Genet.*, **5**, 151–4.

Wood, N.W., Holmans, P., Clayton, D., Robertson, N. & Compston, D.A.S. (1994). No linkage or association between multiple sclerosis and the myelin basic protein gene in affected sibling pairs. *J. Neurol. Neurosurg. Pscyhiat.*, **57**, 1191–4.

Xu, B.Y., Huang, D., Pirkanen, R. & Lefvert, A.K. (2000). Beta2-adrenergic receptor gene polymorphisms in myasthenia gravis (MG). *Clin. Exp. Immunol.*, **119**, 156–60.

Zareparsi, S., Taylor, T.D., Harris, E.L. & Payami, H. (1998). Segregation analysis of Parkinson disease. *J. Med. Genet.*, **4** (80), 410–17.

Zelano, G., Lino, M.M., Evoli, A. et al. (1998). Tumour necrosis factor beta gene polymorphisms in myasthenia gravis. *Eur. J. Immunogenet.*, **25**, 403–8.

Zhang, Y., Chen, H.S., Khanna, V.K. et al. (1993). A mutation in the human ryanodine receptor gene associated with central core disease. *Nat. Genet.*, **5**, 46–50.

Ziegler, D.K., Hur, Y.M., Bouchard, T.J.J., Hassanein, R.S. & Barter, R. (1998). Migraine in twins raised together and apart. *Headache*, **38** (417), 422.

3

Repeat expansion and neurological disease

J. Paul Taylor, Andrew P. Lieberman and Kenneth H. Fischbeck

Neurogenetics Branch, National Institute of Neurological Disorders and Stroke, National Institutes of Health, Bethesda, MD, USA

Repetitive DNA sequences are abundant in the human genome, scattered throughout the regions between genes and, in some cases, within genes. They take the form of minisatellites (repeat sequences ranging in length from tens to hundreds of nucleotides) and microsatellites (repeat sequences consisting of one to several nucleotides in length) and have an intrinsic genetic instability that results in frequent length changes (Charlesworth et al., 1994; Tautz & Schlotterer, 1994). Thus, mini- and microsatellites are highly polymorphic between individuals, a feature which has led to their extensive use in genetic research as markers in positional cloning of genes and also in forensic medicine for DNA-based identification, so-called 'DNA fingerprinting'. While the normal role of these sequences, if any, remains unclear, repeat sequences have gained a great deal of attention over the past decade because of their emerging role in human disease. In particular, expansions of repetitive sequences within genes are increasingly found to underlie hereditary neurological diseases. In this chapter we discuss mechanisms that have been proposed to generate repeat expansion, the relationship between repeat length and disease manifestations, and present a classification scheme for organizing trinucleotide expansion diseases. Finally, we discuss the clinical features, genetics, pathology and molecular pathogenesis of 16 currently recognized trinucleotide expansion diseases.

Anticipation

Neurologists have long recognized the clinical phenomenon of anticipation, the tendency of certain inherited neurological diseases to appear earlier in successive generations, often with more severe clinical manifestations. This phenomenon, which was described as early as 1918 in myo-

tonic dystrophy (Fleischer, 1918) and subsequently observed in other neurodegenerative diseases, was at odds with the classical Mendelian genetic principle that mutations are stably passed on to offspring. Thus, for many years the phenomenon of anticipation was attributed to ascertainment bias. Then, in 1991, spinobulbar muscular atrophy and the fragile X syndrome were found to result from expanded trinucleotide repeats in their respective genes. Furthermore, these expanded repeats were found to be unstable, frequently becoming longer in successive generations. Since longer repeat expansions are generally associated with earlier disease onset and more severe disease, this provided a molecular basis for anticipation. Since then, this dynamic form of genetic mutation has been found to underlie an increasing number of inherited neurological diseases, most of which exhibit anticipation. In general, there is an inverse relationship between age of onset and length of the repeat expansion, and a direct relationship between expansion length and disease severity. In disorders with incomplete penetrance, such as fragile X syndrome, penetrance is also related to length of the expansion.

While anticipation is frequently associated with diseases caused by unstable repeat expansion, it varies markedly in degree, and in some diseases may not occur at all. Anticipation is most pronounced in myotonic dystrophy, but also readily observed in the spinocerebellar ataxias and Huntington's disease. Anticipation is generally not seen in spinobulbar muscular atrophy and oculopharyngeal muscular dystrophy. One feature of anticipation is the 'parent of origin effect'. This is the tendency for anticipation to be observed when the gene is passed on through a specific gender. The tendency may be greater with paternal transmission (e.g. Huntington's disease) or maternal transmission (e.g. myotonic dystrophy), a phenomenon that probably reflects the nature of the expansions underlying the respective diseases.

Mechanisms of repeat expansion

There is an emerging consensus that unusual secondary structures adopted by trinucleotide repeats are responsible for their inherent instability, provoking errors at multiple levels of DNA metabolism (Bowater & Wells, 2000). Errors introduced during DNA replication, DNA repair, and homologous recombination have been implicated as contributing to trinucleotide repeat expansion. The propensity of repetitive DNA sequences to adopt unusual secondary structures (hairpin loops for CAG, CTG, and CGG repeats; triple helices for GAA repeats) provides an explanation for two features of trinucleotide repeat expansion: (i) the threshold effect for repeat instability, and (ii) a greater tendency towards expansion of some trinucleotide repeats than others.

Replication-dependent strand slippage during DNA replication is the mechanism of repeat sequence instability most strongly supported by both in vitro and in vivo evidence. Strand slippage is believed to occur when transient dissociation of the primer and template strands is followed by misaligned reassociation of the complementary strands, resulting in 'slippage' of the nascent DNA to a new position on the template (Wells, 1996). Unusual secondary structures promote primer/template dissociation, probably by causing the DNA replication complex to pause in the vicinity of repeat sequences (Kang et al., 1995).

Nucleotide excision repair systems recognize DNA damage by sensing distortion of helical structure (Wood, 1996). The unusual secondary structures adopted by some trinucleotide repeat sequences are likely to induce this repair pathway. In addition, these structures may be recognized by the mismatch repair system (Modrich & Lahue, 1996). Studies carried out in prokaryotic systems provide evidence that these pathways may contribute to trinucleotide repeat instability (Bowater & Wells, 2000).

An additional mechanism that may contribute to repeat instability is the introduction of errors during homologous recombination. Several human haplotype studies implicated gene conversion and unequal crossing-over as mechanisms that may contribute to the expansions and contractions of CTG trinucleotide repeats observed in myotonic dystrophy (Tsilfidis et al., 1992; O'Hoy et al., 1993; Tishkoff et al., 1998). Three studies investigating the loss of a fragile X mutation between parent and offspring concluded that gene conversion was responsible, suggesting that CGG repeats may also promote errors in homologous recombination (Van den Ouweland et al., 1994; Losekoot et al., 1997; Brown et al., 1996).

Classification of repeat expansion diseases

Trinucleotide repeat expansion disorders may be divided into two types based on the location of the mutation within their respective genes (Paulson & Fischbeck, 1996; see Fig. 3.1). This classification is useful because the location of the mutation may have implications regarding the mechanism of pathogenesis. Type I disorders are those in which the expansion occurs in-frame within the coding region and results in an expanded stretch of amino acids within the gene product. Type II disorders are those in which the expansion occurs outside the coding region: either upstream of the coding sequence, downstream of the coding sequence, or within an intron.

In type I disorders the mutant gene is transcribed and translated normally but leads to production of a protein harboring an expanded repeat of a particular amino acid. The trinucleotide expansions in type I disorders tend to be modest, with a similar threshold for disease (36–40 trinucleotide repeats, with limited exceptions). To date, nine type I diseases have been identified, and in each case the mutant protein is endowed with a toxic 'gain of function'. In general, type I diseases are dominantly inherited (except spinobulbar muscular atrophy), tend to be of late onset, and manifestations are mostly limited to the nervous system.

Conversely, in type II disorders, the coding sequence remains unchanged and the protein product is normal, yet mutations in untranslated regions of the gene lead to abnormal transcription or RNA processing, often resulting in altered levels of gene expression. The trinucleotide expansions leading to type II disorders tend to be large, with hundreds to over one thousand trinucleotides. These mutations often result in 'loss of function' of the relevant gene. To date, seven type II disorders have been identified; most are multisystem disorders and tend to have younger ages of onset than type I disorders.

Type I trinucleotide expansion disorders

Polyglutamine diseases

We currently recognize nine neurodegenerative disorders that result from the same kind of mutation: expansion of a CAG trinuceotide repeat within the coding region of the disease gene. Since CAG is the codon for glutamine, the proteins encoded by these genes carry an expanded polyglutamine tract; thus, these nine disorders are known as the polyglutamine diseases. This list includes Huntington's disease (HD), dentatorubro-pallidoluysian

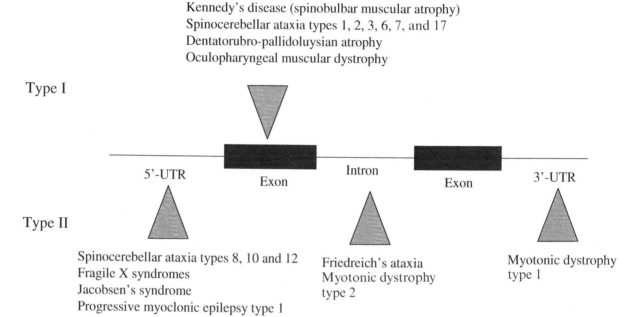

Fig. 3.1. Type I and type II repeat expansion diseases. In type I diseases, the expansion occurs within the coding region (exons) and results in an expanded stretch of amino acids in the mutant protein. In type II diseases, the expansion occurs outside of the coding region in introns, 3' untranslated, or 5' untranslated regions. (Adapted from Paulson & Fischbeck, 1996.)

atrophy (DRPLA), Kennedy's disease (also known as spinobulbar muscular atrophy, SBMA), and six spinocerebellar ataxias (SCAs 1, 2, 3, 6, 7 and 17). Evidence indicates that these eight diseases share a common pathogenic mechanism involving a toxic gain of function by the mutant gene product. Below, we present the clinical features and genetic basis of each of these disorders, followed by a general discussion of polyglutamine disease pathogenesis. The clinical features of HD and the SCAs are covered elsewhere in this book.

Huntington's disease

Huntington's disease (HD) is an autosomal dominant, progressive neurodegenerative disease characterized by disordered movement, intellectual impairment, and emotional disturbance. HD is typically a late-onset illness, and it is invariably fatal (Myers et al., 1988). HD was the first autosomal disorder in which the gene was mapped using polymorphic DNA markers. The initial mapping to chromosome 4p16 was followed by a decade of intensive collaborative research that culminated in the identification of a novel gene (IT15, for 'interesting transcript 15') of unknown function containing a CAG trinucleotide repeat sequence in the first exon (Huntington's Disease

Collaborative Research Group, 1993). The length of this CAG repeat sequence is polymorphic, with 6 to 35 CAGs in normal individuals, and 36 to 121 CAGs in individuals affected by HD. Examination of a large number of individuals carrying 30–40 repeats within IT15 demonstrated that rare individuals become symptomatic with as few as 36 repeats while others show no sign of disease despite two alleles with 40 repeats (Rubinstein et al., 1996). This evidence demonstrates the incomplete penetrance of HD in the range of 35–40 repeats, while repeat lengths greater than 40 are invariably associated with disease.

Huntington's disease frequently demonstrates anticipation, with successive generations experiencing earlier age of onset and more severe disease than their parents. Anticipation is a consequence of intergenerational instability leading to further expansion of CAG repeat in IT15 and is particularly associated with paternal transmission. Eighty per cent of patients with juvenile-onset HD, generally associated with alleles of more than 70 repeats, inherit the mutant gene from their father. A likely explanation for greater repeat instability associated with paternal transmission is the larger number of cellular divisions that take place during spermatogenesis.

Ultrastructural studies of HD brain tissue demonstrate both cytoplasmic and nuclear abnormalities in neurons.

The most notable features are ubiquitinated inclusions that are present in neuronal nuclei and dystrophic neurites throughout the brain regions most affected in HD, including the cortex and neostriatum but not in unaffected regions such as the globus pallidus or cerebellum (DiFiglia et al., 1997). These neuronal inclusions stain with antibodies directed to the amino-terminal portion of huntingtin, the protein product of *IT15*, but not with antibodies to the carboxy-terminus. Moreover, an amino terminal fragment of huntingtin of about 40 kD is detectable in nuclear extracts from patient brain and not in an extract prepared from normal brain (DiFiglia et al., 1997). Huntingtin is cleaved by caspases, cysteine proteases that play a significant role in mediating apoptosis. This observation led to the suggestion that low-grade caspase activation may generate toxic, amino-terminal fragments of mutant huntingtin that aggregate in the nucleus (Wellington et al., 2000).

Dentatorubro-pallidoluysian atrophy

In 1958, Smith et al., described a syndrome of progressive myoclonic epilepsy, ataxia, choreoathetosis, and dementia. They used the term 'dentatorubro-pallidoluysian atrophy' (DRPLA) to describe the most prominent neuropathological features; namely, extensive degeneration of the dentate nucleus, red nucleus, globus pallidus, and subthalamic nucleus of Luys. Rare in most parts of the world, a pocket of relatively high incidence of DRPLA is found in Japan (Naito & Oyanagi, 1982). The gene responsible for DRPLA was mapped to chromosome 12p by linkage analysis. Subsequently, because of phenotypic similarities to HD, genes from chromosome 12 were screened for CAG repeat expansions, a novel approach that culminated in identification of the *DRPLA* gene (Li et al., 1993; Koide et al., 1994; Nagafuchi et al., 1994).

Normal *DRPLA* alleles have 6–36 CAGs, while expanded alleles with 49–84 CAGs have been identified in symptomatic patients. Like Huntington's disease, intergenerational instability is more pronounced with paternal transmission (Koide et al., 1994). The product of the DRPLA gene is a widely expressed protein of approximately 190 kD named 'atrophin-1'. Atrophin-1 shares no homology with other known proteins, and its normal function remains unclear. Like huntingtin, atrophin-1 is cleaved by caspases, producing an amino-terminal fragment. Atrophin-1 is distributed through the cytoplasm in neurons and peripheral tissues of both unaffected and affected individuals (Knight et al., 1997; Yazawa et al., 1995). In addition, nuclear inclusions containing mutant atrophin-1 are found in neurons and glia of affected individuals, especially in degenerating regions of the brain (Hayashi et al., 1998; Igarashi et al., 1998).

Spinobulbar muscular atrophy

Spinobulbar muscular atrophy (SBMA), also known as Kennedy's disease, is an X-linked, slowly progressive disorder resulting from degeneration of motor neurons of the brainstem and spinal cord. Patients with SBMA also frequently exhibit mild signs of feminization (Arbizu et al., 1983). Gynecomastia is present in about half of patients, and some degree of infertility may occur. Pathologically, SBMA is characterized by degeneration of motor neurons in the anterior horn of the spinal cord and lower brainstem motor nuclei. Additionally, there is degeneration of sensory neurons in the dorsal root ganglia. Electrophysiological studies on SBMA patients demonstrate sensory neuropathy as well as neurogenic atrophy with fibrillations and fasciculations. Muscle biopsies show evidence of chronic denervation, often with collateral reinervation (Sobue et al., 1981, 1989; Harding et al., 1982).

In 1991, the cause of SBMA was found to be CAG trinucleotide repeat expansion within the first exon of the androgen receptor (AR) gene (La Spada et al., 1991). Normal alleles exhibit polymorphism with repeat length ranging from 9 to 36, while patients with SBMA have been identified with repeat sizes ranging from 40 to 62. In SBMA, anticipation is usually not observed. There is a correlation between repeat length and clinical manifestations, although as with other repeat expansion diseases, repeat length is not a reliable indicator of age of onset and disease severity (Doyu et al., 1992).

The AR is a member of the nuclear receptor superfamily. Like other steroid hormone receptors, it contains distinct domains for hormone and DNA binding. Upon binding of androgen in the cytoplasm, the receptor/ligand complex is transported to the nucleus where it activates the transcription of hormone responsive genes (Zhou et al., 1994). The AR is expressed widely in the brain, but most extensively in motor neurons of the spinal cord and brainstem where it may mediate a neurotrophic response to androgen (Ogata et al., 1994).

The polyglutamine tract is located at the amino-terminus of AR in a region distinct from the hormone and DNA binding regions. The function of the polyglutamine tract is not known, and it is dispensable for transactivation of hormone responsive genes (Jenster et al., 1991). Expansion of the polyglutamine tract may cause partial loss of receptor function and perhaps underlies the mild androgen insensitivity observed in SBMA. However, loss of function alone cannot account for the neurological features of SBMA, because complete absence of AR leads to androgen insensitivity (testicular feminization) syndrome, with no weakness or motor neuron degeneration. This observation contributes to the argument that SBMA results from a toxic gain of function by mutant AR due to polyglutamine expansion. Heterozygous females carrying a single expanded allele sometimes report mild weakness or muscle cramps and may have subclinical electrophysiological abnormalities. These female carriers may be protected by low androgen levels (if the toxic effect is ligand dependent) or by X-inactivation. Similar to the observations in HD and DRPLA, intranuclear inclusions of mutant AR are found in motor neurons within regions affected by SBMA (Li et al., 1998).

Autosomal dominant spinocerebellar ataxia

The spinocerebellar ataxias (SCAs) are a genetically heterogeneous group of disorders that exhibit substantial overlap in clinical and neuropathological features. We currently recognize 14 genetically distinct forms of autosomal dominant spinocerebellar ataxia (SCA), five of which are caused by CAG repeat expansion and discussed in this section. SCA types 8, 10 and 12 are type II trinucleotide repeat disorders and are presented below. At least five additional genetic loci associated with the SCA phenotype have been identified (SCAs 4, 5, 11, 13 and 14), but the genes and their mutations remain to be determined. The designation SCA 9 remains unassigned.

Degeneration of the cerebellum and brainstem is common to all of the SCAs; consequently, cerebellar ataxia and dysarthria are the hallmark clinical features of these diseases (Zoghbi & Orr, 2000). Additional, variable features may lead the clinician to suspect a particular SCA subtype. For example, SCA1 patients show hyperreflexia, extensor plantar responses, and an increased amplitude of saccadic eye movements, while SCA2 is characterized by reduced saccadic eye movements and depressed or absent reflexes. Protuberant eyes, faciolingual fasciculations, and extrapyramidal signs are features of SCA type 3 (Durr et al., 1996a). SCA type 6 is generally a late-onset, pure cerebellar ataxia. SCA type 7 typically features a pigmentary macular degeneration that accompanies spinocerebellar degeneration. Nevertheless, definitive diagnosis of a particular SCA subtype requires genetic confirmation.

Spinocerebellar ataxia type 1

The SCA1 locus was narrowed by linkage analysis to 6p22–p23 (Zoghbi et al., 1991). When subsequently identified, the *SCA1* gene was found to contain a polymorphic CAG trinucleotide repeat within its coding region (Orr et al., 1993). Normal *SCA1* alleles carry from 6 to as many as 44 CAGs, but those with greater than 20 are interrupted by

several repeats of CAT (Chung et al., 1993). Disease alleles, in contrast, contain longer CAG repeat stretches (39–82) and are uninterrupted by CAT sequences (Goldfarb et al., 1996). Marked intergenerational instability is observed, with paternal transmissions tending to produce expansions, whereas maternal transmissions actually tend to show contractions (Chung et al., 1993; Jodice et al., 1994; Ranum et al., 1994).

The *SCA1* gene encodes a ubiquitously expressed protein named 'ataxin-1' that shares no homology with other known proteins and is normally found in the nucleus and the cytoplasm. Ataxin-1 is highly expressed in the central nervous system including Purkinje cells and brain stem nuclei (Servadio et al., 1995). In SCA1 patients, mutant ataxin-1 localizes to large, solitary, nuclear inclusions in Purkinje cells and brainstem neurons (Skinner et al., 1997; Cummings et al., 1998). These inclusions stain positively for ubiquitin, components of the proteasome, and the molecular chaperone HDJ-2/HSDJ. Ataxin-1 likely plays a role in synaptic plasticity, because mice in which the *SCA1* gene has been disrupted have impaired spatial and motor learning, and decreased paired-pulse facilitation in the CA1 area of the hippocampus (Matilla et al., 1998). These *SCA1* 'knockout' mice do not develop ataxia, supporting the contention that *SCA1* is not caused by loss of normal ataxin-1 function. In an analogous observation in humans, large deletions spanning the *SCA1* gene lead to a syndrome of mental retardation and seizures, but do not result in an ataxic phenotype (Davies et al., 1999).

Spinocerebellar ataxia type 2

The *SCA2* gene was mapped by linkage analysis to chromosome 12q23–24.1 (Gispert et al., 1993), and the gene was subsequently identified by three independent groups and found to contain a CAG repeat (Pulst et al., 1996; Imbert et al., 1996; Sanpei et al., 1996). The CAG repeat in *SCA2* is less polymorphic than in the other genes that are involved in polyglutamine disease. Normal *SCA2* alleles have 15–31 CAGs, but 94% of alleles have 22 CAGs. *SCA2* disease alleles have 36–63 CAGs.

SCA2 encodes a widely expressed protein named 'ataxin-2' of approximately 140 kD that shares no homology with proteins of known function, although an ataxin-2– related protein has been identified (Pulst et al., 1996). Immunostaining of SCA2 brain specimens reveals cytoplasmic inclusions containing the mutant protein in Purkinje cells and dentate neurons, an observation that has also been made in a transgenic mouse model (Huynh et al., 2000).

Spinocerebellar ataxia type 3

Spinocerebellar ataxia type 3 (SCA3), also known as Machado–Joseph disease, was initially described among Portuguese–Azorean emigrants who settled in New England. Since then, this disease has been found worldwide in a variety of ethnic backgrounds, but it is especially prevalent in two islands in the Portuguese Azores (Nakano et al., 1972). The presence of SCA3 in regions with historically active sea-trade such as India, China, and Japan led to speculation that the worldwide distribution of the disease may be attributed to the travels of Azorean sailors in the late fifteenth and sixteenth centuries. In support of this suggestion, a worldwide haplotype study has demonstrated a founder effect, with the majority of non-Portuguese families sharing a disease haplotype with families from one Azorean island (Gaspar et al., 2001).

The *MJD1* gene was mapped to chromosome 14q (Takiyama et al., 1993) and subsequently identified by scanning a human brain library using an oligonucleotide probe designed to detect expanded CAG repeats (Kawaguchi et al., 1994). In normal alleles, the CAG repeat length ranges from 12 to 41, while disease alleles have 62 to 84 CAGs (Durr et al., 1996a; Maruyama et al., 1995). *MJD1* is somewhat unusual among the polyglutamine disease genes in that there is a distinct gap between normal and affected repeat sizes. Intergenerational instability is common and more pronounced with paternal transmission.

The *MJD1* gene encodes an approximately 42 kD protein of unknown function named 'ataxin-3' (Kawaguchi et al., 1994). Ataxin-3 is widely expressed in the brain, and regions of greatest susceptibility to degeneration do not show significantly higher ataxin-3 expression. In SCA3 brain specimens, ataxin-3 localizes to ubiquitinated nuclear inclusions in neurons from affected brain regions (Paulson et al., 1997). In addition, these inclusions are found to colocalize with components of the proteasome and cellular chaperones (Chai et al., 1999).

Spinocerebellar ataxia type 6

The mutation responsible for SCA6 is CAG repeat expansion in the *CACNA14* gene, which encodes the α_{1a}-voltage-dependent Ca^{2+} channel (Zhuchenko et al., 1997). The calcium channels formed by α_{1a} are abundant in the central nervous system, with highest levels in the cerebellum (Fletcher et al., 1996). While the seven other known polyglutamine diseases are associated with expansion beyond 36–40 CAGs, SCA6 has a lower disease threshold. Normal alleles of the *CACNA14* gene have 6–18 CAGs, and disease alleles have 21–33 CAGs (Matsuyama et al., 1997; Zoghbi 1997). SCA6 also differs from the other polyglutamine diseases in that the repeat expansion shows little intergenerational instability and anticipation is not observed.

Other mutations in the *CACNA14* gene are associated with two paroxysmal neurological disorders, episodic ataxia type 2 (EA2) and familial hemiplegic migraine (FHM) (Ophoff et al., 1996). Interestingly, both EA2 and FHM are sometimes associated with persistant, slowly progressive ataxia. In addition, naturally occurring mouse mutants known as *tottering* and *leaner*, which exhibit cerebellar atrophy, ataxia and seizures, have point mutations in the orthologous mouse *Cacna1a* gene (Fletcher et al., 1996). The autosomal dominant nature of these disorders suggests that a toxic gain of function may be responsible, but the mechanistic relationship of these disorders to SCA6 remains to be determined. It is also unclear whether altered function of the voltage-gated Ca^{2+} channel contributes to the pathogenesis.

Spinocerebellar ataxia type 7

Using a technique called 'repeat expansion detection' (RED) in which the polymerase chain reaction is used to scan genomic DNA for large trinucleotide repeats, a candidate region for SCA7 was located at chromosome 3p21.1–p12 (Lindblad et al., 1996). Subsequent positional cloning revealed the genetic basis of SCA7 to be expansion of a CAG repeat in a gene of unknown function (David et al., 1997). In normal *SCA7* alleles, CAG repeat lengths range from 7 to 35; and mutant alleles carry 38–200 CAGs (David et al., 1997; Johansson et al., 1998). SCA7 shows anticipation, with greater genetic instability associated with paternal transmission (Johansson et al., 1998). The protein encoded by the *SCA7* gene has been designated 'ataxin-7' and normally consists of 890 amino acids with a nuclear localization motif. Ataxin-7 is widely expressed in the brain and some peripheral tissues, but it is particularly enriched in regions susceptible to degeneration in SCA7 (Cancel et al., 2000; Lindenberg et al., 2000). Two studies have reported ubiquitinated neuronal intranuclear inclusions in the brain and retina of SCA7 patients (Holmberg et al., 1998; Mauger et al., 1999).

Polyglutamine expansion in TATA-binding protein (*SCA17*)

In addition to the eight genes responsible for the polyglutamine diseases listed above, a number of other human genes are known to contain polymorphic stretches of CAG within the coding region. Many of these genes encode transcription factors in which the polyglutamine tract may mediate protein–protein interactions. The recognition that expanded stretches of polyglutamine can cause neurodegeneration has prompted examination of these genes in otherwise unexplained neurodegenerative disorders. In one Japanese patient, a young girl with progressive cerebellar ataxia, hyperreflexia, extensor plantar responses, atypical absence seizures and intellectual impairment, an expanded series of CAG and CAA repeats was identified in the gene encoding TATA-binding protein (Koide et al., 1999). The mutant allele from this patient encodes a stretch of 63 glutamines. In contrast, the patient's parents, who were neurologically normal, carried alleles encoding 35–39 glutamines. This disorder has now been identified in additional families and has been given the designation *SCA17* (Nakamura et al., 2001).

The molecular pathogenesis of polyglutamine disease

A common mechanism?

Four major lines of evidence suggest that the polyglutamine diseases share a common pathogenesis resulting from gain of function in the disease gene product, i.e. that the expanded polyglutamine confers upon the mutant protein a new property that is toxic to neurons. (i) The expanded polyglutamine tract is the only common feature among the genes responsible for these diseases. They share no other sequence homology, no common subcellular localization, and appear to be functionally unrelated. Yet, the phenotype of each disease is characterized by late-onset, slowly progressive neurodegeneration with clinical overlap. Furthermore, they share common pathological features, most notably ubiquitinated neuronal inclusions containing the mutant protein in brain regions susceptible to neurodegeneration. (ii) With the exception of SBMA, which is X-linked, all of these diseases exhibit dominant inheritance. In SBMA, female carriers may complain of cramps and be found to manifest subclinical electrophysiogical abnormalities suggestive of mild motor neuron disease. As mentioned above, female carriers of SBMA may be protected by X chromosome inactivation or low levels of androgen. (iii) A wide array of model systems has been developed, including cell culture and transgenic animal models, in which expression of the disease genes with repeat expansion recapitulates features of the diseases. Furthermore, transgenic expression of expanded polyglutamine in an unrelated protein (hypoxanthine

phosphoribosyl-transferase) also results in neurodegeneration (Ordway et al., 1997). (iv) Naturally occurring and experimentally introduced mutations that cause loss of function in these genes do not recapitulate features of the diseases.

Targets of expanded polyglutamine

Examination of patient tissue, animal models, and in vitro systems has revealed a variety of biochemical pathways and cellular functions that may be altered by expanded polyglutamine (Fig. 3.2). A major challenge is to distinguish primary biochemical derangements caused by expanded polyglutamine from the secondary effects that surely follow. An added difficulty is to discern which alterations are fundamentally related to neuronal dysfunction and death. A primary molecular target of polyglutamine toxicity would be expected to have a novel or altered interaction with the mutant protein, due to altered physical properties resulting from the expanded polyglutamine. Two cellular processes stand out as particular candidates for primary disruption by expanded polyglutamine: transcription and the ubiquitin-proteasome pathway.

The inclusions formed by expanded polyglutamine recruit and sequester additional proteins, particularly proteins that normally contain polyglutamine tracts. One appealing hypothesis suggests that inclusions in the nucleus sequester and deplete factors critical to neuronal function and survival. Candidate targets in this model are transcription factors that are present in limiting quantities and contain polyglutamine tracts. Various transcription factors have been found to colocalize with nuclear inclusions, including CREB-binding protein (CBP), p53, TATA-binding protein, and nuclear receptor co-repressors (Perez et al., 1998; Boutell et al., 1999; McCampbell et al., 2000; Steffan et al., 2000). Furthermore, cell culture studies suggest that sequestration of CBP and p53 has functional consequences on transcriptional regulation. Depletion or altered function of transcription factors in human disease or animal models has yet to be demonstrated directly. Nonetheless, expression-profiling studies on brain tissue from HD and SCA1 mice suggest that altered transcription is an early event in polyglutamine pathogenesis (Luthi-Carter et al., 2000; Lin et al., 2000).

The ubiquitin–proteasome pathway is the primary biochemical means by which cells eliminate unwanted proteins. Proteins are targeted for degradation by covalent linkage to ubiquitin. Ubiquitination is the molecular signature enabling recognition by a family of chaperone proteins which facilitate the targeted protein's access to, and degra-

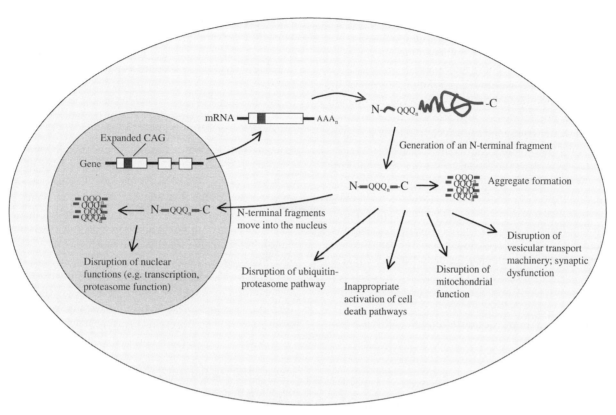

Fig. 3.2. Molecular pathogenesis of polyglutamine disease. The mutant gene with an expanded stretch of CAGs undergoes normal transcription and translation. The mutant gene product contains an expanded polyglutamine tract that confers a toxic gain of function. The mutant protein is susceptible to cleavage, releasing a polyglutamine-containing fragment. The polyglutamine-containing fragments form intracellular aggregates in the cytoplasm and nucleus. It remains unclear whether polyglutamine is toxic as full-length protein, as monomeric fragments, or as aggregate. An array of possible cellular targets is shown and discussed in the text.

dation by, the proteasome, a large macromolecular proteolytic apparatus (Ciechanover, 1997). Normal function of the ubiquitin–proteasome pathway is critical to determining the steady-state levels of many proteins. Additionally, this pathway is charged with rapidly eliminating nascent proteins that fail to adopt their correct structure, thereby protecting the cell from deleterious effects of misfolded proteins. Polyglutamine inclusions in brain specimens from human disease and animal models stain positively for components of the ubiquitin-proteasome pathway, including ubiquitin, chaperone proteins, and proteasome subunits (Paulson et al., 1997; Davies et al., 1997; Hackam et al., 1998). It remains unclear which components of the inclusions are ubiquitinated. The mutant proteins themselves may be ubiquitinated, but resist degradation because of a particular conformation adopted by expanded polyglutamine. Expanded polyglutamine may inhibit the proteasome, resulting in a global accumulation of ubiquitinated substrate with dire consequences for the cell. Neurons may be

particularly susceptible to proteasome dysfunction because they are limited in their ability to dilute accumulating toxic proteins with cell division. Experimental evidence supporting a role for the ubiquitin–proteasome pathway in polyglutamine disease comes from a transgenic mouse study of SCA1. A genetic cross between a SCA1 mouse and a mouse with dysfunctional E6–AP ubiquitin ligase, and impairment of the ubiquitin–proteasome pathway, resulted in exacerbation of the neurodegeneration despite fewer inclusions (Cummings et al., 1999). There are precedents for neurological disease resulting from disruption to the ubiquitin–proteasome pathway: juvenile-onset Parkinson's disease, an autosomal recessive disease, is caused by mutations in the gene for parkin, an E3 ubiquitin ligase (Polymeropoulos, 2000). Angelman's syndrome, a developmental disorder that is characterized by motor and intellectual retardation, ataxia, hypotonia, epilepsy, and dysmorphic features, results from mutation in the gene for E6–AP, which is also an E3 ubiquitin ligase.

Other targets have been proposed for expanded polyglutamine. Ultrastructural examination of brain tissue from Huntington's patients shows mitochondrial abnormalities, and patients with HD have altered energy metabolism in brain and muscle, suggesting a role for mitochondrial dysfunction in this disease (Murphy et al., 2000). Mutant huntingtin has been found to associate with synaptic vesicles and vesicular transport machinery, implicating vesicular transport as a potential target of polyglutamine toxicity (Li et al., 2000). Electrophysiological studies of neurons from HD mice demonstrate abnormalities in synaptic transmission (Murphy et al., 2000). Much attention has focused on the potential role of apoptosis in mediating polyglutamine toxicity. Aside from a single report suggesting that mutant huntingtin activates caspase-8 (Sanchez et al., 1999), evidence is scant that components of the apoptotic machinery serve as a primary target for expanded polyglutamine. On the other hand, evidence is accumulating that caspases may play a role in mediating early events in toxicity. Many of the disease proteins contain consensus caspase cleavage sites. Evidence suggests that an important step in the pathogenesis of HD, SBMA, and DRPLA is caspase-mediated generation of polyglutamine-containing fragments that are more toxic than the parent protein (Ellerby et al., 1999; Wellington et al., 2000).

The deposition of misfolded proteins into neuronal inclusions is a central feature of many neurodegenerative diseases, including Alzheimer's disease, Parkinson's disease, amyotrophic lateral sclerosis and the prion diseases. The importance of aggregation in these disorders has been underscored by the identification of three additional dominantly inherited neurodegenerative disorders that are characterized by intracellular aggregation of mutant α-synuclein (Polymeropoulos, 2000), neuroserpin (Davis et al., 1999), and tau proteins (Lee & Trojanowski, 1999). Deposition of misfolded protein in neuronal inclusions has emerged as a common theme in neurodegenerative diseases, perhaps indicating that these diseases also share common mechanisms.

What is the role of aggregation in the polyglutamine diseases?

One pathological feature shared by the polyglutamine diseases is the presence of intraneuronal, ubiquitinated inclusions in brain regions susceptible to degeneration. At the subcellular level, inclusions may be found in the nucleus (e.g. SCA1), cytoplasm (e.g. SCA2), or both (e.g. Huntington's disease). These inclusions consist of insoluble aggregates of polyglutamine-containing fragments in association with a host of additional proteins. Tracts of polyglutamine aggregate as antiparallel ß-strands linked by additional hydrogen bonding: so-called 'polar zipper' formation. There is a remarkable correlation between the threshold polyglutamine length for aggregation in experimental systems and the CAG repeat length that leads to human disease. These observations form the basis of the argument that self-aggregation by expanded polyglutamine is the acquired property underlying neurodegeneration (Perutz et al., 1994).

But are the inclusions themselves toxic? The dissociation of toxicity from inclusion formation observed in cell culture suggests that they are not (Saudou et al., 1998). A dissociation between inclusion formation and the development of pathology has also been demonstrated in transgenic mice (Klement et al., 1998; Leavitt et al., 1999). Some have suggested that inclusion formation may be a protective mechanism employed by the cell to cope with excess, misfolded polyglutamine, perhaps analogous to so-called 'aggresomes' which form in vitro in response to overexpression of misfolded protein (Johnston et al., 1998).

Oculopharyngeal muscular dystrophy

Oculopharyngeal muscular dystrophy (OPMD) has been recognized as a distinct entity since a report by Victor et al., in 1962, although case reports can be found in the literature dating from the early twentieth century. OPMD is an inherited myopathy that shares with the CAG repeat expansion diseases a similar type of genetic mutation and certain pathologic features. OPMD is inherited as an autosomal dominant disease of late onset. It occurs worldwide, although it is particularly prevalent among French Canadians. Patients typically present in the fifth or sixth decade with bilateral ptosis and dysphagia (Tome & Fardeau, 1994). In an attempt to compensate for severe ptosis, patients may contract the frontalis muscle and throw their head back, a position known as Hutchinson's or astrologist's posture. Unfortunately, this posture often has the unwanted affect of worsening the dysphagia. In late stages of the disease, the eyelids are very thin and transparent, the eyebrows are raised, and the supraorbital ridges are prominent. The disease is slowly progressive, and may eventually impair eye movements, occasionally causing diplopia. Instrinsic eye muscles are always spared. Along with dysphagia, patients may experience decreased palatal mobility, an impaired gag reflex, and laryngeal weakness with dysphonia. Skeletal muscles of the extremities may be affected by the disease, often resulting in shoulder-girdle weakness and atrophy. Involvement of limb muscles is symmetric and is not associated with fasciculations.

Tendon reflexes are typically decreased. Dysphagia predisposes patients to malnutrition and aspiration pneumonia.

The pathologic changes in skeletal muscle are progressive, and parallel the worsening clinical features. Biopsy reveals myopathic features, including increased variation in fibre size, internal nuclei, and interstitial fibrosis. There are often scattered small, angulated fibres that are strongly NADH positive. Two pathologic features help distinguish OPMD. Rimmed vacuoles, first described by Dubowitz and Brooke in 1973, appear as clear spaces lined by a granular basophilic rim. While these spaces are not membrane bound, they are likely derived from autophagic vacuoles. Ultrastructural examination has also revealed the presence of intranuclear inclusions (Tome & Fardeau, 1980). These inclusions are composed of aggregated tubular filaments that measure 8.5 nm in outer diameter and up to 0.25 μm in length. They contain the poly(A)-binding protein 2, the protein mutated in the disease (see below), and sequestered poly(A) RNA (Becher et al., 2000; Calado et al., 2000).

The French Canadian population provided a rich source of OPMD families that was important for the identification of the defective gene. After studying these families, Andre Barbeau concluded that the causative mutation was likely introduced into Quebec by ancestors who emigrated from France in 1634 (Barbeau, 1969). A genome-wide scan pointed to a critical region on 14q11 (Brais et al., 1995), which was further narrowed to a 0.26 cM candidate interval (Brais et al., 1998). Within this interval is the gene encoding poly(A)-binding protein 2 (PABP2), a nuclear protein that increases the efficiency of polyadenylation and specifies the length of the mRNA poly(A) tail (Barabino & Keller, 1999). The first exon of the PABP2 gene encodes a stretch of ten alanines, the first six of which are encoded by a GCG repeat. Rouleau and colleagues (Brais et al., 1998) demonstrated an expansion of this repeat in 144 families with OPMD, with the mutated tract containing 8 to 13 GCG triplets. This group of families came from 15 different countries, indicating that cases of OPMD occurring worldwide are caused by the same genetic mutation. Rare cases with two pathologically expanded alleles presented with an earlier onset of the disease (Blumen et al., 1999). This short repeat expansion differs from the longer CAG expansions in SBMA and other polyglutamine diseases in that it is meiotically stable, and therefore families with OPMD do not show genetic anticipation.

Two per cent of the French Canadian population carry a $(GCG)_7$ allele. This allele acts as a modifier of the disease phenotype by worsening symptoms in heterozygotes carrying one pathologically expanded allele. The $(GCG)_7$ allele also functions as a recessive mutation, causing late-onset disease in homozygotes (Brais et al., 1998). Thus, changes in GCG repeat length in the PABP2 gene account for cases of OPMD that are inherited in both a dominant and a recessive fashion.

The mechanism by which an expanded alanine tract leads to OPMD is unknown. One attractive hypothesis is that the mutated protein is prone to form insoluble aggregates, particularly in the nucleus where PABP2 is normally located. These aggregates may then disrupt cell function by mechanisms similar to those proposed for the polyglutamine disorders. Alternatively, as with the polyglutamine disorders, these intranuclear aggregates may be markers of disease that are not mechanistically related to cell injury. It may be that dominantly inherited cases of OPMD are due to haploinsufficiency. Intranuclear aggregates and rimmed vacuoles are also present in other muscle diseases that occur without a GCG expansion in the PABP2 gene, such as inclusion body myositis (Mezei et al., 1999). This may indicate that similar pathways leading to muscle injury are triggered in these diseases, although further studies are required to define this relationship.

Type II repeat expansion disorders

We currently recognize seven type II trinucleotide expansion disorders (see Table 3.1). These are inherited neurological diseases in which a trinucleotide repeat expansion occurs outside the coding region of the mutated gene. The expansions in this diverse group tend to be longer than those observed in the Type 1 diseases. Most often, these repeat expansions lead to reduced expression of the affected genes resulting in loss of gene function and a recessively inherited phenotype that may present early in life. In other instances, the disease phenotype is dominantly inherited, likely reflecting a toxic gain of function. The molecular mechanisms by which these expansions exert their effects are varied and complex.

Myotonic dystrophy

Myotonic dystrophy (DM) is a dominantly inherited multisystem disorder that was first described in the early twentieth century. It has a prevalence of approximately 1 in 8000 worldwide. The clinical presentation is highly variable, reflecting the diverse effects that the underlying mutation has on gene expression. Adult patients with DM often present in the second or third decade with slowly progressive disease. Typical cases are characterized by muscle weakness and wasting particularly involving the face and distal limbs, and by myotonia. Patients may have

Table 3.1. Trinucleotide repeat expansion diseases

Disorder	Gene/locus	Chromosomal location	Protein	Repeat Sequence	Repeat location	Inheritance
Type I						
Huntington's disease	IT15	4p16.3	Huntingtin	CAG	Coding	AD
Dentatorubro-pallidoluysian atrophy	DRPLA	12p13.31	Atrophin-1	CAG	Coding	AD
Spinobulbar muscular Atrophy (Kennedy's disease)	AR	Xq13–21	Androgen receptor	CAG	Coding	X-linked
Spinocerebellar ataxia Type 1	SCA1	6p23	Ataxin-1	CAG	Coding	AD
Spinocerebellar ataxia Type 2	SCA2	12.24.1	Ataxin-2	CAG	Coding	AD
Spinocerebellar ataxia Type 3	SCA3/MJD1	14q32.1	Ataxin-3	CAG	Coding	AD
Spinocerebellar ataxia Type 6	CACNA14	19p13	α_{1A} Subunit of voltage-dependent calcium channel	CAG	Coding	AD
Spinocerebellar ataxia Type 7	SCA7	3p12–13	Ataxin-7	CAG	Coding	AD
Spinocerebellar ataxis Type 17	SCA17	6q27	TATA binding protein	CAG	Coding	AD
Oculopharyngeal dystrophy	PABP2	14q11	Poly-A binding protein	GCG	Coding	AD
Type II						
Fragile X syndrome	FMR1 (FRAXA)	Xq27.3	FMRP	CGG	5′-UTR	X-linked
Fragile XE mental retardation	FMR2 (FRAXE)	Xq28	FMR2	GCC	5′-UTR	X-linked
Spinocerebellar ataxia Type 8	SCA8	13q21	KLH1	CTG	5′-UTR	AD
Spinocerebellar ataxia Type 10	SCA10	22q13	Ataxin-10	ATTCT	9th intron	AD
Spinocerebellar ataxia Type 12	PPP2R2B	5q31–33	PP2A regulatory protein	CAG	5′-UTR	AD
Friedreich's ataxia	X25	9q13–21.1	Frataxin	GAA	1st intron	AR
Myotonic dystrophy	DMPK	19q13.3	Myotonic dystrophy protein kinase	CTG	3′-UTR	AD
Myotonic dystrophy Type 2	ZNF9	3q13–24	Zinc finger protein 9	CCTG	1st intron	AD

a characteristic facial appearance due to atrophy of the masseters, sternocleidomastiods, and temporalis muscle, with involvement of the extraocular muscles that produces ptosis, weakness of eyelid closure, and limited extraocular movements. In addition, the disease often has systemic manifestations, including cataracts, cardiac conduction defects, male frontal balding, testicular atrophy, insulin resistance, pilomatrixomas, and intellectual impairment. Congenital myotonic dystrophy has a more severe presentation with profound hypotonia and weakness from birth, poor feeding and respiratory distress. Cataracts and clinical myotonia are not evident at presentation. Congenital cases typically occur in the setting of maternal transmission from mildly to moderately affected female patients (Harper & Rudel, 1994). Muscle biopsies show an increased number of internal nuclei that are often arrayed in chains, sarcoplasmic masses, ring fibres, and type 1 fibre atrophy. Other myopathic changes may be present, especially in biopsies from patients with advanced disease.

DM is caused by a CTG repeat expansion in the 3′ untranslated region of a cAMP-dependent serine–threonine protein kinase, named 'DM protein kinase' (DMPK) or 'myotonin', one of several genes found at the disease locus 19q13.3 (Brook et al., 1992; Buxton et al., 1992; Fu et al., 1993; Mahadevan et al., 1992). The CTG repeat length is polymorphic in the normal population, varying between 5 and 37 CTGs. Patients with DM have between 50 and several thousand CTGs. The age of onset is inversely correlated with repeat length (Brook et al., 1992; Harley et al., 1992; Hunter et al., 1992; Mahadevan et al., 1992).

The mechanism by which this repeat expansion leads to disease is complex. It was initially hypothesized that loss of DMPK function led to DM, but mice with null mutations in the DMPK gene did not replicate the disease phenotype (Jansen et al., 1996; Reddy et al., 1996). When knockout mice were bred to homozygosity, complete loss of expression did result in a mild myopathy and cardiac conduction abnormalities, but not other features of DM, such as the hallmark myotonia (Berul et al., 1999). Several studies have found that expression levels of DMPK protein and mRNA are also decreased in patient muscle (Carango et al., 1993; Fu et al., 1992; Hofmann-Radvanyi et al., 1993). These data suggest that loss of DMPK function contributes to the disease, but is insufficient to account for the full spectrum of clinical manifestations observed in DM.

In addition to loss of DMPK function, the CTG repeat expansion alters the expression of other genes by various mechanisms, including disruption of RNA processing. DMPK transcripts that harbour expanded repeats accumulate in intranuclear clusters (Davis et al., 1997; Hamshere et al., 1997; Taneja et al., 1995). This abnormal retention of transcripts is associated with decreased DMPK RNA splicing and polyadenylation (Hamshere et al., 1997; Krahe et al., 1995; Wang et al., 1995). Defects in RNA processing may be caused by altered function of RNA-binding proteins that normally recognize CUG repeats. Several CUG-binding proteins have been identified (Timchenko et al., 1996). One of these proteins, CUGBP1, is involved in pre-mRNA splicing and has altered function in DM (Philips et al., 1998). Sequestration of this, or other RNA-binding proteins, may have widespread effects on gene expression, possibly contributing to the varied manifestations of the disease. In support of this RNA gain of function model, mice in which an untranslated CUG repeat is expressed as a transgene develop certain features of DM, including myotonia and myopathy (Mankodi et al., 2000).

The CTG expansion may also interfere with expression of genes near DMPK on chromosome 19. DM-locus-associated homeodomain protein (DMAHP/Six5) is a homeobox gene located close to the expanded repeat in exon 15 of the DMPK gene. DMAHP/Six5 mRNA expression in fibroblasts and myoblasts from DM patients is significantly decreased (Klesert et al., 1997; Thornton et al., 1997). This decreased expression may be mediated by methylation of a CpG island adjacent to the expanded repeat (Steinbach et al., 1998). Mice in which the DMAHP/Six5 gene is disrupted develop cataracts but no apparent skeletal muscle abnormalities (Klesert et al., 2000; Sarkar et al., 2000), suggesting that DM is a contiguous gene disorder caused by altered expression of more than one gene. The CTG repeat expansion may also influence the expression of other nearby genes, including DMR-N9/59, a WD-repeat gene located telomeric to DMPK (Alwazzan et al., 1999; Jansen et al., 1995).

A phenocopy of myotonic dystrophy was described in a large family that lacks a CTG expansion in the DMPK gene (David et al., 1997; Ranum et al., 1998). This disease locus, called DM2, maps to chromosome 3q. Other patients with disease manifestations similar to DM but lacking an expansion in the DMPK gene also have been described (Ricker et al., 1994; Thornton et al., 1994). Some of these patients have been classified as having proximal myotonic myopathy (PROMM) to highlight clinical differences with DM (Ricker et al., 1994). The gene mutated in this disorder was recently identified as the zinc finger protein 9 gene (Liquori et al., 2001). The responsible mutation is an intronic tetranucleotide CCTG repeat expansion that results in RNA sequestration, consistent with a messenger RNA gain of function mechanism for both DM and DM2.

Fragile X syndrome

Fragile X syndrome, one of the most common forms of inherited mental retardation, has an estimated incidence of 1 in 4000 males and 1 in 8000 females (Warren & Nelson, 1994). It is inherited as an X-linked dominant trait with reduced penetrance. Those affected have mild to moderate mental retardation, with IQ scores ranging as low as 20 to 60. Clinical features may include hyperkinetic behaviour and concentration problems, and systemic manifestations such as macro-orchidism in males, and abnormal facial features with large ears and a prominent jaw.

Fragile X syndrome is associated with a folate sensitive fragile site at Xq27.3 (Giraud et al., 1976; Harvey et al., 1977; Sutherland, 1977). This cytogenetically defined alteration is caused by an expansion of a CGG trinucleotide repeat. The repeat falls within the 5′ untranslated region of the gene fragile X mental retardation-1 (FMR1) (Kremer et al., 1991; Yu et al., 1991; Verkerk et al., 1991; Oberle et al., 1991). The FMR1 gene, encompassing 17 exons and spanning approximately 38 kb of DNA, is widely expressed in mammalian tissues (Ashley et al, 1993; Eichler et al., 1994b). In the normal population, the CGG repeat is polymorphic both in length, ranging from seven to 60 triplets, and in content, as it is variably punctuated by AGG triplets. These AGG interruptions contribute to the stability of the CGG repeat length, and their loss is associated with tracts that are prone to expansion (Fu et al., 1991; Eichler et al., 1994a, b; Kunst & Warren, 1994; Snow et al., 1993, 1994).

Full mutations in patients with fragile X syndrome contain over 230 CGG triplets. These large expansions are associated with DNA hypermethylation and decreased expression of the *FMR1* gene. Somatic mosaicism may affect both repeat length and methylation status. That loss of FMR1 protein (FMRP) is causative of fragile X syndrome is supported by the identification of patients who lack a cytogenetically identified fragile site, and who have deletions or point mutations in the *FMR1* gene (De Boulle et al., 1993; Wohrle et al., 1992). Full mutations are generally inherited through maternal transmission and arise from expansion of an unstable premutation that contains 60 to 230 repeats. These premutations expand during gametogenesis or very early embryonic development (Malter et al., 1997). In carrier females, premutations are unmethylated and give rise to normal levels of *FMR1* transcript and protein. The risk of premutation expansion to full mutation increases exponentially as the number of repeats increases from 65 to 100. Males with full mutations do not, as a rule, transmit alleles with very long expansions, and sperm from these patients have premutation length repeat expansions. These unusual genetics provide a mechanistic explanation of the Sherman paradox (Sherman et al., 1984, 1985; Fu et al., 1991), which states that fragile X transmission occurs through normal males, that their heterozygous daughters are not mentally retarded and have few or no fragile sites, but that by the next generation, a third of heterozygous females are mentally subnormal and contain fragile sites.

Loss of FMRP causes fragile X syndrome in humans, and its targeted deletion causes macro-orchidism and subtle learning and memory deficits in mice (Dutch–Belgian Fragile X Consortium, 1994). FMRP is located primarily in the cytoplasm, but it contains both a nuclear localization signal and a nuclear export signal, suggesting that it shuttles between these two compartments (Eberhart et al., 1996). The protein contains two types of RNA-binding protein motifs, two ribonucleotide K homology domains (KH domains), and clusters of arginine and glycine residues known as RGG boxes (Ashley et al., 1993; Siomi et al., 1993). These RNA-binding domains enable the binding of FMRP to RNA, as demonstrated by in vitro assays where it preferentially associates with poly(G) or poly(U). Its in vivo binding specificity and native targets remain unknown.

FMRP associates with ribosomes as a component of messenger ribonucleoprotein (mRNP) particles. Additional components of these mRNP particles include two autosomal homologues of FMRP, designated FXR1P and FXR2P, nucleolin, and at least three other proteins (Siomi et al, 1995; Zhang et al., 1995). In this context, FMRP may play a role in the export of specific mRNAs from the nucleus to the cytoplasm. Alternatively, FMRP may regulate the stability or translation of the mRNAs with which it associates. In either case, FMRP likely plays an important role in protein synthesis, and its loss may severely impact neuronal function during development and learning.

FRAXE, FRAXF, and Jacobsen syndrome

In addition to the folate-sensitive fragile site associated with fragile X syndrome (FRAXA), two other fragile sites are present distally on Xq. FRAXE at Xq28 is caused by amplification of a CCG repeat (Knight et al., 1993). In normal individuals, this region contains 6 to 25 triplets, whereas in FRAXE-positive mentally retarded patients there are more than 200 triplets. The expansion is associated with methylation of a nearby CpG island, and decreased expression of a putative transcription factor, designated FMR2 (Gu et al., 1996; Gecz et al., 1996). Distal to both FRAXA and FRAXE is a third folate-sensitive fragile site, designated FRAXF (Hirst et al., 1993). This site results from the expansion of a GCC repeat that is polymorphic in the normal population, ranging from 6 to 29 triplets (Parrish et al., 1994). Rarely, an expansion to several hundred triplets has been associated with developmental delay (Ritchie et al., 1994), but there is not a well-established correlation between FRAXF and human disease.

Mental retardation may be associated with fragile sites on autosomes as well. One such example is Jacobsen syndrome, a clinically complex disorder with manifestations that include psychomotor retardation and trigonocephaly (Jacobsen et al., 1973). The disorder is due to deletions of the long arm of chromosome 11, typically from 11q23 to the telomere, with subsequent loss of numerous genes. Jacobsen syndrome is associated with a folate-sensitive fragile site at 11q23.3, designated FRA11B. As with other fragile sites, this cytogenetic abnormality is caused by the expansion and hypermethylation of CCG repeats. For Jacobsen syndrome, the triplets fall within the 5′ end of the gene encoding the proto-oncogene *CBL2* (Jones et al., 1995). Here, the fragile site may predispose to chromosome breakage, resulting in profound clinical consequences.

Progressive myoclonus epilepsy type 1

Progressive myoclonus epilepsy type 1 (EPM1), also known as Unverricht–Lundborg disease or Baltic myoclonus, was separately described by Unverricht and Lundborg in cases from Estonia and Sweden, respectively, near the turn of the last century. It is an autosomal recessive disorder that occurs worldwide, but is particularly prevalent in the Baltic and western Mediterranean regions. EPM1 is also the major cause of progressive myoclonus epilepsy in North America (Lehesjoki & Koskiniemi, 1998).

EPM1 has its onset in childhood, typically between the ages of 6 and 13 years (Lehesjoki & Koskiniemi, 1998). The myoclonus may generalize to shaking attacks and usually progresses to tonic–clonic seizures. Later in the course of the disease, patients may exhibit ataxia, intention tremor, and dysarthria. A slow cognitive decline and emotional lability are often seen. EEG abnormalities are present in patients even before the onset of symptoms, and characteristically manifest as symmetric, generalized and high-voltage spike and wave and polyspike and wave paroxysms. Other laboratory tests are generally unrevealing, except for increased urinary excretion of indican.

EPM1 is associated with severe diffuse Purkinje cell loss and Bergmann's gliosis (Hanovar & Meldrum, 1997). Surviving Purkinje cells are swollen and vacuolated. Mild to moderate neuron loss also occurs in the cerebral cortex, striatum, medial thalamic nucleus, brainstem nuclei, and spinal motor neurons. No Lafora bodies are present, indicating that EPM1 and Lafora disease are both pathologically and genetically distinct (Labauge et al., 1995).

EPM1 is caused by mutations in the *CSTB* gene, which encodes cystatin B, a cysteine protease inhibitor. Uncommonly, point mutations in the coding region result in protein truncation (Pennacchio et al., 1996). More often, expansions of a 12-nucleotide repeat in the 5′ untranslated region result in reduced mRNA expression (Lalioti et al., 1997; Lefreniere et al., 1997, Virtaneva et al., 1997). While normal alleles contain two to three copies of this 12-mer repeat unit, mutant alleles contain more than 60 copies. Unstable premutations containing 12–17 repeats are prone to expansion but do not cause clinical symptoms. That EPM1 is caused by the loss of cystatin B expression is further supported by the targeted disruption of this gene in mice, which causes progressive ataxia and myclonic epilepsy (Pennacchio et al., 1998).

Spinocerebellar ataxia type 8

The spinocerebellar ataxia type 8 (SCA8) locus at 13q21 was identified in a family with an undefined form of adult-onset, autosomal dominant spinocerebellar ataxia (Koob et al., 1998, 1999). The identified expansion consisted of 80 CAG triplets followed by 11 TAG triplets. DNA from a collection of ataxia families was then screened, leading to the identification of seven other affected kindreds carrying this expansion. The largest of these families, with 7 generations and 84 members, was evaluated clinically and genetically. All affected family members were found to have the expansion, yielding a maximum lod score for linkage between ataxia and the expansion of 6.8 at $\theta = 0.00$. In this and other kindreds (Ikeda et al., 2000), disease onset was in adulthood, ranging from 18 to 73 years, with symptoms including limb and truncal ataxia, ataxic dysarthria, and horizontal nystagmus. Disease manifestations were slowly progressive, and only severely affected individuals were non-ambulatory by the fourth to sixth decades. MRI scans revealed marked cerebellar atrophy.

Characterization of transcripts from the SCA8 locus indicate that the repeat expansion is near the 3′ end of an RNA that lacks an extended open reading frame (Nemes et al., 2000). The expansion is transcribed in the CTG orientation, complementary to the CAG repeat found in other spinocerebellar ataxias and reminiscent of the expansion in myotonic dystrophy (Koob et al., 1999). The 5′ exon of the SCA8 transcript is complementary to the first exon of another gene that is transcribed in the opposite orientation. This gene encodes a novel actin-binding protein that is primarily expressed in brain, named Kelch-like 1 (KLH1). The arrangement of these two genes suggests that the SCA8 transcript may be an endogenous antisense RNA that regulates the expression of KLH1.

Caution should be observed in interpreting whether expansion at the SCA8 locus is causative for the disease. In the large SCA8 kindred originally described, both the CTG and adjacent CTA repeats were polymorphic, and were expanded to 110–130 combined repeats in affected individuals. Normal alleles were found to carry 16–91 combined repeats. Several studies (Stevanin et al., 2000; Worth et al., 2000; Vincent et al., 2000) have since confirmed that the vast majority of control alleles (over 97%) have a small combined CTG/CTA repeat length, ranging from 3–31. However, in each of these studies, rare expanded alleles were also identified in the control population and in patients with other neurologic disorders. Very large expansions to hundreds of repeats were also observed in unaffected members of SCA8 kindreds and in a CEPH reference family. These data have raised the question whether the repeat expansion is causative for the disease or only linked to the causative mutation. If the expansion is involved in disease pathogenesis, then the reduced penetrance of the SCA8 phenotype and ranges for normal and pathologic expansions need to be explained.

Spinocerebellar ataxia type 10

Spinocerebellar ataxia type 10 (SCA10) is an autosomal dominant form of spinocerebellar ataxia associated with seizures. The disease locus was originally mapped to a 15 cM region at 22q13 (Zu et al., 1999). Matsuura et al., (2000) identified large expansions of an ATTCT pentanucleotide repeat in five Mexican SCA10 families. This pentanucleotide repeat is polymorphic in normal controls of European, Japanese and Mexican descent, and ranges in length from 10 to 22. In patients with the disease, there is a marked expansion to upwards of 4500 repeats. The pentanucleotide repeat is present within intron 9 of a gene of unknown function, designated *SCA10*, that is widely expressed within the mammalian brain. The mechanism by which the repeat expansion causes the diseases is unknown, and the possibility that it represents a rare polymorphism in linkage disequilibrium to the true pathogenic mutation has not been formally excluded.

Spinocerebellar ataxia type 12

Spinocerebellar ataxia type 12 (SCA12) is an autosomal dominant form of spinocerebellar ataxia identified in a single, large pedigree of German descent (Holmes et al., 1999). Clinical onset ranged from 8 to 55 years. Most patients presented in the fourth decade with a slowly progressive illness initially characterized by upper extremity tremor. The disease typically progressed to include head tremor, gait ataxia, dysmetria, dysdiadokinesis, hyperreflexia, paucity of movement, abnormal eye movements, and, in the oldest patients, dementia. MRI and CT scans of five cases revealed cortical and cerebellar atrophy. No pathological studies have been reported.

Like other autosomal dominant spinocerebellar ataxias, SCA12 is defined based on the involvement of a distinct genetic locus. Using a PCR-based strategy (Schalling et al., 1993; Koob et al., 1998; Holmes et al., 1999), a novel CAG repeat expansion was identified in the proband and other affected family members of the German pedigree. The range of expansion was relatively narrow (66–78 CAGs), and distinct from that observed in 394 normal subjects and 1099 disease controls (7–28 CAGs). In affected individuals, there was no apparent correlation between repeat length and age of onset, although the precise age of onset was often difficult to define and the expansion range in this pedigree was narrow.

The SCA12 CAG repeat is located 133 nucleotides 5′ of the apparent transcriptional start site of the gene encoding a brain-specific regulatory subunit of protein phosphatase PP2A, known as *PPP2R2B*, which has been mapped to 5q31–5q33. The use of an alternative transcriptional start site 5′ of the CAG repeat was suggested by the identification of a mouse brain EST derived from this region, and by the identification of promoter elements upstream of the repeat. As such, the repeat expansion may affect expression of this PP2A regulatory subunit, thereby altering PP2A function in the brain. Alternatively, the repeat may lie within an as yet unidentified overlapping or adjacent gene, or it may be in linkage disequilibrium with the causative mutation.

Friedreich's ataxia

Friedreich's ataxia (FRDA) is an autosomal recessive, multisystem degenerative disorder affecting approximately 1 in 40 000 individuals in the United States. The principal feature of FRDA is progressive gait and limb ataxia (Harding, 1981). Other commonly associated neurological features include cerebellar dysarthria, sensory loss, distal weakness, pyramidal signs, and absent reflexes in the lower limbs (Durr et al., 1996b). Disease onset is usually before age 25, and the symptoms are progressive. Skeletal deformities, diabetes, and progressive hypertrophic cardiomyopathy are found in many patients (Sanchez-Casis et al., 1977). This later aspect of the disease often contributes to mortality.

The neurological manifestations of FRDA reflect the distribution of pathology within the nervous system. FRDA is characterized by widespread neuronal degeneration within the central nervous system, but the hallmarks are atrophy of the posterior columns of the spinal cord, loss of deep cerebellar nuclei and efferent cerebellar pathways and degeneration of distal corticospinal tracts. In the peripheral nervous system, loss of sensory neurons is observed in the dorsal root ganglia (Hewer, 1968; Lamarche et al., 1993).

FRDA results from mutations causing loss of function of the *FRDA* gene at chromosome 9q13 (Campuzano et al., 1996). The vast majority of these mutations (more than 95%) are expansions of a guanine–adenine–adenine (GAA) trinucleotide repeat in the first intron of *FRDA*. The causative nature of *FRDA* mutations was verified by the identification of patients carrying one expanded allele and one allele with a point mutation (Campuzano et al., 1996; Durr et al., 1996b). No patients with point mutations in both alleles have yet been reported. The length of the GAA trinucleotide repeat in the *FRDA* gene is polymorphic, with normal chromosomes carrying fewer than 42 triplets (Cossee et al., 1997). FRDA chromosomes, in contrast, carry from 80 up to 1200 GAA repeats. Through a mechanism that remains unclear, but which likely involves defective transcriptional elongation, the expanded GAA repeat results in reduced *FRDA* expression.

The *FRDA* gene encodes a widely expressed 210-amino acid protein, frataxin, which localizes to the mitochondria (Campuzano et al., 1996, 1997) and likely contributes to iron homeostasis (Koutnikova et al., 1997; Babcock et al., 1997). In model systems, loss of frataxin results in overload of mitochondrial iron accompanied by reduced activity of key mitochondrial enzymes, hypersensitivity to oxidative stress, and defective oxidative phosphorylation (Wilson & Roof, 1997; Babcock et al., 1997; Rotig, 1997; Radisky et al., 1999). Mitochondria are a major source of reactive oxygen species, catalysed by iron via the Fenton reaction. These reactive oxygen species are believed to be the principal mediators of mitochondrial injury.

In patients with FRDA, loss of frataxin expression and function also results in accumulation of iron within mitochondria. This iron overload is especially pronounced in the tissues that are most severely affected in FRDA, including cardiac muscle, pancreatic islet cells, and the nervous system (Sanchez-Casis et al., 1977; Campuzano et al., 1997). Examination of tissues from patients with FRDA confirms that excess iron accumulation is associated with a reduction in mitochondrial enzyme function, increased susceptibility to oxidative stress, and defective oxidative phosphorylation (Lamarche et al., 1993; Waldvogel et al., 1999; Lodi et al., 1999; Delatycki et al., 1999; Rotig, 1999). Iron-induced injury in FRDA tissues is diminished by free radical scavengers such as ubiquinone (coenzyme Q_{10}) and idebenone, supporting the contention that the injury is mediated by reactive oxygen species (Wong et al., 1999). Elevated levels of urinary 8-hydroxy-2′-deoxyguanosine (a byproduct of oxidative damage to DNA) and plasma malondialdehyde (a byproduct of lipid peroxidation) are found in patients with FRDA, lending further support to the hypothesis that iron overload is associated with oxidative injury (Schultz et al., 2000; Edmond et al., 2000). The emerging consensus regarding the pathogenesis of FRDA is that loss of frataxin expression leads to a loss of iron homeostasis. The resulting overload of iron in mitochondria, in turn, results in increased steady-state levels of reactive oxygen species which cause oxidative damage and decreased ATP production causing injury to tissues – particularly those with a high energy demand (Beal, 2000).

In conclusion, the last decade of research in neurology has resulted in recognition of an entirely new class of hereditary disease. Progress in understanding these diseases will probably proceed hand in hand with a better understanding of underlying biochemical and cellular processes. Beyond the specific mechanisms at work in each of these disorders, there are a number of shared characteristics. First, all known repeat expansion diseases affect the nervous system. This may be related to specific molecular targets that are expressed only in neurons, or to a deficiency in some compensatory mechanism relative to non-neuronal cells. That neurons are long-lived cells with limited regenerative capacity probably contributes to their selective vulnerability. Secondly, naturally occurring repeat expansion diseases have thus far only been found in humans. Perhaps this is related to the long duration between birth and age of procreation in humans, which allows a large numbers of cell divisions in spermatogenesis, resulting in a greater opportunity for these dynamic mutations to occur. Also, since many of these diseases appear late in life, it is likely that the long lifespan of humans favours a higher incidence of disease. Ascertainment probably also plays a role. Finally, the repeat expansion diseases may be related to other non-expansion neurodegenerative diseases. Parallels exist between the polyglutamine diseases and more common neurodegenerative proteinopathies such as Parkinson's disease, Alzheimer's disease, prion diseases and amyotrophic lateral sclerosis. It is possible that protein deposition is an epiphenomenon representative of a morbid state in neurons. But the recent recognition of additional dominantly inherited neurodegenerative disorders that are characterized by intraneuronal aggregation of the mutant gene product, and the emerging evidence that defects in the ubiquitin–proteasome pathway may underlie neurodegenerative disease, argue that many of these diseases share a common pathogenesis. If the next decade of neurological research is as productive as the last, then a better understanding of this pathogenesis may lead to effective treatment for these disorders.

References

Alwazzan, M., Newman, E., Hamshere, M.G. & Brook, J.D. (1999). Myotonic dystrophy is associated with a reduced level of RNA from the DMWD allele adjacent to the expanded repeat. *Hum. Mol. Genet.*, **8**, 1491–7.

Arbizu, T., Santamaria, J., Gomez, J.M., Quilez, A. & Serra, J.P. (1983). A family with adult spinal and bulbar muscular atrophy, X-linked inheritance and associated testicular failure. *J. Neurol. Sci.*, **59**, 371–82.

Ashley, C.T., Wilkinson, K.D., Reines, D. & Warren, S.T. (1993). FMR1 protein: conserved RNP family domains and selective RNA binding. *Science*, **262**, 563–6.

Babcock, M., DeSilva, D., Oaks, R. et al. (1997). Regulation of mito-chondrial iron accumulation by Yfh1, a putative homolog of fra-taxin. *Science*, **276**, 1709–12.

Barabino, S.M.L. & Keller, W. (1999). Last but not least: regulated poly(A) tail formation. *Cell*, **99**, 9–11.

Barbeau, A. (1969). Oculopharyngeal muscular dystrophy in French Canada. In *Progress in Neuro-ophthalmology*, ed. J.R. Burnette & A. Barbeau, Vol. 2, p. 3. Amsterdam: Excerpta Medica.

Beal, M.F. (2000). Energetics in the pathogenesis of neurodegener-ative diseases. *Trends Neurosci.*, **23**, 298–304.

Becher, M.W., Kotzuk, J.A., Davis, L.E. & Bear, D.G. (2000). Intranuclear inclusions in oculopharyngeal muscular dystrophy contain poly(A) binding protein 2. *Ann. Neurol.*, **48**, 812–15.

Berul, C.I., Maguire, C.T., Aronovitz, M.J. et al. (1999). DMPK dosage alterations result in atrioventricular conduction abnor-malities in a mouse myotonic dystrophy model. *J. Clin. Invest.*, **103**, R1–7.

Blumen, S.C., Brais, B., Korczyn, A.D. et al. (1999). Homozygotes for oculopharyngeal muscular dystrophy have a severe form of the disease. *Ann. Neurol.*, **46**, 115–18.

Boutell, J.M., Thomas, P., Neal, J.W. et al. (1999). Aberrant interac-tions of transcriptional repressor proteins with the Huntington's disease gene product, huntingtin. *Hum. Mol. Genet.*, **8**, 1647–55.

Bowater, R.P. & Wells, R.D. (2000). The intrinsically unstable life of DNA triplet repeats associated with human hereditary disorders. *Prog. Nucl. Acids Res. and Mol. Biol.*, **66**, 159–202.

Brais, B., Xie, Y.G., Sanson, M. et al. (1995). The oculopharyngeal muscular dystrophy locus maps to the region of the cardiac α and β myosin heavy chain genes on chromosome 14q11.2–q13. *Hum. Mol. Genet.*, **4**, 429–34.

Brais, B., Bouchard, J.P., Xie, Y.G. et al. (1998). Short GCG expan-sions in the PABP2 gene cause oculopharyngeal muscular dys-trophy. *Nat. Genet.*, **18**, 164–7.

Brook, J.D., McCurrach, M.E., Harley, H.G. et al. (1992). Molecular basis of myotonic dystrophy: expansion of a trinucleotide (CTG) repeat at the 3′ end of a transcript encoding a protein kinase family member. *Cell*, **77**, 799–808.

Brown, W.T., Houck, G.E., Jr., Ding, X. et al. (1996). Reverse muta-tions in the fragile X syndrome. *Am. J. Med. Genet.*, **64**, 287–92.

Buxton, J., Shelbourne, P., Davies, J. et al. (1992). Detection of an unstable fragment of DNA specific to individuals with myotonic dystrophy. *Nature*, **355**, 547–8.

Calado, A., Tome, F.M.S., Brais, B. et al. (2000). Nuclear inclusions in oculopharyngeal muscular dystrophy consist of poly(A) binding protein 2 aggregates which sequester poly(A) RNA. *Hum. Mol. Genet.*, **9**, 2321–8.

Campuzano, V., Montermini, L., Molto, M.D. et al. (1996). Friedreich ataxia: autosomal recessive disease caused by an intronic GAA triplet repeat expansion. *Science*, **271**, 1423–6.

Campuzano, V., Montermini, L., Lutz, Y. et al. (1997). Frataxin is reduced in Friedreich ataxia patients and is associated with mit-ochondrial membranes. *Hum. Mol. Genet.*, **6**, 1771–80.

Cancel, G., Duyckaerts, C., Holmberg, M. et al. (2000). Distribution of ataxin-7 in normal human brain and retina. *Brain*, **123**, 2519–30.

Carango, P., Noble, J.E., Marks, H.G. & Funanage, V.L. (1993). Absence of myotonic dystrophy protein kinase (DMPK) mRNA as a result of a triplet repeat expansion in myotonic dystrophy. *Genomics*, **18**, 340–8.

Chai, Y., Koppenhafer, S.L., Shoesmith, S.J., Perez, M.K. & Paulson, H.L. (1999). Evidence for proteasome involvement in polygluta-mine disease: localization to nuclear inclusions in SCA3/MJD and suppression of polyglutamine aggregation in vitro. *Hum. Molec. Genet.*, **8**, 673–82.

Charlesworth, B. Sniegowski, P. & Stephan, W. (1994). The evolu-tionary dynamics of repetitive DNA in eucaryotes. *Nature*, **371**, 215–20.

Chung, M-Y., Ranum, L.P.W., Duvick, L., Servadio, A., Zoghbi, H. & Orr, H.T. (1993). Analysis of the CAG repeat expansion in spino-cerebellar ataxia type 1: evidence for a possible mechanism pre-disposing to instability. *Nat. Genet.*, **5**, 254–8.

Ciechanover, A. (1997). The ubiquitin–proteasome proteolytic pathway. *Cell*, **79**, 13–21.

Cossee, M., Schmitt, M., Campuzano, V. et al. (1997). Evolution of the Friedreich's ataxia trinucleotide repeat expansion: founder effect and permutations. *Proc. Natl. Acad. Sci., USA*, **94**, 7452–7.

Cummings, C.J., Mancini, M.A., Antalffy, B., DeFranco, D.B., Orr, H.T. & Zoghbi, H.Y. (1998). Chaperone suppression of aggrega-tion and altered subcellular proteasome localization imply protein misfolding in SCA1. *Nat. Genet.*, **19**, 148–54.

Cummings, C.J., Reinstein, E., Sun, Y. et al. (1999). Mutation of the E6–AP ubiquitin ligase reduces nuclear inclusion frequency while accelerating polyglutamine-induced pathology in SCA1 mice. *Neuron*, **24**, 879–92.

David, G., Abbas, N., Stevanin, G. et al. (1997). Cloning the SCA7 gene reveals a highly unstable CAG repeat expansion. *Nat. Genet.*, **17**, 65–70.

Davies, S.W., Beardsall, K., Turmaine, M., DiFiglia, M., Aronin, N. & Bates, G.P. (1998). Are neuronal intranuclear inclusions the common neuropathology of triplet-repeat disorders with polyg-lutamine-repeat expansions? *Lancet*, **351**, 131–3.

Davies, A.F., Mirza, G., Sekhon, G. et al. (1999). Delineation of two distinct 6p deletion syndromes. *Hum. Genet.*, **104**, 64–72.

Davis, B.M., McCurrach, M.E., Taneja, K.L., Singer, R.H. & Housman, D.E. (1997). Expansion of a CUG trinucleotide repeat in the 3′ untranslated region of myotonic dystrophy protein kinase transcripts results in nuclear retention of transcripts. *Proc. Natl. Acad. Sci., USA*, **94**, 7388–93.

Davis, R.L., Shrimpton, A.E., Holohan, P.D. et al. (1999). Familial dementia caused by polymerization of mutant neuroserpin. *Nature*, **401**, 376–9.

De Boulle, K., Verderk, A.J., Reyniers, E. et al. (1993). A point muta-tion in the *FMR-1* gene associated with fragile X mental retarda-tion. *Nat. Genet.*, **3**, 31–5.

Delatycki, M.B., Camakaris, J., Brooks, H. et al. (1999). Direct evi-dence that mitochondrial iron accumulation occurs in Friedreich ataxia. *Ann. Neurol.*, **45**, 673–5.

DiFiglia M., Sapp, E., Chase, K.O. et al. (1997). Aggregation of hun-tingtin in neuronal intranuclear inclusions and dystrophic neu-rites in brain. *Science*, **277**, 1990–3.

Doyu, M., Sobue, G., Mukai, E. et al. (1992). Severity of X-linked recessive bulbospinal neuropathy correlates with size of the tandem CAG repeat in androgen receptor gene. *Ann. Neurol.*, **32**, 707–10.

Dubowitz, V. & Brooke, M.H. (1973). *Muscle Biopsy: A Modern Approach*, pp. 231–41. Philadelphia: Saunders.

Durr, A., Stevanin, G., Cancel, G. et al. (1996a). Spinocerebellar ataxia 3 and Machado–Joseph disease: clinical, molecular and neuropathological features. *Ann. Neurol.*, **39**, 490–9.

Durr, A., Cossee, M., Agid, Y. et al. (1996b). Clinical and genetic abnormalities in patients with Friedreich's ataxia. *N. Engl. J. Med.*, **335**, 1169–75.

Dutch–Belgium Fragile X Consortium. (1994). *Fmr1* knockout mice: a model to study fragile X mental retardation. *Cell*, **78**, 23–33.

Eberhart, D.E., Malter, H.E., Feng, Y. & Warren, S.T. (1996). The fragile X mental retardation protein is a ribonucleoprotein containing both nuclear localization and nuclear export signals. *Hum. Mol. Genet.*, **5**, 1083–91.

Edmond, M., Lepage, G., Vanasse, M. & Pandolfo, M. (2000). Increased levels of plasma malondialdehyde in Friedreich ataxia. *Neurology*, **55**, 1752–1753.

Eichler, E.E., Richards, S., Gibbs, R.A. & Nelson, D.L. (1994a). Fine structure of the human *FMR1* gene. *Hum. Mol. Genet.*, **3**, 684–5.

Eichler, E.E., Holden, J.J., Popovich, B.W. et al. (1994b). Length of uninterrupted CGG repeats determines instability in the *FMR1* gene. *Nat. Genet.*, **8**, 88–94.

Ellerby, L.M., Hackam, A.S., Propp, S.S. et al. (1999). Kennedy's disease: caspase cleavage of the androgen receptor is a crucial event in cytotoxicity. *J. Neurochem.*, **72**, 185–95.

Fleischer, B. (1918). Uber myotonische Dystrophie mit katarakt. *Graefes Arch. Exp. Ophthalmol.*, **96**, 91–133.

Fletcher, C.F., Lutz, C.M., O'Sullivan, T.N. et al. (1996). Absence epilepsy in Tottering mutant mice is associated with calcium channel defects. *Cell*, **87**, 607–17.

Fu, Y.H., Kuhl, D.P., Pizzuti, A. et al. (1991). Variation of the CGG repeat at the fragile X site results in genetic instability: resolution of the Sherman paradox. *Cell*, **67**, 1047–58.

Fu, Y.H., Friedman, D.L., Richards, S. et al. (1993). Decreased expression of myotonin-protein kinase messenger RNA and protein in adult form of myotonic dystrophy. *Science*, **260**, 235–8.

Gaspar, C., Lopes-Cendes, I., Hayes, S. et al. (2001). Ancestral origins of the Machado–Joseph disease mutation: a worldwide haplotype study. *Am. J. Hum. Genet.*, **68**, 523–8.

Gecz, J., Gedeon, A.K., Sutherland, G.R. & Mulley, J.C. (1996). Identification of the gene FMR2, associated with FRAXE mental retardation. *Nat. Genet.*, **13**, 105–8.

Giraud, F., Ayme, S., Mattei, J.F. & Mattei, M.G. (1976). Constitutional chromosomal breakage. *Hum. Genet.*, **34**, 125–36.

Gispert, S., Twells, R., Orozco, G. et al. (1993). Chromosomal assignment of the second locus for autosomal dominant cerebellar ataxia (SCA2) to chromosome 12q23–24.1. *Nat. Genet.*, **4**, 295–9.

Goldfarb, L.G., Vasconcelos, O., Platonov, F.A. et al. (1996). Unstable triplet repeat and phenotypic variability of spinocerebellar ataxia type 1. *Ann. Neurol.*, **39**, 500–6.

Gu, Y., Shen, Y., Gibbs, R.A. & Nelson, D.L. (1996). Identification of FMR2, a novel gene associated with the FRAXE CCG repeat and CpG island. *Nat. Genet.*, **13**, 109–13.

Hackam, A.S., Singaraja, R., Wellington, C.L. et al. (1998). The influence of Huntingtin protein size on nuclear localization and cellular toxicity. *J. Cell Biol.* **141**, 1097–105

Hamshere, M.G., Newman, E.E., Alwazzan, M., Athwal, B.S. & Brook, J.D. (1997). Transcriptional abnormality in myotonic dystrophy affects DMPK but not neighboring genes. *Proc. Natl. Acad. Sci., USA*, **94**, 7394–9.

Hanovar, M. & Meldrum, B.S. (1997). Epilespsy. In *Greenfield's Neuropathology*, ed. D.T. Graham & P.L. Lantos, Vol. 1, pp. 954–955. London: Arnold.

Harding, A. (1981). Friedreich's ataxia: a clinical and genetic study of 90 families with an analysis of early diagnostic criteria and intrafamilial clustering of clinical features. *Brain*, **104**, 598–620.

Harding, A.E., Thomas, P.K., Baraitser, M., Bradbury, P.G., Morgan-Hughes, J.A. & Ponsford, J.R. (1982). X-linked recessive bulbospinal neuronopathy: a report of ten cases. *J. Neurol. Neurosurg. Psychiat.*, **45**, 1012–19.

Harley, H.G., Brook, J.D., Rundle, S.A. et al. (1992). Expansion of an unstable DNA region and phenotypic variation in myotonic dystrophy. *Nature*, **355**, 545–6.

Harper, P.S. & Rudel, R. (1994). Myotonic dystrophy. In *Myology*, ed. A.G. Engel & C. Franzini-Armstrong, 2nd edn, Vol 2, pp. 1192–219. New York: McGraw-Hill.

Harvey, J., Judge, C. & Wiener, S. (1997). Familial X-linked mental retardation with an X-chromosome abnormality. *J. Med. Genet.*, **14**, 46–50.

Hayashi, Y., Kakita, A., Yamada, M. et al. (1998). Hereditary dentatorubral-pallidoluysian atrophy: detection of widespread ubiquitinated neuronal and glial intranuclear inclusions in the brain. *Acta Neuropath.*, **96**, 547–52.

Hewer, R.L. (1968). Study of fatal cases of Friedreich's ataxia. *Br. Med. J.*, **3**, 649–52.

Hirst, M.C., Barnicoat, A., Flynn, G. et al. (1993). The identification of a third fragile site, FRAXF, in Xq27–q28 distal to both FRAXA and FRAXE. *Hum. Mol. Genet.*, **2**, 197–200.

Hofmann-Radvanyi, H., Lavedan, C., Rabes, J.P. et al. (1993). Myotonic dystrophy: absence of CTG enlarged transcript in congenital forms, and low expression of normal allele. *Hum. Mol. Genet.*, **2**, 1263–6.

Holmberg, M., Duyckaerts, C., Durr, A. et al. (1998). Spinocerebellar ataxia type 7 (SCA7): a neurodegenerative disorder with neuronal intranuclear inclusions. *Hum. Mol. Genet.*, **7**, 913–18.

Holmes, S.E., O'Hearn, E.E., McInnis, M.G. et al. (1999). Expansion of a novel CAG trinucleotide repeat in the 5' region of *PPP2R2B* is associated with SCA12. *Nat. Genet.*, **23**, 391–2.

Hunter, A., Tsilfidis, C., Mettler, G. et al. (1992). The correlation of age of onset with CTG trinucleotide repeat amplification in myotonic dystrophy. *J. Med. Genet.*, **29**, 774–9.

Huntington's Disease Collaborative Research Group. (1993). A novel gene containing a trinucleotide repeat that is expanded and unstable on Huntington's disease chromosomes. *Cell*, **72**, 971–83.

Huynh, D.P., Del Bigio, M.R., Ho, D.H. & Pulst, S.M. (2000). Expression of ataxin-2 in brains from normal individuals and patients with Alzheimer's disease and spinocerebellar ataxia type 2. *Ann. Neurol.*, **45**, 232–41.

Igarashi, S., Koide, R., Shimohata, T. et al. (1998). Suppression of aggregate formation and apoptosis by transglutaminase inhibitors in cells expressing truncated DRPLA protein with an expanded polyglutamine stretch. *Nat. Genet.*, **18**, 111–17.

Ikeda, Y., Shizuka, M., Watanabe, M., Okamoto, K. & Shoji, M. (2000). Molecular and clinical analysis of spinocerebellar ataxia type 8 in Japan. *Neurology*, **54**, 950–5.

Imbert, G., Saudou, F., Yvert, G. et al. (1996). Cloning of the gene for spinocerebellar ataxia 2 reveals a locus with high sensitivity to expanded CAG/glutamine repeats. *Nat. Genet.*, **14**, 285–91.

Jacobsen, P., Hauge, M., Henningsen, K., Hobolth, N., Mikkelsen, M. & Philip, J. (1973). An (11; 21) tranlocation in four generations with chromosome 11 abnormalities in the offspring: a clinical, cytogenetical, and gene marker study. *Hum. Hered.*, **23**, 580–5.

Jansen, G., Bachner, D., Coerwinkel, M., Wormskamp, N., Hameister, H. & Wieringa, B. (1995). Structural organization and developmental expression pattern of the WD-repeat gene DMR-N9 immediately upstream of the myotonic dystrophy locus. *Hum. Mol. Genet.*, **4**, 843–52.

Jansen, G., Groenen, P.J., Bachner, D. et al. (1996). Abnormal myotonic dystrophy protein kinase levels produce only mild myopathy in mice. *Nat. Genet.*, **13**, 316–24.

Jenster, G., van der Korput, H.A., van Vroonhoven, C., van der Kwast, T.H., Trapman, J. & Brinkman, A.O. (1991). Domains of the human androgen receptor involved in steroid binding, transcriptional activation, and subcellular localization. *Mol. Endocrinol.*, **5**, 1396–404.

Jodice, C., Malaspina, P., Persichetti, F. et al. (1994). Effect of trinucleotide repeat length and parental sex on phenotypic variation in spinocerebellar ataxia type 1. *Am. J. Hum. Genet.*, **54**, 959–65.

Johansson, J. Forsgren, L., Sandgren, O., Brice, A., Holmgren, G. & Holmberg, M. (1998). Expanded CAG repeats in Swedish spinocerebellar ataxia type 7 (SCA7) patients: effect of CAG repeat length on the clinical manifestation. *Hum. Mol. Genet.*, **7**, 171–6.

Johnston, J.A., Ward, C.L. and Kopito, R.R. (1998). Aggresomes: a cellular response to misfolded proteins. *J. Cell Biol.* **143**, 1883–98.

Jones, C., Penny, L., Mattina, T. et al. (1995). Association of a chromosome deletion syndrome with a fragile site within the proto-oncogene CBL2. *Nature*, **376**, 145–9.

Kang, S.M., Ohshima, K., Shimizu, S., Amirhaeri, S. & Wells, R.D. (1995). Pausing of DNA synthesis *in vitro* at specific loci in CTG and CGG triplet repeats from human hereditary disease genes. *J. Biol. Chem.*, **270**, 27014–21.

Kawaguchi, Y., Okamoto, T., Taniwaki, M. et al. (1994). CAG expansions in a novel gene for Machado–Joseph disease at chromosome 14q32.1. *Nat. Genet.*, **8**, 221–8.

Klement, I.A., Skinner, P.J., Kaytor, M.D. et al. (1998). Ataxin-1 nuclear localization and aggregation: role in polyglutamine-induced disease in SCA1 transgenic mice. *Cell*, **95**, 41–53.

Klesert, T.R., Otten, A.D., Bird, T.D. & Tapscott, S.J. (1997).

Trinucleotide repeat expansion at the myotonic dystrophy locus reduces expression of DMAHP. *Nat. Genet.*, **16**, 402–6.

Klesert, T.R., Cho, D.H., Clark, J.I. et al. (2000). Mice deficient in Six5 develop cataracts: implications for myotonic dystrophy. *Nat. Genet.*, **25**, 105–9.

Knight, S.J.L., Flannery, A.V., Hirst, M.C. et al. (1993). Trinucleotide repeat amplification and hypermethylation of a CpG island in FRAXE mental retardation. *Cell*, **74**, 127–34.

Knight, S.P., Richardson, M.M., Osmand, A.P., Stakkestad, A. & Potter, N.T. (1997). Expression and distribution of the dentatorubral–pallidoluysian atrophy gene product (atrophin1/drplap) in neuronal and non-neuronal tissues. *J. Neurol. Sci.*, **146**, 19–26.

Koide, R., Ikeuchi, T., Onodera, O. et al. (1994). Unstable expansion of CAG repeat in hereditary dentatorubral–pallidoluysian atrophy (DRPLA). *Nat. Genet.*, **6**, 9–13.

Koide, R., Kobayashi, S., Shimohata, T. et al. (1999). A neurological disease caused by an expanded CAG trinucleotide repeat in the TATA-binding protein gene: a new polyglutamine disease? *Hum. Mol. Genet.*, **8**, 2047–53.

Koob, M.D., Benzow, K.A., Bird, T.D., Day, J.W., Moseley, M.L. & Ranum, L.P.W. (1998). Rapid cloning of expanded trinucleotide repeat sequences from genomic DNA. *Nat.Genet.*, **18**, 72–5.

Koob, M.D., Moseley, M.L., Schut, L.J. et al. (1999). An untranslated CTG expansion causes a novel form of spinocerebellar ataxia (SCA8). *Nat. Genet.*, **21**, 379–84.

Koutnikova, H., Campuzano, V., Foury, F., Dolle, P., Cazzalini, O. & Koenig, M. (1997). Studies of human, mouse and yeast homologue indicate a mitochondrial function for frataxin. *Nat. Genet.*, **16**, 345–51.

Krahe, R., Ashizawa, T., Abbruzzese, C. et al. (1995). Effect of myotonic dystrophy trinucleotide repeat expansion on DMPK transcription and processing. *Genomics*, **28**, 1–14.

Kremer, E.J., Pritchard, M., Lynch, M. et al. (1991). Mapping of DNA instability at the fragile X to a trinucleotide repeat sequence p(CGG)n. *Science*, **252**, 1711–14.

Kunst, C.B. & Warren, S.T. (1994). Cryptic and polar variation of the fragile X repeat could result in predisposing normal alleles. *Cell*, **77**, 853–61.

Labauge, P., Beck, C., Bellet, H. et al. (1995). Lafora disease is not linked to the Unverricht–Lundborg locus. *Am. J. Med. Genet.*, **60**, 80–4.

Lalioti, M.D., Scott, H.S., Buresi, C. et al. (1997). Dodecamer repeat expansion in cystatin B gene in progressive myoclonus epilepsy. *Nature*, **386**, 847–51.

Lamarche, J.B., Shapcott, D., Cote, M. & Lemieux, B. (1993). Cardiac iron deposits in Friedreich's ataxia. In *Handbook of Cerebellar Diseases*, ed. R. Lechtenberg, pp. 453–8. New York: Marcel Dekker.

La Spada, A.R., Wilson, E.M., Lubahn, D.B., Harding, A.E. & Fischbeck, K.H. (1991). Androgen receptor gene mutations in X-linked spinal and bulbar muscular atrophy. *Nature*, **352**, 77–9.

Leavitt, B.R., Wellington, C.L. & Hayden, M.R. (1999). Recent insights into the molecular pathogenesis of Huntington disease. *Semin. Neurol.*, **19**, 385–95.

Lee, V.M. & Trojanowski, J.Q. (1999). Neurodegenerative tauopathies: human disease and transgenic mouse models. *Neuron*, **24**, 751–62.

Lefreniere, R.G., Rochefort, D.L., Chretien, N. et al. (1997). Unstable insertion in the 5′ flanking region of the cystatin B gene is the most common mutation in progressive myoclonus epilepsy type 1, EPM1. *Nat. Genet.*, **15**, 298–302.

Lehesjoki, A-E. & Koskiniemi, M. (1998). Clinical features and genetics of progressive myoclonus epilepsy of the Unverricht–Lundborg type. *Ann. Med.*, **30**, 474–80.

Li, H., Li, S.H., Johnston, H., Shelbourne, P.F. & Li, X.J. (2000). Amino-terminal fragments of mutant huntingtin show selective accumulation in striatal neurons and synaptic toxicity. *Nat. Genet.*, **25**, 385–9.

Li, M., Kobayashi, Y., Merry, D.E. et al. (1998). Nuclear inclusions of the androgen receptor protein in spinal and bulbar muscular atrophy. *Ann. Neurol.*, **44**, 249–54.

Li, S.-H., Mcinnis, M.G., Margolis, R.L., Antonarakis, S.E. & Ross, C.A. (1993). Novel triplet repeat containing genes in human brain: cloning, expression, and length polymorphisms. *Genomics*, **16**, 572–9.

Lin, X., Antalffy, B., Kang, D., Orr, H.T. & Zoghbi, H.Y. (2000). Polyglutamine expansion down-regulates specific neuronal genes before pathologic changes in SCA1. *Nat. Neurosci.*, **3**, 157–63.

Lindblad, K., Savontaus, M.L., Stevanin, G. et al. (1996). An expanded CAG repeat sequence in spinocerebellar ataxia type 7. *Genet. Res.*, **10**, 965–71.

Lindenberg, K., Yvert, G., Muller, K. & Landwehrmeyer, B. (2000). Expression of ataxin-7 mRNA and protein in human brain: evidence for a widespread distribution and focal protein accumulation. *Brain Pathol.*, **10**, 385–94.

Liquori, C.L., Ricker, K., Moseley, M.L. et al. (2001). Myotonic dystrophy type 2 caused by a CCTG expansion in intron 1 of ZNF9. *Science* **293**, 864–7.

Lodi, R., Cooper, J.M., Bradley, J.L. et al. (1999). Deficit of in vitro ATP production in patients with Friedreich ataxia. *Proc. Natl. Acad. Sci., USA*, **96**, 11492–5.

Losekoot, M., Hoogendoorn, E., Olmer, R. et al. (1997). *J. Med. Genet.*, **34**, 924–6.

Luthi-Carter, R., Strand, A., Peters, N.L. et al. (2000). Decreased expression of striatal signaling genes in a mouse model of Huntington's disease. *Hum. Mol. Genet.*, **9**, 1259–71.

McCampbell, A., Taylor, J.P., Taye, A.A. et al. (2000). CREB-binding protein sequestration by expanded polyglutamine. *Hum. Mol. Genet.*, **9**, 2197–202.

Mahadevan, M., Tsilfidis, C., Sabourin, L. et al. (1992). Myotonic dystrophy mutation: an unstable CTG repeat in the 3′ untranslated region of the gene. *Science*, **255**, 1253–5.

Malter, H.E., Iber, J.C., Wilemsen, R. et al. (1997). Characterization of the full fragile X syndrome mutation in fetal gametes. *Nat. Genet.*, **15**, 165–9.

Mankodi, A., Logigian, E., Callahan, L. et al. (2000). Myotonic dystrophy in transgenic mice expressing an expanded CUG repeat. *Science*, **289**, 1769–72.

Maruyama, H., Nakamura, S., Matsuyama, Z. et al. (1995). Molecular features of the CAG repeats and clinical manifestation of Machado–Joseph disease. *Hum. Molec. Genet.*, **4**, 807–12.

Matilla, A., Roberson, E.D., Banfi, S. et al. (1998). Mice lacking ataxin-1 display learning deficits and decreased hippocampal paired-pulse facilitation. *J. Neurosci.*, **18**, 5508–16.

Matsuura, T., Yamagata, T., Burgess, D.L. et al. (2000). Large expansion of the ATTCT pentanucleotide repeat in spinocerebellar ataxia type 10. *Nat. Genet.*, **26**, 191–4.

Matsuyama, Z., Kawakami, H., Maruyama, H. et al. (1997). Molecular features of the CAG repeats of spinocerebellar ataxia 6 (SCA6). *Hum. Mol. Genet.*, **6**, 1283–7.

Mauger, C., Del-Favero, J., Ceuterick, C., Lubke, U., van Broeckhoven, C. & Martin, J. (1999). Identification and localization of ataxin-7 in brain and retina of a patient with cerebellar ataxia type II using anti-peptide antibody. *Mol. Brain Res.*, **74**, 35–43.

Mezei, M.M., Mankodi, A., Brais, B. et al. (1999). Minimal expansion of the GCG repeat in the PABP2 gene does not predispose to sporadic inclusion body myositis. *Neurology*, **52**, 669–70.

Modrich, P. & Lahue, R. (1996). Mismatch repair in replication fidelity, genetic recombination and cancer biology. *Ann. Rev. Biochem.*, **65**, 101–33.

Murphy, K.P., Carter, R.J., Lione, L.A. et al. (2000). Abnormal synaptic plasticity and impaired spatial cognition in mice transgenic for exon 1 of the human Huntington's disease mutation. *J. Neurosci.*, **20**, 5115–23.

Myers, R.H., Vonsattel, J.P., Stevens, T.J., Cupples, L.A., Richardson, E.P. & Bird, E.D. (1988). Clinical and neuropathological assessment of severity in Huntington's disease. *Neurology*, **38**, 341–7.

Nagafuchi, S., Yanagisawa, H., Sata, K. et al. (1994). Dentatorubral and pallidoluysian atrophy expansion of an unstable CAG trinucleotide repeat on chromosome 12p. *Nat. Genet.*, **6**, 14–18.

Naito, H. & Oyanagi, S. (1982). Familial myoclonus epilepsy and choreoathetosis: hereditary dentatorubral–pallidoluysian atrophy. *Neurology*, **32**, 798–807.

Nakano, K.K., Dawson, D.M. & Spence, A. (1972). Machado disease: a hereditary ataxia in Portuguese emigrants to Massachussetts. *Neurology*, **22**, 49–55.

Nakamura, K., Jeong, S.Y., Uchihara, T. (2001). SCA17, a novel autosomal dominant cerebellar ataxia caused by an expanded polyglutamine in TATA-binding protein. *Hum. Mol. Genet.*, **10**, 1441–8.

Nemes, J.P., Benzow, K.A. & Koob, M.D. (2000). The *SCA8* transcript is an antisense RNA to a brain-specific transcript encoding a novel actin-binding protein (KLHL1). *Hum. Mol. Genet.*, **9**, 1543–51.

Oberle, I., Rousseau, F., Heitz, D. et al. (1991). Instability of a 550-base pair DNA segment and abnormal methylation in fragile X syndrome. *Science*, **252**, 1097–102.

Ogata, A., Matsuura, T., Tashiro, K. et al. (1994). Expression of androgen receptor in X-linked spinal and bulbar muscular atrophy and amyotrophic lateral sclerosis. *J. Neurol. Neurosurg. Psychiat.*, **63**, 1274–5.

O'Hoy, K.L., Tsilfidis, C., Mahadevan, M.S. et al. (1993). Reduction in size of the myotonic dystrophy trinucleotide repeat mutation during transmission. *Science*, **259**, 809–10.

Ophoff, R.A., Terwindt, G.M., Vergouwe, M.N. et al. (1996). Familial hemiplegic migraine and episodic ataxia type-2 are caused by mutations in the Ca^{2+} channel gene CACNL1A4. *Cell*, **87**, 543–52.

Ordway, J.M., Tallaksen-Greene, S., Gutekunst, C.A. et al. (1997). Ectopically expressed CAG repeats cause intranuclear inclusions and a progressive late onset neurological phenotype in the mouse. *Cell*, **91**, 753–63.

Orr, H.T., Chung, M.Y., Banfi, S. et al. (1993). Expansion of an unstable trinucleotide CAG repeat in spinocerebellar ataxia type 1. *Nat. Genet.*, **4**, 221–6.

Parniewski, P., Bacolla, A., Jawarski, A. & Wells, R.D. (1999). Nucleotide excision repair affects the stability of long transcribed (CTG·CAG) tracts in an orientation dependent manner in *Escherichia coli*. *Nucl. Acids Res.*, **27**, 616–23.

Parrish, J.E., Oostra, B.A., Verkerk, A.J.M.H. et al. (1994). Isolation of a GCC repeat showing expansion in FRAXF, a fragile site distal to FRAXA and FRAXE. *Nat. Genet.*, **8**, 229–35.

Paulson, H.L. & Fischbeck, K.H. (1996). Trinucleotide repeats in neurogenetic disorders. *Annu. Rev. Neurosci.*, **19**, 79–107.

Paulson, H.L., Perez, M.K., Trottier, Y. et al. (1997). Intranuclear inclusions of expanded polyglutamine protein in spinocerebellar ataxia type 3. *Neuron*, **19**, 333–44.

Pennacchio, L.A., Lehesjoki, A.E., Stone, N.E. et al. (1996). Mutations in the gene encoding cystatin B in progressive myoclonus epilepsy (EPM1). *Science*, **271**, 1731–4.

Pennacchio, L.A., Bouley, D.M., Higgins, K.M., Scott, M.P., Noebels, J.L. & Myers, R.M. (1998). Progressive ataxia, myoclonic epilepsy and cerebellar apoptosis in cystatin B-deficient mice. *Nat. Genet.*, **20**, 251–8.

Perez, M.K., Paulson, H.L., Pendse, S.J., Saionz, S.J., Bonini, N.M. & Pittman, R.N. (1998). Recruitment and the role of nuclear localization in polyglutamine-mediated aggregation. *J. Cell Biol.*, **143**, 1457–70.

Perutz, M.F., Johnson, T., Suzuki, M. & Finch, J.T. (1994). Glutamine repeats as polar zippers: their possible role in inherited neurodegenerative diseases. *Proc. Natl. Acad. Sci., USA*, **91**, 5355–8.

Philips, A.V., Timchenko, L.T. & Cooper, T.A. (1998). Disruption of splicing regulated by a CUG-binding protein in myotonic dystrophy. *Science*, **280**, 737–41.

Polymeropoulos, M.H. (2000). Genetics of Parkinson's disease. *Ann. NY Acad. Sci.*, **920**, 28–32.

Pulst, S-M., Nechiporuk, T., Gispert, S. et al. (1996). Moderate expansion of a normally biallelic trinucleotide repeat in spinocerebellar ataxia type 2. *Nat. Genet.*, **14**, 269–76.

Radisky, D.C., Babcock, M. & M.C., Kaplan, J. (1999) The yeast frataxin homologue mediates mitochondrial iron efflux. Evidence for a mitochondrial iron cycle. *J. Biol. Chem.*, **274**, 4497–9.

Ranum, L.P.W., Chung, M-Y., Banfi, S. et al. (1994). Molecular and clinical correlations in spinocerebellar ataxia type 1 (SCA1): evidence for familial effects on the age of onset. *Am. J. Hum. Genet.*, **55**, 244–52.

Ranum, L.P.W., Rasmussen, P.F., Benzow, K.A., Koob, M.D. & Day,

J.W. (1998). Genetic mapping of a second myotonic dystrophy locus. *Nat. Genet.*, **19**, 196–8.

Reddy, S., Smith, D.B., Rich, M.M. et al. (1996). Mice lacking the myotonic dystrophy protein kinase develop a late onset progressive myopathy. *Nat. Genet.*, **13**, 325–35.

Ricker, K., Koch, M.C., Lehmann-Horn, F. et al. (1994). Proximal myotonic myopathy: a new dominant disorder with myotonia, muscle weakness, and cataracts. *Neurology*, **44**, 1448–52.

Ritchie, R.J., Knight, S.J.L., Hirst, M.C. et al. (1994). The cloning of FRAXF: trinucleotide repeat expansion and methylation at a third fragile site in distal Xqter. *Hum. Mol. Genet.*, **3**, 2115–21.

Rotig, A. (1997). Aconitase and mitochondrial iron–sulphur protein deficiency in Friedreich ataxia. *Nat. Genet.*, **17**, 215–17.

Rubinstein, D.C., Leggo, J., Coles, R. et al. (1996). Phenotype characterization of individuals with 30–40 CAG repeats in the Huntington's Disease (HD) gene reveals HD cases with 36 repeats and apparently normal elderly individuals with 36–39. *Am. J. Hum. Genet.*, **59**, 16–22.

Sanchez, I., Xu, C.J., Kakizaka, A., Blenis, J. & Yuan, J. (1999). Caspase-8 is required for cell death induced by expanded polyglutamine repeats. *Neuron*, **22**, 623–33.

Sanchez-Casis, G., Cote, M. & Barbeau, A. (1997). Pathology of the heart in Friedreich's ataxia: review of the literature and report of one case. *Can. J. Neurol. Sci.*, **3**, 349–54.

Sanpei, K., Takano, H., Igarashi, S. et al. (1996). Identification of the spinocerebellar ataxia type 2 gene using a direct identification of repeat expansion and cloning technique, DIRECT. *Nat. Genet.*, **14**, 277–84.

Sarker, P.S., Appukuttan, B., Han, J. et al. (2000). Heterozygous loss of *Six5* in mice is sufficient to cause ocular cataracts. *Nat. Genet.*, **25**, 110–14.

Saudou, F., Finkbeiner, S., Devys, D. & Greenberg, M.E. (1998). Huntingtin acts in the nucleus to induce apoptosis but death does not correlate with the formation of intranuclear inclusions. *Cell*, **95**, 55–66.

Schalling, M., Hudson, T.J., Buetow, K.H. & Housman, D.E. (1993). Direct detection of novel expanded trinucleotide repeats in the humone genome. *Nat. Genet.*, **4**, 135–9.

Schultz, J.B., Dehmer, T., Schols, L. et al. (2000). Oxidative stress in patients with Friedreich's ataxia. *Neurology*, **55**, 1719–21.

Servadio, A., Koshy, B., Armstrong, D., Antalfy, B., Orr, H.T. & Zoghbi, H.Y. (1995). Expression analysis of the ataxin-1 protein in tissues from normal and spinocerebellar ataxia type 1 individuals. *Nat. Genet.*, **19**, 94–8.

Sherman, S.L., Morton, N.E., Jacobs, P.A. & Turner, G. (1984). The marker (X) syndrome: a cytogenetic and genetic analysis. *Ann. Hum. Genet.*, **48**, 21–37.

Sherman, S.L., Jacobs, P.A., Morton, N.E. et al. (1985). Further segregation analysis of the fragile X syndrome with special reference to transmitting males. *Hum. Genet.*, **69**, 289–99.

Siomi, H., Siomi, M.C., Nussbaum, R.L. & Dreyfuss, G. (1993). The protein product of the fragile X gene, *FMR1*, has characteristics of an RNA-binding protein. *Cell*, **74**, 291–8.

Siomi, M.C., Siomi, H., Sauer, W.H., Srinivasan, S., Nussbaum, R.L.

& Dreyfuss, G. (1995). FXR1, an autosomal homolog of the fragile X mental retardation gene. *EMBO J.*, **14**, 2401–8.

Skinner, P.J., Koshy, B., Cummings, C. et al. (1997). Ataxin-1 with extra glutamines induces alterations in nuclear matrix-associated structures. *Nature*, **389**, 971–4.

Smith, J.K., Conda, V.E. & Malamud, N. (1958). Unusual form of cerebellar ataxia: combined dentato-rubral and pallido-Luysian degeneration. *Neurology*, **8**, 205–9.

Snow, K., Doud, L.K., Hagerman, R., Pergolizzi, R.G., Erster, S.H. & Thibodeau, S.N. (1993). Analysis of a CGG sequence at the FMR-1 locus in fragile X families and in the general population. *Am. J. Hum. Genet.*, **53**, 1217–28.

Snow, K., Tester, D.J., Kruckelberg, K.E., Schaid, D.J. & Thibodeau, S.N. (1994). Sequence analysis of the fragile X trinucleotide repeat: implications for the origin of the fragile X mutation. *Hum. Mol. Genet.*, **3**, 1543–51.

Sobue, G., Matsuoka, Y., Mukai, E., Takayanagi, T., Sobue, I. & Hashizume, Y. (1981). Spinal and cranial motor nerve roots in amyotrophic lateral sclerosis and X-linked recessive bulbospinal muscular atrophy: a morphometric and teased-fiber study. *Acta Neuropath.*, **55**, 227–35.

Sobue, G., Hashizume, Y., Mukai, E., Itsuma, T. & Takahashi, A. (1989). X-linked recessive bulbospinal neuronopathy: a clinicopathological study. *Brain*, **112**, 209–32.

Steffan, J.S., Kazantsev, A., Spasic-Boskovic, O. et al. (2000). The Huntington's disease protein interacts with p53 and CREB-binding protein and represses transcription. *Proc. Natl. Acad. Sci., USA*, **97**, 6763–8.

Steinbach, P., Glaser, D., Vogel, W., Wolf, M. & Schwemmle, S. (1998). The DMPK gene of severely affected myotonic dystrophy patients is hypermethylated proximal to the largely expanded CTG repeat. *Am. J. Hum. Genet.*, **62**, 278–85.

Stevanin, G., Herman, A., Durr, A. et al. (2000). Are $(CTG)_n$ expansions at the SCA8 locus rare polymorphisms? *Nat. Genet.*, **24**, 213.

Sutherland, GR. (1977). Fragile sites on human chromosomes: demonstration of their dependence on the type of tissue culture medium. *Science*, **197**, 265–6.

Takiyama, Y., Oyanagi, S., Kawashima, S. et al. (1993). The gene for Machado–Joseph disease maps to human chromosome 14q. *Nat. Genet.*, **4**, 300–4.

Taneja, K.L., McCurrach, M., Schalling, M., Housman, D. & Singer, R.H. (1995). Foci of trinucleotide repeat transcripts in nuclei of myotonic dystrophy cells and tissues. *J. Cell Biol.*, **128**, 995–1002.

Tautz, D. & Schlotterer, C. (1994). Simple sequences. *Curr. Opin. Genet Dev.*, **4**, 832–7.

Thornton, C.A., Griggs, R.C &, Moxley, R.T. (1994). Myotonic dystrophy with no trinucleotide repeat expansion. *Ann. Neurol.*, **35**, 269–72.

Thornton, C.A., Wymer, J.P., Simmons, Z., McClain, C. & Moxley, R.T. (1997). Expansion of the myotonic dystrophy CTG repeat reduces expression of the flanking DMAHP gene. *Nat. Genet.*, **16**, 407–9.

Timchenko, L.T., Timchenko, N.A., Caskey, C.T. & Roberts, R. (1996). Novel proteins with binding specificity for DNA CTG and RNA CUG repeats: implications for myotonic dystrophy. *Hum. Mol. Genet.*, **5**, 115–21.

Tishkoff, S.A., Goldman, A., Calafell, F. et al. (1998). A global haplotype analysis of the myotonic dystrophy locus: implications for the evolution of modern humans and for the origin of myotonic dystrophy mutations. *Am. J. Hum. Genet.*, **62**, 1389–402.

Tome, M.S. & Fardeau, M. (1980). Nuclear inclusions in oculopharyngeal dystrophy. *Acta Neuropathol.*, **49**, 85–7.

Tome, F.M.S. & Fardeau, M. (1994). Oculopharyngeal muscular dystrophy. In *Myology*, ed. A.G. Engel & C. Franzini-Armstrong, 2nd edn, Vol. 2, pp. 1233–45, New York: McGraw-Hill.

Tsilfidis, C., MacKenzie, A.E., Mettler, G., Barcelo, J. & Korneluk, R.G. (1992). Correlation between CTG trinucleotide repeat length and frequency of severe congenital myotonic dystrophy. *Nat. Genet.*, **1**, 192–5.

Van den Ouweland, A.M.W., Deelan, W.H., Kunst, C.B. et al. (1994). Correlation between CTG trinucleotide repeat length and frequency of severe congenital myotonic dystrophy. *Hum. Mol. Genet.*, **3**, 1823–7.

Verkerk, A.J., Pieretti, M., Sutcliffe, J.S. et al. (1991). Identification of a gene (FMR-1) containing a CGG repeat coincident with a breakpoint cluster region exhibiting length variation in fragile X syndrome. *Cell*, **65**, 905–14.

Victor, M., Hayes, R. & Adams, R.D. (1962). Oculopharyngeal muscular dystrophy. A familial disease of late life characterized by dysphagia and progressive ptosis of the eyelids. *N. Engl. J. Med.*, **267**, 1267–72.

Vincent, J.B., Neves-Pereira, M.L., Paterson, A.D. et al. (2000). An unstable trinucleotide-repeat region on chromosome 13 implication in spinocerebellar ataxia: a common expansion locus. *Am. J. Hum. Genet.*, **66**, 819–29.

Virtaneva, K., D'Amato, E., Miao, J. et al. (1997). Unstable minisatellite expansion causing recessively inherited myoclonus epilepsy, EPM1. *Nat. Genet.*, **15**, 393–6.

Waldvogel, D., van Gelderen, P. & Hallett, M. (1999). Increased iron in the dentate nucleus of patients with Friedreich's ataxia. *Ann. Neurol.*, **46**, 123–5.

Wang, J., Pegoraro, E., Menegazzo, E. et al. (1995). Myotonic dystrophy: evidence for a possible dominant-negative RNA mutation. *Hum. Mol. Genet.*, **4**, 599–606.

Warren, S.T. & Nelson, D.L. (1994). Advances in molecular analysis of fragile X syndrome. *J. Am. Med. Assoc.*, **271**, 536–42.

Wellington, C.L., Leavitt, B.R. & Hayden, M.R. (2000). Inhibiting caspase cleavage of huntingtin reduces toxicity and aggregate formation in neuronal and nonneuronal cells. *J. Biol. Chem.*, **275**, 19831–8.

Wells, R.D. (1996). Molecular basis of genetic instability of triplet repeats. *J. Biol. Chem.*, **271**, 2875–8.

Wilson, R.B. & Roof, D.M. (1997). Respiratory deficiency due to loss of mitochondrial DNA in yeast lacking the frataxin homologue. *Nat. Genet.*, **16**, 352–7.

Wohrle, D., Kotzot, D., Hirst, M.C. et al. (1992). A microdeletion of less than 250 kb, including the proximal part of FMR-1 gene and the fragile-X site, in a male with the clinical phenotype of fragile X syndrome. *Am. J. Hum. Genet.*, **51**, 299–306.

Wong, A., Yang, J., Cavadini, P. et al. (1999). The Friedreich's ataxia mutation confers cellular sensitivity to oxidant stress, which is rescued by chelators of iron and calcium and inhibitors of apoptosis. *Hum. Mol. Genet.*, **8**, 425–30.

Wood, R.D. (1996). DNA repair in eukaryotes. *Annu. Rev. Biochem.*, **65**, 135–67.

Worth, P.F., Houlden, H., Giunti, P., Davis, M.B. & Wood, N.W. (2000). Large, expanded repeats in *SCA8* are not confined to patients with cerebellar ataxia. *Nat. Genet.*, **24**, 214–15.

Yazawa, I., Nukina, N., Hashida, H., Goto, J., Yamada, M. & Kanazawa, I. (1995). Abnormal gene product identified in hereditary dentatorubral–pallidoluysian atrophy (DRPLA) brain. *Nat. Genet.*, **10**, 99–103.

Yu, S., Pritchard, M., Kremer, E. et al. (1991). Fragile X genotype characterized by an unstable region of DNA. *Science*, **252**, 1179–81.

Zhang, Y., O'Connor, J.P., Siomi, M.C. et al. (1995). The fragile X mental retardation syndrome protein interacts with novel homologs FXR1 an FXR2. *EMBO J.*, **14**, 5358–66.

Zhou, Z.X., Wong, C.I., Sar, M. & Wilson, E.M. (1994). The androgen receptor: an overview. *Recent Prog. Horm. Res.*, **49**, 249–74.

Zhuchenko, O., Bailey, J., Bonnen, P. et al. (1997). Autosomal dominant cerebellar ataxia (SCA6) associated with small polyglutamine expansions in the α_{1A}-voltage-dependent calcium channel. *Nat. Genet.*, **15**, 62–9.

Zoghbi, H.Y. (1997). CAG Repeats in SCA6: anticipating new clues. *Neurology*, **49**, 1196–9.

Zoghbi, H.Y. & Orr, H.T. (2000). Glutamine repeats and neurodegeneration. *Annu. Rev. Neurosci.*, **23**, 217–47.

Zoghbi, H.Y., Jodice, C., Sandkuijl, L.A. et al. (1991). The gene for autosomal dominant spinocerebellar ataxia (SCA1) maps telomeric to the HLA complex and is closely linked to the D6S89-locus in 3 large kindreds. *Am. J. Hum. Genet.*, **49**, 23–30.

Zu, L., Figueroa, K.P., Grewal, R. & Pulst, S.M. (1999). Mapping of a new autosomal dominant spinocerebellar ataxia to chromosome 22. *Am. J. Hum. Genet.*, **64**, 594–9.

4

Cell birth and cell death in the central nervous system

Samuel J. Pleasure[1] and David E. Pleasure[2]

[1] Department of Neurology, University of California, San Francisco, USA
[2] Children's Hospital of Philadelphia, USA

Formation of the neural tube and control of cell fate by dorsal–ventral signalling centres

One of the most remarkable features of mammalian neural development is the production of the complicated end product, the brain, spinal cord and peripheral nervous system, from a simple one-cell layer thick sheet of neuro-epithelial cells. The first step in this process is the formation and patterning of the neural tube through a process termed neural induction (Kandel et al., 2000). This involves the formation of a specialized region of columnar epithelium, called the neural plate, from the embryonic dorsal ectoderm. Soon after its formation the neural plate folds and becomes a tube (Fig. 4.1). In this process the most medial regions of the neural plate form the ventral neural tube and the more lateral regions of the neural plate form the dorsal neural tube. At the neural plate stage, signals from the mesoderm underlying it pattern the neural plate so that there are molecular differences between the rostral and caudal regions of the neural plate. Therefore, these early patterning events are fundamental to the later production of specialized regions and cells of the nervous system from the neural tube.

Neural induction is not completely understood at the molecular level but significant recent progress has been made (Harland, 2000). Current thinking is that the ectoderm at this stage of embryogenesis has a default neural fate except that the action of bone morphogenetic proteins (BMPs) and Wnts (a family of secreted glycoproteins similar to the *wingless* gene in *Drosophila*) expressed widely in the embryo suppress the acquisition of neural fate. Neural induction then occurs in the neural plate because of the release of soluble BMP and Wnt inhibitors from the underlying mesoderm. The inhibition of BMP and Wnt effects allows the default neural fate pathway to operate and the neural plate forms. The rostral–caudal patterning of the neural plate is further affected by the actions of molecules such as retinoic acid (which induces a caudal neural pattern).

After the neural tube forms, the rostral–caudal subdivisions (that will become the telencephalon, diencephalon, mesencephalon, metencephalon and spinal cord) become visible anatomically. At this stage, at each level from rostral to caudal, the fate of individual neural precursors begins to be controlled by dorsal and ventral signalling centres present in the neural tube called the roofplate and the floorplate, respectively. The roofplate produces a variety of molecules in the Wnt and BMP families, while the floorplate produces sonic hedgehog (SHH). There is now persuasive evidence that signaling by BMPs and Wnts regulates the proliferation, differentiation and migration of derivatives of the dorsal neural tube (Lee & Jessell, 1999). These include dorsal spinal interneurons and neural crest cells, which go on to generate the entire peripheral nervous system. Similarly, the differentiation of spinal motor neurons and ventral spinal interneurons is directly controlled by SHH secreted from the floorplate (Kandel et al., 2000). The roofplate and floorplate also secrete a host of other factors that regulate later events such as axon guidance decisions made by cells at all levels of the developing nervous system. Structures analogous to the roofplate and floorplate are present at rostral levels of the nervous system as well but their role in differentiation is much less completely understood in these more morphologically complex regions. Failure of the proper dorsal–ventral patterning events in the developing prosencephalon leads to major brain malformations such as holoprosencephaly. A number of hereditary cases of this syndrome have been linked to genes involved in dorsal–ventral patterning, including mutations in SHH itself (Wallis & Muenke, 2000). Cyclopamine, a teratogenic chemical, appears to cause holoprosencephaly by interfering with SHH signalling (Cooper et al., 1998).

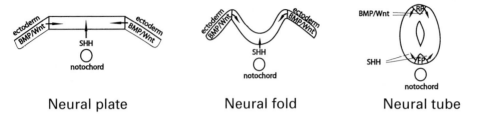

Neural plate   Neural fold   Neural tube

Fig. 4.1. Schematic diagram of the stages of formation of the neural tube from the neural plate. Initially the neuroectoderm is specified from the ectoderm and is a flat sheet of epithelial cells. It begins to fold and finally forms a tube. During this entire time the medial neural plate (which becomes the ventral neural tube) and the lateral neural plate (which becomes the dorsal neural tube) are patterned by secreted molecules. Abbreviations – SHH = sonic hedgehog, RP = roofplate; FP = floorplate.

Cellular and molecular correlates of neurogenesis and gliogenesis during development

Once the neural tube forms and the actions of the dorsal–ventral signalling centres have had their initial effects on the patterning of the neural tube, the process of cellular differentiation begins. Within the ventricular zone, mitotic multipotential cells begin to produce differentiated neuronal and glial cell types following a sequential programme. This process is best understood in the six-layered neocortex. Initially, mitotic stem cells undergo repeated cycles of so-called 'symmetric' cell divisions that yield two daughter cells with the same potential as the parent cell (Lu et al., 2000). These mitoses occur in a characteristic to-and-fro migratory pattern termed interkinetic migration. In this pattern stem cells have cellular processes that span the cortical wall from ventricular to pial surface, and their soma is in an intermediate position. As the stem cell prepares to divide, its cell body descends to the ventricular surface where mitosis occurs. At the appropriate stage of development for the production of differentiated neurons, neural stem cells begin to undergo 'asymmetric' cell divisions that yield a daughter cell that goes on to further differentiate and a daughter cell that remains a stem cell (Lu et al., 2000). The differentiated daughter cell then migrates radially into the cortical plate. As development goes on, progressively more cell divisions are asymmetric and waves of differentiated cells are produced, and less and less stem cells remain in the ventricular zone. Disorders such as tuberous sclerosis and focal cortical dysplasia may arise because of dysfunction in the processes regulating the decision whether to adopt a neuronal or glial fate within the ventricular zone (Walsh, 1999).

In the ventricular zone, neurons with particular laminar fates are produced in a characteristic 'inside-out' manner so that cells destined for the deeper cortical layers are born first and cells destined for superficial cortical layers are born later and migrate past the earlier born cells. The migrating of cells from the ventricular zone using radial glial cells as the scaffolding to reach their final laminar position in a so-called radial pattern of migration. Lissencephalies, periventricular nodular heterotopias and periventricular band heterotopias are all disorders of this process of radial migration and are caused by mutations in genes controlling various steps of migration (Walsh, 1999; Gleeson & Walsh, 2000).

The molecular regulation of the events occurring in the ventricular zone during this period is starting to be elucidated. The decisions made by neural stem cells are controlled in part by the actions of the Notch family of transmembrane receptors. These receptors interact with their ligands, the Delta and Jagged proteins, in a cell contact-dependent manner. Activation of the Notch receptor leads to a decision to remain an undifferentiated stem cell or to become a radial glial cell (Lu et al., 2000). Inhibition of Notch signalling occurs in part by the inheritance of a protein called Numb that is asymmetrically distributed between daughter cells of asymmetric cell divisions. Numb blocks the downstream effects of the Notch receptor and releases the cell to differentiate into a neuron (Lu et al., 2000).

The differentiation of glial progenitors to mature oligodendroglia and astroglia in the developing CNS is also subject to extrinsic regulation. Basic fibroblast growth factor (bFGF) inhibits maturation of glial progenitors to either oligodendroglia or astroglia (McKinnon et al., 1990; Grinspan et al., 2000). Platelet-derived growth factor-alpha (PDGFα) drives recruitment into the oligodendroglial lineage (Fruttiger et al, 1999), whereas the BMPs enhance differentiation of glial progenitors to glial fibrillary acidic protein (GFAP) positive astroglia (Grinspan et al., 2000).

Apoptosis during normal brain development

Immature animals remodel CNS and other tissues by apoptotic removal of redundant cells. Morphological features of apoptosis include nuclear fragmentation, cell shrinkage, membrane blebbing, and phagocytosis by macrophages. Apoptosis is triggered by activation of target cell plasma membrane death receptors (e.g. CD95, the tumor necrosis factor (TNF) receptors, and the low affinity neurotrophin receptor, p75NTR), by unsuccessful competition of the target cell for critical survival factors, or by inability of the target cell to establish and maintain contact with critical extracellular matrix constituents ('anoikis') (Savill & Fadok, 2000; Meier et al., 2000).

A superfamily of cysteine proteases, the caspases, are responsible for apoptotic execution. These proteins are synthesized as procaspases, which require proteolytic clipping in order to activate their catalytic sites. This activation can be initiated by their aggregation with a plasma membrane death receptor or with proteins (cytochrome c and Apaf-1) released through mitochondrial membrane pores. Once begun, a chain reaction of proteolytic caspase activation follows. The caspases cleave target proteins at aspartate residues. In some instances, this cleavage results in protein activation (e.g. other members of the caspase family, and interleukin-1). More commonly, the target protein (e.g. gelsolin, and an inhibitor of a nuclease capable of intranuclear double-stranded DNA nicking) is inactivated. Together, these proteolytic events are responsible for the DNA nicking and cytoplasmic and plasma membrane remodelling that characterize apoptosis, and culminate in cell digestion by macrophages (Hengartner, 2000).

The Bcl-2 family of proteins modulate caspase activation. Pro-apoptotic members of this family (e.g. Bax and Bak) facilitate release of cytochrome c and Apaf-1 from target cell mitochondria, whereas anti-apoptotic members (e.g. Bcl-2 and Bcl-x_L) inhibit this release. Expression of this Bcl-2 family of proteins is developmentally regulated in the CNS (Kelekar & Thompson, 1998; Hengarter, 2000).

Apoptosis is prominent in both neuronal and macroglial lineages in the CNS. In the cat retina, for example, more than 80% of the ganglion cells do not survive long after birth (Meier et al., 2000), and more than 50% of the late oligodendroglial progenitors formed in perinatal rat optic nerve do not survive to maturity (Barres & Raff, 1994). This apoptotic culling of neural cells unable to obtain the survival factors they require provides a powerful and precise means by which normal CNS tissue structure and function can be ensured. An illuminating example of this is provided by examination of transgenic mice that overexpress PDGF$_{AA}$ in CNS. PDGF$_{AA}$ is a growth factor for oligodendroglial progenitors, and these mice accumulate many more oligodendroglial progenitors in the perinatal period than do their normal littermates. Yet, as these transgenic mice mature, the numbers of oligodendroglia and their levels of myelination in the CNS are normal (Calver et al., 1998). Conversely, in mice in which CNS apoptosis is prevented by knocking out caspase-9 or caspase-3, there are ectopic accumulations of supernumerary neurons (Yuan & Yankner, 2000).

Neurogenesis in the normal adult brain

Up to this point only the mechanisms of developmental production of cells have been discussed. It has been known for many years that continued production of glial cells occurs in the adult brain. Most of these are thought to be generated from the striatal and cortical subventricular zones. What has been less widely appreciated, although also well established in the 1960s, is that there is continued production of neurons in the adult brain of mammals in two locations, the dentate gyrus and olfactory bulb (Gage, 2000).

In the dentate gyrus of the hippocampal formation there is a layer of mitotically active cells at the border of the hilus and dentate granule cell layers that has been proven to produce new neurons throughout life in both rodents and primates (Gage, 2000) (Fig. 4.2). The function of the newly born granule cells is unknown, but it is known that at least some of these cells extend axons that integrate into the normal circuitry of the hippocampus. Recent studies have shown that environmental stimuli, including visuospatial learning and physical activity, can have substantial effects on the birth and survival of new dentate granule cells in adult rodents (Kempermann et al., 1997a; Gould et al., 1999a, b; van Praag et al., 1999). Also, there is an age-related decrease in the production of new neurons in the dentate gyrus (Kuhn et al., 1996).

The phenomenon of dentate granule neurogenesis in the adult is being intensively studied since it is a paradigm for the regulation of new neuron production in adult mammals. Many studies have addressed exogenous influences that regulate the rate of proliferation of granule cell precursors, and have shown that granule cell neurogenesis is inhibited by excess glucocorticoids and by excitotoxins (Cameron & Gould, 1994; Cameron et al., 1995). A particularly interesting set of studies has characterized the balance of cell production and granule cell number in inbred strains of mice. These studies demonstrated that various inbred strains of mice may have a low or high basal

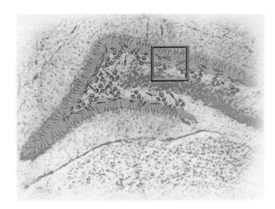

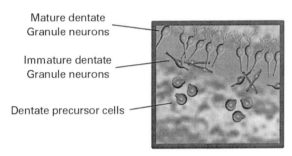

Mature dentate
Granule neurons

Immature dentate
Granule neurons

Dentate precursor cells

Fig. 4.2. Schematic diagram showing the organization of neurogenesis in the adult dentate gyrus. Mitotic dentate precursor cells are located in the zone just under the granule cell layer. Newborn immature cells are at the inner border and more mature granule cells are in the outer domains of the granule cell layer. (Artwork by Erin Browne.)

rate of new granule cell production (Kempermann et al., 1997b). Some strains have basal rates of granule cell death that match the production of granule cells very closely, while others have a lower rate of death leading to an increasing number of granule neurons as the animals mature (Kempermann et al., 1997b).

The granule and periglomerular interneurons of the olfactory bulb are also produced in adult mammals. These cells are generated in a small region of the anterior subventricular zone. They reach the olfactory bulb by migrating long distances in a direction tangential to the radial migration seen during development (Gage, 2000). Once in the bulb, they appose themselves to radial glial-like cells and migrate radially to take up their final position. What functional role the production of new neurons has in the olfactory bulb is currently unknown. In non-human primates, a recent controversial study demonstrated ongoing neurogenesis from the subventricular zone of neurons that migrated to association areas of neocortex (Gould et al., 1999b). This type of adult neurogenesis has never been seen in rodents and thus may be a primate specialization. Again, the function of these new cells is unknown presently

but, if this type of neurogenesis is ongoing in humans, it may have important implications for plasticity of higher cortical functions.

Neurogenesis and gliogenesis in pathologic states

The production of neurons from the dentate subgranular zone and the subventricular zone in the adult nervous system of rodents has been studied in a number of pathologic contexts. The most extensively studied of these is following status epilepticus (Bengzon et al., 1997; Parent et al., 1997). In rodent models of status epilepticus following systemic administration of pilocarpine or kainic acid, there is a dramatic up-regulation of granule cell neurogenesis starting several days after the prolonged seizure and continuing for about 2 weeks. Similar increases in neurogenesis have been seen in the dentate gyrus following transient global ischemia in gerbils (Liu et al., 1998). The functional significance of this response is unclear, but there is some reason to believe that the increased neurogenesis is somehow coupled to increased cell death of granule cells following the same insults (Bengzon et al., 1997). If there is a mechanism for linking the birth of new neurons in the dentate gyrus to cell death, it may also be possible to activate this mechanism in other brain regions that suffer extensive cell death in response to pathologic stimuli like excitotoxicity or neurodegenerative processes. This might serve as a basis for novel therapeutic strategies to help repair the effects of these pathologic insults.

Focal traumatic lesions in the cortex have been shown to up-regulate the rate of proliferation of astrocyte precursors in the subventricular zone. It is possible that this represents the main source of cells contributing to gliosis in the cortex following focal or diffuse injuries (Szele & Chesselet, 1996). In the subventricular zone, increased cell birth of cells with properties of glial cells has been demonstrated in response to experimental allergic encephalomyelitis (Calza et al., 1998). Oligodendroglial progenitors are also identifiable in chronic multiple sclerosis plaques, but often have exited the mitotic cycle (Wolswijk, 1998). Treatment strategies need to be developed that enhance proliferation of these progenitors, and their differentiation to myelin-forming oligodendroglia.

Apoptosis and necrosis in pathologic states

The death of neurons and macroglia caused by deprivation of oxygen and glucose (e.g. in an ischemic infarction) occurs by two apparently distinct mechanisms. Where oxygen/glucose deprivation is most severe, ATP generation is blocked, and the cells lose the capacity to regulate intracellular Ca^{2+} and Na^+ concentrations. Cell necrosis results, characterized by perikaryal swelling, loss of plasma membrane integrity, and cell fragmentation. Ionotropic glutamate receptors (GluR), activated by increased extracellular glutamate concentrations, are of central importance in the pathophysiology of ischemic necrosis of neurons and oligodendroglia, and inhibitors of these GluR minimize the extent of ischemic necrosis (Dugan & Choi, 1999). Where oxygen/glucose deprivation is less severe (e.g. in the 'ischemic penumbra'), neurons and macroglia die by apoptosis, and can be rescued by caspase inhibitors (Yuan & Yankner, 2000).

The contribution of apoptosis to neural cell loss in chronic neurological diseases is less clearcut. While cells undergoing apoptosis are common in active multiple sclerosis plaques, most are lymphocytes rather than cells of the oligodendroglial lineage (Bonetti & Raine, 1997). In respect of Alzheimer's disease, amyloid-β can activate neuronal caspases, but most degenerating neurons in this disorder do not show apoptotic features. In mice expressing the human mutant superoxide dismutase-1 gene that causes a familial form of amyotrophic lateral sclerosis (ALS), inhibition of caspase-1 or overexpression of Bcl-2 delays disease progression, and caspase inhibition also delays disease progression in a transgenic model of human Huntington's disease, but neuronal apoptosis is difficult to demonstrate morphologically in these mouse models (Yuan & Yankner, 2000)

Stem cells in the adult brain

The existence of neurogenesis and gliogenesis in the subventricular zone and dentate gyrus of adult animals implies that there must be precursors for these cells (Gage, 2000). The usual terminology applied to progenitor cells for neurons and glia divides them into stem cells and committed precursor cells. A stem cell is multipotential and capable of numerous self-renewing mitoses. A committed precursor cell will be limited to one or a small number of ultimate fates and has a limited capacity for self-renewal. The clear presence of neurogenesis and gliogenesis and the in situ and in vitro demonstration of dividing precursor cells have led to the search for the elusive multipotential neural stem cells that are assumed to be present in the adult nervous system.

In the early 1990s, several cell culture systems that are capable of maintaining multipotential (cells capable of making neurons and glia) stem cells were described. Following these initial studies, there have been a great number of studies that have demonstrated the properties of these cells and their requirements for trophic factors and mitotic factors (such as basic FGF and epidermal growth factor (EGF)) to be maintained in culture (Gage, 2000). Other studies have demonstrated that treating these cultures with factors like retinoic acid can force these cells into producing neurons, while serum and ciliary neurotrophic factor (CNTF) induce the cells to become astrocytes (Gage, 2000). The use of these culture systems has demonstrated that there are quiescent stem cells in all regions of the nervous system rather that just in the areas known to produce new neurons (Gage, 2000). Are these cells placed in a distributed manner in order to produce new glial cells in areas away from the germinative zones? Are there ways to induce them to become neurons in situ and replace neurons killed or injured by pathologic insults?

The scientific question of the location and identity of the neural stem cells in vivo has recently been addressed. Several laboratories have reported that either the ependymal cells lining the adult ventricles or astrocyte-like glial cells adjacent to them are likely to be the in vivo stem cells responsible for the production of olfactory interneurons and glial cells in the adult subventricular zone (Doetsch et al., 1999; Johansson et al., 1999). The relationship of these two populations of stem cells to each other (e.g. are they transitional forms of the same population?), and their relationship to the multipotential cells in the dentate gyrus and elsewhere in the CNS are unknown.

Until recently it was believed that neural stem cells were capable of producing exclusively neurons and glia. Recent exciting experiments have shown that this view may be too limited. In one set of studies, investigators transplanted mouse neural stem cells that were marked with an enzymatic tag to other mice whose bone marrow had been destroyed by irradiation. In these mice, amazingly, the neural stem cells were able to generate hematopoetic stem cells that populated the bone marrow and produced differentiated blood elements and immune cells that expressed the enzymatic tag (Bjornson et al., 1999). Another, even more startling result was obtained when neural stem cells were injected into mouse blastocysts and were able to contribute differentiated cells to all three germ layers of the developing embryo, albeit less efficiently than true embryonic stem cells (Clarke et al., 2000). These experiments blur the distinctions between neural stem cells and other stem cells in the body and perhaps imply that the immediate molecular milieu may be as important as any developmental history in contributing to the multipotentiality of stem cells.

Therapeutic approaches based on neurogenesis

How can we utilize the new understanding of neurogenesis and gliogenesis in the nervous system to treat neurological diseases? One approach is to generate cells for therapeutic purposes in vitro and transplant them into the diseased host (Bjorklund & Lindvall, 2000a). The other approach is to attempt to harness the regenerative capacity of the nervous system to facilitate functional recovery from insults (Lowenstein & Parent, 1999; Bjorklund & Lindvall, 2000b). In the future it is likely that both approaches will be useful.

The approaches that are based on the in vitro production of neural cells are being investigated most intensively for the treatment of Parkinson's disease, Huntington's disease, stroke and epilepsy (Bjorklund & Lindvall, 2000a). In each of these cases the approach depends on the ability to culture pure populations of the appropriate neurons from identified sources. The sources being investigated include xenografts from porcine sources, expanded human neural stem cells, human bone marrow stromal stem cells, and immortalized human cell lines (Bjorklund & Lindvall, 2000a). Each of these sources has its own perils and promises. Xenotransplants may have a higher potential for rejection or infection with zoonotic organisms. Expanded human neural stem cells are still incapable of producing sufficient quantities of pure cells to meet clinical needs. All immortalized cell lines have the potential to lead to neoplasm. The next 10 years will almost certainly lead to solutions to these problems and will allow the clinical efficacy of these treatments to be tested.

The potential for harnessing the native regenerative capacity of the nervous system is perhaps the most exciting future possibility. A recent series of experiments utilizing a clever technique to deliver focal cell type specific injury to the nervous system has emphasized the heretofore unrecognized ability of the nervous system to replace certain types of cells (Snyder et al., 1997). This technique allows the selective photoablation of cells in the cortex in a layer specific manner. These experiments reveal that, after the selective ablation of cortical pyramidal neurons, the rodent brain is capable of using endogenous precursors to replace these cells, despite the fact that these cells are never normally produced in the adult animal (Magavi et al., 2000). If we can understand the cues that regulate these events then these signals may allow regulatable repairs to be performed in the nervous system (Lowenstein & Parent, 1999; Bjorklund & Lindvall, 2000b).

References   * denotes key references

Barres, B.A. & Raff, M.C. (1994). Control of oligodendrocyte number in the developing rat optic nerve. *Neuron*, **12**, 935–42.

Bengzon, J., Kokaia, Z., Elmer, E. et al. (1997). Apoptosis and proliferation of dentate gyrus neurons after single and intermittent limbic seizures. *Proc. Natl. Acad. Sci., USA*, **94**, 10432–7.

*Bjorklund, A. & Lindvall, O. (2000a). Cell replacement therapies for central nervous system disorders. *Nat. Neurosci.*, **3**, 537–44.

*Bjorklund, A. & Lindvall, O. (2000b). Self-repair in the brain. *Nature*, **405**, 892–5.

Bjornson, C.R., Rietze, R.L., Reynolds, B.A. et al. (1999). Turning brain into blood: a hematopoietic fate adopted by adult neural stem cells in vivo. *Science*, **283**, 534–7.

Bonetti, B. & Raine, C.S. (1997). Multiple sclerosis: oligodendrocytes display cell death-related molecules in situ but do not undergo apoptosis. *Ann. Neurol.*, **42**, 74–84.

Calver A.R., Hall, A.C., Yu, W.P. et al. (1998). Oligodendrocyte population dynamics and the role of PDGF in vivo. *Neuron*, **20**, 869–82.

Calza, L., Giardino, L., Pozza, M. et al. (1998). Proliferation and phenotype regulation in the subventricular zone during experimental allergic encephalomyelitis: in vivo evidence of a role for nerve growth factor. *Proc. Natl. Acad. Sci., USA*, **95**, 3209–14.

Cameron, H.A. & Gould, E. (1994). Adult neurogenesis is regulated by adrenal steroids in the dentate gyrus. *Neuroscience*, **61**, 203–9.

Cameron, H.A., McEwen, B.S. & Gould, E. (1995). Regulation of adult neurogenesis by excitatory input and NMDA receptor activation in the dentate gyrus. *J. Neurosci.*, **15**, 4687–92.

*Clarke, D.L., Johansson, C.B., Wilbertz, J. et al. (2000). Generalized potential of adult neural stem cells. *Science*, **288**, 1660–3.

Cooper, M.K., Porter, J.A., Young, K.E. & Beachy, P.A. (1998). Teratogen-mediated inhibition of target tissue response to Shh signaling. *Science*, **280**, 1603–7.

Doetsch, F., Caille, I., Lim, D.A. et al. (1999). Subventricular zone astrocytes are neural stem cells in the adult mammalian brain. *Cell*, **97**, 703–16.

Dugan, L.L. & Choi, D.W. (1999). Hypoxic–ischemic brain injury and oxidative stress. In *Basic Neurochemistry: Molecular, Cellular and Medical Aspects*, 6th edn, G.J. Siegel et al., eds, Chapter 34, pp. 711–29. Lippincott-Raven Publishers.

*Gage, F.H. (2000). Mammalian neural stem cells. *Science*, **287**, 1433–8.

*Gleeson, J.G. & Walsh, C.A. (2000). Neuronal migration disorders: from genetic diseases to developmental mechanisms. *Trends Neurosci.*, **23**, 352–9.

Gould, E., Beylin, A., Tanapat, P. et al. (1999a). Learning enhances adult neurogenesis in the hippocampal formation. *Nat. Neurosci.*, **2**, 260–5.

Gould, E., Reeves, A.J., Garziano, M.S. & Gross, C.G. (1999b). Neurogenesis in the neocortex of adult primates. *Science*, **286**, 548–52.

Grinspan, J.B., Edell, E., Carpio, D.F. et al. (2000). Stage-specific effects of bone morphogenetic proteins on the oligodendroglial lineage. *J. Neurobiol.*, **43**, 1–17.

Harland, R. (2000). Neural induction. *Curr. Opin. Genet. Dev.*, **10**, 357–62.

*Hengartner M.O. (2000). The biochemistry of apoptosis. *Nature*, **407**, 770–6.

Johansson, C.B., Momma, S., Clarke, D.L. et al. (1999). Identification of a neural stem cell in the adult mammalian central nervous system. *Cell*, **96**, 25–34.

Kandel, E., Schwartz, J.H. et al. (2000). *Principles of Neural Science*, 4th edn, Chapter 52, The induction and patterning of the nervous system, pp. 1019–40.

Kelekar, A. & Thompson, C.B. (1998). Bcl-2-family proteins: the role of the BH3 domain in apoptosis. *Trends in Cell Biol.*, **8**, 324–30.

Kempermann, G., Kuhn, H.G. & Gage, F.H. (1997a). Genetic influence on neurogenesis in the dentate gyrus of adult mice. *Proc. Natl. Acad. Sci., USA*, **94**, 10409–14.

*Kempermann, G., Kuhn, H.G. & Gage, F.H. (1997b). More hippocampal neurons in adult mice living in an enriched environment. *Nature*, **386**, 493–5.

Kuhn, H.G., Dickinson-Anson, H. & Gage, F.H. (1996). Neurogenesis in the dentate gyrus of the adult rat: age-related decrease of neuronal progenitor proliferation. *J. Neurosci.*, **16**, 2027–33.

Lee, K.J. & Jessell, T.M. (1999). The specification of dorsal cell fates in the vertebrate central nervous system. *Ann. Rev. Neurosci.*, **22**, 261–94.

Liu, J., Solway, K., Messing, R.O. et al. (1998). Increased neurogenesis in the dentate gyrus after transient global ischemia in gerbils. *J. Neurosci.*, **18**, 7768–78.

*Lowenstein, D.H. & Parent, J.M. (1999). Brain, heal thyself. *Science*, **283**, 1126–7.

Lu, B., Jan, L. & Jan, Y.N. (2000). Control of cell divisions in the nervous system: symmetry and asymmetry. *Ann. Rev. Neurosci.*, **23**, 531–56.

McKinnon R., Matsui, T., Dubois-Dalcq, M. & Aaronson, S.A. (1990). FGF modulates the PDGF-driven pathway of oligodendrocyte development. *Neuron*, **5**, 603–14.

*Magavi, S.S., Leavitt, B.R. & Macklis, J.D. (2000). Induction of neurogenesis in the neocortex of adult mice. *Nature*, **405**, 951–5.

*Meier P, Finch, A. & Evan, G. (2000). Apoptosis in development. *Nature*, **407**, 796–801.

Parent, J.M., Yu, T.W., Leibowitz, R.T. et al. (1997). Dentate granule cell neurogenesis is increased by seizures and contributes to aberrant network reorganization in the adult rat hippocampus. *J. Neurosci.*, **17**, 3727–38.

*Savill, J. & Fadok, V. (2000). Corpse clearance defines the meaning of cell death. *Nature*, **407**, 784–8.

Snyder, E.Y., Yoon, C., Flax, J.D. & Macklis, J.D. (1997). Multipotent neural precursors can differentiate toward replacement of neurons undergoing targeted apoptotic degeneration in adult mouse neocortex. *Proc. Natl. Acad. Sci., USA*, **94**, 11663–8.

Szele, F.G. & Chesselet, M.F. (1996). Cortical lesions induce an increase in cell number and PSA–NCAM expression in the subventricular zone of adult rats. *J. Comp. Neurol.*, **368**, 439–54.

van Praag, H., Kempermann, G. & Gage, F.H. (1999). Running increases cell proliferation and neurogenesis in the adult mouse dentate gyrus. *Nat. Neurosci.*, **2**, 266–70

*Wallis, D. & Muenke, M. (2000). Mutations in holoprosencephaly. *Hum. Mutat.*, **16**, 99–108.

*Walsh, C.A. (1999). Genetic malformations of the human cerebral cortex. *Neuron*, **23**, 19–29.

Wolswijk, G. (1998). Chronic stage multiple sclerosis lesions contain a relatively quiescent population of oligodendrocyte precursor cells. *J. Neurosci.*, **18**, 601–9.

*Yuan, J. & Yankner, B.A. (2000). Apoptosis in the nervous system. *Nature*, **407**, 802–9.

5

Neuroprotection in cerebral ischemia

Jin-Moo Lee[1] and Dennis W. Choi[2]

[1] Washington University School of Medicine, St Louis, MO, USA
[2] Department of Neurosciences, Merck Research Laboratories, West Point, PA, USA

Ischemic stroke is a consequence of transient or permanent reduction of blood flow to a focal region of the brain, usually caused by the occlusion of an artery by an embolus or thrombus. Cerebral ischemia may also occur globally in the setting of cardiac arrest and resuscitation. While historically brain damage has been considered to be an inexorable consequence of focal or global ischemic insults, in recent years a growing understanding of the underlying mechanisms responsible for brain cell death has led to the identification of new therapeutic approaches. Two main approaches have emerged. The first aims to restore lost blood flow by dissolving the thrombus responsible for cerebral artery obstruction (in ischemic stroke). Thrombolysis has become an established treatment for ischemic stroke after the efficacy of intravenous tissue plasminogen activator (tPA) was demonstrated in a landmark study (The NINDS rt-PA Stroke Study Group, 1995). Promising results have also been reported for the thrombolytic agent pro-urokinase, delivered by intra-arterial catheter directly to the site of intravascular thrombus (Furlan et al., 1999). The second approach, neuroprotection, aims to reduce the intrinsic vulnerability of brain tissue to ischemia; it will be the topic of this chapter.

Mechanisms of ischemic neuronal death

The brain is more vulnerable to ischemia than many other tissues, so it seems plausible that the cellular mechanisms of this heightened vulnerability could be delineated and blocked. Over the last 15 years evidence has accumulated indicating that normal brain signaling and immune defense mechanisms may become harmful after ischemic insults (Rothman & Olney, 1986; Choi, 1988; del Zoppo et al., 2000). In particular, substantial evidence now implicates excitotoxicity, programmed cell death, and inflammation in the pathogenesis of ischemic neuronal death.

Excitotoxicity

The excitatory transmitter glutamate normally mediates most fast synaptic transmission throughout the CNS, but it also has a surprising ability to trigger central neuronal death upon prolonged exposure, a phenomenon called 'excitotoxicity' by Olney (1969). Excitotoxicity now appears to be involved in the pathogenesis of several CNS diseases including ischemic brain injury (Rothman & Olney, 1986; Choi, 1988). Under ischemic conditions, neurons deprived of oxygen and glucose rapidly lose ATP and become depolarized, leading to abnormally high levels of glutamate release (initially mediated by vesicular release from nerve terminals, and later by reverse transport from astrocytes). Once in the extracellular space, glutamate activates three major families of ionophore-linked receptors identified by their preferred agonists: N-methyl-D-aspartate (NMDA) alpha-amino-3-hydroxy-5-methyl-4-isoxazolepropionic acid (AMPA) and kainate. The channels gated by all three receptors subtypes are permeable to both Na^+ and K^+. Channels gated by NMDA receptors, but only a small number of channels gated by AMPA or kainate receptors (see below), additionally possess high permeability to Ca^{2+}. Marked neuronal cell body and dendrite swelling occur, as Na^+ and Ca^{2+} enters the cell joined by the influx of Cl^- and water. Excessive Ca^{2+} influx mediated predominately by NMDA receptors (but also triggered secondarily by Na^+ influx through AMPA-, kainate-, and NMDA-receptor-gated channels via activation of voltage-gated Ca^{2+} channels and reverse operation of the Na^+/Ca^{2+} exchanger), leads to elevated intracellular free Ca^{2+} concentrations and lethal metabolic derangements (Choi, 1988; Kim et al., 2001).

In neuronal cultures, selective NMDA-receptor blockade prevents most of the Ca^{2+} influx and cell death induced by brief intense glutamate exposures, and also markedly attenuates the death of cultured neurons subjected to oxygen and/or glucose deprivation. These observations are consistent with studies conducted with selective agonists: exposure to NMDA for as little as 3–5 minutes triggers widespread necrosis of cultured cortical neurons ('rapidly triggered excitotoxicity'), whereas exposure to high concentrations of kainate typically requires hours to do the same ('slowly triggered excitotoxicity'). NMDA antagonists are also highly neuroprotective in animal models of focal brain ischemia (Albers et al., 1992), but not consistently in models of transient global ischemia (Buchan, 1990).

Profoundly elevated intracellular Ca^{2+} concentrations, resulting from ischemia and excitotoxicity, are thought to initiate many potentially lethal derangements in cellular processes. Work in recent years has assigned particular responsibility for ensuing cellular death to the Ca^{2+}-dependent activation of catabolic enzymes, generation of free radicals including nitric oxide (NO), impairment of mitochondrial function, and excessive utilization of energy by the DNA repair enzyme poly(ADP–ribose) polymerase (PARP) (see below).

Ca^{2+} may not be the only divalent cation whose excessive entry mediates excitotoxic neuronal death after ischemic insults. The excessive influx of Mg^{2+} through NMDA–receptor-gated channels and its toxic intracellular accumulation has been proposed as a potential component of excitotoxic injury (Hartnett et al., 1997). Furthermore, growing evidence suggests that glutamate receptor overactivation may promote the toxicity of neurotransmitter Zn^{2+} (Choi & Koh, 1998). Zn^{2+} is concentrated in synaptic vesicles at excitatory terminals throughout the forebrain and is released upon neuronal stimulation; it can alter the behaviour of several transmitter receptors and voltage-gated channels, including the NMDA receptor (Frederickson, 1989). Cell culture experiments showed that exposure to concentrations of extracellular Zn^{2+} plausibly attained in the ischemic brain could kill central neurons, especially if the neurons were depolarized. Subsequent studies have indicated that the first step in Zn^{2+}-mediated neuronal death, like Ca^{2+}-mediated neuronal death, is excess entry across the plasma membrane, facilitated by membrane depolarization and consequently enhanced influx through several routes, in particular, voltage-gated Ca^{2+} channels (see below). The idea that Zn^{2+} neurotoxicity might contribute specifically to ischemic brain damage was raised by Tonder et al. (1990), who showed that transient global ischemia in rats was associated with depletion of Zn^{2+} from hippocampal mossy fibres, and the abnormal appearance of Zn^{2+} in the cell bodies of degenerating target CA3 or hilar neurons (dubbed 'zinc translocation', Frederickson et al., 1989). This idea was strengthened by the observation that Zn^{2+} translocated into selectively vulnerable postsynaptic neuronal cell bodies throughout the forebrain, and did so prior to neuronal degeneration. Furthermore, intracerebroventricular injection of the membrane-impermeant chelator CaEDTA (EDTA saturated with equimolar Ca^{2+}, so that it does not affect extracellular Ca^{2+} or Mg^{2+} but still avidly binds Zn^{2+}) before transient global ischemia in rats markedly reduced Zn^{2+} translocation into selectively vulnerable neurons throughout the hippocampus, cortex, thalamus and amygdala, and also reduced the delayed death of these neurons (Koh et al., 1996).

Recently, the idea that toxic Zn^{2+} originates primarily from synaptic vesicles has been challenged by intriguing observations suggesting that Zn^{2+}-mediated neuronal death may still occur after kainate-induced seizures in Zn^{2+} transporter 3 gene (*znt-3*)-null mice, which lack histochemically reactive vesicular Zn^{2+} in nerve terminals (Lee et al., 2000; Cole et al., 1999). These observations raise the possibility that at least some of the toxic Zn^{2+} may originate from intracellular sources, perhaps released from protein binding sites by oxidative stress (Aizenman et al., 2000).

The morphology of cells dying after intense glutamate receptor overactivation and Ca^{2+} and/or Zn^{2+} influx typically has characteristics of necrosis, a fulminant form of cell death associated with failure of the plasma membrane and swelling of both the cell and internal organelles. However, milder levels of toxic glutamate receptor stimulation on cells with preserved energy metabolism may lead to an alternative, more orderly death: apoptosis (Ankarcrona et al., 1995).

Apoptosis

Cerebral ischemia seems an obvious example of a violent 'environmental perturbation' capable of producing necrosis; however, growing evidence indicates that many brain cells undergo apoptosis after ischemic insults (Choi, 1996; Dirnagl et al., 1999). Apoptosis is the end result of a genetically regulated program that induces cells to die in an 'altruistic' fashion, with minimal release of genetic material and other proinflammatory intracellular constituents (Kondo, 1988). In normal physiological settings such as during development, apoptosis has a characteristic morphological appearance, featuring chromatin condensation and aggregation to the nuclear margin, cell and internal organelle shrinkage, and fragmentation of the nucleus and cytoplasm into membrane-bound vesicles (apoptotic bodies, Kerr et al., 1972). In the past, it has been characterized biochemically by internucleosomal fragmentation of genomic DNA in 185–200 base pair intervals, resulting in 'DNA laddering' detected on agarose gel electrophoresis, or by TdT-mediated biotinylated dUTP nick end-labeling (TUNEL) of nuclei. It is now becoming clear that DNA fragmentation and TUNEL of nuclei also occurs in cells undergoing necrosis, and thus cannot be the sole criterion for identifying apoptosis.

Recent investigations have yielded insights into the molecular mechanisms underlying programmed cell death. It is now apparent that this process is under tight regulatory control at several checkpoints. One checkpoint occurs on the outer membrane of mitochondria and is regulated by a group of proteins belonging to the bcl-2 family, composed of three groups based on structural and functional similarities. Members of group 1 (including bcl-2 and bcl-x_L) which share four conserved bcl-2 homology domains (BH) BH1–4 and a C-terminal hydrophobic tail (anchoring the protein to the outer mitochondrial membrane), are anti-apoptotic, whereas members of group 2 (including bax and bak), which contain BH1–3 and the hydrophobic tail, are proapoptotic. Members of group 3, which share only the BH3 domain, are pro-apoptotic and include bid and bik (Adams & Cory, 1998). Through a process that is currently poorly understood, pro- and anti-apoptotic members of the bcl-2 family interact on the outer mitochondrial membrane to regulate the release of the electron carrier cytochrome c from the intramembranous compartment (Jurgensmeier et al., 1998). Once in the cytoplasm, cytochrome c binds with another apoptosis regulator, Apaf-1, and dATP to form part of the 'apoptosome' (Cecconi, 1999), which activates the effector arm of programmed cell death carried out by a class of cysteine proteases, termed caspases. Caspases can also be activated by cell surface death receptors such as TNF receptors via caspase-8 (see below). Evidence is also emerging for a caspase-independent pathway of mammalian cell apoptosis, mediated by the mitochondrial release of apoptosis-inducing factor (Joza et al., 2001).

Highly conserved through evolution, more than a dozen caspases have been identified; a majority appear to participate in apoptosis, while others are responsible for the proteolytic activation of proinflammatory cytokines. Caspases are activated by proteolytic cleavage at caspase recognition sites. Thus, activation can occur autocatalytically, or through proteolysis by another caspase family member (Thornberry & Lazebnik, 1998). The apoptosome complex provides the initial stimulus for the autocatalytic activation of apical caspase-9, which subsequently cleaves and activates other downstream caspases including caspase-3, -6, and -7; these in turn cleave several proteins vital to survival (Slee et al., 1999). For example, caspase-3-mediated cleavage of the inhibitory subunit of caspase-activated DNase (CAD) results in internucleosomal DNA cleavage and 'DNA laddering' (Nagata, 2000). In addition, cleavage of nuclear lamins results in nuclear shrinking and budding (Buendia et al., 1999), and cleavage of cytoskeletal proteins such as fodrin and gelsolin result in loss of overall cell shape (Kothakota et al., 1997), characteristic of apoptotic cellular morphology.

Potassium efflux and resultant cell shrinkage may also play an important role in apoptosis. It is well established that raising extracellular K^+ inhibits neuronal apoptosis in vitro, an observation attributed historically to the activation of voltage-gated Ca^{2+} channels (Johnson & Deckwerth, 1993). However, the protective effect of raising extracellular K^+ against cortical neuronal apoptosis induced by staurosporine or serum deprivation was not eliminated by blocking voltage gate Ca^{2+} channels and associated increases in intracellular Ca^{2+} concentrations (Yu et al., 1997). Furthermore, these forms of neuronal apoptosis were associated with an early enhancement of the delayed rectifier current I_K, and depletion of cellular K^+ content; and blocking I_K with tetraethylammonium (TEA) attenuated subsequent neurodegeneration (Yu et al., 1997). Similarly, lymphocytes undergoing apoptosis were found to have intracellular K^+ concentrations of 50 mM (normally 140 mM), and blockade of K^+ efflux by raising extracellular K^+ inhibited apoptosis in these cells (Hughes et al., 1997). Such reductions in the concentration of intracellular K^+ may promote apoptosis by facilitating the proteolytic activation of caspase-3 and Ca^{2+}-activated endonuclease (Bortner et al., 1997).

Early evidence implicating apoptosis in the pathogenesis of brain damage after ischemic insults included findings of condensed nuclei with sharply delineated chromatin, apoptotic bodies, and evidence of internucleosomal DNA fragmentation (Li et al., 1995; Linnik et al., 1993; MacManus et al., 1993). While the precise morphology of ischemic neuronal death does not correspond exactly to that of pure apoptosis, for example, seen during development, it is quite plausible that contributions from excitotoxicity and other concurrent pathogenic events would lead to mixed morphological patterns. More recently, specific molecular markers of apoptosis have been identified in ischemic brain tissue. For example, increased expression of anti-apoptotic regulators bcl-2, bcl-x and bcl-w was shown in neurons that survived focal ischemia (Chen et al., 1995; Isenmann et al., 1998; Minami et al., 2000), while proapoptotic bax expression was increased selectively in vulnerable CA1 neurons following transient global ischemia (Krajewski et al., 1995). The activation of caspase-3 was demonstrated in cortical neurons several hours after a focal ischemic insult (Namura et al., 1998) and after transient global ischemia (Chen et al., 1998). Furthermore, as will be discussed further below, genetic or pharmacological interventions designed to block apoptosis can reduce cell death in cell culture or animal models of brain ischemia.

Inflammation

Cerebral ischemia induces an inflammatory reaction that may exacerbate initial levels of tissue injury in the hours to days after the initial insult. Within hours after transient global ischemia in gerbils, the expression of several proinflammatory cytokines is increased within the hippocampus and thalamus, including tumor necrosis factor (TNF)-α, primarily secreted by microglia, and IL-1β, primarily released from astrocytes. Mounting evidence suggests that the acute expression of these cytokines contributes to brain injury after ischemia, as blockade of their receptors or neutralization with antibodies reduces infarct volumes in rodent models of focal ischemia (for review see Barone & Feuerstein, 1999, and see below). Several actions of TNF-α may contribute to its deleterious effects in the ischemic brain, including a constrictive effect on pial arteries that can exacerbate ischemia, stimulation of matrix-degrading metalloproteinase activity, oligodendrocyte toxicity, and activation of leukocytes (Beutler & Cerami, 1987). However, the effects of TNF-α following cerebral ischemia are not all injurious, as rather surprisingly, mice lacking TNF receptors developed larger infarcts than wild-type controls (Bruce et al., 1996). It has been proposed that this cytokine has dual roles in brain injury, exacerbating toxicity at early time points, but promoting recovery at later times (Shohami et al., 1999).

TNF-α belongs to a family of ligands that activate the TNF superfamily of receptors (so called death receptors), which includes fas ligand (fasL, aka CD-95-L or APO-1-L) and TNF-related apoptosis-inducing ligand (TRAIL). In some cell-types, activation of these death receptors leads to the cleavage and activation of apical pro-caspase-8 (Ashkenazi & Dixit, 1998), which then can activate downstream effector caspases including caspase-3, leading to apoptosis independent of bcl-2-regulated cytochrome c release (Srinivasula et al., 1996). Recent evidence implicates this death receptor pathway of apoptosis in ischemic neuronal death, as fasL and TRAIL were found to be upregulated after transient focal ischemia. Furthermore, *lpr* mice expressing dysfunctional fasL

receptors (fas) had smaller infarct volumes than wild-type animals after transient focal ischemia (Martin-Villalba et al., 1999).

TNF-α and IL-1 also have important effects on leukocyte infiltration. Both cytokines 'prime' endothelium for cellular adherence, probably by increasing the expression of adhesion molecules (e.g. intercellular adhesion molecule 1 [ICAM-1], P-selectins, and E-selectins), enhancing neutrophil adhesion and subsequent infiltration (Barone & Feuerstein, 1999). Macrophages and monocytes follow, guided by chemokines such as IL-8, monocyte chemoattractant protein-1 (MCP-1), and interferon inducible protein-10 (IP-10), which are upregulated in the ischemic brain (del Zoppo et al., 2000). The infiltrating leukocytes probably contribute to ischemic brain injury through several mechanisms, including microvascular occlusion and release of cytotoxic products. One particularly damaging product of infiltrating macrophages is nitric oxide (NO), synthesized inside these cells by inducible NO synthase (iNOS or type II NOS). Under ischemic conditions NO can react with superoxide anion to form the powerfully destructive free radical, peroxynitrite. Other deleterious consequences of NO production include DNA damage (and subsequent activation of PARP, with resultant energy failure), and inhibition of DNA synthesis; both apoptosis and excitotoxic necrosis may be enhanced as a result (Iadecola, 1997; Hewett et al., 1994). Neuronal NOS (nNOS or type I NOS), a second isoform of NOS which is activated by elevated intracellular Ca^{2+}, may be a major mediator of brain cell death following ischemia (see below). In contrast, NO synthesized by a third isoform of NOS in endothelial cells (eNOS or type III NOS) may play a protective role early after ischemia onset, relaxing vascular smooth muscle cells and helping to preserve blood flow (Samdani et al., 1997).

Postischemic inflammation is further augmented by the excessive activation of the Ca^{2+}-activated catabolic enzymes, phospholipase A2 and C (PLA2 and PLC) in neurons, endothelial cells and leukocytes, which promote membrane phospholipid breakdown, producing platelet activating factor (PAF) and arachidonic acid. PAF exerts a variety of deleterious actions in ischemic brain including platelet and leukocyte activation, breakdown of the blood–brain barrier with resultant edema, and direct neurotoxicity at high concentrations (Stanimirovic & Satoh, 2000). Cyclooxygenase-2 (COX-2) is also upregulated following ischemia in close proximity to cells expressing iNOS, probably stimulated by NO (Nogawa et al., 1998), and further metabolizes arachidonic acid to a variety of toxic prostanoids; free radicals are also produced by arachidonic acid metabolism.

Neuroprotective interventions

Antiexcitotoxic approaches

Reducing extracellular glutamate

One approach to decreasing ischemic injury may be to reduce glutamate efflux from presynaptic nerve terminals and astrocytes. The most powerful method of accomplishing this so far may be mild hypothermia, which sharply limits the build-up of extracellular glutamate induced by ischemia (Busto et al., 1989). Both intra- and postischemic hypothermia produce lasting neuroprotective effects in animal cerebral ischemia studies (Barone et al., 1997b). At present, the clinical use of hypothermia is limited to surgical procedures that require concomitant cardiac arrest and neurosurgical procedures such as cerebral aneurysm clipping (Tommasino & Picozzi, 1998). Although hypothermia in patients with traumatic brain injury has been reported to improve outcomes in small clinical studies, a recent randomized trial of hypothermia after acute brain injury initiated within 6 hours did not demonstrate improved outcomes (Clifton et al., 2001).

Neurotransmitters (other than glutamate) released to the extracellular space during ischemia can also influence resultant brain injury, in part by altering circuit excitability and vesicular glutamate release from nerve terminals. GABA is the major inhibitory neurotransmitter in the mammalian brain; agonists at postsynaptic GABA receptors activating Cl^- channels ($GABA_A$ receptors) such as muscimol or benzodiazepines attenuate brain injury in rodent models (Sternau et al., 1989; Lyden & Hedges, 1992; Schwartz-Bloom et al., 1998). However, a phase III trial of the GABA agonist, clomethiazole, failed to show efficacy in patients with acute ischemic stroke (Lyden et al., 2002). One possible explanation for this disappointment might be a surprising ability of $GABA_A$ receptor activation to promote neuronal death induced by oxygen-glucose deprivation, perhaps because it hyperpolarizes neuronal cell membranes and thus enhances the voltage gradient for Ca^{2+} entry (Muir et al., 1996). In addition, it may well be that much of the glutamate accumulating in the extracellular space after ischemic insults is not mediated by circuit activation and vesicular release, but rather by transport from tonically de-energized and depolarized astrocytes (Szatkowski et al., 1990). Agonists of the $5-HT_{1A}$ serotonin receptor subtype have also been reported to reduce brain injury in rodent models of focal and global ischemia (Prehn et al., 1993; Piera et al., 1995), and a phase III clinical trial of the agonist, Bay x 3702, is currently under way (Goldberg, 2001).

A second general approach to reducing membrane excitability and vesicular glutamate release would be to manipulate various membrane ion channels. For example, several K^+ channel openers reduced endogenous glutamate release following brief ischemia in hippocampal slices (Zini et al., 1993) and have shown some promising effects in animal studies (Takaba et al., 1997; Heurteaux et al., 1993). However, BMS-204352, an opener of large-conductance Ca^{2+}-activated K^+ channels (BK channels) failed to show efficacy in a clinical trial for acute ischemic stroke (Goldberg, 2001). A possible explanation for this failure is raised by the potential of K^+ efflux to promote apoptosis (see above). Blocking voltage-gated Na^+ channels may provide another strategy to reduce circuit excitation. Na^+ channel blockers such as tetrodotoxin, phenytoin, and riluzole exhibit neuroprotective effects in vitro against both excitotoxic neuronal cell death (Lustig et al., 1992) and axonal damage (see below), as well as in vivo in both focal and global ischemia models (Yamasaki et al., 1991; Cullen et al., 1979; Pratt et al., 1992), but a recent clinical trial of fosphenytoin failed (Goldberg, 2001). Newer Na^+ channel blockers such as BIII 890 CL, that demonstrate increased activity in depolarized tissue and reduced interference with normal physiologic function, remain promising (Carter et al., 2000). Lastly, blocking voltage-gated Ca^{2+} channels would be a way to reduce glutamate release, as well as postsynaptic Ca^{2+} or Zn^{2+} influx, although more postsynaptic Ca^{2+} influx into neurons is probably mediated by NMDA receptors, and there might also be risk of potentiating apoptosis (see below). In any case, clinical trials with dihydropyridines in ischemic stroke have so far not been encouraging (American Nimodipine Study Group, 1992; Horn et al., 2001).

Manipulating glutamate receptors

Once released into the extracellular space, glutamate activates its ionophore-linked receptors, in addition to a family of metabotropic receptors linked to second messenger systems. These different glutamate receptors subtypes do not participate equally in excitotoxicity, but several receptor subtypes may be manipulated to reduce glutamate-induced Ca^{2+} overload in the ischemic brain.

Consistent with the prominent role of NMDA receptors in mediating glutamate-induced Ca^{2+} overload and rapidly triggered excitotoxic neurodegeneration in vitro, NMDA antagonists can reduce the death of cultured cortical neurons induced by hypoxia and glucose deprivation (Choi, 1992), and a substantial literature indicates that NMDA antagonists can reduce neuronal death in ischemic brain injury in vivo (Simon et al., 1984; McCulloch, 1992). Unfortunately, several recent clinical trials of NMDA antagonists in stroke patients have been disappointing (see Table 5.1); side effects including hallucinations, ataxia, or hypertension were prominent with several drugs (Lees,

Table 5.1. Agents recently tested as acute treatments for brain ischemia

Drug Category	Mechanism	Drug Name	Trial Status
Manipulate glutamate receptors			
Glutamate antagonists	AMPA antagonists	YM872	Phase III: ongoing
		ZK-200775 (MPQX)	Phase IIa: abandoned
	Competitive NMDA antagonists	CGS 19755 (Selfotel®)	Phase III: no efficacy
	NMDA channel blockers	aptiganel (Cerestat®)	Phase III: no efficacy
		dextrorphan	Phase II: abandoned
		dextromethorphan	abandoned
		magnesium	Phase III: ongoing
		NPS 1506	Phase Ib/IIa: suspended
		remacemide	Phase III in cardiopulmonary bypass: borderline efficacy
	NMDA glycine site antagonist	ACEA 1021 (Licostinel®)	Phase I: abandoned
		GV 150526	Phase III: no efficacy
	NMDA polyamine site antagonist	SL 82-0715 (eliprodil)	Phase III: abandoned
Reduce extracellular glutamate			
GABA agonists	↓ excitation, ↓ glutamate release	clomethiazole (Zendra®)	Phase III: no efficacy
Opiate antagonists		nalmefene (Cervene®)	Phase III: no efficacy
Serotonin agonists		Bay x 3702 (Repinotan®)	Phase III: ongoing
Sodium channel antagonists		Fosphenytoin (Cerebryx®)	Phase III: no efficacy
		BW619C89	Phase II: abandoned
Voltage-gated calcium channel antagonists	↓ Ca^{2+} influx, ↓ glutamate release	nimodipine (Nimotop®)	Phase III: no efficacy
		flunarizine (Sibelium®)	Phase III: no efficacy
Voltage-dependent potassium channel agonists		BMS-204352	Phase III: no efficacy
Unknown	↓ glutamate release, ↓ neuronal excitability, or ↓ NO-mediated injury	lubeluzole (Prosynap®)	Phase III: no efficacy
Block downstream mediators			
Free radical scavengers	↓ free radical-mediated injury	tirilazad mesylate (Freedox®)	Phase III: abandoned
		ebselen	Phase III: borderline efficacy
Phosphatidylcholine precursor	Membrane stabilizer	citicoline (Ceraxon®)	Phase III: no efficacy
Anti-apoptotic			
Growth factor	Anti-apoptotic?, ↑ NMDA receptor inactivation	Fibroblast growth factor (Fiblast®)	Phase II / III: abandoned
Anti-inflammatory			
Leukocyte adhesion inhibitor	Reduction of leukocyte infiltration	anti-ICAM antibody (Enlimomab®)	Phase III: no efficacy
		Hu23F2G	Phase III: no efficacy

Source: From Goldberg (2001).

1997). It remains to be seen whether efficacy can be established with this strategy, perhaps with the aid of enhancements in dosage regimens or drug characteristics, or whether utility in human stroke will prove to be fundamentally constrained (see below).

NMDA receptor blockade can be achieved in a variety of ways, using agents that act at distinct molecular sites within the receptor complex. Competitive antagonists bind the glutamate recognition site; channel blockers (or uncompetitive antagonists), bind sites within the channel pore; glycine antagonists bind the glycine recognition site; and noncompetitive antagonists bind other sites on NMDA receptors (e.g. polyamines, Zn^{2+}, redox site), downmodulating receptor activation via remote actions, for example, via allosteric changes. One might envision trying to improve the therapeutic index of NMDA antagonists in several ways. One strategy might be to find compounds capable of preferentially blocking overactivated NMDA receptors relative to physiologically activated receptors. Memantine, such an activity-dependent NMDA channel blocker, has shown promise in attenuating excitotoxic neuronal loss in vitro as well as brain damage in a rodent model of stroke, at potentially tolerable concentrations (Chen et al., 1992). Another approach might be to limit antagonism with partial antagonists, such as cycloserine (Hood et al., 1989), or by partial reduction in the endogenous glycine-site agonist D-serine (Snyder & Kim, 2000). A third approach might be to develop NMDA receptor subunit-selective antagonists along the lines of ifenprodil, an NR2B-selective antagonist with neuroprotective efficacy in vivo against focal ischemia (Gotti et al., 1988; Kemp et al., 1999). NR2B-containing NMDA receptors are expressed preferentially in the adult forebrain, so blocking these may give adequate neuroprotection against forebrain ischemia with relatively fewer side effects mediated by antagonism of hindbrain receptors. A novel approach to NMDA receptor antagonism was explored using an oral adeno-associated virus vaccine against the NR1 subunit; strong neuroprotection was demonstrated against focal ischemia-induced injury after a single-dose vaccine (During et al., 2000). This strategy could presumably be adapted to yield subtype-selective NMDA receptor blockade; but on the other hand, the resulting blockade cannot be easily controlled, and there is a risk of developing compensatory changes in the NMDA receptor system.

While NMDA antagonists may reduce the toxic influx of Ca^{2+} following cerebral ischemia in certain neurons, there is a risk that NMDA blockade may concurrently increase the likelihood of apoptosis in other neurons (Lee et al., 1999). Several studies have indicated that there can be an inverse relationship between intracellular Ca^{2+} concentration and the propensity to undergo apoptosis (Ca^{2+} setpoint hypothesis, Koike & Tanaka, 1991). One unsettling corollary of this hypothesis is that NMDA-antagonist drugs may act as double-edged swords, attenuating excitotoxic necrosis in cells that are in a state of relative Ca^{2+} overload, but promoting apoptosis in Ca^{2+}-starved neurons. While Ca^{2+} overload and Ca^{2+} starvation are opposite states, both could be triggered by the same ischemic event, separated in space or time: for example, excitotoxic Ca^{2+} overload might predominate acutely, close to the ischemic core, whereas at later time intervals and further from the core, Ca^{2+} starvation and apoptosis might predominate. Supporting this idea is the recent observation that NMDA antagonists reduced primary excitotoxic injury in a rodent head trauma model at the impact site, but increased the severity of secondary apoptotic injury at distant sites (Pohl et al., 1999).

As discussed above, AMPA/kainate receptors can directly mediate excitotoxic cell death, albeit less powerfully than NMDA receptors. Besides promoting toxic Ca^{2+} entry, depolarization mediated by AMPA/kainate receptor activation may be a key factor promoting toxic levels of Zn^{2+} entry (see above). The competitive AMPA/kainate receptor antagonist NBQX is effective in reducing neuronal loss following both global (Sheardown et al., 1990) and focal (Buchan et al., 1991) cerebral ischemia. Likewise, the noncompetitive antagonist GYKI-52466 has also exhibited neuroprotective effects in studies of global (Le-Peillet et al., 1992) or focal (Smith & Meldrum, 1992) ischemia. Several factors that operate in the ischemic brain, in particular a shift towards acid pH due to buildup of lactic acid, may attenuate NMDA-receptor function and so reduce the prominence of NMDA-receptor-mediated neurotoxicity relative to AMPA- or kainate-receptor-mediated neurotoxicity. Acid pH may also enhance AMPA receptor-mediated neurotoxicity, perhaps by slowing recovery of cellular calcium homeostasis (McDonald et al., 1998b).

Another mechanism that has been proposed to enhance the contribution of AMPA/kainate receptor-mediated toxicity to ischemic neuronal death is an ischemia-induced enhancement of the expression of Ca^{2+} (and Zn^{2+}) permeable AMPA receptors, due to an alteration in subunit composition (reduced expression of AMPA receptor subunit GluR2/GluR-B (Pellegrini-Giampietro et al., 1997). However, on the downside, AMPA/kainate receptor blockade may be inadequate to reduce calcium overload on neurons where NMDA receptors have been strongly activated, and conversely, AMPA/kainate receptor blockade also has some potential to enhance apoptosis in the setting of relative calcium starvation. Will the strategy work? A phase III trial of the AMPA antagonist YM872 in acute ischemic stroke is currently ongoing.

Although not directly mediating excitotoxicity, the metabotropic glutamate receptors can modify excitotoxicity and thus may be useful targets for therapeutic manipulation. These receptors, which are linked to G-proteins rather than ion channels, have been identified and segregated into three groups based on sequence similarity and mechanisms of signal transduction (Nakanishi & Masu, 1994; Conn & Pin, 1997). The first clue to neuroprotective actions was the demonstration that the nonselective mGluR agonist, trans-1-aminocyclopentane-1, 3-dicarboxylic acid (tACPD), could attenuate glutamate-induced neuronal death (Koh et al., 1991); non-selective activation of mGluRs also reduced infarct volume in vivo after focal ischemia (Chiamulera et al., 1992). Growing evidence suggests that activation of mGluR group II and III receptors, which typically have inhibitory effects on circuit excitation and glutamate release (Conn & Pin, 1997; Cartmell & Schoepp, 2000), may have more powerful antiexcitotoxic effects than non-selective agonists. A recent study suggests that the excitatory effects of group I mGluR activation may be harnessed to reduce neuronal apoptosis (Allen et al., 2000).

Blocking downstream mediators

Many enzymes including proteases, endonucleases, kinases, and phosphatases are activated directly or indirectly by increases in intracellular Ca^{2+} concentration and may contribute to cellular damage after ischemic insult. Compared with glutamate-receptor antagonists, interventions directed at blocking the downstream intracellular mediators of excitotoxicity may have a longer therapeutic window. For example, calpain inhibition by MDL 28170 decreased infarct volume after transient focal ischemia even when administered 6 hours after ischemia onset (Markgraf et al., 1998). Cytoplasmic phospholipase A2 ($cPLA_2$) is activated following NMDA receptor stimulation and promotes membrane phospholipid breakdown, liberating arachidonic acid (Dumuis et al., 1988) and producing free radicals. Pharmacological inhibition (Phillis, 1996) or genetic ablation (Bonventre et al., 1997) of $cPLA_2$ reduced brain injury in animal models of cerebral ischemia. Blocking PAF, a product of phospholipid breakdown, with gingkolide B or BN 52021 also reduced ischemic injury (Lindsberg et al., 1991).

Adding to the injury occurring during a given ischemic insult, postischemic reperfusion induces further tissue damage in the brain, probably mediated by the accelerated formation of several reactive oxygen species including superoxide, hydroxyl, and NO radicals (Kuroda & Siesjo, 1997). Free radical production is likely a specific downstream mediator of glutamate-induced neuronal death. As noted above, nNOS which is activated by elevated intracellular Ca^{2+} forms the weak oxidant, NO (Dawson & Snyder, 1994), but in the presence of superoxide anion can be converted to peroxynitrite (Beckman & Koppenol, 1996). Inhibiting nNOS either pharmacologically or genetically (via gene deletion) renders cultured neurons resistant to NMDA-induced death, and also reduces infarct volume in rodent models of transient focal ischemia (Samdani et al., 1997). Blockade of iNOS in inflammatory cells after ischemia will be discussed below. COX-mediated metabolism of arachidonic acid to a prostaglandin intermediate can also lead to the production of toxic superoxide anion (Chan et al., 1985). In cortical neuronal cultures, NMDA-induced excitotoxicity was decreased by a specific COX-2 inhibitor (Hewett et al., 2000) which also afforded neuroprotection against focal ischemia when administered to rats postocclusion (Nogawa et al., 1997). Another link between excitotoxicity and free radicals is through excessive Ca^{2+} accumulation in mitochondria which uncouples energy production from electron transport and the formation of toxic levels of free radicals (Dugan et al., 1995; Reynolds & Hastings, 1995).

Beneficial results have been obtained with several free radical scavenger drugs in animal studies of ischemic or traumatic brain injury (Clemens et al., 1994), although the magnitude of neuroprotection observed has typically not been very large. Two phase III clinical trials involving free radical scavengers in acute ischemic stroke were conducted recently. One trial testing the lipid peroxidation inhibitor tirilazad mesylate was prematurely terminated due to concerns about the safety of the drug (Haley, 1998). The second trial involved treatment with ebselen, a selenoorganic compound with antioxidant activity, and did not demonstrate definitive efficacy (Yamaguchi et al., 1998). It is possible that more powerful antioxidant agents may yield greater therapeutic benefits. The spin trapping agent α-phenyl-N-tert-butyl nitrone (PBN) reduced infarct volume following focal ischemia in rats even when administered up to 3 hours after ischemia onset (Zhao et al., 1994).

One especially important consequence of reactive oxygen species formation may be single-stranded DNA breakage, leading to activation of the repair enzyme, PARP, and consequent depletion of cellular NAD^+ and energy stores (Szabo & Dawson, 1998). Pharmacological inhibition or gene deletion of PARP attenuated neuronal death induced by glutamate receptor agonists in vitro (Zhang et al., 1994; Eliasson et al., 1997), and decreased infarct size in rodent focal ischemia studies (Zhang et al., 1994; Eliasson et al., 1997; Endres et al., 1997).

Antiapoptotic strategies

As noted above, accumulating evidence suggests that many brain cells undergo apoptosis following ischemic insults, including evidence that blocking apoptosis reduces ischemic brain damage in vivo or in vitro. Transgenic overexpression of *bcl-2* (Martinou et al., 1994) or its delivery via herpes virus vector (Linnik et al., 1995) were both found to reduce infarct volume in mice subjected to focal ischemia; and the survival of hippocampal CA1 neurons after transient global ischemia was enhanced in transgenic mice overexpressing bcl-2 (Kitagawa et al., 1998). Likewise, overexpression of *bcl-x*$_L$ in transgenic mice reduced infarct volume following permanent focal ischemia (Wiessner et al., 1999). In experiments in our laboratory, mice lacking the *bax* gene exhibited reduced infarct volumes after transient focal ischemia (F. Gottron & D.W.C., unpublished data). While genetic manipulation of the Bcl-2 family of genes may not be a practical approach to antiapoptotic therapy in the human, future development of strategies to suppress or enhance this family of proteins (e.g. using antisense oligonucleotides) or to disrupt interactions between family members may prove beneficial (Nicholson, 2000).

A more immediately viable approach to antiapoptotic therapy might be via pharmacological caspase inhibitors. Intracerebroventricular (icv) infusion of the relatively non-specific caspase-3 inhibitor (*N*-benzyloxycarbonyl-Asp(OMe)-Glu(OMe)-Val-Asp(OMe)-fluoromethylketone or z-DEVD.FMK) decreased infarct size after transient focal ischemia (Hara et al., 1997) and reduced hippocampal CA1 cell death in transient global ischemia (Chen et al., 1998). In addition, the pan-caspase inhibitor, boc-aspartyl(OMe)-fluoromethylketone (BAF) given icv or systemically, was markedly neuroprotective in a rat model of neonatal hypoxia-ischemia even when administered 3 hours after the insult (Cheng et al., 1998). It is plausible that non-specific caspase inhibitors may be more effective at stopping the effector arm of apoptosis, owing to the broad-spectrum inhibition of all caspases in the cascade. Several caspases other than effector caspase-3 have been implicated in ischemic brain injury including the upstream caspases, caspase-9 (Krajewski et al., 1999), and caspase-8 which is activated via the death receptor pathway (Martin-Villalba et al., 1999). In addition, recent work suggests that caspase-11, a novel upstream caspase activated only under pathological conditions, is also activated after cerebral ischemia (Kang et al., 2000). Although concerns about the systemic blockade of all caspase activity are warranted, given the importance of apoptosis in normal physiologic processes, short-term administration after acute stroke may be tolerable. Another approach to inhibiting caspases may be modelled by the inhibitor of apoptosis (IAP) family of proteins, which bind and inhibit both initiator and effector caspases (Reed & Tomaselli, 2000). Included in this family is neuronal AIP (NAIP); inactivation by a hereditary mutation underlies motor neuron degeneration in spinal muscular atrophy (Roy et al., 1995). While antiapoptotic caspase inhibitors have not yet reached the clinic, drugs that block caspase-1 (or interleukin-1 converting enzyme, ICE) have recently been introduced for the treatment of rheumatoid arthritis (Nicholson, 2000).

The recent finding that the death receptor-mediated pathway to apoptosis may be involved in ischemic injury opens other potential targets for intervention. Development of means to suppress fasL or to block its receptor fas may be of benefit. The immunosuppressant FK506, a known neuroprotective agent following focal ischemia, suppresses the upregulation of fasL following ischemia (Martin-Villalba et al., 1999). In addition, one might try to mimic or augment the action of a naturally occurring protein known as FLICE-inhibitory protein (FLIP), which blocks the recruitment and activation of caspase-8 (formerly known as FLICE) and inhibits apoptosis induced by several death ligands (Thome et al., 1997).

As outlined above, transmembrane ionic fluxes may play a role in the regulation of programmed cell death, with Ca^{2+} starvation and K^+ efflux promoting apoptosis. Addressing these derangements through therapeutic intervention is plausible, but will have to be done in such a way that death due to excitotoxic calcium overload is not augmented. We have speculatively suggested a 'pull–push' approach to manipulating neuronal calcium homeostasis during ischemic insults: initially reducing calcium influx, with drugs like NMDA antagonists, to reduce excitotoxicity, and then later enhancing calcium influx to reduce calcium starvation and apoptosis (Lee et al., 1999). Similarly, targeting K^+ depletion in cells at risk for apoptosis, for example by augmenting K^+ influx or blocking upregulation of the neuronal delayed rectifier current, has to be accomplished with specificity, as this may also enhance circuit excitability and excitotoxicity.

Growth factors may be valuable in reducing apoptosis following cerebral ischemia. The expression of several growth factors increases in ischemic tissue, likely as a protective response. In addition, exogenous administration of growth factors including nerve growth factor (NGF), brain-derived neurotrophic factor (BDNF), neurotrophins 4/5 (NT-4/5), basic fibroblast growth factor (bFGF), and type-1 insulin-like growth factor (IGF-1) reduces brain damage in rats subjected to cerebral ischemia (Hefti, 1997). Some growth factors may also enhance nerve fibre sprouting and synapse formation after ischemic injury, thereby promoting functional recovery. Delivery issues are substantial obstacles to practical use, but may be surmountable through the development of small-molecule agonists that bind immunophilins, and have neurotrophic and neuroprotective actions that can be separated from immunosuppressant effects (Snyder et al., 1998). Unfortunately, the first trial of a growth factor for treatment of ischemia, bFGF in acute ischemic stroke, was unsuccessful (Goldberg, 2001). In addition, in a fashion akin to the situation with manipulation of calcium homeostasis, a downside risk of at least the neurotrophins and IGF-1 may be the enhancement of excitotoxic necrosis (Koh et al., 1995).

Anti-inflammatory approaches

Interference with inflammatory cascades is another general approach likely to aid neural cell survival. A key early event amenable to therapeutic intervention may be the suppression of key cytokines which are induced shortly after ischemia onset. For example, delivery of the IL-1 receptor antagonist (IL-1ra, which is a naturally occurring inhibitor in the brain) by intracerebroventricular injection (Loddick & Rothwell, 1996) or by adenoviral vector (Betz et al., 1995) reduced brain injury following focal ischemia in rats. Although clinically impractical, these interventions underscore the potential of this pathway as a target for neuroprotection. The peripheral administration of IL-1ra (a more clinically relevant route) reduced infarct volume in a rodent focal ischemia model (Relton et al., 1996). Likewise, interfering with TNF-α signalling using an anti-TNF-α monoclonal antibody or soluble TNF-α receptor I (which acts by competing with membrane receptors) resulted in attenuation of brain injury after focal ischemia (Barone et al., 1997a), likely by improving microvascular perfusion in ischemic cortex (Dawson et al., 1996). These effects must be interpreted with caution, as cerebral ischemia in mice lacking TNF receptors demonstrated larger infarct volumes than their wild-type counterparts (Bruce et al., 1996).

One of the detrimental effects of TNF-α is the upregulation of endothelial cell adhesion molecules and leukocyte adherence to blood vessels, another potential target for intervention. Administration of antibodies to either ICAM-1 or the β-integrins (CD11a/CD18) expressed on leukocytes decreased infarct size in rodent transient (Chopp et al., 1996), but not permanent focal ischemia (Zhang et al., 1995). In addition, mice lacking the ICAM-1 gene were less susceptible to ischemia-reperfusion injury (Connolly et al., 1996). A phase III clinical trial using anti-ICAM antibodies failed, possibly due to murine antibody-induced complications; however, another trial using humanized antibodies directed against CD11/CD18 also failed to show efficacy in patients with acute ischemic stroke (Enlimomab Acute Stroke Trial Investigators and Sherman, 1997; Goldberg, 2001).

Following cerebral ischemia infiltrating leukocytes increase expression of iNOS, peaking 12–48 hours after ischemia onset (del Zoppo et al., 2000). The relatively selective iNOS inhibitor, aminoguanidine, reduced infarct volume following focal ischemia even if given 24 hours after MCA occlusion (Nagayama et al., 1998). Confirming the pharmacological effect, mice lacking the iNOS gene also had smaller infarcts than their wild-type littermates (Iadecola et al., 1997). The delayed expression of iNOS following cerebral ischemia makes it an attractive target for intervention in human stroke with a potentially long therapeutic window.

The secretion of vasoactive mediators by endothelial cells is another consequence of ischemia-induced inflammation, and may lead to vasoconstriction and microvascular thrombosis, resulting in further exacerbation of ischemic damage (del Zoppo et al., 2000). Two classes of agents, attractive because they are currently in clinical use, may be able to reduce ischemic brain damage by altering vasoactive mediators. The cholesterol-lowering agents, 3-hydroxy-3-methylglutaryl (HMG)-CoA reductase inhibitors (or statins) decreased cerebral infarct size in mice by upregulating eNOS, resulting in increased cerebral blood flow (CBF) during ischemia (Endres et al., 1998). In addition, the estrogens have been shown to have neuroprotective properties in rodent cerebral ischemia models. Although the mechanism of action is not as well defined as that of the statins, it is believed that improvement in CBF may contribute, in part by up-regulation of NOS. Other proposed neuroprotective mechanisms include antioxidant actions, induction of *bcl-2* and neurotrophic factors, and modulation of excitotoxicity (Hurn & Macrae, 2000).

White matter injury

While much of the current work in neuroprotection has focused on blocking injury mechanisms relevant to dendrites and neuronal perikarya (grey matter), myelinated fibre tracts (white matter) are also damaged by ischemic insults and could benefit from targeted neuroprotective approaches. Many antiexcitotoxic treatments, such as NMDA receptor antagonists, would not be expected to protect white matter. Experiments using isolated rat optic nerve as an in vitro model for myelinated CNS tracts have revealed that compound action potentials disappear after 8–10 minutes of anoxia, evidence that white matter tracts are critically dependent on oxidative metabolism to maintain energy for excitability (Waxman et al., 1991). Hypoxic–ischemic energy depletion leads to failure of the membrane Na^+–K^+-ATPase, leading to membrane depolarization and accumulation of axoplasmic free Na^+, largely due to influx through tetrodotoxin-sensitive, voltage-gated Na^+ channels subserving action potentials. This elevation in axonal $[Na^+]_i$ stimulates the Na^+/Ca^{2+} exchanger, resulting in Ca^{2+} influx and toxic elevations in $[Ca^{2+}]_i$ (Stys, 1998), leading to consequences presumably similar to those outlined in studies of cultured neurons. Agents that block voltage-gated Na^+ channels, including local anesthetics, antiarrhythmics and certain anticonvulsants, are protective in the optic nerve anoxia model, as are the Na^+/Ca^{2+} exchange inhibitors, bepridil and benzamil (Stys, 1998).

Oligodendrocytes, responsible for myelinating nerve fibres in the CNS, express Ca^{2+}-permeable AMPA receptors and are highly vulnerable to AMPA-receptor-mediated injury in vitro (Matute et al., 1997). In addition, cultured oligodendrocytes deprived of oxygen and glucose were protected by an AMPA receptor antagonist, and injection of AMPA into rat brain white matter induced widespread oligodendrocyte death (McDonald et al., 1998a). Although most oligodendrocytes are remote from synapses, they may be exposed to excess extracellular glutamate, released by adjacent neurons or astrocytes following ischemic insults. Glutamate may also be released along axons through a non-synaptic process mediated by reversal of the Na^+/K^+-glutamate transporter (Nicholls & Attwell, 1990).

Clinical trials and future directions

Despite the wealth of preclinical data supporting the efficacy of many neuroprotective agents, why have these agents failed so far in human trials? The answer to this vexing question probably lies partly in the difficulty of conducting human clinical trials of neuroprotective agents, and partly in limitations of neuroprotective efficacy in the agents tested to date. Clinical trials have many more variables than studies with experimental animals in controlled laboratory settings. While most laboratory investigations are conducted on young healthy animals, patients suffering strokes or cardiac arrest typically are elderly and have concomitant diseases such as hypertension or diabetes; etiology, severity, and lesion location (cortical vs. subcorti-

cal infarction) typically vary widely. The endpoint used to determine efficacy is another important difference between human and experimental studies: most animal studies have utilized lesion size measured hours to days after ischemia, whereas human clinical studies have relied upon functional outcome as measured by clinical assessment scales (Barthel Index, Rankin Score, etc.) usually several months after ischemia. A drug that reduces lesion size may or may not produce a detectable improvement in functional outcome, depending upon multiple other factors, in particular lesion location. In the future, enhanced neuroimaging techniques may be able to provide sufficient quantitation of lesion volume to be able to serve as surrogate outcome measures for assessing neuroprotective interventions. Furthermore, techniques for imaging at-risk tissue, such as diffusion- and perfusion-weighted magnetic resonance imaging, may permit each patient to serve as his/her own control (comparing the brain volume initially at risk, to the volume of damage that ultimately evolves with or without intervention).

Most clinical trials of neuroprotective agents to date share, at least in part, a common rationale of reducing excitotoxicity. The future of neuroprotective approaches for brain ischemia will likely lie in broader aims, specifically encompassing strategies to limit ischemic apoptosis and post-ischemic inflammation. Indeed, as discussed above, the postulate that the prominence of apoptosis in the brain after ischemic insults approximates that of excitotoxicity, supported by substantial emerging evidence, places many anti-excitotoxic treatments on a dangerous balance point (Fig. 5.1). Many approaches useful in limiting excitotoxicity, reducing circuit activation, glutamate release, membrane depolarization, calcium entry, etc., may have a downside, enhancement of apoptosis. Perhaps the key difference between experimental studies, for the most part conducted with lissencephalic rodent brains and sharply controlled ischemic insults, and human stroke, involving a gyrencephalic brain and sometimes fluctuating levels of ischemia, is a greater prominence of mild ischemia and apoptosis in the latter setting.

One path ahead may thus be to combine approaches, so that excitotoxicity and apoptosis might be simultaneously reduced. Two experimental studies have so far tested the concurrent administration of NMDA antagonists and inhibitors of apoptosis. Coadministration of dextrorphan and cycloheximide produced greater than 80% reduction of infarct volume after transient focal ischemia in rats, better than the effect of optimal doses of either agent alone (Du et al., 1996). Furthermore, the combination of MK-801 and z-VAD.fmk demonstrated neuroprotective synergy in reducing infarction, and an extended therapeu-

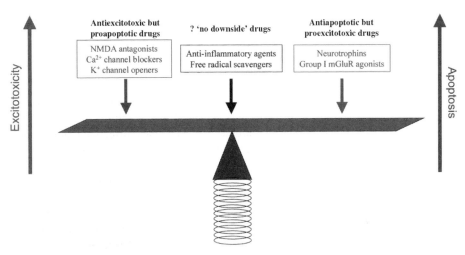

Fig. 5.1. Balancing antiexcitotoxic and antiapoptotic approaches to neuroprotection in the ischemic brain. Speculative diagram depicting the possibility that some approaches may reduce excitotoxicity but enhance apoptosis, or vice-versa; whereas some 'no downside' approaches may reduce both forms of death (or at least reduce one without enhancing the other).

tic window compared to that of either drug alone (Ma et al., 1998).

Alternatively, it may be possible to target antiexcitotoxic and anti- apoptotic approaches in time or space to maximize benefits and minimize deleterious consequences. With progressive enhancements in brain imaging, both in terms of resolution and in terms of yielding information about functional state, one can envision a time when imaging techniques are used to select and direct the optimal neuroprotective strategies for a given specific clinical situation. For example, the development of methods for identifying the early activation of the apoptosis cascades, or levels of intracellular free calcium, might enable clinicians to know when to stop delivery of acutely initiated NMDA antagonist drugs, and begin treatment with caspase inhibitors or neurotrophins.

A third path ahead might be to prioritize the deployment of 'no downside' drugs: capable of limiting excitotoxicity or apoptosis, but lacking concurrent ability to enhance the other form of death. Examples of such drugs might be PARP inhibitors for excitotoxicity or caspase inhibitors for apoptosis; antioxidants or anti-inflammatory drugs might be able to reduce both forms of death (Fig. 5.1).

References

Adams, J. M. & Cory, S. (1998). The Bcl-2 protein family: arbiters of cell survival. *Science*, **281**, 1322–6.

Aizenman, E., Stout, A.K., Hartnett, K.A., Dineley, K.E., McLaughlin, B. & Reynolds, I.J. (2000). Induction of neuronal apoptosis by thiol oxidation: putative role of intracellular zinc release. *J. Neurochem.*, **75**, 1878–88.

Albers, G.W., Goldberg, M.P. & Choi, D.W. (1992). Do NMDA antagonists prevent neuronal injury? Yes. *Arch. Neurol.*, 49: 418–20.

Allen, J.W., Knoblach, S.M. and Faden, A.I. (2000). Activation of group I metabotropic glutamate receptors reduces neuronal apoptosis but increases necrotic cell death in vitro. *Cell Death Differ.*, **7**, 470–6.

American Nimodipine Study Group. (1992). Clinical trial of nimodipine in acute ischemic stroke. *Stroke*, **23**, 3–8.

Ankarcrona, M., Dypbukt, J.M., Bonfoco, E. et al. (1995). Glutamate-induced neuronal death: a succession of necrosis or apoptosis depending on mitochondrial function. *Neuron*, **15**, 961–73.

Ashkenazi, A. & Dixit, V. (1998). Death receptors: signaling and modulation. *Science*, **281**, 1305–8.

Barone, F.C. & Feuerstein, G.Z. (1999). Inflammatory mediators and stroke: new opportunities for novel therapeutics. *J. Cereb. Blood Flow Metab.*, **19**, 819–34.

Barone, F.C., Arvin, B., White, R.F. et al. (1997a). Tumor necrosis factor-alpha. A mediator of focal ischemic brain injury. *Stroke*, **28**, 1233–44.

Barone, F.C., Feuerstein, G.Z. & White, R.F. (1997b). Brain cooling during transient focal ischemia provides complete neuroprotection. *Neurosci. Biobehav. Rev.*, **21**, 31–44.

Beckman, J.S. & Koppenol, W.H. (1996). Nitric oxide, superoxide, and peroxynitrite: the good, the bad, and ugly. *Am. J. Physiol.*, **271**, C1424–37.

Betz, A.L., Yang, G.Y. & Davidson, B.L. (1995). Attenuation of stroke size in rats using an adenoviral vector to induce overexpression of interleukin-1 receptor antagonist in brain. *J. Cereb. Blood Flow Metab.*, **15**, 547–51.

Beutler, B. & Cerami, A. (1987). Cachectin: more than a tumor necrosis factor. *N. Engl. J. Med.*, **316**, 379–85.

Bonventre, J.V., Huang, Z., Taheri, M.R. et al. (1997). Reduced fertility and postischaemic brain injury in mice deficient in cytosolic phospholipase A2. *Nature*, **390**, 622–5.

Bortner, C.D., Hughes, F.M.J. & Cidlowski, J.A. (1997). A primary role for K+ and Na+ efflux in the activation of apoptosis. *J. Biol. Chem.*, **272**, 32436–42.

Bruce, A.J., Boling, W., Kindy, M.S. et al. (1996). Altered neuronal and microglial responses to excitotoxic and ischemia brain injury in mice lacking TNF receptors. *Nat. Med.*, **2**: 788–94.

Buchan, A.M. (1990). Do NMDA antagonists protect against cerebral ischemia: are clinical trials warranted? *Cerebrovasc. Brain Metab. Rev.*, **2**, 1–26.

Buchan, A.M., Xue, D., Huang, Z.G., Smith, K.H. & Lesiuk, H. (1991). Delayed AMPA receptor blockade reduces cerebral infarction induced by focal ischemia. *Neuroreport*, **2**, 473–6.

Buendia, B., Santa-Maria, A. & Courvalin, J.C. (1999). Caspase-dependent proteolysis of integral and peripheral proteins of nuclear membranes and nuclear pore complex proteins during apoptosis. *J. Cell. Sci.*, **112**, 1743–53.

Busto, R., Globus, M.Y., Dietrich, W.D., Martinez, E., Valdes, I. & Ginsberg, M.D. (1989). Effect of mild hypothermia on ischemia-induced release of neurotransmitters and free fatty acids in rat brain. *Stroke*, **20**, 904–10.

Carter, A.J., Grauert, M., Pschorn, U. et al. (2000). Potent blockade of sodium channels and protection of brain tissue from ischemia by BIII 890 CL. *Proc. Natl. Acad. Sci., USA*, **97**, 4944–9.

Cartmell, J. & Schoepp, D.D. (2000). Regulation of neurotransmitter release by metabotropic glutamate receptors. *J. Neurochem.*, **75**, 889–907.

Cecconi, F. (1999). Apaf1 and the apoptotic machinery. *Cell Death Differ.*, **6**, 1087–98.

Chan, P.H., Fishman, R.A., Longar, S., Chen, S. & Yu, A. (1985). Cellular and molecular effects of polyunsaturated fatty acids in brain ischemia and injury. *Prog. Brain Res.*, **63**, 227–35.

Chen, H.S., Pellegrini, J.W., Aggarwal, S.K. et al. (1992). Open-channel block of *N*-methyl-D-aspartate (NMDA) responses by memantine: therapeutic advantage against NMDA receptor-mediated neurotoxicity. *J. Neurosci.*, **12**, 4427–36.

Chen, J., Graham, S.H., Chan, P.H., Lan, J., Zhou, R.L. & Simon, R.P. (1995). Bcl-2 is expressed in neurons that survive focal ischemia in the rat. *Neuroreport*, **6**, 394–8.

Chen, J., Nagayama, T., Jin, K. et al. (1998). Induction of caspase-3-like protease may mediate delayed neuronal death in the hippocampus after transient cerebral ischemia. *J. Neurosci.*, **18**, 4914–28.

Cheng, Y., Deshmukh, M., D'Costa, A. et al. (1998). Caspase inhibitor affords neuroprotection with delayed administration in a rat model of neonatal hypoxic-ischemic brain injury. *J. Clin. Invest.*, **101**, 1992–9.

Chiamulera, C., Albertini, P., Valerio, E. & Reggiani, A. (1992). Activation of metabotropic receptors has a neuroprotective effect in a rodent model of focal ischaemia. *Europ. J. Pharmacol.*, **216**, 335–6.

Choi, D.W. (1988). Calcium-mediated neurotoxicity: relationship to specific channel types and role in ischemic damage. *Trends Neurosci.*, **11**, 465–9.

Choi, D.W. (1992). Excitotoxic cell death. *J. Neurobiol.*, **23**, 1261–76.

Choi, D.W. (1996). Ischemia-induced neuronal apoptosis. *Curr. Opin. Neurobiol.*, **6**, 667–72.

Choi, D.W. & Koh, J.Y. (1998). Zinc and brain injury. *Annu. Rev. Neurosci.*, **21**, 347–75.

Chopp, M., Li, Y., Jiang, N., Zhang, R.L. & Prostak, J. (1996). Antibodies against adhesion molecules reduce apoptosis after transient middle cerebral artery occlusion in rat brain. *J. Cereb. Blood Flow Metab.*, **16**, 578–84.

Clemens, J.A., Smalstig, E.B., Bhagwandin, B. & Panetta, J.A. (1994). Preservation of a functionally intact neuronal network after global ischemia. *Neurosci. Lett.*, **170**, 244–6.

Clifton, G.L., Miller, E.R., Choi, S.C. et al. (2001). Lack of effect of induction of hypothermia after acute brain injury. *N. Engl. J. Med.*, **344**, 556–63.

Cole, T.B., Wenzel, H.J., Kafer, K.E., Schwartzkroin, P.A. & Palmiter, R.D. (1999). Elimination of zinc from synaptic vesicles in the intact mouse brain by disruption of the ZnT3 gene. *Proc. Natl. Acad. Sci., USA*, **96**, 1716–21.

Conn, P.J. & Pin, J.P. (1997). Pharmacology and functions of metabotropic glutamate receptors. *Annu. Rev. Pharmacol. Toxicol.*, **37**, 205–37.

Connolly, E.S., Winfree, C.J., Springer, T.A. et al. (1996). Cerebral protection in homozygous null ICAM-1 mice after middle cerebral artery occlusion. Role of neutrophil adhesion in the pathogenesis of stroke. *J. Clin. Invest.*, **97**, 209–16.

Cullen, J.P., Aldrete, J.A., Jankovsky, L. & Romo-Salas, F. (1979). Protective action of phenytoin in cerebral ischemia. *Anesth. Analg.*, **58**, 165–9.

Dawson, D.A., Martin, D. & Hallenbeck, J.M. (1996). Inhibition of tumor necrosis factor-alpha reduces focal cerebral ischemic injury in the spontaneously hypertensive rat. *Neurosci. Lett.*, **218**, 41–4.

Dawson, T.M. & Snyder, S.H. (1994). Gases as biological messengers: nitric oxide and carbon monoxide in the brain. *J. Neurosci.*, **14**, 5147–59.

del Zoppo, G., Ginis, I., Hallenbeck, J.M., Iadecola, C., Wang, X. & Feuerstein, G.Z. (2000). Inflammation and stroke: putative role for cytokines, adhesion molecules and iNOS in brain response to ischemia. *Brain Pathol.*, **10**, 95–112.

Dirnagl, U., Iadecola, C. & Moskowitz, M.A. (1999). Pathobiology of ischaemic stroke: an integrated view. *Trends Neurosci.*, **22**, 391–7.

Du, C., Hu, R., Csernansky, C.A., Liu, X.Z., Hsu, C.Y. & Choi, D.W. (1996). Additive neuroprotective effects of dextrorphan and cycloheximide in rats subjected to transient focal cerebral ischemia. *Brain Res.*, **718**, 233–6.

Dugan, L.L., Sensi, S.L., Canzoniero, L.M.T. et al. (1995). Mitochondrial production of reactive oxygen species in cortical neurons following exposure to *N*-methyl-D-aspartate. *J. Neurosci.*, **15**, 6377–88.

Dumuis, A., Sebben, M., Haynes, L., Pin, J.P. & Bockaert, J. (1988). NMDA receptors activate the arachidonic acid cascade system in striatal neurons. *Nature*, **336**, 68–70.

During, M.J., Symes, C.W., Lawlor, P.A. et al. (2000). An oral vaccine against NMDAR1 with efficacy in experimental stroke and epilepsy. *Science*, **287**, 1453–60.

Eliasson, M.J., Sampei, K., Mandir, A.S. et al. (1997). Poly(ADP-ribose) polymerase gene disruption renders mice resistant to cerebral ischemia. *Nat. Med.*, **3**, 1089–95.

Endres, M., Wang, Z.Q., Namura, S., Waeber, C. & Moskowitz, M.A. (1997). Ischemic brain injury is mediated by the activation of poly(ADP–ribose)polymerase. *J. Cereb. Blood Flow Metab.*, **17**, 1143–51.

Endres, M., Laufs, U., Huang, Z. et al. (1998). Stroke protection by 3-hydroxy-3-methylglutaryl (HMG)-CoA reductase inhibitors mediated by endothelial nitric oxide synthase. *Proc. Natl. Acad. Sci., USA*, **95**, 8880–5.

Enlimomab Acute Stroke Trial Investigators & Sherman, D.G. (1997). The enlimomab acute stroke trial: final results. *Neurology*, **48**, A270.

Frederickson, C.J. (1989). Neurobiology of zinc and zinc-containing neurons. *Int. Rev. Neurobiol.*, **31**, 145–238.

Frederickson, C.J., Hernandez, M.D. & McGinty, J.F. (1989). Translocation of zinc may contribute to seizure-induced death of neurons. *Brain Res.*, **480**, 317–21.

Furlan, A., Higashida, R., Wechsler, L. et al. (1999). Intra-arterial prourokinase for acute ischemic stroke. The PROACT II study: a randomized controlled trial. Prolyse in Acute Cerebral Thromboembolism. *JAMA*, **282**, 2003–11.

Goldberg, M. (2001). Washington University School of Medicine Internet Stroke Clinical Trials Database. *http://www.neuro.wustl.edu/stroke/stroke-trials.htm*.

Gotti, B., Duverger, D., Bertin, J. et al. (1988). Ifenprodil and SL 82.0715 as cerebral anti-ischemic agents. I. Evidence for efficacy in models of focal cerebral ischemia. *J. Pharmacol. Exp. Therap.*, **247**, 1211–21.

Haley, E.C. (1998). High-dose tirilazad for acute stroke (RANTTAS II). RANTTAS II Investigators. *Stroke*, **29**, 1256–7.

Hara, H., Friedlander, R.M., Gagliardini, V. et al. (1997). Inhibition of interleukin 1beta converting enzyme family proteases reduces ischemic and excitotoxic neuronal damage. *Proc. Natl Acad. Sci., USA*, **94**, 2007–12.

Hartnett, K.A., Stout, A.K., Rajdev, S., Rosenberg, P.A., Reynolds, I.J. & Aizenman, E. (1997). NMDA receptor-mediated neurotoxicity: a paradoxical requirement for extracellular Mg^{2+} in Na^{+}/Ca^{2+}-free solutions in rat cortical neurons in vitro. *J. Neurochem.*, **68**, 1836–45.

Hefti, F. (1997). Pharmacology of neurotrophic factors. *Annu. Rev. Pharmacol. Toxicol.*, **37**, 239–67.

Heurteaux, C., Bertaina, V., Widmann, C. & Lazdunski, M. (1993). K^{+} channel openers prevent global ischemia-induced expression of c-fos, c-jun, heat shock protein, and amyloid beta-protein precursor genes and neuronal death in rat hippocampus. *Proc. Natl Acad. Sci., USA*, **90**, 9431–5.

Hewett, S.J., Csernansky, C.A. & Choi, D.W. (1994). Selective potentiation of NMDA-induced neuronal injury following induction of actrocytic iNOS. *Neuron*, **13**, 487–94.

Hewett, S.J., Uliasz, T.F., Vidwans, A.S. & Hewett, J.A. (2000). Cyclooxygenase-2 contributes to *N*-methyl-D-aspartate-mediated neuronal cell death in primary cortical cell culture. *J. Pharmacol. Exp. Therp.*, **293**, 417–25.

Hood, W.F., Compton, R.P. & Monahan, J.B. (1989). D-cycloserine: a ligand for the *N*-methyl-D-aspartate coupled glycine receptor has partial agonist characteristics. *Neurosci. Lett.*, **98**, 91–5.

Horn, J., de Haan, R.J., Vermeulen, M. & Limburg, M. (2001). Very Early Nimodipine Use in Stroke (VENUS): a randomized, double-blind, placebo-controlled trial. *Stroke*, **32**, 461–5.

Hughes, F.M., Jr., Bortner, C.D., Purdy, G.D. & Cidlowski, J.A. (1997). Intracellular K^{+} suppresses the activation of apoptosis in lymphocytes. *J. Biol. Chem.*, **272**, 30567–76.

Hurn, P.D. & Macrae, I.M. (2000). Estrogen as a neuroprotectant in stroke. *J. Cereb. Blood Flow Metab.*, **20**, 631–52.

Iadecola, C. (1997). Bright and dark sides of nitric oxide in ischemic brain injury. *Trends Neurosci.*, **20**, 132–9.

Iadecola, C., Zhang, F., Casey, R., Nagayama, M. & Ross, M.E. (1997). Delayed reduction of ischemic brain injury and neurological deficits in mice lacking the inducible nitric oxide synthase gene. *J. Neurosci.*, **17**, 9157–64.

Isenmann, S., Stoll, G., Schroeter, M., Krajewski, S., Reed, J.C. & Bahr, M. (1998). Differential regulation of Bax, Bcl-2, and Bcl-X proteins in focal cortical ischemia in the rat. *Brain Pathol.*, **8**, 49–62; discussion 62–3.

Johnson, J. & Deckwerth, T.L. (1993). Molecular mechanisms of developmental neuronal death. *Ann. Rev. Neurosci.*, **16**, 31–46.

Joza, N., Susin, S. A., Daugas, E. et al. (2001). Essential role of the mitochondrial apoptosis-inducing factor in programmed cell death. *Nature*, **410**, 549–54.

Jurgensmeier, J., Xie, Z., Deveraux, Q., Ellerby, L., Bredesen, D. & Reed, J. (1998). Bax directly induces release of cytochrome c from isolated mitochondria. *Proc. Natl. Acad. Sci., USA*, **95**, 4997–5002.

Kang, S.J., Wang, S., Hara, H. et al. (2000). Dual role of caspase-11 in mediating activation of caspase-1 and caspase-3 under pathological conditions. *J. Cell Biol.*, **149**, 613–22.

Kemp, J.A., Kew, J.N.C. & Gill, R. (1999). NMDA receptor antagonists and their potential as neuroprotective agents. In *Ionotropic Glutamate Receptors in the CNS*, ed. P. Jonas & H. Monyer, pp. 495–527. Berlin, Hiedelberg, New York: Springer.

Kerr, J., Wyllie, A. & Currie, A. (1972). Apoptosis: a basic biological phenomenon with wide-ranging implications in tissue kinetics. *Br. J. Cancer*, **26**, 239–57.

Kim, A.H., Kerchner, G.A. & Choi, D.W. (2001). Blocking excitotoxicity. In *CNS Neuroprotection*, ed. F.W. Marcoux, & D.W. Choi, Heidelberg: Springer-Verlag, in press.

Kitagawa, K., Matsumoto, M., Tsujimoto, Y. et al. (1998). Amelioration of hippocampal neuronal damage after global ischemia by neuronal overexpression of BCL-2 in transgenic mice. *Stroke*, **29**, 2616–21.

Koh, J.Y., Palmer, E. & Cotman, C.W. (1991). Activation of the metabotropic glutamate receptor attenuates *N*-methyl-D-aspartate neurotoxicity in cortical cultures. *Proc. Natl Acad. Sci., USA*, **88**, 9431–5.

Koh, J.Y., Gwag, B.J., Lobner, D. & Choi, D.W. (1995). Potentiated necrosis of cultured cortical neurons by neurotrophins. *Science*, **268**, 573–5.

Koh, J.Y., Suh, S.W., Gwag, B.J., He, Y.Y., Hsu, C.Y. & Choi, D.W. (1996). The role of zinc in selective neuronal death after transient global cerebral ischemia. *Science*, **272**, 1013–16.

Koike, T. & Tanaka, S. (1991). Evidence that nerve growth factor dependence of sympathetic neurons for survival in vitro may be determined by levels of cytoplasmic free Ca^{2+}. *Proc. Natl. Acad. Sci., USA*, **88**, 3892–6.

Kondo, S. (1998). Altruistic cell suicide in relation to radiation hormesis. *Int. J. Radiat. Biol. Relat. Stud. Phys. Chem. Med.*, **53**, 95–102.

Kothakota, S., Azuma, T., Reinhard, C. et al. (1997). Caspase-3-generated fragment of gelsolin: effector of morphological change in apoptosis. *Science*, **278**, 294–8.

Krajewski, S., Mai, J.K., Krajewska, M., Sikorska, M., Mossakowski, M.J. & Reed, J.C. (1995). Upregulation of bax protein levels in neurons following cerebral ischemia. *J. Neurosci.*, **15**, 6364–76.

Krajewski, S., Krajewska, M., Ellerby, L.M et al. (1999). Release of caspase-9 from mitochondria during neuronal apoptosis and cerebral ischemia. *Proc. Natl Acad. Sci., USA*, **96**, 5752–7.

Kuroda, S. & Siesjo, B.K. (1997). Reperfusion damage following focal ischemia: pathophysiology and therapeutic windows. *Clin. Neurosci.*, **4**, 199–212.

Lee, J.M., Zipfel, G.J. & Choi, D.W. (1999). The changing landscape of ischaemic brain injury mechanisms. *Nature*, **399**, A7–14.

Lee, J.Y., Cole, T.B., Palmiter, R.D. & Koh, J.Y. (2000). Accumulation of zinc in degenerating hippocampal neurons of ZnT3-null mice after seizures: evidence against synaptic vesicle origin. *J. Neurosci. (Online)*, **20**, RC79.

Lees, K.R. (1997) Cerestat and other NMDA antagonists in ischemic stroke. *Neurology*, **49**, S66–9.

Le-Peillet, E., Arvin, B., Moncada, C. & Meldrum, B.S. (1992). The non-NMDA antagonists, NBQX and GYKI 52466, protect against cortical and striatal cell loss following transient global ischaemia in the rat. *Brain Res.*, **571**, 115–20.

Li, Y., Sharov, V.G., Jiang, N., Zaloga, C., Sabbah, H.N. & Chopp, M. (1995). Ultrastructural and light microscopic evidence of apoptosis after middle cerebral artery occlusion in the rat. *Am. J. Pathol.*, **146**, 1045–51.

Lindsberg, P.J., Hallenbeck, J.M. & Feuerstein, G. (1991). Platelet-activating factor in stroke and brain injury. *Ann. Neurol.*, **30**, 117–29.

Linnik, M., Zobrist, R. & Hatfield, M. (1993). Evidence supporting a role for programmed cell death in focal cerebral ischemia in rats. *Stroke*, **24**, 2002–8.

Linnik, M.D., Zahos, P., Geschwind, M.D. & Federoff, H.J. (1995). Expression of bcl-2 from a defective herpes simplex virus-1 vector limits neuronal death in focal cerebral ischemia. *Stroke*, **26**, 1670–4.

Loddick, S.A. & Rothwell, N.J. (1996). Neuroprotective effects of human recombinant interleukin-1 receptor antagonist in focal cerebral ischaemia in the rat. *J. Cereb. Blood Flow Metab.*, **16**, 932–40.

Lustig, H. S., von Brauchitsch, K.L., Chan, J. & Greenberg, D.A. (1992). A novel inhibitor of glutamate release reduces excitotoxic injury in vitro. *Neurosci. Lett.*, **143**, 229–32.

Lyden, P.D. & Hedges, B. (1992). Protective effect of synaptic inhibition during cerebral ischemia in rats and rabbits. *Stroke*, **23**, 1463–9; discussion 1469–70.

Lyden, P., Shuaib, A., Ng,K et al. (2002). Clomethiazole acute stroke study in ischemic stroke (Class I): final results. *Stroke*, **33**, 122–9.

Ma, J., Endres, M. & Moskowitz, M.A. (1998). Synergistic effects of caspase inhibitors and MK-801 in brain injury after transient focal cerebral ischaemia in mice. *Br. J. Pharmacol.*, **124**, 756–62.

McCulloch, J. (1992). Excitatory amino acid antagonists and their potential for the treatment of ischaemic brain damage in man. *Br. J. Clin. Pharmacol.*, **34**, 106–14.

McDonald, J.W., Althomsons, S.P., Hyrc, K.L., Choi, D.W. & Goldberg, M.P. (1998a). Oligodendrocytes from forebrain are highly vulnerable to AMPA/kainate receptor-mediated excitotoxicity. *Nat. Med.*, **4**, 291–7.

McDonald, J.W., Bhattacharyya, T., Sensi, S.L. et al. (1998b). Extracellular acidity potentiates AMPA receptor-mediated cortical neuronal death. *J. Neurosci.*, **18**, 6290–9.

MacManus, J.P., Buchan, A.M., Hill, I.E., Rasquinha, I. & Preston, E. (1993). Global ischemia can cause DNA fragmentation indicative of apoptosis in rat brain. *Neurosci. Lett.*, **164**, 89–92.

Markgraf, C.G., Velayo, N.L., Johnson, M.P. et al. (1998). Six-hour window of opportunity for calpain inhibition in focal cerebral ischemia in rats. *Stroke*, **29**, 152–8.

Martinou, J., Dubois-Dauphin, M., Staple, J. et al. (1994). Overexpression of BCL-2 in transgenic mice protects neurons from naturally occurring cell death and experimental ischemia. *Neuron*, **13**, 1017–30.

Martin-Villalba, A., Herr, I., Jeremias, I. et al. (1999). CD95 ligand (Fas-L/APO-1L) and tumor necrosis factor-related apoptosis-inducing ligand mediate ischemia-induced apoptosis in neurons. *J. Neurosci.*, **19**, 3809–17.

Matute, C., Sanchez-Gomez, M.V., Martinez-Millan, L. & Miledi, R. (1997). Glutamate receptor-mediated toxicity in optic nerve oligodendrocytes. *Proc. Natl Acad. Sci., USA*, **94**, 8830–5.

Minami, M., Jin, K.L., Li, W., Nagayama, T., Henshall, D.C. & Simon, R.P. (2000). Bcl-w expression is increased in brain regions affected by focal cerebral ischemia in the rat. *Neurosci. Lett.*, **279**, 193–5.

Muir, J.K., Lobner, D., Monyer, H. & Choi, D.W. (1996). GABAA receptor activation attenuates excitotoxicity but exacerbates oxygen-glucose deprivation-induced neuronal injury in vitro. *J. Cereb. Blood Flow Metab.*, **16**, 1211–18.

Nagata, S. (2000). Apoptotic DNA fragmentation. *Exp. Cell Res.*, **256**, 12–18.

Nagayama, M., Zhang, F. & Iadecola, C. (1998). Delayed treatment with aminoguanidine decreases focal cerebral ischemic damage and enhances neurologic recovery in rats. *J. Cereb. Blood Flow Metab.*, **18**, 1107–13.

Nakanishi, S. & Masu, M. (1994). Molecular diversity and functions of glutamate receptors. [Review]. *Annu. Rev. Biophys. Biomol. Struct.*, **23**, 319–48.

Namura, S., Zhu, J., Fink, K. et al. (1998). Activation and cleavage of caspase-3 in apoptosis induced by experimental cerebral ischemia. *J. Neurosci.*, **18**, 3659–68.

National Institute of Neurological Disorders and Stroke rt-PA Stroke Study Group. (1995). Tissue plasminogen activator for acute ischemic stroke. *N. Engl. J. Med.*, **333**, 1581–7.

Nicholls, D. & Attwell, D. (1990). The release and uptake of excitatory amino acids. *Trends Pharmacol. Sci.*, **11**, 462–8.

Nicholson, D.W. (2000). From bench to clinic with apoptosis-based therapeutic agents. *Nature*, **407**, 810–16.

Nogawa, S., Zhang, F., Ross, M.E. & Iadecola, C. (1997). Cyclo-oxygenase-2 gene expression in neurons contributes to ischemic brain damage. *J. Neurosci.*, **17**, 2746–55.

Nogawa, S., Forster, C., Zhang, F., Nagayama, M., Ross, M.E. & Iadecola, C. (1998). Interaction between inducible nitric oxide synthase and cyclooxygenase-2 after cerebral ischemia. *Proc. Natl. Acad. Sci., USA*, **95**, 10966–71.

Olney, J.W. (1969). Brain lesion, obesity and other disturbances in mice treated with monosodium glutamate. *Science*, **164**, 719–21.

Pellegrini-Giampietro, D.E., Gorter, J.A., Bennett, M.V. & Zukin, R.S. (1997). The GluR2 (GluR-B) hypothesis: Ca^{2+}-permeable AMPA receptors in neurological disorders. *Trends Neurosci.*, **20**, 464–70.

Phillis, J.W. (1996). Cerebroprotective action of the phospholipase inhibitor quinacrine in the ischemia/reperfused gerbil hippocampus. *Life Sci.*, **58**, L97–101.

Piera, M.J., Beaughard, M., Michelin, M.T. & Massingham, R. (1995). Effects of the 5-hydroxytryptamine1A receptor agonists, 8–OH-DPAT, buspirone and flesinoxan, upon brain damage induced by transient global cerebral ischaemia in gerbils. *Arch. Int. Pharmacodyn. Ther.*, **329**, 347–59.

Pohl, D., Bittigau, P., Ishimaru, M.J. et al. (1999). N-Methyl-D-aspartate antagonists and apoptotic cell death triggered by head trauma in developing rat brain. *Proc. Natl Acad. Sci., USA*, **96**, 2508–13.

Pratt, J., Rataud, J., Bardot, F. et al. (1992). Neuroprotective actions of riluzole in rodent models of global and focal cerebral ischaemia. *Neurosci. Lett.*, **140**, 225–30.

Prehn, J.H., Welsch, M., Backhauss, C. et al. (1993). Effects of serotonergic drugs in experimental brain ischemia: evidence for a protective role of serotonin in cerebral ischemia. *Brain Res.*, **630**, 10–20.

Reed, J.C. & Tomaselli, K.J. (2000). Drug discovery opportunities from apoptosis research. *Curr. Opin. Biotechnol.*, **11**, 586–92.

Relton, J.K., Martin, D., Thompson, R.C. & Russell, D.A. (1996). Peripheral administration of Interleukin-1 Receptor antagonist inhibits brain damage after focal cerebral ischemia in the rat. *Exp. Neurol.*, **138**, 206–13.

Reynolds, I.J. & Hastings, T.G. (1995). Glutamate induces the production of reactive oxygen species in cultured forebrain neurons following NMDA receptor activation. *J. Neurosci.*, **15**, 3318–27.

Rothman, S.M. & Olney, J.W. (1986). Glutamate and the pathophysiology of hypoxic–ischemic brain damage. *Ann. Neurol.*, **19**, 105–11.

Roy, N., Mahadevan, M.S., McLean, M. et al. (1995). The gene for neuronal apoptosis inhibitory protein is partially deleted in individuals with spinal muscular atrophy. *Cell*, **80**, 167–78.

Samdani, A.F., Dawson, T.M. & Dawson, V.L. (1997). Nitric oxide synthase in models of focal ischemia. *Stroke*, **28**, 1283–8.

Schwartz-Bloom, R.D., McDonough, K.J., Chase, P.J., Chadwick, L.E., Inglefield, J.R. & Levin, E.D. (1998). Long-term neuroprotection by benzodiazepine full versus partial agonists after transient cerebral ischemia in the gerbil [corrected]. *J. Cereb. Blood Flow Metab.*, **18**, 548–58.

Sheardown, M., Nielsen, E., Hansen, A., Jacobsen, P. & Honore, T. (1990). 2,3-Dihydroxy-6-nitro-7-sulfamoyl-benzo(F)quinoxaline: a neuroprotectant for cerebral ischemia. *Science*, **247**, 571–4.

Shohami, E., Ginis, I. & Hallenbeck, J.M. (1999). Dual role of tumor necrosis factor alpha in brain injury. *Cytokine Growth Factor Rev.*, **10**, 119–30.

Simon, R.P., Swan, J.H., Griffiths, T. & Meldrum, B.S. (1984). Blockade of N-methyl-D-aspartate receptors may protect against ischemic damage in the brain. *Science*, **226**, 850–2.

Slee, E., Adrain, C. & Martin, S. (1999). Serial killers: ordering caspase activation events in apoptosis. *Cell Death Differ.*, **6**, 1067–74.

Smith, S.E. & Meldrum, B.S. (1992). Cerebroprotective effect of a non-N-methyl-D-aspartate antagonist, GYKI 52466, after focal ischemia in the rat. *Stroke*, **23**, 861–4.

Snyder, S.H. & Kim, P.M. (2000). D-amino acids as putative neurotransmitters: focus on D-serine. *Neurochem. Res.*, **25**, 553–60.

Snyder, S.H., Lai, M.M. & Burnett, P.E. (1998). Immunophilins in the nervous system. *Neuron*, **21**, 283–94.

Srinivasula, S.M., Ahmad, M., Fernandes-Alnemri, T., Litwack, G. & Alnemri, E.S. (1996). Molecular ordering of the Fas-apoptotic pathway: the Fas/APO-1 protease Mch5 is a CrmA-inhibitable protease that activates multiple Ced-3/ICE- like cysteine proteases. *Proc. Natl. Acad. Sci., USA*, **93**, 14486–91.

Stanimirovic, D. & Satoh, K. (2000). Inflammatory mediators of cerebral endothelium: a role in ischemic brain inflammation. *Brain Pathol.*, **10**, 113–26.

Sternau, L.L., Lust, W.D., Ricci, A.J. & Ratcheson, R. (1989). Role for gamma-aminobutyric acid in selective vulnerability in gerbils. *Stroke*, **20**, 281–7.

Stys, P.K. (1998). Anoxic and ischemic injury of myelinated axons in CNS white matter: from mechanistic concepts to therapeutics. *J. Cereb. Blood Flow Metab.*, **18**, 2–25.

Szabo, C. & Dawson, V.L. (1998). Role of poly(ADP-ribose) synthetase in inflammation and ischaemia-reperfusion. *Trends Pharmacol. Sci.*, **19**, 287–98.

Szatkowski, M., Barbour, B. & Attwell, D. (1990). Non-vesicular release of glutamate from glial cells by reversed electrogenic glutamate uptake. *Nature*, **348**, 443–6.

Takaba, H., Nagao, T., Yao, H., Kitazono, T., Ibayashi, S. & Fujishima, M. (1997). An ATP-sensitive potassium channel activator reduces infarct volume in focal cerebral ischemia in rats. *Am. J. Physiol.*, **273**, R583–6.

Thome, M., Schneider, P., Hofmann, K. et al. (1997). Viral FLICE-inhibitory proteins (FLIPs) prevent apoptosis induced by death receptors. *Nature*, **386**, 517–21.

Thornberry, N.A. & Lazebnik, Y. (1998). Caspases: enemies within. *Science*, **281**, 1312–16.

Tommasino, C. & Picozzi, P. (1998). Mild hypothermia. *J. Neurosurg. Sci.*, **42**, 37–8.

Tonder, N., Johansen, F.F., Frederickson, C.J., Zimmer, J. & Diemer, N.H. (1990). Possible role of zinc in the selective degeneration of dentate hilar neurons after cerebral ischemia in the adult rat. *Neurosci. Lett.*, **109**, 247–52.

Waxman, S.G., Ransom, B.R. & Stys, P.K. (1991). Non-synaptic mechanisms of Ca^{2+}-mediated injury in CNS white matter. *Trends Neurosci.*, **14**, 461–8.

Wiessner, C., Allegrini, P.R., Rupalla, K. et al. (1999). Neuron-specific transgene expression of Bcl-XL but not Bcl-2 genes reduced lesion size after permanent middle cerebral artery occlusion in mice. *Neurosci. Lett.*, **268**, 119–22.

Yamaguchi, T., Sano, K., Takakura, K. et al. (1998). Ebselen in acute ischemic stroke: a placebo-controlled, double-blind clinical trial. Ebselen Study Group. *Stroke*, **29**, 12–17.

Yamasaki, Y., Kogure, K., Hara, H., Ban, H. & Akaike, N. (1991). The possible involvement of tetrodotoxin-sensitive ion channels in ischemic neuronal damage in the rat hippocampus. *Neurosci. Lett.*, **121**, 251–4.

Yu, S.P., Yeh, C.H., Sensi, S.L. et al. (1997). Mediation of neuronal apoptosis by enhancement of outward potassium current. *Science*, **278**, 114–17.

Zhang, J., Dawson, V.L., Dawson, T.M. & Snyder, S.H. (1994). Nitric oxide activation of poly(ADP-ribose) synthetase in neurotoxicity. *Science*, **263**, 687–9.

Zhang, R.L., Chopp, M., Jiang, N. et al. (1995). Anti-intercellular adhesion molecule-1 antibody reduces ischemic cell damage after transient but not permanent middle cerebral artery occlusion in the Wistar rat. *Stroke*, **26**, 1438–42; discussion 1443.

Zhao, Q., Pahlmark, K., Smith, M.L. & Siesjo, B.K. (1994). Delayed treatment with the spin trap alpha-phenyl-*N*-tert-butyl nitrone (PBN) reduces infarct size following transient middle cerebral artery occlusion in rats. *Acta Physiol. Scand.*, **152**, 349–50.

Zini, S., Roisin, M.P., Armengaud, C. & Ben-Ari, Y. (1993). Effect of potassium channel modulators on the release of glutamate induced by ischaemic-like conditions in rat hippocampal slices. *Neurosci. Lett.*, **153**, 202–5.

6

Promoting recovery of neurological function

Ted Abel[1] and Michael E. Selzer[2]

Department of [1]Biology and [2]Neurology, University of Pennsylvania, Philadelphia, PA, USA

This chapter focuses on the biologically driven strategies that are being developed to enhance that recovery following neural injury. It is beyond the scope of this chapter to review the entire field of neurologic rehabilitation, much of which involves orthotic, prosthetic, behavioural, psychological and sociological approaches. Many of these approaches are accumulating substantial evidence for their effectiveness and their omission here should not be interpreted as an indication of lack of importance. Several recent monographs on neurologic rehabilitation cover them in greater detail (Dobkin, 1996; Lazar, 1998; Ozer, 2000). Here, the behavioural, physiological and structural mechanisms by which the nervous system adapts spontaneously to injury will be reviewed. Then some promising current approaches to optimizing recovery by utilizing the nervous system's own adaptive processes will be discussed. Finally the mechanisms that limit the ability of the nervous system to reconstitute the lost neural circuitry will be examined, and strategies that are being developed to overcome these limitations will be summarized.

Mechanisms of spontaneous recovery

Following injury to the nervous system, it is usual for patients to recover to a variable degree. This is a consequence of three processes. First, depending on the type of injury, an ischemic/traumatic penumbra (Heiss & Graf, 1994; Tator, 1995) results in temporary dysfunction of neuronal elements due to pressure from edema, excitotoxicity with intracellular (intramitochondrial) calcium accumulation (Stout et al., 1998), extracellular accumulation of potassium and magnesium, and inflammation (Carlson et al., 1998) (Fig. 6.1). If they do not kill the neurons, these changes eventually resolve and neuronal function is restored. Secondly, patients can employ a variety of behav-

ioural adaptations to restore equivalent functions to those lost as a consequence of the structural and physiological alterations brought about by the injury. Thirdly, physiological changes and short distance anatomic rearrangements in spared neural pathways may result in compensatory enhancement in transmission through those pathways to reproduce or substitute for lost functions. A fourth mechanism, frank regeneration of injured axons and replacement of lost neurons to reconstitute the interrupted synaptic circuits, is currently believed not to occur to a significant degree in the mammalian CNS. Strategies to promote such neural repair are discussed later in the chapter.

Behavioural adaptation

Behavioural adaptation refers to the conscious substitution of behaviours, based on spared physiological functions for the lost more natural or commonly utilized functions, aimed at producing the same desired result. For example, a right-handed person who has suffered a left hemispheric stroke might begin using his left hand to perform functions previously performed with the right hand. To a large extent, occupational therapy is involved in teaching patients to utilize effective behavioural adaptations (see below). To the extent that the newly acquired behaviours must be learned and learning involves physiological plasticity, most behavioural adaptations involve physiological plasticity as well.

Cortical remodelling

Experiments utilizing electrophysiological, stimulation and imaging techniques have demonstrated that injuries to both the peripheral and central nervous systems result in alterations in the central representations of sensory and motor functions in such a way as to suggest effective

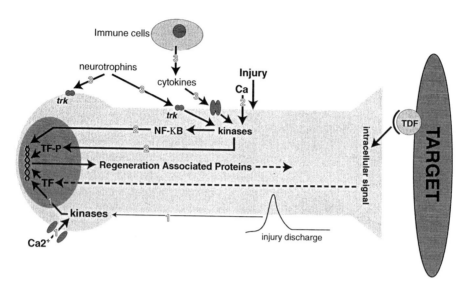

Fig. 6.1. Molecular responses to axon injury leading to regeneration. Neural injury gives rise to an injury-related discharge (1) that back-propagates towards the cell body where it leads to the opening of voltage-dependent calcium channels. This calcium influx activates kinases, including CaMKII, PKA, PKA and MAP kinase, that phosphorylate a variety of target proteins. Especially important targets of these kinases are transcription factors such as CREB and NF-κB. These transcription factors induce the expression of regeneration-associated proteins such as GAP-43, CAP-23 and several cytoskeletal proteins. Injury also results in bulk calcium influx at the site of injury (2). The longer-term response to injury involves the release of neurotrophins (NGF, BDNF, NT-3, NT-4/5) and cytokines (CNTF, LIF, IGF, IL-6) that activate intracellular signalling pathways via specific receptors (3).

compensation for the injury. These changes following injury resemble in many ways the cortical changes that are observed following learning or other experiences. A common term used to describe these altered physiological responses following injury and training is 'neural plasticity'. Many plastic processes result from alterations in intracellular signalling cascades but, in many cases, ultrastructural or immunohistological alterations also are observed.

Reorganization of synaptic contacts is especially prevalent in the cortex, where sensory and motor maps undergo extensive reorganization and remapping as a result of experience (Buonomano & Merzenich, 1998). One well-known example of neural plasticity within the cortex is the rearrangement of hand representation in the somatosensory cortex following injury to a peripheral nerve or amputation of a digit. Following such deafferentation, the cortical representation of adjacent regions expands over the surface of the cortex for a distance of approximately 1.5 mm, an area that encompasses the distribution of terminals of thalamocortical neurons (Rausell & Jones, 1995). Because this initial expansion occurs rapidly, it might be the result of the unmasking of formerly inactive synaptic connections that were previously masked by inhibition from the lost afferent pathway (Jones, 1993). At longer

recovery times, the area covered by the shifting sensory map increases substantially beyond that covered by the distribution of thalamic afferents (Pons et al., 1991).

Cortical plasticity may contribute to functional recovery following a CNS injury such as stroke. A region of the sensory cortex to which behaviourally important portions of the finger tips project was destroyed by microlesions, the behaviour of monkeys in a learned sensorimotor task at first deteriorated, but then improved (Xerri et al., 1998). Concomitantly, the central projection for those finger tips shifted to neighbouring regions of cortex. These findings are consistent with 'substitution' and 'vicariation' models of recovery from brain damage and stroke. In these models, adaptive reorganization of the cortex takes place following a lesion in such a way that other regions of the cortex that may not have been originally involved in the function of the injured area now directly compensate for the dysfunctional area (Xerri et al., 1998).

Afferent input to the cortex can also be modulated by experience, including environmental enrichment and training. Increases in dendritic arbourization and synaptic contacts in the cerebellar and cerebral cortices have been observed in many environmental enrichment studies and after extensive training (van Praag et al., 2000). These alterations are thought to result from the induction of use-dependent patterns of neural activity that lead to the selective reshaping of neuronal connections. Whether similar mechanisms act following injury is not known, but the similarity between the two processes suggests that they may share overlapping molecular mechanisms. Repeated sensory overstimulation and training on digital dexterity tasks can increase the receptive fields of the involved digits within the primary somatosensory cortex in primates (Buonomano & Merzenich, 1998). Enlarged representation of relevant movements is also observed in the primary motor cortex after training (Buonomano & Merzenich, 1998). Such remapping results in a much finer representational grain than normal. Thus, for both sensory and motor cortices, experience alters the cortical map in a way that correlates with the behavioural demands of the task.

Using transcranial magnetic stimulation (TMS), functional imaging, magnetoencephalography or high resolution electroencephalography, many examples have been documented of cortical remapping in normal human subjects as well as in patients with peripheral or central nervous system lesions (Classen et al., 1998; Karni et al., 1995). For example, focal stimulation of the motor cortex using TMS was used to evoke thumb movements before and after the practising of thumb movements. Focal TMS more often evoked movements in the recently practised direction than in other directions (Classen et al., 1998). Thus, in humans, training rapidly and transiently induces a change in the cortical network representing the movement of the thumb, thereby encoding the details of the practised movement.

What molecular mechanisms are responsible for this newly emergent representation of sensory information or motor maps within the cortex? There are several mechanisms that might be responsible for the neural plasticity that underlies the long-term alterations in cortical maps that follow injury or training. Two major mechanisms are the restructuring of neuronal morphology and changes in the strength of synaptic connections. It is important to note that these mechanisms may be inter-related. The induction of synaptic plasticity is accompanied by morphological changes in neurons (Segal & Andersen, 2000). Morphological changes might result from the sprouting of collateral axon branches, the extension of dendritic arbours, the creation of dendritic spines, and the creation of new synapses. The expansions of sensory receptive fields produced by long-term alterations in afferent input are probably due to physiological and/or anatomical plastic changes (Buonomano & Merzenich, 1998). Activity-dependent modifications in synaptic strength may play a critical role in cortical remapping, perhaps via NMDA receptor mediated long-term potentiation (Garraghty & Muja, 1996), as has been described for synaptic plasticity in the hippocampus (Bliss & Collingridge, 1993).

To investigate the hypothesis that synaptic plasticity underlies cortical map reorganization, researchers have used pharmacological, electrophysiological and genetic approaches. Recent experiments in humans have used the changes in TMS-evoked thumb movements after training (Classen et al., 1998) to explore the effects of drugs that block synaptic plasticity in the motor cortex in vitro on cortical map plasticity in vivo. An NMDA receptor antagonist, dextromethorphan, and a GABA-A receptor modulator, lorazepam, both of which block the induction of long-term potentiation (LTP) in the motor cortex in vitro, block the use-dependent reorganization of the cortical thumb representation in human subjects (Butefisch et al., 2000). By contrast, lamotrigine, a drug that modifies sodium and calcium channels without altering LTP induction, does not alter cortical map reorganization. Thus, these findings point to a striking similarity between use-dependent cortical plasticity and the cellular mechanisms of LTP, which is thought to underlie learning and memory (Martin et al., 2000; Rioult-Pedotti et al., 2000). Genetic approaches in mice have been used to study plasticity in the barrel (somatosensory) cortex, which receives input from the whiskers. Removal of all facial whiskers (vibrissae) except for one results in the expansion of the spared whisker's functional representation in the somatosensory cortex. Mutant mice with impairments in LTP, including those with alterations in CaMKII or CREB, exhibit impairments in this form of experience dependent cortical plasticity (e.g. Glazewski et al., 2000). Thus, understanding the molecular mechanisms underlying forms of synaptic plasticity, such as LTP, may provide insights into the molecular basis of cortical remodelling following injury.

Physiological plasticity

Since its introduction over a century ago by Santiago Ramón y Cajal, the word 'plasticity' has been used in many ways by neuroscientists studying a variety of processes ranging from recovery from neural injury to learning and memory to drug addiction and psychiatric disorders (Nestler & Hyman, 1999). We will focus our discussion on two broad forms of plasticity: physiological plasticity, in which patterns of use and disuse modify synaptic strength (synaptic plasticity) and modulate neuronal firing (neural plasticity), and anatomical plasticity, which involves structural alterations (e.g. sprouting, pruning, regeneration) following injury or use. Many of these forms of plasticity share

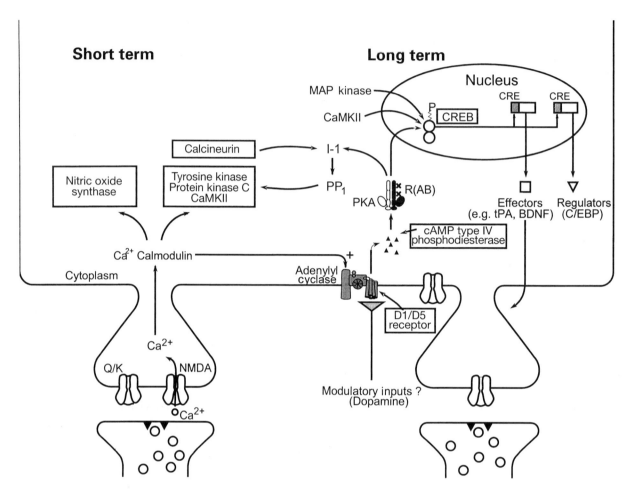

Fig. 6.2. Molecular mechanisms of synaptic plasticity. Studies of long-term potentiation in the hippocampus have revealed the signaling pathways that mediate changes in synaptic strength. Activation of the NMDA type of glutamate receptor leads to calcium influx and the activation of calcium sensitive enzymes such as CaMKII, PKC and calcineurin. Other signaling pathways involved in the early phase of LTP include tyrosine kinases and nitric oxide synthase, which may give rise to a retrograde messenger in the form of the diffusible gas NO. Long-term changes in synaptic strength result from the activation of adenylyl cyclase by calcium or modulatory neurotransmitters that stimulate G protein coupled receptors. This activation of adenylyl cyclase leads to the synthesis of the second messenger cAMP, which, in turn, activates PKA. PKA plays a central role in initiating the events that lead to long-lasting changes in synaptic strength by acting on a variety of targets, including the transcription factor CREB. CREB, which is also the target of other kinases such as CaMKIV and MAP kinase, turns on a variety of effector and regulatory genes whose gene products include tPA and BDNF. (Adapted with permission from Abel et al., 1997.)

common underlying molecular mechanisms mediated by intracellular signal transduction cascades (Girault and Greengard, 1999). The responses of a neuron to neurotransmitters or neuromodulators, or to neural injury are mediated by intracellular signal transduction pathways that include a large variety of protein kinases, protein phosphatases and adapter molecules (Fig. 6.2). Kinases play a particularly important role in signalling cascades that respond to alterations in synaptic input. These kinases include tyrosine kinase receptors that are activated by the binding of a growth factor or a neurotrophic factor such as

BDNF or NGF, as well as cytoplasmic Src family tyrosine kinases, such as Fyn. In other cases, serine/threonine kinases, such as protein kinase A (PKA) or protein kinase C (PKC), may be activated by second messenger molecules, such as cAMP or IP_3, respectively. These second messengers are formed when a neurotransmitter (e.g. norepinephrine or dopamine) or hormone (e.g. insulin) binds to a receptor that is linked by a GTP-binding-protein. These G proteins activate enzymes such as adenylyl cyclase or phospholipase C, thus leading to the production of cAMP or IP_3. Calcium is another second messenger molecule that activates calcium-dependent enzymes, including certain isoforms of adenylyl cyclase and PKC. Once kinases are activated, they modulate the activity of a number of target proteins ranging from ion channels to metabolic enzymes to transcription factors. These transcription factors are potentially important candidates to mediate long-term changes in neural function that might occur following injury and during the recovery from neural injury. Transcription factors bind to DNA and regulate the expression of one or more genes, whose protein products may mediate long-term changes in the physiology and structure of the neuron, including processes such as programmed cell death (apoptosis), increased synthesis and release of neurotransmitter, or the sprouting of extra branches by spared axons.

Although we will consider physiological and anatomical plasticity in separate sections, it is worth noting that there has been a convergence of these two processes in recent years (Squire & Kandel, 1999). Kandel's work on the mollusk *Aplysia* has revealed that long-term memory for sensitization is accompanied by the increased strength of particular synaptic connections as well as the growth of new synaptic connections between neurons mediating the reflex that has undergone sensitization (Abel & Kandel, 1998). These long-term changes in behaviour, neural anatomy and synaptic function are mediated by the activation of genes containing cAMP response elements (CRE) through the phosphorylation of the transcription factor CRE-binding protein (CREB). A critical challenge is to see if such transcription-mediated changes in neural function and structure underlie the recovery from neural injury.

Long-term potentiation

Synaptic plasticity, the use-dependent change in the strength of neuronal connections in the brain, is thought to underlie memory storage and may play a crucial role in a variety of neurological and mental disorders, including Alzheimer's disease, mental retardation, epilepsy and depression. During recovery following neural injury, the changed pattern of activity in the remaining synaptic connections may alter the strength of these connections and perhaps contribute to recovery. Repeated high frequency stimulation of excitatory glutamatergic pathways to the pyramidal cells of the CA1 region of hippocampus results in a large increase in synaptic efficacy of those pathways that may last hours or even days, a phenomenon termed LTP (Martin et al., 2000). LTP has been observed in many locations in the brain, and the cellular mechanism may vary from location to location. Further, some synapses in the brain undergo long-term depression, depending on the pattern and intensity of stimulation (Linden & Connor, 1995). Our discussion will focus on LTP in the CA1 region of the hippocampus because of the extensive knowledge of the signal transduction mechanisms that mediate this form of synaptic plasticity (Fig. 6.2). This form of LTP depends critically on the NMDA subtype of glutamate receptor, a receptor that serves as a 'coincidence detector' because it is activated in response to both neurotransmitter and membrane depolarization. Once activated, the NMDA receptor is permeant to calcium, and thus calcium is a critical second messenger mediating LTP in hippocampal area CA1.

Genetically modified mice have been particularly useful in the study of the molecular basis of hippocampal LTP. The analysis of genetically modified mice provides a way to test whether a particular gene product is important for synaptic plasticity and provides a useful bridge between molecules and synaptic plasticity, on the one hand, and systems of neurons and behaviour, on the other. Many of these studies have focused on an early, transient phase of LTP (E-LTP) that lasts 1 to 2 hours in hippocampal slices. These studies have shown that genetic manipulation of any one of several kinases, including calcium/calmodulin-dependent protein kinase II (CaMKII) and fyn, interferes with E-LTP, and also often results in impaired short-term memory (Fig. 6.2; Martin et al., 2000). The influx of calcium that occurs during the induction of LTP also appears to result in the creation of a retrograde chemical signal directed back to the presynaptic terminal, where it may regulate neurotransmitter release. The nature of the retrograde signal is not known, but both nitric oxide and carbon monoxide have been suggested as candidate retrograde signals (Zhuo et al., 1999).

The study of amnesic patients and experimental animals has revealed, however, that the role of the hippocampus in memory storage extends from weeks to months (Squire & Alvarez, 1995), suggesting that longer lasting forms of hippocampal synaptic plasticity may be required. LTP in the CA1 region of hippocampal slices, like many other forms of synaptic plasticity and memory, has distinct temporal phases (Huang et al., 1996). In contrast to E-LTP, the late phase of LTP (L-LTP) lasts for up to 8 hours in hippocampal slices and for days in the intact animal. Long-term memory storage is sensitive to disruption by inhibitors of protein synthesis, and L-LTP in the CA1 region of hippocampal slices, unlike E-LTP, shares with long-term memory a requirement for translation and transcription (Huang et al., 1996; Silva et al., 1998).

Although extensive information is available about E-LTP and its relation to behaviour, less is known about L-LTP. Pharmacological experiments have suggested that PKA plays a critical role in L-LTP (Fig. 6.2) (Huang et al., 1996). One of the nuclear targets of PKA is CREB, and CRE-mediated gene expression is induced in response to stimuli that generate L-LTP and long-term memory. Behavioural studies of mice lacking the α and Δ isoforms of CREB have suggested that this transcription factor plays a role in long-term memory storage (Silva et al., 1998). The deficits in long-lasting forms of LTP and in long-term memory observed in transgenic mice with alterations in PKA suggest that this signal transduction pathway plays a role in initiating the molecular events leading to long-lasting changes in neuronal function in mammals (Abel et al., 1997). The importance of the cAMP/PKA pathway is further underscored by recent work examining mutant mice lacking calcium/calmodulin activated isoforms of adenylyl cyclases, AC1 and AC8 (Wong et al., 1999). These mutant mice exhibit deficits in long-lasting forms of LTP and in long-term memory that are strikingly similar to those observed in the R(AB) transgenics.

Alterations in the subunit composition of NMDA receptors in the hippocampus can also modulate synaptic strength and hippocampal function. This is shown by the study of mice overexpressing the 2B subtype of NMDA receptor (Tang et al., 1999). In these transgenic mice, the NMDAR2B subunit is expressed in neurons within the forebrain using the CaMKIIα promoter, resulting in increased activation of the NMDA receptor and increased long-term potentiation. These mice also exhibit increased performance on a number of behavioural tasks. This study has received much attention, both in the scientific literature and in the popular press and it would seem to suggest that the 2B subunit of the NMDA receptor would be an interesting candidate for enhancing neuronal function.

Memory suppressor genes

The study of synaptic plasticity in a number of systems has revealed the existence of proteins that act as inhibitory constraints to block increases in synaptic strength and impede memory storage. These inhibitory constraints have been termed memory suppressor genes by analogy to tumour suppressor genes that restrict cell proliferation (Abel et al., 1998; Cardin & Abel, 1999). The study of memory suppressor genes is important not only for understanding the link between synaptic plasticity and learning, but also for identifying potential targets for future pharmaceuticals to treat memory disorders. In *Aplysia*, memory suppressor gene products act at each step in long-term facilitation: in the cytoplasm to regulate kinase activity, in the nucleus to alter the activity of transcriptional regula-

tory proteins, and on the cell surface to modulate cell–cell interactions. During long-term facilitation following serotonin treatment, the activity of PKA is constitutively enhanced as a result of the proteasome-mediated degradation of the regulatory subunit of PKA. A cell adhesion molecule, apCAM, is internalized via a MAP kinase-mediated process thus allowing for defasiculation and synaptic growth. In the nucleus, a transcriptional repressor, CREB-2, is inactivated, thus enabling the induced expression of a number of effector genes.

One potential memory suppressor gene product in mammalian systems is cAMP phosphodiesterase. Rolipram, an inhibitor of type IV cAMP phosphodiesterase, induces persistent long-term potentiation in hippocampal area CA1 after a single tetanic train of stimulation, which normally gives rise to a transient potentiation in untreated slices (Barad et al., 1998). Behaviourally, rolipram treatment prior to training increased long-term memory for contextual fear conditioning, without altering short-term memory. Further, rolipram is able to overcome the deficits in synaptic plasticity and spatial memory that are observed with aging in rodents (Bach et al., 1999). Thus, memory suppressor genes may be particularly attractive targets for therapies designed to enhance neural function.

Denervation supersensitivity

Following the loss of a synaptic input, a neuron generally becomes more responsive to that transmitter, a phenomenon termed 'denervation supersensitivity'. This supersensitivity is usually specific to the neurotransmitter at that synapse. At the neuromuscular junction, an increase in the number of extrajunctional acetylcholine receptors is observed due to loss of electrical activity in the muscle (Lomo & Rosenthal, 1972). In the CNS, the depletion of dopamine in the nigra-striatal tract results in supersensitivity to dopamine in the basal ganglia (Rioux et al., 1991). A similar receptor hyperactivity has been observed in some patients with Parkinson's disease and this may explain some of the dyskinesias observed after chronic L-dopa treatment of Parkinson's disease patients (Nguyen et al., 2000). Such changes in receptor responsiveness may also play a role in the response of schizophrenics to neuroleptics (Seeman & Van Tol, 1995). The upregulation of receptors or the signal transduction pathways that they activate may also be the basis for the behavioural changes induced by chronic exposure to drugs of abuse such as cocaine or morphine (Nestler, 1997). Denervation supersensitivity appears to be a widespread phenomenon seen in many neurotransmitter and neuromodulator systems. Thus, it may play a role in the response to injury and the subsequent recovery of function. Such supersensitivity of α-adrenergic receptors in peripheral nociceptors has been proposed as a mechanism for the causalgic pain that follows partial nerve injuries (Perl, 1999). Whether supersensitivity plays a role in the hyper-reflexia or functional recovery seen after partial spinal cord injury represents an important direction of future research.

Anatomical plasticity

Some of the molecular mechanisms of neural plasticity result in changes of neuron structure, such as axonal sprouting and dendritic remodelling. These changes are important, not only because they have functional consequences; they may represent a potential for more profound regenerative responses.

Collateral sprouting

Ideally, injured axons would regenerate towards their appropriate targets and form functional synapses, thereby restoring the connection severed by the lesion. This type of regeneration is seen in the CNS of amphibia, fish and lampreys (Cohen et al., 1998), but is not seen in birds and mammals. However, during development and during regeneration of peripheral nerve, the sprouting of collateral branches of axons plays an important role in the establishment and refinement of neuronal circuitry. This sprouting occurs when new motile structures, filopodia and lamellae, form along previously quiescent regions of the axon. In the peripheral nervous system (PNS), partial denervation of muscle is followed by sprouting of neurites from neighbouring spared axons and reinnervation of the denervated muscle fibres by the sprouts (Brown et al., 1981). Collateral sprouting is different in several ways from regenerative growth. First, collateral sprouting occurs from unlesioned axon fibres near the lesioned axons. Secondly, collateral sprouting occurs close to the denervated target cells, so axon fibres do not have to extend over long distances. In this way, collateral sprouting in response to injury is similar to the terminal branching that occurs near the target region during development. Thirdly, the regions near targets are often less myelinated and thus provide less impedance to axon elongation. As discussed below, myelin associated neurite growth inhibitors appear to be present in the CNS. Thus collateral sprouting is increased in rats in which myelination has been suppressed by neonatal X-irradiation (Schwegler et al., 1995). Fourthly, at the neuromuscular junction, Schwann cells that cap degenerated nerve terminals send out processes to adjacent neuromus-

cular junctions that may also serve to guide sprouts to the denervated muscle and thus help establish a new neuromuscular junction (Son et al., 1996).

Collateral sprouting has been observed in the spinal cord (Liu & Chambers, 1958) and in several locations within the brain, including the septal nucleus, the CA3 region of hippocampus and the dentate gyrus, where it has been studied most extensively. Entorhinal cortical lesions result in sprouting of as much as 2–3 mm within the contralateral entorhinal cortical projection to the dentate gyrus (Steward et al., 1974). Sprouting of the mossy fibre projection from the dentate gyrus to hippocampal area CA3 has been observed following electroconvulsive, pharmacological or kindling induced seizures (McKinney et al., 1997).

The functional role of sprouting remains unclear. In the spinal cord, the time course of sprouting correlates with the development of hyper-reflexia and increased muscle tone following spinal transection, suggesting that sprouting might be of functional benefit in spinal cord injured animals by enhancing their ability to support their weight (Goldberger & Murray, 1974; Murray & Goldberger, 1974). Sprouting in the spinal cord after peripheral nerve lesions may also underlie chronic pain conditions. Here, sprouting often involves the expansion of axons into inappropriate target areas, perhaps leading to severe pain syndromes because sprouting axons derive from low threshold mechanoreceptors (Woolf & Doubell, 1994). In the hippocampus, mossy fibre sprouting develops in parallel with recurrent seizures. It has been suggested that sprouting contributes to post-traumatic epileptogenesis in the hippocampus by eliciting 'reactive synaptogenesis', which may contribute to the formation of a functional excitatory feedback circuit (McKinney et al., 1997). Alternatively, sprouting might be protective against seizures as a result of sprouting mossy fibres synapsing onto inhibitory interneurons.

The molecular mechanisms underlying sprouting in the CNS are not known, but as at the neuromuscular junction, sprouting appears to involve interactions between cells in the region of axon terminal degeneration and the neighbouring spared axons. In addition to inhibitory proteins in myelin, the intrinsic growth potential of the axon also appears to be a determinant of the extent of axonal outgrowth. Axonal sprouting is increased in the peripheral and central nervous system in adult mice that overexpress the growth associated protein GAP-43 (Aigner et al., 1995). Moreover, the neurotrophins nerve growth factor (NGF) and brain derived neurotrophic factor (BDNF) are often up-regulated following seizures (Ernfors et al., 1991) and may provide a signal for collateral sprouting of mossy fibres (Patel & McNamara, 1995). Neurotrophins promote axon collateral formation in vivo, modulate growth cone morphology in culture and mediate developmental processes involving collateral sprouting (Cohen-Cory & Fraser, 1995). Further, neurotrophins produced by target tissues can modulate axon branching (Hoyle et al., 1993). During regeneration of DRG cell axons, NGF promotes the formation of collateral branches (Diamond et al., 1987). Neurotrophins act directly on the axon of DRG cells to promote the formation of collaterals (Gallo & Letourneau, 1998). This sprouting is mediated by the activation of actin-dependent motility via a phosphoinositide-3 kinase pathway initiated by the trk A receptor. Although neurotrophins can initiate and stabilize branching, other factors may be responsible for stabilizing collaterals and allowing them to mature (Bastmeyer & O'Leary, 1996).

Cell adhesion molecules (CAMs) may also regulate axon outgrowth and synapse formation. In *Aplysia*, long-term memory storage and long-term changes in synaptic strength are accompanied by increases in axonal branching and in the number of synaptic contacts (Abel et al., 1998). This is paralleled by a decrease in the levels of apCAM as a result of endocytosis of this molecule. This downregulation of apCAM suggests that cell adhesion molecules may normally act to block synaptic growth. Thus a CAM may act as a 'memory suppressor' gene product, normally inhibiting memory storage (Abel et al., 1998). The removal of these inhibitory constraints may provide a mechanism to enhance axon outgrowth and new synapse formation during memory storage and recovery from neural injury.

Dendritic remodelling

The loss of input to a postsynaptic neuron leads to changes in neuronal morphology, including the loss of dendritic spines, the simplification of the dendritic arbour and atrophy of the postsynaptic neuron, processes that are termed dendritic pruning. The mechanisms underlying this dendritic plasticity are unknown but changes in intracellular calcium may play a crucial role (Segal, 2001). Calcium may act to regulate protein synthesis within the spines because clusters of polyribosomes have been demonstrated associated with cysternae at the base of dendritic spines (Steward & Reeves, 1988). Denervation results in loss of these polyribosomes, whereas reinnervation is associated with their return (Steward & Fass, 1983). Thus synaptic activity localized to one spine could rapidly influence protein synthesis in that portion of dendrite and thereby affect the size, shape and function of the dendritic tree.

The communication between the dendritic spine, the dendrite itself and the soma are crucial issues. The dendritic spine is often thought of as a relatively isolated environment in which calcium can reach sufficient levels to activate intracellular signal transduction pathways, but this depends critically on spine head and spine neck geometry. Further, the activation of calcium release from intracellular stores can have dramatic effects on calcium levels throughout the cell, leading to the activation of transcriptional processes (Berridge, 1988). This complexity of calcium signalling may potentially explain the many contradictory findings in studies of dendritic morphology (Segal, 2001): at very low calcium levels, spines are eventually eliminated, moderate increases in calcium cause the elongation of spines and the formation of new ones and large increases in calcium, such as occur during trauma or an epileptic seizure, cause the shrinkage and collapse of spines.

A crucial issue is how new dendritic processes form in response to collateral sprouting and axonal outgrowth. The formation of new synapses has been observed after environmental enrichment, learning and long-term potentiation (Segal, 2001). Recent studies have used organotypic cultures of hippocampal slices combined with a local superfusion technique to restrict the site of LTP induction to a small dendritic region. Using two-photon laser scanning microscopy, three-dimensional images of the postsynaptic neuron can be obtained. In these studies, new spines are observed on the postsynaptic dendrite of the CA1 pyramidal cell after the induction of long-term synaptic potentiation (Engert & Bonhoeffer, 1999). No changes in dendritic morphology are observed after short-lasting potentiation or in control regions that were not potentiated. Are such newly formed dendritic spines functional? This is a difficult and important question. Quantal analysis of synaptic transmission does suggest that cAMP-induced long-lasting forms of LTP are accompanied by an increase in the number of quanta released in response to a single presynaptic action potential (Bolshakov et al., 1997). This increase may be due to an increase in the number of sites of synaptic transmission, an idea supported by studies using the fluorescent dye FM 1–43, which suggest that cAMP-induced synaptic potentiation is accompanied by an increase in the number of active presynaptic terminals (Ma et al., 1999).

Although much of the discussion of anatomical plasticity has focused on morphological changes in axonal arbourization or dendritic spines, it is important to note that molecular changes can make previously 'silent' (or, perhaps more precisely, 'deaf') synapses functional. Studies of LTP in hippocampal area CA1 have revealed intracellular trafficking processes in the postsynaptic neuron by which AMPA receptors are rapidly redistributed after NMDA receptor activation (Shi et al., 1999). The redistribution of AMPA receptors provides a striking mechanism by which synapses may be strengthened.

Therapeutic approaches to recovery

In order to promote recovery from neural injury, it is necessary to optimize the nervous system's own adaptive responses as well as to intervene in those mechanisms that inhibit full neurophysiological restoration. Promising approaches include: (i) teaching patients adaptive behaviours; (ii) harnessing the physiological plasticity of the CNS through cutting edge physical therapies; (iii) promoting regeneration of axons by neutralizing environmental inhibitory influences, upregulating the intraneuronal molecular regeneration program and supplying growth promoting factors; (iv) replacing lost neurons. By using one or a combination of these approaches, researchers have already made progress in eliciting functional recovery in animals, and even in some human patients.

Behavioural adaptation (occupational therapy)

The field of occupational therapy is targeted toward promoting recovery of vocational, recreational and self-care functions by teaching patients adaptive strategies to substitute for lost physiologic functions. The focus is mostly on upper extremity and cognitive/perceptual functions. For example, a person with a homonymous hemianopia can be taught to scan the written page to be certain that she is not ignoring written material on the hemianopic side. Much of conventional practice in occupational therapy has been based on common empirical experience, *a priori* reasoning and theories that have not been subjected to controlled clinical trials. Increasingly, the practices in the field are coming under experimental test. In any case, there is little doubt that retraining of patients with neurological injuries and diseases, by any number of strategies, results in significant functional improvement (Cheung & Broman, 2000). A generalization that can be drawn from a variety of studies is that functional improvement is most likely to occur when the training is task specific. Thus, relearning words after an aphasic injury requires that the words to be learned be repeated. Learning one word has little effect on the ability to learn another word. Similarly, the effect of exercise in improving a particular function is greatest when the exercise task closely resembles the function (Kwakkel et al., 1999; Taub et al., 1999).

Physical therapies

Conventional practice methods

Although there is considerable overlap in the potential roles of occupational therapists and physical therapists in the rehabilitation of patients with neurological impairments, physical therapists tend to be concerned more with issues of gait retraining, strengthening and cardiovascular conditioning. Thus they more often address lower extremity functions than upper extremity functions or cognition. The comments made above regarding occupational therapy are also true for the therapist-assisted, staged retraining of gait following stroke, spinal cord injury and other CNS injuries using parallel bars, walkers, canes and braces. However, specific types of training targeted at inducing plastic changes in the motor output warrant special consideration.

Constraint-induced forced use

In an attempt to test the theory that learned non-use contributes to upper limb disability in stroke patients, Ostendorf and Wolf constrained the unaffected left arm in a sling in a patient 18 months after a right hemiplegic stroke, forcing her to use the affected right arm (Ostendorf & Wolf, 1981). During a 1-week trial, there was no change in the function of the restrained arm but the patient used the affected arm more frequently and more effectively. Subsequently, several studies of patients with chronic hemiparesis due to stroke or head trauma confirmed that constraint-induced, forced use of the impaired arm for a period of 2 weeks or less results in functional improvement of that arm for many months (Miltner et al., 1999; Wolf et al., 1989). A recent randomized, single blind, controlled study of constraint-induced forced use vs. conventional rehabilitation was carried out on 20 patients within 14 days of an ischemic stroke (Dromerick et al., 2000). Measurements during acute inpatient rehabilitation suggested that the constraint technique provides improved recovery on some tests of arm function. How this would affect long-term recovery remains to be determined. Electrophysiological studies have shown that forced use of the limb results in long-lasting plastic changes in the CNS. In four hemiparetic stroke patients, movement-related cortical potentials before and immediately after training and at 3 months follow-up suggested that movement of the affected hand was associated with activation not only of the contralateral hemisphere but also the ipsilateral hemisphere in the absence of mirror movements of the unaffected hand (Kopp et al., 1999). By contrast, TMS before and after a 12-day-period of constraint-induced movement therapy in 13 chronic stroke patients showed an increase in the motor representation of the test muscle on the affected side and a displacement of the center of the motor output area of that muscle to adjacent cortex (Liepert et al., 2000). As with the changes seen in functional imaging of recovery from stroke, the significance of the shifts, particularly the activation of cortex ipsilateral to the affected arm, is not clear. However, these studies do suggest that functional recovery by application of constraint-induced forced use of a paretic limb is associated with electrophysiological evidence of cortical plasticity.

Partial body weight supported treadmill training

The spinal cord of all vertebrates studied thus far contains intrinsic circuitry, called central pattern generators (CPGs), that produce rhythmic locomotor efferent discharges to synergistic groups of muscles (Cazalets et al., 1995; Grillner, 1975). There is evidence that the spinal CPG is subject to experience-induced plastic changes, i.e. the spinal cord is capable of a form of learning that is now under investigation as a possible means by which impaired locomotion due to stroke or spinal cord injury may be improved (Dobkin, 1999). Experiments in thoracic spinal transected cats indicated that treadmill training with early support of the hindlimbs could permit the animals to develop rhythmic stepping of the previously paralysed hindlimbs, and eventually to do so while supporting their own weight (Barbeau & Rossignol, 1987; Lovely et al., 1986). Although the hindlimb stepping was not coordinated with that of the forelimbs, the hindlimb stepping persisted for 6 weeks after cessation of training, declining by 12 weeks (De Leon et al., 1999a). Retraining resulted in an accelerated acquisition of full weight-bearing stepping. These observations suggest that the spinal cord pattern generator for locomotion is subject to a form of learning. Of interest, training for weight bearing caused a loss of previously attained ability to step. This loss could be reversed immediately by strychnine, suggesting a role for glycinergic inhibition in the ability of locomotor circuits to interpret sensory input to drive stepping (De Leon et al., 1999b).

There is also EMG and visual observation evidence for spinal cord rhythmic motor output in paralysed humans (Bussel et al., 1996; Calancie et al., 1994), suggesting that a locomotor central pattern generator exists in the human lumbosacral enlargement. As in animals, the human pattern generator appears to be subject to modulation by sensory input (Harkema et al., 1997). If so, then the human pattern generating circuitry might also be subject to use-dependent and pharmacological enhancement (Fung et al., 1990). Given the widespread acceptance of the principle of task-specific training, a difficulty with attempting to retrain the central pattern generator in paralysed patients is that weakness in patients' antigravity muscles prevents them from practising the task (locomotion) that is to be recovered. In order to get around this problem patients have been placed in harnesses that partially support their weight, permitting them to practise locomotion on a treadmill. Preliminary clinical trials have suggested that such training can enhance recovery in chronic and acute patients with incomplete spinal cord injury (Dietz et al., 1995; Gazzani et al., 1999; Wernig et al., 1995) and hemiparetic stroke (Hesse et al., 1995; Visintin et al., 1998). In one follow-up study on spinal cord injured patients, improvement persisted for 6 months to 6 years (Wernig et al., 1998). While promising, all these studies have been limited in some degree by small sample size, lack of prospective design, non-randomization of controls, lack of blinding in outcomes measurements or non-uniformity of rehabilitation protocol, including time of intervention after injury (for critical review, see Dobkin, 1999). An NIH-supported, prospective, randomized, multicenter trial of body weight supported treadmill training in spinal cord injured patients is currently under way (Dobkin, 1999).

Promotion of regeneration

Although there is great promise in approaches that harness the endogenous plasticity of the CNS, maximal recovery will require reconstitution of lost neuronal connections. The peripheral and central nervous systems both show evidence for regenerative potential but they have different strengths and limitations in this regard.

Spontaneous axonal regeneration in PNS

Wallerian degeneration
Injury to peripheral nerve results in variable effectiveness of regeneration, depending on the type of injury, the distance from the perikaryon and the distance from the target. Proximal lesions result in faster regeneration (3–6 mm/day) than distal lesions (1 mm/day; reviewed in Selzer, 1987). When an axon is interrupted by physical trauma, a process called 'Wallerian degeneration' ensues (Scherer & Salzer, 2001). This consists of breakdown of the axon distal to the lesion, and the separation of myelin sheaths at the incisures of Schmidt–Lanterman into ovoids that are phagocytosed primarily by macrophages that invade the degenerating nerve. Schwann cells also participate in the phagocytosis and proliferate within the denervated connective tissue sheath, forming linear arrays called 'bands of Büngner'. The molecular signals that trigger the Schwann cell proliferation are not known, but

correlative data suggest involvement of neuregulin-1, a constituent of axons that is a potent Schwann cell mitogen in vitro. Denervated Schwann cells express a receptor for neuregulin 1, consisting of a heterodimer of ErbB2/ErbB3. During Schwann cell proliferation, ErbB2 is activated by phosphorylation (Kwon et al., 1997).

The degenerated distal nerve stump supports regeneration

The bands of Büngner form a particularly fertile environment for regeneration of the peripheral axons. This appears to be due to a combination of complex factors including the nature of the basal lamina sheath, which includes extracellular matrix molecules such as laminin-2, fibronectin and type IV collagen and several others that are excellent substrates for axon elongation in vitro (Fu & Gordon, 1997). Denervated Schwann cells contribute importantly to the regenerative ability of peripheral nerve fibres by synthesizing these extracellular matrix molecules and a variety of cell adhesion molecules, including the Ig-like cell adhesion molecules (CAMs) N-CAM, P_0, L1 and MAG. The axon binds to extracellular matrix molecules by expressing a family of heterodimeric receptors called integrins, which connect the extracellular matrix molecules to the axon cytoskeleton (Helmke et al., 1998; Schmidt et al., 1995) and may mediate activation of intracellular signaling cascades, as suggested primarily by studies in non-neuronal cells (Boudreau & Jones, 1999; Clark & Brugge, 1995). However, the axon growth cone appears to grow along Schwann cells in preference to the basal lamina, when given a choice in vitro (reviewed by Martini, 1994). As with extracellular matrix molecules, CAMs not only provide an adhesive surface for axons to grow along, but also mediate the activation of intracellular signalling pathways (Walsh et al., 1997). In this way, the extracellular matrix and cell adhesion molecules synthesized by denervated Schwann cells may contribute to the elongation and navigation of growing axon tips during regeneration. These conclusions are based primarily on studies of embryonic neurons growing in vitro. The degree to which they apply to regeneration of peripheral nerve in vivo is not clear.

Denervated Schwann cells, together with macrophages and fibroblasts in the denervated nerve, also manufacture a variety of trophic molecules and their receptors, many of which appear to be important for both axonal regeneration and Schwann cell proliferation. Among these factors are the neurotrophins NGF, BDNF, neurotrophin 3 (NT-3) and NT-4, transforming growth factors β (TGF-βs), glial cell line derived neurotrophic factors (GDNFs), the cytokines ciliary neurotrophic factor (CNTF), leukemia inhibitory factor (LIF), interleukin 6 (IL-6), and the insulin-like growth factors (IGFs) and fibroblast growth factors (FGFs). Their possible role in regeneration of peripheral nerve has recently been reviewed (Scherer & Salzer, 2001).

Specificity of regeneration

Although the precise roles of all of these molecules in regeneration are not known, the denervated distal stump of injured peripheral nerve provides an especially welcoming environment for regenerating axons to grow in. Yet, many injuries to peripheral nerve are not followed by regeneration that is adequate to result in satisfactory functional recovery. The distance of regeneration might be further enhanced by the application of extrinsic trophic factors but the main reason for incomplete functional restoration is that the degree to which regenerating axons find their correct targets is limited (Lee & Farel, 1988; Scherer, 1986). The anasthomotic fascicular structure of peripheral nerve is such that the individual axons of a severed nerve do not regenerate to their original destinations unless they find their original endoneurial tubes. Even if the fascicles are matched perfectly by microsurgical repair, the preponderance of experimental evidence (Aldskogius et al., 1987) and clinical experience has indicated that the specificity of reinnervation is still limited. The further the injury from the target, the greater the number of nerve branches the regenerating axons might enter and the more likely that a mismatch will occur between the axon and its eventual target. On the other hand, when the axon is interrupted by a compressive injury that does not interrupt the Schwann cell basal lamina endoneurial sheath, the nerve can regenerate along its original path and innervate its original muscle or sensory target (Brown & Hardman, 1987; Selzer, 1987).

Despite the above observations of inaccuracy in regeneration of severed peripheral nerve, more recent studies suggest that a certain degree of specificity does occur. In tadpoles before the Schwann cells have elaborated a basal lamina tube, severed motor axons tended to reinnervate their correct muscles selectively. It is only after a basal lamina tube is formed that axons are forced to innervate incorrect muscles if the axons enter an incorrect tube (Meeker & Farel, 1993). In neonatal but not adult rats, transection of facial nerve is followed by selective reinnervation of correct muscles (Aldskogius & Thomander, 1986). Even in adult rats, transected nerves reinnervate portions of the serratus anterior and diaphragm muscles in a somatotopically correct, though imperfect way (Laskowski & Sanes, 1988). This positional selectivity may involve the expression of ephrins by muscle fibres (and presumably complementary receptors on the motor axons) (Feng et al., 2000) and competition among regenerating axons for correct synaptic targets (Laskowski et al., 1998). Thus, in some circumstances, synaptic competition and pruning of incorrectly regenerated axons may compensate for randomness in reinnervation of Schwann cell tubes. A form of secondary pruning also accounts for selective reinnervation of motor and sensory branches by motor and sensory axons respectively, during regeneration of severed rat femoral nerve (Brushart et al., 1998; Madison et al., 1996). Unlike the selectivity in the reinnervation of the serratus anterior, the selectivity of motor vs. sensory nerve reinnervation appears to involve guidance signals associated with the Schwann cells (Martini, 1994). Unfortunately, the specificity in regeneration of some peripheral nerve axons is not absolute but reflects statistical trends that still are not robust enough to result in functional recovery in most cases.

Spontaneous axonal regeneration in CNS

By contrast with the PNS, regeneration is quantitatively much less successful. Paradoxically, where regeneration does occur, it appears much more specific. Thus if ways can be found to enhance the probability and distance of regeneration in CNS, sufficient specificity in pathway selection and synapse formation would occur that the regeneration would yield functional recovery. Some of the molecular mechanisms that block regeneration in CNS and also contribute to its specificity are summarized below. For additional details, see Chapter 47 by J. McDonald.

Extracellular determinants

Growth cone collapsing factors

During regeneration, axons come in contact with molecules in their environment that inhibit their growth. An understanding of this phenomenon requires an understanding of the mechanisms of axon elongation.

Mechanisms of axon growth in the regenerating CNS

The leading edge of axons belonging to embryonic or invertebrate neurons grown on conventional adhesive substrates such as laminin or polo-L-lysine takes the form of a specialized structure, the 'growth cone' (Gordon-Weeks, 1989; Lankford et al., 1990; Lin et al., 1994; Rivas et al., 1992). The proximal flattened portion of the growth cone is the 'lamellipodium', which contains microtubules and short actin and myosin filaments in a relatively disorganized orientation. Extending along the leading edge of the lamellipodium are fine projections called 'filopodia'. These contain bundles of fibrous actin (f-actin) microfila-

ments and elongate on the extracellular matrix through target activated polymerization of the actin filaments at their distal end (Lin & Forscher, 1993). The elongation of filopodia translates into tension on the more proximal growth cone by actin-myosin linkages to the microtubules (Lin et al., 1996). This results in the rapid (1–3 mm/day) growth that characterizes early embryonic development. While much of the thinking about mechanisms underlying axon regeneration assumes that this mechanism obtains in axonal regeneration in the mature CNS, work in the lamprey suggests that this may not be true (Conti & Selzer, 2000). In this species, the growth cones of cut spinal cord axons lack filopodia (Lurie et al., 1994), have little f-actin (Hall et al., 1997) and regenerate more slowly (Yin & Selzer, 1983) than vertebrate and invertebrate embryonic axons. Observations on the morphology and cytoskeletal contents of growth cones regenerating in the CNS of mammals and other vertebrates in vivo have been scant. Thus it is not known whether the differences between regenerating lamprey growth cones and growth cones of embryonic neurons are due to species differences or to differences between axon development and regeneration.

Myelin associated growth inhibitors

Cells in the mature CNS express several molecules that inhibit axon growth in tissue culture by causing collapse of the growth cone. Because most knowledge concerning axon elongation has been derived from studies in vitro, work on the molecular mechanisms involved in growth inhibition have usually employed tissue culture assays. Perhaps most well known of these growth inhibitors was described by Caroni and Schwab (1988a, b), who observed that neurons can grow long processes when cultured on peripheral myelin fractions but not on fractions of CNS myelin. They identified two molecules with MW 35 000 and 250 000 (NI-35/NI-250) on the surfaces of oligodendrocytes, but not Schwann cells, that cause growth cones to collapse on contact (Caroni & Schwab, 1988b). Both molecules were bound by a single mAb, IN-1 (Caroni & Schwab, 1988a). These molecules appear to cause growth cone collapse by activating a G protein (Igarashi et al., 1993) and releasing calcium from intracellular stores (Bandtlow et al., 1993). The excess calcium might activate breakdown of microtubules and actin microfilaments and thus turn off growth cone motility. For years, the identities of NI-35/250 remained a mystery. However, similar molecules have now been sequenced from rats (Chen et al., 2000) and humans (GrandPre et al., 2000) and renamed 'Nogo'. Three members of the Nogo family have been identified, of which Nogo A appears to be the one responsible for the oligodendrite associated growth inhibition (Chen et al., 2000). Several lines of in vivo experimentation suggest that neutralizing Nogo with IN-1 can enhance the regenerative capacity of CNS axons but the role of Nogo as the main cause of regenerative failure in the CNS is still debated (see below and Chapter 47 by McDonald).

Myelin-associated glycoprotein (MAG) has also been shown to have neurite outgrowth inhibiting and growth cone collapsing activity in vitro (McKerracher et al., 1994; Mukhopadhyay et al., 1994). This activity can be overcome by prior administration of neurotrophins or dibutyryl cAMP, which is elevated by neurotrophins (Cai et al., 1999). It has been suggested that in the presence of appropriate neurotrophins, cAMP levels in neurons are elevated, activating PKA, which blocks subsequent inhibition of regeneration. MAG activates a Gai protein, which blocks increases in cAMP, thus voiding the neurotrophin effect (Cai et al., 1999). The significance of MAG for regeneration in vivo has been questioned because axon outgrowth was not better on CNS myelin of MAG-deficient mice than on myelin of wild-type mice (Bartsch et al., 1995).

Two chondroitin sulfate proteoglycans, each having neurite growth inhibiting properties, have been demonstrated on the surfaces of bovine spinal cord oligodendrocytes (Niederost et al., 1999). Treatment with beta-xylosides, which inhibited synthesis of both proteoglycans, reversed the growth cone collapse seen during encounters of neurites with oligodendrocytes. Since chondroitin sulfate proteoglycans had previously been suggested to be inhibitors of regeneration associated with glial scars (Bovolenta et al., 1997) (see below), these molecules might also account for part of the regeneration inhibiting effect of CNS myelin.

Another molecule that has neurite growth inhibiting properties in vitro and is produced by oligodendrocytes is tenascin-R. In the salamander, optic nerves regenerate after they are cut, even though the myelinated optic nerve contains tenascin-R and retinal ganglion cells of salamander do not grow on a surface of tenascin-R in vitro. This may be explained by the disappearance of myelin, MAG and tenascin-R from the optic nerve by phagocytosing cells within 8 days after transection (Becker et al., 1999). In rats, optic nerves do not regenerate and tenascin-R is not removed after optic nerve transection (Becker et al., 2000). Thus tenascin-R may be a significant inhibitor of axonal regeneration in CNS, but thus far the evidence is only correlational.

It is not clear how universal the inhibitory effect of oligodendrocytes is. Contact with oligodendrocytes in vitro inhibited the growth of dorsal root ganglion (DRG) cell axons but not those of retinal cells (Kobayashi et al., 1995). Growth cone collapsing activities require not only the presence of an inhibitory molecule but also the presence of receptors on the surfaces of susceptible neurons. It is assumed that axons grow readily during embryogenesis because the late development of myelin delays contact with myelin-associated growth inhibitors. However, embryonic neurons from hippocampus, neocortex and superior colliculus were able to grow long axons when transplanted by atraumatic microinjection into various white matter tracts in the adult mouse (Davies et al., 1994). This may reflect an absence in these immature neurons of receptors for myelin-associated inhibitory molecules. On the other hand, myelin-associated growth inhibitors might not be as potent when encountered by growing axons in vivo as in vitro and other molecules normally introduced at the site of injury might be more important (Davies et al., 1997).

Neuron-associated growth inhibitors
Growth cone collapsing activity is also associated with neuronal membranes (Kapfhammer & Raper, 1987). Axons from the nasal side of the developing retina grow selectively to the posterior part of the optic tectum, while temporal retinal axons grow to the anterior tectum. This is due to a growth cone collapsing activity on cell membranes from the posterior tectum that act only on temporal but not nasal retinal axons (Cox et al., 1990). This is now ascribed to the interaction between ephrins on the surfaces of posterior tectal membranes and Eph receptors on the surfaces of growth cones of temporal retinal neurons (Ciossek et al., 1998). Ephrin signalling may also be involved in the development of the spinal cord (Yue et al., 1999). Re-expression of Eph B3 after spinal cord injury (Miranda et al., 1999) suggests the possibility that ephrin signalling may inhibit regeneration of some spinal cord axons (see section on Specificity of Regeneration below). Similarly, the persistence of netrins and their chemorepellent receptor molecule UNC-5 in the CNS of postembryonic animals suggests that netrin may act as a chemorepellent to some growth cones during regeneration (Shifman & Selzer, 2000).

Astrocyte-derived extracellular matrix molecules
It was long assumed that axons did not regenerate through an astrocytic injury scar because of the scar's hard consistency and other mechanical features. However, although membrane fractions from grey matter support axon growth in vitro, membrane fractions from astrocytic scars do not (Bovolenta et al., 1993). This growth-inhibiting activity appears to be associated with one or more cell surface sulfated glycoproteins, especially chondroitin sulfate proteoglycans. Secretion of proteoglycans by reactive astrocytes is

one proposed mechanism by which the glial scar inhibits axonal regeneration in the CNS (McKeon et al., 1991). Thus adult DRG cells grew long processes when microinjected atraumatically into spinal cord white matter (Davies et al., 1997). In a few cases, the injection was traumatic enough to activate secretion of proteoglycans, and this was associated with failure of axon growth. Such observations have suggested that CNS myelin is not significantly inhibitory to regeneration in vivo, but rather it is the proteoglycans secreted at the site of injury that inhibits regeneration. Until now, it has not been possible to repeat the microinjection experiments with adult neurons other than DRG cells.

Intraneuronal determinants

Within a species, the ability of axons to regenerate decreases with age. For example, spinal axons regenerate in tadpoles, but not in postmetamorphic frogs (Beattie et al., 1990; Clarke et al., 1986; Forehand & Farel, 1982). Fetal spinal cord transplants are more successful in restoring anatomic connectivity and locomotor function to a spinal cord injury when performed in neonatal mammals than in adults (Miya et al., 1997). Most explanations for the failure of regeneration in the mature CNS have focused on the delayed appearance of myelin and its growth inhibiting molecules discussed above. The importance of environmental causes for failure of regeneration may have been overemphasized as a result of the striking observations that some axons of mature CNS can regenerate into peripheral nerve grafts (David & Aguayo, 1981; Richardson et al., 1980; Vidal-Sanz et al., 1987). However, in these and subsequent experiments on retinal ganglion cells, environmental influences were insufficient to explain the decline in regenerative ability in postembryonic mammals. For example, only a minority of injured axons regenerate into peripheral nerve grafts (Villegas-Perez et al., 1988). This issue has been investigated in cocultures of retina and optic tectum in rat (Chen et al., 1995). Embryonic retinal cells were able to extend axons into adult tectum, but postnatal retinas were unable to send axons into embryonic tecta. Thus the age of the neuron rather than that of its host environment most influenced the regenerative ability of axons. Similar conclusions were drawn when cocultures of entorhinal cortex and hippocampus were used to test the influence of postnatal age on regeneration of the entorhino-dentate pathway of rats (Li et al., 1995). Perhaps the most convincing evidence for the importance of intraneuronal factors is the great heterogeneity in regenerative abilities of axons growing in the same part of the CNS in the same animal. Following spinal cord transection in the lamprey, identified reticulospinal

neurons vary greatly in their ability to regenerate through the same spinal cord environment (Davis & McClelland, 1994; Jacobs et al., 1997; Yin & Selzer, 1983). The same axons regenerated better following axotomy close to the perikaryon than more distally (Yin & Selzer, 1983). Similarly in the rat, supraspinal axons did not regenerate as well into peripheral nerve grafts inserted into the spinal cord at thoracic or lumbar levels as into cervical levels (Richardson et al., 1984). It is also well known that adult neurons are difficult to grow in culture in the absence of myelin and on the same substrates that support extensive survival and neurite outgrowth in embryonic neurons. Thus neuron intrinsic factors must contribute greatly to the limitations on regeneration in the CNS. Recent therapeutic approaches have attempted to enhance the intrinsic regenerative abilities of neurons through the use of supplemental trophic factors. Several examples of neuron intrinsic influences on regeneration and of the effects of trophic factors are reviewed below.

Conditioning lesion effects

A conditioning axotomy can accelerate regeneration after a second lesion (Lanners & Grafstein, 1980). Although environmental changes at the injury site may contribute, the conditioning lesion effect is attributed mainly to intracellular changes of the injured neuron (Lankford et al., 1998). That this is true can be deduced from experiments using DRG neurons, which have two processes originating from a unipolar axon. One process travels with the peripheral nerve and the second enters the spinal cord with the dorsal root. Injury of the peripheral process initiates a robust metabolic response that leads to regeneration. The regenerative response to injury of the central process in the dorsal root is weaker (Chong et al., 1994; Oblinger & Lasek, 1988). Although the axons regenerate within the dorsal root, they do not penetrate the spinal cord at the dorsal root entry zone (Liuzzi & Lasek, 1987; Pindzola et al., 1993). Nor do the central processes ascending in the dorsal columns regenerate after spinal cord injury. However, regeneration of the central processes of DRG cells can be enhanced by a preceding peripheral nerve injury that boosts the growth-associated metabolic response in the cell body (Neumann & Woolf, 1999; Richardson & Issa, 1984). The conditioning lesion may upregulate the expression of growth-associated genes and decrease the synthesis of receptors for inhibitory molecules within the spinal cord (for review see Chong et al., 1999).

GAP-43

An early strategy to identify molecules that may be important in regeneration was to look for proteins whose concentrations are greatly increased in neurons during regeneration of their axon. The best known of these proteins, growth-associated protein of 43 kDa (GAP-43), was discovered in the frog retina during regeneration of the optic nerve (Skene & Willard, 1981). GAP-43 is transported to the growth cone, where it is preferentially concentrated during development and synaptic remodelling (Goslin et al., 1988). Although the precise mechanism is still unknown, GAP-43 may mediate signal transduction for the reorganization of the cytoskeleton in growth cones and synaptic terminals in response to extrinsic stimuli (Igarashi et al., 1995) that activate axon growth and synaptic plasticity, e.g. LTP (Namgung et al., 1997). There is also correlative evidence for a role of GAP-43 in regeneration (Chong et al., 1996; Kobayashi et al., 1997; Ng et al., 1995; Schaden et al., 1994). Direct evidence for a role of GAP-43 in axon regeneration has been difficult to obtain, although a role in axon development has been fairly well supported. Some of the ambiguities concerning the role of GAP-43 in regeneration may ultimately be cleared up by recent studies suggesting that a second growth associated protein, CAP-23, acts in concert with GAP-43 in promoting subplasmalemmal accumulation of actin in the growth cone (Frey et al., 2000). Thus, although overexpressing GAP-43 alone does not enhance regeneration of DRG axons, coexpression of GAP-43 and CAP-23 in DRG cells resulted in enhanced process outgrowth in vitro and increased regeneration of DRG axons after spinal cord injury (Bomze et al., 2001).

Cytoskeletal proteins

The neuronal cytoskeleton consists of three major elements: (i) microtubules, molecularly complex structures that mediate axonal transport of molecules and organelles; (ii) microfilaments, f-actin strands composed of polymers of g-actin; and (iii) intermediate filaments, heteropolymers of three neurofilament subunits NF-L, NF-M and NF-H. Axotomy of motoneurons in peripheral nerve results in decreased synthesis of neurofilament and increased synthesis of actin and tubulin (for review see Bisby & Tetzlaff, 1992; Conti & Selzer, 2000). After the nerve has regenerated to its target, the changes are reversed (Muma et al., 1990; Oblinger & Lasek, 1988), but they are permanent if regeneration is prevented (Tetzlaff et al., 1988). Thus regeneration of peripheral nerve may depend on the transport and assembly of actin and microtubules, while neurofilaments are important to the subsequent maturation and enlargement of the regenerated fibres.

Even less is known about the role of cytoskeletal proteins in regeneration of axons in the CNS. Arguments against the applicability of developmental growth cone mechanisms to regeneration in the CNS have been made in the lamprey,

which recover normal appearing swimming and other behaviours after spinal transection (Selzer, 1978). Unlike growth cones of embryonic neurons, the growth cones of regenerating lamprey axons lack lamellipodia and filopodia (Lurie et al., 1994) and contain densely packed neurofilaments (Pijak et al., 1996) but little f-actin (Hall et al., 1997). Moreover, neurons whose axons regenerate well showed only a transient downregulation of neurofilament mRNA expression, while neurons that regenerate poorly showed a permanent downregulation (Jacobs et al., 1997). This has suggested a hypothesis that regeneration involves a protrusive force generated by the transport of cytoskeletal elements such as neurofilaments into the growing tip (Jacobs et al., 1997; Pijak et al., 1996). However, it will be necessary to manipulate expression of cytoskeletal proteins in vivo in order to test any specific hypothesis concerning their roles in regeneration.

Specificity of axonal regeneration

In recent years, substantial progress has been made in understanding how developing axons choose their paths (Goodman, 1996). Much less is known about the degree to which axons are guided during regeneration, the specificity with which they form synapses, or the molecular mechanisms of any specificity that they show. Regeneration in the CNS of several lower vertebrates does appear to be specific to a significant degree. The severed optic nerves of fish and frogs regenerate to their proper target regions of the optic tectum, restoring accurate vision (Gaze & Jacobson, 1963; Sperry, 1948). Retinotectal regeneration in reptiles is much less specific and does not restore correct vision (Dunlop et al., 2000). Cut or crushed dorsal roots in the frog regenerate into the spinal cord and muscle sensory neurons form synaptic contacts selectively with appropriate agonist motoneurons (Sah & Frank, 1984). In the lamprey, axons cut by a spinal transection regenerate selectively in their original paths (Lurie & Selzer, 1991; Yin et al., 1984). During regeneration, these axons behave as if they were following local environmental guidance cues (Mackler et al., 1986). Moreover, they form functioning synapses selectively with correct neurons distal to the lesion (Mackler & Selzer, 1987).

Much less is known about the specificity of axonal regeneration in mammalian CNS. Rat retinal ganglion cell axons regenerate through peripheral nerve grafts into the superior colliculus and terminate in correct layers, forming synapses with normal ultrastructural features (Vidal-Sanz et al., 1991). In similar experiments, peripheral nerve grafts connected the cut optic nerve with the rostral brainstem or diencephalon. In one-third of such animals, retinal axons had regenerated up to 6 mm within the brainstem, terminating selectively in normally retinorecipient pretectal nuclei, i.e. the nucleus of the optic tract and the olivary pretectal nucleus (Aviles-Trigueros et al., 2000). Thus even in mammals, there is evidence for at least limited specificity in the regeneration of optic nerve when inhibitory effects of the adult CNS environment are circumvented by peripheral nerve grafts.

The molecular mechanisms underlying specificity in CNS axon regeneration are still unknown. Several developmental guidance molecules are expressed in postembryonic CNS of lower vertebrates and mammals (Aubert et al., 1995; Shifman & Selzer, 2001). Expression of some guidance molecules is upregulated in the spinal cord or supraspinal projecting neurons following spinal cord injury. These include: Eph B3 (Miranda et al., 1999), a member of the Eph family of protein tyrosine kinase receptors for the chemorepellent molecules of the ephrin family; netrins (Shifman & Selzer, 2000), molecules that can act as either chemorepellents or chemoattractants, depending on the receptor with which they interact; and the chemorepellent netrin receptor UNC-5 (Shifman & Selzer, 2000). In the lamprey, netrin mRNA expression has been demonstrated widely throughout the spinal cord, while UNC-5 is expressed by some reticulospinal neurons. Following spinal cord transection, UNC-5 may be upregulated selectively in neurons that are bad regenerators, suggesting that netrin signaling might be involved in modulating the regeneration of these axons (Shifman & Selzer, 2000). In adult zebrafish, rostral-low to caudal-high gradients of ephrine-A2 and ephrin-A5b mRNA expression have been found in the tecta of normal animals and during retinotopically correct regeneration of optic nerve (Becker & Becker, 2000). It has not yet been established that the retinal ganglion cells express the corresponding Eph receptors. Thus far, evidence that guidance molecules influence the pathfinding of regenerating axons in the CNS is only correlative.

Potential therapeutic approaches based on repairing the injured nervous system

Substantial progress has been made in developing methods to repair the injured nervous system. These are reviewed briefly below. Additional details may be found in Chapter 47 by McDonald.

Enhance neuronal survival and regenerative capacity

Secondary neuronal death in acute CNS injury
Part of the functional loss that follows CNS injury is attributable to the secondary death of neurons near the site of injury due to a complex interplay among glutamate excitotoxicity, edema, vascular changes and possibly cytokine toxicity (for reviews see Martin et al., 1998; Schwab & Bartholdi, 1996; Tator & Koyanagi, 1997). This is especially problematic in spinal cord injury, where the process of secondary neuronal damage is especially virulent. Despite a large number of interventions that have been successful in reducing excitotoxic and other modes of secondary neuronal injury in experimental animals (Anderson et al., 1985), the only treatment of acute spinal cord injury that has proven successful in humans is high dose methylprednisolone (Bracken et al., 1992), which is thought to act primarily by suppressing lipid peroxidation and opposing the effects of free radicals (Anderson et al., 1988).

Neurotrophic factors
Additional functional loss is attributable to atrophy or apoptotic death of axotomized neurons due to loss of target derived trophic support (Himes & Tessler, 2000; Martin et al., 1998). In addition to eliminating the possible involvement of surviving neurons in compensatory neuronal circuits, neuron death precludes the application of strategies designed to promote regeneration. Thus there is a rationale for developing pharmacological strategies to sustain the viability and vigor of axotomized neurons until a more definitive reparative manipulation can be instituted.

Peripheral nerve bridges

The ability of some CNS axons to regenerate in peripheral nerve grafts has been employed to reconnect transected optic nerve to the superior colliculus (Carter et al., 1989; Vidal-Sanz et al., 1987). Schwann cells in the nerve grafts produce growth-permissive extracellular matrix molecules such as laminin. The grafts also release trophic factors necessary for the survival of the injured neurons, in particular brain-derived neurotrophic factor (BDNF) and neurotrophin 4/5 (NT-4/5) (Cohen et al., 1994; Jelsma et al., 1993; Mansour-Robaey et al., 1994). The neurotrophic effect was enhanced when the nerve grafts predegenerated for 7 days (Golka et al., 2001), presumably because the denervated Schwann cells upregulate their production of trophic factors and extracellular matrix. These nerve grafts were reported to mediate light–dark discrimination in hamsters (Sasaki et al., 1993) and pupillary light reflexes in rats (Whiteley et al., 1998). Peripheral nerve grafts might be used to enhance recovery in spinal cord injury and other cases of interruption of compact long white matter tracts.

However, peripheral nerve grafts attract axons primarily from neurons situated close to the grafts (Richardson et al., 1984), as opposed to axons of supraspinal projection neurons such as the corticospinal or rubrospinal tracts.

Neutralize inhibitory factors

Antibodies directed at oligodendrocyte-associated growth cone collapsing factors have been used to promote regeneration (Schnell & Schwab, 1990). IN-1 secreting hybridomas were transplanted into the parietal lobes of rats, which were then subjected to spinal cord dorsal over-hemisection, interrupting both corticospinal tracts. Corticospinal axons grew up to 15 mm around and beyond the hemisection. Contact placing reflexes were restored in the hindlimbs and stride length was partly normalized (Bregman et al., 1995). In control rats, regeneration did not exceed 1 mm. Similar regeneration has been achieved by infusion of a partially humanized, recombinant Fab fragment derived from IN-1 directly into the injury site (Brosamle et al., 2000). However, in such experiments, only approximately 10% of corticospinal axons regenerate, possibly due to the presence of additional myelin-associated growth inhibitory molecules. A novel approach to dealing with this limitation has been developed by immunizing mice against myelin, using incomplete Freund's adjuvent to avoid the development of experimental allergic encephalomyelitis (Huang et al., 1999). This presumably resulted in neutralizing several inhibitory molecules. Immunized animals showed regeneration of large numbers of corticospinal axons and recovery of hindlimb motor functions after spinal cord dorsal over-hemisection.

Fetal tissue transplants

Transplants of fetal spinal cord can reduce both retrograde death of axotomized neurons (Himes et al., 1994; Shibayama et al., 1998) and the amount of glial scarring that occurs at the site of a spinal cord injury (Houle, 1992). The axons of corticospinal and bulbospinal neurons regenerate through fetal spinal cord transplants and into caudal host spinal cord, where they enhance the development of locomotion and other motor functions in newborn animals (Bregman et al., 1993; Diener & Bregman, 1998; Kim et al., 1999; Miya et al., 1997). By contrast, in adult hosts long axon tracts regenerate poorly through the transplant and regeneration of CNS axons is almost exclusively from neurons close to the transplants. Even these axons do not extend into the distal host spinal cord (Jakeman & Reier, 1991). Administration of exogenous neurotrophic factors increases growth of supraspinal axons into the transplant (Bregman et al., 1997). By combining fetal spinal cord transplants with exogenous neurotrophic factors or with the IN-1 antibody against Nogo, it was possible to increase sprouting adjacent to the transplants, enhance long distance regeneration and promote recovery of hindlimb locomotor function (for review see Bregman et al., 1998).

Modulate intraneuronal factors

As we learn more about the neuron-intrinsic factors that modulate axonal regeneration, it will become possible to manipulate expression of these factors such as growth associated and cytoskeletal proteins, as well as the proteins important for synaptic plasticity. However, intraneuronal growth programs are modulated by environmental factors such as guidance molecules and neurotrophic factors. For the moment, most manipulations of the intrinsic regenerative capacities of neurons has been achieved through extrinsic application of trophic factors, as described above.

Neuronal replacement

Fetal neurons

Embryonic neurons have been used to promote recovery by transplanting them into the brains of patients with neurodegenerative diseases (Bjorklund & Lindvall, 2000). The most extensive experience has been with Parkinson's disease (Lindvall, 1998; Olanow et al., 1996). This approach is reviewed in more detail in chapters on the relevant diseases. Challenges associated with this approach include (i) addressing the ethical and practical difficulties associated with the use of human fetal tissue; (ii) enhancing survival of grafted cells; (iii) enhancing the degree of innervation of the host striatum. Theoretically, the difficulties associated with the use of human fetal tissues can be addressed by the substitution of stem cells and immortalized cell lines. In practice, using xenografts of fetal porcine dopaminergic neurons has already shown promise (Schumacher et al., 2000), with clinical improvement comparable to that reported with human allografts. On the basis of animal studies, survival of the graft may be improved by the use of trophic factors, antiapoptotic drugs, calcium channel blockers and inhibitors of lipid peroxidation (Brundin et al., 2000). Porcine xenografts of striatal cells have now been inserted into several patients with Huntington's disease (Fink et al., 2000). It is too soon to know whether there will be a therapeutic response.

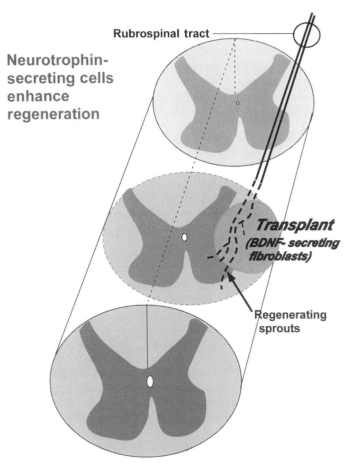

Neurotrophin-secreting cells enhance regeneration

Rubrospinal tract

Transplant (BDNF- secreting fibroblasts)

Regenerating sprouts

Fig. 6.3. Use of genetically modified cell lines to deliver trophic factors. Fibroblasts can be genetically modified to release molecules that enhance regeneration and clonally expanded (Blesch et al., 1999). This would have the advantage that a patient's own fibroblasts could be used for transplantation into the CNS, thus reducing the risk of immune rejection. An example of this strategy is illustrated in the work of Liu et al. (1999a), who transplanted BDNF-expressing fibroblasts into a spinal hemisection lesion that severed the rubrospinal tract, among others. Anterograde tracing from the red nucleus revealed regeneration of rubrospinal axons through the transplant into the spinal cord caudal to the lesion. This was accompanied by evidence of enhanced functional recovery.

Stem cells, neuronal progenitors and other cell lines
Because of the limited effectiveness of fetal transplants in many circumstances, the limited availability of human fetal tissue and the ethical considerations that their use has raised, alternative sources of neurons have been explored. The most promising approaches are based on cell lines that can be genetically modified to express desirable molecules, such as trophic factors. One attractive approach is to use cells from the patient's own body. Fibroblasts and Schwann cells engineered to synthesize trophic factors have been transplanted in rats to rescue axotomized neurons, promote regeneration and remyelination, and even enhance functional recovery (c.f. Blesch et al., 1999; Jin et al., 2000; Liu et al., 1999a; McTigue et al., 1998) (Fig. 6.3).

Neural stem cells and progenitor cells are particularly attractive for use as transplants (McKay, 1997). They have been isolated from the brain and spinal cord of adult as well as developing animals (Gage, 1998), including humans (Eriksson et al., 1998). Neural progenitors can be genetically modified to make neurotrophic factors (Liu et al., 1999b) and may be able to generate neurons to replace those lost to trauma and to furnish oligodendrocytes (Liu et al., 2000) that can remyelinate surviving and regenerating axons.

The olfactory nerve is constantly regenerating in life. Adult olfactory bulb ensheathing glia, which form the environment for this natural regeneration, can be transplanted into the injured spinal cord to promote axonal regeneration (Ramon-Cueto et al., 1998) and even functional recovery (Li et al., 1997).

Combination approaches

It is unlikely that any individual treatment will restore function completely and combinations of therapeutic approaches will probably be required. For example, Schnell and Schwab combined the IN-1 antibody and fetal spinal cord tissue inserted into the lesion to enhance the distance and profusion of regeneration (Schnell & Schwab, 1993). Local injections of NGF, BDNF or NT-3 were effective substitutes for the fetal transplants (Schnell et al., 1994). Olson's group in Sweden combined multiple peripheral nerve grafts, fibrin tissue glue, acidic fibroblast growth factor (aFGF) and compressive wiring of the dorsal spines in dorsiflexion to bridge a gap of 5 mm of spinal cord produced in rats by excision of the T_8 segment. Anterograde tracing demonstrated evidence for anatomic regeneration of ascending and descending pathways (Cheng et al., 1996) and improvement in open-field walking scores and in more elaborate measures of gait coordination (Cheng et al., 1997). These striking observations and other recent experiments suggest that combinations of surgical manipulations, trophic factors and growth inhibitor neutralization measures may be more effective than single therapies. Moreover, as the mechanisms of spontaneous recovery are better understood, new therapeutic approaches will incorporate strategies that optimize these mechanisms into the combination approach.

References

Abel, T. & Kandel, E. (1998). Positive and negative regulatory mechanisms that mediate long-term memory storage. *Brain Res. Rev.*, **26**, 360–78.

Abel, T., Nguyen, P.V., Barad, M., Deuel, T.A., Kandel, E.R. & Bourtchouladze, R. (1997). Genetic demonstration of a role for PKA in the late phase of LTP and in hippocampus-based long-term memory. *Cell*, **88**, 615–26.

Abel, T., Martin, K.C., Bartsch, D. & Kandel, E.R. (1998). Memory suppressor genes: inhibitory constraints on the storage of long-term memory. *Science*, **279**, 338–41.

Aigner, L., Arber, S., Kapfhammer, J.P. et al. (1995). Overexpression of the neural growth-associated protein GAP-43 induces nerve sprouting in the adult nervous system of transgenic mice. *Cell*, **83**: 269–78.

Aldskogius, H. & Thomander, L. (1986). Selective reinnervation of somatotopically appropriate muscles after facial nerve transection and regeneration in the neonatal rat. *Brain Res.*, **375**, 126–34.

Aldskogius, H., Molander, C., Persson, J. & Thomander, L. (1987). Specific and nonspecific regeneration of motor axons after sciatic nerve injury and repair in the rat. *J. Neurol. Sci.*, **80**, 249–57.

Anderson, D.K., Demediuk, P., Saunders, R.D., Dugan, L.L., Means, E.D. & Horrocks, L.A. (1985). Spinal cord injury and protection. *Ann. Emerg. Med.*, **14**, 816–21.

Anderson, D.K., Braughler, J.M., Hall, E.D., Waters, T.R., McCall, J.M. & Means, E.D. (1988). Effects of treatment with U-74006F on neurological outcome following experimental spinal cord injury. *J. Neurosurg.*, **69**, 562–7.

Aubert, I., Ridet, J.L. & Gage, F.H. (1995). Regeneration in the adult mammalian CNS: guided by development. *Curr. Opin. Neurobiol.*, **5**, 625–35.

Aviles-Trigueros, M., Sauve, Y., Lund, R.D. & Vidal-Sanz, M. (2000). Selective innervation of retinorecipient brainstem nuclei by retinal ganglion cell axons regenerating through peripheral nerve grafts in adult rats. *J. Neurosci.*, **20**, 361–74.

Bach, M.E., Barad, M., Son, H. et al. (1999). Age-related defects in spatial memory are correlated with defects in the late phase of hippocampal long-term potentiation in vitro and are attenuated by drugs that enhance the cAMP signaling pathway. *Proc. Natl. Acad. Sci., USA*, **96**, 5280–5.

Bandtlow, C.E., Schmidt, M.F., Hassinger, T.D., Schwab, M.E. & Kater, S.B. (1993). Role of intracellular calcium in NI-35-evoked collapse of neuronal growth cones. *Science*, **259**, 80–3.

Barad, M., Bourtchouladze, R., Winder, D.G., Golan, H. & Kandel, E. (1998). Rolipram, a type IV-specific phosphodiesterase inhibitor, facilitates the establishment of long-lasting long-term potentiation and improves memory. *Proc. Natl Acad. Sci., USA*, **95**, 15020–5.

Barbeau, H. & Rossignol, S. (1987). Recovery of locomotion after chronic spinalization in the adult cat. *Brain Res.*, **412**, 84–95.

Bartsch, U., Bandtlow, C.E., Schnell, L., et al. (1995). Lack of evidence that myelin-associated glycoprotein is a major inhibitor of axonal regeneration in the CNS. *Neuron*, **15**, 1375–81.

Bastmeyer, M. & O'Leary, D.D. (1996). Dynamics of target recognition by interstitial axon branching along developing cortical axons. *J. Neurosci.*, **16**, 1450–9.

Beattie, M.S., Bresnahan, J.C. & Lopate, G. (1990). Metamorphosis alters the response to spinal cord transection in Xenopus laevis frogs. *J. Neurobiol.*, **21**, 1108–22.

Becker, C.G. & Becker, T. (2000). Gradients of ephrin-A2 and ephrin-A5b mRNA during retinotopic regeneration of the optic projection in adult zebrafish. *J. Comp. Neurol.*, **427**, 469–83.

Becker, C.G., Becker, T., Meyer, R.L. & Schachner, M. (1999). Tenascin-R inhibits the growth of optic fibers in vitro but is rapidly eliminated during nerve regeneration in the salamander Pleurodeles waltl. *J. Neurosci.*, **19**, 813–27.

Becker, T., Anliker, B., Becker, C.G. et al. (2000). Tenascin-R inhibits regrowth of optic fibers in vitro and persists in the optic nerve of mice after injury. *Glia*, **29**, 330–46.

Berridge, M.J. (1988). Neuronal calcium signaling. *Neuron*, **21**, 13–26.

Bisby, M.A. & Tetzlaff, W. (1992). Changes in cytoskeletal protein synthesis following axon injury and during axon regeneration. *Molec. Neurobiol.*, **6**, 107–23.

Bjorklund, A. & Lindvall, O. (2000). Cell replacement therapies for central nervous system disorders. *Nat. Neurosci.*, **3**, 537–44.

Blesch, A., Uy, H.S., Grill, R.J., Cheng, J.G., Patterson, P.H. & Tuszynski, M.H. (1999). Leukemia inhibitory factor augments neurotrophin expression and corticospinal axon growth after adult CNS injury. *J. Neurosci.*, **19**, 3556–66.

Bliss, T.V.P. & Collingridge, G.L. (1993). A synaptic model of memory: long-term potentiation in the hippocampus. *Nature*, **361**, 31–9.

Bolshakov, V.Y., Golan, H., Kandel, E.R. & Siegelbaum, S.A. (1997). Recruitment of new sites of synaptic transmission during the cAMP-dependent late phase of LTP at CA3–CA1 synapses in the hippocampus. *Neuron*, **19**, 635–51.

Bomze, H.M., Bulsara, K.R., Iskandar, B.J., Caroni, P. & Skene, J.H. (2001). Spinal axon regeneration evoked by replacing two growth cone proteins in adult neurons. *Nat. Neurosci.*, **4**, 38–43.

Boudreau, N.J. & Jones, P.L. (1999). Extracellular matrix and integrin signalling: the shape of things to come. *Biochem. J.*, **339**, 481–8.

Bovolenta, P., Wandosell, F. & Nieto-Sampedro, M. (1993). Characterization of a neurite outgrowth inhibitor expressed after CNS injury. *Eur. J. Neurosci.*, **5**, 454–65.

Bovolenta, P., Fernaud-Espinosa, I., Mendez-Otero, R. & Nieto-Sampedro, M. (1997). Neurite outgrowth inhibitor of gliotic brain tissue. Mode of action and cellular localization, studied with specific monoclonal antibodies. *Eur. J. Neurosci.*, **9**, 977–89.

Bracken, M.B., Shepard, M.J., Collins, W.F.J. et al. (1992). Methylprednisolone or naloxone treatment after acute spinal cord injury: 1-year follow-up data. Results of the second National Acute Spinal Cord Injury Study. *J. Neurosurg.*, **76**, 23–31.

Bregman, B.S., Kunkel-Bagden, E., Reier, P.J., Dai, H.N., McAtee, M. & Gao, D. (1993). Recovery of function after spinal cord injury: mechanisms underlying transplant-mediated recovery of function differ after spinal cord injury in newborn and adult rats. *Exp. Neurol.*, **123**, 3–16.

Bregman, B.S., Broude, E., McAtee, M. & Kelley, M.S. (1998). Transplants and neurotrophic factors prevent atrophy of mature CNS neurons after spinal cord injury. *Exp. Neurol.*, **149**, 13–27.

Bregman, B.S., Kunkel-Bagden, E., Schnell, L., Dai, H.N., Gao, D. & Schwab, M.E. (1995). Recovery from spinal cord injury mediated by antibodies to neurite growth inhibitors. *Nature*, **378**, 498–501.

Bregman, B.S., McAtee, M., Dai, H.N. & Kuhn, P.L. (1997). Neurotrophic factors increase axonal growth after spinal cord injury and transplantation in the adult rat. *Exp. Neurol.*, **148**, 475–94.

Brosamle, C., Huber, A.B., Fiedler, M., Skerra, A. & Schwab, M.E. (2000). Regeneration of lesioned corticospinal tract fibers in the adult rat induced by a recombinant, humanized IN-1 antibody fragment. *J. Neurosci.*, **20**, 8061–8.

Brown, M.C. & Hardman, V.J. (1987). A reassessment of the accuracy of reinnervation by motoneurons following crushing or freezing of the sciatic or lumbar spinal nerves of rats. *Brain*, **110**, 695–705.

Brown, M.C., Holland, R.L. & Hopkins, W.G. (1981). Motor nerve sprouting. *Ann. Rev. Neurosci.*, **4**, 17–42.

Brundin, P., Karlsson, J., Emgard, M. et al. (2000). Improving the survival of grafted dopaminergic neurons: a review over current approaches. *Cell Transpl.*, **9**, 179–95.

Brushart, T.M., Gerber, J., Kessens, P., Chen, Y.G. & Royall, R.M. (1998). Contributions of pathway and neuron to preferential motor reinnervation. *J. Neurosci.*, **18**, 8674–81.

Buonomano, D.V. & Merzenich, M.M. (1998). Cortical plasticity: from synapses to maps. *Ann. Rev. Neurosci.*, **21**, 149–86.

Bussel, B., Roby-Brami, A., Neris, O.R. & Yakovleff, A. (1996). Evidence for a spinal stepping generator in man. Electrophysiological study. *Acta Neurobiol. Exp.*, **56**, 465–8.

Butefisch, C.M., Davis, B.C., Wise, S. et al. (2000). Mechanisms of use-dependent plasticity in the human motor cortex. *Proc. Natl Acad. Sci., USA*, **97**, 3661–5.

Cai, D., Shen, Y., De Bellard, M., Tang, S. & Filbin, M.T. (1999). Prior exposure to neurotrophins blocks inhibition of axonal regeneration by MAG and myelin via a cAMP-dependent mechanism. *Neuron*, **22**, 89–101.

Calancie, B., Needham-Shropshire, B., Jacobs, P., Willer, K., Zych, G. & Green, B.A. (1994). Involuntary stepping after chronic spinal cord injury. Evidence for a central rhythm generator for locomotion in man. *Brain*, **117**, 1143–59.

Cardin, J.A. & Abel, T. (1999). Memory suppressor genes: enhancing the relationship between synaptic plasticity and memory storage. *J. Neurosci. Res.*, **58**, 10–23.

Carlson, S.L., Parrish, M.E., Springer, J.E., Doty, K. & Dossett, L. (1998). Acute inflammatory response in spinal cord following impact injury. *Exp. Neurol.*, **151**, 77–88.

Caroni, P. & Schwab, M.E. (1988a). Antibody against myelin-associated inhibitor of neurite growth neutralizes nonpermissive substrate properties of CNS white matter. *Neuron*, **1**, 85–96.

Caroni, P. & Schwab, M.E. (1988b). Two membrane protein fractions from rat central myelin with inhibitory properties for neurite growth and fibroblast spreading. *J. Cell Biol.*, **106**, 1281–88.

Carter, D.A., Bray, G.M. & Aguayo, A.J. (1989). Regenerated retinal ganglion cell axons can form well-differentiated synapses in the superior colliculus of adult hamsters. *J. Neurosci.*, **9**, 4042–50.

Cazalets, J.R., Borde, M. & Clarac, F. (1995). Localization and organization of the central pattern generator for hindlimb locomotion in newborn rat. *J. Neurosci.*, **15**, 4943–51.

Chen, D.F., Jhaveri, S. & Schneider, G.E. (1995). Intrinsic changes in developing retinal neurons result in regenerative failure of their axons. *Proc. Natl. Acad. Sci., USA*, **92**, 7287–91.

Chen, M.S., Huber, A.B., van der Haar, M.E. et al. (2000). Nogo-A is a myelin-associated neurite outgrowth inhibitor and an antigen for monoclonal antibody IN-1. *Nature*, **403**, 434–9.

Cheng, H., Cao, Y. & Olson, L. (1996). Spinal cord repair in adult paraplegic rats: partial restoration of hind limb function. *Science*, **273**, 510–3.

Cheng, H., Almstrom, S., Gimenez-Llort, L. et al. (1997). Gait analysis of adult paraplegic rats after spinal cord repair. *Exp. Neurol.*, **148**, 544–57.

Cheung, M.E. & Broman, S.H. (2000). Adaptive learning: Interventions for verbal and motor deficits. *Neurorehabil. Neural Repair*, **14**, 159–69.

Chong, M.S., Reynolds, M.L., Irwin, N. et al. (1994). GAP-43 expression in primary sensory neurons following central axotomy. *J. Neurosci.*, **14**, 4375–84.

Chong, M.S., Woolf, C.J., Turmaine, M., Emson, P.C. & Anderson, P.N. (1996). Intrinsic versus extrinsic factors in determining the regeneration of the central processes of rat dorsal root ganglion neurons: the influence of a peripheral nerve graft. *J. Comp. Neurol.*, **370**, 97–104.

Chong, M.S., Woolf, C.J., Haque, N.S. & Anderson, P.N. (1999). Axonal regeneration from injured dorsal roots into the spinal cord of adult rats. *J. Comp. Neurol.*, **410**, 42–54.

Ciossek, T., Monschau, B., Kremoser, C. et al. (1998). Eph receptor-ligand interactions are necessary for guidance of retinal ganglion cell axons in vitro. *Eur. J. Neurosci.*, **10**, 1574–80.

Clark, E.A. & Brugge, J.S. (1995). Integrins and signal transduction pathways: the road taken. *Science*, **268**, 233–9.

Clarke, J.D., Tonge, D.A. & Holder, N.H. (1986). Stage-dependent restoration of sensory dorsal columns following spinal cord transection in anuran tadpoles. *Proc. R. Soc. Lond. B, Biol Sci.*, **227**, 67–82.

Classen, J., Liepert, J., Wise, S.P., Hallett, M. & Cohen, L.G. (1998). Rapid plasticity of human cortical movement representation induced by practice. *J. Neurophysiol.*, **79**, 1117–23.

Cohen, A., Bray, G.M. & Aguayo, A.J. (1994). Neurotrophin-4/5 (nt-4/5) increases adult-rat retinal ganglion-cell survival and neurite outgrowth in-vitro. *J. Neurobiol.*, **25**, 953–9.

Cohen, A.H., Mackler, S.A. & Selzer, M.E. (1998). Behavioral recovery following spinal transection: functional regeneration in the lamprey CNS. *Trends Neurosci.*, **11**, 227–31.

Cohen-Cory, S. & Fraser, S.E. (1995). Effects of brain-derived neurotrophic factor on optic axon branching and remodelling in vivo. *Nature*, **378**, 192–6.

Conti, A. & Selzer, M.E. (2000). The role of cytoskeleton in regeneration of central nervous system axons. In *Degeneration and*

Regeneration in the Nervous System, ed. N.R. Saunders & K.M. Dziegielewska, pp. 153–69. Amsterdam: Harwood Academic Publishers.

Cox, E.C., Muller, B. & Bonhoeffer, F. (1990). Axonal guidance in the chick visual system: posterior tectal membranes induce collapse of growth cones from the temporal retina. *Neuron*, **4**, 31–7.

David, S. & Aguayo, A.J. (1981). Axonal elongation into peripheral nervous system 'bridges' after central nervous system injury in adult rats. *Science*, **214**, 931–3.

Davies, S.J., Field, P.M. & Raisman, G. (1994). Long interfascicular axon growth from embryonic neurons transplanted into adult myelinated tracts. *J. Neurosci.*, **14**, 1596–612.

Davies, S.J., Fitch, M.T., Memberg, S.P., Hall, A.K., Raisman, G. & Silver, J. (1997). Regeneration of adult axons in white matter tracts of the central nervous system. *Nature*, **390**, 680–3.

Davis, G.R. & McClelland, A.D. (1994). Extent and time course of restoration of descending brainstem projections in spinal cord-transected lamprey. *J. Comp. Neurol.*, **344**, 65–82.

De Leon, R.D., Hodgson, J.A., Roy, R.R. & Edgerton, V.R. (1999a). Retention of hindlimb stepping ability in adult spinal cats after the cessation of step training. *J. Neurophysiol.*, **81**, 85–94.

De Leon, R.D., Tamaki, H., Hodgson, J.A., Roy, R.R. & Edgerton, V.R. (1999b). Hindlimb locomotor and postural training modulates glycinergic inhibition in the spinal cord of the adult spinal cat. *J. Neurophysiol.*, **82**, 359–69.

Diamond, J., Coughlin, M., Macintyre, L., Holmes, M. & Visheau, B. (1987). Evidence that endogenous beta nerve growth factor is responsible for the collateral sprouting, but not the regeneration, of nociceptive axons in adult rats. *Proc. Natl. Acad. Sci., USA*, **84**, 6596–600.

Diener, P.S. & Bregman, B.S. (1998). Fetal spinal cord transplants support the development of target reaching and coordinated postural adjustments after neonatal cervical spinal cord injury. *J. Neurosci.*, **18**, 763–78.

Dietz, V., Colombo, G., Jensen, L. & Baumgartner, L. (1995). Locomotor capacity of spinal cord in paraplegic patients. *Ann. Rev. Neurol.*, **37**, 574–82.

Dobkin, B.H. (1996). *Neurologic Rehabilitation*. Philadelphia: F. A. Davis.

Dobkin, B.H. (1999). An overview of treadmill training with partial body weight support: a neurophysiologically sound approach whose time has come for randomized clinical trials. *Neurorehabil. Neural Repair*, **13**, 157–65.

Dromerick, A.W., Edwards, D.F. & Hahn, M. (2000). Does the application of constraint-induced movement therapy during acute rehabilitation reduce arm impairment after ischemic stroke? *Stroke*, **31**, 2984–8.

Dunlop, S.A., Tran, N., Tee, L.B., Papadimitriou, J. & Beazley, L.D. (2000). Retinal projections throughout optic nerve regeneration in the ornate dragon lizard, Ctenophorus ornatus. *J. Comp. Neurol.*, **416**, 188–200.

Engert, F. & Bonhoeffer, T. (1999). Dendritic spine changes associated with hippocampal long-term synaptic plasticity. *Nature*, **399**, 66–70.

Eriksson, P.S., Perfilieva, E., Bjork-Eriksson, T. et al. (1998).
Neurogenesis in the adult human hippocampus. *Nat. Med.*, **4**, 1313–7.

Ernfors, P., Bengzon, J., Kokaia, Z., Persson, H. & Lindvall, O. (1991). Increased levels of messenger RNAs for neurotrophic factors in the brain during kindling epileptogenesis. *Neuron*, **7**, 165–76.

Feng, G., Laskowski, M.B., Feldheim, D.A. et al. (2000). Roles for ephrins in positionally selective synaptogenesis between motor neurons and muscle fibers. *Neuron*, **25**, 295–306.

Fink, J.S., Schumacher, J.M., Ellias, S.L. et al. (2000). Porcine xeno-grafts in Parkinson's disease and Huntington's disease patients: preliminary results. *Cell Transpl.*, **9**, 273–8.

Forehand, C.J. & Farel, P.B. (1982). Anatomical and behavioral recovery from the effects of spinal cord transection: dependence on metamorphosis in anuran larvae. *J. Neurosci.*, **2**, 654–62.

Frey, D., Laux, T., Xu, L., Schneider, C. & Caroni, P. (2000). Shared and unique roles of CAP23 and GAP43 in actin regulation, neurite outgrowth, and anatomical plasticity. *J. Cell Biol.*, **149**, 1443–54.

Fu, S.Y. & Gordon, T. (1997). The cellular and molecular basis of peripheral nerve regeneration. *Mol. Neurobiol.*, **14**, 67–116.

Fung, J., Stewart, J.E. & Barbeau, H. (1990). The combined effects of clonidine and cyproheptadine with interactive training on the modulation of locomotion in spinal cord injured subjects. *J. Neurol. Sci.*, **100**, 85–93.

Gage, F.H. (1998). Stem cells of the central nervous system. *Curr. Opin. Neurobiol.*, **8**, 671–6.

Gallo, G. & Letourneau, P.C. (1998). Localized sources of neuro-trophins initiate axon collateral sprouting. *J. Neurosci.*, **18**, 5403–14.

Garraghty, P.E. & Muja, N. (1996). NMDA receptors and plasticity in adult primate somatosensory cortex. *J. Comp. Neurol.*, **367**, 319–26.

Gaze, R.M. & Jacobson, M. (1963). A study of the retino-tectal projection during regeneration of the optic nerve in the frog. *Proc. Roy. Soc. (Lond.)*, **157**, 420–48.

Gazzani, F., Bernardi, M., Macaluso, A. et al. (1999). Ambulation training of neurological patients on the treadmill with a new Walking Assistance and Rehabilitation Device (WARD). *Spinal Cord*, **37**, 336–44.

Girault, J-A. & Greengard, P. (1999). Principles of signal transduction. In *Neurobiology of Mental Illness*, ed. D.S. Charney, E.J. Nestler & B.S. Bunney, pp. 37–60. Oxford, GB: Oxford University Press.

Glazewski, S., Giese, K.P., Silva, A. & Fox, K. (2000). The role of alpha-CaMKII autophosphorylation in neocortical experience-dependent plasticity. *Nat. Neurosci.*, **3**, 911–18.

Goldberger, M.E. & Murray, M. (1974). Restitution of function and collateral sprouting in the cat spinal cord: The deafferented animal. *J. Comp. Neurol.*, **158**, 37–54.

Golka, B., Lewin-Kowalik, J., Swiech-Sabuda, E., Larysz-Brysz, M., Gorka, D. & Malecka-Tendera, E. (2001). Predegenerated peripheral nerve grafts rescue retinal ganglion cells from axotomy-induced death. *Exp. Neurol.*, **167**, 118–25.

Goodman, C.S. (1996). Mechanisms and molecules that control growth cone guidance. *Ann. Rev. Neurosci.*, **19**, 341–77.

Gordon-Weeks, P.R. (1989). Growth at the growth cone. *Trends Neurosci.*, **12**, 238–40.

Goslin, K., Schreyer, D.J., Skene, J.H. & Banker, G. (1988). Development of neuronal polarity: GAP-43 distinguishes axonal from dendritic growth cones. *Nature*, **336**, 672–4.

GrandPre, T., Nakamura, F., Vartanian, T. & Strittmatter, S.M. (2000). Identification of the Nogo inhibitor of axon regeneration as a Reticulon protein. *Nature*, **403**, 439–44.

Grillner, S. (1975). Locomotion in vertebrates: Central mechanisms and reflex interaction. *Physiol. Rev.*, **55**, 247–304.

Hall, G.F., Yao, J., Selzer, M.E. & Kosik, K.S. (1997). Cytoskeletal changes correlated with the loss of neuronal polarity in axotomized lamprey central neurons. *J. Neurocytol.*, **26**, 733–53.

Harkema, S.J., Hurley, S.L., Patel, U.K., Requejo, P.S., Dobkin, B.H. & Edgerton, V.R. (1997). Human lumbosacral spinal cord interprets loading during stepping. *J. Neurophysiol.*, **77**, 797–811.

Heiss, W.D. & Graf, R. (1994). The ischemic penumbra. *Curr. Opin. Neurol.*, **7**, 11–19.

Helmke, S., Lohse, K., Mikule, K., Wood, M.R. & Pfenninger, K.H. (1998). SRC binding to the cytoskeleton, triggered by growth cone attachment to laminin, is protein tyrosine phosphatase-dependent. *J. Cell Sci.*, **111**, 2465–75.

Hesse, S., Bertelt, C., Jahnke, M.T. et al. (1995). Treadmill training with partial body weight support compared with physiotherapy in nonambulatory hemiparetic patients. *Stroke*, **26**, 976–81.

Himes, B.T., Goldberger, M.E. & Tessler, A. (1994). Grafts of fetal central-nervous-system tissue rescue axotomized Clarke nucleus neurons in adult and neonatal operates. *J. Comp. Neurol.*, **339**, 117–31.

Himes, B.T. & Tessler, A. (2001). Neuroprotection from cell death following axotomy. In *Nerve Regeneration*, ed. N. Ingoglia & M. Murray, pp. 477–503. New York: Marcel Dekker.

Houle, J. (1992). The structural integrity of glial scar tissue associated with a chronic spinal cord lesion can be altered by transplanted fetal spinal cord tissue. *J. Neurosci. Res.*, **31**, 120–30.

Hoyle, G.W., Mercer, E.H., Palmiter, R.D. & Brinster, R.L. (1993). Expression of NGF in sympathetic neurons leads to excessive axon outgrowth from ganglia but decreased terminal innervation within tissues. *Neuron*, **10**, 1019–34.

Huang, D.W., McKerracher, L., Braun, P.E. & David, S. (1999). A therapeutic vaccine approach to stimulate axon regeneration in the adult mammalian spinal cord. *Neuron*, **24**, 639–47.

Huang, Y.Y., Nguyen, P.V., Abel, T. & Kandel, E.R. (1996). Long-lasting forms of synaptic potentiation in the mammalian hippocampus. *Learn Mem.*, **3**, 74–85.

Igarashi, M., Strittmatter, S.M., Vartanian, T. & Fishman, M.C. (1993). Mediation by G proteins of signals that cause collapse of growth cones. *Science*, **259**, 77–9.

Igarashi, M., Li, W.W., Sudo, Y. & Fishman, M.C. (1995). Ligand-induced growth cone collapse: amplification and blockade by variant GAP-43 peptides. *J. Neurosci.*, **15**, 5660–7.

Jacobs, A.J., Swain, G.P., Snedeker, J.A., Pijak, D.S., Gladstone, L.J. & Selzer, M.E. (1997). Recovery of neurofilament expression selectively in regenerating reticulospinal neurons. *J. Neurosci.*, **17**, 5206–20.

Jakeman, L.B. & Reier, P.J. (1991). Axonal projections between fetal spinal cord transplants and the adult rat spinal cord: a neuroanatomical tracing study of local interactions. *J. Comp. Neurol.*, **307**, 311–34.

Jelsma, T.N., Friedman, H.H., Berkelaar, M., Bray, G.M. & Aguayo, A.J. (1993). Different forms of the neurotrophin receptor *trk*b messenger-RNA predominate in rat retina and optic nerve. *J. Neurobiol.*, **24**, 1207–14.

Jin, Y., Tessler, A., Fischer, I. & Houle, J.D. (2000). Fibroblasts genetically modified to produce BDNF support regrowth of chronically injured serotonergic axons. *Neurorehabil. Neural Repair*, 14.

Jones, E.G. (1993). GABAergic neurons and their role in cortical plasticity in primates. *Cereb. Cortex*, **3**, 361–72.

Kapfhammer, J.P. & Raper, J.A. (1987). Interactions between growth cones and neurites growing from different neural tissues in culture. *J. Neurosci.*, **7**, 1595–600.

Karni, A., Meyer, G., Jezzard, P., Adams, M.M., Turner, R. & Ungerleider, L.G. (1995). Functional MRI evidence for adult motor cortex plasticity during motor skill learning. *Nature*, **377**, 155–8.

Kim, D., Adipudi, V., Shibayama, M. et al. (1999). Direct agonists for serotonin receptors enhance locomotor function in rats that received neural transplants after neonatal spinal transection. *J. Neurosci.*, **19**, 6213–24.

Kobayashi, H., Watanabe, E. & Murikami, F. (1995). Growth cones of dorsal root ganglion but not retina collapse and avoid oligodendrocytes in culture. *Dev. Biol.*, **168**, 383–94.

Kobayashi, N.R., Fan, D.P., Giehl, K.M., Bedard, A.M., Wiegand, S.J. & Tetzlaff, W. (1997). BDNF and NT-4/5 prevent atrophy of rat rubrospinal neurons after cervical axotomy, stimulate GAP-43 and Talpha1-tubulin mRNA expression, and promote axonal regeneration. *J. Neurosci.*, **17**, 9583–95.

Kopp, B., Kunkel, A., Muhlnickel, W., Villringer, K., Taub, E. & Flor, H. (1999). Plasticity in the motor system related to therapy-induced improvement of movement after stroke. *Neuroreport*, **10**, 807–10.

Kwakkel, G., Wagenaar, R.C., Twisk, J.W., Lankhorst, G.J. & Koetsier, J.C. (1999). Intensity of leg and arm training after primary middle-cerebral-artery stroke: a randomised trial. *Lancet*, **354**, 191–6.

Kwon, Y.K., Bhattacharyya, A., Alberta, J.A. et al. (1997). Activation of ErbB2 during wallerian degeneration of sciatic nerve. *J. Neurosci.*, **17**, 8293–9.

Lankford, K., Cypher, C. & Letourneau, P. (1990). Nerve growth cone motility. *Curr. Opin. Cell Biol.*, **2**, 80–5.

Lankford, K.L., Waxman, S.G. & Kocsis, J.D. (1998). Mechanisms of enhancement of neurite regeneration in vitro following a conditioning sciatic nerve lesion. *J. Comp. Neurol.*, **391**, 11–29.

Lanners, H.N. & Grafstein, B. (1980). Effect of a conditioning lesion on regeneration of goldfish optic axons: ultrastructural evidence of enhanced outgrowth and pinocytosis. *Brain Res.*, **196**, 547–53.

Laskowski, M.B. & Sanes, J.R. (1988). Topographically selective reinnervation of adult mammalian skeletal muscles. *J. Neurosci.*, **8**, 3094–9.

Laskowski, M.B., Colman, H., Nelson, C. & Lichtman, J.W. (1998).

Synaptic competition during the reformation of a neuromuscular map. *J. Neurosci.*, **18**, 7328–35.

Lazar, R.B., ed. (1998). *Principles of Neurologic Rehabilitation.* New York: McGraw Hill.

Lee, M.T. & Farel, P.B. (1988). Guidance of regenerating motor axons in larval and juvenile bullfrogs. *J. Neurosci.*, **8**, 2430–7.

Li, D., Field, P.M. & Raisman, G. (1995). Failure of axon regeneration in postnatal rat entorhinohippocampal slice coculture is due to maturation of the axon, not that of the pathway or target. *Eur. J. Neurosci.*, **7**, 1164–71.

Li, Y., Field, P.M. & Raisman, G. (1997). Repair of adult rat corticospinal tract by transplants of olfactory ensheathing cells. *Science*, **277**, 2000–2.

Liepert, J., Bauder, H., Wolfgang, H.R., Miltner, W.H., Taub, E. & Weiller, C. (2000). Treatment-induced cortical reorganization after stroke in humans. *Stroke*, **31**, 1210–16.

Lin, C.H. & Forscher, P. (1993). Cytoskeletal remodeling during growth cone-target interactions. *J. Cell Biol.*, **121**, 1369–83.

Lin, C.H., Thompson, C.A. & Forscher, P. (1994). Cytoskeletal reorganization underlying growth cone motility. *Curr. Opin. Neurobiol.*, **4**, 640–7.

Lin, C.H., Espreafico, E.M., Mooseker, M.S. & Forscher, P. (1996). Myosin drives retrograde F-actin flow in neuronal growth cones. *Neuron*, **16**, 769–82.

Linden, D.J. & Connor, J.A. (1995). Long-term synaptic depression. *Ann. Rev. Neurosci.*, **18**, 319–57.

Lindvall, O. (1998). Update on fetal transplantation: the Swedish experience. *Mov. Disord.*, **13**, 83–7.

Liu, C.N. & Chambers, W.W. (1958). Intraspinal sprouting of dorsal root axons. *Arch. Neurol. Psychiat.*, **79**, 46–61.

Liu, S., Qu, Y., Stewart, T.J. et al. (2000). Embryonic stem cells differentiate into oligodendrocytes and myelinate in culture and after spinal cord transplantation. *Proc. Natl. Acad. Sci., USA*, **97**, 6126–31.

Liu, Y., Kim, D., Himes, B.T. et al. (1999a). Transplants of fibroblasts genetically modified to express BDNF promote regeneration of adult rat rubrospinal axons and recovery of forelimb function. *J. Neurosci.*, **19**, 4370–87.

Liu, Y., Himes, B.T., Solowska, J. et al. (1999b). Intraspinal delivery of neurotrophin-3 using neural stem cells genetically modified by recombinant retrovirus. *Exp. Neurol.*, **158**, 9–26.

Liuzzi, F.J. & Lasek, R.J. (1987). Astrocytes block axonal regeneration in mammals by activating the physiological stop pathway. *Science*, **237**, 642–5.

Lomo, T. & Rosenthal, J. (1972). Control of ACh sensitivity by muscle activity in the rat. *J. Physiol.*, **221**, 493–513.

Lovely, R.G., Gregor, R.J., Roy, R.R. & Edgerton, V.R. (1986). Effects of training on the recovery of full-weight-bearing stepping in the adult spinal cat. *Exp. Neurol.*, **92**, 421–35.

Lurie, D.I. & Selzer, M.E. (1991). Axonal regeneration in the adult lamprey spinal cord. *J. Comp. Neurol.*, **306**, 409–16.

Lurie, D.I., Pijak, D.S. & Selzer, M.E. (1994). Structure of reticulospinal axon growth cones and their cellular environment during regeneration in the lamprey spinal cord. *J. Comp. Neurol.*, **344**, 559–80.

Ma, L., Zablow, L., Kandel, E.R. & Siegelbaum, S.A. (1999). Cyclic AMP induces functional presynaptic boutons in hippocampal CA3–CA1 neuronal cultures. *Nat. Neurosci.*, **2**, 24–30.

McKay, R. (1997). Stem cells in the central nervous system. *Science*, **276**, 66–71.

McKeon, R.J., Schreiber, R.C., Rudge, J.S. & Silver, J. (1991). Reduction of neurite outgrowth in a model of glial scarring following CNS injury is correlated with the expression of inhibitory molecules on reactive astrocytes. *J. Neurosci.*, **11**, 3398–411.

McKerracher, L., David, S., Jackson, D.L., Kottis, V., Dunn, R.J. & Braun, P.E. (1994). Identification of myelin-associated glycoprotein as a major myelin-derived inhibitor of neurite growth. *Neuron*, **13**, 805–11.

McKinney, R.A., Debanne, D., Gahwiler, B.H. & Thompson, S.M. (1997). Lesion-induced axonal sprouting and hyperexcitability in the hippocampus in vitro: implications for the genesis of post-traumatic epilepsy. *Nat. Med.*, **3**, 990–6.

McTigue, D.M., Horner, P.J., Stokes, B.T. & Gage, F.H. (1998). Neurotrophin-3 and brain-derived neurotrophic factor induce oligodendrocyte proliferation and myelination of regenerating axons in the contused adult rat spinal cord. *J. Neurosci.*, **18**, 5354–65.

Mackler, S.A. & Selzer, M.E. (1987). Specificity of synaptic regeneration in the spinal cord of the larval sea lamprey. *J. Physiol. (Lond.)*, **388**, 183–98.

Mackler, S.A., Yin, H.S. & Selzer, M.E. (1986). Determinants of directional specificity in the regeneration of lamprey spinal axons. *J. Neurosci.*, **6**, 1814–21.

Madison, R.D., Archibald, S.J. & Brushart, T.M. (1996). Reinnervation accuracy of the rat femoral nerve by motor and sensory neurons. *J. Neurosci.*, **16**, 5698–703.

Mansour-Robaey, S., Clarke, D.B., Wang, Y.C., Bray, G.M. & Aguayo, A.J. (1994). Effects of ocular injury and administration of brain-derived neurotrophic factor on survival and regrowth of axotomized retinal ganglion cells. *Proc. Natl. Acad. Sci., USA*, **91**, 1632–6.

Martin, L.J., Al-Abdulla, N.A., Brambrink, A.M., Kirsch, J.R., Sieber, F.E. & Portera-Cailliau, C. (1998). Neurodegeneration in excitotoxicity, global cerebral ischemia, and target deprivation: a perspective on the contributions of apoptosis and necrosis. *Brain Res. Bull.*, **46**, 281–309.

Martin, S.J., Grimwood, P.D. & Morris, R.G. (2000). Synaptic plasticity and memory: an evaluation of the hypothesis. *Annu. Rev. Neurosci.*, **23**, 649–711.

Martini, R. (1994). Expression and functional roles of neural cell surface molecules and extracellular matrix components during development and regeneration of peripheral nerves. *J. Neurocytol.*, **23**, 1–28.

Meeker, M.L. & Farel, P.B. (1993). Coincidence of Schwann cell-derived basal lamina development and loss of regenerative specificity of spinal motoneurons. *J. Comp. Neurol.*, **329**, 257–68.

Miltner, W.H., Bauder, H., Sommer, M., Dettmers, C. & Taub, E. (1999). Effects of constraint-induced movement therapy on patients with chronic motor deficits after stroke: a replication. *Stroke*, **30**, 586–92.

Miranda, J.D., White, L.A., Marcillo, A.E., Willson, C.A., Jagid, J. & Whittemore, S.R. (1999). Induction of Eph B3 after spinal cord injury. *Exp. Neurol.*, **156**, 218–22.

Miya, D., Giszter, S., Mori, F., Adipudi, V., Tessler, A. & Murray, M. (1997). Fetal transplants alter the development of function after spinal cord transection in newborn rats. *J. Neurosci.*, **17**, 4856–72.

Mukhopadhyay, G., Doherty, P., Walsh, F.S., Crocker, P.R. & Filbin, M.T. (1994). A novel role for myelin-associated glycoprotein as an inhibitor of axonal regeneration. *Neuron*, **13**, 757–67.

Muma, N.A., Hoffman, P.N., Slunt, H.H., Applegate, M.D., Lieberburg, I. & Price, D.L. (1990). Alterations in levels of mRNAs coding for neurofilament protein subunits during regeneration. *Exp. Neurol.*, **107**, 230–5.

Murray, M. & Goldberger, M.E. (1974). Restitution of function and collateral sprouting in the cat spinal cord: The partially hemisected animal. *J. Comp. Neurol.*, **158**, 19–36.

Namgung, U., Matsuyama, S. & Routtenberg, A. (1997). Long-term potentiation activates the GAP-43 promoter: selective participation of hippocampal mossy cells. *Proc. Natl. Acad. Sci., USA*, **94**, 11675–80.

Nestler, E.J. (1997). Molecular mechanisms of opiate and cocaine addiction. *Curr. Opin. Neurobiol.*, **7**, 713–19.

Nestler, E.J. & Hyman, S.E. (1999). Mechanisms of neural plasticity. In *Neurobiology of Mental Illness*, ed. D.S. Charney, E.J. Nestler & B.S. Bunney, pp. 61–72. Oxford: Oxford University Press.

Neumann, S. & Woolf, C.J. (1999). Regeneration of dorsal column fibers into and beyond the lesion site following adult spinal cord injury. *Neuron*, **23**, 83–91.

Ng, T.F., So, K.F. & Chung, S.K. (1995). Influence of peripheral nerve grafts on the expression of GAP-43 in regenerating retinal ganglion cells in adult hamsters. *J. Neurocytol.*, **24**, 487–96.

Nguyen, T.V., Brownell, A.L., Iris Chen, Y.C. et al. (2000). Detection of the effects of dopamine receptor supersensitivity using pharmacological MRI and correlations with PET. *Synapse*, **36**, 57–65.

Niederost, B.P., Zimmermann, D.R., Schwab, M.E. & Bandtlow, C.E. (1999). Bovine CNS myelin contains neurite growth-inhibitory activity associated with chondroitin sulfate proteoglycans. *J. Neurosci.*, **19**, 8979–89.

Oblinger, M.M. & Lasek, R.J. (1988). Axotomy-induced alterations in the synthesis and transport of neurofilaments and microtubules in dorsal root ganglion cells. *J. Neurosci.*, **8**, 1747–58.

Olanow, C.W., Kordower, J.H. & Freeman, T.B. (1996). Fetal nigral transplantation as a therapy for Parkinson's disease. *Trends Neurosci.*, **19**, 102–9.

Ostendorf, C.G. & Wolf, S.L. (1981). Effect of forced use of the upper extremity of a hemiplegic patient on changes in function. A single-case design. *Phys. Ther.*, **61**, 1022–8.

Ozer, M., ed. (2000). *Management of Persons with Chronic Neurological Illness*. Boston: Butterowth-Heinemann.

Patel, M.N. & McNamara, J.O. (1995). Selective enhancement of axonal branching of cultured dentate gyrus neurons by neurotrophic factors. *Neuroscience*, **69**, 763–70.

Perl, E.R. (1999). Causalgia, pathological pain, and adrenergic receptors. *Proc. Natl. Acad. Sci., USA*, **96**, 7664–7.

Pijak, D.S., Hall, G.F., Tenicki, P.J., Boulos, A.S., Lurie, D.I. & Selzer, M.E. (1996). Neurofilament spacing, phosphorylation, and axon diameter in regenerating and uninjured lamprey axons. *J. Comp. Neurol.*, **368**, 569–81.

Pindzola, R.R., Doller, C. & Silver, J. (1993). Putative inhibitory extracellular matrix molecules at the dorsal root entry zone of the spinal cord during development and after root and sciatic nerve lesions. *Dev. Biol.*, **156**, 34–48.

Pons, T.P., Garraghty, P.E., Ommaya, A.K., Kaas, J.H., Taub, E. & Mishkin, M. (1991). Massive cortical reorganization after sensory deafferentation in adult macaques. *Science*, **252**, 1857–60.

Ramon-Cueto, A., Plant, G.W., Avila, J. & Bunge, M.B. (1998). Long-distance axonal regeneration in the transected adult rat spinal cord is promoted by olfactory ensheathing glia transplants. *J. Neurosci.*, **18**, 3803–15.

Rausell, E. & Jones, E.G. (1995). Extent of intracortical arborization of thalamocortical axons as a determinant of representational plasticity in monkey somatic sensory cortex. *J. Neurosci.*, **15**, 4270–88.

Richardson, P.M. & Issa, V.M. (1984). Peripheral injury enhances central regeneration of primary sensory neurones. *Nature*, **309**, 791–3.

Richardson, P.M., McGuinness, U.M. & Aguayo, A.J. (1980). Axons from CNS neurons regenerate into PNS grafts. *Nature*, **284**, 264–5.

Richardson, P.M., Issa, V.M. & Aguayo, A.J. (1984). Regeneration of long spinal axons in the rat. *J. Neurocytol.*, **13**, 165–82.

Rioult-Pedotti, M.S., Friedman, D. & Donoghue, J.P. (2000). Learning-induced LTP in neocortex. *Science*, **290**, 533–6.

Rioux, L., Gaudin, D.P., Gagnon, C., Di, P.T. & Bedard, P.J. (1991). Decrease of behavioral and biochemical denervation supersensitivity of rat striatum by nigral transplants. *Neuroscience*, **44**, 75–83.

Rivas, R.J., Burmeister, D.W. & Goldberg, D.J. (1992). Rapid effects of laminin on the growth cone. *Neuron*, **8**: 107–15.

Sah, D.W. & Frank, E. (1984). Regeneration of sensory-motor synapses in the spinal cord of the bullfrog. *J. Neurosci.*, **4**, 2784–91.

Sasaki, H., Inoue, T., Iso, H., Fukuda, Y. & Hayashi, Y. (1993). Light-dark discrimination after sciatic nerve transplantation to the sectioned optic nerve in adult hamsters. *Vision Res.*, **33**, 877–80.

Schaden, H., Stuermer, C.A. & Bahr, M. (1994). GAP-43 immunoreactivity and axon regeneration in retinal ganglion cells of the rat. *J. Neurobiol.*, **25**, 1570–8.

Scherer, S.S. (1986). Reinnervation of the extraocular muscles in goldfish is nonselective. *J. Neurosci.*, **6**, 764–73.

Scherer, S.S. & Salzer, J.L. (2001). Axon–Schwann cell interactions during peripheral nerve degeneration and regeneration. In *Glial Cell Development*, ed. K.R. Jessen & W.D. Richardson, 2nd edn, pp. 299–330. Oxford, UK: Oxford University Press.

Schmidt, C.E., Dai, J., Lauffenburger, D.A., Sheetz, M.P. & Horwitz, A.F. (1995). Integrin–cytoskeletal interactions in neuronal growth cones. *J. Neurosci.*, **15**, 3400–7.

Schnell, L. & Schwab, M.E. (1990). Axonal regeneration in the rat spinal cord produced by an antibody against myelin-associated neurite growth inhibitors. *Nature*, **343**, 269–72.

Schnell, L. & Schwab, M.E. (1993). Sprouting and regeneration of lesioned corticospinal tract fibres in the adult rat spinal cord. *Eur. J. Neurosci.*, **5**, 1156–71.

Schnell, L., Schneider, R., Kolbeck, R., Barde, Y.A. & Schwab, M.E. (1994). Neurotrophin-3 enhances sprouting of corticospinal tract during development and after adult spinal cord lesion. *Nature*, **367**, 170–3.

Schumacher, J.M., Ellias, S.A., Palmer, E.P. et al. (2000). Transplantation of embryonic porcine mesencephalic tissue in patients with PD. *Neurology*, **54**, 1042–50.

Schwab, M.E. & Bartholdi, D. (1996). Degeneration and regeneration of axons in the lesioned spinal cord. *Physiol. Rev.*, **76**, 319–70.

Schwegler, G., Schwab, M.E. & Kapfhammer, J.P. (1995). Increased collateral sprouting of primary afferents in the myelin-free spinal cord. *J. Neurosci.*, **15**, 2756–67.

Seeman, P. & Van Tol, H.H. (1995). Dopamine D4-like receptor elevation in schizophrenia: cloned D2 and D4 receptors cannot be discriminated by raclopride competition against [³H]nemonapride. *J. Neurochem.*, **64**, 1413–15.

Segal, M. (2001). Rapid plasticity of dendritic spine: hints to possible functions? *Prog. Neurobiol.*, **63**, 61–70.

Segal, M. & Andersen, P. (2000). Dendritic spines shaped by synaptic activity. *Curr. Opin. Neurobiol.*, **10**, 582–6.

Selzer, M.E. (1978). Mechanisms of functional recovery and regeneration after spinal cord transection in larval sea lamprey. *J. Physiol. (Lond.)*, **277**, 395–408.

Selzer, M.E. (1987). Nerve regeneration. *Semin. Neurol.*, **7**, 88–96.

Shi, S.H., Hayashi, Y., Petralia, R.S. et al. (1999). Rapid spine delivery and redistribution of AMPA receptors after synaptic NMDA receptor activation. *Science*, **284**, 1811–16.

Shibayama, M., Hattori, S., Himes, B.T., Murray, M. & Tessler, A. (1998). Neurotrophin-3 prevents death of axotomized Clarke's nucleus neurons in adult rat. *J. Comp. Neurol.*, **390**, 102–11.

Shifman, M.I. & Selzer, M.E. (2000). Expression of netrin receptor UNC-5 in lamprey brain; modulation by spinal cord transection. *Neurorehabil. Neural Repair*, **14**, 49–58.

Silva, A.J., Kogan, J.H., Frankland, P.W. & Kida, S. (1998). CREB and memory. *Ann. Rev. Neurosci.*, **21**, 127–48.

Skene, J.H. & Willard, M. (1981). Characteristics of growth-associated polypeptides in regenerating toad retinal ganglion cell axons. *J. Neurosci.*, **1**, 419–26.

Son, Y.J., Trachtenberg, J.T. & Thompson, W.J. (1996). Schwann cells induce and guide sprouting and reinnervation of neuromuscular junctions. *Trends Neurosci.*, **19**, 280–5.

Sperry, R.W. (1948). Orderly patterning of synaptic associations in regeneration of intracentral fiber tracts mediating visuomotor coordination. *Anat. Rec.*, **102**, 63–75.

Squire, L.R. & Alvarez, P. (1995). Retrograde amnesia and memory consolidation: a neurobiological perspective. *Curr. Opin. Neurobiol.*, **5**, 169–77.

Squire, L.R. & Kandel, E.R. (1999). *Memory*. New York, NY: W. H. Freeman and Co.

Steward, O. & Fass, B. (1983). Polyribosomes associated with dendritic spines in the denervated dentate gyrus: evidence for local regulation of protein synthesis during reinnervation. *Prog. Brain Res.*, **58**, 131–6.

Steward, O. & Reeves, T.M. (1988). Protein-synthetic machinery beneath postsynaptic sites on CNS neurons: association between polyribosomes and other organelles at the synaptic site. *J. Neurosci.*, **8**, 176–84.

Steward, O., Cotman, C.W. & Lynch, G.S. (1974). Growth of a new fiber projection in the brain of adult rats: re-innervation of the dentate gyrus by contralateral entorhinal cortex following ipsilateral entorhinal lesions. *Exp. Brain Res.*, **20**, 45–66.

Stout, A.K., Raphael, H.M., Kanterewicz, B.I., Klann, E. & Reynolds, I.J. (1998). Glutamate-induced neuron death requires mitochondrial calcium uptake. *Nat. Neurosci.*, **1**, 366–73.

Tang, Y.P., Shimizu, E., Dube, G.R. et al. (1999). Genetic enhancement of learning and memory in mice. *Nature*, **401**, 63–9.

Tator, C.H. (1995). Update on the pathophysiology and pathology of acute spinal cord injury. *Brain Pathol.*, **5**, 407–13.

Tator,, C.H. & Koyanagi, I. (1997). Vascular mechanisms in the pathophysiology of human spinal cord injury. *J. Neurosurg.*, **86**, 483–92.

Taub, E., Uswatte, G. & Pidikiti, R. (1999). Constraint-induced movement therapy: a new family of techniques with broad application to physical rehabilitation – a clinical review. *J. Rehabil. Res. Dev.*, **36**, 237–51.

Tetzlaff, W., Bisby, M.A. & Kreutzberg, G.W. (1988). Changes in cytoskeletal proteins in the rat facial nucleus following axotomy. *J. Neurosci.*, **8**, 3181–9.

van Praag, H., Kempermann, G. & Gage, F.H. (2000). Neural consequences of environmental enrichment. *Nat. Rev. Neurosci.*, **1**, 191–8.

Vidal-Sanz, M., Bray, G.M., Villegas-Perez, M.P., Thanos, S. & Aguayo, A.J. (1987). Axonal regeneration and synapse formation in the superior colliculus by retinal ganglion cells in the adult rat. *J. Neurosci.*, **7**, 2894–909.

Vidal-Sanz, M., Bray, G.M. & Aguayo, A.J. (1991). Regenerated synapses persist in the superior colliculus after the regrowth of retinal ganglion cell axons. *J. Neurocytol.*, **20**, 940–52.

Villegas-Perez, M.P., Vidal-Sanz, M., Bray, G.M. & Aguayo, A.J. (1988). Influences of peripheral nerve grafts on the survival and regrowth of axotomized retinal ganglion cells in adult rats. *J. Neurosci.*, **8**, 265–80.

Visintin, M., Barbeau, H., Korner-Bitensky, N. & Mayo, N.E. (1998). A new approach to retrain gait in stroke patients through body weight support and treadmill stimulation. *Stroke*, **29**, 1122–8.

Walsh, F.S., Meiri, K. & Doherty, P. (1997). Cell signalling and CAM-mediated neurite outgrowth. *Soc. Gen. Physiol. Ser.*, **52**, 221–6.

Wernig, A., Muller, S., Nanassy, A. & Cagol, E. (1995). Laufband therapy based on 'rules of spinal locomotion' is effective in spinal cord injured persons. *Eur. J. Neurosci.*, **7**, 823–9.

Wernig, A., Nanassy, A. & Muller, S. (1998). Maintenance of locomotor abilities following Laufband (treadmill) therapy in para- and tetraplegic persons: follow-up studies. *Spinal Cord*, **36**, 744–9.

Whiteley, S.J., Sauve, Y., Aviles-Trigueros, M., Vidal-Sanz, M. & Lund, R.D. (1998). Extent and duration of recovered pupillary light reflex following retinal ganglion cell axon regeneration through peripheral nerve grafts directed to the pretectum in adult rats. *Exp. Neurol.*, **154**, 560–72.

Wolf, S.L., Lecraw, D.E., Barton, L.A. & Jann, B.B. (1989). Forced use of hemiplegic upper extremities to reverse the effect of learned nonuse among chronic stroke and head-injured patients. *Exp. Neurol.*, **104**, 125–32.

Wong, S.T., Athos, J., Figueroa, X.A. et al. (1999). Calcium-stimulated adenylyl cyclase activity is critical for hippocampus-dependent long-term memory and late phase LTP. *Neuron*, **23**, 787–98.

Woolf, C.J. & Doubell, T.P. (1994). The pathophysiology of chronic pain—increased sensitivity to low threshold A beta-fibre inputs. *Curr. Opin. Neurobiol.*, **4**, 525–34.

Xerri, C., Merzenich, M.M., Peterson, B.E. & Jenkins, W. (1998). Plasticity of primary somatosensory cortex paralleling sensori-motor skill recovery from stroke in adult monkeys. *J. Neurophysiol.*, **79**, 2119–48.

Yin, H.S. & Selzer, M.E. (1983). Axonal regeneration in lamprey spinal cord. *J. Neurosci.*, **3**, 1135–44.

Yin, H.S., Mackler, S.A. & Selzer, M.E. (1984). Directional specificity in the regeneration of lamprey spinal axons. *Science*, **224**, 894–6.

Yue, Y., Su, J., Cerretti, D.P., Fox, G.M., Jing, S. & Zhou, R. (1999). Selective inhibition of spinal cord neurite outgrowth and cell survival by the eph family ligand ephrin-A5. *J. Neurosci.*, **19**, 10026–35.

Zhuo, M., Laitinen, J.T., Li, X.C. & Hawkins, R.D. (1999). On the respective roles of nitric oxide and carbon monoxide in long-term potentiation in the hippocampus. *Learn. Mem.*, **6**, 63–76

7

Measurement of neurological outcomes

Jeremy Hobart[1] and Alan J. Thompson[2]

[1] Department of Neurology, The Peninsula Medical School, Derriford Hospital,
Plymouth, Devon, UK and Institute of Neurology, London, UK
[2] Neurological Outcome Measures Unit, Institute of Neurology, Queen Square, London, UK

Increasingly, clinical trials in neurology are using rating scales of patient-based outcomes to evaluate the effectiveness of therapeutic interventions and, therefore, influence patient care and the expenditure of public funds. To justify this important role in research and clinical practice, these measurement methods must demonstrate that they are rigorous indicators of abstract and unobservable variables such as disability and health-related quality of life.

This chapter, divided into five major sections, is about rating scales for measuring health. The first section examines the history underpinning the science of health measurement and psychometrics, demonstrates that the scientific foundations of this new medical discipline are deeply rooted in education and psychology, and discusses how clinical variables can be rigorously measured. Sections two to four discuss frameworks for evaluating, choosing and developing measures. This approach, rather than recommending a list of instruments, has been chosen because the clinical neurologist is often faced with a choice of instruments. No instrument has universal usefulness, it is therefore important to identify the strengths and weaknesses of individual measures. Section five introduces some of the new developments in health measurement.

Health measurement and psychometrics

History

Although health measurement as a distinct discipline emerged in the 1980s (Ware et al., 1980; McDowell & Newell, 1987; Streiner & Norman, 1989), it is derived from well-established theories and methods of measurement in the field of social sciences whose origins can be traced to the mid-1800s. The basic scientific principles of measurement were established by mathematical psychologists interested in the human being as a measuring instrument. By studying how people make subjective judgements about measurable physical stimuli (e.g. length, weight, loudness), they developed the science of psychophysics: the precise and quantitative study of how human judgements are made (Guilford, 1954). The investigation of overt responses to physical stimuli requires precise methods, referred to as psychophysical methods, for presenting the stimuli and for measuring responses (Nunnally, 1959).

The work of psychophysicists seems far removed from health measurement. It established the fundamental principles of subjective measurement which are as equally relevant to judgements about health as to judgements about physical stimuli. The psychophysicists demonstrated that: subjective judgement is a valid approach to measurement; humans make judgements about abstract comparisons in an internally consistent manner; and accurate judgements can be made on ratio rather than simple ordinal scales. It is notable that psychophysical methods are still used in neurology; thermal threshold testing is based on the principle of the just noticeable differences in temperature detection and audiometry on a person's response to different sound frequencies.

Whilst the psychophysicists were measuring subjective judgements about physical stimuli that could be independently and objectively measured and verified, experimental psychologists were attempting to measure human attributes for which there were no independent physical scales of measurement (e.g. intelligence, personality, attitudes) (Nunnally, 1959). Darwin's empirical demonstration of evolution in the *Origin of Species* in 1859 was the impetus behind the study of individual differences in psychology (Rogers, 1995). It was reasoned that, if animals inherit ancestral characteristics, and if individual differences influence their ability to adapt and survive, so individual differences in humans would have functional significance and could be inherited. Galton, who followed Darwin and believed that the human race could be bettered through controlled mating (eugenics), realized that human characteristics must be measured in a standardized manner before their inheritance could be studied. He coined the term 'mental test' for any measure of a human attribute (this explains why this term appears in the original literature, e.g. Gulliksen (1950), Lord & Novick (1968), and set about the large-scale testing of sensory discrimination and motor function in the belief that people with the most acute senses would be the most gifted and most knowledgeable (Rogers, 1995). However, when Galton's colleague Pearson developed and applied the correlation coefficient, it became clear that results from these simple sensory and motor tests bore almost no relationship to measures of intellectual achievement, such as school grades (Nunnally, 1970). This finding prompted the development of the mental test movement, i.e. the widespread interest in the development and application of mental testing, and the measurement of individual differences.

A major advance in mental testing (Torgerson, 1958) was made when Thurstone demonstrated that psychophysical scaling methods could be used to accurately measure psychological attributes (Thurstone, 1925; Thurstone & Chave, 1929). This finding prompted the development of psychological (or psychometric) scaling methods, which are defined as procedures for constructing scales for the measurement of psychological attributes (Guilford, 1954). Spurred on by the practical need to measure diverse outcomes, the mental test movement flourished between 1930 and 1950 with the spread of standardized testing for assessing educational achievement, measuring attitudes and personality and selecting and screening personnel. In addition, scientific interest in methods of testing led to the development of psychometrics as a prominent discipline within psychology and established the cornerstones of the scientific evaluation of measuring instruments based on reliability and validity testing (Guilford, 1954; Nunnally, 1967).

Thus, when health care evaluation needed methods for measuring patient-oriented outcomes, the technology already existed. Since the 1970s, the focus of health care evaluation has moved to the measurement of function (the ability of patients to perform the daily activities of their lives), how patients feel, and their own personal evaluation of their health in general (Stewart & Ware, 1992). The primary source of this information is standardized surveys (Ware et al., 1980), for which psychometric techniques of scale construction are highly appropriate (Stewart & Ware, 1992). Two studies in the US confirmed the value of psychometric methods for measuring health variables.

The Health Insurance Experiment (Brook et al., 1979), a randomized experiment conducted by The RAND Corporation between 1974 and 1981, demonstrated that psychometric methods can be used to generate reliable and valid measures for assessing changes in health status for both adults and children in the general population. Following on from this, the Medical Outcomes Study (Stewart et al., 1989; Stewart & Ware, 1992) demonstrated that psychometric methods of scale construction and data collection were successful for measuring health status in samples of sick and elderly people. This study also demonstrated that psychometrically equivalent short-form measures could be constructed from the original longer-forms (McHorney et al., 1992), thereby reducing respondent and administrative burden and improving measurement efficiency. These two pivotal studies confirmed that psychometric methods, borrowed from the social sciences, generated scientifically sound and clinically useful health measures.

Psychometric methods, however, have been slow to transfer to clinical practice. Perhaps because many clinicians do not have the time to learn about instrument development and evaluation, and the literature, which is directed primarily towards educationalists and psychologists, is incomprehensible (Streiner & Norman, 1995). Consequently, awareness of psychometric methods is limited, despite a rapid expansion of the health measurement literature since the mid-1980s. Although the principles and standards developed in psychology and education are highly applicable to health, it is important to note that they may not be wholly appropriate as measurement of health differs from measurement of psychological and educational constructs (McDowell & Jenkinson, 1996). McDowell and Jenkinson argue that 'as health is based on biological processes it includes a factual element and a consistent internal logical structure that is absent in ratings of political opinions or economic preferences' (McDowell & Jenkinson, 1996, page 238). Important health-specific methodological work is still needed (Hunt, 1997).

Measuring clinical variables

Traditionally, medicine has evaluated the effectiveness of therapeutic interventions using measurements made by machines or by documenting simple clinical end points. For example, studies of interferons in MS have measured MRI abnormalities and relapse rates; studies of interventions in stroke have measured mortality rates, recurrence of stroke rates, and incidence of cerebral haemorrage as a complication of treatments; studies in epilepsy have meas-

0   No increase in tone

1   Slight increase in tone giving a "catch" when the limb is moved in flexion or extension

[1+* Slight increase in tone, manifested by a catch, followed by minimal resistance throughout the remainder (less than half) of the range of movement]

2   More marked increase in tone but the limb easily flexed

3   Considerable increase in tone, passive movement difficult

4   Limb rigid in flexion or extension

* The modified Ashworth scale includes the 1+ rating

Fig. 7.1. Ashworth scale of spasticity.

ured seizure frequency; studies of neurological cancers have measured mortality rates, duration of survival and 5-year survival rates.

Two limitations of traditional outcomes have recently been highlighted. They provide little information about the diverse consequences of disease, and they fail to incorporate the patient perspective. Consequently, there is a need to measure more pertinent but abstract health status concepts such as disability/activities, handicap/participations, and health-related quality of life. As neurology is a specialty with few cures and a large proportion of chronic disorders, this change in focus from measuring quantity of life towards assessing aspects of the quality of life is particularly appropriate. However, this change has brought new challenges because abstract health status concepts, unlike concrete physical entities such as height, weight, and blood pressure, are impossible to measure explicitly because they are unobservable (Bland & Altman, 1997). In the social sciences unobservable variables are know as theoretical constructs or latent variables. Reliable and valid rating scales must be devised to measure these variables. (A construct is a variable that is relatively abstract as opposed to concrete, and is defined or operationalized in terms of observed indicators (Stewart & Ware, 1992)).

Latent variables can be measured indirectly by asking questions intended to capture empirically the essential meaning of the construct. The simplest way to do this is to ask a single straightforward question (item). For example, rate patient X's degree of disability on a scale of 1 (no disability) to 5 (extremely disabled). The Ashworth scale (Fig. 7.1), which grades spasticity from 0 (no increase in tone) to 4 (limb rigid in flexion or extension), is an example of a single item measure (Ashworth, 1964; Bohannon & Smith,

1987). Although single item measures are simple, user friendly, and appropriate for measuring some individual properties, they have a number of scientific limitations when measuring complex clinical variables. Single items are unlikely to represent well the broad scope of a complex theoretical construct and, are likely to interpreted in many different ways by respondents. In addition, single items are imprecise as they cannot discriminate fine degree of an attribute (the Ashworth scale categorises patients into five levels only), and are notoriously unreliable (prone to random error) as they do not produce consistent answers over time (Nunnally, 1978). Finally, it is difficult to estimate the measurement properties of single item measures (McIver & Carmines, 1981).

Multi-item instruments, where each item addresses a different aspect of the same underlying construct, are able to overcome the scientific limitations of single items and are superior methods of measuring latent variables. More items increase the scope of the measure, are less open to variable interpretation, enable better precision, and improve reliability by allowing random errors of measurement to average out (Nunnally, 1978). The Barthel Index (Mahoney & Barthel, 1965) is an example of a multi-item measure. Its ten items measure feeding, grooming, dressing, bathing, walking, transfers, stairs, toilet use, bladder, and bowels. Item scores are summed to generate a total score, which is an estimate of dependency in activities of daily living.

There are many methods, termed scaling models, for combining multiple items into scales depending on the purpose the resulting scale is to serve (Thurstone, 1925; Guttman, 1945; Gulliksen, 1950; Edwards, 1957; Torgerson, 1958). The most widely used scaling model in health measurement is the method of summated rating proposed by

Likert in 1932 (Likert, 1932; Likert et al., 1934). Four characteristics constitute a summated rating scale. First, there are multiple items whose scores are summed, without weighting, to generate a total score. Secondly, each item measures a property that can vary quantitatively (e.g. difficulty walking ranges from none to unable to walk). Thirdly, each item has no right answer. Fourthly, each item in the scale can be rated independently. Examples of Likert scales in health measurement are: the Barthel Index (BI) (Mahoney & Barthel, 1965), functional independence measure (FIM) (Granger et al., 1986), Medical Outcomes Study 36-item Short Form Health Survey (SF-36) (Ware et al., 1993, 1994), General Health Questionnaire (GHQ) (Goldberg, 1978), Hospital Anxiety and Depression Scale (HADS) (Zigmond & Snaith, 1983), and the Parkinson's Disease Questionnaire (PDQ-39) (Peto et al., 1995). Likert scales are popular because they are simple, easy to administer, user friendly, cheap, relatively straightforward to develop, and can be reliable and valid.

Evaluating health rating scales

In this section we discuss the process of evaluating rating scales. We make the assumption that a neurologist has chosen to use a particular scale but there is no published evidence concerning its measurement properties. This is a common scenario…what should be done?

There are two compelling reasons why it is important for clinicians to consider formally evaluating health rating scales. First, the properties of a scale are sample dependent (not simply disease dependent) and, therefore, the performance of a measure in a specific application is more important than its performance generally (McHorney et al., 1994). Secondly, data are only as strong as the instruments used to collect them. Sophisticated statistical methods and advances in study design will do little to overcome the damage done by poor quality measures (Fleiss, 1986; Cone & Foster, 1991), despite opinions to the contrary (Wade, 1999). It is sobering to think that vast amounts of money have been spent evaluating the impact of interferons on disability in MS using a measure, the Expanded Disability Status Scale (Kurtzke, 1983). Prior to these studies there had been limited evaluation of the EDSS using formal psychometric methods. Subsequently, evaluations have demonstrated its limited ability to discriminate between individuals and groups known to differ in their levels of disability and poor responsiveness (Sharrack et al., 1999; Hobart et al., 2000).

The aim of scale evaluation is to determine whether an instrument satisfies criteria for rigorous measurement.

Much of this information can be gained from the retrospective analysis of data if they have already have been collected. However, prospective studies are often required. We recommend evaluating five measurement properties: data quality, scaling assumptions, acceptability, reliability, validity and responsiveness.

Data quality

Indicators of data quality, such as percentage item non-response and percentage computable scores, determine the extent to which an instrument can be incorporated into a clinical setting. These indicators, like all psychometric properties, vary across samples (McHorney et al., 1994). If the measure is patient report, these indicators reflect respondents' understanding and acceptance of a measure and help to identify items that may be irrelevant, confusing, or upsetting to patients (McHorney et al., 1994). If the measure is clinician report, these indicators reflect the ability to incorporate a measure into a clinical setting. When there are large amounts of missing data for items, scores for scales cannot be reliably estimated.

Scaling assumptions

Tests of scaling assumptions determine whether it is legitimate to generate scores for an instrument using the algorithms proposed by the developers. For example, the Medical Outcomes Study 36-item Short-Form Health Survey (SF-36; Ware et al., 1993), a generic measure of health status, has 36 items grouped into eight scales. A score is generated for each SF-36 scale by summing scores across groups of items. However, few investigators examine whether the assumptions that underpin the summing of items to generate scores are satisfied. Items can be summed without weighting or standardization when they measure at the same point on the scale (have similar mean scores), contribute similarly to the variance of the total score (have similar variances), measure a common underlying construct (the items must be internally consistent), and are correctly grouped into scales (hypothesized item groupings are supported by techniques including factor analysis and examination of item convergent and discriminant validity).

Acceptability

Acceptability is the extent to which the spectrum of health measured by a scale matches the distribution of health in the study sample and is determined simply by examining score distributions (Lohr et al., 1996). Ideally, the observed scores from a sample should span the entire range of the

Table 7.1. Score ranges, means, standard deviations, floor and ceiling effects for EDSS[a], Barthel Index, and FIM[b] ($n = 64$)

Instrument	Admission score			Floor effect n (%)	Ceiling effect n (%)
	Range				
	Scale	Sample	Mean (SD)		
EDSS	0–10	5.0–9.0	7.1 (0.9)	0 (0)	0 (0)
Barthel Index	0–20	0–20	12.02 (5.7)	5 (2.5)	10 (5.4)
FIM	18–126	24–122	89.42 (23.6)	0 (0)	0 (0)

Notes:

[a] EDSS = Kurtzke Expanded Disability Status Scale.

[b] FIM = Functional Independence Measure.

scale, the mean score should be near the scale midpoint, and floor and ceiling effects (percentage of the sample having the minimum and maximum score, respectively) should be small. McHorney recommends floor and ceiling effects should be <15% (McHorney & Tarlov, 1995).

Table 7.1 presents results from an unpublished study and illustrates the importance of examining score distributions. Score distributions for 64 MS patients undergoing inpatient neuro-rehabilitation are presented for three disability measures, the EDSS, Barthel Index, and Functional Independence Measure (FIM). Neither scale has floor or ceiling effects. These results indicate that the range of disability in the sample is adequately covered by all three instruments. However, the sample spans the whole range of the Barthel Index and FIM but only 50% of the EDSS scale range. These results indicate that the EDSS covers a greater range of disability than the Barthel and FIM. More importantly, these findings indicate that the EDSS does not discriminate as well as the Barthel Index and FIM between different levels of disability. This is further exemplified by examining Table 7.2, which reports the range of Barthel and FIM scores for each EDSS score in the study sample.

Reliability

Reliability is defined as the extent to which a measure is free from random error, and is expressed as a reliability coefficient. However, reliability is a generic term, multiple types (and therefore many reliability coefficients) exist for each instrument. Each type of reliability addresses a different source (or sources) of random error. Ideally, all relevant types of reliability should be quantified.

For health measures the most important (but not the only) types of reliability are internal consistency and reproducibility (test–retest, inter-rater, and intrarater). Other

Table 7.2. Barthel Index and FIM score ranges and means for each EDSS score ($n = 311$)

EDSS score	n	Barthel Index score		FIM score	
		Range	Mean	Range	Mean
5.0	3	19–20	N/A[a]	114–122	NA
5.5	6	14–19	17.7	99–119	112.0
6.0	49	8–20	17.9	80–122	110.3
6.5	80	8–20	15.6	71–122	103.8
7.0	48	5–20	12.3	64–117	93.6
7.5	37	2–18	10.1	37–114	83.3
8.0	54	2–16	8.1	38–113	75.9
8.5	23	0–11	3.7	33–93	56.5
9.0	11	0–5	N/A	24–57	n/A

Notes:

[a] Not applicable due to small sample.

types of reliability are beyond the scope of this chapter but are detailed in standard texts (Cronbach, 1949; Nunnally, 1978; Anastasi & Urbina, 1997). Internal consistency is the extent to which items within a scale are reliable measures of the same construct. This type of reliability only applies to multi-item measures like the SF-36 and Barthel Index and is determined using Cronbach's alpha coefficient (Cronbach, 1951). Reproducibility is the agreement between two or more ratings on the same person. Test–retest reliability is the agreement between two or more self-report ratings for the same patient. Intrarater reproducibility is the agreement between two or more ratings for the same patient made by the same observer. Inter-rater reproducibility is the agreement between two or more ratings for the same patient made by the different

Table 7.3. Product–moment correlations between the FIM, other measures of disability, and measures of handicap, psychological well-being, health status and age

	Barthel Index	EDSS[a]	LHS[b]	GHQ[c]	SF-36 PCS[d]	SF-36 MCS[e]	Age
FIM[f]	0.94	0.87	0.42	0.13	0.14	0.28	−0.05

Notes:

[a] EDSS = Kurtzke expanded disability status scale.

[b] LHS = London handicap scale.

[c] GHQ = general health questionnaire.

[d] SF-36 PCS = medical outcomes study 36-item short form health survey physical component summary score.

[e] SF-36 MCS = medical outcomes study 36-item short form health survey mental component summary score.

[f] FIM = functional independence measure.

observers. Reproducibility should be reported as an intraclass correlation coefficient for continuous data (Shrout & Fleiss, 1979), and Kappa coefficients for dichotomous data (Cohen, 1960).

Validity

The validity of a health measure is the extent to which it measures what it purports to measure (Nunnally, 1978). Determining the validity of a health measure is difficult for three reasons: validity cannot be proven it can only be supported, there is no consensus as to the minimum requirement of evidence to satisfy validity, and evidence supporting validity in one context does not guarantee validity for another.

Although any evidence that an instrument measures the construct it is purported to measure supports its validity, the strongest evidence is provided by examining its correlations with other measures collected at the same time (convergent and discriminant construct validity; Cronbach & Meehl, 1955). Validity is supported by the extent to which correlations conform with the direction, pattern, and magnitude of predictions. For example, Table 7.3 presents correlations between the FIM and a selection of other scales in 64 MS patients undergoing inpatient rehabilitation. If the FIM measures disability, we would predict: high correlations with other measures of physical disability (BI, EDSS); higher correlation with measures of disability than with measures of handicap (LHS), and psychological well-being (GHQ); low correlations with age. The data in Table 7.3 conform with these predictions and therefore provide strong evidence for the validity of the FIM as a measure of disability in MS patients. Studies of convergent and discriminant construct validity are limited if the validating instruments themselves have not been comprehensively validated. Consequently, it is important to have results from multiple studies.

Responsiveness

Responsiveness is the ability of an instrument to detect clinically significant change in the attribute measured (Guyatt et al., 1987). Responsiveness methodology is less well advanced than that for reliability and validity, and whilst several methods have been proposed for determining the responsiveness of health measures there is no clear consensus as to which method is optimal (Liang, 1995). Most methods examine scores at two points in time, usually before and after an intervention thought to alter the attribute being measured. Responsiveness is reflected by the magnitude of the standardised change score (effect size). Simply reporting raw change scores as indices of responsiveness is limited because these do not take into account the sample studied nor allow comparison between different instruments. Only reporting the statistical significance of change scores as an index of instrument responsiveness is also limited because this is heavily dependent upon the sample size. Moreover, statistical significance doesn't guarantee clinical significance (Cohen, 1994; Cortina & Dunlap, 1997). For these reasons it is recommended that responsiveness is reported in the form of an effect size (standardized change score). The formula for the most commonly reported effect size is: mean change score divided by the standard deviation of the baseline scores (Kazis et al., 1989). The larger the effect size, the greater the responsiveness of an instrument. To aid the clinical interpretation of effect size values it has been recommended that Cohen's arbitrary criteria are applied: 0.20 = small; 0.50 = medium; 0.80 = large (Cohen, 1988; Kazis et al., 1989). However, when comparing instruments, the strongest evidence for the superior responsiveness of an instrument comes from head-to-head comparisons of instruments.

Practical aspects of scale evaluation

Data quality, scaling assumptions, and internal consistency reliability can be examined from a single administration of a rating scale to a sample of people. Some aspects of validity, for example intercorrelations between scales and group differences validity, can also be examined. Convergent and discriminant validity can be examined from a single administration when other scales are administered at the same time.

Reproducibility (test–retest, inter-rater, intrarater) and responsiveness require an instrument to be administered on two or more occasions. The time interval between the two administrations for reproducibility estimation is important. Whilst some authors recommend around two weeks (Streiner & Norman, 1995), the most appropriate interval is study dependent. The aim is to achieve the optimum balance between raters (patient of clinicians) remembering their answers and therefore observed reliability being an overestimate, and true change occurring in the person being rated. Memory effect leads to overestimates of reliability and change results in underestimates of reliability. Nevertheless, more conservative estimates are best. Responsiveness studies require that an instrument is re-administered after change has occurred.

As many measurement properties can be evaluated from the single administration of a scale, psychometric studies can often be undertaken on the data arising from clinical trials. Whilst we do not encourage the retrospective evaluation of scales as the primary approach to determining the psychometric properties of an instrument, such data are important evidence of the value of a rating scale in a given clinical setting.

There is no consensus or even published guidelines for sample size calculations for psychometric studies. However, there are two rules of thumb. First, the sample studied should be representative of the population in whom the rating scale is going to be used. Secondly, the larger the sample the greater the confidence of the results. It is also important to consider clinical practicality. It may be impossible to study large samples of people with rare or uncommon diseases. Finally, some evidence is better than none.

Choosing a rating scale

Clinical trialists often have to choose one scale from among many potential candidates (Bowling, 1991, 1995; Wade, 1992; Wilkin et al., 1992; McDowell & Newell, 1996; Herndon, 1997). Unfortunately, no one scale exhibits all desirable qualities, different scales have different virtues, and instruments that are useful for one clinical trialist may not be useful for others. Therefore, scales must be selected for the particular purpose for which they are to be used and the scale user must be able to choose measures intelligently based on their needs.

For success in clinical trials, instruments must be clinically useful and scientifically sound. Clinical usefulness refers to the successful incorporation of an instrument into clinical practice and its appropriateness to the study sample. Scientific soundness refers to the demonstration of reliable, valid, and responsive measurement of the outcome of interest. Clinical usefulness does not guarantee scientific soundness, and vice versa. Below is a list of questions that we think should be addressed when selecting a rating scale.

Does the scale measure the appropriate health entity?

This is a fundamental question that must be addressed head on. Instruments selection should be based on a clear hypothesis of the impact of the intervention under study. Choosing scales simply because of their popularity, or because they were developed locally, is likely to result in the measurement of outcomes that are distal to the ideal. Under these circumstances the effectiveness of an intervention may be misrepresented.

Is the method of administration appropriate for the study?

The method of administration of an instrument should not be changed from that recommended by the instrument developers in order to suit the needs of a study. This is because altering the method of administration may affect the scientific properties (reliability and validity) of a measure. If an alternative method of administration is considered necessary, the validity of this method needs to be evaluated before the instrument is used. This can be achieved by correlating scores for patients obtained by the two methods, the higher the correlation the greater the validity of the alternative method of administration.

Is the rating scale acceptable to patients?

User acceptability is important in obtaining the cooperation of persons in the study. Patients in clinical trials are often ill or disabled and their tolerance for completing long and complex questionnaires may be limited. Seemingly irrelevant items arouse criticism. Busy clinicians with no ownership of a study have little personal gain from the results. These factors influence the interest of patients and clinicians in participating in clinical trials, affect the reliability and validity of scores, and also the relationships between the investigators, clinicians and patients.

Does the spectrum of health measured by the scale match the level of health in the study sample?

The range of health addressed by a rating scale needs to match the distribution of scores in the sample otherwise there will be notable floor and ceiling effects (percentage of subjects scoring the minimum and maximum possible scores, respectively). Floor and ceiling effects represent subsamples of patients for whom actual changes in health will be underestimated (floor) or not recorded (ceiling) by a rating scale. The acceptability of a scale can be determined by examining score distributions for the sample of interest. Ideally, scores should span the entire scale range, means scores should be near the scale midpoint, and floor and ceiling effects should be small (<15%) (McHorney & Tarlov, 1995).

Does the rating scale generate reliable estimates?

When evaluating reliability data available for instruments, investigators should try and answer three questions:

Have the appropriate types of reliability been assessed?

Internal consistency can be examined in all multi-item measures. Test–retest reproducibility should be examined for self-report measures. Inter-rater and intrarater reproducibility should be examined for observer report measures. It is unusual to find instruments were the assessment of reliability is comprehensive. For multi-item measures the most useful index of reliability is the internal consistency because the major source of error is item sampling. A full explanation of this can be found in standard texts (Nunnally, 1978). Also, there is good evidence that estimates of internal consistency and reproducibility are similar (Ware et al., 1978, 1979) and that Cronbach's alpha tends to provide a conservative reliability estimate (Bravo & Potvin, 1991). Finally, high test–retest reliability with low internal consistency is much more likely than low internal consistency with high test–retest reliability.

Were the reliability studies conducted in appropriate samples?

All psychometric properties are dependent upon the samples from which they were determined. Therefore, results can only be generalised from one sample to another

if the reliability in the two samples is expected to be similar. For example, demonstration of high reliability for a self-report health measure in persons with cervical myelopathy cannot be assumed to indicate high reliability in persons with dementia. However, evidence of reliability from multiple studies in different groups suggests reliability is a stable property for the instrument. There is no consensus as to the sizes of samples for reliability studies. However, it is important that the sample is representative of the larger sample in which the rating scale is to be used.

Has adequate reliability been demonstrated?

Widely recommended minimum requirements are 0 .80 (ideally 0.85 (Nunnally & Bernstein, 1994)) for group comparison studies, and 0.90 (ideally >0.95) for individual comparison studies (Nuyens et al., 1994; Lohr et al., 1996). The need for high reliability in individual comparison studies is clear when confidence intervals around individual scores are calculated using the standard error of measurement (SEM). This estimates the standard deviation of scores obtained if an instrument were administered repeatedly to the same individual using the following formula:

$$SEM = SD \times \sqrt{(1 - reliability)};$$
$$95\% \text{ confidence intervals } (+/- 1.96 \text{ SEM}).$$

Table 7.4 illustrates the effect of decreasing reliability on the confidence intervals of Barthel Index scores and demonstrates why scores for individual patients should be interpreted with extreme caution.

Is the rating scale valid?

To determine whether an instrument is valid for a specific purpose, clinical trialists must assess the strength of empirical evidence available. Evidence for content validity

Table 7.4. Effect of different levels of reliability on the confidence intervals around individual patient scores for the Barthel Index

Reliability	95% confidence interval
0.95	+/−2.6
0.90	+/−3.7
0.80	+/−5.2
0.70	+/−6.3
0.60	+/−7.3
0.50	+/−8.2

Notes:

Barthel Index scores: $n = 149$; mean score = 11.5; SD = 5.9; sample range 0–20; floor effect = 2.5%; ceiling effect = 5.4%.

is weak validity evidence. Stronger evidence is provided by studies of group differences. Even stronger validity evidence is provided by studies of convergent and discriminant construct validity.

Is there evidence that the scale will detect change?

When evaluating responsiveness data, the most useful studies are head-to-head comparisons of instruments purported to measure the same health construct. These data are rare. The most likely scenario, if responsiveness has been examined, is that the statistical significance of the change scores is reported. These results can be misleading as P values are sample size dependent. Are the raw data available to compute effect sizes?

Developing scales

Developing clinical scales is a labour-intensive process requiring considerable expertise in health measurement (Spector, 1992). Therefore, clinical trialists are advised to carefully evaluate available measures before abandoning them. The psychometric properties of available measures can be determined more quickly. Here, we present an overview on instrument development.

Development of a measurement instrument in accordance with psychometric theory involves four stages: first, defining a conceptual model; secondly, generation of an item pool; thirdly, reduction the item pool to form an instrument; fourthly, testing the reliability, validity and responsiveness of the final instrument.

A conceptual model is the rationale for, and description of the concept(s) that the measure is intended to assess (Lohr et al., 1996). The importance of a conceptual basis for the measurement of latent variables cannot be overemphasized (DeVellis, 1991; Kopec et al., 1995). However, this is often absent or poorly defined for health measurement instruments (McDowell & Newell, 1996). For example, a clinical trialist may wish to develop a measure of disability for MS. The trialist must first define disability in MS and decide which aspects to measure. Only when this has been done can a comprehensive approach to item generation be undertaken.

There are four sources from which candidate items can be generated: semistructured interviews of patients with the disorder under study, consensus opinion of experts in the field, literature review, and examination of available measures. Patient interviews are very valuable as they help to identify areas that are important to them, a process that maximizes the validity of an instrument. From these four sources, items are devised aiming to address the appropriate range and depth of concept/s to be measured. These items are then pretested on a small sample to assess how easily they can be understood and completed. Appropriate alterations are made and this version is used in the preliminary field test.

The purpose of the preliminary field test phase is to reduce the number of items and to develop a scale. The instrument is administered to a large sample of patients and the results are analysed using standard psychometric techniques for item analysis (Nunnally & Bernstein, 1994; Streiner & Norman, 1995). The aim of item reduction is to select, on an empirical basis, the items that measure the construct of interest, that is items that discriminate between individuals, are stable over time, and measure the same underlying construct. The importance of selecting items on an empirical basis is that approaches to measurement on an intuitive basis often fail to produce the desired empirical results (Nunnally, 1970). After items have been reduced, they may need to be grouped into scales if it is anticipated that the instrument may measure more than one related but different construct. Items can be grouped in two ways: first, on a theoretical basis and, secondly on an empirical basis using item-level exploratory factor analysis. Item groupings, both hypothesized and empirically defined, are then tested using multitrait scaling techniques to define which method of grouping items produces the best empirical measurement instrument (Ware et al., 1997). When items have been reduced and scales formed, the final instrument must be tested on an independent sample for its clinical usefulness and scientific soundness (reliability, validity and responsiveness) using the techniques outlined above.

It is encouraging to see that traditional psychometric methods are being used increasingly in the neurosciences (Peto et al., 1995; Jenkinson et al., 1999; Williams et al., 1999; Hobart et al., 2001).

New development in psychometrics

The methods we have described above are termed traditional psychometric methods. These methods have been used successfully to develop reliable and valid patient-based health outcome measures (Stewart & Ware, 1992). Most of these measures are multi-item rating scales in which scores across several items or questions are summed to generate a total (raw) score that quantifies the health variable of interest (e.g. physical function). Nevertheless, the raw scores generated by these rating scales have important limitations that restrict the impact of patient-based outcomes on clinical trials, epidemiological studies and routine clinical practice.

The first limitation is that raw scores are non-linear counts and not interval measures. This potentially biases the interpretation of scores and score changes, and may result in treatment effectiveness being underestimated (Wright & Linacre, 1989; Wright, 1997). A second limitation is that raw scores are scale dependent. Therefore, different scales purporting to measure the same health construct cannot be accurately equated, or their results combined for systematic reviews and meta-analyses (Bjorner & Ware, 1998). A third limitation is that the psychometric properties of scales are sample dependent and, therefore, not necessarily stable across different samples (McHorney et al., 1994). A fourth limitation is that rating scales tend to cover a limited spectrum of health. Samples in clinical studies often extent outside of the range of the scale resulting in floor and ceiling effects. These represent subsamples of patients for whom health changes will not be detected, or be underestimated by scales. A final limitation is that raw scores are not precise enough for individual patient clinical decision-making. Therefore, rating scales cannot be used in routine clinical practice (McHorney & Tarlov, 1995).

These limitations of summed rating scales were recognized years ago in education and psychology. Research led to the development of Rasch item analysis (Rasch, 1960) and Item Response Theory (IRT; Lord & Novick, 1968) models. These new psychometric methods convert raw scores into interval measures using a log odds-ratio transformation (Wright & Stone, 1979). Moreover, these methods claim to generate sample-free item calibrations and scale-free person measures, thereby enabling the accurate cocalibration of measures of the same health construct and the formation of calibrated item banks from which any subsets of items can be chosen to solve measurement problems (Wright, 1977). Calibrated item banks lay the foundation for rapid and efficient individual-patient measurement using computer algorithms (Wainer et al., 1990).

Since 1990 there has been considerable interest in applying Rasch analysis and IRT to health measurement. Initially, studies concentrated on using these methods to evaluate (Linacre et al., 1994; Tennant et al., 1996a, b), and refine (Prieto et al., 1998) existing rating scales. More recently, studies have successfully used Rasch and IRT to equate rating scales in oncology (Chang & Cella, 1997), elderly adults (McHorney & Cohen, 2000), and headache (Ware et al., 2000). Although many believe that Rasch item analysis and IRT have the potential to take the health outcomes field to a new plateau (Cella & Chang, 2000; Hambleton, 2000; Hays et al., 2000; McHorney & Cohen,

2000; Ware et al., 2000), these methods have been criticized (Divgi, 1986; Rust & Golombok, 1999) and are not as widely used as their apparent advantages would suggest they should be (Embretson & Hershberger, 1999). These facts have been attributed, in part, to a misunderstanding of the models and ill-considered applications (Linacre, 2000). Nevertheless, there have been surprisingly few empirical studies critically evaluating these methods in health measurement and comparing them with traditional psychometric approaches.

Conclusions

Latent variables can be measured rigorously using Likert scales and should be used as outcomes in the evaluation of therapeutic interventions in neurology. When assessing available instruments, clinical trialists must evaluate their clinical usefulness and scientific soundness with respect to a particular study. First, find instruments that can be incorporated into the study design, whose items look like they measure the required constructs for the study (don't be misled by instrument names), and are appropriate to the study sample. Next, examine the empirical evidence that these measures are reliable, valid and responsive in the study sample. Start with evidence for reliability as this is a prerequisite for (but not sufficient for) validity and responsiveness. Have the important types of reliability been determined in appropriate samples, and have minimum criteria for the type of study (group or individual comparisons) been satisfied? Next, examine the empirical evidence that the instrument measures what it purports to measure. What type of evidence supports the instrument's validity and how strong is this evidence? Finally, what evidence is there that the instrument has the ability to detect change over time?

The trialist is commonly left with no instrument fulfilling all the above criteria. Can further evaluative studies be undertaken on available instruments, or does the study design need to be reconsidered? If no instrument exists and no compromise is acceptable, a new instrument may need to be developed. Be sure to collaborate with a health measurement expert, but also be sure that they have one foot in clinical reality (Aaronson, 1988). Finally, new methods of data analysis have the potential to overcome the limitations of summed rating scales and improve the value of health measurement to clinical practice.

References

Aaronson, N.K. (1988). Quantitative issues in health-related quality of life assessment. *Health Policy*, **10**, 217–30.

Anastasi, A. & Urbina, S. (1997). *Psychological Testing*. Upper Saddle River, New Jersey: Prentice-Hall.

Ashworth, B. (1964). Preliminary trial of carisoprodol in multiple sclerosis. *Practitioner*, **192**, 540–2.

Bjorner, J.B. & Ware, J.E.J. (1998). Using modern psychometric methods to measure health outcomes. *Med. Outcomes Trust Monitor*, **3**(2), 1–5.

Bland, J.M. & Altman, D.G. (1997). Cronbach's alpha. *Br. Med. J.*, **314**, 572.

Bohannon, R.W. & Smith, M.B. (1987). Inter-rater reliability of a modified Ashworth scale of spasticity. *Physical Therapy*, **67**, 206–7.

Bowling, A. (1991). *Measuring Health: A Review of Quality of Life Measurement Scales*. Milton Keynes: Open University Press.

Bowling, A. (1995). *Measuring Disease: A Review of Disease-specific Quality of Life Measurement Scales*. Buckingham: Open University Press.

Bravo, G. & Potvin, L. (1991). Estimating the reliability of continuous measures with Cronbach's alpha or the intraclass correlation coefficient: toward the integration of two traditions. *J. Clin. Epidemiol.*, **44**(4/5), 381–90.

Brook, R.H., Ware, J.E. Jr et al. (1979). Overview of adult health status measures fielded in Rand's Health Insurance Study. *Med. Care*, **17**(7 Suppl.), 1–131.

Cella, D. & Chang, C-H. (2000). A discussion of item response theory and its application in health status measurement. *Med. Care*, **38**(9 Suppl. 11), 66–72.

Chang, C-H. & Cella, D. (1997). Equating health-related quality of life instruments in applied oncological settings. *Physical Medicine and Rehabilitation: State of the Art Reviews. Outcomes Measurement*, ed. R. Smith, pp. 397–406. Phildelphia: Hanley & Belfus, Inc.

Cohen, J. (1960). A coefficient of agreement for nominal scales. *Educ. Psychol. Measurem.*, **20**(1), 37–46.

Cohen, J. (1988). *Statistical Power Analysis for the Behavioural Sciences*. Hillsdale, New Jersey: Lawrence Erlbaum Associates.

Cohen, J. (1994). The earth is round (*P*<0.05). *Am. Psychol.*, **49**(12), 997–1003.

Cone, J.D. & Foster, S.L. (1991). Training in measurement: always the bridesmaid. *Am. Psychol.*, **46**(6), 653–4.

Cortina, J.M. & Dunlap, W.P. (1997). On the logic and purpose of significance testing. *Psychol. Methods*, **2**(2), 161–72.

Cronbach, L.J. (1949). *Essentials of Psychological Testing*. New York: Harper and Row.

Cronbach, L.J. (1951). Coefficient alpha and the internal structure of tests. *Psychometrika*, **16**(3), 297–334.

Cronbach, L.J. & Meehl, P.E. (1955). Construct validity in psychological tests. *Psychol. Bull.*, **52**(4), 281–302.

DeVellis, R.F. (1991). *Scale Development: Theory and Applications*. London: Sage Publications.

Divgi, D. (1986). Does the Rasch model really work for multiple choice items? Not if you look closely. *J. Educ. Measurem.*, **23**(4), 283–98.

Edwards, A.L. (1957). *Techniques of Attitude Scale Construction*. New York: Appleton-Century-Crofts.

Embretson, S.E. & Hershberger, S.L. eds. (1999). *The New Rules of Measurement*. Mahwah, New Jersey: Lawrence Erlbaum Associates.

Fleiss, J.L. (1986). *The Design and Analysis of Clinical Experiments*. New York: Wiley.

Goldberg, D.P. (1978). *Manual of the General Health Questionnaire*. Windsor: NFER-Nelson.

Granger, C.V., Hamilton, B.B. et al. (1986). Advances in functional assessment for medical rehabilitation. *Topics Geriat. Rehabil.*, **1**(3), 59–74.

Guilford, J.P. (1954). *Psychometric Methods*. New York: McGraw-Hill.

Gulliksen, H. (1950). *Theory of Mental Tests*. New York: Wiley.

Guttman, L. (1945). A basis for analysing test-retest reliability. *Psychometrika*, **10**(4), 255–82.

Guyatt, G.H., Walter, S. et al. (1987). Measuring change over time: assessing the usefulness of evaluative instruments. *J. Chronic Dis.*, **40**(2), 171–8.

Hambleton, R.K. (2000). Item response theory modeling in instrument development and data analysis. *Med. Care*, **38**(9 Suppl. 11), 60–5.

Hays, R.D., Morales, L.S. et al. (2000). Item response theory and health outcomes measurement in the 21st century. *Med. Care*, **38**(9 Suppl. 11), 28–42.

Herndon, R.M., ed. (1997). *Handbook of Neurological Rating Scales*. New York: Demos.

Hobart, J.C., Freeman, J.A. et al. (2000). Kurtzke scales revisited: the application of psychometric methods to clinical intuition. *Brain*, **123**, 1027–40.

Hobart, J.C., Lamping, D.L. et al. (2001). The Multiple Sclerosis Impact Scale (MSIS-29): a new patient-based outcome measure. *Brain*, **124**, 962–73.

Hunt, S.M. (1997). The problem of quality of life. *Qual. Life Res.*, **6**, 205–12.

Jenkinson, C., Fitzpatrick, R. et al. (1999). Development and validation of a short measure of health status for individuals with ALS/MND. *J. Neurol.*, **246**(Suppl. 3), 16–21.

Kazis, L.E., Anderson, J.J. et al. (1989). Effect sizes for interpreting changes in health status. *Med. Care*, **27**(3 Suppl), S178–89.

Kopec, J.A., Esdaile, J.M. et al. (1995). The Quebec Back Pain Disability Scale: measurement properties. *Spine*, **20**(3), 341–52.

Kurtzke, J.F. (1983). Rating neurological impairment in multiple sclerosis: an expanded disability status scale (EDSS). *Neurology*, **33**, 1444–52.

Liang, M.H. (1995). Evaluating instrument responsiveness. *J. Rheumatol.*, **22**(6), 1191–2.

Likert, R.A. (1932). A technique for the development of attitudes. *Arch. Psychol.*, **140**, 5–55.

Likert, R.A., Roslow, S. et al. (1934). A simple and reliable method of scoring the Thurstone attitude scales. *J. Soc. Psychol.*, **5**, 228–38.

Linacre, J. (2000). Historic misunderstandings of the Rasch model. *Rasch Measurem. Trans.*, **14**(2), 748–9.

Linacre, J.M., Heinemann, A.W. et al. (1994). The structure and stability of the Functional Independence Measure. *Arch. Phys. Med. Rehabil.*, **75**(2), 127–32.

Lohr, K.N., Aaronson, N.K. et al. (1996). Evaluating quality of life and health status instruments: development of scientific review criteria. *Clin. Ther.*, **18**(5), 979–92.

Lord, F.M. & Novick, M.R. (1968). *Statistical Theories of Mental Test Scores*. Reading, Massachusetts: Addison-Wesley.

McDowell, I. & Jenkinson, C. (1996). Development standards for health measures. *J. Health Serv. Res. Policy*, **1**(4), 238–46.

McDowell, I. & Newell, C. (1987). *Measuring Health: A Guide to Rating Scales and Questionnaires*. Oxford: Oxford University Press.

McDowell, I. & Newell, C. (1996). *Measuring Health: A Guide to Rating Scales and Questionnaires*. Oxford: Oxford University Press.

McHorney, C.A. & Cohen, A.S. (2000). Equating health status measures with item response theory: illustrations with functional status items. *Med. Care*, **38**(9 Suppl. 11), 43–59.

McHorney, C.A. & Tarlov, A.R. (1995). Individual-patient monitoring in clinical practice: are available health status surveys adequate? *Qual. Life Res.*, **4**, 293–307.

McHorney, C.A., Ware, J.E. Jr et al. (1992). The validity and relative precision of MOS short- and long-form health status scales and Dartmouth COOP charts. *Med. Care*, **30**(5), MS253–65.

McHorney, C.A., Ware, J.E. Jr et al. (1994). The MOS 36–Item Short-Form Health Survey (SF-36): III. Tests of data quality, scaling assumptions and reliability across diverse patient groups. *Med. Care*, **32**(1), 40–66.

McIver, J.P. & Carmines, E.G. (1981). *Unidimensional Scaling*. Newbury Park, California: Sage.

Mahoney, F.I. & Barthel, D.W. (1965). Functional evaluation: the Barthel Index. *Maryland State Med. J.*, **14**, 61–5.

Nunnally, J.C. Jr (1970). *Introduction to Psychological Measurement*. New York: McGraw-Hill.

Nunnally, J.C. (1967). *Psychometric Theory*. New York: McGraw-Hill.

Nunnally, J.C. Jr (1959). *Tests and Measurements: Assessment and Prediction*. New York: McGraw-Hill.

Nunnally, J.C. (1978). *Psychometric Theory*. New York: McGraw-Hill.

Nunnally, J.C. & Bernstein, I.H. (1994). *Psychometric Theory*. New York: McGraw-Hill.

Nuyens, G., De Weerdt, W. et al. (1994). Inter-rater reliability of the Ashworth scale in multiple sclerosis. *Clin. Rehabil.*, **8**, 286–92.

Peto, V., Jenkinson, C. et al. (1995). The development and validation of a short measure of functioning and well-being for individuals with Parkinson's Disease. *Qual. Life Res.*, **4**, 241–8.

Prieto, L., Alonso, J. et al. (1998). Rasch measurement for reducing the items of the Nottingham Health Profile. *J. Outcome Measurem.*, **2**, 285–301.

Rasch, G. (1960). *Probabilistic Models for Some Intelligence and Attainment Tests*. Chicago: University of Chicago Press.

Rogers, T. (1995). *The Psychological Testing Enterprise: An Introduction*. Pacific Grove, California: Brooks/Cole.

Rust, R. & Golombok, S. (1999). *Modern Psychometrics: The Science of Psychological Assessment*. London: Routledge.

Sharrack, B., Hughes, R.A.C. et al. (1999). The psychometric properties of clinical rating scales used in multiple sclerosis. *Brain*, **122**, 141–59.

Shrout, P.E. & Fleiss, J.L. (1979). Intraclass correlations: uses in assessing rater reliability. *Psychol. Bull.*, **86**(2), 420–8.

Spector, P.E. (1992). *Summated Rating Scale Construction: An Introduction*. Newbury Park, California: Sage.

Stewart, A.L. & Ware, J.E.J. eds. (1992). *Measuring Functioning and Well-being: The Medical Outcomes Study Approach*. Durham, North Carolina: Duke University Press.

Stewart, A.L., Greenfield, S. et al. (1989). Functional Status and well-being of patients with chronic conditions. Results from the medical outcomes study. *J. Am. Med. Assoc.*, **262**(7), 907–13.

Streiner, D.L. & Norman, G.R. (1989). *Health Measurement Scales: A Practical Guide to Their Development and Use*. Oxford: Oxford University Press.

Streiner, D.L. & Norman, G.R. (1995). *Health Measurement Scales: A Practical Guide to Their Development and Use*. Oxford: Oxford University Press.

Tennant, A., Geddes, J. et al. (1996a). The Barthel Index: an ordinal score or interval measure. *Clin. Rehabil.*, **10**, 301–8.

Tennant, A., Hillman, M. et al. (1996b). Are we making the most of the Stanford Health Assessment Questionnaire? *Br. J. Rheumatol.*, **35**, 574–8.

Thurstone, L.L. (1925). A method for scaling psychological and educational tests. *J. Educat. Psychol.*, **16**(7), 433–51.

Thurstone, L.L. & Chave, E.J. (1929). *The Measurement of Attitude*. Chicago, Illinois: The University of Chicago Press.

Torgerson, W.S. (1958). *Theory and Methods of Scaling*. New York: John Wiley.

Wade, D.T. (1992). *Measurement in Neurological Rehabilitation*. Oxford: Oxford University Press.

Wade, D.T. (1999). Outcome measurement and rehabilitation (editorial). *Clin. Rehabil.*, **13**, 93–5.

Wainer, H., Dorans, N.J. et al., eds. (1990). *Computerized Adaptive Testing: A Primer*. Hillsdale, New Jersey: Lawrence Erlbaum Associates.

Ware, J.E. Jr, Davies-Avery, A. et al. (1978). *Conceptualization and Measurement of Health for Adults in the Health Insurance Study*. Vol. V. *General Health Perceptions*. Santa Monica, California: The Rand Corporation.

Ware, J.E. Jr, Johnson, S.A. et al. (1979). *Conceptualization and Measurement of Health for Adults in the Health Insurance Study*. Vol. III. *Mental Health*. Santa Monica, California: The Rand Corporation.

Ware, J.E. Jr, Brook, R.H. et al. (1980). *Conceptualization and Measurement of Health for Adults in the Health Insurance Study*. Vol. I. *Model of Health and Methodology*. Santa Monica, California: The Rand Corporation.

Ware, J.E. Jr, Snow, K.K. et al. (1993). *SF-36 Health Survey Manual and Interpretation Guide*. Boston, Massachusetts: Nimrod Press.

Ware, J.E. Jr, Kosinski, M.A. et al. (1994). *SF-36 Physical and Mental*

Health Summary Scales: A User's Manual. Boston, Massachusetts: The Health Institute, New England Medical Centre.

Ware, J.E. Jr, Harris, W.J. et al. (1997). *MAP-R for Windows: Multitrait/Multi-item Analysis Program – Revised User's Guide.* Boston, MA: Health Assessment Lab.

Ware, J.E. Jr, Bjorner, J.B. et al. (2000). Practical implications of item response theory and computer adaptive testing. A brief summary of ongoing studies of widely used headache impact scales. *Med. Care*, **38**(9 Suppl. 11), 73–82.

Wilkin, D., Hallam, L. et al. (1992). *Measures of Need and Outcome for Primary Health Care.* Oxford: Oxford University Press.

Williams, L., Weinberger, M. et al. (1999). Development of a stroke specific quality of life scale. *Stroke*, **30**(7), 1362–9.

Wright, B.D. (1977). Solving measurement problems with the Rasch model. *J. Educ. Measurem.*, **14**(2), 97–116.

Wright, B.D. (1997). Fundamental measurement for outcome evaluation. *Physical Medicine and Rehabilitation: State of the Art Reviews*, ed. R.M. Smith, Vol. 11(2), pp. 261–88. Philadelphia: Hanley & Belfus, Inc.

Wright, B.D. & Linacre, J.M. (1989). Observations are always ordinal: measurements, however must be interval. *Arch. Phys. Med. Rehabil.*, **70**, 857–60.

Wright, B.D. & Stone, M.H. (1979). *Best Test Design: Rasch Measurement.* Chicago: MESA.

Zigmond, A.S. & Snaith, R.P. (1983). The hospital anxiety and depression scale. *Acta Psychiat. Scand.*, **67**, 361–70.

8

Principles of clinical neuro-epidemiology

Michael D. Hill and Thomas E. Feasby

Department of Clinical Neurosciences, University of Calgary, Alberta, Canada

Epidemiology is 'the study of the distribution and determinants of health-related states or events in specified populations, and the application of this study to the control of health problems' (Last, 1995). Historically, the science of epidemiology began with the study of outbreaks of infectious disease. It has since progressed in parallel with a shift, in the Western world, from infectious disease to chronic diseases as the major causes of morbidity and mortality. New branches have developed, such as clinical epidemiology, which again have spawned the concept of evidence-based medicine. The modern neurologist must now have both an understanding of the traditional concepts of epidemiology, such as incidence and prevalence of major diseases, and also a solid understanding of clinical research methods and how results of clinical trials apply to their patients. This chapter is designed, with brevity in mind, to provide an initial overview of these fundamentals.

Population-based research in neurological disease

Populations and sampling

There is no substitute for good natural history data. In some cases, society has legislated that all instances of a disease be reported. Both rare diseases, such as rabies or previously more common diseases such as poliomyelitis, are reportable in most jurisdictions in the western world. Legislated data collection results in population-based information. It is no coincidence that these examples are both infectious diseases. With the shift to chronic or degenerative diseases such as atherosclerosis, cancer, arthritis as the leading killing and disabling illnesses, we have not made the same commitments to collecting data as with infectious diseases. We rely upon extrapolation from much smaller samples drawn from the population.

If one could study every human being, it would be unnecessary to understand sampling. Even in very large studies, researchers can only study a tiny proportion of the population; pragmatism dictates it. The principle of sampling is to select from the population a truly representative group for study. A population is any group of persons described as generally or as specifically as appropriate. One may study the entire population of the Western hemisphere, the population of North American First Nations peoples, or the population born in a particular year or years, e.g. the 'baby boomers'. A sampling unit is the basic unit of sampling, e.g. individual, family, city, etc. This entire list of sampling units is called the sampling frame. The sample is derived from the sampling frame.

Samples may, or may not, be random. For example, in studying individual patients, a simple random sample is one in which each person in the population has an equal probability of being chosen for the sample. Sampling may be stratified according to some characteristic or done in a clustered fashion, e.g. by household. The choice of sampling methodology is governed by such things as cost, convenience, generalizability and has an important bearing on the interpretation of the results of the study.

Causation and causal inference

Determination of the causative factors in human disease is not a facile exercise. This is particularly true in the western world where diseases with long latency between exposure and disease onset have replaced shorter latency infectious diseases as the major causes of morbidity and mortality. Koch postulated that in determining the cause of disease, the following conditions should be met: (i) the agent must be found in every case, i.e. it was a necessary

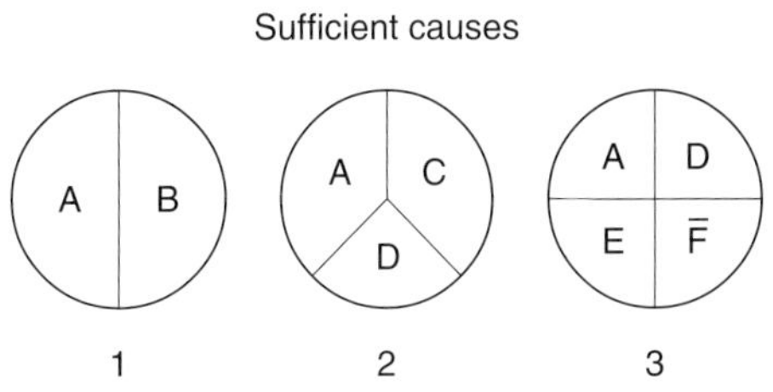

Sufficient causes

Fig. 8.1.

cause; (ii) the agent should occur in no other situation; and (iii) the agent must be isolated from a case and induce disease when transferred to a susceptible host. These were reasonable for the time but, in fact, do not apply even to most infectious diseases. For instance, the tubercle bacillus does not necessarily comply with postulates 2 or 3. It is a necessary but not sufficient cause. Disease causes are multifactorial.

Rothman described a modern deterministic model of disease causation, suggesting that sets of one or more factors act as sufficient causes (Rothman & Greenland, 1998). Each sufficient cause has an independent effect on disease causation, being responsible for a number of cases. Consider, for example, that there are six factors involved in the cause of a disease, and that these combine to form three sufficient causes (Fig. 8.1).

The effects of each component cause within each sufficient cause are mutually interdependent. For instance, in sufficient cause 2, A does not cause the disease unless C and D are present. If the sufficient cause is complete, the disease becomes inevitable, and the latent period begins. A component cause which appears in each sufficient cause, is known as a necessary cause. For instance, herpes simplex virus type 1 is a necessary but not sufficient cause for herpes simplex encephalitis. That is, many people carry the virus but some additional factor (s) is necessary to produce a sufficient cause. Because of the impossibility of determining the component causes in individuals, it is necessary to study samples of populations and use a probabilistic approach to determine causal relationships between exposure and disease. Factors shown to have a causal relationship with a disease are known as risk factors.

Several criteria have been proposed to strengthen the concept of causal inference, since the probabilistic approach lacks the finality of a true experiment, such as a clinical trial. Doll and Hill (1950) proposed six criteria based upon their work examining cigarette smoking and lung cancer. To conclude that an exposure is a causative factor in human illness, they suggested that the following be considered:

(i)   the strength of the statistical association
(ii) the biological credibility
(iii) the consistency with other investigations
(iv) the temporal relationship between exposure and disease
(v)   the dose–response relationship
(vi) the effect of removal of exposure

The two most important statistical ratio measures of association are the odds ratio (OR) and the relative risk (RR). These describe, in different ways, the difference in the risk of disease occurrence between those exposed and not exposed. Thus, the higher the RR or OR, the stronger the association. Because inferring causation for many of the determinants of health and disease is not simplistic, many so-called 'causes' of disease are really only associations. Based upon the above criteria, we assume with a leap of faith, that they are causative.

Study designs and interpretation

Epidemiologic studies can be descriptive, examining the distribution of disease or analytic, uncovering the determinants of disease. Descriptive epidemiology encompasses both individual level studies and population level research. Analytic epidemiology involves highly selected groups of subjects and exposures.

Descriptive: case reports, case series, cross-sectional studies and ecologic studies

The simplest observational studies are case reports and case series. These represent clinical observations and may be the first step toward an important understanding of neurological disease. Cross-sectional studies are designed usually to assess prevalence. They may examine the burden of disease, prevalence of risk factors, resource utilization, demographics, etc. They do not provide evidence for causation. The fallacy of reverse causality may occur when two factors A and B are identified in a cross-sectional survey and A is imputed to be the cause of the B. This may be a false deduction as B could just as easily be the cause of A, or both could be influenced by something else. Similarly, one must recognize that all prevalence studies are a reflection of disease duration as well as disease incidence. Nevertheless, these study designs are useful as hypothesis generating tools.

Ecological studies generally analyse groups, such as regions or worksites. Administrative and/or public health data such as mortality data are often used. Comparison of the incidence of multiple sclerosis and rate of seropositivity to HHV-6 across several cities would be an example of an ecological study. It would be erroneous to link a possible exposure, e.g. HHV-6, with the disease (MS) on an individual basis in this kind of study since it is impossible to control for confounding. This error of logic is named the ecological fallacy. Similarly, temporal association between putative risk factors cannot be assessed by this study design.

Analytic: case-control and cohort studies and clinical trials

Case-control methodology was devised in response to a shift from acute to chronic diseases as major causes of morbidity and mortality in the western world. A case-control study is best used to study rare diseases or events. Subjects are classified according to disease status. The cases and non-cases (controls) are sampled separately and the proportions of subjects with a given exposure in each group are compared. From this type of analysis, an odds ratio (OR) can be derived as an expression of the magnitude of association between the disease and the exposure (risk factor).

The advantages of case control studies include low cost, rapid completion, suitability for studying rare outcomes, the possibility of examining multiple exposures and the quantification of the magnitude of association. Case-control studies are subject to selection bias. It is imperative that the controls be chosen, preferably randomly, from the same population as the cases. Similarly, the information collected and setting should be the same for both cases and controls. Research personnel should be blinded to case or control status and if possible, to the study hypothesis. It may be difficult to establish temporal relationships and it may not be possible to derive incidence rates unless the study is population based.

A recent case-control study assessed the risk of a rare outcome – hemorrhagic stroke – in association with a common exposure – phenylpropanolamine in commonly available cold remedies and appetite suppressants (Kernan et al., 2000). There was an increased odds of hemorrhagic stroke in women (OR = 16.6) but not in men.

Cohort studies are longitudinal studies of a defined group or population, stratified on the basis of exposure status. A well-known example of a prospective cohort study is the Framingham study. In this study, an inception cohort was defined from one geographic location (Framingham, MA) and subjects, divided into groups on the basis of exposures such as hypertension, were studied at baseline and sequentially over time. This type of study is expensive, lengthy and labour intensive; it is not easy to follow people prospectively over time. Undertaking representative sampling, minimizing loss to follow-up, standardizing follow-up and blinding outcome assessment are important measures to be taken in reducing potential bias. This type of study design is robust in that it can assess risk factors which were measured premorbidly, allowing the calculation of relative risk (RR).

Clinical trials

A clinical trial is an interventional cohort study. This is a prospective study in which the subjects are randomly assigned to the exposure (treatment) at the outset, with blinded follow-up for the measurement of outcome. This design is thought to be the ideal method of eliminating selection bias and unknown confounding factors. Successful randomization should result in equal distribution of any premorbid factors in each group or groups. Several design variations on the clinical trial include crossover vs. parallel group design, factorial design and pseudorandomization. Most clinical trials are analysed on an intention-to-treat basis. This implies that outcomes are assessed based upon the initial assignment of exposure group, regardless of whether patients dropped out or switched treatment regimens. Such studies are expensive and labour intensive. Additionally, it is not clear that results of randomized trials can be generalized to the usual situation in day-to-day medical practice, since the study subjects are not necessarily representative of the population. Nevertheless, because it is the epidemiological gold standard methodology, the randomized clinical trial has been adopted as the standard by which new pharmacotherapies and surgical interventions are tested.

Several important issues arise at the inception of any intervention trial. Perhaps, the most important is ethical. Is there sufficient uncertainty to withhold a treatment from one half of the cohort? The ethical underpinnings of RCTs have been recently readdressed in the literature (Weijer et al., 2000; Shapiro & Glass, 2000; Ellenberg & Temple, 2000a, b).

Neurology has become a specialty in which therapy plays an increasing role. New treatments for stroke, Guillain–Barré syndrome, multiple sclerosis, amyotrophic lateral sclerosis, and Alzheimer's disease have all been proven to have efficacy based upon randomized clinical trials (National Institute, 1995; Plasma Exchange, 1997; IFNB Multiple Sclerosis Study Group, 1995; Lacomblez et al., 1996; Rogers et al., 1998).The clinician needs to be able to understand the clinical trial and how it might apply to his/her patients and the neurology community must assess the effectiveness of a given therapy in the community once it has passed the test of a clinical trial. The magnitude of effect of tested agent or procedure in a clinical trial can be measured in several ways. Both ratio measures and difference measures can be used (Table 8.1).

Table 8.1.

		Outcome		
		+	−	
Treated	+	a	b	a + b
Placebo	−	c	d	c + d
		a + c	b + d	a + b + c + d

The relative risk (RR) is the risk of disease in the exposed (treated) group compared to the non-exposed (placebo or usual care) group.

$$RR = [a/(a+b)]/[c/(c+d)]$$

The risk difference (RD) is the incidence of the outcome in the exposed group less the incidence in the non-exposed group. This difference is also called the absolute risk reduction (ARR) and should be carefully distinguished from the relative risk reduction (RRR).

$$ARR = a/(a+b) - c/(c+d)$$

These are known as measures of efficacy. Where the exposure and outcome are causal, the ARR can be interpreted as the attributable risk – the risk attributable to the exposure.

$$NNT = 1/ARR$$

In understanding clinical trial results, the reciprocal of the absolute risk reduction (1/ARR) is used to derive the number need to treat (NNT) to prevent one occurrence of the outcome. For example, in the NASCET study (1991) of carotid endarterectomy to prevent stroke, the ARR in favour of surgery for symptomatic carotid stenosis with 70% or greater narrowing measured on angiography was 0.17 or 17%. This results in an NNT of 6 implying that, in order to prevent one ipsilateral stroke or death over 2 years of follow-up, six patients must be treated with endarterectomy compared to medical therapy. Alternatively, the number of patients who benefit per 1000 patients can be expressed at the ARR% × 10. Both methods of understanding the ARR are useful but limited by what they measure. They only provide an indication of the benefit or lack of it according to the outcome measure chosen by the study designers. For instance, an NNT of 9 for tPA treatment of acute ischemic stroke does not imply that the eight patients who did not achieve an excellent functional outcome did not benefit. Additionally, one must consider the time of follow-up. The NASCET study was instructive in showing that the event rate in the medical group waned considerably after 2 years. Extrapolating constant event

rates from short term follow-up data may not be valid. In Table 8.2, we have listed some examples of major trials in clinical neurosciences and the NNT.

Guyatt et al. (1993, 1994) have provided criteria for reviewing and interpreting the results of clinical trials as part of a series on evidence-based medicine, published in the *JAMA*. The reader is encouraged to review the series.

The concept of effectiveness is beginning to gain credence in contemporary medicine. Despite solid evidence that the treatment of hypertension reduces the risk of stroke, MI and vascular death, it is common parlance (without tongue in cheek), that only half of hypertensives know they are hypertensive, half of those who know are treated and half of those who are treated actually comply with their prescribed medicine. Similarly, the rate of treatment of atrial fibrillation with anticoagulation is poor (Leckey et al., 2000). Two recent reports suggest that carotid endarterectomy for both asymptomatic and even symptomatic carotid stenosis may be vastly overused because community-based effectiveness does not measure up to the standard established in clinical trials (Chaturvedi et al., 2000; O'Neill et al., 2000). These are examples where the benefit established as efficacy of therapy in tightly controlled clinical trials has not been generalisable to the community as effectiveness of therapy. This distinction becomes particularly relevant where the risk–benefit ratio of any given therapy is close to one. Often, in 'real-life' the risks are higher and the benefit achieved lower than in clinical trials. If the demonstrated benefit is obliterated by the elevated risk observed in community practice, the treatment cannot be routinely justified. This may be the case for carotid endarterectomy for asymptomatic carotid stenosis in many jurisdictions in North America (Perry et al., 1997; Feasby, 2000).

Diagnostic and screening tests for neurologic diseases

Sensitivity, specificity, positive-predictive value (PPV) and negative-predictive value (NPV) are conditional probabilities and are best understood using a 2 × 2 table (Table 8.3).

The sensitivity of a test is the probability that the test is positive given that the patient has the disease [a/(a + c)]. Specificity is the probability that the test is negative, given that the patient does not have the disease [d/(b + d)]. The positive predictive value is the probability that the patient has the disease given that the test is positive [a/(a + b)] and the negative predictive value is the probability that the patient does not have the disease given that the test is negative [d/(c + d)].

Table 8.2.

Trial	Outcome measure	Absolute RR	NNT
Carotid endarterectomy for ≥70% symptomatic stenosis (NASCET Collaborators, 1991)	Ipsilateral stroke or death over 2 years	17%	6 – treat 6 pts and follow for 2 years to prevent 1 outcome
Carotid endarterectomy for ≥60% asymptomatic stenosis (Exec. Comm. ACAS, 1995)	Ipsilateral stroke or death over 5 years	5.9%	17 – treat 17 patients and follow for 5 years to prevent 1 outcome
Intravenous tPA for acute ischemic stroke (Nat. Inst., 1995)	Excellent functional outcome at 90 days	11%	9 – treat 9 patients and follow for 3 months to get 1 outcome
β-interferon for relapsing–remitting MS (IFNB MS Study Group, 1993)	Proportion of symptom-free subjects in the high-dose treatment group at 2 years	15%	7 – treat 7 patients for 2 years to prevent 1 outcome
Treatment of isolated systolic hypertension in the elderly (SHEP) (1991)	Incidence of total stroke over 5 years	3%	33 – treat 33 patients for 5 years to prevent 1 outcome

Table 8.3.

		Disease (truth)		
		+	−	
Test	+	a	b	a+b
	−	c	d	c+d
		a+c	b+d	a+b+c+d

Table 8.4.

		Disease (truth)		
		+	−	
Test	+	2	4	6
	−	1	93	94
		3	97	100

In clinical practice, the interpretation of diagnostic testing is most informed by the use of PPV and NPV. This is because one does not know whether the patient has the disease or not, while one does know the test result. Both sensitivity and specificity are functions of the test itself. However, PPV and NPV depend upon the patients and the population from which they arise and therefore will vary as the prevalence of disease within a population. Calculation of PPV and NPV when the characteristics of a test are known (sensitivity and specificity), is a function of Bayesian theory (Table 8.4).

In the foregoing example, the prevalence of the disease is only 3%. The result is that the PPV = 0.5 and NPV = 0.99. Therefore, when the prevalence of a disease is low, a positive test may not be helpful since there may be a significant probability that the test is a false positive. A negative test adds only minimally to the diagnostic process since the prior probability of the diagnosis was only 3%.

The usefulness of any test depends very much upon what its intended use is. One can deduce from the above explanations of sensitivity and specificity that increased sensitivity comes at the expense of decreased specificity and vice versa. For example, when selecting a test for the diagnosis of a disease, a test with high specificity, which results in the highest positive predictive value, will be most useful. Alternately, if you wish to exclude a disease then a test with high sensitivity is best. For tests used in screening, similar considerations apply.

Graphically, this relationship is shown in a receiver–operator characteristic (ROC) curve. A ROC curve provides a visual method to examine the sensitivity and specificity of a diagnostic or screening tool at every possible cut-off point (Murphy et al., 1987). It is created by plotting the sensitivity of a diagnostic or screening tool as a function of (1 − specificity). This reveals a function that, at each point in the distribution of the screening test, yields a sensitivity and specificity for identifying those with disease. For tests where no clear cut-off for identification exists, the point of maximal sensitivity and specificity can be found.

Burden of neurologic disease

Major neurologic diseases

Neurological illness routinely creates long-term disability; it is therefore important to understand the differences between incidence and prevalence. Incidence is the number of new cases of a disease in a specified time in a population. Prevalence is the number of existing cases of a disease in a population. When a disease has either a high mortality or high resolution rate, the prevalence and incidence will be approximately equal. For example the incidence of Bell's palsy is 15–40 cases per 100 000 population. The prevalence is the same because mortality from Bell's palsy is nil and there is a high rate of spontaneous resolution. For chronic illnesses, such as multiple sclerosis, which have low mortality and low spontaneous cure rates and therefore long durations, the prevalence will be higher than the incidence.

Stroke is numerically the most important neurological disease. The incidence and prevalence are significantly higher than any of the other major neurological diseases and neurological mortality is highest for stroke. Stroke may increasingly account for the rising incidence of epilepsy in the older population. Indeed, as the population ages, brain neoplasms and dementia will play an increasing role in population neurological morbidity and mortality.

In the developing world AIDS plays an increasingly devastating role. Much of the continent of Africa continues to be and will be for the foreseeable future, bludgeoned by the virus. Neurological manifestations of AIDS resulting both from the virus (e.g. progressive multifocal leukoencephalopathy, primary CNS lymphoma, HIV dementia) and from the treatment (e.g. myopathy, painful neuropathy) are very important components of the overall morbidity and mortality from the virus.

Stroke

Stroke is a major cause of both mortality and morbidity. It is the third leading cause of death in North America and Canada and a leading cause of acquired adult disability. US data suggests that there are seven to eight times more stroke survivors than stroke deaths. The age-adjusted incidence of stroke, determined from the Framingham study, is 603 per 100 000 men and 453 per 100 000 women. There is a clear association of increasing stroke incidence with increasing age. As with other diseases, there is substantial regional variability in stroke incidence.

Of interest in stroke epidemiology has been the dramatic decline in age-adjusted mortality rates from stroke. Parallel declines have been seen in other atherosclerotic diseases such as coronary heart diseases. However, the impending aging of the population in many countries will more than make up for the declining mortality and we will see increasing numbers of patients with stroke over the next several decades.

The cost and burden of stroke are enormous because of the sheer numbers of persons affected. Estimates of societal cost in the US approach tens of billions of dollars per annum (Taylor et al., 1996). This is therefore an exciting period, with the introduction of the first new and cost-effective therapy (tPA) for acute ischemic stroke, bringing the potential for reduced cost and suffering (Kwiatkowski et al., 1999; Fagan et al., 1998).

Brain cancer

Brain tumours are second after stroke as a cause of neurological death. There are wide geographical variations in incidence ranging from 1.0 to 14.3 per 100 000 population (Bahemuka, 1988). However, older studies are marred by incomplete ascertainment due to the lack of modern imaging techniques. Indeed, an ongoing issue in the epidemiology of brain tumours is lead-time bias. Studies that suggest longer survival after brain tumour therapy may be biased by earlier diagnosis due to increased use of CT and MRI scanning. A corollary to this concept is that more asymptomatic tumours are uncovered in life rather than as incidental findings at autopsy (Nakasu et al., 1987).

The age-adjusted incidence of brain neoplasms was 14.1 in Olmstead County, Minnesota (Annegers et al., 1981). Incidence of primary brain neoplasms clearly rises with age. Types of brain tumours vary by gender. For example, meningiomas are more common in females and glioma more common in males (Preston-Martin, 1989).

Despite several reports suggesting that the incidence of primary brain tumours is rising rapidly, it appears that, with the exception of primary CNS lymphoma, brain tumour incidence is stable. The dissemination and widespread use of CT and MR imaging has resulted in greater diagnostic accuracy and increased case recognition rates (Radhakrishnan et al., 1995).

Primary CNS lymphoma, accounting for only 1% of CNS neoplasms, has shown an increasing incidence (threefold) over the last several decades. Although the AIDS epidemic has dramatically increased the absolute number of cases, it appears that the trends to increasing numbers began before the AIDS epidemic accelerated. Increased case acquisition also does not explain the rising incidence (Eby et al., 1988).

Dementia

Dementia, like stroke, is an enlarging public health issue because of aging populations in many parts of the world. Dementia, of which Alzheimer's disease is the most common, occurs with steeply increasing incidence and prevalence with age. Data on the descriptive epidemiology of dementia is quite consistent across the world, where it has been gathered. However, the prevalence of the disease in older age groups is more variable because small sample sizes in the oldest old produce more variation in these age brackets (Fratiglioni et al., 1999).

While Alzheimer's disease is the most common form of dementia, differing case definitions of vascular dementia allow for variations in the proportion of cases attributable to each and in which age brackets (Hebert & Brayne, 1995). Recent work suggests that there is a very strong synergy between cerebrovascular disease and Alzheimer's disease (Snowdon et al., 1997). Because of difficulties in premorbid clinical diagnosis, it remains unclear how commonly other forms of dementia, e.g. diffuse Lewy body disease, the fronto-temporal dementias, progressive supranuclear palsy, etc., are found across the world.

Multiple sclerosis (MS)

Interest in the epidemiology of MS is piqued by the non-random distribution of the disease with increasing prevalence according to increasing latitude in both hemispheres (Kurtze, 1975, 1977; Hammond et al., 1988). In addition, smaller migration studies have suggested that migrants take on the prevalence of the disease in the indigenous population of the new country. These observations 'favour an environmentally-based latitude effect' upon MS prevalence (Ebers & Sadornick, 1998). Genetic influences have generally not been controlled for in these studies such that, despite enthusiasm for viral and other infectious causes of MS, genetic predisposition with a non-specific inciting environmental agent may be the most plausible ontogenic theory of MS.

The prevalence of MS varies from 5/100 000 to as high as 120/100 000 population. The incidence of the disease is much harder to estimate for several reasons. The biology of the disease suggests that it exists well before a clinically definite diagnosis can be reached, and this lag time may be quite variable among patients. Improving diagnostic strategies may improve this situation but they also cast doubt upon research done prior to routine magnetic resonance imaging. Data from Olmstead County, Minnesota suggest an annual incidence rate of 3.6 per 100 000 (Percy et al., 1971).

The burden of MS upon patients, families and society is tremendous. A majority of patients are unemployed either inside or outside of the home after 10 years. Depression and other psychiatric conditions occur in MS due to both the disease itself and its effects upon the psyche. Cost estimates including both direct and indirect medical care as well as lost wages suggest that MS is an expensive disease. Although there is excess mortality from MS, particularly the malignant, rapidly progressive forms (e.g. Marburg variant) and from suicide, the societal impact is due to chronic morbidity and reduced quality of life rather than increased mortality (Swingler & Compston, 1992).

Epilepsy

Epilepsy is a disease of the extremes of age in the developed world. While the overall incidence varies between 34 and 53/100 000/y, children (<20 y) and older adults (>60 y) have two to four times that incidence. In Africa and South America, this U-shaped curve is flatter and an increase in incidence in the elderly has not been observed (Rwiza et al., 1992; Lavados et al., 1992). The prevalence of epilepsy worldwide is much higher, ranging from 400–800 per 100 000 population (Hauser & Hesdorffer, 1990).

Epilepsy is slightly more common in males and its overall incidence in the western world has been stable. However, data from Rochester suggest that overall stability reflects significant declines in the pediatric age group and increases in incidence in the group over 60 y (Hauser et al., 1993) (Table 8.5).

In conclusion, a solid comprehension of basic clinical epidemiology is invaluable to the practicing clinician. Particularly as clinical neuroscience practice becomes more and more subject to the results of clinical trials, clinicians will need to know how to interpret the literature for both therapeutic and diagnostic modalities. The concepts

Table 8.5.

Disease[a]	Estimated age-adjusted annual incidence per 100 000 population
Stroke	603 (men); 453 (women)
Dementia[b]	80–400 for the age-group 60–64 4980–13 570 for the age group >95
Epilepsy	24–53
Primary brain neoplasms	9.0
MS	3.6
Guillain–Barré syndrome	1–2

Notes:
[a] Referenced in the text.
[b] Not age adjusted.

outlined here are only the tip of the iceberg and further exploration is suggested (Sackett et al., 1991).

Review of some of the major neurological diseases is helpful in placing both ourselves as treating physicians and our patients in context. From a public policy point of view, interventions to prevent stroke will have the most chance of reducing neurological morbidity and mortality. From the viewpoint of physicians and patients, knowledge of disease prevalence aids in the interpretation of diagnostic testing and awareness of risk factors aids preventative management. Understanding from where and how these data are derived can only further the practice of good clinical medicine.

Acknowledgements

M.D. Hill was supported in part by grants from the Heart and Stroke Foundation of Canada, the Canadian Institutes of Health Research and the Alberta Heritage Foundation of Medical Research.

T.E. Feasby was supported in part by grants from the Heart and Stroke Foundation of Canada, the Canadian Institutes of Health Research and the Canadian Stroke Network

References

Annegers, J.F., Schoenberg, B.S., Okazaki, H. & Kurland, L.T. (1981). Epidemiologic study of primary intracranial neoplasms. *Arch. Neurol.*, **38**, 217–19.

Bahemuka, M. (1988). Worldwide incidence of primary nervous system neoplasms: geographical, racial and sex differences, 1960–1977. *Brain*, **111**, 737–55.

Chaturvedi, S., Aggarwa, R. & Murugappan, A. (2000). Results of carotid endarterectomy with prospecive neurologist follow-up. *Neurology*, **55**, 769–72.

Doll, G. & Hill, A.B. (1950). Smoking and carcinoma of the lung: preliminary report. *Brit. Med. J.*, **2**, 739.

Ebers, G.C. & Sadovnick, A.D. (1998). *Epidemiology*. In *Multiple Sclerosis*, ed. W. Paty & G.C. Ebers, Chapter 2, pp. 5–28. Philadelphia, USA: F.A. Davis Company.

Eby, N.L., Grufferman, S., Flannelly, C.M., Schold, S.C. Jr., Vogel, F.S. & Burger, P.C. (1988). Increasing incidence of primary brain lymphoma in the US. *Cancer*, **62**, 2461–5.

Ellenberg, S.S. & Temple, R. (2000a). Placebo-controlled trials and active-control trials in the evaluation of new treatments. Part 1: Ethical and scientific issues. *Ann. Intern. Med.*, **133**, 455–63.

Ellenberg, S.S. & Temple, R. (2000b). Placebo-controlled trials and active-control trials in the evaluation of new treatments. Part 2: Practical issues and specific cases. *Ann. Intern. Med.*, **133**, 464–70.

Executive Committee for the ACAS. (1995). Endarterectomy for asymptomatic carotid artery stenosis. *J. Am. Med. Assoc.*, **273**, 1421–8.

Fagan, S.C., Morgenstern, L.B., Petitta, A. et al. (1998). Cost-effectiveness of tissue plasminogen activator for acute ischemic stroke. NINDS rt-PA Stroke Study Group. *Neurology*, **50**, 883–90.

Feasby, T.E. (2000). Endarterectomy for asymptomatic carotid stenosis in the real (editorial). *Can. J. Neurol. Sci.*, **27**, 95–6.

Fratiglioni, L., De Ronchi, D. & Agüero-Torres, H. (1999). Worldwide prevalence and incidence of dementia. *Drugs Aging*, **15**, 365–75.

Guyatt, G.H., Sackett, D.L. & Cook, D.J. for the Evidence-based medicine working group. (1993). Users' Guides to the Medical Literature. IIA. How to use an article about therapy or prevention. *J. Am. Med. Assoc.*, **270**, 2598–601.

Guyatt, G.H., Sackett, D.L. & Cook, D.J. for the Evidence-based medicine working group. (1994). Users' Guides to the Medical Literature. IIB. How to use an article about therapy or prevention. *J. Am. Med. Assoc.*, **271**, 59–63.

Hammond, S.R., McLeod, J.G., Millingen, K.S. et al. (1988). The epidemiology of multiple sclerosis in three Australian cities: Perth, Newcastle and Hobart. *Brain*, **111**, 1–25.

Hauser, W.A. & Hesdorffer, D.H. (1990). *Epilepsy: Frequency, Causes and Consequences*. New York: Demos Press.

Hauser, W.A., Annegers, J.F. & Kurland, L.T. (1993). The incidence of epilepsy and unprovoked seizures in Rochester, Minnesota, 1935–1984. *Epilepsia*, **34**, 453–68.

Hebert, R. & Brayne, C. (1995). Epidemiology of vascular dementia. *Neuroepidemiology*, **14**, 240–57.

Kernan, W.N., Viscoli, C.M., Brass, L.M. et al. (2000). Phenylpropanolamine and the Risk of Hemorrhagic Stroke. *N. Eng. J. Med.*, **343**, 25: (in press) *http: //www.nejm.org/ content/kernan/1.asp.*

Kurtze, J.F. (1975). A reassessment of the distribution of multiple sclerosis. *Acta Neurol. Scand.*, **51**, 110–57.

Kurtze, J.F. (1977). Geography in multiple sclerosis. *J. Neurol.*, **215**, 1–26

Kwiatkowski, T.G., Libman, R.B., Frankel, M. et al. (1999). Effects of tissue plasminogen activator for acute ischemic stroke at one year. National Institute of Neurological Disorders and Sroke Recombinant Tissue Plasminogen Activator Stroke Study Group. *N. Eng. J. Med.*, **340**, 1781–7.

Lacomblez, L., Bensimon, G., Leigh, P.N., Guillet, P. & Meininger, V. (1996). Dose-ranging study of riluzole in amyotrophic lateral sclerosis. Amyotrophic Lateral Sclerosis/Riluzole Study Group II. *Lancet*, **347**, 1425–31.

Last, J.A. (1995). *A Dictionary of Epidemiology*, 3rd edn, Oxford: Oxford University Press.

Lavados, J., Germain, L., Morales, A., Campero, M. & Lavados, P. (1992). A descriptive study of epilepsy in the district of El Salvador, Chile, 1984–1988. *Acta Neurol. Scand.*, **85**(4), 249–56.

Leckey, R.G., Aguilar, E. & Phillips, S.J. (2000). Atrial fibrillation and the use of warfarin in patients admitted to an acute stroke unit. *Can. J. Cardiol.*, **16**, 481–5.

Murphy, J.M., Berwick, D.M., Weinstein, M.C., Borus, J.F., Budman, S.H. & Klaman, G.L. (1987). Performance of screening and diagnostic tests: application of receiver-operating charac-teristics analysis. *Arch. Gen. Psychiatry*, **44**, 550–5.

Nakasu, S., Hirano, A., Shimura, T. & Llena, J.F. (1987). Incidental meningioma in autopsy study. *Surg. Neurol.*, **27**, 319–22.

NASCET Collaborators. (1991). Beneficial effect of carotid endarterectomy in symptomatic patients with high-grade carotid stenosis. *N. Engl. J. Med.*, **325**, 445–53.

O'Neill, L., Lanska, D.J. & Hartz, A. (2000). Surgeon characteristics associated with mortality and morbidity following carotid endarterectomy. *Neurology*, **55**, 773–81.

Percy, A.K., Nobrega, F.T., Okazaki, H., Glattre, E. & Kurland, L.T. (1971). Multiple sclerosis in Rochester, Minn: a 60-year appraisal. *Arch. Neurol.*, **25**, 105–11.

Perry, J.R., Szalai, J.P. & Norris, J.W. for the Canadian Stroke Consortium. (1997). Consensus against both endarterectomy and routine screening for asymptomatic carotid stenosis. *Arch. Neurol.*, **54**, 25–8.

Plasma Exchange/Sandoglobulin Guillain–Barré Syndrome Trial Group. (1997). Randomised trial of plasma exchange, intravenous immunoglobulin, and combined treatments in Guillain–Barré syndrome. *Lancet*, **349**, 225–30.

Preston-Martin, S. (1989). Descriptive epidemiology of primary tumours of the brain, cranial nerves and cranial meninges in Los Angeles county. *Neuroepidemiology*, **8**, 283–95.

Radhakrishnan, K., Mokri, B., Parisi, J.E., O'Fallon, W.M., Sunku, J. & Kurland, L.T. (1995). The trends in incidence of primary brain tumours in the population of Rochester, MN. *Ann. Neurol.*, **37**, 67–73

Rogers, S.L., Farlow, M.R., Doody, R.S., Mohs, R. & Friedhoff, L.T. (1998). A 24-week, double-blind, placebo-controlled trial of donepezil in patients with Alzheimer's disease. Donepezil Study Group. *Neurology*, **50**, 136–45.

Rothman, K.J. & Greenland, S. (1998). Causation and causal inference. In *Modern Epidemiology*, K.J. Rothman & S. Greenland, 2nd edn, pp. 7–28. USA: Lippincott-Raven.

Rwiza, H.T., Kilonzo, G.P., Haule, J. et al. (1992). Prevalence and incidence of epilepsy in Ulanga, a rural Tanzanian district: a community-based study. *Epilepsia*, **33**, 1051–6.

Sackett, D.L., Haynes, R.B., Guyatt, G.H. & Tugwell, P. (1991). *Clinical Epidemiology: A Basic Science for Clinical Medicine*, 2nd edn. USA: Little, Brown & Co.

Shapiro, S.H. & Glass, K.C. (2000). Why Sackett's analysis of randomized controlled trials fails, but needn't. *CMAJ*, **163**, 834–5.

SHEP co-ordinating research group. (1991). Prevention of stroke by antihypertensive drug treatment in older persons with isolated systolic hypertension. *J. Am. Med. Assoc.*, **265**, 3255–64.

Snowdon, D.A., Greiner, L.H., Mortimer, J.A., Riley, K.P., Greiner, P.A. & Markesbery, W.R. (1997). Brain infarction and the clinical expression of Alzheimer's disease. The Nun Study. *J. Am. Med. Assoc.*, **277**, 813–17.

Swingler, R.J. & Compston, D.A.S. (1992). The morbidity of multiple sclerosis. *Quart. J. Med.*, **83**, 325–37.

Taylor, T., Davis, P.H., Torner, J.C., Holmes, J., Meyer, J.W. & Jacobson, M.F. (1996). Lifetime cost of stroke in the United States. *Stroke*, **27**, 1459–66.

The IFNB MS study group. (1993). Interferon beta-1b is effective in relapsing-remitting multiple sclerosis. *Neurology*, **43**, 655–61.

The IFNB Multiple Sclerosis Study Group and The University of British Columbia MS/MRI Analysis Group. (1995). Interferon beta-1b in the treatment of multiple sclerosis: final outcome of the randomized controlled trial. *Neurology*, **45**, 1277–85.

The National Institute of Neurological Disorders and Stroke rtPA Stroke Study Group. (1995). Tissue plasminogen activator for acute ischaemic stroke. *N. Engl. J. Med.*, **14**(333), 1581–7.

Weijer, C., Shapiro, S.H., Glass, K.C. & Enkin, M.W. (2000). For and against: clinical equipoise and not the uncertainty principle is the moral underpinning of the randomised controlled trial. *Br. Med. J.*, **321**, 756–8.

9

Principles of therapeutics

Peter J. Goadsby

Institute of Neurology, The National Hospital for Neurology and Neurosurgery, Queen Square, London, UK

Traditional neurology has been dominated by a focus on diagnosis with accurate neuroanatomical localization of the lesion or pathophysiological definition of the underlying disease process. With some notable exceptions, such as changes in the pattern of infectious diseases in the Western world, neurological diseases have not altered much since Gowers (1888) set out the problem. The process of diagnosis, certainly for structurally based conditions, has been immeasurably served by brain imaging, first with X-ray computerized tomography and most recently with magnetic resonance imaging. Pathological study remains a cornerstone of accurate disease classification for some brain disorders, notably tumours, while the pathophysiological basis of many diseases has been elucidated by techniques including molecular biology, clinical neurophysiology and functional brain imaging. However, therapeutics in neurology can be barren, indeed neurology has often suffered the tag of being expert on diagnosis and wanting in treatment. While there can be no doubt that patients seek a label, or explanation, for their problems, treatments, indeed cures, for neurological maladies must be our aim.

Several areas of neurology have seen substantial advances in their therapeutic armamentarium in recent times and it seems appropriate to consider some of the underlying principles that drive neurological therapy and how new therapies may fit such a framework. First, some principles will be covered, after which some specific generic issues will be considered, clinical trial evaluation, dose selection, drug metabolism and interactions, and some issues of special populations.

Some principles

While everything in neurology, indeed medicine, can be individualized there are some underlying themes. The emphasis on these themes will vary with the condition being considered, and the needs of the patient. However, some part of these principles can be applied in many clinical conditions.

- Patients need an explanation of the condition from which they suffer and how their symptoms fit that diagnosis.
- Patients need to know the natural history of their condition so they can judge the likely benefit of treatments.
- Patients need to know the treatment options, both complementary if they exist, and orthodox.
- It should be made clear whether a treatment will address symptoms or the underlying disease process.
- Realistic goals need to be set for treatment: if the best that can be expected is a 50% improvement this needs to be stated clearly.
- Commonly expected or potentially serious side effects need to be stated and explained.

Naturally, these principles simply state what most neurologists do, coming as no surprise to the clinician. In the modern, ever more technologically driven and litigious environment in which we practice one might add some expectations of patients. Therapeutics should not be a battle, with tension between treatments and side effects, but a partnership. Most practitioners seek to do good and it is a shame that this is not the starting point in all clinical interactions. Notwithstanding the best intentions an adequate record of the management plan, including side effects explained and options offered needs to be recorded in the case notes for the many good reasons that such records are made.

Evaluating clinical trials

The cornerstone of modern neurotherapeutics is the controlled trial. The importance of proper, scientifically sound clinical studies cannot be overemphasized. Many neurological disorders have such remarkable variability with time or between ictal events that uncontrolled studies are unacceptable. This does not imply that good clinical observation has no place in modern therapeutics; indeed many important developments come from the careful observer noting change where it was not expected, but this approach generates hypotheses not textbook advice. Some conditions lend themselves to clinical study and some do not. For rare conditions the *N*-of-1 approach (Jones & Kenward, 1989) deserves more exploration, often overcoming the problem of recruitment.

Ideally therapeutic studies need a control group and must be randomized and double-blinded. Clinicians need to understand the many biases of single blinding, of the patient without the clinician, and generally reject such designs. If it is undesirable to offer treatments without evidence, it is even more unhelpful to conduct studies that cannot by their design yield useful information. The control group needs careful consideration, it should be contemporaneous, not historical, carefully matched for obvious variables: age, sex and disease, and consider other issues of matching, such as weight, that may effect the study outcome. Often a placebo control group is desirable but for some indications in which there are established treatments an active control group, in addition or instead of the placebo group, may be desirable. An active control group can help clinicians position a new treatment, whereas a placebo control can facilitate comparison with previous studies in a therapeutic area.

A special problem arises when, as in the case of multiple sclerosis, several treatments are licensed to modify the course of the disease but none is more than modestly effective and better treatments are clearly needed. Because there are licensed treatments available, it may no longer be ethically justified to perform large, double blind, placebo controlled, randomized clinical trials. In this context historical controls may be necessary; mathematical modelling of disease course utilizing data from the placebo arms of previous clinical trials and from epidemiological studies may provide a basis for comparison of the effects of new agents. The Sylvia Lawry Centre for Multiple Sclerosis Research in Munich set up by the Multiple Sclerosis Federation is an attempt to develop such an approach.

Study analysis and data presentation is an area that is often found lacking when new data are published. Study size is crucial; how was the study powered and to what end-point? When new treatments are being evaluated against established therapies and equivalence is claimed, was the study powered adequately for equivalence? What clinical difference is being evaluated? Is a difference of 5% of any

clinical relevance? What was the primary end-point and was it significant? How many hypotheses have been tested to obtain a positive result? In our clinical desire to have new treatments it is important that substandard studies do not end up driving clinical practice inappropriately.

Some principles in evaluating clinical trials

These include:

- Has the therapy been studied in randomized controlled double-blinded studies?
- Is the control group appropriate and suitably matched?
- Is the primary end-point clear and was it statistically significant?
- Was the study adequately powered?
- Are the reported differences and benefits clinically important?
- Were the adverse events clearly stated, and were there any serious adverse events that will be important to mention in clinical practice?

Dose selection

The pharmaceutical industry has often taken the view that simplicity is best and one dose should fit all patients. It is borne of the perception that anything too complex will not be used and dose titration is too much trouble. It is a nonsense to expect that a treatment studied in 70–80 kg patients would necessarily be of any use to those weighing 100 kg, or that tolerability will not be a problem in those weighing 40 kg. Weight is a simple but clear example of the need to consider dose carefully. Patients can often be engaged in such a process of dose selection understanding that one is trying to do what is best for the individual rather than applying a *herd-based* therapeutic approach.

If individualization, where possible, is one guiding principle, the other must be the often-quoted medicinal aphorism: start low and go slow. Patient responses may be idiosyncratic, indeed side effects may be unpredictable on the base of dose so that giving a low dose and making small increments will greatly aid compliance and alert the clinician to a problem when the drug load is low. Many drugs that are used in neurology have significant central nervous system side effects that can be tolerated if patients are gradually exposed. It is a shame to lose a useful treatment in the rush for a response. Again, it is important to make it clear to the patient why one is taking this approach so that their expectations for a response are suitably modified.

An obvious general exception to the slow and steady principle is the neurological emergency. In some situations, such as acute stroke or giant cell arteritis, dosing must reflect the significant morbidity, indeed mortality, of the condition being treated.

Pharmacokinetics: giving drugs safely and effectively

When prescribing a treatment, the clinician needs to consider how the substance might interact with the patient, in terms of metabolism and drug interactions. Such interactions vary from trivial alterations in drug metabolism to profound change, as may be seen with some of the older anticonvulsants.

Issues of drug metabolism have become more complex as our treatment options expand, and those of other specialties conspire to make administration much harder in some individuals. It is beyond the scope of this chapter to discuss every aspect of pharmacokinetics but as a checklist one might consider:

- absorption issues in oral medications vs. other routes of administration;
- bioavailability and the effect of feeding or interactions with the disease on absorption, such as impaired oral absorption in acute migraine;
- drug metabolism involving monoamine oxidase (MAO) or cytochrome P450 pathways that can cause potential interactions with other medications;
- drug delivery issues, such a protein binding or special brain issues, such as whether a medication is a substrate for the brain P-glycoprotein (PGP) pump (Wacher *et al.*, 1995), which can specifically promote efflux of medicines out of the brain, or the state of blood–brain barrier itself;
- drug half-life issues that may drive dosing considerations, and thus affect compliance;
- drug elimination issues such as those seen in hepatic impairment or renal failure.

The list is not exhaustive, but illustrates the challenges we face as we seek to employ new medications into daily practice. On-line and various electronic PDA solutions will help alert clinicians to potentially fatal interactions but will not replace the thoughtful, well-trained neurologist who plays the pivotal role in bringing innovative medicines to daily clinical practice.

Special populations

Some populations are so special that therapeutics can be a particular challenge, which deserves particular attention.

Females of child-bearing age and pregnancy

For very good reasons females of child-bearing age and pregnant women are generally excluded from clinical studies of new therapeutic agents. While it is easier to include females in the child-bearing age by adequate screening and discussion, pregnant women are a complex therapeutic proposition. Generally, females of child-bearing age should not be denied the potential benefits of treatments for their neurological conditions. Contraceptive issues can be discussed and the lack of experience of any treatment in pregnancy explained. Indeed clinical trials should seek actively to include patients in the demographic distribution of the target condition. Pregnancy is a more complex issue.

Given that most therapeutics studies will exclude pregnant females, there can be no data concerning the effects of a new agent on the pregnant female or the fetus. The possibility of teratogenicity or abortion must be mentioned even though it is effectively impossible to give any reliable estimates of the chance of an adverse event. Often the clinical condition will assist in making these decisions in that the disease itself may adversely affect the fetus; situations such as a prolonged seizure or acute migraine with vomiting and dehydration, weigh into the risk–benefit of treating pregnant females. Ideally treatments whose risks are minimal, or at least clearly understood, can be presented to the patient. It is attractive and often helpful to have both parents, when possible, hear the same information and certainly to document what is said.

It is worth remarking that effects of the pregnancy on a treatment should be considered. Metabolic, hormonal or simply blood volume changes should be considered when dosing the pregnant female. Having taken a decision to treat, that treatment must be adequate to prevent or control symptoms, as desired.

Younger patients and the elderly

Neurological disorders clearly affect children and adolescents, as well as the elderly. The general issues surround dosing and desirability to treat these groups. Dosing is an obvious issue with simple weight adjustments being a minimal consideration in the young, while in the elderly drug metabolism needs to be factored into dosing considerations. The route of elimination of a compound is important, particularly for renal excretion in the elderly, and if dose adjustment is recommended this needs action.

Some conditions, perhaps most notably stroke and degenerative diseases, affect the population more with time, and development programmes for new treatments will reflect this reality. However, some conditions of younger patients also affect the elderly, and are no less disabling. Where the age cut-off for studies should be, and what constitutes elderly, is no simple decision. Many patients over 65 years, and particularly under the age of 75, are remarkably biologically agile, while many adolescents acquire both the physiology and responsibility of adulthood before their 18th birthday. Lack of exposure of a new therapy to an older or younger age must be weighed against the disability that is attendant the disease process. For the young, perhaps school attendance and performance, and for the elderly issues of quality of life need to be considered when planning treatment. For children careful involvement of the parents or care-givers is essential.

In conclusion, neurotherapeutics is likely to be the next great change to neurological practice. Increasingly neurologists will be required to treat what has been untreatable, to palliate where only suffering was previously on offer, and eventually to alter the course of neurological diseases as modifying and curative approaches become available.

The challenges are substantial and the rewards considerable. Neurotherapeutics will drive subspecialization in neurology as patient expectations grow and the number of options becomes more complex. Careful attention to the principles will help the clinician bring the fruits of the post-human genome translational therapeutic revolution to the group of diseases that neurologists are charged with managing.

References

Gowers, W.R. (1988). *A Manual of Diseases of the Nervous System.* Philadelphia: P. Blakiston, Son & Co.

Jones, B. & Kenward, M.G. (1989). *Design and Analysis of Cross-Over Trials.* 1st edn. London: Chapman & Hall.

Wacher, V.J., Wu, C-Y. & Benet, L.Z. (1995). Overlapping substrate specifiities and tissue distribution of cytochrome P450 3A and P-glycoprotein: implications for drug delivery and activity in cancer chemotherapy. *Molecular Carcinogenesis,* **13**, 129–34.

10

Windows on the working brain: functional imaging

John A. Detre[1,2] and Paul D. Acton[2]

[1] Department of Neurology and [2] Department of Radiology, University of Pennsylvania, PA, USA

Functional imaging encompasses methods used for visualizing a variety of aspects of cerebral physiology ranging from cerebral blood flow and metabolism to neurotransmitter binding and turnover. Functional imaging has numerous applications in basic and clinical neuroscience, many of which are now in routine clinical use. These techniques may be used to image physiological alterations in the brain that cannot be detected by structural assessment, or to elucidate metabolic changes which underlie structural lesions. The major modalities used for functional imaging of the brain include positron emission tomography (PET), single photon emission tomography (SPECT), and magnetic resonance imaging (MRI). PET and SPECT methods measure the distribution of exogenously administered radioactive tracers, while functional MRI (fMRI) studies primarily utilize endogenous contrast and as such are completely non-invasive. For this reason, over the past 5 years fMRI has begun to replace PET as the technique of choice for mapping regional brain function in response to sensorimotor and cognitive tasks, as well as for imaging alterations in cerebral blood flow and metabolism. However, because of the extreme sensitivity of radioactive tracer techniques, PET and SPECT remain the only means of mapping changes occurring at very low concentrations, such as receptor binding. This chapter will provide an overview of these approaches to physiological imaging of the brain. Applications to neurological diagnosis and management as well as to cognitive neuroscience will also be addressed.

Physiology of regional brain function

A number of cellular and metabolic processes in the brain can be monitored using functional imaging methods, and have relevance to basic and clinical neuroscience. Figure 10.1 illustrates these processes which include neurotransmitter binding and reuptake, glucose utilization (CMRGlu), oxygen metabolism (CMRO$_2$), and hemodynamic parameters of cerebral blood flow (CBF), cerebral blood volume (CBV), and mean transit time (MTT) and time to peak (TTP) for intravascular tracers. Depending on the specific application, some of these parameters may be more relevant than others. For example, studies in cerebrovascular disease have focused on hemodynamic parameters and their effects on oxidative metabolism, as well as on the apparent diffusion coefficient (ADC) in brain, a biophysical parameter available in MRI that reflects early cytotoxic injury. By contrast, functional imaging studies in epilepsy have primarily examined ictal hyperperfusion using CBF imaging and interictal hypometabolism using CMRGlu imaging, and in Parkinson's disease, where brain dysfunction is better understood at a neurochemical level, much of the functional imaging has involved receptor mapping of the dopaminergic system.

In cognitive and systems neuroscience, there has been great interest in using functional neuroimaging to map regional brain function in response to cognitive or sensorimotor tasks. In patients these approaches may also be used to map eloquent function as part of preoperative evaluation for neurosurgical procedures, and for studying reorganization of function following focal brain injury. Nearly all studies of task-specific activation using functional neuroimaging rely on the existence of a coupling between regional changes in brain metabolism and regional cerebral blood flow (CBF), herein referred to as activation-flow coupling (AFC). Changes in blood flow and metabolism occur with excitatory or inhibitory neurotransmission, both of which are energy consuming processes. Surprisingly little is known about the physiology underlying AFC, which was originally described in 1890 by Roy and Sherrington. Studies over the intervening century have yet

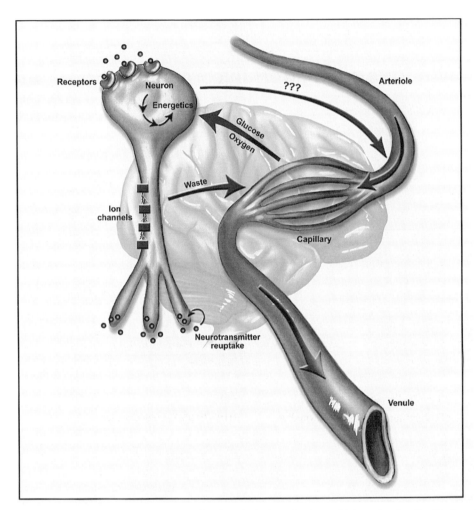

Fig. 10.1. Schematic diagram illustrating the physiological mechanisms which can be visualized by functional imaging. Brain function is represented by a neuron that receives synaptic input, conducts electrical signals by an energy dependent process, and has synaptic output with transmitter recycling. The adjacent microvasculature provides oxygen and glucose to support these functions through perfusion, which also affects local blood volume and blood oxygenation.

to fully characterize the mechanisms and mediators of AFC (Villringer & Dirnagl, 1995). The extent to which non-neuronal constituents of brain parenchyma contribute to the overall metabolic rate is also uncertain, and may be variable. Nonetheless, regional blood flow changes have typically colocalized with known functional specialization.

Functional imaging using radioactive tracers; PET and SPECT

The techniques of PET and SPECT enable the three-dimensional distribution of a radioactively labeled tracer to be measured in vivo. Radioisotopes used in PET imaging decay with the emission of positrons, which travel only a short distance in tissue before annihilating with an electron to form two colinear photons, each with 511 keV energy. In contrast, SPECT tracers emit just a single gamma ray, with energies dependent on the specific radioisotope used. The technology for detecting these gamma rays differs between the two systems, with PET generally having superior spatial resolution and system sensitivity, although SPECT is considerably less expensive, and much more widely available.

The spatial resolution of PET is limited by the range of positrons in tissue, and the slight acolinearity of the emitted gamma rays. Depending on the radioisotope, the absolute limit of resolution is approximately 1.5–2.5 mm, though generally this is not achieved in routine clinical practice. SPECT resolution is limited by the design of the

Table 10.1. Selected radiotracers for PET and SPECT imaging of the brain

Measurement	PET tracers	SPECT tracers
Cerebral blood flow	$H_2^{15}O$	[^{123}I]IMP, [^{99m}Tc]HMPAO, [^{99m}Tc]ECD
Cerebral blood volume	^{11}CO, $C^{15}O$	[^{99m}Tc]red blood cells
Oxygen metabolism	$^{15}O_2$	
Glucose metabolism	^{18}FDG	
Dopamine D$_1$ receptors	[^{11}C]SCH23390, [^{11}C]NNC756	[^{123}I]TISCH
Dopamine D$_2$ receptors	[^{11}C]raclopride, [^{11}C]NMSP	[^{123}I]IBZM, [^{123}I]IBF, [^{123}I]epidepride
Dopamine synthesis	[^{18}F]DOPA	
Dopamine transporters	[^{11}C]cocaine, [^{11}C]β-CIT, [^{11}C]FP-CIT, [^{11}C]CFT, [^{11}C]methylphenidate	[^{123}I]β-CIT, [^{123}I]FP-CIT, [^{123}I]IPT, [^{99m}Tc]TRODAT, [^{123}I]altropane
Serotonin 5-HT$_{1A}$ receptors	[^{11}C]WAY100635, [^{18}F]MPPF	
Serotonin 5-HT$_{2A}$ receptors	[^{11}C]MDL100907	[^{123}I]R-91150
Serotonin transporters	[^{11}C](+)McN5652	[^{123}I]β-CIT, [^{123}I]5-iodo-6-nitroquipazine, [^{123}I]IDAM, [^{123}I]ADAM
GABA receptors	[^{11}C]flumazenil	[^{123}I]iomazenil
NMDA receptors	[^{18}F]AFA	[^{123}I]MK801, [^{123}I]CNS1261
Nicotine receptors	[^{11}C]nicotine	[^{123}I]nicotine
Opioid receptors	[^{11}C]carfentanil, [^{11}C]diprenorphine	
Gene expression	[^{18}F]FIAU, [^{18}F]FGCV	[^{123}I]FIAU
Brain tumours (various types and modes of action)	^{18}FDG, [^{11}C]methionine, [^{11}C]thymidine	^{201}Tl, [^{123}I]MIBG, [^{111}In]octreotide

collimator, and the distance from the subject to the detector. Most clinical systems can attain a resolution of 6–7 mm, though better resolution is possible with more specialized collimators. The temporal resolution of both systems is poor, as it can take several minutes of scanning to acquire sufficient statistics to form an image. However, despite the poorer spatial and temporal resolution of PET and SPECT compared with other modalities, such as fMRI, their tremendous advantage is their exquisite sensitivity. PET and SPECT can measure picomolar (10^{-12} M) concentrations of tracer, many orders of magnitude less than can be detected with MRI. The quantity of radiotracer injected is tiny, and generally has no effect on the biological system under study.

Radiotracers for PET and SPECT

Many radioisotopes for PET imaging are found naturally in living organisms and are amenable to labeling biologically interesting molecules. These include carbon (^{11}C), nitrogen (^{13}N), oxygen (^{15}O), and fluorine (^{18}F). SPECT radioisotopes tend to be much larger, such as technetium (^{99m}Tc)

and iodine (^{123}I), and are more difficult to incorporate into a radiotracer without disturbing the biochemical properties of the molecule. However, SPECT tracers generally have longer half-lives, and are therefore much more widely available than PET radioisotopes, which usually require an on-site cyclotron and production facility. Applications of these imaging technologies have gone hand-in-hand with developments in radiopharmaceutical chemistry. Both PET and SPECT are now capable of imaging biological systems with unprecedented accuracy and sensitivity, mainly due to the tremendous advances in the development of novel radiopharmaceuticals (Table 10.1).

Cerebral blood flow and metabolism

Originally, PET and SPECT were used to measure cerebral blood flow and metabolism. A number of tracers exist which can measure regional cerebral blood flow (rCBF), such as [^{123}I]IMP, [^{99m}Tc]HMPAO and [^{99m}Tc]ECD for SPECT, and $H_2^{15}O$ for PET. The SPECT tracers are examples of the 'trapping' mechanism for measuring cerebral function. For a molecule to enter the brain, it must be neutral and lipophilic which enables it to pass by passive diffusion through the lipid bilayer in the blood–brain barrier (BBB). Once across the BBB, the molecule may become trapped if it interacts with an intracellular component that either reduces its lipophilicity or restricts further free diffusion of the tracer. Chemical instabilities in the ^{99m}Tc-complex in [^{99m}Tc]HMPAO result in the conversion to a less lipophilic species causing sustained retention in brain tissue. Hence, the concentration of tracers such as [^{99m}Tc]HMPAO in the brain are determined by the rate of tracer delivery by the blood supply, giving an indirect measure of rCBF at the time of injection of the tracer. Imaging of rCBF can be carried out at a later time, for example allowing rCBF during brief neurological events such as seizures to be determined without requiring immediate access to the scanner. Conversely, radioactive water, $H_2^{15}O$, used for PET measurements of rCBF is unchanged within the brain, freely diffusing across the BBB, and will concentrate in brain tissue at a rate proportional to rCBF. Unlike [^{99m}Tc]HMPAO, which only provides a single 'snapshot' of rCBF, the uptake of $H_2^{15}O$ changes over time as the demands for blood flow alter in the brain. This has led to its use as a sensitive and quantitative indicator of changes in rCBF in sensorimotor and cognitive tasks, though fMRI is now becoming more popular in this application.

Blood volume can be measured using a tracer that binds to red blood cells and remains within the vasculature of the brain. For PET, carbon monoxide can be labelled with either ^{11}C or ^{15}O and inhaled, where it will bind tightly to the hemoglobin in red blood cells. Alternatively, SPECT measurements of blood volume can be made using the subject's own red blood cells labelled with ^{99m}Tc. Both techniques give a quantitative measure of regional cerebral blood volume (rCBV). In a similar manner, equilibrium images of inhaled $^{15}O_2$ obtained in conjunction with these measures can yield the rate of cerebral oxygen metabolism (CMRO$_2$).

Another powerful indicator of cerebral function is the measurement of regional cerebral glucose metabolism. Glucose provides approximately 95–99% of the brain's energy requirement under normal conditions, and the rate at which glucose is utilized in different regions of the brain is an excellent indicator of local energy-requiring functions. Glucose is transported across the BBB where it is phosphorylated by the enzyme hexokinase to glucose-6–PO$_4$. The glucose analogue ^{18}F-labelled fluorodeoxyglucose (^{18}FDG) is a competitive substrate for this phosphorylation stage, where it, too, is converted to ^{18}FDG-6–PO$_4$. However, while glucose-6–PO$_4$ undergoes further metabolism, ^{18}FDG-6–PO$_4$ does not, and becomes trapped in brain tissue, as it cannot diffuse back across cell membranes. The metabolic trapping of ^{18}FDG can be used to derive the cerebral metabolic rate of glucose utilization (CMRGlu).

Measurements of cerebral blood flow and metabolism have been used widely to study a variety of disorders, ranging from cerebral infarct to drug addiction, and Alzheimer's disease (AD) to mood disorders. Large-scale changes in cerebral function can be detected with high sensitivity using blood flow tracers, and remains the gold standard in many diagnostic imaging applications, such as epilepsy (Spencer et al., 1995). However, structural and hemodynamic changes induced by many neurological and psychiatric disorders are generally small, and often only evident when the disease is into an advanced stage. In addition, the changes in cerebral activity measured using rCBF, rCBV, CMRO$_2$, CMRGlu, or any other index of cerebral blood flow or metabolism are highly non-specific. This has led to the further development of specialized radiotracers that enable PET and SPECT to image directly various neurotransmitter systems and the complex interactions between them.

Neuroligand binding studies

Neuroreceptors are proteins in the membrane of neurons, which are sensitive to neurotransmitters, chemicals that transmit signals from one nerve cell to another. Receptors play two key roles; they recognize only certain neurotransmitter(s), and they activate additional events based on that recognition. The interaction of the neurotransmitter with the specific receptor mimics the effects of nerve stimulation, and begins a sequence of events that either excite or inhibit further neuronal firing. The concentration of neurotransmitter within the synaptic cleft is controlled by other transmembrane transporter proteins, which reuptake the chemical back into the presynaptic nerve terminal.

To study receptor binding sites in vivo, several radiolabelled ligands have been developed which selectively bind to specific neuroreceptors or presynaptic reuptake sites (Table 10.1). The uptake and retention of a radioligand depends on a number of factors, such as its lipophilicity, the presence of non-specific binding, the affinity of the tracer for the receptor, and the concentration of available receptors. Most importantly, these radioligands are active competitors with other exogenous and endogenous chemicals for the binding site, a situation that has been used to great effect in many neurotransmitter studies. A compartmental kinetic model can describe neuroligand imaging. The free, unmetabolized tracer present in plasma crosses the BBB into cerebral tissue, where it can bind selectively to the receptor under study. Simplifications of this kinetic model have been developed, most notably to eliminate the necessity of performing rapid arterial blood sampling (Lammertsma & Hume, 1996). Techniques also have been developed which use a continuous infusion of radiotracer to maintain a constant equilibrium state between specific binding and plasma activity (Laruelle et al., 1993).

Studies of neuroreceptor concentrations in disease initially focused on measuring differences between healthy control subjects and subjects with neurological and psychiatric disorders. In some cases the findings have been unequivocal, such as PET and SPECT measurements of dopaminergic neuronal degeneration in Parkinson's disease (PD) using radioligands which bind to the dopamine transporter (Brooks et al., 1990; Innis et al., 1993; Mozley et al., 2000). More recently, the availability of radioligands for imaging the serotonergic neurotransmitter system have given many insights into depression and other mood disorders (D'Haenen et al., 1992; Malison et al., 1998). However, many disorders, such as schizophrenia, have failed to exhibit the expected changes in receptor densities. This has led investigators away from studies of static receptor systems, in the belief that these disorders may be a result of neurotransmitter system dynamics, rather than simple alterations in receptor concentrations.

Drug challenge studies, using both exogenous and endogenous chemicals to stimulate the neurotransmission process, have yielded new information on several diseases. Many drugs occupy the same binding sites in the brain as the radioligand; reductions in specific binding of a tracer can be interpreted as an increase in the concentration of a competing drug. For example, the modes of action of antipsychotic drugs have been investigated in vivo by measuring the competition between the radioligand and the drug, which both bind to the same dopamine and serotonin receptors (Farde et al., 1992; Pilowsky et al., 1992).

While many interesting results have been obtained by introducing an exogenous drug that competes with the same binding sites as the radioligand, some of the most exciting recent developments have occurred using the endogenous neurotransmitter as the competing drug. If the levels of endogenous neurotransmitter can be manipulated, either chemically or using a cognitive or sensorimotor task, the degree of specific binding of the tracer will change to reflect the alterations in neurotransmitter. Other studies have used drugs to manipulate one neuroreceptor while studying the effects 'downstream' on another, revealing the modulatory effect neurotransmitters have on each other (Smith et al., 1997). Most recently the chemical manipulation of neurotransmitter behaviour was replaced by a cognitive task, where the release of endogenous dopamine as a result of playing a video game was measured using [^{11}C]raclopride and PET (Koepp et al., 1998). This potentially provides an opportunity to study cerebral activation at the neuronal level, where the involvement of each individual neurotransmitter system can be examined during a cognitive or sensorimotor task.

Other PET and SPECT studies

Recent developments in radiopharmaceutical chemistry have opened up entirely new applications for PET and SPECT imaging in the brain. For example, novel radiopharmaceuticals are being created which bind selectively to amyloid plaques in Alzheimer's disease, providing an early diagnostic tool for detecting amyloid deposition long before structural changes become apparent (Zhen et al., 1999). Imaging of gene expression is now possible, particularly in tumors, using reporter genes labelled by reporter probes (MacLaren et al., 1999). The ability to quantitatively and repeatedly measure the expression of particular genes in vivo will become a powerful tool in the study of genetic contributions to disease, and to monitor gene therapy.

Functional imaging using magnetic resonance

Magnetic resonance utilizes electromagnetic rather than ionizing radiation to probe structure and function. The vast majority of MRI utilizes the nuclear magnetic resonance signal of water protons that are present in high concentration in biological systems. Image contrast is derived from variations in the molecular environment of water in various structures and compartments. These contrast mechanisms are summarized in Table 10.2. FMRI simply refers to MRI scanning in which significant tissue contrast can be attributed to changes in blood flow and/or metabolism. For measurement of task activation, such changes are typically of the order of only a few per cent or less of the overall signal intensity. The primary contrast mechanisms used for detecting task activation with fMRI are blood oxygenation level dependent (BOLD) contrast and perfusion contrast obtained using arterial spin labelling (ASL). Because BOLD contrast is easier to obtain and generally provides higher signal-to-noise for task specific activation, it has been widely adopted as the method of choice for imaging regional brain activation using MRI. In contrast to PET methods for mapping task activation which have often relied on a multisubject design, BOLD fMRI provides sufficient sensitivity to reliably carry out studies in single subjects. To maximize temporal resolution and slice coverage

Table 10.2. Contrast mechanisms for functional MRI (fMRI)

MRI contrast	Imaging sequence	Physiological parameter
Dynamic susceptibility contrast (DCS)	T_2^*-weighted during administration of MRI contrast agent, typically echoplanar or spiral.	Cerebral blood volume and mean transit time. CBF calculated through central volume principle
Arterial spin labeling	Preparatory radiofrequency labelling of arterial water. Any imaging sequence can be used, typically short TE echoplanar or spiral.	Cerebral perfusion in ml/g min or relative perfusion change
Blood oxygenation level dependent (BOLD)	T_2^*-weighted, typically echoplanar or spiral.	Deoxyhemoglobin concentration (represents a complex interaction between CBF, CBV, and oxygen utilization)
Diffusion	T_2-weighted with and without diffusion sensitization gradients, typically echoplanar or spiral.	Apparent diffusion coefficient (ADC) reflects water mobility within voxel; ADC is reduced in cytotoxic injury and across myelinated fiber tracts

as well as to minimize image degradation by subject motion, most fMRI studies utilize ultrafast imaging methods such as echoplanar or spiral techniques in which each imaging slice is obtained in 100 ms or less using a single radiofrequency excitation (Vlaardingerbroek & den Boer, 1996).

For clinical applications, hemodynamic measurements can also be made by following the initial passage of an exogenously administered susceptibility contrast agent through the cerebral vasculature, termed dynamic susceptibility contrast (DSC) perfusion MRI. Since these agents remain intravascular, only mean transit time, time to peak, and blood volume can be precisely measured, while CBF must be estimated using the central volume principle (Sorensen et al., 1997). This approach was used to generate the first report of fMRI in humans during photic stimulation (Belliveau et al., 1991). However, since contrast administration is required for each measurement, its use for task activation studies in humans has waned.

The practical spatial resolution limits of fMRI are currently unknown. While MRI is capable of imaging structures in the micron range, signal-to-noise varies directly with voxel size and signal-averaging time for extremely small voxels would likely be prohibitive for most human applications. In addition, degradation by motion becomes a very significant problem with high-resolution imaging, particularly since even normal physiological motion such as that induced by arterial pulsatility can be of the order of millimeters. The spatial extent of AFC is also unknown, but current thinking is that flow effects are considerably less localized than metabolic effects. However, at least in some brain regions, the vascular supply is organized in a functionally significant manner. This has been demonstrated

for rat whisker barrel cortex where the cortical region subserving each whisker appears to have a dedicated microvascular supply (Woolsey et al., 1996). Although these regions are less than 1 mm, it has been possible to visualize them using fMRI in the rat brain at high fields (Yang, Hyder & Shulman, 1996). It has also been possible to visualize similarly sized ocular dominance columns in calcarine cortex in cats (Kim et al., 1999) and in humans (Menon et al., 1997).

Blood oxygenation level dependent (BOLD) contrast

BOLD contrast reflects a complex interaction between blood flow, blood volume, and hemoglobin oxygenation (Ogawa et al., 1998). Functional contrast is obtained because the iron present in hemoglobin becomes paramagnetic only when it is deoxygenated, producing a local susceptibility increase manifested as a change in T2*, among other effects. This change in hemoglobin oxygenation is usually monitored using gradient echo echoplanar sequences which particularly emphasize T2* effects and allow multiple slices to be acquired at rapid intervals. With regional brain activation, a reduction in T2* is observed, reflecting a decrease in regional deoxyhemoglobin which has been attributed to increases in CBF which exceed increases in oxygen metabolism, though the universality and precise basis for this mismatch is uncertain.

A typical BOLD response consists of a 0.5–5% change in regional image intensity which develops over 3–8 s following task initiation. This peak latency of several seconds represents a major limiting factor in the temporal resolution of functional imaging methods that rely on AFC. There is growing evidence that prior to the increase in regional CBF, there is a more localized decrease in hemoglobin oxygenation, presumably due to a more rapid increase in oxygen utilization than in blood flow (Malonek & Grinvald, 1996), however this subtle effect has been difficult to detect reliably. Sensitivity to T2* increases at higher magnetic field strengths, such that at 4.0 Tesla BOLD peak signal changes may approach 25% with sensorimotor tasks. This increased signal can be used to improve sensitivity or spatial resolution. Higher field strengths may also increase the sensitivity for detecting the initial decrease in BOLD signal. Task specific BOLD signal changes are not directly quantifiable in physiological units, but rather are expressed as a percentage signal change or as a statistical significance level based on a particular statistical model. Absolute or resting function cannot be easily assessed, and for clinical studies it may be difficult to know whether any observed abnormalities are due to baseline or task-specific effects.

Perfusion MRI

Classical perfusion can also be measured directly using endogenous contrast with ASL (Detre & Alsop, 1998). This class of techniques utilizes electromagnetically labelled arterial blood water as a diffusible tracer for blood flow measurements, in a manner analogous to that used for ^{15}O PET scanning. The 'electromagnetic' tracer has a decay rate of T1, which is sufficiently long to allow perfusion of the microvasculature and tissue to be detected. This form of image contrast can be sampled with any imaging sequence. ASL techniques are capable of quantifying cerebral blood flow in well-characterized physiological units of ml/100 g min, or may be used in a qualitative fashion similar to that used in BOLD fMRI. The development of multislice ASL (Alsop & Detre, 1998) has considerably enhanced its utility. The use of ASL methods for imaging task activation has been less widespread than BOLD methods because these techniques produce a lower signal change for activation and are somewhat more difficult to implement. However, potential advantages of ASL approaches include greater temporal stability due to absolute quantification of flow changes, direct comparison with PET rCBF studies, and the possibility of detecting activation in the presence of high static magnetic susceptibility.

Diffusion MRI

Diffusion weighted MRI (DWI) uses large magnetic field gradient pulses to spatially label tissue water, allowing its microscopic motion over tens of milliseconds to be measured (Le Bihan et al., 1986). The resulting apparent diffusion coefficient (ADC) reflects a weighted average of intracellular and extracellular water, and the shift from extracellular to intracellular water which occurs during early cytotoxic injury results in a large signal change using this contrast (Moseley et al., 1990). DWI and perfusion MRI are now in fairly routine use in hyperacute stroke evaluation (Baird & Warach, 1998; Neumann-Haefelin et al., 2000). Directional effects also occur in DWI due to anisotropy of microscopic diffusion of water in white matter tracts, an effect that has high sensitivity to changes in fibre tract myelination. By separately measuring diffusion effects using orthogonal gradients for diffusion sensitization, a diffusion tensor image can be generated which reflects fibre orientation (Pierpaoli et al., 1996) and may be used to examine connectivity between brain regions.

Mapping cognition with functional imaging

Perhaps the greatest promise for functional neuroimaging is to elucidate mechanisms of higher cognitive function. This pursuit has intensified with the advent of fMRI because it affords a sensitive and inexpensive means of detecting task-specific regional brain activation. Since hemodynamic changes occur on a drastically longer timescale and with considerably poorer spatial localization than neuronal firing, and since the mechanisms of coupling between neural activity and hemodynamic changes remain to be completely understood, cognitive mapping using functional imaging remains an indirect link to neural function. While considerable effort is now being given to determining the relationship between neural activity and hemodynamic effects as well as the spatial and temporal resolution limits of functional imaging, the strategies for making inferences about cognitive function based on imaging experiments are still being developed. At present, cognitive brain mapping experiments are most effective for determining the locations of task activation rather than their magnitude or relative contributions to overall task performance. Identification of the ventral 'what' and dorsal 'where' streams in visual function is an example of cognitive processing mechanisms that were elucidated at least partly through functional neuroimaging (Ungerleider & Haxby, 1994).

Paradigm design for cognitive brain mapping

Because PET studies of regional brain activation have poorer temporal resolution than fMRI, most PET activation studies have examined differences in regional brain activation during blocks of repetitive stimuli of differing types. Subtraction of blocks of stimuli differing in a single cognitive process is then used to determine the localization of that process. For example, activation during reading of pseudofont words might be subtracted from reading true font words to determine brain region involved in written language processing. Based on this tradition, early fMRI studies also used blocked-trial designs with alternating epochs of task and control conditions, each consisting of multiple trials. This approach maximizes sensitivity, since large signal changes are sustained, and also minimizes the requirement of an accurate estimate of the hemodynamic response.

More recently, many investigators have explored techniques that allow fMRI responses to individual task stimuli to be segregated (Buckner et al., 1996). These approaches allow different classes of stimuli to be randomized, reducing habituation effects, and also facilitate retrospective analysis of fMRI data based on subject performance on individual trials (Brewer et al., 1988; Wagner et al., 1998). Thus, regional brain activation following only correctly or incorrectly performed trials can be compared across subjects or across control and patient groups, independent of overall performance on the task. However, the results of individual trial analysis may depend heavily on the assumed neural activity and AFC response.

A fundamentally different approach to functional brain imaging in clinical populations which circumvents the issue of task performance is to correlate specific neurocognitive deficits with alterations in resting brain function using quantitative functional imaging such as CBF measurements using ASL techniques (Alsop et al., 2000). Since only resting perfusion is measured, the interpretation of the imaging data is not confounded by task performance. This approach is also applicable to structural imaging data (Mummery et al., 2000).

Analysis of functional activation data

Task-specific functional activation is typically determined by statistical analyses of time series data with respect to the administered task. This can be accomplished using a simple correlation analysis, though multiple linear regression methods (Friston et al., 1994) including a variety of confounds now more common, and non-parametric approaches as well as task-independent approaches are being developed. Linearity between neural activity and AFC responses is often assumed in these analyses, though deviations from linearity clearly occur. For both resting and activation studies, time series data must be examined and corrected for motion effects. Task-correlated motion

may be particularly difficult to distinguish from functional activation. A thresholded statistical map is ultimately superimposed upon high-resolution anatomical images or other representations of the brain. Thresholding for significance is complicated, and requires consideration of spatial and temporal autocorrelation in the data as well as false positive activation that may result from multiple comparisons, since three-dimensional images may contain thousands of pixels.

Comparison of functional localization across subjects presents yet additional challenges in the interpretation of clinical functional neuroimaging studies. Many such comparisons have been accomplished through the use of transformation into standard neuroanatomical spaces such as Talairach space (Talairach & Tournoux, 1988), though more complicated algorithms are available, including those which attempt to unfold cerebral gyri. These algorithms rely on characteristic signal intensities of gray matter, white matter, and cerebrospinal fluid that can be altered in the presence of lesions such as tumours, strokes, or focal atrophy. When lesions are large, they may distort the brain sufficiently to make automated or semiautomatic morphing into a standard space impossible.

Functional imaging in neurological diagnosis and management

Functional imaging techniques have been applied to nearly every category of central nervous system disorder, with variable results (Detre & Floyd, 2000). This section will focus on selected applications in which functional imaging has successfully contributed to neurological differential diagnosis or patient management.

Presurgical localization of function

Since fMRI provides sufficient sensitivity to map functional activation within a single subject, one of the earliest clinical applications of fMRI was the localization of motor cortices with respect to brain tumours requiring neurosurgical resection. In several studies, fMRI localization of finger tapping paradigms has been compared with cortical stimulation. Since cortical stimulation is essentially a 'lesion' study confined to the superficial cortex while BOLD fMRI measures endogenous function throughout the brain, these modalities may be expected to differ somewhat in functional localization. Nonetheless, an excellent correlation has been consistently found between regions of motor activation seen on BOLD-fMRI and intraoperative cortical stimulation (Yetkin et al., 1997).

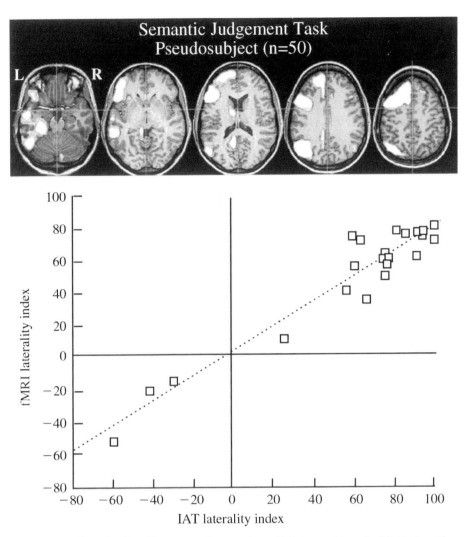

Fig. 10.2. FMRI lateralization of language and comparison with intracarotid amobarbital testing. These studies utilized a semantic judgement task with a tone sequence judgement task as a baseline. The top panel shows averaged fMRI task activation from 50 normal right-handed subjects, demonstrating left hemisphere lateralization of language-related activity. The scatter plot below shows the strong correlation ($r = 0.96$, $P < 0.0001$) between an IAT language laterality index and an analogous index based on fMRI in 22 epilepsy patients. (These data are presented courtesy of Dr Jeffrey Binder.)

FMRI has also been compared to intracarotid amobarbital testing (IAT) for presurgical lateralization of language and memory in several studies. While the IAT has been the gold standard for identifying lateralization of language and memory function preoperatively, it is invasive and carries significant risks. Further, fMRI offers the capability of spatially resolving functional activation within each hemisphere, potentially guiding tailored resections to spare eloquent cortex. Successful functional activation studies using motor and language tasks have been reported in partial complex epilepsy by several groups. Binder et al. (1996) reported a cross validation study comparing language

dominance determined by both fMRI and IAT in 22 epilepsy patients. Examples of fMRI lateralization of language are illustrated in Fig. 10.2. A semantic decision task was used to activate a distributed network of brain regions involved in language specialization. Excellent agreement in language laterality was observed in this and other studies, though there has been some controversy concerning the optimum task for lateralizing language. A complex visual scene encoding task has been used to lateralize mesial temporal lobe memory dysfunction in patients with temporal lobe epilepsy, and showed a good correlation with memory lateralization by IAT in preliminary studies (Detre et al., 1998).

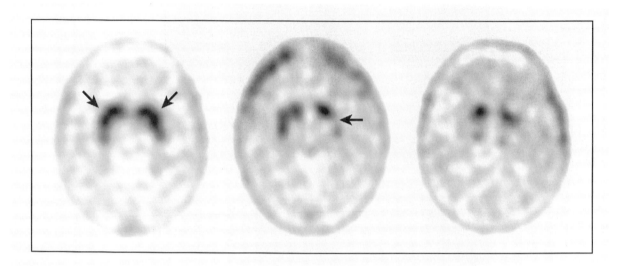

Fig. 10.3. SPECT images of [99mTc]TRODAT-1 binding to dopamine transporters in the striatum. The healthy subject (*left*) shows high uptake in the striatum (arrows), while patients with progressively more severe Parkinson's disease exhibit unilateral (arrow, *centre*) and bilateral (*right*) degeneration of dopaminergic neurons, and a reduction in tracer binding. (Images courtesy of Dr David Mozley, University of Pennsylvania.)

Functional imaging has also contributed to the localization of seizure foci. Interictal hypometabolism measured using FDG-PET is now widely accepted in clinical lateralization of temporal lobe epilepsy (Duncan, 1997). Ictal events can be localized using HMPAO-SPECT, as noted above, as well by fMRI with (Krakow et al., 1999) or without EEG triggering (Detre et al., 1995). Localized changes in tissue diffusion have also been observed in patients with focal status epilepticus (Lansberg et al., 1999).

Parkinsonian syndromes

PET and SPECT imaging of the dopaminergic system in the differential diagnosis of parkinsonian disorders may become the first routine clinical application of neuroligand imaging (Fig. 10.3). Studies of neuronal degeneration in the nigrostriatal pathway, using tracers that bind to dopamine transporters, have nearly 100% accuracy in diagnosing some forms of neurodegenerative disease (Brooks, 1997). The diagnosis at an early stage in the progression of PD, even before clinical symptoms have become apparent, is possible, although differentiating PD from other parkinsonian disorders, such as multiple system atrophy, progressive supranuclear palsy, or Huntington's disease, may require multiple imaging modalities or combinations of tracers.

Early diagnosis may become increasingly important once the genetic contribution to parkinsonian disorders is fully understood. PET and SPECT imaging are beginning to make important contributions to the understanding of the pathogenesis of PD, and may be able to elucidate the role of other neurotransmitter systems, such as NMDA and GABA, in the onset and progression of PD (Acton & Mozley, 2000). Longitudinal studies of patients undergoing treatment, whether by neuroprotective drugs or surgical intervention, will become increasingly important in the assessment of treatment efficacy, and also to determine the exact mode of action of each therapy.

Dementia

Post mortem studies have shown a high degree of misdiagnosis of dementia using clinical symptoms alone. This has led to a growing trend to use imaging techniques to provide a more accurate, unbiased diagnosis, and to assess treatment efficacy. PET and SPECT imaging in dementia generally measure reductions in cerebral blood flow or metabolism resulting from the disease, using tracers such as $H_2^{15}O$, [99mTc]HMPAO and ^{18}FDG (Frey et al., 1998). A pattern of hypoperfusion and hypometabolism in temporoparietal brain regions, with frontal changes occurring as the condition deteriorates, has been established in Alzheimer's disease (Fig. 10.4). Abnormalities on functional images may precede cognitive defects, raising the possibility of using PET and

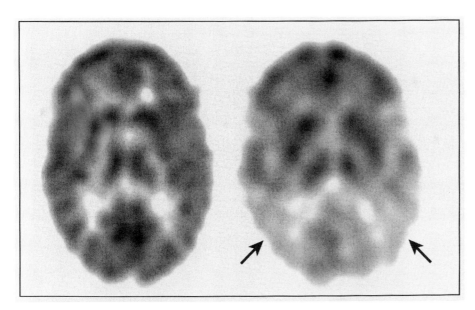

Fig. 10.4. Comparison of cerebral glucose metabolism, measured using [18]FDG and PET, in a normal healthy subject (*left*) and a patient with Alzheimer's disease (*right*). The pattern of hypometabolism reflects neuronal degeneration in the temporoparietal regions (arrows), which is consistently found in AD. (Images courtesy of Dr David Mozley, University of Pennsylvania.)

SPECT in the early, presymptomatic diagnosis of dementia (Rapoport, 1997). Some studies suggest that functional imaging with PET or SPECT is superior to structural imaging in the diagnosis of some dementias, particularly Alzheimer's disease.

Tumour imaging

Functional imaging plays an important role in brain tumour management due to the difficulty in differentiating post-therapy residual viable tumour tissue from local recurrence and necrosis using structural imaging. One of the most useful radiotracers for imaging tumours of almost any kind is [18]FDG, which takes advantage of the dramatic increase in glucose metabolism in tumour cells. PET imaging of the brain with [18]FDG is capable of the early detection of tumours, provides information on the staging and response to therapy, and is a good prognostic indicator. However, due to the high uptake of [18]FDG in normal brain tissue, the tumour-to-background ratios can be quite low. Alternatively, labelled amino acids, such as [^{11}C]methionine, or indicators of excessive DNA fabrication, such as [^{11}C]thymidine, provide high contrast images of many brain tumours, and can distinguish between viable tumour and radiation necrosis.

Radioactive thallium (^{201}Tl) has been used extensively for SPECT imaging of tumours. While the exact mechanism of thallium uptake by tumour cells is not clear, it provides very high contrast images of brain tumours. Thallium imaging provides good diagnosis and staging of malignant disease, clear delineation between viable tumour and cell necrosis, and is used to assess the response to chemotherapy and radiation treatment. Other SPECT tracers, such as MIBG, have been shown to be effective diagnostic tools for neuroblastomas and other neural crest tumours, and even can be administered in much larger radiation doses for radiotherapy. More recently, attention has focused on the overexpression of certain types of receptors by tumours. In particular, many tumours express somatostatin receptors, which has been used to great advantage in the development of radiolabelled somatostatin analogues, which bind selectively to these receptors and can be used to image many types of brain tumour.

Cerebrovascular disease

Functional imaging has been used extensively in cerebrovascular disease and acute stroke in an attempt to better characterize physiological changes accompanying brain ischemia, identify brain tissue at risk for infarction, and predict outcome. Studies of patients with stroke using [15]O PET measures of CBF, CBV, and oxygenation characterized the pathophysiology of cerebral ischemia, with initial autoregulation of CBF though vasodilatation, followed by hypoperfusion with increased oxygen extraction fraction (OEF) and finally decreased $CMRO_2$ and infarction (Heiss &

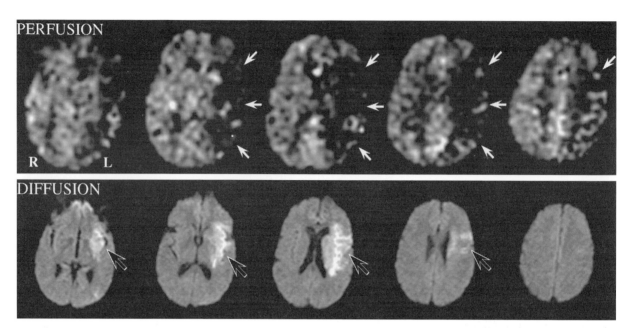

Fig. 10.5. Perfusion and diffusion MRI in a patient presenting with acute right hemiparesis and aphasia. Top panel: Perfusion MRI obtained using ASL demonstrates hypoperfusion throughout the left middle cerebral artery distribution (white arrows). Bottom panel: Diffusion MRI demonstrates a somewhat smaller region of cytotoxic injury (black arrows). Images are in radiological orientation (left is on the right).

Podreka, 1993). In chronic cerebrovascular disease, an increased OEF predicts an increased stroke risk (Grubb et al., 1998) and suggests a need for therapeutic intervention such as revascularization. Since PET scanning remains limited to only a few academic centres, over the past decade much interest has been focused on more widely available imaging modalities. A reduced CBF response to acetazolamide or carbon dioxide measured using computer-assisted tomographic (CAT) scanning with xenon or perfusion MRI has recently been used as an indication of hemodynamic compromise, and also indicates an increased stroke risk (Webster et al., 1995). While the relative contribution of primary hypoperfusion versus thromboembolism to stoke incidence remains controversial, it is hoped that these approaches can also be used to improve patient selection for interventions such as angioplasty or carotid endarterectomy.

The demonstration of effective thrombolytic therapy for hyperacute stroke has intensified the need for rapid assessment of regional brain physiology in stroke patients. This application of functional imaging would ideally be obtained in only a few minutes and would confirm the presence of ongoing ischemia, indicate the risk of hemorrhage following thrombolysis, and replace symptom duration as the determinant of reversible versus irreversible brain injury. There is also a rationale for using functional

imaging to measure the effects of novel neuroprotective therapies in acute stroke, since clinical measures have thus far failed to detect any incremental benefits. MRI scanning with diffusion and perfusion contrast, along with magnetic resonance angiography, currently appears best suited for these purposes (Tong & Albers, 2000), though CT scanning with xenon perfusion and computed tomographic angiography also shows promise in this regard. An example of MRI scanning in a patient with acute stroke is illustrated in Fig. 10.5.

Recovery of function

Several groups have used functional neuroimaging to explore changes in functional brain organization in response to focal lesions such as stroke. Utilizing PET in humans after deep capsular infarcts, Weiller and Chollet (Chollet & Weiller, 1994) identified increased cerebral blood flow in bilateral premotor and supplementary motor areas, in unaffected primary motor cortex and along the rim of the cortical infarct, suggesting a hierarchical network of compensatory function. Some of this activation was ultimately attributed to mirror movements in the unaffected limb. FMRI studies in motor recovery have largely confirmed prior PET results with activation of a motor network in the unaffected hemisphere to a greater extent than found in controls, increased degree of supplementary motor area activation, and perilesional activation. The location of ipsilateral motor cortex activation both in normals and following stroke appears to be ventrolateral to the region which is activated by contralateral movements (Cramer et al., 1999), suggesting that it may correspond to a separate motor homunculus. Although perilesional recovery of function has been confirmed by cortical and cellular electrophysiological methods in animals and using transcranial stimulation in humans, it remains difficult to conclusively prove that all of the perilesional effects observed with fMRI are functionally significant. Some apparent activation observed using blood flow as a surrogate marker for neural function might actually reflect vascular reorganization following ischemic brain injury.

In patients with stroke and aphasia, spontaneous redistribution of function to the right hemisphere has frequently been observed within days of the stroke. However, a prospective PET study of language activation in patients with acute left hemispheric stroke concluded that although right hemispheric activation clearly occurred, recovery of useful language only correlated with left hemispheric activation (Heiss et al., 1997). These results highlight the difficulties of interpreting regional activation in terms of being either necessary or sufficient for supporting a given cognitive or sensorimotor function.

Neuroimaging techniques have also been used to study the dynamic reorganization of function following amputation. In animal models, cortical sensory organization has been shown to occur within minutes. In human amputees, the somatotopic representation of the phantom limb may be activated by stimulation of other body regions such as the face. Since phantom limb effects probably occur independently of any alteration in cerebral vasculature, interpretation of fMRI findings in terms of neural reorganization is perhaps more convincing.

An emerging application of fMRI is in brain bionics. Implantable stimulators are now used in the management of a variety of neurological syndromes including Parkinson's disease, epilepsy, and chronic pain. It is possible to use fMRI to visualize the hemodynamic effects of neurostimulation (Rezai et al., 1999). FMRI can also be used to guide the placement of electrodes into brain regions under conscious control such as motor cortex. Such electrodes have been used to control computerized robotics in paralyzed patients (Kennedy & Bakay, 1998), and fMRI should also be of use in monitoring functional reorganization resulting from brain-electrode interactions.

In conclusion, functional imaging techniques provide numerous approaches to visualizing regional brain activity non-invasively, and are sensitive to a broad range of physiological and neurochemical processes. These techniques have numerous applications in basic and clinical neuroscience and should provide new insights into brain organization and function. Because the technology for functional imaging of the brain is now widely available, its impact on neurological diagnosis and management could be substantial.

References   * denotes key references

Acton, P.D. & Mozley, P.D. (2000). Single photon emission tomography imaging in parkinsonian disorders: a review. *Behav. Neurol.*, **12**, 11–27.

Alsop, D.C. & Detre, J.A. (1998). Multisection cerebral blood flow MR imaging with continuous arterial spin labeling. *Radiology*, **208**, 410–16.

Alsop, D.C., Detre, J.A. & Grossman, M. (2000). Assessment of cerebral blood flow in Alzheimer's disease by spin-labeled magnetic resonance imaging. *Ann.. Neurol.*, **47**, 93–100.

Baird, A.E. & Warach, S. (1998). Magnetic resonance imaging of acute stroke. *J. Cereb. Blood Flow Metab.*, **18**, 583–609.

Belliveau, J.W., Kennedy, D.W., McKinstry, R.C. et al. (1991). Functional mapping of the human visual cortex by magnetic resonance imaging. *Science*, **254**, 716–18.

*Binder, J.R., Swanson, S.J., Hammeke, T.A. et al. (1996). Determination of language dominance using functional MRI: A comparison with the Wada test. *Neurology*, **46**, 978–84.

Brewer, J.B., Zhao, Z., Desmond, J.E. et al. (1988). Making memories: brain activity that predicts how well visual experience will be remembered. *Science*, **281**, 1185–7.

Brooks, D.J. (1997). PET and SPECT studies in Parkinson's disease. *Baillières Clin. Neurol.*, **6**, 69–87.

*Brooks, D.J., Ibanez, V., Sawle, G.V. et al. (1990). Differing patterns of striatal ^{18}F-dopa uptake in Parkinson's disease, multiple system atrophy, and progressive supranuclear palsy. *Ann. Neurol.*, **28**, 547.

Buckner, R.L., Bandettini, P.A., O'Craven, K.M. et al. (1996). Detection of cortical activation during averaged single trials of a cognitive task using functional magnetic resonance imaging. *Proc. Natl Acad. Sci., USA*, **93**, 14878–83.

Chollet, F. & Weiller, C. (1994). Imaging recovery of function following brain injury. *Curr. Opin. Neurobiol.*, **4**, 226–30.

Cramer, S.C., Finklestein, S.P., Schaechter, J.D. et al. (1999). Distinct regions of motor cortex control ipsilateral and contralateral finger movements. *J. Neurophysiol.*, **81**, 383–7.

D'Haenen, H., Bossuyt, A., Mertens, J. et al. (1992). SPECT imaging of 5-HT2 receptors in depression. *Psychiatry Res.*, **45**, 227–37.

Detre, J.A. & Alsop, D.C. (1998). Perfusion fMRI with arterial spin labeling (ASL). In *Functional MRI*, ed. C. Moonen & P. Bandettini. Heidelberg: Springer-Verlag.

*Detre, J.A. & Floyd, T.F. (2000). Functional MRI and its applications to the clinical neurosciences. *Neuroscientist*, **7**, 64–79.

Detre, J.A., Sirvan, J.I., Alsop, D.C. et al. (1995). Localization of sub-clinical ictal activity by functional MRI: correlation with invasive monitoring. *Ann. Neurol.*, **38**, 618–24.

Detre, J.A., Maccotta, L., King, D. et al. (1998). Functional MRI lateralization of memory in temporal lobe epilepsy. *Neurology*, **50**, 926–32.

Duncan, J.S. (1997). Imaging and epilepsy. *Brain*, **120**, 339–77.

*Farde, L., Nordström, A.L., Wiesel, F.A. et al. (1992). Positron emission tomographic analysis of central D_1 and D_2 dopamine receptor occupancy in patients treated with classical neuroleptics and clozapine: relation to extrapyramidal side effects. *Arch. Gen. Psychiatry*, **49**, 538–44.

Frey, K.A., Minoshima, S. & Kuhl, D.E. (1998). Neurochemical imaging of Alzheimer's disease and other degenerative dementias. *Quart. J. Nucl. Med.*, **42**, 166–78.

Friston, K.J., Jezzard, P. & Turner, R. (1994). Analysis of functional MRI time-series. *Hum. Brain Mapping*, **1**, 153–74.

Grubb, R.L., Jr., Derdeyn, C.P., Fritsch, S.M. et al. (1998). Importance of hemodynamic factors in the prognosis of symptomatic carotid occlusion. *J. Am. Med. Ass.*, **280**, 1055–60.

Heiss, W.D. & Podreka, I. (1993). Role of PET and SPECT in the assessment of ischemic cerebrovascular disease. *Cerebrovasc. Brain Metab. Rev.*, **5**, 235–63.

Heiss, W.D., Karbe, H., Weber-Luxenburger, G. et al. (1997). Speech-induced cerebral metabolic activation reflects recovery from aphasia. *J. Neurol. Sci.*, **145**, 213–17.

Innis, R.B., Seibyl, J.P., Scanley, B.E. et al. (1993). Single photon emission computed tomographic imaging demonstrates loss of striatal dopamine transporters in Parkinson's disease. *Proc. Natl Acad. Sci., USA*, **90**, 11965–9.

Kennedy, P.R. & Bakay, R.A. (1998). Restoration of neural output from a paralyzed patient by a direct brain connection. *Neuroreport*, **9**, 1707–11.

Kim, D-S., Duong, T.Q. & Kim, S-G. (1999). Magnetic resonance imaging of iso-orientation domains in cat visual cortex using early negative BOLD signals (abstract). *Soc. Neurosci. Abstr.*, **25**, 783.

*Koepp, M.J., Gunn, R.N., Lawrence, A.D. et al. (1998). Evidence for striatal dopamine release during a video game. *Nature*, **393**, 266–8.

Krakow, K., Woermann, F.G., Symms, M.R. et al. (1999). EEG-triggered functional MRI of interictal epileptiform activity in patients with partial seizures. *Brain*, **122**, 1679–88.

Lammertsma, A.A. & Hume, S.P. (1996). Simplified reference tissue model for PET receptor studies. *Neuroimage*, **4**, 153–8.

Lansberg, M.G., O'Brien, M.W., Norbash, A.M. et al. (1999). MRI abnormalities associated with partial status epilepticus. *Neurology*, **52**, 1021–7.

Laruelle, M.A., Abi-Dargham, A., Rattner, Z. et al. (1993). Single photon emission tomography measurement of benzodiazepine receptor number and affinity in primate brain: a constant infusion paradigm with [^{123}I]iomazenil. *Europ. J. Pharmacol.*, **230**, 119–23.

Le Bihan, D., Breton, E., Lallemand, D. et al. (1986). MR imaging of intravoxel incoherent motions: application to diffusion and perfusion in neurologic disorders. *Radiology*, **161**, 401–7.

*MacLaren, D.C., Gambhir, S.S., Satyamurthy, N. et al. (1999). Repetitive, non-invasive imaging of the dopamine D2 receptor as a reporter gene in living animals. *Gene Therapy*, **6**, 785–91.

Malison, R.T., Price, L.H., Berman, R. et al. (1998). Reduced brain serotonin transporter availability in major depression as measured by [^{123}I]-2b-carbomethoxy-3b-(4-iodophenyl)tropane and single photon emission computed tomography. *Biol. Psychiatry*, **11**, 1090–8.

Malonek, D. & Grinvald, A. (1996). Interactions between electrical activity and cortical microcirculation revealed by imaging spectroscopy: implications for functional brain mapping. *Science*, **272**, 551–4.

*Menon, R.S., Ogawa, S., Strupp, J. et al. (1997). Ocular dominance in human V1 demonstrated by functional magnetic resonance imaging. *J. Neurophys.*, **77**, 2780–7.

Moseley, M.E., Cohen, Y., Mintotovitch, J. et al. (1990). Early detection of regional cerebral ischemia in cats: comparison of diffusion- and T_2-weighted MRI and spectroscopy. *Magn. Reson. Med.*, **14**, 330–46.

Mozley, P.D., Schneider, J.S., Acton, P.D. et al. (2000). Binding of [Tc-99m]TRODAT-1 to dopamine transporters in patients with Parkinson's disease and healthy volunteers. *J. Nucl. Med.*, **41**, 584–9.

Mummery, C.J., Patterson, K., Price, C.J. et al. (2000). A voxel-based morphometry study of semantic dementia: relationship between temporal lobe atrophy and semantic memory. *Ann. Neurol.*, **47**, 36–45.

Neumann-Haefelin, T., Moseley, M.E. & Albers, G.W. (2000). New magnetic resonance imaging methods for cerebrovascular disease: emerging clinical applications. *Ann. Neurol.*, **47**, 559–70.

Ogawa, S., Menon, R.S., Kim, S.G. et al. (1998). On the characteristics of functional magnetic resonance imaging of the brain. *Ann. Rev. Biophys. Biomolec. Struct.*, **27**, 447–74.

Pierpaoli, C., Jezzard, P., Basser, P.J. et al. (1996). Diffusion tensor MR imaging of the human brain. *Radiology*, **201**, 637–48.

Pilowsky, L.S., Costa, D.C., Ell, P.J. et al. (1992). Clozapine, single photon emission tomography, and the D_2 dopamine receptor blockade hypothesis of schizophrenia. *Lancet*, **340**, 199–202.

Rapoport, S.I. (1997). Discriminant analysis of brain imaging data identifies subjects with early Alzheimer's disease. *Int. Psychogeriat.*, **9**, 229–35; discussion 247–52.

Rezai, A.R., Lozano, A.M., Crawley, A.P. et al. (1999). Thalamic stimulation and functional magnetic resonance imaging: localization of cortical and subcortical activation with implanted electrodes. Technical note. *J. Neurosurg.*, **90**, 583–90.

Roy, C.S. & Sherrington, C.S. (1890). On the regulation of the blood-supply of the brain. *J. Physiol.*, **11**, 85–108.

Smith, G.S., Dewey, S.L., Brodie, J.D. et al. (1997). Serotonergic modulation of dopamine measured with [^{11}C]raclopride and PET in normal human subjects. *Am. J. Psychiatry*, **154**, 490–6.

Sorensen, A.G., Tievsky, A.L., Ostergaard, L. et al. (1997). Contrast agents in functional MR imaging. *J. Mag. Res. Imag.* **7**, 47–55.

Spencer, S.S., Theodore, W.H. & Berkovic, S.F. (1995). Clinical applications: MRI, SPECT, and PET. *Magn. Res. Imaging*, **13**, 1119–24.

Talairach, J. & Tournoux, P. (1988). *Co-planar Stereotaxic Atlas of the Human Brain*. Stuttgart: Thieme.

Tong, D.C. & Albers, G.W. (2000). Diffusion and perfusion magnetic resonance imaging for the evaluation of acute stroke: potential use in guiding thrombolytic therapy. *Curr. Opin. Neurol.*, **13**, 45–50.

Ungerleider, L.G. & Haxby, J.V. (1994). 'What' and 'where' in the human brain. *Curr. Opin. Neurobiol.*, **4**, 157–65.

Villringer, A. & Dirnagl, U. (1995). Coupling of brain activity and cerebral blood flow: basis of functional neuroimaging. *Cereb. Brain Metab. Rev.*, **7**, 240–76.

Vlaardingerbroek, M.T. & den Boer, J.A. (1996). *Magnetic Resonance Imaging: Theory and Practice.* New York: Springer-Verlag.

Wagner, A.D., Schacter, D.L., Rotte, M. et al. (1998). Building memories: remembering and forgetting of verbal experiences as predicted by brain activity. *Science*, **281**, 1188–91.

Webster, M.W., Makaroun, M.S., Steed, D.L. et al. (1995). Compromised cerebral blood flow reactivity is a predictor of stroke in patients with symptomatic carotid artery occlusive disease. *J. Vasc. Surg.*, **21**, 338–44.

Woolsey, T.A., Rovainen, C.M., Cox, S.B. et al. (1996). Neuronal units linked to microvascular modules in cerebral cortex: response elements for imaging the brain. *Cereb. Cortex*, **6**, 647–60.

Yang, X., Hyder, F. & Shulman, R.G. (1996). Activation of single whisker barrel in rat localized by functional magnetic resonance imaging. *Proc. Natl. Acad. Sci., USA*, **93**, 475–8.

*Yetkin, F.Z., Mueller, W.M., Morris, G.L. et al. (1997). Functional MR activation correlated with intraoperative cortical mapping. *Am. J. Neuroradiol.*, **18**, 1311–15.

Zhen, W., Han, H., Anguiano, M. et al. (1999). Synthesis and amyloid binding properties of rhenium complexes: preliminary progress toward a reagent for SPECT imaging of Alzheimer's disease brain. *J. Med. Chem.*, **42**, 2805–15.

11

Windows on the working brain: magnetic resonance spectroscopy

James W. Prichard,[1] Jeffrey R. Alger,[2] Douglas Arnold,[3] Ognen A. C. Petroff [1] and Douglas L. Rothman[4]

[1] Department of Neurology, Yale Medical School, New Haven, CT, USA
[2] Department of Radiology, University of California at Los Angeles, CA, USA
[3] Department of Neurology, Montreal Neurological Institute, Canada
[4] Department of Diagnostic Radiology, Yale Medical School, New Haven, CT, USA

Nuclear magnetic resonance (NMR) spectroscopy is an observational technique based on detection of signals from magnetic atomic nuclei such as ^1H, ^{31}P, ^{13}C, ^{15}N, and ^{17}O. It is most familiar to physicians and the public as magnetic resonance imaging (MRI), which uses the strong signal from water protons to make the most highly detailed pictures of living tissue available from any non-invasive method. In consequence, MRI, including its special forms magnetic resonance angiography, diffusion-weighted imaging, and magnetization transfer imaging – quickly became a major tool for medical diagnosis and research on living creatures. Its applications to neurological disease are described in several other chapters of this book.

Magnetic resonance spectroscopy (MRS) is the designation used in the biomedical world for measurement of NMR signals from non-water protons and other magnetic nuclei. The usage is not accurate, MRI is the MRS of water, but it is convenient. MRS signals detectable in living brain are thousands of times weaker than the water proton signal; hence observing them requires extra time and special procedures. The reward for the effort is an abundance of chemically specific information which can be acquired as often as necessary, since the measurement process is non-invasive. In the living human brain, ^1H signals can be obtained from N-acetyl aspartate, creatine, choline moieties, glutamate, glutamine, lactate, and several other small molecules. Phosphocreatine, adenosine triphosphate, and inorganic phosphate can be measured directly by their ^{31}P signals, and intracellular pH calculated from its effect on these signals. Information from the ^{31}P spectrum allows calculation of the rate of the creatine kinase reaction. The spectra of ^{13}C, ^{15}N, ^{17}O, and other magnetic nuclei contain many more small signals from a variety of molecules which will become detectable as technology advances.

This unprecedented measurement capability provides an opportunity for characterization of human neurological diseases along several axes of chemical variation throughout their natural histories. The data are obtained without hazard to the patient, are free from artefacts of tissue preparation, and can be compared in as much detail as necessary to identically acquired information from normal subjects. As MRS matures technically over the first decades of the twenty-first century, it can be expected to take a place among the principal technologies contributing to illumination of disease processes and evaluation of new treatments.

For these reasons, MRS had become well established as an important research technology in neurology and neuroscience by 2001, but not yet as a diagnostic resource necessary for much of neurological practice, as MRI had been for some years. That is likely to change. The wealth of MRS data accumulated on diseases of the human brain since the mid-1980s indicates several possible avenues to routine diagnostic application. As this literature is far too extensive to review here, we emphasize three aspects of MRS which we believe will flourish during the years following publication of this volume, producing novel data of interest to most neurologists. These are: spectroscopic imaging (SI), a way of mapping anatomical distribution of specific compounds in the brain; measurement of γ-aminobutyric acid (GABA) in the ^1H spectrum; and labeling of brain metabolite pools with ^{13}C.

We first present a brief account of how NMR measurements are made, the signals available in the ^1H spectrum, localization methods, and some highlights of ^1H MRS findings in neurological disease.

The physical basis of NMR measurements

Figures 11.1 and 11.2 (see colour plate section) illustrate in cartoon form one common way of making basic NMR

1 Certain atomic nuclei are magnetic; ^1H, ^{31}P, ^{13}C, ^{15}N & ^{17}O are examples of biological interest. They behave like small compass needles which spin around their own long axis, even when bound to other atoms in molecular structures:

2 In the strong magnetic field of an NMR spectrometer, they line up along the flux lines in a Boltzmann distribution, a few more with the field than against it, and their spins cause them to precess around the flux lines:

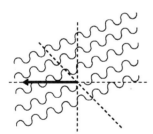

3 The net magnetization of such a spin population is a vector parallel to the flux lines, along the magnet's Z axis:

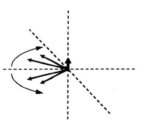

4 For measurements by the common spin echo method, an additional small magnetic field rotating near the precession frequency of the spins is applied briefly to tip the vector in the X–Y plane:

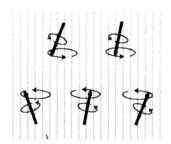

5 Slight differences in precession frequency due to magnetic field inhomogeneities cause spins to spread out in the X–Y plane (dephase), up spins one way, down spins the other (T2 relaxation), while some return to the Z axis (T1 relaxation):

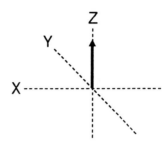

6 Another kind of brief magnetic pulse flips spins still in the X–Y plane by 180 degrees:

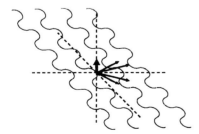

7 Because spins still in the X–Y plane continue to precess in the same direction, their net magnetization refocuses as a vector along –X:

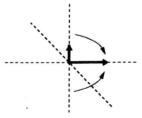

Fig. 11.1. NMR principles.

measurements, the spin echo technique, and the general procedure by which images are generated from NMR data. Many variations on these basic techniques exist, and new ones are constantly being developed.

Several aspects of NMR technology not evident in the cartoons are important for understanding both its power and its limitations:

MRS sensitivity is low

The Boltzmann distribution illustrated in panel 2 of Fig. 11.1 actually produces a difference between up and down spins not in the 2:3 ratio shown, but only about 1 part in 10^6. The strength of NMR signals is proportional to the size of the difference, which is why they are weak. For this reason, MRS of the human brain cannot detect compounds below the millimolar range under most circumstances. Methods for temporarily increasing the polarization difference of spin populations are under development, but so far only for increasing the signal obtainable from inhalable gases used as MRI contrast agents.

MRS signals come from small, mobile chemical entities

Only molecules which tumble freely in solution or especially mobile parts of large fixed molecules yield signals large enough to detect in living tissue. Hence free glutamate and aspartate can be detected, but the same molecules are invisible when their movement is constrained by incorporation into proteins. Together with the inherent insensitivity mentioned above, this limitation precludes MRS measurement of many important brain substances, such as biogenic amines, acetylcholine, and most membrane structural elements.

MRS and MRI are sessile, motion-sensitive techniques

All measurements must be made in a large, heavy magnet which usually remains in a fixed location. Subjects must lie nearly motionless in the magnet bore while measurements are made, which can be an hour or more for MRS, due to the small size of the signals. These conditions circumscribe the range of physical activity that can be incorporated into study design essentially to small finger and toe movements.

MRS and MRI are safe

Because the Boltzmann difference between up and down spins is so small, only a small amount of energy is neces-

sary to perturb the spin population for measurements. Neither that injected magnetic energy nor the static magnetic field used to align the spin population has any deleterious effect on living tissue. The major hazard to subjects is from movement of ferromagnetic objects within or near their bodies caused by the static field and is easily avoided by adherence to safety procedures.

Stronger magnetic fields give better measurements

The static magnetic field represented by vertical lines in panel 2 of Fig. 11.1 determines the strength of NMR signals and the degree to which signals from different chemical entities are resolved (separated) from each other. For most biomedical applications, the stronger the field, the higher the quality of the information that can be obtained. By 2001, the standard field for clinical MRI machines had reached 1.5 tesla, or about 30 000 times as strong as the terrestrial field which aligns a compass needle. Much stronger fields have been used for in vivo animal research for years with no indication that they damage tissue. Several dozen human research instruments with fields ranging from 2 to 8 tesla exist and have been shown to improve brain MRS signal quality. The outer limit of practical field strength is not yet known; it may be dictated more by instrument cost than by safety considerations.

The ^{1}H spectrum

Figure 11.3 is a ^{1}H spectrum acquired from a small volume of cat brain in a 2 tesla instrument. With special effort, spectra showing this degree of detail can be obtained from human brain at 1.5 tesla, but they are routine in the 2–7 tesla machines that were becoming available in research facilities by 2001. The figure therefore illustrates what can reasonably be expected from ^{1}H MRS over the decade or so following publication of this volume.

The spectroscopic signatures of several distinct molecules are evident in Fig. 11.3. The strongest determinant of signal intensity is the tissue concentration of the molecule that generates it, although the relaxation times T1 and T2 (see panel 5 of Fig. 11.1) of each signal also influence signal intensity and depend on conditions of signal acquisition. Apart from the water signal, which was selectively reduced by acquisition procedures, the strongest signal in the figure is from N-acetylaspartate (NAA). This amino acid of unknown function is present in neurons but not glia of normal mature brain at a concentration of 7–10 mmole/kg of tissue. The other labelled signals identify compounds that are consistently detectable in ^{1}H spectra of human

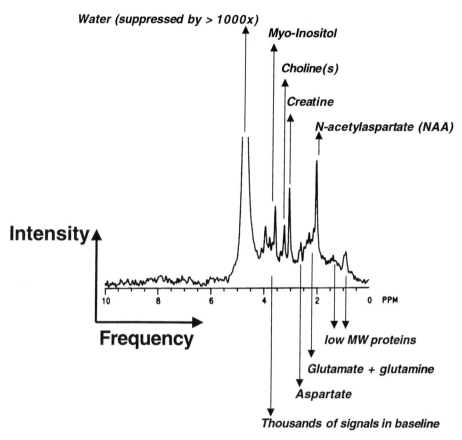

Fig. 11.3. Proton (^{1}H) spectrum of living cat brain obtained at 2 tesla. PPM: parts per million; standard units for expressing 'chemical shift', the displacement of resonant signals relative to that of a reference compound.

brain in standard 1.5 tesla clinical instruments equipped with MRS capability.

Spectral noise defines one ultimate limit on signal detection. This can be appreciated by comparing the NAA signal to the noise level that is most obvious in the leftmost portion of Fig. 11.3. Signals from a molecule with the same spectral properties but present at a concentration only 1/10th that of NAA would be barely discernible above noise, and signals only a little weaker would not be detectable at all. Metabolite detection threshold can be lowered by signal-to-noise ratio improvements achieved by time averaging or enlargement of the sampled volume. Averaging of repeated signal acquisitions tends to cancel the noise while accentuating signals that are the same every time. A bigger sampled volume increases the number of nuclei which contribute to the signal. Both procedures are quite useful in practice, but each brings its own new set of limitations: averaging degrades temporal resolution and increases the risk of movement artifact; larger volumes reduce anatomical resolution and may mix together

signals that actually have different properties. The optimum balance among these factors must be matched specifically to each application.

Spectral crowding also complicates isolation of signals from individual molecular species. Many atomic nuclei transmit on very nearly the same frequency, and their signals overlap each other. The broad hump from about 0.5 to 5.5 ppm in Fig. 11.3 is the sum of thousands of small signals from a variety of molecules. Selective extraction of a single signal from many overlapping ones is sometimes possible by spectral editing procedures which exploit some property possessed only by the desired signal. The GABA detection scheme illustrated in Fig. 11.6 is an example of such a strategy, in that case based on selective magnetic perturbation of the C3 protons in a way that changes their influence on the C4 protons and distinguishes the signal of the latter from overlapping ones. Glutamate, lactate, and some other molecules can be detected selectively in similar fashion, but many more, including NAA, creatine, cholines, and myo-inositol among the large signal sources in the ^{1}H spectrum, lack features of chemical structure which make editing of their signals possible. When signals of that kind change during brain activity or under the influence of disease, any combination of changes in the overlapping signals may be responsible; interpretation must therefore be guided by independent information about of how many overlapping signals are present and how the molecules generating them behave under the particular circumstances of the observation.

Signals from larger and less mobile molecules such as proteins, nucleic acid polymers and proteolipid aggregates are of special importance in this regard. Compounds with molecular weights greater than about 1000 daltons usually produce signals with very short T2 and very long T1. Because of short T2, their signals do not persist long enough to be measured accurately without a great deal of averaging of responses to repeated stimulations, and even when they are detectable, they are very broad, overlapping each other and the narrow signals from smaller, more mobile molecules. At the same time, their long T1s require long waiting times between successive stimulations. Both factors reduce the signal-to-noise ratios that can be achieved in a given time and thereby limit the ability of MRS to detect macromolecular signals selectively.

In one way, the low signal-to-noise ratio of macromolecular resonances is an advantage for measurement of the narrow signals in Fig. 11.3. If the intensity of myelin signals were proportional to myelin concentration, ^{1}H spectra from brain would be overwhelmed by them, and most of the observations described in this chapter would be extremely difficult or impossible. This does not happen because myelin protons have an extremely short T2 relaxation time.

But in another way, broad macromolecular signals complicate quantitative measurement of narrow ones, because they are a potentially variable baseline on which the latter are superimposed. Methods are under development for determining whether an apparent change in a narrow signal is actually due in whole, or in part, to changes in macromolecular signals underlying it.

Signal localization

Matching the spatial resolution of MRS to the anatomical heterogeneity of the brain well enough to permit reliable measurement of localized functional and disease effects on brain chemistry has absorbed the effort of many spectroscopists since human MRS research began. The problems are the same in principle as the ones encoun-

tered in the quest for ever greater anatomical resolution in MRI, which is below 1 mm; but because MRS signals are so much smaller than the water proton signal, resolution in the millimetre range is hard to achieve.

For most of its history, MRS was possible only on single volumes of brain. Recently, acquisition from multiple volumes simultaneously has become practical by techniques usually referred to as chemical shift imaging or spectroscopic imaging. The characteristics of the single volume approach make the advantages of the multiple volume approach clear.

Single volume MRS

Spectra can be acquired from single cubic or rectangular tissue volumes down to about 2 cubic centimetres, localized to a region of interest with the help of a guiding MRI. Appropriately equipped commercial MRI machines can acquire localized spectra from volumes of that size or larger in automated fashion, once the desired volume is selected.

Localized single volume MRS has distinct advantages and disadvantages. The principal advantage is that it provides a single spectrum from a tissue volume defined by MRI in a few minutes. The characteristics of the acquisition can be adjusted to permit a number of spectroscopic features to be accentuated. For example, it is usually possible to collect the spectroscopic information at relatively short echo time which provide the full array of detectable tissue signals without excessive loss associated with T2 relaxation. Alternatively, if less complex spectra are desired, the echo time may be lengthened to suppress signals with short T2s.

The principal disadvantages of localized single volume MRS are its inherent time inefficiency, poor conformance of acquisition volume to brain anatomy, and the difficulty of localizing signal to precisely the same volume in different subjects or in the same subject at different times. Acquisition of spectra from more than one brain location requires separate measurements, each taking several minutes. When several regions are to be compared, the limits of subject tolerance are quickly reached. Volumes of interest must be bounded by planes; practical methods for defining volumes with curved surfaces are not available. Therefore, fitting the acquisition volume to a region of interest is usually only approximate. Finally, the goal of detecting signal from a particular anatomical region in consistently reproducible fashion is an elusive one. Small variations in placement of the volume in different subjects or in the same subject from one examination to the next can easily confound comparison of subjects and monitoring of changes over time in an individual.

Spectroscopic imaging (SI)

This method of localizing MRS signals works by acquiring spectra simultaneously from a grid of tissue regions within a brain volume. The techniques are similar to some of those used in conventional MRI. The entire volume of interest is excited by stimulating cues which induce the magnetic nuclei within it to broadcast their signals. Additional manipulations extract spatially localized information from the complicated signal by a series of measurements in which the cueing pulse sequence is altered slightly in a systematic manner. Analysis of how the total signal varies with alterations in the cueing process permits the signal contributions of each volume element in the grid to be determined.

SI has not yet come into routine use because of its technical complexity. However, it has been shown to be practical for research and diagnosis in several brain diseases, it is much more powerful than single volume methods in dealing with the heterogeneity of brain anatomy and pathology, and it offers significant gains in time efficiency. Accordingly, its clinical applications can be expected to increase rapidly.

MRS findings in neurological disease

Thousands of MRS studies covering all major categories of human brain disease were published in the first 15 years after the technique became available. More extensive consideration of this literature than can be given here is available in a recent book (Danielsen & Ross, 1999), where the reader can also find numerous examples of how an experienced research group has applied early MRS techniques to specific diagnostic problems in clinical neurology.

Most MRS studies of brain disease show some combination of three changes: loss of NAA signal, interpreted to signify loss of neurons; elevation of lactate, signifying lack of tissue oxygen or infiltration of high-lactate cells such as macrophages; and an elevated choline signal, thought to reflect acceleration of metabolic pathways involving components of biological membranes. As these changes appear to come about by different mechanisms in different diseases, they reflect general pathophysiological processes more often than disease-specific phenomena. In some instances, however, they have stimulated new thinking about particular diseases and shown promise for refinement of diagnosis and treatment evaluation. Space limits the examples we can offer to a few.

Stroke

Loss of NAA and elevation of lactate in acute stroke was predicted by decades of earlier work, and they were confirmed in human patients when ^{1}H MRS became available (Graham et al., 1992). However, persistence of lactate elevation for months after a stroke was not anticipated (Graham et al., 1993); the fact that it could be labelled with ^{13}C from infused glucose showed that it was metabolically active, not trapped in dead tissue (Rothman et al., 1991). Other MRS work suggested that persistently high lactate is in macrophages and other cells participating in the infarcted tissue's response to injury (Petroff et al., 1992).

An interesting body of data indicates that changes in ^{1}H spectra of hemispheres perfused by diseased carotids precedes clinical symptoms of cerebral ischemia (Klijn et al., 2000). If this finding is confirmed, MRS may one day help distinguish patients who need surgical intervention from those who can safely be treated by medical means.

Epilepsy

Decreased NAA in one or both temporal lobes compares well with lateralization of seizure foci and positron emission tomography in identifying the correct side for surgical treatment of intractable temporal lobe epilepsy (Cendes et al., 1997a). It may emerge as the single most useful laboratory technique for that purpose, due to its favourable combination of specificity with non-invasiveness.

Loss of NAA signal is apparently not always due to permanent loss of neurons. Normalization of temporal NAA during seizure-free periods in temporal lobe epileptics indicates that reversible neuronal dysfunction associated with the ictal state is a significant pathophysiological factor in this condition (Cendes et al., 1997b).

Multiple sclerosis

Decreased NAA is regularly observed in acute plaques, implying that more axonal damage occurs in such lesions than had been thought; as in the seizure-free temporal lobes mentioned above, NAA recovers partially in demyelinating lesions in a manner that correlates with clinical recovery, confirming the role of reversible axonal dysfunction in the disease (Matthews et al., 1991; Arnold et al., 1992; Davie et al., 1994). More recently, decreased NAA has been observed in white matter that is normal on MRI, and in patients with chronic illness, this change correlates better with clinical disability than the MRI lesions (Fu et al., 1998).

Childhood ataxia with diffuse central nervous system hypomyelination (CACH)

This is a rare genetic disorder with variable clinical manifestations. A ^{1}H MRS study showed changes (low NAA, choline, and creatine in heterogeneous distribution) that were more consistent than the clinical data (Tedeschi et al., 1995). The result is an early example of what may become a prominent role for MRS in disease classification.

MRS observations have also been made repeatedly in Alzheimer's disease and other dementias, parkinsonism, motor neuron disease, HIV encephalopathy and metabolic disorders which affect the brain. New findings may bring it to the front line of diagnosis, treatment monitoring, or research in any of these areas as the technology matures.

Spectroscopic imaging of brain tumours

Intracranial neoplasia is a historically intractable clinical problem, which is much in need of new approaches. Accordingly, when magnetic resonance instrumentation capable of doing MRS on human brain became available in the mid-1980s, investigators almost immediately began using it to evaluate human intracranial neoplasms, and interest in the possibility that chemically specific data obtained non-invasively can facilitate brain tumour management has remained high ever since.

Single volume ^{31}P and, later, ^{1}H methods were the first available for this purpose, and in a short time they confirmed that a number of common biochemical characteristics of brain tumours could be detected in undisturbed lesions by MRS. However, these single volume measurements were subject to the same sampling problem that bedevils brain tumour biopsy data, the cellular heterogeneity of the lesions. MRI and X-ray computed tomography can document the vascular changes and edema associated with a particular brain tumour with a high degree of precision, but they cannot reliably identify the tumour's predominant cell type or detect anatomical variations in its chemistry.

One promising way to probe those areas is by positron and single photon emission tomography of radionuclide binding patterns specific for tumour type, once appropriate ligands are developed. Another is ^{1}H SI. Non-invasively obtained information about chemical variation within brain tumours has considerable potential for individual patient management and as a surrogate endpoint for evaluation of new treatments. Being free of hazard to the patient, the measurements can be repeated and correlated with MRI studies as often as necessary. With further technical development already under way, their anatomical resolution will be competitive with that of radionuclide methods.

The results of a ^{1}H SI study done on a patient with a tumour shortly afterward identified at surgery as a glioblastoma multiforme are shown in Fig. 11.4 (see colour plate section). The technique used long echo time (TE 272 ms) and multiple slices. Fig. 11.4(a) shows MRI scans of the three slices that were chosen for SI measurements. The white grids on the images in Fig. 11.4(b) show all the brain volume elements that generated an interpretable ^{1}H spectrum.

Figure 11.4(c) illustrates the characteristic chemical differences between the tumour (left spectrum and image) and adjacent normal tissue (right). In the tumour, choline-containing compounds (Cho) are greatly elevated, N-acetylaspartate (NAA) is undetectable, and a large lactate signal (Lac) is present. In the spectrum from normal tissue, these resonances appear as they would in a brain undisturbed by pathology. Of the prominent resonances, only the one from creatine (Cre) is the same in both spectra.

Figures 11.4(d) and 11.4(e) are the main point of this illustration. In the same way that the water proton signal was used to make the images in Fig. 11.4(a), the Cho and NAA signals were used to make (d) and (e). The metabolite images are much coarser, because the metabolite signals are so much weaker than that of water. Colour coding is commonly added to coarse images to emphasize variations, which are less obvious in grey-scale display of the same information. Elevated Cho in the tumour region and the void of NAA there are clearly evident in the images.

Single volume MRS cannot detect anatomical variations on the scale of Fig. 11.4(d) and 11.4(e). For chemical analysis of anatomically heterogeneous lesions in an anatomically heterogeneous organ, the future lies with SI.

Figure 11.5 (see colour plate section) shows ^{1}H SI results from another patient with a glioblastoma multiforme, also untreated at the time of study. The metabolite images demonstrate four distinct biochemical features of the lesion: Elevation of the choline signal in and near the tumour; relative diminution of the creatine and NAA signals; and elevation of lactate and lipid signals. The lactate signal appears in the same portion of the spectrum as signals generated by mobile lipid molecules and is therefore difficult to separate from them in the raw spectra, although spectral editing techniques mentioned elsewhere in this chapter can extract it cleanly when necessary.

Caveat spectator!

The metabolite images in Fig. 11.5 (see colour plate section) appear to be more finely resolved than the ones in Fig. 11.4 (see colour plate section). In fact, they were acquired in the same time with the same pulse sequences. Although the signal changes were actually somewhat larger in the Fig. 11.5 patient, most of the difference from Fig. 11.4 is due to postacquisition SI signal processing, for which no standards currently exist. Efforts to establish standards are under way. Meanwhile, SI interpretation for clinical purposes must be done with explicit awareness of how the data were processed.

The biochemical differences between tumours and normal brain illustrated in Figs. 11.4 and 11.5 (see colour plate section) are most pronounced in aggressive brain tumours, but they occur in various combinations in more slowly growing tumours of several histological types. By current biological interpretation, they reflect the reduced neuronal fraction of tumour cell mass (decreased NAA), anaerobic metabolism (elevated lactate), and acceleration of membrane metabolism (increased signals from cholines and small lipid molecules free to tumble in solution). To become useful in brain tumour management, the changes must be correlated quantitatively with tumour histology, treatment responsiveness, or both. These are active areas of current research.

Spectroscopic images are naturally registered with MRI scans and therefore offer an opportunity for chemical analysis of tumours and the tissue around them at the anatomical resolution of ^{1}H SI, currently about 0.2 cubic centimetres. As its anatomical and biochemical resolutions are improved yet further by intense technical development efforts under way in several countries, the rich store of chemically specific information from non-invasive SI can be expected to figure prominently in brain tumour research and therapy.

^{1}H MRS studies of GABA in the living human brain

GABA is the major inhibitory neurotransmitter in the cerebral cortex. It is synthesized from glutamate in specialized neurons, which release it from synaptic terminals that are intimately integrated into most cortical networks. Extensive studies in animals, isolated brain cells, and brain slices have shown that GABAergic function is altered in a variety of models of neurological and psychiatric disease (Roberts, 1986; Meldrum, 1989; Olsen & Avoli, 1997). Several antiepileptic and psychiatric drugs are targeted on GABAergic systems. Non-invasive measurements of GABA are therefore of interest to a wide range of neuroscientists, neurologists, and psychiatrists. Novel ^{1}H MRS techniques have made such measurements possible in recent years.

The most useful GABA resonance in the ^{1}H spectrum of living brain is overlapped by more intense resonances from glutathione and creatine (Behar & Boehm, 1994). Spectral editing techniques which permit separation of the GABA resonance from the others created a new opportunity for non-invasive study of GABA metabolism and GABAergic function in animals and humans (Rothman et al., 1984, 1993).

Figure 11.6 illustrates the current GABA editing technique. The remarkable signal-to-noise ratio of the GABA resonance in the difference spectrum allows measurement of rather small variations in GABA concentration caused by drugs and disease.

GABA studies in epileptics receiving vigabatrin

Impaired GABAergic function has been implicated in the etiology of epilepsy (Meldrum, 1989). Consistent with this proposal, ^{1}H MRS editing studies have found decreased brain GABA in adult (Petroff et al., 1996c, 2000) and pediatric (Novotny et al., 1999) epilepsy. Release of cytosolic GABA has been proposed as an important mechanisms for seizure suppression (Kocsis & Mattson, 1996; Richerson & Gaspary, 1997). The finding that low GABA concentration was strongly associated with poor seizure control in epileptics supports the idea that the relationship is causal rather than coincidental. An opportunity to test the idea by direct GABA measurements in the human brain was afforded by development of the ^{1}H MRS methods described above.

Vigabatrin is a drug which irreversibly inhibits the enzyme GABA transaminase (GABA-T), which catalyses breakdown of GABA in GABAergic neurons and in astrocytes, and thereby causes an elevation in GABA concentration. Animal studies indicate that vigabatrin reduces cortical excitability by this mechanism. Non-invasive measurement by ^{1}H MRS editing of GABA elevations caused by GABA-T inhibitors was first demonstrated in the rat brain (Behar & Boehm, 1994; Preece et al., 1994).

MRS editing studies of GABA have subsequently illuminated several aspects of vigabatrin action in the brains of epileptic patients. These include the following.

(i) The effectiveness of vigabatrin in controlling seizures depends upon elevating GABA concentration above the mean level found in non-epileptic subjects, and,

(ii) chronic dosing above 3 grams per day does not increase GABA concentration further (Petroff et al., 1996a; b, c).

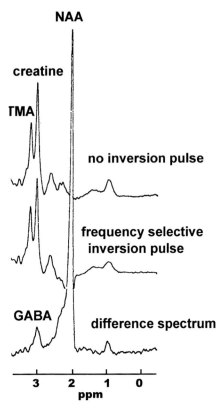

Fig. 11.6. GABA signal detection by spectral editing in human brain. The top spectrum is unmodified. During acquisition of the middle spectrum, the GABA C3 proton resonance near 1 ppm was selectively inverted by frequency-specific magnetic pulses. The C3 resonance itself is not visible due to a larger signal at the same chemical shift; the inversion pulse reduces the intensity of the larger signal in the middle spectrum compared to the top one. Magnetic interaction between the inverted C3 proton signal and the C4 proton resonance near 3 ppm alters the latter, transferring to it part of the effect of the inversion pulses at 1 ppm. When one spectrum is subtracted from the other, all of the metabolite signals drop out except the ones affected directly by the inversion pulses and the GABA C4 proton signal affected indirectly by them (difference spectrum). The GABA C4 proton signal is thereby isolated from larger coresonant signals, and its high signal-to-noise ratio allows accurate measurement of its intensity, which reflects GABA concentration. The residual water signal does not drop out because it is slightly affected by the inversion pulses and its high intensity magnifies the effect. TMA – tetramethylamines. (Unpublished data, similar to Rothman, 1993.)

(iii) GABA concentration reaches a maximum level within two hours of initial drug administration, and,

(iv) GABA concentration remains elevated over 48 hours after a single dose of vigabatrin (Petroff et al., 1999a, b).

(v) No down-regulation of GABA-A receptors occurs during chronic dosing with vigabatrin (Petroff & Rothman, 1998).

These data correspond well with other information about the clinical pharmacology of vigabatrin in epileptic patients. They imply strongly that the antiepileptic effect is due to elevation of brain GABA.

Data like these are available only from human brain MRS. They expose the human neuropharmacology of vigabatrin to a new standard of precise analysis, and they point the way to similar studies of other drugs which affect MRS-measurable resonances.

Some of these observations are of immediate practical significance. The finding that brain GABA concentration increases with vigabatrin dose up to, but not above, 3 grams per day suggests that, in general, better seizure control need not be sought above that dose. Figure 11.7 illustrates the phenomenon in quantitative form.

Such insights achieved by non-invasive observation of drug action directly in the brain can be expected to take clinical management of epilepsy to higher level of effectiveness, much as measurements of antiepileptic drug concentrations in the blood did by revealing individual differences in drug metabolism a generation ago. That earlier advance came about through better understanding of what happened to the drug outside the blood–brain barrier. Non-invasive MRS allows the analysis to be continued on the other side of that barrier, in the brain itself.

GABA studies of other antiepileptic drugs

MRS studies similar to the ones described above have found that several antiepileptic drugs with unknown mechanisms of action also cause rapid elevation of brain GABA concentration. These include gabapentin, topirimate, and lamotragine (Petroff et al., 1996b, c, 1999a, b, 2000; Hetherington et al., 1998; Kuzniecky et al., 1998). Their effects on GABA may be the mechanism of their antiepileptic action, as appears to be the case with vigabatrin. Data now available certainly motivate experiments to test that idea, but until a correlation between GABA elevation and seizure control is actually demonstrated, as was done for vigabatrin in the studies mentioned above, the idea is but an interesting possibility. Some antiepileptic drugs may elevate brain GABA and thereby prevent seizures. Others may elevate GABA but prevent seizures by a different mechanism. Drugs which elevate GABA but do not prevent seizures may be found. The point here is that non-invasive MRS measurements of GABA in the human brain allow a more direct approach to such questions than is possible by any other means.

GABA studies of depression and other brain disorders

Reduced GABA concentration has been found in unipolar depression (Sanacora et al., 1999), alcohol withdrawal, and hepatic encephalopathy (Behar et al., 1999). Results from the depression study are shown in Fig. 11.8.

These disorders are associated with an alteration in inhibitory GABAergic function. The finding of low GABA associated with them is additional evidence that the brain metabolic GABA pool is closely related to GABAergic function.

Low cortical GABA in unipolar depression appears para-doxical since the condition is not associated with enhanced cortical excitability. A potential explanation is that the low GABA concentration is a compensation for the reduction in excitatory glutamatergic activity (Sanacora et al., 1999). Future studies using ^{13}C MRS to monitor the flow of ^{13}C through observable metabolic pools in the brain (see below) may be able to test this hypothesis.

Parsing the edited GABA resonance

Both GABA and the GABA derivative homocarnosine, a condensation product of GABA and histidine, contribute to this signal. Homocarnosine is a neuromodulator present in a specific subclass of GABAergic neurons in the primate brain. Short TE ^{1}H MRS with macromolecule suppression may be used to measure the homocarnosine histidine proton resonances in the downfield region of the short TE spectrum (Behar et al., 1994; Rothman et al., 1997). Combining the homocarnosine measurement and the total GABA editing measurements allows separate meas-urement of homocarnosine and GABA. By additional mod-ification of editing selectivity the GABA derivative pyrrolidinone can also be measured in the edited spectrum (Hyder et al., 1999). Changes in concentrations of GABA, homocarnosine, and pyrrolidinone have been found to have different time courses in response to a first-time chal-lenge with vigabatrin (Petroff et al., 1999a, b).

The homocarnosine resonance titrates with pH. Hence the cytosolic pH of the GABAergic neurons where it is prin-cipally localized can be measured in the ^{1}H spectrum (Rothman et al., 1997). Together with measurement by ^{31}P MRS of cytosolic pH in the large fraction of brain cells

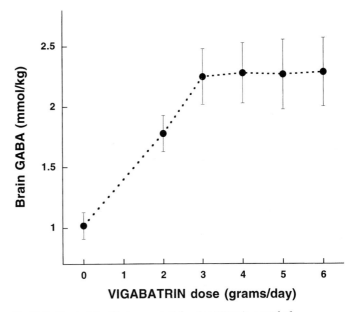

Fig. 11.7. Vigabatrin effect on occipital cortex GABA in a total of 26 patients with complex partial epilepsy. Doses above 3 grams/day caused no further GABA elevation, as the figure shows, and seizure control was not further improved either. Means ± standard deviation. (Redrawn with permission from Petroff et al., 1996a, 1999a.)

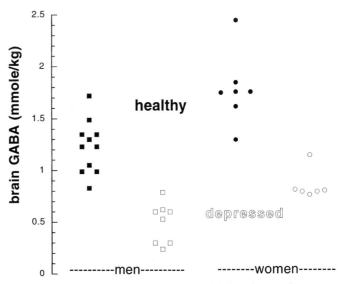

Fig. 11.8. Occipital cortex GABA in 18 normal (filled markers) and 14 medication-free depressed (open markers) men (squares) and women (circles). Analysis of covariance showed a highly significant 52% overall reduction of GABA in depressed patients. Significant age and sex interactions with GABA, but not diagnosis, were also present. (Redrawn with permission from Sanacora et al., 1999, Fig. 2. © American Medical Association.)

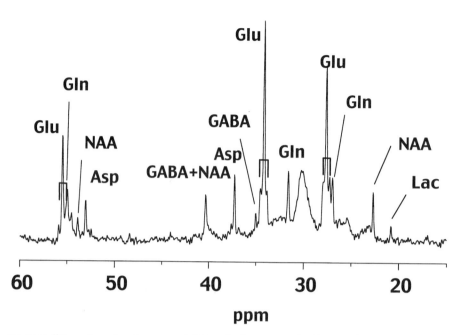

Fig. 11.9. [13]C spectrum from human occipital–parietal cortex acquired in a 4 tesla instrument after infusion of 1-^{13}C-glucose for 50 minutes. Only the resonances from NAA and the broad one at 30 ppm were present in the natural abundance spectrum prior to the infusion. The others reveal metabolic incorporation of ^{13}C into various positions of glutamate (Glu), glutamine (Gln), aspartate (Asp), and lactate (Lac), as well as GABA. Although the metabolite resonances are better resolved (separated) in ^{13}C than in ^{1}H spectra (see Figs 11.3 and 11.6), the long acquisition times required by the lower sensitivity of the ^{13}C nucleus make indirect detection of ^{13}C metabolites through the ^{1}H spectrum more useful for most metabolic studies, particularly if labelling time course is to be measured (see text and Fig. 11.10). (Reproduced with permission from Gruetter, 1998.)

which contain inorganic phosphate, this capability offers new opportunities for analysis of how pH is related to brain function and pathology (Prichard et al., 1998).

Metabolic rate studies by ^{13}C and ^{1}H-^{13}C MRS

The ^{13}C nucleus is a stable (non-radioactive) isotope of carbon which is 1.1% abundant in nature; the nearly 99% abundant ^{12}C nucleus is not magnetic. Thus, about 11 carbon atoms in every 1000 are potentially detectable directly by ^{13}C MRS. The isotopic fraction of ^{13}C in brain metabolic pools observable in vivo can be raised above 1.1% by infusion of ^{13}C enriched substrates, usually 1–[13]C-glucose.

The presence of ^{13}C in brain metabolic pools can in some cases be measured with enhanced sensitivity by indirect detection of ^{13}C by ^{1}H MRS, which can report the presence of a ^{13}C atom covalently bonded to protons. Among the carbon atoms in important molecules that can be studied in this way are C1 of glucose, C3 of lactate, C4 of glutamate, and C2 of GABA. Measurements of ^{13}C flow through these positions yield estimates of glycolytic and oxidative fluxes

which have been shown to agree with data from other techniques and to vary appropriately with changes in metabolic demand.

Building on methods developed in animal research, several groups have demonstrated the feasibility of using rates of ^{13}C incorporation into brain metabolic pools to measure metabolic flux, enzyme activity, and metabolic regulation in the living human brain (Rothman et al., 1992; Gruetter et al., 1994, 1998; Mason et al., 1995; Shen et al., 1999).

Figure 11.9 shows the ^{13}C-labelled resonances in a ^{13}C spectrum obtained from occipital/parietal region of the brain of a human subject after infusion of 1–[13]C-glucose for 50 minutes. Only the NAA signals and the broad one at 30 ppm were present before the infusion.

As is evident from the figure, separation of resonances along the frequency axis is much greater in ^{13}C than in ^{1}H spectra. However, ^{13}C MRS is not the most effective way to do ^{13}C-labelling studies in vivo. The spectra take much longer to acquire, because ^{13}C gives a much weaker signal than ^{1}H, and they give information only about the fraction of a metabolite pool which contains [13]C. The combined ^{1}H/^{13}C method solves these problems.

Observation of the brain by ^{1}H techniques which reveal the presence of ^{13}C at certain positions of glutamate, glutamine, lactate, and other detectable metabolites (Rothman et al., 1992) opens a new era in the study of brain metabolism, both as it operates during normal brain function and as it is altered by disease.

Figure 11.10 shows the time course of ^{13}C labelling from 1–[13]C-glucose of glutamate and glutamine in the human occipital region obtained with the ^{1}H/^{13}C method (Shen et al., 1999). The high sensitivity of ^{1}H MRS allowed a data point to be acquired every 5 minutes. Detection of the unlabelled portions of the metabolite pools allowed calculation of the time course of increase in their isotopic fractions (not shown). Data like these provide direct access to dynamic aspects of brain metabolism with time and space resolutions which surpass those available from any other non-invasive technology. Improvements in both kinds of resolution and detection of additional compounds are possible by use of higher magnetic fields and other technical advances which are known to be feasible. These facts ensure that MRS technology will figure prominently in metabolic research on the living human brain for years to come.

The future

Much of the achievement of brain MRS before 2001 was demonstration that it can observe, in the living organ, in an hour or less, phenomena that decades of invasive research had laboriously established to be true of brain function occurring normally and altered by disease. With confirmation of its capabilities now firmly in hand, MRS can be used with increasing confidence to acquire information about normal and pathological brain function that is beyond the reach of any other observational technology.

Books focused as this one is on mechanisms of neurological disease invite consideration of where precisely the boundary between normal and pathological brain function lies and how it may be defined. Most of the methods mentioned in this chapter can be used to improve that definition in novel ways.

An early example was demonstration of a lactate rise in human visual cortex during stimulation by flashing lights (Prichard et al., 1991; Sappey-Marinier et al., 1992). Previously, lactate elevations had been universally regarded as a sign of distress in brain tissue. This MRS-enabled finding provided new insight concerning how glycolytic and oxidative metabolism are integrated during normal brain activity, and it fuelled a controversy on the

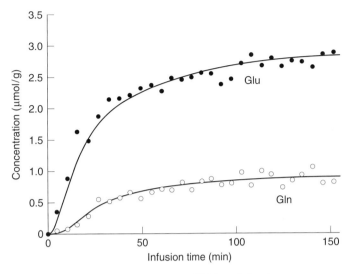

Fig. 11.10. Time course of incorporation of ^{13}C from infused 1-^{13}C-glucose into the C4 positions of glutamate (Glu) and glutamine (Gln) in human occipital cortex. Data were obtained by a combined ^{1}H/^{13}C method (see text) in a 2.1 tesla instrument. Curves were fitted by a model which allows rate calculations of glucose oxidation, the tricarboxylic acid cycle, and the glutamate/glutamine cycle. (Reproduced with permission from Shen, 1999 © 1999, National Academy of Sciences, USA.)

subject that can end nowhere but in improved understanding of how the brain works normally.

MRS methods have the potential to probe such matters much more deeply. The information gained is certain to anchor new data on brain disease mechanisms to a firm background of steadily improving insight into normal brain function.

Acknowledgements

The authors' own work was supported by the United States Public Health Service (CA76524, NS06208, NS32518), the Medical Research Council of Canada, and the Multiple Sclerosis Society of Canada.

References

Arnold, D.L., Matthews, M.D., Francis, G.S., O'Connor, J. & Antel, J.P. (1992). Proton magnetic resonance spectroscopic imaging for metabolic characterization of demyelinating plaques. *Ann. Neurol.*, **31**, 235–41.

Behar, K.L. & Boehm, D. (1994). Measurement of GABA following GABA-transaminase inhibition by gabaculine: a ^{1}H and ^{31}P NMR spectroscopic study of rat brain in vivo. *Magn. Reson. Med.*, **31**(6), 660–7.

Behar, K.L., Rothman, D.L., Spencer, D.D. & Petroff, O.A. (1994). Analysis of macromolecule resonances in ^{1}H NMR spectra of human brain. *Magn. Reson. Med.*, **32**(3), 294–302.

Behar, K.L., Rothman, D.L., Petersen, K.F. et al. (1999). Preliminary evidence of low cortical GABA levels in localized [1]H-MR spectra of alcohol-dependent and hepatic encephalopathy patients. *Am. J. Psychiatry*, **156**(6), 952–4.

Cendes, F., Andermann, F., Dubeau, F., Matthews, P.M. & Arnold, D.L. (1997a). Normalization of neuronal metabolic dysfunction after surgery for temporal lobe epilepsy. Evidence from proton MR spectroscopic imaging. *Neurology*, **49**(6), 1525–33.

Cendes, F., Stanley, J.A., Dubeau, F., Andermann, F. & Arnold, D.L. (1997). Proton magnetic resonance spectroscopic imaging for discrimination of absence and complex partial seizures. *Ann. Neurol.*, **41**(1), 74–81.

Danielsen, E.R. & Ross, B. (1999). *Magnetic Resonance Spectroscopy Diagnosis of Neurological Diseases*. New York: Marcel Dekker, Inc.

Davie, C.A., Hawkins, C.P., Barker, G.J. et al. (1994). Serial proton magnetic resonance spectroscopy in acute multiple sclerosis lesions. *Brain*, **117**(1), 49–58.

Fu, L., Matthews, P.M., De Stefano, N. et al. (1998). Imaging axonal damage of normal-appearing white matter in multiple sclerosis. *Brain*, **121**(1), 103–13.

Graham, G.D., Blamire, A.M. Howseman, A.M. et al. (1992). Proton magnetic resonance spectroscopy of cerebral lactate and other metabolites in stroke patients. *Stroke*, **23**(3), 333–40.

Graham, G.D., Blamire, A.M. Rothman, D.L. et al. (1993). Early temporal variation of cerebral metabolites after human stroke. *Stroke*, **24**, 1891–6.

Gruetter, R., Novotny, E.J., Boulware, S.D. et al. (1994). Localized ^{13}C NMR spectroscopy in the human brain of amino acid labeling from D-[1-13C]glucose. *J. Neurochem.*, **63**(4), 1377–85.

Gruetter, R., Seaquist, E.R., Kim, S. & Ugurbil, K. (1998). Localized in vivo ^{13}C-NMR of glutamate metabolism in the human brain: initial results at 4 tesla. *Dev. Neurosci.*, **20**(4–5), 380–8.

Hetherington, H.P., Newcomer, B.R. & Pan, J.W. (1998). Measurements of human cerebral GABA at 4.1 T using numerically optimized editing pulses. *Magn. Reson. Med.*, **39**(1), 6–10.

Hyder, F., Petroff, O.A., Mattson, R.H. & Rothman, D.L. (1999). Localized 1H NMR measurements of 2-pyrrolidinone in human brain in vivo. *Magn. Reson. Med.*, **41**(5) 889–96.

Klijn, C.J., Kappelle, L.J., van Der Grond, J., Algra, A., Tulleken, C.A. & van Gijn, J. (2000). Magnetic resonance techniques for the identification of patients with symptomatic carotid artery occlusion at high risk of cerebral ischemic events. *Stroke*, **31**(12), 3001–7.

Kocsis, J.D. & Mattson, R.H. (1996). GABA levels in the brain: a target for new antiepileptic drugs. *Neuroscientist*, **6**, 326–34.

Kuzniecky, R., Hetherington, H., Ho, S. et al. (1998). Topiramate increases cerebral GABA in healthy humans. *Neurology*, **51**(2), 627–9.

Mason, G.F., Gruetter, R., Rothman, D.L., Behar, K.L., Shulman, R.G. & Novotny, E.J. (1995). Simultaneous determination of the rates of the TCA cycle, glucose utilization, alpha-ketoglutarate/glutamate exchange, and glutamine synthesis in human brain by NMR. *J. Cereb. Blood Flow Metab.*, **15**(1), 12–25.

Matthews, P.M., Francis, G., Antel, J. & Arnold, D.L. (1991). Proton magnetic resonance spectroscopy for metabolic characterization of plaques in multiple sclerosis. *Neurology*, **41**, 1251–6.

Meldrum, B.S. (1989). GABAergic mechanisms in the pathogenesis and treatment of epilepsy. *Br. J. Clin. Pharmacol.*, **27**(Suppl. 1), 3S–11S.

Novotny, E.J., Jr., Hyder, F., Shevell, M. & Rothman, D.L. (1999). GABA changes with vigabatrin in the developing human brain. *Epilepsia*, **40**(4), 462–6.

Olsen, R.W. & Avoli, M. (1997). GABA and epileptogenesis. *Epilepsia*, **38**(4), 399–407.

Petroff, O.A. & Rothman, D.L. (1998). Measuring human brain GABA in vivo: effects of GABA-transaminase inhibition with vigabatrin. *Mol. Neurobiol.*, **16**(1), 97–121.

Petroff, O.A., Graham, G.D., Blamire, A.M. et al. (1992). Spectroscopic imaging of stroke in humans: histopathology correlates of spectral changes. *Neurology*, **42**(7), 1349–54.

Petroff, O.A., Behar, K.L., Mattson, R.H. & Rothman, D.L. (1996a). Human brain gamma-aminobutyric acid levels and seizure control following initiation of vigabatrin therapy. *J. Neurochem.*, **67**(6), 2399–404.

Petroff, O.A., Rothman, D.L., Behar, K.L., Lamoureux, D. & Mattson, R.H. (1996b). The effect of gabapentin on brain gamma-aminobutyric acid in patients with epilepsy. *Ann. Neurol.*, **39**(1), 95–9.

Petroff, O.A., Rothman, D.L., Behar, K.L. & Mattson, R.H. (1996c). Low brain GABA level is associated with poor seizure control. *Ann. Neurol.*, **40**(6), 908–11.

Petroff, O.A., Behar, K.L. & Rothman, D.L. (1999a). New measurements in epilepsy. Measuring brain GABA in patients with complex partial seizures. *Adv. Neurol.*, **79**, 939–45.

Petroff, O.A., Hyder, F., Collins, T., Mattson, R.H. & Rothman, D.L. (1999b). Acute effects of vigabatrin on brain GABA and homocarnosine in patients with complex partial seizures. *Epilepsia*, **40**(7), 958–64.

Petroff, O.A., Hyder, F., Mattson, R.H. & Rothman, D.L. (1999c). Topiramate increases brain GABA, homocarnosine, and pyrrolidinone in patients with epilepsy [see comments]. *Neurology*, **52**(3), 473–8.

Petroff, O.A., Hyder, F., Rothman, D.L. & Mattson, R.H. (2000). Effects of gabapentin on brain GABA, homocarnosine, and pyrrolidinone in epilepsy patients. *Epilepsia*, **41**(6), 675–80.

Preece, N.E., Jackson, G.D., Houseman, J.A., Duncan, J.S. & Williams, S.R. (1994). Nuclear magnetic resonance detection of increased cortical GABA in vigabatrin-treated rats in vivo. *Epilepsia*, **35**(2), 431–6.

Prichard, J., Rothman, D., Novotny, E. et al. (1991). Lactate rise detected by 1H NMR in human visual cortex during physiologic stimulation. *Proc. Natl. Acad. Sci., USA*, **88**, 5829–31.

Prichard, J.W., Rothman, D.L. & Petroff, O.A.C. (1998). Brain pH measurements by NMR spectroscopy. In *pH and Brain Function*, ed. K. Kaila & B.R, pp. 149–65. Ransom. New York: John Wiley.

Richerson, G B. & Gaspary, H.L. (1997). Carrier-mediated GABA release: is there a functional role? *Neuroscientist*, **3**, 151–7.

Roberts, E. (1986). Failure of GABAergic inhibition: a key to local and global seizures. *Adv. Neurol.*, **44**, 319–41.

Rothman, D.L., Behar, K.L., Hetherington, H.P. & Shulman, R.G. (1984). Homonuclear 1H double-resonance difference spectroscopy of the rat brain in vivo. *Proc. Natl. Acad. Sci., USA*, **81**(20), 6330–4.

Rothman, D.L., Howseman, A.M., Graham, G.D. et al. (1991). Localized proton NMR observation of [3–13C]lactate in stroke after [1–13C]glucose infusion. *Magn. Reson. Med.*, **21**(2), 302–7.

Rothman, D.L., Novotny, E.J., Shulman, G.I. et al. (1992). 1H-[13C] NMR measurements of [4-13C]glutamate turnover in human brain. *Proc. Natl. Acad. Sci., USA*, **89**(20), 9603–6.

Rothman, D.L., Petroff, O.A., Behar, K.L. & Mattson, R.H. (1993). Localized 1H NMR measurements of gamma-aminobutyric acid in human brain in vivo. *Proc. Natl. Acad. Sci., USA*, **90**(12), 5662–6.

Rothman, D.L., Behar, K.L., Prichard, J.W. & Petroff, O.A. (1997). Homocarnosine and the measurement of neuronal pH in patients with epilepsy. *Magn. Reson. Med.*, **38**(6), 924–9.

Sanacora, G., Mason, G.F., Rothman, D.L. et al. (1999). Reduced cortical gamma-aminobutyric acid levels in depressed patients determined by proton magnetic resonance spectroscopy. *Arch. Gen. Psychiatry*, **56**(11), 1043–7.

Sappey-Marinier, D., Calabrese, G., Fein, G., Hugg, J., Biggins, C. & Weiner, M. (1992). Effect of photic stimulation on human visual cortex lactate and phosphates using ¹H and ³¹P magnetic resonance spectroscopy. *J. Cereb. Blood Flow Metab.*, **12**, 584–92.

Shen, J., Petersen, K.F., Behar, K.L. et al. (1999). Determination of the rate of the glutamate/glutamine cycle in the human brain by in vivo 13C NMR. *Proc. Natl. Acad. Sci., USA*, **96**(14), 8235–40.

Tedeschi, G., Schiffmann, R., Barton, N.W. et al. (1995). Proton magnetic resonance spectroscopic imaging in childhood ataxia with diffuse central nervous system hypomyelination. *Neurology*, **45**(8), 1526–32.

12

Windows on the working brain: evoked potentials, magnetencephalography and depth recording

Hans-Joachim Freund[1] and Hans Joachen Heinze[2]

[1] University of Dusseldorf Neurology Clinic, Germany
[2] University of Magdeburg, Germany

A number of techniques have been developed for the study of human brain functions in normal and disordered states. Each of them monitors function from a selective point of view. Whereas functional imaging techniques are based on neurovascular coupling (functional magnetic resonance imaging (fMRI), positron emission tomography (PET), near-infrared spectroscopy (NIRS) and optical imaging), electrophysiological methods directly reflect neuronal activity. Electroencephalography (EEG) and magnetencephalography (MEG) provide information about global as well as regional activity under stationary conditions or for evoked or event related responses. Subdural or epicortical recordings for the identification of epileptogenic foci and microelectrode recordings for functional target identification during stereotactic neurosurgery complement the spectrum of the clinical application of neurophysiological tools.

Taken together, the neurovascular and neurophysiological methods provide largely complementary information that allows better insights in normal and disturbed brain function. The superimposition of MEG data on MR images combines the high spatial and temporal resolution of the respective methods. EEG recordings can now be conducted inside the MR scanner allowing the recognition of epileptogenic foci during EEG-defined seizure episodes.

Towards an integrative MEG and EEG study of cognitive brain functions

EEG and MEG measures arise from the same cortical source, namely from ordered intracellular currents in the pyramidal cells (Okada, 1982). Since the pyramidal cells in a circumscribed area show basically the same orientation orthogonal to the surface, the superimposed neural currents may result in macroscopically measurable electromagnetic fields. The electric and magnetic fields have orthogonal orientation and bear formally equivalent information; however, it may well be that stimulus-triggered event related potentials (ERPs) or magnetic fields (MFs) reveal different aspects of the underlying neural sources depending, for example on the nature of the task and the anatomy of the cortical region of interest. For several reasons, source estimation based on MFs is often superior to ERP based fits. First, opposite to electrical currents MF remain almost unchanged when passing through anatomical structures between the cortex and the sensor sets. Hence, the MFs are less susceptible to inadequate head models, both regarding anatomical shape and tissue conductivities (CSF space, scull, scalp). Secondly, the superficially observed MF originate from the primary neuronal currents (i.e. currents inside the dendrites) whereas volume currents do not contribute for physical reasons. In contrast, ERPs reflect both primary and volume currents. As a consequence, in comparison to the MEG, the electrical signal shows spatial blurring that necessarily increases uncertainties during source localization. Thirdly, the magnetic field distribution outside the head arises mainly from source currents that flow tangentially to the head surface (Williamsen & Kaufman, 1987); radially oriented source components do not significantly contribute to the observed MEG for physical reasons. This contrasts with the ERP component distribution that reflects both tangential and radial current sources. In anatomical terms, measurable magnetic activity arises almost exclusively from the sulcal part of the cortical grey matter. Accordingly, the extracranial magnetic fields are linked to a selective part of the cortical sources and not obscured by overlying fields generated by radial sources.

The role of attention in visual perception

Higher visual functions involve a number of potentially overlapping radial and tangential electromagnetic sources in the visual cortex. For instance, visual attention can modulate the signal flow in adjacent early visual areas and is a good example to illustrate the MEG/EEG comparison. Convergent input to subsequently higher cortical processing levels (V1 to V4, IT, MT) entails progressively enlarging receptive fields with a coarser representation of visual input at higher cortical levels. An increasing portion of stimuli competes inside receptive fields and, therefore, necessitates effective disambiguation mechanisms. There is evidence from brain imaging, human electrophysiology and single-cell recording that a competition bias on different cortical levels provides a solution for this coarse coding problem (Reynolds et al., 1999; Luck & Hillyard, 1994). For instance, recording ERPs triggered by a search array that contains a target feature or feature conjunction gives rise to a negative voltage of approximately 200–300 ms over posterior scalp electrodes contralateral to the field where the target occurs. This N2pc component (negativity in the N2 time range posterior contralateral) appears to be a common correlate of attentional selection across different feature types in visual search and is thought to represent a manifestation of cortical processes related to the suppression of interfering visual input from distractor items (Luck et al., 1997). So far, efforts to characterize the neural origin of the N2pc using ERP source analysis have not been successful.

In a recent study, the neural origin of this component was investigated by using a combined EEG and MEG analysis (Hopf et al., 2000). MEG data were recorded using a 148 whole-head magnetometer, and EEG data were simultaneously acquired from 32 electrode sites. As an experimental task, subjects had to identify a predefined target stimulus in the left or right visual field (LVF or RVF) among a number of randomly distributed distractor items. To derive the N2pc component, ERP-/MF-responses triggered by the RVF targets were subtracted from responses triggered by LVF targets. By this subtraction the electric and magnetic activity specifically related to the focusing of attention was obtained. Figure 12.1 (see colour plate section) illustrates the ERP scalp distribution (*a*) and magnetic field distribution (*b*) for two subsequent time windows that cover the early (180–200 ms) and late (220–240 ms) portion of the N2pc component. Shown are the average data over four independent experimental sessions of one subject. As can be seen, ERP voltage distributions in the early and late time window (Fig. 12.1(*a*)) are roughly identical showing the previously known bilateral occipital topography (Luck & Hillyard, 1994). Contrastingly, a comparison of magnetic field distributions in the early and late time range (Fig. 12.1(*b*)) reveals qualitatively different patterns. Between 180 and 200 ms the magnetic field configuration suggests a generating source in the parietal cortex as indicated by a parietal flux transition zone between the maximum magnetic outflux- and influx regions (arrow). The field config-

uration between 220 and 240 ms, however, shows two major transition zones over left and right inferior temporal sensors implying the presence of two independent posterior–temporal sources. A distributed source analysis using the minimum norm least square method in combination with a realistic volume conductor model derived from structural MR data indicates the presence of two qualitatively different source configurations for this late magnetic attention effect (Fig. 12.2(*b*), see colour plate section). In contrast, source density estimates of the ERP data revealed a similar pattern for the early and late attention effect with a broadly distributed scalp topography over the posterior cortex (Fig. 12.2(*a*), see colour plate section).

The source estimates for MF and ERP data differ in two major respects. First, there is no indication in the ERP data for a separation into early (parietal) and late (temporal) sources, and, secondly, source configurations between 220 and 240 ms are qualitatively different for both data sets. The first difference may be related to spatial blurring of ERPs leading to a confluence of scalp topographies of a weak early and stronger late field components. The second difference may result from inverse dipole modelling of the ERP data as illustrated in Fig. 12.3 (see colour plate section). In this case, ERP source modelling erroneously links two independent field components (Fig. 12.3(*a*) and (*c*), see colour plate section) to a common underlying source (Fig. 12.3, green dipole, see colour plate section) probably due to suboptimal field projections (Fig. 12.3(*b*) and (*d*)) of the underlying sources (Fig. 12.3, black dipoles, see colour plate section). Note, the problem of suboptimal field projections is not inherently linked to ERP data and may in other experiments also be relevant for MEG data. Taken together, the present example clearly demonstrates that the validity of inverse source modelling considerably benefits from a comparison of complementary electrophysiological measures like ERP and MEG. This is because EEG and MEG provide different electromagnetic views onto the same underlying current source. A combination of both datasets necessarily draws a more complete picture and clearly diminishes the risk of source mislocalization during inverse modelling.

The study of memory functions

The study of memory functions in humans is another example of how MF analysis can improve our analysis of higher brain functions. MEG sensors can detect hippocampal postsynaptic activity (Tesche et al., 1988; Wu & Okada, 1998; Okada et al., 1997). They selectively measure the tangential source components of the closed field and, therefore, are able to measure hippocampal pyramidal cell activity. MEG sensors are now being used to record non-invasively stimulus-evoked neural population responses in human hippocampal structures (Tesche et al., 1996; Nishitani et al., 1999; Tesche & Karhu, 1999). These studies describe ongoing oscillatory 4–12 Hz activity (Tesche & Karhu, 1999) and P300-like activity in oddball tasks (Nishitani et al., 1999) generated by hippocampal structures of healthy humans.

Combined ERP and MF analysis can differentiate electrophysiological indices of episodic memory in humans. Cognitive models of recognition converge on the notion that normal recognition has two qualitatively different bases. Recollection-based recognition or 'remembering' is accompanied by contextual information about the episode in which an item was encountered, whereas familiarity-based recognition, or 'knowing' is devoid of such information (Tulving, 1985). Remembering and knowing, in turn, can be considered as characterizing episodic and semantic memory, respectively. There is experimental evidence from behavioural studies that recollection and familiarity-based judgements cannot be reduced to a quantitative difference, but, instead, reflect two qualitatively different aspects of recognition memory (Knowlton & Squire, 1995). This distinction is supported by ERP findings which have revealed qualitatively distinct electrical brain patterns associated with recollection and familiarity. Recollecting recognized words causes an increase in ERP positivity between 500 and 700 ms after the onset of word presentation, a shift sometimes referred to as the late positive component or LPC effect (Rugg et al., 1998). On the other hand, familiarity-based recognition causes an earlier shift in ERP positivity between 300 and 500 ms, referred to as the N400 effect (Duzel, 1997; Paller et al., 1995). These two ERP effects have a different scalp topography suggesting that they are generated by different neuronal populations.

It remains unclear from ERP studies, however, where the corresponding neural populations are located. Lesion studies in animals and humans raise the possibility that both recognition effects should receive contributions from different structures within the temporal lobes (Murray & Mishkin, 1998; Vargha-Khadem et al., 1997b). We used combined EEG and MF recordings to localize the generators of the N400 and LPC effects of recognition in 11 healthy young subjects. EEG and MF were recorded simultaneously for correctly recognized old (repeated) words (hits) and new words (correct rejections) in 11 subjects. Current sources were computed separately for hits and correct rejections for each single subject taking into account their individual brain anatomy. Figure 12.4 (upper part, see colour plate section) shows the current source results obtained for a single subject for correct rejections and hits in the N400 and

LPC time window. It can be seen that in the N400 time window, correct rejections induce stronger current flows than hits in the anterior temporal lobe. In contrast, hits induce stronger current flows in the posterior inferior temporal lobe than correct rejections. To further quantify whether this relationship was significant across subjects, the current source maps were transformed into Talairach space. Scatter plots (lower part, Fig. 12.4) illustrate the current flow of each individual subject in the anterior inferior temporal cortex and for the LPC time window the same is illustrated for the posterior inferior temporal cortex. It can be seen that, in the anterior inferior temporal cortex, all but two subjects show higher currents for correct rejections than for hits. In contrast, in the posterior inferior temporal cortex all but two subjects show higher current flow for hits than for correct rejections. These findings suggest that the N400 old/new effect reflects mainly decremental current strengths during repetition while the LPC old/new effect reflects mainly incremental current strengths during repetition and these two types of processes are spatially dissociated in the left human inferior temporal cortex. So far, this conclusion was not possible on the basis of ERPs alone.

The investigation of sequential cerebral processing stages

A major potential of the MEG is to identify subsequent processing stages of the neural activations during well-defined behavioural states. The neurovascular imaging methods cannot only specify the multiple areas contributing to the functional network but by means of event related fMRI (efMRI) also separate subsequent activations if they are separated by long enough time spans. But efMRI cannot resolve fast sequential processing and the dynamic interactions of these structures. The advantage of the combination of the reasonably good spatial and excellent temporal resolution of the MEG can be illustrated by a study on single word reading in developmental stutterers (Salmelin et al., 2000). Stuttering represents a temporal disorder of still unknown pathophysiology and is therefore of considerable interest for such an inquiry. The task in this study was that normal subjects and stutterers read 7–8 letter words presented for 300 ms. After a blank interval of 500 ms a question mark appeared 2000 ms later prompting the subject to read the word aloud. Mouth movement and speech onset were used for motor related analyses. Figure 12.5 shows the source areas in fluent subjects and stutterers whereas the time histories of the neural activations as revealed by event related changes in the spectral power of distinct frequency bands are shown in Fig. 12.6. Although

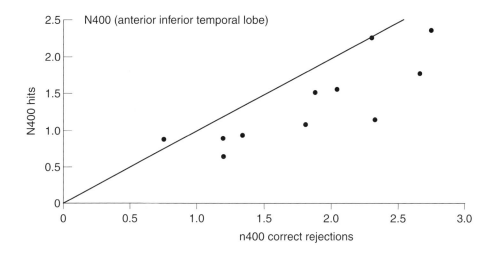

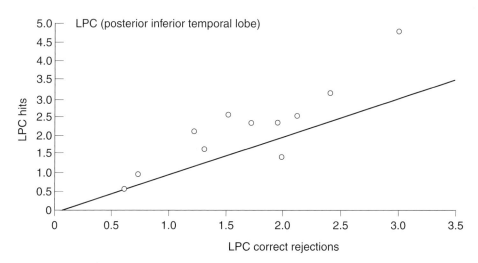

Fig. 12.4. *Lower part:* Scatter plots of the current source strengths for correctly rejected new words and hits measured in the N400 time window in the anterior inferior temporal lobe (upper diagram) and in the LPC time window in the posterior inferior temporal lobe (lower diagram). All but two subjects showed higher current flows for correctly rejected new words than hits in the anterior inferior temporal lobe in the N400 time window. In contrast, current flow was higher for hits in all but two subjects in the posterior inferior temporal lobe in the LPC time window.

the overt performance was essentially identical in the two groups, the stutterers were fluent in this task, cortical activation patterns showed clear differences for the evoked responses and the suppression of 20 Hz oscillation.

As shown in Fig. 12.6 cortical processing proceeded in the following stages:

(i) The overall temporal activation patterns showed occipital and parieto-occipital responses starting 100–150 ms after word onset (visual analysis, continuing until the appearance of the question mark) and in the left and right inferior occipito-temporal cortex (letterstring specific analysis).

(ii) Between 200 and 600 ms left more than right inferior frontal cortex responses probably reflect articulatory aspects of phonological processing, and in left middle superior temporal cortex semantic activation.

(iii) 200–800 ms following word onset, responses in the left and right posterior parietal cortices may reflect phonological aspects of linguistic processing or attentional factors of visual perception. In the third stage the left and right fronto-parietal cortices became involved and remained active throughout vocalization prompt and speech onset.

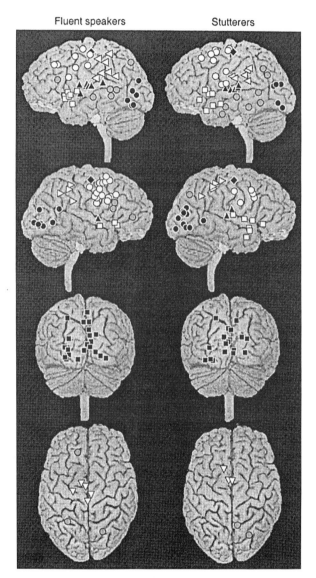

Fig. 12.5. Source areas in fluent subjects (left) and stutterers (right), when the MEG signals were averaged with respect to word onset. The different shapes and colours of the symbols (white and black circles, triangles, squares and arrows) depict the grouping of sources into distinct regions of interest. The grey circles denote sources which do not belong to any well-defined cluster. The black diamond indicates the location of the hand sensorimotor cortex. The size of the symbols equals the mean accuracy of localization (6 mm) (from Salmelin et al., 2000).

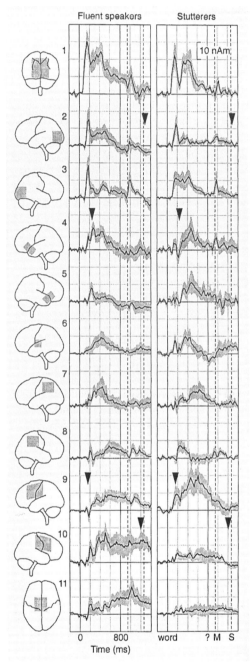

Fig. 12.6. Mean ± standard error of the mean (black curve and shading) source strengths as a function of time in fluent subjects (left) and stutterers (right). The word and question mark onsets are indicated with solid vertical lines and mouth movement (M) and speech (S) onsets with dashed lines. The black arrowheads denote the regions (ROI) and time windows of interest where the responses of stutterers and fluent speakers differed significantly from each other. The studied ROIs are illustrated on the schematic drawings of brains on the left. (From Salmelin et al., 2000.)

It follows that the normal subjects' activity proceeds from the left inferior frontal cortex (articulatory programming) to the lateral part of the left central sulcus and to the dorsolateral premotor cortex (motor preparation) within the first 400 ms after seeing the word. This sequence was reversed in the stutterers who showed an early left motor cortical activation followed by the inferior frontal signal. Stutterers thus appeared to initiate motor programmes before the preparation of the articulatory code. During speech production the right motor area was active in fluent subjects but was silent in stutterers. These findings disclose the nature of such a temporal disorder and demarcate the altered functional connectivity in the respective network, in this case between the left inferior frontal cortex and the right motor/premotor cortex, a circuitry supposed to be relevant for merging linguistic and affective prosody with articulation during fluent speech. This example is meant to illustrate the unique contribution of the MEG to our understanding of the pathophysiology of brain disorders that cannot be accomplished by any other method.

Parallel vs. sequential processing

The combination of relatively high spatial and superb temporal resolution opens new avenues for the study of brain physiology and pathophysiology. For somatosensation it was unclear how the processing of tactile and pain information proceeds in the postcentral primary somatosensory areas, each containing separate body representations for the different submodalities. The comparison of nociceptive as compared to tactile processing showed that the nociceptive sources in the postcentral gyrus were located 10 mm more medially than the early tactile responses arising from area 3b. Whereas tactile stimuli activate sequentially peaking sources in area 3b and 1, nociceptive stimuli activate area 1 indicating that this input does not share the complex hierarchical tactile processing chain (Ploner et al., 2000). MEG data further provided evidence for serial processing from SI to SII and from SI to posterior parietal cortex for tactile input. In contrast nociceptive afferents from the hand are projected to SI and SII in parallel (Ploner et al., 1999). Along these lines the channelling of information processing can be explored for other systems.

MEG in the evaluation of patients with epilepsy

Comparative recordings with MEG and invasive electrical recordings showed excellent agreement for the location of the interictal spike zones and of the spatial relationship of the irritative zone and the structural lesion (Baumgartner et al., 2000a). MEG is also helpful to guide the placement of subdural grid electrodes in patients with non-lesional neocortical epilepsies. For temporal lobe epilepsy (TLE) two types of MEG spike dipoles have been identified: an anterior vertical and an anterior horizontal dipole attributing spike activity to different temporal lobe compartments. This allows differentiation between patients with mesial and lateral temporal seizure onset (Baumgartner et al., 2000b). The disadvantage of the MEG, that it cannot be used for long-term recordings, may be counterbalanced by combined MEG/EEG recordings. The EEG can now even be recorded within the MRI scanner. This allows the use of functional MRI for the localization of EEG identified seizures in patients with focal or partial epilepsy.

The comparison between simultaneous MEG and invasive EEG recordings showed that epileptic foci in mesial temporal structures cannot be detected by MEG if they do not exceed an epileptogenic area of 6–8 cm^2. By contrast, lateral neocortical temporal lobe generators can better be detected. In a prospective study comparing several diagnostic methods (ictal and interictal scalp and intracranial EEG, MRI and MEG) in 58 patients with refractory partial epilepsy the main outcome measure was the efficacy of these methods to identify the resected epileptogenic zone (Simos et al., 2000). MEG (52%) was second only to ictal intracranial EEG in predicting the epileptogenic zone for the entire group of patients who had an excellent surgical outcome. For temporal lobe surgery this relation was MEG 57%, and ictal intracranial EEG 62%. For extratemporal resections ictal (81%) and interictal (75%) intracranial EEG were superior to MEG (44%) in predicting the surgery site in patients with excellent outcome. As compared with video-EEG, MEG was better than ictal (33%) or interictal (45%) scalp VEEG. In another series comprising 53 epilepsy surgery candidates MEG foci were identified in 47 patients in 46 of whom the lesions were resected (20 of the anterior temporal lobe and 26 of the extratemporal lobe cases) (Wheless et al., 1999). Results of this kind implicate that the MEG may obviate the need for invasive EEG in many cases. In cases selected for pediatric epilepsy surgery, the comparison with invasive intracranial EEG showed that both methods colocalized the epileptogenic focus (Minassian et al., 1999).

MEG for presurgical mapping

MEG can also be used for presurgical mapping in tumour cases in order to delineate eloquent areas (Ganslandt et al.,

1999). Comparative studies based on MEG/MRI comparisons indicate that both methods are suitable for mapping eloquent cortex in relation to tumour-invaded tissue. As a general result activations are almost exclusively seen outside the tumour invaded area (Wunderlich et al., 1998). Reliable mapping of the functionally active zone is particularly useful in the many cases with considerable displacement distorting the regional anatomy. Presurgical mapping is usually performed for the sensorimotor strip but also for the language areas. When comparing language lateralization by word-matching tasks or other language paradigms in the MEG the results are similar to those obtained to the Wada test (Simos et al., 2000).

The data on presurgical mapping are also of interest for the assessment of tumour induced plasticity following tumour resection. The rearrangement of the displaced activations can be monitored and the changes in functional maps related to functional recovery. Cortical plasticity may be associated with functional improvement but may also be maladaptive. An example for the latter case are the extensive changes in somatosensory cortical maps following amputation or somatosensory deafferentation. It has been shown (Flor et al., 1995) that the amount of cortical alteration and the magnitude of a phantom pain in amputees reveal a positive relationship ($r = 0.93$). But there was no correlation between non-painful phantom phenomena and the amount of cortical reorganization. This, and related data, indicate that phantom limb pain goes along with plastic changes in primary somatosensory cortex and its afferent stages.

Combination of electromagnetic and hemodynamic measures

The idea behind this approach is to relate the areas of functionally relevant brain activations, as identified by regional blood flow changes, to the time course of associated neural processes, as reflected by successive ERP or MF components. For a linear sequence of discrete cognitive events, for example, one would expect a corresponding sequence of electric or magnetic components mapped onto a distinct pattern of hemodynamic brain activations. However, our experiences suggest that these relationships are highly complex and usually do not allow for simple solutions. In this respect, an important question is whether and to what extent it is reasonable to assume that electromagnetic and hemodynamic parameters are related, given that ERP and MF components reflect postsynaptic activity and blood flow change might occur seconds after the electromagnetic events. Evidently, electrophysiological and hemodynamic

indices of cortical activation do not necessarily match. For instance, cognitive ERP components in the later time range may reflect the integrated activity of multiple and broadly distributed sources and, therefore, are difficult to relate to few circumscribed hemodynamic sources as revealed by standard statistical mapping neuroimaging procedures. Therefore, some neural processes may be hidden in these results because the corresponding data just do not reach significance due to a poor signal-to-noise ratio or because of a too rigid significance thresholding. On the other hand, an activated area identified by hemodynamic measurements may generate electromagnetic signals that cannot be recorded at scalp locations because the fields cancel locally due to the cortical geometry. Together, the combined imaging approach does not aim for a complete integration of different physiological parameters; rather, the goal is to obtain complementary information about different aspects of the same neural process.

An important step towards a combined analysis of neural functions implies a physiologically, anatomically and mathematically profound approach to the so-called inverse problem. This term denotes the estimation of the intracranial sources of electromagnetic activity sampled at various scalp locations given the fact that a scalp recorded pattern of electromagnetic parameters does not have a unique intracranial solution. At present, most studies apply the so-called equivalent dipole model or the distributed cortical surface model. The dipole model simulates the neuroelectric activity as generated by a single point source with a certain location, an orientation and an amplitude, as can be assumed for a relatively small activated cortical region. The distributed source approach is suitable for the estimation of more widely spread activity sources. It assumes a multitude of dipoles distributed over the brain. For an improved solution, they may be constrained by restricting their location to the MR-based cortical surface and their orientation perpendicular to it; with the location and orientation of the dipoles fixed, only their strength needed to be solved. As a result, the solution resembles a distributed electrical solution of the cortical surface.

The source estimation provided by these different algorithms is only a first step in the combination of electromagnetic and hemodynamic parameters. Consider an experiment in which parallel recording of ERPs and fMRI in the same subject under the same experimental conditions has identified a number of electromagnetic sources and MR signal changes related to a particular performance. What kind of evidence substantiates the assumption that these different parameters reflect the same or different neural processes? There are different approaches to answer this question. One is called the 'seeded forward solution' (Heinze et al., 1994). This solution implies that the equivalent dipoles of electromagnetic activity are placed within the anatomical areas defined by MR signal change to test whether these dipoles could have generated the electrical patterns that were recorded from the scalp. If this is the case, the next step is to show that other possible locations of these dipoles provide a worse or at least not significantly better (in terms of goodness of fit) solution than the seeded dipole fit. Another approach is to test the covariation of MR and electrical signals when the task changes. The logic is that if both signals reflect the same cognitive event, one would expect a covariation over task manipulations. New developments in combined neuroimaging incorporate statistical approaches for estimating the most probable numbers, locations, orientations and strength of active cortical regions.

To illustrate such a comparative approach and the advantage of MEF measurements over EEG data a combined EEG, MEG and fMRI study assessing the neural indices of word fragment completion can be used. Seven subjects completed four-letter fragments to German words whose length varied between 7 and 9 letters and indicated the time point of completion with a right hand, index-finger button press. EEG and MF data were analysed response locked to the motor response that indicated completion. With both EEG and MF, response-locked waveforms deviated from zero starting at approximately 500 ms before the motor response. The current density solution of this 500 ms time window was derived using the MF data, and for comparison also using the EEG data alone. Both types of solutions were compared to the fMRI measurements (different subjects) obtained during the same task. In accord with the fMRI findings, the combined EEG and MF current density analyses revealed a left frontal and two bilateral temporal sources of activity (Fig. 12.7, see colour plate section). In contrast, current density performed with EEG data alone, misallocated the bilateral parietal sources to a single, widely distributed source located over the convexity of the parieto-central scalp. Both types of source analyses, however, correctly revealed activity in the left motor cortex starting from 20 ms prior to the motor response. These data provide fMRI supported evidence that source analysis based on EEG data alone can provide wrong solutions in the case of more complex, bilateral neural activity, and the MEG data can help to substantially improve the spatial resolution in these cases.

The study of cortical rhythms

EEG/MEG studies have provided evidence that the mixed frequency content of the human brain oscillations can be fractionated into several region specific intrinsic rhythms. The functional significance of these rhythms is still unclear, but there is increasing evidence that some of them respond to peripheral sensory or motor events. This can be shown by calculating the event related modulation in the spectral power of these cortical rhythms (Hari & Salmelin, 1997; Pfurtscheller & Aranibar, 1979).

Sources around the parieto-occipital sulcus generate the well known α-rhythm. They show dampening of the α-rhythm within 200 ms after the presentation of visual stimuli and also during visual imagery. The Rolandic Mu-rhythm consists of 10 and 20 Hz components with different source locations. The 10 Hz component is supposed to be somatosensory in origin, whereas the 20 Hz signal originates mainly from motor cortex (Hari & Salmelin, 1997) with clearly detectable somatotopy of the oscillatory sources. These components are suppressed by either somatosensory input or movement. The human auditory cortex shows spontaneous oscillations around 10 Hz (tau rhythm) that is transiently suppressed during auditory input (Lehtala et al., 1997). Oscillatory responses in the γ-band (25–50 Hz) also showed differences in relation to the perception of auditory stimuli.

The spatial analysis of these rhythms and their interdependence is of considerable significance for a better understanding of the pathophysiology of cortico-cortical and cortico-thalamic interaction, but also for cortico-muscular coupling. Llinas and coworkers (1999) have recently proposed that patients with neurogenic pain, Parkinson's disease or depression show increased low frequency theta rhythmicities associated with a pronounced increase in coherence between high and low frequency oscillations. This was supposed to indicate thalamo-cortical dysrhythmia as a common principle underlying the abnormal coherence in the theta range.

New approaches for the study of coherence

The understanding of the synchronization of neuronal firing within and across areas is pivotal for the understanding of brain function and dysfunction. Coherence between signals of sensors or electrodes covering different scalp areas is usually taken as a measure of functional coupling. This approach was hitherto limited by methodical constraints. A new method, dynamic imaging of coherent sources (DICS), has been introduced by Gross et al., (2001). Since MEG and EMG signals are non-stationary, this new tool has been implemented for the detection of phase synchronization in non-stationary noisy data (Tass et al., 1998). In contrast to classical coherence, this method allows the separation of amplitude and phase information by means of the Hilbert transform. DICS allows different approaches to the study of coherence. One is to identify a cortical area showing the strongest coherence with a peripheral signal and to take this as a reference for calculating cortico-cortical coherences. Another strategy is to calculate coherences between all sensor pairs and then select the strongest coherence between non-adjacent sensors. Finally a *priori* information can be used to define a reference region based on knowledge of anatomical structures or pathways or results from other functional imaging studies.

The examination of cortico-muscular coherence during static isometric muscle contraction and simultaneous electromyographic and MEG recordings revealed significant coherence in the 15–33 Hz frequency range (Conway et al., 1995; Salenius et al., 1997). This corresponds to the 20–30 Hz coherence between local field potentials in primary motor cortex and rectified EMG from the contralateral hand and forearm muscles in monkey (Baker et al., 2000). The coupling of central oscillatory activity to peripheral muscle activity is apparent in the MEG signal averaged to the onset of motor unit potentials (Fig. 12.8(*a*)) and in the coherence (Fig. 12.8(*b*)) between rectified EMG signal and the neural activity of the contralateral primary motor cortex (Fig. 12.8(*c*)). The delays between the oscillatory motor cortical and EMG signals computed from their phase difference provide information about conduction times. Figure 12.9 shows the close agreement with the conduction times as determined by transcranial magnetic stimulation.

For the clinic this method opens new applications. One is the measurement of conduction times and conduction velocities in normal conditions and demyelinating disorders. Another possibility is the detection of abnormal synchronization. This is not only at issue for hypersynchronized states such as tremor, myoclonus or epilepsy but also for disclosing abnormal interareal coupling or changes due to afferent pathology. The latter has recently been demonstrated in cases with pseudo-chorea-athetosis, a condition characterized by continuous involuntary finger movements following partial or complete deafferentation. Whereas the coherence during isometric muscle contraction was normal, the involuntary finger movements during rest exhibited an abnormally strong 12 Hz coherence between motor cortex and EMG reflecting a disinhibition of rhythmic cortical output. This coherence was not seen during voluntary finger movements (Timmermann et al., 2001).

A major difference between MEG and fMRI lies in the detection of dynamic and static behavioural states. fMRI is well suited to detect dynamic changes of behaviour. When examining the relationship between the fMRI signal during a static finger flexion task and dynamic finger flexions no or inconsistent small fMRI responses were recorded during the static task (Thickbroom et al., 1999). In contrast, the MEG is well suited to continuously record cortico-muscular or cortico-cortical coherences during static muscle contractions or behavioural states (Gross et al., 2000).

Microelectrode recordings

Microelectrode recordings can specify pathophysiology at a finer grain than macropotentials. They can reveal changes characteristic for certain disorders such as altered neuronal discharge patterns and rates or abnormal synchronization as they occur in movement disorders. Although such recordings have been employed for the study of cortical functions, the major field for microelectrode studies in the human brain is functional target localization during stereotactic surgery for the treatment of Parkinson's disease (STN), tremor (thalamus) and dystonia (thalamus, GPi). One major issue is the determination of the borders of the target nuclei and of the somatotopy therein, thus improving the precision of electrode placement. Beside somatotopy the discharge behaviour, firing pattern and rate, are characteristic for different basal ganglia compartments along the trajectory to the target as illustrated in Fig. 12.10. The adequate interpretation of these discharge patterns rests on comparisons with data recorded from non-human primates because normal data cannot be obtained from human subjects.

Recordings in Parkinson's disease

Gold-standard for our understanding of the pathophysiology of Parkinson's disease is the comparison with its animal model, the MPTP monkey where recordings in the basal ganglia show typical changes in discharge rates and pattern. Intraoperative microelectrode recordings in Parkinsonian patients show similar abnormalities. Spontaneous discharge rates in the STN that normally lie around 40 Hz are increased in Parkinson's disease and decreased in Huntington's chorea (Fig. 12.11). The increased firing rates of the excitatory glutamatergic STN neurons elicit increased firing rates in the inhibitory GABA-ergic output neurons of the GPi resulting in strong inhibition of their thalamic or brainstem target neurons. This inhibition is thought to arrest the ongoing motor activity in the thalamo-cortical loops involved in the regulation of motor behaviour. In contrast, intraoperative micro-

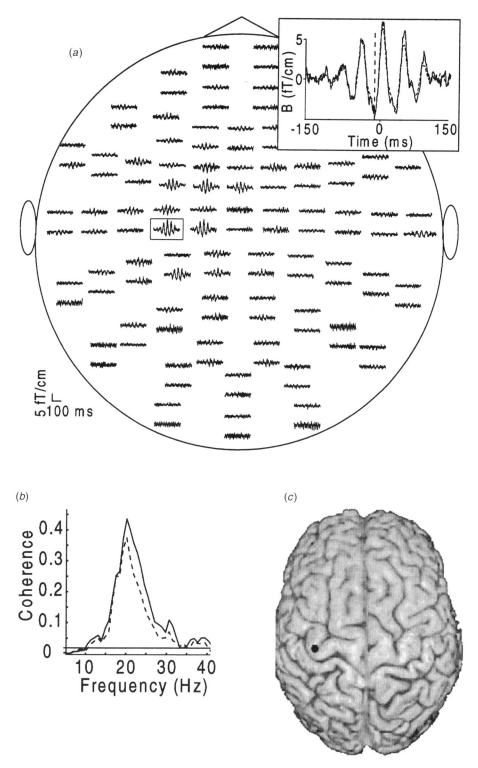

Fig. 12.8. (*a*) Unfiltered averaged MEG signals timelocked to onsets of the motor unit potentials (phase-triggered average). The dashed vertical line at −15 ms in the inset marks the minimum in the signal and the dashed trace shows the part of the signal that is accounted for by the dipole. (*b*) Coherence as function of frequency between EMG and M1 (solid line) and between EMG and the MEG signal with the highest coherence (dotted line). (*c*) The dipole superimposed on the subject's brain. (From Gross et al., 2000.)

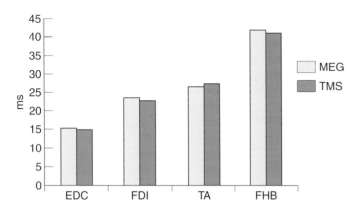

Fig. 12.9. Latencies calculated from cortico-muscular phase differences between MEG sources and EMG of the respective muscle (left column). The right column denotes the cortico-muscular conduction times determined by transcranial magnetic stimulation. (From Rothwell et al., 1991.)

electrode recordings from the GPi in dystonic patients revealed abnormally low spontaneous discharge rates of the pallidal neurons along with changes in the discharge characteristics from tonic to phasic discharge patterns (Lenz et al., 1999). The lower than normal firing rates in the GPi imply decreased inhibition of thalamic throughput to motor and premotor cortex.

The identification of the actual changes in firing rates and patterns along with the determination of increased synchronization between neurons, which is now possible with the use of multielectrodes, is of prime importance for disclosing the relevant aspects of the pathophysiology of the disease. They further provide the basis for a better understanding of the effects of deep brain stimulation (DBS) on these disordered neuronal states. DBS is assumed to act by desynchronizing and decreasing abnormal discharge rates thus counteracting the pathological discharge characteristics resulting from dopamine depletion.

What is presently unknown is the impact of DBS on neuronal discharge behaviour as it relates to the processing of motor but also limbic or complex loop information. Investigating the functional anatomy of these different basal ganglia loops in the monkey has shown that these segregated channels are funnelled through the basal ganglia via distinct microcircuitries. Accordingly, recordings in the human GPi or STN revealed that only a relatively small proportion of the neurons are motor related. Alterations in the discharge characteristics of the limbic and complex loop neurons will provide a more comprehensive picture of these complex relationships and hopefully allow a better understanding of the non-motor aspects of basal ganglia disorders.

Thalamic recordings

The thalamus is a major target for the treatment of tremor, but also for dystonia and pain (Hua et al., 2000). Thalamic recordings mainly in Vim show tremor related rhythmic burst activities possibly representing the neural drive for the motor network generating rhythmic motor output (Magnin et al., 2000). The thalamic oscillations are in part generated by the electrical properties of the neurons with the slow oscillatory tendency that is reinforced by the re-entry properties of the network connecting cortex and thalamus. Thalamic cells are barely activated by voluntary movements.

Recordings in the ventral caudal thalamus in dystonic patients showed large scale modifications of sensory maps with increased receptive fields of the somatosensory afferents showing extensive overlap and distortions of the somatotopic map (Hua et al., 2000). These changes are similar to those described in a monkey model where dystonia-like movements were induced by overuse of certain repetitive hand movements. Representations of the hand surface showed distinct remodelling in S1 with cutaneous receptive field extending across multiple digits and the whole hand, a somatotopic reorganization grossly different from the normal small distinct topographically ordered distribution (Byl et al., 1997). These alterations in thalamic somatotopic maps are particularly interesting with respect to receptive field enlargements in patients with amputations who show increases in the thalamic area from which stimulation evokes sensations in the stump area.

In conclusion, the microelectrode recordings are not only useful tools for improving the remaining inaccuracy of anatomical targeting but they provide new insights in the characteristic pathophysiological features. This information can solely be obtained by microphysiological exploration. For these reasons microphysiological recordings that are increasingly employed are relevant for new applications of DBS for the treatment of other disorders such as dystonia, bulimia and epilepsy.

Cortical recordings

Microelectrode recordings from the right and left superior, middle and inferior temporal gyri in conscious humans during open brain surgery for the treatment of epilepsy showed no significant differences between the right and left hemisphere with respect to neuronal responses to words and sentences (Creutzfeld et al., 1989a). All neurones in the superior temporal gyrus (STG) of both sides responded to various aspects of spoken language either by

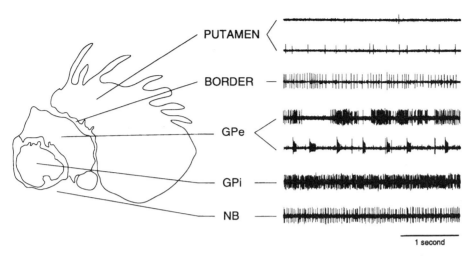

Fig. 12.10. Different patterns of neural activity encountered in the basal ganglia during a single penetration with the microelectrode. GPe: globus pallidus pars externa, GPi: globus pallidus pars interna, NB: nucleus basalis. (From Vitek et al., 1997.)

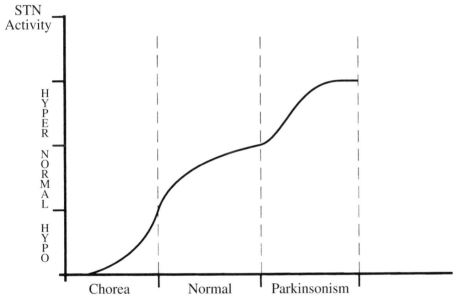

Fig. 12.11. Schematic explanation of how differences in the activity of the subthalamic nucleus (STN) modify the threshold for the appearance of chorea/ballism. In the parkinsonian state, STN activity is greatly augmented so that its lesion reduces basal ganglia output towards normal levels without necessarily reaching the threshold for dyskinesias. The normal state has a relatively wide range. Thus, a small focal lesion of the STN may not induce ballism. However, a large lesion will always be associated with ballism because it reduces the activity to well below the dyskinesia threshold. (From Guridi & Obeso, 1997.)

activation or inhibition without obvious changes in firing pattern or rate in response to non-linguistic acoustic input. Most neurones in the middle and inferior temporal gyri showed only minor modifications by listening to words or sentences.

Neuronal activity in response to the subject's own voice during overt naming or reading words or short sentences was also equally modified in the temporal lobes on both sides. Again, neurons in the STG responded clearly and in a characteristic manner (Creutzfeld et al., 1989b). These data demonstrate symmetrical language-related neuronal activity in both hemispheres of the adult brain. This opens new perspectives for discussing concepts on asymmetries as known from clinical evidence and neuroimaging. The recordings are of particular interest with respect to the capacity of the minor hemisphere to take over language functions, as exemplified in children after left-sided hemispherectomies (Vargha-Khadem et al., 1997a).

In conclusion MEG and MEG/EEG combinations can identify event-related changes thus complementing fMRI and PET on a finer timescale. New developments overcame some previous limitations and now allow for reliable spatial localizations of multiple independent coherent sources. These maps can be compared with those established by fMRI and superimpose the fourth dimension of functional imaging, the high temporal resolution. For clinical neurology, MEG is a robust method for presurgical mapping, for the detection of epileptic foci and for the monitoring of postlesional plasticity. The examination of brain rhythms and coherences opens new inroads into the study of cortico-cortical and cortico-muscular coupling along with the determination of the respective conduction times. In contrast to the neurovascular methods they also provide information about this relationship in steady state conditions. Microelectrode recordings can assess regional pathophysiology in a unique way and help to understand how disturbed functions emerge and may be corrected.

References   * denotes key references

Baker, S.N., Olivier, E. & Lemon, R.N. (2000). Coherent oscillations in monkey motor cortex and hand muscle EMG show task-dependent modulation. *J. Physiol.*, **501**, 225–41.

Baumgartner, C., Pataraia, E., Lindinger, G. & Deecke, L. (2000a). Magnetoencephalography in focal epilepsy. *Epilepsia*, **41**, 39–47.

Baumgartner, C., Pataraia, E., Lindinger, G. & Deecke, L. (2000b). Neuromagnetic recordings in temporal lobe epilepsy. *J. Clin. Neurophysiol.*, **17**, 177–89.

Byl, N.N., Merzenich, M.M., Cheung, S., Bedenbaugh, P., Nagarajian, S.S. & Jenkins, W.M. (1997). A primate genesis model of focal dystonia and repetitive strain injury: II. The effect of movement strategy on the de-differentiation of the hand representation in the primary somatosensory cortex of owl monkeys. *Soc. Neurosci. Abstr.*, **22**, 1055.

Conway, B.A., Halliday, D.M., Farmer, S.F. et al. (1995). Synchronization between motor cortex and spinal motoneuronal pool during the performance of a maintained motor task in man. *J. Physiol.*, **489**, 917–24.

Creutzfeld, O., Ojemann, G. & Lettich, E. (1989a). Neuronal activity in the human lateral temporal lobe. I. Responses to speech. *Exp. Brain Res.*, **77**, 451–75.

Creutzfeld, O., Ojemann, G. & Lettich, E. (1989b). Neuronal activity in the human lateral temporal lobe. II. Responses to the subjects own voice. *Exp. Brain Res.*, **77**, 476–89.

Duzel, E., Kaufmann, J., Kanowski, M., Tempelman, C. & Heinze, H.J. (2000). Effects of unilateral hippocampal pathology on brain activity during episodic retrieval. A combined H-Spectroscopy, diffusion weighted imaging and MEG/EEG study in patients with temporal lobe epilepsy. Abstract, Cognitive Neuroscience Meeting, San Francisco.

Flor, H., Elbert, T., Knecht, S. et al. (1995). Phantom-limb pain as a perceptual correlate of cortical reorganization following arm amputation. *Nature*, **375**, 482–4.

Ganslandt, O., Fahlbusch, R., Nimsky, C. et al. (1999). Functional neuronavigation with magnetoencephalography: outcome in 50 patients with lesions around the motor cortex. *J. Neurosurg.*, **91**, 73–9.

Gross, J., Tass, P., Salenius, S., Hari, R., Freund, H-J. & Schnitzler, A. (2000). Cortico-muscular synchronization during isometric muscle contraction in humans as revealed by magnetoencephalography. *J. Physiol.*, **527**, 623–31.

*Gross, J., Kujala, J., Hämäläinen, M., Timmermann, L., Schnitzler, A. & Salmelin, R. (2001). Dynamic imaging of coherent sources: studying neural interactions in the human brain. *Proc. Nat. Acad. Sci., USA*, **98**, 694–99.

Guridi, J. & Obeso, J.A. (1997). The role of the subthalamic nucleus in the origin of hemiballism and parkinsonism: new surgical perspectives. In *Advances in Neurology*, Vol. 74, ed. J.A. Obeso, M.R. DeLong, C. Ohye & C.D. Marsden, pp. 183–98. Philadelphia: Lippincott-Raven Publishers.

*Hari, R. & Salmelin, R. (1997). Human cortical oscillations: a neuromagnetic view through the skull. *Trends Neurosci.*, **20**, 44–9.

*Heinze, H.J., Mangun, G.R., Burchert, W. et al. (1994). Combined spatial and temporal imaging of brain activity during visual selective attention in humans. *Nature*, **372**, 543–6.

*Hopf, J.-M., Luck, S.J., Girelli, M. et al. (2000). Neural sources of focused attention in visual search. *Cereb. Cortex*, **10**, 1233–41.

Hua, S.E., Garonzik, I.M., Lee, J.I. & Lenz, F.A. (2000). Microelectrode studies of normal organization and plasticity of human somatosensory thalamus. *J. Clin. Neurophysiol.*, **17**, 559–74.

Knowlton, B.J. & Squire, L.R. (1995). Remembering and knowing: two different expressions of declarative memory. *J. Exp. Psychol. Learn. Mem. Cogn.*, **21**, 699–710.

Lehtela, L., Salmelin, R. & Hari, R. (1997). Evidence for reactive magnetic 10 Hz rhythm in the human auditory cortex. *Neurosci. Lett.*, **222**, 111–14.

*Lenz, F.A., Seike, M.S., Jaeger, C.J. et al. (1999). Thalamic single neuron activity in patients with dystonia: dystonia-related activity and somatic sensory reorganization. *J. Neurophysiol.*, **82**, 2372–92.

Llinás, R.R., Ribary, U., Jeanmonod, D., Kronberg, E. & Mitra, P.P. (1999). Thalamocortical dysrhythmia: A neurological and neuropsychiatric syndrome characterized by magnetoencephalography. *Proc. Natl. Acad. Sci., USA*, **96**, 15222–7.

Luck, S.J. & Hillyard, S.A. (1994). Electrophysiological correlates of feature analysis during visual search. *Psychophysiology*, **31**.

*Luck, S.J., Girelli, M., McDermott, M.T. & Ford, M.A. (1997).

Bridging the gap between monkey neurophysiology and human perception: an ambiguity resolution theory of visual selective attention. *Cogn. Psychol.*, **33**, 64–87.

Magnin, M., Morel, A. & Jeanmonod, D. (2000). Single-unit analysis of the pallidum, thalamus and subthalamic nucleus in parkinsonian patients. *Neuroscience*, **96**, 549–64.

Minassian, B.A., Otsubo, H., Weiss, S., Elliott, I., Rutka, J.T. & Snead, O.C. (1999). Magnetoencephalographic localization in pediatric epilepsy surgery: comparison with invasive intracranial electroencephalography. *Ann. Neurol.*, **46**, 627–33.

Murray, E.A. & Mishkin, M. (1998). Object recognition and location memory in monkeys with excitotoxic lesions of the amygdala and hippocampus, *J. Neurosci.*, **18**, 6568–82.

Nishitani, N., Ikeda, A., Nagamine, T. et al. (1999). The role of the hippocampus in auditory processing studied by event-related electric potentials and magnetic fields in epilepsy patients before and after temporal lobectomy. *Brain*, **122**, 687–707.

Okada, Y. (1982). Neurogenesis of evoked magnetic fields. In *Biomagnetism: An Interdisciplinary Approach*, ed. S.J. Williamson, G.L. Romani, L. Kaufman & I. Modena, pp. 399–408. New York and London: Plenum Press.

Okada, Y.C., Wu, J. & Kyuhou, S. (1997). Genesis of MEG signals in a mammalian CNS structure. *J. Electroencephalogr. Clin. Neurophysiol.*, **103**, 474–85.

Olichney, J.M., Van Petten, C., Paller, K.A. et al. (2000). Word repetition in amnesia. Electrophysiological measures of impaired and spared memory. *Brain*, **123**, 1948–63.

Paller, K.A., Kutas, M. & McIsaac, H.K. (1995). Monitoring conscious recollection via the electrical activity of the brain. *Psychol. Sci.*, **6**, 107–111.

*Pfurtscheller, G. & Aranibar, A. (1979). Evaluation of event-related desynchronization (ERD) preceding and following voluntary self-paced movement. *J. Electroencephalogr. Clin. Neurophysiol.*, **46**, 138–46.

Ploner, M., Schmitz, F., Freund, H-J. & Schnitzler, A. (1999). Parallel activation of primary and secondary somatosensory cortices in human pain processing. *J. Neurophysiol.*, **81**, 3100–4.

Ploner, M., Schmitz, F., Freund, H-J. & Schnitzler, A. (2000). Differential organisation of touch and pain in human primary somatosensory cortex. *J. Neurophysiol.*, **83**, 1770–6.

Reynolds, J.H., Chelazzi, L. & Desimone, R. (1999). Competititve mechanisms subserve attention in macaque areas V2 and V4. *J. Neurosci.*, **19**, 1736–53.

Rothwell, J.C., Thompson, P.D., Day, B.L., Boyd, S. & Marsden, C.D. (1991). Stimulation of the human motor cortex through the scalp. *Exp. Physiol.*, **76**, 159–200.

*Rugg, M.D., Mark, R.E., Walla, P., Schloerscheidt, A.M., Birch, C.S. & Allan, K. (1998). Dissociation of the neural correlates of implicit and explicit memory. *Nature*, **392**, 595–8.

Salenius, S., Portin, K., Kajola, M., Salmelin, R. & Hari, R. (1997). Cortical control of human motoneuron firing during isometric contraction. *Neurophysiology*, **77**, 3401–5

Salmelin, R., Hämäläinen, M., Kajola, M. & Hari, R. (1995). Functional segregation of movement-related rhythmic activity in the human brain. *Neuroimage*, **2**, 237–43.

Salmelin, R., Schnitzler, A., Schmitz, F. & Freund, H-J. (2000). Single word reading in developmental stutterers and fluent speakers. *Brain*, **123**, 1184–202.

Simos, P.G., Papanicolaou, A.C., Breier, J.I. et al. (2000). Insights into brain functional and neural plasticity using magnetic source imaging. *J. Clin. Neurophysiol.*, **17**, 143–62.

*Tass, P., Rosenblum, M.G., Weule, J. et al. (1998). Detection of n: m phase locking from noisy data: Application to magnetoencephalography. *Phys. Rev. Lett. Rev.*, **81**, 3291–4.

Tesche, C.D. & Karhu, J. (1999). Interactive processing of sensory input and motor output in the human hippocampus. *J. Cogn. Neurosci.*, **11**, 424–36.

Tesche, C.D., Krusin-Elbaum, L. & Knowles, W.D. (1988). Simultaneous measurement of magnetic and electric responses of in vitro hippocampal slices. *Brain Res.* **462**, 190–3.

Tesche, C.D., Karhu, J. & Tissari, S.O. (1996). Non-invasive detection of neuronal population activity in human hippocampus. *Brain Res. Cogn. Brain Res.*, **4**, 39–47.

Thickbroom, G.W., Phillips, B.A., Morris, I., Byrnes, M.L., Sacco, P. & Mastaglia, F.L. (1999). Differences in functional magnetic resonance imaging of sensorimotor cortex during static and dynamic finger flexion. *Exp. Brain Res.*, **126**, 431–8.

Timmermann, L., Gross, J., Schmitz, F., Freund, H-J. & Schnitzler, A. (2001). Pathologically enhanced corticomuscular coupling in pseudochoreoathetosis. *Movement Disorders*, **16**(5), 876–81.

Tulving, E. (1985). Memory and consciousness. *Canad. Psychol.*, **26**, 1–12.

Vargha-Khadem, F., Carr, L. J., Isaacs, E., Brett, E., Adams, C. & Mishkin, M. (1997a). Onset of speech after left hemispherectomy in a nine-year-old boy. *Brain*, **120**, 159–82.

Vargha-Khadem, F., Gadian, D.G., Watkins, K.E., Connelly, A., Van Paesschen, W. & Mishkin, M. (1997b). Differential effects of early hippocampal pathology on episodic and semantic memory, *Science*, **277**, 376–80.

Vitek, J.L., Bakay, R.A.E. & DeLong, M.R. (1997). Microelectrode-guided pallidotomy for medically intractable Parkinson's disease. In *Advances in Neurology*, Vol. 74, ed. J.A. Obeso, M.R. DeLong, C. Ohye & C.D. Marsden, pp. 183–98. Philadelphia: Lippincott-Raven Publishers.

Wheless, J.W., Willmore, L.J., Breier, J.I. et al. (1999). A comparison of magnetoencephalography, MRI, and V-EEG in patients evaluated for epilepsy surgery. *Epilepsia*, **???**, 931–41.

Williamsen, S.J. & Kaufman, L. (1987). Analysis of neuromagnetic signals. In *Methods of Analysis of Brain and Magnetic Signals*, ed. A.S. Gevins & A. Remond, pp. 405–48. BV: Elsevier Science Publishers.

Wu, J. & Okada, Y.C. (1998). Physiological bases of the synchronized population spikes and slow wave of the magnetic field generated by a guinea-pig longitudinal CA3 slice preparation. *J. Electroencephalogr. Clin. Neurophysiol.*, **107**, 361–73.

Wunderlich, G., Knorr, U., Herzog, H., Kiwit, J.C., Freund, H-J. & Seitz, R.J. (1998). Precentral glioma location determines the displacement of cortical hand representation. *J. Neurosurg.*, **42**, 18–26.

Part II

Disorders of higher functions

13

Congenital disorders of cerebral cortical development

Ganeshwaran H. Mochida[1,2,3] and Christopher A. Walsh[1,3]

[1] Department of Neurology, Beth Israel Deaconess Medical Center, Boston, MA, USA
[2] Pediatric Neurology Unit, Department of Neurology, Massachusetts General Hospital, USA
[3] Harvard Medical School, Boston, MA, USA

Developmental malformations of the cerebral cortex represent a heterogeneous group of disorders that are individually rare, but that collectively account for a large number of cases of epilepsy, mental retardation and other cognitive disorders. Though many of the disorders discussed in this chapter have been known for decades, our view of them has been revolutionized in recent years. Two recent major advances facilitated our understanding of these disorders. First is the use of non-invasive brain imaging techniques, particularly MRI, in clinical neurological practice (Osborn et al., 1988). This has enabled accurate diagnosis of disorders of cortical development, which had only been diagnosed by post mortem examinations in the past. Improved imaging techniques have also led to the recognition of new clinical entities and the recognition of mendelian inheritance of many cortical malformations. Second are the advances in molecular genetics, which have allowed identification of genes responsible for inherited diseases using methods of positional cloning (Walsh, 1999). Identification of genes responsible for cortical malformations has led to molecular diagnosis in many cases. Furthermore, genes identified as responsible for human disorders have provided us with important clues to understand the mechanisms of normal brain development.

With these advances in our knowledge, the traditional classification scheme of cortical malformations, which is solely based on morphological abnormalities, has been reassessed. Several attempts have recently been made to classify the disorders of cortical development, reflecting new insights into their pathogenesis. A classification based on the time that the derangement is presumed to have occurred has been proposed (van der Knaap & Valk, 1988). Another classification system devised by Barkovich et al., (1996) is based on a combination of embryology, genetics, imaging and pathology. Because our understanding of these disorders is still incomplete, any classification is somewhat provisional. In this chapter, the disorders are categorized according mainly to the disturbed developmental process. As our knowledge about their pathogenesis evolves, the classification systems will inevitably be modified and refined.

Normal development of the cerebral cortex

The neurons of the cerebral cortex are formed in the ventricular zone, which consists of a specialized proliferative region along the wall of the lateral ventricles. The postmitotic neurons then leave the ventricular zone and migrate over considerable distances to reach the cortex. The first postmitotic neurons to leave the ventricular zone form a pioneer layer called the primordial plexiform layer (Marín-Padilla, 1971). This layer is later split into an outer marginal zone and a deeper subplate layer by later arriving neurons, which form the cortical plate. The cortical plate subsequently increases its thickness as it is populated by arriving neurons. Neurons are added to the cortical plate in an 'inside-out' fashion so that newly arriving neurons always migrate past older cortical plate neurons until they arrest immediately underneath the marginal zone. Consequently, the deeper cortical layers contain neurons born earlier in gestation, while more superficial cortical layers contain neurons born later in gestation (Fig. 13.1). In the marginal zone, Cajal–Retzius cells secrete a large extracellular protein, Reelin, which appears to act as a 'stop signal' for migrating neurons (Dulabon et al., 2000). The long-range migration of cortical neurons is guided by long, radially aligned glial cells, termed radial glial cells (Rakic, 1971, 1972). These cells extend from the ventricular zone to the pial surface, and serve as a 'scaffold' for the migrating neurons (see Fig. 13.1, in colour plate section).

Recently, it became clear that a large fraction of cortical neurons, particularly inhibitory interneurons, actually originate outside of the cortex itself (Anderson et al., 1997; Tamamaki et al., 1997; Lavdas et al., 1999). These neurons are generated in the ganglionic eminence, which gives rise to the basal ganglia, and then migrate into the developing cortex moving tangentially. This mode of migration is called 'tangential' migration in contrast to the classic 'radial' migration (Walsh & Cepko, 1992). Tangentially migrating neurons do not appear to be guided by radial glial fibres in their course from the ganglionic eminence to the cortex.

In human cortex, postmitotic neurons start to migrate out of the ventricular zone into the primordial plexiform layer between the sixth and seventh fetal week (Marín-Padilla, 1983). Initial formation of the cortical plate occurs from the seventh to tenth fetal week (Sidman & Rakic, 1973; Marín-Padilla, 1983). Migration of neurons into the cortical plate appears to peak between the eleventh and fifteenth week of gestation (Sidman & Rakic, 1973). A majority of neurons have entered the cortical plate by around the twenty-fourth week of gestation (Marín-Padilla, 1990), although it is not clear when migration is finally completed. Distal processes of the radial glia disappear between the fifth and seventh month of gestation (Marín-Padilla, 1970), suggesting that little or no glia-guided migration occurs after this stage. With this general background we will briefly review the major developmental disorders in the rough sequence in which they disrupt patterning, proliferation, specification, and later stages of cortical neuronal development.

Disorders of pattern formation in the forebrain

Holoprosencephaly

The left and right cerebral hemispheres derive from the prosencephalon, which represents the rostral end of the neural tube. Holoprosencephaly (HPE) is a malformation characterized by failure of the normal cleavage of the prosencephalon to form two cerebral hemispheres. HPE shows a wide spectrum of severity, and clinically is categorized into three subgroups, namely, alobar, semilobar and lobar types. Alobar HPE refers to cases with complete or almost complete lack of cleavage. A single ventricle in the midline is seen in these cases. In semilobar HPE, there is often cleavage in the posterior aspect of the hemispheres, but the anterior portion lacks a separation. Lobar HPE shows formation of an interhemispheric fissure in both posterior and anterior aspects, and only a mild degree of incomplete separation is seen. The prevalence of HPE has been estimated to be 5–12/100 000 live births (Croen et al.,

1996; Rasmussen et al., 1996; Olsen et al., 1997), but this may underestimate the true incidence, as milder cases are increasingly recognized. Also, in one large series, HPE was found in 0.4 % of embryos (Matsunaga & Shiota, 1977).

The clinical manifestations of HPE cover a wide spectrum, reflecting the wide range of structural abnormalities. Microcephaly is the rule. Dysfunction of the hypothalamic–pituitary axis, including diabetes inspidus and growth hormone deficiency, can be seen. Children with alobar HPE have profound developmental delay, but even these children can often acquire new skills and interact with the environment, albeit slowly and in limited fashion (Barr & Cohen, 1999). Associated facial anomalies also vary widely. Alobar HPE can be accompanied by cyclopia, ethmocephaly (ocular hypotelorism with proboscis, which is a rudimentary nose-like structure), cebocephaly (ocular hypotelorism and a blind-ended, single-nostril nose) or a median cleft lip. In contrast, semilobar HPE or lobar HPE are often accompanied by milder facial phenotypes, including ocular hypotelorism, hypertelorism, a unilateral or bilateral cleft lip, or a single midline incisor (Cohen, 1989).

The etiology of HPE is complex, and both genetic and environmental factors seem to play a role. Approximately 20–40% of children with HPE have chromosome anomalies, with trisomy 13 being most common, followed by trisomy 18 (Kinsman et al., 2000). HPE can also be seen in association with various genetic syndromes, such as the Smith–Lemli–Opitz syndrome. These observations, as well as autosomal dominant inheritance in some families, strongly suggested genetic causes of HPE. A recent extensive search for causative genes has implicated at least 12 different loci in 11 chromosomes (Roessler & Muenke, 1998). So far, four genes have been identified as causative genes for HPE. The first one to be identified was the *Sonic Hedgehog* (*SHH*) gene on chromosome 7q36, which is homologous to the *Drosophila melanogaster* segment polarity gene *hedgehog* (Roessler et al., 1996). *SHH* is highly expressed in the ventral neural tube, and considered a critical molecule in dorsoventral patterning of the neural tube. *SIX3* (Wallis et al., 1999) and *ZIC2* (Brown et al., 1998), localized on chromosomes 2p21 and 13q32, respectively, are transcription factors that are implicated in forebrain development. More recently, a homeobox gene on chromosome 18p11.3, named *TGIF*, has been found to be mutated in HPE (Gripp et al., 2000). Cellular mechanisms by which mutations in these genes cause HPE are being studied intensely. Environmental factors also seem to be crucial in some cases, and maternal gestational diabetes has been associated with increased risk of HPE in the offspring (Martínez-Frías et al., 1998).

Disorders of cell fate, proliferation and specification

Microcephaly

Overview

Microcephaly is a condition in which the size of the cranial vault, measured by the occipito-frontal head circumference (OFC), is significantly smaller than the standard for the person's age and sex. OFC of less than 2 standard deviations below the mean is often used as a definition, although some researchers use other cut-off points such as 3 standard deviations. The etiology of microcephaly is extremely diverse, posing challenges to clinicians dealing with this condition, but can be broadly divided into environmental and genetic causes. Common environmental causes include congenital infection, intra-uterine exposure to teratogenic agents, and hypoxic–ischemic injury. The clinical history usually provides important diagnostic clues in these cases. On the other hand, even the genetic causes of microcephaly are quite diverse (Table 13.1; Mochida & Walsh, 2001). For example, hereditary metabolic disorders, which cause neuronal degeneration, usually cause the postnatal onset of micro-cephaly (acquired microcephaly) and are not discussed here.

Genetic causes of microcephaly associated with micro-cephaly at birth (congenital microcephaly) frequently reflect developmental malformations of the cerebral cortex. For example, microcephaly is frequently seen in association with chromosomal abnormalities or other well-defined genetic syndromes (e.g. Smith–Lemli–Opitz syndrome). These disorders are not reviewed here. An overview of 'syndromal' microcephaly has also been pro-vided by Opitz and Holt (1990). In these cases, the charac-teristic patterns of involvement of other organ systems and/or the presence of specific dysmorphic features often help make the diagnosis. Other well-characterized CNS disorders such as neuronal migration disorders (e.g. lissen-cephaly) can be associated with microcephaly without other organ involvement, and these conditions are described below. Finally, there are an increasing number of syndromes and genetic loci in which the central nervous system is typically the only affected organ system and in which the brain is characteristically quite small but the normal pattern is relatively well preserved ('isolated microcephaly'). The prototype of this group of disorders is microcephaly vera, which is discussed next. Other forms of isolated microcephaly are also briefly mentioned in the section.

Table 13.1. Genetic forms of microcephaly

I. Isolated microcephaly
A. Autosomal recessive microcephaly
(i) Microcephaly vera
(ii) Microcephaly with simplified gyral pattern
B. Autosomal dominant microcephaly
C. X-linked microcephaly
II. Microcephaly associated with major brain malformations
A. Holoprosencephaly
B. Schizencephaly
C. Lissencephaly
D. Others
III. Chromosomal disorders
A. Down's syndrome and other trisomies
B. Chromosome deletions/duplications
C. Others
IV. Microcephaly associated with genetic syndromes
A. Smith–Lemli–Opitz syndrome
B. Rubinstein–Taybi syndrome
C. Angelman syndrome
D. Rett syndrome
E. Cornelia de Lange syndrome
F. Others
V. Microcephaly associated with hereditary metabolic disorders

Notes:
This table briefly summarizes genetic conditions associated with microcephaly. Only major disorders are listed in the categories II through IV, and the existence of additional syndromes that are not included is indicated by 'others'. The vast assortment of degenerative metabolic disorders associated with postnatal onset of microcephaly are described in other chapters and are not listed here.

Microcephaly vera

Introduction

This term, meaning 'true' microcephaly, was coined by Giacomini in 1885 to denote a condition in which no gross pathological abnormality other than smallness of the brain was observed (Friede, 1989a). When this term is used in a broader sense, it may include a wide variety of isolated microcephaly. Here we use a narrower definition, implying a subgroup of isolated microcephaly with certain clinical features described below.

Clinical features

Microcephaly vera is characterized by microcephaly at birth, relatively normal early motor milestones and mental retardation of variable severity. Usually, there are few dysmorphic features, except narrow, sloping forehead and relative prominence of ears. Seizures are relatively uncommon. On imaging studies, there are little or no gross abnormalities of the brain architecture, except its smallness. Other subtypes of isolated microcephaly are often associated with different clinical manifestations (see below).

Pathology

Grossly, the gyral pattern is relatively well preserved despite the often striking smallness of the brain. Histopathological study of the brain may reveal no microscopic abnormality in cortical laminar formation (McCreary et al., 1996). In some cases, depletion of neurons in cortical layers II and III (i.e. later-born neurons), as well as early depletion of cells in the germinative zone near the ventricles have been observed (Evrard et al., 1989). This led to a hypothesis that premature exhaustion of neuronal progenitors in the ventricular zone might be responsible for microcephaly vera (Evrard et al., 1989).

Genetics

Microcephaly vera is often inherited as an autosomal recessive trait, and has recently become a subject of active linkage analysis. Microcephaly is frequently seen in geographical areas with high consanguinity rates, such as the Middle East (Farag et al., 1993). Recently, five genetic loci for autosomal recessive microcephaly have been mapped. These loci, termed *MCPH 1, 2, 3, 4* and *5*, map to chromosomes 8p22-pter (Jackson et al., 1998), 19q13.1–13.2 (Roberts et al., 1999), 9q34 (Moynihan et al., 2000), 15q (Jamieson et al., 1999) and 1q25–32 (Jamieson et al., 2000; Pattison et al., 2000), respectively. The clinical presentation of the patients in pedigrees that map to these five distinct loci is similar enough to suggest that there will be significant genetic heterogeneity in autosomal recessive microcephaly.

Some cases of isolated microcephaly, however, are distinguished on the basis of imaging studies and clinical phenotypes. For example, there are patients who show an abnormally simplified gyral pattern, namely too few and often shallow sulci (Barkovich et al., 1998), and some of these cases are consistent with an autosomal recessive mode of inheritance(Peiffer et al., 1999; Sztriha et al., 1999). This group of patients tend to show more severe neurological signs and symptoms, such as spasticity, severe developmental delay and seizures. An autosomal dominant form of microcephaly has also been described, and is perhaps relatively common; however, this form is often associated with normal intelligence and may not come to clinicians' attention very often (Ramírez et al., 1983).

The assessment of recurrence risk of microcephaly is often challenging because of the heterogeneous nature of this condition. Unless the mode of inheritance is evident from family history and examination, accurate assessment may be difficult. In one population-based study in British Columbia, Canada, the recurrence risk of mental retardation in the siblings of microcephalic individuals was estimated to be 5.9%, one-third of whom also had microcephaly (Herbst & Baird, 1982). Another study estimated the recurrence risk of microcephaly in siblings of microcephalic individuals to be 19% (Tolmie et al., 1987), more suggestive of an autosomal recessive trait. This large difference may reflect differences in the percentage of autosomal recessive forms of microcephaly in each population studied.

Biological basis

Since no genes responsible for this condition have been found yet, the exact pathogenesis remains unclear. Although a decreased number of neurons in the cerebral cortex is considered to be primarily responsible for the smallness of the brain in microcephaly vera, there are many potential ways in which the number of cortical neurons can be subnormal. For example, decreased proliferation of neuronal progenitors, decreased production of mature neurons by each neuronal progenitor, or excessive cell death of neuronal progenitors or of mature neurons may all lead to an eventual decrease in the number of neurons. One or more of these mechanisms may be involved in the pathogenesis of microcephaly vera, but these mechanisms will not be clear until genes are identified.

Schizencephaly

Introduction

The term 'schizencephaly', originally coined by Yakovlev and Wadsworth in 1946, refers to a full-thickness cleft of the cerebral mantle (Yakovlev & Wadsworth, 1946a, b). The cleft extends from the pial surface to the lateral ventricle, and the walls of the cleft are usually lined by abnormal polymicrogyric cortex. Schizencephaly can be divided into two subtypes, namely, closed-lip type and open-lip type. When two walls, or lips, are in apposition, it is called closed-lip schizencephaly. On the other hand, in open-lip schizencephaly, the two walls are separated by a cerebrospinal fluid space (Fig. 13.2). Although the word schizencephaly has gained wide acceptance, the term 'porencephaly' is often favoured by pathologists in describing the same anatomical abnormality.

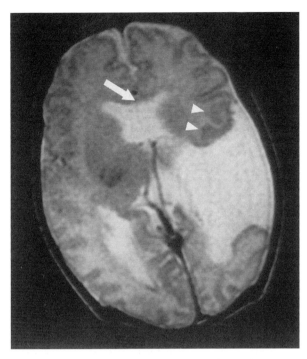

Fig. 13.2. Open-lip schizencephaly. Axial MRI shows a large schizencephalic cleft, which is lined by polymicrogyric cortex (arrowheads). Absence of the septum pellucidum is also noted (arrow).

Clinical features

The clinical presentation of patients with schizencephaly varies depending upon the type and extent of malformation, as well as the location of the cleft. The closed-lip type often presents with hemiparesis or seizures. The open-lip type can present with motor delay or seizures, but hydrocephalus may be the first presentation (Packard et al., 1997). In open-lip schizencephaly, sometimes large amounts of cerebral mantle, spanning more than one lobe, may be absent, and affected patients generally have poor neurodevelopmental outcome compared to the closed-lip variety. Seizures are commonly seen, and the seizure types can be either focal or generalized. Some cases may present with infantile spasms. Seizures can be refractory, but there are no good early predictors of seizures that are difficult to control.

Pathology

The walls, or lips, of the cleft are usually lined with polymicrogyric cortex (see Fig. 13.2). The areas of abnormal cortex may extend outside the cleft. Where the walls are in apposition, they form a so-called pia-ependymal seam. When followed from outer surface into the cleft, cells of the pia show transition to ependymal cells of the ventricular

surface via this 'seam'. There are often other associated developmental abnormalities, such as absence of the septum pellucidum or focal cortical dysplasia.

Genetics

Schizencephaly is usually sporadic, but there have been case reports of recurrence in siblings, suggesting a possible genetic origin in at least some cases (Hosley et al., 1992; Hilburger et al., 1993; Haverkamp et al., 1995). In 1996, heterozygous mutations in a homeobox gene, *EMX2*, were reported in three patients with severe cases of schizencephaly (Brunelli et al., 1996). Subsequent reports described additional patients with mutations, including a family with two affected siblings (Faiella et al., 1997; Granata et al., 1997). These mutations were *de novo*, namely not present in the parents. At this point, it is not clear what proportion of patients with schizencephaly has mutations in *EMX2*. It is possible that there are other genes that can cause schizencephaly.

Biological basis

The role of *EMX2* in brain development is yet to be fully elucidated, but recent reports suggest it has a role in determining area identity in the neocortex. *EMX2* is expressed highly in caudal and medial areas of developing mouse neocortex, and in *EMX2* knockout mice, areas of neocortex with caudal and medial identity are found to be contracted (Bishop et al., 2000; Mallamaci et al., 2000). These mice, as well as heterozygous mutant mice, do not have a phenotype that resembles human schizencephaly.

There is also a strong argument for the presence of non-genetic causes of schizencephaly. Hypoxic–ischemic insult early in fetal life has been considered to be a strong possibility. Schizencephalic clefts are usually lined by polymicrogyric cortex, and this may argue for a common pathogenesis of schizencephaly and polymicrogyria. Since there is evidence suggesting hypoxic–ischemic injury as a cause of polymicrogyria in some cases (see below), it is conceivable that some cases of schizencephaly may be a result of a similar insult. This notion of shared pathogenesis between schizencephaly and polymicrogyria may further be supported by the observation that areas of cortical dysplasia in schizencephalic brains often appear to be polymicrogyria (Barkovich & Kjos, 1992c).

Focal cortical dysplasia

Introduction

Focal cortical dysplasia (FCD) refers to a localized area of disorganized cortex, which interrupts a morphologically normal cortex. This concept was originally proposed by Taylor et al., (1971). They reported ten patients who underwent lobectomy for epilepsy and were found to have similar histopathologic features. Microscopic examination of the resected specimens showed 'localized disruption of the normal cortical lamination by an excess of large aberrant neurones scattered randomly through all but the first layer'. In most cases, 'grotesque cells, probably glial in origin, were also present in the depths of the affected cortex and in the subjacent white matter'. These bizarre cells are called 'balloon cells', and their origin is not clear.

Clinical features

Common clinical manifestations include seizures, focal neurological signs, and when the abnormality is extensive, developmental delay. FCD is a well-known cause of intractable epilepsy, and it is reported to be found in 15–40% of cases of extratemporal lobe resection (Wolf et al., 1993; Frater et al., 2000). MRI is useful in detecting FCD. Characteristic findings include blurring of the grey–white junction, widening of gyri, thickening of the cortical ribbon and increased T_2-weighted signal in subcortical white matter underlying the abnormal cortex (Yagishita et al., 1997; Chan et al., 1998; Lee et al., 1998). Detection of FCD by MRI frequently requires the use of specialized techniques and data reformatting (Barkovich et al., 1995; Grant et al., 1997). The term 'focal transmantle dysplasia' has recently been coined to describe a subtype of FCD, in which the area of dysplasia spans the entire thickness of the cerebral mantle (Barkovich et al., 1997).

Pathology

Histological changes in FCD include cortical laminar disorganization, neuronal cytomegaly (enlargement of the neuronal cell body), increased neurons in the molecular layer (layer I), heterotopic neurons in the white matter and balloon cell change (Mischel et al., 1995; Frater et al., 2000). Often two or more of these findings are seen in combination within a single lesion. The histological changes may be mild and, for example, limited to disorganization of cortical architecture, or marked with all of the features described in the original report by Taylor et al. The latter is sometimes called 'Taylor-type' FCD, and balloon cells are often considered its hallmark. These cells are typically located in the deep cortical layers or in the white matter underneath the abnormal cortex. They have a large cell body with glassy, eosinophilic cytoplasm and pleomorphic, eccentric nuclei. Immunohistochemical stains reveal variable staining with neuronal markers, glial markers or both (Vinters et al., 1992; Vital et al., 1994). In some cases, tumours, such as ganglioglioma or dysembryoplastic neuroepithelial tumour, may be found to coexist with an area of FCD (Prayson et al., 1993; Frater et al., 2000).

Genetics

FCD is usually encountered as a sporadic, non-inherited condition. Although one pedigree has been reported with apparently familial FCD, this is quite unusual (Muntaner et al., 1997).

Biological basis

The pathogenesis of FCD is not yet clear. However, it has been suggested that cell fate determination and differentiation are deranged in this condition. Balloon cells are known to express markers for neuronal and/or glial lineage, which may suggest failure of appropriate cell fate determination. Recently, altered staining patterns of proteins in the Wnt/Notch signalling pathway, which is important in neuronal cell fate determination and differentiation, was also reported, further suggesting abnormality in commitment of progenitor cells (Cotter et al., 1999).

The histopathological features of FCD show similarity to cortical tubers seen in tuberous sclerosis. Within the tubers, normal laminar structure is lost, and enlarged, dysmorphic neurons as well as 'giant cells' (or 'balloon cells') with abundant eosinophilic cytoplasm are seen. These giant cells variably express neuronal and glial markers (Hirose et al., 1995). These similarities have led to a debate whether FCD represents a 'forme fruste' of tuberous sclerosis, though this has not been settled yet (Andermann et al., 1987).

Disorders of neuronal migration

Classical lissencephaly

Overview

The term 'lissencephaly' derives from the Greek words '*lissos*', meaning 'smooth', and '*enkephalos*', meaning 'brain'. As the name implies, lissencephaly refers to a brain with a lack or severe paucity of normal gyri, and as a result, it appears smooth on the surface (Fig. 13.3). Related terms include 'agyria' and 'pachygyria'. Agyria refers to a complete lack of gyri, whereas pachygyria refers to a broadening of gyri. As many patients with lissencephaly have mixed agyric and pachygyric areas, some people prefer 'agyria/pachygyria'. Several clinical entities are associated with this type of malformation, including Miller–Dieker syndrome, isolated lissencephaly and double cortex/X-

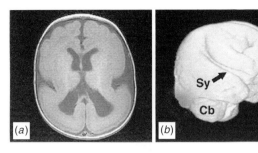

Fig. 13.3. Classical lissencephaly. Axial MRI image of classical lissencephaly (*a*) shows paucity of gyri and typical 'figure-eight' appearance. 3D-reconstruction of MRI images (*b*) illustrates lack of gyration, with posterior aspects of the brain being more severely affected, and a few rudimentary gyri remaining anteriorly. The sylvian fissure is exposed because of poor development of the operculum. Fp = frontal pole, Sy = sylvian fissure, Cb = cerebellum. (Courtesy of Dr P. Ellen Grant.)

linked lissencephaly syndrome. These disorders will be discussed below.

Miller–Dieker syndrome and isolated lissencephaly sequence

Introduction

The prototype of the disorders with classical lissencephaly is Miller–Dieker syndrome (MDS), which consists of classical lissencephaly and characteristic dysmorphic facial features. Even though the cases reported by Miller (1963) and Dieker et al., (1969) were familial, most cases of MDS are sporadic. Patients with classical lissencephaly, but without characteristic facial features of MDS, are classified as having isolated lissencephaly sequence (ILS) (Dobyns et al., 1984).

Clinical features

Essentially all children with classical lissencephaly have profound developmental delay. About half achieve essentially no developmental milestones, and the rest acquire some social and motor skills (Dobyns et al., 1993). The majority of the patients have seizures, which often start during the first 6 months of life (de Rijk-van Andel et al., 1990). Various seizure types are seen, but infantile spasms are common. Only a minority of patients are microcephalic at birth, but almost all fall within the microcephalic range during the first year of life due to a lack of normal brain growth (Dobyns et al., 1993). Patients with MDS have characteristic facial features, which include a prominent forehead, bitemporal narrowing, widely spaced eyes with upward slanting palpebral fissures, short nose with ante-

verted nares, thin vermilion border of the upper lip, and small chin (Jones et al., 1980; Dobyns et al., 1993). Some patients with MDS also have digital abnormalities (e.g. syndactyly), congenital heart disease and other visceral abnormalities (Jones et al., 1980; de Rijk-van Andel et al., 1990).

On imaging studies, the cerebral hemispheres have decreased convolutions. Often agyric areas coexist with pachygyric areas in a given patient. There is a lack of development of the frontal and parietal opercula, which leads to a characteristic 'figure-eight' shape of the brain on axial images. The lateral ventricles, particularly posterior aspects, are enlarged. Absence or hypoplasia of corpus callosum may be seen. Small midline calcifications in the region of the septum pellucidum may be present in patients with MDS (Dobyns et al., 1993).

Pathology

The cerebral cortex of classical lissencephaly is abnormally thick, and the ratio of grey to white matter is greatly increased. The cortex comprises four layers instead of the normal six layers (Crome, 1956). These four layers are (i) marginal layer, (ii) superficial cellular layer, (iii) sparsely cellular layer, and (iv) deep cellular layer. Whereas the cell-sparse subpial marginal layer corresponds to layer I of the normal cortex, the precise relationship of the three other lissencephalic layers to the five other normal cortical layers is not certain. In the brainstem, dysplastic inferior olivary nuclei with large heterotopias are characteristic (Kuchelmeister et al., 1993). On the other hand, the cerebellum in MDS is typically remarkably normal.

Genetics

Identification of patients with MDS and monosomy of chromosome 17p suggested that this locus might harbour a gene responsible for this condition (Dobyns et al., 1983). A decade later, the causative gene for MDS was found in this locus, and was named *LIS1* (Reiner et al., 1993). Subsequent analyses showed more than 90% of patients with MDS and approximately 40% of patients with ILS have deletions of the *LIS1* gene (Pilz et al., 1998). Point mutations of *LIS1* have also been identified among patients with ILS (Lo Nigro et al., 1997). As the deletions are generally larger in patients with MDS than those with ILS, it has been suggested that MDS may represent a contiguous gene syndrome, in which deletion of additional genes is responsible for the dysmorphic features of MDS (Dobyns et al., 1993).

Most of the mutations of *LIS1* that cause MDS and ILS seem to arise *de novo*. Therefore, if a deletion or a mutation of *LIS1* is found in a patient, the risk of recurrence in siblings is considered to be very low (Leventer et al., 2000). An exception to this is when one of the parents harbours a balanced translocation involving the *LIS1* locus. In such a situation, the risk is considerably higher, with up to 33% of the offspring having an abnormal genotype (i.e. deletion or duplication of chromosome 17p) and/or phenotype (Pollin et al., 1999). Translocations involving chromosome 17p were later found in both families originally reported by Miller (1963) and Dieker et al., (1969), explaining recurrence in these families (Dobyns et al., 1984).

Biological basis

After identification as the causative gene for MDS, *LIS1* was found to encode a regulatory subunit of platelet activating factor acetylhydrolase, an enzyme which inactivates platelet activating factor (PAF) (Hattori et al., 1994). However, the role of PAF in neuronal migration has not been well established. It has been suggested that the LIS1 protein may regulate neuronal migration through pathways other than PAF. For example, LIS1 has been shown to associate with microtubules directly and to stabilize them (Sapir et al., 1997), and to interact with other protein components of the microtubule organizing center (Feng et al., 2000). As microtubules are important in cell motility, this function is probably pertinent to the control of neuronal migration.

Double cortex/X-linked lissencephaly syndrome

Introduction

In this unusual condition, males and females are both clinically affected, but show very different disorders due to mutation in a common, X-linked gene. Males with mutation of the *doublecortin* (*DCX*) gene show classical lissencephaly that is generally similar to that seen in *LIS1* mutation. On the other hand, affected heterozygous females show a different malformation called 'double cortex' syndrome (DC; also known as 'subcortical band heterotopia' or 'laminar heterotopia'), where there is a band of heterotopic neurons in between the cortex and the lateral ventricles (Fig. 13.4). Even though DC has been known for many years from autopsy studies (Matell, 1893; Friede, 1989b), its recognition as an X-linked disorder, which causes lissencephaly in males, did not come until recently. In 1994, two families were reported, in which mothers with DC had sons with lissencephaly and daughters with DC (Pinard et al., 1994). This established the mode of inheritance, and also led to the recognition that there is a second genetic locus for classical lissencephaly.

Clinical features

The main clinical features of the affected females are epilepsy and mental retardation. Seizures often start during

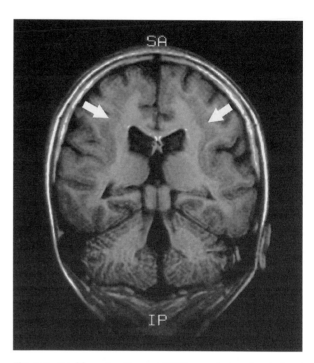

Fig. 13.4. Double cortex. Coronal MRI image shows a band of heterotopic grey matter (arrows) between the cortex and the lateral ventricles.

the first decade. Various seizure types have been documented, including generalized tonic–clonic, complex partial, myoclonic, atypical absence and atonic (Palmini et al., 1991; Barkovich et al., 1994; Gleeson et al., 2000a). Response to anticonvulsant therapy varies widely. Mental retardation is often mild to moderate. There is some suggestion that cognitive development may slow after the onset of seizures (Palmini et al., 1991). Imaging studies of the females usually show a symmetric, thick band of grey matter deep to the cortex (see Fig. 13.4; Barkovich et al., 1989). The overlying cortex often shows mild pachygyria (Barkovich et al., 1989; Palmini et al., 1991). On the other hand, the affected males show similar neurological manifestation as Miller–Dieker syndrome and isolated lissencephaly sequence, with profound developmental delay and epilepsy. Imaging findings of the males are also very similar to that of Miller–Dieker syndrome. However, the pattern of malformation is slightly different. In the X-linked lissencephaly (XLIS), anterior aspects of the brain tend to be more severely affected, in contrast to the lissencephaly due to *LIS1* mutations, where posterior aspects of the brain are almost always more severely affected (Pilz et al., 1998; Dobyns et al., 1999).

Pathology

Brains with DC show a symmetric band of grey matter between the cortex and the lateral ventricles. Microscopically, the overlying cortex shows a normal six-layered structure (Friede, 1989b). Heterotopic grey matter consists of coalescent clusters of unlaminated, well-differentiated neurons (Palmini et al., 1991). Males with XLIS show brain pathology similar to Miller–Dieker syndrome (Berg et al., 1998).

Genetics

Linkage analysis of familial cases and studies of a patient with lissencephaly and a translocation involving the X-chromosome localized the DC/XLIS locus in chromosome Xq22.3–q23 (des Portes et al., 1997; Ross et al., 1997). Subsequently, a novel gene in this region was cloned as the causative gene, and was named *doublecortin* (*DCX*) (des Portes et al., 1998; Gleeson et al., 1998). While most cases of DC or XLIS represent *de novo* mutations, families with multiple affected children can occur if the mother has subtle clinical signs or is a somatic mosaic for *DCX* mutation (Gleeson et al., 2000b). Mutation analysis of a large number of patients with DC revealed that there are patients who do not harbor a mutation in *DCX* gene (Gleeson et al., 2000a). This suggests that DC is a genetically heterogeneous disorder, and other genetic loci may be responsible for some cases of DC. Mutation analysis of patients with isolated lissencephaly sequence, who did not show deletion of *LIS1* locus detectable by fluorescence *in situ* hybridization, revealed mutations of *LIS1* gene in 40% of the cases and mutations of *DCX* gene in 20% (Pilz et al., 1998). Thus, these two genes are thought to be responsible for the majority of cases with isolated lissencephaly sequence.

Biological basis

Doublecortin is a protein that is specific to the developing nervous system, and that is widely expressed by migrating neurons (Francis et al., 1999; Gleeson et al., 1999). It has been shown to interact with microtubules, and to increase the stability of microtubules (Francis et al., 1999; Gleeson et al., 1999; Horesh et al., 1999), and the amino acid substitution mutations that cause DC/XLIS occur in the microtubule binding domain of the protein (Sapir et al., 2000; Taylor et al., 2000). It is interesting to note that two proteins that are associated with classical lissencephaly, LIS1 and Doublecortin, have been shown to interact with microtubules and possibly regulate them. This supports the hypothesis that regulation of microtubule dynamics is essential in neuronal migration, and that interruption of this process contributes to the pathogenesis of classical lissencephaly.

Lissencephaly with cerebellar hypoplasia

Lissencephaly with cerebellar hypoplasia is an autosomal recessive condition characterized by an abnormally thick and simplified gyral pattern of the cerebral cortex and hypoplasia of the cerebellum. Clinical features include hypotonia, severe developmental delay, seizures, and nystagmus (Hourihane et al., 1993; Al Shawan et al., 1996). Recently, mutations in the *RELN* gene were identified as a cause of this malformation (Hong et al., 2000). The protein product, Reelin, is a human homologue of a mouse protein, which was originally identified as the gene product that is mutated in the '*reeler*' mouse (D'Arcangelo et al., 1995). The anatomical abnormalities of the *reeler* mouse include disorganized lamination of the cerebral cortex, as well as severe hypoplasia of the cerebellum (de Rouvroit & Goffinet, 1998). Reelin is a protein secreted by Cajal–Retzius cells, which are early-born neurons that populate the embryonic marginal zone. Several molecules such as lipoprotein receptors (D'Arcangelo et al., 1999; Hiesberger et al., 1999; Trommsdorff et al., 1999), cadherin-related neuronal receptors (Senzaki et al., 1999) and $\alpha 3\beta 1$ integrin (Dulabon et al., 2000) have all been shown to act as potential receptors for Reelin. Although there is some evidence that Reelin functions in arresting migrating neurons at their proper cortical location (Dulabon et al., 2000), the precise molecular pathways through which Reelin regulates neuronal migration have not been completely elucidated.

Periventricular heterotopia

Introduction

Periventricular heterotopia (PH) is a malformation in which heterotopic nodules of grey matter are seen in the subependymal region (Fig. 13.5). Several familial cases of PH were recently reported, and this led to the recognition that this entity is genetic (DiMario et al., 1993; Kamuro & Tenokuchi, 1993; Huttenlocher et al., 1994). It was noted that typically only females were affected, and there was a high rate of miscarriages among affected females. These observations suggested that periventricular heterotopia was an X-linked disorder with prenatal lethality in affected males (Huttenlocher et al., 1994). It is now recognized that many of these cases reflect mutations of the X-linked gene, *FLN1*.

Clinical features

The most common presentation of PH in affected females is epilepsy. Common seizure types include generalized tonic–clonic and complex partial (Barkovich & Kjos, 1992a; Huttenlocher et al., 1994). Onset of the seizures is most

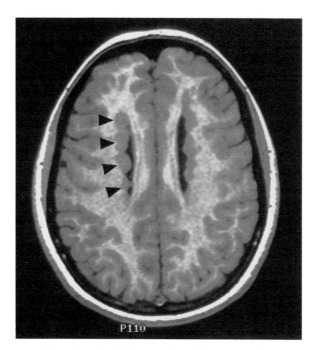

Fig. 13.5. Periventricular heterotopia. Axial MRI image shows nodular masses of grey matter (arrowheads) lining the wall of the lateral ventricles. Note that the nodules have the same signal characteristics as the normal grey matter.

commonly before the mid-20s, with an average of around 15 years (Ekşioğlu et al., 1996). Seizures may be infrequent and easily controlled, or intractable. Most individuals with PH have normal intelligence, and a minority have borderline mental retardation (Dobyns et al., 1996); 25% of affected patients may have no obvious neurological manifestations (Ekşioğlu et al., 1996). An increased incidence of patent ductus arteriosus and strokes at younger age has been reported (Fox et al., 1998).

MRI imaging characteristically shows nodular, subependymal masses, which are isointense with cortical grey matter in all imaging sequences (see Fig. 13.5; Barkovich & Kjos, 1992a). The heterotopic nodules are usually bilateral, though they may occur unilaterally. The overlying cortex is typically normal appearing. Enlargement of the cisterna magna, which may represent subtle cerebellar hypoplasia, is also common.

Pathology

The heterotopic grey matter lines the lateral ventricles as round nodules separated from each other by myelinated fibres. Microscopically, the nodules consist of highly differentiated neurons, which are haphazardly oriented (Ekşioğlu et al., 1996).

Genetics

PH may be familial or sporadic. Familial cases show X-linked dominant inheritance with presumed prenatal lethality in affected males. Most of the sporadic cases are also females, though sporadic male patients with a similar clinical presentation to females have been known (Huttenlocher et al., 1994; Dobyns et al., 1996).

Linkage analysis in familial cases identified the disease locus in chromosome Xq28 (Ekşioğlu et al., 1996). Subsequently, mutations in *FLN1* gene were identified as the cause of this disorder (Fox et al., 1998). Some of the sporadic cases have also been found to harbor mutations in *FLN1* (Fox et al., 1998).

Biological basis

The *FLN1* gene encodes Filamin 1, a large cytoplasmic actin-binding protein that is also known as actin binding protein 280 (ABP-280). It was originally identified as a high molecular weight protein isolated from macrophages that precipitated actin (Hartwig & Stossel, 1975). Subsequently, Filamin 1 was shown to be essential for migration in malignant melanoma cells (Cunningham et al., 1992) and macrophages (Stendahl et al., 1980) in vitro, but its role in neuronal migration was not suspected until it was identified as the causative gene in PH. *FLN1* gene is expressed by the cortical neurons during migration (Fox et al., 1998). It probably acts as a link between extracellular signals and the actin cytoskeleton, thereby controlling actin cross-linking, which is critical to the neuronal migration. Filamin 1 has been suggested to have roles in hemostasis and vascular remodelling, which may explain the high prevalence of strokes at young ages and patent ductus arteriosus in females, and the apparent prenatal lethality of affected males (Fox et al., 1998).

How the presence of heterotopic nodules leads to epilepsy is poorly understood. The heterotopic neurons were shown to form synapses, but the source of this innervation is unclear (Ekşioğlu et al., 1996). Knowledge of the functional connectivity of the heterotopic neurons will most likely help understand the pathogenesis of epilepsy in this disorder.

Disorders of the integrity of the pial surface

Cobblestone dysplasia

Introduction

Cobblestone dysplasia is characterized by disorganized cortical lamination and the proliferation of gliovascular tissue, which contains ectopic neurons on the pial surface of the brain. This surface abnormality gives rise to a nodular appearance, therefore the term 'cobblestone dysplasia' is applied. It is also called 'type II lissencephaly' (in contrast to 'type I' or 'classical' lissencephaly) or 'cobblestone lissencephaly', because normal gyration is often absent and as a result, the brain appears smooth on its surface. However, cobblestone dysplasia often shows various abnormal gyral patterns, including agyria, pachygyria and polymicrogyria. Therefore, it is probably better to avoid applying the term lissencephaly in this condition, and the term cobblestone dysplasia has been developed to describe it more precisely.

Cobblestone dysplasia is seen in association with three human genetic disorders: Fukuyama-type congenital muscular dystrophy (FCMD), Walker–Warburg syndrome (WWS) and muscle–eye–brain disease (MEB). FCMD is primarily seen in Japan, and MEB is most commonly seen in Finland. WWS has been reported from various parts of the world.

Clinical features

Brain and muscle involvement is common to all three disorders, but the clinical features are more or less unique in each disorder. FCMD presents with early (before 8 or 9 months) hypotonia, generalized weakness (including facial muscles), mental retardation and occasional seizures, and the condition appears to be very slowly progressive (Fukuyama et al., 1981). WWS generally has a much more severe phenotype. Often, affected children present with severe hypotonia and lethargy during the neonatal period. Median survival for live-born infants in one study was 18 weeks, although some children survive beyond 5 years (Dobyns et al., 1989). Various forms of eye and retinal abnormalities are seen, including microphthalmia, coloboma, retinal dysplasia, retinal non-attachment/detachment (Pagon et al., 1983; Dobyns et al., 1989). Occipital encephalocele may be occasionally seen. The clinical features of MEB were reported by Santavuori et al., (1989). The patients often present during the neonatal period with hypotonia and weakness, and later develop spasticity and contracture to a various degrees. Mental retardation is severe. Eye abnormalities usually manifest as severe visual failure and myopia.

On imaging studies, cobblestone dysplasia usually appears as an agyric or pachygyric area. It should be noted, however, that even though the lesions may be described as agyria or pachygyria, these are entirely different from agyria and pachygyria seen in classical (type I) lissencephaly in histologic appearance. A thick outer layer of grey matter and a thinner, irregular inner layer may be distinguished (Barkovich, 1998). In FCMD, the frontal lobe typically shows polymicrogyria, and cobblestone dysplasia is limited to the temporo-occipital area (Barkovich, 1998; Aida, 1998). In WWS, abnormalities are more striking, coinciding with severe clinical manifestations. These include diffuse agyric or pachygyric cobblestone cortex, enlarged ventricles, hypoplasia of the pons and cerebellar vermis, and fusion of the superior and inferior colliculi (Barkovich, 1998; van der Knaap et al., 1997). Diffuse abnormality of the cerebral white matter signal is the rule in WWS, reflecting almost complete lack of myelination (van der Knaap et al., 1997; Barkovich, 1998). Imaging findings of MEB are similar to those of WWS, but usually less extensive, and the white matter abnormality is often patchy (van der Knaap et al., 1997; Valanne et al., 1994; Barkovich, 1998). Cerebellar polymicrogyria with or without small cysts may be seen in all three conditions.

Pathology

Pathological features of cobblestone dysplasia, that are common to all three disorders, include gliovascular proliferation near the surface and disorganized lamination with disoriented neurons (Takada et al., 1984; Williams et al., 1984; Dobyns et al., 1985; Haltia et al., 1997). The gliovascular tissue often obliterates the subarachnoid space, and may penetrate inward to separate the cortex into 'islands' of grey matter (Dobyns et al., 1985; Haltia et al., 1997). Although it is difficult to speculate about the pathogenesis of the cobblestone dysplasia from these findings, recent pathologic studies of fetal cases of FCMD (which presumably show the cobblestone dysplasia in evolution) have suggested that the basic defect may be abnormalities in the pial–glial barrier (the outermost surface of the brain composed of the pia, basement membrane and glial endfeet) (Takada et al., 1987; Nakano et al., 1996; Yamamoto et al., 1997). Overmigration of the neurons through 'breaches' in the pial–glial barrier into the subarachnoid space may be the fundamental pathogenetic mechanism for all three conditions. Muscle pathology in all three disorders is consistent with muscular dystrophy.

Genetics

FCMD, WWS and MEB are all inherited as autosomal recessive traits. FCMD was localized to chromosome 9q31 (Toda et al., 1993, 1994, 1996), and subsequently, the causative gene was cloned. This gene encodes futukin a novel secreted protein (Kobayashi et al., 1998). In 87% of the FCMD chromosomes, the mutation was the same insertion of retrotransposon sequence in the 3' untranslated region, suggesting a Japanese founder mutation (Kobayashi et al., 1998). It has been suggested that this mutation only partly inhibits the function of the gene, whereas other reported mutations cause an even more severe phenotype that can be prenatally lethal (Kondo-Iida et al., 1999). Thus, this single mutant allele is virtually solely responsible for the existence of FCMD. The biological function of fukutin in relation to the pial–glial barrier is not understood.

It has been debated whether these three conditions share the same genetic etiology, and this has been clarified recently. MEB has recently been shown to map to chromosome 1p32–p34 (Cormand et al., 1999), and hence is not allelic to FCMD. The locus for WWS has not been found, but a family with three siblings showing either FCMD or WWS phenotype has been reported (Toda et al., 1995). This might argue for genetic identity between these two disorders, though this still remains controversial.

Disorders of less certain pathogenetic mechanisms

Polymicrogyria

Introduction
Polymicrogyria refers to an area of the cortex with numerous small meandering gyri. It is heterogeneous both in clinical presentation and etiology. For example, as mentioned above, polymicrogyria can be seen in cobblestone dysplasia or schizencephaly. Traditionally, polymicrogyria has been regarded as a result of environmental insults, such as hypoxic–ischemic injury during fetal life or congenital infection, but recently genetic etiologies have been implicated in some cases.

Clinical features
The clinical presentation of polymicrogyria depends on the anatomical distribution and extent of the abnormality. Patients with bilateral, diffuse polymicrogyria often have severe developmental delay, seizures and hypotonia with subsequent development of spasticity (Barkovich & Kjos, 1992b). Patients with unilateral, focal polymicrogyria are more likely to present with less severe developmental delay, seizures and contralateral hemiplegia (Barkovich & Kjos, 1992b). On MRI imaging, polymicrogyric cortex appears as thickened cortex with shallow sulci, mimicking pachygyria. However, with high-resolution imaging, irregularity of the grey–white junction is usually apparent (Barkovich & Kuzniecky, 1996).

Pathology
Grossly, numerous small gyri are visible. However, because the molecular layers of the adjacent gyri often fuse, it may give an appearance of abnormally thick and broad gyri in low resolution MRI or even grossly (Friede, 1989b). There are two histological subtypes of polymicrogyria. One is called 'four-layered' type, and the other is called 'unlayered' type. Four-layered polymicrogyria consists of (i) molecular layer, (ii) outer cellular layer, (iii) cell-sparse layer, and (iv) inner cellular layer (Richman et al., 1974). Even though a four-layered lamination is also seen in classical lissencephaly, they are quite distinct entities. For example, the thickness of the cortex in polymicrogyria is much less than that of lissencephaly. In unlayered polymicrogyria, no cell-sparse layer is seen.

Genetics
Usually, polymicrogyria is encountered as a sporadic condition. However, genetic forms of polymicrogyria also appear to exist. For example, possible X-linked inheritance of a unique subtype of polymicrogyria called congenital bilateral perisylvian syndrome, in which polymicrogyria is seen in perisylvian region, has been documented in some cases (Guerreiro et al., 2000). Also, several reported patients with bilateral frontal or frontoparietal polymicrogyria were born to consanguineous parents, possibly suggesting autosomal recessive inheritance (Straussberg et al., 1996; Guerrini et al., 2000; Sztriha & Nork, 2000). Cases of polymicrogyria associated with chromosome 22q11 deletions have been reported as well (Cramer et al., 1996; Bingham et al., 1998).

Biological basis
There is convincing evidence that environmental insults such as hypoxic-ischemic injury to the developing cortex can lead to polymicrogyria. There are several cases with well-documented, dated prenatal insults leading to polymicrogyria. For example, a case of a child born with polymicrogyria after carbon monoxide poisoning of the mother during the 5th month of the pregnancy has been reported (Hallervorden, 1949). Richman et al., (1974) suggested that four-layered polymicrogyria resulted from post-mitotic laminar necrosis. They demonstrated by a detailed pathological analysis of a 27-week fetus with four-layered polymicrogyria that the cell-sparse layer corresponded to layer V of normal cortex, with normal topographical relationships retained in layers II, III, IV and VI. This finding was supported by a Golgi analysis of another case (Williams et al., 1976). On the other hand, animal models have produced four-layered polymicrogyria only when cortical injury was induced during the course of neuronal migration (Dvořák and Feit, 1977; Dvořák et al., 1978). Further studies are necessary to identify the relationship between the nature and the timing of injury and development of polymicrogyria.

Other types of intrauterine insults, in particular cytomegalovirus infection, have been associated with polymicrogyria. The pathogenetic mechanism of polymicrogyria in cases with cytomegalovirus infection is not clear.

Conclusions

With the combination of genetic and radiographic analysis, disorders of cerebral cortical development are increasingly coming into focus as a series of well-defined disorders. While their clinical features are often not distinctive, consisting of epilepsy and mental retardation, imaging studies are often distinctive, and give important keys to prognosis and recurrence risk. The near future promises clearer information and the broader application of DNA-based, as well as MRI-based, diagnosis.

Acknowledgements

This work is supported by grants from NINDS (RO1 NS35129 and PO1 NS39404) and the March of Dimes.

G.H.M. is a Howard Hughes Medical Institute Physician Postdoctoral Fellow and a former fellow of the Clinical Investigator Training Program (Beth Israel Deaconess Medical Center – Harvard MIT Health Sciences and Technology).

The authors thank Jun Shen for providing helpful information and references about holoprosencephaly, and Dr Kalpathy S. Krishnamoorthy for helpful suggestions in preparing the figures.

References

Aida, N. (1998). Fukuyama congenital muscular dystrophy: a neuroradiologic review. *J. Magn. Reson. Imaging*, **8**, 317–26.

Al Shawan, S.A., Bruyn, G.W. & Al Deeb, S.M. (1996). Lissencephaly with pontocerebellar hypoplasia. *J. Child Neurol.*, **11**, 241–4.

Andermann, F., Olivier, A., Melanson, D. & Robitaille, Y. (1987). Epilepsy due to focal cortical dysplasia with macrogyria and the forme fruste of tuberous sclerosis: a study of fifteen patients. *Adv. Epilepsy*, **16**, 35–8.

Anderson, S.A., Eisenstat, D.D., Shi, L. & Rubenstein, J.L. (1997). Interneuron migration from basal forebrain to neocortex: dependence on *Dlx* genes. *Science*, **278**, 474–6.

Barkovich, A.J. (1998). Neuroimaging manifestations and classification of congenital muscular dystrophies. *Am. J. Neuroradiol.*, **19**, 1389–96.

Barkovich, A.J. & Kjos, B.O. (1992a). Gray matter heterotopias: MR characteristics and correlation with developmental and neurologic manifestations. *Radiology*, **182**, 493–9.

Barkovich, A.J. & Kjos, B.O. (1992b). Nonlissencephalic cortical dysplasias: correlation of imaging findings with clinical deficits. *Am. J. Neuroradiol.*, **13**, 95–103.

Barkovich, A.J. & Kjos, B.O. (1992c). Schizencephaly: correlation of clinical findings with MR characteristics. *Am. J. Neuroradiol.*, **13**, 85–94.

Barkovich, A.J. & Kuzniecky, R.I. (1996). Neuroimaging of focal malformations of cortical development. *J. Clin. Neurophysiol.*, **13**, 481–94.

Barkovich, A.J., Jackson, D.E., Jr. & Boyer, R.S. (1989). Band heterotopias: a newly recognized neuronal migration anomaly. *Radiology*, **171**, 455–8.

Barkovich, A.J., Guerrini, R., Battaglia, G. et al. (1994). Band heterotopia: correlation of outcome with magnetic resonance imaging parameters. *Ann. Neurol.*, **36**, 609–17.

Barkovich, A.J., Rowley, H.A. & Andermann, F. (1995). MR in partial epilepsy: value of high-resolution volumetric techniques. *Am. J. Neuroradiol.*, **16**, 339–43.

Barkovich, A.J., Kuzniecky, R.I., Dobyns, W.B., Jackson, G.D., Becker, L.E. & Evrard, P. (1996). A classification scheme for malformations of cortical development. *Neuropediatrics*, **27**, 59–63.

Barkovich, A.J., Kuzniecky, R.I., Bollen, A.W. & Grant, P.E. (1997). Focal transmantle dysplasia: a specific malformation of cortical development. *Neurology*, **49**, 1148–52.

Barkovich, A. J., Ferriero, D.M., Barr, R.M. et al. (1998). Microlissencephaly: a heterogeneous malformation of cortical development. *Neuropediatrics*, **29**, 113–19.

Barr, M., Jr. & Cohen, M.M., Jr. (1999). Holoprosencephaly survival and performance. *Am. J. Med. Genet. (Semin. Med. Genet.)*, **89**, 116–20.

Berg, M.J., Schifitto, G., Powers, J.M. et al. (1998). X-linked female band heterotopia-male lissencephaly syndrome. *Neurology*, **50**, 1143–6.

Bingham, P.M., Lynch, D., McDonald-McGinn, D. & Zackai, E. (1998). Polymicrogyria in chromosome 22 deletion syndrome. *Neurology*, **51**, 1500–2.

Bishop, K.M., Goudreau, G. & O'Leary, D.D. (2000). Regulation of area identity in the mammalian neocortex by *Emx2* and *Pax6*. *Science*, **288**, 344–9.

Brown, S.A., Warburton, D., Brown, L.Y. et al. (1998). Holoprosencephaly due to mutations in *ZIC2*, a homologue of *Drosophila odd-paired*. *Nat. Genet.*, **20**, 180–3.

Brunelli, S., Faiella, A., Capra, V. et al. (1996). Germline mutations in the homeobox gene *EMX2* in patients with severe schizencephaly. *Nat. Genet.*, **12**, 94–6.

Chan, S., Chin, S.S., Nordli, D.R., Goodman, R.R., DeLaPaz, R.L. & Pedley, T.A. (1998). Prospective magnetic resonance imaging identification of focal cortical dysplasia, including the non-balloon cell subtype. *Ann. Neurol.*, **44**, 749–57.

Cohen, M.M., Jr. (1989). Perspectives on holoprosencephaly: Part III. Spectra, distinctions, continuities, and discontinuities. *Am. J. Med. Genet.*, **34**, 271–88.

Cormand, B., Avela, K., Pihko, H. et al. (1999). Assignment of the muscle–eye–brain disease gene to 1p32–p34 by linkage analysis and homozygosity mapping. *Am. J. Hum. Genet.*, **64**, 126–35.

Cotter, D., Honavar, M., Lovestone, S. et al. (1999). Disturbance of Notch-1 and Wnt signalling proteins in neuroglial balloon cells and abnormal large neurons in focal cortical dysplasia in human cortex. *Acta Neuropathol. (Berl.)*, **98**, 465–72.

Cramer, S.C., Schaefer, P.W. & Krishnamoorthy, K.S. (1996). Microgyria in the distribution of the middle cerebral artery in a patient with DiGeorge syndrome. *J. Child Neurol.*, **11**, 494–7.

Croen, L.A., Shaw, G.M. & Lammer, E.J. (1996). Holoprosencephaly: epidemiologic and clinical characteristics of a California population. *Am. J. Med. Genet.*, **64**, 465–72.

Crome, L. (1956). Pachygyria. *J. Pathol. Bacteriol.*, **71**, 335–52.

Cunningham, C.C., Gorlin, J.B., Kwiatkowski, D.J. et al. (1992). Actin-binding protein requirement for cortical stability and efficient locomotion. *Science*, **255**, 325–7.

D'Arcangelo, G., Miao, G.G., Chen, S.C., Soares, H.D., Morgan, J.I. & Curran, T. (1995). A protein related to extracellular matrix proteins deleted in the mouse mutant *reeler*. *Nature*, **374**, 719–23.

D'Arcangelo, G., Homayouni, R., Keshvara, L., Rice, D.S., Sheldon, M. & Curran, T. (1999). Reelin is a ligand for lipoprotein receptors. *Neuron*, **24**, 471–9.

de Rijk-van Andel, J.F., Arts, W.F.M., Barth, P.G. & Loonen, M.C.B. (1990). Diagnostic features and clinical signs of 21 patients with lissencephaly type I. *Dev. Med. Child Neurol.*, **32**, 707–17.

de Rouvroit, C.L. & Goffinet, A.M. (1998). The reeler mouse as a model of brain development. *Adv. Anat. Embryol. Cell Biol.*, **150**, 1–106.

des Portes, V., Pinard, J.M., Smadja, D. et al. (1997). Dominant X linked subcortical laminar heterotopia and lissencephaly syndrome (XSCLH/LIS): evidence for the occurrence of mutation in males and mapping of a potential locus in Xq22. *J. Med. Genet.*, **34**, 177–83.

des Portes, V., Pinard, J.M., Billuart, P. et al. (1998). A novel CNS gene required for neuronal migration and involved in X-linked subcortical laminar heterotopia and lissencephaly syndrome. *Cell*, **92**, 51–61.

Dieker, H., Edwards, R.H., ZuRhein, G., Chou, S. & Opitz, J.M. (1969). The lissencephaly syndrome. *Birth Defects Orig. Artic. Ser.*, **5**, 53–64.

DiMario, F.J., Jr., Cobb, R.J., Ramsby, G.R. & Leicher, C. (1993). Familial band heterotopias simulating tuberous sclerosis. *Neurology*, **43**, 1424–6.

Dobyns, W.B., Stratton, R.F., Parke, J.T., Greenberg, F., Nussbaum, R.L. & Ledbetter, D.H. (1983). Miller–Dieker syndrome: lissencephaly and monosomy 17p. *J. Pediatr.*, **102**, 552–8.

Dobyns, W.B., Stratton, R.F. & Greenberg, F. (1984). Syndromes with lissencephaly. I: Miller–Dieker and Norman–Roberts syndromes and isolated lissencephaly. *Am. J. Med. Genet.*, **18**, 509–26.

Dobyns, W.B., Kirkpatrick, J.B., Hittner, H.M., Roberts, R.M. & Kretzer, F.L. (1985). Syndromes with lissencephaly. II: Walker–Warburg and cerebro-oculo-muscular syndromes and a new syndrome with type II lissencephaly. *Am. J. Med. Genet.*, **22**, 157–95.

Dobyns, W.B., Pagon, R.A., Armstrong, D. et al. (1989). Diagnostic criteria for Walker–Warburg syndrome. *Am. J. Med. Genet.*, **32**, 195–210.

Dobyns, W.B., Reiner, O., Carrozzo, R. & Ledbetter, D.H. (1993). Lissencephaly. A human brain malformation associated with deletion of the *LIS1* gene located at chromosome 17p13. *J. Am. Med. Ass.*, **270**, 2838–42.

Dobyns, W.B., Andermann, E., Andermann, F. et al. (1996). X-linked malformations of neuronal migration. *Neurology*, **47**, 331–9.

Dobyns, W.B., Truwit, C.L., Ross, M.E. et al. (1999). Differences in the gyral pattern distinguish chromosome 17-linked and X-linked lissencephaly. *Neurology*, **53**, 270–7.

Dulabon, L., Olson, E.C., Taglienti, M.G. et al. (2000). Reelin binds $\alpha 3\beta 1$ integrin and inhibits neuronal migration. *Neuron*, **27**, 33–44.

Dvořák, K. & Feit, J. (1977). Migration of neuroblasts through partial necrosis of the cerebral cortex in newborn rats – contribution to the problems of morphological development and developmental period of cerebral microgyria. Histological and autoradiographical study. *Acta Neuropathol. (Berl.)*, **38**, 203–12.

Dvořák, K., Feit, J. & Juránková, Z. (1978). Experimentally induced focal microgyria and status verrucosus deformis in rats – pathogenesis and interrelation. Histological and autoradiographical study. *Acta Neuropathol. (Berl.)*, **44**, 121–9.

Ekşioğlu, Y.Z., Scheffer, I.E., Cardenas, P. et al. (1996). Periventricular heterotopia: an X-linked dominant epilepsy locus causing aberrant cerebral cortical development. *Neuron*, **16**, 77–87.

Evrard, P., de Saint-Georges, P., Kadhim, H.J. & Gadisseux, J. F. (1989). Pathology of prenatal encephalopathies. In *Child Neurology and Developmental Disabilities: Selected Proceedings of the Fourth International Child Neurology Congress*, ed. J.H. French, S. Harel, P. Casaer, M.I. Gottlieb, I. Rapin & D.C. De Vivo, pp. 153–76. Baltimore, MD: Paul H. Brookes.

Faiella, A., Brunelli, S., Granata, T. et al. (1997). A number of schizencephaly patients including 2 brothers are heterozygous for germline mutations in the homeobox gene EMX2. *Eur. J. Hum. Genet.*, **5**, 186–90.

Farag, T.I., Al-Awadi, S.A., El-Badramary, M.H. et al. (1993). Disease profile of 400 institutionalized mentally retarded patients in Kuwait. *Clin. Genet.*, **44**, 329–34.

Feng, Y., Olson, E.C., Stukenberg, P.T., Flanagan, L.A., Kirschner, M.W. & Walsh, C.A. (2000). Interactions between LIS1 and mNudE, a central component of the centrosome, are required for CNS lamination. *Neuron*, **28**, 665–79.

Fox, J.W., Lamperti, E.D., Ekşioğlu, Y.Z. et al. (1998). Mutations in *filamin 1* prevent migration of cerebral cortical neurons in human periventricular heterotopia. *Neuron*, **21**, 1315–25.

Francis, F., Koulakoff, A., Boucher, D. et al. (1999). Doublecortin is a developmentally regulated, microtubule-associated protein expressed in migrating and differentiating neurons. *Neuron*, **23**, 247–56.

Frater, J.L., Prayson, R.A., Morris, H.H. & Bingaman, W.E. (2000). Surgical pathologic findings of extratemporal-based intractable epilepsy: a study of 133 consecutive resections. *Arch. Pathol. Lab. Med.*, **124**, 545–9.

Friede, R.L. (1989a). Disturbances in bulk growth: megalencephaly, micrencephaly, atelencephaly and others. In *Developmental Neuropathology*, 2nd edn, pp. 296–308. Berlin: Springer-Verlag.

Friede, R.L. (1989b). Dysplasias of cerebral cortex. In *Developmental Neuropathology*, 2nd edn, pp. 330–46. Berlin: Springer-Verlag.

Fukuyama, Y., Osawa, M. & Suzuki, H. (1981). Congenital progressive muscular dystrophy of the Fukuyama type – clinical, genetic and pathological considerations. *Brain Dev.*, **3**, 1–29.

Gleeson, J.G., Allen, K.M., Fox, J.W. et al. (1998). *doublecortin*, a brain-specific gene mutated in human X-linked lissencephaly and double cortex syndrome, encodes a putative signaling protein. *Cell*, **92**, 63–72.

Gleeson, J.G., Lin, P.T., Flanagan, L.A. & Walsh, C.A. (1999). Doublecortin is a microtubule-associated protein and is expressed widely by migrating neurons. *Neuron*, **23**, 257–71.

Gleeson, J.G., Luo, R.F., Grant, P.E. et al. (2000a). Genetic and neuroradiological heterogeneity of double cortex syndrome. *Ann. Neurol.*, **47**, 265–9.

Gleeson, J.G., Minnerath, S., Kuzniecky, R.I. et al. (2000b). Somatic and germline mosaic mutations in the *doublecortin* gene are associated with variable phenotypes. *Am. J. Hum. Genet.*, **67**, 574–81.

Granata, T., Farina, L., Faiella, A. et al. (1997). Familial schizencephaly associated with *EMX2* mutation. *Neurology*, **48**, 1403–6.

Grant, P.E., Barkovich, A.J., Wald, L.L., Dillon, W.P., Laxer, K.D. & Vigneron, D. (1997). High-resolution surface-coil MR of cortical lesions in medically refractory epilepsy: a prospective study. *Am. J. Neuroradiol.*, **18**, 291–301.

Gripp, K.W., Wotton, D., Edwards, M.C. et al. (2000). Mutations in *TGIF* cause holoprosencephaly and link NODAL signalling to human neural axis determination. *Nat .Genet.*, **25**, 205–8.

Guerreiro, M.M., Andermann, E., Guerrini, R. et al. (2000). Familial perisylvian polymicrogyria: a new familial syndrome of cortical maldevelopment. *Ann. Neurol.*, **48**, 39–48.

Guerrini, R., Barkovich, A.J., Sztriha, L. & Dobyns, W.B. (2000). Bilateral frontal polymicrogyria: a newly recognized brain malformation syndrome. *Neurology*, **54**, 909–13.

Hallervorden, J. (1949). Über eine Kohlenoxydvergiftung im Fetalleben mit Entwicklungsstörung der Hirnrinde. *Allg. Z. Psychiatr.*, **124**, 289–98.

Haltia, M., Leivo, I., Somer, H. et al. (1997). Muscle–eye–brain disease: a neuropathological study. *Ann. Neurol.*, **41**, 173–80.

Hartwig, J.H. & Stossel, T.P. (1975). Isolation and properties of actin, myosin, and a new actin-binding protein in rabbit alveolar macrophages. *J. Biol. Chem.*, **250**, 5696–705.

Hattori, M., Adachi, H., Tsujimoto, M., Arai, H. & Inoue, K. (1994). Miller-Dieker lissencephaly gene encodes a subunit of brain platelet-activating factor acetylhydrolase. *Nature*, **370**, 216–18.

Haverkamp, F., Zerres, K., Ostertun, B., Emons, D. & Lentze, M.J. (1995). Familial schizencephaly: further delineation of a rare disorder. *J. Med. Genet.*, **32**, 242–4.

Herbst, D.S. & Baird, P.A. (1982). Sib risks for nonspecific mental retardation in British Columbia. *Am. J. Med. Genet.*, **13**, 197–208.

Hiesberger, T., Trommsdorff, M., Howell, B.W. et al. (1999). Direct binding of Reelin to VLDL receptor and ApoE receptor 2 induces tyrosine phosphorylation of disabled-1 and modulates tau phosphorylation. *Neuron*, **24**, 481–9.

Hilburger, A.C., Willis, J.K., Bouldin, E. & Henderson-Tilton, A. (1993). Familial schizencephaly. *Brain Dev.*, **15**, 234–6.

Hirose, T., Scheithauer, B.W., Lopes, M.B. et al. (1995). Tuber and subependymal giant cell astrocytoma associated with tuberous sclerosis: an immunohistochemical, ultrastructural, and immunoelectron microscopic study. *Acta Neuropathol.*, **90**, 387–99.

Hong, S.E., Shugart, Y.Y., Huang, D.T. et al. (2000). Autosomal recessive lissencephaly with cerebellar hypoplasia is associated with human *RELN* mutations. *Nat. Genet.*, **26**, 93–6.

Horesh, D., Sapir, T., Francis, F. et al. (1999). Doublecortin, a stabilizer of microtubules. *Hum. Mol. Genet.*, **8**, 1599–610.

Hosley, M.A., Abroms, I.F. & Ragland, R.L. (1992). Schizencephaly: case report of familial incidence. *Pediatr. Neurol.*, **8**, 148–50.

Hourihane, J.O'B., Bennett, C.P., Chaudhuri, R., Robb, S.A. & Martin, N.D.T. (1993). A sibship with a neuronal migration defect, cerebellar hypoplasia and congenital lymphedema. *Neuropediatrics*, **24**, 43–6.

Huttenlocher, P.R., Taravath, S. & Mojtahedi, S. (1994). Periventricular heterotopia and epilepsy. *Neurology*, **44**, 51–5.

Jackson, A.P., McHale, D.P., Campbell, D.A. et al. (1998). Primary autosomal recessive microcephaly (MCPH1) maps to chromosome 8p22-pter. *Am. J. Hum. Genet.*, **63**, 541–6.

Jamieson, C.R., Govaerts, C. & Abramowicz, M.J. (1999). Primary autosomal recessive microcephaly: homozygosity mapping of MCPH4 to chromosome 15. *Am. J. Hum. Genet.*, **65**, 1465–9.

Jamieson, C.R., Fryns, J.P., Jacobs, J., Matthijs, G. & Abramowicz, M.J. (2000). Primary autosomal recessive microcephaly: *MCPH5* maps to 1q25–q32. *Am. J. Hum. Genet.*, **67**, 1575–7.

Jones, K.L., Gilbert, E.F., Kaveggia, E.G. & Opitz, J.M. (1980). The Miller–Dieker syndrome. *Pediatrics*, **66**, 277–81.

Kamuro, K. & Tenokuchi, Y. (1993). Familial periventricular nodular heterotopia. *Brain Dev.*, **15**, 237–41.

Kinsman, S.L., Plawner, L.L. & Hahn, J.S. (2000). Holoprosencephaly: recent advances and new insights. *Curr. Opin. Neurol.*, **13**, 127–32.

Kobayashi, K., Nakahori, Y., Miyake, M. et al. (1998). An ancient retrotransposal insertion causes Fukuyama-type congenital muscular dystrophy. *Nature*, **394**, 388–92.

Kondo-Iida, E., Kobayashi, K., Watanabe, M. et al. (1999) Novel mutations and genotype-phenotype relationships in 107 families with Fukuyama-type congenital muscular dystrophy (FCMD). *Hum. Mol. Genet.*, **8**, 2303–9.

Kuchelmeister, K., Bergmann, M. & Gullotta, F. (1993). Neuropathology of lissencephalies. *Childs Nerv. Syst.*, **9**, 394–9.

Lavdas, A.A., Grigoriou, M., Pachnis, V. & Parnavelas, J.G. (1999). The medial ganglionic eminence gives rise to a population of early neurons in the developing cerebral cortex. *J. Neurosci.*, **19**, 7881–8.

Lee, B.C., Schmidt, R.E., Hatfield, G.A., Bourgeois, B. & Park, T.S. (1998). MRI of focal cortical dysplasia. *Neuroradiology*, **40**, 675–83.

Leventer, R.J., Pilz, D.T., Matsumoto, N., Ledbetter, D.H. & Dobyns, W.B. (2000). Lissencephaly and subcortical band heterotopia: molecular basis and diagnosis. *Mol. Med. Today*, **6**, 277–84.

Lo Nigro, C., Chong, S.S., Smith, A.C.M., Dobyns, W.B., Carrozzo, R. & Ledbetter, D.H. (1997). Point mutations and an intragenic deletion in *LIS1*, the lissencephaly causative gene in isolated lissencephaly sequence and Miller-Dieker syndrome. *Hum. Mol. Genet.*, **6**, 157–64.

McCreary, B.D., Rossiter, J.P. & Robertson, D.M. (1996). Recessive (true) microcephaly: a case report with neuropathological observations. *J. Intellect. Disabil. Res.*, **40**, 66–70.

Mallamaci, A., Muzio, L., Chan, C.H., Parnavelas, J. & Boncinelli, E. (2000). Area identity shifts in the early cerebral cortex of *Emx2-/-* mutant mice. *Nat. Neurosci.*, **3**, 679–86.

Marín-Padilla, M. (1970). Prenatal and early postnatal ontogenesis of the human motor cortex: a Golgi study. I. The sequential development of the cortical layers. *Brain Res.*, **23**, 167–83.

Marín-Padilla, M. (1971). Early prenatal ontogenesis of the cerebral cortex (neocortex) of the cat (*Felis domestica*). A Golgi study. I. The primordial neocortical organization. *Z. Anat. Entwicklungsgesch.*, **134**, 117–45.

Marín-Padilla, M. (1983). Structural organization of the human cerebral cortex prior to the appearance of the cortical plate. *Anat. Embryol.*, **168**, 21–40.

Marín-Padilla, M. (1990). Origin, formation, and prenatal maturation of the human cerebral cortex: an overview. *J. Craniofac. Genet. Dev. Biol.*, **10**, 137–46.

Martínez-Frías, M.L., Bermejo, E., Rodríguez-Pinilla, E., Prieto, L. & Frías, J.L. (1998). Epidemiological analysis of outcomes of pregnancy in gestational diabetic mothers. *Am. J. Med. Genet.*, **78**, 140–5.

Matell, M. (1893). Ein Fall von Heterotopie der grauen Substanz in den beiden Hemisphären des Grosshirns. *Arch. Psychiatr. Nervenkr.*, **25**, 124–36.

Matsunaga, E. & Shiota, K. (1977). Holoprosencephaly in human embryos: epidemiologic studies of 150 cases. *Teratology*, **16**, 261–72.

Miller, J. Q. (1963). Lissencephaly in 2 siblings. *Neurology*, **13**, 841–50.

Mischel, P.S., Nguyen, L.P. & Vinters, H.V. (1995). Cerebral cortical dysplasia associated with pediatric epilepsy. Review of neuropathologic features and proposal for a grading system. *J. Neuropathol. Exp. Neurol.*, **54**, 137–53.

Mochida, G.H. & Walsh, C.A. (2001). Molecular genetics of human microcephaly. *Curr. Opin. Neurol.*, **14**, 151–6.

Moynihan, L., Jackson, A.P., Roberts, E. et al. (2000). A third novel locus for primary autosomal recessive microcephaly maps to chromosome 9q34. *Am. J. Hum. Genet.*, **66**, 724–7.

Muntaner, L., Pérez-Ferrón, J.J., Herrera, M., Rosell, J., Taboada, D. & Climent, S. (1997). MRI of a family with focal abnormalities of gyration. *Neuroradiology*, **39**, 605–8.

Nakano, I., Funahashi, M., Takada, K. & Toda, T. (1996). Are breaches in the glia limitans the primary cause of the micropolygyria in Fukuyama-type congenital muscular dystrophy (FCMD)? Pathological study of the cerebral cortex of an FCMD fetus. *Acta Neuropathol. (Berl.)*, **91**, 313–21.

Olsen, C.L., Hughes, J.P., Youngblood, L.G. & Sharpe-Stimac, M. (1997). Epidemiology of holoprosencephaly and phenotypic characteristics of affected children: New York State, 1984–1989. *Am. J. Med. Genet.*, **73**, 217–26.

Opitz, J.M. & Holt, M.C. (1990). Microcephaly: general considerations and aids to nosology. *J. Craniofac. Genet. Dev. Biol.*, **10**, 175–204.

Osborn, R.E., Byrd, S.E., Naidich, T.P., Bohan, T.P. & Friedman, H. (1988). MR imaging of neuronal migrational disorders. *Am. J. Neuroradiol.*, **9**, 1101–6.

Packard, A.M., Miller, V.S. & Delgado, M.R. (1997). Schizencephaly: correlations of clinical and radiologic features. *Neurology*, **48**, 1427–34.

Pagon, R.A., Clarren, S.K., Milam, D.F., Jr. & Hendrickson, A.E. (1983). Autosomal recessive eye and brain anomalies: Warburg syndrome. *J. Pediatr.*, **102**, 542–6.

Palmini, A., Andermann, F., Aicardi, J. et al. (1991). Diffuse cortical dysplasia, or the 'double cortex' syndrome: the clinical and epileptic spectrum in 10 patients. *Neurology*, **41**, 1656–62.

Pattison, L., Crow, Y.J., Deeble, V.J. et al. (2000). A fifth locus for primary autosomal recessive microcephaly maps to chromosome 1q31. *Am. J. Hum. Genet.*, **67**, 1578–80.

Peiffer, A., Singh, N., Leppert, M., Dobyns, W.B. & Carey, J.C. (1999). Microcephaly with simplified gyral pattern in six related children. *Am. J. Med. Genet.*, **84**, 137–44.

Pilz, D.T., Matsumoto, N., Minnerath, S. et al. (1998). *LIS1* and *XLIS* (*DCX*) mutations cause most classical lissencephaly, but different patterns of malformation. *Hum. Mol. Genet.*, **7**, 2029–37.

Pinard, J-M., Motte, J., Chiron, C., Brian, R., Andermann, E. & Dulac, O. (1994). Subcortical laminar heterotopia and lissencephaly in two families: a single X linked dominant gene. *J. Neurol., Neurosurg. Psychiatry.*, **57**, 914–20.

Pollin, T.I., Dobyns, W.B., Crowe, C.A. et al. (1999). Risk of abnormal pregnancy outcome in carriers of balanced reciprocal translocations involving the Miller–Dieker syndrome (MDS) critical region in chromosome 17p13.3. *Am. J. Med. Genet.*, **85**, 369–75.

Prayson, R.A., Estes, M.L. & Morris, H.H. (1993). Coexistence of neoplasia and cortical dysplasia in patients presenting with seizures. *Epilepsia*, **34**, 609–15.

Rakic, P. (1971). Guidance of neurons migrating to the fetal monkey neocortex. *Brain Res.*, **33**, 471–6.

Rakic, P. (1972). Mode of cell migration to the superficial layers of fetal monkey neocortex. *J. Comp. Neurol.*, **145**, 61–83.

Ramírez, M.L., Rivas, F. & Cantú, J.M. (1983). Silent microcephaly: a distinct autosomal dominant trait. *Clin. Genet.*, **23**, 281–6.

Rasmussen, S.A., Moore, C.A., Khoury, M.J. & Cordero, J.F. (1996). Descriptive epidemiology of holoprosencephaly and arhinencephaly in metropolitan Atlanta, 1968–1992. *Am. J. Med. Genet.*, **66**, 320–33.

Reiner, O., Carrozzo, R., Shen, Y. et al. (1993). Isolation of a Miller–Dieker lissencephaly gene containing G protein β-subunit-like repeats. *Nature*, **364**, 717–21.

Richman, D.P., Stewart, R.M. & Caviness, V.S., Jr. (1974). Cerebral microgyria in a 27-week fetus: an architectonic and topographic analysis. *J. Neuropathol. Exp. Neurol.*, **33**, 374–84.

Roberts, E., Jackson, A.P., Carradice, A.C. et al. (1999). The second locus for autosomal recessive primary microcephaly (*MCPH2*) maps to chromosome 19q13.1–13.2. *Eur. J. Hum. Genet.*, **7**, 815–20.

Roessler, E. & Muenke, M. (1998). Holoprosencephaly: a paradigm for the complex genetics of brain development. *J. Inherit. Metab. Dis.*, **21**, 481–97.

Roessler, E., Belloni, E., Gaudenz, K. et al. (1996). Mutations in the human *Sonic Hedgehog* gene cause holoprosencephaly. *Nat. Genet.*, **14**, 357–60.

Ross, M.E., Allen, K.M., Srivastava, A.K. et al. (1997). Linkage and physical mapping of X-linked lissencephaly/SBH (*XLIS*): a gene causing neuronal migration defects in human brain. *Hum. Mol. Genet.*, **6**, 555–62.

Santavuori, P., Somer, H., Sainio, K. et al. (1989). Muscle–eye–brain disease (MEB). *Brain Dev.*, **11**, 147–53.

Sapir, T., Elbaum, M. & Reiner, O. (1997). Reduction of microtubule catastrophe events by LIS1, platelet-activating factor acetylhydrolase subunit. *EMBO J.*, **16**, 6977–84.

Sapir, T., Horesh, D., Caspi, M. et al. (2000). Doublecortin mutations cluster in evolutionarily conserved functional domains. *Hum. Mol. Genet.*, **9**, 703–12.

Senzaki, K., Ogawa, M. & Yagi, T. (1999). Proteins of the CNR family are multiple receptors for Reelin. *Cell*, **99**, 635–47.

Sidman, R.L. & Rakic, P. (1973). Neuronal migration, with special reference to developing human brain: a review. *Brain Res.*, **62**, 1–35.

Stendahl, O.I., Hartwig, J.H., Brotschi, E.A. & Stossel, T.P. (1980). Distribution of actin-binding protein and myosin in macrophages during spreading and phagocytosis. *J. Cell Biol.*, **84**, 215–24.

Straussberg, R., Gross, S., Amir, J. & Gadoth, N. (1996). A new autosomal recessive syndrome of pachygyria. *Clin. Genet.*, **50**, 498–501.

Sztriha, L. & Nork, M. (2000). Bilateral frontoparietal polymicrogyria and epilepsy. *Pediatr. Neurol.*, **22**, 240–3.

Sztriha, L., Al-Gazali, L.I., Várady, E., Goebel, H.H. & Nork, M. (1999). Autosomal recessive micrencephaly with simplified gyral pattern, abnormal myelination and arthrogryposis. *Neuropediatrics*, **30**, 141–5.

Takada, K., Nakamura, H. & Tanaka, J. (1984). Cortical dysplasia in congenital muscular dystrophy with central nervous system involvement (Fukuyama type). *J. Neuropathol. Exp. Neurol.*, **43**, 395–407.

Takada, K., Nakamura, H., Suzumori, K., Ishikawa, T. & Sugiyama, N. (1987). Cortical dysplasia in a 23-week fetus with Fukuyama congenital muscular dystrophy (FCMD). *Acta Neuropathol. (Berl.)*, **74**, 300–6.

Tamamaki, N., Fujimori, K.E. & Takauji, R. (1997). Origin and route of tangentially migrating neurons in the developing neocortical intermediate zone. *J. Neurosci.*, **17**, 8313–23.

Taylor, D.C., Falconer, M.A., Bruton, C.J. & Corsellis, J.A.N. (1971). Focal dysplasia of the cerebral cortex in epilepsy. *J. Neurol., Neurosurg. Psychiatry*, **34**, 369–87.

Taylor, K.R., Holzer, A.K., Bazan, J.F., Walsh, C.A. & Gleeson, J. G. (2000). Patient mutations in doublecortin define a repeated tubulin-binding domain. *J. Biol. Chem.*, **275**, 34442–50.

Toda, T., Segawa, M., Nomura, Y. et al. (1993). Localization of a gene for Fukuyama type congenital muscular dystrophy to chromosome 9q31–33. *Nat. Genet.*, **5**, 283–6.

Toda, T., Ikegawa, S., Okui, K. et al. (1994). Refined mapping of a gene responsible for Fukuyama-type congenital muscular dystrophy: evidence for strong linkage disequilibrium. *Am. J. Hum. Genet.*, **55**, 946–50.

Toda, T., Yoshioka, M., Nakahori, Y., Kanazawa, I., Nakamura, Y. & Nakagome, Y. (1995). Genetic identity of Fukuyama-type congenital muscular dystrophy and Walker–Warburg syndrome. *Ann. Neurol.*, **37**, 99–101.

Toda, T., Miyake, M., Kobayashi, K. et al. (1996). Linkage-disequilibrium mapping narrows the Fukuyama-type congenital muscular dystrophy (FCMD) candidate region to <100 kb. *Am. J. Hum. Genet.*, **59**, 1313–20.

Tolmie, J.L., McNay, M., Stephenson, J.B., Doyle, D. & Connor, J.M. (1987). Microcephaly: genetic counselling and antenatal diagnosis after the birth of an affected child. *Am. J. Med. Genet.*, **27**, 583–94.

Trommsdorff, M., Gotthardt, M., Hiesberger, T. et al. (1999). Reeler/Disabled-like disruption of neuronal migration in knockout mice lacking the VLDL receptor and ApoE receptor 2. *Cell*, **97**, 689–701.

Valanne, L., Pihko, H., Katevuo, K., Karttunen, P., Somer, H. & Santavuori, P. (1994). MRI of the brain in muscle–eye–brain (MEB) disease. *Neuroradiology*, **36**, 473–6.

van der Knaap, M.S. & Valk, J. (1988). Classification of congenital abnormalities of the CNS. *Am. J. Neuroradiol.*, **9**, 315–26.

van der Knaap, M.S., Smit, L.M., Barth, P.G. et al. (1997). Magnetic resonance imaging in classification of congenital muscular dystrophies with brain abnormalities. *Ann. Neurol.*, **42**, 50–9.

Vinters, H.V., Fisher, R.S., Cornford, M.E. et al. (1992). Morphological substrates of infantile spasms: studies based on surgically resected cerebral tissue. *Childs Nerv. Syst.*, **8**, 8–17.

Vital, A., Marchal, C., Loiseau, H. et al. (1994). Glial and neuronoglial malformative lesions associated with medically intractable epilepsy. *Acta Neuropathol. (Berl.)*, **87**, 196–201.

Wallis, D.E., Roessler, E., Hehr, U. et al. (1999). Mutations in the homeodomain of the human *SIX3* gene cause holoprosencephaly. *Nat. Genet.*, **22**, 196–8.

Walsh, C.A. (1999). Genetic malformations of the human cerebral cortex. *Neuron*, **23**, 19–29.

Walsh, C. & Cepko, C.L. (1992). Widespread dispersion of neuronal clones across functional regions of the cerebral cortex. *Science*, **255**, 434–40.

Williams, R.S., Ferrante, R.J. & Caviness, V.S., Jr. (1976). The cellular pathology of microgyria. A Golgi analysis. *Acta Neuropathol. (Berl.)*, **36**, 269–83.

Williams, R.S., Swisher, C.N., Jennings, M., Ambler, M. & Caviness, V.S., Jr. (1984). Cerebro-ocular dysgenesis (Walker–Warburg syndrome): neuropathologic and etiologic analysis. *Neurology*, **34**, 1531–41.

Wolf, H.K., Zentner, J., Hufnagel, A. et al. (1993). Surgical pathology of chronic epileptic seizure disorders: experience with 63 specimens from extratemporal corticectomies, lobectomies and functional hemispherectomies. *Acta Neuropathol. (Berl.)*, **86**, 466–72.

Yagishita, A., Arai, N., Maehara, T., Shimizu, H., Tokumaru, A.M. & Oda, M. (1997). Focal cortical dysplasia: appearance on MR images. *Radiology*, **203**, 553–9.

Yakovlev, P.I. & Wadsworth, R.C. (1946a). Schizencephalies. A study of the congenital clefts in the cerebral mantle. I. Clefts with fused lips. *J. Neuropathol. Exp. Neurol.*, **5**, 116–30.

Yakovlev, P.I. & Wadsworth, R.C. (1946b). Schizencephalies. A study of the congenital clefts in the cerebral mantle. II. Clefts with hydrocephalus and lips separated. *J. Neuropathol. Exp. Neurol.*, **5**, 169–206.

Yamamoto, T., Toyoda, C., Kobayashi, M., Kondo, E., Saito, K. & Osawa, M. (1997). Pial–glial barrier abnormalities in fetuses with Fukuyama congenital muscular dystrophy. *Brain Dev.*, **19**, 35–42.

14

The aging brain: morphology, imaging and function

Marilyn S. Albert[1] and Guy M. McKhann[2]

[1]Department of Psychiatry and Neurology, Harvard Medical School, Boston, MA, USA
[2]Department of Neurology, Johns Hopkins School of Medicine, Baltimore, MD, USA

Not too many years ago, the concept by both physicians and the general public was that your brain deteriorated as you got older. It was believed that, with aging, the brain shrank, there was significant drop out of nerve cells throughout the brain, and that once lost, those cells could not be replaced. In addition, at a subcellular level, data suggested that synaptic contacts markedly decreased. Moreover, it was thought that these changes began among individuals in young adulthood and progressed inexorably across the adult life span. As we will emphasize, among individuals who are optimally healthy these previously held concepts are wrong. The information that allows us to draw this conclusion is based on modern technologies for studying postmortem tissue, imaging the living brain, careful cognitive evaluations, and the innovative use of animal models.

Methodologic and technical issues

Focus on optimally healthy older individuals

One of the major changes to occur in the study of brain–behaviour relationships in aging is the focus on optimally healthy participants. This permits one to differentiate changes related to disease from those related to age. Among human subjects, this requires careful exclusion of subjects in the early stages of dementia. However, many medical diseases are common in older individuals (e.g. hypertension, respiratory or cardiac disease, vitamin deficiency), all of which may impair intellectual function. Ideally, if one wants to study healthy individuals, these disorders should be excluded as well. Subjects selected without evidence of clinical disease will differ greatly from a group of older persons that is chosen at random from a population, containing many individuals with serious medical illness. Some of these illnesses will include those with considerable impact on cognitive function, such as Alzheimer's disease (Odenheimer et al., 1994). Thus, optimally healthy individuals, although non-representative, can be of heuristic value, and may ultimately make it easier to identify interventions that can minimize age-related cognitive change.

Inter-individual differences and aging

In recent years, when researchers have focused their attention on animal models and human studies of aging, it has become clear that, even among optimally healthy subjects, there is considerable variability in both cognitive and physical abilities. Within a group of healthy older individuals, there are invariably individuals whose brain structure and function appears similar to that of persons many decades younger than themselves. Thus, the general statements about age-related changes in function apply to the changes for the average individual in the group, but cannot be said to apply to all individuals. For example, as shown in Fig. 14.1, the ability to recall information after reading a paragraph is better on average in younger subjects than in older ones; however, many older individuals perform just as well as their younger colleagues. The cause of this inter-individual difference is an area of intense interest, as it suggests that there may be ways of reducing change among a larger number of older persons.

Approaches to studying aging populations

In general, there are two approaches to the study of aging populations. The most commonly used, and certainly the easiest, is the cross-sectional approach. In this method, a group of younger people is compared to a group of older people at a particular point in time. The problem is that

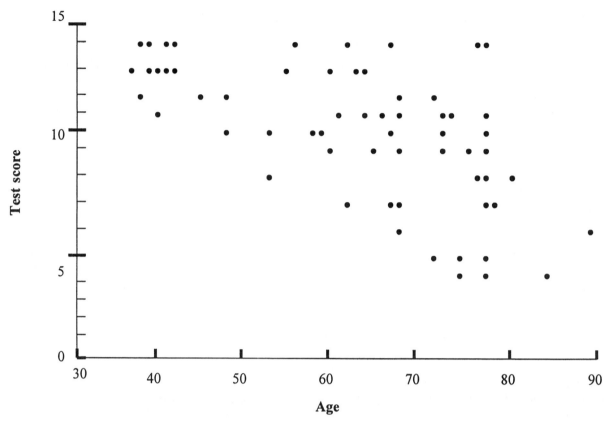

Fig. 14.1. Test scores by optimally healthy subjects 30–80 years of age on recall of a lengthy paragraph. Subjects were selected so that the level of education is not significantly different across the decades. Each dot represents the score of an individual subject.

humans born and raised at different time points have experienced different life events that can have long-term consequences on them. For example, individuals born in the 1920s to 1930s typically constitute the aging subjects in any current cross-sectional study of aging, and those born and raised in the 1970s to 1980s would constitute the sample of young adult subjects. During the 70+-year period from the 1920s, countless improvements in health care have taken place that have resulted in a dramatic change in the average human. For example, the improvements in prenatal care, postnatal care, nutrition and antibiotics have resulted in a population of young adults that not only are taller and heavier in body weight than their grandparents or great-grandparents but who also have bigger brains.

In addition, major worldwide events that have taken place at particular time points in history have had profound impacts on particular segments of a cohort. For example, large numbers of males were killed at relatively young ages by various wars. At the time of these wars, the screening process for determining who was potentially placed at greatest risk was not always socioeconomically or socioeducationally unbiased, suggesting that the remain-

ing population of males, in particular, may have been biased by this selection process.

Longitudinal studies are designed to reduce these secular trends. While such studies must overcome the difficulties associated with the loss of subjects due to drop out, they nonetheless provide us with greater insights into the direct affects of age. Longitudinal studies have suggested that age-related declines occur slightly later in the life span than do cross-sectional ones. There is one area, as we will discuss, where longitudinal studies are essential, that is, the definition and establishment of predictive factors of change.

Postmortem examination of carefully screened subjects

Another change that has produced a dramatic revision of our concepts of brain aging derives from new techniques for the study of postmortem tissue. Postmortem examination of well-studied individuals represent the most long-standing method for establishing brain–behaviour relationships. The major technological advance pertains to the development of non-biased stereological techniques, which permit investigators to accurately count neurons within a prescribed volume of tissue. It is this technological advance, combined with careful screening to assure that subjects with evidence of any relevant disease are excluded from examination, that has changed our concepts of the amount and nature of neuronal loss with advancing age, as described below.

Non-invasive imaging techniques

The advent of modern imaging techniques, beginning in about the mid-1970s, provided another major advance in the ability to study aging and structure–function relationships. For the first time it was possible to study the living brain. This was particularly advantageous for the study of aging, because it became possible to examine optimally healthy individuals and determine whether changes in the brain occurred in the absence of clinical disease and, if so, how this related to changes in cognition. These imaging techniques can loosely be divided into two basic types, structural scans and functional scans. The structural scans produce highly detailed images of the anatomical features of the brain. In fact, the images produced by the most advanced of these techniques look very similar in detail to that seen on postmortem examination of brain tissue. Examples of this type of structural scan include computerized tomography (CT) and magnetic resonance imaging (MRI). Functional scans, on the other hand, provide an indication of the activity of the brain, but do not tend to produce high anatomical detail. Examples of functional imaging scans include positron emission tomography (PET) and functional MRI (fMRI). When these functional methods are combined with structural scans, as is now commonly done, considerable localization of function is possible. Non-invasive imaging procedures have demonstrated that changes in the brain are, at least in part, responsible for age-related declines in cognition. However, a comprehensive explication of the reasons for these declines has not yet been provided by either the structural imaging procedures currently available, or by the initial functional methods that have been applied to this question, as will be discussed below.

Changes in brain structure and function with age

Neuronal studies

Neuronal number
Recent morphological data in humans (Haug, 1984; Leuba & Garey, 1989; Terry et al., 1987), indicate that, with advancing age, neuronal loss in the cortex is either not significant or not as extensive as reports prior to 1984 had suggested (Brody, 1955, 1970; Colon, 1972; Shefer, 1973; Henderson et al., 1980; Anderson et al., 1983). While large neurons appear to shrink, few are lost (Terry et al., 1987).

There are, in addition, comparable data in monkeys. Minimal neuronal cortical loss with age in monkeys has now been demonstrated in the striate cortex (Vincent et al., 1989), motor cortex (Tigges et al., 1992), frontal cortex (Peters et al., 1994), and the entorhinal cortex (Amaral, 1993). These general conclusions have been reached not only on the basis of a comparison of counts of neurons in young (5 to 6 years) and old (over 25 years of age) monkeys but also on the basis of an examination of the cortical tissue by electron microscopy (Peters et al., 1994). Beyond an accumulation of lipofuscin granules in the cell body of some neurons and some cellular debris in neuroglial cells, there is very little evidence of changes with age in the neurons of these cortical regions (Peters et al., 1991).

Given the intense interest in age-related changes in memory, it is important to emphasize that the weight of the evidence from postmortem studies supports the conclusion that the hippocampus also shows minimal structural change with advancing age. The postmortem data in humans and monkeys indicate that neuronal loss is surprisingly low in most subfields of the hippocampus. For example, the subiculum shows a significant age-related loss in humans, with a similar trend in monkeys, however, the CA1, CA2 and CA3 subfields of the hippocampus show no evidence of age-related neuronal loss (Amaral, 1993; Rosene, 1993; West et al., 1994; Gomez-Isla et al., 1996). Equivalent data have recently been reported in rodents, where it was shown that even in the subset of animals with declines on a memory task, there was no decrease in the number of neurons in the various hippocampal subfields (Rapp & Gallagher, 1996). (See Morrison & Hof, 1997, for a more detailed discussion of these issues.)

Neuronal loss and neurotransmitter changes
There is substantial neuronal loss in selected subcortical regions that is likely responsible for decreases in the production of neurotransmitters important for cognitive function, such as in the basal forebrain and the locus coeruleus (e.g. Chan-Palay & Asan, 1989; Rosene, 1993). For example, in humans and monkeys there is approximately a 50% neuronal loss with age in the basal forebrain and 35–40% loss in the locus coeruleus and dorsal raphe (Kemper, 1993). This compares with an approximate loss of 5% in the CA1 subfield of the hippocampus. The neuronal loss in these subcortical nuclei may be very important for memory function, as these brain regions influence the

production of several neurotransmitters important for memory (such as acetylcholine and serotonin). Though subcortical, these nuclei have extensive connections with the cortex, and thus are responsible for the level of many neurotransmitters within the cortex.

It should also be noted that there are alterations in at least one receptor type (i.e. NMDA receptors) within the hippocampus that play an important role in cognitive change, particularly in memory function (Gazzaley et al., 1996; Barnes et al., 1977).

Synaptic integrity

Even though there does not appear to be enough neuronal loss to account for age-related cognitive change, there could be changes in other aspects of neuronal function, specifically the number and/or function of synapses. Most of the studies that have explored this question with respect to aging pertain to learning and memory in rodents. Modern theories of memory mechanisms imply changing strengths of connections between neurons, based on activity-dependent synaptic plasticity in particular regions of the brain (Martin et al., 2000). It has been demonstrated that there are synaptic changes in the CA3 region of the hippocampus when one compares older rodents who are memory-impaired to younger rodents (Smith et al., 2000). Specifically, older rodents with spatial learning deficits display significant reductions in synaptophysin immunoreactivity in the CA3 region of the hippocampus, but not in other subfields. This region receives its input from layer II of the entorhinal cortex. Thus, it has been hypothesized that there are circuit-specific changes involving the entorhinal input to CA3 that influence the computational function of the hippocampus and are thereby related to age-related memory change (Smith et al., 2000). This hypothesis is consistent with electrophysiological alterations in aged rodents with learning deficits (Barnes et al., 1997; Tanila et al., 1977). Though comparable studies are not possible in humans, these results suggest that the variability seen in memory changes with advancing age among healthy individuals might be related to variations in synaptic integrity in specific brain circuits related to learning and memory.

Neuronal proliferation in the adult brain

One of the most strongly held dogmas of neurobiology was the concept that once nerve cells were formed they could only die. There was no such thing as endogenous neuronal replacement. There is increasing evidence that that concept is incorrect. The work of Altman over 30 years ago suggested that, in the rodent, neurogenesis could continue in selected regions of the brain into adulthood, particularly in the dentate region of the hippocampus, the olfactory system and cerebellum (Altman & Das, 1965). In recent years, this issue has been revisited in rodents and there is ample evidence, based on the DNA marker, bromodeoxyuridine, that neurogenesis occurs in the hippocampus and olfactory system. Similar findings have also been demonstrated in old world monkeys (Kornack & Rakic, 1999; Gould et al., 1999), and even in the human (Eriksson et al., 1998).

In the dentate gyrus of the macaque monkey, labelled cells are thought to proliferate in the border zone between the hilus and granular cell layer, and then to migrate and differentiate in the granule cell layer. The proliferation of new neurons decreases with age. In the rodent there appears to be a gradual increase in total numbers of neurons; in primates, such an accumulation is less certain. It has been suggested (Kornack & Rakic, 1999) that the number of neurons in the hippocampus is constant, but with a fixed replacement rate: neurogenesis balanced by the rate of apoptosis and cell removal. They even invoke the intriguing analogy of neurons being replaced 'like successive rows of shark teeth'.

The source of these new neurons may be pluripotential stem cells or neural progeniture cells. In the rodent it has been shown that physical activity stimulates this neurogenesis from stem cells (Kemperman et al., 2000). Investigators are exploring ways to cause these cells to produce new neurons. This is an active area of research in neuroregeneration.

White matter changes

In addition, age-related alterations in the white matter have recently been described in some detail (Peters et al., 1994; Peters, 1996; Neilson & Peters, 2000). At first glance, the data suggesting loss of white matter in the brain without a loss of grey matter can be difficult to understand. Conventional knowledge suggests that white matter consists of the axons of neurons and that if there is a loss of axons, there should be cell death and a loss of grey matter. However, the white matter of the brain is also composed of a number of glial elements, particularly oligodendrocytes. Evidence from the non-human primate suggests that the oligodendrocytes, that are responsible for forming the myelin sheath surrounding the axons, may be less efficient with age. For example, when the oligodendrocytes of old and young monkeys were compared (Peters, 1996) it was found that the myelin sheaths in the old monkeys were abnormal and appeared to be degenerating. However, when the number of axons in old and young monkeys was compared by the same investigators (Nielsen & Peters, 2000) relatively few degenerating axons were found in the

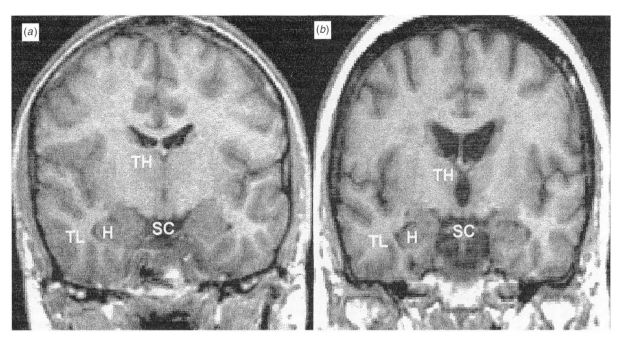

Fig. 14.2. An example of a structural MRI (*a*) in a healthy young and (*b*) healthy older individual. H = hippocampus, TH = thalamus, SC = suprasellar cistern

old monkeys. Taken together, these findings suggest changes in myelin, rather than axonal loss, are at least in part responsible for age-related changes in white matter observed with advancing age.

Imaging studies

Structural imaging

The first striking finding to emerge from computerized tomography (CT) studies of healthy adults across the age range was that there is clear evidence of decreases in the amount of brain tissue in older individuals compared with younger ones, i.e. atrophy. In general, CT studies have concluded that the average individual above 55 to 65 years of age demonstrates brain atrophy and increasing amounts of atrophy are seen as people get older. Thus, as people get older, the volume of CSF within the ventricles increases and the volume of brain tissue decreases (Roberts & Caird, 1976; Hughes & Gado, 1981; Barrow et al., 1976; Brinkman et al., 1981; de Leon et al., 1989; Gado et al., 1982, 1983; Huckman et al., 1975; Kaszniak et al., 1979; Stafford et al., 1988; Zatz et al., 1982).

CT studies conducted in the same individuals over time have demonstrated this phenomenon as well. Longitudinal evaluation over a 1-year period (Gado et al., 1983) and a 3-year period (e.g. de Leon et al., 1989) have

demonstrated an approximate rate of atrophy of 2% per year among healthy older individuals over the age of 64. This rate of change is relatively low compared to the 9% rate of atrophy seen in the brains of patients with Alzheimer's disease (de Leon et al., 1989).

MRI studies of healthy adults across the age range have confirmed the findings described above for CT. That is, regardless of the sequence type, overall brain volume shows a decrease with age, while the amount of CSF increases, even if individuals are healthy (Christiansen et al., 1994; Coffey et al., 1992; Harris et al., 1994; Jernigan et al., 1990, 1991; Lim et al., 1992; Murphy et al., 1992; Matsumae et al., 1996; Pfefferbaum et al., 1994; Tanna et al., 1991).

Visual examination of an MRI image from a healthy young and older individual exemplifies some of the changes described above. Figure 14.2 shows an MRI image, taken at approximately the same anatomical level, in a healthy, young adult (see Fig. 14.2(*a*)) and a healthy, older adult (see Fig. 14.2(*b*)). As can be seen, the general shape and size of the bone around the brain is nearly equal in both subjects. However, the image on the right appears to have less tissue than the image on the left. The cavities within the brain that contain CSF are also larger in the older individual than in the young. The largest CSF spaces in the brain, the lateral and third ventricles, clearly appear larger in the older person, but it is more difficult to determine visually whether the lower portion of the lateral ventricle (known as the 'inferior horn of the lateral ventricle') is enlarged. In addition, sulci on the cortical surface appear to be more spread apart in the older than in the younger subject. The space between the temporal lobes (i.e. the supracellar cistern, [SC]) also appears to be wider in the older person than the young.

However, the grey matter of the brain does not appear to be as changed as the CSF spaces. The ribbon of grey matter forming the outer surface of the cortex appears as thick in the older subject as it does in the young. The hippocampal formation (H) is of nearly equal size in the two subjects. The deep grey matter structures, such as the thalamus (TH), also appear to be of approximately equivalent size in the two individuals. Close inspection of the images suggests that the white matter of the brain may be changed in the older person. Overall, there appears to be less white matter in the older individual than in the young, however, this is difficult to assess convincingly with visual inspection.

Functional imaging

One of the most important innovations for the study of brain–behaviour relationships has been the development of functional imaging, using PET and fMRI. In PET scanning, a radioactive isotope is either injected or inhaled by the subject, and the scanning machine evaluates the differential decay of radioactivity in order to assess regional changes in blood flow in the brain. The blood flow is considered a surrogate for neuronal activity. Likewise, fMRI uses the magnetic qualities of water molecules to evaluate the differential distribution of oxygenated blood in the brain, and the ratio of oxygenated to deoxygenated blood is thought to be an indirect measure of neuronal activity.

To obtain information about how the brain performs cognitive tasks, these imaging techniques are combined with cognitive paradigms, which produce a range of brain activations. Through careful design of such paradigms, it becomes possible to obtain information about the brain regions that are involved in a specific cognitive activity. Perceptual and emotional experience can also be interrogated in a similar manner. When such functional imaging procedures are combined with structural imaging, one can obtain data with highly accurate anatomical detail.

Positron emission tomography

Most PET studies that have included older individuals have focused on the examination of memory changes with age. Due to the technological limitations of PET, these studies have generally focused on either the encoding or the retrieval phase of memory.

The most important general concept to emerge from such studies is that multiple brain regions are essential for encoding or retrieving new information. Moreover, some of the brain regions that appear to be integral to 'memory networks' have not been easy to evaluate by other imaging modalities. The most important in this regard is the frontal lobes, which are activated during both encoding and retrieval in normal young individuals (Kapur et al., 1994, 1996; Demb et al., 1995; Fletcher et al., 1995; Wagner et al., 1998a; Madden et al., 1999; Buckner et al., 1999).

The hippocampus, known to be essential for normal memory based primarily on lesion studies (Squire et al., 1988), is more difficult to activate than many other brain regions, for reasons that are not entirely clear. Nevertheless, many recent PET studies have shown that significant activations of the hippocampus may be demonstrated when an individual is attempting to learn or retrieve new information. The parahippocampal gyrus, a cortical region adjacent to the hippocampus, is also frequently activated in cognitive paradigms focused on explicit memory (Schacter & Wagner, 1999; Gabrielli et al., 1997; Brewer et al., 1998; Martin et al., 1997; Stern et al., 1996; Wagner et al., 1998a), as is the prefrontal cortex (e.g. Haxby et al., 1996; Wagner et al., 1998b).

The most consistent finding to emerge from PET studies of aging is that there are alterations in the activation of the frontal lobes during encoding and/or retrieval of new information, (e.g. Cabeza et al., 1997, 2000; Hazlett et al., 1998; Grady et al., 1999), although the specific nature of these age-related differences remains to be clarified. Some have found increased activity, while others have found decreases. However, the nature of the activation paradigms have differed considerably among these studies, no doubt contributing to the differential findings.

There has been even less agreement about age-related changes in the hippocampus. For example, a PET study in which young subjects demonstrated significant hippocampal and prefrontal activation during an encoding task failed to produce similar activations in the elderly (Grady et al., 1995). Conversely, a PET study that examined subjects during a recall task reported similar activations in the hippocampus and/or parahippocampal gyrus in both young and elderly subjects, but substantial differences between the age groups in other brain regions, particularly the frontal lobes (Schacter et al., 1996). Differences between the cognitive paradigms in the two studies, particularly in the degree to which the subjects learned the to-be-remembered material, are the most likely cause of these discrepancies.

Functional magnetic resonance imaging

Since fMRI does not involve exposure to radioactivity, and measurements are closer to real time, many investigators who previously employed PET are turning to fMRI. Though few such studies have been published, a number have been reported at meetings. They concur with the PET studies in finding altered prefrontal activity during encoding, mentioned above. Most of these fMRI studies have demonstrated decreased activation of the prefrontal lobe when older individuals are trying to learn new information (e.g. Sperling et al., 1999, Logan et al., 2002). It has been hypothesized that the differences in prefrontal activation between the young and the elderly subjects may reflect the fact that the two age groups use differing strategies to perform the task (e.g. Cabeza et al., 1997; Grady et al., 1999). This is consistent with numerous reports showing that elderly individuals are less likely to spontaneously use mnemonic strategies than the young, when trying to learn new information (for reviews see Craik, 1977; Arenberg & Robertson-Tchabo, 1977). An alternate possibility is that the same strategy is being applied in different ways by the two age groups.

Increased activation in the elderly compared with the young has also been demonstrated. For example, in tasks where the stimuli to-be-remembered are visual in nature, older individuals have shown greater activity than the young in the parietal cortex (one of the brain regions involved with spatial organization) (Bates et al., submitted; Sperling et al., 1999). This may also be a reflection of the differential deployment of cognitive strategies during the task, as mentioned above.

It should also be noted that some investigators have reported differences between the young and the elderly in hemodynamic response (D'Esposito et al., 1999; Ross et al., 1997; Taoka et al., 1998). While the nature of these changes is still controversial, ranging from the possibility of decreased hemodynamic response (and therefore signal change) in the elderly, to increased noise with no absolute reduction in the magnitude of signal change, it is clearly possible that these differences are, at least in part, responsible for some of the fMRI differences between healthy young and older individuals. It is, however, reasonable to hypothesize that, if such underlying hemodynamic changes exist, they might affect the ability to remember new information.

Domains of cognitive function

Although one could fractionate cognitive function into an almost unlimited number of components, most investigators in the field of neuropsychology view higher cortical function as composed of a relatively small number of major categories. For the purposes of this chapter, we will discuss changes in cognitive function with age within the following domains: (i) attention, (ii) memory, (iii) executive function, (iv) language, (v) visuospatial processing, and (vi) general intelligence.

Memory performance and aging

Workers in the field of memory have accepted the conclusion that memory is not a unitary phenomenon, and most models of memory function hypothesize that memory consists of a series of specific yet interactive stores (e.g. Waugh & Norman, 1965; Tulving, 1972). They include, at a minimum: sensory memory, primary memory, and secondary memory. In addition, a distinction has been made between information that is consciously learned (called explicit or declarative memory) and information that is acquired over time, unrelated to specific conscious effort of episodes (called implicit or procedural memory) (Reber & Squire, 1994).

Sensory memory

Sensory memory, also called registration, represents the earliest stage of information processing. It is modality specific (i.e. visual, auditory, tactile), highly unstable, and characterized by rapid decay.

Primary memory

The component of the memory system referred to as primary memory (or alternatively, immediate memory or short term memory) permits one to hold spans of auditory and/or visual information for relatively long periods of time by active rehearsal. The ability to concentrate on, rehearse, and recall a span of digits, words or visual features is perhaps the best example of this capacity. Any disruption to the rehearsal process results in the information being lost from immediate memory. Experiments by Petersen and Petersen (1959) have demonstrated that normal subjects forget a significant proportion of new information in less than 1 minute when distractions are present. The amount of information that immediate memory can store is limited to about five to seven items, as mentioned earlier. There is not complete consensus among neuropsychologists and memory researchers as to whether immediate memory should be considered a form of memory at all. Primary or immediate memory, as described here, may rely more on attentional skills. Thus, Spitz (1972), among others, has argued that digit span forward is actually a measure of attention rather than of memory.

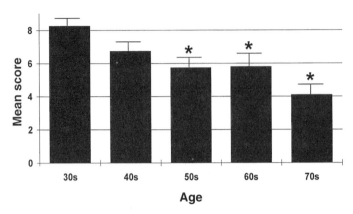

Fig. 14.3. Delayed recall performance of healthy subjects 30 to 80 years old. The subjects are asked to report what they remember of two lengthy paragraphs after a 15-minute delay.

Secondary memory

Secondary memory (also referred to as long-term memory) is involved when information must be retained over a long period of time. Thus, information from immediate memory must be assembled into multimodal units to be placed in storage. Storage of information by the memory system appears to take place differentially. As early as 1949, Hebb postulated that two processes were necessary for the brain to retain information. The first process, analogous to what we have termed primary memory, required the continual reverberation of a neural circuit. The second process, equivalent to secondary memory, required an actual structural change in the neural pattern of the central nervous system.

Sensory memory and age

There is considerable information to indicate that changes in explicit sensory memory are minimal with age. For example, the time necessary to identify a single letter does not change significantly between the late teens and early 70s. When seven-letter strings are used, the rate of letter identification increases with age by a factor of 1.3 (Cerella et al., 1982). These and other data indicate that there is a minimal decline in sensory memory with age (see Craik, 1977; for detailed review, see Poon, 1985).

Primary memory and age

Primary explicit memory also shows little decline with age. Most studies report no significant age differences in digit span forward (Drachman & Leavitt, 1972), no age differences in word span (Talland, 1967), and only moderate differences in letter span (Botwinick & Storandt, 1974). Older subjects show as much of a recency effect (i.e.

retrieval of the last few items on a list in a word list learning task) as younger subjects (Raymond, 1971).

Secondary memory and age

However, there are substantial changes in explicit secondary memory, in contrast to the minimal age changes in sensory and primary memory (for a review, see Craik, 1977; Poon, 1985). The age at which changes in secondary memory occur depends upon the methods that are used to test the memory store. Difficult explicit memory tasks (e.g. delayed recall) demonstrate statistically significant differences by subjects in their 50s, in comparison to younger individuals (Albert et al., 1987a). Age decrements are greater on recall than recognition tasks. This is true whether words or pictures are used. Cueing during encoding or retrieval also alters the appearance of an age decline. Cueing at both encoding and retrieval produces the smallest age differences, whereas no cueing at either stage of the task maximizes age differences (Craik et al., 1987). However, even with cued recall and recognition, there are often declines. Rabinowitz (1986) reported a 33% age-related decrement in cued recall, and an 11% age-related decrement in recognition, when comparing young and old subjects (mean age 19 vs. 68).

Figure 14.3 shows the performance of subjects across the age range on delayed recall of two lengthy paragraphs. That is, each subject read two lengthy paragraphs and, immediately after hearing each one, and then again after 20 min, the subject is asked to state what he/she can recall of the paragraphs.

A close examination of these data indicates that the older individuals are not more rapidly forgetting what they learned, but rather they are taking longer to learn the new information. For example, if one compares the difference between immediate and delayed recall over the lifespan, there are no statistically significant age differences (Petersen et al., 1992). Thus, if one allows older subjects to learn material well (i.e. to the point where few errors are made), they do not forget what they have learned more rapidly than the young (see Fig. 14.3). However, if older subjects are not given the ability to learn material to the same level of proficiency as younger individuals, after a delay, less information will be retained by the average older person.

However, there is considerable variability among older subjects on tasks of this sort. There are many healthy older subjects who have test scores that overlap those of subjects many years younger than themselves, e.g. about one-third of healthy 70-year-old humans have delayed recall scores that overlap those of 30-year-olds (equated for education).

Executive function

The complex set of abilities sometimes referred to as 'executive functions' include: concurrent manipulation of information (e.g. cognitive flexibility), concept formation and cue-directed behaviour. The wide variety of abilities that are sometimes included under the term 'executive function' is therefore striking.

Tests evaluating concept formation and set shifting uniformly show significant changes with age, primarily when subjects are in their late 60s or 70s. For example, the similarities subtest of the Wechsler Adult Intelligence Scale (WAIS), which asks subjects to identify how two objects (e.g. a table and a chair) are similar to each other, is the subtest on the Verbal scale of the WAIS that shows the greatest decline with age (Heaton et al., 1986). Education appears to be a modifier of this decline, in that subjects with lower amounts of education demonstrate declines at younger ages, however, all subjects in the oldest group (mean age 68 years), regardless of educational level, show significant declines in performance.

Series completion tests also show substantial age declines. These tests generally require the subject to examine a series of letters or numbers and determine the rule that governed the sequencing of the items in the series. Cross-sectional and longitudinal data demonstrate age-related declines on tasks of this sort (e.g. Lachman & Jelalian, 1984; Schaie, 1983).

Proverb interpretation tests, which require the subject to provide the general meaning of a proverb (e.g. 'barking dogs seldom bite'), also demonstrate age-related declines (Albert et al., 1990). This is true whether or not subjects are asked to provide the meaning of the proverb themselves or are given alternate choices among which to choose. Similarly, set shifting tasks, such as the visual–verbal test (in which subjects are asked to look at a series of cards and indicate how three of the four objects on each card are alike in one way, and then how three of the objects are alike in another way), also show substantial age-related declines. These changes appear to be related to the fact that older subjects have difficulty switching from one abstract answer to another (i.e. they tend to get the first item in the set correct but the second one wrong). Slowness in establishing mental set (i.e. getting the first item in the set wrong but the second one right) and failure to establish set (i.e. getting both items in the set wrong) did not increase differentially with age (Albert et al., 1990).

Visuospatial function

Visuospatial function is characterized by the ability to produce, and recognize figures and to form relationships among spatial locations. Specific visual functions include the ability to recognize familiar faces, the ability to copy or match objects or pictures, and the ability to translate spatial elements from one mode to another. Translation of mirror image spatial arrangements into self-oriented positions is an example of a task that requires intact and efficient visuospatial abilities.

Visuospatial ability therefore can be assessed by (i) constructional tasks, such as the assembly of blocks, sticks or puzzles; (ii) drawing tasks that involve copying; or (iii) matching tasks that require the subject to identify pictures with similar elements.

The most complex three-dimensional construction task in common use is the block design subtest of the WAIS. The subject is presented with a two-dimensional drawing in red and white of a target design, and a set of blocks (some sides of the blocks are all red, some are all white, and some are half red and half white). The subject is asked to arrange the blocks, which are, of course, three dimensional, so that they mimic the two-dimensional design. To receive credit, the subject must assemble the blocks correctly within a specified time limit. This task shows substantial declines with age (Doppelt & Wallace, 1955), perhaps because it is a timed task, and involves perception of three-dimensional space (see below) as well as a shifting and monitoring of behaviour.

Performance on figure drawing tasks is also affected by age. Older subjects are impaired, in comparison to the young, in depicting and perceiving three-dimensional drawings. Plude et al., (1986) asked a group of young and old adults (mean ages 21 and 67, respectively, and equated for static visual acuity) to draw a cube to command. The cubes were then rated by ten independent raters, with an interrater reliability of 0.98. The drawings of the young adults were rated as significantly better than those of the old. The older subjects were also less accurate than the young in judging the adequacy of drawings of cubes that were distorted to varying degrees. The elderly were less accurate than the young in discriminating between distorted and undistorted cubes. They were, however, equally able to copy a cube when landmarks were provided regarding the size of the lines. Comparable reports of the depiction and perception of two-dimensional drawings are not available.

Language

Linguistic ability is thought to encompass at least four domains: phonological, lexical, syntactic and semantic. It was previously assumed that linguistic ability is preserved into very old age, primarily because performance on the vocabulary subtest of the WAIS, the best general estimate of verbal intelligence, is well maintained until individuals are in their 80s (Schaie, 1983). However, within the last decade, a number of studies have shown that some aspects of linguistic knowledge decline with age, although not until relatively late in the lifespan (i.e. >70).

Phonology

Phonologic knowledge refers to the use of the sounds of language and the rules for their combination. Phonologic capabilities are well preserved with age (Bayles & Kaszniak, 1987).

Lexicon

Psycholinguists distinguish between the lexical representation of a word, i.e. the name of an item, and its semantic representation, i.e. the meaning of a word (Clark & Clark, 1977). The lexicon of healthy older individuals appears to be intact, as are the semantic relationships of the lexicon.

Syntax

Syntactic knowledge refers to the ability to meaningfully combine words. A large number of studies have shown that age has little effect on syntax. Obler et al., (1985) found that syntactic forms that were difficult for older individuals were also difficult for younger ones.

Semantic knowledge

Older individuals appear to have difficulty with the semantic aspects of word retrieval. Several groups of investigators have reported that scores on a test of confrontation naming decrease with age (Borod et al., 1980; LaBarge et al., 1986; Albert et al., 1987b). However, declines in naming ability do not become statistically significant until subjects are in their 70s (Albert et al., 1987b). When subjects could not correctly name an item, the most common error they committed was semantic in nature, i.e. they produced semantically related associates, circumlocutions, and nominalizations. The nature of these semantic errors suggests that older individuals have a great deal of knowledge about the target word. For example, a semantically related associate ('dice' for 'dominoes') can only be produced if the subject apprehends the general category associated with the stimulus item.

Verbal fluency also assesses semantic ability. In a verbal fluency task a subject is asked to name as many examples of a category (e.g. animals or vegetables) as possible in specified period of time (e.g. 1 min) or as many words beginning with a particular letter (e.g. F) within a specified period of time. Several studies report a decline in verbal fluency with age (Obler et al., 1985; Albert et al., 1987b). These changes also occur relatively late in the life span (>70). Thus, semantic linguistic ability appears to change with advancing age, while other aspects of linguistic ability are relatively well preserved.

General intelligence

Although intelligence tests measure most of the abilities previously discussed, they do so in a complex way. Intelligence tests were designed to predict with a reasonable degree of certainty how a person would function in an academic environment, not to provide a complete assessment of cognitive function. Thus, intelligence tests do not assess all aspects of cognitive ability. For example, the Wechsler Adult Intelligence Scale does not include an evaluation of memory. In addition, IQ tests do not assess cognitive abilities in relative isolation from one another. Many of the tasks require a complex interaction of abilities and often depend upon speed for an adequate level of performance. Nevertheless, intelligence testing has been one of the most widely explored topics in the psychology of aging.

There is widespread agreement that there are changes in intelligence test performance with age. There has, however, been considerable debate about the point at which declines occur and the magnitude of the declines. The age at which declines are observed appears to depend upon the methodology employed. There is some consensus that relatively little decline in performance occurs prior to the time that people are in their 50s (Schaie & Labouvie-Vief, 1974). After this age, results differ depending upon whether cross-sectional or longitudinal testing designs were employed. The cross-sectional method shows declines of 1 SD or more beginning about age 60 (Doppelt & Wallace, 1955; Schaie, 1983), over the age of 70 scores drop sharply. The longitudinal method shows declines beginning in the late 60s. Both methods find substantial declines after individuals are in their mid-70s. Thus, the major difference between cross-sectional and longitudinal investigations is observed between subjects in their late 50s and early 60s. In this age range, the cross-sectional method shows greater age declines than the longitudinal method.

Summary

In summary, changes in cognitive function with age occur only in specific domains and in specific components of these domains, as indicated in Table 14.1.

Table 14.1. Cognitive changes with age

Domain	No change	Change	Age range
Memory			
sensory memory	*		
primary explicit memory	*		
secondary explicit memory		*	50s and over
Executive function		*	60s–70s
Visuospatial ability		*	60s and over
Language			
phonology	*		
lexicon	*		
syntax	*		
semantic knowledge		*	70s
General intelligence		*	60s–70s

Prediction of future cognitive status

Maintenance of cognitive function

As the aging population grows, there is increasing interest in maintaining cognitive function at its maximum. One of the major studies that sought to answer this question followed approximately 1000 participants who were 70 to 80 when the study began. These individuals had been selected because they fell within the top third of the population in terms of both physical and mental function (Berkman et al., 1993). Over time (i.e. 5–10 years), some of these individuals maintained their high level of cognitive performance and others declined. Thus, it was possible to determine what behaviours differentiated these two groups. Those who maintained cognitive function had higher levels of education, physical activity, lung function, and feelings of self-efficacy (Albert et al., 1995). It is hypothesized that each of these four variables directly influence the status of the brain and thereby, cumulatively, influence maintenance of cognition.

Prediction of decline in cognitive function

The concern of many older people, when they are unable to find their car keys or blank on attempting to recall a name, is that they have the first indication of a serious and progressive problem with memory. Thus, the ability to predict who has the expected cognitive changes with age, and who may go on to Alzheimer's disease or some other dementing process, it of utmost importance. Studies to

answer this question have also employed a longitudinal approach, using data from baseline to predict subsequent outcomes. This baseline information has included cognitive performance, imaging and genetics (Albert et al., 2001a). Some of these studies compare those without significant memory complaints with those with mild memory complaints. Over time, some in each category may progress or 'convert' to the clinical symptoms of dementia. Predictions are based on comparing the baseline characteristics of the Converters with the non-Converters and with those who continue to have memory problems but do not have evidence of dementia. The cognitive measures that are predictive of conversion are tests of memory and executive function (Albert et al., 2001b). The imaging measures that are useful in this regard include volumetric measures of the entorhinal cortex, the anterior cingulate, and the hippocampus (Killiany et al., 2000), and perfusion measures of hippocampal-amygdaloid complex, the posterior cingulate and related structures (Johnson et al., 1998).

Another approach has been to compare individuals with a genetic risk for AD, based on their apolipoprotein E status (see Chapter 17), and to examine cognitive and imaging differences among them. These studies have not followed individuals to the point where a substantial number have converted to AD, however, they have demonstrated imaging differences, particularly using PET scanning, in posterior cingulate and superior parietal regions (Small et al., 1995; Reiman et al., 1996).

Based on these preliminary observations, it is likely that predictive paradigms for who will and who will not convert to dementia will be developed and validated. Such paradigms will be useful not only clinically, but in the design of intervention studies.

References

Albert, M., Duffy, F. & Naeser, M. (1987a). Non-linear changes in cognition with age and neurophysiological correlates. *Canad. J. Psychol.*, **41**, 141–57.

Albert, M., Heller, H. & Milberg, W. (1987b). Changes in naming ability with age. *Psychol. Aging*, **41**, 141–57.

Albert, M., Wolfe, J. & Lafleche, G. (1990). Differences in abstraction ability with age. *Psychol. Aging*, **5**, 94–100.

Albert, M., Jones, K., Savage, C. et al. (1995). Predictors of cognitive change in older persons: MacArthur studies of successful aging. *Psychol. Aging*, **10**, 578–89.

Albert, M., Killiany, R., Johnson, K., Tanzi, R. & Jones, K. (2001a). Preclinical prediction of AD: Relation between neuropsychological and neuroimaging findings. In *Alzheimer's Disease: Advances in Etiology, Pathogenesis and Therapeutics*, ed. K. Iqbal, S. Sisodia & B. Winblad, pp. 99–110. London: John Wiley.

Albert, M., Moss, M., Tanzi, R. & Jones, K. (2001b). Preclinical prediction of AD using neuropsychological tests. *J. Int. Neuropsychol. Soc.*, **7**, 631–9.

Altman, J. & Das, G.D. (1965). Autoradiographic and histologic evidence of postnatal hippocampal neurogenesis. *J.Comp. Neurol.*, **124**, 319–36.

Amaral, D. (1993). Morphological analyses of the brains of behaviorally characterized aged nonhuman primates. *Neurobiol. Aging*, **14**, 671–2.

Anderson, J.M., Hubbard, B.M., Coghill, G.R. & Slidders, W. (1983). The effect of advanced old age on the neurone content of the cerebral cortex. Observations with an automatic image analyser point counting method. *J. Neurol. Sci.*, **58**, 233–44.

Arenberg, D. & Robertson-Tchabo, E. (1977). Learning and aging. In *Handbook of the Psychology of Aging*, ed. J. Birren & K. Schaie, pp. 421–49. New York: Van Nostrand Reinhold.

Barnes, C.A., Suster, M.S., Shen, J. & McNaughton, B.L. (1977). Multistability of cognitive maps in the hippocampus of old rats. *Nature*, **388**, 272–5.

Barrow, S. A., Jacobs, L. & Kinkel, W.R. (1976). Changes in size of normal lateral ventricles during aging determined by computerized tomography. *Neurology*, **26**, 1011–13.

Bayles, K. & Kaszniak, A. (1987). *Communication and Cognition in Normal Aging and Dementia*. Boston: Little Brown.

Berkman, L., Seeman, T., Albert, M. et al. (1993). High, usual and impaired functioning in community-dwelling older men and women: findings from the MacArthur foundation network on successful aging. *J. Clin. Epidemiol.*, **46**, 1129–40.

Borod, J., Goodglass, H. & Kaplan, E. (1980). Normative data on the Boston diagnostic aphasia examination, parietal lobe battery, and Boston naming test. *J. Clin. Neuropsychol.*, **2**, 209–15.

Botwinick, J. & Storandt, M. (1974). *Memory, Related Functions and Age*. Springfield, IL: Charles C. Thomas.

Brewer, J., Zhao Z., Desmond, J., Glover, G. & Gabrieli, J. (1998). Making memories: brain activity that predicts how well visual experience will be remembered. *Science*, **281**, 1185–7.

Brinkman, A.D., Sarwar, M., Levin, H.S. & Morris, H.H. (1981). Quantitative indexes of computed tomography in dementia and normal aging. *Radiology*, **138**, 89–92.

Brody, H. (1955). Organization of cerebral cortex. III. A study of aging in the human cerebral cortex. *J. Comp. Neurol.*, **102**, 511–56.

Brody, H. (1970). Structural changes in the aging nervous system. *Interdiscipl. Top. Gerontol.*, **7**, 9–21.

Buckner, R., Kelley, W. & Petersen, W. (1999). Frontal cortex contributes to human memory formation. *Nature Neurosci.*, **2**, 1–4.

Cabeza, R., Grady, C., Nyberg, L. et al. (1997). Age-related differences in neural activity during memory encoding and retrieval: a positron emission tomography study. *J. Neurosci.*, **17**, 391–400.

Cabeza, R., Anderson, N., Houle, S., Mangels, J. & Nyberg, L. (2000). Age-related differences in neural activity during item and temporal-order memory retrieval: a positron emission tomography study. *J. Cogn. Neurosci.*, **12**, 197–206.

Cerella, J., Poon, L. & Fozard, J. (1982). Age and iconic read-out. *J. Gerontol.*, **37**, 197–202.

Chan-Palay, V. & Asan, E. (1989). Quantitation of catecholamine neurons in the locus ceruleus in human brains of normal young and older adults in depression. *J. Comp. Neurol.*, **287**, 357–72.

Christiansen, P., Larsson, H.B., Thomsen, C., Wieslander, S.B. & Henriksen, O. (1994). Age dependent white matter lesions and brain volume changes in healthy volunteers. *Acta Radiol.*, **35**, 117–22.

Clark, H. & Clark, E. (1977). *Psychology and Language: An Introduction to Psycholinguistics*. New York: Harcourt, Brace, Jovanovich.

Coffey, C.E., Wilkinson, W.E., Parashos, I.A. et al. (1992). Quantitative cerebral anatomy of the aging human brain: a cross-sectional study using magnetic resonance imaging. *Neurology*, **42**, 527–36.

Colon, E.J. (1972). The elderly brain. A quantitative analysis of the cerebral cortex in two cases. *Psych. Neurol. Neurochir.*, **75**, 261–70.

Craik, F. (1977). Age differences in human memory. In *Handbook of the Psychology of Aging*, ed. J. Birren & K. Schaie, pp. 384–420. New York: Van Nostrand Reinhold.

Craik, F., Byrd, M. & Swanson, J. (1987). Patterns of memory loss in three elderly samples. *Psychol. Aging*, **2**, 79–86.

de Leon, M. J., George, A.E., Reisberg, B et al. (1989). Alzheimer's disease: Longitudinal CT studies of ventricular change. *Am. J. Neurorad.*, **10**, 371–6.

Demb, J., Desmond, J., Wagner, A., Waidya, C., Glover, G. & Gabrieli, J. (1995). Semantic encoding and retrieval in the left inferior prefrontal cortex: a functional MRI study of task difficulty and process specificity. *J. Neurosci.*, **15**, 5870–8.

D'Esposito, M., Zarahn, E., Aguirre, G. & Rypma, B. (1999). The effect of normal aging on the coupling of neural activity to the BOLD hemodynamic response. *Neuroimage*, **10**, 6–14.

Doppelt, J. & Wallace, W. (1955). Standardization of the Wechsler Adult Intelligence Scale for older persons. *J. Abnorm. Soc. Psychol.*, **51**, 312–30.

Drachman, D. & Leavitt, J. (1972). Memory impairment in the aged: storage versus retrieval deficit. *J. Exper. Psychol.*, **93**, 302–8.

Eriksson, P.S., Perfilieva, E., Bjork-Eriksson, T. et al. (1988). *Nat. Med.*, **4**, 1313–17.

Fletcher, P., Frith, C., Grasby, P., Shallice, T., Frackowiack, R. & Dolan, R. (1995). Brain systems for encoding and retrieval of auditory-verbal memory: an in vivo study in humans. *Brain*, **118**, 401–16.

Gabrielli, J. Brewer, J., Desmond, J. & Glover, G. (1997). Separate neural bases of two fundamental memory processes in the human medial temporal lobe. *Science*, **276**, 264–6.

Gado, M., Hughes, C. P., Danziger, W., Chi, D., Jost, G. & Berg, L. (1982). Volumetric measurements of cerebrospinal fluid spaces in demented subjects and controls. *Radiology*, **144**, 535–8.

Gado, M., Hughes, C. P. Danziger, W. & Chi, D. (1983). Aging, dementia, and brain atrophy: a longitudnal computed tomographic study. *Am. J. Neurorad.*, **4**, 699–702.

Gazzaley, A., Siegel, R., Kordowe, J., Mufson, E. & Morrison, J.

(1996). Circuit-specific alterations of *N*-methyl-D-aspartate receptor subunit 1 in the dentate gyrus of aged monkeys. *Proc. Natl. Acad. Sci., USA*, **93**, 3121–5.

Gomez-Isla, T., Price, J.L., McKeel, D.W., Jr. Morris, J.C., Growdon, J.H. & Hyman, B.T. (1996). Profound loss of layer II entorhinal cortex neurons occurs in very mild Alzheimer's disease. *J. Neurosci.*, **16**, 4491–500.

Gould, E., Reeves, A., Fallah, M., Tanapat, P., Gross, C. & Fuchs, E. (1999). Hippocampal neurogenesis in old world primates *Proc. Natl. Acad. Sci., USA*, **27**, 5263–7.

Grady, C., Masoig, J., Horwitz, B. et al. (1995). Age-related reductions in human recognition memory due to impaired encoding. *Science*, **269**, 218–21.

Grady, C., McIntosh, A., Rajah, N., Beig, S. & Craik, F. (1999). The effects of age on the neural correlates of episodic encoding. *Cereb. Cortex*, **9**, 805–14.

Harris, G.J., Schlaepfer, T.E., Peng, L.W., Lee, S., Federman, E.B. & Pearlson, G. (1994). Magnetic resonance imaging evaluation of the effects of ageing on grey–white ratio in the human brain. *Neuropath. Appl. Neurobiol.*, **20**, 290–3.

Haug, H. (1984). Macroscopic and microscopic morphometry of the human brain and cortex. A survey in the light of new results. *Brain Pathol.*, **1**, 123–49.

Haxby, J., Ungerleider, L., Horwitz, B., Maisog, J., Rapaport, S. & Grady, C. (1996). Face encoding and recognition in human brain. *PNAS*, **93**, 922–7.

Hazlett, E., Buchsbaumm, M., Mohs, R. et al. (1998). Age-related shift in brain region activity during successful memory performance. *Neurobiol. Aging*, **19**, 437–45.

Heaton, R., Grant, I. & Matthes, C. (1986). Differences in neuropsychological function test performance associated with age, education, and sex. In *Neuropsychological Assessment of Neuropsychiatric Disorders*, ed. I. Grant & K. Adams, pp. 100–20. New York: Oxford University Press.

Henderson, G., Tomlinson, B. & Gibson, P. (1980). Cell counts in human cerebral cortex in normal adults throughout life, using an image analysing computer. *J. Neurol. Sci.*, **46**, 113–36.

Huckman, M.S., Fox, J. & Topel, J. (1975). The validity of criteria for the evaluation of cerebral atrophy by computed tomography. *Radiology*, **116**, 85–92.

Hughes, C.P. & Gado, M.H. (1981). Computed tomography and aging of the brain. *Radiology*, **139**, 391–6.

Jernigan, T.L., Press, G.A. & Hesselink, J.R. (1990). Methods for measuring brain morphologic features on magnetic resonance images. *Arch. Neurol.*, **47**, 27–32

Jernigan, T.L. Archibald, S., Berhow, M., Sowell, E., Foster, D. & Hesselink, J. (1991). Cerebral structure on MRI. I. Localization of age-related changes. *Biol. Psychiatr.*, **29**, 55–67.

Johnson, K., Jones, K., Holman, B.L. et al. (1998). Preclinical prediction of Alzheimer's disease using SPECT. *Neurology*, **50**, 1563–71.

Kapur, S., Craik, F., Tulving, E., Wilson, A., Houle, S. & Brown, G. (1994). Neuroanatomical correlates of encoding in episodic memory: levels of processing effects. *Proc. Natl. Acad. Sci., USA*, **91**, 2008–11.

Kapur, S., Tulving, E., Cabeza, R., McIntosh, A., Houle, S. & Craik, F.

(1996). The neural correlates of intentional learning of verbal materials: a PET study in humans. *Cogn. Brain Res.*, **4**, 243–9.

Kaszniak, A.W., Garron, D.C., Fox, J.H., Bergen, D. & Huckman, M.S. (1979). Cerebral atrophy, EEG slowing age, education and cognitive functioning in suspected dementia. *Neurology*, **29**, 1273–9.

Kemper, T. (1993). The relationship of cerebral cortical changes to nuclei in the brainstem. *Neurobiol. Aging*, **14**, 659–60.

Kemperman, G., vanPraag, H. & Gage, F. (2000). Activity-dependent regulation of neuronal plasticity and self repair. *Progr. Brain Res.*, **127**, 35–48.

Killiany, R.J., Gomez-Isla, T., Moss, M. et al. (2000). Use of structural magnetic resonance imaging to predict who will get Alzheimer's disease. *Ann. Neurol.*, **47**, 430–9.

Kornack, D. & Rakic, P. (1999). Continuation of neurogenesis in the hippocampus of the adult macaque monkey. *Proc. Natl. Acad. Sci., USA*, **96**, 5768–73.

Lachman, M. & Jelalian, E. (1984). Self-efficacy and attributions for intellectual performance in young and elderly adults. *J. Gerontol.*, **39**, 577–82.

LaBarge, E., Edwards, D. & Knesevich, J. (1986). Performance of normal elderly on the Boston Naming Test. *Brain Lang.*, **27**, 380–4.

Leuba, B. & Garey, L. (1989). Comparison of neuronal and glial numerical density in primary and secondary visual cortex. *Exp. Brain Res.*, **77**, 31–8.

Lim, K.O., Zipursky, R.B., Watts, M.C. & Pfefferbaum, A. (1992). Decreased gray matter in normal aging: an in vivo magnetic resonance study. *J. Gerontol.*, **47**, B26–30.

Logan, J., Sanders, A., Snyder, A., Morris, J. & Buckner, R. (2002). Under-recruitment and nonselective recruitment dissociate neural mechanisms associated with aging. *Neuron*, **33**, 827–40.

Madden, D.J., Turkington, T.G., Provenzale, J.M. et al. (1999). Adult age differences in the functional neuroanatomy of verbal recognition memory. *Hum. Brain Mapp.*, **7**, 115–35.

Martin, A., Wiggs, C. & Weisberg, J. (1997). Modulation of human medial temporal lobe activity by form, meaning and experience. *Hippocampus*, **7**, 587–93.

Martin, S., Grimwood, P. & Morris, R. (2000). Snyaptic plasticity and memory: an evaluation of the hypothesis. *Ann. Rev. Neurosci.*, **23**, 649–711.

Matsumae, M., Kikinis, R., Morocz, I.A. et al. (1996). Age-related changes in intracranial compartment volumes in normal adults assessed by magnetic resonance imaging. *J. Neurosurg.*, **84**, 982–91.

Morrison, J.H. & Hof, R.P. (1997). Life and death of neurons in the aging brain. *Science*, **278**, 412–19.

Murphy, D.G., DeCarli, C., Schapiro, M. B., Rapoport, S.I. & Horwitz, B. (1992). Age-related differences in volume of subcortical nuclei, brain matter, and cerebrospinal fluid in healthy men as measured with magnetic resonance imaging. *Arch. Neurol.*, **49**, 839–45.

Neilsen, K. & Peters, A. (2000). The effects on the frequency of nerve fibers in rhesus monkey striate cortex. *Neurobiol. Aging*, **21**, 621–8.

Obler, L., Nicholas, M., Albert, M.L. & Woodward, S. (1985). On comprehension across the adult life span. *Cortex*, **21**, 273–80.

Odenheimer, G., Funkenstein, H., Beckett, L. et al. (1994). Comparison of neurologic changes in successfully aging persons vs the total aging population. *Arch. Neurol.*, **51**, 573–80.

Peters, A. (1996). Age-related changes in oligodendrocytes in monkey cerebral cortex. *J. Comp. Neurol.*, **371**, 153–63.

Peters, A., Josephson, K. & Vincent, S. (1991). Effects of aging on the neuroglial cells and pericytes within area 17 of the rhesus monkey (*Macaca mulatta*). *Anat. Rec.*, **229**, 384–98.

Peters, A., Leahu, D., Moss, M.B. & McNally, K. (1994). The effects of aging on area 46 of the frontal cortex of the aging monkey. *Cereb. Cortex*, **6**, 621–35.

Petersen, L. & Petersen, M. (1959). Short term retention of individual items. *J. Exp. Psych.*, **91**, 341–3.

Petersen, R., Smith, G., Kokmen, E., Ivnik, R. & Tangalos, E. (1992). Memory function in normal aging. *Neurology*, **42**, 396–401.

Pfefferbaum, A., Mathalon, D.H., Sullivan, E.V., Rawles, J.M., Zipursky, R.B. & Lim, K.O. (1994). A quantitative magnetic resonance imaging study of changes in brain morphology from infancy to late adulthood. *Arch. Neurol.*, **51**, 874–87.

Plude, D., Milberg, W. & Cerella, J. (1986). Age differences in depicting and perceiving tridimensionality in simple line drawings. *Exper. Aging Res.*, **12**, 221–5.

Poon, L. (1985). Differences in human memory with aging. In *Handbook of the Psychology of Aging*, ed. J.E. Birren & K.W. Schaie, pp. 427–62. New York: Van Nostrand Reinhold.

Rabinowitz, J. (1986). Priming in episodic memory. *J. Gerontol.*, **41**, 204–13.

Rapp, P.R. & Gallagher, M. (1996). Preserved neuron number in the hippocampus of aged rats with spatial learning deficits. *Proc. Natl. Acad. Sci., USA*, **93**, 9926–30.

Raymond, B. (1971). Free recall among the aged. *Psychol. Rep.*, **29**, 1179–82.

Reber, P. & Squire, L. (1994). Parallel brain systems for learning with and without awareness. *Learn Mem.*, **4**, 217–19.

Reiman, E.M., Caselli, R.J., Yun, L.S. et al. (1996). Preclinical evidence of Alzheimer's disease in persons homozygous for the epsilon 4 allele for apolipoprotein Ev. *N. Engl. J. Med.*, **334**, 752–8.

Roberts, M.A. & Caird, F.I. (1976). Computerized tomography and intellectual impairment in the elderly. *J. Neurol. Neurosurg. Psychiat.*, **39**, 986–9.

Rosene, D. (1993). Comparing age-related changes in the basal forebrain and hippocampus of the rhesus monkey. *Neurobiol. Aging*, **14**, 669–70.

Ross, P, Yurgelon-Todd, D., Renshaw, P. et al. (1997). Age-related reduction in functional MRI response to photic stimulation. *Neurology*, **48**, 173–6.

Schacter, D. & Wagner, A. (1999). Medial temporal lobe activations in fMRI and PET studies of episodic encoding and retrieval. *Hippocampus*, **9**, 7–24.

Schacter, D.L., Savage, C.R., Alpert, N.M., Rauch, S.L. & Albert, M.S. (1996). The role of the hippocampus and frontal cortex in age-related memory changes: a PET study. *Neuroreport*, **7**, 1165–1169.

Schaie, K. (1983). The Seattle longitudinal study: a 21 year exploration of psychometric intelligence in adulthood. In *Longitudinal Studies of Adult Psychological Development*, ed. K.W. Schaie, pp. 64–135. New York: Guilford.

Schaie, K. & Labouvie-Vief, G. (1974). Generational vs. ontogenetic changes in adult cognitive behavior: a fourteen year cross-sequential study. *Dev. Psychol.*, **10**, 305–20.

Shefer, V. (1973). Absolute number of neurons and thickness of cerebral cortex during aging, senile and vascular dementia and Pick's and Alzheimer's disease. *Neurosci. Behav. Physiol.*, **6**, 319–24.

Small, G.W., Mazziotta, J.C., Collins, M.T. et al. (1995). Apolipoprotein E type 4 allele and cerebral glucose metabolism in relatives at risk for familial Alzheimer disease. *J. Am. Med. Ass.*, **273**, 942–7.

Smith, T., Adams, M., Gallagher, M., Morrison, J. & Rapp. P. (2000). Circuit-specific alterations in hippocampal synaptophysin immunoreactivity predict spatial learning impairment in aged rats. *J. Neurosci.*, **20**, 6587–93.

Sperling, R., Bates, J., Cocchiarella, A. et al. (1999). fMRI of face-name association in healthy young and older subjects. *Soc. Neurosci.*, **25**, 646.

Spitz, H. (1972). Note on immediate memory for digits: invariance over the years. *Psych. Bull.*, **78**, 183–5.

Squire, L., Zola-Morgan, S. & Chen, K. (1988). Human amnesia and animal models of amnesia: performance of amnesic patients on tests designed for the monkey. *Behav. Neurosci.*, **11**, 210–21.

Stafford, J., Albert, M.S., Naeser, M., Sandor, T. & Garvey, A. (1988). Age related differences in CT scan measurements. *Arch. Neurol.*, **45**, 409–19.

Stern, C., Corkin, S., Gonzalez, R. et al. (1996). The hippocampus participates in novel picture encoding: Evidence from functional magnetic resonance imaging. *Proc. Natl. Acad. Sci., USA*, **93**, 8660–5.

Talland, G. (1967). Age and the immediate memory span. *The Gerontologist*, **7**, 4–9.

Tanila H, Shapiro M, Gallagher M. & Eichenbaum H. (1997). Brain aging: changes in the nature of information encoding in the hippocampus. *J. Neurosci.*, **17**, 5155–66.

Tanna, N.K., Kohn, M.I., Horwich, D.N. et al. (1991). Analysis of brain and cerebrospinal fluid volumes with MR imaging: impact on PET data correction for atrophy. Part II. Aging and Alzheimer's dementia. *Radiology*, **178**, 123–30.

Taoka, T., Iwasaki, S., Uchida, H. et al. (1998). Age correlation of the time lag in signal change on EPI–fMRI. *J. Comp. Assist. Tomog.*, **22**, 514–17.

Terry, R.D., DeTeresa, R. & Hansen, L.A. (1987). Neocortical cell counts in normal human adult aging. *Ann. Neurol.*, **21**, 530–9.

Tigges, J., Herndon, J. & Peters, A. (1992). Neuronal population of area 4 during life span of rhesus monkeys. *Neurobiol. Aging*, **11**, 201–8.

Tulving, E. (1972). Episodic and semantic memory. In *Organization of Memory*, ed. E. Tulving & W. Donaldson, pp. 381–403. New York: Academic Press.

Vincent, S., Peters, A. & Tigges J. (1989). Effects of aging on neurons within area 17 of rhesus monkey cerebral cortex. *Anat. Rec.*, **223**, 329–41.

Wagner, A., Poldrack, R., Eldridge, L., Desmond, J., Glover, G. & Gabrieli, J. (1998a). Material-specific lateralization of prefrontal activation during episodic encoding and retrieval. *Neuroreport*, **9**, 3711–17.

Wagner, A., Schacter, D., Rotte M. et al. (1998b). Building memories: remembering and forgetting verbal experiences as predicted by brain activity. *Science*, **281**, 1188–91.

Waugh, N. & Norman, D. (1965). Primary memory. *Psychol. Rev.*, **72**, 89–104.

West, M., Coleman, P., Flood, D. & Troncoso, J. (1994). Differences in the pattern of hippocampal neuronal loss in normal aging and Alzheimer's disease. *Lancet*, **344**, 769–72.

Zatz, L., Jernigan, T.L. & Ahumada, A.J. (1982). Changes on computed cranial tomography with aging: intracranial fluid volume. *Am. J. Neuroradiol.*, **3**, 1–11.

15

Neurodegenerative diseases

Stanley B. Prusiner

Institute for Neurodegenerative Diseases and Departments of Neurology and of Biochemistry and Biophysics, University of California, San Francisco, CA, USA

Twenty-five years ago, there was little understanding of the causes of neurodegeneration. In fact, the term degenerative disease was used as a wastebasket for illnesses of unknown etiology. But progress over the past quarter of a century in research focused on degenerative disorders of the central nervous system (CNS) has been impressive. It is now clear that neurodegenerative diseases are caused by the misprocessing of proteins. In each disease, one or more specific proteins have been identified that are misprocessed; this results in the accumulation of one or more particular proteins.

The proteins that accumulate in the CNS of patients with neurodegenerative diseases were initially identified by purifying these polypeptides from the brains of animals or humans with these diseases (Glenner & Wong, 1984; Masters et al., 1985; Prusiner et al., 1982). Subsequently, molecular genetics was used to identify the genes responsible for the familial forms of Alzheimer's and Parkinson's diseases as well as amyotrophic lateral sclerosis (ALS) and frontotemporal dementia (FTD). Similarly, molecular genetic investigations of Huntington's disease (HD) and the spinocerebellar ataxias have led to the identification of the genes responsible for the pathogenesis of these illnesses.

Of all the studies on neurodegenerative diseases, the discovery of prions has been most unexpected. The finding that a protein can act as an infectious pathogen and cause degeneration of the CNS was unprecedented (Prusiner, 1998b). The prion concept was so novel that achieving acceptance required a long and arduous battle (Prusiner, 1999). The prion concept not only explained how a disease can be both infectious and genetic, but it has also created new disease paradigms and revolutionized thinking in biology.

Although progress in the study of neurodegeneration has been impressive, there are still no curative treatments.

Only for patients with Parkinson's disease is there a palliative drug with reasonable efficacy (Cotzias et al., 1967). L-dopa and related drugs do not stop the underlying degeneration, which often renders patients refractory to pharmacologic treatment in the later stages of Parkinson's disease (Marsden & Parkes, 1977). Stereotactic surgery has produced limited success in ameliorating the symptoms of Parkinson's disease when L-dopa becomes ineffective. Transplantation of cells secreting dopamine into the brains of patients with advanced Parkinson's disease is the subject of much research. It is noteworthy that many patients with Parkinson's disease develop dementia in the later stages of this disorder.

This chapter is not intended as an exhaustive review of neurodegenerative diseases and as such the bibliography is regrettably limited. Rather, it is an attempt to view the many common features of these degenerative illnesses from the perspective of the prion diseases (Prusiner, 1984). Progress in deciphering the etiologies of many neurodegenerative diseases has greatly strengthened the unifying concepts presented here. Based on the common features of these maladies, I suggest a new definition for the neurodegenerative diseases.

Aging and neurodegeneration

Age is the single most important risk factor for degenerative diseases of the CNS (Holman et al., 1996; Kawas & Katzman, 1999; Lilienfield, 1993). Many, but not all, cases of neurodegenerative diseases are sporadic in that no heritable, toxic, or infectious etiology can be discerned. These disorders are often characterized by a chronic, progressive deterioration of the CNS lasting from several months to more than a decade. Although the disease process is relentless, the immune system seems to remain quiescent.

Table 15.1. *Epidemiology of neurodegenerative diseases*[a]

Disease	Number of US patients	US prevalence per 100 000[b]
Prion diseases	400	0.1
Alzheimer's disease	4 000 000	1200
Parkinson's disease	1 000 000	300
FTD	40 000	14
Pick's disease	5000	2
PSP	15 000	5
ALS	20 000	7
Huntington's disease	30 000	10
Spinocerebellar ataxias	12 000	4

Notes:

[a] Abbreviations: FTD = frontotemporal dementia, PSP = progressive supranuclear palsy, ALS = amyotrophic lateral sclerosis.

[b] Population of United States is approximately 275 million in the year 2000.

Table 15.2. Sporadic, genetic and infectious etiologies of neurodegenerative diseases

Disease	Etiologic frequency (%)		
	Sporadic	Genetic	Infectious
Prion diseases	85	>10	<1
Alzheimer's disease	90	10	
Parkinson disease	95	<5	
FTD	90	10	
Pick's disease	95	<5	
PSP	95	<5	
ALS	90	10	
Huntington's disease		100	
Spinocerebellar ataxias		100	

Patients are afebrile and exhibit neither leukocytosis in blood nor pleocytosis in the cerebrospinal fluid (CSF).

While a complete compendium of neurodegenerative diseases is quite long, a brief list composed of the more common disorders and a few less common maladies, which have been particularly amenable to investigation, are discussed here (Table 15.1). Alzheimer's and Parkinson's diseases are the most common neurodegenerative diseases. Over four million people suffer from Alzheimer's disease (AD) in the United States and another million have Parkinson's disease (Kawas & Katzman, 1999; Lilienfield, 1993; Tanner & Goldman, 1996). Far less common are ALS, FTD, prion diseases, Huntington's disease and spinocerebellar ataxias. The vast majority of the first five neurodegenerative diseases are sporadic with 10% or less of cases being inherited (Table 15.2). In contrast, virtually all cases of Huntington's disease and the spinocerebellar ataxias are inherited disorders.

Because people are living longer, there is now considerable concern about the increasing numbers of individuals who are developing Alzheimer's and Parkinson's diseases. At age 60, the risk of developing AD is approximately 1 in 10 000 but by age 85 the risk is greater than 1 in 3 (Evans et al., 1989). Such statistics argue that, by the year 2025, more than 10 million people will suffer from AD in the United States and by the year 2050, the number of afflicted individuals will approach 20 million (Kawas & Katzman, 1999). Just as staggering as the number of people with AD is the cost of caring for these patients. It is estimated that AD currently costs the United States as much as $200 billion annually for the care of these people as well as in lost productivity of both the patients and caregivers.

Like Alzheimer's disease, age is the most important risk factor for Parkinson's disease. By age 85, nearly 50% of people exhibit at least one symptom or sign of Parkinsonism (Bennett et al., 1996).

Prions

Prions are infectious proteins. In mammals, prions reproduce by recruiting the normal, cellular isoform of the prion protein (PrP^C) and stimulating its conversion into the disease-causing isoform (PrP^{Sc}).

A major feature that distinguishes prions from viruses is the finding that both PrP isoforms are encoded by a chromosomal gene (Prusiner, 1998b). In humans, the PrP gene is designated *PRNP* and is located on the short arm of chromosome 20. Limited proteolysis of PrP^{Sc} produces a smaller, protease-resistant molecule of ~142 amino acids, designated PrP 27–30; under the same conditions, PrP^C is completely hydrolyzed (Fig. 15.1). In the presence of detergent, PrP 27–30 polymerizes into amyloid (McKinley et al., 1991). Prion amyloid formed by limited proteolysis and detergent extraction is indistinguishable from the filaments that aggregate to form PrP amyloid plaques in the CNS. Both the rods and the PrP amyloid filaments found in brain tissue exhibit similar ultrastructural morphology and green-gold birefringence after staining with Congo red dye.

PrP^C is rich in α-helix and has little β-sheet while PrP^{Sc} has less α-helix and a high β-sheet content. Comparisons

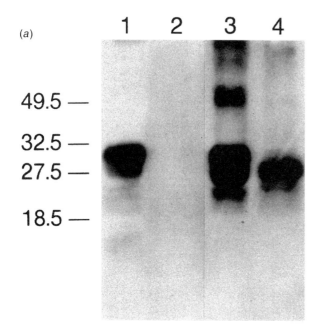

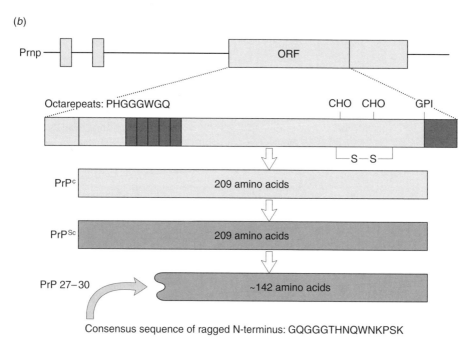

Fig. 15.1. Prion protein isoforms. (*a*) Western immunoblot of brain homogenates from uninfected (lanes 1 and 2) and prion-infected (lanes 3 and 4) Syrian hamsters (SHa). Samples in lanes 2 and 4 were digested with 50 μg/ml of proteinase K for 30 min at 37 °C. PrP^C in lanes 2 and 4 was completely hydrolyzed under these conditions whereas approximately 67 amino acids were digested from the NH$_2$-terminus of PrP^{Sc} to generate PrP 27–30. After polyacrylamide gel electrophoresis (PAGE) and electrotransfer, the blot was developed with anti-SHaPrP R073 polyclonal rabbit antiserum (Serban et al. 1990). Molecular size markers are in kilodaltons (kDa). (*b*) Bar diagram of SHaPrP gene which encodes a protein of 254 amino acids. After processing of the NH$_2$- and COOH- termini, both PrP^C and PrP^{Sc} consist of 209 residues. After limited proteolysis, the NH$_2$-terminus of PrP^{Sc} is truncated to form PrP 27–30 that is composed of approximately 142 amino acids, the N-terminal sequence of which was determined by Edman degradation.

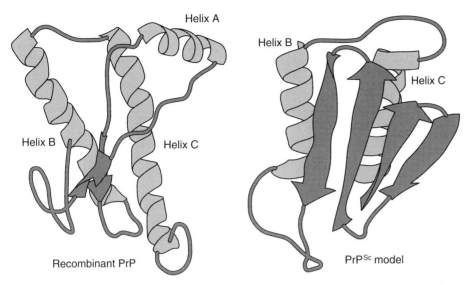

Fig. 15.2. Structures of prion protein isoforms. (*a*) NMR structure of Syrian hamster (SHa) recombinant (rec) PrP(90–231). Presumably, the structure of the α-helical form of recPrP(90–231) resembles that of PrP^C. recPrP(90–231) is viewed from the interface where PrP^{Sc} is thought to bind to PrP^C. α-helices A (residues 144–157), B (172–193), and C (200–227) residues 129–134 encompassing strand S1 and residues 159–165 in strand S2; the arrows span residues 129–131 and 161–163, as these show a closer resemblance to β-sheet. (*b*) Plausible model for the tertiary structure of human PrP^{Sc}. S1 β-strands are residues 108–113 and 116–122 in red; S2 β-strands are residues 128–135 and 138–144; α-helices B (residues 178–191) and C (residues 202–218). (Illustrations prepared by Fred E. Cohen.)

of secondary structures of PrP^C and PrP^{Sc} were performed on the proteins purified from Syrian hamster (SHa) brains (Pan et al., 1993). Based on these data, structural models for PrP^C and PrP^{Sc} were proposed (Huang et al., 1995). Subsequently, solution NMR structures of recombinant SHa and mouse PrPs produced in bacteria showed that it is likely that PrP^C has three α-helices and not four as predicted by molecular modelling (Fig. 15.2) (Liu et al., 1999; Riek et al., 1996). The computational model of PrP^{Sc} is supported by studies with recombinant antibody fragments, which have been used to map the surfaces of PrP^C and PrP^{Sc} (Peretz et al., 1997). This α- to-β transition in PrP structure is the fundamental event underlying prion diseases, which are disorders of protein conformation.

Much has been learned about the basic biology of prions using yeast in which two different proteins, unrelated to PrP, form prions (Sparrer et al., 2000; Wickner, 1994).

Four new concepts

Four new concepts have emerged from studies of prions. First, prions are the only known example of infectious pathogens that are devoid of nucleic acid. All other infectious agents possess genomes composed of either RNA or DNA that direct the synthesis of their progeny. Secondly, prion diseases may be manifest as infectious, genetic, and sporadic disorders. No other group of illnesses with a single etiology presents with such a wide spectrum of clinical manifestations. Thirdly, prion diseases result from the accumulation of PrP^{Sc}, the conformation of which differs substantially from that of its precursor PrP^C. Fourthly, PrP^{Sc} can exist in a variety of different conformations, each of which seems to indicate a specific disease phenotype. How a specific conformation of a PrP^{Sc} molecule is imparted to PrP^C during prion replication to produce nascent PrP^{Sc} with the same conformation is unknown. Additionally, it is unclear what factors determine where in the CNS a particular PrP^{Sc} molecule will be deposited, which results in neurologic dysfunction.

Common themes define neurodegeneration

With the recognition that a common feature of all well studied neurodegenerative diseases is the misprocessing of proteins, it is reasonable to propose a new definition of neurodegenerative disease based on this unifying etiologic characteristic. I suggest the following: 'neurodegenerative diseases are progressive nervous system disorders of protein processing. Aberrant protein processing includes misfolding, altered post-translational modification, aberrant proteolytic cleavage, anomalous gene splicing, improper expression, and diminished clearance. The misprocessed proteins often accumulate because the cellular mechanisms for removing these proteins are ineffective. Neurodegenerative diseases typically present as sporadic and genetic maladies of delayed onset, but can also be infectious illnesses with prolonged incubation times. The particular protein that undergoes misprocessing determines the disease-specific phenotype, which results from the malfunction of distinct sets of neurons.'

In the past, degenerative diseases of the CNS have often been defined as idiopathic disorders accompanied by mental deterioration. Neuropathologically, they have been defined in terms of region-specific retrogressive changes in cells resulting in impaired function. Such pathologic changes have also been equated with the death of specific neuronal populations (Martin, 1999).

The broad spectrum of presenting clinical deficits in the prion diseases illustrates how ineffective a clinical classification scheme can be; these diseases can present with dementia, ataxia, insomnia, paraplegia, paresthesias and deviant behaviour (Will et al., 1999a). While none of the clinical presentations of prion diseases are diagnostic, patients who present with a rapidly progressive dementia accompanied by myoclonus often have Creutzfeldt–Jakob disease (CJD). The spectrum of neuropathologic changes in prion diseases ranges from none to widespread atrophy, from rare to frequent neuronal loss, from sparse to severe vacuolation or spongiform change, from mild to intense reactive astrocytic gliosis, and from none to abundant PrP amyloid plaques (DeArmond & Prusiner, 1997). None of these neuropathologic changes except the presence of PrP amyloid plaques is unequivocally diagnostic. Past attempts to classify and characterize other neurodegenerative diseases (Table 15.1) based on the clinical presentations or neuropathologic manifestations have been equally unsatisfying.

The discovery of amyloid in brain fractions enriched for prion infectivity was completely unexpected (Prusiner et al., 1983). The amyloid plaques in prion diseases and AD as well as large intracellular structures such as Lewy and Pick bodies were not considered to be of etiologic importance. Once anti-PrP 27–30 antibodies were raised, the amyloid plaques in prion diseases were found to stain readily (Bendheim et al., 1984; DeArmond et al., 1985).

It seems likely that the mechanisms, by which misprocessed proteins disrupt cellular functions such as signal transduction and gene transcription, are diverse. The

Table 15.3. Protein deposition in neurodegenerative diseases

Disease	Protein	Aggregate
Prion diseases	PrP^{Sc}	PrP amyloid
Alzheimer's disease	Aβ	Aβ amyloid
	tau	PHF in NFT[a]
Parkinson disease	α-synuclein	Lewy bodies
FTD	tau	straight filaments and PHF
Pick's disease	tau	Pick bodies
PSP	tau	straight filaments in NFT
ALS	neurofilament	neuronal aggregates
Huntington's disease	huntingtin	nuclear inclusions
Spinocerebellar ataxia 1	ataxin 1	nuclear inclusions
Spinocerebellar ataxia 2	ataxin 2	cytoplasmic inclusions
Machado–Joseph disease	ataxin 3	nuclear inclusions

[a] PHF, paired helical filaments; NFT, neurofibrillary tangles.

secondary responses to misprocessed proteins may amplify the damage done by these macromolecules by activation of cytokine release, reactive gliosis, apoptosis, and oxidative injury (Cotman et al., 1999; Markesbery & Ehmann, 1999). In some neurodegenerative diseases, the misprocessed proteins might cause CNS dysfunction when they are monomers or oligomers while in other disorders, larger aggregates may prove to be the culprits (Chiti et al., 1999). In the case of PrP^{Sc}, the protein accumulates and fragments sometimes polymerize to form amyloid fibrils that are deposited in the extracellular space as plaques. With α-synuclein, tau and mutant huntingtin proteins, ubiquitinated deposits are found as Lewy bodies, Pick bodies and nuclear aggregates, respectively (Table 15.3). As discussed below, the aggregates may not cause cellular dysfunction but simply represent the attempt of cells to sequester these misprocessed proteins in a form that is less deleterious. Finding ubiquitinated deposits of α-synuclein, tau and mutant huntingtin argues that these proteins were destined for clearance but the process was incomplete. The covalent attachment of ubiquitin, which is a 76-residue polypeptide, to particular proteins targets them for degradation (Hershko & Ciechanover, 1998).

In sporadic cases, which account for more than 85% of all human prion disease (Table 15.2), the prion concept explains how wild-type (wt) PrP^{C} is progressively converted into PrP^{Sc}. Although the mechanism of prion replication is unclear, the stimulation of this process by PrP^{Sc} provides the driving force for the misfolding of PrP^{C} into PrP^{Sc}. No similar formulation exists to explain the progressive deterioration of the nervous system that follows the misprocessing of proteins in sporadic cases of AD, FTD, Parkinson's disease, and ALS. For example, factors driving the accumulation of the Aβ peptide in the CNS of people destined to develop sporadic AD are unknown except for the allelic variants of ApoE. Likewise, factors driving the accumulation of the α-synuclein to form Lewy bodies within the neurons of the substantia nigra of people destined to develop sporadic Parkinson's disease are unknown.

In the inherited neurodegenerative diseases, the same problem attends in the sense that these diseases are usually of late onset even though the mutations are present from conception. With few exceptions, the inherited neurodegenerative diseases are autosomal dominant disorders so the mutations are unlikely to produce disease through loss of function. Instead, such dominant mutations are likely to act as gain of dysfunction or as dominant negatives. Even though the mutant protein is expressed in the CNS early in life, no damage is detected clinically for decades in the inherited cases of AD, Parkinson's disease, FTD, ALS, and the prion diseases. Only in the triplet repeat diseases, such as HD, do children manifest neurologic disease when the repeat expansions become very large.

How the aging process features in these diseases is unclear. Is the misprocessing of a particular protein simply a stochastic process, which happens with a much higher probability when it is mutated? In such a model, prolonged periods of time are required for either the mutant or wt protein to be misprocessed into a disease-causing form. But perhaps, the milieu of the aging brain provides a more permissive environment for the misprocessing of proteins. The accumulation of proteins modified by oxidation has been suggested as a possible factor in virtually every degenerative disease (Markesbery & Ehmann, 1999). Clearance of misprocessed proteins may diminish with age and thus, may be responsible for their accumulation.

The neurodegenerative diseases elude detection by the immune and interferon defense systems: patients remain afebrile throughout the courses of their illness and show no leukocytosis in blood or pleocytosis in the CSF. Grossly, the brain can be atrophic with enlarged ventricles as in many cases of AD; alternatively, the basal ganglia may show selective atrophy as in HD. The degree of neuronal loss and the extent of reactive astrocytic gliosis can be quite variable for a particular disease. Although microglia often accumulate and cytokines are released late in the various neurodegenerative diseases, no inflammatory response characterized by accumulation of antigen–antibody complexes, lymphocytic infiltration or the perivascular accumulation of monocytes is generally seen.

Prion biology and diseases

Because prions and the mechanism of disease pathogenesis are without precedent, the classification of the prion diseases has been quite varied. For many years, the human prion diseases were classified as idiopathic degenerative disorders of the CNS based upon pathologic changes confined to the CNS. With the transmission of kuru and CJD to apes, investigators began to view these diseases as CNS infectious illnesses caused by 'slow viruses' (Gibbs et al., 1968).

The sporadic form of CJD is the most common prion disorder in humans and typically presents with dementia and myoclonus (Table 15.4). Sporadic CJD (sCJD) accounts for ~85% of all cases of human prion disease while inherited prion diseases account for 10–15% of all cases (Tables 15.2 and 15.4). Familial CJD (fCJD), Gerstmann–Sträussler–Scheinker disease (GSS), and fatal familial insomnia (FFI) are all dominantly inherited prion diseases caused by mutations in the PrP gene (Table 15.5) (Dlouhy et al., 1992; Gabizon et al., 1993; Hsiao et al., 1989a; Petersen et al., 1992; Poulter et al., 1992).

Even though the familial nature of a subset of CJD cases had been well described (Kirschbaum, 1968), the significance of this observation became more obscure with the transmission of CJD to animals (Gibbs et al., 1968). The conundrum that faced investigators reporting transmission of familial cases of CJD and GSS to apes and monkeys (Masters et al., 1981; Roos et al., 1973) is of considerable interest. They offered three hypotheses to explain fCJD and GSS. First the 'CJD virus' was transmitted to family members living in close proximity. Secondly, patients with fCJD or GSS carried a genetic predisposition to the ubiquitous CJD virus. Thirdly, the CJD virus was transmitted from parent to offspring either in utero or during birth as was later seen with HIV. All three of these explanations proved to be incorrect: the CJD virus does not exist and the familial prion diseases are caused by mutations in the PrP gene (Hsiao et al., 1989b).

The prion concept readily explains how a disease can be manifest as a heritable or sporadic disorder as well as an infectious illness. Moreover, the hallmark common to all of the prion diseases, whether sporadic, dominantly inherited, or acquired by infection, is that they involve the aberrant metabolism of the prion protein.

Table 15.4. The prion diseases

Disease	Host	Mechanism of pathogenesis
Kuru	Fore people	Infection through ritualistic cannibalism
iCJD*	Humans	Infection from prion-contaminated HGH, dura mater grafts, etc.
vCJD	Humans	Infection from bovine prions
fCJD	Humans	Germline mutations in PrP gene
GSS	Humans	Germline mutations in PrP gene
FFI	Humans	Germline mutation in PrP gene (D178N, M129)
sCJD	Humans	Somatic mutation or spontaneous conversion of PrP^C into PrP^{Sc}?
sFI	Humans	Somatic mutation or spontaneous conversion of PrP^C into PrP^{Sc}?
Scrapie	Sheep	Infection in genetically susceptible sheep
BSE	Cattle	Infection with prion-contaminated MBM
TME	Mink	Infection with prions from sheep or cattle
CWD	Mule deer, elk	Unknown
FSE	Cats	Infection with prion-contaminated beef
Exotic ungulate encephalopathy	Greater kudu, nyala, oryx	Infection with prion-contaminated MBM

Notes:

* Abbreviations: BSE, bovine spongiform encephalopathy; CJD, Creutzfeldt–Jakob disease; sCJD, sporadic CJD; fCJD, familial CJD; iCJD, iatrogenic CJD; vCJD, (new) variant CJD; CWD, chronic wasting disease; FFI, fatal familial insomnia; FSE, feline spongiform encephalopathy; sFI, sporadic fatal insomnia; GSS, Gerstmann–Sträussler–Scheinker disease; HGH, human growth hormone; MBM, meat and bone meal; TME, transmissible mink encephalopathy.

Table 15.5. Mutant genes in familial neurodegenerative diseases

Inherited disease	Gene	Mutation
Prion diseases	PrP	point mutations and octarepeat expansions
Alzheimer's disease	APP	point mutations
	PS1	point mutations
	PS2	point mutations
Parkinson's disease	α-synuclein	point mutations
	Parkin	point mutations
FTD	tau	point mutations deletions
Pick's disease	tau	point mutations
ALS	SOD1	point mutations
Huntington's disease	HD	polyglutamine expansions
Spinocerebellar ataxia 1	SCA1	polyglutamine expansions
Spinocerebellar ataxia 2	SCA2	polyglutamine expansions
Machado–Joseph disease	SCA3	polyglutamine expansions

In both the sporadic and inherited prion diseases, infectious prions are generated *de novo* within the host. In the sporadic prion diseases, wt PrP^C is converted into wt PrP^{Sc}, which is infectious. In the inherited prion diseases, mutant PrP^C is converted into mutant PrP^{Sc}, which in some cases appears to be able to stimulate the conversion of wt PrP^C into wt PrP^{Sc}. In these diseases, the process of prion formation begins endogenously. The accumulation of sufficient wt PrP^{Sc} to establish a slow infection and ultimately disease is a rare event and is presumably governed by both the frequency of PrP^{Sc} formation and the rate of PrP^{Sc} clearance. In contrast, the accumulation of sufficient mutant PrP^{Sc} to establish a slow infection and ultimately disease is a much more frequent event since all people carrying a PrP mutation will develop disease if they live long enough (Chapman et al., 1994; Spudich et al., 1995). Whether some pathologic PrP mutations act primarily by increasing the frequency of PrP^{Sc} formation and others by decreasing the rate of PrP^{Sc} clearance remains to be established.

Six diseases of animals are caused by prions (Table 15.4). Scrapie of sheep and goats is the prototypic prion disease. Mink encephalopathy, bovine spongiform encephalopathy (BSE), feline spongiform encephalopathy, and exotic ungulate encephalopathy are all thought to occur after the consumption of prion-infected foodstuffs.

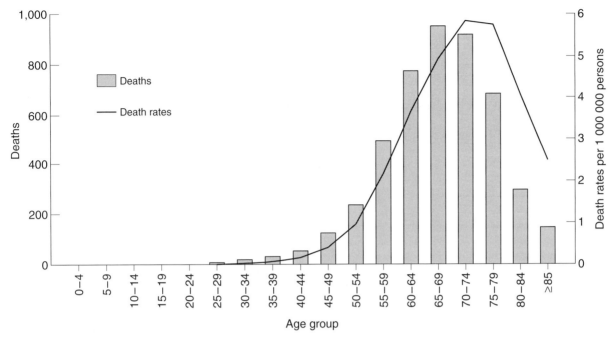

Fig. 15.3. Age-specific incidence of Creutzfeldt-Jakob disease in the United States. Total numbers of deaths for the period 1979 to 1998 are shown by the open bars and the death rates per million population are depicted by the solid line. (Graph prepared by Lawrence Schonberger.)

Epidemiology

Prions cause CJD in humans throughout the world. The incidence of sporadic CJD is approximately one case per million population (Masters et al., 1978), but is nearly five per million people between the ages of 60 to 74 (Fig. 15.3) (Holman et al., 1996). Patients as young as 17 years and as old as 83 have been recorded (Cathala & Baron, 1987; Masters et al., 1978). CJD is a relentlessly progressive malady that results in death usually within a year of onset. Each geographic cluster of prion disease was initially thought to be a manifestation of the communicability of the CJD virus (Kahana et al., 1974), but each was later shown to be due to a *PRNP* gene mutation, which results in a non-conservative substitution. Although infectious prion diseases account for less than 1% of all cases and infection does not seem to play an important role in the natural history of these illnesses, the transmissibility of prions is an important biologic feature. Attempts to identify common exposure to some etiologic agent have been unsuccessful for both the sporadic and familial cases (Cousens et al., 1990). Ingestion of scrapie-infected sheep or goat meat as a cause of CJD in humans has not been demonstrated by epidemiologic studies although speculation about this potential route of infection continues (Johnson & Gibbs, 1998). Studies with

Syrian hamsters demonstrated that oral infection by prions can occur, but the process is quite inefficient compared to intracerebral inoculation (Prusiner et al., 1985).

Why the human prion diseases are so rare compared to the more common disorders of AD and Parkinson's disease is unknown. AD is about four times more common than Parkinson's disease and approximately 10 000 times more common than CJD (Table 15.1). Deciphering the mechanism of these remarkable differences in prevalence may help elucidate the factors underlying the etiologies and pathogenesis of these maladies.

Neuropathology

Frequently, the brains of patients with CJD show no recognizable abnormalities upon gross examination. In patients surviving several years, variable degrees of cerebral atrophy are likely to result in brain weights as low as 850 g.

The pathologic hallmarks of CJD at the light microscopic level are spongiform degeneration and astrogliosis (Fig. 15.4(*a*) and (*b*), see colour plate section) (DeArmond & Ironside, 1999). The lack of an inflammatory response in CJD and other prion diseases is an important pathologic feature of these degenerative disorders. Generally, the spongiform changes occur in the cerebral cortex, putamen, caudate nucleus, thalamus, and molecular layer of the cerebellum. Spongiform degeneration is characterized by many 5–20 μm vacuoles in the neuropil between nerve cell bodies. Astrocytic gliosis is a constant but nonspecific feature of prion diseases (DeArmond & Prusiner, 1997). Widespread proliferation of fibrous astrocytes is found throughout the grey matter of brains infected with CJD prions. Astrocytic processes filled with glial filaments form extensive networks.

Amyloid plaques have been found in ∼10% of CJD cases. Purified CJD prions from humans and animals exhibit the ultrastructural and histochemical characteristics of amyloid (Prusiner et al., 1983). In first passage to mice from some human Japanese CJD cases, amyloid plaques were found in the mouse brains (Tateishi et al., 1996). These plaques were stained with antisera raised against PrP.

The amyloid plaques of GSS are distinct from those seen in kuru, AD, or scrapie. GSS plaques consist of a central dense core of amyloid surrounded by smaller globules of amyloid (Fig. 15.4(c) and (d)). Ultrastructurally, they consist of a radiating fibrillar network of amyloid fibrils with scant or no neuritic degeneration. The plaques can be distributed throughout the brain but are most frequently found in the cerebellum. They are often located adjacent to blood vessels. Congophilic angiopathy has been noted in some cases of GSS. In addition to the multicentric plaques of GSS, unicentric kuru plaques may also be seen (Masters et al., 1981). In GSS caused by the F198S mutation, neurofibrillary tangles (NFT) composed of paired helical filaments (PHF) are frequently seen surrounding PrP amyloid plaques (Dlouhy et al., 1992; Gambetti et al., 1999).

In new variant CJD (vCJD), a characteristic feature is the presence of 'florid plaques'. These are composed of a central core of PrP amyloid surrounded by vacuoles in a pattern suggesting petals of a flower (Fig. 15.4(e) and (f)).

Species barrier

Studies on the role of the primary and tertiary structures of PrP in the transmission of prion disease have given new insights into the pathogenesis of these maladies. In general, transmission of prion disease from one species to another is inefficient, in that not all intracerebrally inoculated animals develop disease, and those that fall ill, do so only after long incubation times, which can approach the natural lifespan of the animal (Pattison, 1965). This 'species barrier' to transmission is correlated with the degree of homology between the amino acid sequence of PrP^C in the inoculated host and of PrP^{Sc} in the prion inoculum (Prusiner et al., 1990). Thus, the amino acid sequence of PrP encodes the species of the prion, and the prion derives its PrP^{Sc} sequence from the last mammal in which it was

passaged (Scott et al., 1997). The importance of sequence homology between the host and donor PrP argues that PrP^C directly interacts with PrP^{Sc} in the prion conversion process; PrP^{Sc} seems to function as a template in determining the tertiary structure of nascent PrP^{Sc} molecules as they are formed from PrP^C.

Prion strains

The existence of prion strains raised the question of how heritable biological information can be enciphered in a molecule other than nucleic acid (Bruce & Dickinson, 1987; Dickinson et al., 1968; Ridley & Baker, 1996). Strains or varieties of prions have been defined by incubation times and the distribution of neuronal vacuolation (Dickinson et al., 1968). Subsequently, the patterns of PrP^{Sc} deposition were found to correlate with vacuolation profiles and these patterns were also used to characterize strains of prions (Bruce et al., 1989; DeArmond et al., 1987).

Mounting evidence supports the hypothesis that prion diversity is enciphered in the conformation of PrP^{Sc} (Prusiner, 1991); thus, prion strains seem to represent different conformers of PrP^{Sc} (Bessen & Marsh, 1994; Safar et al., 1998; Scott et al., 1997; Telling et al., 1996). Persuasive evidence that strain-specific information is enciphered in the tertiary and quaternary structure of PrP^{Sc} comes from transmission of two different inherited human prion diseases to mice expressing a chimeric human-mouse PrP transgene (Telling et al., 1996). In FFI, the protease-resistant fragment of PrP^{Sc} after deglycosylation has a molecular size of 19 kDa, whereas in fCJD with a substitution of a lysine (K) for glutamate (E) at residue 200 (E200K) and most sporadic prion diseases, it is 21 kDa (Table 15.6) (Parchi et al., 1996). This difference in molecular size was shown to be due to different sites of proteolytic cleavage at the NH$_2$-termini of the two human PrP^{Sc} molecules, reflecting different tertiary structures. These distinct conformations were not unexpected because the amino acid sequences of the PrPs differ.

Extracts from the brains of FFI patients transmitted disease into mice expressing a chimeric human-mouse PrP transgene about 200 days after inoculation and induced formation of the 19 kDa PrP^{Sc}, whereas fCJD(E200K) and sCJD extracts produced the 21 kDa PrP^{Sc} in mice expressing the same transgene (Telling et al., 1996). On second passage, transgenic (Tg) mice inoculated with FFI prions showed an incubation time of ∼130 days and a 19 kDa PrP^{Sc}, whereas those inoculated with fCJD(E200K) prions exhibited an incubation time of ∼170 days and a 21 kDa PrP^{Sc} (Prusiner, 1998b). The experimental data demonstrate that chimeric PrP^{Sc} can exist in two different conformations based on the sizes of the pro-

Table 15.6. Distinct prion strains generated in humans with inherited prion diseases and transmitted to transgenic mice[a]

Inoculum	Host Species	Host PrP Genotype	Incubation time [days ± SEM] (n/n$_0$)	PrP^{Sc}(kDa)
None	Human	FFI(D178N, M129)		19
FFI	Mouse	Tg(MHu2M)	206 ± 7(7/7)	19
FFI→Tg(MHu2M)	Mouse	Tg(MHu2M)	136 ± 1 (6/6)	19
None	Human	fCJD(E200K)		21
fCJD	Mouse	Tg(MHu2M)	170 ± 2 (10/10)	21
fCJD→Tg(MHu2M)	Mouse	Tg(MHu2M)	167 ± 3 (15/15)	21

Notes:

[a] Data from references (Prusiner, 1998a,b; Telling et al., 1996). Tg(MHu2M) mice express a chimeric human-mouse PrP gene. Clinicopathologic phenotype is determined by the conformation of PrP^{Sc} in accord with the results of the transmission of human prions from patients with FFI to Tg mice (Telling et al., 1996).

tease-resistant fragments; yet the amino acid sequence of PrP^{Sc} is invariant.

This analysis was extended when patients with sporadic fatal insomnia (sFI) were found. Although they did not carry a PrP gene mutation, the clinical and pathologic phenotype was indistinguishable from that of FFI patients. Furthermore, 19 kDa PrP^{Sc} was found in their brains and upon passage of these human prions to mice expressing a chimeric human-mouse PrP transgene, the 19 kDa PrP^{Sc} was also found (Mastrianni et al., 1999). These findings contend that the disease phenotype is dictated by the conformation of PrP^{Sc} and not by the amino acid sequence. The results also demand that PrP^{Sc} acts as a template for the conversion of PrP^{C} into nascent PrP^{Sc}.

Sporadic and genetic neurodegenerative diseases

Prion diseases

Initiation of sporadic disease may follow from a somatic mutation and thus, develop in a manner similar to that for germline mutations in inherited disease (Table 15.5). In this situation, the mutant PrP^{Sc} must be capable of recruiting wt PrP^{C}, a process known to be possible for some mutations (e.g. E200K, D178N) but less likely for others (e.g. P102L) (Telling et al., 1995). Alternatively, the activation barrier separating wt PrP^{C} from PrP^{Sc} could be crossed on rare occasions when viewed in the context of a large population (Fig. 15.3) (Cohen & Prusiner, 1998).

More than 20 different mutations in the human PrP gene resulting in non-conservative substitutions have been found to segregate with inherited human prion diseases, to date (Gambetti et al., 1999). Missense mutations and expansions in the octapeptide repeat region of the gene are responsible for familial forms of prion disease. Five different mutations of the PrP gene have been linked genetically to heritable prion disease (Dlouhy et al., 1992; Gabizon et al., 1993; Hsiao et al., 1989a; Petersen et al., 1992; Poulter et al., 1992).

Although phenotypes may vary dramatically within families, there is a tendency for certain phenotypes to associate with specific mutations (Gambetti et al., 1999). A clinical phenotype indistinguishable from typical CJD is usually seen with substitutions at codons 180, 183, 200, 208, 210, and 232. Substitutions at codons 117, 102, 105, 198, and 217 are associated with the clinicopathological variant of prion disease known as GSS disease. The normal human PrP sequence contains five repeats of an octapeptide sequence. Insertions of an additional 2 to 9 extra octapeptide repeats are associated with variable phenotypes ranging from a condition indistinguishable from CJD to a slowly progressive dementing illness of many years' duration. A mutation at codon 178, resulting in substitution of asparagine for aspartate, produces FFI if a methionine is encoded at the polymorphic 129 residue on the same allele (Goldfarb et al., 1992). Typical CJD is seen if a valine is encoded at position 129 of the mutant allele.

Particularly puzzling are the factors that determine the disease phenotype. As noted above, there is excellent evidence that the tertiary structure of PrP^{Sc} determines whether this disease-causing protein is deposited in subsets of thalamic neurons producing fatal insomnia or it is deposited more widely and resulting in a dementing illness labeled CJD. As more cases of inherited prion diseases have been studied, multiple exceptions have been recorded in which a mutation that produces GSS with ataxia also results in a dementing illness and vice versa (Hsiao et al., 1990, Mastrianni et al., 1999). Within a single family carrying a PrP mutation, some patients develop peripheral neuropathologies while others do not. Elucidating all of the factors that govern the clinical and neuropathologic phenotypes will be challenging.

PrP gene polymorphisms and dominant negative inhibition

Polymorphisms influence the susceptibility to sporadic, inherited, and infectious forms of prion disease. The methionine/valine polymorphism at position 129 not only determines the clinical phenotype as noted above but it also modulates the age of onset of some inherited prion diseases (Gambetti et al., 1999; Palmer et al., 1991). The finding that homozygosity at codon 129 predisposes to sCJD supports a model of prion production that favours PrP interactions between homologous proteins, as appears to occur in Tg mice expressing SHaPrP inoculated with either hamster prions or mouse prions (Prusiner et al., 1990) as well as in Tg mice expressing a chimeric SHa/Mo PrP transgene inoculated with 'artificial' prions.

A lysine residue at 219 has been found in 12% in the Japanese population and this group seems to be resistant to prion disease (Shibuya et al., 1998). Substitution of the basic residue lysine at position 219 produced dominant negative inhibition of prion replication. In scrapie-infected neuroblastoma (ScN2a) cells and Tg mice, substitution of lysine at position 219 prevented PrP^C from being converted into PrP^{Sc} (Kaneko et al., 1997; Zulianello et al., 2000) (V. Perrier, K. Kaneko, S.J. DeArmond, F.E. Cohen and S.B. Prusiner, in preparation). Not only was PrP^C(219K) unable to support prion replication but it also prevented wt PrP^C from being converted into PrP^{Sc}. Dominant negative inhibition of prion replication has also been found in sheep with substitution of the basic residue arginine at position 171. The sheep with arginine are resistant to scrapie (Hunter et al., 1997; Westaway et al., 1994). Both the inability of PrP^C(171R) to support prion replication and exhibit dominant negative inhibition have been demonstrated in ScN2a cells and Tg mice.

Alzheimer's disease

In AD, Aβ amyloid plaques and NFT are found whether the disease is sporadic or inherited (Table 15.3). Like the familial prion diseases, the inheritance of familial AD is autosomal dominant. In contrast to the prion diseases in which only mutations in the PrP gene have been identified to cause familial prion disease, familial AD can be caused by a mutation in one of at least three different genes: amyloid precursor protein (APP), presenilin 1 (PS1), and presenilin 2(PS2) (Table 15.5) (St. George-Hyslop, 1999). Cleavage of APP at residue 671 by β-secretase and at either residue 711 or 713 by γ-secretase produces Aβ(1-40) or Aβ(1-42), respectively. Aβ(1-40) is soluble and its levels do not correlate with AD whereas Aβ(1-42) readily forms fibrils and is thought to cause CNS dysfunction prior to being deposited in plaques (De Strooper and Annaert, 2000; Selkoe, 1999; Wilson et al., 1999). The cleavage of APP by γ-secretase within the plasma membrane is a highly regulated, complex process (Brown et al., 2000; De Strooper & Annaert, 2000). Cleavage at residue 687 by α-secretase prevents Aβ peptide formation. Six different mutations of the APP gene have been implicated in familial AD. More than 30 mutations of the PS1 gene and two of the PS2 gene in familial AD have been found (St. George-Hyslop, 1999). PS1 and PS2 are thought to form complexes with at least one other protein, nicastrin, and these complexes have γ-secretase activity (Yu et al., 2000). Mutations in PS1 have been shown to increase the amount of Aβ(1-42) peptide.

NFT in AD are composed of PHF that are composed of hyperphosphorylated tau (Goedert et al., 1988; Lee et al., 1991; Wolozin et al., 1986). The tau protein binds to microtubules and facilitates assembly of these polymers but hyperphosphorylated tau isolated from AD brains does not bind to microtubules. Six different isoforms of tau are produced by alternative splicing of a single copy gene expressed in brain. Although mutations of the tau gene cause neurodegeneration as described below, they do not cause AD.

The age of onset of both the sporadic and familial AD is modulated by the allelic variants of apolipoprotein E (ApoE) (Saunders et al., 1993). Three alternative allelic products of ApoE, denoted ε2, ε3 and ε4, differ at amino acid residues 112 and 158. Many people with two ε4 alleles can expect to develop AD at least a decade before those with two copies of ε2, whereas those with ε3 exhibit an intermediate age of onset (Farrer et al., 1997). How ApoE modulates the onset of AD is unknown but one hypothesis suggests that ApoE features in the clearance of the Aβ(1-42) peptide. A less compelling hypothesis argues that ApoE modulates the formation of NFTs that are composed of PHF (Roses, 1994).

Frontotemporal dementia

Mutations in the tau gene are responsible for inherited cases of FTD and Pick's disease (Clark et al., 1998; Hutton et al., 1998; Spillantini et al., 1998b). Like AD, about 90% of FTD cases are sporadic and approximately 10% are familial (Table 15.2). In familial FTD, straight filaments composed of hyperphosphorylated mutant tau have been found (Table 15.3) (Hong et al., 1998). In patients from some families with FTD, NFT composed of PHF have been found; the formation of PHF seems to depend upon the specific tau mutation and the expression of specific isoforms that are determined by alternative splicing (Table 15.5) (Buée et al., 2000). In sporadic FTD, aggregates of tau are rarely found.

Approximately 15% of FTD cases coming to autopsy were found to have Pick bodies (Brun, 1993), which are the neuropathologic hallmark of Pick's disease. Pick bodies are intracellular collections of ubiquitinated tau fibrils (Kertesz & Munoz, 1998). Like FTD, most cases of Pick's disease are sporadic.

In some familial cases of FTD caused by tau mutations, Parkinson's disease and disinhibition have been found (Wilhelmsen et al., 1994). Additional disorders thought to be caused by the aberrant processing of tau include progressive supranuclear palsy (PSP), progressive subcortical gliosis, and corticobasal degeneration (Buée et al., 2000; Conrad et al., 1997; Goedert et al., 1999; Kertesz & Munoz, 1998).

Parkinson's disease

In Parkinson's disease, the same theme of protein deposits in the CNS of patients with sporadic and familial forms of the disease has been discovered. Although most patients with Parkinson's disease have a sporadic form of the disease (Nussbaum & Polymeropoulos, 1997; Tanner et al., 1999), mutations have been discovered in the α-synuclein gene of patients with familial Parkinson's disease (Polymeropoulos et al., 1997). When antibodies were raised to α-synuclein, they were found to stain intracellular aggregates of protein in the malfunctioning neurons of the substantia nigra called Lewy bodies (Spillantini et al., 1997). Lewy bodies are present in both the sporadic and familial forms of Parkinson's disease. While the inheritance of Parkinson's disease caused by mutations in the α-synuclein gene is autosomal dominant, a childhood form of Parkinson's disease caused by mutations in the ubiquitin-protein ligase gene (*parkin*) is a recessive disorder (Table 15.5) (Shimura et al., 2000). The recessive inheritance Parkinson's disease caused by mutations in the *parkin* gene is currently the only familial neurodegenerative disease that is not dominantly inherited. Whether people carrying mutations in the *parkin* gene develop Parkinson's disease due to decreased ubiquitination of α-synuclein is unknown, but the ubiquitin pathway is known to participate in the degradation of α-synuclein. There is considerable interest in the possible role of oxidative metabolism in the etiology of Parkinson's disease and selective nitration of α-synuclein in Lewy bodies has been found (Giasson et al., 2000).

The onset of Parkinson's disease in people age 70 or older is associated with a high incidence of dementia (Hughes et al., 2000). At autopsy, the brains of these people often display the neuropathologic hallmarks of both AD and Parkinson's disease. Ubiquitin and α-synuclein immunostaining to identify cortical Lewy bodies has helped resolve the conundrum of how a patient could have insufficient numbers of plaques and NFTs for diagnosis of AD but still be demented. It is estimated that α-synuclein deposition as Lewy bodies in cortical neurons may by itself or in combination with AD changes be the second most common form of neurodegeneration, accounting for 20 to 30% of dementia cases over the age of 60 (Hansen et al., 1990; Hashimoto & Masliah, 1999). A small group of younger people with Parkinson's disease become demented due to diffuse Lewy body disease, in which Lewy bodies are found throughout the cerebral cortex (Spillantini et al., 1998a).

For nearly two decades, some investigators have argued that Parkinson's disease is acquired by the accumulation of toxic molecules in neurons of the substantia nigra (Tanner et al., 1999). The dramatic ability of the synthetic heroin derivative MPTP to produce the symptoms and signs of Parkinson's disease in humans and apes provided seductive evidence in favour of the toxin hypothesis (Langston et al., 2000) as did the possibility that a molecule in cycad plants causes an ALS-Parkinson's disease complex in the indigenous people of Guam (Spencer et al., 1990). Studies of the etiology of Parkinson's disease have also been complicated by Parkinsonism (or the symptoms of Parkinson's disease) that is seen in a variety of neurologic disorders, including post-encephalitis lethargica following the influenza pandemic of 1916–1926 and post-hypoxic encephalopathy.

ALS

While most cases of ALS are sporadic, familial cases have been identified (Table 15.2) (Bobowick & Brody, 1973; Hudson, 1981; Swash, 2000). Approximately 20% of all familial ALS cases has been shown to be due to mutations in the cytoplasmic superoxide dismutase (SOD1) (Table 15.5) (Rosen et al., 1993). Deposits of SOD1 have been found in the CNS of some patients with sporadic and familial forms of ALS (Cleveland & Liu, 2000). Of note, some mutant SOD1 molecules exhibit increased SOD activity compared to wt SOD while others display activities that are similar or decreased compared to wt SOD (Wong et al., 1995). In some cases of ALS, abnormal collections of neurofilaments have been seen in degenerating motor neurons but no familial cases of ALS have been shown to be due to mutations in any of the neurofilament genes (Cleveland & Liu, 2000). In a few cases of sporadic ALS and one family with ALS, deletions in the tail domain of the large neurofilament subunit (NF-H) have been reported.

Huntington's disease and spinocerebellar ataxias

HD and the spinocerebellar ataxias (SCA) provide important contrasts and similarities to the foregoing neurodegenerative diseases. In contrast to AD, FTD, Parkinson's disease, ALS, and the prion diseases, in which most of the cases are sporadic, both HD and the SCAs are exclusively genetic diseases (Table 15.2) (Reed & Neel, 1959) caused by expanded polyglutamine repeats (Table 15.5) (Lin et al., 1999; Martin, 1999; Paulson, 1999). But like the inherited forms of AD, FTD, Parkinson's disease, ALS, and the prion diseases, most cases of HD and the SCAs present with neurologic deficits in adulthood despite the mutant gene products being expressed in the CNS from early in life. Childhood forms of HD and the SCAs are known to be due to enlarged expansions of the triplet repeats that cause these diseases (Lin et al., 1999; The Huntington's Disease Collaborative Research Group, 1993; Zoghbi & Orr, 2000).

In both HD and SCA, the mutant gene products appear to be deposited in the CNS of patients. These misprocessed mutant proteins seem to accumulate in malfunctioning neurons and to be responsible for the neurologic deficits that these patients exhibit. In HD, SCA1, and Machado-Joseph disease (SCA3) as well as in some cases of SCA2, nuclear inclusions of the mutant proteins, which are ubiquitinated, have been found (Koyano et al., 1999; Lin et al., 1999).

Additional disorders caused by the misprocessing of proteins with expanded polyglutamine repeats include spinobulbar muscular atrophy (SBMA) also called Kennedy's syndrome, in which the androgen receptor carries the expanded repeat (LaSpada et al., 1991), as well as dentatorubropallidoluysian atrophy (DRPLA), and the spinocerebellar ataxias 6 and 7 (Martin, 1999; Paulson, 1999).

The neurodegenerative diseases described here represent only a small fraction of the total number of neurologic maladies given this label. Undoubtedly, many of these disorders will require reclassification as the molecular basis of each is elucidated.

Infectious prion diseases

Although infectious prion diseases constitute less than 1% of all cases, the circumstances surrounding these infectious illnesses are often dramatic (Table 15.4) (Will et al., 1999a). The ritualistic cannibalism involved the transmission of kuru among the Fore people of New Guinea, the industrial cannibalism responsible for 'mad cow disease' in Europe, and the growing group of patients with vCJD contracted from prion-tainted beef products are all examples of infectious prion diseases that almost defy imagination.

Kuru

Kuru has disappeared, but the impact of this illness on medical science remains immense. Kuru was the first human prion disease to be transmitted to experimental animals (Gajdusek et al., 1966). Based on the similarities of the neuropathologic lesions of scrapie and kuru (Hadlow, 1959), transmission studies to apes were performed and similar investigations followed with CJD (Gibbs et al., 1968; Klatzo et al., 1959). The transmissibility of kuru suggested that the disease resulted from ritualistic cannibalism among the Fore people living in the highlands of New Guinea (Alpers, 1968). Presumably, kuru began with a person who had developed a sporadic case of prion disease; at death, the brain was removed and distributed to relatives in order to immortalize the spirit of the deceased.

Iatrogenic prion disease

Accidental transmission of CJD to humans appears to have occurred with corneal transplantation (Duffy et al., 1974) and contaminated EEG electrode implantation (Bernouilli et al., 1977). Corneas removed from donors who unknowingly had CJD have been transplanted to apparently healthy recipients who developed CJD after prolonged incubation periods. The same improperly decontaminated EEG electrodes that caused CJD in two young patients with intractable epilepsy were found to cause CJD in a chimpanzee 18 months after their experimental implantation (Gibbs et al., 1994).

Surgical procedures may have resulted in accidental inoculation of patients with prions during their operations (Collins et al., 1999; Gajdusek, 1977; Will & Matthews, 1982), presumably because some instrument or apparatus in the operating theatre became contaminated when a CJD patient underwent surgery. Although the epidemiology of these studies is highly suggestive, no proof for such episodes exists.

Dura mater grafts

More than 70 cases of CJD after implantation of dura mater grafts have been recorded (Centers for Disease Control, 1997). All of the grafts were thought to have been acquired from a single manufacturer whose preparative procedures were inadequate to inactivate human prions. One case of CJD occurred after repair of an eardrum perforation with a pericardium graft (Tange et al., 1989).

Human growth hormone therapy

The possibility of transmission of CJD from contaminated human growth hormone (HGH) preparations derived from human pituitaries has been raised by the occurrence of fatal cerebellar disorders with dementia in more than 100 patients ranging in age from 10 to 41 years (Fradkin et al., 1991; Will et al., 1999a). These patients received injections of HGH every 2 to 4 days for 4 to 12 years (PHS, 1997). Assuming these patients developed CJD from injections of prion-contaminated HGH preparations, the possible incubation periods range from 4 to 30 years. Even though several investigations argue for the efficacy of inactivating prions in HGH fractions prepared from human pituitaries using 6 M urea, it seems doubtful that such protocols will be used for purifying HGH because recombinant HGH is available. Four cases of CJD have occurred in women receiving human pituitary gonadotropin (Cochius et al., 1990).

New variant Creutzfeldt–Jakob disease

The restricted geographical occurrence and chronology of vCJD have raised the possibility that BSE prions have been transmitted to humans. Over 80 vCJD cases have been recorded, but the incidence has been too low to be useful in establishing the origin of vCJD (Balter, 2000; Will et al., 1999b). No set of dietary habits distinguishes vCJD patients from apparently healthy people. Moreover, there is no explanation for the predilection of vCJD for teenagers and young adults. It is noteworthy that epidemiological studies over the past three decades have failed to find evidence for transmission of sheep prions to humans (Cousens et al., 1990). Attempts to predict the future number of cases of vCJD, assuming exposure to bovine prions prior to the offal ban, have been questioned because so few cases of vCJD have occurred (Ghani et al., 2000). Are we at the beginning of a human prion disease epidemic in Great Britain like those seen for BSE and kuru, or will the number of vCJD (vCJD) cases remain small as seen with iatrogenic CJD (iCJD) caused by cadaveric HGH?

Although the mechanism of infection of vCJD has not been yet established, mounting evidence argues for transmission of bovine prions to humans. This conclusion is based on multiple lines of inquiry including: (i) the spatial-temporal clustering of vCJD (Will et al., 1996; Zeidler et al., 1997), (ii) the successful transmission of BSE to macaques with induction of PrP plaques similar to those seen in vCJD (Lasmézas et al., 1996), (iii) the similarity of the glycoform pattern of brain but not tonsil PrP^{Sc} in vCJD to that in cattle, mice, domestic cats, and macaques infected with BSE prions (Hill et al., 1997, 1999), and (iv) transmission studies in non-Tg mice suggesting that vCJD and BSE represent the same prion strain (Bruce et al., 1997). The prolonged incubation periods and inefficient transmission of prions that is seen after inoculation of foreign prions into non-Tg mice can readily confuse the interpretation of the findings (Lasmézas et al., 1997; Prusiner, 1998a).

The most compelling evidence that vCJD is caused by BSE prions has come from experiments using mice expressing the bovine (Bo) PrP transgene (Scott et al., 1999). The incubation times, neuropathologic profiles, and patterns of PrP^{Sc} deposition in Tg mice expressing the BoPrP gene are indistinguishable whether the inocula originated from the brains of cattle with BSE or humans with vCJD (Scott et al., 1999). Neither CJD nor fCJD(E200K) prions have transmitted disease to the Tg(BoPrP) mice. In contrast to CJD and CJD(E200K) prions, which transmit disease efficiently to mice expressing a chimeric human-mouse PrP transgene, vCJD prions do not. Interestingly, none of the Tg mice expressing the chimeric human-mouse PrP developed disease after more than 600 days when inoculated with BSE prions from cattle.

Since the Tg(BoPrP) mice are also excellent hosts for transmission of natural sheep scrapie, this raises the possibility that sheep carry several strains of prions, including the BSE strain (M. Scott and S.B. Prusiner, in preparation). But the BSE strain might replicate more slowly in sheep than many scrapie strains and thus, is present at low levels. If the scrapie strains were more heat labile than the BSE strain, then the rendering process used in the late 1970s and most of the next decade might have selected for the BSE strain. This BSE strain might have then been reselected multiple times as cattle were infected by ingesting prion-contaminated meat and bone meal (MBM). In this situation, the infected cattle were slaughtered and their offal rendered into more MBM, which was subsequently fed to more cattle.

The foregoing scenario suggests that the BSE strain may be widely distributed in sheep and these prions composed of sheep PrP^{Sc} are non-pathogenic for humans. Once the BSE prions are passaged through cattle, they acquire bovine PrP^{Sc} and become pathogenic for humans.

Diagnostic tests

The attempts to develop diagnostic tests for prion diseases are instructive with respect to the other neurodegenerative diseases. The need for accurate, sensitive diagnostic tests for neurodegenerative diseases, preferably blood- or urine-based, is extreme. Advances in imaging the CNS may also aid in the early diagnosis of neurodegeneration. When effective treatments for neurodegenerative diseases are eventually developed as discussed later, early accurate detection of the disease will be critical in order to institute therapies before CNS function is substantially compromised. The difficulty in distinguishing between early AD and depression in older people would benefit from a diagnostic test since both disorders are so common.

With the exception of brain biopsy, there are no specific tests for CJD. If the constellation of pathologic changes frequently found in CJD is seen in a brain biopsy, then the diagnosis is reasonably secure (Fig. 15.4(a) and (b)). The rapid and reliable diagnosis of CJD postmortem can be accomplished by using antisera to PrP. Numerous Western blotting studies have consistently demonstrated PrP immunoreactive proteins that are proteinase K-resistant in the brains of patients with CJD. It is noteworthy that PrP^{Sc} is not uniformly distributed throughout the CNS so that the apparent absence of PrP^{Sc} in a limited sample, such as a biopsy, does not rule out prion disease (Serban et al., 1990; Taraboulos et al., 1992).

A highly sensitive and quantitative immunoassay was developed based upon epitopes that are exposed in PrP^{C} but buried in PrP^{Sc} (Fig. 15.5(a)). Unlike all other immunoassays for PrP^{Sc}, this conformation-dependent immunoassay (CDI) does not require limited proteolysis to hydrolyze PrP^{C} prior to measuring the protease-resistant core of PrP^{Sc} (PrP 27–30) (Safar et al., 1998). Using the CDI, a new form of PrP^{Sc} has been identified, which is protease-sensitive and is denoted sPrP^{Sc}. The levels of sPrP^{Sc} are proportional to the length of the incubation time (Fig. 15.5(b)) and are often much higher than those of protease-resistant PrP^{Sc}. Why levels of sPrP^{Sc} should be directly proportional to the length of the incubation time is unclear. Whether measurement of sPrP^{Sc} will become the basis of diagnostic tests for prion diseases remains to be established.

If the patient has a family history suggestive of inherited CJD, sequencing the PrP gene may facilitate the diagnosis. Sometimes, the PrP sequence is helpful in even seemingly non-familial cases. Obviously, DNA sequencing is a crucial diagnostic tool in all of the inherited neurodegenerative diseases. In the sporadic form of AD, ApoE allelic typing is a necessary adjunct to any clinical study. Moreover, sporadic neurodegenerative diseases require that both alleles encoding the etiologic, misprocessed protein possess the wt sequence.

In the prion diseases, AD, FTD, and Parkinson's disease, the CT or MRI may be normal or show cortical atrophy. In the prion diseases, the MRI scan may show a subtle increase in intensity in the basal ganglia with T2 or diffusion-weighted imaging, but this finding is neither sensitive nor specific enough to make a diagnosis. In AD, widespread atrophy with enlarged ventricles is often seen, especially late in the disease, but this finding is not diagnostic. Many cognitively intact elderly people have similar radiographic findings (Gertz et al., 1988; Kitagaki et al., 1998). In FTD, atrophy is confined to the frontal and temporal lobes while in HD, profound atrophy of the basal ganglia is commonly seen. In all of the neurodegenerative diseases, the CSF is nearly always normal but may show a minimal protein elevation (Cathala & Baron, 1987). Although the protein 14-3-3 is elevated in the CSF of many CJD patients, similar elevations of 14-3-3 are found in patients with herpes simplex virus encephalitis, multi-infarct dementia, and stroke (Johnson & Gibbs, 1998; Zerr et al., 1998). In Alzheimer's disease, 14-3-3 is generally not elevated. In the serum of some patients with CJD, the S-100 protein is elevated, but like 14-3-3, this elevation is not specific (Zerr et al., 1998). Attempts to use Aβ(1–40) levels in blood and urine have been unrewarding (Ghiso et al., 1997) but use of fluorescence correlation spectroscopy with CSF may provide a reliable diagnostic test for AD (Pitschke et al., 1998).

In contrast to AD, FTD, and Parkinson's disease, the electroencephalogram (EEG) is often useful in the diagnosis of CJD. During the early phase of CJD, the EEG is usually normal or shows only scattered theta activity. In most advanced cases, repetitive, high voltage, triphasic, and polyphasic sharp discharges are seen but, in many cases, their presence is transient. The presence of these stereotyped periodic bursts of <200 ms duration, occurring every 1 to 2 sec, makes the diagnosis of CJD very likely (Cathala & Baron, 1987; Johnson & Gibbs, 1998; Kirschbaum, 1968; Nevin et al., 1960). These discharges are frequently but not always symmetrical; there may be a one-sided predominance in amplitude. As CJD progresses, normal background rhythms become fragmentary and slower.

The possibility of Hashimoto's thyroiditis should always be considered in the differential diagnosis of CJD (Seipelt et al., 1999) since this autoimmune disease is treatable and CJD is not. That the clinical and neuropathologic findings can be so similar in Hashimoto's thyroiditis and CJD is striking; moreover, it raises the possibility that protein misprocessing may underlie both degenerative and autoimmune diseases.

Transgenic models of neurodegeneration

Prion diseases

The development of Tg mouse models that reproduce virtually every aspect of naturally occurring prion disease has created a firm foundation upon which to decipher

(a)

Conformation dependent immunoassay (CDI) for PrP^{Sc}

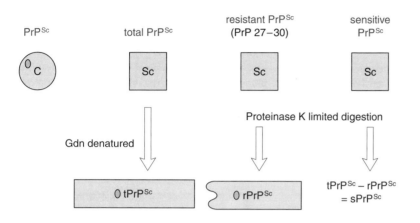

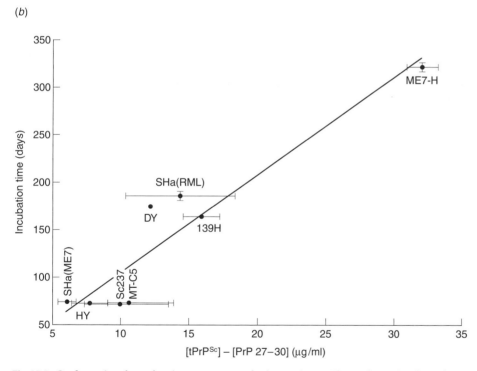

Fig. 15.5. Conformation-dependent immunoassay and prion strains. (a) The conformation dependent immunoassay (CDI) permits measurement of PrP^{Sc} without limited digestion by protease to eliminate PrP^{C}; instead, antibodies to epitopes that are exposed in PrP^{C} but buried in PrP^{Sc} are used to distinguish between the two isoforms. Using the CDI, it became possible to detect two different forms of PrP^{Sc}: one which is resistant to limited digestion by protease and the other which is readily digested. Using one fraction of a sample, total (t) PrP^{Sc} is measured while another aliquot is digested prior to determining the protease-resistant (r) PrP^{Sc} level. rPrP^{Sc} is equivalent to PrP 27–30. By subtracting rPrP^{Sc} from the tPrP^{Sc}, the amount of protease-sensitive (s) PrP^{Sc} can be determined. (b) When the levels of sPrP^{Sc} in brain for eight different prion strains were plotted as a function of the incubation times in Syrian hamsters, a straight line was obtained with an r value of 0.94. (Data from Safar et al., 1998.)

the molecular pathogenesis of prion disease. Tg mice expressing mutant PrP develop CNS degeneration spontaneously and transmit disease to inoculated recipients (Hsiao et al., 1994). Tg mice expressing wt PrP from foreign hosts have been rendered susceptible to foreign prions with abrogation of species barriers (Prusiner et al., 1990), which manifest as a prolongation of the incubation time upon first passage in a foreign host (Pattison, 1965). As the level PrP transgene expression was increased, the incubation time decreased (Prusiner et al., 1990). The species barrier was reproduced in Tg mice expressing a mouse PrP molecule of 106 amino acids with two large deletions accounting for almost 50% of the residues. In these mice, a transmission barrier was observed after inoculation with prions from wt mice, but was abolished once miniprions composed of PrP^{Sc} with 106 residues were used as the inoculum (Supattapone et al., 1999a).

Tg mice expressing the P102L mutation causing GSS the mice developed signs of CNS dysfunction from 50 to 200 days of age (Hsiao et al., 1994). Although little protease-resistant PrP was found, widespread deposition of PrP amyloid and reactive astrocytic gliosis were observed. Extracts from the brains of these ill mice transmitted disease to Tg196 mice expressing the same mutant transgene at a low level that infrequently produces spontaneous disease. The Tg196 mice developed neurologic signs about 240 days after receiving the brain extract and the disease could be serially transmitted. A synthetic peptide of 55 residues carrying the P102L mutation produced disease in Tg196 mice about 360 days after inoculation and the illness could be serially transmitted (Kaneko et al., 2000). Only the mutant peptide in a β-sheet conformation induced by exposure to acetonitrile produced neurologic disease.

Some lines of PrP-deficient ($Prnp^{0/0}$) mice developed ataxia at about 18 months of age (Sakaguchi et al., 1996), while other lines did not (Büeler et al., 1992). Subsequent studies showed that those developing ataxia and Purkinje cell degeneration overexpress an adjacent gene designated Prnd, which encodes the protein doppel (Dpl) (Moore et al., 1999). PrP and Dpl represent an ancient gene duplication with considerable sequence divergence but structural conservation. In mice developing cerebellar degeneration, high levels of an intergenic mRNA were found where the two untranslated exons of the PrP gene were spliced to the Dpl exon containing the open reading frame (ORF) or protein coding region. High levels of Dpl protein expression were found to be toxic for Purkinje cells, but overexpression of PrP rescued the ataxic phenotype (Nishida et al., 1999).

Alzheimer's disease

Tg mice expressing mutant APP have been found to develop amyloid plaques filled with the Aβ peptide (Games et al., 1995; Hsiao et al., 1996). In some cases, these mice show behavioural abnormalities while in others, such changes have not been reported. The development of Aβ plaques was accelerated when extracts from the brains of patients with AD were injected into Tg mice expressing mutant APP (Kane et al., 2000). In earlier studies, AD brain fractions enriched for tau induced deposits of Aβ in the brains of rats (Shin et al., 1993). In uninjected bigenic mice, development of Aβ plaques was hastened by expression of mutant APP and PS1 transgenes (Borchelt et al., 1997). In other bigenic mice expressing human mutant APP and human ApoEε4 but not ε3, cognitive deficits were identified at 6 months of age even though no Aβ plaques could be found (Raber et al., 2000). These findings argue that the neuronal dysfunction in Alzheimer's disease may not be due to the Aβ plaques, but to events occurring prior to the sequestration of Aβ and other molecules into the plaques (Mucke et al., 2000). Such a scenario would be in accord with the findings for prion diseases in which PrP amyloid plaques are not obligatory for disease pathogenesis. In fruit flies, disruption of the APP-like gene or presenilin causes nervous system dysfunction, and overexpression of wt presenilin in flies causes cell death. In worms, suppression of nicastrin expression induces a phenotype similar to that seen with disruption of the presenilin-like genes (Yu et al., 2000).

Nicastrin and the presenilins are thought to form complexes that have γ-secretase activity, which may function in regulated intramembrane proteolysis (Rip) to produce the Aβ peptide from APP (De Strooper et al., 1999). Several other examples in intramembrane proteases acting in diverse metabolic processes have been discovered (Brown et al., 2000; De Strooper & Annaert, 2000).

Frontotemporal dementia

Expression of human tau with the P301L mutation in Tg mice produced neurofibrillary tangles and Pick bodies in neurons throughout the CNS (Lewis et al., 2000). By 10 months of age, ~90% of these Tg mice developed progressive neurologic dysfunction resulting in death within a month.

Parkinson's disease

The expression of either wt or mutant human α-synuclein in fruit flies produced adult onset loss of dopaminergic neurons and locomotor dysfunction (Feany & Bender, 2000). Additionally, filamentous, intraneuronal inclusions of α-synuclein were found. In Tg mice expressing mutant and wt human α-synuclein, intraneuronal inclusions of human α-synuclein were found in the neocortex and hippocampus as well as substantia nigra where a significant loss of dopaminergic neurons was observed (Masliah et al., 2000; van der Putten et al., 2000).

ALS

In Tg mice expressing mutant SOD1, vacuolation, neuronal death, and reactive gliosis in the spinal cord have been found as well as cytoplasmic inclusions of SOD1 in motor neurons (Cleveland & Liu, 2000). Tg mice overexpressing the human large neurofilament subunit (NF-H) produced altered function in large myelinated motor neurons (Kriz et al., 2000). Of particular interest are bigenic mice in which wt NF-H and mutant SOD1(G37R) have been expressed. The overexpression of NF-H extended the lifespan of mice expressing mutant SOD1 by ~6 months (Couillard-Després et al., 1998). The results of these experiments suggest that much of the neurofilament protein was trapped in the cell bodies and thus, was prevented from being transported into the axons where altered neurofilaments would cause dysfunction. Less striking is the increase in survival by ~40 days in Tg mice expressing mutant SOD1(G37R) due to disruption of the neurofilament genes (Williamson et al., 1998).

Huntington's disease

Tg mice expressing the mutant huntingtin protein with 48 or 89 repeating Gln residues develop neurologic dysfunction and striated degeneration (Reddy et al., 1998). In attempts to reproduce all aspects of HD, a large number of Tg mice has been produced using different vectors and varying numbers of CAG repeats (Shelbourne et al., 1999). Notably, YAC clones of the huntingtin gene with 46 or 72 repeating Gln residues have been used to produce selective striatal degeneration (Hodgson et al., 1999). Using the tetracycline inducible transgene system, regulated expression of exon 1 of the huntingtin gene with 94 polyglutamine residues has been used to produce an HD model with reversible neurodegeneration (Yamamoto et al., 2000). Using exon 1 with 92 and 111 repeating Gln residues, gene targeting has been used to produce knockin mice that show accumulation of mutant huntingtin in the nuclei of spiny neurons of the striatum (Wheeler et al., 2000). In Drosophila, expression of the huntingtin protein carrying a polyglutamine repeat of 75 amino acids pro-

duced striking neuronal degeneration (Jackson et al., 1998).

Using cultured neurons from the striatum and hippocampus of the rat, expression of a fragment of the huntingtin protein with 68 repeating Gln residues produced nuclear inclusions of the mutant protein and apoptosis (Saudou et al., 1998). When the nuclear inclusions were diminished by inhibiting ubiquitination, apoptosis increased, arguing that aggregation of the mutant protein helps protect cells. Although some investigators argue that aggregation is an essential feature of the polyglutamine repeat diseases (Perutz, 1996), these results and those discussed below for Tg mice expressing mutant ataxin 1 argue that the misfolding of monomers or oligomers of proteins with Gln expansions is responsible for disease and that nuclear inclusions, which are often seen in humans and Tg models, may reflect sequestration of potentially pathogenic proteins.

Spinocerebellar ataxias

Expanded Gln repeats in ataxin 1 causing SCA1 have been expressed in Tg mice and shown to cause ataxia and Purkinje cell degeneration. Mutation of the nuclear localization signal in ataxin 1 with 82 repeating Gln residues prevented disease in Tg mice (Klement et al., 1998; Lin et al., 1999). In contrast, deletion of 122 amino acids comprising the self-aggregation domain in ataxin 1 with 77 repeating Gln residues did cause disease when expressed in Tg mice. These results argue that nuclear localization is required for disease pathogenesis but aggregation is not. In Tg mice, expression of ataxin 2 with an expanded glutamine repeat of 58 residues resulted in impaired motor skills and cytoplasmic but not nuclear aggregates of the protein in Purkinje cells (Huynh et al., 2000). Tg mice expressing ataxin 3 with an expanded glutamine repeat of 79 residues failed to develop neurologic dysfunction as well as degeneration of cerebellar dentate neurons and the basal ganglia that is seen in Machado–Joseph disease (MJD), also known as SCA3 (Ikeda et al., 1996). When the 79 Gln residues were expressed with adjacent 42 amino acids that are found immediately at the C-terminal of the repeat, they developed ataxia by four weeks of age and showed widespread degeneration of the cerebellum by eight weeks. In Drosophila, expression of the ataxin 3 carrying a polyglutamine repeat of 78 amino acids resulted in degeneration of the eye (Warrick et al., 1999).

The ability to reproduce virtually every aspect of the human prion diseases in Tg mice has proved to be a useful goal for studies of other neurodegenerative diseases. The progress in modelling other neurodegenerative disorders in Tg mice, flies, and worms is impressive. When the CNS dysfunction accompanied by region-specific neuropathology mimicking the human disease is produced in organisms expressing mutant transgenes, it is reasonable to assume that significant progress in understanding the disease process is being made.

Oligomers vs. large aggregates

In a cell culture model of HD and Tg mice expressing mutant ataxin 1, formation of nuclear aggregates was separated from cell death as described above. The issue of whether large aggregates of misprocessed proteins or misfolded monomers (or oligomers) cause CNS degeneration has been addressed in several studies of prion diseases in humans as well as in Tg mice. In humans, the frequency of PrP amyloid plaques varies from 100% in GSS and vCJD to ~70% (Will et al., 1996) in kuru (Klatzo et al., 1959) and ~10% in CJD, arguing that these plaques are a non-obligatory feature of the disease (DeArmond & Prusiner, 1997). In Tg mice expressing both mouse and SHa PrP, those animals inoculated with hamster prions produced hamster prions and developed amyloid plaques composed of SHaPrP (Prusiner et al., 1990). In contrast, those Tg mice inoculated with mouse prions did not develop plaques even though they produced mouse prions and died of scrapie.

While intracellular collections of misprocessed proteins, such as Lewy bodies, nuclear inclusions and Pick bodies, may represent a mechanism whereby cells sequester proteins that cannot be readily degraded, PrP and $A\beta$ amyloid plaques may play a similar role in the extracellular space of the CNS (Table 15.4).

Prevention and therapeutics

There is no known effective therapy for treating or preventing CJD or any of the other neurodegenerative diseases. Only in Parkinson's disease does an effective treatment exist that ameliorates the symptoms (Cotzias et al., 1967; Marsden & Parkes, 1977) but it does not halt the underlying degeneration. Because the prion diseases progress more rapidly than the other neurodegenerative disorders, fatalities from these maladies are more readily measured. There are no well-documented cases of patients with CJD showing recovery either spontaneously or after therapy, with one possible exception (Manuelidis et al., 1976), for which there is no confirmatory example. In the highlands of New Guinea, individuals who were thought to have recovered from kuru were eventually shown to have hysterical illnesses.

The difficulty of developing effective drugs for the prevention and treatment of the neurodegenerative diseases should not be underestimated. New principles of pharmacotherapeutics will undoubtedly emerge from development of drugs for treating neurodegeneration. The history of successful therapeutics for preventing or reversing protein misprocessing is extremely limited. As more is learned about the molecular pathogenesis of the neurodegenerative diseases, more opportunities for drug targets will emerge (Orr & Zoghbi, 2000). Directing these new drugs to specific regions of the CNS will also be challenging.

Preventing misprocessing

Structure-based drug design focused on dominant negative inhibition of prion formation has produced several lead compounds (Perrier et al., 2000). Prion replication depends on protein–protein interactions and a subset of these interactions gives rise to dominant negative phenotypes produced by single residue substitutions (Kaneko et al., 1997; Zulianello et al., 2000). The task of exchanging polypeptide scaffolds for small heterocyclic structures without loss of biological activity remains difficult. Whether this approach, designed to prevent the misfolding and aberrant processing of proteins, will provide general methods for developing novel therapeutics for Alzheimer's and Parkinson's diseases, as well as ALS and other neurodegenerative diseases, remains to be established.

The γ-secretase, which catalyses the hydrolytic cleavage of APP in the production of the $A\beta$ peptide, continues to be a focus with respect to possible therapeutics for AD (Selkoe, 1999). Inhibitors of γ-secretase have been identified and are being evaluated for their efficacy in slowing the ravages of AD. Recent studies suggest that anti-inflammatory and cholesterol-reducing drugs can significantly reduce the risk of AD (Jick et al., 2000).

Enhanced clearance

Several compounds have been demonstrated to eliminate prions from prion-infected cultured cells. A class of compounds known as 'dendrimers' seems particularly efficacious in this regard (Supattapone et al., 1999b). Numerous drugs have been demonstrated to delay the onset of disease in animals inoculated with prions if the drugs are given around the time of the inoculation (Priola et al., 2000). The most common scenario in which one would want to treat humans is either patients showing signs of disease or presymptomatic patients carrying mutations predisposing them to develop prion disease. No treatment has shown any efficacy in animal models of these two scenarios.

A novel approach to treating AD has been developed using Tg mice overexpressing a mutant APP gene. Immunization of these Tg mice with the Aβ peptide resulted in a profound decrease in the Aβ amyloid in the CNS, presumably by accelerating the clearance of Aβ peptides (Schenk et al., 1999). Whether this approach will prove fruitful in patients suffering from AD or applicable to other neurodegenerative disorders is unknown.

Replacement therapy

Because the neurodegeneration in Parkinson's disease is confined largely to the substantia nigra, especially early in the disease process, replacement therapy has proved to be useful; however, many patients eventually become refractory to L-dopa therapy (Marsden & Parkes, 1977).

Similar approaches to AD have been disappointing in large part because the disease process is so widespread. The widespread neuropathology in ALS, FTD, and prion diseases also makes replacement therapy an approach that is unlikely to be successful.

Speculation on the spectrum of degenerative diseases

Besides the neurodegenerative diseases that were discussed previously, it is tempting to speculate that protein misprocessing features in other common diseases of the CNS, such as schizophrenia, bipolar disorders, and autism. Most cases of schizophrenia, bipolar disorders, and autism are sporadic but a substantial minority appear to be familial. The lack of consistent neuropathologic changes in the brains of people with these diseases has impeded studies and complicated phenotypic analysis. Not unlike these diseases are alcoholism and other forms of addiction in which most cases are sporadic but a minority are familial. In one group of patients with inherited FTD, alcoholism and Parkinson's disease are prominent features; these people carry a mutation in the tau gene (Wilhelmsen et al., 1994).

Whether diseases, such as multiple sclerosis (MS), that are frequently classified as neurodegenerative diseases, are caused by protein misprocessing is unknown (Seboun et al., 1997). In MS, the immune system features prominently in the pathogenesis of the disease and thus, it is often argued that MS should be classified as a T-cell mediated autoimmune disorder. In some MS cases, antibody-mediated demyelination has been found (Genain et al., 1999) and in other cases, degeneration of oligodendrocytes has been observed with little or no evidence for immune-mediated damage (Lucchinetti et al., 2000).

Whether the misprocessing of proteins features in neurodegeneration that is independent of the inflammatory process in MS or it initiates an aberrant immune response is unknown. Like the neurodegenerative diseases discussed above, most cases of MS are sporadic while a minority are familial. The inheritance of MS is polygenic but to date, no single mutant gene causing MS has been identified (Haines et al., 1998). Molecular mimicry has been suggested as the mechanism that initiates the immune-mediated demyelination of the CNS in MS, in which an antigenic site on the protein of an infectious pathogen, such as a virus, provokes an immune response directed at an epitope of a myelin protein (Fujinami and Oldstone, 1985; Wucherpfenning and Strominger, 1995). The participation of an infectious pathogen in MS remains an attractive hypothesis that could explain the geographically isolated clusters as well as how the risk for MS is acquired during childhood.

Systemic diseases such as juvenile type I and adult onset type II diabetes mellitus are likely to be caused by protein misprocessing. Juvenile diabetes seems to be an autoimmune disease; despite control of the insulin deficiency, progressive degeneration of peripheral nerves, the retinas, and kidneys often proceeds (Taylor, 1995). In the β-islet cells of patients with type II diabetes, the protein amylin frequently accumulates as amyloid fibrils. Like the juvenile form of diabetes, control of the insulin deficiency does not prevent the development of polyneuropathy, retinopathy, and renal disease in adult onset diabetes. When reflecting on MS, perhaps illnesses like ulcerative colitis, Crohn's disease, rheumatoid arthritis and lupus ought to be considered as possible disorders of protein misprocessing in which misfolded proteins might evoke an autoimmune response. Like the neurodegenerative disorders (Table 15.2), a minority of cases of these autoimmune diseases are familial while the majority are sporadic.

The systemic amyloidoses share important features with the neurodegenerative diseases. In primary amyloidosis, immunoglobulin light chains form amyloid deposits that can cause cardiomyopathy, renal failure and polyneuropathy (Benson, 1995). In response to chronic inflammatory diseases, the serum amyloid A protein is cleaved to form the amyloid A protein, which is deposited as fibrils in the kidney, liver, and spleen. The most common systemic hereditary amyloidosis is caused by the deposition of mutant transthyretin. More than 40 mutations of transthyretin gene have been found to result in proteins causing familial amyloidotic polyneuropathy.

While speculation about the possible role of protein misprocessing in many diseases presents a series of attractive and, in some instances, provocative hypotheses, other mechanisms that compromise cell function need to be entertained. For example, apoptosis can be initiated by a variety of pathways, in which protein misprocessing is likely to play little or no role.

The future

As the lifespan of humans continues to increase through the efforts of modern medical science, an increasing burden of degenerative diseases is emerging. Developing effective means of preventing these disorders and treating them when they do occur are paramount to the personal, political, and economic future of our planet. The problems caused by AD and Parkinson's disease are already so large that if these maladies continue to increase in accord with the changing demographics of the world population, they will bankrupt both the developed and underdeveloped nations over the next 50 years. It is remarkable to think that by the year 2025, more than 65% of people over the age of 65 will be living in countries that are now designated as the developing nations (United Nations, 1999). Unless effective treatments and methods of prevention are developed, this immense group of people will be subject to the same risk for AD, Parkinson's disease, and other neurodegenerative disorders as people who are currently living in the most affluent of nations.

In summary, the discovery of prions and many other findings now permit a molecular definition and classification of the neurodegenerative diseases. Alzheimer's and Parkinson's diseases as well as ALS, FTD and the prion diseases are all disorders of protein processing as are Huntington's disease and the spinocerebellar ataxias. Until recently, clinical signs and neuropathologic lesions were the primary means of describing these disorders. While these characteristics remain useful in diagnosis, the etiologies can now be attributed to the misprocessing of particular proteins. In each of the neurodegenerative disorders, the particular protein that undergoes misprocessing determines the disease-specific phenotype, which results from the malfunction of distinct sets of neurons.

The remarkable progress in elucidating the etiologies of the major neurodegenerative diseases over the past two decades argues that the time has come to intensify the search for drug targets and develop compounds that interrupt the disease processes. In some of the neurodegenera-

tive diseases, it may be most efficacious to design drugs that specifically block the misprocessing of a particular protein while in other cases, drugs that enhance the clearance of an aberrant protein or fragment may prove to be more useful. Regardless of the therapeutic approach, the need for accurate, early detection of neurodegeneration will be extremely important so that drugs can be given before significant damage to the CNS has occurred.

The task of developing useful diagnostic tests and effective therapeutics for neurodegenerative diseases should not be underestimated. Past experience with cardiovascular disease and cancer should be a forewarning of the difficult paths that lie ahead. Nevertheless, the remarkable progress in deciphering the etiologies of the neurodegenerative diseases and the urgency to prevent these age-dependent disorders should provide vigorous encouragement.

Acknowledgements

This work was supported by grants from the National Institutes of Health (NS14069, AG02132 and AG10770) and the American Health Assistance Foundation as well as a gift from the G. Harold and Leila Y. Mathers Foundation. I thank Drs Fred Cohen, Stephen DeArmond, Kirk Wilhemsen, Robert Edwards, Warren Olanow, Steve Finkbiener, and Steve Hauser for their important criticisms and valuable suggestions.

References

Alpers, M.P. (1968). Kuru: implications of its transmissibility for the interpretation of its changing epidemiological pattern. In *The Central Nervous System: Some Experimental Models of Neurological Diseases*, ed. O.T. Bailey and D.E. Smith, pp. 234–51. Baltimore: Williams and Wilkins Co..

Balter, M. (2000). Tracking the human fallout from 'mad cow disease'. *Science*, **289**, 1452–4.

Bendheim, P.E., Barry, R.A., DeArmond, S.J., Stites, D.P. & Prusiner, S.B. (1984). Antibodies to a scrapie prion protein. *Nature*, **310**, 418–21.

Bennett, D.A., Beckett, L.A., Murray, A.M. et al. (1996). Prevalence of Parkinsonian signs and associated mortality in a community population of older people. *N. Engl. J. Med.*, **334**, 71–6.

Benson, M.D. (1995). Amyloidosis. In *The Metabolic and Molecular Bases of Inherited Disease*, 7th edn., ed. C.R. Scriver, A.L. Beaudet, W.S. Sly & D. Valle, pp. 4159–91. New York: McGraw-Hill, Inc.

Bernouilli, C., Siegfried, J., Baumgartner, G. et al. (1977). Danger of accidental person to person transmission of Creutzfeldt-Jakob disease by surgery. *Lancet*, 1, 478–9.

Bessen, R.A. & Marsh, R.F. (1994). Distinct PrP properties suggest the molecular basis of strain variation in transmissible mink encephalopathy. *J. Virol.*, **68**, 7859–68.

Bobowick, A.R. & Brody, J.A. (1973). Epidemiology of motor-neuron diseases. *N. Engl. J. Med.* **288**, 1047–5.

Borchelt, D.R., Ratovitski, T., van Lare, J. et al. (1997). Accelerated amyloid deposition in the brains of transgenic mice coexpressing mutant presenilin 1 and amyloid precursor proteins. *Neuron*, **19**, 939–45.

Brown, M.S., Ye, J., Rawson, R.B. & Goldstein, J.L. (2000). Regulated intramembrane proteolysis: A control mechanism conserved from bacteria to humans. *Cell*, **100**, 391–8.

Bruce, M.E. & Dickinson, A.G. (1987). Biological evidence that the scrapie agent has an independent genome. *J. Gen. Viol.*, **68**, 79–89.

Bruce, M.E., McBride, P.A. & Farquhar, C.F. (1989). Precise targeting of the pathology of the sialoglycoprotein, PrP, and vacuolar degeneration in mouse scrapie. *Neurosci. Lett.* **102**, 1–6.

Bruce, M.E., Will, R.G., Ironside, J.W. et al. (1997). Transmissions to mice indicate that 'new variant' CJD is caused by the BSE agent. *Nature*, **389**, 498–501.

Brun, A. (1993). Frontal lobe degeneration of non-Alzheimer type revisited. *Dementia*, **4**, 126–31.

Buée, L., Bussière, T., Buée-Scherrer, V., Delacourte, A. & Hof, P.R. (2000). Tau protein isoforms, phosphorylation and role in neuro-degenerative disorders. *Brain Res. Brain. Res. Rev.*, **33**, 95–130.

Büeler, H., Fisher, M., Lang, Y. et al. (1992). Normal development and behaviour of mice lacking the neuronal cell-surface PrP protein. *Nature*, **356**, 577–82.

Cathala, F. & Baron, H. (1987). Clinical aspects of Creutzfeldt–Jakob disease. In *Prions – Novel Infectious Pathogens Causing Scrapie and Creutzfeldt–Jakob Disease*, ed. S.B. Prusiner & M.P. McKinley, pp. 467–509. Orlando: Academic Press.

Centers for Disease Control (1997). Creutzfeldt–Jakob disease associated with cadaveric dura mater grafts – Japan, January 1979–May 1996. *MMWR Morb. Mortal Wkly Rep.*, **46**, 1066–9.

Chapman, J., Ben-Israel, J., Goldhammer, Y. & Korczyn, A.D. (1994). The risk of developing Creutzfeldt–Jakob disease in subjects with the *PRNP* gene codon 200 point mutation. *Neurology*, **44**, 1683–6.

Chiti, F., Webster, P., Taddei, N. et al. (1999). Designing conditions for *in vitro* formation of amyloid protofilaments and fibrils. *Proc. Natl. Acad. Sci., USA*, **96**, 3590–4.

Clark, L.N., Poorkaj, P., Wszolek, Z. et al. (1998). Pathogenic implications of mutations in the tau gene in pallido-ponto-nigral degeneration and related neurodegenerative disorders linked to chromosome 17. *Proc. Natl. Acad. Sci., USA*, **95**, 13103–7.

Cleveland, D.W. & Liu, J. (2000). Oxidation versus aggregation – how do SOD1 mutants cause ALS? *Nat. Med.* **6**, 1320–21.

Cochius, J.I., Mack, K., Burns, R.J., Alderman, C.P. & Blumbergs, P.C. (1990). Creutzfeldt–Jakob disease in a recipient of human pituitary-derived gonadotrophin. *Aust. N.Z.J. Med.*, **20**, 592–3.

Cohen, F.E. & Prusiner, S.B. (1998). Pathologic conformations of prion proteins. *Annu. Rev. Biochem.*, **67**, 793–819.

Collins, S., Law, M.G., Fletcher, A., Boyd, A., Kaldor, J. & Masters, C.L. (1999). Surgical treatment and risk of sporadic Creutzfeldt–Jakob disease: a case-control study. *Lancet*, **353**, 693–7.

Conrad, C., Andreadis, A., Trojanowski, J.Q. et al. (1997). Genetic evidence for the involvement of tau in progressive supranuclear palsy [see comments]. *Ann. Neurol.*, **41**, 277–81.

Cotman, C.W., Ivins, K.J. & Anderson, A.J. (1999). Apoptosis in Alzheimer disease. In *Alzheimer Disease*, 2nd edn., ed. R.D. Terry, R. Katzman, K.L. Bick & S.S. Sisodia, pp. 347–57. Philadelphia: Lippincott Williams & Wilkins.

Cotzias, G.C., Van Woert, M.H. & Schiffer, L.M. (1967). Aromatic amino acids and modification of parkinsonism. *N. Engl. J. Med.* **276**, 374–9.

Couillard-Després, S., Zhu, Q., Wong, P.C., Price, D.L., Cleveland, D.W. & Julien, J-P. (1998). Protective effect of neurofilament heavy gene overexpression in motor neuron disease induced by mutant superoxide dismutase. *Proc. Natl. Acad. Sci., USA*, **95**, 9626–30.

Cousens, S.N., Harries-Jones, R., Knight, R., Will, R.G., Smith, P.G. & Matthews, W.B. (1990). Geographical distribution of cases of Creutzfeldt–Jakob disease in England and Wales 1970–84. *J. Neurol. Neurosurg. Psychiatry*, **53**, 459–65.

De Strooper, B. & Annaert, W. (2000). Proteolytic processing and cell biological functions of the amyloid precursor protein. *J. Cell. Sci.*, **113**, 1857–70.

De Strooper, B., Annaert, W., Cupers, P. et al. (1999). A presenilin-1-dependent γ-secretase-like protease mediates release of Notch intracellular domain. *Nature*, **398**, 518–22.

DeArmond, S.J. & Ironside, J.W. (1999). Neuropathology of prion diseases. In *Prion Biology and Diseases*, ed. S.B. Prusiner, pp. 585–652. Cold Spring Harbor, Cold Spring Harbor Laboratory Press.

DeArmond, S.J. & Prusiner, S.B. (1997). Prion diseases. In *Greenfield's Neuropathology*, 6th edn., P. Lantos & D. Graham, pp. 235–80. London, Edward Arnold.

DeArmond, S.J., McKinley, M.P., Barry, R.A., Braunfeld, M.B., McColloch, J.R. & Prusiner, S.B. (1985). Identification of prion amyloid filaments in scrapie-infected brain. *Cell*, **41**, 221–35.

DeArmond, S.J., Mobley, W.C., DeMott, D.L., Barry, R.A., Beckstead, J.H. & Prusiner, S.B. (1987). Changes in the localization of brain prion proteins during scrapie infection. *Neurology*, **37**, 1271–80.

Dickinson, A.G., Meikle, V.M.H. & Fraser, H. (1968). Identification of a gene which controls the incubation period of some strains of scrapie agent in mice. *J. Comp. Pathol.* **78**, 293–9.

Dlouhy, S.R., Hsiao, K., Farlow, M.R. et al. (1992). Linkage of the Indiana kindred of Gerstmann–Sträussler–Scheinker disease to the prion protein gene. *Nat. Genet.*, **1**, 64–7.

Duffy, P., Wolf, J., Collins, G., Devoe, A., Streeten, B. & Cowen, D. (1974). Possible person to person transmission of Creutzfeldt–Jakob disease. *N. Engl. J. Med.*, **290**, 692–3.

Evans, D.A., Funkenstein, H.H., Albert, M.S. et al. (1989). Prevalence of Alzheimer's disease in a community population of older persons – Higher than previously reported. *J. Am. Med. Ass.*, **10**, 2551–6.

Farrer, L.A., Cupples, L.A., Haines, J.L. et al. (1997). Effects of age, sex, and ethnicity on the association between apolipoprotein E genotype and Alzheimer disease. *J. Am. Med. Ass.*, **278**, 1349–56.

Feany, M.B. & Bender, W.W. (2000). A *Drosophila* model of Parkinson's disease. *Nature*, **404**, 394–8.

Fradkin, J.E., Schonberger, L.B., Mills, J.L. et al. (1991). Creutzfeldt–Jakob disease in pituitary growth hormone recipients in the United States. *J. Am. Med. Ass.*, **265**, 880–4.

Fujinami, R.S. & Oldstone, M.B.A. (1985). Amino acid homology between the encephalitogenic site of myelin basic protein and virus: mechanism for autoimmunity. *Science*, **230**, 1043–5.

Gabizon, R., Rosenmann, H., Meiner, Z. et al. (1993). Mutation and polymorphism of the prion protein gene in Libyan Jews with Creutzfeldt–Jakob disease (CJD). *Am. J. Hum. Genet.*, **53**, 828–35.

Gajdusek, D.C. (1977). Unconventional viruses and the origin and disappearance of kuru. *Science*, **197**, 943–60.

Gajdusek, D.C., Gibbs, C.J., Jr. & Alpers, M. (1966). Experimental transmission of a kuru-like syndrome to chimpanzees. *Nature*, **209**, 794–6.

Gambetti, P., Peterson, R.B., Parchi, P. et al. (1999). Inherited prion diseases. In *Prion Biology and Diseases*, ed. S.B. Prusiner, pp. 509–83. Cold Spring Harbor, Cold Spring Harbor Laboratory Press.

Games, D., Adams, D., Alessandrini, R. et al. (1995). Alzheimer-type neuropathology in transgenic mice overexpressing V717F β-amyloid precursor protein. *Nature*, **373**, 523–7.

Genain, C.P., Cannella, B., Hauser, S.L. & Raine, C.S. (1999). Identification of autoantibodies associated with myelin damage in multiple sclerosis. *Nat. Med.*, **5**, 170–5.

Gertz, H.J., Henkes, H., & Cervos-Navarro, J. (1988). Creutzfeldt–Jakob disease: correlation of MRI and neuropathologic findings. *Neurology*, **38**, 1481–2.

Ghani, A.C., Ferguson, N.M., Donnelly, C.A. & Anderson, R.M. (2000). Predicted vCJD mortality in Great Britain. *Nature*, **406**, 583–4.

Ghiso, J., Calero, M., Matsubara, E. et al. (1997). Alzheimer's soluble amyloid β is a normal component of human urine. *FEBS Lett.*, **408**, 105–8.

Giasson, B.I., Duda, J.E., Murray, I.V.J. et al. (2000). Oxidative damage linked to neurodegeneration by selective α-synuclein nitration in synucleinopathy lesions. *Science*, **290**, 985–9.

Gibbs, C.J., Jr., Gajdusek, D.C., Asher, D.M. et al. (1968). Creutzfeldt–Jakob disease (spongiform encephalopathy): transmission to the chimpanzee. *Science*, **161**, 388–9.

Gibbs, C.J., Jr., Asher, D.M., Kobrine, A., Amyx, H.L., Sulima, M.P., & Gajdusek, D.C. (1994). Transmission of Creutzfeldt–Jakob disease to a chimpanzee by electrodes contaminated during neurosurgery. *J. Neurol. Neurosurg. Psychiatry*, **57**, 757–8.

Glenner, G.G. & Wong, C.W. (1984). Alzheimer's disease: initial report of the purification and characterization of a novel cerebrovascular amyloid protein. *Biochem. Biophys. Res. Commun.*, **120**, 885–90.

Goedert, M., Wischik, C.M., Crowther, R.A., Walker, J.E. & Klug, A. (1988). Cloning and sequencing of the cDNA encoding a core protein of the paired helical filament of Alzheimer disease: identification as the microtubule-associated protein tau. *Proc. Natl. Acad. Sci. USA*, **85**, 4051–5.

Goedert, M., Spillantini, M.G., Crowther, R.A. et al. (1999). *Tau* gene mutation in familial progressive subcortical gliosis. *Nat. Med.*, **5**, 454–7.

Goldfarb, L.G., Petersen, R.B., Tabaton, M. et al. (1992). Fatal familial insomnia and familial Creutzfeldt–Jakob disease: disease phenotype determined by a DNA polymorphism. *Science*, **258**, 806–8.

Hadlow, W.J. (1959). Scrapie and kuru. *Lancet*, **ii**, 289–90.

Haines, J.L., Terwedow, H.A., Burgess, K. et al. (1998). Linkage of the MHC to familial multiple sclerosis suggests genetic heterogeneity. *Hum. Mol. Genet.*, **7**, 1229–34.

Hansen, L., Salmon, D., Galasko, D. et al. (1990). The Lewy body variant of Alzheimer's disease: a clinical and pathologic entity. *Neurology*, **40**, 1–8.

Hashimoto, M. & Masliah, E. (1999). α-synuclein in Lewy body disease and Alzheimer's disease. *Brain Pathol.*, **9**, 707–20.

Hershko, A. & Ciechanover, A. (1998). The ubiquitin system, *Annu. Rev. Biochem.*, **67**, 425–79.

Hill, A.F., Desbruslais, M., Joiner, S. et al. (1997). The same prion strain causes vCJD and BSE. *Nature*, **389**, 448–50.

Hill, A.F., Butterworth, R.J., Joiner, S. et al. (1999). Investigation of variant Creutzfeldt–Jakob disease and other human prion diseases with tonsil biopsy samples. *Lancet*, **353**, 183–9.

Hodgson, J.G., Agopyan, N., Gutekunst, C. et al. (1999). A YAC mouse model for Huntington's disease with full-length mutant huntingtin, cytoplasmic toxicity, and selective striatal neurodegeneration. *Neuron*, **23**, 181–92.

Holman, R.C., Khan, A.S., Belay, E.D. & Schonberger, L.B. (1996). Creutzfeldt–Jakob disease in the United States, 1979–1994: using national mortality data to assess the possible occurrence of variant cases. *Emerg. Infect. Dis.*, **2**, 333–7.

Hong, M., Zhukareva, V., Vogelsberg-Ragaglia, V. et al. (1998). Mutation-specific functional impairments in distinct tau isoforms of hereditary FTDP-17. *Science*, **282**, 1914–17.

Hsiao, K., Baker, H.F., Crow, T.J. et al. (1989a). Linkage of a prion protein missense variant to Gerstmann–Sträussler syndrome. *Nature*, **338**, 342–5.

Hsiao, K.K., Doh-ura, K., Kitamoto, T., Tateishi, J. & Prusiner, S.B. (1989b). A prion protein amino acid substitution in ataxic Gerstmann–Sträussler syndrome. *Ann. Neurol.*, **26**, 137.

Hsiao, K.K., Cass, C., Schellenberg, G., Dwine-Gage, E., Bird, T. & Prusiner, S.B. (1990). Correlation of specific prion protein mutations with different forms of prion diseases. *Neurology*, **40**, 388.

Hsiao, K.K., Groth, D., Scott, M. et al. (1994). Serial transmission in rodents of neurodegeneration from transgenic mice expressing mutant prion protein. *Proc. Natl. Acad. Sci., USA*, **91**, 9126–30

Hsiao, K., Chapman, P., Nilsen, S. et al. (1996). Correlative memory deficits, Aβ elevation, and amyloid plaques in transgenic mice. *Science*, **274**, 99–102.

Huang, Z., Prusiner, S.B. & Cohen, F.E. (1995). Scrapie prions: a three-dimensional model of an infectious fragment. *Folding Design*, **1**, 13–19.

Hudson, A.J. (1981). Amyotrophic lateral sclerosis and its association with dementia, parkinsonism and other neurological disorders: a review. *Brain*, **104**, 217–47.

Hughes, T.A., Ross, H.F., Musa, S. et al. (2000). A 10-year study of the incidence of and factors predicting dementia in Parkinson's disease. *Neurology*, **54**, 1596–624.

Hunter, N., Moore, L., Hosie, B.D., Dingwall, W.S. & Greig, A. (1997). Association between natural scrapie and PrP genotype in a flock of Suffolk sheep in Scotland. *Vet. Rec.*, **140**, 59–63.

Hutton, M., Lendon, C.L., Rizzu, P. et al. (1998). Association of missense and 5′-splice-site mutations in tau with the inherited dementia FTDP-17. *Nature*, **393**, 702–5.

Huynh, D.P., Figueroa, K., Hoang, N. & Pulst, S-M. (2000). Nuclear localization or inclusion body formation of ataxin-2 are not necessary for SCA2 pathogenesis in mouse or human. *Nat. Genet.* **26**, 44–50.

Ikeda, H., Yamaguchi, M., Sugai, S., Aze, Y., Narumiya, S. & Kakizuka, A. (1996). Expanded polyglutamine in the Machado–Joseph disease protein induces cell death *in vitro* and *in vivo*. *Nat. Genet.*, **13**, 196–202.

Jackson, G.R., Salecker, I., Dong, X. et al. (1998). Polyglutamine-expanded human huntingtin transgenes induce degeneration of *Drosophila* photoreceptor neurons. *Neuron*, **21**, 633–42.

Jick, H., Zornberg, G.L., Jick, S.S., Seshadri, S. & Drachman, D.A. (2000). Statins and the risk of dementia. *Lancet*, **356**, 1627–31.

Johnson, R.T. & Gibbs, C.J., Jr. (1998). Creutzfeldt–Jakob disease and related transmissible spongiform encephalopathies. *N. Engl. J. Med.*, **339**, 1994–2004.

Kahana, E., Milton, A., Braham, J. & Sofer, D. (1974). Creutzfeldt–Jakob disease: focus among Libyan Jews in Israel. *Science*, **183**, 90–1.

Kane, M.D., Lipinski, W.J., Callahan, M.J. et al. (2000). Evidence for seeding of beta-amyloid by intracerebral infusion of Alzheimer brain extracts in beta-amyloid precursor protein-transgenic mice. *J. Neurosci.*, **20**, 3606–11.

Kaneko, K., Zulianello, L., Scott, M. et al. (1997). Evidence for protein X binding to a discontinuous epitope on the cellular prion protein during scrapie prion propagation. *Proc. Natl. Acad. Sci. USA*, **94**, 10069–74.

Kaneko, K., Ball, H.L., Wille, H. et al. (2000). A synthetic peptide initiates Gerstmann–Sträussler–Scheinker (GSS) disease in transgenic mice. *J. Mol. Biol.* **295**, 997–1007.

Kawas, C.H. & Katzman, R. (1999). Epidemiology of dementia and Alzheimer disease. In *Alzheimer Disease*, 2nd edn., ed. R.D. Terry, R. Katzman, K.L. Bick & S.S. Sisodia, pp. 95–116. Philadelphia, PA: Lippincott Williams & Wilkins.

Kertesz, A. & Munoz, D.G. (eds.) (1998). *Pick's Disease and Pick Complex*. New York, Wiley-Liss.

Kirschbaum, W.R. (1968). *Jakob–Creutzfeldt Disease*. Amsterdam: Elsevier.

Kitagaki, H., Mori, E., Yamaji, S. et al. (1998). Frontotemporal dementia and Alzheimer disease: evaluation of cortical atrophy with automated hemispheric surface display generated with MR images. *Radiology*, **208**, 431–9.

Klatzo, I., Gajdusek, D.C. & Zigas, V. (1959). Pathology of kuru. *Lab. Invest.*, **8**, 799–847.

Klement, I.A., Skinner, P.J., Kaytor, M.D. et al. (1998). Ataxin-1 nuclear localization and aggregation: role in polyglutamine-induced disease in *SCA1* transgenic mice. *Cell*, **95**, 41–53.

Koyano, S., Uchihara, T., Fujigasaki, H., Nakamura, A., Yagishita, S.

& Iwabuchi, K. (1999). Neuronal intranuclear inclusions in spinocerebellar ataxia type 2: triple-labeling immunofluorescent study. *Neurosci. Lett.*, **273**, 117–20.

Kriz, J., Meier, J., Julien, J-P. & Padjen, A.L. (2000). Altered ionic conductances in axons of transgenic mouse expressing the human neurofilament heavy gene: a mouse model of amyotrophic lateral sclerosis. *Exp. Neurol.*, **163**, 414–21.

Langston, J.W., Quik, M., Petzinger, G., Jakowec, M. & Di Monte, D.A. (2000). Investigating Levodopa-induced dyskinesias in the Parkinsonian primate. *Ann. Neurol.*, **47**, S79–89.

Lasmézas, C.I., Deslys, J-P., Demaimay, R. et al. (1996). BSE transmission to macaques. *Nature*, **381**, 743–4.

Lasmézas, C.I., Deslys, J-P., Robain, O. et al. (1997). Transmission of the BSE agent to mice in the absence of detectable abnormal prion protein. *Science*, **275**, 402–5.

LaSpada, A.R., Wilson, E.M., Lubahn, D.B., Harding, A.E. & Fischbeck, K.H. (1991). Androgen receptor gene mutations in X-linked spinal and bulbar muscular atrophy. *Nature*, **352**, 77.

Lee, V. M-Y., Balin, B.J., Orvos, I.J. & Trojanowski, J.Q. (1991). A68: a major subunit of paired helical filaments and derivatized forms of normal tau. *Science*, **251**, 645–78.

Lewis, J., McGowan, E., Rockwood, J. et al. (2000). Neurofibrillary tangles, amyotrophy and progressive motor disturbance in mice expressing mutant (P301L) tau protein. *Nat. Genet.*, **25**, 402–5.

Lilienfield, D.E. (1993). An epidemiological overview of amyotrophic lateral sclerosis, Parkinson's disease, and dementia of the Alzheimer's type. In *Neurodegenerative Diseases*, ed. D.B. Calne, pp. 399–425. New York, W.B. Saunders.

Lin, X., Cummings, C.J. & Zoghbi, H.Y. (1999). Expanding our understanding of polyglutamine diseases through mouse models. *Neuron*, **24**, 499–502.

Liu, H., Farr-Jones, S., Ulyanov, N.B., Llinas, M. et al. (1999). Solution structure of Syrian hamster prion protein rPrP (90–231). *Biochemistry*, **38**, 5362–77.

Lucchinetti, C., Brück, W., Parisi, J., Scheithauer, B., Rodriguez, M. & Lassmann, H. (2000). Heterogeneity of multiple sclerosis lesions: implications for the pathogenesis of demyelination. *Ann. Neurol.*, **47**, 707–17.

McKinley, M.P., Meyer, R.K., Kenaga, L. et al. (1991). Scrapie prion rod formation *in vitro* requires both detergent extraction and limited proteolysis. *J. Virol.*, **65**, 1340–51.

Manuelidis, E., Kim, J., Angelo, J. & Manuelidis, L. (1976). Serial propagation of Creutzfeld–Jakob disease in guinea pigs. *Proc. Natl. Acad. Sci. USA*, **73**, 223–7.

Markesbery, W.R. & Ehmann, W.D. (1999). Oxidative stress in Alzheimer disease. In *Alzheimer Disease*, 2nd edn., ed. R.D. Terry, R. Katzman, K.L. Bick & S.S. Sisodia, pp. 401–14. Philadelphia, Lippincott Williams & Wilkins.

Marsden, C.D. & Parkes, J.D. (1977). Success and problems of long-term levodopa therapy in Parkinson's disease. *Lancet*, **1**, 345–9.

Martin, J.B. (1999). Molecular basis of the neurodegenerative disorders. *N. Engl. J. Med.*, **340**, 1970–80.

Masliah, E., Rockenstein, E., Veinbergs, I. et al. (2000). Dopaminergic loss and inclusion body formation in α-synuclein mice: Implications for neurodegenerative disorders. *Science*, **287**, 1265–9.

Masters, C.L., Harris, J.O., Gajdusek, D.C., Gibbs, C.J., Jr., Bernouilli, C. & Asher, D.M. (1978). Creutzfeldt–Jakob disease: patterns of worldwide occurrence and the significance of familial and sporadic clustering. *Ann. Neurol.*, **5**, 177–88.

Masters, C.L., Gajdusek, D.C. & Gibbs, C.J., Jr. (1981). Creutzfeldt–Jakob disease virus isolations from the Gerstmann–Sträussler syndrome, *Brain*, **104**, 559–88.

Masters, C.L., Simms, G., Weinman, N.A., Multhaup, G., McDonald, B.L. & Beyreuther, K. (1985). Amyloid plaque core protein in Alzheimer disease and Down syndrome. *Proc. Natl. Acad. Sci., USA*, **82**, 4245–9.

Mastrianni, J.A., Nixon, R., Layzer, R. et al. (1999). Prion protein conformation in a patient with sporadic fatal insomnia. *N. Engl. J. Med.*, **340**, 1630–8.

Moore, R.C., Lee, I.Y., Silverman, G.L. et al. (1999). Ataxia in prion protein (PrP) deficient mice is associated with upregulation of the novel PrP-like protein doppel. *J. Mol. Biol.*, **292**, 797–817.

Mucke, L., Masliah, E., Yu, G-Q. et al. (2000). High-level neuronal expression of Aβ_{1-42} in wild-type human amyloid protein precursor transgenic mice: Synaptotoxicity without plaque formation. *J. Neurosci.*, **20**, 4050–8.

Nevin, S., McMenemy, W.H., Behrman, S. & Jones, D.P. (1960). Subacute spongiform encephalopathy – a subacute form of encephalopathy attributable to vascular dysfunction (spongiform cerebral atrophy). *Brain*, **83**, 519–64.

Nishida, N., Tremblay, P., Sugimoto, T. et al. (1999). A mouse prion protein transgene rescues mice deficient for the prion protein gene from Purkinje cell degeneration and demyelination. *Lab. Invest.*, **79**, 689–97.

Nussbaum, R.L. & Polymeropoulos, M.H. (1997). Genetics of Parkinson's disease. *Hum. Mol. Genet.*, **6**, 1687–91.

Orr, H.T. & Zoghbi, H.Y. (2000). Reversing neurodegeneration: a promise unfolds. *Cell*, **101**, 1–4.

Palmer, M.S., Dryden, A.J., Hughes, J.T. & Collinge, J. (1991). Homozygous prion protein genotype predisposes to sporadic Creutzfeldt–Jakob disease. *Nature*, **352**, 340–2.

Pan, K-M., Baldwin, M., Nguyen, J. et al. (1993). Conversion of α-helices into β-sheets features in the formation of the scrapie prion proteins. *Proc. Natl. Acad. Sci. USA*, **90**, 10962–6.

Parchi, P., Castellani, R., Capellari, S. et al. (1996). Molecular basis of phenotypic variability in sporadic Creutzfeldt–Jakob disease. *Ann. Neurol.*, **39**, 767–78.

Pattison, I.H. (1965). Experiments with scrapie with special reference to the nature of the agent and the pathology of the disease. In *Slow, Latent and Temperate Virus Infections*, NINDB Monograph 2, ed. D.C. Gajdusek, C.J. Gibbs, Jr. & M.P. Alpers, pp. 249–57. Washington, DC, US Government Printing.

Paulson, H.L. (1999). Protein fate in neurodegenerative proteinopathies: polyglutamine diseases join the (mis)fold. *Am. J. Hum. Genet.*, **64**, 339–45.

Peretz, D., Williamson, R.A., Matsunaga, Y. et al. (1997). A conformational transition at the N terminus of the prion protein features in formation of the scrapie isoform. *J. Mol. Biol.*, **273**, 614–22.

Perrier, V., Wallace, A.C., Kaneko, K., Safar, J., Prusiner, S.B. & Cohen, F.E. (2000). Mimicking dominant negative inhibition of prion replication through structure-based drug design. *Proc. Natl. Acad. Sci., USA*, **97**, 6073–8.

Perutz, M.F. (1996). Glutamine repeats and inherited neurodegenerative diseases: molecular aspects. *Curr. Opin. Struct. Biol.*, **6**, 848–58.

Petersen, R.B., Tabaton, M., Berg, L. et al. (1992). Analysis of the prion protein gene in thalamic dementia. *Neurology*, **42**, 1859–63.

PHS (1997). Report on human growth hormone and Creutzfeldt–Jakob disease. Public Health Service Interagency Coordinating Committee, pp. 1–11.

Pitschke, M., Prior, R., Haupt, M. & Reisner, D. (1998). Detection of single amyloid beta-protein aggregates in the cerebrospinal fluid of Alzheimer's patients by fluorescence correlation spectroscopy. *Nat. Med.*, **4**, 832–4.

Polymeropoulos, M.H., Lavedan, C., Leroy, E. et al. (1997). Mutation in the α-synuclein gene identified in families with Parkinson's disease. *Science*, **276**, 2045–7.

Poulter, M., Baker, H.F., Frith, C.D. et al. (1992). Inherited prion disease with 144 base pair gene insertion. 1. Genealogical and molecular studies, *Brain*, **115**, 675–85.

Priola, S.A., Raines, A. & Caughey, W.S. (2000). Porphyrin and phthalocyanine antiscrapie compounds. *Science*, **287**, 1503–6.

Prusiner, S.B. (1984). Some speculations about prions, amyloid, and Alzheimer's disease. *N. Engl. J. Med.*, **310**, 661–3.

Prusiner, S.B. (1998a). Molecular neurology of prion diseases. In *Molecular Neurology*, ed. J.B. Martin. New York: Scientific American.

Prusiner, S.B. (1998b). Prions. *Proc. Natl. Acad. Sci. USA*, **95**, 13363–83.

Prusiner, S.B. (1991). Molecular biology of prion diseases, *Science*, **252**, 1515–22.

Prusiner, S.B. (1999). Development of the prion concept. In *Prion Biology and Diseases*, ed. S.B. Prusiner, pp. 67–112. Cold Spring Harbor: Cold Spring Harbor Laboratory Press.

Prusiner, S.B., Bolton, D.C., Groth, D.F., Bowman, K.A., Cochran, S.P. & McKinley, M.P. (1982). Further purification and characterization of scrapie prions. *Biochemistry*, **21**, 6942–50.

Prusiner, S.B., McKinley, M.P., Bowman, K.A. et al. (1983). Scrapie prions aggregate to form amyloid-like birefringent rods. *Cell*, **35**, 349–58.

Prusiner, S.B., Cochran, S.P. & Alpers, M.P. (1985). Transmission of scrapie in hamsters. *J. Infect. Dis.*, **152**, 971–8.

Prusiner, S.B., Scott, M., Foster, D. et al. (1990). Transgenetic studies implicate interactions between homologous PrP isoforms in scrapie prion replication. *Cell*, **63**, 673–86.

Raber, J., Wong, D., Yu, G.Q., Buttini, M., Mahley, R.W., Pitas, R.E. & Mucke, L. (2000). Apolipoprotein E and cognitive performance. *Nature*, **404**, 352–4.

Reddy, P.H., Williams, M., Charles, V. et al. (1998). Behavioural abnormalities and selective neuronal loss in HD transgenic mice expressing mutated full-length *HD* cDNA. *Nat. Genet.*, **20**, 198–202.

Reed, T.E. & Neel, J.V. (1959). Huntington's Chorea in Michigan. *Am. J. Hum. Genet.*, **11**, 107–36.

Ridley, R.M. & Baker, H.F. (1996). To what extent is strain variation evidence for an independent genome in the agent of the transmissible spongiform encephalopathies? *Neurodegeneration*, **5**, 219–31.

Riek, R., Hornemann, S., Wider, G., Billeter, M., Glockshuber, R. & Wüthrich, K. (1996). NMR structure of the mouse prion protein domain PrP(121–231). *Nature*, **382**, 180–2.

Roos, R., Gajdusek, D.C. & Gibbs, C.J., Jr. (1973). The clinical characteristics of transmissible Creutzfeldt–Jakob disease. *Brain*, **96**, 1–20.

Rosen, D.R., Siddique, T., Patterson, D. et al. (1993). Mutations in Cu/Zn superoxide dismutase gene are associated with familial amyotrophic lateral sclerosis. *Nature*, **362**, 59–62.

Roses, A.D. (1994). Apolipoprotein E affects the rate of Alzheimer disease expression: β-amyloid burden is a secondary consequence dependent on APOE genotype and duration of disease. *J. Neuropathol. Exp. Neurol.*, **53**, 429–37.

Safar, J., Wille, H., Itri, V. et al. (1998). Eight prion strains have PrP^{Sc} molecules with different conformations. *Nat. Med.* **4**, 1157–65.

Sakaguchi, S., Katamine, S., Nishida, N. et al. (1996). Loss of cerebellar Purkinje cells in aged mice homozygous for a disrupted PrP gene. *Nature*, **380**, 528–31.

Saudou, F., Finkbeiner, S., Devys, D. & Greenberg, M. (1998). Huntingtin acts in the nucleus to induce apoptosis but death does not correlate with the formation of intranuclear inclusions. *Cell*, **95**, 55–66.

Saunders, A.M., Strittmatter, W.J., Schmechel, D. et al. (1993). Association of apolipoprotein E allele ε4 with late-onset familial and sporadic Alzheimer's disease. *Neurology*, **43**, 1467–72.

Schenk, D., Barbour, R., Dunn, W. et al. (1999). Immunization with amyloid-beta attenuates Alzheimer-disease-like pathology in the PDAPP mouse. *Nature*, **400**, 173–7.

Scott, M.R., Groth, D., Tatzelt, J. et al. (1997). Propagation of prion strains through specific conformers of the prion protein. *J. Virol.*, **71**, 9032–44.

Scott, M.R., Will, R., Ironside, J. et al. (1999). Compelling transgenetic evidence for transmission of bovine spongiform encephalopathy prions to humans. *Proc. Natl. Acad. Sci., USA*, **96**, 15137–42.

Seboun, E., Oksenberg, J.R. & Hauser, S.L. (1997). Molecular and genetic aspects of multiple sclerosis. In *The Molecular and Genetic Basis of Neurological Disease*, 2nd edn., ed. R.N. Rosenberg, S.B. Prusiner, S. DiMauro & R.L. Barchi, pp. 631–60. Boston: Butterworth-Heinemann.

Seipelt, M., Zerr, I., Nau, R. et al. (1999). Hashimoto's encephalitis as a differential diagnosis of Creutzfeldt–Jakob disease. *J. Neurol. Neurosurg. Psychiatry*, **66**, 172–6.

Selkoe, D.J. (1999). Translating cell biology into therapeutic advances in Alzheimer's disease. *Nature*, **399**, A23–31.

Serban, D., Taraboulos, A., DeArmond, S.J. & Prusiner, S.B. (1990). Rapid detection of Creutzfeldt–Jakob disease and scrapie prion proteins. *Neurology*, **40**, 110–17.

Shelbourne, P.F., Killeen, N., Hevner, R.F. et al. (1999). A Huntington's disease CAG expansion at the murine *Hdh* locus is unstable and associated with behavioural abnormalities in mice. *Hum. Mol. Genet.*, **8**, 763–74.

Shibuya, S., Higuchi, J., Shin, R-W., Tateishi, J. & Kitamoto, T. (1998). Codon 219 Lys allele of PRNP is not found in sporadic Creutzfeldt–Jakob disease. *Ann. Neurol.*, **43**, 826–8.

Shimura, H., Hattori, N., Kubo, S-I. et al. (2000). Familial Parkinson disease gene product, parkin, is a ubiquitin-protein ligase. *Nat. Genet.*, **25**, 302–5.

Shin, R-W., Bramblett, G.T., Lee, V. M-Y. & Trojanowski, J.Q. (1993). Alzheimer disease A68 proteins injected into rat brain induce codeposits of β-amyloid, ubiquitin, and α1-antichymotrypsin. *Proc. Natl. Acad. Sci., USA*, **90**, 6825–8.

Sparrer, H.E., Santoso, A., Szoka, F.C., Jr. & Weissman, J.S. (2000). Evidence for the prion hypothesis: induction of the yeast [*PSI*+] factor by in vitro-converted Sup35 protein. *Science*, **289**, 595–9.

Spencer, P.S., Allen, R.G., Kisby, G.E. & Ludolph, A.C. (1990). Excitotoxic disorders. *Science*, **248**, 144.

Spillantini, M.G., Schmidt, M.L., Lee, V. M-Y., Trojanowski, J.Q., Jakes, R. & Goedert, M. (1997). α-Synuclein in Lewy bodies. *Nature*, **388**, 839–40.

Spillantini, M.G., Crowther, R.A., Jakes, R., Hasegawa, M. & Goedert, M. (1998a) α-Synuclein in filamentous inclusions of Lewy bodies from Parkinson's disease and dementia with Lewy bodies. *Proc. Natl. Acad. Sci., USA*, **95**, 6469–73.

Spillantini, M.G., Murrell, J.R., Goedert, M., Farlow, M.R., Klug, A. & Ghetti, B. (1998b). Mutation in the tau gene in familial multiple system tauopathy with presenile dementia. *Proc. Natl. Acad. Sci., USA*, **95**, 7737–41.

Spudich, S., Mastrianni, J.A., Wrensch, M. et al. (1995). Complete penetrance of Creutzfeldt–Jakob disease in Libyan Jews carrying the E200K mutation in the prion protein gene, *Mol. Med.* **1**, 607–13.

St. George-Hyslop, P.H. (1999). Molecular genetics of Alzheimer disease. In *Alzheimer Disease*, 2nd edn., ed. R.D. Terry, R. Katzman, K.L. Bick & S.S. Sisodia, pp. 311–26. Philadelphia: Lippincott Williams & Wilkins.

Supattapone, S., Bosque, P., Muramoto, T. et al. (1999a). Prion protein of 106 residues creates an artificial transmission barrier for prion replication in transgenic mice. *Cell*, **96**, 869–78.

Supattapone, S., Nguyen, H-O.B., Cohen, F.E., Prusiner, S.B. & Scott, M.R. (1999b). Elimination of prions by branched polyamines and implications for therapeutics. *Proc. Natl. Acad. Sci., USA*, **96**, 14529–34.

Swash, M. (2000). Clinical features and diagnosis of amyotrophic lateral sclerosis. In *Amyotrophic Lateral Sclerosis*, ed. R.H. Brown, Jr., V. Meininger & M. Swash, pp. 3–30. London: Martin Dunitz, Ltd.

Tange, R.A., Troost, D. & Limburg, M. (1989). Progressive fatal dementia (Creutzfeldt–Jakob disease) in a patient who received homograft tissue for tympanic membrane closure. *Eur. Arch. Otorhinolaryngol.*, **247**, 199–201.

Tanner, C.M. & Goldman, S.M. (1996). Epidemiology of Parkinson's disease. *Neuroepidemiology*, **14**, 317–35.

Tanner, C.M. Ottman, R., Goldman, S.M. et al. (1999). Parkinson disease in twins: an etiologic study. *J. Am. Med. Ass.*, **281**, 341–6.

Taraboulos, A., Jendroska, K., Serban, D., Yang, S-L., DeArmond, S.J. & Prusiner, S.B. (1992). Regional mapping of prion proteins in brains. *Proc. Natl. Acad. Sci., USA*, **89**, 7620–4.

Tateishi, J., Kitamoto, T., Hoque, M.Z. & Furukawa, H. (1996). Experimental transmission of Creutzfeldt–Jakob disease and related diseases to rodents. *Neurology*, **46**, 532–7.

Taylor, S.I. (1995). Diabetes mellitus. In *The Metabolic and Molecular Bases of Inherited Disease*, 7th edn., ed. C.R. Scriver, A.L. Beaudet, W.S. Sly & D. Valle, pp. 843–96. New York: McGraw-Hill, Inc.

Telling, G.C., Scott, M., Mastrianni, J. et al. (1995). Prion propagation in mice expressing human and chimeric PrP transgenes implicates the interaction of cellular PrP with another protein. *Cell*, **83**, 79–90.

Telling, G.C., Parchi, P., DeArmond, S.J. et al. (1996). Evidence for the conformation of the pathologic isoform of the prion protein enciphering and propagating prion diversity. *Science*, **274**, 2079–82.

The Huntington's Disease Collaborative Research Group (1993). A novel gene containing a trinucleotide repeat that is expanded and unstable on Huntington's disease chromosomes. *Cell*, **72**, 971–83.

United Nations. (1999). World population prospects the 1998 revision volume II: The sex and age distribution of the world population, Vol 2, New York, United Nations Department of Economic and Social Affairs Population Division.

van der Putten, H., Wiederhold, K-H., Probst, A. et al. (2000). Neuropathology in mice expressing human α-synuclein, *J. Neurosci.*, **20**, 6021–9.

Warrick, J.M., Chan, H.Y.E., Gray-Board, G.L., Chai, Y., Paulson, H.L. & Bonini, N.M. (1999). Suppression of polyglutamine-mediated neurodegeneration in *Drosophila* by the molecular chaperone HSP70, *Nat. Genet.*, **23**, 425–8.

Westaway, D., Zuliani, V., Cooper, C.M. et al. (1994). Homozygosity for prion protein alleles encoding glutamine-171 renders sheep susceptible to natural scrapie. *Genes Dev.*, **8**, 959–69.

Wheeler, V.C., White, J.K., Gutekunst, C-A. et al. (2000). Long glutamine tracts cause nuclear localization of a novel form of huntingtin in medium spiny striatal neurons in Hdh^{Q92} and Hdh^{Q111} knock-in mice. *Hum. Mol. Genet.*, **9**, 503–13.

Wickner, R.B. (1994). Evidence for a prion analog in *S. cerevisiae*: the [URE3] non-Mendelian genetic elements as an altered *URE2* protein. *Science*, **264**, 566–9.

Wilhelmsen, K.C., Lynch, T., Pavlou, E., Higgins, M. & Nygaard, T.G. (1994). Localization of disinhibition-dementia-parkinsonism-amyotrophy complex to 17q21–22. *Am. J. Hum. Genet.*, **55**, 1159–65.

Will, R.G. & Matthews, W.B. (1982). Evidence for case-to-case transmission of Creutzfeldt–Jakob disease. *J. Neurol. Neurosurg. Psychiatry*, **45**, 235–8.

Will, R.G., Ironside, J.W., Zeidler, M. et al. (1996). A new variant of Creutzfeldt–Jakob disease in the UK. *Lancet*, **347**, 921–5.

Will, R.G., Alpers, M.P., Dormont, D., Schonberger, L.B. & Tateishi, J. (1999a). Infectious and sporadic prion diseases. In *Prion Biology and Diseases*, ed. S.B. Prusiner, pp. 465–507. Cold Spring Harbor: Cold Spring Harbor Laboratory Press.

Will, R.G., Cousens, S.N., Farrington, C.P., Smith, P.G., Knight, R.S.G. & Ironside, J.W. (1999b). Deaths from variant Creutzfeldt–Jakob disease. *Lancet*, **353**, 979.

Williamson, T.L., Bruijn, L.I., Zhu, Q. et al. (1998). Absence of neurofilaments reduces the selective vulnerability of motor neurons and slows disease caused by a familial amyotrophic lateral sclerosis-linked superoxide dismutase 1 mutant. *Proc. Natl. Acad. Sci., USA*, **95**, 9631–6.

Wilson, C.A., Doms, R.W. & Lee, V.M-Y. (1999). Intracellular APP processing and Aβ production in Alzheimer disease, *J. Neuropathol. Exp. Neurol.*, **58**, 787–94.

Wolozin, B.L., Pruchniki, A., Dickson, D. & Davies, P. (1986). A neuronal antigen in the brain of Alzheimer's disease. *Science*, **232**, 648–50.

Wong, P.C., Pardo, C.A., Borchelt, D.R. et al. (1995). An adverse property of a familial ALS-linked SOD1 mutation causes motor neuron disease characterized by vacuolar degeneration of mitochondria. *Neuron*, **14**, 1105–16.

Wucherpfenning, K.W. & Strominger, J.L. (1995). Molecular mimicry in T-cell mediated autoimmunity: viral peptides activate human T-cell clones specific for myelin basic protein. *Cell*, **80**, 695–705.

Yamamoto, A., Lucas, J.J. & Hen, R. (2000). Reversal of neuropathology and motor dysfunction in a conditional model of Huntington's disease. *Cell*, **101**, 57–66.

Yu, G., Nishimura, M., Arawaka, S. et al. (2000). Nicastrin modulates presenilin-mediated *notch/glp-1* signal transduction and βAPP processing. *Nature*, **407**, 48–54.

Zeidler, M., Stewart, G.E., Barraclough, C.R. et al. (1997). New variant Creutzfeldt–Jakob disease: neurological features and diagnostic tests. *Lancet*, **350**, 903–7.

Zerr, I., Bodemer, M., Gefeller, O. et al. (1998). Detection of 14-3-3 protein in the cerebrospinal fluid supports the diagnosis of Creutzfeldt–Jakob disease. *Ann. Neurol.*, **43**, 32–40.

Zoghbi, H.Y. & Orr, H.T. (2000). Glutamine repeats and neurodegeneration. *Annu. Rev. Neurosci.*, **23**, 217–47.

Zulianello, L., Kaneko, K., Scott, M. et al. (2000). Dominant-negative inhibition of prion formation diminished by deletion mutagenesis of the prion protein. *J. Virol.*, **74**, 4351–60.

16

Aging and dementia: principles, evaluation and diagnosis

Sudha Seshadri[1] and David A. Drachman[2]

[1] Framingham Heart Study, Department of Neurology, Boston University School of Medicine, Framingham, MA, USA
[2] Department of Neurology, University of Massachusetts Medical School, Worcester, MA, USA

'Aging', or 'senescence' usually refers to the involutional changes that occur after an individual has reached full structural and functional maturity (Masoro, 1995). While it is clearly related to the passage of time, there is considerable variability among individuals in when the declines in function occur, the extent of the changes and the selective involvement of specific structures. The onset of impairment due to senescent changes, as well as the overall longevity of individuals, may vary by 50% or more. Senescent changes may involve the heart, joints, skin, brain or other organs in different individuals; and both the organ(s) involved and the degree of decline may be related to genetic and/or experiential factors. Adults between the ages of 65 and 85 years are classified as the 'young-old'; those over age 85 as the 'oldest-old' (Suzman et al., 1992). As the elderly are the fastest growing segment of the population, there is much interest in the causes of senescence, and potential medical means of preventing or delaying their effects, many of which constitute the 'degenerative diseases' of the elderly.

Because of the variability in senescent decline, the concept of 'normal' aging has been controversial, and the term has been used in at least three different ways:

- The optimal level of function seen in individuals of a given age;
- The level of function seen in individuals of a given age in the absence of disease; and
- The mean level of function of all individuals of a given age.

Each of these concepts of 'normal aging', used in the appropriate context, is of value in recognizing and defining the usual expectation, specific disorders, and maximum potential of individuals with advancing age (Rowe & Kahn, 1987). The genetic endowment, the accidents of chance, and the wear and tear of lifetime experience assure that no one definition is necessarily the correct one. Regardless, all three definitions endorse the fact that some decline in function occurs over time; and the relationship between gradual decrements in performance with age, and more rapid and significant impairment of function with disease, is a key issue in understanding the neurologic basis of dementia.

In this chapter we will review:

- anatomic, physiologic and pharmacologic changes that occur in the aging brain;
- cognitive changes with advancing age;
- the molecular basis for age-related changes (ARCs) that cause senescent decline;
- the relationship between aging and dementia;
- clinical manifestations of dementia; and
- a brief classification of dementing disorders.

Anatomical and physiological changes with aging

Gross changes in the aging brain

Autopsy studies have shown that brain weight declines increasingly after age 50, at a rate of about 2% per decade (Miller et al., 1980); by the age of 80 the brain weight is typically decreased by about 10% compared with young adults. CT and MRI studies on aging populations show a linear decrease in brain volume with increasing age (Murphy et al., 1992), and a proportionally more marked increase in ventricular and sulcal volume with age. There is more shrinkage of grey matter than white matter (Pfefferbaum et al., 1994), but gyral atrophy affects predominantly the association and limbic cortices, sparing the primary sensory and motor cortices. On MRI scans, atrophy is seen most prominently in the frontal lobes, less so in the temporal lobes and least in the parieto-occipital lobes; frontal atrophy is more marked in males and parietal atrophy in females (Murphy et al., 1996). In the temporal lobes, medial temporal and hippocampal atrophy predominates, particularly on the left side. The rate of hippocampal atrophy over time correlates with the risk of developing dementia (Jack et al., 1998).

Age-related myelin loss in the brain involves predominantly the small myelinated fibers (Tang et al., 1997). On MRI imaging, white-matter hyperintensities increase exponentially in aging subjects, with only 4.4% of a large, community-dwelling elderly population being entirely free of these changes (Longstreth et al., 1996). The pathological basis and clinical significance of these MRI changes are uncertain; some are ischemic in nature, while periventricular 'caps' may be due to subependymal gliosis (Fazekas et al., 1993).

Microscopic pathology of the aging brain

Changes in the aging brain include neuronal loss, synaptic loss, gliosis and often the accumulation of neuritic plaques and neurofibrillary tangles. Neurons are primarily postmitotic cells and although some may be replaced by neural stem cells (Roy et al., 2000), the vast majority are believed to be irreplaceable. Different neuronal systems have differential vulnerability to aging; the neuronal systems most vulnerable to aging are located in the basal forebrain nuclei, hippocampus, entorhinal cortex, neocortex and brainstem monoaminergic systems. Neuronal loss appears to be regional and lamina specific rather than global, however, and modern stereologic counting techniques show less severe neuronal loss than was previously thought (Coleman & Flood, 1987). The regional pattern of neuronal loss appears to differ in normal aging and Alzheimer's disease: the number of neurons in the entorhinal cortex (layer II), hippocampal CA1 region and the locus ceruleus is not reduced in normal aging, while these regions lose up to 70% of their neurons in Alzheimer's disease (West et al., 1994; Gomez-Isla et al., 1996; Mouton et al., 1994). Similarly, losses of dendrites and synapses are not inevitable correlates of aging. Certain cortical areas show a decline in synaptic density (Lippa et al., 1992; Masliah et al., 1993) while in others there may even be an increase in the synaptic density with aging. While the increase in local synaptic density with aging may be an effort to compensate for regional neuronal loss (Arendt et al., 1995), it may reflect a decrease in neuropil volume. Loss of synapses correlates better with the severity of cognitive impairment in an aging brain than other changes, such as the accumulation of senile plaques and neurofibrillary tangles (NFTs), described below (Terry et al., 1991). Age-related changes

also include granulovacuolar degeneration (1–5 μ intracytoplasmic, neuronal vacuoles with a 1 μ central, basophilic granule) and the appearance of Hirano bodies (eosinophilic, spindle-shaped, intracytoplasmic inclusions), both occurring predominantly in the hippocampus.

With aging, glial proliferation occurs (Hansen et al., 1987), and both neuritic plaques and neurofibrillary tangles are often found, sometimes in large numbers (Fukumoto et al., 1996; Wisniewski et al., 1979). Amyloid is the core constituent of the plaques, where it is surrounded by dystrophic neurites and glial proliferation. Amyloid may also be deposited in and around the walls of aging cerebral arterioles (amyloid angiopathy) or as diffuse plaques without a surrounding glial response. Neurofibrillary tangles (NFT) are intraneuronal silver-staining bodies, seen as paired helical filaments ultrastructurally, and consisting of hyperphosphorylated tau – a microtubule-associated protein, which may also be deposited as intracellular or as extracellular neuropil threads. While amyloid plaques and NFTs increase in frequency and number with normal aging, they are also considered the hallmark of Alzheimer's disease in demented patients (Ball & Murdoch, 1997), using semiquantitative counts of plaques or NFTs as well as their distribution (Khachaturian, 1985; Braak et al., 1993) to distinguish normal from disease. The quantitative histologic distinction between age-related and disease-related findings is still uncertain, especially in the oldest-old, however.

Age-related changes in neurophysiology

In older subjects, resting cerebral blood flow decreases frontally on MR angiography, PET and to a lesser degree SPECT studies (Buijs et al., 1998; Martin et al., 1991); while decreased parietal metabolism may be seen as a marker of early Alzheimer's dementia (Reiman et al., 1996). On EEG, 'healthy aging' by itself causes few EEG changes, such as diminished alpha reactivity and an increase in beta activity (Roubicek, 1977; Koyama et al., 1997). Other changes often seen with aging, such as a decrease in mean alpha frequency and focal temporal slowing, may be correlated with declines in performance on memory and cognitive tests (Drachman & Hughes, 1971).

Age-related changes in neurotransmitter function

Decline in neurotransmitter function is an important factor in the cerebral impairment of aging and dementia (Drachman, 1977; Strong, 1998). In Alzheimer's disease, loss of cholinergic projections from the nucleus basalis of Meynert to the hippocampus and cortex correlate with the loss of memory (Bierer et al., 1995), and the visual hallucinations seen in Lewy body dementia are associated with decreased neocortical cholinergic activity (Perry et al., 1999). It is less certain that acetylcholine levels decline significantly in disease-free aging (Muller et al., 1991; Sarter & Bruno, 1998). A decline in nigral dopamine levels is also well documented in normal aging (Martin et al., 1989), and decreased serotonergic and peptidergic function have been invoked to explain mild age-related memory loss (Buccafusco & Terry, 2000). Response to neurotransmitters may be altered as well; even in the healthy, aging neurons become more susceptible than younger neurons to excessive extracellular glutamate or dopamine levels, and are more likely to suffer excitotoxic cell death (Beal, 1992).

Cognitive changes with aging

Some cognitive changes are nearly universal in the elderly, including a decline in memory storage (i.e. the ability to learn new information), and a decline in the speed of mental processing. Schofield found that 31% of healthy older adults reported memory complaints, such as difficulty remembering names and misplacing of commonly used objects such as keys (Schofield et al., 1997a). Conscious recall (declarative memory) is more often impaired than is motor memory for previously learned skills, such as playing the piano (procedural memory) (Fuld, 1980; Drachman, 1986). Recall of context-specific information (episodic memory) is more affected than the recall of general information (semantic memory); and retrieval is more impaired than recognition. Immediate memory span (what can be recalled after a single hearing) and long-term memory for events in the remote past are preserved. In patients who become demented, this pattern of memory impairment is exaggerated.

Cognitive tasks involving speed of processing begin to show impairment in the fourth decade, and as processing speed continues to slow (Salthouse, 1996), this affects many tests of cognitive function. Actual performance on global intelligence tests, such as the Wechsler Adult Intelligence Scale (WAIS), declines with age, although IQ scores are age corrected, thus numerically masking this decline. To achieve an IQ of 100 at age 75, for example, one need be correct on only half as many items as at age 21 (Wechsler, 1981). The greatest age-related decline in scores is noted in the timed 'performance' subtests (picture completion, digit symbol substitution, block design), with smaller, declines on the untimed 'verbal' subtests (vocabulary, digit span). The time required to perceive a stimulus increases, as measured by tests involving 'backward masking', i.e. the delivery of a second stimulus so close to the first, that the

initial stimulus is not perceived (Kline & Szafran, 1975). The central processing time increases, as shown by a disproportionate increase in choice reaction time (Fozard et al., 1994), and documented by increased latency in the central component of event-related P300 evoked responses (Polich, 1996). Visuospatial construction ability decreases with age, but this does not typically affect daily function. 'Crystallized intelligence', accumulated knowledge as measured, e.g. in tests of vocabulary, tends to be retained, while 'fluid intelligence', the ability to manipulate new information to solve problems, declines with aging (Horn & Cattell, 1967). Cognitive decline with aging is more likely to be seen in elderly subjects with systemic disorders such as hypertension and diabetes mellitus, although the mechanism of causality is uncertain (Skoog, 1997; Skoog et al., 1996). The norms of cognitive function in the oldest-old, those above age 85, are inadequately defined, with only a few studies, such as the Mayo Clinic's Older Americans Normative Study, extended to include subjects in this age range (Ivnik et al., 1997; Lucas et al., 1998).

Other neurological changes with aging

A decrease in special senses is common. Visual acuity declines due to presbyopia and cataract formation (Kini et al., 1978); altered blue perception due to yellowing of the lens; decreased pupillary size and reactivity; and diminished upward gaze. Hearing, especially for high frequencies, decreases (presbyacusis) (Critchley, 1931; Kaye et al., 1994). Olfactory perception (Doty, 1991) and odour identification decrease (Larsson et al., 1999). Motor system changes include diminished muscle bulk and power (a consequence of decreased activity and atrophy of fast-twitch type II fibres) (Aniansson et al., 1986), mild increase in muscle tone (Kaye et al., 1994), slowing of movement (Waite et al., 1996) and an increased frequency of both essential and extrapyramidal tremors (Skre, 1972). Changes in gait include impairment of postural reflexes, a decrease in stride length, gait velocity and arm swing, and gait changes due to orthopedic problems (Murray et al., 1969; Larish et al., 1988) such as osteoarthritis and changes in the spine. The ankle jerks are often hypoactive (Prakash & Stern, 1973). The perception of vibratory and proprioceptive sensation is diminished in the lower limbs.

Molecular mechanisms for age-related changes (ARCs)

Senescence is the consequence of specific biological mechanisms that cause the progressive accumulation of 'age-related changes' (ARCs). Many of these ARCs originate at a molecular or cellular level; they result in clinically evident disorders when sufficient attrition in neural numbers or function occurs so that brain systems can no longer work effectively. ARCs result from both intrinsic events: those due to the inherent attrition of critical survival elements, and those designed to dispose of imperfect components, and from random, extrinsic adverse events. Genetic differences among individuals modify both the timing and the rate of progression of intrinsic events, and the susceptibility to, and effect of, extrinsic events. The precise point at which accumulating ARCs increase the vulnerability to neurodegenerative disorders, or may reach a threshold and become manifest as clinical 'disease', is as yet unclear.

Intrinsic ARCs

The nature of intrinsic ARCs is clearly exemplified by the finite survival of cells and their limited ability to divide in tissue culture, first demonstrated by Hayflick and Moorhead in the early 1960s (Hayflick & Moorhead, 1961). Until that time, it was widely believed that cells grown in culture were immortal. Rigorous studies by Hayflick and his colleagues showed that cells in culture could undergo only a limited number of divisions, then underwent growth arrest at the G_1-S boundary, became dormant and eventually died (Hayflick & Moorhead, 1961; Hayflick, 1965, 1980). Human fetal fibroblasts have the capacity to divide about 50 times, while adult cells can divide only about 20–30 times, the number of replications decreasing with advancing age. The capacity to divide resides in the cellular nucleus, rather than the cytoplasm. When nuclei taken from young cells were transplanted into the cell bodies of older cells, the number of subsequent divisions was increased, based on the age of the young donors; while nuclei from old cells transplanted into young cells bodies reduced the number of divisions and survival to that of the donors.

The nature of the mechanism enabling cells to 'keep count' of the number of divisions they have undergone is largely explained by *telomeric shortening*. The telomere, or chromosome tail, consists of hundreds of TTAGGG repeat sequences, found on each end of every chromosome. Each time a cell divides, its chromosomes lose part of their telomeric tails; when the tails become too short the cell can no longer divide. Most human cells undergo telomeric shortening with advancing age; although this does not apply to adult neurons which are postmitotic, it affects both glial cells and stem cells (Ostenfeld et al., 2000). The enzyme telomerase is present in normal cells but inactive; when

activated, it allows cells to regenerate their telomeres. In germinal cells, cancer cells and 'immortalized cells' telomerase is active, and reactivation of telomerase may increase cell longevity (Greider 1990, 1998; Zhu et al., 2000).

Early concepts regarding the molecular mechanisms contributing to ARCs were the 'somatic mutation theory', proposed by the atomic physicist, Leo Szilard, and the 'error catastrophe theory' of Leslie Orgel. Szilard hypothesized that aging might be due to the accumulation of random mutations in DNA (Szilard, 1959); while Orgel suggested that errors occurring in key functional proteins, such as enzymes, might initiate a cascade of cumulative, increasingly destructive biochemical errors, resulting in senescence and death (Orgel, 1963). Neither of these theories has found direct experimental support, however (Norwood et al., 1990); chemically abnormal proteins are found only occasionally in cell cultures and rarely in vivo.

A novel process, thought to be restricted to aging cells and first described in neurons, is the incorrect conversion of genomic information from normal DNA into nonsense RNA transcripts with subsequent translation into mutant, non-functional proteins. This process has been called 'molecular misreading' and causes some errors unrelated to DNA damage (van Leeuwen et al., 2000).

Accumulation of catabolized structural protein products in increased amounts is found in normal aging and several dementias. The cerebral amyloid precursor protein (APP) normally undergoes enzymatic degradation to form β-amyloid 1–40 and 1–42 (Glenner & Wong, 1984) which accumulates in senile plaques with advancing age. In Alzheimer's disease the exaggerated deposition of β-amyloid 1–42 (Sisodia et al., 1990) results in the hallmark increase in cerebral plaque formation and may cause dementia (Jarrett et al., 1993). Tau, a microtubule associated protein (MAP) normally abundant in the axon stabilizes polymerized microtubules and plays a role in axonal transport. Excessive hyperphosphorylated tau is found in neurofibrillary tangles (Lee et al., 1991), which are found in aging, and are increased in Alzheimer's disease, frontotemporal dementia and other dementing disorders. Other protein products that accumulate in the brain and are associated with age-related degenerations include: α-synuclein (Parkinson's disease and Lewy body dementia) (Spillantini et al., 1998) and ubiquitin (Lewy bodies).

While genetic mutations producing chemical changes in key proteins are probably not an important aging mechanism, conformational changes in proteins may be (Danner & Holbrook, 1990; Johnson et al., 1996; Taubes, 1996; Gafni, 1997). These are post-translational structural changes due to initial misfolding of proteins, or alteration of their normal functional shapes due to cross-linking, covalent bonding, phosphorylation, glycation or other changes (Gafni, 1997; Levine et al., 1996; Richardson & Holbrook, 1996). It is known, for example, that 0.1% of the body's proteins undergo dextrorotation each year, forming right-handed conformations that are non-functional. The chaperone systems, such as the heat-shock proteins (HSPs) of the HSP 70 group, normally both aid in the initial folding of proteins, and in the recognition and refolding, or removal, of conformationally abnormal proteins. The functional capacity of the chaperone systems declines with age, however, related in part to the energy requirements of the process, and the decline in available energy (see below).

Damage to DNA, proteins and membrane lipids may be a result of oxidative stress (Beal, 1995; Venarucci et al., 1999). As a byproduct of oxidative metabolism and normal energy production, oxygen alone or in combined forms (hydroxyl or peroxide radicals) may be produced with an extra unpaired electron. These volatile radicals rapidly oxidize adjacent molecules by donating their extra electrons. Mitochondrial DNA is particularly vulnerable to oxidative stress since it is close to the site of oxidative energy production via phosphorylation; and mitochondrial DNA lacks the repair capability of nuclear DNA. This initiates a cascade of destructive events: impaired mitochondrial function causes decreased energy production, with its consequences: calcium influx into cells, excitotoxic cellular damage, failure of chaperone repair mechanisms, and eventual cellular death (Harman, 1992; Nagley et al., 1992; Julius et al., 1994; Fletcher & Fletcher, 1994; Mattson, 1994). It is not clear whether oxygen free radicals play a major role in senescence, or whether they have an important etiological role in causing parkinsonism, Alzheimer's disease, amyotrophic lateral sclerosis or other degenerative neurologic disorders of aging (Beal, 1995; Mattson, 1994; Harman, 1996; Knight, 1995; Chiueh et al., 1994; Floyd, 1991; Wolozin et al., 1996).

In an experimental model, the brains of aged gerbils contained twice the amount of oxidized protein as those of young gerbils, and the levels of two enzymes helpful in disposing of oxidized products (neutral protease and glutamine synthetase) were reduced with age (Carney et al., 1991). Older gerbils made more errors than younger adult gerbils in running radial mazes, but this difference was abolished if N-tert-butyl-α-phenylnitrone (PBN), a powerful 'spin-trapping' agent that removes free radicals, was administered to both groups of animals (Carney et al., 1991). Accumulation of metals such as aluminium and ferrous iron may facilitate oxidative damage while Vitamins C and E, both antioxidants, are postulated to retard age-related changes. In the Honolulu–Asia aging study of 3385 men aged 71–93 years, use of vitamin C or E supplements was associated with better performance on tests of cognitive function (Masaki et al., 2000).

Caloric restriction (CR), limiting food intake of animals by 50–70%, consistently prolongs the lifespan of many experimental species by up to 40% and postpones most age-related pathology, possibly by reducing oxidative stress (Masoro, 2000; Eckles-Smith et al., 2000). A recent study with an experimental yeast model demonstrated a potential mechanism of this antiaging effect (Lin et al., 2000; Campisi, 2000). Caloric restriction in yeast prolonged survival, but only if genetic pathways for production of Sir2 protein were intact. Sir2p is a 'silencing protein' which maintains compactness of chromosomes by preventing recombination during cell cycling, and requires an energy-providing compound (NAD), which is decreased as a result of oxygen free radicals.

Thus, the cellular basis of aging appears to involve free oxygen radicals, chromosomal integrity, protein conformational accuracy and telomeric adequacy, in addition to as yet unknown changes that occur over time.

Apoptosis is an intrinsically (i.e. genetically) coded and regulated process that results in cell death by means of a predetermined degenerative pathway, in contrast to necrosis. Apoptotic cell death is characterized by a lack of inflammatory changes, the appearance of bullae in the apoptotic cells, and eventually segmentation of the nuclear DNA into small pieces to produce a 'laddered' appearance on electrophoretic gels. During normal cellular function there is an array of opposing factors that can promote or prevent cell survival or division. When the balance tilts sufficiently to invoke the cell death sequence, the apoptotic program begins. Ordinarily, oncogene proteins (e.g. Bcl-2, p35) promote survival and division, and antioncogene proteins (e.g. Rb, p53,) oppose cell division; cell cyclins vary in their roles (Monti et al., 1992). A vast array of opposing factors regulates the survival, growth and division of cells (Steller, 1995; Bump et al., 1995; Rubin et al., 1994). As cells age, these balanced regulatory controls are weakened, and the cells are more readily tipped towards excessive growth (malignancy) or death by apoptotic pathways. The final executioner for most neural apoptotic mechanisms appears to be caspase (Braun et al., 1999); caspase inhibitors may prevent neural degeneration in some age-related disorders such as Huntington's disease (Kim et al., 1999).

Lack of growth factors and generation of proinflammatory cytokines may also play a role in degeneration. Neural growth factors generate 'survival signals' for the neuron; for insulin-like growth factor this 'survival signal' is known to be phosphatidylinositol 3' kinase (PI3 kinase).

Cytokines, such as TNF-α and interleukin-1β, can induce cell-death because TNF receptor activation causes 'silencing of survival signals' (SOSS) (Venters et al., 2000), which may be an important mechanism of neuronal loss in ischemic brain injury and other conditions. Similarly, the interaction of nerve growth factor (NGF) with tyrosine kinase A (*trkA)*, a receptor for this growth factor, promotes survival, differentiation and growth of basal forebrain cholinergic neurons in mouse models; BDNF (brain derived neurotrophic factor) promotes survival and neuronal function in the substantia nigra (Hefti, 1986; Hyman et al., 1991).

Regulation of vascular function by vascular endothelial growth factor (VEGF) and nitric oxide may affect neuronal aging (Kalaria et al., 1998; Rivard et al., 1999; McCann, 1997). Recent reports suggest that dementia may be dramatically reduced in patients treated with HMGCoA reductase inhibitors (statins) for hyperlipidemia, probably independent of the lipid-lowering effects of these drugs, and due to their improvement of microvascular function by increasing endothelial nitric oxide synthetase (eNOS) and reducing endothelin-1, thereby increasing endothelial dilatation and cerebral blood flow (Jick et al., 2000; Wolozin et al., 2000).

The rate of brain aging is affected by the condition of the organ systems that nourish the brain. Systemic disorders can accelerate brain aging through a variety of mechanisms, some of these putative pathways including glycation or cross-linking of proteins (Masoro, 1991), lack of estrogen (Yaffe et al., 1998) and/or dihydroepiandrosterone (DHEA) (Huppert et al., 2000; Moffat et al., 2000), immune failure, or an exaggerated inflammatory response (Maes et al., 1999). Estrogen may improve cerebral circulation, allow brain cells to form and maintain synaptic connections, reduce amyloid deposition and increase brain levels of acetylcholine (McEwen, 1999).

The relationship between aging and dementia

Aging, with the progressive accumulation of ARCs, is the most important risk factor for the development of dementia (Drachman, 1994; Bierer et al., 1995). The annual incidence of dementia rises exponentially with age from less than 1% at age 60 to more than 12% above age 85 (Jorm et al., 1987); the prevalence at 85 is 30-fold greater than at 65. The adverse effects of any brain insult, such as a subarachnoid hemorrhage or a brain tumour, are also greater in older adults (Lanzino et al., 1996; Recht et al., 1989). Women are more likely to develop dementia than men, in part because they live longer. For a 65-year-old woman, the remaining lifetime risk for dementia is approximately 17%, nearly twice the risk of a man the same age (9%); higher than her risk for breast cancer, and equivalent to her lifetime risk of sustaining a hip fracture (Seshadri et al., 1997). Elderly subjects demonstrate a spectrum of cognitive decline, ranging from the normal changes in memory, response speed and channel capacity described earlier, through 'mild cognitive impairment' (MCI) of uncertain clinical significance, to progressive clinical dementia. The extent to which these degrees of impairment represent a spectrum of change, or a series of distinctive disorders, is as yet not entirely clear.

Mild cognitive impairment

Several terms have been used to describe mild decline in cognition in the elderly. In 1962, Kral termed stable minor memory impairment with preserved insight 'benign, senescent forgetfulness' (Kral, 1962). In 1986, Crook and colleagues (Crook et al., 1986) defined age-associated memory impairment (AAMI) as subjective memory loss in the elderly with performance more than 1 S.D. below mean values for young adults on formal memory tests. Aging-associated cognitive decline (AACD) was defined using age-adjusted norms, rather than normal values for young adults, and involved cognitive domains besides memory (Levy, 1994); it is used as a functional category in the DSM-IV classification.

Some investigators take the position that all cognitive decline with age is a consequence of disease, either systemic or involving the brain, and that the standard of 'normal' is optimal cognitive function. Neuropathological changes and measurable neuropsychological declines invariably occur to some extent with aging; yet in some individuals, these changes may represent the beginning of a progressive dementia (Elias et al., 2000). The early stage of cognitive impairment, with impaired memory or cognitive functioning for age, but preserved ability to function in daily life, has been called mild cognitive impairment (MCI) (Zaudig, 1992; Petersen et al., 1999), a diagnosis restricted to older adults when no systemic, psychiatric or neurological disease explaining the memory impairment can be identified. MCI, defined in this way, may represent a preclinical stage of Alzheimer's disease, and a predisposition to clinical dementia following unrelated neurological insults, such as a stroke. A 10–15% annual rate of progression to clinical dementia has been documented in some studies (Petersen et al., 1997). At autopsy the brains in subjects with MCI appear to have significantly more Alzheimer-type changes than those of cognitively intact age-matched subjects (Haroutunian et al., 1999; Price &

Morris, 1999). There is considerable interest in the development of drugs for this group that would delay dementia; but it is not clear what proportion of subjects with MCI would eventually develop dementia, or how to distinguish those who will show progressive deterioration. Accepting MCI as a clearly identifiable diagnostic entity has legal, ethical and financial implications and currently is of use primarily in a research setting.

Dementia

Dementia is defined as a clinical syndrome characterized by the acquired loss of cognitive abilities severe enough to interfere with work or usual social activities, including family obligations. The definition of dementia requires a decline from a prior level of cognitive function and persistence of the condition, the duration being defined in months and years rather than days or weeks. Usually, though not always, the condition is progressive. It requires a diffuse disturbance affecting multiple domains of intellectual function. The DSM-IV criteria require involvement of short-term and long-term memory and at least one of the following spheres of mental activity: language, praxis, executive function (abstract thought, judgment and problem solving) and cortical perception (gnosis) (American Psychiatric Association, 1994). Finally, the diagnosis presupposes an alert patient, without clouding of consciousness (thus excluding the acute confusional states or delirium).

Epidemiology of dementia

Estimates of the prevalence of dementia vary greatly depending on the criteria used to define dementia and the life expectancy of the population. In developed countries, fewer than 1% of the population aged 65 or younger are demented; the prevalence increases exponentially, doubling approximately every 5 years (Molsa et al., 1982; Rocca et al., 1986). Over the age of 85, between 25% and 50% of all subjects are at least mildly demented (Evans et al., 1989), and 20% are completely incapacitated (Wernicke et al., 1994). The incidence of dementia probably increases indefinitely with age; but because of shorter survival in patients over age 90 the prevalence tends to level off at about 45–50% (Ebly et al., 1994; Drachman, 1994). In population-based studies more than 50% of all dementia is due to Alzheimer's disease; a further 15% to vascular dementia; and another 15% to a combination of the two ('mixed dementia') (Schoenberg et al., 1987). Other causes of progressive degenerative dementia of the aged are listed in Table 16.1.

Genetic basis of aging and dementia

Most late-onset dementia is sporadic, with a few identified polymorphisms that modify the risk of dementia, most notably the Apolipoprotein E ε4 allele (Pericak-Vance et al., 1991; Seshadri et al., 1995). The APOE ε4 allele increases the risk of late-onset Alzheimer's disease two- or threefold when present, and halves the risk if absent. Some dementias have an autosomal dominant inheritance, including Huntington's disease; early-onset AD with mutations on chromosome 14 (S182/ PS1) (Sherrington et al., 1995), chromosome 21 (trisomy and APP mutations) (St George-Hyslop et al., 1987), or chromosome 1 (STM2/ PS2) (Rogaev et al., 1995); and frontotemporal dementia with chromosome 17 mutations (tau) (Hutton et al., 1998).

Survival to old-age is not entirely a chance event; the gene pool in very-old subjects differs from that in young adults, (e.g. there is a lower incidence of the APOE ε4 allele) (Yashin et al., 1999; Sobel et al., 1995). Among the oldest-old survivors there may be different etiologies of dementia, and pathological series suggest that 'dementia of unknown etiology' increases to nearly 50% in nonagenarians (Crystal et al., 2000), although clinical Alzheimer's disease remains a major cause of dementia.

Environmental risk factors for dementia

Head injury and minimal education are reported to increase the risk of dementia (Stern et al., 1994; Schofield et al., 1997b). The effect of education may be due to socio-economic disadvantages, a cohort effect (Cobb et al., 1995), an artefact of culturally biased testing, or to an actual beneficial effect of education on brain development. A cerebrovascular accident increases the risk of dementia fivefold in the first year following stroke and doubles the control risk thereafter (Tatemichi et al., 1990). Risk factors for vascular disease have been recognized as risk factors for dementia: e.g., hypertension and diabetes (Breteler et al., 1998; Swan et al., 1998). Physical activity may improve cognitive function and reduce the risk of dementia (Kramer et al., 1999).

Approach to the diagnosis and differential diagnosis of dementia

Screening for dementia and scales used in the assessment of dementia

Simple cognitive screening tests are useful to evaluate cognitive function and establish a performance baseline in

Table 16.1. Disorders that may produce adult-onset dementia

1. Static dementia due to a known cause of brain injury

a. Traumatic brain injury
b. Post anoxic syndrome
c. Single stroke
d. Post infectious sequelae (after recovery from meningitis, encephalitis, ADEM)
e. Dementia pugilistica

2. Symptomatic dementias (some potentially reversible)

a. Endocrine disturbances: hypothyroidism, hyperthyroidism, hyperparathyroidism, Cushing's syndrome, insulinoma
b. Nutritional deficiencies: Wernicke–Korsakoff syndrome, Vitamin B12 or folate deficiency
c. Malignancy (primary or secondary brain tumour, para-neoplastic syndromes, radiation dementia)
d. Chronic subdural hematoma
e. Normal pressure hydrocephalus
f. Multiple sclerosis, adult-onset leukoencephalopathies
g. Systemic lupus erythematosis, cerebral vasculitides
h. AIDS-associated dementias
i. Creutzfeldt–Jakob disease, fatal familial insomnia and other prion diseases
k. Other CNS infections (tuberculous and fungal meningitis, neurosyphilis, neurocysticercosis)
l. Alcoholic dementia, drug or toxin-induced dementias
m. Metabolic encephalopathy: hepatic failure, renal insufficiency, dialysis dementia, hypoxia
n. Inherited metabolic causes of dementia: Wilson's disease, cerebrotendinous xanthomatosis, Kuf's disease, mitochondrial disorders: MELAS, MERRF, lysosomal storage disorders, adult polyglucosan body disease

3. Vascular dementia

4. Alzheimer's disease

5. Non- Alzheimer degenerative dementias with extrapyramidal features

a. Dementia with Lewy bodies
b. Progressive supranuclear palsy
c. Huntington's disease
d. Multisystem atrophy

6. Non-Alzheimer degenerative dementias with focal lobar involvement

a. Frontotemporal dementias (including Pick's disease)
b. Corticobasal ganglionic degeneration

Source: Modified from Rossor (1992).

those over 75. Such screening tests include the Folstein Mini-Mental Status Examination (MMSE) (Folstein et al., 1975), the self-administered Cognitive Assessment Screening Test (CAST) (Drachman & Swearer, 1996; Drachman et al., 1996), and Clock-drawing. More extensive psychometric tests are useful in research settings, or when screening tests signal the need for more detailed clinical evaluation.

Standardized cognitive and functional batteries are used to measure the severity of cognitive impairment (e.g. the Blessed Dementia Rating Scale (Blessed et al., 1968) and Mattis Dementia Rating Scale (DRS) (Mattis, 1988)), and assess both cognitive function and the patient's ability to perform adequately in activities of daily living. The Clinical Dementia Rating Scale (CDR) (Berg, 1988) is a functional rating scale that derives scores from a clinical interview with the patient and caregiver regarding performance in six functional domains (memory, orientation, judgement, home and hobbies, community affairs and personal care). The Index of Activities of Daily Living (IADL) (Lawton & Brody, 1969) and the Physical Self-Maintenance Scale (PSMS) (Lawton & Brady, 1969; Lawton et al., 1982) are used to document impairment in daily activities. These scales document both the diagnosis of dementia and progression of deterioration. There are also well-validated scales to address behavioural changes in dementia, such as the Neuropsychiatric Inventory (NPI) (Cummings et al., 1994), the BEHAVE-AD (Reisberg et al., 1987) and the caregiver obstreperous behaviour rating assessment (COBRA) (Swearer & Drachman, 1996), and to assess depression in the setting of dementia (Cornell Scale for depression in dementia (Alexopoulos et al., 1988); Hamilton Depression Rating Scale (HAM-D) (Hamilton, 1967)). The Hachinski Ischemic Score (HIS) (Hachinski et al., 1975), is used to evaluate the probability of vascular dementia.

Clinical evaluation of a patient with suspected dementia

Individuals may be evaluated for dementia because of self-expressed concerns, referral by a family member or by a physician. The history, obtained from a reliable family member, should include the duration of symptoms, the nature of initial complaints, the rate and pattern of deterioration, and specific areas of cognitive and behavioural impairment including memory, orientation, judgement and problem solving, affect and behaviour. The subject's financial, work, driving, shopping, homemaking and recreational abilities and interests should be documented, as well as the ability to handle personal ADLs (dressing, grooming, bathing, toileting and feeding) compared to prior performance. The instrumental ADLs (cooking, laundry, using a telephone, etc.) are typically impaired before basic ADLs.

Entirely normal performance on office screening tests makes significant dementia less likely; but at times, despite even a detailed clinical and neuropsychological evaluation, the diagnosis may remain uncertain. In these subjects, repeat testing after 6 months or a year can often clarify the diagnosis.

Differential diagnosis of dementia

Once the presence of dementia has been established, the specific underlying dementing disorder is based on the clinical picture: the subject's age, family history, initial symptoms, rate and pattern of progression, findings on systemic and neurological examination, cognitive deficits and behavioural patterns, laboratory evaluation and imaging studies.

The various etiologies of dementia are listed in Table 16.1. Evaluating patients and distinguishing among these numerous causes is facilitated by using a stepwise approach (Drachman et al., 1994). Static dementias, those due to a single event such as a head injury or encephalitis, without progressive deterioration, can be distinguished by the history from progressive dementias. Progressive dementias may be divided into symptomatic dementias, due to an identifiable, and often reversible, cause; and the degenerative dementias. Table 16.2 lists a battery of investigations that permit the identification of most sympto-

Table 16.2. Investigations in patients with dementia

Laboratory:	CBC and differential
	BUN/Creatinine
	Electrolytes (sodium, potassium, calcium)
	Liver function tests
	Thyroid function tests
	Serum B12
Imaging:	MRI scan
When indicated:	EEG (CJD, metabolic encephalopathy, recurrent CPS)
	CSF examination
	Screening for malignancy
	Carotid and cardiac evaluation
	HIV serology; serological tests for syphilis, Lyme disease
	Urine for drug studies, heavy metals
	Brain biopsy

matic dementias. A detailed discussion of the differential diagnosis of dementia is found in Chapter *xxx*.

The degenerative dementias are divided into three groups: (i) Alzheimer's disease and its variants; (ii) the extrapyramidal dementias such as Lewy body dementia; and (iii) focal cortical dementias. Consensus clinical criteria have been published for several etiologies of progressive dementia. Widely accepted clinical criteria exist for the diagnosis of Alzheimer's dementia (McKhann et al., 1984); and more recently criteria have been proposed for dementia with Lewy bodies (McKeith et al., 1996), progressive supranuclear palsy (Litvan et al., 1996), frontotemporal dementia (Neary et al., 1998), and corticobasal ganglionic degeneration (Grimes et al., 1999). Definite diagnosis of dementia type is often possible only by using clinicopathological correlation of clinical and postmortem findings. Some subjects with clinical dementia do not fit pathological diagnostic criteria for any of the classical degenerative dementias, and a number of new disease entities have been proposed, including: argyrophilic grain disease (Braak & Braak, 1998); dementia lacking distinctive histology (Knopman et al., 1990); and hippocampal sclerosis (Dickson et al., 1994; Corey-Bloom et al., 1997). The clinical categorization of some patients with degenerative dementia may be difficult, because of an atypical presentation or unusual overlap of symptoms.

The entity of vascular dementia (VaD) has remained difficult to define. In the first half of the twentieth century, 'cerebral arteriosclerosis' was considered the commonest cause of dementia in the elderly (Mayer-Gross et al., 1960). In 1970, Tomlinson and colleagues showed that, in patients with 'senile dementia' the most frequently found patho-logic changes were those of Alzheimer's disease (Tomlinson et al., 1970). Hachinski coined the term 'multi-infarct dementia', and defined criteria for this entity (Hachinski et al., 1974); it was generally accepted that brain tissue loss due to cerebral infarction was the cause of VaD. More recently, the criteria for the diagnosis of VaD have been debated (Drachman, 1993; Roman et al., 1993); and it has become evident that vascular compromise may play a major role in much dementia of the elderly, including Alzheimer's disease (Jick et al., 2000).

In conclusion, chronological aging, with its associated senescent age-related changes (ARCs) is the single most important risk factor for the development of sporadic dementias. The cumulative effect of a number of known and as yet unknown ARCs produce molecular, cellular, anatomical, physiological and pharmacological changes that render the aging brain vulnerable to neuronal and functional loss, and to degenerative disorders that produce more rapidly progressive cognitive impairment. Although mild declines in cognitive function are inevitable with aging, the factors that transform the vulnerable, aging brain into one with a progressive dementing disorder are not as yet well understood. Genetic, environmental, vascular and experiential factors undoubtedly interact with the normal ARCs to lead to progressive degenerative dementias. Prevention and treatment of Alzheimer's disease, vascular dementia, fronto-temporal dementia, Lewy body dementia and others will depend both on elucidating the specific mechanisms of each of these diseases, and on developing strategies to forestall the ARCs that make the aging brain so vulnerable to these disorders.

References

Alexopoulos, G.S., Abrams, R.C., Young, R.C. & Shamoian, C.A. (1988). Cornell Scale for Depression in Dementia. *Biol. Psychiatry*, **23**(3), 271–84.

American Psychiatric Association (1994). *Diagnostic and Statistical Manual of Mental Disorders*. 4th edn, pp. 143–6. Washington, DC: American Psychiatric Association.

Aniansson, A., Hedberg, M., Henning, G.B. & Grimby, G. (1986). Muscle morphology, enzymatic activity, and muscle strength in elderly men: a follow-up study. *Muscle Nerve*, **9**(7), 585–91.

Arendt, T., Bruckner, M.K., Bigl, V. & Marcova, L. (1995). Dendritic reorganisation in the basal forebrain under degenerative conditions and its defects in Alzheimer's disease. II. Ageing, Korsakoff's disease, Parkinson's disease, and Alzheimer's disease. *J. Comp. Neurol.*, **351**(2), 189–222.

Ball, M.J. & Murdoch G.H. (1997). Neuropathological criteria for the diagnosis of Alzheimer's disease: are we really ready yet? *Neurobiol. Aging*, **18**(Suppl. 4): S3–12.

Beal, M.F. (1992). Does impairment of energy metabolism result in excitotoxic neuronal death in neurodegenerative illnesses? *Ann. Neurol.*, **31**(2), 119–30.

Beal, M.F. (1995). Aging, energy, and oxidative stress in neurode-generative diseases. *Ann. Neurol.*, **38**(3), 357–66.

Berg, L. (1988). Clinical Dementia Rating (CDR). *Psychopharmacol. Bull.*, **24**(4), 637–9.

Bierer, L.M., Haroutunian, V., Gabriel, S. et al. (1995). Neurochemical correlates of dementia severity in Alzheimer's disease: relative importance of the cholinergic deficits. *J. Neurochem.*, **64**(2), 749–60.

Blessed, G., Tomlinson, B.E. & Roth, M. (1968). The association between quantitative measures of dementia and of senile change in the cerebral grey matter of elderly subjects. *Br. J. Psychiatry*, **114**(512), 797–811.

Braak, H. & Braak, E. (1998). Argyrophilic grain disease: frequency of occurrence in different age categories and neuropathological diagnostic criteria. *J. Neural. Transm.*, **105**(8–9), 801–19.

Braak, H., Braak, E. & Bohl, J. (1993). Staging of Alzheimer-related cortical destruction. *Eur. Neurol.*, **33**(6), 403–8.

Braun, J.S., Tuomanen, E.I. & Cleveland, J.L. (1999). Neuroprotection by caspase inhibitors. *Expert Opin. Investig. Drugs*, **8**(10), 1599–610.

Breteler, M.M., Bots, M.L., Ott, A. & Hofman, A. (1998). Risk factors for vascular disease and dementia. *Haemostasis*, **28**(3–4), 167–73.

Buccafusco, J.J. & Terry, A.V., Jr. (2000). Multiple central nervous system targets for eliciting beneficial effects on memory and cognition. *J. Pharmacol. Exp. Ther.*, **295**(2), 438–46.

Buijs, P.C., Krabbe-Hartkamp, M.J., Bakker, C.J. et al. (1998). Effect of age on cerebral blood flow: measurement with ungated two-dimensional phase-contrast MR angiography in 250 adults. *Radiology*, **209**(3), 667–74.

Bump, N.J., Hackett, M., Hugunin, M. et al. (1995). Inhibition of ICE family proteases by baculovirus antiapoptotic protein p35. *Science*, **269**(5232), 1885–8.

Campisi, J. (2000). Aging, chromatin, and food restriction – connecting the dots [comment]. *Science*, **289**(5487), 2062–3.

Carney, J.M., Starke-Reed, P.E., Oliver, C.N. et al. (1991). Reversal of age-related increase in brain protein oxidation, decrease in enzyme activity, and loss in temporal and spatial memory by chronic administration of the spin-trapping compound *N*-tert-butyl-alpha-phenylnitrone. *Proc. Natl. Acad. Sci., USA*, **88**(9), 3633–6.

Chiueh, C.C., Wu, R.M., Mohanakumar, K.P. et al. (1994). In vivo generation of hydroxyl radicals and MPTP-induced dopaminergic toxicity in the basal ganglia. *Ann. NY Acad. Sci.*, **738**, 25–36.

Cobb, J.L., Wolf, P.A., Au, R., White, R. & D'Agostino, R.B. (1995). The effect of education on the incidence of dementia and Alzheimer's disease in the Framingham Study. *Neurology*, **45**(9), 1707–12.

Coleman, P. & Flood, D. (1987). Neuron numbers and dendritic extent in normal aging and Alzheimer's disease. *Neurobiol. Aging*, **8**, 521.

Corey-Bloom, J., Sabbagh, M.N., Bondi, M.W. et al. (1997). Hippocampal sclerosis contributes to dementia in the elderly. *Neurology*, **48**(1), 154–60.

Critchley, M. (1931). The neurology of old age. *Lancet*, **1**, 1221–30.

Crook, T., Bartus, R., Ferris, S. et al. (1986). Age associated memory impairment: Proposed diagnostic criteria and measures of clinical change – report of a National Institute of Mental Health work group. *Dev. Neuropsychol.*, **2**, 261–76.

Crystal, H.A., Dickson, D., Davies, P., Masur, D., Grober, E. & Lipton, R. B. (2000). The relative frequency of 'dementia of unknown etiology' increases with age and is nearly 50% in nonagenarians. *Arch. Neurol.*, **57**(5), 713–19.

Cummings, J.L., Mega, M., Gray, K., Rosenberg-Thompson, S., Carusi, D.A. & Gornbein, J. (1994). The Neuropsychiatric Inventory: comprehensive assessment of psychopathology in dementia. *Neurology*, **44**(12), 2308–14.

Danner, D. & Holbrook, N. (1990). Alterations in gene expression with aging. In *Handbook of the Biology of Aging*, ed. R.J. Schneider, vol. 3, pp. 97–115. San Diego: Academic Press, Inc.

Dickson, D., Davies, W.P., Bevona, C. et al. (1994). Hippocampal sclerosis: a common pathological feature of dementia in very old (≥80 years of age) humans. *Acta Neuropathol.*, **88**(3), 212–21.

Doty, R.L. (1991). Olfactory capacities in aging and Alzheimer's disease. Psychophysical and anatomic considerations. *Ann. NY Acad. Sci.*, **640**, 20–7.

Drachman, D.A. (1977). Memory and cognitive function in man: does the cholinergic system have a specific role? *Neurology*, **27**(8), 783–90.

Drachman, D.A. (1986). Memory and cognitive function in normal aging. *Dev. Neuropsychol.*, **2**, 277–85.

Drachman, D.A. (1993). New criteria for the diagnosis of vascular dementia: do we know enough yet? [editorial; comment]. *Neurology*, **43**(2), 243–5.

Drachman, D.A. (1994). If we live long enough, will we all be demented? [editorial; comment]. *Neurology*, **44**(9), 1563–5.

Drachman, D.A. & Hughes, J.R. (1971). Memory and the hippocampal complexes. 3. Aging and temporal EEG abnormalities. *Neurology*, **21**(1), 1–14.

Drachman, D A. & Swearer, J.M. (1996). Screening for dementia: cognitive assessment screening test (CAST). *Am. Fam. Physician*, **54**(6), 1957–62.

Drachman, D.A., Long, R. & Swearer, J. (1994). Neurological examination of the elderly patient. In *Clinical Neurology of Aging*, ed. J.E. Knoefel & M.L. Albert, pp. 159–80. New York: Oxford University Press.

Drachman, D.A., Swearer, J.M., Kane, K., Osgood, D., O'Toole, C. & Moonis, M. (1996). The cognitive assessment screening test (CAST) for dementia. *J. Geriatr. Psychiatry Neurol.*, **9**(4), 200–8.

Ebly, E.M., Parhad, I.M., Hogan, D.B. & Fung, T.S. (1994). Prevalence and types of dementia in the very old: results from the Canadian Study of Health and Aging. *Neurology*, **44**(9), 1593–600.

Eckles-Smith, K., Clayton, D., Bickford, P. & Browning, M.D. (2000). Caloric restriction prevents age-related deficits in LTP and in NMDA receptor expression. *Brain Res. Mol. Brain Res.*, **78**(1–2), 154–62.

Elias, M.F., Beiser, A., Wolf, P.A., Au, R., White, R.F. & D'Agostino, R.B. (2000). The preclinical phase of Alzheimer disease: a 22-year prospective study of the Framingham Cohort. *Arch. Neurol.*, **57**(6), 808–13.

Evans, D.A., Funkenstein, H.H., Albert, M.S. et al. (1989). Prevalence of Alzheimer's disease in a community population of older persons. Higher than previously reported. *J. Am. Med. Assoc.*, **262**(18), 2551–6.

Fazekas, F., Kleinert, R. Offenbacher, H. et al. (1993). Pathologic correlates of incidental MRI white matter signal hyperintensities. *Neurology*, **43**(9), 1683–9.

Fletcher, R.H. & Fletcher, S.W. (1994). Glutathione and ageing: ideas and evidence. *Lancet*, **344**(8934), 1379–80.

Floyd, R.A. (1991). Oxidative damage to behavior during aging. *Science*, **254**(5038), 1597.

Folstein, M.F., Folstein, S.E. & McHugh, P.R. (1975). 'Mini-mental state'. A practical method for grading the cognitive state of patients for the clinician. *J. Psychiatr. Res.*, **12**(3), 189–98.

Fozard, J.L., Vercryssen, M., Reynolds, S.L., Hancock, P.A. & Quilter, R.E. (1994). Age differences and changes in reaction time: the Baltimore Longitudinal Study of Aging. *J. Gerontol.*, **49**(4), 179–89.

Fukumoto, H., Asami-Odaka, A., Suzuki, N., Shimada, H., Ihara, Y. & Iwatsubo, T. (1996). Amyloid beta protein deposition in normal aging has the same characteristics as that in Alzheimer's disease. Predominance of A beta 42(43) and association of A beta 40 with cored plaques. *Am. J. Pathol.*, **148**(1), 259–65.

Fuld, P.A. (1980). Guaranteed stimulus-processing in the evaluation of memory and learning. *Cortex*, **16**(2), 255–71.

Gafni, A. (1997). Structural modifications of proteins during aging. *J. Am. Geriatr. Soc.*, **45**(7), 871–80.

Glenner, G.G. & Wong, C.W. (1984). Alzheimer's disease: initial report of the purification and characterization of a novel cerebrovascular amyloid protein. *Biochem. Biophys. Res. Commun.*, **120**(3), 885–90.

Gomez-Isla, T., Price, J.L., McKeel, D.W., Jr., Morris, J.C., Growdon, J.H. & Hyman, B.T. (1996). Profound loss of layer II entorhinal cortex neurons occurs in very mild Alzheimer's disease. *J. Neurosci.*, **16**(14), 4491–500.

Greider, C.W. (1990). Telomeres, telomerase and senescence. *Bioessays*, **12**(8), 363–9.

Greider, C.W. (1998). Telomeres and senescence: the history, the experiment, the future. *Curr. Biol.*, **8**(5), R178–81.

Grimes, D.A., Lang, A.E. & Bergeron, C.B. (1999). Dementia as the most common presentation of cortical–basal ganglionic degeneration. *Neurology*, **53**(9), 1969–74.

Hachinski, V.C., Lassen, N.A. & Marshall, J. (1974). Multi-infarct dementia. A cause of mental deterioration in the elderly. *Lancet*, **ii**(7874), 207–10.

Hachinski, V.C., Iliff, L.D., Zilhka, E. et al. (1975). Cerebral blood flow in dementia. *Arch. Neurol.*, **32**(9), 632–7.

Hamilton, M. (1967). Development of a rating scale for primary depressive illness. *Br. J. Soc. Clin. Psychol.*, **6**(4), 278–96.

Hansen, L.A., Armstrong, D.M. & Terry, R.D. (1987). 'An immunohistochemical quantification of fibrous astrocytes in the aging human cerebral cortex. *Neurobiol. Aging*, **8**(1), 1–6.

Harman, D. (1992). Role of free radicals in aging and disease. In *Physiopathological Processes of Aging*, ed. N. Fabris, D. Harman, D. Knook, E. Steinhagen-Thiessen & I. Zs.-Nagy, vol. **673**, pp. 126–141. New York: New York Academy of Sciences.

Harman, D. (1996). Aging and disease. In *Pharmacological Intervention in Aging and Age-Associated Disorders*, ed. K. Kitani, A. Aoba & S. Goto, vol. 786, pp. 321–36. New York: New York Academy of Sciences.

Haroutunian, V., Purohit, D.P., Perl, D.P. et al. (1999). Neurofibrillary tangles in nondemented elderly subjects and mild Alzheimer disease. *Arch. Neurol.*, **56**(6), 713–18.

Hayflick, L. (1965). The limited in vitro lifetime of human diploid cell strains. *Exp. Cell Res.*, **37**, 614–36.

Hayflick, L. (1980). The cell biology of human aging. *Sci. Am.*, **242**(1), 58–65.

Hayflick, L. & Moorhead, P. (1961). The serial cultivation of human diploid cell strains. *Exp. Cell Res.*, **25**, 585–621.

Hefti, F. (1986). Nerve growth factor promotes survival of septal cholinergic neurons after fimbrial transections. *J. Neurosci.*, **6**(8), 2155–62.

Horn, J.L. & Cattell, R.B. (1967). Age differences in fluid and crystallized intelligence. *Acta Psychobiol.*, **26**, 107.

Huppert, F.A., Van Niekerk, J.K. & Herbert, J. (2000). Dehydroepiandrosterone (DHEA) supplementation for cognition and well- being. *Cochrane Database Syst. Rev.*, **2**.

Hutton, M., Lendon, C.L., Rizzu, P. et al. (1998). Association of missense and 5′-splice-site mutations in tau with the inherited dementia FTDP-17. *Nature*, **393**(6686), 702–5.

Hyman, C., Hofer, M., Barde, Y. A. et al. (1991). BDNF is a neurotrophic factor for dopaminergic neurons of the substantia nigra. *Nature*, **350**(6315), 230–2.

Ivnik, R.J., Smith, G.E., Lucas, J.A., Tangalos, E.G., Kokmen, E. & Petersen, R.C. (1997). Free and cued selective reminding test: MOANS norms. *J. Clin. Exp. Neuropsychol.*, **19**(5), 676–91.

Jack, C.R., Jr., Petersen, R.C., Xu, Y. et al. (1998). Rate of medial temporal lobe atrophy in typical aging and Alzheimer's disease. *Neurology*, **51**(4), 993–9.

Jarrett, J.T., Berger, E.P., Lansbury, P.T., Jr. et al. (1993). The C-terminus of the beta protein is critical in amyloidogenesis. *Ann. NY Acad. Sci.*, **695**, 144–8.

Jick, H., Zornberg, G.L., Jick, S.S. et al. (2000). Statins and the risk of dementia. *Lancet*, **356**(9242), 1627–31.

Johnson, T., Lithgow, G., Murakami, S. et al. (1996). Genetics of aging and longevity in lower organisms. In *Cellular Aging and Cell Death*, ed. N. Holbrook, G. Martin & R. Lockshin, vol. **16**, pp. 1–17. New York: Wiley-Liss.

Jorm, A.F., Korten, A E. & Henderson, A.S. (1987). The prevalence of dementia: a quantitative integration of the literature [see comments]. *Acta Psychiatr. Scand.*, **76**(5), 465–79.

Julius, M., Lang, C.A., Gleiberman, L., Harburg, E., DiFranceisco, W. & Schork, A. (1994). Glutathione and morbidity in a community-based sample of elderly. *J. Clin. Epidemiol.*, **47**(9), 1021–6.

Kalaria, R.N., Cohen, D.L., Premkumar, D.R., Nag, S., LaManna, J.C. & Lust, W.D. (1998). Vascular endothelial growth factor in Alzheimer's disease and experimental cerebral ischemia. *Brain Res. Mol. Brain Res.*, **62**(1), 101–5.

Kaye, J.A., Oken, B.S., Howieson, D.B., Howieson, J., Holm, L.A. & Dennison K. (1994). Neurologic evaluation of the optimally healthy oldest old. *Arch. Neurol.*, **51**(12), 1205–11.

Khachaturian, Z. (1985). Diagnosis of Alzheimer's disease. *Arch. Neurol.*, **42**, 1097–105.

Kim, M., Lee, H.S., LaForet, G. et al. (1999). Mutant huntingtin expression in clonal striatal cells: dissociation of inclusion formation and neuronal survival by caspase inhibition. *J. Neurosci.*, **19**(3), 964–73.

Kini, M.M., Leibowitz, H.M., Colton, T., Nickerson, R.J., Ganley, J. & Dawber, T.R. (1978). Prevalence of senile cataract, diabetic retinopathy, senile macular degeneration, and open-angle glaucoma in the Framingham eye study. *Am. J. Ophthalmol.*, **85**(1), 28–34.

Kline, D.W. & Szafran, J. (1975). Age differences in backward monoptic visual noise masking. *J. Gerontol.*, **30**(3), 307–11.

Knight, J A. (1995). Diseases related to oxygen-derived free radicals. *Ann. Clin. Lab. Sci.*, **25**(2), 111–21.

Knopman, D.S., Mastri, A.R., Frey, W.H., Sung, J.H., & Rustan, T. (1990). Dementia lacking distinctive histologic features: a common non-Alzheimer degenerative dementia. *Neurology*, **40**(2), 251–6.

Koyama, K., Hirasawa, H., Okubo, Y. & Karasawa, A. (1997). Quantitative EEG correlates of normal aging in the elderly. *Clin. Electroencephalogr.*, **28**(3), 160–5.

Kral, V. (1962). Senescent forgetfulness: Benign and malignant. *Canad. Med. Assoc. J.*, **86**, 257–60.

Kramer, A.F., Hahn, S., Cohen, N.J. et al. (1999). Ageing, fitness and neurocognitive function [letter]. *Nature*, **400**(6743), 418–19.

Lanzino, G., Kassell, N.F., Germanson, T.P. et al. (1996). Age and outcome after aneurysmal subarachnoid hemorrhage: why do older patients fare worse? *J. Neurosurg.*, **85**(3), 410–18.

Larish, D.D., Martin, P.E. & Mungiole, M. (1988). Characteristic patterns of gait in the healthy old. *Ann. NY Acad. Sci.*, **515**, 18–32.

Larsson, M., Semb, H., Winblad, B., Amberla, K., Wahlund, L.O. & Backman, L. (1999). Odor identification in normal aging and early Alzheimer's disease: effects of retrieval support. *Neuropsychology*, **13**(1), 47–53.

Lawton, M.P. & Brody, E.M. (1969). Assessment of older people: self-maintaining and instrumental activities of daily living. *Gerontologist*, **9**(3), 179–86.

Lawton, M.P., Moss, M., Fulcomer, M. & Kleban, M.H. (1982). A research and service oriented multilevel assessment instrument. *J. Gerontol.*, **37**(1), 91–9.

Lee, V.M., Balin, B.J., Otvos, L., Jr. & Trojanowski, J.Q. (1991). A68: a major subunit of paired helical filaments and derivatized forms of normal Tau. *Science*, **251**(4994), 675–8.

Levine, R. & Stadtman, E. (1996). Protein modifications with aging. In *Handbook of the Biology of Aging*, ed. E. Scheider & J. Rowe, pp. 184–97. San Diego: Academic Press, Inc.

Levy, R. on behalf of the Aging-Associated Cognitive Decline Working Party. (1994). Aging-associated cognitive decline. *Int. Psychogeriatr.*, **6**: 63–8.

Lin, S.J., Defossez, P.A. & Guarente, L. (2000). Requirement of NAD and SIR2 for life-span extension by calorie restriction in *Saccharomyces cerevisiae* [see comments]. *Science*, **289**(5487), 2126–8.

Lippa, C.F., Hamos, J.E., Pulaski-Salo, D., DeGennaro, L.J. & Drachman, D.A. (1992). Alzheimer's disease and aging: effects on perforant pathway perikarya and synapses. *Neurobiol. Aging*, **13**(3), 405–11.

Litvan, I., Agid, Y., Calne, D. et al. (1996). Clinical research criteria for the diagnosis of progressive supranuclear palsy (Steele–Richardson–Olszewski syndrome): report of the NINDS-SPSP international workshop. *Neurology*, **47**(1), 1–9.

Longstreth, W.T., Jr., Manolio, T.A., Arnold, A, et al. (1996). Clinical correlates of white matter findings on cranial magnetic resonance imaging of 3301 elderly people. The Cardiovascular Health Study [see comments]. *Stroke*, **27**(8), 1274–82.

Lucas, J.A., Ivnik, R.J., Smith, G.E. et al. (1998). Mayo's older Americans normative studies: category fluency norms. *J. Clin. Exp. Neuropsychol.*, **20**(2), 194–200.

McCann, S.M. (1997). The nitric oxide hypothesis of brain aging. *Exp. Gerontol.*, **32**(4–5), 431–40.

McEwen, B.S. (1999). Clinical review 108: The molecular and neuroanatomical basis for estrogen effects in the central nervous system. *J. Clin. Endocrinol. Metab.*, **84**(6), 1790–7.

McKeith, I.G., Galasko, D., Kosaka, K. et al. (1996). Consensus guidelines for the clinical and pathologic diagnosis of dementia with Lewy bodies (DLB): report of the consortium on DLB international workshop. *Neurology*, **47**(5), 1113–24.

McKhann, G., Drachman, D., Folstein, M., Katzman, R., Price, D. & Stadlan, E.M. (1984). Clinical diagnosis of Alzheimer's disease: report of the NINCDS-ADRDA Work Group under the auspices of Department of Health and Human Services Task Force on Alzheimer's Disease. *Neurology*, **34**(7), 939–44.

Maes, M., DeVos, N., Wauters, A. et al. (1999). Inflammatory markers in younger vs elderly normal volunteers and in patients with Alzheimer's disease. *J. Psychiatr. Res.*, **33**(5), 397–405.

Martin, W.R., Palmer, M.R., Patlak, C.S. & Calne, D.B. (1989). Nigrostriatal function in humans studied with positron emission tomography. *Ann. Neurol.*, **26**(4), 535–42.

Martin, A.J., Friston, K.J., Colebatch, J.G. & Frackowiak, R.S. (1991). Decreases in regional cerebral blood flow with normal aging. *J. Cereb. Blood Flow Metab.*, **11**(4), 684–9.

Masaki, K.H., Losonczy, K.G., Izmirlian, G. et al. (2000). Association of vitamin E and C supplement use with cognitive function and dementia in elderly men. *Neurology*, **54**(6), 1265–72.

Masliah, E., Mallory, M., Hansen, L., DeTeresa, R. & Terry, R.D. (1993). Quantitative synaptic alterations in the human neocortex during normal aging. *Neurology*, **43**(1), 192–7.

Masoro, E.J. (1991). Biology of aging: facts, thoughts, and experimental approaches. *Lab. Invest.*, **65**(5), 500–10.

Masoro, E.J. (1995). (ed.) Aging: current concepts. *Handbook of Physiology: Aging*, pp. 3–24. New York: Oxford University Press.

Masoro, E.J. (2000). Caloric restriction and aging: an update. *Exp. Gerontol.*, **35**(3), 299–305.

Mattis, S. (1988). *DRS: Dementia Rating Scale Manual*. Odessa, FL: Psychological Assessment Resources.

Mattson, M.P. (1994). Calcium and neuronal injury in Alzheimer's disease. Contributions of beta-amyloid precursor protein mismetabolism, free radicals, and metabolic compromise. *Ann. NY Acad. Sci.*, **747**, 50–76.

Mayer-Gross, W., Slater, E. & Roth, M. (1960). *Clinical Psychiatry*. London: Bailliere, Tindall and Cassell.

Miller, A.K., Alston, R.L. & Corsellis, J.A. (1980). Variation with age in the volumes of grey and white matter in the cerebral hemispheres of man: measurements with an image analyser. *Neuropathol. Appl. Neurobiol.*, **6**(2), 119–32.

Moffat, S.D., Zonderman, A.B., Harman, S.M., Blackman, M.R., Kawas, C. & Resnick, S.M. (2000). The relationship between longitudinal declines in dehydroepiandrosterone sulfate concentrations and cognitive performance in older men. *Arch. Intern. Med.*, **160**(14), 2193–8.

Molsa, P.K., Marttila, R.J. & Rinne, U.K. (1982). Epidemiology of dementia in a Finnish population. *Acta Neurol. Scand.*, **65**(6), 541–52.

Monti, D., Grassilli, E. & Troiano, L. (1992). Senescence, immortalization, and apoptosis. In *Physiopathological Processes of Aging*, ed. N. Fabris, D. Harman, D. Knook, E. Steinhagen-Thiessen & I. Zs.-Nagy, vol. 673, 70–82. New York: New York Academy of Sciences.

Mouton, P.R., Pakkenberg, B., Gundersen, H.J. & Price, D.L. (1994). Absolute number and size of pigmented locus coeruleus neurons in young and aged individuals. *J. Chem. Neuroanat.*, **7**(3), 185–90.

Muller, W.E., Stoll, L., Schubert, T. & Gelbmann, C.M. (1991). Central cholinergic functioning and aging. *Acta Psychiatr. Scand. Suppl.*, **366**, 34–9.

Murphy, D.G., DeCarli, C., Schapiro, M.B., Rapoport, S.I. & Horwitz, B. (1992). Age-related differences in volumes of subcortical nuclei, brain matter, and cerebrospinal fluid in healthy men as measured with magnetic resonance imaging [published erratum appears in *Arch. Neurol.* 1994 Jan; 51(1): 60]. *Arch. Neurol.*, **49**(8), 839–45.

Murphy, D.G., DeCarli, C., McIntosh, A.R. et al. (1996). Sex differences in human brain morphometry and metabolism: an in vivo quantitative magnetic resonance imaging and positron emission tomography study on the effect of aging. *Arch. Gen. Psychiatry*, **53**(7), 585–94.

Murray, M.P., Kory, R.C. & Clarkson, B.H. (1969). Walking patterns in healthy old men. *J. Gerontol.*, **24**(2), 169–78.

Nagley, P., Mackay, I. & Baumer, A. (1992). Mitochondrial DNA mutation associated with aging and degenerative disease. In *Physiopathological Processes of Aging*, ed. N. Fabris, D. Harman, D. Knook, E. Steinhagen-Thiessen & I. Zs.-Nagy, vol. 673, pp. 92–102. New York: New York Academy of Sciences.

Neary, D., Snowden, J.S., Gustafson, L. et al. (1998). Frontotemporal lobar degeneration: a consensus on clinical diagnostic criteria [see comments]. *Neurology*, **51**(6), 1546–54.

Norwood, T., Smith, J. & Stein, G. (1990). Aging at the cellular level: the human fibroblastlike cell model. In *Handbook of the Biology of Aging*, ed. R.J. Schneider, pp. 131–54. San Diego: Academic Press, Inc.

Orgel, L. (1963). The maintenance of the accuracy of protein synthesis and its relevance to ageing. *Proc. Natl. Acad. Sci., USA*, **49**, 517–21.

Ostenfeld, T., Caldwell, M.A., Prowse, K.R., Linskens, M.H., Jauniaux E. & Svendsen, C.N. (2000). Human neural precursor cells express low levels of telomerase in vitro and show diminishing cell proliferation with extensive axonal outgrowth following transplantation. *Exp. Neurol.*, **164**(1), 215–26.

Pericak-Vance, M.A., Bebout, J.L., Gaskell, P.C., Jr. et al. (1991). Linkage studies in familial Alzheimer disease: evidence for chromosome 19 linkage. *Am. J. Hum. Genet.*, **48**(6), 1034–50.

Perry, E., Walker, M., Grace, J. & Perry, R. (1999). Acetylcholine in mind: a neurotransmitter correlate of consciousness? [see comments]. *Trends Neurosci.*, **22**(6), 273–80.

Petersen, R.C., Smith, G.E., Waring, S.C., Ivnik, R.J., Kokmen, E. & Tangelos, E.G. (1997). Aging, memory, and mild cognitive impairment. *Int. Psychogeriatr.*, **9**(Suppl. 1), 65–9.

Petersen, R.C., Smith, G.E., Waring, S.C. et al. (1999). Mild cognitive impairment: clinical characterization and outcome [published erratum appears in *Arch. Neurol.* 1999 Jun; 56(6): 760]. *Arch. Neurol.*, **56**(3), 303–8.

Pfefferbaum, A., Mathalon, D.H., Sullivan, E.V., Rawles, J.M., Zipursky, R.B. & Lim, K.O. (1994). A quantitative magnetic resonance imaging study of changes in brain morphology from infancy to late adulthood. *Arch. Neurol.*, **51**(9), 874–87.

Polich, J. (1996). Meta-analysis of P300 normative aging studies. *Psychophysiology*, **33**(4), 334–53.

Prakash, C. & Stern, G. (1973). Neurological signs in the elderly. *Age Ageing*, **2**(1), 24–7.

Price, J.L. & Morris, J.C. (1999). Tangles and plaques in nondemented aging and 'preclinical' Alzheimer's disease. *Ann. Neurol.*, **45**(3), 358–68.

Recht, L.D., McCarthy, K., O'Donnell, B.F., Cohen, R. & Drachman, D.A. (1989). Tumor-associated aphasia in left hemisphere primary brain tumors: the importance of age and tumor grade. *Neurology*, **39**(1), 48–50.

Reiman, E.M., Caselli, R.J., Yun, L.S. et al. (1996). Preclinical evidence of Alzheimer's disease in persons homozygous for the epsilon 4 allele for apolipoprotein E [see comments]. *N. Engl. J. Med.*, **334**(12), 752–8.

Reisberg, B., Borenstein, J., Salob, S.P., Ferris, S.H., Franssen, E. & Georgotas, A. (1987). Behavioral symptoms in Alzheimer's disease: phenomenology and treatment. *J. Clin. Psychiatry*, **48 Suppl.**, 9–15.

Richardson, A. & Holbrook, N. (1996). Aging and the cellular response to stress: Reduction in the heat shock response. In *Cellular Aging and Cell Death*, ed. N. Holbrook, G. Martin & R. Lockshin, vol. 16, pp. 67–80. New York: Wiley-Liss.

Rivard, A., Fabre, J.E., Silver, M. et al. (1999). Age-dependent impairment of angiogenesis. *Circulation*, **99**(1), 111–20.

Rocca, W.A., Amaducci, L.A. & Schoenberg, B.S. (1986). Epidemiology of clinically diagnosed Alzheimer's disease. *Ann. Neurol.*, **19**(5), 415–24.

Rogaev, E.I., Sherrington, R., Rogaeva, E.A. et al. (1995). Familial Alzheimer's disease in kindreds with missense mutations in a gene on chromosome 1 related to the Alzheimer's disease type 3 gene. *Nature*, **376**(6543), 775–8.

Roman, G.C., Tatemichi, T.K., Erkinjutti, T. et al. (1993). Vascular dementia: diagnostic criteria for research studies. Report of the NINDS-AIREN International Workshop. *Neurology*, **43**(2), 250–60.

Rossor, M. (1992). Disorders of psychic function: dementia. In *Diseases of the Nervous System: Clinical Neurobiology*, ed. A.K. Asbury, G.M. McKhann & W.I. McDonald, pp. 788–94. Philadelphia: Saunders.

Roubicek, J. (1977). The electroencephalogram in the middle-aged and the elderly. *J. Am. Geriatr. Soc.*, **25**(4), 145–52.

Rowe, J.W. & Kahn, R.L. (1987). Human aging: usual and successful. *Science*, **237**(4811), 143–9.

Roy, N. S., Wang, S., Jiang, L. et al. (2000). In vitro neurogenesis by progenitor cells isolated from the adult human hippocampus. *Nat. Med.*, **6**(3), 271–7.

Rubin, L.L., Gatchalian, C.L., Rimon, G. & Brooks, S.F. (1994). The molecular mechanisms of neuronal apoptosis. *Curr. Opin. Neurobiol.*, **4**(5), 696–702.

Salthouse, T.A. (1996). The processing-speed theory of adult age differences in cognition. *Psychol. Rev.*, **103**(3), 403–28.

Sarter, M. & Bruno, J.P. (1998). Age-related changes in rodent cortical acetylcholine and cognition: main effects of age versus age as an intervening variable. *Brain Res. Rev.*, **27**(2), 143–56.

Schoenberg, B.S., Kokmen, E. & Okazaki, H. (1987). Alzheimer's disease and other dementing illnesses in a defined United States population: incidence rates and clinical features. *Ann. Neurol.*, **22**(6), 724–9.

Schofield, P.W., Marder, K., Dooneief, G., Jacobs, D.M., Sano, M. & Stern, Y. (1997a). Association of subjective memory complaints with subsequent cognitive decline in community-dwelling elderly individuals with baseline cognitive impairment. *Am. J. Psychiatry*, **154**(5), 609–15.

Schofield, P.W., Tang, M., Marder, K. et al. (1997b). Alzheimer's disease after remote head injury: an incidence study. *J. Neurol., Neurosurg. Psychiatry*, **62**(2), 119–24.

Seshadri, S., Drachman, D.A. & Lippa, C.F. (1995). Apolipoprotein E epsilon 4 allele and the lifetime risk of Alzheimer's disease. What physicians know, and what they should know. *Arch. Neurol.*, **52**(11), 1074–9.

Seshadri, S., Wolf, P.A., Beiser, A. et al. (1997). Lifetime risk of dementia and Alzheimer's disease. The impact of mortality on risk estimates in the Framingham Study. *Neurology*, **49**(6), 1498–504.

Sherrington, R., Rogaev, E.I., Liang, Y. et al. (1995). Cloning of a gene bearing missense mutations in early-onset familial Alzheimer's disease [see comments]. *Nature*, **375**(6534), 754–60.

Sisodia, S.S., Koo, E.H., Beyrenthes, K., Unterbeck, A. & Price, D.L. (1990). Evidence that beta-amyloid protein in Alzheimer's disease is not derived by normal processing. *Science*, **248**(4954), 492–5.

Skoog, I. (1997). The relationship between blood pressure and dementia: a review. *Biomed. Pharmacother.*, **51**(9), 367–75.

Skoog, I., Lernfelt, B., Landahl, S., et al. (1996). 15-year longitudinal study of blood pressure and dementia [see comments]. *Lancet*, 347(9009), 1141–5.

Skre, H. (1972). Neurological signs in a normal population. *Acta Neurol. Scand.*, 48(5), 575–606.

Sobel, E., Louhija, J., Sulkava, R. et al. (1995). Lack of association of apolipoprotein E allele epsilon 4 with late- onset Alzheimer's disease among Finnish centenarians. *Neurology*, 45(5), 903–7.

Spillantini, M.G., Crowther, R.A., Jakes, R., Hasegawa, M. & Goedert, M. (1998). Alpha-Synuclein in filamentous inclusions of Lewy bodies from Parkinson's disease and dementia with lewy bodies. *Proc. Natl. Acad. Sci., USA*, 95(11), 6469–73.

St George-Hyslop, P.H., Tanzi, R.E., Polinsky, R.J. et al. (1987). The genetic defect causing familial Alzheimer's disease maps on chromosome 21. *Science*, 235(4791), 885–90.

Steller, H. (1995). Mechanisms and genes of cellular suicide. *Science*, 267(5203), 1445–9.

Stern, Y., Gurland, B., Tatemichi, T.K., Tang, M.X., Wilder, D. & Mayeux, R. (1994). Influence of education and occupation on the incidence of Alzheimer's disease. *J. Am. Med. Assoc.*, 271(13), 1004–10.

Strong, R. (1998). Neurochemical changes in the aging human brain: implications for behavioral impairment and neurodegenerative disease. *Geriatrics*, 53, S9–S12.

Suzman, R., Manton, K., Willis, D. (1992). Oldest old. In *Oldest Old*, ed. K. Manton, R.M. Suzman & D.P. Willis, p. 3. New York: Oxford University Press.

Swan, G.E., DeCarli, C., Miller, B.L. et al. (1998). Association of midlife blood pressure to late-life cognitive decline and brain morphology. *Neurology*, 51(4), 986–93.

Swearer, J.M. & Drachman, D.A. (1996). Caretaker Obstreperous Behavior Rating Scale. *Int. Psychogeriatr.*, 8(Suppl. 3), 321–4.

Szilard, L. (1959). On the nature of the aging process. *Proc. Natl. Acad. Sci., USA*, 45, 30–45.

Tang, Y., Nyengaard, J.R., Pakkenberg, B. & Gundersen, H.J. (1997). Age-induced white matter changes in the human brain: a stereological investigation. *Neurobiol. Aging*, 18(6), 609–15.

Tatemichi, T.K., Foulkes, M.A., Mohr, J.P. et al. (1990). Dementia in stroke survivors in the Stroke Data Bank cohort. Prevalence, incidence, risk factors, and computed tomographic findings. *Stroke*, 21(6), 858–66.

Taubes, G. (1996). Misfolding the way to disease [news]. *Science*, 271(5255), 1493–5.

Terry, R.D., Masliah, E., Salmon, D.P. et al. (1991). Physical basis of cognitive alterations in Alzheimer's disease: synapse loss is the major correlate of cognitive impairment. *Ann. Neurol.*, 30(4), 572–80.

Tomlinson, B.E., Blessed, G. & Roth, M. (1970). Observations on the brains of demented old people. *J. Neurol. Sci.*, 11(3), 205–42.

van Leeuwen, F.W., Fischer, D.F., Benne, R. & Hol, E.M. (2000). Molecular misreading. A new type of transcript mutation in gerontology. *Ann. NY Acad. Sci.*, 908, 267–81.

Venarucci, D., Venarucci, V., Vallese, A. et al. (1999). Free radicals: important cause of pathologies refer to ageing. *Panminerva Med.*, 41(4), 335–9.

Venters, H.D., Dantzer, R. & Kelley, K.W. (2000). A new concept in neurodegeneration: TNFalpha is a silencer of survival signals. *Trends Neurosci.*, 23(4), 175–80.

Waite, L.M., Broe, G.A., Creasey, H., Grayson, D., Edelbrock, D. & O'Toole, B. (1996). Neurological signs, aging, and the neurodegenerative syndromes. *Arch. Neurol.*, 53(6), 498–502.

Wechsler, D. (1981). *Manual for the Wechsler Adult Intelligence Scale – Revised*. New York: The Psychological Corporation.

Wernicke, T.F. & Reischies, F.M. (1994). Prevalence of dementia in old age: clinical diagnoses in subjects aged 95 years and older. *Neurology*, 44(2), 250–3.

West, M.J., Coleman, P.D., Flood, D.G. & Troncoso, J.C. (1994). Differences in the pattern of hippocampal neuronal loss in normal ageing and Alzheimer's disease. *Lancet*, 344(8925), 769–72.

Wisniewski, K., Jervis, G.A., Moretz, R.C. & Wisniewski, H.M. (1979). Alzheimer neurofibrillary tangles in diseases other than senile and presenile dementia. *Ann. Neurol.*, 5(3), 288–94.

Wolozin, B., Luo, Y. & Wood, K. (1996). Neuronal loss in aging and disease. In *Cellular Aging and Cell Death*, ed. N. Holbrook, G. Martin & R. Lockshin, vol. 16, pp. 283–302.New York: Wiley-Liss.

Wolozin, B., Kellman, W., Ruosseau, P., Celesia, G.G. & Siegel, G. (2000). Decreased prevalence of Alzheimer disease associated with 3-hydroxy-3-methyglutaryl coenzyme A reductase inhibitors. *Arch. Neurol.*, 57(10), 1439–43.

Yaffe, K., Grady, D., Pressman, A. & Cummings, S. (1998). Serum estrogen levels, cognitive performance, and risk of cognitive decline in older community women [see comments]. *J. Am. Geriatr. Soc.*, 46(7), 816–21.

Yashin, A.I., De Benedictis, G., Vaupel, J.W. et al. (1999). Genes, demography, and life span: the contribution of demographic data in genetic studies on aging and longevity. *Am. J. Hum. Genet.*, 65(4), 1178–93.

Zaudig, M. (1992). A new systematic method of measurement and diagnosis of 'mild cognitive impairment' and dementia according to ICD-10 and DSM-III-R criteria. *Int. Psychogeriatr.*, 4(Suppl. 2), 203–19.

Zhu, H., Fu, W., Mattson, M.P. et al. (2000). The catalytic subunit of telomerase protects neurons against amyloid beta-peptide-induced apoptosis. *J. Neurochem.*, 75(1), 117–24.

17

Alzheimer's disease

Raymond J. Kelleher III[1,2] and John H. Growdon[1]

[1] Memory Disorders Unit, Neurology Service, Massachusetts General Hospital, and Department of Neurology, Harvard Medical School, Boston, MA, USA
[2] Center for Learning and Memory, Department of Brain and Cognitive Sciences, Massachusetts Institute of Technology, Cambridge, MA, USA

Alzheimer's disease (AD) is an age-related, neurodegenerative disorder that represents the most common cause of dementia and is one of the leading causes of medical morbidity and mortality in the developed world. The implications of increasing longevity and shifting population demographics have led to the recognition of AD as a public health problem of major proportions. The percentage of the US population over age 65 will more than double over the next 30 to 40 years. According to these projections, as many as 10 million persons will be afflicted with dementia, the majority of whom will suffer from AD, with associated annual health care costs of over $100 billion (Cummings, 1995). On a personal level, the insidious but relentless decline in the affected individual's cognitive and functional abilities imposes a particularly heavy burden on patient, caregivers and family members alike. These considerations have greatly increased public awareness of AD during the past 20 years, and have stimulated the increasingly rapid pace of scientific progress directed toward the development of effective, disease-modifying treatments.

Historical perspective

In 1907, Alois Alzheimer published the initial report of the clinical and pathologic features of the disease that was soon named after him by Emil Kraepelin (Alzheimer, 1907; Kraepelin, 1910; Maurer et al., 1997). This report summarized a lecture he had given the prior year on the case of 'Auguste D', a 51-year-old woman admitted in 1901 to the Hospital for the Mentally Ill and Epileptics in Frankfurt, Germany. Alzheimer described a syndrome of 'rapidly increasing memory impairments', aphasia, disorientation, paranoia, and auditory hallucinations. His detailed histopathological analysis upon her death in 1906, which was aided by the new staining techniques introduced by his colleague Franz Nissl, revealed 'numerous small miliary

foci . . . caused by the deposition of a peculiar substance in the cortex'. These 'foci' or neuritic plaques, as they came to be called, were accompanied by extensive loss of cortical neurons and striking neurofibrillary changes: 'In the center of an otherwise normal cell there stand out one or several fibrils due to their characteristic thickness and peculiar impregnability.' Alzheimer provided a more thorough description of this original case, along with an account of a second case ('Johann F'.) from his Munich clinic, in a subsequent publication that included numerous illustrations of the characteristic neuritic plaques and neurofibrillary tangles (Alzheimer, 1911).

Alzheimer's description of the key pathologic features, along with contemporaneous reports of similar findings by Fischer (1907), Bonfiglio (1908) and Perusini (1909), promoted the acceptance of 'Alzheimer's disease' as a distinct and important disease entity. Despite the relatively young age of Alzheimer's original two patients, it gradually became apparent that the clinical and pathologic features of presenile and senile cases were essentially indistinguishable. For example, Perusini stated in 1909: 'The pathological process recalls the main features of senile dementia; however, the alterations in the cases described are more far-reaching, although some of them represent presenile diseases.' (cf. Maurer et al., 1997). In the eighth edition of his influential textbook *Psychiatrie*, published in 1910, Kraepelin was the first to attribute the definitive description of the disease to Alzheimer, who was then his colleague in Munich: 'The clinical interpretation of this Alzheimer's disease [*Alzheimersche Krankheit*] is still unclear. Although the anatomical findings suggest that we are dealing with a particularly serious form of senile dementia, the fact is that this disease sometimes starts as early as in the late forties.' The following year, Alzheimer himself accordingly entered the postmortem diagnosis of Johann F. in the Munich clinic records as '*Alzheimersche Krankheit*' (Graeber et al., 1997). From this modest initial description of two case reports, AD has come to be recognized as the most important cause of intellectual deterioration in adult life, and the underlying neuropathological abnormalities described by Alzheimer represent the most common disease process leading to progressive cerebral atrophy, neuronal death and dementia.

Epidemiology and risk factors

Age is the single greatest risk factor for AD. Estimates of the prevalence of dementia among individuals older than age 65 in population-based studies from the US, Europe, and Asia have ranged from approximately 2% to 10% (Rocca et al., 1986; Schoenberg et al., 1987; Evans et al., 1989; Zhang et al., 1990), with the variability probably attributable to differences in study design and diagnostic criteria. AD is uncommon before the age of 60 years, but increases exponentially thereafter, with incidence and prevalence estimates doubling every 5 years after age 65 (Ott et al., 1995; Jorm et al., 1987; Ritchie et al., 1992; Hebert et al., 1995). The proportion of individuals affected by dementia thus increases from 1% in the age group 65–69 years to greater than 40% among nonagenarians, with AD accounting for the majority of cases regardless of age, sex or ethnic group. Incidence estimates increase from 0.6% among those 65–69 years old to 8.4% among persons over age 85. Inasmuch as prevalence estimates remain well short of 100%, even among the oldest old, dementia is not an inevitable consequence of the aging process, at least not within the current limits of human lifespan.

The next most significant risk factor for AD is a positive family history of the disease. Familial aggregation of AD has been recognized for many years; 20–40% of AD patients have an affected first-degree relative, and increases in the cumulative incidence of dementia among first-degree relatives of AD patients ranging from two- to sixfold have been reported in various studies (Heston et al., 1981; Heyman et al., 1983; Breitner & Folstein, 1984; Nee et al., 1987; Breitner et al., 1988; Farrer et al., 1989; Mayeux et al., 1991; Silverman et al., 1994). In a small number of families, perhaps 150–200 worldwide, there is a clear, autosomal-dominant mode of disease transmission, with early onset between 30 and 60 years of age. In the majority of these early-onset familial AD pedigrees, the disease is caused by point mutations in one of three chromosomal loci: the amyloid precursor protein (APP) gene on chromosome 21; the presenilin-1 (PS1) gene on chromosome 14; and the presenilin-2 (PS2) gene on chromosome 1 (see below). In contrast to these early-onset pedigrees, 90% of AD cases exhibit onset after age 65 and occur in a sporadic

fashion without any clear familial pattern of transmission.

More than 25 genetic risk factors have been associated with late-onset AD, including polymorphisms in the genes encoding apolipoprotein E (ApoE), α2-microglobulin, cystatin C, LDL receptor-related protein (LRP), and interleukin-1 (for review see Price et al., 1998; St.George-Hyslop, 1999). Of these, the best-characterized susceptibility locus for sporadic AD is the gene on chromosome 19 encoding ApoE, a lipid transport protein (for review see Roses, 1996). The *APOE* gene was initially identified as a susceptibility locus for late-onset familial AD by positional cloning strategies, but was subsequently shown to represent a major risk factor for sporadic AD as well (Corder et al., 1993; Poirier et al., 1993; Rebeck et al., 1993; Saunders et al., 1993; Strittmatter et al., 1993). Polymorphisms in the *APOE* gene define three distinct alleles, designated ε2, ε3, and ε4, which influence the relative risk and age of onset for the development of AD. Inheritance of the ε4 allele confers an increased risk and earlier age of onset for both familial and sporadic AD, while the ε2 allele appears to be protective in both respects.

Additional minor risk factors for AD identified in some but not all studies include prior head trauma (Heyman et al., 1984; Mortimer et al., 1985) and low educational level (Katzman, 1993; Stern et al., 1994; Ott et al., 1995). The roles of these potential risk factors have been disputed due to their confounding effects on cognitive performance. There is some evidence for a higher prevalence of AD among women, independent of longer life expectancy (Kay, 1986; Katzman et al., 1989). Various environmental exposures have been proposed as predisposing factors for AD, particularly aluminium and other heavy metals (Basun et al., 1991; Perl & Good, 1987), but the weight of evidence has fallen against a causative role for such exposures. Retrospective analyses have identified several factors that may exert a protective effect against the development of AD, most notably the use of non-steroidal anti-inflammatory drugs (NSAIDS) (Breitner, 1996), estrogen replacement therapy (Paganini-Hill & Henderson, 1996), the use of HMG-CoA reductase inhibitors (Jick et al., 2000; Wolozin et al., 2000) and wine consumption (Orgogozo et al., 1997).

Clinical features and course

AD is characterized clinically by prominent impairments in cognition, often accompanied by neuropsychiatric behavioural disturbances, in the face of an otherwise bland elementary neurologic examination. Clinical criteria for the diagnosis of AD (DSM-IV, ICD-10, and NINCDS–ADRDA) all share common features: onset between ages 40 and 90; progressive dementia, as defined by prominent memory loss plus impairment in at least one other cognitive domain (such as language or praxis) sufficiently severe to impair social and/or occupational function; no disturbance of consciousness; and absence of other brain and systemic diseases that can cause dementia (McKhann et al., 1984). The NINCDS–ADRDA criteria further subdivide the diagnosis into definite (autopsy-proven), probable (meets all clinical criteria) and possible (some atypical features). The accuracy of these criteria relative to the neuropathological diagnosis of AD has been validated in clinicopathologic studies (Joachim et al., 1988; Tierney et al., 1988). Staging schemes for AD generally incorporate ratings of the severity of impairments in both cognitive and functional abilities; the systems in widest use are the Global Deterioration Scale (GDS) and the Clinical Dementia Rating scale (CDR) (Reisberg et al., 1988; Hughes et al., 1982). The CDR, for example, defines the severity of dementia as questionable (CDR 0.5), mild (CDR 1.0), moderate (CDR 2.0) or severe (CDR 3.0) based upon the scores in subcategories for memory, orientation, judgment, problem solving, community affairs, home and hobbies, and personal care.

AD typically begins with the gradual onset of forgetfulness (amnesia). Impairment of explicit memory for recent events is the most prominent early deficit. The observation that patients have difficulty learning or retaining new information reflects the early involvement of medial temporal lobe structures, including the entorhinal cortex and hippocampal formation, in the disease process. Forgetfulness for recent events or conversations, misplacement of objects, and repetitive questions are gradually noticed by family members or friends, even though patients themselves may be unaware of the problem (anosognosia). Word-finding difficulty (anomia) is the next most common manifestation. This feature generally emerges after the onset of amnesia, and reflects dysfunction of the temporal and frontal neocortices. An important practical index of the significance of reported cognitive disturbances is the extent to which they interfere with everyday functional abilities in the home or workplace. Difficulty with organizational tasks that were previously easily accomplished, such as management of the household finances or occupational duties, may become evident during the early stages of the illness and prompt neurologic evaluation. A change in personality is common: some patients become anxious or irritable, while others become quiet, withdrawn, and lose interest in their surroundings. These behavioural changes may resemble depression, but most often stem from apathy related to frontal lobe dysfunction. In spite of these limitations, social graces and other automatic behaviours are generally well preserved in the early stages of AD.

As the disease progresses, the impairments in memory and language become more profound, and the patient is no longer able to work. Visuospatial difficulties and trouble with dressing or the use of utensils (apraxia) become evident to varying degrees. The patient may become lost when out of the house, and assistance with the activities of daily living becomes necessary. Eventually, daily supervision may be required to prevent wandering or protect the patient from harm. Neuropsychiatric manifestations become more frequent and may include disinhibition, agitation, disruption of the sleep–wake cycle, hallucinations and frank delusions. These features probably arise as a primary consequence of the neurodegenerative process, and are thus 'organic' in nature. In the latter stages of the disease, speech disintegrates and functional abilities are progressively lost. Ultimately the patient is left in a mute, rigid, bedridden state requiring complete care; death usually results from a superimposed infection or medical illness. The average duration of AD is approximately 8 years from onset to death (Barclay et al., 1985), with a range of 1 to 25 years. There is considerable variation in the rate of progression; the clinical course is often marked by long periods of apparent stability, while in other cases patients can experience a rapid, relentless decline.

The elementary neurologic examination is generally unremarkable in the early stages of AD. The presence of primitive reflexes, such as snout, palmomental, grasping or suck responses, is frequently noted as the disease progresses to involve the frontal lobes. Olfactory deficits have been reported in a small number of patients (Serby et al., 1985). Focal neurologic signs are not observed unless the disease has been complicated by a discrete parenchymal lesion, such as a stroke, tumour or hemorrhage. Late in the course, patients may develop parkinsonian extrapyramidal signs of bradykinesia and rigidity, but rarely tremor. Some exhibit myoclonus, and a small fraction develop generalized seizures. The presence of prominent parkinsonism early in the course of dementia should prompt consideration of the alternative diagnosis of diffuse Lewy body disease (DLBD), while prominent early myoclonus should suggest the possibility of metabolic encephalopathy or Creutzfeld–Jakob disease.

Neuropathologic features

The gross appearance of the brain in AD is marked by diffuse cerebral atrophy, gyral atrophy with thinning of the cortical grey matter ribbon and secondary ventricular enlargement. These features are not specific for AD, however, since considerable age-associated atrophy can be seen in the absence of dementia or AD pathology. The cerebral atrophy in AD reflects the underlying neuronal degeneration and is most prominent in the temporal lobes, hippocampi and association areas of the frontal and parietal lobes. Primary motor and sensory cortices are relatively spared, as are subcortical structures, with the notable exception of the amygdala, basal forebrain nuclei and locus ceruleus.

The microscopic hallmarks of AD are the presence of numerous extracellular neuritic or senile amyloid plaques (SPs), intraneuronal neurofibrillary tangles (NFTs), neuropil threads and cerebral vascular amyloid deposits. These changes are accompanied by selective neuronal and synaptic loss in the cerebral cortex and certain subcortical regions. Microscopically, neuronal loss is evident in the subiculum and CA1 fields of the hippocampus, the neocortex of the frontal and temporal lobes, the cholinergic nucleus basalis of Meynert, septal nuclei, amygdala, noradrenergic locus ceruleus, serotonergic dorsal raphé nucleus, and dorsal tegmental nucleus. In some regions, such as the entorhinal cortex and superior temporal sulcus, 50% of the neurons are lost (Gomez-Isla et al., 1996). Synaptic loss, revealed by electron microscopy and immunostaining with markers for synaptic terminals, has been described in many of these regions, particularly in the hippocampus and neocortex (Masliah et al., 1989; Hamos et al., 1989; Scheff et al., 1990). Although the SPs and NFTs are the most readily detected pathologic features, neuronal loss and decreased synaptic contacts are the proximate causes of the clinical manifestations of dementia in AD.

The mature SP has a dense central core of amyloid surrounded by dystrophic neuronal processes ('neurites') interspersed with the processes of activated microglia and reactive astrocytes, indicating an inflammatory response and neuronal injury associated with the amyloid deposition (Fig. 17.1(*a*) and (*b*)). Ultrastructurally, the plaque core consists of ordered arrays of amyloid fibrils, and the binding of Congo red dye to the core indicates that these fibrils possess a β-pleated sheet structure (this feature is the basis of the descriptive term amyloid, as in the case of other diseases characterized by extracellular, Congo red-positive deposits). In the brains of normal elderly individuals, diffuse deposits of amyloid lacking neuritic features are a common finding. These diffuse, non-neuritic plaques stain weakly with Congo red and ultrastructurally exhibit little fibrillary character. The principal molecular constituents of both neuritic and non-neuritic plaques are 40 to 42 amino acid β-amyloid (Aβ) peptides derived from proteolytic processing of the large amyloid precursor protein, a

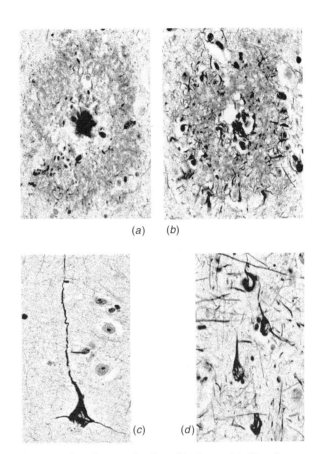

(*a*)   (*b*)

(*c*)   (*d*)

Fig. 17.1. Microphotographs of neuritic plaques (*a*), (*b*) and neurofibrillary tangles (*c*), (*d*) in the brain of a 65-year-old woman with end-stage Alzheimer's disease. (*a*) Neuritic plaque involving the amygdala. The discrete, centrally located amyloid core is surrounded by a clear halo, with argyrophilic dystrophic neurites scattered at the periphery of the plaque (Bielschowsky stain, original maginification 500×). (*b*) Neuritic plaque involving the neocortex (third layer of Brodmann area 9). The centrally located amyloid core is fragmented and dystrophic neurites are abundant (Bielschowsky, 500×). (*c*) Argyrophilic neurofibrillary tangles involving the uncus. Note the presence of three apparently normal neurons alongside the tangle (Bielschowsky, 500×). (*d*) Four argyrophilic neurofibrillary tangles involving the third cortical layer of the superior parietal lobule (Brodmann area 40; Bielschowsky, 500×). (Photomicrographs courtesy of Dr Jean-Paul Vonsattel, Massachusetts General Hospital.)

finding which led to the identification of mutations in APP as the first known genetic cause of AD (see *Etiology*, below). Biochemical analyses have revealed that the diffuse plaques are primarily composed of the slightly longer and more hydrophobic 42-amino acid form of Aβ, whereas neuritic plaques contain both Aβ42 and the more soluble, abundant Aβ40 peptide (Iwatsubo et al., 1994). Amyloid deposition in the form of diffuse plaques can thus clearly precede the onset of the clinical manifestations of AD, particularly in the case of Down's syndrome (Rumble et al., 1989), suggesting that diffuse plaques may represent a substrate for the formation of neuritic plaques. The deposition of Aβ42 may therefore be an initiating event that in some circumstances leads to the further deposition of Aβ40 and neuritic plaque formation. Aβ oligomers also form within neurons, and may contribute directly to cell dysfunction and death (Walsh et al., 2000).

NFTs are composed primarily of hyperphosphorylated, ubiquitinated forms of the microtubule-associated axonal protein tau (Fig. 17.1(c) and (d)). These cytoplasmic deposits also have an ultrastructural fibrillary appearance, consisting of dense bundles of long, twisted filaments. Such paired helical filaments are also found in the dystrophic neurites of neuritic plaques. Like amyloid deposits, NFTs are not specific to AD, as they can occur in much smaller numbers with normal aging. Moreover, NFTs with slight variations in ultrastructural and biochemical features characterize a number of neurodegenerative diseases, including Pick's disease, progressive supranuclear palsy, and corticobasal degeneration. This observation has prompted the conceptualization of these diseases as 'tauopathies', postulating a central role for NFTs in their pathogenesis (Goedert, 1998; Lee & Trojanowski, 1999).

SPs and NFTs exhibit distinct topographic distributions within the AD brain (Arnold et al., 1991). NFTs initially and preferentially affect the structures of the medial temporal lobe, including the amygdala, hippocampal formation, and parahippocampal regions, whereas amyloid plaques are more uniformly distributed throughout the neocortex of the frontal, temporal and parietal lobes. In late-stage AD, NFTs are plentiful in temporal, parietal and frontal neocortices. Given this hierarchical distribution, NFTs are a better pathological correlate of the pattern of neuronal loss and the severity of dementia than are amyloid plaques, and a pathological staging system has been proposed based on NFTs alone (Braak & Braak, 1991; NIA/Reagan criteria, 1997). In contrast to the NFT criteria, CERAD criteria for the neuropathological diagnosis for AD depend on an assessment of the frequency of amyloid plaques in three specific neocortical regions, the superior temporal gyrus, the prefrontal cortex, and the inferior parietal lobule, with an emphasis placed on the presence of neuritic plaques. In conjunction with the clinical findings, the 'plaque scores' for these areas define AD as possible, probable, or definite. The correspondence between the NIA/Reagan and CERAD criteria is high (Newell et al., 1999).

Multiple neurochemical abnormalities have been identified in the AD brain, reflecting the depletion of specific neuronal subpopulations (Francis et al., 1985; Mann & Yates, 1986; Bowen et al., 1994). Decreases in indices of the neurotransmitter acetylcholine in hippocampus and neocortex reflect atrophy and loss of cholinergic neurons in the ventral forebrain (Whitehouse, 1998). Similarly, neuronal loss in the noradrenergic locus ceruleus and the serotonergic dorsal raphé nuclei correlates with deficiencies in the corresponding neurotransmitters, and the depletion of excitatory pyramidal neurons in association neocortex contributes to a reduction in cortical glutamate levels. The deficiencies in multiple neurotransmitter systems suggest that pharmacologic therapies based on transmitter replacement will be of limited benefit, and that effective treatment will require prevention of the underlying neuronal loss.

Etiology

Molecular genetics and the amyloid hypothesis

Genetic studies based on large, multigenerational families with early-onset AD have identified causative mutations in three genes that can cause autosomal-dominant AD: the genes encoding APP, PS1 and PS2 (for review see Selkoe, 1996; Wasco & Tanzi, 1997; St. George Hyslop, 2000). The observation that pathogenic mutation in all three of these genes increases the production of β-amyloid underlies the amyloid hypothesis of AD, which postulates that amyloid deposition in the brain initiates a cascade of events that eventually leads to neuronal dysfunction and death. Additional chromosomal loci responsible for familial AD also apparently exist, since FAD pedigrees without mutations in these genes have been reported.

The *APP* gene encodes a type I integral membrane glycoprotein whose normal function remains unclear. Proteolytic processing of APP around its C-terminal transmembrane domain gives rise to a complex array of secreted and membrane-associated fragments (Fig. 17.2). APP cleavage by α-secretase splits the β-amyloid region and generates a long, soluble N-terminal fragment that possesses neurotrophic properties. Aβ peptides, which have neurotoxic properties (Yankner et al., 1989), are produced by the sequential action of two other proteases: β-secretase, which cleaves the juxtamembranous extracellular region of APP to yield the N-terminal end of Aβ, and γ-secretase, which cleaves the transmembrane portion of APP at two distinct positions to yield secreted Aβ peptides of either 40 or 42 amino acids (for review, see Vassar & Citron, 2000).

Although the cleavage of APP within the Aβ region by α-secretase predominates, Aβ peptides are produced at low

APP

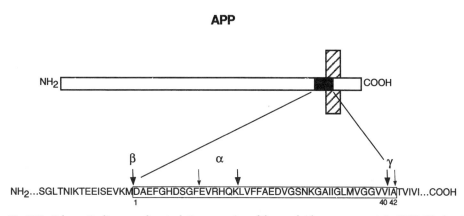

Fig. 17.2. Schematic diagram of proteolytic processing of the amyloid precursor protein (APP). The hatched box represents the plasma membrane, and the solid area of APP represents the β-amyloid region, whose amino-acid sequence is expanded below. The cleavage sites of the α-, β- and γ-secretases are indicated by the corresponding arrows. The boxed area of the β-amyloid region corresponds to the 40–42 residue Aβ peptides produced by the sequential action of β- and γ-secretase. Note that α-secretase cleaves within the β-amyloid region, thereby precluding the generation of Aβ species. The alternative intramembranous cleavage sites for γ-secretase produce either Aβ40 or Aβ42.

levels during normal cellular metabolism, and increased Aβ production (or an increased ratio of the levels of Aβ42 to Aβ40) has been consistently associated with the genetic lesions in familial AD (for summary, see Selkoe, 1997, 1999). All known FAD-linked mutations in APP occur at or near the sites of β- and γ-secretase cleavage that release the Aβ fragment, increasing the generation of Aβ42, and elevation of the Aβ42: Aβ40 ratio can be detected presymptomatically in carriers of an FAD mutation. Similarly, patients with Down's syndrome show increased levels of Aβ production, and the invariant association of the classic neuropathology of AD with adult cases of Down's syndrome is likely explained by the presence of an additional copy of the APP gene.

In addition to overproduction of Aβ, it is possible that alterations in degradation or clearance mechanisms may contribute to amyloid deposition in AD. Endogenous pathways for the degradation of Aβ and its clearance from brain tissue, which may antagonize cerebral amyloid deposition, have been identified. Several metalloendopeptidases have been implicated in the proteolytic degradation of Aβ, including insulin-degrading enzyme (IDE) (Vekrellis et al., 2000; Qiu et al., 1998) and neprilysin (NEP) (Iwata et al., 2000). NEP, which was shown to degrade Aβ42 in vivo, is a zinc–metalloprotease that inactivates several biologically active brain peptides, including enkaphalins, tachykinins, bradykinin and endothelins. Interaction of Aβ with ApoE and α-macroglobulin may provide another major clearance route. Both of these molecules are internalized by low-density lipoprotein receptor related protein, which is hypothesized to regulate the complex metabolic cascades

that balance Aβ synthesis and clearance (Hyman et al., 1984).

Reproduction of the genetic alterations associated with familial AD in animal models has provided important experimental support for the 'amyloid hypothesis.' Overexpression of APP-bearing FAD-linked mutations in transgenic mice is sufficient to cause persistently elevated levels of soluble Aβ and an age-dependent accumulation of amyloid plaques in the cerebral cortex that closely resemble those in the brains of AD patients (Games et al., 1995; Hsiao et al., 1996). In contrast, mice in which both copies of the APP gene have been inactivated (APP 'knockout' mice) exhibit only slight phenotypic abnormalities, and do not develop AD-like neuropathological changes (Zheng et al., 1995). Consistent with the autosomal-dominant inheritance pattern of FAD, the results from mouse model systems suggest that APP mutations do not result in a loss of protein function, but rather promote the abnormal accumulation of cerebral amyloid through a gain-of-function mechanism.

While APP mutations have been found in fewer than 2–3% of reported AD pedigrees, mutations in the PS1 gene on chromosome 14 account for the majority of early-onset, familial AD. The PS1 gene was initially identified by positional cloning based on genetic linkage to a region of the long arm of chromosome 14 (Sherrington et al., 1995), and more than 50 pathogenic mutations in the PS1 coding region have subsequently been identified (Wasco & Tanzi, 1997; Fraser et al., 2000). Mutations in the highly related PS2 gene on chromosome 1, which was originally identified on the basis of homology with PS1, have been linked to familial AD in a small number of pedigrees (Rogaev et al., 1995; Levy-Lahad et al., 1995a, b). (An annotated compendium of the mutations in APP, PS1 and PS2 linked to FAD is available at http: //www.alzforum.org.)

The presenilins are integral membrane proteins that are involved in the proteolytic processing of both APP and Notch (for review see Selkoe, 1998; Haass & De Strooper, 1999). Studies in cell culture and transgenic mice have demonstrated that pathogenic mutations in PS1 and PS2 enhance Aβ production (particularly the production of the more amyloidogenic species, Aβ42). Conversely, Aβ levels are considerably reduced in cultured neurons derived from *PS1* knockout mice, with the reduction primarily attributable to decreased γ-secretase activity (De Strooper et al., 1998). As in the case of APP, mutations in the presenilins thus appear to contribute to the pathogenesis of AD through a gain-of-function mechanism. Analysis of *PS1* knockout mice and studies of PS1-deficient cultured cells have further shown that PS1 regulates the activity of the Notch transmembrane receptor protein, a key regulator of cellular differentiation during development (Shen et al., 1997; De Strooper et al., 1999; Song et al., 1999; Handler et al., 2000).

Presenilin mutations produce effects on APP processing in the brains of affected individuals that are consistent with their apparent role in γ-secretase cleavage: levels of Aβ are elevated in patients bearing PS1 or PS2 mutations, even at presymptomatic stages; the density of plaques containing Aβ42 is increased in the brains of such patients; expression of mutant presenilin genes in cultured cells causes increased Aβ (Aβ42) production; overexpression of mutant PS1 in transgenic mice results in increased brain levels of Aβ42, and causes accelerated formation of amyloid plaques in the presence of a mutant APP transgene. On the basis of these observations and additional structure-function studies, it has been proposed that presenilins may themselves possess γ-secretase activity (Wolfe et al., 1999). At the very least, PS1 is a component of a multiprotein complex necessary for γ-secretase activity (Yu et al., 2000).

Beyond amyloid: tau pathology and neurodegeneration

The amyloid hypothesis may paint an incomplete picture of the pathogenesis of AD, as major unanswered questions remain concerning the connection between Aβ deposition and the other neuropathological features of AD. With respect to neuronal loss, it has been proposed that Aβ may exert a direct neurotoxic effect, or that it may injure neurons indirectly through the activation of an inflammatory response mediated by microglia and astrocytes (Yankner, 1996). The inflammatory response is associated with the formation of dystrophic neuronal processes in the neuritic plaques, and may contribute to derangement of neuronal metabolism, alterations in the cytoskeleton and the formation of neurofibrillary tangles. One limitation of the amyloid hypothesis, however, has been the failure to observe neurofibrillary changes as a result of experimental manipulations that increase Aβ production or deposition in any of the systems studied. In addition, significant neuronal loss has not been observed in the transgenic mouse models of AD, despite massive amyloid deposition in older animals (Irizarry et al., 1997). These considerations lead to the interpretation that amyloid accumulation, while likely a critical step in the pathogenesis of AD, is not sufficient to produce the full neuropathological picture of AD (Fig. 17.3).

The significance of neurofibrillary changes in the mechanistic process leading to neuronal loss has been emphasized by the discovery that mutations in the tau protein are sufficient to cause neurodegeneration and dementia in the absence of Aβ deposition. A variety of mutations occurring in and around the microtubule-binding repeats of the tau protein have been identified in autosomal-dominant pedigrees with frontotemporal dementia and parkinsonism linked to chromosome 17 (FTDP-17; for review see Goedert, 1998; Lee & Trojanowski, 1999). The neuropathology of some FTDP-17 cases resembles that of Pick's disease, with prominent circumscribed atrophy and neuronal loss in the frontal and temporal lobes, accompanied by intraneuronal filamentous deposits of hyperphosphorylated tau. Additional subcortical changes and intraglial tau deposits are sometimes seen, but significant amyloid pathology is absent. These findings provided strong evidence linking tau dysfunction and deposition to the pathogenesis of the large group of neurodegenerative diseases ('tauopathies') characterized by neurofibrillary lesions independent of Aβ accumulation. Exonic tau mutations associated with FTDP-17 have been shown to decrease the binding of tau to microtubules, impairing its ability to promote microtubule assembly (Hong et al., 1998). Hyperphosphorylation of tau also inhibits its binding to microtubules, though the relationship between hyperphosphorylation and tau deposition is unclear (Goedert, 1998). These observations suggest that biochemical alterations in tau structure and function may contribute to neuronal dysfunction through destabilization of the neuronal cytoskeleton and disruption of axonal transport. In addition, an increase in cytoplasmic levels of tau that is not bound to microtubules may promote its aggregation, possibly conferring an additional 'toxic' gain of function. In support of this notion, overproduction of wild-type tau or tau bearing an FTDP-17-linked mutation (P301L) in the brains of transgenic mice resulted in an age-

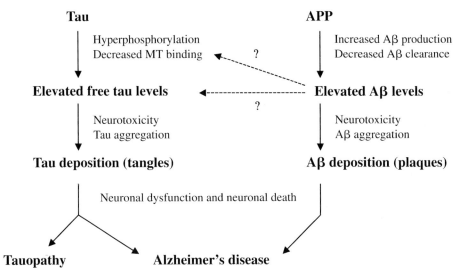

Fig. 17.3. A model for the pathogenesis of Alzheimer's disease (AD). The central roles of tau and the amyloid precursor protein (APP) in the molecular and cellular events leading to neurodegeneration are highlighted. Tau hyperphosphorylation and decreased microtubule binding may promote tau aggregation by elevating the levels of free unbound tau, possibly resulting in neurotoxicity as a result of cytoskeletal dysfunction. Elevated levels of β-amyloid (Aβ) peptides, particularly the more amyloidogenic species Aβ42, may result from either increased β- and/or γ-secretase cleavage of APP or decreased Aβ degradation and clearance. Increased soluble Aβ and Aβ aggregation, either intracellularly or in the form of amyloid plaques, are thought to promote neurotoxicity and neurodegeneration. Tau pathology and neuronal death in the absence of Aβ pathology characterize the 'tauopathies', whereas the neuronal death in AD is associated with the presence of both NFTs and amyloid deposition. Although the connections between tau and amyloid pathology (indicated by dashed lines) in AD remain unclear, a sustained increase in the levels of Aβ may be the initiating event that activates multiple cellular pathways leading to neuronal dysfunction and death, including tau aggregation and NFT formation.

and dose-dependent accumulation of filamentous deposits containing phosphorylated tau (Ishihara et al., 1999; Lewis et al., 2000). In two recent reports, overexpression of a mutant human APP transgene or intracerebral injection of Aβ_{42} fibrils enhanced the formation of tau deposits in the brains of mutant tau transgenic mice (Lewis et al., 2001; Götz et al., 2001), providing experimental evidence that Aβ can influence the development of tau neurofibrillary pathology (see Fig. 17.3).

Despite advances in understanding the molecular basis of AD, the events that ultimately precipitate neuronal death remain uncertain. Programmed cell death, or apoptosis, is a potential mechanism for the neuronal loss in a variety of neurodegenerative diseases (Rinkenberger & Korsmeyer, 1997; Nijhawan et al., 2000). Apoptosis is a cellular suicide pathway, largely operative during embryogenesis and in the immune system, that induces characteristic molecular and cellular alterations leading rapidly and irreversibly to cell death, such as activation of specific death proteases, endonucleolytic degradation of DNA and dissolution of cellular membranes. It has not been convincingly shown, however, that the neuronal loss in AD and other neurodegenerative diseases occurs via an apoptotic mechanism. In addition, studies in a variety of cell culture systems have produced conflicting results on the effects of the presenilins on sensitivity to apoptosis, suggesting both pro- and anti-apoptotic functions. Lack of PS1 function in the embryonic brain of *PS1* knockout mice, however, does not lead to increased neuronal cell death (Handler et al., 2000). Other avenues of investigation into the mechanisms of neuronal death in neurodegenerative disease have implicated free radical injury and mitochondrial dysfunction, which can produce neuronal death through both apoptosis and necrosis (Beal, 2000). Such pathways may represent primary causes of neurodegeneration, or alternatively, they may be activated as downstream events subsequent to some other initiating event, such as amyloid deposition.

Diagnostic evaluation

There are more than 50 medical, psychiatric, and neurological diseases considered in the differential diagnosis of dementia (Mayeux et al., 1993). Alzheimer's disease is by far the most common cause of dementia; DSM-IV and ICD-10 criteria follow closely on the NINDS-ADRDA guidelines first published in 1984 (McKhann et al., 1984).

Because of these common international standards, diagnostic procedures for AD are remarkably uniform throughout the world. In a survey of 26 centres specialized for AD care in the U.S., Europe, and Japan, six items out of a menu of 17 were specified as essential steps in the diagnosis of AD (Growdon, 2001). These procedures were: history of illness, physical examination, laboratory blood tests, a mental status test, psychometric testing, and a CT or MR brain scan. There was a high (>50%) frequency of use and importance ascribed to results obtained from these six measures, regardless of the geographic region. All other procedures, including many proposed as biomarkers of AD, were much less frequently used. Thus, there is worldwide consensus regarding the core features of the diagnostic evaluation for AD-type dementia.

The history is always obtained from an informant who knows the patient well, e.g. spouse or adult child. While interviewing the family members, it is always necessary to conduct the diagnostic assessment with the differential diagnosis of dementia in mind, so that history can be obtained to support or exclude diagnostic possibilities. The physical examination, including a compulsory neurological evaluation and a psychiatric examination as indicated, seeks to identify signs that might point to causes of dementia that might be confused with AD, such as Huntington's disease or Parkinson's disease. Laboratory blood tests are conducted to exclude underlying medical or metabolic derangements that can produce dementia. For example, it is necessary to exclude liver or kidney failure, or thyroid abnormality as a contributing cause of dementia. Mental status testing is recommended to document the presence of dementia and to estimate its severity. The three most common tests employed: the Information, Memory and Concentration subscale of the Blessed Dementia Score (Blessed et al., 1968), the Mini-Mental State Examination (Folstein et al., 1975), and the Alzheimer's Disease Assessment Scale (Rosen et al., 1984), are comparable rating scales. These tests require five to ten minutes to administer, and have a high intertest correlation (Solomon et al., 1999).

Psychometric tests explore aspects of cognition that are affected in AD in greater detail than mental status testing. Results of psychometric tests give confidence to the diagnosis of dementia by showing that AD patients have impairments in multiple cognitive domains. Cognitive tests range from such standard neuropsychiatric measures as the Wechsler Adult Intelligence Scale and the Wechsler Memory Scale to sets of tests that have been developed specifically for AD patients, such as the CERAD set of tests (Welsh et al., 1992) and the set of tests administered in the Massachusetts Alzheimer's Disease Research Center (Locascio et al., 1995). These latter specialized tests assess memory, language capacity, visual-spatial function, abstract reasoning, and frontal lobe function. Regardless of the set of cognitive tests, the findings are similar: in AD, there is an early and pronounced deficit in explicit memory, as tested by delayed recall. In addition, there are variable impairments in the other cognitive domains that decline over time. The decline in explicit memory is rapid and curvilinear; the decline in other functions, such as verbal fluency and naming objects, tends to be more linear and steady (Fig. 17.4). The results of cognitive tests provide an index of brain function and reflect the underlying pathology in AD. The pathologic bases of impaired delayed recall are atrophy of cholinergic ventral forebrain neurons (Whitehouse, 1998) and deafferentation of the hippocampus (Hyman et al., 1984), both of which occur early in the course of AD. Worsening language and visual-spatial abilities likely reflect progressive loss of neocortical neurons and their connections.

Neuroimaging is the sixth standard procedure. Standard CT or MRI scans are performed to search for brain lesions that could account for dementia or contribute to it; examples include hydrocephalus, stroke, and brain tumour. Conventional interpretations of these morphologic brain images do not add to the positive diagnosis of AD, but serve to exclude these and other conditions that can masquerade as AD. To extract more diagnostic information from the images, quantitative methods are being developed to measure brain regions vulnerable to AD pathology, such as the medial temporal lobe. There is ample experimental data now that atrophy of the medial temporal lobe, and hippocampal structures in particular, is greater in AD than in age-matched non-demented control subjects (de Leon et al., 1993; Jack et al., 1997). With sophisticated MR quantification, even greater precision is possible: in one study (Killiany et al., 2000), baseline MRI measures of atrophy in the entorhinal cortex, superior temporal sulcus and anterior cingulate were characteristic of AD, and identified with 95% sensitivity and 90% specificity non-demented individuals with mild memory difficulty who converted to Alzheimer's disease after three years. These findings are internally consistent with what is known about the pathophysiology of memory loss in AD: the deficit in explicit memory is usually the first sign of AD dementia (Locascio et al., 1995); explicit memory depends heavily upon the entorhinal–hippocampal–medial temporal lobe region (Corkin et al., 1997); and there is massive loss of neurons in the entorhinal cortex in AD (Gomez-Isla et al., 1996).

As dementia worsens, deficits in cognitive domains other than memory emerge or worsen, even if they had been normal at initial examination. The neuropathological substrate for further cognitive decline is decreased

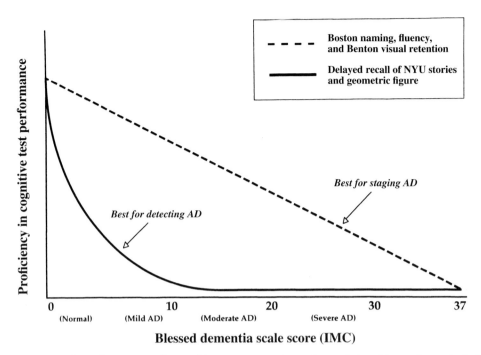

Fig. 17.4. Relation between specific cognitive test scores and a continuous index of dementia severity in AD patients: the information, memory and concentration (IMC) score of the Blessed Dementia Scale. Performance on tests of explicit memory, such as delayed recall of stories and geometric figures, falls precipitously early in the course of AD, and is therefore helpful in detecting the presence of dementia. Since performance on other measures, such as language tests, declines in a steady linear fashion over time, the Boston Naming and verbal fluency tasks are best for staging the severity of dementia and tracking its course. (Reproduced by permission from Locascio et al. 1995).

number of cortical synaptic contacts and neuronal loss (Gomez-Isla et al., 1997). Based upon serial MRI examinations, total brain volume in AD was found to decrease by about 2–3% per year compared to less than 1% per year in normal control subjects (Fox et al., 1999). Physiological brain imaging with positron emission tomography (PET) or single photon computed tomography (SPECT) brain scans has made it possible to detect neuronal dysfunction in life, even when the brain structure is normal on conventional CT or MR scan. Bilateral posterior parietal/temporal hypometabolism and hypoperfusion are characteristic of AD and found in 80–85% of cases (Kennedy, 1998). This pattern of deficit matches the distribution of pathological lesions in AD, which affects the multimodal association neocortices in temporal and parietal lobes out of proportion to the somatosensory and occipital regions (Arnold et al., 1991).

In centres that specialize in the diagnosis and care of patients with dementia and Alzheimer's disease, these six diagnostic procedures lead to a clinical diagnosis of AD that is confirmed pathologically in about 90% of cases. Diagnostic accuracy may be lower in practices outside of specialized academic centres, and regardless of site, these conventional diagnostic procedures are labour-intensive,

time-consuming, and expensive. Thus, there is a need for a biomarker or set of biomarkers that would quickly and accurately diagnose AD and circumvent the current practice of expensive and time-consuming testing. The search for biomarkers builds upon advances in understanding the biology of AD, and ranges from uncovering genetic risk factors to documenting the pathology of AD and describing the resultant molecular and biochemical changes that result from the AD process. These advances have sparked the hope of detecting some of these characteristic changes, especially those noted in brain tissue, during life (NIA/Reagan workshop 1998).

Although there are scores of biological correlates of Alzheimer's disease, no biological marker has yet gained full acceptance in practice as the sole test needed to diagnose AD. Several biomarkers, however, show promise, usually as a confirmatory aid in the conventional diagnostic assessment of a patient with dementia. Detecting a mutation in the *APP*, *PS1* or *PS2* gene carries high specificity for the diagnosis of AD, but such screening cannot be recommended as a routine measure because of extremely low sensitivity (infrequent number of affected individuals) in the total AD population. Thus, searching for a mutation should generally be limited to instances of familial AD cases under the age of 50 years. Detecting the ε4 allele of *APOE* can add a small increment of confidence to the AD diagnosis when used in conjunction with conventional diagnostic workup, but by itself has low diagnostic sensitivity and specificity.

Given the central position of cerebral amyloid deposition as the potential toxic event initiating a cascade of neurodegeneration, many molecular biomarkers centre on amyloid fragments in blood and CSF. Characteristic findings are increased levels of Aβ42 in plasma of patients with familial AD due to mutations in the *APP*, *PS1* and *PS2* genes (Scheuner et al., 1996); increased Aβ42 levels in some non-familial cases (Mayeux et al., 1999); and reduced APP isoform ratio in platelets of AD patients compared to control subjects (Baskin et al., 2000). CSF levels of Aβ42 are reduced in AD whereas CSF levels of the hyperphosphorylated tau protein are increased (Motter et al., 1995; Hulstaert et al., 1999). These tests have not achieved widespread diagnostic use either because they lack sufficient diagnostic sensitivity and specificity, or because they are available only in an experimental setting. Neuroimaging procedures appear most promising in the diagnosis of AD, especially quantitative measures of medial temporal lobe structures and whole brain volume. Because conventional brain scans are part of the standard diagnostic evaluation, quantitative measures can be readily adapted to the image data that are collected. In contrast to MRI, the use of PET scans will likely be limited to confirmatory or experimental studies performed in academic centres because of limited availability and expense.

Therapy

Currently available therapies for AD are symptomatic in nature, and ameliorate the cognitive or neuropsychiatric impairments without altering the course of the disease. Drugs that inhibit acetylcholinesterase are the current mainstays of treatment for the cognitive abnormalities of AD. Their use is based on the cholinergic hypothesis of memory dysfunction, which links pathological, biochemical and pharmacological evidence for a deficit in cholinergic neurotransmission with impaired memory (Bartus et al., 1982). The initial drug of this class, tacrine (Cognex®), improved memory in some patients but is now rarely prescribed due to its associated hepatotoxicity and the availability of safe alternative agents. Aricept® (donepezil), the cholinesterase inhibitor presently in widest use, produces modest improvement in memory performance when given as a single daily dose of 5 or 10 mg (Rogers & Friedhoff, 1996; Greenberg et al., 2000). Rivastigmine (Exelon®) is available in twice-daily dosing and has similar efficacy to donepezil (Corey-Bloom et al., 1998).

Apathy, depression, agitation, delusions and hallucinations are common neuropsychiatric alterations in AD. The selective serotonin reuptake inhibitors (SSRIs) are the drugs of choice to treat depression in the context of AD due to their favourable side effect profile, and particularly the absence of significant anticholinergic effects. Low doses of sedative or anxiolytic drugs may be used to treat agitation, but should be monitored closely to avoid possible side effects such as increased confusion or even a paradoxical increase in agitation. Paranoia, hallucinations and agitation generally respond to antipsychotic therapy, and the newer atypical neuroleptics (e.g. risperidone, olanzepine) are preferred because of their low risk of causing extrapyramidal side effects.

Agents that simply replace, or bypass, a neurotransmitter deficit will produce at most only short-term symptomatic benefit. The next generation of therapies for AD will attempt to correct the underlying pathogenic processes that lead to dementia. The first step in this effort was to administer high doses (2000 I.U./day) of the anti-oxidant vitamin E, which reportedly slowed the rate of deterioration in AD patients (Sano et al., 1997). Attempts to develop more effective disease-modifying therapies for AD have focused on antiamyloidogenic approaches that either block Aβ production or reduce its deposition in brain. The clinical implementation of such strategies will thus represent a formal test of the amyloid hypothesis of AD. Promising lines of development include small molecules that inhibit β- and γ-secretase, which should decrease Aβ production (Vassar & Citron, 2000). Another proposed approach is immunization against Aβ peptide, which is postulated to increase immune-mediated clearance of soluble Aβ (Schenk et al., 1999). Such strategies to decrease brain levels of soluble Aβ may also promote the dissolution of insoluble Aβ deposits by shifting the equilibrium in favour of solubility.

Future approaches to AD therapy may exploit other aspects of our understanding of the pathogenesis of AD. For example, stimulation of endogenous pathways for the degradation and clearance of Aβ may offer an alternative approach to antiamyloidogenic therapy. Inhibition of tau aggregation and NFT formation, possibly through modulation of tau phosphorylation, may help to promote neuronal survival in AD and other tauopathies. Strategies that block the pathways leading to neuronal death, whether apoptotic or otherwise, may provide benefit in neurodegenerative disorders of diverse etiologies. Finally, therapies relying on implantation of neural stem cells (Erickson et al., 1996) or stimulation of endogenous adult neurogenesis

(Björklund & Lindvall, 2000) may help to combat neuronal loss and restore or preserve cognitive function in AD.

References

Alzheimer, A. (1907). Über eine eigenartige Erkrankung der Hirnrinde. *Allg. Zeitschr. Psychiat. Psych.-Gerichtl. Med.*, **64**, 146–8.

Alzheimer, A. (1911). Über eigenartige Krankheitsfälle des späteren Alters. *Zeitschr. ges. Neurol. Psych.*, **4**, 356–85.

Arnold, S.E., Hyman, B.T., Flory, J., Damasio, A.R. & Van Hoesen, G.W. (1991). The topographical and neuroanatomical distribution of neurofibrillary tangles and neuritic plaques in the cerebral cortex of patients with Alzheimer's disease. *Cereb. Cortex*, **1**(1), 103–16.

Barclay, L.L., Zemcov, A., Blass, J.P. & Sansone, J. (1985). Survival in Alzheimer's disease and vascular dementias. *Neurology*, **35**(6), 834–40.

Bartus, R.T., Dean, R.L. d., Beer, B. & Lippa, A.S. (1982). The cholinergic hypothesis of geriatric memory dysfunction. *Science*, **217**(4558), 408–14.

Baskin, F., Rosenberg, R.N., Iyer, L., Hynan, L. & Cullum, C.M. (2000). Platelet APP isoform ratios correlate with declining cognition in AD. *Neurology*, **54**(10), 1907–9.

Basun, H., Forssell, L.G., Wetterberg, L. & Winblad, B. (1991). Metals and trace elements in plasma and cerebrospinal fluid in normal aging and Alzheimer's disease. *J. Neural. Transm. Park Dis. Dement. Sect.*, **3**(4), 231–58.

Beal, M.F. (2000). Energetics in the pathogenesis of neurodegenerative diseases. *Trends Neurosci.*, **23**(7), 298–304.

Blessed, G., Tomlinson, B.E. & Roth, M. (1968). The association between quantitative measures of dementia and senile change in the cerebral grey matter of elderly subjects. *Br. J. Psychiat.*, **114**, 797–811.

Bjöklund, A. & Lindvall, O. (2000). Cell replacement therapies for central nervous system disorders. *Nat. Neurosci.*, **3**, 537–44.

Bonfiglio, F. (1908). Di speciali reperti in un caso di probabile sifilde cerebrale. *Riv. Sperim. Freniatria*, **34**, 196–206.

Bowen, D.M., Francis, P.T., Chessell, I.P. & Webster, M.T. (1994). Neurotransmission – the link integrating Alzheimer research? *Trends Nuerosci.*, **17**, 149–50.

Braak, H. & Braak, E. (1991). Neuropathological stageing of Alzheimer-related changes. *Acta Neuropathol.*, **82**(4), 239–59.

Breitner, J.C. (1996). The role of anti-inflammatory drugs in the prevention and treatment of Alzheimer's disease. *Ann. Rev. Med.*, **47**, 401–11.

Breitner, J.C. & Folstein, M.F. (1984). Familial Alzheimer Dementia: a prevalent disorder with specific clinical features. *Psychol. Med.*, **14**(1), 63–80.

Breitner, J.C., Silverman, J.M., Mohs, R.C. & Davis, K.L. (1988). Familial aggregation in Alzheimer's disease: comparison of risk among relatives of early- and late-onset cases, and among male and female relatives in successive generations. *Neurology*, **38**(2), 207–12.

Corder, E.H., Saunders, A.M., Strittmatter, W.J. et al. (1993). Gene dose of apolipoprotein E type 4 allele and the risk of Alzheimer's disease in late onset families. *Science*, **261**(5123), 921–3.

Corey-Bloom, J., Anand, R. & J. Veach for the ENA 713 B352 Study Group (1998). A randomized trial evaluating the efficacy and safety of ENA 713 (rivastigmine tartrate), a new acetylcholinesterase inhibitor, in patients with mild to moderately severe Alzheimer's disease. *Int. J. Ger. Psychopharm.*, **1**, 55–65.

Corkin, S., Amaral, D.G., Gonzalez, R.G., Johnson, K.A. & Hyman, B.T. (1997). H. M.'s medial temporal lobe lesion: findings from magnetic resonance imaging. *J. Neurosci.*, **17**(10), 3964–79.

Cummings, J.L. (1995). Dementia: the failing brain. *Lancet*, **345**, 1481–4.

de Leon, M.J., Golomb, J., Convit, A., DeSanti, S., McRae, T.D. & George, A.E. (1993). Measurement of medial temporal lobe atrophy in diagnosis of Alzheimer's disease. *Lancet*, **341**(8837), 125–6.

De Strooper, B., Annaert, W., Cupers, P. et al. (1999). A presenilin-1-dependent gamma-secretase-like protease mediates release of Notch intracellular domain. *Nature*, **398**(6727), 518–22.

De Strooper, B., Saftig, P., Craessaerts, K. et al. (1998). Deficiency of presenilin-1 inhibits the normal cleavage of amyloid precursor protein. *Nature*, **391**, 387–90.

Eriksson, P.S., Perfilieva, E., Bjork-Eriksson, T. et al. (1998). Neurogenesis in the adult human hippocampus. *Nat. Med.*, **4**(11), 1313–17.

Evans, D.A., Funkenstein, H.H., Albert, M.S. et al. (1989). Prevalence of Alzheimer's disease in a community population of older persons. Higher than previously reported. *J. Am. Med. Assoc.*, **262**, 2551.

Farrer, L.A., O'Sullivan, D.M., Cupples, L.A., Growdon, J.H. & Myers, R.H. (1989). Assessment of genetic risk for Alzheimer's disease among first-degree relatives. *Ann. Neurol.*, **25**(5), 485–93.

Fischer, O. (1907). Miliare Nekrosen mit drusigen Wucherungen der Neurofibrillen, eine regelmäßige Veränderung der Hirnrinde bei seniler Demenz. *Monatsschr. Psychiatr. Neurol.*, **22**, 361–72.

Folstein, M.F., Folstein, S.E. & McHugh, P.R. (1975). 'Mini-mental state'. A practical method for grading the cognitive state of patients for the clinician. *J. Psychiatr. Res.*, **12**(3), 189–98.

Fox, N.C., Warrington, E.K. & Rossor, M.N. (1999). Serial magnetic resonance imaging of cerebral atrophy in preclinical Alzheimer's disease. *Lancet*, **353**(9170), 2125.

Francis, P.T., Palmer, A.M., Sims, N.R. et al. (1985). Neurochemical studies of early-onset Alzheimer's disease. Possible influence on treatment. *N. Engl. J. Med.*, **313**, 7–11.

Fraser, P.E., Yang, D.S., Yu, G. et al. (2000). Presenilin structure, function and role in Alzheimer disease. *Biochim. Biophys. Acta*, **1502**(1), 1–15.

Games, D., Adams, D., Alessandrini, R. et al. (1995). Alzheimer-type neuropathology in transgenic mice overexpressing V717F β-amyloid precursor protein. *Nature*, **373**, 523–7.

Goedert, M. (1998). Tau mutations cause frontotemporal dementias. *Neuron*, **21**, 955–8.

Gomez-Isla, T., Price, J.L., McKeel, D.W., Jr., Morris, J.C., Growdon, J.H. & Hyman, B.T.(1996). Profound loss of layer II entorhinal cortex neurons occurs in very mild Alzheimer's disease. *J. Neurosci.*, **16**(14), 4491–500.

Gomez-Isla, T., Hollister, R., West, H. et al. (1997). Neuronal loss correlates with but exceeds neurofibrillary tangles in Alzheimer's disease. *Ann. Neurol.*, **41**(1), 17–24.

Götz, I., Chen, F., van Dorpe, J. & Nitsch, R.M. (2001). Formation of neurofibrillary tangles in P301L tau transgenic mice induced by Aβ 42 fibrils. *Science*, **293**, 1491–5.

Graeber, M.B., Kosel, S., Egensperger, R. et al. (1997). Rediscovery of the case described by Alois Alzheimer in 1911: historical, histological and molecular genetic analysis. *Neurogenetics*, **1**(1), 73–80.

Greenberg, S.M., Tennis, M.K., Brown, L.B. et al. (2000). Donepezil therapy in clinical practice: a randomized crossover study. *Arch. Neurol.*, **57**(1), 94–9.

Growdon, J.H. (2001). Evaluating CNS biomarkers for Alzheimer's disease. In *Alzheimer's Disease: Biology, Diagnosis and Therapeutics*, ed. K. Iqbal, S. Sisodia & B. Winblad, pp. 265–73. UK: John Wiley.

Haass, C. & De Strooper, B. (1999). The presenilins in Alzheimer's disease – proteolysis holds the key. *Science*, **286**, 916–19.

Hamos, J.E., DeGennaro, L.J. & Drachman, D.A. (1989). Synaptic loss in Alzheimer's disease and other dementias. *Neurology*, **39**(3), 355–61.

Handler, M., Yang, X. & Shen, J. (2000). Presenilin-1 regulates neuronal differentiation during neurogenesis. *Development*, **127**, 2593–606.

Hebert, L.E., Scherr, P.A., Beckett, L.A. et al. (1995). Age-specific incidence of Alzheimer's disease in a community population. *J. Am. Med. Assoc.*, **273**(17), 1354–9.

Heston, L.L., Mastri, A.R., Anderson, V.E. & White, J. (1981). Dementia of the Alzheimer type. Clinical genetics, natural history, and associated conditions. *Arch. Gen. Psychiatry*, **38**(10), 1085–90.

Heyman, A., Wilkinson, W.E., Hurwitz, B.J. et al. (1983). Alzheimer's disease: genetic aspects and associated clinical disorders. *Ann. Neurol.*, **14**(5), 507–15.

Heyman, A., Wilkinson, W.E., Stafford, J.A., Helms, M.J., Sigmon, A.H. & Weinberg, T. (1984). Alzheimer's disease: a study of epidemiological aspects. *Ann. Neurol.*, **15**(4), 335–41.

Hong, M., Zhukareva, V., Vogelsberg-Ragaglia, V. et al. (1998). Mutation-specific functional impairments in distinct tau isoforms of hereditary FTDP-17. *Science*, **282**, 1914–17.

Hsiao, K., Chapman, P., Nilsen, S. et al. (1996). Correlative memory deficits, Aß elevation, and amyloid plaques in transgenic mice. *Science*, **274**, 99–102.

Hughes, C.P., Berg, L., Danziger, W.L., Coben, L.A. & Martin, R.L. (1982). A new clinical scale for the staging of dementia. *Br. J. Psychiatry*, **140**, 566–72.

Hulstaert, F., Blennow, K., Ivanoiu, A. et al. (1999). Improved discrimination of AD patients using β-amyloid(1–42) and tau levels in CSF. *Neurology*, **52**(8), 1555–62.

Hyman, B.T., Van Horsen, G.W., Damasio, A.R. & Barnes, C.L. (1984). Alzheimer's disease: cell-specific pathology isolates the hippocampal formation. *Science*, **225**(4667), 1168–70.

Irizarry, M.C., Soriano, F., McNamara, M. et al. (1997). Aβ deposition is associated with neuropil changes, but not with overt neuronal loss in the human amyloid precursor protein V717F (PDAPP) transgenic mouse. *J. Neurosci.*, **17**(18), 7053–9.

Ishihara, T., Hong, M., Zhang, B. et al. (1999). Age-dependent emergence and progression of a tauopathy in transgenic mice overexpressing the shortest human tau isoform. *Neuron*, **24**, 751–62.

Iwata, N., Tsubuki, S., Takaki, Y. et al. (2000). Identification of the major Aβ1–42-degrading catabolic pathway in brain parenchyma: suppression leads to biochemical and pathological deposition. *Nat. Med.*, **6**(2), 143–50.

Iwatsubo, T., Odaka, A., Suzuki, N., Mizusawa, H., Nukina, H. & Ihara, Y. (1994). Visualization of Aβ 42(43) and A beta 40 in senile plaques with end-specific Aβ monoclonals: evidence that an initially deposited species is Aβ 42(43). *Neuron*, **13**, 45–53.

Jack, C.R., Jr., Petersen, R.C., Xu, Y.C. et al. (1997). Medial temporal atrophy on MRI in normal aging and very mild Alzheimer's disease. *Neurology*, **49**(3), 786–94.

Jick, H., Zornberg, G.L., Jick, S.S., Seshadri, S. & Drachman, D.A. (2000). Statins and the risk of dementia. *Lancet*, **356**, 1627–31.

Joachim, C.L., Morris, J.H. & Seloke, D.J. (1988). Clinically diagnosed Alzheimer's disease: autopsy results in 150 cases. *Ann. Neurol.*, **24**(1), 50–6.

Jorm, A.F., Korten, A.E. & Henderson, A.S. (1987). The prevalence of dementia: a quantitative integration of the literature. *Acta Psychiatr. Scand.*, **76**(5), 465–79.

Katzman, R. (1993). Education and the prevalence of dementia and Alzheimer's disease. *Neurology*, **43**(1), 13–20.

Katzman, R., Aronson, M., Fuld, P. et al. (1989). Development of dementing illnesses in an 80-year-old volunteer cohort. *Ann. Neurol.*, **25**(4), 317–24.

Kay, D.W. (1986). The genetics of Alzheimer's disease. *Br. Med. Bull.*, **42**(1), 19–23.

Kennedy, A.M. (1998). Functional neuroimaging in dementia. In *The Dementias*, ed. J.H. Growdon & M.N. Rossor, pp. 219–55. Boston: Butterworth Heinemann.

Killiany, R.J., Gomez-Isla, T., Moss, M. et al. (2000). Use of structural magnetic resonance imaging to predict who will get Alzheimer's disease [see comments]. *Ann. Neurol.*, **47**(4), 430–9.

Kraepelin, E. (1910). *Psychiatrie: Ein Lehrbuch für Studierende und Ärzte.* Verlag J.A. Barth, Leipzig.

Lee, V.M. & Trojanowski, J.Q. (1999). Neurodegenerative tauopathies: human disease and transgenic mouse models. *Neuron*, **24**(3), 507–10.

Levy-Lahad, E., Wasco, W., Poorkaj, P. et al. (1995a). Candidate gene for the chromosome 1 familial Alzheimer's disease locus. *Science*, **269**, 973–7.

Levy-Lahad, E., Wijsman, E.M., Nemens, E. et al. (1995b). A familial Alzheimer's disease locus on chromosome 1. *Science*, **269**, 970–3.

Lewis, J., McGowan, E., Rockwood, J. et al. (2000). Neurofibrillary tangles, amyotrophy and progressive motor disturbance in mice expressing mutant (P301L) tau protein. *Nat. Genet.*, **25**, 402–5.

Lewis, J., Dickson, D.W., Lin, W-L, et al. (2001). Enhanced neurofibrillary degeneration in transgenic mice expressing mutant tau and APP, *Science*, **293**, 1487–91.

Locascio, J.J., Growdon,J.H. & Corkin, S. (1995). Cognitive test performance in detecting, staging, and tracking Alzheimer's disease. *Arch. Neurol.*, **52**(11), 1087–99.

McKhann, G., Drachman, D., Folstein, M., Katzman, R., Price, D. & Stadlan, E.M. (1984). Clinical diagnosis of Alzheimer's disease: report of the NINCDS–ADRDA Work Group under the auspices of Department of Health and Human Services Task Force on Alzheimer's Disease. *Neurology*, **34**(7), 939–44.

Mann, D.M. & Yates, P.O. (1986). Neurotransmitter deficits in Alzheimer's disease and in other dementing disorders. *Hum. Neurobiol.*, **5**, 147–58.

Masliah, E., Terry, R.D., DeTeresa, R.M. & Hansen, L.A. (1989). Immunohistochemical quantification of the synapse-related protein synaptophysin in Alzheimer disease. *Neurosci. Lett.*, **103**(2), 234–9.

Maurer, K., Volk, S. & Gerbaldo, H. (1997). Auguste D and Alzheimer's disease. *Lancet*, **349**(9064), 1546–9.

Mayeux, R., Sano, M., Chen, J., Tatemichi, T. & Stern, Y. (1991). Risk of dementia in first-degree relatives of patients with Alzheimer's disease and related disorders. *Arch. Neurol.*, **48**(3), 269–73.

Mayeux, R., Foster, N.L. & Whitehouse, P.J. (1993). The clinical evaluation of patients with dementia. In *Dementia*, ed. P.J. Whitehouse, pp. 92–129. Philadelphia: F.A. Davis.

Mayeux, R., Tang, M.X., Jacobs, D.M. et al. (1999). Plasma amyloid beta-peptide 1–42 and incipient Alzheimer's disease. *Ann. Neurol.*, **46**(3), 412–16.

Mortimer, J.A., French, L.R., Hutton, J.T. & Schuman, L.M. (1985). Head injury as a risk factor for Alzheimer's disease. *Neurology*, **35**(2), 264–7.

Motter, R., Vigo-Pelfrey, C., Kholodenko, D. et al. (1995). Reduction of beta-amyloid peptide 42 in the cerebrospinal fluid of patients with Alzheimer's disease. *Ann. Neurol.*, **38**(4), 643–8.

The National Institute on Aging and Reagan Institute Working Group on Diagnostic Criteria for the Neuropathological Assessment of Alzheimer's Disease. Consensus recommendations for the postmortem diagnosis of Alzheimer's disease. (1997). *Neurobiol. Aging*, **18**(Suppl. 4), S1–2.

Nee, L.E., Eldridge, R., Sunderland, T. et al. (1987). Dementia of the Alzheimer type: clinical and family study of 22 twin pairs. *Neurology*, **37**(3), 359–63.

Newell, K.L., Hyman, B.T., Growdon, J.H. & Hedley-Whyte, E.T. (1999). Application of the National Institute on Aging (NIA)-Reagan Institute criteria for the neuropathological diagnosis of Alzheimer disease. *J. Neuropathol. Exp. Neurol.*, **58**(11), 1147–55.

Nijhawan, D., Honarpour, N. & Wang, X. (2000). Apoptosis in neural development and disease. *Ann. Rev. Neurosci.*, **23**, 73–87.

Orgogozo, J.M., Dartigues, J.F., Lafont, S. et al. (1997). Wine consumption and dementia in the elderly: a prospective community study in the Bordeaux area. *Rev. Neurol. (Paris)*, **153**(3), 185–92.

Ott, A., Breteler, M.M., van Karskamp, F., Claus, J.J., van der Cammen, T.J., Grobbee, D.E. & Hofman, A. (1995). Prevalence of Alzheimer's disease and vascular dementia: association with education. The Rotterdam study. *Br. Med. J.*, **310**(6985), 970–3.

Paganini-Hill, A. & Henderson, V.W. (1996). Estrogen replacement therapy and risk of Alzheimer disease. *Arch. Intern. Med.*, **156**(19), 2213–17.

Perl, D.P. & Good, P.F. (1987). The association of aluminum, Alzheimer's disease and neurofibrillary tangles. *J. Neural Transm.*, Suppl, **24**, 205–11.

Perusini, G. (1909). Über klinisch und histologisch eigenartige psychische Erkrankungen des höheren Lebensalters. In *Histologische und Histopathologische Arbeiten*, ed. F. Nissl & A. Alzheimer, vol. 3, pp. 297–351. Jena: Verlag G. Fischer.

Poirier, J., Davignon,J., Bouthillier, D., Kogan, S., Bertrand, P. & Gauthier, S. (1993). Apolipoprotein E polymorphism and Alzheimer disease. *Lancet*, **342**, 697–9.

Price, D.L., Tanzi, R.E., Borchelt, D.R. & Sisodia, S.S. (1998). Alzheimer's disease: genetic studies and transgenic models. *Ann. Rev. Genet.*, **32**, 461–93.

Qiu, W.Q., Walsh, D.M., Ye, Z. et al. (1998). Insulin-degrading enzyme regulates extracellular levels of amyloid beta- protein by degradation. *J. Biol. Chem.*, **273**(49), 32730–8.

Rebeck, G.W., Reiter, J.S., Strickland, D.K. & Hyman, B.T. (1993). Apolipoprotein E in sporadic Alzheimer's disease: allelic variation and receptor interactions. *Neuron*, **11**, 575–80.

Reisberg, B., Ferris, S.H., de leon, M.J. & Crook, T. (1988). Global Deterioration Scale (GDS). *Psychopharmacol. Bull.*, **24**(4), 661–3.

Rinkenberger, J.L. & Korsmeyer,S.J. (1997). Errors of homeostasis and deregulated apoptosis. *Curr. Opin. Genet. Dev.*, **7**(5), 589–96.

Ritchie, K., Kildea, D. & Robine, J.M. (1992). The relationship between age and the prevalence of senile dementia: a meta-analysis of recent data. *Intern. J. Epidemiol.*, **21**, 763–9.

Rocca, W.A., Amaducci, L.A. & Schoenberg, B.S. (1986). Epidemiology of clinically diagnosed Alzheimer's disease. *Ann. Neurol.*, **19**(5), 415–24.

Rogaev, E.I., Sherrington, R., Rogaeva, E.A. et al. (1995). Familial Alzheimer's disease in kindreds with missense mutations in a gene on chromosome 1 related to the Alzheimer's disease type 3 gene. *Nature*, **376**, 775–8.

Rogers, S.L. & Friedhoff, L.T. (1996). The efficacy and safety of donepezil in patients with Alzheimer's disease: results of a US Multicentre, Randomized, Double-Blind, Placebo-Controlled Trial. The Donepezil Study Group. *Dementia*, **7**(6), 293–303.

The Ronald and Nancy Reagan Research Institute of the Alzheimer's Association and the National Institute on Aging Working Group (1998) Consensus Report of the Working Group on: Molecular and Biochemical Markers of Alzheimer's Disease. *Neurobiol. Aging*, **19**, 109–16.

Rosen, W.G., Mohs, R.C. & Davis, K.L. (1984). A new rating scale for Alzheimer's disease. *Am. J. Psychiatry*, **141**(11), 1356–64.

Roses, A.D. (1996). Apolipoprotein E alleles as risk factors in Alzheimer's disease. *Ann. Rev. Med.*, **47**, 387–400.

Rumble, B., Retallack, R., Hilbich, C. et al. (1989). Amyloid A4 protein and its precursor in Down's syndrome and Alzheimer's disease. *N. Engl. J. Med.*, **320**(22),1446–52.

Sano, M., Ernesto, C., Thomas, R.G. et al. (1997). A controlled trial of selegiline, alpha-tocopherol, or both as treatment for Alzheimer's disease. The Alzheimer's Disease Cooperative Study. *N. Engl. J. Med.*, **336**(17), 1216–22.

Saunders, A.M., Strittmatter, W.J., Schmechel, D. et al. (1993). Association of apolipoprotein E allele epsilon 4 with late-onset familial and sporadic Alzheimer's disease. *Neurology*, **43**(8) 1467–72.

Scheff, S.W., DeKosky, S.T. & Price, D.A. (1990). Quantitative assessment of cortical synaptic density in Alzheimer's disease. *Neurobiol. Aging*, **11**(1), 29–37.

Schenk, D., Barbour, R., Dunn, W. et al. (1999). Immunization with amyloid-ß attenuates Alzheimer-disease-like pathology in the PDAPP mouse. *Nature*, **400**, 173–7.

Scheuner, D., Eckman, C., Jernsen, M. et al. (1996). Secreted amyloid ß protein similar to that in the senile plaques of Alzheimer's disease is increased *in vivo* by the presenilin 1 and 2 and *APP* mutations linked to familial Alzheimer's disease. *Nature Med.*, **2**, 864–70.

Schoenberg, B.S., Kokmen, E. & Okazaki, H. (1987). Alzheimer's disease and other dementing illnesses in a defined United States population: incidence rates and clinical features. *Ann. Neurol.*, **22**(6), 724–9.

Selkoe, D.J. (1996). Amyloid beta-protein and the genetics of Alzheimer's disease. *J. Biol. Chem.*, **271**(31), 18295–8.

Selkoe, D.J. (1997). Alzheimer's disease: genotypes, phenotypes, and treatments. *Science*, **275**(5300), 630–1.

Selkoe, D.J. (1998). The cell biology of beta-amyloid precursor protein and presenilin in Alzheimer's disease. *Trends Cell Biol.*, **8**(11), 447–53.

Selkoe, D.J. (1999). Translating cell biology into therapeutic advances in Alzheimer's disease. *Nature*, **399**(Suppl. 6738), A23–31.

Serby, M., Corwin, J., Conrad, P. & Rotrosen, J. (1985). Olfactory dysfunction in Alzheimer's disease and Parkinson's disease. *Am. J. Psychiatry*, **142**(6), 781–2.

Shen, J., Bronson, R.T., Chen, D.F., Zia, W., Selkoe, D.J. & Tonegawa, S. (1997). Skeletal and CNS defects in Presenilin-1-deficient mice. *Cell*, **89**(4), 629–39.

Sherrington, R., Rogaev, E.I., Liang, Y. et al. (1995). Cloning of a novel gene bearing missense mutations in early onset familial Alzheimer disease. *Nature*, **375**, 754–60.

Silverman, J.M., Raiford, K., Edland, S. et al. (1994). The Consortium to Establish a Registry for Alzheimer's Disease (CERAD). Part VI. Family history assessment: a multicenter study of first-degree relatives of Alzheimer's disease probands and nondemented spouse controls. *Neurology*, **44**(7), 1253–9.

Solomon, P.R., Adams, F.A., Groccia, M.E., DeVeaux, R., Growdon, J.H. & Pendlebury, W.W. (1999). Correlational analysis of five commonly used measures of mental status/functional abilities in patients with Alzheimer disease. *Alzheimer Dis. Assoc. Disord.*, **13**(3), 147–50.

Song, W., Nadeau, P., Yuanm M., Ynag, X., Shen, J. & Yankner, B.A. (1999). Proteolytic release and nuclear translocation of Notch-1 are induced by presenilin-1 and impaired by pathogenic presenilin-1 mutations. *Proc. Natl. Acad. Sci., USA*, **96**(12), 6959–63.

St.George-Hyslop, P.H. (1999). Molecular genetics of Alzheimer disease. *Semin. Neurol.*, **19**(4), 371–83.

St. George Hyslop, P.H. (2000). Molecular genetics of Alzheimer's disease. *Biol. Psychiatry*, **47**(3), 183–99.

Stern, Y., Gurland, B., Tatemachi, T.K., Tang, M.X., Wilder, D. & Mayeux, R. (1994). Influence of education and occupation on the incidence of Alzheimer's disease. *J. Am. Med. Assoc.*, **271**(13), 1004–10.

Strittmatter, W.J., Saunders, A.M., Schmechel, D. et al. (1993). Apolipoprotein E: high-avidity binding to β-amyloid and increased frequency of type 4 allele in late-onset familial Alzheimer disease. *Proc. Natl. Acad. Sci., USA*, **90**, 1977–81.

Tierney, M.C., Fisher, R.H., Lewis, A.J. et al. (1988). The NINCDS–ADRDA Work Group criteria for the clinical diagnosis of probable Alzheimer's disease: a clinicopathologic study of 57 cases. *Neurology*, **38**(3), 359–64.

Vassar, R. & Citron, M. (2000). Aβ-Generating enzymes: recent advances in β- and γ-secretase research. *Neuron*, **27**, 419–22.

Vekrellis, K., Ye, Z., Qiu, W. Q. et al. (2000). Neurons regulate extracellular levels of amyloid beta-protein via proteolysis by insulin-degrading enzyme. *J. Neurosci.*, **20**(5), 1657–65.

Walsh, D.M., Tseng, B.P., Rydel, R.E., Podlisny, M.B. & Selkoe, D.J. (2000). The oligomerization of amyloid ?-protein begins intracellularly in cells derived from human brain. *Biochemistry*, **39**, 10831–9.

Wasco, W. & Tanzi, R.E. (1997). Etiological clues from gene defects causing early onset familial Alzheimer's disease. In *Molecular Mechanisms of Dementia*. NJ: Humana Press.

Welsh, K.A., Butters, N., Hughes, J.P., Mohs, R.C. & Heyman, A. (1992). Detection and staging of dementia in Alzheimer's disease. Use of the neuropsychological measures developed for the Consortium to Establish a Registry for Alzheimer's Disease. *Arch. Neurol.*, **49**(5), 448–52.

Whitehouse, P.J. (1998). The cholinergic deficit in Alzheimer's disease. *J. Clin. Psychiatry*, **59**(Suppl. 13), 19–22.

Wolfe, M.S., Xia, W., Ostaszewski, B.L., Diehl, T.S., Kimberly, W.T. & Selkoe, D.J. (1999). Two transmembrane aspartates in presenilin-1 required for presenilin endoproteolysis and γ-secretase activity. *Nature*, **398**, 513–17.

Wolozin, B., Kellman, W., Ruosseau, P., Celesia, G-G. & Siegel, G. (2000). Decreased prevalence of Alzheimer disease associated with 3-hydroxy-3-methylglutaryl coenzyme A inhibitors. *Arch. Neurol.* **57**, 1439–43.

Yankner, B.A. (1996). Mechanisms of neuronal degeneration in Alzheimer's disease. *Neuron*, **16**(5), 921–32.

Yankner, B.A., Dawes, L.R., Fisher, S., Vila-Komaroff, L., Oster-Granite, M.L. & Neve, R.L. (1989). Neurotoxicity of a fragment of the amyloid precursor associated with Alzheimer's disease. *Science*, **245**, 417–20.

Yu, G., Nishimura, M., Arawaka, S. et al. (2000). Nicastrin modulates presenilin-mediated notch/glp-1 signal transduction and betaAPP processing. *Nature*, **407**(6800), 48–54.

Zhang, M.Y., Katzman, R., Salmon, D. et al. (1990). The prevalence of dementia and Alzheimer's disease in Shanghai, China: impact of age, gender, and education. *Ann. Neurol.*, **27**(4), 428–37.

Zheng, H., Jiang, M., Trumbauer, M.E. et al. (1995). β-amyloid precursor protein-deficient mice show reactive gliosis and decreased locomotor activity. *Cell*, **81**: 525–31.

18

Dementia with Lewy bodies

Pamela J. McLean,[1] Estrella Gómez-Tortosa,[1,2] Michael C. Irizarry[1] and Bradley T. Hyman[1]

[1] Department of Neurology, Massachusetts General Hospital East, Charlestown, MA, USA
[2] Servicio de Neurología, Fundación Jiménez Díaz, Madrid, Spain

History

The concept of the clinical syndrome of 'dementia with Lewy bodies' arose within the context of correlations with the pathological descriptions of Lewy body inclusions. These inclusions were first described by F. H. Lewy in 1912 in the dorsal motor nucleus of the vagus and substantia innominata (Lewy, 1912), and Lewy bodies in the substantia nigra were postulated to be specific for Parkinson's disease by Tretiakoff in 1919 (Tretiakoff, 1919). Cortical Lewy bodies were initially described in association with postencephalitic parkinsonism (Lipkin, 1959), in elderly with incidental nigral Lewy bodies (Forno, 1969), in severe dementia (Okazaki et al., 1961), and in institutionalized psychiatric patients (Woodward, 1962). From a clinicopathologic study of 20 cases in 1980, K. Kosaka proposed that the neuroanatomical spectrum of Lewy bodies ranged from isolated substantia nigra inclusions to widespread cortical inclusions; he coined the term 'diffuse Lewy body disease' to describe a clinical syndrome of parkinsonism, dementia, and/or psychosis associated pathologically with Lewy bodies in cortical and limbic regions in addition to subcortical nuclei (Kosaka et al., 1980). In more recent nomenclature, the clinicopathological syndrome has been termed 'Dementia with Lewy bodies' (DLB).

Epidemiology

DLB has been recognized as the second most common form of degenerative dementia, after Alzheimer's disease, occurring in 15–36% of pathological series of dementia (Hansen et al., 1990; Holmes et al., 1999; Perry et al., 1990), with an estimated prevalence of 10–25% in hospital and community elderly with dementia (Ballard et al., 1995; Shergill et al., 1994). Furthermore, cortical Lewy bodies are found in more than 25% of AD cases (Bergeron & Pollanen, 1989; Ditter & Mirra, 1987; Forno & Langston, 1993). In a review of autopsy-confirmed cases of DLB and AD, the frequency of males was greater in DLB (M:F 1.7 in DLB vs. 0.53 in AD), the average age of onset was similar (70 years old in DLB, 71 years old in AD), with a trend toward more rapidly progressive illness in DLB (duration 6.25 of years in DLB vs. 7.3 of years in AD) (McKeith & O'Brien, 1999).

Clinical features

The clinical features of DLB have been incorporated into consensus criteria for the clinical diagnosis of DLB (Table 18.1) (McKeith et al., 1996). The criteria list dementia in association with fluctuating mental status, visual hallucinations, and parkinsonism as required or core features of DLB; supportive features are repeated falls, syncope, transient loss of consciousness, sensitivity to extrapyramidal side effects of neuroleptics, delusions and other hallucinations. Additional proposed supportive features include depression and REM sleep behavioural disorder (McKeith et al., 1999). Several studies have addressed the accuracy of the clinical criteria for DLB. The specificity (proportion of non-DLB cases correctly identified) of the clinical criteria for probable DLB compared to neuropathological diagnosis ranges from 0.84–1.00 in prospective and retrospective studies (Holmes et al., 1999; Litvan et al., 1998; Luis et al., 1999; McKeith et al., 2000a; Mega et al., 1996; Verghese et al., 1999). The sensitivity of the clinical criteria for probable DLB has been more variable, as high as 0.83–0.89 in prospective studies (McKeith et al., 2000a; McShane et al., 1998), and ranging from 0.40–0.65 in retrospective studies (Litvan et al., 1998; Luis et al., 1999; Mega et al., 1996; Verghese et al., 1999).

Dementia (slowly progressive global cognitive impairment) is a mandatory feature of DLB, and is the presenting

Table 18.1. Clinical and pathological features in dementia with Lewy bodies

Clinical features	Pathological features
1. Central feature: Progressive dementia	1. Essential for diagnosis: Lewy bodies
2. Probable (2/3)[a] or possible (1/3) if:	2. Associated but not essential
– fluctuating cognition and alertness	Lewy-related neurites
– recurrent visual hallucinations	Amyloid plaques (all types)
– spontaneous parkinsonism	Neurofibrillary tangles
3. Supportive features: repeated falls, syncopes,	Neuronal loss / synapse loss
neuroleptic hypersensitivity, delusions,	Spongiform change (temporal)
hallucinations in other modalities, REM – sleep,	Neurotransmitter abnormalities
behaviour disorder, depression	

Notes:

[a] Two of the three features are required for a diagnosis of probable DLB, one for possible DLB.

Source: From McKeith et al. (1996).

feature in about 82% (range 40–100%) (McKeith & O'Brien, 1999). Psychometric features of the cognitive dysfunction in DLB such as amnesia, dyscalculia, and aphasia, overlap those of AD, not surprising given the frequently coexisting pathology. However, several studies suggest that, compared to AD patients of comparable global severity of dementia, patients with DLB perform less poorly on tests of verbal memory, and worse in tests of attention, visuospatial and visuoconstructive function, and fluency (Galasko et al., 1996; Gnanalingham et al., 1997; Hansen et al., 1990; Mori et al., 2000; Shimomura et al., 1998; Walker et al., 1997). Early in the illness, memory deficits may be minimal, or consist of selective deficits of memory retrieval, with recall significantly improved by prompting. This may be distinct from the deficits in memory acquisition and consolidation characteristic of AD (Ballard et al., 1999a; Walker et al., 1997). Frontal lobe dysfunction and visuospatial impairment may be more prominent early on in DLB. Language dysfunction of dysnomia progressing to dysphasia tends to parallel the clinical course of AD, although speech block has been described early in the illness. The rate of cognitive decline is faster in DLB compared to AD (Ballard et al., 1996; Olichney et al., 1998), and DLB has been associated with shorter survival, 7.7 ± 3.0 years after onset of cognitive symptoms versus 9.3 ± 3.5 years in AD (Olichney et al., 1998), although in a prospective study, no differences were found between age of onset, age of death, or survival between AD and DLB (Walker et al., 2000a, b).

A particular feature of the mental status in DLB is fluctuations, including periods of confusion, inattention, somnolence, or worsening cognitive impairment alternating with more lucid periods. These periods of variation may last from minutes to days (McKeith et al., 1996), and are unrelated to exogenous factors such as anxiety or unfamiliar surroundings; they are distinct from 'sundowning' episodes of evening confusion common in Alzheimer's disease. The prevalence of fluctuation in cognition in autopsy-proven DLB has ranged from 40–86% (Hohl et al., 2000; McKeith et al., 1992b; Verghese et al., 1999), and can be noted early in the course of the illness (McKeith & O'Brien, 1999). Episodes of syncope or transient loss of consciousness may be more extreme forms of the fluctuations. In the elderly, these symptoms must be differentiated from delirium from infection or toxic–metabolic encephalopathy, transient ischemic attacks, focal seizures, orthostasis, and cardiac disease.

Spontaneous, complex visual hallucinations occur in 40–75% of DLB patients, typically early in the illness and unrelated to medications (Galasko et al., 1996; Klatka et al., 1996; McKeith & O'Brien, 1999; Mega et al., 1996; Weiner et al., 1996). Delusional misidentification is also common early in DLB (Ballard et al., 1999b). Auditory hallucinations are less common, noted in an average of 19% of patients at presentation or during the entire course of illness (McKeith & O'Brien, 1999).

Parkinsonism is common as an early or initial feature of DLB, occurring at presentation in 43% (range 10–78%), and during the entire course in 77% (range 50–100%) (McKeith & O'Brien, 1999). The parkinsonism is usually symmetric, consisting of parkinsonian gait with reduced arm swing and *en bloc* turning, bradykinesia, rigidity, and hypomimia. Parkinsonian resting tremor is less common. Parkinsonism may contribute to falls, which occur in 28% of DLB patients at presentation, and 37% of DLB patients during the entire course of illness (McKeith & O'Brien, 1999). Patients with DLB also are sensitive to the extrapyramidal side effects of neuroleptic medications, including severe rigidity and obtundation at low doses of neuroleptics that persist after drug withdrawal. Neuroleptic sensitivity is noted in an average of 61% of DLB patients relative to 15% of AD patients (McKeith & O'Brien, 1999).

Depressive features are nearly twice as common in DLB relative to AD, noted in an average of 29% of DLB patients at presentation, and 38% during the course of illness (McKeith & O'Brien, 1999).

Atypical Lewy body syndromes include primary autonomic failure, associated with Lewy bodies in the sympathetic neurons of the spinal cord, and Lewy body dysphagia, associated with Lewy bodies in the dorsal vagal nuclei.

The differential diagnosis of DLB involves other parkinsonian and/or dementia syndromes in addition to Parkinson's disease and Alzheimer's disease, such as multiple system atrophy, progressive supranuclear palsy, cortical basal degeneration, Pick's disease and frontal lobe dementias, Creutzfeld–Jakob disease, normal pressure hydrocephalus, multi-infarct dementia and Binswanger's disease, and Hallervorden–Spatz disease.

Imaging and laboratory investigations

There has been considerable interest in the use of CT and MRI imaging studies to differentiate the dementias. A CT measure of minimum temporal lobe width was significantly reduced in dementia (10.4–10.9 mm) relative to depression (13.7 mm), but could not distinguish DLB from AD or vascular dementia (VD) (O'Brien et al., 2000). MRI imaging in DLB is non-specific. While both AD and DLB brain show generalized atrophy relative to non-demented brains (Hashimoto et al., 1998), medial temporal atrophy tends to be intermediate between non-demented cases and AD (Barber et al., 1999b; Harvey et al., 1999; Hashimoto et al., 1998). White matter hyperintensities on MRI, which occur with increased aging, are more extensive in dementia than controls, although they do not differentiate AD from DLB (Barber et al., 1999a).

Metabolic studies of DLB using SPECT and PET suggest a more global pattern of hypermetabolism compared to the typical temporal–parietal hypometabolism of AD. This may be reflected in reduced frontal (Defebvre et al., 1999) or occipital perfusion (Donnemiller et al., 1997; Ishii et al., 1999) by SPECT in DLB relative to AD, and reduced occipital glucose metabolism by PET in DLB relative to AD (Higuchi et al., 2000; Ishii et al., 1998). Dopamine transporter function as assessed by CIT SPECT may also be more impaired in DLB than AD (Donnemiller et al., 1997). PET measures of occipital glucose utilization in particular

could differentiate DLB from AD with relatively high sensitivity (86–92%) and specificity (91–92%) in a small clinical studies (Higuchi et al., 2000; Ishii et al., 1998). Nonetheless, conventional SPECT scan is limited in its diagnostic utility in distinguishing AD from DLB given the heterogeneity of perfusion patterns, semiquantitive nature, and low sensitivity and specificity (Pasquier et al., 1997; Talbot et al., 1998).

Electrophysiologic studies with EEG in DLB show slowing with loss of alpha activity as the dominant rhythm and temporal slow wave transients. EEG slowing is common in DLB, characterized by loss of alpha activity as the dominant rhythm, and may be correlated to MMSE (Barber et al., 2000; Briel et al., 1999). Temporal lobe slow wave transients have also been described, correlated to reported episodes of loss of consciousness in DLB (Briel et al., 1999). Fluctuating cognition may correlate with fluctuation in mean EEG frequency over 1.5 minutes by EEG brain mapping (Walker et al., 2000a, b). While slowing of alpha rhythm and temporal slow wave transients are common in DLB, they are not specific, and may be seen in AD (Briel et al., 1999).

The usefulness of CSF biochemical markers in DLB is unclear, as most studies have looked at small clinical samples. Some studies show elevated CSF tau in DLB similar to AD (Arai et al., 1997; Higuchi et al., 2000), while others demonstrate normal CSF tau and low Aß42 (Kanemaru et al., 2000).

Genetics

Genetic factors in the etiology of DLB are suggested by pedigrees of familial DLB (Hardy et al., 1998; Ohara et al., 1999) or PD in which members have developed dementia. Furthermore, some studies find an increased risk of dementia in first-degree relatives of PD patients (Van Duijn et al., 1991), and of PD in first-degree relatives of AD patients (Amaducci et al., 1986; Hofman et al., 1989), although other studies have disputed these findings (Mickel et al., 1997). Genetic studies in DLB have assessed genetic risk factors and causative genes that are important in PD and AD.

AD related polymorphisms that have been evaluated in DLB include apolipoprotein E (*APOE*), butyrylcholinesterase, α1-antichymotrypsin (*AACT*), presenilin-1 (*PS1*), and α2-macroglobulin (*A2M*). The *APOE* ϵ4 allele is a risk factor for late-onset sporadic and familial AD (Rebeck et al., 1993; Saunders et al., 1993). The *APOE* ϵ4 allele is over-represented in DLB cases to a lesser degree than in AD (Benjamin et al., 1994a; Lamb et al., 1998; Morris et al.,

1996). Under-representation of the *APOE* ϵ2 allele, which may be protective for AD (Benjamin et al., 1994b; Corder et al., 1994; West et al., 1994), has not been found in DLB (Lamb et al., 1998; Morris et al., 1996).

The butyrylcholinesterase K allele is not over-represented in DLB; however, an increased number of homozygotes for the K allele was found in a small number of DLB cases (Singleton et al., 1998). No association with DLB was found with the *PS1* allele 1 intronic polymorphism (Singleton et al., 1997), the *AACT* A allele (Lamb et al., 1998), the *A2M* Val1000Ile polymorphism, or the *A2M* pentanucleotide deletion, although a trend toward increased homozygotes for the pentanucleotide deletion polymorphism was noted in DLB and AD (Singleton et al., 1999).

PD related genes evaluated in DLB include α-synuclein and the cytochrome P450 CYP2D6 (*CYP2D6*). α-Synuclein mutations have been identified in five pedigrees of autosomal dominant familial Parkinson's disease, but have not been found in sporadic PD or DLB (Higuchi et al., 1998). While allele 4 of the *CYP2D6* gene has been associated with PD, it is not associated with AD or DLB (Atkinson et al., 1999). Finally, a pentanucleotide repeat polymorphism in the promoter region of nitrogen oxide synthase 2A gene (*NOS2A*) has been linked to DLB but not AD in a single report (Xu et al., 2000).

Clinical management

Management of DLB targets motor, cognitive and behavioural symptoms. General principles of dementia management should be employed, including regular assessment of functional capabilities, family education, social service support, environmental modification, optimization of medications, and aggressive recognition and treatment of delirium. In addition, specific medication therapy may be required for treatment of motor, cognitive and behavioral symptoms. Trials of L-dopa or dopaminergic agonists may ameliorate motor symptoms of parkinsonism; however, patients with DLB are less likely to respond than PD patients, and are more sensitive to side effects of hallucinations, delusions, and agitation.

Similar to patients with AD, cholinergic agents can improve memory and behaviour in DLB. A double-blind, placebo- controlled study of the cholinesterase inhibitor rivastigmine (Exelon) 3–12 mg/d in DLB demonstrated greater improvement relative to placebo in the Neuropsychiatric Inventory (McKeith et al., 2000b).

Behavioural symptoms may require drug therapy if they are unresponsive to environmental modification and are disturbing to the patient and caregiver. Agitation may

Table 18.2

Pathological features in DLB

1. Essential for diagnosis: Lewy bodies in cortical areas
2. Associated but not essential:
Lewy-related neurites
Amyloid plaques (all types)
Neurofibrillary tangles
Neuronal loss/synapse loss
Spongiform change (temporal)
Neurotransmitter abnormalities

respond to non-neuroleptic medications such as anxiolytics (benzodiazepines, buspar), antidepressants (trazadone) or anticonvulsants (gabapentin, valproate). Hallucinations and delusions may require carefully monitored treatment with atypical neuroleptics. High potency neuroleptics such as haloperidol should be avoided, as patients with DLB are particularly susceptible to severe extrapyramidal side effects (McKeith et al., 1992a). Low doses of atypical neuroleptics such as risperidone, olanzepine, seroquel, and clozaril are preferable; however, even these may potentiate extrapyramidal symptoms in DLB.

Pathological features in DLB

The hallmark and the essential pathological requirement for the diagnosis of DLB is the presence of Lewy bodies. Other pathological features are frequently associated with the Lewy bodies (Table 18.2).

Lewy bodies

Lewy bodies (LB) are eosinophilic intracytoplasmic inclusions with hematoxilin and eosin stain, that can be recognized with more sensitivity with ubiquitin immunostaining (Kuzuhara et al., 1988; Lennox et al., 1989b) and with great specificity with α-synuclein antibodies (Irizarry et al., 1998; Spillantini et al., 1997). The presence of this presynaptic protein seems to be so specific for the LB that α-synuclein intraneuronal immunoreactivity is considered now parallel to Lewy-related pathology. However, more than 20 different antigens have been detected in the LB (Gómez-Tortosa et al., 1998; Pollanen et al., 1993). The appearance of the LB varies slightly depending on their location in brainstem or in cortical regions (Fig. 18.1). Classic LB, as seen in brainstem, are compact,

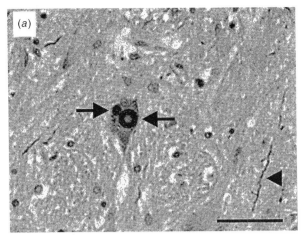

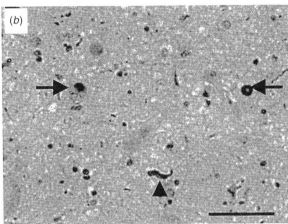

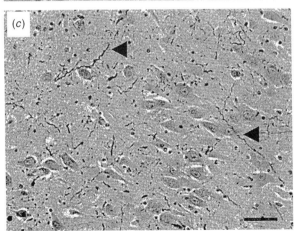

Fig. 18.1. Lewy bodies (arrows) and Lewy neurites (arrowheads) in substantia nigra (*a*), entorhinal cortex (*b*), and hippocampal CA2/3 subfields (*c*) in DLB by α-synuclein immunostaining (hematoxylin and eosin counterstain.) Scale bars = 50 μm.

with a well defined halo. When double immunostained for α-synuclein and ubiquitin, the first shows a tendency to be distributed in an outer rim, while ubiquitin is present more towards the core. In substantia nigra, α-synuclein immunoreactivity also shows a wide spectrum of intracytoplasmic inclusions with variable ubiquitin costaining that may represent progressive stages of aggregation and LB formation (Gómez-Tortosa et al., 2000). Cortical LB are less well defined, lack the halo (Lowe, 1994), and the pattern of double immunostaining is more homogenous.

The distribution of the LB in cases with DLB shows a very consistent hierarchical vulnerability to LB formation across brain regions. Substantia nigra and other brainstem nuclei are affected with the highest density of LB, followed by paralimbic regions (basal forebrain nuclei, entorhinal, cingulate and insular cortices) and neocortical regions having the lowest density (Gómez-Tortosa et al., 1999; Rezaie et al., 1996) (Fig. 18.2, see colour plate section). Depending on the more or less widespread distribution of the LB, the spectrum of Lewy body disorders is classified into three types (McKeith et al., 1996). LB restricted to brainstem and basal forebrain nuclei define the brainstem type which is basically the pathology of idiopathic PD. In the transitional type, LB are found in limbic and paralimbic regions, but not in neocortex. When LB are also present in neocortex, it is the neocortical type. The density of LB in substantia nigra does not necessarily correlate with the density of LB in paralimbic and neocortical areas (Gómez-Tortosa et al., 1999) which suggests that DLB does not simply reflect severe or long-lasting PD. In cortical regions, LB frequently occur in the deep cortical layers V and VI as if only certain subpopulations of neurons are vulnerable to develop the inclusions.

Lewy neurites

Lewy neurites in the CA2–3 regions of the hippocampus are a pathological feature frequently associated with the presence of LB (Dickson et al., 1991). They show the same immunohistochemical profile as the LB, in terms of containing α-synuclein, ubiquitin and neurofilaments (Dickson et al., 1994; Irizarry et al., 1998). Lewy neurites are found in about two-thirds to three-quarters of the cases with Lewy bodies and their presence is very specific for Lewy body diseases, because they do not appear in other neurodegenerative diseases with nigral degeneration but without LB (Kim et al., 1995). Thus, CA2–3 neuritic degeneration seems a manifestation of the same process that leads to LB formation. Double immunostaining against α-synuclein and either SMI-32 (non-phosphorylated neurofilament present in dendrites) or SMI-312 (axonal phosphorylated neurofilament) suggests that Lewy neurites are mostly axonal fibres. Because the cell bodies in the hippocampus generally lack α-synuclein inclusions, these neurites are likely to derive from axonal afferents to CA2–3. The absence of tyrosine hydroxylase immunoreactivity suggests that CA2–3 neuritic processes do not derive from brainstem dopaminergic afferents to the hippocampus (Dickson et al., 1994). Thus, the origin of these neurites may be entorhinal cortex or septal nuclei, regions projecting to the CA2–3 fields of the hippocampus and usually affected by α-synuclein inclusions. Recent studies show that hippocampal pathology in PD and DLB is more extensive than recognized with α-synuclein immunostaining, as revealed by abnormal neurites immunostained with antibodies against β- and γ-synucleins in the dentate gyrus and mossy fibres that synapse on hilar neurons (Galvin et al., 1999).

In DLB, scattered neurites are also found in other regions, especially in the nigra, basal forebrain nuclei, amygdala, entorhinal and cingulate cortices (Braak et al., 1999; Gómez-Tortosa et al., 2000; Pellise et al., 1996).

Alzheimer changes

Concomitant Alzheimer changes, that is amyloid plaques and neurofibrillary tangles (NFT), are very common in DLB, but the frequency of this association varies depending on the criteria used to define neuropathological AD. About 30% of cases fulfilling neuropathological criteria for definitive or probable AD have some cortical LB and constitute what is called the Lewy body variant of AD. Thirty-two to 89% (depending on the criteria used) of the DLB cases have concomitant Alzheimer-type changes (Hansen, 1996). In general, the Alzheimer changes found in DLB are characterized by the predominance of senile plaques, mostly of diffuse type rather than neuritic, with more $A\beta$42 than $A\beta$40, and fewer NFT, especially in the neocortex (Hansen, 1996; Hansen et al., 1993; Heyman et al., 1999; Mann et al., 1998; Samuel et al., 1997b). A simplified but useful schema would be to consider AD with LB or the Lewy body variant of AD those cases having enough neocortical tangles to meet a Braak stage V or VI, while cases with only entorhinal and paralimbic tangles (Braak I to IV) would be considered as DLB (Gearing et al., 1999; Hansen, 1996).

In DLB, Alzheimer and LB pathology seem to be independent of each other, both in terms of distribution and quantity. The distribution of LBs does not coincide with that of neurofibrillary tangles, which are most abundant in the hippocampus and layers III and V of association cortex.

There is no correlation between LB density and the degree of neurofibrillary tangle involvement or the amount of cortical senile plaques, which suggests an independence in the formation or in the dynamic turnover of these pathological structures (Gómez-Isla et al., 1999).

Neuronal loss

Neuronal loss in DLB is significant in brainstem and nucleus basalis of Meynert associated with Lewy-pathology (Lippa et al., 1999), but it seems that cortical neuronal loss is just modest, which is consistent with the lack of gross atrophy of DLB brains (Hashimoto et al., 1998; Lippa et al., 1998). Several studies have examined neuronal loss in different cortical regions. In the temporal cortex, DLB brains showed a 10 to 20% (non-significant) neuronal loss in comparison with controls, while DLB cases with concomitant AD changes had pronounced neuronal loss (around 40 to 50%), comparable to that of pure AD cases (Gómez-Isla et al., 1999; Lippa et al., 1994; Wakabayashi et al., 1995). The study of specific neuronal subpopulations characterized by the expression of neurofilaments (pyramidal neurons) and several calcium binding proteins (gabaergic interneurons) in the superior temporal sulcus cortex, also shows no differences in neuronal densities between DLB cases and controls (Gómez-Tortosa et al., 2001).

In entorhinal cortex, neuronal loss has been examined in specific layers and it is not significant in comparison with controls unless Alzheimer changes are present. Lippa et al. (1997) did not find neuronal loss in layer II, origin of the perforant pathway and a group of neurons affected very early by neuronal loss in AD (Gómez-Isla et al., 1996b). Nor is there neuronal loss in pure DLB cases in layers V/VI, where the LB are mainly found, compared to controls. The number of LB does not correlate with neuronal loss, suggesting that they are not directly implicated in widespread neuronal death in pure DLB. Other studies have not found neuronal or synapse loss in frontal cortex (Hansen et al., 1998; Lippa et al., 1994; Samuel et al., 1997a) or hippocampus (Ince et al., 1991; Lippa et al., 1994) of DLB compared with control brains. Thus, in contrast with AD, widespread cortical neuronal loss is not a major feature in the pathology of DLB. However, there is still the possibility of a selective or restricted neuronal loss, not yet recognized.

Other neuropathological features in DLB

Circumscribed spongiform change occurs in some DLB cases in layers II–III of the perirhinal cortex and in the accessory basal amygdaloid nucleus (Iseki et al., 1997). This pathological feature is usually associated with a more aggressive disease with rapid onset of symptoms and a rapid course with a total duration of illness of less than three years (Hansen et al., 1989).

Finally, because of the involvement of basal forebrain and brainstem nuclei there are widespread neurotransmitter deficits in cortical regions. Monoamines and, especially, acetylcholine are severely depleted in the cortex of DLB brains in comparison with controls and AD (Langlais et al., 1993; Samuel et al., 1997a; Tiraboshi et al., 2000). Marked losses in midfrontal choline acetyltransferase (ChAT) activity occurs in DLB independently of coexistent AD changes (Tiraboshi et al., 2000). Reduced cortical ChAT correlates with neuronal loss and LB densities in the nucleus basalis of Meynert (Lippa et al., 1999).

Clinico-pathological correlations

It is not clear yet to what extent each of the above neuropathological features contributes to the clinical phenotype in DLB. It is also not known whether cortical LB are directly responsible for neuronal injury and, therefore, for the clinical syndrome; or whether the α-synuclein deposits within the Lewy neurites interfere with normal neurotransmission. Pathological changes coexisting with the Lewy pathology, such as Alzheimer-type changes, may also contribute to the clinical phenotype.

Lewy-related pathology

The contribution of the LB to the clinical phenotype has been studied with different approaches. The first has been to examine whether PD cases with dementia consistently have cortical LB that may account for the cognitive decline. What seems clear from clinicopathologic studies of PD patients is that there is not a clear threshold for cortical LB density that distinguishes between demented and nondemented PD. Among the 30 to 40% of idiopathic PD patients who develop dementia not all have cortical LB. In one study, cortical LB were considered to be the likely cause of dementia in only 10% of the demented cases (Hughes et al., 1993). AD changes seem to be the major determinant of the cognitive decline in PD patients (de Vos et al., 1995; Hughes et al., 1993).

The second is to correlate LB densities with the severity of the disease as assessed by a cognitive or functional score close to the time of death. The results with this approach are not uniform. Some studies have found a significant correlation between dementia severity and cortical LB counts (Lennox et al., 1989a; Mattila et al., 1998; Samuel et al., 1997a; Samuel et al., 1996), while others have failed to find any correlation (Churchyard & Lees, 1997; Gómez-Isla et al., 1999; Perry et al., 1990, 1996). There are several differences among these studies in terms of the clinical data used to represent severity of the disease, the degree of concomitant AD in the DLB cases, and the methodology used to quantitate LB, that may account for the different results. In several studies finding a significant correlation between cortical LB and severity of the disease, the significance seems to rely mainly upon the most severely demented cases having the highest LB densities (Lennox et al., 1989a; Mattila et al., 1998). Thus, there is the possibility that LB may be just a marker or be in parallel with a more widespread pathology underlying the disease and not necessarily be the cause of the cognitive decline.

The third approach is to correlate the density of LB in certain brain regions with specific clinical phenotypes. A plausible hypothesis would be that the presence in DLB cases of motor symptoms (such as parkinsonism or recurrent falls) would be associated with higher LB densities in substantia nigra and that the presence of psychiatric symptoms, such as delusions or hallucinations, would be related with a higher density of LB in paralimbic or neocortical regions, in comparison with cases who did not present these symptoms. However, no significant differences have been found in LB densities in substantia nigra, paralimbic regions and neocortex comparing patients with or without specific symptoms (Gómez-Tortosa et al., 1999). It is surprising that DLB patients with or without clinical parkinsonism had similar LB densities in nigra. There was a slight tendency for cases with hallucinations and delusions to have a higher density of LB in paralimbic regions versus those without these symptoms, but the differences were not statistically significant. One group has found an association between the presence of cortical Lewy body pathology and persistent hallucinations (McShane et al., 1995, 1996) but other studies have failed to demonstrate any correlation (Perry et al., 1990). Therefore, the distribution and number of cortical LB do not seem to be clearly associated with the clinical symptoms. In most clinico-pathological studies the density of cortical LB also does not correlate with the duration of the disease (Gómez-Isla et al., 1999; Gómez-Tortosa et al., 1999; Mattila et al., 1998).

The contribution of the Lewy neurites to the cognitive impairment is not understood yet, but they may well play a prominent role. Churchyard & Lees (1997) found a positive correlation between the density of hippocampal CA2–3 neurites and cognitive impairment (MMSE) in Parkinson's disease patients, even when in this same study there was no correlation with the density of LB. The CA2–3 regions of the hippocampus receive major inputs from the dentate gyrus, entorhinal cortex, septal nuclei, amygdala and hypothalamus, and then project to the CA1 field, which in turn projects to the subiculum. These connections are crucial for memory and cognition, suggesting that the neuritic inclusions may disrupt hippocampal function by interfering with inputs to the CA1 field and contribute to the cognitive deficits in DLB. Furthermore, more extensive hippocampal neuritic abnormalities can be revealed with β- and γ-synuclein immunostaining in the dentate gyrus and mossy fibres that synapse on hilar neurons (Galvin et al., 1999). These abnormal processes are likely to impair synaptic transmission in the perforant pathway, which is a critical network for memory and cognition, known to be severely affected in AD. Therefore, the same hippocampal circuitry may be involved in Alzheimer and DLB diseases. As widespread α-synuclein-positive neuritic processes are revealed in DLB brains, there is a growing impression that abnormal neurites, not only in hippocampus but also in other cortical regions, may impair neuronal connectivity and play a significant role in the progression of the cognitive deficits in DLB.

Neuronal loss/Alzheimer changes

Alzheimer-type pathology likely has an additive or synergistic effect in producing the clinical phenotype of DLB, but cannot be the sole cause. First, there is a well documented number of DLB cases that represent pure LB pathology (Armstrong et al., 1997; Perry et al., 1996). Secondly, Alzheimer changes do not correlate with the severity of cognitive impairment in DLB (Gómez-Isla et al., 1999; Samuel et al., 1996). This is not surprising considering that there are few neurofibrillary tangles, which are most strongly correlated with neuronal loss and cognitive impairment in AD (Gómez-Isla et al., 1996a, 1997), and that amyloid plaques are mostly of the diffuse type, which are not associated with cognitive impairment and are present in cognitively preserved elderly (Crystal et al., 1993; Dickson et al., 1992). Furthermore, DLB cases are equally demented as AD cases with many fewer neurofibrillary tangles and senile plaques, which suggests that other pathological features besides the Alzheimer changes are contributing to the clinical phenotype. On the other hand, DLB cases are less demented than cases with the Lewy body variant of AD for equal LB densities and ChAT loss, which suggests that when present, AD changes have an additive effect in the clinical phenotype (Samuel et al., 1997a).

Neurochemical deficits

There is severe ACh depletion in DLB cases all through cortical regions (temporal, parietal, midfrontal, septal). This ACh depletion correlates with dementia severity, and its role in the cognitive phenotype is supported by the good response some DLB cases have to treatment with cholinesterase inhibitors. The most robust neurobiological correlate of the dementia so far identified appears to be extensive cholinergic deficits in the neocortex (Perry et al., 1997).

Finally, impairment of the mesocortical and mesoneocortical dopaminergic projections may be also implicated in cognitive dysfunction. The lesion of these connections in animals produces behavioural changes and it has been suggested that in humans such lesions may be responsible for the cognitive manifestations in PD, and for some neuropsychiatric disorders such as schizophrenia or Tourette's syndrome.

Underlying biochemical abnormalities reflected in Lewy bodies: the role of alpha-synuclein

An abundant component of Lewy bodies in dementia with Lewy bodies and related disorders is the presynaptic protein, α-synuclein (Irizarry et al., 1998; Spillantini et al., 1997). α-Synuclein is a highly conserved 140 amino acid phosphoprotein of unknown function that was originally isolated from *Torpedo californica* (Maroteaux et al., 1988). The name synuclein was coined on the basis of both synaptic and nuclear localization in *Torpedo*, however, nuclear localization has not been consistently observed in subsequent studies (George et al., 1995; Iwai et al., 1995; Jakes et al., 1994; Maroteaux et al., 1988). Although the normal function of α-synuclein is unknown, studies of song-learning in the zebra-finch have implicated a role for the protein in neuronal plasticity. In juvenile birds just learning their song, α-synuclein is especially abundant in the glutamatergic presynaptic terminals of the key regulatory projection essential for song memorization (George et al., 1995).

The structure of α-synuclein may provide clues to its possible function. The amino-terminal region contains 7 degenerate 11 amino acid imperfect repeat sequences predicted to form 5 amphipathic alpha helices. α-Synuclein is predicted to have a random coil conformation in solution (Weinreb et al., 1996), however, when studied in the presence of synthetic membranes, lipid binding is accompanied by an increase in alpha helicity (Davidson et al., 1998), suggesting that, in an isolated system, α-synuclein may be membrane associated.

Studies into the genetic basis of familial Parkinson's disease have led to the identification of two missense mutations in the gene encoding α-synuclein (Ala53Thr and Ala30Pro) in some families with early onset familial Parkinson's disease (Krüger et al., 1998; Polymeropoulos et al., 1997). It is unclear how the mutations effect the normal function of α-synuclein but it has been hypothesized that the normal localization of the protein is disrupted, causing α-synuclein to accumulate in the cell bodies of degenerating neurons as a component of Lewy bodies.

Research aimed at understanding the role of α-synuclein in normal and parkinsonian cell function have led to the identification of several potential interacting species. α-Synuclein was found to bind synthetic vesicles containing acidic phospholipids in vitro (Davidson et al., 1998), and investigators have reported interactions of α-synuclein with the structural protein tubulin (Alim et al., 2002), tau (Jensen et al., 1999), microtubule-associated protein 1B (MAP-1B) (Jensen et al., 2000), and with a previously unknown protein called 'synphilin-1' (Engelender et al., 1999). Subsequently, MAP-1B (Jensen et al., 2000) and synphilin-1 (Wakabayashi et al., 2000) have been identified as components of Lewy bodies suggesting that interactions of α-synuclein with these proteins may be a critical component of Lewy body formation.

Studies into the effects of the Parkinson's disease associated mutations have revealed that the Ala30Pro mutation abolishes the binding of α-synuclein to brain vesicles in vitro (Jensen et al., 1998) suggesting that this may lead to the accumulation of the protein and, as a result, its assembly into Lewy bodies. By contrast, neither the Ala30Pro nor Ala53Thr mutation was found to have an effect on the association of α-synuclein with cellular membranes (McLean et al., 2000). Further examination of the normal function of α-synuclein and the effect of the mutations on subcellular localization will provide insight into the mechanisms that lead to the accumulation of the protein in certain neurodegenerative disorders.

α-Synuclein protein has a demonstrated propensity to aggregate in vitro (Conway et al., 1998; Giasson et al., 1999) with the Ala53Thr mutant seemingly forming fibrils faster than both wild-type and Ala30Pro α-synuclein (Conway et al., 1998). Subsequent studies have suggested that both Parkinson's disease associated mutations (Ala53Thr and Ala30Pro) accelerate the rate of α-synuclein aggregation (Nahri et al., 1999). More recently, it has been suggested that a nonfibrillar oligomer species precedes the formation of fibrils of α-synuclein and that acceleration of oligomerization, rather than acceleration of fibrillization, is a shared property of both mutant proteins (Conway et al., 2000a). Interestingly, the fibrils generated in vitro from both wild-type and mutant α-synuclein have been found to possess features that are characteristic of amyloid fibrils (Conway et al., 2000b; Serpell et al., 2000).

A common mechanism whereby manipulations of the C-terminus lead to aggregation and inclusion body formation is suggested by recent studies where C-terminally truncated forms of α-synuclein more readily formed fibrils in vitro (Crowther et al., 1998). Furthermore, although Lewy bodies contain predominantly full-length α-synuclein, Baba et al. (1998) reported the presence of truncated α-synuclein in purified Lewy bodies which suggests that a truncation event occurs. In addition, α-synuclein aggregation in vitro was recently demonstrated to be a nucleation-dependent event (Wood et al., 1999) which raises the possibility that a C-terminally modified form of the protein acts as a seed for fibril formation. SH-SY5Y cells overexpressing C-terminally truncated α-synuclein, particularly the 1–120 residue protein, have been shown to be more susceptible to oxidative stress following exposure to hydrogen peroxide or to the dopaminergic neurotoxin MPP+ (Kanda et al., 2000).

Chemical manipulations have also been determined to promote α-synuclein aggregation in vitro. Coincubation of recombinant α-synuclein with cytochrome c/hydrogen peroxide or hemin/hydrogen peroxide induced α-synuclein aggregation that could be blocked by anti-oxidant agents such as N-acetyl-L-cysteine (Hashimoto et al., 1999a). Likewise, human α-synuclein was found to aggregate in the presence of ferric ion and this was inhibited by the iron chelator, deferoxamine (Hashimoto et al., 1999b). Consistent with the in vitro study by Hashimoto et al. (1999b), Osterova-Golts and colleagues demonstrated aggregation of α-synuclein in neuroblastoma cells in culture following exposure to iron or iron plus either hydrogen peroxide or dopamine, which generate free radicals (Osterova-Golts et al., 2000). Moreover, they observed that the Ala53Thr α-synuclein mutation had an increased tendency to aggregate, consistent with observations in vitro (Conway et al., 1998, 2000a; Giasson et al., 1999).

It is unclear at this time if the aggregation of α-synuclein into Lewy bodies is neurotoxic, which would suggest that Lewy bodies are analogous to amyloid plaques in Alzheimer's disease, which have been proposed to be toxic. Alternatively, Lewy bodies could be a result of neuronal damage, but are in themselves, not toxic. Finally, it has been proposed that Lewy bodies may be an inert end point in a process that, early on, produces a neurotoxic species, and that Lewy body formation may actually protect against cell death by sequestering the toxic species (Conway et al., 2000a).

It has yet to be determined what role, if any, α-synuclein plays in neurotoxicity however, several studies have examined the effect of α-synuclein overexpression on cell death. Overexpression of human mutant α-synuclein (Ala53Thr) selectively induced apoptotic programmed cell death of primary dopamine neurons as well as mesencephalon-derived N27 cells (Zhou et al., 2000), with the mutant protein also potentiating the neurotoxicity of 6-hydroxy-dopamine (6–OHDA). Likewise, human dopaminergic neuroblastoma SH-SY5Y cells overexpressing Ala 53 Thr α-synuclein were significantly more vulnerable to oxidative stress following exposure to hydrogen peroxide or to the dopaminergic neurotoxin MPP$^+$ (Kanda et al., 2000). Similarly, aggregates of NAC and α-synuclein proteins induced apoptotic cell death in SH-SY5Y cells (El-Agnaf et al., 1998) and preaggregated NAC was toxic to rat primary mesencephalic neurons and to a PC12 cell line differentiated with nerve growth factor (Forloni et al., 2000).

Transgenic models

Animal models aimed at addressing the fundamental aspects of α-synucleinopathy have yielded some clues as to the normal function of α-synuclein and the effect of overexpression of the Parkinson's disease associated mutations. Mice lacking α-synuclein (α-syn$^{-/-}$) do not display any gross pathological abnormalities and possess a normal complement of dopaminergic cell bodies, fibres and synapses (Abeliovich et al., 2000). However, the α-syn$^{-/-}$ mice exhibit altered stimulus-dependent dopamine release, which suggest that α-synuclein is an activity-dependent negative regulator of dopamine neurotransmission. Neuronal expression of human α-synuclein and the Ala30Pro mutant in mice results in a progressive, abnormal accumulation of α-synuclein in neuronal cell bodies and neurites in several regions of the brain (Kahle et al., 2000; Masliah et al., 2000). Behavioural deficits are observed only in mice expressing the highest levels of wild-type α-synuclein (Masliah et al., 2000) and correspond to increased amounts of α-synuclein immunoreactive neuronal inclusions. Such an observation suggests that a critical threshold of α-synuclein accumulation is required before dopaminergic and behavioural deficits become apparent.

Analogous phenotypes have also been observed in a *Drosophila* model of Parkinson's disease where expression of wild-type and mutant forms of α-synuclein in *Drosophila melanogaster* produce adult-onset loss of dopaminergic neurons, filamentous intraneuronal inclu-

sions containing α-synuclein, and locomotor dysfunction (Feany & Bender, 2000). These recent mouse and drosophila models of Parkinson's disease support a central role for the process of α-synuclein aggregation in the pathogenesis of α-synucleinopathies.

In conclusion, Lewy body dementia has emerged as a major clinical and pathological entity contributing to dementia. Although substantial data have been presented regarding the clinical and pathological features of this illness, and the identity of some of the proteins involved in the neuronal inclusions has been uncovered, major questions remain unanswered. The vast majority of instances of Lewy body dementia show at least some pathological overlap with Alzheimer's disease-related changes. This concordance far exceeds that which might be expected by chance alone; it suggests strongly that the disease processes are interrelated. This impression is reinforced by the observation that certain cases of early onset autosomal-dominant familial Alzheimer's disease show, in addition to marked Alzheimer changes, Lewy bodies in the cortex (Lantos et al., 1994; Lippa et al., 1995). It is uncertain whether this represents a common genetic predisposition to neurodegenerative diseases, common environmental influences that predispose to both diseases, or a more fundamental intertwining of these pathophysiological processes.

Although most cases of Lewy body dementia overlap with Alzheimer-type pathology, some cases exist where the Lewy bodies in widespread cortical regions are the sole neuropathological alterations. Clinically, these cases are essentially indistinguishable from those that overlap with Alzheimer's disease. Nonetheless, there is minimal or no neuronal loss, and the absolute number of Lewy bodies seems small in comparison to the devastating nature of the severe dementia syndrome. Thus, a major unanswered question remains 'what effect does the presence of Lewy bodies have on the cortex to impair neural systems so profoundly?'

Perhaps better understanding of the protein constituents that precipitate in Lewy body formation would be revealing. α-Synuclein appears to be the major protein constituent, and the presence of the mutations in α-synuclein that lead to autosomal dominantly inherited Parkinson's disease encourages the belief that α-synuclein dysfunction lies at the heart of the illness. Unfortunately, the neuronal functional role of α-synuclein remains unknown. α-Synuclein knockout mice have only a subtle phenotype and minimal electrophysiological dysfunction, suggesting that the impact of α-synuclein alterations in Lewy body diseases is not a simple loss of function (Abeliovich et al., 2000).

It has been suggested that protein misfolding, and thereby potential gain of function, lies at the heart of synuclein aggregation into Lewy bodies and, perhaps more generally, is a cause of synaptic dysfunction in Lewy body dementias. This is an appealing idea from the perspective of other neurodegenerative diseases in that similar mechanisms have been evoked in prion diseases, triplet repeat disorders, and Alzheimer's disease. Nonetheless, direct experimental evidence to support this idea remains elusive.

Thus, while the clinical, neuropathological, genetic, and even biochemical characterization of dementia with Lewy bodies is well underway, definitive understanding of the pathophysiology and therapy await answers to some of these remaining questions. The recent development of a transgenic mouse model of dopaminergic loss and inclusion body formation after overexpression of α-synuclein (Masliah et al., 2000) and the Drosophila model also based on genetic manipulation of α-synuclein (Feany & Bender, 2000), provide important tools for future studies.

Acknowledgements

Supported by the MGH-MIT Parkinson's Disease Research Center, PONS 38372, MBRC Tosteson postdoctoral fellowship award to PJM, AG00793 to MCI and Merin Family Foundation award to BTH.

References

Abeliovich, A., Schmitz, Y., Farinas, I. et al. (2000). Mice lacking α-synuclein display functional deficits in the nigrostriatal dopamine system. *Neuron*, **25**, 239–52.

Alim, M.A., Hossain, M.S., Arima, K. et al. (2002). Tubulin seeds alpha-synuclein fibril formation. *J. Biol. Chem.*, **277**, 2112–17.

Amaducci, L.A., Fratiglioni, L., Rocca, W.A. et al. (1986). Risk factors for clinically diagnosed Alzheimer's disease: a case-control study of an Italian population. *Neurology*, **36**, 922–31.

Arai, H., Morikawa, Y., Higuchi, M. et al. (1997). Cerebrospinal fluid tau levels in neurodegenerative diseases with distinct tau-related pathology. *Biochem. Biophys. Res. Commun.*, **236**, 262–4.

Armstrong, R., Cairns, N. & Lantos, P. (1997). Beta-Amyloid (A beta) deposition in the medial temporal lobe of patients with dementia with Lewy bodies. *Neurosci. Lett.*, **227**, 193–6.

Atkinson, A., Singleton, A.B., Steward, A. et al. (1999). CYP2D6 is associated with Parkinson's disease but not with dementia with Lewy Bodies or Alzheimer's disease. *Pharmacogenetics*, **9**, 31–5.

Baba, M., Nakajo, S., Tu, P-H. et al. (1998). Aggregation of α-synuclein in Lewy bodies of sporadic Parkinson's disease and dementia with Lewy bodies. *Am. J. Pathol.*, **152**, 879–84.

Ballard, C.G., Saad, K., Patel, A. et al. (1995). The prevalence and phenomenology of psychotic symptoms in dementia sufferers. *Int. J. Geriatr. Psychiatry*, **10**, 477–85.

Ballard, C., Patel, A., Oyebode, F. & Wilcock, G. (1996). Cognitive decline in patients with Alzheimer's disease, vascular dementia and senile dementia of Lewy body type. *Age Ageing*, **25**, 209–13.

Ballard, C.G., Ayre, G., O'Brien, J. et al. (1999a). Simple standardised neuropsychological assessments aid in the differential diagnosis of dementia with Lewy bodies from Alzheimer's disease and vascular dementia. *Dement. Geriatr. Cogn. Disord.*, **10**, 104–8.

Ballard, C.G., Holmes, C., McKeith, I. et al. (1999b). Psychiatric morbidity in dementia with Lewy bodies: a prospective clinical and neuropathological comparative study with Alzheimer's disease. *Am. J. Psychiatry*, **156**, 1039–45.

Barber, R., Scheltens, P., Gholkar, A. et al. (1999a). White matter lesions on magnetic resonance imaging in dementia with Lewy bodies, Alzheimer's disease, vascular dementia, and normal aging. *J. Neurol., Neurosurg. Psychiatry*, **67**, 66–72.

Barber, R., Gholkar, A., Scheltens, P., Ballard, C., McKeith, I.G. & O'Brien, J. T. (1999b). Medial temporal lobe atrophy on MRI in dementia with Lewy bodies. *Neurology*, **52**, 1153–8.

Barber, P.A., Varma, A.R., Lloyd, J.J., Haworth, B., Snowden, J.S. & Neary, D. (2000). The electroencephalogram in dementia with Lewy bodies. *Acta Neurol. Scand.*, **101**, 53–6.

Benjamin, R., Leake, A., Edwardson, J.A. et al. (1994a). Apolipoprotein E genes in Lewy body and Parkinson's disease. *Lancet*, **343**, 1565.

Benjamin, R., Leake, A., McArthur, F.K. et al. (1994b). Protective effect of apoE epsilon 2 in Alzheimer's disease. *Lancet*, **344**, 473.

Bergeron, C. & Pollanen, M. (1989). Lewy bodies in Alzheimer's disease – One or two diseases. *Alzheimer Dis. Assoc. Disord.*, **3**, 197–204.

Braak, H., Sandmann-Keil, D., Gai, W. & Braak, E. (1999). Extensive axonal Lewy neurites in Parkinson's disease: a novel pathological feature revealed by alpha-synuclein immunocytochemistry. *Neurosci. Lett.*, **265**, 67–9.

Briel, R.C., McKeith, I.G., Barker, W.A. et al. (1999). EEG findings in dementia with Lewy bodies and Alzheimer's disease. *J. Neurol., Neurosurg. Psychiatry*, **66**, 401–3.

Churchyard, A. & Lees, A.J. (1997). The relationship between dementia and direct involvement of the hippocampus and amygdala in Parkinson's disease. *Neurology*, **49**, 1570–6.

Conway, K.A., Harper, J.D. & Lansbury, P.T. (1998). Accelerated in vitro fibril formation by a mutant α-synuclein linked to early-onset Parkinson disease. *Nat. Med.*, **4**, 1318–20.

Conway, K.A., Lee, S-J., Rochet, J-C., Ding, T.T., Williamson, R.E. & Lansbury, P.T. (2000a). Acceleration of oligomerization, not fibrillization, is a shared property of both α-synuclein mutations limked to early-onset Parkinson's disease: implications for pathogenesis and therapy. *Proc. Natl. Acad., Sci. USA*, **97**, 571–6.

Conway, K.A., Harper, J.D. & Lansbury, P.T. (2000b). Fibrils formed in vitro from α-synuclein and two mutant forms linked to Parkinson's disease are typical amyloid. *Biochemistry*, **39**, 2552–63.

Corder, E.H., Saunder, A.M., Risch, N.J. et al. (1994). Apolipoprotein

E type 2 allele decreases the risk of late onset Alzheimer disease. *Nat. Genet.*, **7**, 180–4.

Crowther, R.A., Jakes, R., Spillantini, M.G. & Goedert, M. (1998). Synthetic filaments assembled from C-terminally truncated α-synuclein. *FEBS Lett.*, **436**, 309–12.

Crystal, H.A., Dickson, D.W., Sliwinski, M.J. et al. (1993). Pathological markers associated with normal aging and dementia in the elderly. *Ann. Neurol.*, **34**, 566–73.

Davidson, W.S., Jonas, A., Clayton, D.F. & George, J.M. (1998). Stabilization of α-synuclein secondary structure upon binding to synthetic membranes. *J. Biol. Chem.*, **273**, 9443–9.

de Vos, R., Jansen, E., Stam, F., Ravid, R. & Swaab, D. (1995). Lewy body disease: clinico-pathological correlations in 18 consecutive cases of Parkinson's disease with and without dementia. *Clin. Neurol. Neurosurg.*, **97**, 13–22.

Defebvre, L.J., Leduc, V., Duhamel, A. et al. (1999). Technetium HMPAO SPECT study in dementia with Lewy bodies, Alzheimer's disease and idiopathic Parkinson's disease. *J. Nucl. Med.*, **40**, 956–62.

Dickson, D.W., Ruan, D., Crystal, H. et al. (1991). Hippocampal degeneration differentiates diffuse Lewy body disease (DLBD) from Alzheimer's disease: light and electron microscopic immunocytochemistry of CA2–3 neurites specific to DLBD. *Neurology*, **41**, 1402–9.

Dickson, D.W., Crystal, H., Mattiace, L.A. et al. (1992). Identification of normal and pathological aging in prospectively studied nondemented elderly humans. *Neurobiol. Aging*, **13**, 179–89.

Dickson, D., Schmidt, M., Lee, Y.M-Y., Zhao, M-L., Yen, S. & Trojanowski, J. (1994). Immunoreactivity profile of hippocampal CA2/3 neurites in diffuse Lewy body disease. *Acta Neuropathol. (Berl.)*, **87**, 269–76.

Ditter, S.M. & Mirra, S.S. (1987). Neuropathologic and clinical features of Parkinson's disease in Alzheimer's disease patients. *Neurology*, **37**, 754–60.

Donnemiller, E., Heilmann, J., Wenning, G.K. et al. (1997). Brain perfusion scintigraphy with 99mTc-HMPAO or 99mTc-ECD and 123I-beta-CIT single-photon emission tomography in dementia of the Alzheimer-type and diffuse Lewy body disease. *Eur. J. Nucl. Med.*, **24**, 320–5.

El-Agnaf, O.M.A., Jakes, R., Curran, M.D. et al. (1998). Aggregates from mutant and wild-type α-synuclein proteins and NAC peptide induce apoptotic cell death in human neuroblastoma cells by formation of β-sheet and amyloid-like filaments. *FEBS Lett.*, **440**, 71–5.

Engelender, S., Kaminsky, Z., Guo, X. et al. (1999). Synphilin-1 associates with α-synuclein and promotes the formation of cytosolic inclusions. *Nat. Genet.*, **22**, 110–14.

Feany, M.B. & Bender, W.W. (2000). A drosophila model of Parkinson's disease. *Nature*, **404**, 394–7.

Forloni, G., Bertani, I., Calella, A.M., Thaler, F. & Invernizzi, R. (2000). α-Synuclein and Parkinson's disease: selective neurodegerative effect of α-synuclein fragment on dopaminergic neurons in vitro and in vivo. *Ann. Neurol.*, **47**, 632–40.

Forno, L.S. (1969). Concentric hyalin intraneuronal inclusions of Lewy type in the brains of elderly persons (50 incidental cases): relationship to parkinsonism. *J. Am. Geriatr. Soc.*, **17**, 557–75.

Forno, L.S. & Langston, J.W. (1993). Lewy bodies and aging: relation to Alzheimer's and Parkinson's disease. *Neurodegeneration*, **2**, 19–24.

Galasko, D., Katzman, R., Salmon, D.P. & Hansen, L. (1996). Clinical and neuropathological findings in Lewy body dementias. *Brain Cogn.*, **31**, 166–75.

Galvin, J., Uryu, K., Lee, V.M-Y. & Trojanowski, J. (1999). Axon pathology in Parkinson's disease and Lewy body dementia hippocampus contains α-, β- and γ-synuclein. *Proc. Natl. Acad. Sci., USA*, **96**, 13450–5.

Gearing, M., Lynn, M. & Mirra, S. (1999). Neurofibrillary pathology in Alzheimer disease with Lewy bodies: two subgroups. *Arch. Neurol.*, **56**, 203–8.

George, J.M., Jin, H., Woods, W.S. & Clayton, D.F. (1995). Characterization of a novel protein regulated during the critical period for song learning in the zebra finch. *Neuron*, **15**, 361–72.

Giasson, B.I., Uryu, K., Trojanowski, J.Q. & Lee, V.M-Y. (1999). Mutant and wild-type human α-synucleins assemble into elongated filaments with distinct morphologies *in vitro*. *J. Biol. Chem.*, **274**, 7619–22.

Gnanalingham, K.K., Byrne, E.J., Thornton, A., Sambrook, M.A. & Bannister, P. (1997). Motor and cognitive function in Lewy body dementia: comparison with Alzheimer's and Parkinson's diseases. *J. Neurol., Neurosurg. Psychiatry*, **62**, 243–52.

Gómez-Isla, T., West, H.L., Rebeck, G.W et al. (1996a). Clinical and pathological correlates of apolipoprotein E epsilon4 in Alzheimer's disease. *Ann. Neurol.*, **39**, 62–70.

Gómez-Isla, T., Price, J.L., McKeel, D.W. Jr., Morris, J.C., Growdon, J.H. & Hyman, B.T. (1996b). Profound loss of layer II entorhinal cortex neurons occurs in very mild Alzheimer's disease. *J. Neurosci.*, **16**, 4491–500.

Gómez-Isla, T., Hollister, R., West, H. et al. (1997). Neuronal loss correlates with but exceeds neurofibrillary tangles in Alzheimer's disease. *Ann. Neurol.*, **41**, 17–24.

Gómez-Isla, T., Growdon, W.B., McNamara, M. et al. (1999a). Clinicopathologic correlates in temporal cortex in dementia with Lewy bodies. *Neurology*, **53**, 2003–9.

Gómez-Tortosa, E., Ingraham, A.O., Irizarry, M.C. & Hyman, B.T. (1998). Dementia with Lewy bodies. *J. Am. Geriatr. Soc.*, **46**, 1449–58.

Gómez-Tortosa, E., Newell, K., Irizarry, M.C., Albert, M., Growdon, J.H. & Hyman, B.T. (1999). Clinical and quantitative pathologic correlates of dementia with Lewy bodies. *Neurology*, **53**, 1284–91.

Gómez-Tortosa, E., Newell, K., Irizarry, M.C., Sanders, J.L. & Hyman, B.T. (2000). Alpha-synuclein immunoreactivity in dementia with Lewy bodies: morphological staging and comparison with ubiquitin immunostaining. *Acta Neuropathol. (Berl.)*, **99**, 352–7.

Gómez-Tortosa, E., Sanders, J., Newell, K. & Hyman, B. (2001). Cortical neurons expressing calcium binding proteins are spared in dementia with Lewy bodies. *Acta Neuropathol. (Berl.)*, **101**, 36–42.

Hansen, L. (1996). Tautological tangles in neuropathological criteria for dementias associated with Lewy bodies. In *Dementia with Lewy Bodies. Clinical, Pathological and Treatment Issues*, ed. M.I. Perry & R, Perry E, pp. 204–11. Cambridge, UK: Cambridge University Press.

Hansen, L.A., Masliah, E., Terry, R.D. & Mirra, S.S. (1989). A neuropathological subset of Alzheimer's disease with concomitant Lewy body disease and spongiform change. *Acta Neuropathol. (Berl.)*, **78**, 194–201.

Hansen, L., Salmon, D., Galasko, D. et al. (1990). The Lewy body variant of Alzheimer's disease: a clinical and pathologic entity. *Neurology*, **40**, 1–8.

Hansen, L., Masliah, E., Galasko, D. & Terry, R. (1993). Plaque-only Alzheimer disease is usually the Lewy body variant, and vice versa. *J. Neuropathol. Exp. Neurol.*, **52**, 648–54.

Hansen, L., Daniel, S., Wilcock, G. & Love, S. (1998). Frontal cortical synaptophysin in Lewy body diseases: relation to Alzheimer's disease and dementia. *J. Neurol., Neurosurg. Psychiatry*, **64**, 653–6.

Hardy, J., Perez-Tur, J., Baker, M. et al. (1998). Exclusion of genetic linkage to 4q21–23 and 17q21 in a family with Lewy body parkinsonism. *Am. J. Med. Genet.*, **81**, 166–71.

Harvey, G.T., Hughes, J., McKeith, I.G. et al. (1999). Magnetic resonance imaging differences between dementia with Lewy bodies and Alzheimer's disease: a pilot study. *Psychol. Med.*, **29**, 181–7.

Hashimoto, M., Kitagaki, H., Imamura, T. et al. (1998). Medial temporal and whole-brain atrophy in dementia with Lewy bodies: a volumetric MRI study. *Neurology*, **51**, 357–62.

Hashimoto, M., Takeda, A., Hsu, J., Takenouchi, T. & Masliah, E. (1999a). Role of cytochrome *c* as a stimulator of α-synuclein aggregation in Lewy body disease. *J. Biol. Chem.*, **274**, 28849–52.

Hashimoto, M., Hsu, L. J., Xia, Y. et al. (1999b). Oxidative stress induces amyloid-like aggregate formation of NACP/α-synuclein *in vitro*. *Neuroreport*, **10**, 717–21.

Heyman, A., Fillenbaum, G., Gearing, M. et al. (1999). Comparison of Lewy body variant of Alzheimer's disease with pure Alzheimer's disease. *Neurology*, **52**, 1839–44.

Higuchi, S., Arai, H., Matsushita, S. et al. (1998). Mutation in the alpha-synuclein gene and sporadic Parkinson's disease, Alzheimer's disease, and dementia with Lewy bodies. *Exp. Neurol.*, **153**, 164–6.

Higuchi, M., Tashiro, M., Arai, H. et al. (2000). Glucose hypometabolism and neuropathological correlates in brains of dementia with Lewy bodies. *Exp. Neurol.*, **162**, 247–56.

Hofman, A., Schulte, W., Tanja, T.A. et al. (1989). History of dementia and Parkinson's disease in 1st-degree relatives of patients with Alzheimer's disease. *Neurology*, **39**, 1589–92.

Hohl, U., Tiraboschi, P., Hansen, L.A., Thal, L.J. & Corey-Bloom, J. (2000). Diagnostic accuracy of dementia with Lewy bodies. *Arch. Neurol.*, **57**, 347–51.

Holmes, C., Cairns, N., Lantos, P. & Mann, A. (1999). Validity of current clinical criteria for Alzheimer's disease, vascular dementia and dementia with Lewy bodies. *Br. J. Psychiatry*, **174**, 45–50.

Hughes, A., Daniel, S., Blankson, S. & Lees, A. (1993). A clinicopathologic study of 100 cases of Parkinson's disease. *Arch. Neurol.*, **50**, 140–8.

Ince, P., Irving, D., MacArthur, F. & Perry, R. (1991). Quantitative neuropathological study of Alzheimer-type pathology in the hippocampus: comparison of senile dementia of Alzheimer type, senile dementia of Lewy body type, Parkinson's disease and nondemented elderly control patients. *J. Neurol. Sci.*, **106**, 142–52.

Irizarry, M.C., Growdon, W., Gomez-Isla, T. et al. (1998). Nigral and cortical Lewy bodies and dystrophic nigral neurites in Parkinson's disease and cortical Lewy body disease contain α-synuclein immunoreactivity. *J. Neuropathol. Exp. Neurol.*, **57**, 334–7.

Iseki, E., Li, F. & Kosaka, K. (1997). Close relationship between spongiform change and ubiquitin-positive granular structures in diffuse Lewy body disease. *J. Neurol. Sci.*, **146**, 53–7.

Ishii, K., Imamura, T., Sasaki, M. et al. (1998). Regional cerebral glucose metabolism in dementia with Lewy bodies and Alzheimer's disease. *Neurology*, **51**, 125–30.

Ishii, K., Yamaji, S., Kitagaki, H., Imamura, T., Hirono, N. & Mori, E. (1999). Regional cerebral blood flow difference between dementia with Lewy bodies and AD. *Neurology*, **53**, 413–16.

Iwai, A., Masliah, E., Yoshimoto, M. et al. (1995). The precursor protein of non-Aβ component of Alzheimer's disease amyloid is a presynaptic protein of the central nervous system. *Neuron*, **14**, 467–75.

Jakes, R., Spillantini, M.G. & Goedert, M. (1994). Identification of two distinct synucleins from human brain. *FEBS Lett.*, **345**, 27–32.

Jensen, P.H., Nielsen, M S., Jakes, R., Dotti, C.G. & Goedert, M. (1998). Binding of α-synuclein to brain vesicles is abolished by familial Parkinson's disease mutation. *J. Biol. Chem.*, **273**, 26292–4.

Jensen, P.H., Hager, H., Nielsen, M.S., Højrup, P., Gliemann, J. & Jakes, R. (1999). α-Synuclein binds to tau and stimulates the protein kinase A-catalyzed tau phosphorylation of serine residues 262 and 356. *J. Biol. Chem.*, **274**, 25481–9.

Jensen, P.H., Islam, K., Kenney, J., Nielsen, M.S., Power, J. & Gai, W.P. (2000). Microtubule-associated protein 1B is a component of cortical Lewy bodies and binds α-synuclein filaments. *J. Biol. Chem.*, **275**, 21500–7.

Kahle, P.J., Neumann, M., Ozmen, L. et al. (2000). Subcellular localization of wild-type and Parkinson's disease-associated mutant α-synuclein in human and transgenic mouse brain. *J. Neurosci.*, **20**, 6365–73.

Kanda, S., Bishop, J. F., Eglitis, M.A., Yang, Y. & Mouradian, M.M. (2000). Enhanced vulnerability to oxidative stress by α-synuclein mutations and C-terminal truncation. *Neuroscience*, **97**, 279–84.

Kanemaru, K., Kameda, N. & Yamanouchi, H. (2000). Decreased CSF amyloid beta42 and normal tau levels in dementia with Lewy bodies. *Neurology*, **54**, 1875–6.

Kim, H., Gearing, M. & Mirra, S. (1995). Ubiquitin-positive CA2/3 neurites coexist with cortical Lewy bodies. *Neurology*, **45**, 1768–70.

Klatka, L.A., Louis, E.D. & Schiffer, R.B. (1996). Psychiatric features in diffuse Lewy body disease: a clinicopathologic study using Alzheimer's disease and Parkinson's disease comparison groups. *Neurology*, **47**, 1148–52.

Kosaka, K., Matsushita, M., Oyanagi, S. & Mehraein, P. (1980). [A cliniconeuropathological study of 'Lewy body disease']. *Seishin Shinkeigaku Zasshi*, **82**, 292–311.

Krüger, R., Kuhn, W., Müller, T. et al. (1998). Ala30Pro mutation in the gene encoding α-synuclein in Parkinson's disease. *Nat. Genet.*, **18**, 106–8.

Kuzuhara, S., Mori, H., Izumiyama, N., Yoshimura, M. & Ihara, Y. (1988). Lewy bodies are ubiquitinated. A light and electron microscopic immunocytochemical study. *Acta Neuropathol. (Berl.)*, **75**, 345–53.

Lamb, H., Christie, J., Singleton, A.B. et al. (1998). Apolipoprotein E and alpha-1 antichymotrypsin polymorphism genotyping in Alzheimer's disease and in dementia with Lewy bodies. Distinctions between diseases. *Neurology*, **50**, 388–91.

Langlais, P., Thal, L., Hansen, L., Galasko, D., Alford, M. & Masliah, E. (1993). Neurotransmitters in basal ganglia and cortex of Alzheimer's disease with and without Lewy bodies. *Neurology*, **43**, 1927–34.

Lantos, P.L., Ovenstone, I.M., Johnson, J., Clelland, C.A., Roques, P. & Rossor, M.N. (1994). Lewy bodies in the brain of two members of a family with the 717 (Val to Ile) mutation of the amyloid precursor protein gene. *Neurosci. Lett.*, **172**, 77–9.

Lennox, G., Lowe, J., Landon, M., Byrne, E., Mayer, R. & Godwin-Austen, R. (1989a). Diffuse Lewy body disease, correlative neuropathology using anti-ubiquitin immunocytochemistry. *J. Neurol., Neurosurg. Psychiatry*, **52**, 1236–47.

Lennox, G., Lowe, J., Morrell, K., Landon, M. & Mayer, R. (1989b). Antiubiquitin immunocytochemistry is more sensitive than conventional techniques in the detection of diffuse Lewy body disease. *J. Neurol., Neurosurg. Psychiatry*, **52**, 67–71.

Lewy, F.H. (1912). Paralysis agitans. I pathologische anatomie. In *Handbuch der Neurologie*, ed. M. Lewandowski, pp. 920–33. Berlin: Springer.

Lipkin, L.E. (1959). Cytoplasmic inclusions in ganglion cells associated with parkinsonian states. *Am. J. Pathol.*, **35**, 1117–33.

Lippa, C., Smith, T. & Swearer, J. (1994). Alzheimer's disease and Lewy body disease: a comparative clinicopathological study. *Ann. Neurol.*, **35**, 81–8.

Lippa, C.F., Smith, T.W., Nee, L. et al. (1995). Familial Alzheimer's disease and cortical Lewy bodies: is there a genetic susceptibility factor? *Dementia*, **6**, 191–4.

Lippa, C.F., Pulaski-Salo, D., Dickson, D.W. & Smith, T.W. (1997). Alzheimer's disease, Lewy body disease and aging: a comparative study of the perforant pathway. *J. Neurol. Sci.*, **147**, 161–6.

Lippa, C., Johnson, R. & Smith, T. (1998). The medial temporal lobe in dementia with Lewy bodies: a comparative study with Alzheimer's disease. *Ann. Neurol.*, **43**, 102–6.

Lippa, C., Smith, T. & Perry, E. (1999). Dementia with lewy bodies: choline acetyltransferase parallels nucleus basalis pathology. *J. Neural Transm.*, **106**, 525–35.

Litvan, I., MacIntyre, A., Goetz, C.G. et al. (1998). Accuracy of the clinical diagnoses of Lewy body disease, Parkinson disease, and dementia with Lewy bodies: a clinicopathologic study. *Arch. Neurol.*, **55**, 969–78.

Lowe, J. (1994). Lewy bodies. In *Neurodegenerative Diseases*, pp. 51–69. Philadelphia: WB Saunders.

Luis, C.A., Barker, W.W., Gajaraj, K. et al. (1999). Sensitivity and specificity of three clinical criteria for dementia with Lewy bodies in an autopsy-verified sample. *Int. J. Geriatr. Psychiatry*, **14**, 526–33.

McKeith, I. & O'Brien, J. (1999). Dementia with Lewy bodies. *Aust. NZ J. Psychiatry*, **33**, 800–8.

McKeith, I., Fairbairn, A., Perry, R., Thompson, P. & Perry, E. (1992a). Neuroleptic sensitivity in patients with senile dementia of Lewy body type. *Br. Med. J.*, **305**, 673–8.

McKeith, I., Perry, R., Fairbairn, A., Jabeen, S. & Perry, E. (1992b). Operational criteria for senile dementia of Lewy body type (SDLT). *Psychol. Med.*, **22**, 911–22.

McKeith, I.G., Galasko, D., Kosaka, K. et al. (1996). Consensus guidelines for the clinical and pathological diagnosis of dementia with Lewy bodies (DLB): Report of the consortium on DLB international workshop. *Neurology*, **47**, 1113–24.

McKeith, I.G., Perry, E.K. & Perry, R. H. (1999). Report of the second dementia with Lewy body international workshop: diagnosis and treatment. Consortium on Dementia with Lewy Bodies. *Neurology*, **53**, 902–5.

McKeith, I.G., Ballard, C.G., Perry, R.H. et al. (2000a). Prospective validation of consensus criteria for the diagnosis of dementia with Lewy bodies. *Neurology*, **54**, 1050–8.

McKeith, I., Del Ser, T., Anand, R. et al. (2000b). Rivastigmine provides symptomatic benefit in dementia with Lewy bodies: findings from a placebo-controlled international multicenter study. *Neurology*, **54** (Suppl. 3), A450.

McLean, P.J., Kawamata, H., Ribich, S. & Hyman, B. T. (2000). Membrane association and protein conformation of α-synuclein in intact neurons: effect of Parkinson disease linked mutations. *J. Biol. Chem.*, **275**, 8812–16.

McShane, R., Gedling, K., Reading, M., McDonald, B., Esiri, M. & Hope, T. (1995). Prospective study of relations between cortical Lewy bodies, poor eyesight and hallucinations in Alzheimer's disease. *J. Neurol., Neurosurg. Psychiatry*, **59**, 185–8.

McShane, R., Keene, J., Gedling, K. & Hope, T. (1996). Hallucinations, cortical Lewy body pathology, cognitive function and neuroleptic use in dementia. In *Dementia with Lewy bodies. Clinical, Pathological and Treatment Issues*, ed. M.I. Perry & R.E. Perry, pp. 85–98. Cambridge, UK: Cambridge University Press.

McShane, R.H., Esiri, M. M., Joachim, C., Smith, A.D. & Jacoby, R. J. (1998). Prospective evaluation of diagnostic criteria for dementia with Lewy bodies. *Neurobiol. Aging*, **19** (4S), 204.

Mann, D., Pickering-Brown, S., Owen, F., Baba, M. & Iwatsubo, T. (1998). Amyloid β protein (Aβ) deposition in dementia with Lewy bodies: predominance of Aβ 42(43) and paucity of Aβ 40 compared with sporadic Alzheimer's disease. *Neuropathol. Appl. Neurobiol.*, **24**, 187–94.

Maroteaux, L., Campanelli, J.T. & Scheller, R.H. (1988). Synuclein: A neuron-specific protein localized to the nucleus and presynaptic nerve terminal. *J. Neurosci.*, **8**, 2804–15.

Masliah, E., Rockenstein, E., Veinbergs, I. et al. (2000). Dopaminergic loss and inclusion body formation in α-synuclein mice: implications for neurodegenerative disorders. *Science*, **287**, 1265–9.

Mattila, P., Roytta, M., Torikka, H., Dickson, D. & Rinne, J. (1998). Cortical Lewy bodies and Alzheimer-type changes in patients with Parkinson's disease. *Acta Neuropathol. (Berl.)*, **95**, 576–82.

Mega, M.S., Masterman, D.L., Benson, D.F. et al. (1996). Dementia with Lewy bodies: reliability and validity of clinical and pathologic criteria. *Neurology*, **47**, 1403–9.

Mickel, S.F., Broste, S.K. & Hiner, B.C. (1997). Lack of overlap in genetic risks for Alzheimer's disease and Parkinson's disease. *Neurology*, **48**, 942–9.

Mori, E., Shimomura, T., Fujimori, M. et al. (2000). Visuoperceptual impairment in dementia with Lewy bodies. *Arch. Neurol.*, **57**, 489–93.

Morris, C.M., Massey, H.M., Benjamin, R. et al. (1996). Molecular biology of APO E alleles in Alzheimer's and non-Alzheimer's dementias. *J. Neural Transm. Suppl.*, **47**, 205–18.

Nahri, L., Wood, S.J., Steavenson, S. et al. (1999). Both familial Parkinson's disease mutations accelerate α-synuclein aggregation. *J. Biol. Chem.*, **274**, 9843–6.

O'Brien, J. T., Metcalfe, S., Swann, A. et al. (2000). Medial temporal lobe width on CT scanning in Alzheimer's disease: comparison with vascular dementia, depression and dementia with Lewy bodies. *Dement. Geriatr. Cogn. Disord.*, **11**, 114–18.

Ohara, K., Takauchi, S., Kokai, M., Morimura, Y., Nakajima, T. & Morita, Y. (1999). Familial dementia with Lewy bodies (DLB). *Clin. Neuropathol.*, **18**, 232–9.

Okazaki, H., Lipkin, L.E. & Aronson, S.M. (1961). Diffuse intracytoplasmic ganglionic inclusions (Lewy type) associated with progressive dementia and quadriparesis in flexion. *J. Neuropathol. Exp. Neurol.*, **20**, 237–44.

Olichney, J.M., Galasko, D., Salmon, D.P. et al. (1998). Cognitive decline is faster in Lewy body variant than in Alzheimer's disease. *Neurology*, **51**, 351–7.

Osterova-Golts, N., Petrucelli, L., Hardy, J., Lee, J.M., Farer, M. & Wolozin, B. (2000). The A53T α-synuclein mutation increases iron-dependent aggregation and toxicity. *J. Neurosci.*, **20**, 6048–54.

Pasquier, F., Lavenu, I., Lebert, F., Jacob, B., Steinling, M. & Petit, H. (1997). The use of SPECT in a multidisciplinary memory clinic. *Dement. Geriatr. Cogn. Disord.*, **8**, 85–91.

Pellise, A., Roig, C., Barraquer-Bordas, L. & Ferrer, I. (1996). Abnormal, ubiquitinated cortical neurites in patients with diffuse Lewy body disease. *Neurosci. Lett.*, **206**, 85–8.

Perry, R.H., Irving, D., Blessed, G., Fairbairn, A. & Perry, E.K. (1990). Senile dementia of Lewy body type. A clinically and neuropathologically distinct form of Lewy body dementia in the elderly. *J. Neurol. Sci.*, **95**, 119–39.

Perry, R., Jaros, E., Irving, D. et al. (1996). What is the neuropathological basis of dementia associated with Lewy bodies? In *Dementia with Lewy bodies. Clinical, Pathological and Treatment Issues*, ed. M.I. Perry & R.E. Perry E. pp. 212–23. Cambridge, UK: Cambridge University Press.

Perry, R., McKeith, I. & Perry, E. (1997). Lewy body dementia—clinical, pathological and neurochemical interconnections. *J. Neural Transm. Suppl.*, **51**, 95–109.

Pollanen, M., Dickson, D. & Bergeron, C. (1993). Pathology and biology of the Lewy body. *J. Neuropathol. Exp. Neurol.*, **52**, 183–91.

Polymeropoulos, M.H., Lavedan, C., Leroy, E. et al. (1997). Mutation in the α-synuclein gene identified in families with Parkinson's disease. *Science*, **276**, 2045–7.

Rebeck, G.W., Reiter, J.S., Strickland, D.K. & Hyman, B.T. (1993). Apolipoprotein E in sporadic Alzheimer's disease: allelic variation and receptor interactions. *Neuron*, **11**, 575–80.

Rezaie, P., Cairns, N.J., Chadwick, A. & Lantos, P. L. (1996). Lewy bodies are located preferentially in limbic areas in diffuse Lewy body disease. *Neurosci. Lett.*, **212**, 111–14.

Samuel, W., Galasko, D., Masliah, E. & Hansen, L.A. (1996). Neocortical Lewy body counts correlate with dementia in the Lewy body variant of Alzheimer's disease. *J. Neuropathol. Exp. Neurol.*, **55**, 44–52.

Samuel, W., Alford, M., Hofstetter, C.R. & Hansen, L. (1997a). Dementia with Lewy bodies versus pure Alzheimer disease: differences in cognition, neuropathology, cholinergic dysfunction, and synapse density. *J. Neuropathol. Exp. Neurol.*, **56**, 499–508.

Samuel, W., Crowder, R., Hofstetter, C.R. & Hansen, L. (1997b). Neuritic plaques in the Lewy body variant of Alzheimer disease lack paired helical filaments. *Neurosci. Lett.*, **223**, 73–6.

Saunders, A., Strittmater, W., Schmechel, D. et al. (1993). Association of apolipoprotein E allele e4 with late-onset familial and sporadic Alzheimer's disease. *Neurology*, **43**, 1467–72.

Serpell, L.C., Berriman, J., Jakes, R., Goedert, M. & Crowther, R.A. (2000). Fiber diffraction of synthetic α-synuclein filaments shows amyloid-like cross-β conformation. *Proc. Natl. Acad. Sci., USA*, **97**, 4897–902.

Shergill, S., Mullan, E., Dath, P. & Katona, C. (1994). What is the clinical prevalence of Lewy body dementia? *Int. J. Geriatr. Psychiatry*, **9**, 907–12.

Shimomura, T., Mori, E., Yamashita, H. et al. (1998). Cognitive loss in dementia with Lewy bodies and Alzheimer disease. *Arch. Neurol.*, **55**, 1547–52.

Singleton, A.B., Lamb, H., Leake, A. et al. (1997). No association between a polymorphism in the presenilin 1 gene and dementia with Lewy bodies. *Neuroreport*, **8**, 3637–9.

Singleton, A.B., Gibson, A.M., Edwardson, J.A., McKeith, I.G. & Morris, C.M. (1998). Butyrylcholinesterase K: an association with dementia with Lewy bodies. *Lancet*, **351**, 1818.

Singleton, A.B., Gibson, A.M., McKeith, I.G. et al. (1999). Alpha2-macroglobulin polymorphisms in Alzheimer's disease and dementia with Lewy bodies. *Neuroreport*, **10**, 1507–10.

Spillantini, M.G., Schmidt, M.L., Lee, M-Y., Trowjanowski, J.Q., Jakes, R. & Goedert, M. (1997). α-Synuclein in Lewy bodies. *Nature*, **388**, 839–40.

Talbot, P.R., Lloyd, J.J., Snowden, J.S., Neary, D. & Testa, H.J. (1998). A clinical role for 99mTc-HMPAO SPECT in the investigation of dementia? *J. Neurol., Neurosurg. Psychiatry*, **64**, 306–13.

Tiraboshi, P., Hansen, L., Alford, M. et al. (2000). Cholinergic dysfunction in diseases with Lewy bodies. *Neurology*, **54**, 407–11.

Tretiakoff, C. (1919). Contribution a l'etude de l'anatomie pathologique du locus niger de Soemmering avec quelques deductions relatives a la pathologenie des troubles du tonus musculaires et de la maladie de Parkinson: (University of Paris).

van Duijn, C.M., Clayton, D., Chandra, V. et al. (1991). Familial aggregation of Alzheimer's disease and related disorders: a collaborative re-analysis of case control studies. *Int. J. Epidemiol.*, **20** Suppl., 13–20.

Verghese, J., Crystal, H.A., Dickson, D.W. & Lipton, R.B. (1999). Validity of clinical criteria for the diagnosis of dementia with Lewy bodies. *Neurology*, **53**, 1974–82.

Wakabayashi, K., Hansen, L.A. & Masliah, E. (1995). Cortical Lewy body-containing neurons are pyramidal cells: laser confocal imaging of double-immunolabeled sections with anti-ubiquitin and SMI32. *Acta Neuropathol. (Berl.)*, **89**, 404–8.

Wakabayashi, K., Engelender, S., Yoshimoto, M., Ross, C.A. & Takahashi, H. (2000). Synphilin-1 is present in Lewy bodies in Parkinson's disease. *Ann. Neurol.*, **47**, 521–3.

Walker, Z., Allen, R.L., Shergill, S., and Katona, C.L. (1997). Neuropsychological performance in Lewy body dementia and Alzheimer's disease. *Br. J. Psychiatry*, **170**, 156–8.

Walker, Z., Allen, R.L., Shergill, S., Mullan, E. & Katona, C.L. (2000a). Three years survival in patients with a clinical diagnosis of dementia with Lewy bodies. *Int. J. Geriatr. Psychiatry*, **15**, 267–73.

Walker, M.P., Ayre, G.A., Cummings, J.L., Wesnes, K., McKeith, I.G., O'Brien, J.T. & Ballard, C.G. (2000b). Quantifying fluctuation in dementia with Lewy bodies, Alzheimer's disease, and vascular dementia. *Neurology*, **54**, 1616–25.

Weiner, M.F., Risser, R.C., Cullum, C.M., Honig, L., White, C., 3rd, Speciale, S. & Rosenberg, R. N. (1996). Alzheimer's disease and its Lewy body variant: a clinical analysis of postmortem verified cases. *Am. J. Psychiatry*, **153**, 1269–73.

Weinreb, P.H., Zhen, W., Poon, A.W., Conway, K.A. & P.T. Lansbury, J. (1996). NACP, a protein implicated in Alzheimer's disease and learning, is natively unfolded. *Biochemistry*, **35**, 13709–15.

West, H., Rebeck, G. & Hyman, B. (1994). Frequency of the apolipoprotein E ϵ2 allele is diminished in sporadic Alzheimer disease. *Neurosci. Lett.*, **175**, 46–8.

Wood, S.J., Wypych, J., Steavenson, S., Louis, J-C., Citron, M & Biere, A.L. (1999). α-Synuclein fibrillogenesis is nucleation-dependent: implications for the pathogenesis of Parkinson's disease. *J. Biol. Chem.*, **274**, 19509–512.

Woodward, J.S. (1962). Concentric hyaline inclusion body formation in mental disease. Analysis of twenty-seven cases. *J. Neuropathol. Exp. Neurol.*, **21**, 442–9.

Xu, W., Liu, L., Emson, P. et al. (2000). The CCTTT polymorphism in the NOS2A gene is associated with dementia with Lewy bodies. *Neuroreport*, **11**, 297–9.

Zhou, W., Hurlbert, M.S., Schaack, J., Prasad, K.N. & Freed, C. R. (2000). Overexpression of human α-synuclein causes dopamine neuron death in rat primary culture and immortalized mesencephalon-derived cells. *Brain Res.*, **866**, 33–43.

19

Frontotemporal dementia

Bruce L. Miller,[1] Howard J. Rosen[1] and Michael D. Greicius[2]

[1] Department of Neurology, UCSF School of Medicine, San Francisco, CA, USA
[2] Department of Psychiatry and Behavioral Sciences, Stanford, CA, USA

Historically, classification schemas for degenerative dementias were framed around the clinical and pathological phenomenology of the illness. With improved understanding of the molecular basis for many degenerative conditions, traditional taxonomies are being replaced by molecule-based schemas. Nowhere has this transition been more evident than with frontotemporal dementia (FTD) where, until recently, FTD (or Pick's disease) was used to define a group of patients with selective degeneration of frontotemporal cortex in whom Alzheimer's disease (AD) pathology was absent. With the discovery of tau exon mutations (Poorkaj et al., 1998; Spillantini & Goedert, 1998; Clark et al., 1998) and intron mutations (Hutton et al., 1998) in familial cases with selective frontotemporal degeneration, a clinical/pathological syndrome suddenly had a well-defined molecular and genetic basis. This work clarified the importance of tau protein in the pathogenesis of both sporadic and familial FTD and many hoped that this would lead to a molecule-based diagnostic schema for FTD. However, not all cases with tau pathology have selective frontotemporal anatomic involvement and there are many patients with selective frontotemporal degeneration in whom tau pathology is absent (Kertesz et al., 2000). This has left the field somewhat in limbo with many patients falling in between clinical, pathological or molecule-based diagnostic criteria. Thus, although new insights about abnormalities in tau metabolism are an important piece of the FTD story, it is clear that other factors contribute to producing the clinical syndrome that is recognizable as FTD.

Despite still unresolved issues related to nomenclature, FTD represents an important disorder with distinctive epidemiology, genetics, neuropathology, clinical features and treatment. Importantly, it is possible to diagnose most FTD patients during life (Lopez et al., 1999) and to differentiate them from patients with AD. Because FTD has a distinctive pattern or brain degeneration, it offers many clues to the function of the frontal and anterior cortical regions.

Terminology and epidemiology

In recent years FTD has been recognized as a common cause for degenerative dementia. However, in many clinical settings FTD is rarely, if ever, diagnosed. One problem limiting its recognition is that many patients present with psychiatric symptoms (Gustafson, 1993; Lesser et al., 1989) and do not develop a dementia until much later in the course of their illness. Persistent variability in the diagnostic accuracy and diagnostic suspicion from site to site has compounded the confusion related to the epidemiological features of FTD. Indeed, defining the disease has proven difficult from its very beginnings. The term Pick's disease was coined not by Pick, but by two of his students, Onari and Spatz (Berrios, 1996). Although for many decades Pick's disease has been considered as a frontal lobe degeneration associated with neuronal inclusions, Arnold Pick had more interest in focal temporal than focal frontal atrophy. Similarly, the Pick body that carries Pick's name was first described by Alzheimer, and Pick never focused upon the microscopic features of FTD (Berrios, 1996). For many years after Pick's original discoveries, investigators took a restrictive view of the frontotemporal dementias, limiting the diagnosis to cases that demonstrated the classic neuropathological findings of Pick's disease, frontal atrophy with Pick bodies and Pick cells (silver-staining neuronal inclusions). Basing a diagnosis of a degenerative disorder upon the presence or absence of a sometimes-elusive silver-staining inclusion has always been problematic. Many FTD patients have inclusions that do not stain with silver, while other FTD cases lack any cellular inclusions (Nasreddine et al., 1999).

Beginning in the 1980s, investigators began to take a more inclusive view of FTD. Brun and Gustafson from Lund, Sweden and Neary and Snowden from Manchester, England, began considering all cases of non-AD, presenile dementia with frontal lobe atrophy under the category of frontal dementia (Brun, 1987; Neary et al., 1987). Although most investigators continued to separate patients with classical Pick bodies from those without these inclusions, some suggested an even more unified approach classifying all such cases under the category of Pick-Complex disorder (Kertesz et al., 1999). The term FTD was coined in 1994 by the Lund–Manchester groups in an attempt to establish reliable diagnostic criteria for a clinically heterogeneous group of disorders that still shared many pathological features (Brun et al., 1994). Recent advances in molecular genetics have supported the validity of this more inclusive perspective. In 1998 these criteria were modified further and the new diagnostic criteria for FTD divided frontotemporal dementias into three subgroups; primary progressive aphasia, semantic dementia and frontotemporal dementia.

The most frequently cited prevalence figures for FTD come from Europe. Based on clinical, pathologic, and imaging studies, these groups estimate that 12–16% of presenile dementias suffer from frontal lobe atrophy without AD pathology (Neary et al., 1988; Brun, 1987). Fewer than 20% of these cases show the classic pathologic findings of Pick's disease. FTD's true prevalence remains unknown but the disease is relatively common. If AD has a prevalence of four million (Evans et al., 1989) and is somewhere between 10 to 20 times more common than FTD, this would still leave FTD with a prevalence of somewhere between 200 000 and 400 000 cases.

Genetics

Roughly 40% of FTD cases are familial with up to 80% of these familial cases inherited in an autosomal dominant pattern (Gustafson, 1987; Chow et al., 1999). Wilhelmsen and colleagues made a major stride toward defining the genetic basis for this condition in 1994 with linkage of a familial FTD syndrome to chromosome 17 (Wilhelmsen et al., 1994). In 1998 came the discovery of at least ten new exonic or intronic mutations in at least 20 different families with FTD (Poorkaj et al., 1998; Spillantini & Goedert, 1998; Clark et al., 1998; Hutton et al., 1998). These families were extraordinarily diverse both in their clinical and pathological features, despite the fact that they carried nearly identical genetic mutations. In some families clinical features were dominated by frontal lobe degeneration (Lynch et al.,

1994), while in others the presentation was shaped by loss of function in the amygdala and anterior temporal lobe (Bird et al., 1999). More recently, cases suggestive of corticobasal ganglionic degeneration (Bugiani et al., 1999) or progressive supranuclear palsy (Reed et al., 1998) have been noted, broadening the phenotype of familial-FTD. Remarkably in one family, a tau mutation led to frontotemporal degeneration in a father with a clinical presentation of corticobasal ganglionic degeneration in the son (Bugiani et al., 1999). Based upon clinical features alone, it is difficult to differentiate a sporadic from a genetic case of FTD.

The neuropathological cases with familial FTD linked to tau mutations show neuronal inclusions that stain positively for tau suggesting abnormal cellular processing of tau (Reed et al., 1998). In some families tau-staining neuronal inclusions alone are prominent, while in others, glial inclusions are also present. Even though neuronal inclusions are evident in most of the families, classical silver-staining Pick bodies are uncommon (Nasreddine et al., 1999). Neurofibrillary tangles are present in some cases, but absent in most. The majority of cases of FTD linked to chromosome 17 have demonstrated a mutation in tau (Heutink, 2000), although four kindreds with linkage to chromosome 17 have yet to yield specific mutations in the tau gene. Recently, Lee and colleagues found that in one of these families an absence of brain tau was a characteristic feature: so-called 'no tau tauopathy'. (Zhukareva et al., 2001). In total, these cases suggest that overexpression or underexpression of tau, or expression of mutated tau represent a major risk factor for FTD. Some even suggested that FTD should be considered a tauopathy.

However, the initial excitement for tau has been tempered. Not all familial cases of FTD are caused by tau gene mutations. At least three families have been identified which do not show linkage to the tau region of chromosome 17 (Gasser et al., 1996) and almost no sporadic cases have demonstrated tau mutations (Rizzu et al., 1999). Estimates of familial FTD cases with a known mutation in tau range from less than 10% up to 40% (Houlden et al., 1999; Rizzu et al., 1999). Similarly, other chromosomal locations have been found in familial FTD including chromosome three (Brown et al., 1995). Additionally, the mixture of FTD and amyotrophic lateral sclerosis has been linked to chromosomes 9 (Hosler et al., 2000) and 15 (K.C. Wilhelmsen et al., personal communication).

Pathology and pathogenesis

The more inclusive view of FTD includes patients with classical Pick's disease as well as those with the other non-

AD dementias with frontal or temporal lobe atrophy. The unifying feature across all these cases is the presence of focal atrophy in the frontal lobes, the temporal lobes, or both. The gross pattern of atrophy in FTD can have a unilateral predominance or it can be symmetrical and bilateral. In the temporal lobes the more anterior regions typically show greater pathology than the posterior regions. The amygdala, for example, shows more involvement than does the hippocampus (Brun, 1999), and the posterior parietal and temporal-occipital regions are relatively preserved. Subcortical structures such as the substantia nigra, putamen, and globus pallidus may show marked involvement by microscopy. Those cases with a motor neuron component also show pathological changes in the anterior horn cells.

The microscopic changes in the affected regions include neuronal loss, synaptic loss, gliosis, and spongiosis often most prominent in the first three cortical layers (Brun, 1993). Some cases of FTD demonstrate swollen neurons with inclusion bodies. Only a minority of the cases with cellular inclusions will exhibit the classic silver staining that is typical of a Pick body. However, in many cases 'Pick-like' inclusions in both neurons and glia that are not silver staining are identified (Nasreddine et al., 1999). Recent work has shown that the silver-staining is due to deposition of three repeat tau rather than the four repeat isoform found in the other inclusions (Delacourte, 1999). Tau immunoreactivity is the most common finding in familial and sporadic FTD. Furthermore, the presence of tau-positive inclusions in progressive supranuclear palsy (PSP) and corticobasal ganglionic degeneration (CBD) has even prompted some to view PSP, CBD, and FTD as clinical variants of a 'tauopathy' (van Slegtenhorst et al., 2000).

Tau is a microtubule-associated protein that binds, stabilizes and promotes the assembly of microtubules (Hong et al., 1998). Depending on how the tau gene is transcribed, the microtubule-binding region of the protein can have either 3 or 4 tandem repeats of a 31–32 amino acid sequence yielding 3Rtau or 4Rtau (Spillantini & Goedert, 2000). Mutations in the tau gene can cause either altered binding properties of tau or changes in the ratio of 3R to 4Rtau. With exon mutations, altered binding properties cause a relative loss of function by destabilizing microtubules and disrupting axonal transport (Hong et al., 1998). Alternatively, altered binding properties may result in a toxic gain of function by providing an excess of free, cytoplasmic tau available to form insoluble protein aggregates. A number of tau gene mutations increase the amount of 4Rtau presumably resulting in a toxic gain of function caused by insoluble protein aggregates (Hong et al., 1998). Tau aggregates typically contain the 4R isoform, although the aggregates found in Pick bodies contain the 3R isoform (Delacourte, 1999). The significance of different filament morphologies within tau aggregates (paired helical filaments, straight filaments) and their differential prevalence in AD vs. FTD remains to be elucidated (Spillantini & Goedert, 2000). Transgenic mice with tau abnormalities have recently been developed and offer promise for better understanding the pathogenesis of FTD.

Mice expressing the P301L human mutations and mice overexpressing human tau develop behavioural and motor changes, remarkably similar to those seen in the human forms of this condition (Lewis et al., 2000; Ishihara et al., 1999). These changes develop within 6 months allowing researchers the opportunity of studying interventions related to abnormal tau processing that might accelerate or slow this process. However, there are many cases of FTD where abnormal tau is not visualized in the brain and tau does not unify all of FTD. Munoz (2000) has emphasized that there are tau-negative and ubiquitin positive inclusions in many of the cases of FTD associated with motor neuron disease and none of the families with both prominent FTD and motor neuron disease have shown tau mutations.

A few studies on the neurochemistry of FTD suggest a specific neurochemical profile. In particular, there are severe losses of brain serotonin, of both pre- and post-synaptic receptors (Sparks et al., 1991). In contrast, FTD is one of the few conditions where cholinergic cell concentration in the nucleus basalis of Meynert is normal (Sparks, et al., 1991). The changes with dopamine are more variable. These neuropathological findings suggest that the AD treatments based upon a cholinergic deficit are unlikely to work with FTD. The clinical symptoms of irritability, depression, compulsions and hyperorality may be explained by the loss of brain serotonin seen with FTD (Miller et al., 1995).

Diagnosis

The mean age of onset for FTD is the sixth decade, although formal diagnosis is often delayed for many years due to the insidious course and early predominance of behavioural symptoms. The clinical presentation of FTD can vary depending on where the disorder begins in the brain. The illness starts in the anterior frontal or temporal lobes (Miller et al., 1993; Hodges et al., 1992; Neary et al., 1987). Lifespan following a diagnosis of FTD can vary considerably with an 8–9 years on average (Rossor, 1999).

A consensus group delineated three main cognitive subtypes of FTD (Neary et al., 1998). The first, referred to as

FTD, is characterized mainly by behavioural changes and develops in the patient with degeneration in the frontal lobes bilaterally or unilaterally in the right frontal lobe. Patients with this subtype will demonstrate loss of normal social interactions and may become withdrawn or disinihibited. Other features include lack of insight or empathy for others, blunted affect, decreased grooming, hyperorality, perseverative behaviours and social inappropriateness (Rosen et al., 2000).

The second subtype is referred to as progressive nonfluent aphasia. These patients display expressive language dysfunction with effortful speech, word-finding difficulty, grammatical errors and relatively preserved comprehension. Behaviour and social conduct are often remarkably spared until late in the illness in patients with progressive non-fluent aphasia. Complicating this diagnosis is that some patients with selective left parietal degeneration present with non-fluent aphasia and many of these individuals suffer from AD, not FTD (Galton et al., 2000).

The last subtype outlined by the consensus group is semantic dementia (Snowden et al., 1989). Here, the bulk of the pathology occurs in the left anterior temporal lobe, but most cases also show involvement of the right anterior temporal lobe. These patients progressively lose their semantic knowledge of the world (facts, words, objects, etc.). The content of speech eventually deteriorates with loss of language specificity. Hawks become 'birds', then 'animals' and then 'things' (Graham et al., 1999). Naming and comprehension are impaired due to loss of word knowledge. Many of the semantic dementia cases have right as well as left temporal degeneration. This group shows loss of insight, disinhibition, disregard of interpersonal space, and antisocial behaviour (Miller et al., 1993). Those with the right temporal variant exhibit loss of empathy, irritability, fixed and rigid thinking, poor grooming, and decreased facial expression (Edwards-Lee et al., 1997). These clinical distinctions are most apparent earlier in the course and many ultimately progress to more global impairment in frontal and temporal lobe functions.

The current terminology for FTD is complex, even for the experienced neurologist. In particular, it excessively relies upon language based clinical syndromes such as semantic dementia. However, most FTD patients can be reliably diagnosed during life (McKhann et al., 2001). In one study, hyperorality, loss of personal conduct, disabling compulsions, progressive loss of speech and sparing of drawing separated 30 FTD patients from 30 with AD (Miller et al., 1997). In a recent study of autopsy-proven FTD cases we found that loss of social conduct, relative absence of amnesia and hyperorality separated the vast majority of FTD patients from those with AD.

In addition to the various cortical symptoms, some FTD patients will develop Parkinsonian features or symptoms of motor neuron disease. The Parkinsonian features overlap with progressive supranuclear palsy with falls, axial rigidity and ophthalmoplegia more common than tremor. Knopman and colleagues (Knopman et al., 1990; Munoz, 2000) suggest that nearly 80% of FTD patients demonstrate midbrain degeneration. In our cohort, nearly 15% of FTD patients developed symptoms of motor neuron disease during life.

Given the pronounced variation in initial presentation and the common early prominence of behavioural symptoms, misdiagnosis is a common problem for patients and their families. Clinical criteria alone can be useful in distinguishing FTD from AD. Increasingly, however, neuroimaging is being relied upon to increase both the sensitivity and specificity of the diagnosis. The addition of SPECT to clinical criteria has been shown to improve diagnostic accuracy to as high as 90% (Read et al., 1995). FTD patients tend to show bifrontal and bitemporal hypoperfusion vs. the typical temporal parietal defects seen in AD (Miller et al., 1991). Specific patterns of tissue loss which relate to the clinical presentation can often be appreciated with MRI scanning as well (see Fig. 19.1, in colour plate section). Additionally, FTD patients show global atrophy of the corpus callosum (Kaufer et al., 1997), while AD patients show selective atrophy of the third and fourth segments of the callosum. Structural MRI has also shown promise as a test to help distinguish FTD from AD and other dementias (Miller & Gearhart, 1999).

Treatment

There are few diseases in all of medicine that cause greater difficulties for a family than does FTD. Poor judgement in the work place, financial arena or home environment can lead to loss of income, financial devastation or legal difficulties. Because loss of insight is such a prominent feature of FTD it is often difficult to reason with the FTD patient. When family members are probed, they often describe puzzling social withdrawal and loss of concern in the patient that profoundly disrupts the family unit. This, in turn, can diminish the empathy for these patients that they truly deserve. Because apathy intervenes in nearly all cases, the later stages of FTD can be easier to manage than the initial stages (Levy et al., 1996).

Treatment of FTD is limited to the behavioural disorders and there are no known preventive therapies or therapies that improve cognition. No placebo-controlled studies of FTD have been performed, although open-label studies suggest that selective serotonin reuptake inhibitors may be beneficial in management of the disinhibition, depressive symptoms, carbohydrate craving, and/or compulsions frequently encountered in FTD (Swartz et al., 1997). Support for such an approach can be found in molecular studies showing low serotonin receptor binding in FTD (Sparks et al., 1991). Some behavioural symptoms may require more aggressive pharmacotherapy, including the use of antipsychotics, in which case, as with AD, the newer, atypical agents are favoured in order to minimize Parkinsonian side effects. Anticholinesterase medications do not appear to improve cognitive status and can worsen irritability (Perry, 2001).

References

Ashburner, J. & Friston, K.J. (2000). Voxel-based morphometry – the methods. *Neuroimage*, **11**, 805–21.

Berrios, G.E. (1996). *The History of Mental Symptoms: Descriptive Psychopathology Since the Nineteenth Century*. New York: Cambridge University Press, Cambridge.

Bird, T., Nochlin, D., Poorkaj, P. et al. (1999). A clinical pathological comparison of three families with frontotemporal dementia and identical mutations in the tau gene (P301L). *Brain*, **April**, 741–56.

Brown, J., Ashworth, A., Gydesen, S. et al. (1995). Familial non-specific dementia maps to chromosome 3. *Hum. Mol. Genet.*, **4**, 1625–8.

Brun, A. (1987). Frontal lobe degeneration of non-Alzheimer type. I. Neuropathology. *Arch. Gerontol.Geriatr.*, **6**, 193–208.

Brun, A. (1993). Frontal lobe degeneration of non-Alzheimer type revisited. *Dementia*, **4**, 126–31.

Brun, A. (1999). The emergence of the frontal lobe as opposed to the central lobe. *Dementia Geriat. Cogn. Disord.*, **10**, 3–5.

Brun, A., Englund, B., Gustafson, L. et al. (1994). Clinical and neuropathological criteria for frontotemporal dementia. *J. Neurol. Neurosurg. Psychiatry*, **57**, 416–18.

Bugiani, O., Murrell, J.R., Giaccone, G. et al. (1999). Frontotemporal dementia and corticobasal degeneration in a family with a P301S mutation in tau. *J. Neuropathol. Exper. Neurol.*, **58**, 667–77.

Chow, T.W., Miller, B.L., Hayashi, V.N. et al. (1999). Inheritance of frontotemporal dementia. *Arch. Neurol.*, **56**, 817–22.

Clark, L. N., Poorkaj, P., Wszolek, Z. et al. (1998). Pathogenic implications of mutations in the tau gene in pallido-ponto-nigral degeneration and related neurodegenerative disorders linked to chromosome 17. *Proc. Natl. Acad. Sci., USA*, **95**, 13103–7.

Delacourte, A. (1999). Biochemical and molecular characterization of neurofibrillary degeneration in frontotemporal dementias, *Dement. Geriatr. Cogn. Disord.*, **Suppl. 1**, 75–9.

Edwards-Lee, T., Miller, B.L., Benson, D.F. et al. (1997). The temporal variant of frontotemporal dementia. *Brain*, **120**, 1027–40.

Evans, D A., Funkenstein, H.H. & Albert, M.S. (1989). Prevalence of Alzheimer's disease in a community population of older persons. *J. Am. Med. Assoc.*, **18**, 2551–6.

Galton, C.J., Patterson, K., Xuereb, J.H. et al. (2000). Atypical and typical presentations of Alzheimer's disease: a clinical, neuro-psychological, neuroimaging and pathological study of 13 cases, *Brain*, **123** (3), 484–98.

Gasser, T., Wszolek, Z., Supala, A. et al. (1996). Genetic linkage studies in autosomal dominantly inherited L-DOPA responsive parkinsonism. Evaluation of candidate genes. *Adv. Neurol.*, **69**, 87–95.

Graham, K.S., Patterson, K. & Hodges, J.R. (1999). Episodic memory: new insights from the study of semantic dementia. *Curr. Opin. Neurobiol.*, **9**, 245–50.

Gustafson, L. (1987). Frontal lobe degeneration of non-Alzheimer type. II. Clinical picture and differential diagnosis. *Arch. Gerontol. Geriatr.*, **6**, 209–23.

Gustafson, L. (1993). Clinical picture of frontal lobe degeneration of non-Alzheimer type. *Dementia*, **4**, 143–8.

Heutink, P. (2000). Untangling tau-related dementia. *Hum. Mol. Genet.*, **9**, 979–86.

Hodges, J.R., Patterson, K., Oxbury, S. et al. (1992). Semantic dementia. Progressive fluent aphasia with temporal lobe atrophy. *Brain*, **115**, 1783–806.

Hong, M., Zhukareva, V., Vogelsberg-Ragaglia, V. et al. (1998). Mutation-specific functional impairments in distinct tau iso-forms of hereditary FTDP-17. *Science*, **282**, 1914–17.

Hosler, B.A., Siddique, T., Sapp, P.C. et al. (2000). Linkage of familial amyotrophic lateral sclerosis with frontotemporal dementia to chromosome 9q21–q22. *J. Am. Med. Ass.*, **284**, 1664–9.

Houlden, H., Baker, M., Adamson, J. et al. (1999). Frequency of tau mutations in three series of non-Alzheimer's degenerative dementia. *Ann. Neurol.*, **46**, 243–8.

Hutton, M., Lendon, C.L., Rizzu, P. et al. (1998). Association of mis-sense and 5'-splice-site mutations in tau with the inherited dementia FTDP-17. *Nature*, **393**, 702–5.

Ishihara, T., Hong, M., Zhang, B. et al. (1999). Age-dependent emergence and progression of a tauopathy in transgenic mice overex-pressing the shortest human tau isoform. *Neuron*, **24**, 751–62.

Kaufer, D.I., Miller, B.L., Itti, L. et al. (1997). Midline cerebral morphometry distinguishes frontotemporal dementia and Alzheimer's disease. *Neurology*, **48**, 978–85.

Kertesz, A., Davidson, W. & Munoz, D.G. (1999). Clinical and pathological overlap between frontotemporal dementia, primary progressive aphasia and corticobasal degeneration: the Pick complex. *Dement. Geriatr. Cogn. Disord.*, 10, 46–9.

Kertesz, A., Kawarai, T., Rogaeva, E. et al. (2000). Familial fronto-temporal dementia with ubiquitin-positive, tau-negative inclusions. *Neurology*, **54**, 818–27.

Knopman, D.S., Mastri, A.R., Frey, W.H.D. et al. (1990). Dementia lacking distinctive histologic features: a common non-Alzheimer degenerative dementia. *Neurology*, **40**, 251–6.

Lesser, I., Miller, B., Boone, K. et al. (1989). Psychosis as the first manifestation of degenerative dementia. *Bull. Clin. Neurosci.*, **4**, 59–64.

Levy, M.L., Miller, B.L., Cummings, J.L. et al. (1996). Alzheimer disease and frontotemporal dementias: behavioural distinctions. *Arch. Neurol.*, **53**, 687–90.

Lewis, J., McGowan, E., Rockwood, J. et al. (2000). Neurofibrillary tangles, amyotrophy and progressive motor disturbance in mice expressing mutant (P301L) tau protein. *Nat. Genet.*, **25**, 402–5.

Lopez, O. L., Litvan, I., Catt, K. E. et al. (1999). Accuracy of four clinical diagnostic criteria for the diagnosis of neurodegenerative dementias. *Neurology*, **53**, 1292–9.

Lynch, T., Sano, M., Marder, K. S. et al. (1994). Clinical characteristics of a family with chromosome 17-linked disinhibition–dementia–parkinsonism–amyotrophy complex [see comments]. *Neurology*, **44**, 1878–84.

McKhann, G.M., Albert, M.S., Grossman, M., Miller, B., Dickson, D. & Trojanowski, J.R. (2001). Clinical and pathological diagnosis of frontotemporal dementia: report of the work group on frontotemporal dementia and Pick's disease. *Arch. Neurol.*, **58**, 1803–9.

Miller, B.L. & Gearhart, R. (1999). Neuroimaging in the diagnosis of frontotemporal dementia. *Dement. Geriatr. Cogn. Disord.*, **10**, 71–4.

Miller, B.L., Cummings, J.L., Villanueva-Meyer, J. et al. (1991). Frontal lobe degeneration: clinical, neuropsychological, and SPECT characteristics. *Neurology*, **41**, 1374–82.

Miller, B.L., Chang, L., Mena, I. et al. (1993). Progressive right frontotemporal degeneration: clinical, neuropsychological and SPECT characteristics. *Dementia*, **4**, 204–13.

Miller, B.L., Darby, A.L., Swartz, J.R. et al. (1995). Dietary changes, compulsions and sexual behavior in frontotemporal degeneration. *Dementia*, **6**, 195–9.

Miller, B.L., Ikonte, C., Ponton, M. et al. (1997). A study of the Lund-Manchester research criteria for frontotemporal dementia: clinical and single-photon emission CT correlations. *Neurology*, **48**, 937–42.

Munoz, D. (2000). Neuropathology of frontotemporal dementia. *Neurologia*, **Suppl. 1**, 2–8.

Nasreddine, Z.S., Loginov, M., Clark, L.N. et al. (1999). From genotype to phenotype: a clinical pathological, and biochemical investigation of frontotemporal dementia and parkinsonism (FTDP-17) caused by the P301L tau mutation. *Ann. Neurol.*, **45**, 704–15.

Neary, D., Snowden, J. S., Shields, R. A. et al. (1987). Single photon emission tomography using 99mTc-HM-PAO in the investigation of dementia, *J. Neurol. Neurosurg. Psychiatry*, **50**, 1101–09.

Neary, D., Snowden, J.S., Northen, B. et al. (1988). Dementia of frontal lobe type. *J. Neurol. Neurosurg. Psychiatry*, **51**, 353–61.

Neary, D., Snowden, J.S., Gustafson, L. et al. (1998). Frontotemporal lobar degeneration: a consensus on clinical diagnostic criteria. *Neurology*, **51**, 1546–54.

Perry, R.J. & Miller, B.L. (2001). Behavior and treatment in frontotemporal dementia. *Neurology*, **56** (11Suppl. 4), S46–S51.

Poorkaj, P., Bird, T.D., Wijsman, E. et al. (1998). Tau is a candidate gene for chromosome 17 frontotemporal dementia [published erratum appears in *Ann Neurol* 1998 Sep; 44(3): 428]. *Ann. Neurol.*, **43**, 815–25.

Read, S.L., Miller, B.L., Mena, I. et al. (1995). SPECT in dementia: clinical and pathological correlation, *J. Am. Geriatr. Soc.*, **43**, 1243–7.

Reed, L.A., Schmidt, M.L., Wszolek, Z.K. et al. (1998). The neuropathology of a chromosome 17-linked autosomal dominant parkinsonism and dementia ('pallido-ponto-nigral degeneration'). *J. Neuropathol. Exp. Neurol.*, **57**, 588–601.

Rizzu, P., Van Swieten, J.C., Joosse, M. et al. (1999). High prevalence of mutations in the microtubule-associated protein tau in a population study of frontotemporal dementia in the Netherlands. *Am. J. Hum. Genet.*, **64**, 414–21.

Rosen, H.J., Lengenfelder, J. & Miller, B. (2000). Frontotemporal dementia. *Neurol. Clin.*, **18**.

Rossor, M.N. (1999). Differential diagnosis of frontotemporal dementia: Pick's disease. *Dement. Geriatr. Cogn. Disord.*, **10**, 43–5.

Snowden, J.S., Goulding, P.J. & Neary, D. (1989). Semantic dementia: a form of circumscribed cerebral atrophy. *Behav. Neurol.*, **2**, 167–82.

Sparks, D.L., Woeltz, V.M. & Markesbery, W.R. (1991). Alterations in brain monoamine oxidase activity in aging, Alzheimer's disease, and Pick's disease. *Arch. Neurol.*, **48**, 718–21.

Spillantini, M.G. & Goedert, M. (1998). Tau protein pathology in neurodegenerative diseases, *Trends Neurol. Sci.*, **21**, 428–33.

Spillantini, M.G. & Goedert, M. (2000). Tau mutations in familial frontotemporal dementia. *Brain*, **123**, 857–9.

Swartz, J.R., Miller, B.L., Lesser, I.M. et al. (1997). Frontotemporal dementia: treatment response to serotonin selective reuptake inhibitors [published erratum appears in *J. Clin. Psychiatry*, 1997 Jun; 58(6): 275], *J. Clin. Psychiatry*, **58**, 212–16.

van Slegtenhorst, M., Lewis, J. & Hutton, M. (2000). The molecular genetics of the tauopathies. *Exp. Gerontol.*, **35**, 461–471.

Wilhelmsen, K.C., Lynch, T., Pavlou, E. et al. (1994). Localization of disinhibition–dementia–parkinsonism–amyotrophy complex to 17q21–22, *Am. J. Hum. Genet.*, **55**, 1159–65.

Zhukareva, V., Vogelsberg-Ragaglia, V., Van Deerlin, V.M. et al. (2001). Loss of brain tau defines novel sporadic and familial tauopathies with frontotemporal dementia. *Ann. Neurol.*, **49**, 165–75.

20

Consciousness and its disorders

Antonio R. Damasio

Department of Neurology, University of Iowa College of Medicine, Iowa City, IA, USA

Background and working definition of consciousness

It is generally acknowledged that understanding the neurobiological mechanisms responsible for consciousness is one of the most difficult tasks in the agenda of neuroscience. At first glance, however, the notion of consciousness appears uncontroversial, and it has even been claimed that since everyone is conscious and the notion of consciousness obvious, there is hardly any need to define the phenomenon. Clinicians, neurologists and others tend to believe that determining whether consciousness is present or not is a simple matter. The view presented in this chapter, however, is less optimistic. Although experts and non-experts can come to an agreement on what constitutes the essence of consciousness, the full scope of the phenomena described under that term requires careful consideration and a provisional definition that can guide clinical evaluations and research. Both fundamental scientists and neurologists need a working concept of consciousness, and nothing prevents us from possibly modifying that concept in the future according to new evidence. Moreover, given the particular nature of consciousness, there are no standard neuropsychological tools to assess its impairments, and there may never be. Also, because the study of those phenomena is of recent vintage, we do not have yet available diagnostic imaging procedures for the evaluation of such impairments. For these reasons, the assessment of patients with impairments of consciousness relies primarily on systematic and comprehensive clinical observations, complemented by a good history and by fine structural neuroimaging and electrophysiologic studies.

Whether one consults a good dictionary, a neurology textbook, or a psychology textbook, the current definitions of consciousness one is likely to encounter are fairly similar: the definitions state that consciousness is the ability to be aware of self and surroundings. These are hardly ideal definitions, considering that consciousness is being defined in terms of awareness and that awareness and consciousness are usually regarded as synonyms. In spite of their awkwardness, however, these definitions capture something that we can agree on: 'consciousness is the ability to know of our own existence and of the existence of objects and events, inside and outside our organism'. Our proposed working definition of consciousness is in line with this idea and states that consciousness is 'a momentary creation of mental knowledge which describes a relation between the organism, on the one hand, and an object or event, on the other'; the definition also indicates that 'the presence of consciousness, as a mental phenomenon, is accompanied by certain observable behaviours'. To be conscious, at a given moment, is to have a sense of our own organism in the act of knowing an object (or event). Consciousness is not just about the object being known; it is always about the owner of the organism in the process of knowing. Individuals whom we describe as conscious are generating, continuously, 'moments of consciousness' which conjoin organism and object. They are generating in a seamless manner multiple and consecutive periods of mental knowledge along with the external behaviours that accompany such knowledge. (For more on the cognitive and neuroscientific background for this definition see Damasio, 1998, 2000. For other views on the phenomena of consciousness from philosophical, cognitive and neurobiological perspectives see Baars, 1988; Crick, 1994; Dennett, 1991; Edelman, 1989; Metzinger, 1995, 2000; Searle, 1992.)

A practical consequence of this definition is that consciousness must be considered from two standpoints: the external (or behavioural), and the internal (cognitive or mental). Taking the external standpoint, the human organism can be said to be conscious when it exhibits sustained attention towards objects and events in its environment and when it gives evidence of sustained purposeful behaviour relative to those objects and events. The temporal scale for the qualification of 'sustained' is in the order of minutes, not seconds (a practical yardstick is 10 minutes). From the internal standpoint, a human organism can be said to be conscious if its mental state represents objects and events in relation to itself, in other words, if the representation of objects and events is accompanied by a sense that the organism is in the act of perceiving, that the perception is owned by the organism and established in its perspective.

The fundamental components of consciousness: mind and self

From the internal standpoint, we regard consciousness as a combination of two related processes. The first is the process of generating inside the human organism the mental patterns we call images, relative to an object or event. (By object we mean entities as diverse as a person, a place, a melody, state of localized pain, or a state of feeling; by image we mean a mental pattern in any of the sensory modalities, e.g. a sound image, a tactile image, the image of a state of pain or well being that is conveyed by visceral senses; images convey the physical characteristics of an object or the reaction of like or dislike one may have for an object or the plans one may formulate for it, or the relationships of the object to other objects.) The images that constitute the fabric of the mind are integrated spatially and temporally, across sensory modalities. For example, when we watch a person talking, we generate visual images of the person and also auditory images of her speech, yet those two streams of images are synchronized and spatially coherent, as we can verify by noting that the lip movements are in sync with the speech sounds, and the sound waves come from the appropriate region in space.

This first process of consciousness, then, consists of generating neural patterns in neural circuits and turning those neural patterns into the mental patterns we call images. When we commonly use the term consciousness, however, and certainly when we talk about consciousness according to the working definition provided earlier, we are referring to more than this first process of 'mind', to more than the process of generating spatially and temporally integrated mental images. We are also referring to a second process, that of engendering a sense of 'self in the act of knowing', a process that is parallel to, and combined with that of, engendering mental patterns for an object. This process allows the images of an object and of the complex matrix of relations, reactions, and plans related to it, to be sensed as

the unmistakable mental property of an automatic owner who becomes an observer, a knower and a potential actor. This process allows us to know that we own our minds, and that the contents in our minds are shaped in a particular perspective, that of the individual inside of whom the mind is formed. This second process of consciousness allows us to construct not just the mental patterns of objects and events, the temporally and spatially unified images of persons, places, melodies, and of their relationships, but also the mental patterns which convey, automatically and naturally, the sense of a self in the act of knowing. The process of mind and the process of self are so intimately related that the latter is nested within the former. In effect, the second process is that of generating the appearance of an owner and observer for the mind, within that same mind (Damasio, 2000).

Kinds of consciousness

Consciousness can be separated into simple and complex kinds, and the evidence from neurological patients makes the separation transparent. The simplest kind, which we call core consciousness, provides the organism with a sense of self about one moment, now, and about one place, here. The scope of core consciousness is the here and now. Core consciousness does not illuminate the future, and the only past it vaguely lets us glimpse is that which occurred in the instant just before. The complex kind of consciousness, which we call extended consciousness and of which there are many levels, provides the organism with an elaborate sense of self, and places that self in individual historical time, in a perspective of both the lived past and the anticipated future. Core consciousness is a simple, biological phenomenon; it has one single level of organization; it is stable across the lifetime of the organism; and it is not dependent on conventional memory, working memory, reasoning, or language. Extended consciousness is a complex biological phenomenon; it has several levels of organization; and it evolves across the lifetime of the organism.

Extended consciousness is built on the foundation of core consciousness. Neurological impairments reveal that impairment of extended consciousness allows core consciousness to remain intact. This is exemplified by patients with profound disturbances of autobiographical memory caused by global amnesia. By contrast, impairments of core consciousness entail the collapse of extended consciousness, as happens in akinetic mutisms, absence seizures and epileptic automatisms, persistent vegetative state, coma, deep sleep (dreamless), and deep anesthesia. When core consciousness fails, in keeping with its foundational nature, extended consciousness fails as well.

To the two kinds of consciousness, correspond two kinds of self. The sense of self which emerges in core consciousness is the core self, a transient entity, ceaselessly recreated for each and every object with which the brain interacts. Our traditional notion of self, however, is linked to the idea of personhood and identity, and corresponds to a non-transient collection of unique facts and ways of being which characterize a person, the autobiographical self. The autobiographical self depends on systematized memories of situations in which core consciousness was involved in the knowing of the most invariant characteristics of an organism's biography (Damasio, 2000).

Other components of consciousness

In addition to separating the processes of mind and self within the larger process of consciousness, and in addition to distinguishing kinds of consciousness related to their complexity, it is important to tease apart subcomponents that contribute to consciousness but are not the same as consciousness. This componential analysis is vital both for research and for clinical assessment, and is usually neglected to the peril of proper research and diagnosis. For example, it is possible to separate consciousness in general from functions such as wakefulness, low-level attention, working memory, high-level (focused) attention, conventional memory, language, and reasoning.

Core consciousness is not the same as wakefulness or low-level attention, although it requires both to operate normally. Patients with absence seizures or automatisms or akinetic mutism are technically awake but not conscious. On the other hand, patients who lose wakefulness can no longer be conscious, the only exception to this rule being dream sleep.

Core consciousness is also not the same as holding an image over time, a process known as working memory (see Baddeley, 1992; Smith et al., 1996). The sense of self and of knowing is so brief and so abundantly produced, that there is no need to hold it over time in order for it to be effective. However, working memory is vital for the process of extended consciousness.

Core consciousness does not depend on making a stable memory of an image or recalling it, i.e. it does not depend on the processes of conventional learning and memory. Core consciousness is not based on language either. No less importantly, core consciousness is not the same as manipulating an image intelligently in processes such as planning, problem solving, and creativity. Patients with profound defects of reasoning and planning may exhibit normal core consciousness although the higher levels of extended consciousness may be compromised. In brief,

wakefulness, image making, attention, working memory, conventional memory, language, intelligence, can be separated by appropriate analysis and investigated separately in spite of the fact that they operate in concert to permit consciousness or assist with functions that require consciousness, such as reasoning.

The relation between emotion and core consciousness, on the other hand, is quite different. Emotion and core consciousness are associated. Patients whose core consciousness is impaired do not reveal emotion by facial expression, body expression, or vocalization. The entire range of emotion, from background emotions to secondary emotions, is usually missing in these patients. By contrast, patients with preserved core consciousness but impaired extended consciousness have normal background and primary emotions. This association suggests that some of the neural devices on which both emotion and core consciousness depend are located within the same region.

Consciousness as a central resource

Disturbances of core consciousness affect the whole of mental activity and the full range of sensory modalities. Patients with disturbed core consciousness, from those with coma and persistent vegetative state to those with epileptic automatisms, akinetic mutisms, and absence seizures, have no island of preserved consciousness and the impairment covers mental images originating from all sensory modalities. Core consciousness serves the entire compass of mental images, i.e. of thoughts that can be made conscious. It is a central resource.

By contrast, the impairment of image making within one sensory modality, for example, visual or auditory, compromises only the conscious appreciation of one aspect of an object, e.g. the visual or the auditory, but does not even compromise consciousness of the same object through a different sensory channel, e.g. olfactory or tactile. Naturally, because consciousness operates on images, an impairment of all image-making capability abolishes consciousness altogether. The sensory processing for a sensory modality may be lost in its entirety as in cortical blindness, or one aspect of the modality may be lost, as in achromatopsia, or a substantial part of a process may be disrupted, as in prosopagnosia (Damasio et al., 1990). Those patients have a disturbance of the processing of the object to be known, but they have normal core consciousness for all the images formed in other sensory modalities, and they even have normal core consciousness for the specific stimuli that they fail to process normally. Patients who cannot recognize a previously familiar face have normal core consciousness for the stimulus that confronts them, and are fully aware that they do not recognize a face that others expect them to. Those patients have normal core consciousness, and a normal extended consciousness outside of the island of defective knowledge. Their circumscribed defect underscores the fact that core consciousness and its resulting sense of self is a central resource.

The fact that core consciousness is separable from other cognitive processes does not mean that consciousness does not have an influence on them. On the contrary, core consciousness assists with the focusing and enhancement of attention and working memory; favours the establishment of memories; is indispensable for the normal operations of language; enlarges the scope of intelligent manipulations of images, e.g. planning, problem solving and creativity.

The clinical evaluation of consciousness

One of the notable areas of recent progress in neurology and neuroscience came from the development of standardized neuropsychological testing instruments which allow both clinicians and researchers to measure a large range of cognitive performances, from those related to reasoning, attention, and perceptual abilities, to those related to learning and memory, language, and personality. As noted, however, no comparable tests are available or are likely to become available to assess most impairments of consciousness. More often than not, consciousness is either normal (in which case a large range of other neuropsychological functions can be evaluated and found intact or disturbed), or so impaired that assessment of any neuropsychological functions is only possible indirectly by means of careful clinical observations.

Because the study of human consciousness requires both internal and external views, the investigation of consciousness is partially indirect. Behavioural acts are expressions of the mental process, but they are not the same thing as the mental process that precedes or accompanies them. The same is true of any kind of encephalogram, electrical or magnetic, and of functional imaging scans. All of these methods of analysis capture only correlates of the mental process.; they are not the same as the mental process. The fact that mental processes are only accessible to the organism who owns them, however, does not preclude their characterization through appropriate cognitive approaches, and the connection between the result of those characterizations and the correlates obtained through external approaches.

Table 20.1. The key areas of behavioural observation in the assessment of consciousness

State of wakefulness
Presence of background emotions
Presence of basic and sustained attention
Presence of purposeful behaviour

As noted, although consciousness occurs in the interior of an organism it is associated with a number of external manifestations. Those manifestations do not translate the internal process in the same direct way that a spoken sentence translates a thought, but there they are available to observation as correlates and signs of the presence of consciousness. Based on what we know about private human minds and on what we know and can observe of human behaviour, it is possible to establish a three-way correspondence among: (a) certain external manifestations, e.g. wakefulness, background emotions, attention, specific behaviours; (b) the corresponding internal manifestations of the human being having those behaviours as reported by that human being; and (c) the internal manifestations that we, as observers, can verify in ourselves when we are in circumstances equivalent to those of the observed individual. This three-way correspondence permits us to make reasonable inferences about human internal mental states based on external behaviours.

In brief, the contemporary approach to studying the biological basis of the private human mind involves two steps. The first step consists of observing and measuring the actions of an experimental subject; or collecting and measuring the reports of internal experience offered by a subject or both. The second step consists of relating the collected evidence to the measured manifestation of one of the neurobiological phenomena we are beginning to understand, at the level of molecules, neurons, neural circuits, or systems of circuits.

The evaluation of the state of consciousness in a neurological or psychiatric patient should concentrate on analysing their wakefulness, background emotions, attention, and purposeful behaviour. Let us consider these varied processes individually (Table 20.1).

Wakefulness

Wakefulness is easy to establish on the basis of a few objective signs. The eyes of the subject should be open; the muscular tone should be compatible with movements against gravity; and the electroencephalogram should reveal the characteristic awake EEG pattern. Normal consciousness requires wakefulness, but the presence of wakefulness does not guarantee normal consciousness. As noted below, patients with impaired consciousness in conditions such as persistent vegetative state, epileptic automatisms, and akinetic mutisms, are technically awake. Wakefulness is disrupted in coma, general anesthesia, and during episodes of fainting.

Background emotion

The term emotion usually conjures up the primary emotions, e.g. fear, anger, sadness, happiness, disgust, or the secondary emotions, e.g. embarrassment, guilt, pride, but the field of emotion also includes background emotions, those that occur in continual form when the organism is not engaged in either primary or secondary emotions. Background emotions are experienced in configurations of body movement, in the face, the trunk and the limbs, and suggest to the observer states such as fatigue or energy; discouragement or enthusiasm; malaise or well-being; anxiety or relaxation. The continuity of background emotions is an important fact to consider in our observation of normal human behaviour. When we observe someone with intact consciousness, well before any words are spoken, we find ourselves presuming the subject's state of mind. Correct or not, the presumptions are largely based on the emotional signals available in the subject's behaviour. Importantly, normal consciousness is accompanied by background emotions, and the absence of background emotions usually betrays impairments of consciousness.

Attention

Besides exhibiting wakefulness and background emotions, conscious subjects also exhibit attention. They orient themselves toward objects and concentrate on them as needed. Eyes, head, neck, torso, and arms move about in a coordinated pattern which establishes an unequivocal relationship between subject and certain stimuli in their surround. The mere presence of attention toward an external object usually signifies the presence of consciousness, but there are exceptions. Patients in states of so-called akinetic mutism, whose consciousness is impaired, can pay transient attention to a salient object or event, for example, a phone ringing, a tray with food, an observer calling their name. Attention only guarantees the presence of consciousness when it can be sustained, over a substantial period of time, focused on the objects or events that must be considered for behaviour to be appropriate in a given context. This period of time is measured in many minutes and hours rather than seconds. As noted, a sample of 10 minutes is usually sufficient. Another important qualification is needed. Lack of attention toward an external object may indicate that attention is being directed toward an internally represented mental object and does not necessarily indicate impaired consciousness. This is the basis for absentmindedness. Sustained failure of attention as happens in drowsiness, confusional states, or stupor, is associated with the dissolution of consciousness. Attention is entirely disrupted in coma, general anesthesia, and episodes of fainting.

Conscious subjects are attentive to certain objects and concentrate on them, something that matches our own introspection when we think about our own mental events in comparable situations. Attention and consciousness are thus related, the former being necessary for the latter, but neither attention nor consciousness are monoliths. They occur in levels and grades, and they influence each other as they become more complex. Low-level attention is needed to engage the processes that generate core consciousness, but the process of core consciousness drives higher-level attention toward a focus.

Purposeful behaviour

The presence of adequate and purposeful behaviour is easy to establish in patients who can converse with the observer. When there are impairments of communication, however, the observation requires more detail. Conscious subjects behave purposefully toward the stimuli on which they concentrate, which means that their behaviour is part of an immediately recognizable plan that could only have been formulated by an organism cognizant of its immediate past, present, and anticipated future conditions. The sustained purposefulness and adequateness of behaviour requires the presence of consciousness even if consciousness does not guarantee purposeful and adequate behaviour. By sustained, we mean, once again, minutes to hours. A sample of 10 minutes, complete with evidence from the patient's history may be sufficient.

Sustained and adequate behaviour is accompanied by a flow of emotional states as part of their unfolding. The background emotions discussed above continuously underscore the subject's actions. Telltale signals include the overall body posture and the range of motion of the limbs relative to the trunk; the spatial profile of limb movements, which can be smooth or jerky; the speed of motions; the congruence of movements occurring in different body tiers such as face, hands, and legs; and last, and perhaps most important, the animation of the face. Even when the observed subject speaks, emotional aspects of the communication are separate from the content of the words and sentences spoken. Moreover, specific emotions often succeed stimuli or actions that seemingly motivate them in the subject, as judged from the perspective of the observer. In effect, normal human behaviour exhibits a continuity of emotions induced by a continuity of thoughts.

The impairment of consciousness is not compatible with the maintenance of purposeful behaviour.

Confusing terms

On occasion, terms such as alertness and arousal are incorrectly used as synonyms of wakefulness, attention, and even of consciousness. The term alertness should be used to signify that the subject is both awake and disposed to perceive and act. The proper meaning of alert is somewhere between 'awake' and 'attentive'. The term arousal denotes the presence of signs of autonomic nervous system activation such as changes in skin colour (rubor or pallor), behaviour of skin hair (piloerection), diameter of the pupils, sweating, sexual erection and so on, which correspond to the lay term of excitement. Subjects can be awake, alert, and fully conscious without being aroused, in this sense, and subjects can be aroused, in this sense, during sleep and even coma, obviously when they are not awake, attentive or conscious.

Disorders of consciousness

A clinical classification of the disorders of consciousness

Consciousness is disrupted in a number of neurologic conditions and the profile of impairment varies with the neural systems that are rendered dysfunctional. For practical purposes, we classify the disorders of consciousness according to those profiles. In the largest group of these disorders both core consciousness and extended consciousness are impaired. The impairment or intactness of the other components of consciousness that we discussed earlier permit a further subclassification. In another group of disorders extended consciousness is impaired but not core consciousness.

An overview of the classification we have adopted is as follows.

Disruption of consciousness accompanied by disruption of wakefulness
The examples are coma, the transient loss of consciousness caused by head injury or fainting, and general (deep) anesthesia. The cases of coma caused by structural lesions reveal

that the primary site of dysfunction is in structures of the upper brain stem, hypothalamus, and thalamus (Plum & Posner, 1980), although dysfunction in brainstem entails dysfunction elsewhere in the brain, namely in the cerebral cortex. In a recent study of 50 patients with brainstem stroke, we found that all 12 patients whose coma was caused by a structural lesion, had lesions in the upper brainstem tegmentum, involving either pons or midbrain or both (Parvizi et al., 2000). It is now apparent that, at least in some forms of general anesthesia, for example, propofol anesthesia, the anesthetics act in these same regions (Fiset et al., 1999).

In situations of coma caused by metabolic imbalance, drug overdose, and circulatory collapse, brain dysfunction is far more pervasive and compromises both cortical and subcortical territories (Plum & Posner, 1980).

Disruption of consciousness with preserved wakefulness but defective minimal attention/behaviour
Absence seizures and persistent vegetative state are the prime examples. Absence seizures are related to dysfunction in regions such as the thalamus and the anterior cingulate cortex and have a distinctive electroencephalographic pattern.

Persistent vegetative state can be distinguished from coma in that vegetative patients have cycles of sleep and wakefulness as shown by the opening and closing of their eyes and, sometimes, also by their EEG patterns. Vegetative states are typically caused by dysfunction in the same set of structures of the upper brainstem, hypothalamus, and thalamus that are compromised in coma, and often vegetative states become a stage in the recovery of comatose patients. But vegetative states can also be caused by extensive cortical damage affecting both hemispheres as, for example, in carbon monoxide poisoning (see Plum & Posner, 1980).

Disruption of consciousness with preserved wakefulness and preserved minimal attention/behaviour
The prime examples are akinetic mutisms and epileptic automatisms. Akinetic mutisms are caused by dysfunction in the cingulate cortex, in the basal forebrain, in the thalamus, and in the medial, parietal cortex surrounding the posterior cingulate cortex (see section below and Damasio, 2000, Chapter 8).

Selective disruption of extended consciousness with preserved core consciousness
The prime examples occur with disorders of autobiographical memory, as seen in permanent and transient global amnesia (see below and Damasio, 2000).

Further assessment of patients with impairments of consciousness

The several varieties of impaired consciousness, coma, persistent vegetative state, deep anesthesia, afford little opportunity for behavioural analyses because nearly all behavioural manifestations of consciousness are abolished, and all or nearly all the internal manifestations are presumed abolished as well. The notion that consciousness is suspended, in such situations, is an intuition based on solid reflections on our own condition and on equally solid observations of the behaviour of others. The notion is also supported by the rare but valuable reports of persons who return to consciousness after being in coma, and by reports of being placed under anesthesia and returning to consciousness. Patients can recall the loss of consciousness on the way to coma, much as we can recall the induction of general anesthesia, and both patients and non-patients can recall the return to knowingness. However, nothing at all is recalled of the intervening period, which can span weeks or months in the case of coma or vegetative state. It is reasonable to assume, given all the evidence, that little or nothing was going on in the mind in such circumstances.

Three groups of patients, however, afford some opportunity for behavioural analyses. One group is made up of patients with a complicated phenomenon known as epileptic automatism. The other group brings together patients who, as a result of a variety of neurologic diseases, develop a condition known by the blanket term akinetic mutism. In both groups, core consciousness and extended consciousness are profoundly affected, and yet not all of the manifestations of consciousness are abolished, thus allowing for the analysis of a residual performance. A third group is made up of patients with global amnesia in whom extended consciousness is compromised but core consciousness is intact.

Epileptic automatisms

Epileptic automatisms can appear as part of seizures or immediately following seizures (Penfield & Jasper, 1954; Penry et al., 1975). The most revealing, in relation to the phenomena of consciousness are associated with absence seizures, although automatisms are also seen in association with so-called temporal-lobe seizures. Absence seizures are one of the main varieties of epilepsy, in which consciousness is momentarily suspended along with emotion, attention, and purposeful behaviour. The disturbance is accompanied by a characteristic pattern in the EEG. Absence seizures are of great value to the student of consciousness, and the typical variety of absence seizure is one of the most pure examples of loss of consciousness, the term absence being shorthand for 'absence of consciousness'. The absence automatism that follows an especially long absence seizure is perhaps the purest example of all.

Patients so affected interrupt their behaviours abruptly (e.g. stop in the middle of a sentence) and freeze whatever movement was being performed, and stare blankly, the eyes focused on nothing, the face devoid of any expression, a meaningless mask. The patients remain awake, the eyes remain open and the muscular tone is preserved. The patients do not fall, or have convulsions, or drop whatever they are holding. This state of suspended animation may last for as little as 3 seconds, and for as long as tens of seconds. The longer it lasts, the more likely it is that absence proper will be followed by absence automatism, which can take a few seconds or many. As the automatism starts, the events are not unlike the unfreezing of film images when you release a freeze-frame control. As the patients unfreeze they look about, vacantly, their faces remaining a blank, with no recognizable emotional expression. They may smack their lips, fumble with clothes, get up and move without colliding with objects, and execute correctly a number of isolated actions that will never form a coherent pattern. One of several scenarios might unfold. In the most likely scenario, the patient might stop and stand somewhere in the hallway, appearing confused; or he might sit on a bench, if there were one. But the patient might possibly enter another room or continue walking. In the most extreme variety of such episodes, in what is known as an 'epileptic fugue', the patient might even get out of the building and walk about in a street. To a good observer he would have looked strange and confused, but he might get by without any harm coming to him. Along the trajectory of any of these scenarios, most frequently within seconds, more rarely within a few minutes, when the automatism episodes come to an end, the patients look bewildered. Consciousness returns as suddenly as it disappeared. The patients have no recollection whatsoever of the intervening time. They do not know what their organisms were doing during the episode. They remember what went on before the seizure and can retrieve those contents from memory, an indication that their learning mechanisms were intact prior to the seizure. They immediately learn what goes on after the seizure ends, a sign that the seizure did not produce a permanent impairment of learning. But the events that occur during the period of seizure are not committed to memory (or are not retrievable if they have been).

When the patients are interrupted at any point during the episode, they look bewildered or indifferent. They do

Table 20.2. The main sites of structural brain damage associated with impaired consciousness

Brainstem tegmentum (pons and midbrain)
The hypothalamus
The thalamus
The cingulate cortex
The mesial parietal cortices (especially in precuneus)
The *right* somatosensory cortex complex (insula, SII, and SI)

not know who they or the observers are, spontaneously or upon specific questioning. The contents that make up a conscious mind are missing, and accordingly there are neither verbal reports nor intelligent actions. The patients remain awake and attentive enough to process the object that comes next into their perception, but that may be all that is going on in their minds. There is no evidence of plan, of forethought, of sense of individual wishing, wanting, considering, believing. There is no sense of self.

During such states, the presence of an object promotes the next action and that action may be adequate within the microcontext of the moment, e.g. opening a door. But that action, and other actions, will not be adequate in the broader context of circumstances in which the patient is operating. As one watches actions unfold, one realizes that they are devoid of ultimate purpose and are inappropriate for an individual in that situation (Table 20.2).

Akinetic mutisms

Another important source of information regarding impaired consciousness comes from the study of patients with akinetic mutism, a term suggestive of what goes on externally, but fails to account for the inside view. From all the available evidence, consciousness is severely diminished or even suspended altogether.

Akinetic mutism is often produced by bilateral cerebrovascular lesions in the mesial regions of the frontal lobe. The cingulate cortex, along with nearby regions is almost invariable damaged. Patients become suddenly motionless and speechless, and remain so for weeks or months. They lie in bed with eyes open but with a blank facial expression. When they catch an object in motion, they may track it for a few instants, eyes and head moving along for a moment, but the non-focused staring is rapidly resumed. The term neutral conveys the equanimity of these patients' facial expressions, but their bodies are no more animated than their faces. They may make a normal movement with arm and hand, but in general their limbs are in repose.

Body and face never express any emotion, background, primary, or secondary, in response to the many stimuli that would normally evoke such emotions.

When asked about their situation, the patients are invariably silent, although, after much insistence they may say their names. They have nothing to say about the events leading to their admission, their past or present. They do not react to the presence of relatives or friends. As they emerge from this state and gradually begin to answer some questions, the patients have no recall of any particular experience during their long period of silence; they do not report having fear or anxiety or wishing to communicate. Unlike the patients with locked-in syndrome, akinetic mutes seem not to have had any sense of self and surroundings, any sense of knowing, for most of their akinetic mute period.

In some patients with advanced stages of Alzheimer's disease consciousness is also impaired, and in a manner similar to the one just described for akinetic mutism. Early in the disease, memory loss dominates the clinical presentation and consciousness is intact, but as the ravages of Alzheimer's deepen, one often finds a progressive degradation of consciousness. Unfortunately, textbooks and lay descriptions of Alzheimer's emphasize the loss of memory and the early preservation of consciousness and often fail to mention this important aspect of the disease. The decline first affects extended consciousness by narrowing its scope progressively to the point at which virtually all semblance of autobiographical self disappears. Eventually, it is the turn of core consciousness to be diminished to a degree in which even the simple sense of self is no longer present. Wakefulness is maintained and patients respond to people and objects in elementary fashion, but in a matter of a few seconds, the continuity of the patient's attention is disrupted, and the lack of overall purpose becomes evident. It is interesting to note that several brain regions whose integrity is necessary for normal consciousness are severely damaged in Alzheimer's disease. This is true of nuclei in the brainstem tegmentum, as has been shown recently by Parvizi et al. (2000), who demonstrated a selective involvement in some brainstem nuclei by both neurofibrillary tangles and amyloid plaques. This is also true of the posterior cingulate cortex and surrounding mesial parietal regions (Van Hoesen & Damasio, 1987).

Global amnesia

Loss of core consciousness entails the compromise of extended consciousness, but the converse is not true. Patients in whom extended consciousness is compromised retain core consciousness. The most notable examples of isolated impairments of extended consciousness occur acutely in transient global amnesia (TGA). Beginning acutely and lasting for a period of a few hours, an otherwise normal individual is suddenly deprived of the access to records that have been recently added to the autobiographical memory. The objects and events processed in the instants, minutes and hours before the onset of TGA, are no longer available to the mind. On occasion, nothing that has happened in the days prior to the beginning of TGA is available at all (Damasio, et al., 1983).

Because our memory constantly includes records of the events that we anticipate, it follows that patients struck by TGA do not have available any record of the intended plans for the minutes, hours, or days that lie ahead. Patients with TGA are thus deprived of both personal historical provenance and personal future, but retain core consciousness for the events and objects in the here and now. When patients fail to recognize a particular situation, there is core consciousness for the fact that some aspect of knowledge is no longer present. In spite of adequate consciousness for the current objects and actions the situation fails to make sense to the patient because, without an updated autobiography, the here and now is not meaningful. The predicament of TGA patients reveals the significant limitations of core consciousness. Without a way of explaining where current objects come from along with the motive for the current actions, the here-and-now is an indecipherable puzzle. This is the reason why TGA patients constantly repeat the same anxious questions: Where am I? What am I doing here? How did I come here? What am I supposed to be doing? The patients tend not to ask who they are because they often retain a basic sense of their persons, although even that sense is almost always impoverished. In conclusion, while patients with epileptic automatisms are good examples of the suspension of core consciousness and of everything that depends on it (core self, autobiographical self, extended consciousness), patients with TGA are a good example of suspended extended consciousness and autobiographical self, with the preservation of core consciousness and core self.

The loss of extended consciousness is seen in other conditions. One is the stable global amnesia caused by bilateral temporal lobe damage in patients with herpes simplex encephalitis (Tranel et al., 2000). Another condition is posttraumatic amnesia, one of the frequent consequences of acute head injuries. In such cases, the drama of TGA is frequently played in a matter of minutes. While the amnesia lasts, the patient is confined to core consciousness. Finally, extended consciousness is also impaired in Alzheimer's disease. When the loss of memory for past events is marked enough to compromise autobiographical records, the autobiographical self is gradually reduced and extended consciousness collapses. Only later in the progression of the disease does core consciousness collapse as well.

Ancillary tests

It has long been known that there is an electroencephalographic pattern characteristic of the awake state. Moreover the electroencephalogram can identify patterns characteristic of different types of seizure, of coma, and of persistent vegetative state. The electroencephalogram is thus an important complement to clinical observation in the assessment of consciousness (see Chapter 00).

By far the most important ancillary information for a clinician who is evaluating a patient with impaired consciousness comes from structural imaging, namely from magnetic resonance (MR). Leaving aside the situations of coma due to drug overdose and metabolic imbalance, most significant impairments of consciousness are associated with structural damage in a number of critical territories: (i) the brainstem tegmentum, especially at pontine and midbrain levels; (ii) the diencephalon, i.e. the hypothalamus and thalamus; (iii) the cingulate cortex, in its entirety, and the mesial parietal territories which surround the posterior section of this region, namely in the precuneus; (iv) the right hemisphere complex of somatosensory cortices formed by the insula, and the secondary (SII) and primary somatosensory cortices (SI).

The results of functional imaging tests are somewhat less helpful in clinical management, although they can provide important information especially for research. Cerebral blood flow is generally depressed in the most severe disorders of consciousness, namely, coma and persistent vegetative state, even when the cause is structural and confined to the brainstem (Laureys et al., 1999a, b), although on occasion islands of nearly intact blood flow may be seen (Plum et al., 1998). Notably, conditions such as locked-in syndrome do not reveal significant depressions of cerebral blood flow. Of interest, patients in persistent vegetative state who were studied with functional imaging, revealed activation of inferotemporal areas that are normally engaged by processing faces, when faces were flashed in their retinas (Meno et al., 1998). This result supports the notion that preserving the neural basis for image processing by no means guarantees that the processed images become conscious.

Reflection on the neuropathological correlates of the most frequent impairments of consciousness reveals one important fact. Most of the sites of brain damage associated with a significant disruption of consciousness share one important trait: they are located near the brain's midline, and the left and right sides of these structures are like mirror-images of each other across the midline. At the level of the brainstem and diencephalon, the damaged sites are close to the system of canals and ventricles that defines the midline of the central nervous system. At cortical level, they are located in the mesial surface. These structures are evolutionarily old, they are present in numerous non-human species, and they mature early in individual human development.

The neurobiological basis of consciousness

We defined consciousness in terms of two participants, the organism and the object, and in terms of the relationships those participants hold. In this perspective, consciousness becomes the problem of constructing knowledge about two facts: the fact that the organism is involved in relating to some object, and that the object in the relation is causing a change in the organism. In its normal and optimal operation, consciousness is the process of achieving a particular mental pattern which brings together, in about the same instant, the pattern for the object, the pattern for the organism, and the pattern for the relationship between the two. The emergence of each of these patterns and their conjoining depends on the contributions of individual brain sites working in close cooperation. Elucidating the neurobiology of consciousness consists of identifying those individual contributions, namely discovering how the brain can construct neural patterns that map each of the two participants and the relationships they hold, and how the brain can conjoin the patterns.

Consciousness begins to occur when the brain generates an imaged, non-verbal account of how the organism's representation is affected by the organism's processing of an object, and when this process enhances the image of the causative object, thus placing it saliently in a spatial and temporal context. There are two component mechanisms: the generation of an imaged non-verbal account of the organism–object relationship; and the enhancement of the images of the object.

The imaged account is based on second-order neural patterns generated from structures capable of receiving signals from maps which represent both the organism and the object. The imaged account describes the relationship between the reactive changes in the internal milieu, the viscera, the musculoskeletal frame, and the object that causes those changes. The assembly of the second-order neural pattern describing the object–organism relationship subsequently modulates the neural patterns which describe the object and leads to the enhancement of the image of the object. The feeling of self knowing an object, emerges from the contents of the imaged account, and from the enhancement of the object.

The neural pattern which underlies core consciousness for an object, the sense of self in the act of knowing a particular thing, is a large-scale neural pattern involving activity in two interrelated sets of structures: the set whose cross-regional activity generates an integrated view of the organism (the proto-self) and second-order maps; and the set whose cross-regional activity generates the representation of the object. The latter set has a dual role: it is both the initiator of the changes in the former set and the recipient of its modulating influences.

The neuroanatomical structures required to accomplish these component mechanisms encompass, respectively, (i) the structures needed to map the structure and state of the organism; (ii) those needed to process the object; and (iii) those needed to generate the imaged account of the relationship and produce its consequences. Let us consider each of these anatomical requirements.

Much is known about how the organism is represented in the brain, although the idea that such representations could be linked to the notion of self has received little attention. The brain represents, within itself, varied aspects of the structure and current state of the organism in a large number of neural maps from the level of the brainstem and hypothalamus to that of the somatosensory cortices (insula, SII, SI). The state of the internal milieu, the viscera, the vestibular apparatus, and the musculoskeletal system are thus continuously represented (Damasio, 2000; Parvizi & Damasio, 2001).

There have been considerable efforts to understand the neural basis of object representation. Extensive studies of perception, learning and memory, and language, have given us a workable idea of how the brain processes an object, in sensory and motor terms, and an idea of how knowledge about an object can be stored in memory, categorized in conceptual or linguistic terms, and retrieved in recall or recognition modes. In the relationship process we have proposed for consciousness, the object is exhibited as neural patterns in the sensory cortices appropriate for its nature. For example, in the case of the visual aspects of an object, the appropriate neural patterns are constructed in a variety of regions of the early visual cortices, while memory records pertaining to the past perception of such objects are held in highest-order association cortices located in temporal, parietal, and frontal regions. These cortices are interconnected with the early visual cortices (Damasio & Damasio, 1994). In brief, early sensory cortices, and higher-order cortices are involved (*a*) in signalling the objects and the events which come to be known because of core consciousness; (b) in holding records pertaining to their experience; and (c) in manipulating those records in reasoning and creative thinking. Thus, the early sensory structures are also involved in the process of making consciousness, but in a different manner from the structures involved in representing the organism. The participation of early sensory structures; includes: (a) initiating the process of generating consciousness by influencing the organism-representing structures (b) signalling to second-order structures, and (c) being the recipients of the modulatory influences consequent to the second-order neural patterns. It is because of the latter influence that the enhancement of the neural patterns which support the object does occur, and that varied components of the object being known in consciousness can become integrated.

The neuroanatomy underlying the imaged account of the relationship depends on several structures, the most important of which are the cingulate cortices and the medial parietal cortices which surround their posterior sector. Finally, the subsequent image enhancement is achieved via modulation from basal forebrain/brainstem acetylcholine and monoamine nuclei, as well as thalamo-cortical modulation.

In brief, core consciousness depends most critically on the activity of a restricted number of phylogenetically old brain structures, beginning in the brainstem and ending with the somatosensory and cingulate cortices. The interaction among the structures in this set: (a) supports the creation of an integrated map of the organism state (the proto-self); (b) engenders the second-order neural pattern which describes the relationship between the integrated organism representation (proto-self) and the object representation; and (c) modulates the activity of object-processing regions which are not part of the set.

The specificity with which these neural structures are enumerated should not be taken to mean that any one of them alone can be the basis for consciousness. None of the functions outlined above is executed at the level of a single structure, but emerges, rather, as a result of cross-regional integrations of neural activity.

There is a remarkable overlap of biological functions within the structures which support the integrated mapping of the organism state (the proto-self) and the second-order mappings. For example, the brainstem nuclei and the cingulate cortices are involved in most of the following functions: (a) regulating homeostasis and signalling body structure and state, including the processing of signals related to pain, pleasure, and drives; (b) participating in the processes of emotion and feeling; (c) participating in processes of attention; (d) participating in

the processes of wakefulness and sleep; (e) participating in the learning process.

The meaning of these functional overlaps may be gleaned by focusing on the brainstem, where distinct 'families' of nuclei are closely contiguous, and in spite of their anatomical distinctiveness, the varied families of nuclei are highly interrelated by anatomical connections. It would be functionally convenient to have structures governing attention and emotion in the vicinity of each other. Moreover, it makes good functional sense that such structures should be in the vicinity of those which regulate and signal body states since the causes and consequences of emotion and attention are related to the fundamental process of managing life within the organism, and it is not possible to manage life and maintain homeostatic balance without data on the current state of the organism's body-proper. Finally, if we regard consciousness as another contributor to the regulation of homeostasis, it also makes functional sense to place the critical neural machinery of consciousness within and in the vicinity of the neural machinery involved in basic homeostasis, that is, the machinery of emotion, attention and regulation of body state.

This perspective does not deny that some brainstem structures are involved in wakefulness and attention, and that they modulate the activity of cerebral cortex via the intralaminar thalamic nuclei, via the non-thalamic cortical projections of monamines, and via the thalamic projections of acetylcholine nuclei. The point is that nearby brainstem structures, and perhaps even some of the very same structures, have other activities, namely, managing body states and representing current body states. Those activities are not incidental to the brainstem's well established activation role: they may be the reason why such an activation role has been maintained evolutionarily and why it is primarily operated from the brainstem.

The roles that have been traditionally assigned to the brainstem's 'ascending reticular activating system', and to its extension in the thalamus, as presented in the classical work of Moruzzi and Magoun (1949), Penfield and Jasper (1954), and in the modern work of Llinas and Paré (1991), Llinas and Ribary (1993), Hobson (1994), Steriade (1988, 1993a, b, 1995), Munk et al. (1996), and Singer (1998) is compatible with this interpretation. The activity of the 'ascending reticular activating system' contributes to creating the selective, integrated and unified contents of the conscious mind, although such a contribution is not sufficient to explain consciousness comprehensively.

Although even the simplest form of consciousness requires ensemble activity that involves varied regions of the brain, consciousness depends most critically on regions that are evolutionarily older rather than recent, and are located in the depth of the brain rather than on its surface. These basic mechanisms are anchored on ancient neural structures, intimately interwoven with homeostasis, rather than on the modern structures of the neocortex, those on which fine movement, perception, language and high-reason are based.

References

Baars, B. (1988). *A Cognitive Theory of Consciousness.* Cambridge: Cambridge University Press.

Baddeley, A. (1992). Working memory. *Science,* **255**, 566–9.

Crick, F. (1994). *The Astonishing Hypothesis: the Scientific Search for the Soul.* New York: Charles Scribner's Sons.

Damasio, A.R. (1998). Investigating the biology of consciousness. *Trans. Roy. Soc. (Lond.),* **353**, 1879–82.

Damasio, A.R. (1999/2000). *The Feeling of What Happens: Body and Emotion in the Making of Consciousness.* New York: Harcourt Brace.

Damasio, A.R. & Damasio, H. (1994). Cortical systems for retrieval of concrete knowledge: The convergence zone framework. In *Large-Scale Neuronal Theories of the Brain,* ed. C. Koch & J.L. Davis, pp. 61–74. Cambridge, MA: MIT Press.

Damasio, A.R., Graff-Radford, N.R. & Damasio, H. (1983). Transient partial amnesia. *Arch. Neurol.,* **40**, 656–57.

Damasio, A.R., Tranel, D. & Damasio, H. (1990). Face agnosia and the neural substrates of memory. *Ann. Rev. Neurosci.,* **13**, 89–109.

Dennett, D. (1991). *Consciousness Explained.* Boston: Little Brown.

Edelman, G. (1989). *The Remembered Present.* New York: Basic Books.

Fiset, P., Paus, T., Daloze, T. et al. (1999). Brain mechanisms of propofol-induced loss of consciousness in humans: a positron emission tomographic study. *J. Neurosci.,* **19**, 5506–13.

Hobson, A. (1994). *The Chemistry of Conscious States.* New York: Basic Books.

Laureys, S., Goldman, S., Phillips, C. et al. (1999a). Impaired effective cortical connectivity in vegetative state: preliminary investigation using PET. *Neuroimage,* **9**, 377–82.

Laureys, S., Lemaire, C., Maquet, P., Phillips, C. & Fanck, G. (1999b). Cerebral metabolism during vegetative state and after recovery to consciousness. *J. Neurol. Neurosurg. Psychiatry,* **67**, 121.

Llinas, R. & Paré, D. (1991). Of dreaming and wakefulness. *Neuroscience,* **44**, 521–35.

Llinas, R. & Ribary, U. (1993). Coherent 40-Hz oscillation characterizes dream state in humans. *Proc. Natl. Acad. Sci., USA,* **90**, 2078–81.

Maquet, P., Degueldre, C., Delfiore, G. et al. (1997). Functional neuroanatomy of human slow wave sleep. *J. Neurosci.,* **17**, 2807–12.

Maquet, P., Peters, J-M., Aerts, J. et al. (1996). Functional neuroanatomy of human rapid-eye-movement sleep and dreaming. *Nature,* **383**, 163.

Meno, D.K., Owen, A.M., Williams, E.J. et al. (1998). Cortical processing in persistent vegetative state. *Lancet,* **352**, 800.

Metzinger, T. (1995). *Conscious Experience.* Paderborn, Germany: Imprint Academic/Schoeningh.

Metzinger, T. (2000). *Neural Correlates of Consciousness.* Cambridge: The MIT Press.

Moruzzi, G. & Magoun, H.W. (1949). Brain stem reticular formation and activation of the EEG. *Electroencephalography and Clinical Neurophysiology,* **1**, 455–73.

Munk, M.H.J., Roelfsema, P.R., Konig, P., Engel, A.K. & Singer, W. (1996). Role of reticular activation in the modulation of intracortical synchronization. *Science,* **272**, 271–4.

Parvizi, J. & Damasio, A.R. (2001). Consciousness and the brainstem. *Cognition,* **49**, 135–60.

Parvizi, J., Van Hoesen G.W. & Damasio, A.R. (2000). Selective pathological changes of the periaqueductal gray in Alzheimer's disease. *Ann. Neurol.,* **48**, 344–53.

Penfield, W. & Jasper, H. (1954). *Epilepsy and the Functional Anatomy of the Human Brain.* Boston: Little, Brown.

Penry, J.K., Porter, R. & Dreifuss, F. (1975). Simultaneous recording of absence seizures with video tape and electroencephalography, a study of 374 seizures in 48 patients. *Brain,* **98**, 427–40.

Plum, F. & Posner, J.B. (1980). *The Diagnosis of Stupor and Coma.* Philadelphia: F. A. Davis Company.

Plum, F., Schiff, N., Ribary, U. & Llinas, R. (1998). Coordinated expression in chronically unconscious persons. *Phil. Trans. Roy. Soc. Lond. B,* **353**, 1929–33.

Searle, J. (1992). *The Rediscovery of the Mind.* Cambridge: MIT Press.

Singer, W. (1998). Consciousness and the structure of neuronal representations. *Phil. Trans. Roy. Soc. Lond. B,* **353**, 1829–40.

Smith, E.E., Jonides, J. & Koeppe, R.A.(1996). Dissociating verbal and spatial working memory using PET. *Cerebr. Cortex,* **6**, 11–20.

Steriade, M. (1988). New vistas on the morphology, chemical transmitters and physiological actions of the ascending brainstem reticular system. *Arch. Ital. Biol.,* **126**, 225–38.

Steriade, M. (1993a). Basic mechanisms of sleep generation. *Neurology,* **42**, 9–17.

Steriade, M. (1993b). Central core modulation of spontaneous oscillations and sensory transmission in thalamocortical systems. *Curr. Opin. Neurobiol.,* **3**, 619–25.

Steriade, M. (1995). Brain activation, then (1949) and now: coherent fast rhythms in corticothalamic networks. *Arch. Ital. Biol.,* **134**, 5–20.

Tranel D., Damasio H. & Damasio, A.R. (2000). Amnesia caused by herpes simplex encephalitis, infarctions in basal forebrain, and anoxia/ischemia. In *Handbook of Neuropsychology,* 2nd edn., ed. F. Boller & J. Grafman, pp. 85–110. Amsterdam: Elsevier Science.

Van Hoesen, G. & Damasio, A. (1987). Neural correlates of cognitive impairment in Alzheimer's disease. In *Handbook of Physiology,* ed. V. Mountcastle & F. Plum, pp. 871–98. Bethesda: American Physiological Society.

21

Mechanisms of memory and amnestic syndromes

John D.E. Gabrieli and Silvia A. Bunge

Department of Psychology, Stanford University, Palo Alto, CA, USA

Memory comprises the recording, retention and retrieval of knowledge. All that we know, except for what is genetically predetermined, is acquired through experience. Such knowledge includes the events we remember, the facts we know, and the skills we master. Memory is not a unitary faculty, but rather an ensemble of multiple forms of learning that differ in their uses, their operating characteristics, and the neural networks that mediate their processing (Gabrieli, 1998). A memory system may be defined as a particular neural network that mediates a specific form of mnemonic processing. Neurological and psychiatric diseases result in characteristic mnemonic deficits that reflect which memory systems are injured by a particular disease.

Levels of analysis: cells and systems

Learning and memory reflect experience-induced plasticity in the brain. An experience leaves a memory trace composed of an enduring alteration in the cellular organization of the brain called an engram. Experience-induced plasticity can be examined at many levels of analysis, including molecular events at the cellular and synaptic level, reorganization of local neuronal circuits, and large-scale alterations in the functional neural architecture of memory systems.

Cellular mechanisms of memory

Little is known about neural plasticity in the human brain, but findings from in vitro and invertebrate models offer suggestions about the cellular bases of human memory. Studies of the marine snail *Aplysia* have revealed links between learning and alterations in neurotransmitter release. *Aplysia* have a gill withdrawal reflex that is triggered when the gill is touched by a rod. Repeated stimula-

tion leads to habituation such that the gills are no longer withdrawn in response to the rod. Short-term habituation has been linked to decreased presynaptic transmitter release. Repeated stimulation with a highly noxious stimulus, such as an electric shock, can lead to sensitization, an intensification of the withdrawal response. Short-term sensitization involves increased neurotransmitter release from a facilitating interneuron (Kandel & Schwartz, 1982). Modulation of neurotransmitter release may underlie short-term changes in functional connectivity between neurons.

Long-term memory processes, in contrast, require messenger RNA and protein synthesis (Davis & Squire, 1984) to establish structural changes in synaptic connectivity as a record of experience. Long-term habituation may involve pruning of presynaptic terminals, whereas long-term sensitization may involve proliferation of presynaptic terminals (Bailey & Chen, 1983; Fig. 21.1). The best-studied candidate for a cellular basis of mammalian learning is long-term potentiation (LTP), usually examined in in vitro slice preparations from mammalian brains (Fig. 21.2). A neuron becomes potentiated (i.e. exhibits enhanced response to a given input) when bombarded with brief but rapid series of stimulations. LTP develops rapidly and can last for long periods, and is specific to the activated synapses. LTP has associative properties because it is driven by cooperativity, the simultaneous stimulation of different synapses. LTP has been studied most extensively in hippocampal synapses, in which NMDA glutamate receptors are essential for the establishment, but not the maintenance, of LTP. LTP has also been induced in the amygdala, cerebellum, and cerebral cortex, but differences in LTP properties across brain regions suggest that they are mediated by multiple cellular mechanisms. Mechanisms for long-term depression of synaptic efficacy have also been found in the hippocampus (Malenka, 1994) and cerebral cortex.

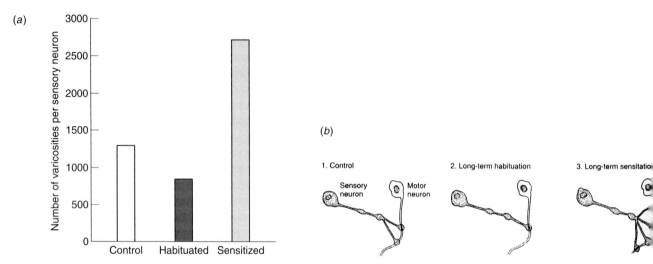

Fig. 21.1. Long-term habituation and sensitization in *Aplysia* involve structural changes in the presynaptic terminals of sensory neurons. (*a*) Number of presynaptic terminals in habituated and sensitized animals relative to control animals. (*b*) Long-term habituation leads to a loss of synapses, whereas long-term sensitization leads to an increase in synapses. (Adapted from Kandel et al., 1991.)

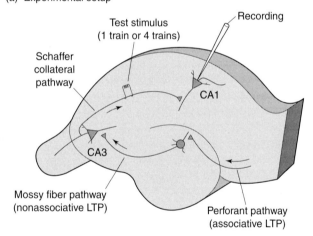

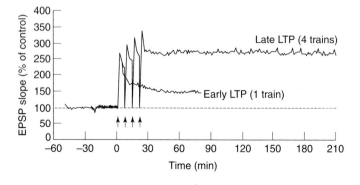

Large-scale memory systems

In humans, the functional neural architecture of memory is best understood in terms of mnemonic functions associated with particular anatomic structures. Studies of patients with brain lesions have provided the foundations of our knowledge about the biological organization of human memory. Lesions have produced dramatic and often unexpected mnemonic deficits that provide clues about the brain regions that are necessary for particular memory processes. The behaviour of memory-impaired patients with brain lesions, however, does not definitively point to the process subserved by the injured tissue. Rather, the behaviour reflects what uninjured brain regions can accomplish after the lesion. Further, naturally occurring lesions often impair multiple brain systems, either by direct insult to a large brain area or through disconnection of interactive brain regions. It is, therefore, difficult to associate particular brain structures with specific memory processes.

Fig. 21.2. LTP in the hippocampus. (*a*) Experimental setup for studying LTP in the CA1 region of the hippocampus. The Schaffer collateral pathway is stimulated electrically and the response of the population of pyramidal neurons is recorded. (*b*) Early and late LTP in a cell in the CA1 region of the hippocampus. Shown is a plot of the slope (rate of rise) of the excitatory postsynaptic potentials in the cell as a function of time. A test stimulus was given every 60 s to the Schaffer collaterals. To elicit early LTP, a single train of stimuli is given for 1 s at 100 Hz. To elicit the late phase of LTP, four trains are given separated by 10 min. The resulting early LTP lasts 2–3 hours, whereas the late LTP lasts 24 or more hours. (Adapted from Kandel et al., 2000.)

Functional neuroimaging studies using positron emission tomography (PET) or functional magnetic resonance imaging (fMRI) now permit the visualization of memory processes in the healthy brain. Functional neuroimaging studies allow for the design of psychological experiments targeted at specific memory processes. They are limited, however, by several factors. PET and fMRI derive their signals not from direct measures of neural activity, but rather from local changes in blood flow or metabolism related to neural activity. These indirect measures of neural activity limit the temporal and spatial fidelity of activations. Additionally, there is a great deal of psychological interpretation involved in understanding the meaning of an activation, i.e. in specifying the mental process signified by an activation. The combination of lesion and neuroimaging studies may overcome the limitations of each source of evidence and provide powerful, mutual constraints on ideas about memory systems.

Types of memory

Distinctions between different kinds of memory are useful from both clinical and neuroscience perspectives. A fundamental distinction is that of declarative versus nondeclarative forms of memory (Cohen & Squire, 1980). Declarative memory refers to the everyday sense of memory, and is responsible for the learning and remembrance of new events, facts and materials. It encompasses both episodic memories (remembrance of personal experiences that occurred at a particular time and place) and semantic memories (knowledge of generic information, such as the meaning of a word) (Tulving, 1983). It is the form of memory that people use to recollect facts and events consciously and intentionally, and is therefore also referred to as explicit memory (Graf & Schacter, 1985). In the clinic or experimental laboratory, declarative memory is usually tested directly by asking a person to recall or recognize information that was presented recently.

Non-declarative memory refers to the many forms of memory that do not depend on the psychological processes or brain regions essential for declarative memory. Non-declarative memories are not retrieved intentionally or explicitly, but rather incidentally or implicitly through behaviour. These forms of memory are established during an experience, and guide future behaviour in a way that is unrelated to any conscious awareness of that experience. Non-declarative forms of memory are tested implicitly or indirectly by measuring the influence of a specific prior experience upon subsequent performance, but without making any direct reference to that prior experience. Such experience-induced alterations in behaviour must reflect the consequence of memories established during the initial experience. Three main classes of non-declarative memory (skill learning, conditioning, and repetition priming) are discussed below.

Temporal properties distinguish one form of memory from another. Immediate memory refers to the recall of information without delay, either immediately after presentation or after uninterrupted rehearsal. Immediate memory is characterized by sharply limited capacities for how much and how long information can be remembered. For example, people can remember no more than about seven random digits, and only as long as they rehearse those digits. Immediate memory often has perception-like characteristics. For example, errors in immediate memory for words are more likely to reflect word sounds than word meanings (e.g. a person might recall 'pound' when they actually heard 'sound').

Working memory is a multi-component psychological system that mediates the temporary processing and storage of internal representations that guide and control action. Information can be held in working memory beyond the span of immediate memory, but only insofar as is useful for solving a problem at hand. Working memory is conceptualized to include immediate memory capacities and the executive or control processes that guide the goal-driven selection of relevant information to be held in immediate memory stores (Baddeley, 1986).

Long-term memory refers to large and permanent stores of episodic and semantic memories. Long-term memories are not, however, passively stored records of experience. Rather, they are constantly used to interpret new experiences. Our knowledge of words and concepts, for example, is used to interpret the meaning of sentences that we hear or see, and past experiences that resemble a current event are used to interpret that event. Long-term memory is often organized by meaning (semantics) or gist rather than by the perceptual characteristics of an experience. For example, people remember the content or gist of a sentence they have read far better than the specific order of words or the font in which the sentence was seen. Similarly, people remember a set of related words (e.g. birds) better than a set of unrelated words.

The rapid application of prior knowledge to interpret the meaning of a novel experience is a powerful mechanism for comprehension, but it can also generate inaccurate memories. Ongoing use of a long-term memory can alter the original memory (retroactive interference); indeed it is thought that forgetting is due much more to subsequent interference (multiple, related experiences are inadvertently blended) than to simple disuse of a memory.

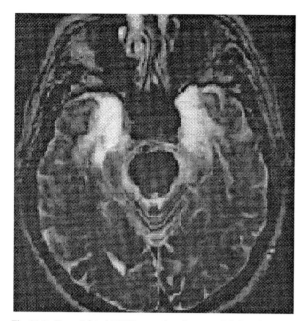

Fig. 21.3. T_2-weighted MRI image showing an axial slice through the temporal lobes of patient E.P. Damage to the bilateral medial temporal lobe extends caudally from the temporal pole and includes the hippocampal region, the entorhinal cortex, the perirhinal cortex, the parahippocampal cortex and the amygdaloid complex. The lesion also extends laterally to include the anterior portion of the fusiform gyrus. (Adapted from Teng & Squire, 1999.)

Remembering the gist of an experience is an efficient way to learn without recording minor details, but it is also prone to errors. For example, one can falsely remember that the name of a particular bird was included in a list of birds when it was not actually presented, simply because one has considered the gist of the set to be about birds.

Long-term memory involves three successive temporal phases. Encoding refers to processes that originally register an experience, including attentional, perceptual, and semantic processes. Storage (or consolidation) refers to the enduring maintenance of that memory. Retrieval refers to recovery of the memory at a later time. Accurate retrieval of a memory requires all three phases to be executed successfully. Long-term memories include those established many years or decades ago, sometimes referred to as remote memories.

The relation between short-term and long-term memory is susceptible to misunderstanding, in part due to various meanings of the term short-term memory. Sometimes short-term memory is used to refer to attention. An individual who cannot repeat back even a single digit or word is better described as having a deficit in atten-

tion than a deficit in any sort of memory. A second use of short-term memory is to refer to a memory mechanism that supports remembrance of a memory after a delay of seconds or minutes without rehearsal. There is, however, no evidence of any anatomical system that has a temporal span intermediate to those of immediate and long-term memory. Rather, there is constant and rapid loss of long-term memory for most events and facts. Therefore, memory for an episode after a brief delay of seconds or minutes will be superior to memory for that episode after a longer delay, just as memory for most episodes that occurred last week is superior to episodes that occurred last year. These differences, however, all reflect the temporal dynamics of long-term memory, and not the existence of a memory store that is intermediate between immediate and long-term memory. It is common to refer to an inability to acquire new long-term memories as a deficit in short-term memory. In this case, failure to learn new information is being contrasted with the preservation of remote memories, but the deficit is really one of failing to establish new long-term memories.

Amnesia and the declarative memory system

Amnesia is a selective disorder of declarative memory. It is defined by a behavioural syndrome rather than by etiology or lesion location. A pure amnesia refers to a relatively circumscribed disorder of declarative memory that cannot be accounted for by non-mnemonic deficits such as attention, perception, language, or motivation, because those abilities are all intact. In amnesia, immediate memory and cognitive abilities are intact. Anterograde amnesia refers to the inability to acquire new declarative memories. Retrograde amnesia refers to the loss of memories acquired prior to the onset of amnesia. Retrograde amnesia is described as flat when it extends back uniformly through an individual's life. More often however, retrograde amnesia is temporally graded, being most severe for, or limited to, a period of time immediately preceding the onset of the amnesia, and less severe or absent for more remote periods. Depending on the size and location of lesions, amnesias can vary considerably in extent and severity of anterograde and retrograde memory loss. Typically, the severity of the anterograde amnesia and the temporal extent of the retrograde amnesia are correlated, such that patients with a complete inability to form new memories have retrograde amnesia extending for long periods, up to decades (Rempel-Clower et al., 1996).

Amnesia results from injury to medial temporal lobe (Scoville & Milner, 1957; Fig. 21.3), diencephalic (von

Cramon et al., 1985; Dusoir et al., 1990), or basal forebrain (Damasio et al., 1985) regions. Bilateral lesions in any of these regions lead to global amnesia, a pervasive declarative memory failure that encompasses both verbal and non-verbal information. Patients with severe global amnesia fail all tests of declarative memory in all modalities, regardless of the difficulty of the test. They do not remember the most famous of public events or the most salient of personal events, such as the deaths of loved ones. Because the patient retains all other mental abilities, severe amnesia can appear to be a relatively minor problem. It is, however, remarkably debilitating because patients cannot take care of themselves, hold jobs, or develop human relations. When asked their age, the current year, or their home address, such patients respond with answers that are many years out of date. They cannot remember goals or intentions for more than a few moments, unless explicitly reminded with instructions. Milder cases of amnesia allow for some learning of especially salient or often repeated information, but even these patients have great trouble at home or at work. Unilateral left- or right-sided lesions typically result in material-specific memory dysfunctions for verbal or non-verbal information, respectively (Milner, 1974). This asymmetry can be more complex, however, in patients with longstanding unilateral injury when there is opportunity for reorganization, as can occur in epilepsy.

The medial temporal lobe region (Fig. 21.4) is comprised of a number of interconnected but anatomically distinct structures: the amygdala, the hippocampal formation, which includes cornu ammonis (CA) fields, dentate gyrus, subiculum, and fornix, the entorhinal cortex; the perirhinal cortex; and the parahippocampal cortex. Research with animals and humans indicates that each of these structures makes a unique contribution to declarative memory, and that they act in complex concert to establish new memories. It is now thought that the amygdala is not critical for most aspects of declarative memory. Rather, this region plays a specific role in the emotional modulation of memories, as reviewed below.

Higher-level olfactory, frontal, parietal, and temporal cortices provide widespread, convergent inputs to the medial temporal lobe region (Fig. 21.5). Two-thirds of these inputs traverse the perirhinal and parahippocampal cortices that surround the hippocampal formation. These regions send major input to the entorhinal cortex, which, in turn, provides major input to the hippocampal formation. The fornix is a major fibre bundle that connects the hippocampal formation to the septum and other subcortical structures.

Damage to medial temporal lobe structures is the most

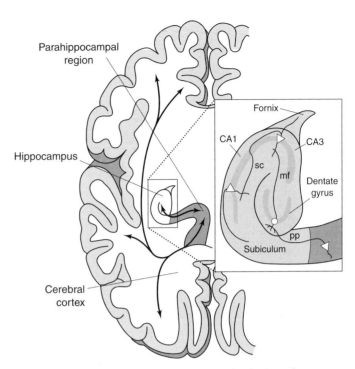

Fig. 21.4. Major pathways of the hippocampus. Left: A horizontal section through the human brain showing major pathways by which the hippocampus is connected with cortical areas. Inset: Diagram of major intra-hippocampal connections. (Adapted from Eichenbaum & Cohen, 2001.)

common etiology for pure amnesia or declarative memory disorders that are part of a more widespread dementia. This region is highly susceptible to a variety of insults, including epilepsy, anoxia, and herpes simplex encephalitis. Postmortem and in vivo imaging studies indicate that the entorhinal cortex and hippocampus are the first structures typically affected by Alzheimer's disease, in which a declarative memory disorder is the most common and severe initial behavioural deficit (Hyman et al., 1984; de Leon et al., 1993).

For many years, it was thought that the hippocampus *per se* was the critical structure among these for declarative memory. Focal damage restricted to the CA1 component of the hippocampus is indeed sufficient to yield a clinically substantial declarative memory deficit (Zola-Morgan et al., 1986). Animal research has shown, however, that perirhinal or other lesions can have at least as great a consequence on memory performance as hippocampal lesions (Murray & Mishkin, 1986; Zola-Morgan et al., 1989). In humans, more widespread damage to entorhinal, perirhinal, and parahippocampal cortices results in an increasingly devastating memory deficit (Rempel-Clower et al., 1996; Corkin et

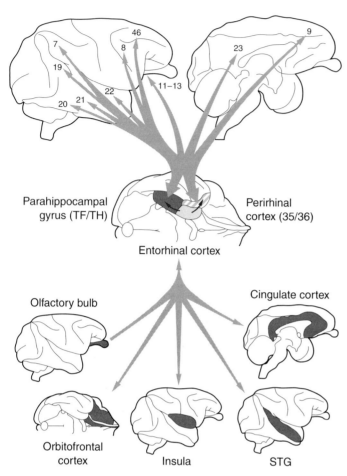

Fig. 21.5. Major cortical areas that compose the afferent sources and efferent targets of information to and from the parahippocampal region in monkeys. (Adapted from Eichenbaum & Cohen, 2001.)

al., 1997). In addition, damage to the fornix can produce global amnesia (Gaffan & Gaffan, 1991). The specific mnemonic roles of particular medial temporal lobe structures have not yet been well characterized in humans, because it is rare for an injury to damage one of these structures without injuring neighbouring structures.

Diencephalic regions linked to declarative memory include the dorsomedial and anterior nuclei of the thalamus, the mammillary bodies, the mammillothalamic fibre tract connecting the medial hippocampal complex to the anterior thalamic nuclei, and the ventroamygdalofugal fibre tract connecting the amygdala to the dorsomedial nuclei (Victor et al., 1971; Fig. 21.6). Damage to these regions is sufficient to produce severe memory impairments even when medial–temporal regions remain anatomically intact (Press et al., 1989). The precise roles of these structures are not well specified, in part because

damage tends to co-occur in multiple structures. For example, the mammillary bodies and dorsomedial nuclei are both greatly affected in alcoholic Korsakoff's amnesia, the most common etiology of diencephalic amnesia. Acute thalamic lesions producing amnesia often injure both the dorsomedial nucleus of the thalamus and the surrounding mammillothalamic and ventroamygdalofugal tracts. The preponderance of evidence favours a critical role in declarative memory for the dorsomedial nucleus, perhaps in combination with the surrounding fibres of the mammillothalamic tract (von Cramon et al., 1985). The consequence of a lesion limited to the mammillary bodies is less certain. Lesions there sometimes appear to account for declarative memory deficits in patients (Dusoir et al., 1990), but do not yield the long-lasting memory impairments seen in monkeys after medial-temporal or dorsomedial thalamic lesions (Zola-Morgan & Squire, 1985). Declarative memory failure after diencephalic lesions appears quite similar to that seen after medial–temporal lesions, although additional non-mnemonic deficits may result from diencephalic lesions.

The basal forebrain is composed of midline structures including the septal nuclei, diagonal band of Broca, and substantia innominata. These regions provide the largest input of acetylcholine, the neurotransmitter most directly implicated as critical for declarative memory, to the hippocampus and many neocortical areas. The basal forebrain also supplies other neurotransmitters to the cerebral cortex that contribute to the modulation of memory, including dopamine, norepinephrine, and serotonin. An extensive lesion to the basal forebrain yields a severe declarative memory impairment (Damasio et al., 1985). Partial damage to this and adjacent ventromedial frontal cortex often occurs after ruptures of anterior communicating artery aneurysms, which often lead to mild but persistent anterograde amnesia.

Amygdala and the emotional modulation of memory

Lesion and functional neuroimaging findings have illuminated the importance of the amygdala in emotional aspects of human (Phelps & Anderson, 1997). Medial temporal lobe lesions are rarely restricted to the amygdala, but valuable information can be gained from a rare congenital dermatological disorder, Urbach–Weithe syndrome. This disorder leads to mineralization of the amygdala that spares the hippocampal formation (Fig. 21.7). It is also possible to study patients who have undergone amygdala resection for treatment of pharmacologically intractable

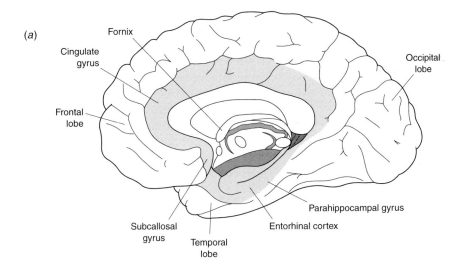

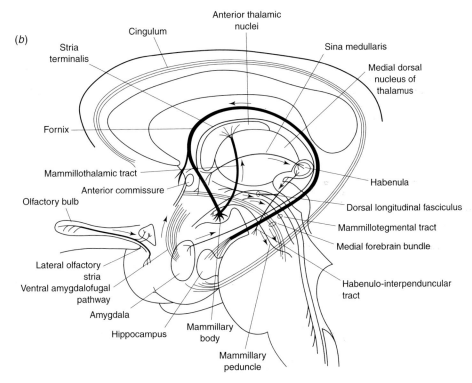

Fig. 21.6. The limbic system, consisting of the limbic lobe and deep-lying structures. (*a*) Medial view of the brain showing the limbic lobe (stippled area). (*b*) Interconnections of the deep-lying limbic structures. The predominant direction of flow of neural activity in each tract is indicated by an arrow, but the designated tracts are typically bidirectional. (Adapted from Kandel et al., 1991.)

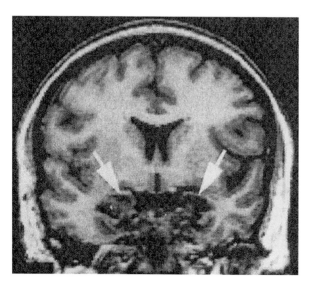

Fig. 21.7. T_1-weighted MRI image showing a coronal slice through the brain of a patient with Urbach–Wiethe disease. Arrows indicate loci where the amygdala would normally be found. (Adapted from Adolphs et al., 1995.)

epilepsy, but the resection usually involves additional medial–temporal structures.

There is convergent evidence of a specific role for the amygdala in emotional declarative memory. Healthy people show superior memory for emotionally disturbing relative to emotionally neutral stimuli. An Urbach–Weithe patient showed normal memory for neutral slides, but failed to show the normal additional memory for the emotionally salient slides (Cahill et al., 1995). In a PET study, amygdala activation correlated with individual differences in subsequent recall for emotional, but not for neutral, film clips (Cahill et al., 1996). In an event-related fMRI study, amygdala activation correlated with how emotionally intense people rated individually presented scenes (Canli et al., 2000). For scenes rated most emotionally intense, the magnitude of amygdala activation predicted later recognition memory. Most studies have examined participation of the amygdala in memory for negative events, but amygdala activation also predicts memory for positive emotional events (Hamann et al., 1999). Patients with amygdala lesions, however, typically report normal emotional evaluation of situations or stimuli, so the amygdala does not appear critical for generating emotions. Rather, the amygdala enables emotional arousal to strengthen memory encoding.

The amygdala participates not only in explicit memory for aversive stimuli, but also in implicit memory for aversive stimuli (reviewed later). Patients with amygdala lesions exhibit emotion-selective deficits in the identifica-

tion of fearful or angry facial expressions (Adolphs et al., 1994) or prosody (Scott et al., 1997). Amygdala activations occur in PET and fMRI studies during the perception of fearful facial expressions or scenes (Morris et al., 1996). Thus, the amygdala appears to have a widespread role in processing negatively salient stimuli. This subcortical structure, however, is composed of multiple nuclei with distinct connectivity, and is adjacent to another brain region important for emotion, the substantia innominata. Thus, it is unclear whether some of these emotional and memory processes are mediated by the same or different specific pathways in that region. It is clear, however, that injury restricted to this region affects emotional memory without resulting in a global amnesia.

Neocortical basis of declarative memory

Declarative memory likely depends on interactions between the domain-independent regions described above, where injury results in broad memory failure, and domain-specific neocortical regions. Long-term episodic and semantic memories are thought to be stored in the neocortex, with different regions representing different types of knowledge. Thus, knowledge about the visual appearance of a tool may be stored near visual cortex, separate from knowledge about its use, which may be stored in areas such as premotor cortex (Martin et al., 1995). There is evidence that semantic memories for the names of people, tools, and animals are represented in distinct, adjacent left temporal lobe regions (Damasio et al., 1996). Damage to a cortical area can result in both the loss of previously acquired memories stored in that area and an inability to acquire new memories involving that kind of knowledge. A patient with a specific anomia for names of people, for example, would be unable to learn a new person's name but able to learn new names for animals or tools.

Personal knowledge also appears to be organized topographically in the neocortex. Some patients with mild anterograde amnesia exhibit a remarkable loss of personal memories concerning major life events or family members (Kapur et al., 1992). These patients typically have sustained damage to lateral temporal cortex, most often in the right hemisphere, which may store long-term autobiographical memory representations. They do not exhibit the temporally graded retrograde amnesia characteristic of patients with medial temporal lobe lesions.

Memory for an event or fact is conceptualized as being widely distributed in the neocortex, with specific perceptual, conceptual, and emotional features of an event represented in specialized cortical regions. It is hypothesized that medial temporal lobe structures bind or relate the multiple features that define memory for an event across physically disparate neocortical regions.

Over time, the features somehow become consolidated in the neocortex and no longer require the medial temporal lobe for binding. It is thought that temporally limited retrograde amnesia reflects the sparing of remote, well-consolidated memories and the disruption of ongoing consolidation for more recent memories.

Immediate memory

Immediate memory, such as the recall of a series of digits that one has just heard or spatial locations that one has just seen, depends on cortical areas specialized for both modality (visual or auditory) and material (verbal or non-verbal). Patients with lesions of the left inferior parietal cortex may be able to repeat only two digits or words immediately after hearing them, in contrast to the normal span of seven items (Warrington et al., 1971). More posterior and inferior lesions at the occipital-temporal boundary can result in reduced visual–verbal immediate memory spans (Kinsbourne & Warrington, 1962). Reduced immediate memory for spatial locations and other visual–spatial displays can result from right occipital–parietal lesions (Warrington & James, 1967). Immediate memory, therefore, does not depend upon a common set of brain structures. Rather, there are distinct cortical regions, specialized both by modality and material, that briefly store information just heard or seen.

The consequences of a greatly reduced immediate memory span are remarkably few. Patients with very limited auditory–verbal immediate memory have trouble comprehending grammatically complex sentences and learning new foreign words, two situations in which a person may have to review carefully the sounds just heard because their meanings were not instantly grasped. Such patients, however, have normal or near-normal long-term memory for auditory–verbal information. This finding counters the expectation that information must pass through short-term memory in order to reach long-term memory. Instead, information from the environment enters immediate-memory and long-term memory stores in parallel rather than serially.

Working memory and strategic declarative memory

The frontal lobes appear to play a critical role in working memory (maintaining and manipulating information in a

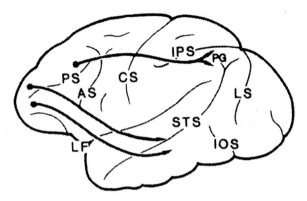

Fig. 21.8. Schematic of long-range projections between prefrontal and posterior association areas in the monkey. (Adapted from Pandya & Yeterian, 1985.)

goal-directed manner for a brief period) and in strategic declarative memory. Frontal regions are thought to select goal-relevant information from immediate and long-term memory stores in posterior cortices (Fig. 21.8). Evidence that working memory depends critically on frontal cortices comes from many sources, including human and animal lesion studies (Goldman-Rakic, 1987; Owen et al., 1996), single-cell recording studies (Funahashi et al., 1989), and neuroimaging studies (e.g. Cohen et al., 1994; Jonides et al., 1993). Functional neuroimaging studies indicate that executive processes (working memory resources beyond immediate spans) in humans may be especially linked to dorsolateral prefrontal cortex (e.g. D'Esposito et al., 1995; Petrides et al., 1993). Patients with frontal-lobe lesions are impaired on tasks that demand substantial working memory resources, such as reasoning (Milner, 1963; Shallice, 1982). These patients do not, however, exhibit the pervasive or severe declarative memory deficit seen in amnesia.

Patients with dorsolateral prefrontal lesions are impaired on declarative memory tasks that have great strategic demands, i.e. memory tasks that demand substantial planning, organization, evaluation, or manipulation of information for accurate performance. Some declarative memory tasks have relatively minimal strategic demands. Recognition tests, in which studied items are re-presented along with novel distracter items, typically require little strategy, as responses can be guided relatively easily and quickly on the basis of stimulus familiarity. Free recall tests, on the other hand, require people to devise their own strategy for recollecting prior experiences without experimenter-supplied assistance.

Lesions to dorsolateral and anterior prefrontal regions lead to specific impairments on tests of source memory

(Janowsky et al., 1989), list discrimination (Butters et al., 1994); frequency of occurrence (Angeles-Jurado et al., 1997; Smith & Milner, 1988); recency (Milner et al., 1991), temporal ordering (Shimamura et al., 1990), and free recall (Wheeler et al., 1995). What is common across these tasks is that a person has to make a difficult memory judgment that requires the active planning and organization of a retrieval strategy. These strategic memory deficits occur even when performance on corresponding recognition tests is normal. Specific impairments in strategic declarative memory may be contrasted with those seen in amnesia. In most cases, amnesic patients perform poorly on both strategic and nonstrategic memory tests. The strategic memory deficit in amnesic patients, however, is the consequence of their global declarative memory deficit.

The working memory and reasoning deficits that result from frontal lesions may be related to the specific failure in strategic memory performance. Difficult memory tasks require that reasoning capacities be brought to bear on, or work with, memory retrieval. Thus, the strategic memory failure may be the consequence of diminished reasoning and working memory resources being applied to otherwise intact declarative memory processes.

Selective deficits of strategic declarative memory have been found also in degenerative or developmental diseases of the basal ganglia, such as Parkinson's disease (PD), Huntington's disease (HD), and Gilles de la Tourette's syndrome (Gabrieli, 1996). Striatal diseases also impair reasoning (Lees & Smith, 1983) and working memory (Gabrieli et al., 1996b), and these deficits are correlated with the strategic memory deficits.

Thus, strategic declarative memory appears to depend on the integrity of corticostriatal circuits (Alexander et al., 1986) that mediate working memory and reasoning. Furthermore, animal (Brozoski et al., 1979; Sawaguchi & Goldman-Rakic, 1991) and human (Luciana et al., 1992; Müller et al., 1998) drug studies indicate that the neurotransmitter dopamine plays a critical role in working memory. PD patients have severely reduced dopamine functioning, and dopamine treatment can enhance their working memory performance (Cooper et al., 1992).

Non-declarative memory systems

Despite their global anterograde amnesia, even the most severely amnesic patients have demonstrated entirely normal learning on a number of skill learning, repetition priming and conditioning tasks. These findings provide compelling evidence for the independence of multiple memory systems in the human brain. Preservation of these

forms of memory in amnesia demonstrates that they do not depend upon the medial temporal lobe or other structures essential for declarative memory. Some of the neural systems underlying non-declarative memory have been identified in neuropsychological and neuroimaging studies. Non-declarative forms of memory do not depend on any common brain regions in the way that all forms of declarative memory depend on medial temporal lobe or diencephalic regions. Rather, each kind of non-declarative memory appears to involve experience-induced plasticity in the neural systems engaged by a particular task (e.g. motor areas for motor tasks, perceptual areas for perceptual tasks).

Skill learning

Skill learning (sometimes referred to as procedural memory) is expressed as the enhancement of accuracy or speed in performing a task across multiple training sessions. Amnesic patients have shown entirely normal and long-lasting skill learning on motor tasks (e.g. mirror tracing and rotary pursuit) (Milner, 1962; Corkin, 1968; Gabrieli et al., 1993), perceptual tasks (e.g. reading mirror-reversed text) (Cohen & Squire, 1980), and cognitive tasks (e.g. probabilistic classification) (Knowlton et al., 1994). Amnesic patients learn how to perform these tasks skillfully without knowing that they have had prior practice. Patients with basal ganglia diseases, especially HD, have shown impaired skill learning on many of these motor (Gabrieli et al., 1997b; Heindel et al., 1989), perceptual (Martone et al., 1984), and cognitive (Knowlton et al., 1996a, b) tasks. Thus, the basal ganglia appear to play an essential and widespread role in human skill learning that extends to cognitive skills.

Functional neuroimaging studies have revealed a dynamic plasticity of brain activations associated with skill learning. Learning a new skill is associated with expansion and reduction of initial activations and shifts in brain areas activated during initial, unskilled performance vs. later, skilled performance. For example, some motor skill learning tasks involve an expansion of activation in primary motor cortex and the basal ganglia (Grafton et al., 1992; Karni et al., 1995; Doyon et al., 1996; Hazeltine et al., 1997). For the perceptual skill of mirror reading, activation has been shown to increase in left inferior occipito-temporal cortex and decrease in bilateral parietal cortex as people improved their reading skill (Poldrack et al., 1998). These shifts in activity may represent a shift from reliance upon visuospatial decoding of mirror-reversed words in unskilled performance to more direct reading in skilled performance. These alterations in activation must reflect alterations in neural connectivity that mediate skilled performance.

Conditioning

The neural circuitry underlying classical and other forms of conditioning has been studied extensively in animals. There appears to be a remarkable conservation of memory mechanisms for conditioning across mammalian species, which provides an opportunity to integrate invasive animal and noninvasive human research about memory systems.

The memory system underlying classical delay eyeblink conditioning has been delineated with great precision in the rabbit, and may be the most precisely understood mammalian memory system (Thompson, 1990; Fig. 21.9). In the typical delay paradigm, a 250–500 ms tone (conditioned stimulus or CS) is repeatedly followed by an air-puff (unconditioned stimulus or US) delivered to the eye that elicits a blink reflex, the unconditioned response (UR). The tone and air-puff coterminate. With repeated CS–US pairings, subjects learn to associate the tone with the air-puff, and initiate an eyeblink (conditioned response or CR) to the CS before the onset of the US. The convergence of CS and US projections in eyeblink conditioning occurs in the cerebellum ipsilateral to the eye receiving the air-puff. Lesions of the cerebellar dentate–interpositus nuclei prevent acquisition or abolish retention of the conditioned association, but lesions of the hippocampus do not affect delay conditioning (Schmaltz & Theios, 1972). In humans, delay eyeblink conditioning is intact in amnesic patients with bilateral medial–temporal (Gabrieli et al., 1995b) or bilateral thalamic lesions (Daum & Ackermann, 1994), but abolished in patients with cerebellar lesions (Daum et al., 1993).

More complex forms of conditioning, however, are impaired after medial–temporal lobe lesions in humans and rabbits. In animals, medial–temporal lesions impair trace eyeblink conditioning, which differs from delay conditioning in that there is a short time period, a second or less, between the offset of the CS and the onset of the US (Solomon et al., 1986). Amnesic patients with medial–temporal lesions who are unimpaired on delay conditioning show impaired trace conditioning with CS–US trace intervals as short as 500 ms (McGlinchey-Berroth et al., 1997). In animals, medial–temporal lesions also impair discrimination reversal, in which the two CS stimuli are switched in terms of their association with the US (Berger & Orr, 1983). Amnesic patients with medial–temporal lesions also have impaired conditioning for discrimination reversal (Daum et al., 1989). These findings suggest that the same medial–temporal lobe structures that are essential for

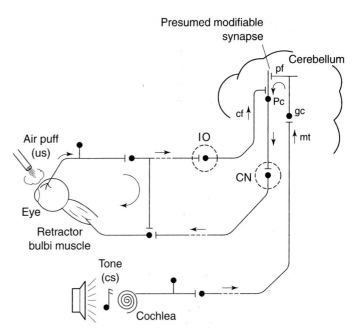

Fig. 21.9. Proposed minimal circuitry for eyeblink conditioning in the rabbit. An airpuff to the eye (us) is signalled to cerebellar Purkinje cells (PC) via the climbing fibres (cf), which originate in the inferior olive (IO). The tone (CS) is also signalled to the Purkinje cells through mossy fibres (mf), the cerebellar granule cells (gc), and the parallel fibres (pf). Modification at the putative plastic synapse (pf to Purkinje cell) would depend on properly timed activity in cf and pf. The Purkinje cells project to the cerebellar dentate–interpositus nuclei and then onto the motor neurons mediating the eyeblink response. (Adapted from Squire, 1987.)

declarative memory also mediate processes required for more complex forms of conditioning in humans and other mammals.

The critical role of the amygdala in fear conditioning to aversive stimuli such as electric shocks has been well established in rats (Hitchcock & Davis, 1986). Amygdala damage also impairs fear conditioning in humans. In two studies, participants were exposed to pairings of initially neutral conditioned visual stimuli (CS) preceding aversive unconditioned auditory stimuli (US), white-noise or boat-horn bursts, which elicited an unconditioned response measured as a change in skin conductance response. Over multiple trials, normal participants showed fear conditioning, as evidenced by conditioned skin conductance responses to the CS. An Urbach–Weithe patient (Bechara et al., 1995) and patients with amygdala resections (LaBar et al., 1995) showed little or no fear conditioning. The fear-conditioning deficit was dissociated from declarative memory because the patients had excellent declarative memory for the experimental experience, including the stimuli. In contrast, amnesic patients without amygdala damage demonstrated intact fear conditioning but impaired declarative memory for the experimental experience (Bechara et al., 1995).

Repetition priming

Repetition priming refers to facilitated processing of a stimulus, such as a word or picture, due to prior exposure to that or a related stimulus. In a typical experiment, participants process a set of stimuli in a study phase. In a subsequent test phase, participants perform a task with 'old' stimuli identical or related to the study-phase stimuli, and with 'new' stimuli that are unrelated to the study-phase and provide a baseline measure of performance. The difference in performance with old and new stimuli, the consequence of memories established during study, constitutes the measure of repetition priming (hereafter referred to as priming). For example, seeing the word STORK or a picture of a stork in a study phase makes people in a test phase more likely to identify that word or picture correctly when it is presented very briefly (e.g. less than one-twentieth of a second) or in a partial, fragmented form. People are also faster to read that word aloud and to name that picture aloud, and more likely to say 'STORK' when asked to complete three letters (STO _ _) with the first word that comes to mind, or to add letters so as to make a fragment (S _ _ R _) into a real word, or to say the first word that goes with BABY, or to provide examples of birds. Some of these examples of priming are primarily perceptual in nature and are linked to stimulus form (e.g. identifying a rapidly presented word); others are primarily conceptual in nature and are linked to stimulus meaning (e.g. listing examples of birds) (Roediger & McDermott, 1993).

Amnesic patients exhibit normal priming on many perceptual and conceptual tasks, despite little or no declarative memory for the stimuli they are identifying or producing with measurable benefits from prior processing (Warrington & Weiskrantz, 1970; Graf et al., 1984, 1985; Shimamura & Squire, 1984; Cermak et al., 1985; Cave & Squire 1992; Vaidya et al., 1995; Verfaellie et al., 1996). Amnesic patients can also show normal priming for novel materials (Gabrieli et al., 1990) and novel associations between materials (Moscovitch et al., 1986; Musen & Squire, 1993; Gabrieli et al., 1997a). Therefore, priming does not depend on medial–temporal lobe or other structures important for declarative memory. HD patients show intact priming (Heindel et al., 1989), so priming is also not dependent upon basal ganglia structures critical for skill learning.

Several lines of evidence indicate that priming is mediated by neocortical areas, with perceptual priming being mediated by modality-specific cortical areas and conceptual priming by amodal language areas. One source of evidence is the performance of AD patients, who exhibit severely reduced conceptual priming (Monti et al., 1996) but intact perceptual priming on visual tasks (Fleischman et al., 1995; Keane et al., 1991, 1995a). This pattern of impaired conceptual and intact perceptual priming may be interpreted in terms of the characteristic neocortical neuropathology in AD. In vivo metabolic imaging studies (e.g. (Frackowiak et al., 1981)) and postmortem studies of late-stage AD patients (Brun & Englund, 1981) find substantial damage to association neocortices in the frontal, parietal, and temporal lobes but relatively little compromise of primary visual, somatosensory, auditory, and motor cortices, the basal ganglia, or the cerebellum. The sparing of modality-specific cortices and the compromise of association cortices may account, respectively, for intact perceptual and impaired conceptual priming observed in AD. More direct evidence that modality-specific neocortex mediates modality-specific perceptual priming comes from patients with right occipital lesions. These patients have exhibited an absence of priming on visual tasks despite intact declarative memory and intact conceptual priming (Fleischman et al., 1995; Gabrieli et al., 1995a, b; Keane et al., 1995a).

Neuroimaging studies also indicate that separate cortical areas mediate perceptual and conceptual priming. Priming on visual tasks is associated with reduced activity in bilateral occipito-temporal regions (Squire et al., 1992; Schacter et al., 1996). Priming on conceptual tasks is associated with reduced activity in left frontal neocortex in healthy subjects (Raichle et al., 1994; Demb et al., 1995; Blaxton et al., 1996; Gabrieli et al., 1996a) and amnesic patients (Gabrieli et al., 1998).

Thus, lesion and imaging studies provide convergent evidence that different forms of priming reflect process-specific plasticity in separate neocortical regions. Visual priming is associated with changes in occipital cortex, whereas conceptual priming is associated with changes in language-related areas in left frontal cortex. Repetition priming in a given domain appears to reflect experience-induced changes in the same neural networks that subserved initial processing in that domain (Gabrieli et al., 1996a; Raichle et al., 1994). These changes facilitate or bias the subsequent reprocessing of the stimuli. The enhanced efficiency of reprocessing may diminish computational demands and thus lead to reduced activations relative to baseline conditions.

In conclusion, the global amnesia resulting from bilateral medial, diencepahlic, or basal forebrain lesions constitutes the most striking and debilitating memory disorder. Clinical and experimental studies have shown, however, that the brain is composed of multiple memory systems that include the cerebral cortex, amygdala, basal ganglia, and cerebellum. Indeed, all brain regions appear to be involved in one sort or another of memory. Further, it is likely that many effective forms of human learning involve collaborative interactions among multiple memory systems. Memory systems may be seen as highly specialized instruments of memory that normally act in seamless concert to allow lessons from the past to guide actions in the future.

Acknowledgement

Writing of this chapter was supported by NIH grants: NIAAG 09466, NH 59940 and NS 26985.

References

Adolphs, R., Tranel, D., Damasio, H. & Damasio, A. (1994). Impaired recognition of emotion in facial expressions following bilateral damage to the human amygdala. *Nature*, **372**, 669–72.

Adolphs, R., Tranel, D., Damasio, H. & Damasio, A.R. (1995). Fear and the human amygdala. *J. Neurosci.*, **15**, 5879–91.

Alexander, G.E., DeLong, M.R. & Strick, P.L. (1986). Parallel organization of functionally segregated circuits linking basal ganglia and cortex. *Ann. Rev. Neurosci.*, **9**, 357–81.

Angeles-Jurado, M., Junique, C., Pujol, J., Oliver, B. & Vendrell, P. (1997). Impaired estimation of word occurence frequency in frontal lobe patients. *Neuropsychologia*, **35**, 635–41.

Baddeley, A. (1986). *Working Memory*. Oxford, Clarendon Press.

Bailey, C.H. & Chen, M. (1983). Morphological basis of long-term habituation and sensitization in Aplysia. *Science*, **220** (4592), 91–3.

Bechara, A., Tranel, D., Damasio, H., Adolphs, R., Rockland, C. & Damasio, A. (1995). Double-dissociation of conditioning and declarative knowledge relative to the amygdala and the hippocampus in humans. *Science*, **269**, 1115–18.

Berger, T.W. & Orr, W.B. (1983). Hippocampectomy selectively disrupts discrimination reversal conditioning of the rabbit nictitating membrane response. *Behav. Brain Res.*, **8**, 49–68.

Blaxton, T.A., Bookheimer, S.Y., Zeffiro, T.A, Figlozzi, C.M., William, D.G. & Theodore, W.H. (1996). Functional mapping of human memory using PET: comparisons of conceptual and perceptual tasks. *Canad. J. Exp. Psychol.*, **50**, 42–56.

Brozoski, T., Brown, R.M., Rosvold, H.E. & Goldman-Rakic, P.S. (1979). Cognitive deficit caused by regional depletion of dopamine in prefrontal cortex of rhesus monkey. *Science*, **205**, 929–32.

Brun, A. & Englund, E. (1981). Regional pattern of degeneration in Alzheimer's disease: neuronal loss and histopathological grading. *Histopathology*, **5**, 549–64.

Butters, M.A., Kaszniak, A.W., Glisky, E.L., Eslinger, P.J. & Schacter, D.L. (1994). Recency discrimination deficits in frontal lobe patients. *Neuropsychology*, **8**, 343–53.

Cahill, L., Babinsky, R., Markowitsch, H. & McGaugh, J. (1995). The amygdala and emotional memory. *Nature*, **377**, 295–6.

Cahill, L., Haier, R., Fallon, J. et al. (1996). Amygdala activity at encoding correlated with long-term, free recall of emotional memory. *Proc. Natl. Acad. Sci., USA*, **93**, 8016–21.

Canli, T., Zhao, Z., Brewer, J., Gabrieli, J.D. & Cahill, L. (2000). Event-related activation in the human amygdala associates with later memory for individual emotional experience. *J. Neurosci.*, **20** (19), RC99.

Cave, C.B. & Squire, L.R. (1992). Intact and long-lasting repetition priming in amnesia. *J. Exp. Psychol.: Learning, Memory Cogn.*, **18**, 509–20.

Cermak, L.S., Talbot, N., Chandler, K. & Wolbarst, L.R. (1985). The perceptual priming phenomenon in amnesia. *Neuropsychologia*, **23**, 615–22.

Cohen, J.D., Forman, S.D., Braver, T.S., Casey, B.J., Servan-Schreiber, D. & Noll, D.C. (1994). Activation of prefrontal cortex in a non-spatial working memory task with functional MRI. *Hum. Brain Mapp.*, **1**, 293–304.

Cohen, N.J. & Squire, L.R. (1980). Preserved learning and retention of pattern-analyzing skill in amnesia: dissociation of knowing how and knowing that. *Science*, **210**, 207–10.

Cooper, J.A., Sagar, H.J., Doherty, S.M., Jordan, N., Tidswell, P. & Sullivan, E.V. (1992). Different effects of dopaminergic and anti-cholinergic therapies on congnitive and motor function in Parkinson's disease. *Brain*, **115**, 1701–25.

Corkin, S. (1968). Acquisition of motor skills after bilateral medial temporal-lobe excision. *Neuropsychologia*, **6**, 255–65.

Corkin, S., Amaral, D., Gonzalez, R., Johnson, K. & Hyman. B. (1997). H.M.'s medial temporal-lobe lesion: Findings from MRI. *J. Neurosci.*, **17**, 3964–79.

D'Esposito, M., Detre, J.A., Alsop, D.C., Shin, R.K., Atlas, S. & Grossman, M. (1995). The neural basis of the central executive system of working memory. *Nature*, **378**, 279–81.

Damasio, A.R., Graff-Radford, N.R., Eslinger, P.J., Damasio, H. & Kassell. N. (1985). Amnesia following basal forebrain lesions. *Arch. Neurol.*, **42**, 263–71.

Damasio, H., Grabowski, T.J., Tranel, D., Hichwa, R.D. & Damasio, A.R. (1996). A neural basis for lexical retrieval. *Nature*, **380**, 499–505.

Daum, I. & Ackermann, H. (1994). Dissociation of declarative and nondeclarative memory after bilateral thalamic lesions: a case report. *Int. J. Neurosci.*, **75** (3–4), 153–65.

Daum, I., Channon, S. & Canavan, A.G.M. (1989). Classical conditioning in patients with severe memory problems. *J. Neurol. Neurosurg. Psychiatry*, **52**, 47–51.

Daum, I., Schugens, M.M., Ackermann, H., Lutzenberger, W., Dichgans, J. & Birbaumer, N. (1993). Classical conditioning after cerebellar lesions in humans. *Behav. Neurosci.*, **107**, 748–56.

Davis, H.P. & Squire, L,R. (1984). Protein synthesis and memory: a review. *Psychol. Bull.*, **96** (3), 518–59.

de Leon, M.J., Golomb, J., George, A.E. et al. (1993). The radiologic prediction of Alzheimer's disease: the atrophic hippocampal formation. *Am. J. Neuroradiol.*, **14**, 897–906.

Demb, J.B., Desmond, J.E., Wagner, A.D., Vaidya, C.J., Glover, G.H. & Gabrieli, J.D.E. (1995). Semantic encoding and retrieval in the left inferior cortex: a functional MRI study of task difficulty and process specificity. *J. Neurosci.*, **15**, 5870–8.

Doyon, J., Owen, A.M., Petrides, M., Sziklas, V. & Evans, A.C. (1996). Functional anatomy of visuomotor skill learning in human subjects examined with positron emission tomography. *Eur. J. Neurosci.*, **8** (4), 637–48.

Dusoir, H., Kapur, N., Byrnes, D.P., McKinstry, S. & Hoare, R.D. (1990). The role of diencephalic pathology in human memory disorder. *Brain*, **113**, 1695–706.

Eichenbaum, H. & Cohen, N.J. (2001). *From Conditioning to Conscious Recollection: Memory Systems of the Brain*. New York: Oxford University Press.

Fleischman, D.A., Gabrieli, J.D.E., Reminger, S., Rinaldi, J., Morrell, F. & Wilson, R. (1995). Conceptual priming in perceptual identification for patients with Alzheimer's disease and a patient with a right occipital lobectomy. *Neuropsychology*, **9**, 187–97.

Frackowiak, R.S.J., Pozzilli, C., Legg, N.J. et al. (1981). Regional cerebral oxygen supply and utilization in dementia: a clinical and physiological study with oxygen-15 and positron tomography. *Brain*, **104**, 753–78.

Funahashi, S., Bruce, C.J. & Goldman-Rakic, P.S. (1989). Mnemonic coding of visual space in the monkey's dorsolateral prefrontal cortex. *J. Neurophysiol.*, **61** (2), 331–49.

Gabrieli, J.D.E. (1996). Memory systems analyses of mnemonic disorders in aging and age-related diseases. *Proc. Natl. Acad. Sci., USA*, **93**, 13534–40.

Gabrieli, J.D.E. (1998). Cognitive neuroscience of human memory. *Ann. Rev. Psychol.*, **49**, 87–115.

Gabrieli, J.D.E., Milberg, W., Keane, M.M. & Corkin, S. (1990). Intact priming of patterns despite impaired memory. *Neuropsychologia*, **28**, 417–27.

Gabrieli, J.D.E., Corkin, S., Mickel, S.F. & Growdon, J.H. (1993). Intact acquisition and long-term retention of mirror-tracing skill in Alzheimer's disease and in global amnesia. *Behav. Neurosci.*, **107**, 899–910.

Gabrieli, J.D.E., Fleischman, D.A., Keane, M.M., Reminger, S.L. & Morrell, F. (1995a). Double dissociation between memory systems underlying explicit and implicit memory in the human brain. *Psychol. Sci.*, **6**, 76–82.

Gabrieli, J.D.E., McGlinchey-Berroth, R., Carillo, M.C., Gluck, M.A., Cermak, L.S. & Disterhoft, J.F. (1995b). Intact delay-eyeblink classical conditioning in amnesia. *Behav. Neurosci.*, **109**, 819–27.

Gabrieli, J.D.E., Desmond, J.E., Demb, J.B. et al. (1996a). Functional magnetic resonance imaging of semantic memory processes in the frontal lobes. *Psychol. Sci.*, **7**, 278–83.

Gabrieli, J.D.E., Singh, J., Stebbins, G.T. & Goetz, C.G. (1996b). Reduced working-memory span in Parkinson's disease: Evidence for the role of a fronto-striatal system in working and strategic memory. *Neuropsychology*, **10**, 322–32.

Gabrieli, J.D.E., Keane, M.M., Zarella, M.M. & Poldrack, R.A. (1997a). Preservation of implicit memory for new associations in global amnesia. *Psychol. Sci.*, **8**, 326–9.

Gabrieli, J.D.E., Stebbins, G.T., Singh, J., Willingham, D.B. & Goetz, C.G. (1997b). Intact mirror-tracing and impaired rotary-pursuit skill learning in patients with Huntington's disease: evidence for dissociable memory systems in skill learning. *Neuropsychology*, **11**, 272–81.

Gabrieli, J.D., Poldrack, R.A. & Desmond, J.E. (1998). The role of left prefrontal cortex in language and memory. *Proc. Natl. Acad. Sci., USA*, **95**, 906–13.

Gaffan, D. & Gaffan, E.A. (1991). Amnesia in man following transection of the fornix. A review. *Brain*, **114** (6), 2611–18.

Goldman-Rakic, P.S. (1987). Circuitry of primate prefrontal cortex and regulation of behavior by representational memory. In *The Handbook of Physiology – The Nervous System*, ed. V. F. Plum, pp. 373–417. New York: Oxford University Press.

Graf, P. & Schacter, D.L. (1985). Implicit and explicit memory for new associations in normal and amnesic subjects. *J. Exp. Psychol.: Learning, Memory Cogn.*, **11**, 501–18.

Graf, P., Squire, L.R. & Mandler, G. (1984). The information that amnesic patients do not forget. *J. Exp. Psychol.: Learning, Memory Cogn.*, **10**, 164–78.

Graf, P., Shimamura, A.P. & Squire, L.R. (1985). Priming across modalities and priming across category levels: extending the domain of preserved function in amnesia. *J. Exp. Psychol.: Learning, Memory Cogn.*, **11**, 386–96.

Grafton, S.T., Mazziotta, J.C., Presty, S., Friston, K.J. & Frackowiak, R.S.J. (1992). Functional anatomy of human procedural learning determined with regional cerebral blood flow and PET. *J. Neurosci.*, **12**, 2542–8.

Hamann, S.B., Ely, T.D., Grafton, S.T. & Kilts, C.D. (1999). Amygdala activity related to enhanced memory for pleasant and aversive stimuli. *Nat. Neurosci.*, **2** (3), 289–93.

Hazeltine, E., Grafton, S.T. & Ivry, R. (1997). Attention and stimulus characteristics determine the locus of motor-sequence encoding. A PET study. *Brain*, **120** (1), 123–40.

Heindel, W.C., Salmon, D.P., Shults, C.W., Walicke, P.A. & Butters, N. (1989). Neuropsychological evidence for multiple implicit memory systems: a comparison of Alzheimer's, Huntington's, and Parkinson's disease patients. *J. Neurosci.*, **9**, 582–7.

Hitchcock, J. & Davis, M. (1986). Lesions of the amygdala, but not of the cerebellum or red nucleus, block conditioned fear as measured with the potentiated startle paradigm. *Behav. Neurosci.*, **100**(1), 11–22.

Hyman, B.T., Van Hoesen, G.W., Damasio, A.R. & Barnes, C.L. (1984). Alzheimer's disease: cell-specific pathology isolates the hippocampal formation. *Science*, **225**, 1168–70.

Janowsky, J.S., Shimamura, A.P. & Squire, L.R. (1989). Source memory impairment in patients with frontal lobe lesions. *Neuropsychologia*, **8**, 1043–56.

Jonides, J., Smith, E.E., Koeppe, R.A., Awh, E., Minoshima, S. & Mintun, M.A. (1993). Spatial working memory in humans as revealed by PET. *Nature*, **363**, 623–5.

Kandel, E.R. & Schwartz, J.H. (1982). Molecular biology of learning: modulation of transmitter release. *Science*, **218**, 433–43.

Kandel, E.R., Schwartz, J.H. & Jessell, T.M. (2000). *Principles of Neural Science*. New York: McGraw-Hill.

Kapur, N., Ellison, D., Smith, M.P., Mclellan, D.L. & Burrows, E.H.

(1992). Focal retrograde amnesia following bilateral temporal lobe pathology: a neuropsychological and magnetic resonance study. *Brain*, **115**, 73–85.

Karni, A., Meyer, G., Jezzard, P., Adams, M.M., Turner, R. & Ungerleider, L.G. (1995). Functional MRI evidence for adult motor cortex plasticity during motor skill learning. *Nature*, **377** (6545), 155–8.

Keane, M.M., Gabrieli, J.D.E. et al. (1991). Evidence for a dissociation between perceptual and conceptual priming in Alzheimer's disease. *Behav. Neurosci.*, **105**, 326–42.

Keane, M.M., Gabrieli, J.D.E. et al. (1995a). Double dissociation of memory capacities after bilateral occipital-lobe or medial temporal-lobe lesions. *Brain*, **118**, 1129–48.

Keane, M.M., Gabrieli, J.D.E., Growdon, J.H. & Corkin. S. (1995b). Normal perceptual priming of orthographically illegal nonwords in amnesia. *J. Int. Neuropsychol. Soci.*, **1**, 425–33.

Kinsbourne, M. & Warrington, E.K. (1962). A disorder of simultaneous form perception. *Brain*, **85** (461–86).

Knowlton, B.J., Squire, L.R. & Gluck, M. (1994). Probabilistic classification learning in amnesia. *Learning Memory*, **1**, 106–20.

Knowlton, B., Mangels, L. & Squire, L. (1996a). A neostriatal habit learning system in humans. *Science*, **273**, 1399–402.

Knowlton, B.J., Squire, L.R., Paulsen, J.S., Swerdlow, N.R., Swenson, M. & Butters, N. (1996b). Dissociations within nondeclarative memory in Huntington's Disease. *Neuropsychology*, **10**, 538–48.

LaBar, K., Le Doux, J., Spencer, D. & Phelps, E. (1995). Impaired fear conditioning following unilateral temporal lobectomy in humans. *J. Neurosci.*, **15**, 6846–55.

Lees, A.J. & Smith, E. (1983). Cognitive deficits in the early stages of Parkinson's disease. *Brain*, **106**, 257–70.

Luciana, M., Depue, R.A., Arbisi, P. & Leon, A. (1992). Facilitation of working memory in humans by a D2 dopamine receptor. *J. Cogn. Neurosci.*, **4** (1), 58–68.

McGlinchey-Berroth, R., Carrillo, M., Gabrieli, J.D.E., Brawn, C.M. & Disterhoft, J.F. (1997). Impaired trace eyeblink conditioning in bilateral medial temporal lobe amnesia. *Behav. Neurosci.*, **111**, 873–82.

Malenka, R.C. (1994). Synaptic plasticity in the hippocampus: LTP and LTD. *Cell*, **78** (4), 535–8.

Martin, A., Haxby, J., Lalonde, F.M., Wiggs, C.L. & Ungerleider, L.G. (1995). Discrete cortical regions associated with knowledge of color and knowledge of action. *Science*, **270**, 102–5.

Martone, M., Butters, N., Payne, M., Becker, J.T. & Sax, D.S. (1984). Dissociations between skill learning and verbal recognition in amnesia and dementia. *Arch. Neurol.*, **41**, 965–70.

Milner, B. (1962). Les troubles de la memoire accompagnant des lesions hippocampiques bilaterales. In *Psychologie de l'hippocampe*. Paris: Centre National de la Recherche Scientifique.

Milner, B. (1963). Effects of different brain lesions on card sorting. *Arch. Neurol.*, **9**, 90–100.

Milner, B. (1974). Hemispheric specialization: scope and limits. In *The Neurosciences: Third Study Program*, ed. F.O. Schmitt & F.G. Wordon, pp. 75–89. Cambridge, MA: MIT Press.

Milner, B., Corsi, P. & Leonard, G. (1991). Frontal-lobe contribution to recency judgements. *Neuropsychologia*, **29**(6), 601–18.

Monti, L.A., Gabrieli, J.D.E., Reminger, S.L., Rinaldi, J.A., Wilson, R.S. & Fleischman, D.A. (1996). Differential effects of aging and Alzheimer's disease upon conceptual implicit and explicit memory. *Neuropsychology*, **10**, 101–12.

Morris, J.S., Frith, C.D,. Perrett, D.I. et al. (1996). A differential neural response in the human amygdala to fearful and happy facial expressions. *Nature*, **383**, 812–15.

Moscovitch, M., Winocur, G. & McLachlan, D. (1986). Memory as assessed by recognition and reading time in normal and memory-impaired people with Alzheimer's disease and other neurological disorders. *J. Exp. Psychol.: Gen.*, **115**, 331–47.

Müller, U., von Cramon, D.Y. & Pollmann, S. (1998). D1 versus D2-receptor modulation of visuospatial working memory in humans. *J. Neurosci.*, **18** (7), 2720–8.

Murray, E.A. & Mishkin, M. (1986). Visual recognition in monkeys following rhinal cortical ablations combined with either amygdalectomy or hippocampectomy. *J. Neurosci.*, **6**, 1991–2003.

Musen, G. & Squire, L.R. (1993). On the implicit learning of novel associations by amnesic patients and normal subjects. *Neuropsychology*, **7** (2), 119–35.

Owen, A.M., Morris, R.G., Sahakian, B.J., Polkey, C.E. & Robbins, T.W. (1996). Double dissociations of memory and executive functions in working memory tasks following frontal lobe excisions, temporal lobe excisions or amygdalo-hippocampectomy in man. *Brain*, **119** (5), 1597–615.

Pandya, D.N. & Yeterian, E.H. (1985). Architecture and connections of cortical association areas. In *Cerebral Cortex*, ed. A.P. Jones, pp. 3–61. New York: Plenum.

Petrides, M., Alivisatos, B., Meyer, E. & Evans, A.C. (1993). Functional activation of the human frontal cortex during the performance of verbal working memory tasks. *Proc. Natl. Acad. Sci, USA*, **90**, 878–82.

Phelps, E.A. & Anderson, A.K. (1997). Emotional memory: What does the amygdala do? *Curr. Opin. Biol.*, **7**, 11–13.

Poldrack, R.A., Desmond, J.E., Glover, G.H. & Gabrieli, J.D.E. (1998). The neural basis of visual skill: an fmri study of mirror reading. *Cereb. Cortex*, **8**, 1–10.

Press, G.A., Amaral, D.G. & Squire, L.R. (1989). Hippocampal abnormalities in amnesic patients revealed by high-resolution magnetic resonance imaging. *Nature*, **341**, 54–7.

Raichle, M.E., Fiez, J.A., Videen, T.O. et al. (1994). Practice-related changes in human brain functional anatomy during nonmotor learning. *Cereb. Cortex*, **4**, 8–26.

Rempel-Clower, N., Zola, S., Squire, L. & Amaral, D. (1996). Three cases of enduring memory impairment after bilateral damage limited to the hippocampal formation. *J. Neurosci.*, **16**, 5233–55.

Roediger, H.L. & McDermott, K.B. (1993). Implicit memory in normal human subjects. In *Handbook of Neuropsychology*, ed. H.S.F. Boller, vol. 8, pp. 63–131. Amsterdam: Elsevier.

Sawaguchi, T. & Goldman-Rakic, P.S. (1991). D1 Dopamine receptors in prefrontal cortex: involvement in working memory. *Science*, **251**, 947–50.

Schacter, D.L., Alpert, N.M., Savage, C.R., Rauch, S.L. & Albert, M.S. (1996). Conscious recollection and the human hippocampal formation: evidence from positron emission topography. *Proc. Natl. Acad. Sci., USA*, **93**, 321–5.

Schmaltz, L.W. & Theios. J. (1972). Acquisition and extinction of a classically conditioned response in hippocampectomized rabbits (oryctolagus cuniculus). *J. Comp. Physiol. Psychol.*, **79**, 328–33.

Scott, S.K., Young, A.W., Calder, A.J., Hellawell, D.J., Aggleton, J.P. & Johnson, M. (1997). Impaired auditory recognition of fear and anger following bilateral amygdala lesions. *Nature*, **385**, 254–7.

Scoville, W.B. & Milner, B. (1957). Loss of recent memory after bilateral hippocampal lesions. *J. Neurol. Neurosurg. Psychiatry*, **20**, 11–21.

Shallice, T. (1982). Specific impairments of planning. *Phil. Trans. Roy. Soc. Lond. B Biol. Sci.*, **298**(1089), 199–209.

Shimamura, A.P. & Squire, L.R. (1984). Paired-associate learning and priming effects in amnesia: a neuropsychological study. *J. Exp. Psychol.: Gen.*, **113**, 556–70.

Shimamura, A.P., Janowsky, J.S. et al. (1990). Memory for the temporal order of events in patients with frontal lobe lesions and amnesic patients. *Neuropsychologia*, **28**, 803–13.

Smith, M.L. & Milner, B. (1988). Estimation of frequency of occurrence of abstract designs after frontal or temporal lobectomy. *Neuropsychologia*, **26**, 297–306.

Solomon, P.R., Vander Schaaf, E.R., Thompson, R.F. & Weisz, D.J. (1986). Hippocampus and trace conditioning of the rabbits classically conditioned nictitating membrane response. *Behav. Neurosci.*, **100**, 729–44.

Squire, L.R. (1987). *Memory and Brain.* New York: Oxford University Press.

Squire, L.R., Ojemann, J.G., Miezin, F.M., Petersen, S.E., Videen, T.O. & Raichle, M.E. (1992). Activation of the hippocampus in normal humans: a functional anatomical study of memory. *Proc. Natl. Acad. Sci, USA*, **89**, 1837–41.

Teng, E. & Squire, L.R. (1999). Memory for places learned long ago is intact after hippocampal damage. *Nature*, **400**, 675–7.

Thompson, R.F. (1990). Neural mechanisms of classical conditioning in mammals. *Phil. Trans. Roy. Soc. Lond. B*, **329**, 161–70.

Tulving, E. (1983). *Elements of Episodic Memory.* London: Oxford University Press.

Vaidya, C.J., Gabrieli, J.D.E., Keane, M.M. & Monti, L.A. (1995). Perceptual and conceptual memory processes in global amnesia. *Neuropsychology*, **9**, 580–91.

Verfaellie, M., Gabrieli, J.D.E., Vaidya, C.J., Croce, P. & Reminger, S.L. (1996). Implicit memory for pictures in amnesia: role of etiology and priming task. *Neuropsychology*, **10**, 517–28.

Victor, M.R., Adams, R.D. & Collins, G.H. (1971). *The Wernicke–Korsakoff Syndrome.* Philadelphia: Davis.

von Cramon, D.Y., Hebel, N. & Schuri, U. (1985). A contribution to the anatomical basis of thalamic amnesia. *Brain*, **108** (4), 993–1008.

Warrington, E.K. & James, M. (1967). Disorders of visual perception in patients with localised cerebral lesions. *Neuropsychologia*, **5**, 253–66.

Warrington, E.K. & Weiskrantz, L. (1970). The amnesic syndrome: consolidation or retrieval? *Nature*, **228**, 628–30.

Warrington, E.K., Logue, V. & Pratt, R.T.C. (1971). The anatomical localisation of selective impairment of auditory verbal short-term memory. *Neuropsychologia*, **9**, 377–87.

Wheeler, M.A., Stuss, D.T. & Tulving, E. (1995). Frontal lobe damage produces episodic memory impairment. *J. Int. Neuropsychol. Soc.*, **1**, 525–36.

Zola-Morgan, S. & Squire, L.R. (1985). Amnesia in monkeys following lesions of the mediodorsal nucleus of the thalamus. *Ann. Neurol.*, **17**, 558–64.

Zola-Morgan, S., Squire, L.R. & Amaral, D.G. (1986). Human amnesia and the medial temporal region: enduring memory impairment following a bilateral lesion limited to field CAI of the hippocampus. *J. Neurosci.*, **6**, 2950–67.

Zola-Morgan, S., Squire, L.R., Amaral, D.G. & Suzuki, W.A. (1989). Lesions of perirhinal and parahippocampal cortex that spare the amygdala and hippocampal formation produce severe memory impairment. *J. Neurosci.*, **9** (12), 4355–70.

22

Acquired disorders of language

John Hart, Jr[1] and Ola A. Selnes[2]

[1] Laboratory of Cognition and Brain Imaging, Donald W. Reynolds Center on Aging, Unversity of Arkansas Medical School, USA
[2] Department of Neurology, School of Medicine and Department of Cognitive Science, Krieger Mind/Brain Institute, The Johns Hopkins University, MD, USA

In 1915, the British neurologist Henry Head commented on recent developments in clinical aphasiology and concluded that: 'It is generally conceded that the views on aphasia and analogous disturbances of speech found in the textbooks of today are of little help in understanding an actual case of disease' (Head, 1915). This may still be true to a certain extent, although perhaps for different reasons from those that Head had in mind. Most textbooks typically describe classical aphasia syndromes that are based on chronic, stable patients; thus by definition different from the patient with acute symptoms that the neurologist typically encounters. It has been estimated that only 20–30% of all patients with aphasia will fit neatly into one of the classical aphasia syndromes (Albert et al., 1991). Nonetheless, the clinical use of the classical syndrome classification as a basis for diagnosis has continued more or less unchanged.

The convenience of this approach in clinical settings notwithstanding, increasing dissatisfaction with the classical taxonomy of aphasia has been expressed by researchers in the field of aphasia, in particular psycholinguistics and cognitive psychologists (Schwartz, 1984). The principal concern is that the classical model does not necessarily generate any meaningful generalizations about the nature of brain-language relationships. Some have argued that the classical aphasia syndromes do not meet standard criteria for a syndrome, in that none of the syndromes can be characterized in terms of invariant features that are shared by all patients given a certain classification and are absent in patients with a different classification (Caramazza, 1984). Classical taxonomy can thus best be characterized as polytypic, implying that any given feature or impairment, for example phonological paraphasias, can be part of more than one syndrome (Schwartz, 1984).

Despite the controversy over classical aphasia taxonomy in research settings and the limited number of aphasic patients it accounts for, the clinical utility of classic aphasia syndromes has rarely been questioned. It appears to have been assumed that the syndromes are associated with a certain degree of anatomical predictability, which may allow the clinician to infer lesion location, etiology, and prognosis (Albert et al., 1991). Recent studies have questioned the validity of these assumptions, however. In particular, the expectation that aphasia syndromes have localizing value does not appear to have stood the test of time (Willmes & Poeck, 1993; Basso et al., 1985; Vignolo et al., 1986). The evidence that classic aphasia syndromes carry prognostic implications is also not compelling. The Boston Diagnostic Aphasia Examination (BDAE) diagnostic classifications are somewhat predictive of outcome for syndromes characterized by mild impairment, such as anomic and conduction aphasia, and for those characterized by severe syndromes, such as global aphasia. This is consistent with the findings from several studies showing that one of the best prognostic indicators for recovery from aphasia is initial degree of severity (Pedersen et al., 1995). Syndromes that are characterized by a greater range in severity, such as Broca's and Wernicke's aphasia, are not predictive of outcomes (Kertesz & McCabe, 1977).

Thus, classic subtyping of aphasia does not appear to offer any particular benefits for either research or clinical purposes. In the absence of a better system for characterizing clinical aphasia subtypes, it is nonetheless likely to persist. One commonly used alternative to the classic aphasia taxonomy is to dichotomize patients on the basis of speech fluency. Fluency can be rated on the basis of conversational speech. The BDAE criteria for fluency are based on the 'longest occasional uninterrupted string of words' that the patient is able to produce. The speech of non-fluent patients may range from complete mutism to slow, halting, and effortful production of individual words. Mutism is a rare finding in aphasia and most often occurs as a transient initial sign. Non-fluent speech is often associated with articulatory problems or dysarthria, but some non-fluent aphasics have normal articulation. A subset of non-fluent patients have a tendency to omit grammatical words from their speech, resulting in telegraphic or agrammatic speech output. The speech of patients with fluent aphasia resembles normal speech in terms of rate of word production and phrase length. Non-fluent aphasia may be somewhat more common in younger patients, whereas fluent aphasia tends to predominate in patients 70 years or older (Ferro & Madureira, 1997). Speech fluency provides an approximate guide to lesion location in that non-fluent aphasia is most commonly associated with lesions that include anterior regions of the perisylvian language areas, whereas fluent aphasia is frequently associated with posterior lesions. This classification by itself does not necessarily carry much prognostic implication, although patients who remain non-fluent at 1 month after stroke are not likely to show substantial future improvement in fluency (Knopman et al., 1983).

Overall, there is no single language symptom that can adequately capture the nature of observed language disorders or provide adequate anatomic specificity to allow for an anatomic classification of aphasic disorders. Nor at this point, does any one language symptom provide a clear theoretical framework to account for what a particular brain region 'subserves' (e.g. there is no brain region that specifically performs a function like 'comprehension'). Thus, clinicians have been faced with performing a systematic evaluation of aphasia by characterizing a group of standard language components (e.g. speech, comprehension, naming, and repetition), assessing the pattern of impaired performance on these components, and inferring anatomic localization resulting in these deficits from these patterns.

Signs and symptoms of aphasia

Most cases of aphasia are secondary to stroke, and the abrupt onset of change in language-related functions may be the most reliable indicator that the symptoms stem from an aphasia. Very few aphasic symptoms are by themselves unique or diagnostic of aphasia. Dysnomia, paraphasias, and dysgraphias may occur in neurologically intact individuals. Therefore, it may be difficult to diagnose cases of aphasia due to causes other than stroke, such as primary progressive aphasia, during the early stages of the disease.

Dysnomia

Of the variety of symptoms associated with aphasia, none is more ubiquitous than dysnomia. A disorder of word finding or retrieval is present in all types of aphasia. In most cases, word finding difficulties are readily apparent in the patient's attempts at spontaneous speech. In milder cases, formal testing with confrontation naming may be required to document the dysnomia. Whereas non-fluent patients struggle to find individual words, the fluent patient often will substitute non-specific grammatical function words for content words. Poor recovery of naming has been associated with lesions involving either the posterior superior temporal lobe or the insula/putamen (Knopman et al., 1984). Unlike patients with Alzheimer's disease, whose naming failure may be principally on the basis of an impairment at the level of semantics, the dysnomia of patients with aphasia typically is on the basis of an impairment at the level of phonological activation. In some patients, the dysnomia may be restricted to certain semantic categories, such as colours, fruits and vegetables or tools (Warrington & Shallice, 1984; Hart et al., 1985). Although cases of category-specific naming deficits are relatively rare, detailed study of these cases may eventually provide critical information about the organization of the normal lexicon and its neural substrates (Caramazza & Shelton, 1998). Dysnomia in the absence of significant impairment in other aspects of speech and language does not appear to carry any specific localizing value.

Paraphasias

These refer to unintended substitutions at the level of individual sounds or words and are common in all types of aphasia. The principal subtypes of verbal substitutions are phonemic, semantic, and neologistic. Phonemic paraphasias refer to substitutions of one *sound* (or phoneme) for another, such as saying 'tork' instead of 'fork'. Phonemic paraphasias are common to most subtypes of aphasia, but are particularly abundant in aphasia secondary to incomplete lesions of the posterior language areas, such as conduction aphasia. Semantic paraphasias, or substitution of another word for an intended one, generally occur with significant involvement of the posterior superior temporal lobe (Wernicke's area). Neologisms are substitutions that are so far removed from the intended word that the target can no longer be recognized as an English word. Neologistic substitutions are most often seen with severe aphasias involving lesions of Wernicke's area and posterior extensions. Although both the frequency and type of paraphasic errors are relevant,

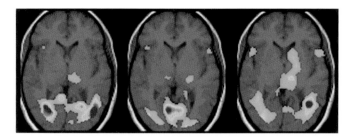

Fig. 1.1. Functional MRI signal changes during performance of a cognitive task. The above images are at the level of the thalamus for three normal controls showing that each of the participants exhibited signal changes in the thalamic hemispheres when they activated an object in memory (Kraut et al., 2001).

...and imaging

8 A coil in the spectrometer detects the vector in -X as an induced voltage, like this one showing 2 resonant frequencies:

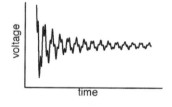

9 Fourier transformation of such a signal into the frequency domain produces a spectrum with two frequency peaks:

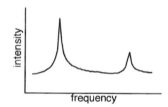

10 Anatomical images can be made from large frequency peaks. A magnetic field gradient placed across the sample causes the peak's resonant frequency to assume a different value at each spatial point. If this is done in 2 or 3 dimensions, a computer can reconstruct a 2D or 3D image of the peak's intensity and relaxation properties, both of which vary due to differences in the local microchemical environment across the compartments of biological tissue. These variations provide the anatomical contrast in images like this one (from Fig. 4A), which is a standard T2-weighted MRI scan made from the water proton signal. A glioma and its surrounding edema are visible because they provide microchemical environments for water different from those of normal brain.

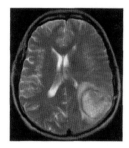

11 Several peaks from other compounds are sufficiently intense and well separated from each other to allow mapping of their anatomical distribution by a similar process. This example (Fig. 11.4D) shows the distribution of the signal from choline-containing compounds; signal intensity is color-coded, red high, blue low. The signal is strongest in the region of the glioma, a finding which is characteristic of many brain tumors and may reflect increased membrane synthesis. The map is coarser than the above MRI of the same brain, because the choline signal is several thousand times smaller than the one from water protons. Comparable maps can currently be made from the signals of N-acetyl aspartate, creatine, and lactate (see Figs. 11.4 and 11.5). Methods under development will extend the list to include glutamate, GABA, and other compounds of neurobiological interest.

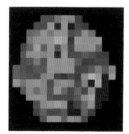

Fig. 11.2. NMR principles continued.

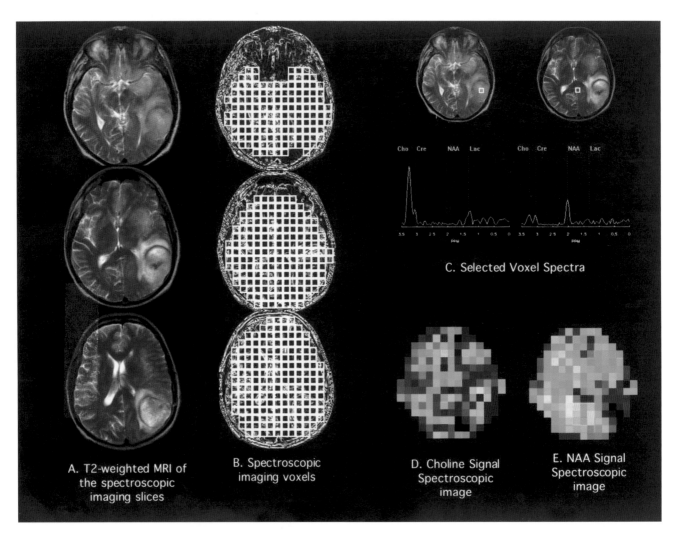

Fig. 11.4. MRI and MRS from a patient later found to have glioblastoma multiforme. (*a*) MRIs at three levels. (*b*) Locations of spectroscopic imaging voxels. (*c*) Images and spectra from voxels in tumour (left) and adjacent normal brain. (*d*), (*e*) Spectroscopic images made from the choline and NAA signals, showing the former elevated in the tumour and the latter depressed.

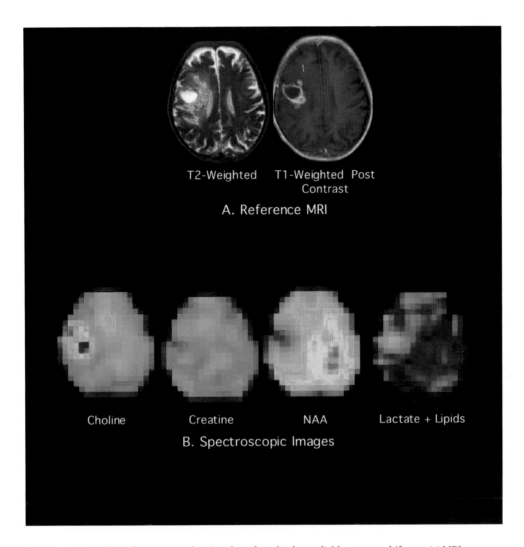

Fig. 11.5. MRI and MRS from a second patient later found to have glioblastoma multiforme. (*a*) MRIs showing the tumour. (*b*) Spectroscopic images showing elevated choline, lactate and lipid signals and depressed creatine and NAA signals associated with the tumour.

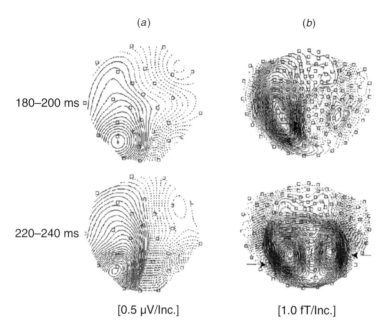

(a) (b)

180–200 ms

220–240 ms

[0.5 µV/Inc.] [1.0 fT/Inc.]

Fig. 12.1. ERP scalp distribution (*a*) and magnetic field distribution (*b*) of the N2pc component in two subsequent time windows (180–200 ms, 220–240 ms). Red lines indicate positive voltage of the potential distribution in (*a*) and magnetic flux leaving the cortex in (*b*). Note, polarities have relative character due to the direction of subtraction (LVF minus RVF targets) that was arbitrarily chosen. Arrows in (*b*) indicate locations of underlying current dipoles.

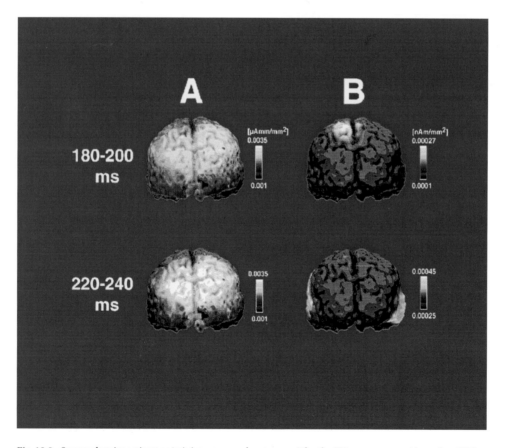

Fig. 12.2. Source density estimates (minimum norm least square) for the N2pc-component based on ERP difference waves (LVF minus RVF targets) (*a*) and MEG difference waves (*b*) in the early (180–200 ms) and late (220–240 ms) time window.

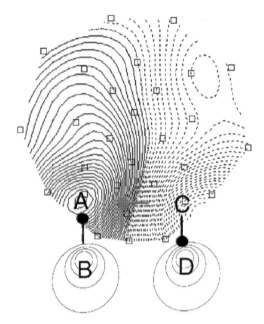

Fig. 12.3. An illustration of the erroneous link between ERP field components that gives rise to the discrepant source density estimates for ERP and MEG data as shown in Fig. 12.2. The measured ERP distribution between 220 and 240 ms is schematically completed by field components (*b*) and (*d*) that could not be picked up with the used electrode array, but are strongly implied by the magnetic field configuration. Specifically, linking field component (*a*) to (*b*) and (*c*) to (*d*) would give rise to source configurations as indicated by black dipoles. In contrast, the green dipole illustrates the potential mislocalization due to erroneous linkage of (*a*) and (*c*).

Current Density Analysis of ERP/MEF in a single subject

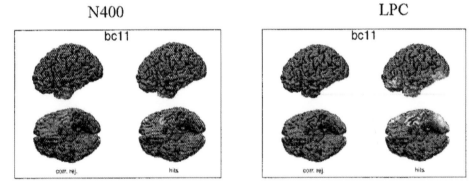

Fig. 12.4. *Upper part:* Single subject current density analysis for hits and correct rejections in the N400 time window and the LPC time window performed by taking into account the subjects 3D MRI. Red colours indicate areas of high current flows on the brain surface that account for the recorded electric and magnetic activity. It can be seen that in the N400 time window, correct rejections induce stronger current flows in the left anterior temporal lobe than hits. In contrast, hits induce stronger current flows in the posterior inferior temporal lobe than correct rejections.

EEG   MEG

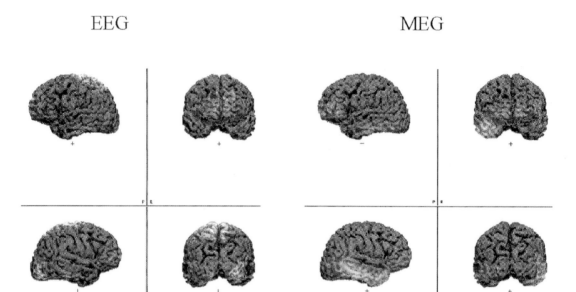

Fig. 12.7. Single subject current density analysis of EEG and MEG measured 200 ms prior to a motor response indicating the completion of a word fragment. While the MEG data reveal, in accord with a concurrent fMRI study, bilateral temporal activity, source analysis based on EEG data alone indicate a prominent parieto-central source.

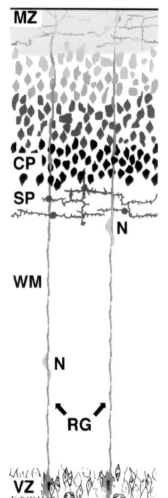

Fig. 13.1. A scheme of glia-guided migration. Postmitotic neurons (N), which are born in the ventricular zone (VZ), migrate along the radial glial fibres (RG) through the developing white matter (WM) and the subplate layer (SP) into the cortical plate (CP). They are added to the cortical plate in an 'inside-out' fashion, and stop immediately underneath the marginal zone (MZ). Reelin protein in the marginal zone (represented by yellow colour) serves as an apparent 'stop signal' for the neurons (see text).

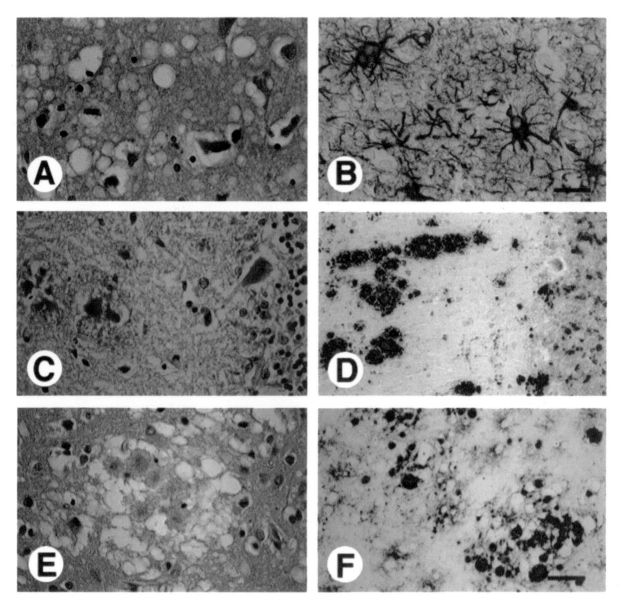

Fig. 15.4. Neuropathology of human prion diseases. Sporadic CJD is characterized by vacuolation of the neuropil of the grey matter, by exuberant reactive astrocytic gliosis, the intensity of which is proportional to the degree of nerve cell loss, and rarely by PrP amyloid plaque formation (not shown). The neuropathology of familial CJD is similar. GSS(P102L), as well as other inherited forms of GSS (not shown), is characterized by numerous deposits of PrP amyloid throughout the CNS. The neuropathological features of nvCJD are unique among CJD cases because of the abundance of PrP amyloid plaques that are often surrounded by a halo of intense vacuolation. (*a*) Sporadic CJD, cerebral cortex stained with hematoxylin and eosin showing widespread spongiform degeneration. (*b*) Sporadic CJD, cerebral cortex immunostained with anti-GFAP antibodies demonstrating the widespread reactive gliosis. (*c*) GSS, cerebellum with most of the GSS-plaques in the molecular layer (left 80% of micrograph), and many but not all are periodic acid Schiff (PAS) reaction positive. Granule cells and a single Purkinje cell are seen in the right 20% of the panel. (*d*) GSS, cerebellum at the same location as panel C with PrP immunohistochemistry after the hydrolytic autoclaving reveals more PrP plaques than seen with the PAS reaction. (*e*) New variant CJD, cerebral cortex stained with hematoxylin and eosin shows the plaque deposits uniquely located within vacuoles. With this histology, these amyloid deposits have been referred to as 'florid plaques'. (*f*) New variant CJD, cerebral cortex stained with PrP immunohistochemistry after hydrolytic autoclaving reveals numerous PrP plaques often occurring in clusters as well as minute PrP deposits surrounding many cortical neurons and their proximal processes. Bar in (*b*) = 50 mm and applies also to panels (*a*), (*c*) and (*e*). Bar in (*f*) is 100 mm and applies also to panel (*d*). Photomicrographs prepared by Stephen DeArmond. (New variant CJD specimens provided by James Ironside, Jeanne Bell, and Robert Will.)

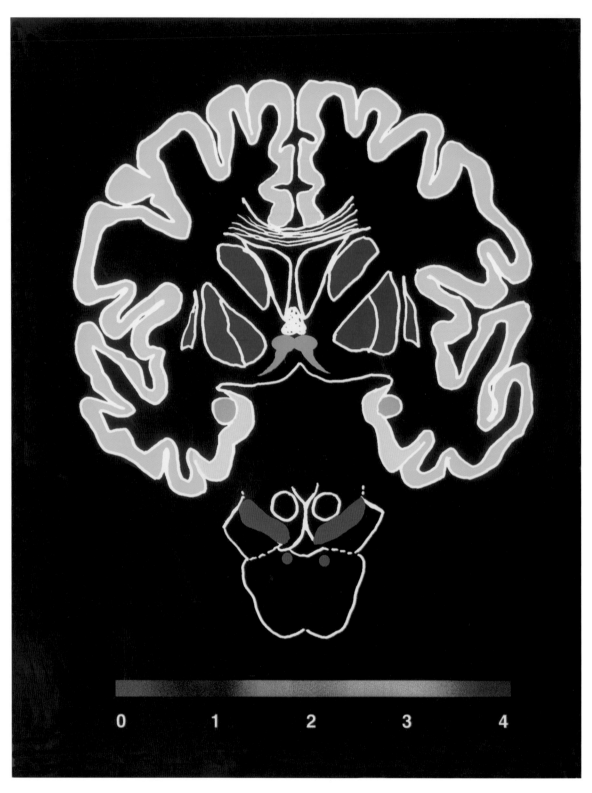

Fig. 18.2. A colour representation of the topography of Lewy bodies plotted onto a coronal human brain section at the level of the amygdala based on Lewy body density data from Gómez-Tortosa et al. (1999). The colour bar indicates red as the greatest quantity and blue as the least.

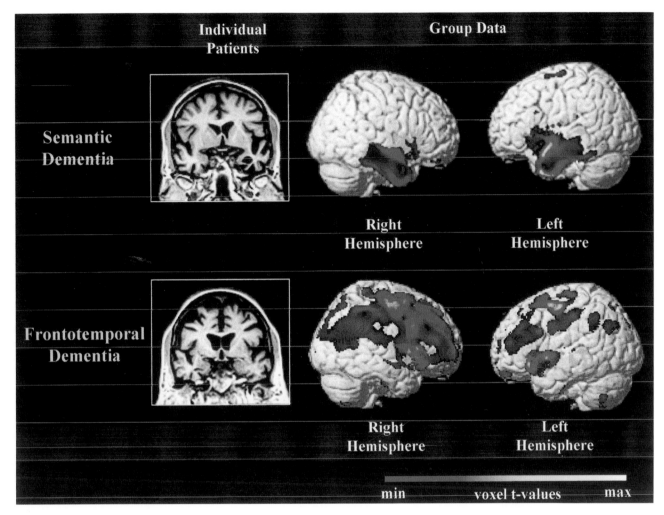

Fig. 19.1. Differing patterns of atrophy in patients with FTD are illustrated. On the left, coronal slices from T1-weighted MRI images in two individual patients are shown. The patient on top shows predominantly frontal atrophy, while the patient on the bottom shows predominantly temporal atrophy, more severe on the left. On the right, group data from a formal analysis of twenty patients with FTD are shown. Twenty patients with FTD were divided into two groups, those with ($N=12$, top) and without ($N=8$, bottom) semantic impairment, and compared with twenty age matched controls subjects. Anatomical analysis was performed using voxel-based morphometry, a technique that allows automated detection of regional atrophy (Ashburner & Friston, 2000). The t-values at the regions where atrophy was significant in each group ($P<0.001$) are superimposed on a normal brain. The group with semantic impairment shows atrophy predominantly in the anterior temporal regions, while the group without semantic impairment shows predominantly frontal atrophy. These data illustrate how specific clinical syndromes are associated with specific patterns of cerebral atrophy in FTD.

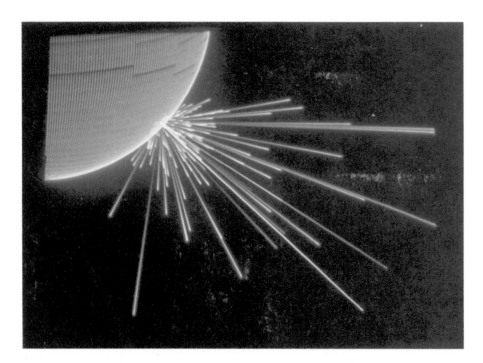

Fig. 31.5. An example of the population coding of movement direction. The blue lines represent the vectorial contribution of individual cells in the population ($N = 475$). The actual movement direction is in yellow and the direction of the population vector is in red. (From Georgopoulos et al., 1986, figure 1.)

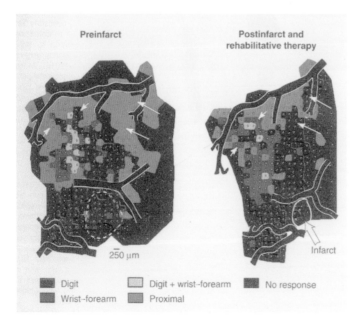

Preinfarct

Postinfarct and rehabilitative therapy

250 μm

Infarct

- ■ Digit
- ■ Wrist–forearm
- ▢ Digit + wrist–forearm
- ■ Proximal
- ■ No response

Fig. 31.8. Reorganization of hand representations in the primary motor cortex associated with rehabilitation following ischemic infarct. The volume circumscribed by a dashed line in the preinfarct map shows the area targeted for infarction, the solid line in the postinfarct map indicates the infarcted region. Digit representations all but disappear from the area of the infarct but after rehabilitation have invaded areas of cortex previously occupied by more proximal arm muscles (long thin arrows). In addition, the representation of the wrist–forearm expanded into areas previously occupied by shoulder (short thick arrows). (Adapted from Nudo et al., 1996, figure 3.)

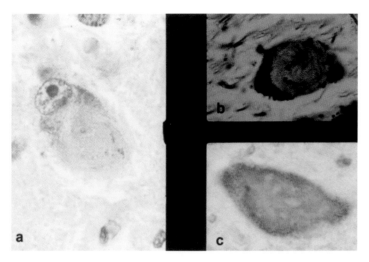

Fig. 34.1. Progressive supranuclear palsy ultrastructural pathology showing a typical globose neurofibrillary tangle in the substantia nigra stained with hematoxylin eosin (*a*); Bieschowsky's silver impregnation (*b*); tau immunohistochemistry (*c*). (Courtesy Dr Tamas Revesz, Dept of Neuropathology, Institute of Neurology, London.)

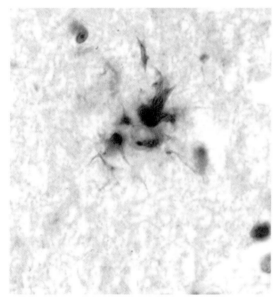

Fig. 34.2. Progressive supranuclear palsy ultrastructural pathology showing a typical tufted astrocyte in the motor cortex. Tau immunohistochemistry. (Courtesy Dr Tamas Revesz, Dept of Neuropathology, Institute of Neurology, London.)

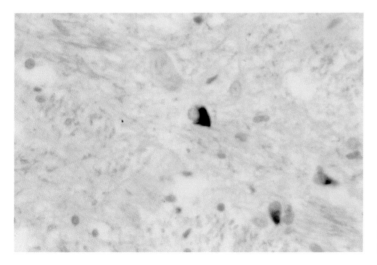

Fig. 34.5. Olgodendroglial inclusion seen in multiple system atrophy. (Gallyas stain). (Courtesy Prof. Francesco Scaravilli Institute of Neurology, London.)

(a)

(b)

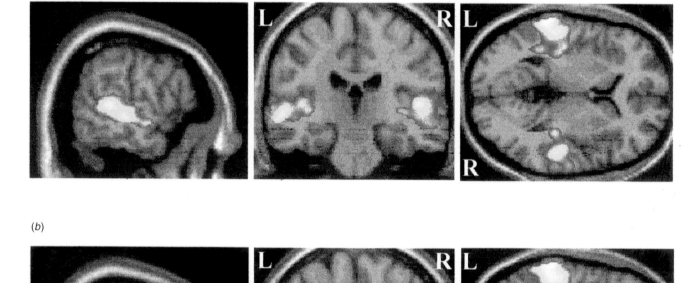

Fig. 45.11. Functional MRI: Activation of temporal cortex during (*a*) passive listening and (*b*) active listening to modulated tones projected into sagittal, coronal and axial planes; both A and B show that the volume of temporal activation is greater on the left side in both passive and active listening; only active listening produces activation in other areas (in this illustration, bilateral postcentral gyri and left insula cortex). (Hall et al., 2000.)

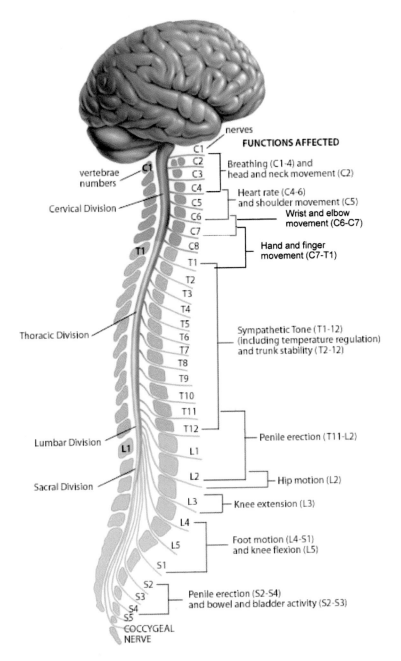

nerves

FUNCTIONS AFFECTED

C1
C2 — Breathing (C1-4) and
C3   head and neck movement (C2)
C4 — Heart rate (C4-6)
C5   and shoulder movement (C5)
C6 — Wrist and elbow
C7   movement (C6-C7)
C8 — Hand and finger
T1   movement (C7-T1)
T2
T3
T4
T5 — Sympathetic Tone (T1-12)
T6   (including temperature regulation)
T7   and trunk stability (T2-12)
T8
T9
T10
T11
T12 — Penile erection (T11-L2)
L1
L2 — Hip motion (L2)
L3 — Knee extension (L3)
L4
L5   Foot motion (L4-S1)
S1   and knee flexion (L5)
S2
S3 — Penile erection (S2-S4)
S4   and bowel and bladder activity (S2-S3)
S5
COCCYGEAL
NERVE

vertebrae numbers

C1

Cervical Division

T1

Thoracic Division

Lumbar Division

L1

Sacral Division

Fig. 47.2. Four divisions of the spinal cord and their associated nerves serve specific areas of the body. In general, the cervical nerves link to the neck, arms and respiratory apparatus; the thoracic nerves control posture and many internal organs; the lumbar nerves work the legs; and the sacral nerves regulate the bladder and bowel and play a role in sexual function.

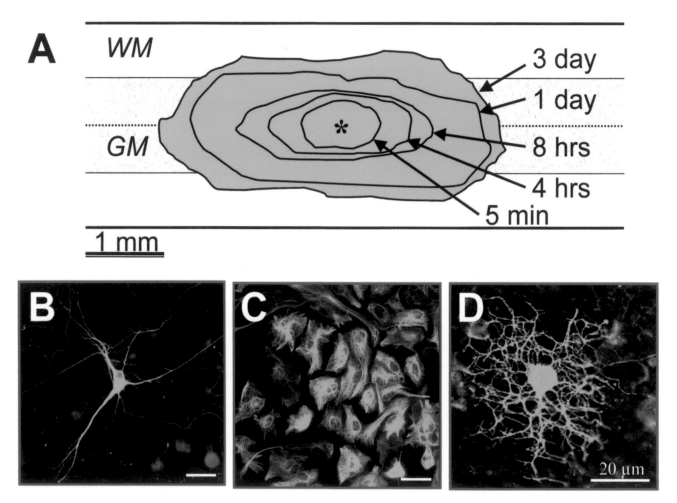

Fig. 47.3. (*a*) Schematic drawing illustrating lesion expansion over time in longitudinal sections through the central canal of rat spinal cords that sustained a moderate contusion injury. The cords were examined at 5 min, 4 and 8 h, and 1 and 3 days after the injury. *WM*, white matter; *GM*, grey matter. * Site of impact. (Adapted from Liu et al., 1997.) Panels (*b*)–(*d*) illustrate the three principal cell types of the central nervous system that are important for function and which are damaged following injury. The (*b*) neuron, (*c*) astrocyte, and (*d*) oligodendrocyte shown were derived from mouse embryonic stem cells, neurally induced with retinoic acid, and grown in culture for 9 days.

Targets for Therapy

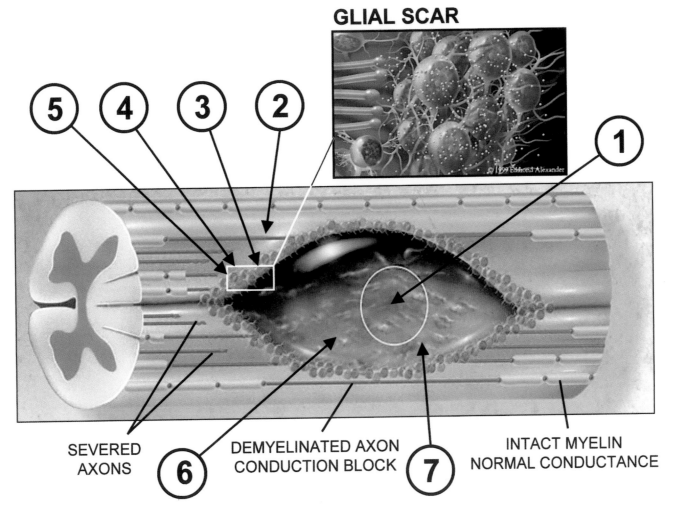

Fig. 47.5. Treatment of spinal cord injury will likely involve several interventions, delivered in an ordered sequence, each with incremental benefits. Illustrated are specific examples representing the different levels of intervention. 1. **Prevent progression of secondary injury**: Prevention of necrotic and apoptotic cell death using anti-excitotoxic drugs (glutamate-receptor blockers) and anti-apoptotic treatments (growth factors such as NT-3, BDNF, and ICE-protease inhibitors). 2. **Compensate for demyelination**: Supply chemicals that prevent action potentials from dissipating at demyelinated areas (prevent conduction block). Provide agents that encourage surviving oligodendrocytes to remyelinate axons. Replenish lost oligodendrocytes. 3. **Overcome inhibition**: Deliver agents that block the actions of natural inhibitors of regeneration (inhibitor neutralizing antibody, IN-1, masks an inhibitory protein) or drugs that down-regulate expression of inhibitory proteins. 4. **Promote axonal regeneration**: Delivery of growth factors that promote regeneration (sprouting) of new axons (e.g. NT-3, BDNF). 5. **Direct axons to proper targets**: Deliver targeting molecules or alter their expression in host cells to guide axons to appropriate targets. 6. **Create bridges**: Implant into the syrinx tissue that can serve as scaffolding for axons and that encourages them to grow (e.g. transplant peripheral nerves or cells competent to support axonal growth, such as ensheathing glia, into the empty syrinx). 7. **Replace lost cells**: Implant cells able to produce all the lost types (e.g. stem cells or ES cells). Deliver substances that can induce undifferentiated cells already in the cord to replace dead cells. In addition to replacing cells, transplanted cells can be used as cellular genetic vectors to deliver regenerative molecules on command (e.g. vectors producing NT-3, bFGF, or PDGF). (Figure reproduced with permission from *Scientific American* (McDonald et al., 1999).)

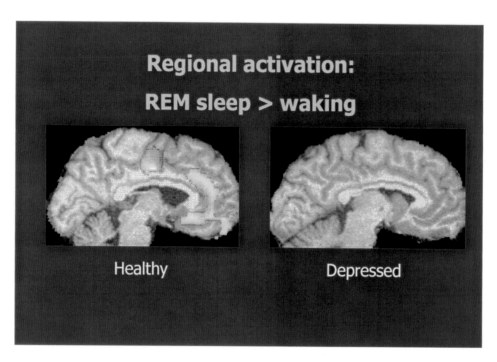

Fig. 55.4. PET studies of REM sleep. See text for description.

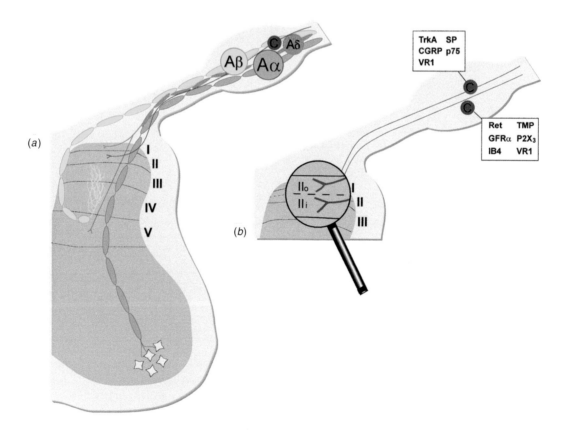

Fig. 58.2. (*a*) Subpopulations of primary sensory neurons synapse in a lamina-specific manner within the dorsal horn. (*b*) Within the C-fibre population of sensory neurons, different chemically defined cells synapse in different parts of lamina II.

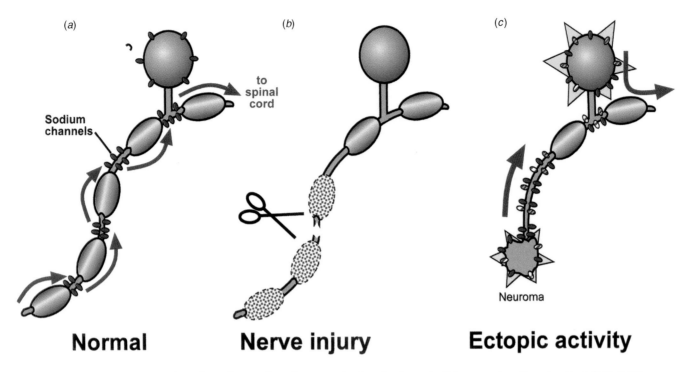

Normal   **Nerve injury**   **Ectopic activity**

Fig. 58.5. (*a*) In sensory neurons with myelinated axons, fast saltatory conduction of action potentials occurs along the axon at speeds up to 100 metres/second, mediated in part by the expression and discrete localization of voltage gated sodium channels (VGSCs) at the Nodes of Ranvier. (*b*) Following nerve injury, the distal axon segment undergoes Wallerian degeneration, and the Schwann cells lining the end of the proximal axon dedifferentiate and stop producing myelin. (*c*) Injured sensory neurons then display ectopic discharge at the neuroma site, proximally on the axon and from the cell body as a consequence of altered ion channel expression, altered ion channel membrane organization and altered ion channel properties. Note that ectopic activity is also observed in adjacent uninjured fibres following nerve injury.

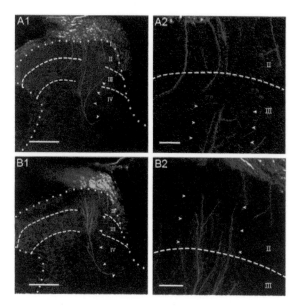

Fig. 58.12. (*a*) Normally, Aβ-fibre central terminals in the ipsilateral dorsal horn synapse within the deeper laminae (II and IV) and those innervating the skin have a characteristic flame shaped central arbour (arrow heads). (*b*) Two weeks after nerve injury in laboratory animals, Aβ-fibre central terminals sprout dorsally into laminae I and II, a region normally innervated only by C-fibres. (Printed with permission from Kohama et al., 2000.)

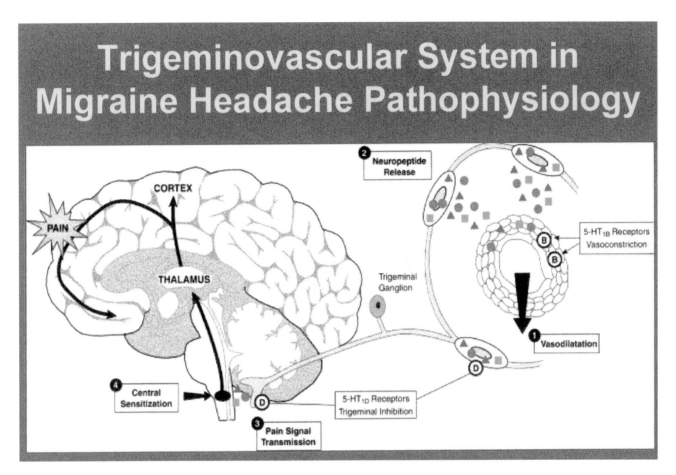

Fig. 61.1. Integrated hypothesis of the pathogenesis of the migraine headache and associated symptoms, and the role of the trigeminovascular system. For explanation, see the various sections in the text.

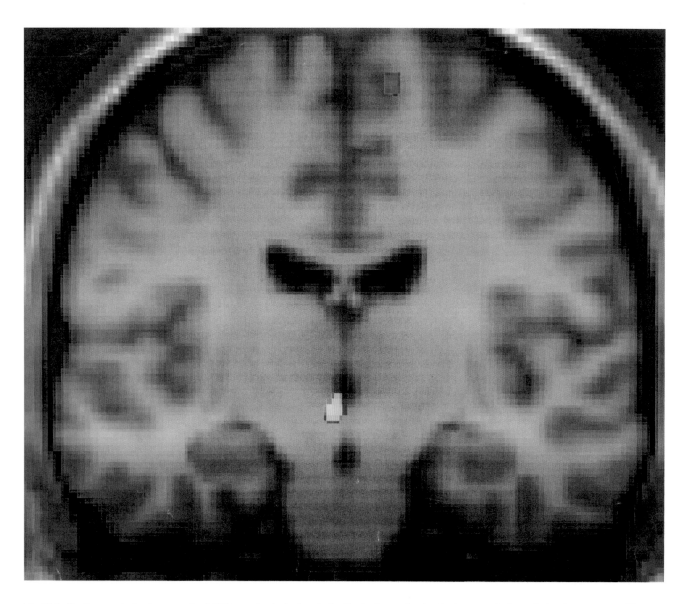

Fig. 62.1. Positron emission tomography (PET) in acute cluster headache illustrating activation in the posterior hypothalamic grey matter. This area is active only in acute cluster headache and not in migraine, nor experimental head pain. It is likely that the crucial neurons responsible for the fundamental pathophysiology of cluster headache are to be found in this region (May et al., 1998).

phonemic paraphasias are typically associated with milder forms of aphasia, while neologisms are associated with more severe forms.

Perseverations

Verbal perseverations, the unintended repetition of a preceding response, are common during the early stages of any acute aphasia syndrome, but occur in non-aphasic brain injured patients as well. Subtypes of verbal perseveration have been described (continuous, recurrent, stuck-in-set), but it is not clear whether these carry any prognostic information. The lesion correlates of perseverations are varied, but a recent study reported an association between head of caudate lesions and perseveration in patients with acute aphasia (Kreisler et al., 2000).

Echolalia

This refers to unsolicited, compulsive repetition (echoing) of verbal stimuli. Patients with echolalia do not echo everything they hear, but only utterances directed towards them. It is typically associated with poor comprehension. Despite this, aphasic patients with echolalia often demonstrate a completion-response (Stengel et al., 1947). If given a simple, but incomplete sentence, the patient will frequently complete the sentence spontaneously. Because of the implied intact repetition, echolalia does not usually occur with perisylvian lesions but is most common in so-called transcortical aphasias (Kornyey, 1975). Echolalia is also frequent in certain non-aphasic conditions, such as degenerative disorders and autism (Rapin & Dunn, 1997).

Stereotypical utterances

The speech of patients with severe non-fluent or global aphasia may sometimes be limited to one or two utterances, repeated in succession. These utterances may be real words or meaningless nonsense syllables. Repetitive stereotypical utterances, first described by Hughlings-Jackson (1880), represent a symptom that typically occurs only in patients with global aphasia (Brunner et al., 1982). The speech of Broca's initial patient Leborgne, who was only capable of uttering the word *Tan*, is one of the first known cases of stereotypical utterances. Curiously, it also suggests that Broca's first patient may, in fact, have had a global rather than what we today think of as Broca's aphasia (Selnes & Hillis, 2000). Stereotypical utterances, which may be one of the few pathognomonic signs of aphasia, invariably carry a poor prognosis.

Aprosody

Prosody, sometimes referred to as melodic line, refers to features such as stress, rhythm and intonational contours that convey both linguistic and non-linguistic information. Impairments of speech prosody are seen most often with non-fluent aphasia. In rare cases, the prosodic and articulatory changes are so prominent that the impression is given that the patient is speaking with a foreign accent. This condition was first described by the Norwegian neurologist Monrad-Krohn (1947), who reported the case of a woman with a war-related shrapnel injury to her left frontal lobe. When she recovered her speech, the rhythm and sentence melody were altered, and she was thought to be speaking with a German accent (Ryalls & Reinvang, 1985). Although an infrequent manifestation of aphasia, the foreign accent syndrome may occur during the recovery from severe non-fluency to a more fluent output. Foreign accent syndrome in the absence of aphasia has also been reported (Takayama et al., 1993). The role of the right hemisphere in prosody still remains controversial (Ryalls, 1986).

Palilalia

This is an acquired speech impairment characterized by recurrent repetition of a word or part of a word. With each recurrence, the rate tends to increase and the loudness decreases until the palilalia fades away. This symptom is relatively rare in aphasias with primarily cortical involvement, but can occur with subcortical involvement. Thus, palilalia with thalamic infarctions has been reported (Abe et al. 1993) and it frequently occurs in patients with Parkinson's disease.

Bedside language examination

At a minimum, the bedside language examination should include the basic elements listed in Table 22.1. Information about the quality of speech fluency and the ability to comprehend conversational speech can be obtained from the clinical interview. For patients with non-fluent aphasia, the use of automatic sequences, such as asking the patient to count from 1–10, reciting the letters of the alphabet, days of the week, and months of the year, can be helpful in eliciting enough speech to allow assessment of articulation and fluency. The critical elements in assessing spontaneous speech include: articulation, fluency, melodic line (prosody), grammatical form (syntax), paraphasic errors, and word-finding. In patients with no verbal output,

Table 22.1. Elements of the bedside language exam

Spontaneous speech
   automatic sequences

Auditory comprehension
   single word
   sentences (commands)

Naming
   objects, body parts, colours

Repetition

Writing
   spontaneous
   dictation
   copying

Reading
   aloud
   comprehension

assessment of writing can help differentiate between aphasia versus aphonia. Auditory comprehension for individual words can be tested by asking the patient to point to body parts, everyday objects, or items in the room. Single word comprehension may be the best index of initial aphasia severity, and thus carries potential prognostic implications (Selnes et al., 1984). Sentence comprehension can be assessed by asking the patient to perform single or multistep commands. The ability to comprehend more complex syntactical relationships can be probed by the use of so-called syntactically reversible sentences. For example, in response to a sentence such as 'the lion was killed by the tiger, ' some patients have difficulty answering the question: 'which animal died?' Regardless of the severity of the aphasia, most patients will be able to demonstrate comprehension of commands that involve the body axis, such as: 'look up, look down, stand up, lean forward.' (Albert et al., 1991).

Naming can be assessed by asking the patient to name objects, body parts, or colors. For more detailed assessment, quantitative tests such as the Boston Naming Test are recommended (Kaplan et al., 1983). Repetition can be screened with sentences such as 'no ifs ands or buts'. Patients who are able to repeat this sentence generally have intact repetition. If the patient does not repeat this sentence correctly, however, additional testing of repetition with single words and simpler sentences should be performed. Writing can be assessed by asking the patient to write a sentence spontaneously. Patients unable to write a sentence should be asked to attempt to copy single words or sentences. In patients with severe motor deficits or apraxic agraphia, testing oral

spelling can be useful. Reading aloud of single words, sentences, and paragraphs should be assessed. Most patients with problems in reading comprehension also have problems when reading aloud, but the converse is not true. A selective deficit of reading words that do not conform to standard sound-to-print rules, such as 'lieutenant, beautiful, steak', is sometimes observed.

Traditional anatomy of aphasia

For decades, our understanding of the anatomy of the left hemisphere language system was constrained by a bias in patient investigation: only patients with 'classic' symptoms of aphasia were investigated. Patients with left hemisphere lesions but no aphasia were rarely subjected to systematic study. Consequently, this resulted in a somewhat biased and restricted view. Advances in neuroimaging technologies over the past several decades have resulted in several modifications of the Wernicke–Lichtheim standard model of the left hemisphere language system. Although contemporary textbooks still feature the standard model of Wernicke's and Broca's areas interconnected by the arcuate fasciculus, evidence from several different lines of inquiry is now accumulating that this model is an oversimplification. There have been three major trends. First, it is now appreciated that lesions restricted to the traditional language areas of Broca and Wernicke are neither necessary nor sufficient to produce the classical syndromes. Secondly, it is now commonly accepted that multiple left hemisphere regions other than Broca's and Wernicke's areas appear to participate in language functions. Thirdly, there is significant variability in the lesion correlates of the so-called traditional syndromes (Basso et al., 1985; Vignolo et al., 1986).

Broca's area (Brodmann's area 44/45)

The first major revision to standard teaching about the role of Broca's area in language came with the studies of J.P. Mohr, who showed that a lesion restricted to Broca's area does not produce the clinical syndrome of Broca's aphasia (Mohr et al., 1999). According to Mohr, the lesion responsible for the clinical picture of Broca's aphasia is a large infarct in the sylvian area, which includes the operculum, the insula, and surrounding deep white matter. Others have shown that although the anterior insula is consistently involved, Broca's area proper need not be part of the lesion (Knopman et al., 1983; Blunk et al., 1981). Thus, a lesion of Broca's area is neither sufficient nor necessary for producing the syndrome of persistent non-fluent aphasia of Broca. More detailed analysis suggests that despite considerable variability, components of the syndrome of Broca's aphasia, such as impaired articulation, delayed initiation of speech, and aprosody can be related to regional involvement of the frontal operculum (Alexander et al., 1992). Although there have been some contemporary studies of the anatomy of this area, more detailed studies of the cytoarchitecture, individual variability, and connectivity of this area are just beginning to emerge (Amunts et al., 1999; Petrides & Pandya, 1988).

Wernicke's area

The anatomical boundaries of the part of the posterior superior temporal lobe that constitutes Wernicke's region have never been specified, because there are no specific cytoarchitectonic or other criteria for supporting such a definition (Bogen & Bogen, 1976). A lesion of the posterior superior temporal lobe is almost always associated with fluent, paraphasic speech and poor comprehension. It has also been demonstrated that the degree of destruction of the posterior superior temporal lobe is correlated with outcome. Partial lesions are associated with favorable outcomes, whereas lesions that include more than 50% of the region are associated with poor outcomes (Selnes et al., 1984). If the lesion is limited to the posterior superior temporal lobe, prognosis for improvement to anomic aphasia is good, but if the lesion includes anterior extensions, prognosis for recovery is poor (Naeser et al., 1987).

Planum temporale

The planum temporale is a triangular structure located on the superior plane of the temporal lobe within the sylvian fissure. The normal anatomy of this region is quite variable, but cytoarchitectonically it consists of auditory association cortex. It has attracted considerable research attention after the discovery by Geschwind and Levitsky (1968) that this particular region of the brain tends to be larger on the left. Although the distribution of the anatomical asymmetry (left larger in 64% of brains) did not exactly fit with estimates of left hemisphere dominance, the assumption was made that the asymmetry somehow reflected the important role of the posterior superior temporal lobe in language. However, a specific role of this area in language, if any, has not yet been demonstrated (Binder et al., 1996).

Insula

The role of the insula in speech and language has been controversial since the time of Pierre Marie. The anterior insula is almost always implicated in patients with persistent non-fluent aphasia. A recent study reported that patients with so-called apraxia of speech all had lesions that involved the anterior insula, while none of the patients without apraxia of speech had a lesion that included this area (Dronkers, 1996). There is also evidence to suggest that some of the connections from the posterior superior temporal lobe to anterior speech areas actually pass through the extreme capsule (Petrides & Pandya, 1988). Lesions of the insula therefore frequently produce impaired repetition (Damasio & Damasio, 1980).

Angular/supramarginal gyri

The angular and supramarginal gyri are part of the inferior parietal lobe, and are strategically located for polymodal association of vision, touch and hearing. These areas may play an important role during language development, because basic linguistic functions, such as object naming, depend on establishing an association between auditory and other sensory modalities. Although there is some evidence that lesions restricted to the angular gyrus may produce an agraphia, the role of the angular gyrus in reading is less clear. Although traditionally implicated in the syndrome of alexia with agraphia, the lesions responsible for this syndrome typically include other structures as well (Sakurai et al., 2000). The so-called Gerstmann syndrome has also been shown to be associated with larger lesions that include the angular gyrus but not restricted to this area (Benton, 1992). With disconnection of visual input to the angular gyrus, alexia without agraphia occurs. Comprehension of written words is impaired, but writing is generally intact. Spelling, and comprehension of spelled words, is generally intact.

Arcuate fasciculus

The long white matter tract known as the arcuate fasciculus has traditionally been conceptualized as the direct pathway between the posterior and anterior language areas. Lesions of the arcuate fasciculus have been thought to be responsible for the repetition deficit observed in patients with conduction aphasia. The presumptive role of the arcuate fasciculus in repetition disorders has been surprisingly resistant to more recent findings suggesting that a lesion of the arcuate fasciculus is neither necessary nor sufficient for the production of the syndrome of conduction aphasia (Selnes et al, 1985; Damasio & Damasio, 1980; Brown, 1975; Shuren et al., 1995; Anderson et al., 1999). Recent anatomical studies also suggest that it is only the most posterior areas of the superior temporal lobe that project to anterior speech areas via the arcuate fasciculus. The anterior two thirds of the posterior superior temporal lobe appear to be connected through white matter tracts that pass through the extreme capsule (Petrides & Pandya, 1988). Thus, there is neither compelling behavioural nor anatomical evidence for a specific role of the arcuate fasciculus in repetition.

Basal temporal language area

Functional localization of language-relevant cortex by using electrical stimulation has become routine in patients who are candidates for epilepsy surgery (Lesser et al., 1986, 1987; Schaffler et al., 1993). This methodology has revealed evidence of interference with language functions in areas outside the classical language areas. Electrical stimulation of the dominant basal temporal area has been shown to produce problems in both comprehension and production in some patients (Luders et al., 1986, 1991). Surgical resection of this area does not produce any lasting language deficits in most patients, but some patients have persistent dysnomia (Krauss et al., 1996). Thus far, the specific role this region subsumes in language functions is unclear.

Supplementary motor area

The anterior part of area 6 on the medial surface of the cerebral hemisphere, the supplementary motor area, has been implicated in speech functions since the work of Penfield and Roberts (1959), but its specific functions are still poorly understood. Stimulation of the supplementary motor area most commonly results in speech arrest (Fried et al., 1991). Surgical lesions of the dominant supplementary motor area may produce moderate to severe initial deficits, but significant lasting speech changes are uncommon (Rostomily et al., 1991).

The basic Wernicke–Geschwind model of the anatomy of language has thus undergone considerable evolution over the past several decades. The following quote from Mesulam is representative of this more contemporary view: 'There are no "centres" dedicated to comprehension, articulation, or grammar but a distributed network in which nodal foci of relative specialization work in concert.' (Mesulam, 1990). The extent to which this updated model will prevail remains to be seen, but as noted by Damasio: 'The time for modernizing the classic view is now, and the past decade has brought forth a number of new findings likely to make the modernization stick.' (Damasio, 1997).

Integrated cognitive neuroscience approach to the neural basis of language

Rapid developments in cognitive neuroscience in the past two decades have allowed us to develop a cognitive neuroscience model that describes how the brain encodes language operations and explains aphasic behaviour. The advantages of these types of models are that they (a) can account for the observed aphasic language disorders, (b) provide more theoretically and clinically relevant language components that correlate with specific brain regions, and (c) take advantage of the multitude of activation studies conducted in control subjects to understand how the normal brain performs language functions. This point raises the important issue that an integrated account of language and aphasia is required to reconcile the findings of activation and lesion studies in describing how the brain performs language operations.

The basic language operations assessed above in the classical approach are still correlated with their associated anatomic regions including this within their framework. The cognitive neuroscience approach supplements the classical approach by assessing the networks of brain regions associated with the linguistic components of semantic, orthographic, and phonological lexicons and syntax. These components are most useful for developing both theoretical and practical explanations for normal and aphasic language function. It is believed that these networks consist of various combinations of circumscribed brain regions subserving processing or access to representation of language units (e.g. words, letters, sounds, among others), some of which may be encoded in spatially distributed representations (Hinton, 1981).

Although the tests for assessing each of these components and their access can be similar to those outlined above, the results are interpreted and framed in terms of linguistic and cognitive components. The following outlines a framework for an integrated cognitive neuroscience approach to language representation in the brain and its application to explaining aphasic behaviour. As further studies are completed, clarification and expansion of the framework will provide a more detailed account of the networks involved.

Semantic lexicon (stores in the brain encoding the linguistic meaning of words)

This component is usually assessed by how a patient performs on comprehension questions (e.g. 'Do birds have wings?'), comprehension of single words, confrontation naming, and the output of spontaneous speech (e.g. error patterns, word-finding difficulties). The pattern of performance across these types of tasks indicates deficits in the lexical semantic system, for example, if the patient has empty speech with word-finding difficulties and impaired comprehension.

Studies of clinical patients and activation studies have both demonstrated behavioural and anatomical aspects of the organization of the semantic lexicon and possible associated processing regions (see Hart et al., 2001). Evidence from focal brain lesions and from degenerative brain conditions has shown that aspects of the lexical semantic system may be organized by semantic category (see Caramazza & Shelton, 1998), because categories can be differentially affected by these neural injuries. Nielsen (1946) was the first to describe a double dissociation between the ability to name living things and non-living things (with opposite patterns of preservation or impairment across different patients). Since then, there have been many individual and group reports of such dissociations for a variety of categories including living things, animals, plants, food, fruits and vegetables, body parts, countries, emotional facial expressions, small manipulable objects, shapes, colours, letters, numbers, action names, verbs, case marking prepositions and tense, girls' and boys' names, family and friends, famous people, proper names, cities, rivers, countries, mountains (Semenza & Zettin 1988, 1989; Goodglass et al., 1966, 1986; Funnell & Sheridan, 1992; Hillis & Caramazza, 1991; Farah et al., 1991, 1996; Silveri et al., 1991; Damasio et al., 1990; Farah & Wallace, 1992; Farah, 1989; Temple, 1986; Warrington & Shallice, 1984; Rapcsak et al., 1989, 1993; McCarthy & Warrington, 1988; Hart et al., 1985; Berndt, 1988; Humphreys & Riddoch, 1987; Damasio, 1990; Silveri & Gainotti, 1988; Warrington & McCarthy, 1983, 1987; Hart & Gordon, 1992; Sartori et al., 1993; Robinson et al., 1996; Gainotti et al., 1995; Mauri et al., 1994; Tippett et al., 1996; Sartori & Job, 1988; Sacchett & Humphreys, 1992; Damasio et al., 1996; Cappa et al., 1998; Garrard et al., 1998; Ferreira et al., 1997; see Grossman et al., 1998 for similar issues in degenerative conditions). In addition, functional imaging studies of the picture naming task have suggested that aspects of this categorical organization may be localized to specific brain regions (e.g. animals selectively activated the left medial occipital lobe and tools selectively activated the left middle temporal gyrus and the left premotor region (Martin et al., 1996) or animals were associated with activation of the left 3rd (inferior) and fourth temporal gyri, whereas naming of tools was associated with activation of the left middle and inferior temporal gyri (Damasio et al., 1996). These distinctions have not yet been fully reconciled (see Spitzer et al., 1995; Moore & Price, 1999a).

In addition, there are distinct brain regions associated with aspects of semantic processing, including the lcft dorsal lateral prefrontal cortex (DLPFC) with selection between multiple semantic stimuli (Thompson-Schill et al., 1997; Posner et al., 1988; Demb et al., 1995; Kapur et al., 1994; Demonet et al., 1992; Ricci et al., 1999), left inferior parietal-posterior superior temporal region (Hart & Gordon, 1990; Vandenberghe et al., 1996) and the left fusiform gyri (Hart et al., 1998; Nobre et al., 1994; Abdullaev & Posner, 1988) with categorization, synonymity and property judgment as well as other semantic processing, and bilateral inferior (ventral) temporo-occipital regions.

As investigative techniques provide greater resolution, and further regions involved in the lexical semantic network are identified with their associated function, the anatomic substrates of the lexical semantic system will be further defined, resulting in descriptions of pure and mixed deficits associated with lexical semantics. In addition, further specification of lexical semantic components will aid in describing the selective language impairments seen in semantic aphasia and semantic dementia (Hodges et al., 1992).

Orthographic lexicons (stores in the brain encoding written version of words)

The most efficacious method of assessing these components is by having the patient write, read, and perform a lexical decision task (e.g. deciding if a letter string is a word or a non-word, 'trest' vs. 'treat'). These tasks readily assess the integrity of the orthographic lexical elements as well as access to them.

Localization of the input and output orthographic lexicons has been a controversial issue in functional imaging studies. Whereas some investigators suspect that the word representations or stores themselves are encoded in a spatially distributed fashion (Hart et al., 2000), others have suggested a more focal circumscribed localization (Petersen et al., 1988). These focal localizations isolated with functional imaging studies, however, have not always been substantiated by similar localizations in numerous lesion studies. Until more definitive studies are performed, at a minimum these activation studies identify regions associated with access to orthographic lexicons. These regions include the superior and middle temporal gyri and inferior parietal lobule (Hart et al., 2000; Moore & Price, 1999b; Simos et al., 2000) for the input lexicon; middle part of the left superior and middle temporal gyri for the input and posterior part of the left middle temporal gyrus for the output orthographic lexicon (Howard et al., 1992); the lateral occipital extrastriate area for the input orthographic lexicon (Petersen et al., 1988); and the left frontal lobe for orthographic to phonological transformation (Fiez et al., 1999).

Extensive lesion studies of patients with alexia have delineated several plausible pathways involved in the three proposed routes to reading (direct access to an orthographic lexicon, orthographic-to-phonologic conversion, and direct access to semantics) and provide converging evidence that the above localizations may be important in accessing the input orthographic lexicon (see Coslett, 2000; Coltheart et al., 1980; Patterson et al., 1985). There is less evidence for anatomic localization of an independent output orthographic lexicon, although aspects of that lexicon have been behaviourally described (Hillis et al., 1999).

Phonological lexicons (stores encoding the sounds of words)

Speech discrimination tasks, repetition, and analysis of spontaneous speech are useful indices of the integrity of the phonological lexicons and their access. Phonemic paraphasic errors have been considered a hallmark feature of damage to the brain's internal storage system for the sounds of words for speech production, but it is also clear that inability to discriminate speech sounds can reflect impairment of an input phonological lexicon. This was demonstrated in the description of patient J.S., whose pure word deafness clinically was shown to stem from a disruption involving the input phonological lexical system (Caramazza et al., 1983).

It is clear that different neural mechanisms support input and output phonology, as well as different routes into these proposed lexical systems (e.g. access to input phonology from reading differs from access from speech perception) (Bub & Kertesz, 1982). As in the orthographic lexicons, it is not yet clear that anatomic localization defines the lexicons themselves or access to them. The localization of regions associated with access to input phonology from speech has been dissociated by focal, circumscribed temporary, reversible lesions produced by cortical electrical interference in left lateral superior temporal gyrus during speech discrimination tasks (Boatman et al. 1995, 1997). These regions bordered the primary auditory cortex, but were distinctly dissociated from it.

The network supporting the output phonologic lexicon has been shown through functional imaging studies to extend from the mouth representation in the primary motor cortex, the supplementary motor area, the inferior lateral premotor cortex (Broca's area), the anterior insula, and the cerebellum (Fox et al., 2000). In addition, the left posterior superior temporal gyrus has been shown to participate in phonemic aspects of speech production, as well as its previously described role in speech perception (Hickok et al., 2000). Distinguishing between the specific cognitive components that each region encodes, if they do function independently, is left to future studies.

Syntax (system of grammar)

Syntactical structures can be examined in both production and comprehension. Typical assessment of syntactic production extends from evaluating spontaneous speech for grammatical complexity (Kaplan et al., 1983), repetition of syntactically complex sentences or sentences with numerous function words (e.g. no ifs, ands, or buts), and reading of concrete and abstract words. Syntactic comprehension is routinely assessed at a basic level in a picture-sentence matching task using semantically reversible passive sentences ('Point to the correct picture describing this sentence, "The car was hit by the truck."')

Anatomical localization of syntactic processes have been variable (see Caplan, 1999). For example, in two patients aphasic syntactic and morphological aspects of grammar were localized to the left frontal lobe and the postcentral perisylvian cortex, respectively (Nadeau, 1988). In an activation study of syntactic processing, however, there was selective involvement of a deep component of Broca's area, a right inferior frontal region, and the left caudate nucleus and insula were activated (Moro et al., 2001). Alternatively, by studying sentences of increasing syntactic complexity, increased blood flow was found in Broca's area during syntactic judgment tasks (Caplan et al., 2000). Part of the variability in localizing syntactic processing may be attributable to different stimuli, testing paradigms, and investigative techniques, although some investigators have suggested that the variability is due to the lack of focal, circumscribed localization to syntactic processes.

Overall, the cognitive neuroscience approach is evolving as both functional imaging studies of normal and aphasic subjects are conducted. The success of this model will likely depend on several factors, not the least of which is to formally reconcile the disparities between activation and lesion studies to best determine the cognitive operation an anatomic region subserves. Another major factor will be the ability to combine experimental paradigms with the evolving investigative techniques to explore, in both spatial and temporal domains, the networks involved in the processing of these various linguistic components. As these techniques evolve, the cognitive neuroscience framework will also need to incorporate in the model the neural mechanisms (for example, electrophysiological coherence, neurotransmitter mediation) that subserves the cognitive operations involved in language. And finally, it will be essential to integrate in this model not only the connections between the linguistic components within language (e.g. the interface between orthography and phonology, and others) but also with other cognitive components outside the language system proper but necessary to its successful operation. For example, while not included directly in the above neural circuits, it has become increasing clear through a variety of functional imaging studies (D'Esposito et al., 1999) that the dorsal lateral prefrontal cortex (DLPFC) is involved in aspects of working memory. As this region and its connections to other linguistic components are explored, it will be useful to integrate working memory and its substrates into the network model of language proposed here.

Aphasia in degenerative conditions

It is well recognized that changes in speech and language may occur during the later stages of most forms of dementing illness. If symptoms of aphasia occur as the presenting symptoms, alternate etiologies should be considered. In 1982, Mesulam described six patients with a history of slowly progressive speech and language symptoms in the absence of any signs of dementia (Mesulam, 1982). Although previous cases of slowly progressive aphasia had been described (Poeck & Luzatti, 1988), Mesulam's publication resulted in widespread recognition of the entity now commonly referred to as primary progressive aphasia (Mesulam, 1982). The epidemiology and risk factors for primary progressive aphasia are not known, in part because the disease is rare. In 1997, Westbury and Bub reviewed the findings from 112 cases published since 1982 (Westbury & Bub, 1997). Most patients with this condition will eventually develop a more generalized dementia syndrome. In rare cases, the patient may remain cognitively intact (except for language) for a number of years, but in most instances, some degree of cognitive impairment can be detected on standardized neuropsychological testing after 2–3 years of progression. Therefore, it has been suggested that a period of 2 years of language-related decline in a patient otherwise free of symptoms of dementia is sufficient for making the diagnosis (Weintraub et al., 1990). The average age of onset of symptoms in progressive aphasia is approximately 59 years, somewhat earlier than for typical Alzheimer's disease. Most patients present with a non-fluent aphasia, making it relatively easy to differentiate from early Alzheimer's disease (Caselli, 1995). The most common initial symptom is word-finding difficulty, but some patients also report early problems with comprehension of spoken language. Phonemic paraphasias and speech hesitancy may also occur relatively early. In rare cases, the patient may present with an otherwise isolated dysarthria (Selnes et al., 1996; Broussolle et al., 1996; Cohen et al., 1993). The degree of agraphia often mirrors the degree of speech impairment. Reading and repetition tend to be relatively preserved, during later stages of the disease. With progression of the disease, all language modalities become impaired, and vocalization may be reduced to single word utterances or complete muteness. MRI findings are not very specific, but often demonstrate bilateral atrophy in the perisylvian regions. Of the cases of primary progressive aphasia with autopsy information, some have shown changes consistent with Alzheimer's disease (Benson & Zaias, 1991), but the most common findings involve gliosis and neuronal loss of superficial cortical layers.

Other degenerative conditions that are sometimes accompanied by prominent speech and language changes include Pick's disease (Holland et al., 1985) and corticobasal degeneration (Sakurai et al., 1996). Detailed neuropsychological testing can be helpful for early differentiation of these syndromes from primary progressive aphasia.

Aphasia recovery and treatment

Recovery from aphasia has traditionally been thought to depend on a complex interaction of lesion size and location with patient characteristics such as age, gender and handedness. Nevertheless, large scale prospective studies of aphasia recovery have not confirmed a significant predictive relationship between demographic variables and degree of recovery. Although methods for assessing initial severity have varied across studies, there is considerable agreement that the most important factor predicting recovery from aphasia after stroke is initial degree of severity of language symptoms (Pedersen et al., 1995). Few systematic studies have compared recovery from aphasia after etiologies other than stroke, but some have found that post-traumatic aphasia has a better prognosis than aphasia due to cerebral infarction (Kertesz & McCabe, 1977).

Although it is well known that small lesions cause milder and shorter lasting impairments, only a handful of studies have examined the effect of lesion volume on aphasia recovery. Selnes and colleagues found that single word comprehension at 6 months after stroke was significantly related to lesion volume (Selnes et al., 1984). One subsequent study has also confirmed the importance of overall lesion volume for degree of recovery (Goldenberg & Spatt, 1994). Furthermore, Naeser and her colleagues demonstrated that region-specific volume is also of importance, in that the degree of destruction within Wernicke's area itself was significantly related to levels of auditory comprehension. Patients with less than 50% destruction of Wernicke's area had good recovery of auditory comprehension at 6 months, whereas patients with destruction of more than half of Wernicke's region had limited recovery even at one year after onset. As with lesions of Broca's area, extension of the lesion beyond Wernicke's area was also associated with poor outcomes (Naeser et al., 1987).

The time course of recovery after aphasia may also depend on the initial level of severity. Patients with mild initial symptoms of aphasia often recover within a few weeks after the onset. With symptoms of moderate initial level, spontaneous recovery may last several months before a stable level of functioning is achieved (Pedersen et al., 1995). Patients with severe Global or Wernicke's aphasia may show some spontaneous recovery during the first 18 months after stroke, but the majority of the improvement takes place during the first 6 months (Nicholas et al., 1993).

There have been a number of studies attempting to quantify the degree of improvement, over and beyond spontaneous recovery, offered by speech therapy. In a recent meta-analysis of the findings from 21 studies, treatment by a speech-language pathologist was found to result in better outcomes (Robey, 1994). Treatment initiated during the acute stages of recovery was found to be significantly more effective than treatment initiated at later stages. In addition to behavioural treatments, pharmacotherapy for the treatment of symptoms of aphasia has also begun to be explored. Some studies have suggested a benefit of catecholaminergic drugs when used as an adjunct to behavioural therapy. At this time, further studies with appropriate controls are needed to assess which patients might potentially benefit from pharmacotherapy (Small, 1994).

References

Abdullaev, Y.G. & Posner, M.I. (1988). Event-related brain potential imaging of semantic encoding during processing single words. *Neuroimage*, **7**, 1–13.

Abe, K., Yokomaya, R. & Yorifuji, S. (1993). Repetitive speech disorder resulting from infarcts in the paramedian thalami and midbrain. *J. Neurol. Neurosurg. Psychiatry*, **56**, 1024–6.

Albert, M.L., Goodglass, H., Helm, N.A., Rubens, A.B. & Alexander M.P. (1991). *Clinical Aspects of Dysphasia*. New York: Springer Verlag.

Alexander, M.P., Naeser, M.A. & Palumbo, C. (1992). Broca's area aphasia: Aphasia after lesions including the frontal operculum. *Neurology*, **40**, 353–62.

Amunts, K., Schleicher, A., Burgel, U., Mohlberg, H., Uylings, H.B. & Zilles K. (1999). Broca's region revisited: Cytoarchitecture and intersubject variability. *J. Comp. Neurol.*, **412**, 319–41.

Anderson, J.M., Gilmore, R., Roper, S. et al. (1999). Conduction aphasia and the arcuate fasciculus: a reexamination of the Wernicke-Geschwind model. *Brain Lang.*, **70**, 1–12.

Basso, A., Lecours, A.R., Moraschini, S. & Vanier M. (1985). Anatomoclinical correlations of the aphasias as defined through computerized tomography: exceptions. *Brain Lang.*, **26**, 201–29.

Benson, D.F. & Zaias, B.W. (1991). Progressive aphasia: a case with postmortem correlation. *Neuropsychiat. Neuropsychol. Behav. Neurol.*, **4**, 215–23.

Benton, A.L. (1992). Gerstmann's syndrome. *Arch. Neurol.*, **49**, 445–7.

Berndt, R.S. (1988). Category-specific deficits in aphasia. *Aphasiology*, **2**, 237–40.

Binder, J.R., Frost, J.A., Hammeke, T.A., Rao, S.M. & Cox, R.W. (1996). Function of the left planum temporale in auditory and linguistic processing. *Brain*, **119**, 1239–47.

Blunk, R., De Bleser, R., Willmes, K. & Zeumer H. (1981). A refined method to relate morphological and functional aspects of aphasia. *Eur. Neurol.*, **20**, 69–79.

Boatman, D., Lesser, R.P. & Gordon, B. (1995). Auditory speech processing in the left temporal lobe: an electrical interference study. *Brain Lang.*, **51**, 269–90.

Boatman, D., Hall, C., Goldstein, M.H., Lesser, R. & Gordon B. (1997). Neuroperceptual differences in consonant and vowel discrimination: as revealed by direct cortical electrical interference. *Cortex*, **33**, 83–98.

Bogen, J.E. & Bogen, G.M. (1976). Wernicke's region: where is it? *Ann. NY Acad. Sci.*, **280**, 834–43.

Broussolle, E., Bakchine, S., Tommasi, M. et al. (1996). Slowly progressive anarthria with late anterior opercular syndrome: a variant form of frontal cortical atrophy syndromes. *J. Neurol. Sci.*, **144**, 44–58.

Brown, J.W. (1975). The problem of repetition: a study of 'conduction' aphasia and the 'isolation' syndrome. *Cortex*, **11**, 37–52.

Brunner, R.J., Kornhuber, H.H., Seemuller, E., Suger, G. & Wallesch, C.W. (1982). Basal ganglia participation in language pathology. *Brain Lang.*, **16**, 281–99.

Bub, D. & Kertesz, A. (1982). Evidence for lexicographic processing in a patient with preserved written over oral single word naming. *Brain*, **105**, 697–717.

Caplan, D. (1999). Activating brain systems for syntax and semantics. *Neuron*, **24**, 292–3.

Caplan, D., Alpert, N., Waters, G. & Olivieri, A. (2000). Activation of Broca's area by syntactic processing under conditions of concurrent articulation. *Hum. Brain Mapp.*, **9**, 65–71.

Cappa, S.F., Frugoni, M., Pasquali, P., Perani, D. & Zorat, F. (1998). Category-specific naming impairment for artefacts: a new case. *Neurocase*, **4/5**, 391–8.

Caramazza A. (1984). The logic of neuropsychological research and the problem of patient classification in aphasia. *Brain Lang.*, **21**, 9–20.

Caramazza, A. & Shelton, J.R. (1998). Domain-specific knowledge systems in the brain: the animate–inanimate distinction. *J. Cogn. Neurosci.*, **10**, 1–34.

Caramazza, A., Berndt, R.S. & Basili, A.G. (1983). The selective impairment of phonological processing: a case study. *Brain Lang.*, **18**, 128–74.

Caselli, R.J. (1995). Focal and asymmetric cortical degeneration syndromes. *Neurologist*, **1**, 1–19.

Cohen, L., Benoit, N., Van Eeckhout, P., Ducarne, B. & Brunet, P. (1993). Pure progressive aphemia. *J. Neurol. Neurosurg. Psychiatry*, **56**, 923–4.

Coltheart, M., Patterson, K. & Marshall, J.C. (1980). *Deep Dyslexia*. Boston: Routledge & Kegan Paul.

Coslett, H.B. (2000). Acquired dyslexia. *Semin. Neurol.*, **20**, 419–26.

Damasio, A.R. (1990). Category-related recognition defects as a clue to the neural substrates of knowledge. *Trends Neurosci.*, **13**, 95–8.

Damasio, A.R. (1997). Brain and language: what a difference a decade makes. *Curr. Opin. Neurol.*, **10**, 177–8.

Damasio, H. & Damasio, A.R. (1980). The anatomical basis of conduction aphasia. *Brain*, **103**, 337–50.

Damasio, A.R., Damasio, H., Tranel, D. & Brandt, J.P. (1990). Neural regionalization of knowledge access: preliminary evidence. *Cold Spring Harbor Symposia on Quantitative Biology*, **55**, 1039–47.

Damasio, H., Grabowski, T.J., Tranel, D., Hichwa, R.D. & Damasio, A.R. (1996). A neural basis for lexical retrieval. *Nature*, **380**, 499–505.

Demb, J.B., Desmond, J.E., Wagner, A.D., Vaidya, C.J., Glover, G.H. & Gabrieli, J.D. (1995). Semantic encoding and retrieval in the left inferior prefrontal cortex: a functional MRI study of task difficulty and process specificity. *J. Neurosci.*, **15**, 5870–8.

Demonet, J.F., Chollet, F., Ramsay, S. et al. (1992). The anatomy of phonological and semantic processing in normal subjects. *Brain*, **115**, 1753–68.

D'Esposito, M., Postle, B.R., Jonides, J. & Smith, E.E. (1999). The neural substrate and temporal dynamics of interference effects in working memory as revealed by event-related functional MRI. *Proc. Natl. Acad. Sci., USA*, **96**, 7514–9.

Dronkers, N.F. (1996). A new brain region for coordinating speech articulation. *Nature*, **384**, 159–61.

Farah, M.J. (1989). The neuropsychology of mental imagery. In *Neuropsychology of Visual Perception*, ed. J.W. Brown. Hillsdale, NJ: Erlbaum.

Farah, M.J. & Wallace, M.A. (1992). Semantically-bounded anomia: implications for the neural implementation of naming. *Neuropsychologia*, **30**, 609–22.

Farah, M.J., McMullen, P. & Meyer, M. (1991). Can recognition of living things be selectively impaired? *Neuropsychologia*, **29**, 85–193.

Farah, M.J., Meyer, M.M. & McMullen, P.A. (1996). The living/non-living dissociation is not an artifact: giving an a priori implausible hypothesis a strong test. *Cogn. Neuropsychol.*, **13**, 137–54.

Ferreira, C.T., Giusiano, B. & Poncet, M. (1997). Category-specific anomia: implication of different neural networks in naming. *Neuroreport*, **8**, 1595–602.

Ferro, J.M. & Madureira, S. (1997). Aphasia type, age and cerebral infarct localisation. *J. Neurol.*, **244**, 505–9.

Fiez, J.A., Balota, D.A., Raichle, M.E. & Petersen, S.E. (1999). Effects of lexicality, frequency, and spelling-to-sound consistency on the functional anatomy of reading. *Neuron*, **24**, 205–18.

Fox, P.T., Ingham, J.C., Zamarripa, F., Xiong, J.H. & Lancaster, J.L. (2000). Brain correlates of stuttering and syllable production: a PET performance-correlation analysis. *Brain*, **123**, 1985–2004.

Fried, I., Katz, A., McCarthy, G. et al. (1991). Functional organization of human supplementary motor cortex studied by electrical stimulation. *J. Neurosci.*, **11**, 3656–66.

Funnell, E. & Sheridan, J. (1992). Categories of knowledge? Unfamiliar aspects of living and nonliving things. *Cogn. Neuropsychol.*, **9**, 135–53.

Gainotti, G., Silveri, M., Daniele, A. & Giustolisi, L. (1995). Neuroanatomical correlates of category-specific semantic disorders: a critical survey. *Memory*, **3/4**, 247–64.

Garrard, P., Patterson, K., Watson, P.C. & Hodges, J.R. (1998). Category-specific semantic loss in dementia of Alzheimer's type: functional-anatomical correlations form cross-sectional analyses. *Brain*, **121**, 633–46.

Geschwind, N. & Levitsky, W. (1968). Human Brain: Left-right asymmetries in temporal speech region. *Science*, **161**, 186–7.

Goldenberg, G. & Spatt, J. (1994). Influence of size and site of cerebral lesions on spontaneous recovery of aphasia and on success of language therapy. *Brain Lang.*, **47**, 684–98.

Goodglass, H., Klein, B., Carey, P. & Jones, K. (1966). Specific semantic word categories in aphasia. *Cortex*, **2**, 74–89.

Goodglass, H., Wingfield, A., Hyde, M. & Theurkauf, J.C. (1986). Category specific dissociations in naming and recognition by aphasic patients. *Cortex*, **22**, 87–102.

Grossman, M., Robinson, K., Biassou, N., White-Devine, T. & D'Esposito, M. (1998). Semantic memory in Alzheimer's disease: Representativeness, ontologic category, and material. *Neuropsychology*, **12**, 34–42.

Hart, J. & Gordon, B. (1990). Delineation of single-word semantic comprehension deficits in aphasia, with anatomical correlation. *Ann. Neurol.*, **27**, 226–31.

Hart, J. & Gordon, B. (1992). Neural subsystems for object knowledge. *Nature*, **359**, 60–4.

Hart, J., Berndt, R.S. & Caramazza, A. (1985). Category-specific naming deficit following cerebral infarction. *Nature*, **316**, 439–40.

Hart, J., Crone, N.E., Lesser, R.P. et al. (1998). Temporal dynamics of verbal object comprehension. *Proc. Natl. Acad. Sci., USA*, **95**, 6498–503.

Hart, J., Kraut, M.A., Kremen, S., Soher, B. & Gordon, B. (2000). Neural substrates of orthographic lexical access as demonstrated by functional brain imaging. *Neuropsychiat. Neuropsychol. Behav. Neurol.*, **13**, 1–7.

Hart, J., Moo, L.R., Segal, J.B., Adkins, E. & Kraut, M.A. (2001). Neural substrates of semantics. In *Handbook of Language Disorders*, ed. A.E. Hillis. Philadelphia: Psychology Press.

Head, H. (1915). Hughlings Jackson on aphasia and kindred affections of speech. *Brain*, **38**, 1–27.

Hickok, G., Erhard, P., Kassubek, J. et al. (2000). A functional magnetic resonance imaging study of the role of left posterior superior temporal gyrus in speech production: implications for the explanation of conduction aphasia. *Neurosci. Lett.*, **287**, 156–60.

Hillis, A. & Caramazza, A. (1991). Category-specific naming and comprehension impairment: a double dissociation. *Brain*, **114**, 2081–94.

Hillis, A.E., Rapp, B.C. & Caramazza, A. (1999). When a rose is a rose in speech but a tulip in writing. *Cortex*, **35**, 337–56.

Hinton, G.E. (1981). Implementing semantic networks in parallel hardware. In *Parallel Models of Associative Memory*, ed. G.E. Hinton & J.A. Anderson. Hillsdale, NJ: Erlbaum.

Hodges, J.R., Patterson, K., Oxbury, S. & Funnell, E. (1992). Semantic dementia. Progressive fluent aphasia with temporal lobe atrophy. *Brain*, **15**, 1783–806.

Holland, A.L., McBurney, D.H., Moossy, J. & Reinmuth, O.M. (1985). The dissolution of language in Pick's disease with neurofibrillary tangles: a case study. *Brain Lang.*, **24**, 36–58.

Howard, D., Patterson, K., Wise, R. et al. (1992). The cortical localization of the lexicons. Positron emission tomography evidence. *Brain*, **115**, 1769–82.

Hughlings-Jackson, J. (1880). On affections of speech from disease of the brain. *Brain*, **2**, 203–20.

Humphreys, G.W. & Riddoch, M.J. (1987). On telling your fruits from your vegetables: a consideration of category-specific deficits after brain damage. *Trends Neurosci.*, **10**, 145–8.

Kaplan, E., Goodglass, H. & Weintraub, S. (1983). *The Boston Naming Test*, 2nd edn. Philadelphia: Lea & Febiger.

Kapur, S., Rose, R., Liddle, P. F., Zipursky, R. B., Brown, G. M. & Stuss, D. (1994). The role of the left prefrontal cortex in verbal processing: Semantic processing or willed action? *Neuroreport*, **5**, 2193–6.

Kertesz, A. & McCabe, P. (1977). Recovery patterns and prognosis in aphasia. *Brain*, **1**, 1–18.

Knopman, D.S., Selnes, O.A., Niccum, N., Rubens, A.B., Yock, D. & Larson, D. (1983). A longitudinal study of speech fluency in aphasia: CT correlates of recovery and persistent nonfluency. *Neurology*, **33**, 1170–8.

Knopman, D.S., Selnes, O.A., Niccum, N. & Rubens, A.B. (1984). Recovery of naming in aphasia: relationship to fluency, comprehension and CT findings. *Neurology*, **34**, 1461–70.

Kornyey, E. (1975). Transcortical aphasia and echolalia; problems of speech initiative. *Rev. Neurol.*, **131**, 347–63.

Krauss, G.L., Fisher, R., Plate, C. et al. (1996). Cognitive effects of resecting basal temporal language areas. *Epilepsia*, **37**, 476–83.

Kreisler, A., Godefroy, O., Delmaire, C. et al. (2000). The anatomy of aphasia revisited. *Neurology*, **54**, 1117–23.

Lesser, R.P., Luders, H., Morris, H.H. et al. (1986). Electrical stimulation of Wernicke's area interferes with comprehension. *Neurology*, **36**, 658–63.

Lesser, R.P., Luders, H., Klem, G. et al. (1987). Extraoperative cortical functional localization in patients with epilepsy. *J. Clin. Neurophysiol.*, **4**, 27–53.

Luders, H., Lesser, R.P., Hahn, J. et al. (1986). Basal temporal language area demonstrated by electrical stimulation. *Neurology*, **36**, 505–10.

Luders, H., Lesser, R.P., Hahn, J. et al. (1991). Basal temporal language area. *Brain*, **114**, 743–54.

McCarthy, R.A. & Warrington, E.K. (1988). Evidence for modality-specific meaning systems in the brain. *Nature*, **334**, 428–30.

Martin, A., Wiggs, C.L., Ungerleider, L.G. & Haxby, J.V. (1996). Neural correlates of category-specific knowledge. *Nature*, **379**, 649–52.

Mauri, A., Daum, I., Sartori, G., Riesch, G. & Birbaumer, N. (1994). Category-specific semantic impairment in Alzheimer's disease and temporal lobe dysfunction: a comparative study. *J. Clin. Exp. Neuropsychol.*, **16**, 689–701.

Mesulam, M-M. (1982). Slowly progressive aphasia without generalised dementia. *Ann. Neurol.*, **11**, 592–8.

Mesulam, M-M. (1990). Large-scale neurocognitive networks and distributed processing for attention, language and memory. *Ann. Neurol.*, **28**, 597–613.

Mohr, J.P., Pessin, M.S., Finkelstein, S., Funkenstein, H.H., Duncan, G.W. & Davis, K.R. (1999). Broca aphasia: pathologic and clinical. *Neurology*, **28**, 311–24.

Monrad-Krohn, G. (1947). Dysprosody or altered 'melody of language'. *Brain*, **70**, 405–15.

Moore, C.J. & Price, C.J. (1999a). A functional neuroimaging study of the variables that generate category-specific object processing differences. *Brain*, **122**, 943–62.

Moore, C.J. & Price, C.J. (1999b). Three distinct ventral occipito-temporal regions for reading and object naming. *Neuroimage*, **10**, 181–92.

Moro, A., Tettamanti, M., Perani, D., Donati, C., Cappa, S.F. & Fazio, F. (2001). Syntax and the brain: disentangling grammar by selective anomalies. *Neuroimage*, **13**, 110–18.

Nadeau, S.E. (1988). Impaired grammar with normal fluency and phonology. Implications for Broca's aphasia. *Brain*, **111**, 1111–37.

Naeser, M.A., Helm-Estabrooks, N., Haas, G., Auerbach, S. & Srinivasan, M. (1987). Relationship between lesion extent in 'Wernicke's area' on computed tomographic scan and predicting recovery of comprehension in Wernicke's aphasia. *Arch. Neurol.*, **44**, 73–82.

Nicholas, M.L, Helm-Estabrooks, N., Ward-Lonergan, J. & Morgan, A.R. (1993). Evolution of severe aphasia in the first two years post onset. *Arch. Phys. Med. Rehabil.*, **74**, 830–6.

Nielsen, J.M. (1946). *Agnosia, Apraxia, Aphasia: Their Value In Cerebral Localization*, 2nd edn. New York: Paul B. Hoeber.

Nobre, A.C., Allison, T. & McCarthy, G. (1994). Word recognition in the human inferior temporal lobe. *Nature*, **372**, 260–3.

Patterson, K.E., Marshall, J.C. & Coltheart, M. (1985). *Surface Dyslexia: Neuropsychological and Cognitive Studies of Phonological Reading*. Hillsdale, NJ: Lawrence Erlbaum Associates.

Pedersen, P.M., Jorgensen, H.S., Nakayama, H., Raaschou, H.O. & Olsen, T.S. (1995). Aphasia in acute stroke: incidence, determinants, and recovery. *Ann. Neurol.*, **38**, 659–66.

Penfield, W. & Robert, L. (1959). *Speech and Brain-Mechanisms*. Princeton, NJ: Princeton University Press.

Petersen, S.E., Fox, P.T., Posner, M.I., Mintun, M. & Raichle, M.E. (1988). Positron emission tomographic studies of the cortical anatomy of single-word processing. *Nature*, **331**, 585–9.

Petersen, S.E., Fox, P.T., Snyder, A.Z. & Raichle, M.E. (1990). Specific extrastriate and frontal cortical areas are activated by visual words and word-like stimuli. *Science*, **249**, 1041–4.

Petrides, M. & Pandya, D.N. (1988). Association fiber pathways to the frontal cortex from the superior temporal region in the rhesus monkey. *J. Comp. Neurol.*, **273**, 52–66.

Poeck, K. & Luzatti, C. (1988). Slowly progressive aphasia in three patients. The problem of accompanying neuropsychological deficit. *Brain*, **111**, 151–68.

Posner, M.I., Petersen, S.E., Fox, P.T. & Raichle, M.E. (1988). Localization of cognitive operations in the human brain. *Science*, **240**, 1627–31.

Rapcsak, S.Z., Comer, J.F. & Rubens, A.B. (1983). Anomia for facial expressions: neuropsychological mechanisms and anatomical correlates. *Brain Lang.*, **45**, 233–52.

Rapcsak, S.Z., Kaszniak, A.W. & Rubens, A.B. (1989). Anomia for facial expressions: evidence for a category specific visual-verbal disconnection syndrome. *Neuropsychologia*, **27**, 1031–41.

Rapin, I. & Dunn, M. (1997). Language disorders in children with autism. *Semin. Pediatr. Neurol.*, **4**, 86–92.

Ricci, P.T., Zelkowicz, B.J., Nebes, R.D., Meltzer, C.C., Mintun, M.A. & Becker, J.T. (1999). Functional neuroanatomy of semantic memory: recognition of semantic associations. *Neuroimage*, **9**, 88–96.

Robey, R.R. (1994). The efficacy of treatment of aphasic persons: a meta-analysis. *Brain Lang.*, **47**, 582–608.

Robinson, K.M., Grossman, M., White-Devine, T. & D'Esposito, M. (1996). Category-specific difficulty naming with verbs in Alzheimer's disease. *Neurology*, **47**, 178–82.

Rostomily, R.C., Berger, M.S., Ojemann, G.A. & Lettich, E. (1991). Postoperative deficits and functional recovery following removal of tumours involving the dominant hemisphere supplementary motor area. *J. Neurosurg.*, **75**, 62–8.

Ryalls, J. (1986). What constitutes a primary disturbance of speech prosody? A reply to Shapiro and Danly. *Brain Lang.*, **29**, 183–7.

Ryalls, J. & Reinvang, I. (1985). Some further notes on Monrad–Krohn's case study of foreign accent syndrome. *Folia Phoniatr. (Basel)*, **37**, 160–2.

Sacchett, C. & Humphreys, G.W. (1992). Calling a squirrel a squirrel but a canoe a wigwam: a category-specific deficit for artefactual objects and body parts. *Cogn. Neuropsychol.*, **9**, 73–86.

Sakurai, Y., Hashida, H., Uesugi, H. et al. (1996). A clinical profile of corticobasal degeneration presenting as primary progressive aphasia. *Europ. Neurol.*, **36**, 134–7.

Sakurai, Y., Takeuchi, S., Takada, T., Horiuchi, E., Nakase, H. & Sakuta, M. (2000). Alexia caused by a fusiform or posterior inferior temporal lesion. *J. Neurol. Sci.*, **178**, 42–51.

Sartori, G. & Job, R. (1988). The oyster with four legs: a neuropsychological study on the interaction of visual and semantic information. *Cogn. Neuropsychol.*, **5**, 105–32.

Sartori, G., Job, R., Miozzo, M., Zago, S. & Marchiori, G. (1993). Category-specific form-knowledge deficit in a patient with herpes simplex virus encephalitis. *J. Clin. Exp. Neuropsychol.*, **15**, 280–99.

Schaffler, L., Luders, H.O., Dinner, D.S., Lesser, R.P. & Chelune, G.J. (1993). Comprehension deficits elicited by electrical stimulation of Broca's area. *Brain*, **116**, 695–715.

Schwartz, M.F. (1984). What the classical aphasia categories can't do for us and why. *Brain Lang.*, **21**, 3–8.

Selnes, O.A. & Hillis, A.E. (2000). Patient Tan revisited: a case of atypical global aphasia? *J. History Neurosci.*, **9**, 233–7.

Selnes, O.A., Niccum, N., Knopman, D.S. & Rubens, A.B. (1984). Recovery of single word comprehension: CT-scan correlates. *Brain Lang.*, **21**, 72–84.

Selnes, O.A., Knopman, D.S., Niccum, N. & Rubens, A.B. (1985). The critical role of Wernicke's area in sentence repetition. *Ann. Neurol.*, **17**, 549–57.

Selnes, O.A., Holcomb, H.H. & Gordon, B. (1996). Progressive dysarthria: structural and functional brain correlations. *Am. J. Psychiat.*, **153**, 309–10.

Semenza, C. & Zettin, M. (1988). Generating proper names: a case of selective inability. *Cogn. Neuropsychol.*, **5**, 711–21.

Semenza, C. & Zettin, M. (1989). Evidence from aphasia for the role of proper names as pure referring expressions. *Nature*, **342**, 678–9.

Shuren, J.E., Schefft, B.K., Yeh, H.S., Privitera, M.D., Cahill, W.T. & Houston, W. (1995). Repetition and the arcuate fasciculus. *J. Neurol.*, **242**, 596–8.

Silveri, M.C. & Gainotti, G. (1988). Interaction between vision and language in category-specific semantic impairment. *Cogn. Neuropsychol.*, **5**, 677–709.

Silveri, M.C., Daniele, A., Giustolisi, L. & Gainotti, G. (1991). Dissociation between knowledge of living and nonliving things in dementia of the Alzheimer type. *Neurology*, **41**, 545–6.

Simos, P.G., Breier, J.I., Wheless, J.W. et al. (2000). Brain mechanisms for reading: the role of the superior temporal gyrus in word and pseudoword naming. *Neuroreport*, **11**, 2443–7.

Small, S.L. (1994). Pharmacotherapy of aphasia. A critical review. *Stroke*, **25**, 1282–9.

Spitzer, M., Kwong, K.K., Kennedy, W., Rosen, B.R. & Bellivean, J.W. (1995). Category-specific brain activation in fMRI during picture naming. *Neuroreport*, **6**, 2109–12.

Stengel, E., Vienna, M.D. & Edin, L.R.C.P. (1947). A clinical and psychological study of echo-reactions. *J. Ment. Sci.*, **93**, 598–612.

Takayama, Y., Sugishita, M., Kido, T., Ogawa, M. & Akiguchi, I. (1993). A case of foreign accent syndrome without aphasia caused by a lesion of the left precentral gyrus. *Neurology*, **43**, 1361–3.

Temple, C. (1986). Anomia for animals in a child. *Brain*, **109**, 1225–42.

Thompson-Schill, S.L., D'Esposito, M., Aguirre, G.K. & Farah, M.J. (1997). Role of left inferior prefrontal cortex in retrieval of semantic knowledge: a reevaluation. *Proc. Natl. Acad. Sci., USA*, **94**, 14792–7.

Tippett, L.J., Glosser, G. & Farah, M.J. (1996). A category-specific naming impairment after temporal lobectomy. *Neuropsychologia*, **34**, 139–46.

Vandenberghe, R., Price, C., Wise, R., Josephs, O. & Frackowiak, R.S. (1996). Functional anatomy of a common semantic system for words and pictures. *Nature*, **383**, 254–6.

Vignolo, L.A., Boccardi, E. & Caverni, L. (1986). Unexpected CT-scan findings in global aphasia. *Cortex*, **22**, 55–69.

Warrington, E.K. & McCarthy, R.A. (1983). Category specific access dysphasia. *Brain*, **106**, 859–78.

Warrington, E.K. & McCarthy, R.A. (1987). Categories of knowledge: further fractionation and an attempted integration. *Brain*, **110**, 1273–96.

Warrington, E.K. & Shallice, T. (1984). Category specific semantic impairments. *Brain*, **107**, 829–54.

Weintraub, S., Rubin, N.P. & Mesulam, M-M. (1990). Primary progressive aphasia. Longitudinal course, neuropsychological profile, and language features. *Arch. Neurol.*, **47**, 1329–35.

Westbury, C. & Bub, D. (1997). Primary progressive aphasia: a review of 112 cases. *Brain Lang.*, **60**, 381–406.

Willmes, K. & Poeck, K. (1993). To what extent can aphasic syndromes be localized? *Brain*, **1527**, 15–40.

23

Neglect

Kenneth M. Heilman

Department of Neurology, University of Florida College of Medicine, Gainesville, FL, USA

A patient with the neglect syndrome fails to report, respond or orient to, novel or meaningful stimuli presented to the side opposite a brain lesion (Heilman, 1979). If this failure can be attributed to either sensory or motor defects, the patient is not considered to have neglect.

The two basic mechanisms that are thought to be responsible for the failure to report, respond, or orient are defects in the systems that mediate sensory attention or motor intention. Whereas attentional defects may be associated with unawareness, intentional disorders may cause a failure to respond despite stimulus awareness. Attention and intention defects may occur in two domains: spatial and personal. Patients with neglect can also have spatial memory defects. This defect can be for new information or old memories (representational defects). This chapter describes tests that may be used to assess patients and behaviourally define these disorders. This chapter also discusses the pathophysiology underlying these disorders and their treatment.

Behavioural testing for the components of neglect

Tests for inattention and extinction

The attentional aspects of the neglect syndrome are detected by observing abnormal responses to sensory stimuli. Stimuli should be given in at least three modalities, somatesthetic, visual, and auditory, but other stimuli, such as gustatory and olfactory, may be used. Examiners often request immediate responses, however, delaying the response and using distractor techniques may help amplify the symptoms.

When testing with somatesthetic stimuli, one may control the intensity of a tactile stimulus by using Von Frei's hairs. However, fingers or cotton applicators are more convenient. Other cutaneous stimuli, such as pins, may be used. For bedside auditory testing, we use sounds made by either rubbing the fingers together or snapping them. When possible, perimetric and tangent screen studies should be used for testing visual fields. However, for bedside testing the confrontational method may be used; the examiner's finger movement can be used as the stimulus. A modified Poppelreuter diagram or written sentences may also be used.

These somatesthetic, auditory and visual stimuli should be presented to the abnormal (contralateral) side and to the normal side of the body in random order. If the patient responds normally to unilateral stimulation, simultaneous bilateral stimulation may be used. Unilateral stimuli should be randomly interspersed with simultaneous bilateral stimuli. Bender (1952) noted that normal subjects may show extinction to simultaneous stimulation when the stimuli are delivered to two different (asymmetric) parts of the body (simultaneous bilateral heterologous stimulation). For example, if the right side of the face and the left hand are stimulated simultaneously, normal subjects sometimes report only the stimulus on the face. Normal subjects do not extinguish symmetric stimuli (simultaneous bilateral homologous stimulation). Simultaneous bilateral heterologous stimulation can sometimes be used to test for milder defects in patients with extinction. For example, when the right side of the face and the left hand are stimulated, patients with left-sided neglect might not report the stimulus on the left hand, but when the left side of the face and right hand are stimulated, they might report both stimuli.

The most frequent response by patients is verbal (i.e. right, left or both). In addition, the patient may be instructed (verbally or non-verbally by gesture) to move the extremity or extremities the examiner has touched.

Patients may be considered to have hemi-inattention when they fail to orient, report, or respond to contralateral stimuli and when it can be demonstrated that the lesion does not interrupt afferent projectors and does not destroy primary sensory cortex or sensory thalamic nuclei. However, unless the site of the lesion is known, it may be difficult to distinguish between hemianesthesia or hemianopsia and severe somatesthetic and visual hemiattention. Occasionally, visual inattention may be distinguished from hemianopsia by changing the hemispace of presentation. Kooistra and Hellman (1989) reported a patient who could not detect single stimuli presented in the left visual field when the eyes were directed straight ahead, but could detect stimuli in the same retinotopic position when the eyes were directed toward right hemispace so that the left visual half-field was in the right hemispace.

Patients with hemianesthesia from unilateral cortical lesions probably suffer from inattention rather than from deafferentation. Elementary somatic sensation such as touch can be subserved by the thalamus. Lesions of the ventral posterolateral and ventral posteromedial thalamic nuclei result in hemianesthesia, but lesions in somatosensory cortex should not. Some patients with cortical lesions who appear to have tactile anesthesia can detect contralesional stimuli when cold water is injected into the contralesional ear. This increases orientation toward the side of the cold ear via vestibular mechanisms, suggesting that the hemianesthesia in fact results from sensory neglect (Vallar et al., 1995). One can also use psychophysiological procedures, such as early evoked potentials and skin conductance responses, to discriminate between inattention and deafferentation.

Although hemianesthesia and hemianopsia are fairly common manifestations of central nervous system lesions, unilateral hearing loss is almost always due to a disturbance in the peripheral hearing mechanisms or in the auditory nerve. Because the auditory pathways that ascend from the brainstem to the cortex are bilateral, each ear projects to both hemispheres. Thus, a unilateral central nervous system lesion will not produce unilateral hearing loss. Consequently, patients without peripheral hearing loss who fail to orient to, or report, unilateral auditory stimulation usually have hemi-inattention. Furthermore, because sound presented on one side of the body projects to both ears, patients with unilateral hearing loss caused by a peripheral lesion usually respond to unilateral auditory stimulation unless the stimulus is extremely close to the ear. Therefore, patients who neglect unilateral auditory stimuli most often have unilateral inattention.

Patients with unilateral neglect are most inattentive to stimuli contralateral to the lesion, but they are often also inattentive to ipsilateral stimuli, although ipsilateral inattention is not so severe.

Tests for personal neglect

Whereas the failure to detect tactile stimuli described in the preceding section may be a sign of personal neglect, patients with flagrant personal inattention may deny that their own limbs belong to them. This deficit is also called asomatognosia. The examiner can demonstrate personal neglect by asking patients to show a limb or by showing them their own limb and asking them to whom the limb belongs. Patients with personal neglect may also fail to groom or dress half of their body. Although anosognosia of a left hemiplegia and allesthesia (misplacing contralesional stimuli to the ipsilesional part of the body) are often associated with personal neglect, these three signs are often dissociable.

Coslett (1998) showed right hemisphere damaged patients diagrams of the palmar or dorsal aspect of the right or left hand and asked them to tell if the picture showed a right or left hand. To perform this task, one has to image one's own right or left hand in either the prone or supine position. Coslett's patients were impaired when shown diagrams of the left hand but not the right hand, suggesting a defect in the left side of a personal representation.

Tests for spatial neglect

Patients fail to act on contralesional stimuli presented in space. They may fail to act on stimuli presented to the left of their body (viewer centred hemispatial neglect), or they may fail to act on the left side of the environment or they may fail to act on the left side of the stimulus (allocentric spatial neglect). The three most frequently used methods for testing spatial neglect are the line bisection, the cancellation tasks and drawing. In the cancellation test, small lines are randomly drawn on a sheet of paper and the patient is asked to cross out all the lines. This can be made more difficult by using a task in which patients must either discriminate or focus their attention (Rapcsak et al., 1989). In the line bisection task an 8- to 10-inch line is presented to the patient, who is asked to bisect the line (find the middle of the line). This task can be made more difficult by using longer lines (Butter et al., 1988a) or by placing lines to the left of the midsagittal plane (Heilman & Valenstein, 1979).

When using very short lines patients with contralesional neglect may place their bisection mark on the side of the line that is contralateral to their hemispheric lesion. This has been termed the cross-over effect (Halligan & Marshall, 1991).

Lastly, one can test for spatial neglect by having a subject copy drawings. Because neglect is often associated with right hemisphere lesions, patients may have constructional apraxia. Therefore, simple drawings (flower, clock) should be used.

Although spatial neglect is most often described in the horizontal plane (left spatial neglect), vertical neglect (Rapcsak et al., 1988) and radial neglect (Shelton et al., 1990) have also been reported. Vertical neglect and radial neglect can be assessed by orienting the line to be bisected in a radial or vertical direction.

Bisiach and Luzzatti (1978) asked patients to describe a familiar scene. Patients with left-sided neglect failed to recall the left side of the scene. Unfortunately, there is no simple bedside test for examining spatial representations. However, one can ask patients to describe the layout of their house, describe the sites on a famous street in their hometown going in a specific direction, or name the cities in the state in which they live. Failure to describe more items on one side than the other may suggest spatial representational neglect. Asking a patient to spell words from memory may also elicit spatial representational neglect but is an insensitive test. Finally, one could ask a patient who can copy drawings to make the same drawings from memory.

There are patients with hemispheric dysfunction who will bisect long lines toward contralesional rather than ipsilesional hemispace (Kwon & Heilman, 1991; Na et al., 1998a). This is called ipsilateral neglect.

Tests for motor-intention deficits: akinesia and motor neglect

Akinesia is the inability to initiate a movement that cannot be attributed to a defect in the motor unit or corticospinal neurons. Milder forms of akinesia may be expressed as a delay in initiating a movement (hypokinesia) or decreased amplitude of movement (hypometria). Akinesia may affect one or more body parts (legs, limbs, eyes, head) and may be spatial or directional. It may be seen only with spontaneously evoked activities (endo-evoked akinesia) or only in response to stimuli (exo-evoked akinesia) or may be mixed. When akinesia is mixed, involves a limb, and is not spatially or directionally specific, it may be difficult to dissociate from a motor defect caused by corticospinal tract damage, and one may have to rely on imaging studies or caloric stimulation.

When examining a patient for akinesia, one must make multiple observations, including watching spontaneous activity to see if the patient moves their eyes, head, and limbs in all directions. After an acute insult to the right hemisphere, it is not unusual for the head and eyes to be deviated to the right and not to move toward the left either spontaneously or in response to stimuli and instructions. However, even in the absence of this florid manifestation, contralesional directional akinesia may be detected using a modification of the crossed response task (Watson et al., 1978). The examiner holds one hand in the patient's right visual half-field and the other in the left visual half-field. In the first series of trials, the index finger of the examiner's right or left hand is moved and the patient is instructed to look at the moving finger. A patient who fails to look at the contralesional stimulus may have hemianopsia, visual inattention, or directional akinesia. These can be dissociated by instructing the patient to look to the side opposite that stimulated, so that when the examiner's right index finger is moved, the patient looks toward the left hand and vice versa. Failure to look at the contralesional hand indicates directional akinesia, and failure to look at the ipsilesional finger suggests inattention or hemianopsia (Butter et al., 1998b). In less severe cases of directional akinesia, patients may move in a contralesional direction by making multiple hypometric saccades (Heilman et al., 1980).

A condition similar to eye deviation may be detected in the arm by asking blindfolded patients with neglect to point to their midsagittal plane (Heilman et al., 1983a). Patients may point toward the ipsilateral hemispace. To detect directional akinesia of the limbs, a blindfolded patient may be placed before a table that has pennies randomly distributed over the top and be asked to pick up all the pennies. Patients with directional akinesia may fail to explore left hemispace. Patients may also have a directional hypokinesia of the limbs, so that movements toward the left are initiated more slowly than movements toward the right (Heilman et al., 1985). Patients may demonstrate hemispatial akinesia of the limbs such that when the limb is in contralateral hemispace it does not move or it moves less than when it is in ipsilateral hemispace (Meador et al., 1986).

Testing for anosognosia

Explicit verbal denial or unawareness of illness is termed anosognosia. Patients with neglect often deny a left hemiplegia, and they may also be unaware of a left hemianopsia. Verbally acknowledging a problem but failing to be concerned is called anosodiaphoria. Anosognosia and anosodiaphoria are best tested by asking patients why they came to the hospital. If they fail to describe their problems,

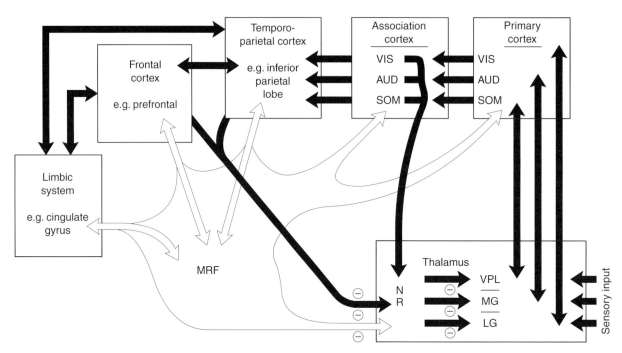

Fig. 23.1. Schematic representation of systems important in attention and arousal (see text for details). NR = nucleus reticularis thalami; MRF = mesencephalic reticular formation; VPL = ventralis posterolateris; MG = medial geniculate; LG = lateral geniculate; VIS = visual; AUD = auditory; SOM = somatosensory.

more specific questions may be asked. If patients have hemispatial inattention, the hemiparetic limbs should be brought into ipsilesional hemispace and the patients should be asked to move the limb and then asked again if they are impaired.

Testing for allesthesia and allokinesia

When stimulated on the side contralateral to a lesion, patients with allesthesia misplace the location of the stimulus to the normal side. Patients with allokinesia respond with the wrong limb or move in the wrong direction. Allesthesia and allokinesia should be distinguished from right–left confusion. Patients with right–left confusion do not make systematic directional errors, whereas patients with allesthesia misattribute left side stimuli to the right, but not vice versa.

Pathophysiology of the components of neglect

Pathophysiology of inattention

Unilateral inattention can be induced in humans by lesions in a variety of loci. Contralateral inattention may be induced by lesions in the temporal–parietal–occipital junction or inferior parietal lobe (Critchley, 1966; Heilman et al., 1983b). In humans, inferior parietal lobe lesions are probably most commonly associated with inattention, but lesions of the dorsolateral frontal lobe may also be associated with inattention (Damasio et al., 1980; Heilman & Valenstein, 1972). In humans and monkeys, lesions in the cingulate gyrus (Heilman & Valenstein, 1972; Watson et al., 1973) and subcortical lesions in such areas as the thalamus and mesencephalic reticular formation (Watson & Heilman, 1979; Watson et al., 1974) may also induce inattention.

Cerebral infarction is the most common cause of cortical lesions associated with neglect. Intracerebral hemorrhage is the cause of most subcortical lesions associated with inattention; however, other disease processes, including tumours, may induce inattention.

Inattention is probably caused by dysfunction in a cortical–limbic–reticular formation network (Heilman & Valenstein, 1972; Watson et al., 1974, 1981) (Fig. 23.1). A discussion of possible mechanisms requires some consideration of the phenomena of arousal, a physiologic state that prepares the organism for sensory and motor processing.

Stimulation of the mesencephalic reticular formation is associated with arousal and also with desynchronization of the electroencephalogram, a physiologic measure of arousal (Moruzzi & Magoun, 1949). Unilateral stimulation induces greater desynchronization of the electroencephalogram in the ipsilateral than in the contralateral hemisphere (Moruzzi & Magoun, 1949). Bilateral mesencephalic reticular formation lesions result in coma. Unilateral lesions result in contralateral inattention, which is probably due to unilateral hemispheric hypoarousal (Reeves & Hagamen, 1971; Watson et al., 1974). The mesencephalic reticular activating system probably projects to the cortex in a diffuse polysynaptic fashion (Schiebel & Schiebel, 1967). This projection may occur through the thalamus (Steriade & Glenn, 1982) or basal forebrain.

There is another way in which the mesencephalic reticular activating system can affect cortical processing of sensory stimuli. Sensory information that reaches the cortex is relayed through specific thalamic nuclei. The nucleus reticularis thalami, a thin reticular nucleus enveloping the thalamus, projects to the thalamic relay nuclei and appears to inhibit thalamic relay to the cortex (Schiebel & Schiebel, 1966). The mesencephalic reticular formation projects to the nucleus reticularis. Rapid stimulation of the mesencephalic reticular formation (or behavioural arousal) inhibits the nucleus reticularis and is thereby associated with enhanced thalamic sensory transmission to the cerebral cortex (Singer, 1977). Unilateral lesions of the mesencephalic reticular formation may induce neglect because in the absence of mesencephalic reticular formation-mediated arousal, the cortex is not prepared for processing sensory stimuli and the thalamic sensory relay nuclei are being inhibited by the nucleus reticularis thalami.

Modality-specific association areas may detect stimulus novelty (Sokolov, 1963). When a stimulus is neither novel nor significant, corticofugal projections to the nucleus reticularis thalami may allow habituation to occur by selectively influencing thalamic relay. When a stimulus is novel or significant, the corticofugal projections may inhibit the nucleus reticularis thalami and allow the thalamus to relay additional sensory input.

Unimodal association areas converge on polymodal association areas (see Fig. 23.1) in the prefrontal cortex and in the posterior superior portion of the temporal lobe and inferior parietal lobe (Pandya & Kuypers, 1969). Polymodal convergence areas may subserve cross-modal associations and polymodal sensory synthesis. Polymodal sensory synthesis may also be important in the detection of stimulus novelty (modelling) and significance. In contrast to the unimodal association cortex that projects to specific parts of the nucleus reticularis thalami and thereby gates sensory input in one modality, these multimodal conver-

gence areas may have a more general inhibitory action on the nucleus reticularis thalami and provide further arousal after cortical analysis. These convergence areas also may project directly to the mesencephalic reticular formation, which may either induce a general state of arousal because of diffuse multisynaptic connections to the cortex or increase thalamic transmission through connections with the nucleus reticularis thalami, or both. Evidence that polymodal areas of the cortex, such as the prefrontal and inferior parietal lobe, are important in arousal comes from neurophysiological studies showing that stimulation of these cortical sites induces a generalized arousal response (Segundo et al., 1955). When similar sites are ablated, there is electroencephalographic evidence of ipsilateral hypoarousal (Watson et al., 1977).

Although the sensory association cortex may mediate determination of stimulus novelty, stimulus significance is determined in part by the needs of the organism (motivational state). Limbic system input into the brain regions important for determining stimulus significance may provide information about biologic needs. The frontal lobes may provide input about needs related to goals that are neither dependent directly on the stimulus nor motivated by an immediate biologic need, because the frontal lobes have a critical role in goal-mediated behaviour and in developing sets.

The inferior parietal lobe has prominent limbic (cingulate) and frontal connections (Baleydier & Mauguiere, 1980; Pandya & Kuypers, 1969; Vogt et al., 1979) that may provide an anatomic substrate through which motivational states (for example, biologic needs, sets, and long-term goals) may influence stimulus processing (Heilman, 1979; Heilman & Valenstein, 1972; Watson et al., 1981).

Investigators have been able to study the physiologic function of specific areas of the nervous system by recording from single neurons in awake animals. In this experimental situation, the firing characteristics of individual neurons can be measured in relation to specific sensory stimulation or motor behaviour. Investigators have thus defined the properties of neurons in the inferior parietal lobule (area 7) of the monkey (Lynch, 1980; Mountcastle et al., 1975). Unlike the activity of single cells in primary sensory cortex, the activity of many neurons in the inferior parietal lobule correlates best with stimuli or responses of importance to the animal, and similar stimuli or responses that are unimportant are associated with either no change or a lesser change in neuronal activity. These cells appear to be critical in directing attention.

The attentional model we have discussed is summarized in Fig. 23.1. Unilateral inattention follows lesions of the unilateral mesencephalic reticular activation system because loss of inhibition of the ipsilateral nucleus reticularis by the mesencephalic reticular activating system decreases thalamic transmission of sensory input to the cortex or because the mesencephalic reticular formation does not prepare the cortex for sensory processing, or both. Unilateral lesions of the primary or association cortices cause contralateral unimodal sensory loss or inability to synthesize contralateral unimodal sensory input. Corticothalamic collaterals from the association cortex to the nucleus reticularis may serve unimodal habituation and attention. Unilateral lesions of multimodal sensory convergence areas that project into mesencephalic reticular activating system and nucleus reticularis induce contralateral inattention because the subject cannot be aroused to, or process, multimodal contralateral stimuli. A lesion of the inferior parietal lobule, because of its reciprocal connections with polymodal areas and the limbic system, may impair the subject's ability to determine the significance of a stimulus.

Pathophysiology of extinction

Although patients may initially have hemi-inattention, most improve. Whereas at first they fail to detect stimuli presented to the side opposite the lesion, they eventually become able to report these stimuli. When given bilateral simultaneous stimulation, however, they often fail to report the stimulus presented to the side contralateral to the lesion (Anton, 1899; Bender, 1952; Loeb, 1885; Poppelreuter, 1917).

Extinction can be seen in normal subjects as well as in patients with central nervous system lesions (Benton & Levin, 1972; Kimura, 1967). The lesions causing extinction are often in the same areas as lesions that cause inattention. However, certain forms of extinction may also occur after lesions of the corpus callosum (Milner et al., 1968; Sparks & Geschwind, 1968), and left-sided extinction has even been reported after left hemisphere lesions (Schwartz et al., 1979).

The mechanisms underlying extinction in normal subjects and in patients with callosal lesions, sensory defects, or hemispheric lesions may differ and, in general, are poorly understood. Several investigators have suggested that extinction and perhaps obscuration in normal subjects and patients with sensory loss result from suppression or reciprocal inhibition. In the case of cerebral damage, the normal hemisphere inhibits the damaged hemisphere more than the damaged hemisphere inhibits the normal hemisphere. Consequently, stimuli contralateral to the damaged hemisphere are not perceived when the normal side is stimulated. The physiologic mechanisms that induce this reciprocal inhibition are unknown. However, as discussed earlier, the thalamic reticular nucleus can selectively inhibit various thalamic sensory nuclei. Each association cortex may not only project to the ipsilateral thalamic reticular nucleus but also influence the contralateral thalamic reticular nucleus. Unlike the ipsilateral connections, which are inhibitory, the contralateral projections may be facilitatory. Therefore, even under normal conditions, a stimulus on one side should induce an increase of threshold for stimuli on the other side. With a lesion of association cortex there should be less ipsilateral inhibition of nucleus reticularis thalami, which in turn should inhibit the thalamic sensory nuclei, thus making the thalamus less sensitive to contralateral stimuli. If the opposite side were simultaneously stimulated, activated attentional cells should further increase contralateral nucleus reticularis thalami activity, further inhibiting the thalamic sensory nuclei and thereby inducing extinction. The pathway by which one association cortex may influence the contralateral nucleus reticularis thalami is unknown.

Birch et al. (1967) proposed and provided support for the hypothesis that the damaged hemisphere processes information more slowly than does the intact hemisphere. Because of this inertia, the damaged side is more subject to interference from the normal side. When stimuli must be processed by a lateralized system, callosal lesions may induce extinction because the information cannot reach the processor or is delayed.

Another explanation for extinction, the limited attention theory, proposes that under normal circumstances bilateral simultaneous stimuli are processed simultaneously, each hemisphere processing the contralateral stimulus. However, a damaged hemisphere may be unable to attend to contralateral stimuli, making the organism inattentive to those stimuli. As the organism recovers, it can attend to contralateral stimuli. This improvement may be mediated by the normal (ipsilateral) hemisphere. The normal hemisphere, however, may have a limited attentional capacity. Therefore, with bilateral simultaneous stimulation the normal hemisphere's attentional mechanism, occupied with the contralateral stimulus, may be unable to attend to the ipsilateral stimulus (Heilman, 1979).

These theories may not be mutually exclusive. Because extinction can be caused by lesions in a variety of anatomically and functionally different areas, the reciprocal inhibition, limited attention, and interference theories may each be correct, but for different lesions.

Pathophysiology of akinesia and motor neglect

Attention and intention (preparation to make a movement) are closely linked, and lesions in many of the areas that induce inattention and extinction may also induce akinesia. For example, unilateral sensory neglect (inattention) has been reported to follow unilateral dorsolateral frontal lesions in monkeys (Bianchi, 1895; Kennard & Ectors, 1938; Welch & Stuteville, 1958) and humans (Heilman & Valenstein, 1972). In most testing paradigms the animal is required to respond to a stimulus contralateral to the lesion either by orienting to the stimulus or by moving the limbs on the side of the stimulus. These animals with frontal lobe lesions were not weak, so it was assumed that they had sensory neglect when they failed to make the appropriate response. Although this neglect was usually assumed to result from inattention to the sensory stimuli, we suggested that it could equally well be caused by unilateral akinesia (Watson et al., 1978). Therefore, we trained monkeys to use the left hand to respond to a tactile stimulus on the right leg and the right hand to respond to a tactile stimulus on the left. After a unilateral frontal arcuate lesion, the monkeys appeared to have contralateral neglect, but when stimulated on their neglected side, they responded normally with the limb on the side of the lesion. When stimulated on the side ipsilateral to the lesion, however, they often failed to respond (with the limb on the neglected side) or responded by moving the limb ipsilateral to the lesion. These results cannot be explained by sensory or perceptual hypotheses and are thought to reflect a defect in intention to make a correct response.

In considering the possible role of the dorsolateral frontal lobes in attention and intention related to multimodal sensory and limbic inputs, it is important to examine their connections. The dorsolateral frontal lobe has reciprocal connections with unimodal and polymodal posterior sensory association cortex (Chavis & Pandya, 1976) and is an area of sensory convergence (Bignall & Imbert, 1969). The dorsolateral frontal lobe has reciprocal connections with medial (non-specific) thalamic nuclei. Projections to the mesencephalic reticular formation (Kuypers & Lawrence, 1967) and non-reciprocal projections to caudate also exist. Also, the dorsolateral frontal lobe receives input from the limbic system, primarily from the anterior cingulate gyrus (Baleydier & Mauguiere, 1980).

Its connections with neocortical sensory association and sensory convergence areas may provide the frontal lobe with information about external stimuli that may call the organism to action. The limbic connections (anterior cingulate gyrus) may provide the frontal lobe with motivational information. Connections with the mesencephalic reticular formation may be important in arousal.

Because the dorsolateral frontal lobe has sensory association cortex, limbic and reticular formation connections, it seems to be ideal for mediating a response to a stimulus to which the subject is attending. Physiologic studies support this hypothesis (Goldberg & Bushnell, 1981).

Motor neglect or akinesia may also accompany lesions of the non-specific intralaminar thalamic nuclei (Watson et al., 1978), which project to both the frontal lobe and the neostriatum. Akinesia may result from basal ganglia and ventral thalamic lesions (ventralis lateralis and ventralis anterior) (Velasco & Velasco, 1979). The basal ganglia project to the ventral thalamus, and this motor portion of the thalamus is also gated by nucleus reticularis thalami. The nucleus reticularis thalami may be inhibited by the mesencephalic reticular formation during an arousal or orienting response and be inhibited by the frontal lobes during a motor set.

Akinetic mute states are often induced by bilateral lesions of the frontal lobes, cingulate gyri, and medial thalamus. These lesions are usually caused by vascular disease (Segarra & Angelo, 1970). A cingulate gyrus lesion may be induced by an infarct in the distribution of the anterior cerebral artery, secondary to thrombosis, embolism, or aneurysm-induced spasm. Akinetic mutism of thalamic origin is most often the result of occlusion of the posterior thalamic–subthalamic paramedian arteries (Segarra & Angelo, 1970).

Degenerative diseases that affect the basal ganglia, limbic system and frontal lobes may also induce akinesia. These include Parkinson's disease, progressive supranuclear palsy, striatonigral degeneration, olivopontocerebellar degeneration and related diseases. Late in the course of several degenerative dementias, including Pick's disease and Alzheimer's disease, akinesia may be a prominent sign.

Lesions that disrupt the connections of the frontal lobes, limbic system, basal ganglia and thalamus may also be associated with akinesia. Hydrocephalus, tumours (such as butterfly gliomas), lacunae and Binswanger's disease are common causes of such lesions.

Pathophysiology of spatial neglect

Lesions associated with contralesional hemispatial neglect are similar to those associated with inattention and extinction. Although hemianopsia may enhance the symptoms of hemispatial neglect, hemianopsia alone cannot account for the deficit because some patients with hemispatial neglect do not have hemianopsia (McFie et al., 1950) and some patients with hemianopsia do not have spatial neglect.

The abnormal performance of patients in contralesional hemispace suggests that brain mechanisms related to the opposite hemispace have been disturbed. It also suggests that each hemisphere is responsible not only for receiving stimuli from the contralateral visual field and for controlling the contralateral limbs but also for attention and intention in and toward contralateral hemispace, independent of which visual field the stimulus enters or which hand is used (Bowers & Heilman, 1980; Heilman, 1979). The postulate that each hemisphere attends to and intends in and toward contralateral hemispace has been supported by studies of normal subjects (Bowers et al., 1981).

Hemispace can be defined according to the visual half-field (eye position), head position, or trunk position. With the eyes and head facing directly ahead, the hemispaces defined by the eyes, head, and body are congruent. But if the eyes are directed to the far right, for example, the left visual field falls in the right hemispace, as defined by the head and body midline. Similarly, if the head and eyes are turned far to the right, the left head and eye hemispaces can both be in the right hemispace of the body. There is evidence that head and body hemispaces are important in determining the symptoms of hemispatial neglect (Bowers & Heilman, 1980; Heilman & Valenstein, 1979). For example, when patients with left hemispatial neglect are asked to bisect a line, their performance is poorer in left body hemispace than in right hemispace even when a strategy is used to ensure that the line is seen in the normal right hemifield (Heilman & Valenstein, 1979). Similarly, independent of visual field and body hemispace, lines are more poorly bisected in left head hemispace than in right head hemispace (Coslett et al., 1985).

Several neuropsychological mechanisms could account for the hemispatial defect associated with neglect. Patients with hemispatial neglect may have a hemispatial sensory-attentional deficit. Although the line is seen in the normal visual field, it is not attended and thus is not fully processed; the percept is therefore not consolidated and the stimulus does not affect the patient's behaviour. Alternatively, the percept can be weakened and appear of less magnitude. The attentional defect may also be associated with a hemispatial memory defect (Heilman et al., 1974).

Patients with neglect may have an attentional bias such that their attention is drawn to the side of space ipsilateral to their lesion (Kinsbourne, 1970) and they are unable to draw their attention away from the ipsilateral part of space. Partial support for the attentional bias hypothesis comes from the observation that, in a cancellation task, erasing lines is associated with better performance than cancelling lines. When lines are erased, they no longer draw attention (Mark et al., 1988).

Hemispatial neglect may be associated with a directional and hemispatial akinesia of the eyes and the arm. The former together with inattention would prevent patients from fully exploring the left side of space, and the latter would prevent patients with neglect from acting with their arms in the left side of space. As previously discussed, patients with neglect may have a directional akinesia of their eyes that is independent of their inattention (Butter et al., 1988b). In regard to the arm, Coslett et al. (1990) prevented patients from looking directly at their hand when performing a line bisection task; instead, a video camera projected the hand and the line to a video monitor. Using this technique, the hemispace where the action took place could be dissociated from the hemispace where visual feedback took place. Some patients did better when the monitor was in ipsilateral hemispace than in contralateral hemispace. Others were not affected by the position of the monitors but did better when the action took place in ipsilateral hemispace than they did when the action took place in contralateral hemispace. Coslett et al. (1990) suggested that patients with intentional neglect had more involvement of the frontal lobes than those with attentional spatial neglect who had involvement of the parietal lobes.

That spatial neglect can be associated with a motor-intentional bias or a sensory attentional bias is also supported by the work of Bisiach et al. (1990). They used a loop of string stretched around two pulleys. An arrow was attached to the top segment of string. Subjects with neglect and control subjects were asked to place the arrow midway between the two pulleys. In the congruent condition, the subject held the arrow on the upper string and in the non-congruent condition, the subject moved the arrow by lateral displacement of the lower string, which moved the arrow in the opposite direction. If neglect was caused by a directional hypokinesia, the error in the congruent and noncongruent conditions should be in opposite directions but if it was caused by an attentional bias it will remain in the same direction. Six of 13 subjects showed a significant reduction of neglect in the noncongruent condition, suggesting that they had a significant motor-intentional bias and these patients had predominately frontal lesions. The other subject showed an attentional bias. Na and coworkers (1998b) also attempted to dissociate attentional and intentional aspects of neglect by having subjects view their performance of a line bisection task on a video monitor on which the task was displayed either normally (direct condition) or right-left reversed (indirect condition). Subjects could not view the work space directly, but only on the monitor. This technique allows the investigator to investigate the relative contribution of attentional and intentional biases in the same subject. Using this apparatus Na et al. (1998a, b) found that most patients with spatial neglect have both intentional and attentional biases, but in patients with frontal lesions the intentional bias dominated, whereas in patients with temporal–parietal lesions the attentional bias predominated. The finding of mixed attentional and intentional bias is consistent with the idea that the networks subserving attention and intention influence one another. Anatomically, the parietal and frontal lobes are involved in both networks.

Pathophysiology of ipsilateral neglect

Butter et al. (1988a, b), studied the eye movements of a patient with left-sided neglect from a right dorsolateral frontal lesion by asking the patient to move his eyes in the direction opposite a lateralized stimulus. When presented with a left-sided stimulus, instead of looking rightward the patient first looked leftward. This has been termed a visual grasp. The patient with ipsilateral neglect reported by Kwon and Heilman (1991) also had a visual grasp from a frontal lesion. Kim et al. (1999) studied a series of patients with ipsilateral neglect and demonstrated that most had frontal lesions. Patients with frontal lesions have manual grasp, sucking, and rooting reflexes. They also may have mitgehen and facilitory paratonia, all approach behaviours. Denny-Brown and Chambers (1958) proposed that the parietal lobes mediate approach behaviours and the frontal lobes mediate avoidance behaviours. Therefore, injury to the frontal lobes disinhibits the parietal lobes and induces aberrant approach. Kwon and Heilman suggested that the left-sided visual grasp and ipsilateral neglect may both be manifestations of inappropriate approach behaviours. Robertson et al. (1994) replicated Kwon and Heilman's observations, but suggested that ipsilateral neglect was related to a learned compensatory strategy. Some of the patients with ipsilateral neglect, however, reported by Kim et al. (1999), demonstrated this phenomenon almost immediately after their stroke suggesting that ipsilateral neglect could not be attributed entirely to a compensatory strategy. Na et al. (1998a) also demonstrated that ipsilateral neglect, like contralateral neglect, can be induced by both a contralesional attentional bias and a contralesional intentional bias.

Pathophysiology of representational defects

Denny-Brown and Banker (1954) described a patient who could not describe from memory the details of the side of a room opposite her cerebral lesion. Bisiach and Luzzatti (1978) asked two patients with right hemisphere damage to describe from memory a familiar scene in Milan from two different perspectives, one facing the cathedral and the other facing away. In both orientations, left-sided details were omitted. On the basis of these findings, the investigators postulated that the mental representation of the environment is structured topographically and is mapped across the brain so that it is split between the two hemispheres (like the projection of a real scene). With hemispheric damage there is a representational disorder for the contralateral half of this image. Brain (1941) proposed that the parietal lobes contain personal (body) and spatial schemata (representations). The two patients of Bisiach and Luzzatti (1978) and the one described by Meador and colleagues (1987) with hemispatial representational disorder all had right temporo-parietal damage.

There are at least three explanations for the failure of Bisiach and Luzzatti's patients to envision one half of the mental image: (i) the representation may have been destroyed, as suggested by Bisiach and Luzzatti; (ii) the representation may have been intact but could not be activated, so an image could not be formed; and (iii) the image was formed, but it could not be fully explored or attended to (e.g. hemispatial inattention to an internal representation). If a representation is destroyed, attentional manipulation should not affect retrieval, but if patients with neglect have an activational or attentional deficit, attentional manipulation may affect retrieval. Meador et al. (1986) not only replicated Bisiach and Luzzatti's observations but also provided evidence that behavioural manipulations could affect performance. When normal subjects are asked to recall an object in space, they move their eyes to the position the object occupied in space (Kahneman, 1973). Moving one's eyes to a specific spatial location may aid recall. Having patients move their eyes toward neglected hemispace may aid recall because the eye movement induces hemispheric activation or helps direct attention. Meador et al. (1986) asked a patient with left hemispatial neglect and defective left hemispatial recall to move his eyes to either right or left hemispace while recalling a scene. The patient's recall of details on the left side was better when he was looking towards the left than towards the right. This finding provides evidence that hemispatial representational deficit may be induced by an activation or an exploratory-attentional deficit.

Pathophysiology of denial of hemiplegia (anosognosia)

Denial or unawareness of hemiplegia is most often seen with right hemisphere lesions. The lesion usually includes both the frontal and parietal regions. There have been many explanations of this dramatic behavioural aberration. Weinstein and Kahn (1955) studied the premorbid personalities of patients with anosognosia and found that, before their strokes, they used denial mechanisms more frequently than did controls. However, Weinstein and Kahn's study cannot explain why denial of hemiplegia is more frequently associated with right hemisphere dysfunction (Gilmore et al., 1992). Denial of hemiplegia is often associated with neglect, and perhaps patients do not recognize that they are hemiplegic because they have personal neglect. However, Bisiach et al. (1986) demonstrated that personal neglect was not always associated with denial of hemiplegia. The disconnection hypothesis has also been used to explain denial of hemiplegia, postulating that the damaged right hemisphere is disconnected from other areas of the brain, including speech–language areas (Geschwind, 1965). It is well established that the left hemisphere speech areas in the absence of input often confabulate a response (Gazzaniga, 1970). Neither the disconnection hypothesis nor the neglect hypothesis can explain why patients still deny hemiplegia when the paretic hand is brought into right hemispace or into the right visual field, where it gains direct access to the left hemisphere (Adair et al., 1995).

Many theories of anosognosia are related to defective feedback. Even though these feedback theories may help explain failure to recognize a hemianopsia, they cannot explain denial of hemiplegia when the arm is brought into a normal visual field and gains access to the normal hemisphere. We propose a 'feed-forward' or 'intentional' theory of denial of hemiplegia, in which the previously discussed intentional system may be responsible not only for activating the motor systems but also for feeding information about motor expectations to comparator systems. When a patient without anosognosia attempts to move a paretic limb, the comparator notes a mismatch between expectations and performance. However, when the intentional system is impaired (independently or along with the motor systems), not only is there inability to activate the motor neurons but also expectations are not fed to the comparator. When the patient fails to move there is no mismatch and, therefore, no awareness of a deficit. Perhaps this is why patients who have denial of left hemiplegia, when asked why they are not moving their arm, call it 'lazy' (Weinstein & Kahn, 1955). As discussed, intentional defects such as akinesia are more commonly associated with right then left hemisphere lesions. If denial of hemiplegia is related to intentional defects, it is not surprising that denial of hemiplegia is also more common with right hemisphere lesions.

Hemispheric asymmetries and the neglect syndrome

Many early investigators noted that inattention is more often associated with right than with left hemisphere lesions (Brain, 1941; Critchley, 1966; McFie et al., 1950). To account for hemispheric asymmetry of attention in humans, it has been postulated that temporo-parietal regions of the human brain have attentional or comparator neurons, but that the neuronal networks in the right hemisphere are more likely to have bilateral receptive fields than those in the left hemisphere. Thus, the networks in the left hemisphere would be activated predominantly by novel or significant stimuli on the right, but the networks in the right hemisphere would be activated by novel or significant stimuli on either or both sides (Heilman & Van Den Abell, 1980). If this were the case, right hemisphere lesions would cause inattention more often than left hemisphere lesions. When the left hemisphere is damaged, the right can attend to ipsilateral stimuli, but the left hemisphere cannot attend to ipsilateral stimuli after right-sided damage. Support for this hypothesis has been provided by electrophysiologic (Heilman & Van Den Abell, 1980) and imaging (Prohovnik et al., 1981; Rosen et al., 1981) studies. Extinction has also been shown to be more frequent with right than left hemisphere dysfunction (Meador et al., 1988) and may also be related to the hemispheric asymmetries in attentional capacity.

Some patients with right hemisphere lesions are also inattentive to right-sided stimuli (Albert, 1973). Although damage to attentional or comparator networks in the right hemisphere may induce an ipsilateral defect, the cortical lesions may also induce an arousal defect. Using a galvanic skin response and electroencephalographic power spectrum recording, it has been shown that right hemisphere lesions reduce arousal to stimuli presented to the hand ipsilateral to the lesion (Heilman et al., 1978) as well as to the opposite hand.

Patients with right hemisphere lesions also have contralateral limb akinesia more often than do patients with left hemisphere lesions (Coslett & Heilman, 1989). Hypokinesia, however, is not always limited to the contralateral extremities. Howe and Boller (1975) found that patients with right hemisphere lesions had slower reaction times than did patients with left hemisphere lesions. In their patients, the right hemisphere lesions associated with this slowing were not larger than those on the left. Although the right parietal lobe lesions appeared to induce the most profound slowing, these investigators did not mention whether the patients with ipsilateral slowing had unilateral neglect. In monkeys, no hemispheric asymmetries in production of the neglect syndrome have been noted. However, monkeys with lesions inducing neglect had slower ipsilateral reaction times than did monkeys with equal-sized lesions that did not induce neglect (Valenstein et al., 1987).

Lansing and colleagues (1959) have shown that warning stimuli may prepare an organism for action and thereby reduce reaction times. Pribram and McGuinness (1975) used the term activation to define the physiologic readiness to respond to environmental stimuli. Because patients with right hemisphere lesions have reduced behavioural evidence of activation (Howe & Boller, 1975), it has been postulated that in humans the right hemisphere dominates in mediating the activation process (Heilman & Van Den Abell, 1979). That is, the left hemisphere prepares the right extremities for action, and the right prepares both. Therefore, with left-sided lesions, left-sided limb akinesia is minimal, but with right-sided lesions there is severe left limb akinesia. In addition, because the right hemisphere is more involved than the left hemisphere in activating the right extremities, there is more ipsilateral hypokinesia with right hemisphere lesions, than with left hemisphere lesions.

That the right hemisphere dominates mediation of activation or intention (physiologic readiness to respond) has been demonstrated in normal subjects. They show more activation (measured behaviourally by the reaction time) with warning stimuli delivered to the right hemisphere than to the left hemisphere. That is, warning stimuli projected to the right hemisphere reduced reaction times of the right hand more than stimuli projected to the left hemisphere reduced left-hand reaction times; warning stimuli projected to the right hemisphere reduced reaction times of the right hand even more than did warning stimuli projected to the left hemisphere. These results support the hypothesis that the right hemisphere dominates activation or intention (Heilman & Van Den Abell, 1979).

Physical therapists and occupational therapists have noted that it is more difficult to rehabilitate patients with right hemisphere damage than those with left hemisphere damage. Right hemisphere-damaged patients have a greater mortality (related to pulmonary emboli and pneumonia) immediately after stroke. Both the difficulties in rehabilitation and the greater mortality after stroke may be related to the akinesia induced by right hemisphere lesions.

Lesions in the right hemisphere more often induce hemispatial neglect than do those in the left hemisphere. The neglect induced by right hemisphere lesions is also more severe (Albert, 1973; Costa et al., 1969; Gainotti et al., 1972). Verbal stimuli might activate the left hemisphere and thereby further enhance attentional–intentional hemispatial asymmetry (Heilman & Watson, 1978). However, when paradigms that do not use verbal stimuli or verbal instructions are tested, right hemisphere lesions induce more severe hemispatial neglect than do those on the left (Albert, 1973). The mechanism of this asymmetry

may be similar to mechanisms already discussed. The left hemisphere may be able to attend and intend only in and toward the right hemispatial field. Therefore, with left hemisphere lesions the right hemisphere will attend and intend in and toward ipsilateral (right) hemispace. However, with right hemisphere lesions, the left hemisphere attends and intends in and toward the right hemispace and the left hemispace is neglected.

Recovery of function and treatment

Recovery

Hier et al. (1983) demonstrated that neglect spontaneously improves in many patients. The mechanism underlying recovery is not completely understood. One hypothesis is that the undamaged hemisphere is involved in recovery.

Crowne et al. (1981) showed that neglect resulting from frontal ablations was worse when the corpus callosum was simultaneously transected than when the callosum was intact, and Watson et al. (1984) demonstrated that monkeys that had a frontal arcuate gyrus ablation several months after a corpus callosum section had worse neglect than did animals with an intact callosum. Although callosal section worsened the severity of neglect, it did not influence the rate of recovery, suggesting that recovery is an intrahemispheric process.

Hughlings Jackson (Taylor, 1932) postulated that certain functions could be mediated at several levels of the nervous system. Lesions of higher areas (e.g. cortex) would release phylogenetically more primitive areas that might take over the function of the lesioned cortical areas. The superior colliculus receives not only optic but also somatesthetic projections (Sprague & Meikle, 1965). Sprague and Meikle thought that the colliculus is more than a reflex centre controlling eye movements: it is a sensory integrative centre. Tectoreticular fibres project to the mesencephalic reticular formation, and ipsilateral fibres are more abundant than contralateral fibres (Truex & Carpenter, 1964). Stimulation of the colliculus (like stimulation of the arcuate gyrus of the frontal lobe) induces an arousal response (Jefferson, 1958). Unilateral lesions of the superior colliculus induce a multimodal unilateral neglect syndrome, and combined cortical–collicular lesions induce a more profound disturbance, regardless of the order of removal (Sprague & Meikle, 1965). On the basis of these observations, we suspect that much of the recovery seen after cortical lesions may be mediated by the colliculus.

Subcortical lesions of ascending dopamine projections in rats induce permanent neglect (Marshall, 1982). The severity and persistence of neglect induced by 6-hydroxydopamine injections into the ventral tegmental area of rats correlate with the amount of striatal dopamine depletion: those with more than 95% loss of striatal dopamine have a permanent deficit. The extent of recovery of these animals is also directly related to the quantity of neostriatal dopamine present when the animal is killed. Non-recovered rats show pronounced contralateral turning after injections of apomorphine, a dopamine receptor stimulant. Recovered rats given methyl-p-tyrosine, a catecholamine synthesis inhibitor, or spiroperidol, a dopamine receptor blocking agent, had their deficits reappear. These results suggest that restoration of dopaminergic activity in dopamine-depleted rats is sufficient to reinstate orientation (Marshall, 1979). Further investigation of these findings indicates that proliferation of dopamine receptors may contribute to pharmacologic supersensitivity and recovery of function (Neve et al., 1982). Implanting dopaminergic neurons from the ventral tegmental area of fetal rats adjacent to the striatum ipsilateral to the lesion induces recovery in rats with unilateral neglect resulting from a 6-hydroxydopamine lesion in the ascending dopamine tracts (Dunnett et al., 1981). This recovery is related to growth of dopamine-containing neurons into the partially denervated striatum.

Incorporation of ^{14}C-labelled 2-deoxy-D-glucose (2-DG) permits a measure of metabolic activity. In rats with 6-hydroxydopamine lesions of the ventral tegmental area that had shown no recovery from neglect, the uptake of labelled 2-DG into the neostriatum, nucleus accumbens septi, olfactory tubercle, and central amygdaloid nucleus was significantly less on the denervated side than on the normal side. Rats that recovered by 6 weeks showed equivalent 2-DG uptake in the neostriatum and central amygdaloid nucleus on the two sides. Recovery is therefore associated with normalization of neostriatal metabolic activity (Kozlowski & Marshall, 1981).

Similar results have been obtained for monkeys recovering from frontal arcuate gyrus-induced neglect (Deuel et al., 1979). Animals with neglect showed depression of ^{14}C-labelled 2-DG in ipsilateral subcortical structures, including the thalamus and basal ganglia. Recovery from neglect occurred concomitantly with reappearance of symmetric metabolic activity.

Treatment

Since neglect and related disorders are behavioural manifestations of underlying cerebral disease, evaluation and treatment of the underlying disease are of primary importance.

There are several behavioural and pharmacologic interventions that can be done to manage and treat some of the symptoms of the neglect syndrome. After he had a large right hemisphere stroke, President Wilson's wife would place him in a room so his left side was against the wall. This placement insured that he would be able to interact with visiting dignitaries. To optimize interactions, we also suggested that patients be positioned such that their 'good' side faces the area where interpersonal actions are most likely to take place. However, Kunkel et al. (1999) treated patients who had a hemiparesis and did not use their weak arm by binding their non-paretic arm and forcing them to use this hemiparetic arm. They found that this procedure induced recovery. It is possible that some of their patients' motor deficit was related to limb akinesia associated with motor neglect, rather than to weakness associated with corticospinal damage. In the last decade, studies have demonstrated that experience can change neuronal networks. It is possible, therefore, that stimulation of the contralesional side may induce functional reorganization and thereby reduce the severity of neglect. Some evidence for this postulate come from treating patients with hemispatial neglect by making them wear special glasses. Patients with neglect often fail to move their eyes to the contralesional (e.g. left) side and miss stimuli on that side because they fail to explore. Both lenses on these glasses are opaque on one side. The opaque half of the lens is ipsilateral to the hemispheric lesion. Thus for patients to see anything they must learn to move their eyes to contralesional hemispace (Arai et al., 1997). In contrast to these stimulation paradigms, studies of rats suggest that acute sensory depravation, such being kept in absolute darkness, may induce recovery from neglect (Corwin & Vargo, 1993). Unlike people, however, rats are nocturnal, and studies in humans have to be performed to help learn if stimulation is beneficial or harmful in the recovery from neglect.

Although we do not know if patients with neglect should be stimulated or sensorily deprived, we do know that we should not allow them to perform activities that may cause injuries to themselves or others. So long as a patient has the neglect syndrome, s/he should not be allowed to drive, or to work with anything that if neglected could cause injury to her himself or to others.

Many patients with neglect have anosognosia which makes rehabilitation difficult. For example, after a right hemisphere stroke Justice Douglas repeatedly checked himself out of hospitals being unaware that he was terribly disabled. In most patients, however, anosognosia is transient. In addition, because patients with neglect remain inattentive to their left side and in general are poorly motivated, training is laborious and in many cases unrewarding. Diller and Weinberg (1977) were able to train patients with neglect to look to their neglected side before they acted; however, it was not clear that these top-down attentional–exploratory treatments generalized to other situations.

In contrast to this top-down treatment Butter et al. (1990) used a bottom-up attentional treatment. Structures such as the superior colliculus may play an important role in recovery from neglect. Dynamic stimuli readily summon attention in normal subjects and are potent activators of the visual colliculi. Butter et al. used dynamic stimuli and demonstrated that, when these stimuli were presented on the contralesional (left) side, the severity of neglect was reduced. Neglect patients with hemianopsia also improved, providing evidence that these dynamic stimuli influence the colliculi. Robertson and North (1993) demonstrated that having patients move their contralesional hand in contralesional hemispace can reduce the severity of hemispatial neglect and these investigators have used a hand movement strategy to manage neglect.

Asymmetrically activating the vestibular system in normal subjects may induce a spatial bias similar to that observed in neglect (Shuren et al., 1998). Rubens (1985) induced asymmetrical vestibular activation in patients with left-sided neglect by injecting cold water into the left ear and noting that unilateral spatial neglect abated. Valler et al. (1995) reported that vestibular stimulation could help sensory inattention, and Rode et al. (1992) found that vestibular stimulation even helped motor neglect. Inducing optokinetic nystagmus, by having patients look at series of stimuli moving in a contralesional direction (Pizzamigialo et al., 1990), and using vibration to stimulate muscle afferents from the neck (Karnath et al., 1995) also reduce neglect. Unfortunately, all these procedures produce only temporary relief, but it is unknown if repeated trials may confer a lasting benefit.

Coslett et al. (1990) demonstrated that patients with the attentional form of hemispatial neglect improved when visual feedback was presented to the ipsilesional side. Rossi et al. (1990) used 15-diopter Fresnel prisms to shift images from the neglected side toward the normal side. After using the prisms for four weeks, the treated group performed better than the control group in tasks such as line bisection or cancellation. However, activities of daily living did not improve. Rossetti et al. (1998) had subjects with neglect adapt to prisms by having them repeatedly point straight ahead while wearing the prisms. After this treatment, on tests of neglect, these treated patients showed a reduction of their ipsilesional bias. Although the effects of this treatment lasted for two hours after the prisms had been removed, it is uncertain how long this effect lasts. It is also unknown if this treatment generalizes to instrumental activities of daily living.

Neglect associated with cortical lesions may be reduced by destroying the ipsilateral colliculus or the intercollicular commisure (Sprague & Meikle, 1965). These findings suggest that the normal colliculus may inhibit the damaged colliculus. Because each colliculus gets greater input from the retina of the contralateral eye than it does from the ipsilateral eye, Posner and Rafal (1987) suggest that patching the ipsilesional eye may reduce neglect because it would deprive the superior colliculus ipsilateral to the intact hemisphere of retinal input and this reduced input may reduce collicular activation. Although some have found this ipsilesional patching procedure useful in reducing the signs of neglect (Butter & Kirsh, 1992) others have found that ipsilateral patching can make neglect more severe (Barrett et al., 1999). Therefore, when patching to treat neglect each eye should be tested before deciding which eye should be patched.

In regard to pharmacological treatment, we discussed the role of dopamine in neglect and recovery. Neglect in rats with unilateral frontal (Corwin et al., 1986) and parietal lesions (Burcham et al., 1997) were treated with apomorphine, a dopamine agonist. Dopamine agonist therapy significantly reduced neglect in these animals. Spiroperidol, a dopamine receptor blocking agent, blocked the therapeutic effect of apomorphine. Fleet et al. (1987) treated two neglect patients with bromocriptine, a dopamine agonist. Both showed dramatic improvements. Subsequently, other investigators have also shown that dopamine agonist therapy may be helpful in the treatment of neglect (Hurford et al., 1998; Geminiani et al., 1998). In addition Geminiani et al. found that dopaminergic agonist treatment helped both the sensory attentional and motor intentional forms of spatial neglect. In contrast, Barrett et al. (1999) and Grujic et al. (1998) found that in some patients dopamine agonist therapy increased rather than decreased the severity of neglect. Barrett et al.'s patient had striatal injury and it was suggested that the paradoxical effect seen in their patient may be related to involvement of the basal ganglia. In patients with striatal injury, dopamine agonists may be unable to activate the striatum on the injured side but instead activate the striatum on the uninjured side and thereby increase the ipsilesional orientation bias. Thus, if a patient has striatal injury, one should probably not use dopamine agonists. In addition, all patients should be repeatedly tested for neglect while these medications are being given. If there is an improvement over baseline, treatment should probably be periodically withdrawn so that one can be certain that the improvement was induced by treatment rather than spontaneous recovery.

References

Adair, J.C., Na, D.L., Schwartz, R.L., Fennell, E.M., Gilmore, R.L. & Heilman, K.M. (1995). Anosognosia for hemiplegia: Test of the personal neglect hypothesis. *Neurology*, **45**, 2195–9.

Albert, M.L. (1973). A simple test of visual neglect. *Neurology (Minneap.)*, **23**, 658–64.

Anton, G. (1899). Uber die Selbstwahrnehmung der Herderkrankungen des Gehirns durch den Kranken der Rindenblindheit und Rindentaubheit. *Arch. Psychiatr.*, **32**, 86–127.

Arai, T., Ohi, H., Sasaki, H., Nobuto, H. & Tanaka, K. (1997). Hemispatial sunglasses: effect on unilateral spatial neglect. *Arch. Phys. Med. Rehabil.*, **78**, 230–2.

Baleydier, C. & Mauguiere, F. (1980). The duality of the cingulate gyrus in monkey – neuroanatomical study in functional hypothesis. *Brain*, **103**, 525–54.

Barrett, A.M., Crucian, G.P., Schwartz, R.L. & Heilman, K.M. (1999). Adverse effect of dopamine agonist therapy in a patient with motor-intentional neglect. *Arch. Phys. Med. Rehabil.*, **80**(5), 600–3.

Bender, M.B. (1952). *Disorders of Perception*. Springfield, IL: Thomas.

Benton, A.L., & Levin, H.S. (1972). An experimental study of obscuration. *Neurology (Minneap.)*, **22**, 1176–81.

Bianchi, L. (1895). The functions of the frontal lobes. *Brain*, **18**, 497–522.

Bignall, K.E. & Imbert, M. (1969). Polysensory and cortico-cortical projections to frontal lobe of squirrel and rhesus monkey. *Electroencephalogr. Clin. Neurophysiol.*, **26**, 206–15.

Birch, H.G., Belmont, I. & Karp, E. (1967). Delayed information processing and extinction following cerebral damage. *Brain*, **90**, 113–30.

Bisiach, E. & Luzzatti, C. (1978). Unilateral neglect of representational space. *Cortex*, **14**, 29–133.

Bisiach, E., Valler, G., Perani, D. et al. (1986). Unawareness of disease following lesions of the right hemisphere: anosognosia for hemiplegia and anosognosia for hemianopsia. *Neuropsychologia*, **24**, 471–82.

Bisiach, E., Geminiani, G., Berti, A. & Rusconi, M.L. (1990). Perceptual and premotor factors of unilateral neglect. *Neurology*, **40**, 1278–81.

Bowers, D. & Heilman, K.M. (1980). Pseudoneglect: effects of hemispace on tactile line bisection task. *Neuropsychologia*, **18**, 491–8.

Bowers, D., Heilman, K.M. & Van Den Abell, T. (1981). Hemispace-VHF compatibility. *Neuropsychologia*, **19**, 757–65.

Brain, W.R. (1941). Visual disorientation with special reference to lesions of the right cerebral hemisphere. *Brain*, **64**, 224–72.

Burcham, K.J., Corwin, J.V., Stoll, M.L. & Reep, R.L. (1997). Disconnection of medial agranular and posterior parietal cortex produces multimodal neglect in rats. *Behav. Brain Res.*, **86**(1), 41–7.

Butter, C.M. & Kirsch, N. (1992). Combined and separate effects of eye patching and visual stimulation on unilateral neglect following stroke. *Arch. Phys. Med. Rehabil.*, **73**(12), 1133–9.

Butter, C.M., Mark, V.W. & Heilman, K.M. (1988a). As an experimental analysis of factors underlying neglect in line bisection. *J. Neurol. Neurosurg. Psychiatry*, **51**, 1581–3.

Butter, C.M., Rapcsak, S.Z., Watson, R.T. et al. (1988b). Changes in sensory attention, directional hypokinesia and release of the fixation reflex following a unilateral frontal lesion: a case report. *Neuropsychologia*, **26**, 533–45.

Butter, C.M., Kirsch, N.L., and Reeves, G. (1990). The effect of lateralized dynamic stimuli on unilateral spatial neglect following right hemisphere lesions. *Restorative Neurol. Neurosci.*, **2**, 39–46.

Chavis, D.A. & Pandya, D.N. (1976). Further observations on cortico-frontal connections in the rhesus monkey. *Brain Res.*, **117**, 369–86.

Corwin, J.V. & Vargo, J.M. (1993). Light deprivation produces accelerated behavioural recovery of function from neglect produced by unilateral medial agranular prefrontal cortex lesions in rats. *Behav. Brain Res.*, **56**(2), 187–96.

Corwin, J.V., Kanter, S., Watson, R.T. et al. (1986). Apomorphine has a therapeutic effect on neglect produced by unilateral dorsomedial prefrontal cortex lesions in rats. *Exp. Neurol.*, **36**, 683–98.

Coslett, H.B. (1998). Evidence for a disturbance of the body schema in neglect. *Brain-Cogn.*, **37**, 527–44.

Coslett, H.B. & Heilman, K.M. (1989). Hemihypokinesia after right hemisphere strokes. *Brain Cogn.*, **9**, 267–78.

Coslett, H.B., Bowers, D. & Heilman, K.M. (1985). An analysis of the determinants of hemispatial performance. Presented at the Meeting of the International Neuropsychological Society, San Diego, February.

Coslett, H.B., Bowers, D., Fitzpatrick, E. et al. (1990). Hemispatial hypokinesia and hemisensory inattention in neglect. *Brain*, **113**, 475–86.

Costa, L.D., Vaughan, H.G., Horwitz, M. et al. (1969). Patterns of behaviour deficit associated with visual spatial neglect. *Cortex*, **5**, 242–63.

Critchley, M. (1966). *The Parietal Lobes*. New York: Hafner Publishers.

Crowne, D.P., Yeo, C.H. & Russell, I.S. (1981). The effects of unilateral frontal eye field lesions in the monkey: visual–motor guidance and avoidance behaviour. *Behav. Brain Res.*, **2**, 165–85.

Damasio, A.R., Damasio, H. & Chui, H.G. (1980). Neglect following damage to frontal lobe or basal ganglia. *Neuropsychologia*, **18**, 123–31.

Denny-Brown, D. & Banker, B.Q. (1954). Amophosynthesis from left parietal lesions. *Arch. Neurol. Psychiatry*, **71**, 302–13.

Denny-Brown, D. & Chambers, R.A. (1958). The parietal lobes and behaviour. *Research Publications Association for Research in Nervous and Mental Disease*, **36**, 35–113.

Deuel, R.K., Collins, R.C., Dunlop, N. et al. (1979). Recovery from unilateral neglect: behavioural and functional anatomic correlations in monkeys. *Soc. Neurosci. Abstr.*, **5**, 624.

Diller, L. & Weinberg, J. (1977). Hemi-inattention in rehabilitation: the evolution of a rational remediation program. *Adv. Neurol.*, **18**, 63–82.

Dunnett, S.B., Bjorklund, A., Stenevi, U. et al. (1981). Behavioral recovery following transplantation of substantia nigra in rats subjected to 6-OHDA lesions of the nigrostriatal pathway. I. Unilateral lesions. *Brain Res.*, **215**, 147–61.

Fleet, W.S. Valenstein, E., Watson, R.T. et al. (1987). Dopamine agonist therapy for neglect in humans. *Neurology*, **37**, 1765–71.

Gainotti, G., Messerli, P. & Tissot, R. (1972). Qualitative analysis of unilateral spatial neglect in relation to laterality of cerebral lesions. *J. Neurol. Neurosurg. Psychiatry*, **35**, 545–50.

Gazzaniga, M.S. (1970). *The Bisected Brain*. New York: Appleton.

Geminiani, G., Bottini, G. & Sterzi, R. (1998). Dopaminergic stimulation in unilateral neglect. *J. Neurol. Neurosurg. Psychiatry*, **65**(3); 344–7.

Geschwind, N. (1965). Disconnexion syndromes in animals and man. *Brain*, **88**, 237–94, 585–644.

Gilmore, R.L., Heilman, K.M., Schmidt, R.P. & Fennell, E.B. (1992). Anosognosia during WADA testing. *Neurology*, **42**, 925–7.

Goldberg, M.E. & Bushnell, M.C. (1981). Behavioral enhancement of visual responses in monkey cerebral cortex: II. Modulation in frontal eye fields specifically related to saccades. *J. Neurophysiol.*, **46**, 773–87.

Grujic, Z., Mapstone, M., Gitelman, D.R. et al. (1998). Dopamine agonists reorient visual exploration away from the neglected hemispace. *Neurology*, **51**(5), 1395–8.

Halligan, P.W. & Marshall, J.C. (1991). Recovery and regression in visuo-spatial neglect: a case study of learning in line bisection. *Brain-Inj.*, **5**(1), 23–31.

Heilman, K.M. (1979). Neglect and related disorders. In *Clinical Neuropsychology*, ed. K.M. Heilman & E. Valenstein, New York: Oxford University Press.

Heilman, K.M. & Valenstein, E. (1972). Frontal lobe neglect in man. *Neurology (Minneap.)*, **22**, 660–4.

Heilman, K.M. & Valenstein, E. (1979). Mechanisms underlying hemispatial neglect. *Ann. Neurol.*, **5**, 166–70.

Heilman, K.M. & Van Den Abell, T. (1979). Right hemispheric dominance for mediating cerebral activation. *Neuropsychologia*, **17**, 315–21.

Heilman, K.M. & Van Den Abell, T. (1980). Right hemisphere dominance for attention: the mechanisms underlying hemispheric asymmetries of inattention (neglect). *Neurology (NY)*, **30**, 327–30.

Heilman, K.M. & Watson, R.T. (1978). Changes in the symptoms of neglect induced by changing task strategy. *Arch. Neurol.*, **35**, 47–9.

Heilman, K. M., Watson, R.T. & Schulman, H.A. (1974). A unilateral memory defect. *J. Neurol. Neurosurg. Psychiatry*, **37**, 790–3.

Heilman, K.M., Schwartz, H.B. & Watson, R.T. (1978). Hypoarousal in patients with the neglect syndrome and emotional indifference. *Neurology (NY)*, **28**, 229–32.

Heilman, K.M., Watson, R.T. & Valenstein, E. (1980). A unidirectional gaze deficit associated with hemispatial neglect (abstract). *Neurology (NY)*, **30**, 360.

Heilman, K.M., Bowers, D. & Watson, R.T. (1983a). Performance on a hemispatial pointing task by patients with neglect syndrome. *Neurology (NY)*, **33**, 661–4.

Heilman, K.M., Valenstein, E. & Watson, R.T. (1983b). Localization of neglect. In *Localization in Neuropsychology*, ed. A. Kertesz, New York: Academic Press.

Heilman, K.M., Bowers, D. & Watson, R.T. (1984). Pseudoneglect in a patient with partial callosal disconnection. *Brain*, **107**, 519–32.

Heilman, K.M., Bowers, D., Coslett, H.B. et al. (1985). Directional hypokinesia in neglect. *Neurology (Cleve.)*, **35** (Suppl.2) 855–60.

Hier, D.B., Mondock, J. & Caplan, L.R. (1983). Recovery of behavioral abnormalities after right hemisphere stroke. *Neurology (NY)*, **33**, 345–50.

Howe, D. & Boller, F. (1975). Evidence for focal impairment from lesions of the right hemisphere. *Brain*, **98**, 317–32.

Hurford, P., Stringer, A.Y. & Jann, B. (1998). Neuropharmacologic treatment of hemineglect: a case report comparing bromocriptine and methyphenidate. *Arch. Phys. Med. Rehabil.*, **79**, 346–9.

Jefferson, G. (1958). Substrates for integrative patterns in the reticular core. In *Reticular Formation*, ed. M.E. Scheibel & A.B. Scheibel, Boston: Little Brown.

Kahneman, D. (1973). *Eye Movement Attention and Effort*. Englewood Cliffs, NJ: Prentice-Hall.

Karnath, H.O. (1995). Transcutaneous electrical stimulation and vibration of neck muscles in neglect. *Exp. Brain Res.*, **105**(2), 321–4.

Kennard, M.A. & Ectors, L. (1938). Forced circling movements in monkeys following lesions of the frontal lobes. *J. Neurophysiol.*, **1**, 45–54.

Kim, M., Na, D.L., Kim, G.M., Adair, J.C., Lee, K.H. & Heilman, K.M. (1999). Ipsilesional neglect: behavioural and anatomical features. *J. Neurol. Neurosurg. Psychiatry*, **67**(1), 35–8.

Kimura, D. (1967). Function asymmetry of the brain in dichotic listening. *Cortex*, **3**, 163–78.

Kinsbourne, M. (1970). A model for the mechanism of unilateral neglect of space. *Trans. Am. Neurol. Assoc.*, **95**, 143.

Kooistra, C.A. & Heilman, K.M. (1989). Hemispatial visual inattention masquerading as hemianopsia. *Neurology*, **39**, 1125–7.

Kozlowski, M.R. & Marshall, J.F. (1981). Plasticity of neostriatal metabolic activity and behavioral recovery from nigrostriatal injury. *Exp. Neurol.*, **74**, 313–23.

Kunkel, A., Kopp, B., Muller, G. et al. (1999). Constraint-induced movement therapy for motor recovery in chronic stroke patients. *Arch. Phys. Med. Rehabil.*, **80**(6), 624–8.

Kuypers, H.G.J.M. & Lawrence, D.G. (1967). Cortical projections to the red nucleus and the brain stem in the rhesus monkey. *Brain Res.*, **4**, 151–88.

Kwon, S.E. & Heilman, K.M. (1991). Ipsilateral neglect in patient following a unilateral frontal lesion. *Neurology*, **41**(12), 2001–4.

Lansing, R.W., Schwartz, E. & Lindsley, D.B. (1959). Reaction time and EEG activation under alerted and nonalerted conditions. *J. Exp. Psychol.*, **58**, 1 and 7.

Loeb. J. (1885). Die elementaren Storungen einfacher Functionen nach oberflachlicher umschriebener Verletzung des Grosshirns. *Pfluegers Arch.*, **37**, 51–6.

Lynch, J.C. (1980). The functional organization of posterior parietal association cortex. *Behav. Brain Sci.*, **3**, 485–534.

McFie, J., Piercy, M.F. & Zangwill, O.L. (1950). Visual spatial agnosia associated with lesions of the right hemisphere. *Brain*, **73**, 167–90.

Mark, V.W., Kooistra, C.A. & Heilman, K.M. (1988). Hemispatial neglect affected by non-neglected stimuli. *Neurology*, **38**, 1207–11.

Marshall, J.F. (1979). Somatosensory recovery and pharmacological control. *Brain Res.*, **177**, 311–24.

Marshall, J.F. (1982). Neurochemistry of attention and attentional disorders. Annual course 214, Behavioral Neurology. Presented at the American Academy of Neurology, April 27.

Meador, K. J., Watson, R.T., Bowers, D. et al. (1986). Hypometria with hemispatial and limb motor neglect. *Brain*, **109**, 293–305.

Meador, K.J., Loring, D.W., Bowers, D. et al. (1987). Remote memory and neglect syndrome. *Neurology*, **37**, 522–6.

Meador, K.J., Loring, D.W., Lee, G.P. et al. (1988). Right cerebral specialization for tactile attention as evidenced by intracarotid sodium amytal. *Neurology*, **38**, 1763–6.

Milner, B., Taylor, L. & Sperry, R.W. (1968). Lateralized suppression of dichotically presented digits after commissural section in man. *Science*, **161**, 184–6.

Moruzzi, G. & Magoun, H.W. (1949). Brainstem reticular formation and activation of the EEG. *Electroencephalogr. Clin. Neurophysiol.*, **1**, 455–73.

Mountcastle, V.B., Lynch, J.C., Georgopoulos, A. et al. (1975). Posterior parietal association cortex of the monkey: command function from operations within extrapersonal space. *J. Neurophysiol.*, **38**, 871–908.

Na, D.L., Adair, J.C., Kim, G.M., Seo, D.W., Hong, S.B. & Heilman, K.M. (1998a). Ipsilateral neglect during intracarotid amobarbital test. *Neurology*, **51**(1), 276–9.

Na, D.L., Adair, J.C., Williamson, D.J.G., Schwartz, R.L., Haws, B. & Heilman, K.M. (1998b). Dissociation of sensor-attention from motor-intentional neglect. *J. Neurol., Neurosurg., Psychiatry*, **64**, 331–8.

Neve, K.A., Kozlowski, M.R. & Marshall, J.F. (1982). Plasticity of neostriatal dopamine receptors after nigrostriatal injury: relationship to recovery of sensorimotor functions and behavioral supersensitivity. *Brain Res.*, **244**, 33–44.

Pandya, D.M. & Kuypers, H.G.J.M. (1969). Cortico-cortical connections in the rhesus monkey. *Brain Res.*, **13**, 13–36.

Pizzamiglio, L., Frasca, R., Guariglia, C., Incoccia, C. & Antonucci, G. (1990). Effect of optokinetic stimulation in patients with visual neglect. *Cortex*, **26**(4), 535–40.

Poppelreuter, W.L. (1917). Die psychischen Schadigungen durch Kopfshuss in Krieg 1914–1916: die Storungen der neideren und hoheren Leistungen durch Verletzungen des Okzipitalhirns. Vol 1. Leipzig, Leopold Voss (Referred to by Critchley, M. *Brain*, **72**, 540, 1949).

Posner, M.I. & Rafal, R.D. (1987). Cognitive theories of attention and rehabilitation of attentional deficits. In *Neuropsychological Rehabilitation*, ed. M.J. Mier, A.L. Benton & L. Diller. New York: Guilford.

Pribram, K.H. & McGuinness, D. (1975). Arousal, activation and effort in the control of attention. *Psychol. Rev.*, **82**, 116–49.

Prohovnik, I., Risberg, J., Hagstadius, S. et al. (1981). Cortical activity during unilateral tactile stimulation: a regional cerebral blood flow study. Presented at the meeting of the International Neuropsychological Society, Atlanta, February.

Rapcsak, S.Z., Cimino, C.R. & Heilman, K.M. (1988). Altitudinal neglect. *Neurology*, **38**, 277–81.

Rapcsak, S.Z., Fleet, W.S., Verfaellie, M. et al. (1989). Selective attention in hemispatial neglect. *Arch. Neurol.*, **46**, 178–82.

Reeves, A.G. & Hagamen, W.D. (1971). Behavioural and EEG asymmetry following unilateral lesions of the forebrain and midbrain of cats. *Electroencephalogr. Clin. Neurophysiol.*, **30**, 83–6.

Robertson, I.H. & North, N. (1993). Active and passive activation of left limbs: influence on visual and sensory neglect. *Neuropsychologia*, **31**, 293–300.

Robertson, I.H., Halligan, P.W., Bergego, C. et al. (1994). Right neglect following right hemisphere damage? *Cortex*, **30**, 199–213.

Rode, G., Charles, N., Perenin, M.T., Vighetto, A., Trillet, M. & Aimard, G. (1992). Partial remission of hemiplegia and somatoparaphrenia through vestibular stimulation in a case of unilateral neglect. *Cortex*, **28**(2), 203–8.

Rosen, A.D., Gur, R.C., Reivich, M. et al. (1981). Preliminary observation of stimulus-related around and glucose metabolism. Presented at the meeting of the International Neuropsychological Society. Atlanta, February.

Rossetti, Y., Rode, G., Pisella, L. et al. (1998). Prism adaptation to a rightward optical deviation rehabilitates left hemispatial neglect. *Nature*, **395**, 166–9.

Rossi, P.W., Kheyfets, S. & Reding, M.J. (1990). Fresnel prisms improve visual perception in stroke patients with homonymous hemianopia unilateral visual neglect. *Neurology*, **40**, 1597–9.

Rubens, A. (1985). Caloric stimulation and unilateral visual neglect. *Neurology*, **35**, 1019–24.

Schiebel, M.E. & Schiebel, A.G. (1966). The organization of the nucleus reticularis thalami: a golgi study. *Brain Res.*, **1**, 43–62.

Schiebel, M.E. & Schiebel, A.B. (1967). Structural organization of nonspecific thalamic nuclei and their projection toward cortex. *Brain*, **6**, 60–94.

Schwartz, A.S., Marchok, P.L., Kreinich, C.J. et al. (1979). The asymmetric lateralization of tactile extinction in patients with unilateral cerebral dysfunction. *Brain*, **102**, 669–84.

Segarra, J.M. & Angelo, J.N. (1970). Presentation I. In *Behavioral Change in Cerebrovascular Disease*, ed. A. Benton. New York: Harper & Row.

Segundo, J.P., Naguet, R. & Buser, P. (1955). Effects of cortical stimulation on electrocortical activity in monkeys. *J. Neurophysiol.*, **18**, 236–45.

Shelton, P.A., Bowers, D. & Heilman, K.M. (1990). Peripersonal and vertical neglect. *Brain*, **113**, 191–205.

Shuren, J., Hartley, T., Heilman, K.M. (1998). The effects of rotation on spatial attention. *Neuropsychiat. Neuropsychol. Behav. Neurol.*, **11**(2), 72–5.

Singer, W. (1977). Control of thalamic transmission by corticofugal and ascending reticular pathways in the visual system. *Physiol. Rev.*, **57**, 386–420.

Sokolov, Y.N. (1963). *Perception and the Conditioned Reflex*. Oxford: Pergamon Press.

Sparks, R. & Geschwind, N. (1968). Dichotic listening in man after section of the neocortical commissures. *Cortex*, **4**, 3–16.

Sprague, J.M. & Meikle, T.H. (1965). The role of the superior colliculus in visually guided behavior. *Exp. Neurol.*, **11**, 115–46.

Steriade, M. & Glenn, L. (1982). Neocortical and caudate projections of intralaminar thalamic neurons and their synaptic excitation from the midbrain reticular core. *J. Neurophysiol.*, **48**, 352–70.

Taylor, J., ed. (1932). *Selected Writings of John Hughlings Jackson.* London: Hodder and Stoughton.

Valenstein, E., Watson, R.T., Van Den Abell, T. et al. (1987). Response time in monkeys with unilateral neglect. *Arch. Neurol.*, **44**, 517–20.

Vallar, G., Papagno, C., Rusconi, M.L. & Bisiach, E. (1995). Vestibular stimulation, spatial hemineglect and dysphasia, selective effects. *Cortex*, **31**(3), 589–93.

Velasco, F. & Velasco, M. (1979). A reticulothalamic system mediating proprioceptive attention and tremor in man. *Neurosurgery*, **4**, 30–6.

Vogt, B.A., Rosene, D.L. & Pandya, D.N. (1979). Thalamic and cortical afferents differentiate anterior from posterior cingulated cortex in the monkey. *Science*, **204**, 205–7.

Watson, R.T. & Heilman, K.M. (1979). Thalamic neglect. *Neurology (NY)*, **29**, 690–4.

Watson, R.T., Heilman, K.M., Cauten, J.C. et al. (1973). Neglect after cingulectomy. *Neurology (Minneap.)*, **23**, 1003–7.

Watson, R.T., Heilman, K.M., Miller, B.D. et al. (1974). Neglect after mesencephalic reticular formation lesions. *Neurology (Minneap.).*, **24**, 294–8.

Watson, R.T., Andriola, M. & Heilman, K.M. (1977). The EEG in neglect. *J. Neurol. Sci.*, **34**, 343–8.

Watson, R.T., Miller, B.D. & Heilman, K.M. (1978). Nonsensory neglect. *Ann. Neurol.*, **3**, 505–8.

Watson, R.T., Valenstein, E. & Heilman, K.M. (1981). Thalamic neglect; possible role of the medial thalamus and nucleus reticularis thalami in behavior. *Arch. Neurol.*, **38**, 501–6.

Watson, R.T., Valenstein, E., Day, A.L. et al. (1984). The effect of corpus callosum lesions on unilateral neglect in monkeys. *Neurology (NY)*, **34**, 812–15.

Weinstein, E.A. & Kahn, R.L. (1955). *Denial of Illness.* Springfield, IL: Thomas.

Welch, K. & Stuteville, P. (1958). Experimental production of neglect in monkeys. *Brain*, **81**, 341–7.

24

Brain death

James L. Bernat

Dartmouth Medical School, Hanover, NH, USA

'Brain death' is the colloquial term for the determination of human death by showing the irreversible cessation of the clinical functions of the brain. It is an unfortunate term because it erroneously implies that there are two types of death: ordinary death and brain death. It also misleadingly implies that only the brain and not the human being is dead. In fact, the term properly refers to a method by which physicians may determine the unitary phenomenon of human death in the relatively rare situation in which ventilation (and hence circulation) are mechanically supported. Because the term 'brain death' is ingrained in common usage, it is essential that we understand and use it correctly. There is evidence that the term and concept of brain death are widely misunderstood by the public and by physicians (Youngner et al., 1989).

Several other terms have been used synonymously or in related contexts. The term 'cerebral death' should be abandoned because it adds nothing and promotes confusion. Some have used it to refer generally to brain death and others specifically to the higher brain formulation of death (discussed below) in which some scholars advocate the unaccepted idea that loss of functions of the cerebrum alone should be sufficient grounds for death. Translations of the term 'brain death' into other languages add to the confusion because it is *morte cerébrale* in French, *muerte cerebrale* in Spanish, and *morte cerebrale* in Italian.

Within the concept of brain death, scholars have argued about how much and what part of the brain must cease to function for a patient to be dead, and have coined the terms 'whole brain death', 'brainstem death', and 'neocortical death' discussed later (Bernat, 1992). These terms may be useful as theories of brain death but should not be used synonymously with the overall concept. The term 'irreversible coma', cited in the title of the Harvard Ad Hoc Committee Report (Ad Hoc Committee 1968), also adds confusion by suggesting that the brain dead patient is simply in a coma; it should be omitted in this context. The clearest statement a physician can make about a patient declared brain dead is 'the patient was declared dead using brain death tests'. This statement clarifies that death is a unitary phenomenon and brain death tests are merely one way to determine death.

History

The concept that the human being is dead when the brain is destroyed or irreversibly ceases functioning is not new but has become prominent in the past 50 years as the development of the mechanical ventilator has permitted such cases to be commonplace. In the ancient Hebrew tradition, the absence of *ruach* or breath was regarded as the primary sign of death, not the absence of heartbeat. Maimonides, the distinguished twelfth-century physician, philosopher, and rabbi, stated that the decapitated human was immediately dead and that the twitches of the limb muscles often present transiently following decapitation were not signs of life because they lacked central direction (Pernick, 1988). Throughout the eighteenth and nineteenth centuries, much fear was expressed over the incorrect medical diagnosis of death and premature burial. Several of the stories of Edgar Allen Poe are noteworthy in that regard.

In the late 1950s, French neurologists first described patients with what later would be called brain death. Several patients had suffered profound and diffuse brain injuries such that they had lost all clinical brain functions. The newly invented mechanical ventilator permitted their ventilation to be supported (which otherwise would have ceased) and hence their heartbeat and circulation could be maintained, at least temporarily. The neurological examination of these patients revealed a complete absence of all clinical brain functions. Their coma was so profound that the neurologists coined the term *coma dépassé* to emphasize that they were in a state beyond coma (Mollaret & Goulon, 1959).

Throughout the next decade, several case reports of similar patients were published. In 1968, a committee of Harvard Medical School faculty published a seminal report that for the first time asserted that these patients were dead and provided tests to demonstrate it (Ad Hoc Committee 1968). They used the term 'brain death' which greatly influenced its subsequent popularity. They did not offer a rigorous philosophical defense of why such patients were dead but instead offered pragmatic reasons for the change, especially the growing need for organ donors and the futility of continued treatment (Giacomini, 1967).

Since 1980, the concept of brain death has been endorsed by American (President's Commission for the Study of Ethical Problems in Medicine and Biomedical and Behavioural Research, 1981), Canadian (Law Reform Commission of Canada, 1979), and British (Conference of Medical Royal Colleges and their Faculties in the United Kingdom, 1976) commissions charged with studying death, as well as numerous others from around the world. Brain death has become codified into law throughout the western and developed world. Medical societies from around the world have formulated and validated batteries of tests to determine brain death and all are remarkably similar (Quality Standards Subcommittee of the American Academy of Neurology, 1995; Canadian Neurocritical Care Group, 1999; Haupt & Rudolf, 1999). The public has accepted brain death as a standard of human death, and has widely supported the current program of multiorgan procurement for transplantation from brain dead donors.

The relatively little controversy that remains is centreed in universities where some scholars continue to argue that brain death is not truly human death but rather is a misunderstanding of the biology of death (Shewmon, 1998a, b), an inconsistent formulation of death (Halevy & Brody, 1993), a legal fiction to permit organ procurement (Taylor, 1997), or an anachronism to permit unilateral termination of life support (Truog, 1997). There is also opposition from some religious authorities who maintain that brain death is not compatible with their religious teachings (discussed below). However, at a recent meeting convened by the National Academy of Sciences Institute of Medicine to study the philosophical, medical, legal, and public policy issues of brain death, there was no support for changing current public laws permitting brain death determination based on the whole-brain criterion (Burt, 1999).

Biophilosophical basis

The concept of brain death became accepted by physicians and codified into law before it was conceptually grounded in rigorous philosophical analysis. Beginning in 1978 with the writings of Julius Korein (1978) and continuing with the papers of my colleagues, Bernard Gert and Charles Culver, and me (Bernat et al., 1981, 1982), brain death was provided a biophilosophical foundation as the most accurate biological representation of human death in our contemporary technological age. While it is beyond the scope of this chapter to provide the complete biophilosophical discussion, interested readers can consult my recently published comprehensive analysis (Bernat, 1998; Bernat, in press) that I briefly review here.

An analysis of death must begin by accepting certain preconditions and assumptions about death. First, death is primarily a biological concept so any definition of it must be compatible with biological reality. Secondly, a concept of death of the human should be consistent with death of other higher animal species. Thirdly, the concept of death should be applied to organisms and not components of organisms. Fourthly, all organisms must be either alive or dead; none can be in neither or in both states. Fifthly, death is an event, not a process, because the transition from alive to dead is necessarily instantaneous, but the timing of the event may not be able to be measured precisely and then only in retrospect. Finally, death is irreversible so no one can return from the dead.

The analysis of death must proceed in three sequential steps. First, one must conduct the philosophical task of defining death by making explicit our consensual concept of death. Secondly, one must conduct the medical and philosophical task of identifying a criterion of death to provide a general, measurable standard showing that the definition has been satisfied. Finally, physicians should construct and validate a set of tests to show that the criterion has been satisfied.

My colleagues and I believe that death is best defined as the irreversible cessation of the critical functions of the organism as a whole. Thus, death refers to the dissolution of the unity of the organism after which all that remains is a group of individual and independent subsystems that may continue functioning because of physiological support. The best criterion of death is the permanent cessation of the clinical functions of the brain because it is these functions that are responsible for the critical functioning of the organism as a whole. The clinical functions encompass those of the entire brain, thus this position has been dubbed 'whole brain death'. The tests for death are divided into two groups. In the most common situation in which there is no mechanical ventilation provided or planned, the prolonged absence of respiration and circulation serves as a valid test of death because it quickly and inevitably produces destruction of the brain. In the rare situation of mechanically maintained ventilation (and hence preserved circulation) the batteries of brain death tests discussed below must be employed.

Some scholars reject outright the concept of brain death. Using philosophical analysis, Alan Shewmon holds that the brain does not provide sufficient integrating functions of the organism as a whole (Shewmon, 1999). Baruch Brody and Robert Truog believe that there is a mismatch between the definition and the criterion of death (Brody, 1999; Truog, 1997). Robert Taylor (1997) holds that brain death is a legal fiction and that the only true death is circulatory failure. Linda Emanuel (1995) holds that there can be no unitary criterion of death because death is an ineluctable process (Emanuel, 1995). I have addressed these criticisms elsewhere (Bernat, 1998).

Other scholars accept brain death on a conceptual basis but disagree on the criterion of death, that is, on precisely how much brain must be destroyed for death to occur. Robert Veatch (1993) advocates for the 'higher brain formulation' which requires only that the neocortex be destroyed ('neocortical death'), a concept that would declare dead patients in persistent vegetative states or with anencephaly (Veatch, 1993). Christopher Pallis holds the concept of 'brainstem death' in which the capacity for consciousness and respiration in the brain stem are the essentials of life (Pallis, 1997). Interestingly, there are only very minor differences in practice between this concept and the 'whole brain death' concept that prevails throughout the majority of the world outside the United Kingdom. I have analysed and critiqued these positions elsewhere (Bernat, 1992). Suffice it to say that despite over a quarter century of these scholars arguing to abandon or change 'whole brain death', its acceptance remains strong in the developed world and is becoming even more widespread in the developing world.

Pathophysiology

The primary pathologic events producing brain death in adults are traumatic brain injury, intracranial hemorrhage, cerebral infarction, brain tumours, and hypoxic–ischemic encephalopathy suffered during cardiopulmonary arrest. In cardiopulmonary arrest, there is evidence that ischemia is a more important cause of neuronal death than hypoxia (Simon, 1999; Miyamoto & Auer, 2000). In children, the most common primary pathologic events are traumatic

brain injury, bacterial meningitis, asphyxia, and drowning (Staworn et al., 1994).

The widespread neuropathologic consequences of these primary illnesses and injuries are responsible for the global neuronal destruction that ensues. Following the direct cellular injury from the primary event, a series of widespread destructive changes are initiated including hypoxia, cerebral acidosis, endothelial swelling, intracranial hypertension, cessation of intracranial blood flow, and transtentorial herniation (Black, 1978). In most cases, as a result of diffuse cerebral edema, intracranial pressure rises until it exceeds mean arterial blood pressure. Intracranial pressure may transiently exceed even systolic blood pressure. In either event, intracranial hypertension produces a cessation of intracranial blood flow. This intracranial circulatory arrest produces global neuronal necrosis at sites distant to the primary pathology. The well-known syndromes of transtentorial herniation inevitably occur, permitting relatively easy clinical confirmation of the irreversibility of the global neuronal destruction by showing signs confirming the complete loss of brain stem clinical functions (Plum & Posner, 1980). Later, intracranial pressure falls and there is reperfusion of the necrotic tissue (Schroder, 1983).

Neuropathologic examination reveals widespread neuronal necrosis that is proportional to the time of continued perfusion following the event of brain death. It takes at least 12 hours for the first neuropathologic signs to be present (Black, 1978). In the early studies of Earl Walker and colleagues, the pathologic *sine qua non* was the 'respirator brain', a state of global liquifactive necrosis of all intracranial contents (Walker et al., 1975). The 'respirator brain' findings are the result of a completely infarcted brain in which liquefactive necrosis has been permitted to evolve by continued warm perfusion. If systemic circulation ceases earlier, these changes do not occur.

Clinical studies of patients admitted with diffuse brain injury who progressed to brain death have been reported in two series of patients admitted with Glasgow Coma Scale scores of 3. The mean progression to brain death was 18 hours in one study (Matuschak, 1993) and 22 hours in another (Cabrer et al., 1992). Prior to brain death, the patients were markedly unstable with profound hypotension, spontaneous cardiac arrest, hypokalemia, temperature dysregulation, diabetes insipidus and coagulopathy (Matuschak, 1993).

The physiologic changes resulting from brain death in patients undergoing organ procurement have been summarized by Power and Van Heerden (1995). The two principal mechanisms are diffuse vascular regulation injury and diffuse metabolic cellular injury. The first phase of the diffuse vascular regulation injury is a massive sympathetic outflow ('autonomic storm') resulting from the Cushing reflex. Organs can be damaged from direct neural stimulation or by catecholamine effect. In the secondary phase, there is a marked drop in sympathetic outflow producing inotropic and chronotropic cardiac effects leading to cardiac failure. In other organs, the loss of sympathetic tone produces generalized vasodilatation and impaired autoregulation (Power & Van Heerden, 1995). Some investigators believe that the sympathetic withdrawal is more important than the autonomic storm in the production of organ damage (Herijigers & Flaming, 1998).

Hemodynamic changes during incipient brain death include cardiac arrhythmia, hypertension, tachycardia, increased contractility and cardiac output, elevations in pulmonary and systemic vascular pressure, and elevation in pulmonary capillary 'wedge' pressure (Powner & Darby, 1999). After the event of brain death, hemodynamic changes include profound hypotension, vasodilatation and decreased cardiac contractility (Powner & Darby, 1999). Some hemodynamic responses may persist after brain death, including transient elevations in blood pressure and heart rate observed during organ procurement (Wetzel et al., 1985), but cold pressor tests usually detect no changes (Goldstein et al., 1993). In a recent series of brain dead organ donors treated to maintain hemodynamic stability, whereas 78% were hemodynamically stable on admission, only 30% remained stable by the time of procurement (Lagiewska et al., 1996).

Pituitary and hypothalamic function have been studied extensively in brain dead patients. Anterior pituitary releasing tests show severe hypothalamic failure whereas posterior pituitary secretion measurements suggest only partial hypothalamic failure of antidiuretic hormone secretion (Arita et al., 1993). It long has been observed that most brain dead patients develop diabetes insipidus, but some do not (Outwater & Rockoff, 1984; Fiser et al., 1987). These finding suggest that there may be a separate circulation for antidiuretic hormone secretion or that only a tiny residual function is sufficient to prevent diabetes insipidus.

Animal experimental models of brain death have been created to study its pathophysiology and its effects on other organs. Experimental models in the baboon and other species have been devised using an epidural balloon catheter that can be inflated to gradually or suddenly raise intracranial pressure (Novitsky et al., 1989; Shivalkar et al., 1993; Chen et al., 1996). The cardiac, pulmonary, renal and endocrine abnormalities have been summarized and analysed, and used as a basis to plan supportive therapy for brain dead organ donors prior to procurement to max-imize success (Power & Van Heerden, 1995). For example, there is evidence that judicious administration of vasopressin and epinephrine (Yoshioka et al., 1986) and thyroid hormone (Randell & Hockerstedt, 1992) improves brain dead donor prolonged physiologic maintenance.

'Prolonged somatic survival'

In the early writings on brain death, it was asserted that, irrespective of treatment, no patients correctly declared brain dead could maintain heartbeat or circulation longer than two weeks because of refractory hypotension and cardiac failure (President's Commission for the Study of Ethical Problems in Medicine and Biomedical and Behavioural Research, 1981). Beginning in the early 1980s, reports began being published of cases of 'prolonged somatic survival': patients whose heartbeat and circulation were supported for months following a diagnosis of brain death as the result of aggressive medical treatment (Parisi et al., 1982). Many of the cases were reported as technologic *tours de force*, documenting the immense ICU effort made to physiologically maintain the patients using advanced ventilation techniques, vasopressors, hormones, temperature control, antibiotics, anticoagulants, and other advanced-technology intensive care therapies (Catanzarite et al., 1997).

Alan Shewmon recently reported a remarkable series of such cases he has termed 'chronic brain death' (Shewmon, 1998a, b). He described 56 cases of brain dead patients with circulatory persistence for greater than one week that were culled from his experience, that of colleagues, and a review of over 12000 published articles describing cases or series of brain dead patients. Half the group retained circulatory function at 2 months following brain death declaration. He concluded that the medical instability of the brain dead patient is temporary and, if aggressively supported, some patients can enter a period of relative quiescence in which their circulation can be maintained for prolonged periods.

The Shewmon series is a mix of well-documented cases in which the patients clearly were brain dead and less well-documented cases in which the patients were presumed to be brain dead. Although all of them apparently received the clinical diagnosis of brain death, the documentation for many of them remains questionable or absent. Although Shewmon correctly points out that they are no less well documented than many other cases encountered in clinical neurology, there is a well-known but unfortunately great variation in the practice of brain death determination on adults and children (Earnest et al., 1986; Mejia & Pollack, 1995), and as a result, there are undoubtedly false-positive diagnostic errors. The standard for making a serious claim such as Shewmon has made, that the presence of these cases invalidates the concept of brain death, requires documentation that the patients were clearly and convincingly brain dead. This standard is higher than that achieved in the presentation of many of his cases (Wijdicks & Bernat, 1999). In any event, the persistence of circulation in even those unequivocally documented cases remains a relatively rare occurrence.

Epidemiology

There are relatively little data on the incidence and prevalence of brain death. A large study from the United Kingdom found that approximately 10% of all patients dying in hospital ICUs were declared brain dead (Gore et al., 1992). A similar study in Spain found that 14% of patients dying in ICUs were brain dead (Navarro, 1996). In two reported large series of children in the United States, brain death accounted for 0.9% of pediatric ICU admissions (Staworn et al., 1994) and 37% of all pediatric ICU deaths (Mejia & Pollack, 1995).

Diagnosis

The determination of brain death has been a critical question since 1968 when the Harvard committee published the first battery of tests (Ad Hoc Committee, 1968). Throughout the next 15 years, several other medical centres and organizations proposed similar test batteries, which were reviewed in 1984 by Julius Korein (1984). The current definitive tests are those proposed by the President's Commission medical consultants in 1981 (Medical Consultants to the President's Commission, 1981) and by the American Academy of Neurology in 1995 (Quality Standards Subcommittee of the American Academy of Neurology, 1995), generated by the evidence-based review by Eelco Wijdicks (1995).

The diagnosis of brain death should be considered in the ventilated patient with profound, irreversible brain damage, apnea, unresponsiveness, and cranial nerve areflexia. A diagnosis of brain death requires that: (i) a structural lesion is present that can account for the clinical findings; (ii) no evidence of clinical brain functions can be found on repeated neurological examinations, by demonstrating utter unresponsiveness, apnea in the presence of hypercapnia and cranial nerve areflexia; and (iii) all potentially reversible metabolic and toxic factors have been excluded. If these conditions cannot be met, the diagnosis

of brain death should be withheld until a confirmatory laboratory test can prove the irreversible absence of all clinical brain functions by showing an absence of intracranial circulation. The diagnosis should be made by an experienced physician, usually a neurologist, neurosurgeon, or intensivist. A diagnostic algorithm for the less experienced physician has been published (Kaufman & Lynn, 1986).

The first condition requires the presence of a structural lesion sufficient to account for the clinical findings. This condition usually is easy to fulfil in cases of massive head trauma, intracranial hemorrhage, stroke, and meningitis complicated by intracranial hypertension. Diffuse hypoxic–ischemic neuronal injury during cardiopulmonary arrest or asphyxia may be less obvious, and therefore, generally requires a longer period of observation.

Unresponsiveness

The coma of the brain dead patient is the deepest coma possible. Patients lie absolutely motionless when the ventilator is stopped. They make no response to any sensory stimuli including bright lights, loud noises, and noxious stimuli. They do not posture or make any other response to stimulation. Deep tendon reflexes usually are absent but may be retained. Because tendon reflexes are integrated at a spinal level, their presence or absence is not necessarily indicative of brain functioning.

A group of spontaneous movements rarely have been observed in brain dead patients. In the best-described movement, called the 'Lazarus' sign, the patient may slowly elevate both arms and adduct them across the chest (Ropper, 1984). Because this movement has been seen most often during apnea testing in the brain-destroyed patient with an intact spinal cord, it has been hypothesized to result from ischemia to cervical spinal cord motor neurons (Turmel et al., 1991). A series of other odd movements occasionally may be encountered, including automatic stepping (Hanna & Frank, 1995), decerebrate-like posturing (Marti-Fabregas et al., 2000), and finger jerks (Saposnik et al., 2000).

Apnea

Testing for apnea must be done while maximally stimulating the brainstem respiratory centres through hypercapnia while protecting against hypoxia. Although there are accepted standards for conducting apnea tests, they are often not followed in practice (Earnest et al., 1986; Mejia & Pollack, 1995). The impulse to breathe is generated in medullary respiratory centres stimulated by chemoreceptors sensitive to rises in pCO_2 (Bruce & Cherniak, 1987).

Intubated, brain-damaged patients in ICUs often are maintained with low pCO_2, however, so merely disconnecting them from the ventilator for a few minutes to see if they breathe is an inadequate test for apnea. To prove true apnea, the pCO_2 must be permitted to rise to a level high enough to maximally stimulate the medullary breathing centres. The optimal target pCO_2 is unknown, but most authorities state it is 60 torr (Schafer & Caronna, 1978; Ropper et al., 1981; Marks & Zisfein, 1990). In patients with chronic CO_2 retention from chronic obstructive lung disease, the target pCO_2 is higher (Prechter et al., 1990) and such patients often breathe primarily by their hypoxemic drive.

The technique of apneic oxygenation assures the preservation of the O_2 level while allowing the pCO_2 to climb to high levels (Ivanov & Nunn, 1969; Marks & Zisfein, 1990). The pCO_2 is permitted to normalize to the 40 torr range by adjusting the ventilator rate and volume. The inspired air is made 100% O_2 and the pO_2 is permitted to rise. In the absence of pulmonary edema or other pulmonary disorders blocking gas exchange, the PO_2 usually rises to the 350–400 torr range. At this point, the ventilator is stopped and 100% O_2 is permitted to passively exchange by introducing a catheter down the endotracheal tube and infusing the O_2 at 8 l/minute, or using blow-by. Because the pCO_2 climbs at a mean rate of 3–4 torr/minute of apnea, depending on the rate of CO_2 production (Schafer & Caronna, 1978; Ropper et al., 1981), the duration of apnea necessary to permit the pCO_2 to climb to 60 torr may be calculated. For true apnea to be present, there should be no respiratory effort, sighing, or hiccuping. The major complications of the apnea test are hypotension, acidosis, and hypoxemia, but usually it can be conducted safely (Belsh et al., 1986; Ebata et al., 1991; Jeret & Benjamin, 1994). An alternative apnea test shortening the duration of disconnection from the ventilator may be conducted by increasing the pCO_2 in the inspired air (Lang, 1995).

Cranial nerve areflexia

The brain dead patient must have unreactivity of all cranial nerve reflexes including those of the pupil to light, the cornea to touch, the vestibulo-ocular, gag, and cough reflexes. Pupils in brain dead patients usually are mid-position and irregular in shape, reflecting simultaneous denervation of sympathetic and parasympathetic supply. They should be tested with a bright point light source. Pupillary reactivity may be absent from pre-existing disorders such as diabetes. Pupillary reflexes are usually unaffected by atropine given intravenously during resuscitation (Goetting & Conteras, 1991). Pupillary light reflexes similarly are unaffected by neuromuscular blockade in

therapeutic dosages such as that given during general anesthesia (Gray et al., 1997).

The vestibulo-ocular reflex should be tested with the technique of maximal cold caloric stimulation. After inspecting the external auditory canals to exclude canal impaction with wax and punctured tympanic membrane, the canals are irrigated sequentially with 50 ml ice water with the head elevated 30 degrees and an assistant holding the eyelids open (Hicks & Torda, 1979). There should be neither reflex eye movement, grimace, limb movement, nor any response from the patient. Patients who have previously received large doses of vestibulotoxic drugs, such as aminoglycoside antibiotics, may have permanently lost vestibulo-ocular reflexes.

Corneal reflexes should be tested with a cotton-tipped applicator and should be completely absent. The gag and cough reflexes can be tested by observing the nurses cannulating the endotracheal tube with deep tracheal suctioning of the patient. There should be no coughing or 'bucking' movements of the chest.

Death declaration

The presence of unresponsiveness, apnea, and cranial nerve areflexia shows the absence of clinical brain functions. To prove that the absence is irreversible, a structural lesion accounting for the findings should be identifiable by CT scan, and potentially reversible metabolic and toxic factors must be excluded. In the case of asphyxia or hypoxic–ischemic encephalopathy from cardiopulmonary arrest, the test battery should be repeated after an interval of time and show the same results. The interval between tests varies as a function of the age of the patient and whether a laboratory confirmatory test has been done. In the latter circumstance, an interval of 4 hours is sufficient. As noted below, in children it is desirable to wait at least 24 hours between tests.

It is essential to exclude potentially reversible metabolic and toxic factors such as depressant drug toxicity, neurmuscular blockade, and severe hypothermia ($T < 32.2\ °C$). For example, barbiturate intoxication and profound hypothermia can mimic the clinical features of brain death yet be completely reversible. Neuromuscular blockade can produce nearly all the signs, except for the pupillary reflex absence. If there is a question of reversibility, it is best to treat the patient, allow time to elapse, and order toxicologic studies. Confirmatory tests are essential for a diagnosis of brain death in the presence of significant toxic and metabolic effects.

The patient ordinarily is declared dead upon completion of the second set of tests. This practice is consistent with declaring death using cardiopulmonary tests. If the patient is an organ donor, following the second apnea test, the ventilator is reattached and the newly declared dead patient is taken to the organ procurement suite with respiratory support and intact circulation. If the patient is not an organ donor, the patient is not reattached to the ventilator following the second apnea test.

If the above tests are performed and interpreted correctly, there is no differential diagnosis; the patient is dead. Avoidance of the pitfalls noted above is critical to eliminate false-positive determinations (Posner, 1978).

Infants and children

The application of brain death tests to infants and children remains controversial, because of the greater tendency for young people to recover from illnesses and injuries. The Task Force for the determination of Brain Death in Children published guidelines in 1987 that have been generally though not universally accepted (Task Force for the Determination of Brain Death in Children, 1987). The guidelines prohibit brain death determination on premature infants or on infants under the age of one week. Infants between age one week and two months require two examinations separated by a 48-hour interval and a confirmatory test. Infants aged two to 12 months require two examinations separated by a 24-hour interval and a confirmatory test. Children over the age of 12 months are treated as adults. The experience of declaring brain death in children and infants reported from pediatric ICUs is similar to that in adults (Staworn et al., 1994; Parker et al., 1995). The specific considerations of neonatal brain death declaration have been reported (Kohrman, 1993; Ashwal, 1997).

Confirmatory tests

Brain death is a clinical diagnosis but the determination may be validated by several laboratory procedures called confirmatory tests. Confirmatory tests are useful in several situations. First, in some cases the clinical tests cannot be performed. Many patients with massive head trauma also have suffered facial trauma to the extent that it is impossible to assess pupillary reflexes, corneal reflexes and vestibulo-ocular reflexes. In many patients with severe pulmonary disease it is unsafe to perform an apnea test because of simultaneously producing severe hypoxemia. Secondly, the tests may be necessary to conform to regulations for the determination of brain death imposed by some authorities. This situation is true in some hospitals, several countries, and when declaring brain death on infants in the United States. Thirdly, the tests are useful in

expediting organ donation by reducing the mandated interval between examinations. Finally, they may be useful in potentially medicolegal situations in which it may be desirable to have objective test data to supplement the physician's examination.

Laboratory tests to confirm brain death are of two types: those showing an absence of electrical activity from the brain, and those showing a cessation of intracranial blood flow. In general, the blood flow tests are more useful but the decision of which to order should be based upon their availability and on the experience and confidence of the clinician in their interpretation. Wijdicks has provided an evidence-based critique of the available studies as of 1995 (Wijdicks, 1995).

Electrical potentials

If electrical tests are chosen, it is desirable to choose both EEG and evoked potentials. The EEG assesses cerebral electrical activity and the brainstem auditory and somatosensory-evoked potentials assess brainstem electrical activity. While electrical activity also may be suppressed by metabolic and toxic disorders, the evoked potentials are less likely to be affected. Technical standards for the performance and interpretation of the EEG in brain death have been published by the American EEG Society (American Electroencephalographic Society, 1994). The EEG should show 'electrocerebral silence' with no recordable potentials greater than 2 µV at a gain of 2 µV/mm, using appropriate filters, and allowing at least a 30-minute recording. All experienced electroencephalographers are aware of the troublesome artefacts that occur at such a high gain (Hughes, 1978). The sensitivity of this study is limited. Grigg and colleagues found that 20% of brain dead patients continued to have rudimentary but measurable EEG activity for a week (Grigg et al., 1987). The specificity of EEG is also limited because electrocerebral silence has been reported in non-brain-dead patients after a variety of drug intoxications (Powner, 1976) and in the severest forms of persistent vegetative state (Brierley et al., 1971; Boutros & Henry, 1982).

Several studies have shown the absence of brainstem auditory-evoked potentials in brain death (Starr 1976; Goldie et al., 1981; Garcia-Larrea et al., 1987; Firsching, 1989; Machado et al., 1991; Hantson et al., 1997; Ruiz-Lopez et al., 1999). For example, Goldie and colleagues showed that all potentials except the cochlear microphonic potential (a peripheral potential) were absent in brain death. All potentials were easily recordable in patients in a persistent vegetative state (Goldie et al., 1981). The small series of published cases permits no clear estimate of the positive and negative predictive value of these tests. Because they are not susceptible to metabolic and toxic suppression, they are useful in declaring brain death in patients with depressant drug intoxication (Hantson et al., 1997).

Short-latency somatosensory evoked responses in brain dead patients have been found to be absent beyond Erb's point in several studies (Anziska & Cracco, 1980; Goldie et al., 1981; Belsh & Chokroverty, 1987; Stohr et al., 1987; Chancellor et al., 1988; Wagner, 1996; Hantson et al., 1997; Ruiz-Lopez et al., 1999; Sonoo et al., 1999). For example, Wagner found that the median nerve-stimulated P14 evoked potential recorded at Fz-Pgz was absent in 100% of 108 brain dead patients but preserved in 100% of the 108 comatose but living patients. Chiappa has reviewed and critiqued the evoked potential studies up to 1997 (Chiappa, 1997).

Blood flow

The demonstration of cessation of intracranial blood flow is a sufficient confirmatory test for brain death because it proves there can be no surviving clinical functions of the brain. At some point in nearly all brain dead patients, intracranial pressure rises to exceed mean arterial blood pressure, at which time there can be no intracranial blood flow. Historically, contrast angiography was the first test used to demonstrate absent intracranial flow of the contrast medium as the internal carotid and vertebral arteries penetrate the dura (Bradac & Simon, 1974). Contrast angiography to confirm brain death is rarely performed in the United States now because it is cumbersome and other technologies can confirm brain death as accurately and more easily.

Intravenous radionuclide angiography is used widely for this purpose. Several studies have employed serum albumin-tagged technetium 99m injected intravenously with static and dynamic images of the brain recorded by a portable gamma camera. In brain death there is no observable intracranial blood flow, but blood is seen to flow into the face and scalp through the patent external carotid arterial system (Korein et al., 1977; Goodman et al., 1985; Flowers & Patel, 1997). There is an excellent correlation with conventional contrast angiography (Korein et al., 1977). One limitation is that slight flow through the posterior circulation may be difficult to detect.

More recently, single photon emission computed tomography (SPECT) scintigraphy using technetium-99m hexamethylpropyleneamineoxime (HMPAO) has been studied in several reports (Reid et al., 1989; Wilson et al., 1993; Yoshikai et al., 1997). The isotope is injected intravenously and a portable gamma camera records images. The images must be recorded immediately after the isotope is injected. The 'hollow skull' sign is seen in brain death revealing the absence of intracranial blood flow (Yoshikai et al., 1997).

Transcranial Doppler (TCD) ultrasound has been studied widely. Skull insonation and recording of the pulses of the intracranial arteries provides a highly specific recording of arterial blood flow in the brain. Several abnormal patterns have been described in brain death, depending upon the ratio of systemic blood pressure to intracranial pressure (Ropper et al., 1987; Powers et al., 1989; Petty et al., 1990; Ducrocq et al., 1998; Razumovsky et al., 1999). When intracranial pressure exceeds systolic blood pressure, no systolic pulses can be recorded. In the more usual circumstance, in which intracranial pressure exceeds mean arterial blood pressure but is lower than systolic blood pressure, the pattern of 'reverberating flow' is seen. It is called reverberating (or oscillating) because there is a forward progression of blood flow during systole but an equal reversal of blood flow to the original starting point during diastole. Multiple vessel insonations must be recorded to confirm the cessation of intracranial blood flow and the results are operator dependent. The American Academy of Neurology Therapeutics and Technology Assessment Subcommittee has published a statement supporting the use of TCD ultrasound in this circumstance (American Academy of Neurology Therapeutics and Technology Assessment Subcommittee, 1990). The reported sensitivity is 91.3% and the specificity is 100% (Petty et al., 1990).

Other techniques used to assess intracranial blood flow in brain death include xenon-enhanced CT scanning (Darby et al., 1987; Ashwal et al., 1989) and diffusion-weighted magnetic resonance imaging (Lovblad & Bassetti, 2000). The former requires specially equipped CT units not generally available. The latter has been reported in only a single case but is worthy of further study because of the wide availability and ease of this technology.

Ethical issues

The introduction of the concept of brain death has raised a series of challenging ethical issues that result from the unique circumstance of our technologic capacity to physiologically maintain certain bodily systems despite death of the human organism. Like many contemporary ethical issues, the question can be framed 'should we perform an intervention simply because we have the technologic capacity to do it'. I have considered these issues in further depth elsewhere (Bernat, 2002) and briefly review them here.

Brain death during pregnancy

Several reports have been published over the past two decades of pregnant women rendered brain dead by head trauma or intracranial hemorrhage in whom the decision to continue physiologic support was made, permitting the Ceasarian delivery of healthy infants (Dillon et al., 1982; Field et al., 1988; Bernstein et al., 1989; Nuutinen et al., 1989; Antonini et al., 1992; Catanzarite et al., 1997). Success in these cases required heroic efforts in the ICU to treat and compensate for myriad metabolic disturbances including respiratory failure, cardiac failure, hypothermia, diabetes insipidus, disseminated intravascular coagulation, infection, and hypopituitarism, as well as management of the pregnancy and nutritional support. Aside from the technical issues, the essential question is whether the good of salvaging a human life justifies subjecting the dead patient to the indignity of prolonged physiologic support, the family to the enormous emotional distress of suspending closure of a loved one's life, and society to the expense of such treatment (Kantor & Hoskins, 1993).

The first question is who should make such a decision. It is most reasonable that in the setting of a stable conjugal relationship in which the father intends to raise the child, the father should decide. In other situations in which grandparents or other family members may be raising the child, the decision should be made jointly among those with the greatest interest in the welfare of the dead mother and the fetus. Hospital ethics committees can assist families and physicians in the decision making in such difficult cases (Spike, 1999).

The ethical duty to try to rescue the fetus in this circumstance has been the subject of several analyses (Loewy 1987; Field et al., 1988; Kantor & Hoskins, 1993; Spike, 1999). In obstetrical practice, there is an ethical duty to insure the welfare of both the pregnant woman and the fetus (Mattingly, 1992). When the two goals come into conflict, ordinarily the welfare of the fetus is sacrificed for the welfare of the mother. But when there is no hope to save the mother, the primary goal is to rescue the fetus. Loewy has argued that the ethical duty to rescue the fetus in these cases increases with increasing fetal maturity because of the growing probability of therapeutic success and the diminishing harms to the mother resulting from the reduction of time for physiologic maintenance (Loewy, 1987).

Religious acceptance and rejection

Organized religions have not remained silent on the brain death issue. In the early writing on brain death, Frank Veith and colleagues asserted that brain death was consistent with the teachings of Roman Catholicism, Protestantism, and Judaism (Veith et al., 1977). This assertion remains mostly true. For the religious groups comprising Protestantism, including the most fundamentalist sects, this acceptance is universal (Campbell, 1999). For Roman Catholics, the acceptance is also strong. In an August 2000 address, Pope John Paul II asserted that the Roman Catholic Church formally regarded brain death as human death. Further, three Vatican Pontifical Councils and Academies assigned to study this topic over the past two decades have opined that brain death is consistent with Catholic teachings (White et al., 1992; Pontifical Council for Pastoral Assistance, 1994; Pontifical Academy of Life, Vatican City, Msgr. Elio Sgreccia, personal communication). In the United States, the National Catholic Bioethics Center (formerly known as the Pope John Center) has published opinions strongly supportive of the concept of brain death (Furton, 1999). Brain death determination and multiorgan procurement for transplantation are permitted at Roman Catholic hospitals throughout the world.

In Judaism, the acceptance of brain death is less uniform and it remains a point of heated rabbinic debate (Rosner, 1999). In general, Reform Judaism and most of Conservative Judaism accept the concept of brain death. But many Orthodox rabbis reject the concept insisting that ancient Jewish law dictates that the human being is not dead until breathing and circulation stop irreversibly, as required by the Talmud (Bleich, 1979; Soloveichik, 1979). But other Orthodox rabbis hold that brain death is consistent with ancient Jewish law because it is the functional equivalent of decapitation (Tendler, 1978; Rosner & Tendler, 1989). As a practical matter, brain death determination is accepted by a large majority of Jews in the United States and only the strictest Orthodox sects, such as Chasidim, reject it.

Islam has embraced the concept of brain death by a ruling of the Council of Islamic Jurisprudence Academy, and now permits multiorgan procurement for transplantation. In Saudi Arabia, for example, the Ullamah Council has authorized physicians to permit brain death determination (Yaqub & Al-Deeb, 1996). The recommended brain death tests are identical to those used elsewhere in the world (Abomelha & Al Kawi, 1992). The Sixth International Conference of Islamic Jurists addressed the various issues of determining brain death and facilitating organ procurement (Albar, 1991).

The acceptance by other religions in the world is varied. Hinduism, as expressed by the official practice in India, permits brain death (Jain & Maheshawari, 1995). In Japan, a cultural battle has been raging during the last quarter-century over the acceptance of brain death advocated by western influences pitted against traditional Shinto, Confucian, and Buddhist religious and cultural practices (Kimura, 1991; Lock, 1995). The western influences appear to be winning because in 1997, Japanese law for the first time explicitly permitted brain death determination and organ transplantation (Akabayashi, 1997).

Research and teaching on brain-dead subjects

Brain-dead patients have been used as subjects for research and teaching purposes. As research subjects, brain-dead patients are ideal for experiments requiring normal organ system physiology in those organ subsystems remaining intact, particularly for dangerous experiments that could not be performed safely on living subjects. The ethical question is whether it is justified to continue physiologic support of dead subjects, with its attendant harms to the patient and family, solely for the purpose of experimentation (Martyn, 1986). Some have argued that it is acceptable because the dead may not have interests (Nelkin & Andrews, 1998).

Thoughtful investigators have proposed guidelines for using the brain dead as research subjects. Coller and associates stated that the research team should not participate in the brain death determination, the research protocol should be approved by the institutional review board, and the research protocol should not bar the possibility of organ procurement (Coller et al., 1988). La Puma added several conditions. The dignity of the human body should be preserved. The experiment should be brief. The consent of an authorized proxy decision maker should be obtained. The importance of the experiment should be great. And any resultant clinical charges should be borne by the investigators (La Puma, 1988).

Similarly, newly dead patients, including brain dead patients, have been used as subjects on whom physicians in-training may practice endotracheal intubation and other resuscitation techniques (Iserson & Culver, 1986). A few scholars have argued that the benefit to society of training young physicians in lifesaving procedures that cannot be learned effectively by any other means eliminates the duty to obtain consent from the patient's next-of-kin for this activity (Orlowski et al., 1988). Others have insisted that consent is necessary and should be requested, despite the awkwardness of such a request (Burns et al., 1994).

Organ procurement

The principal utility of brain death determination is to permit multiorgan procurement for transplantation. Except for the relatively new and not widespread practice of 'non-heart-beating organ donation' (Youngner & Arnold, 1993), and the evolving practice of 'partial donation' of liver and lungs from living donors (Singer et al., 1989), the brain-dead patient comprises the only acceptable donor for unpaired vital organs. There are ethical duties and legal requirements (in the United States) for physicians to identify potential organ donors from among brain-dead patients, and to ask families if they are willing to consent for their dead loved one to be an organ donor, the so-called 'required request' laws (Tolle et al., 1987; Darby et al., 1989). The ethical duty to encourage organ procurement stems from the lives potentially saved of the organ recipients.

Currently, and for the foreseeable future, the number of dying patients in need of vital organ transplants far outpaces the number of organ donors (Evans et al., 1992). Several strategies have been implemented to increase donation. The required request laws have not had the hoped-for effect of increasing organ donation rates (Caplan & Welvang, 1989). Organ procurement rates have been shown to increase with more expeditious brain death determination using confirmatory tests (Jenkins et al., 1998), and when the request for organ donation is made by trained organ procurement personnel (Gortmaker et al., 1998). Traumatic brain-injured patients deemed unsalvageable in emergency rooms should be admitted and declared brain dead to permit organ procurement, rather than be extubated (Riad & Nicholls, 1995). The criteria for the identification and management of the ideal multiorgan donor have been reviewed (Darby et al., 1989; Soifer & Gelb, 1989).

When brain-dead patients had completed organ donor cards, their families should be strongly encouraged to consent to donation to permit the autonomy of the patient to be respected, even after death. There must be a strict separation of the process of brain death determination and the request for organ donation. No member of the organ donor team should participate in the death determination. There is evidence that 'uncoupling the brain death determination from the organ procurement process in the family's mind improves the donation consent rate' (Hauptman & O'Connor, 1997). Families should understand that the benefit of organ donation is not restricted to the organ recipients. There is evidence that family members granting consent for donation experience transcendent meaning that renders the otherwise meaningless tragedy of illness or injury into a profound personal good (Douglass & Daly, 1995).

Legal issues

Laws in the United States, Canada, Mexico, Australia, and in nearly all European and in many South American, Asian, and African countries permit physicians to declare brain death as a test of death. Nearly all use the 'whole-brain' criterion, except for the United Kingdom that uses a brainstem criterion. As noted previously, the brainstem tests are essentially identical to the whole-brain tests, except the brain stem tests cannot use confirmatory tests showing EEG electrocerebral silence (Pallis, 1983) or intracranial blood flow studies showing an absence of intracranial circulation (Kosteljanetz et al., 1988) because these findings are not necessary for 'brainstem' death declaration.

In the United States, since Kansas enacted the first brain death statute in 1970, all states have enacted similar statutes or have issued administrative regulations permitting brain death declaration (Beresford, 1999). Most states employ the Uniform Determination of Death Act, sponsored in 1981 by the President's Commission, that provides:

An individual who has sustained either (i) irreversible cessation of circulatory and respiratory functions, or (ii) irreversible cessation of all functions of the entire brain, including the brain stem, is dead. A determination of death must be made in accordance with accepted medical standards (President's Commission for the Study of Ethical Problems in Medicine and Biomedical and Behavioural Research, 1981).

There are similar statutes or regulations in other countries permitting brain death declaration.

In the United States, the question of accommodating religious disagreement with brain death has been drafted into law in two states: New Jersey and New York. New Jersey amended its death statute (New Jersey Declaration of Death Act, 1991) whereas New York issued administrative regulations through the State Department of Health (NY Comp Codes, Rules and Regs, 1992). The New Jersey statute prohibits physicians from using brain death tests when they 'violate the personal religious beliefs of the individual' (Olick, 1991) whereas the New York regulations require physicians to 'mandate notification of an individual's next of kin' and allow for a 'reasonable accommodation to an individual's religious or moral objections to the use of neurologic criteria to diagnose death' (Beresford, 1999). An important future public policy question for our society is the amount of latitude our public laws should permit in the determination of death (Veatch, 1999).

A clinical problem, encountered more commonly than a religious objection, is the family that for emotional reasons, cannot bear to see the ventilator discontinued on their loved one, despite the determination of brain death. Although there are legal precedents in the United States authorizing physicians to discontinue ventilators is such cases over the objection of the family (*In re Bowman* 1980; *Matter of Haymer* 1983), compassionate physicians try to help the family accept the inevitable futility of further treatment attempts (Cranford, 1999). Many physicians will continue the ventilator temporarily pending acceptance of the family, but the length and extent of such futile treatment to accommodate family wishes remains debatable (Hardwig, 1991; Miedema, 1991).

References

Abomelha, M.S. & Al Kawi, M.Z. (1992). Brain death. *Saudi Kidney Dis. Transpl. Bull.*, **3**, 177–9.

Ad Hoc Committee. (1968). A definition of irreversible coma. Report of the Ad Hoc Committee of the Harvard Medical School to Examine the Definition of Brain Death. *J. Am. Med. Assoc.*, **205**, 337–40.

Akabayashi, A. (1997). Finally done – Japan's decision on organ transplantation. *Hastings Center Rep.*, **27**(5), 47.

Albar, M.A. (1991). Organ transplantation – an Islamic perspective. *Saudi Med. J.*, **12**, 280–4.

American Academy of Neurology Therapeutics and Technology Assessment Subcommittee. (1990). Assessment: transcranial Doppler. *Neurology*, **40**, 680–1.

American Electroencephalographic Society. (1994). Guideline Three: minimal technical standards for EEG recording in suspected cerebral death. *J. Clin. Neurophysiol.*, **11**, 10–13.

Antonini, C., Campailla, M.T., Pelosi, G. et al. (1992). Morte cerebrale e sopravvivenza fetale prolungata. *Minerva Anesthesiol.*, **58**, 1247–52.

Anziska, B.J. & Cracco, R.Q. (1980). Short latency somatosensory evoked potentials in brain-dead patients. *Arch. Neurol.*, **37**, 222–5.

Arita, K., Uozimi, T., Kurisu, K., Ohtani, M. & Mikami, T. (1993). The function of the hypothalamo-pituitary axis in brain dead patients. *Acta Neurochir. (Wien).*, **123**, 64–75.

Ashwal, S. (1997). Brain death in the newborn. Current perspectives. *Clin. Perinatol.*, **24**, 859–82.

Ashwal, S., Schneider, S. & Thompson, J. (1989). Xenon computed tomography measuring cerebral blood flow in the determination of brain death in children. *Ann. Neurol.*, **25**, 539–46.

Belsh, J.M. & Chokroverty, S. (1987). Short-latency somatosensory evoked potentials in brain-dead patients. *Electroencephalogr. Clin. Neurophysiol.*, **68**, 75–8.

Belsh, J.M., Blatt, R. & Schiffman, P.R. (1986). Apnea testing in brain death. *Arch. Intern. Med.*, **146**, 2385–8.

Beresford HR. (1999). Brain death. *Neurol. Clin.* **17** (1999). 295–306.

Bernat, J.L. (1992). How much of the brain must die in brain death? *J. Clin. Ethics*, **3**, 21–6.

Bernat, J.L. (2002). *Ethical Issues in Neurology*. 2nd. edn. Boston: Butterworth-Heinemann.

Bernat, J.L. (1998). A defense of the whole-brain concept of death. *Hastings Cent. Rep.*, **28**(2), 14–23.

Bernat, J.L. (2002). The biophilosophical basis of whole brain death. *Social Philosophy and Policy*, **??**, ???

Bernat, J.L., Culver, C.M. & Gert, B. (1981). On the definition and criterion of death. *Ann. Intern. Med.*, **94**, 389–94.

Bernat, J.L., Culver, C.M. & Gert, B. (1982). Defining death in theory and practice. *Hastings Cent. Rep.*, **12**(1), 5–9.

Bernstein, I.M., Watson, M., Simmons, G.M., Catalano, P.M., Davis, G. & Collins, R. (1989). Maternal brain death and prolonged fetal survival. *Obstet. Gynecol.*, **74**, 434–7.

Black, P.M. (1978). Brain death. Parts 1 and 2. *N. Engl. J. Med.*, **299**, 338–44, 393–401.

Bleich, J.D. (1979). Establishing criteria of death. In *Jewish Bioethics*, ed. F. Rosner & J.D. Bleich, pp. 277–95. New York: Sanhedrin Press.

Boutros, A.R. & Henry, C.E. (1982). Electrocerebral silence associated with adequate spontaneous ventilation in a case of fat embolism: a clinical and medicolegal dilemma. *Arch. Neurol.*, **39**, 314–16.

Bradac, G.B. & Simon, R.S. (1974). Angiography in brain death. *Neuroradiology*, **7**, 25–8.

Brierley, J.B., Adams, J.H., Graham, D.I. & Simpsom, J.A. (1971). Neocortical death after cardiac arrest: a clinical, neurophysiological, and neuropathological report of two cases. *Lancet*, **ii**, 560–5.

Brody, B. (1999). How much of the brain must be dead?? In *The Definition of Death: Contemporary Controversies*, ed. S.J. Youngner, R.M. Arnold & R. Schapiro, pp. 71–82. Baltimore: Johns Hopkins University Press.

Bruce, E.N. & Cherniak, N.S. (1987). Central chemoreceptors. *J. Appl. Physiol.*, **62**, 389–402.

Burns, J.P., Reardon, F.E. & Truog, R.D. (1994). Using newly deceased patients to teach resuscitation procedures. *N. Engl. J. Med.*, **331**, 1652–5.

Burt, R.A. (1999). Where do we go from here? In *The Definition of Death: Contemporary Controversies*, ed. S.J. Youngner, R.M. Arnold & R. Schapiro, pp. 332–9. Baltimore: Johns Hopkins University Press.

Cabrer, C., Manyalich, M., Valero, R. & Garcia-Fahes, L.C. (1992). Timing used in the different phases of the organ procurement process. *Transpl. Proc.*, **24**, 22–3.

Campbell, C.S. (1999). Fundamentals of life and death: Christian fundamentalism and medical science. In *The Definition of Death: Contemporary Controversies*, ed. S.J. Youngner, R.M. Arnold & R. Schapiro, pp. 194–209. Baltimore: John Hopkins University Press.

Canadian Neurocritical Care Group. (1999). Guidelines for the diagnosis of brain death. *Can. J. Neurol. Sci.*, **26**, 64–6.

Caplan, A.L. & Welvang, P. (1989). Are required request laws working? *Clin. Transpl.*, **3**, 170–6.

Catanzarite, V.A., Willms, D.C., Holdy, K.E., Gardner, S.E., Ludwig, D.M. & Cousins, L.M. (1997). Brain death during pregnancy: toc-olytic therapy and aggressive maternal support on behalf of the fetus. *Am. J. Perinatol.*, **14**, 431–4.

Chancellor, A.M., Frith, R.W. & Shaw, N.A. (1988). Somatosensory evoked potentials following severe head injury: loss of the thalamic potential with brain death. *J. Neurol. Sci.*, **87**, 255–63.

Chen, E.P., Bittner, H.B., Kendall, S.W. & Van Trigt, P. (1996). Hormonal and hemodynamic changes in a validated animal model of brain death. *Crit. Care Med.*, **24**, 1352–9.

Chiappa, K. (1997). *Evoked Potentials in Clinical Practice*, 3rd edn. Philadelphia: Lippincott Williams & Wilkins.

Coller, B.S., Scudder, L.E., Berger, H.J. & Iuliucci, J.D. (1988). Inhibition of human platelet function in vivo with a monoclonal antibody: with observations on the newly dead as experimental subjects. *Ann. Intern. Med.*, **109**, 635–8.

Conference of Medical Royal Colleges and their Faculties in the United Kingdom. (1976). Diagnosis of brain death. *Br. Med. J.*, **2**, 1187–8.

Cranford, R.E. (1999). Discontinuation of ventilation after brain death. Policy should be balanced with concern for the family. *Br. Med. J.*, **318**, 1754–5.

Darby, J.M., Yonas, H., Gur, D. & Latchaw, R.E. (1987). Xenon-enhanced computed tomography in brain death. *Arch. Neurol.*, **44**, 551–4.

Darby, J.M., Stein, K., Grenvik, A. & Stuart, S.A. (1989). Approach to the management of the heartbeating 'brain dead' organ donor. *J. Am. Med. Assoc.*, **261**, 2222–8.

Dillon, W.P., Lee, R.V. & Tronolone, M.J. (1982). Life-support and maternal brain death during pregnancy. *J. Am. Med. Assoc.*, **248**, 1089–91.

Douglass, G.E. & Daly, M. (1995). Donor families' experience of organ donation. *Anaesth. Intens. Care*, **23**, 96–8.

Ducrocq, X., Braun, M., Debouverie, M., Junges, C., Hummer, M. & Vespignani, H. (1998) Brain death and transcranial Doppler: experience in 130 cases of brain dead patients. *J. Neurol. Sci.*, **160**, 41–6.

Earnest, M.P., Beresford, H.R. & McIntyre, H.B. (1986). Testing for apnea in brain death: methods used by 129 clinicians. *Neurology*, **36**, 542–4.

Ebata, T., Watanabe, Y., Amaha, K., Hosaka, Y. & Takagi, S. (1991). Haemodynamic changes during the apnoea test for diagnosis of brain death. *Can. J. Anaesth.*, **38**, 436–40.

Emanuel, L.L. (1995). Reexamining death: the asymptotic model and a bounded zone definition. *Hastings Cent. Rep.*, **25**(3), 27–35.

Evans, R.W., Orians, C.E. & Ascher, N.L. (1992). The potential supply of organ donors: an assessment of the efficiency of organ procurement efforts in the United States. *J. Am. Med. Assoc.*, **267**, 239–46.

Field, D.R., Gates, E.A., Creasey, R.K., Jonsen, A.R. & Laros, R.K. Jr. (1988). Maternal brain death during pregnancy. Medical and ethical issues. *J. Am. Med. Assoc.*, **260**, 816–20.

Firsching, R. (1989). The brain-stem and 40 Hz middle latency auditory evoked potentials in brain death. *Acta Neurochir.* (Wien), **101**, 52–5.

Fiser, D.H., Jimenez, J.F., Wrape, V. & Woody, R. (1987). Diabetes insipidus in children with brain death. *Crit. Care Med.*, **15**, 551–3.

Flowers, W.M., Jr & Patel, B.R. (1997). Radionuclide angiography as a confirmatory test for brain death: a review of 229 studies in 219 patients. *South Med. J.*, **90**, 1091–6.

Furton, E.J. (1999). Reflections on the status of brain death. *Ethics Medics*, **24**(10), 2–4.

Garcia-Larrea, B.O., Artu, F., Pernier, J. & Mauguiere, F. (1987). Brain-stem monitoring. II. Preterminal BAEP changes observed until brain death in deeply comatose patients. *Electroencephalogr. Clin. Neurophysiol.*, **69**, 446–57.

Giacomini, M. (1997). A change of heart and a change of mind? Technology and the redefinition of death in 1968. *Soc. Sci. Med.*, **44**, 1465–82.

Goetting, M.G. & Conteras, E. (1991). Systemic atropine administration during cardiac arrest does not cause fixed and dilated pupils. *Ann. Emerg. Med.*, **20**, 55–7.

Goldie, W.D., Chiappa, K.H., Young, R.R. & Brooks, R.B. (1981). Brainstem auditory and short-latency somatosensory evoked responses in brain death. *Neurology*, **31**, 248–56.

Goldstein, B., DeKing, D., DeLong, D.J. et al. (1993). Autonomic cardiovascular state after severe brain injury and brain death in children. *Crit. Care Med.*, **21**, 228–33.

Goodman, J.M., Heck, L.L. & Moore, B. (1985). Confirmation of brain death with portable isotope angiography: a review of 204 consecutive cases. *Neurosurgery*, **16**, 492–7.

Gore, S.M., Cable, D.J. & Holland, A.J. (1992). Organ donation from intensive care units in England and Wales: two year confidential audit of deaths in intensive care. *Br. Med. J.*, **304**, 349–55.

Gortmaker, S.L., Beasley, C.L., Sheehy, L. et al. (1998). Improving the request process to increase family consent for organ donation. *J. Transpl. Coord.*, **8**, 210–17.

Gray, A.T., Krejci, S.T. & Larson, M.D. (1997). Neuromuscular blocking drugs do not alter the pupillary light reflex of anesthetized humans. *Arch. Neurol.*, **54**, 579–84.

Grigg, M.M., Kelly, M.A., Celesia, G.G., Ghobrial, M.W. & Ross, E.R. (1987). Electroencephalographic activity after brain death. *Arch. Neurol.*, **44**, 948–54.

Halevy, A. & Brody, B. (1993). Brain death: reconciling definitions, criteria, and tests. *Ann. Intern. Med.*, **119**, 519–25.

Hanna, J.P. & Frank, J.I. (1995). Automatic stepping in the pontomedullary stage of central herniation. *Neurology*, **45**, 985–6.

Hantson, P., de Tourtchaninoff, M., Guerit, J.M., Vanormelingen, P. & Mahieu, P. (1997). Multimodality evoked potentials as a valuable technique for brain death diagnosis in poisoned patients. *Transpl. Proc.*, **29**, 3345–6.

Hardwig, J. (1991). Treating the brain dead for the benefit of the family. *J. Clin. Ethics*, **2**, 53–6.

Haupt, W.F. & Rudolf, J. (1999). European brain death codes: a comparison of national guidelines. *J. Neurol.*, **246**, 432–7.

Hauptman, P.J. & O'Connor, K.J. (1997). Procurement and allocation of solid organs for transplantation. *N. Engl. J. Med.*, **336**, 363–72.

Herijigers, P. & Flaming, W. (1998). The effect of brain death on cardiovascular function in rats. Part II: the cause of the in vivo hemodynamic changes. *Circ. Res.*, **38**, 107–15.

Hicks, R.G. & Torda, T.A. (1979). The vestibulo-ocular (caloric) reflex in the diagnosis of cerebral death. *Anaesth. Intens. Care*, **7**, 169–73.

Hughes, J.R. (1978). Limitations of the EEG in coma and brain death. *Ann. NY Acad. Sci.*, **315**, 121–36.

In re Bowman, 617, P2d 731 (WN Sup Ct 1980).

Iserson, K.V. & Culver, C.M. (1986). Using a cadaver to practice and teach. *Hastings Cent. Rep.*, **16** (3), 28–9.

Ivanov, S.D. & Nunn, J.F. (1969). Methods of elevation of pCO_2 for restoration of spontaneous breathing after artificial ventilation of anaesthetized patients. *Br. J. Anaesth.*, **41**, 28–37.

Jain, S. & Maheshawari, M.C. (1995). Brain death – the Indian perspective. In *Brain Death*, ed. C. Machado, pp. 261–3. Amsterdam: Elsevier.

Jenkins, D.H., Reilly, P.M., Shapiro, M.B. et al. (1998). Effect of rapid brain death determination on organ donation rates: a preliminary report. *Crit. Care Med.*, **26**, Suppl., A31.

Jeret, J.S. & Benjamin, J.L. (1994). Risk of hypotension during apnea testing. *Arch. Neurol.*, **51**, 595–9.

Kantor, J.E. & Hoskins, I.A. (1993). Brain death in pregnant women. *J. Clin. Ethics*, **4**, 308–14.

Kaufman, H.H. & Lynn, J. (1986). Brain death. *Neurosurgery*, **19**, 850–6.

Kimura, R. (1991). Japan's dilemma with the definition of death. *Kennedy Inst. Ethics J.*, **1**, 123–31.

Kohrman, M.H. (1993). Brain death in neonates. *Semin. Neurol.*, **13**, 116–22.

Korein, J. (1978). The problem of brain death: development and history. *Ann. NY Acad. Sci.*, **315**, 19–38.

Korein, J. (1984). The diagnosis of brain death. *Semin. Neurol.*, **4**, 52–72.

Korein, J., Braunstein, P., George, A. et al. (1977). Brain death I. Angiographic correlation with a radioisotopic bolus technique for evaluation of critical defect of cerebral blood flow. *Ann. Neurol.*, **2**, 195–205.

Kosteljanetz, M., Ohrstrom, J.K., Skjodt, S. & Teglbjaerg, P.S. (1988). Clinical brain death with preserved cerebral arterial circulation. *Acta Neurol. Scand.*, **78**, 418–21.

La Puma, J. (1988). Discovery and disquiet: research on the brain dead. *Ann. Intern. Med.*, **109**, 606–8.

Lagiewska, B., Pacholczyk, M., Szostek, M. et al. (1996). Hemodynamic and metabolic disturbances observed in brain dead organ donors. *Transpl. Proc.*, **28**, 165–6.

Lang, C.J.G. (1995). Apnea testing by artificial CO_2 augmentation. *Neurology*, **45**, 966–9.

Law Reform Commission of Canada. (1979). *Criteria for the Determination of Death*. Ottawa: Law Reform Commission of Canada.

Lock, M. (1995). Contesting the natural in Japan: moral dilemmas and technologies of dying. *Culture, Med. Psychiatry*, **19**, 1–38.

Loewy, E.H. (1987). The pregnant brain dead and the fetus: must we always try to wrest life from death? *Am. J. Obstet. Gynecol.*, **157**, 1097–101.

Lovblad, K-O. & Bassetti, C. (2000). Diffusion-weighted magnetic resonance imaging in brain death. *Stroke*, **31**, 539–42.

Machado, C., Valdes, P., Garcia-Tigera, J. et al. (1991). Brain stem auditory evoked potentials and brain death. *Electroencephalogr. Clin. Neurphysiol.*, **80**, 392–8.

Marks, S.J. & Zisfein, J. (1990). Apneic oxygenation in apnea tests for brain death: a controlled trial. *Arch. Neurol.*, **47**, 1066–8.

Marti-Fabregas, J., Lopez-Navidad, A., Caballero, F. & Otermin, P. (2000). Decerebrate-like posturing with mechanical ventilation in brain death. *Neurology*, **54**, 224–7.

Martyn, R.M. (1986). Using the brain dead for medical research. *Utah Law Rev.*, **1**, 1–28.

Matter of Haymer, 450 NE2d 940 (Ill App Ct 1983).

Mattingly, S.S. (1992). The maternal-fetal dyad: exploring the two-patient obstetrical model. *Hastings Cent. Rep.*, **22**(1), 13–18.

Matuschak, G.M. (1995). Presented at the 13th International Symposium on Intensive Care and Emergency Medicine, Brussels, March, 1993, as quoted in Power and Van Heerde.

Medical Consultants to the President's Commission. (1981). Report of the Medical Consultants on the Diagnosis of Death to the President's Commission for the Study of Ethical Problems in Medicine and Biomedical and Behavioral Research. Guidelines for the determination of death. *J. Am. Med. Assoc.*, **246**, 2184–6.

Mejia, R.E. & Pollack, M.M. (1995). Variability in brain death determination practices in children. *J. Am. Med. Assoc.*, **274**, 550–3.

Miedema, F. (1991). Medical treatment after brain death: a case report and ethical analysis. *J. Clin. Ethics*, **2**, 50–2.

Miyamoto, O. & Auer, R.N. (2000). Hypoxia, hyperoxia, ischemia, and brain necrosis. *Neurology*, **54**, 362–71.

Mollaret, P. & Goulon, M. (1959). Le coma dépassé (mémoire préliminaire). *Rev. Neurol.*, **101**, 3–15.

Navarro, A. (1996). Brain death epidemiology: the Madrid Study. *Transpl. Proc.*, **28**, 102–4.

Nelkin, D. & Andrews, L. (1998). Do the dead have interests? Policy issues for research after life. *Am. J. Law Med.*, **24**, 261–91.

New Jersey Declaration of Death Act. (1991). *NJ Stat Ann* 26, Ch 6, A1–8.

Novitsky, D., Horak, A., Cooper, D.K. & Rose, A.G. (1989). Electro-cardiographic and histologic changes developing during experimental brain death in the baboon. *Transpl. Proc.*, **21**, 2567–9.

Nuutinen, L.S., Alahuta, S.M. & Heikkinen, J.E. (1989). Nutrition during ten-week life support with successful fetal outcome in a case with fatal maternal brain damage. *J. Parent. Ent. Nutrit.*, **13**, 432–5.

NY Comp Codes, Rules & Regs. (1992). Title 10, section 400.16(d), (e)(3).

Olick, R.S. (1991). Brain death, religious freedom, and public policy: New Jersey's landmark legislative initiative. *Kennedy Inst. Ethics J.*, **4**, 275–88.

Orlowski, J.P., Kanoti, G.A. & Mehlman, M.J. (1988). The ethics of using newly dead patients for teaching and practicing intubation techniques. *N. Engl. J. Med.*, **319**, 439–41.

Outwater, K.M. & Rockoff, M.A. (1984). Diabetes insipidus accompanying brain death in children. *Neurology*, **34**, 1243–6.

Pallis, C. (1983). ABC of brain stem death: the arguments about the EEG. *Br. Med. J.*, **286**, 284–7.

Pallis, C. (1997). *ABC of Brainstem Death*, 2nd edn. London: British Medical Journal Publishers.

Parisi, J.E., Kim, R.C., Collins, G.H. & Hilfinger, M.F. (1982). Brain death with prolonged somatic survival. *N. Engl. J. Med.*, **306**, 14–16.

Parker, B.L., Frewen, T.C., Levin, S.D. et al. (1995). Declaring brain death: current practice in a Canadian pediatric critical care unit. *Can. Med. Assoc. J.*, **153**, 909–16.

Pernick, M.S. (1988). Back from the grave: recurring controversies over defining and diagnosing death in history. In *Death: Beyond Whole-Brain Criteria*, ed. R.M. Zaner, pp. 17–74. Dordrecht: Kluwer Academic Publishers.

Petty, G.W., Mohr, J.P., Pedley, T.A. et al. (1990). The role of transcranial Doppler in confirming brain death: sensitivity, specificity, and suggestions for performance and interpretation. *Neurology*, **40**, 300–3.

Plum, F. & Posner, J.B. (1980). *The Diagnosis of Stupor and Coma*, 3rd edn, pp. 87–151. Philadelphia: F A Davis Co.

Pontifical Council for Pastoral Assistance. (1994). *Charter for Health Care Workers*. Boston: St. Paul Books and Media.

Posner, J.B. (1978). Coma and other states of consciousness: the differential diagnosis of brain death. *Ann. NY Acad. Sci.*, **315**, 215–27.

Power, B.M. & Van Heerden, P.V. (1995). The physiological changes associated with brain death – current concepts and implications for treatment of the brain dead organ donor. *Anaesth. Intens. Care*, **23**, 26–36.

Powers, A.D., Graeber, M.C. & Smith, R.R. (1989). Transcranial Doppler ultrasonography in the determination of brain death. *Neurosurgery*, **24**, 884–9.

Powner, D.J. (1976). Drug-associated isoelectric EEGs: a hazard in brain-death certification. *J. Am. Med. Assoc.*, **236**, 1123.

Powner, D.J. & Darby, J.M. (1999). Current considerations in the issue of brain death. *Neurosurgery*, **45**, 1222–7.

Prechter, G.C., Nelson, C.B. & Hubmayr, R.D. (1990). The ventilatory recruitment threshold for carbon dioxide. *Am. Rev. Respir. Dis.*, **141**, 758–64.

President's Commission for the Study of Ethical Problems in Medicine and Biomedical and Behavioral Research. (1981). *Defining Death. Medical, Ethical, and Legal Issues in the Determination of Death*. Washington, DC: US Government Printing Office.

Quality Standards Subcommittee of the American Academy of Neurology. (1995). Practice parameters for determining brain death in adults [summary statement]. *Neurology*, **45**, 1012–14.

Randell, T.T. & Hockerstedt, K.A.V. (1992). Triiodothyronine treatment in brain dead multi-organ donors – a controlled study. *Transplantation*, **54**, 736–8.

Razumovsky, A.Y., Czosnyka, M., Williams, M.A. & Hanley, D.F. (1999). Intensive care unit monitoring. In *Transcranial Doppler Ultrasonography*, ed. V.L. Babikian & L.R. Wechsler, 2nd edn, pp. 191–6. Boston: Butterworth-Heinemann.

Reid, R.H., Gulenchyn, K.Y. & Ballinger, J.R. (1989). Clinical use of technetium-99m HM-PAO for determination of brain death. *J. Nucl. Med.*, **30**, 1621–6.

Riad, H. & Nicholls, A. (1995). Elective ventilation of potential organ donors. *Br. Med. J.*, **310**, 714–15.

Ropper, A. (1984). Unusual spontaneous movements in brain-dead patients. *Neurology*, **34**, 1089–92.

Ropper, A.H., Kennedy, S.K. & Russell, L. (1981). Apnea testing in the diagnosis of brain death: clinical and physiological observations. *J. Neurosurg.*, **55**, 942–6.

Ropper, A.H., Kehne, S.M. & Wechsler, L. (1987). Transcranial Doppler in brain death. *Neurology*, **37**, 1733–5.

Rosner, F. (1999). The definition of death in Jewish law. In *The Definition of Death: Contemporary Controversies*. ed. S.J. Youngner, R.M. Arnold & R. Schapiro, pp. 210–21. Baltimore: John Hopkins University Press.

Rosner, F. & Tendler, M.D. (1989). Definition of death in Judaism. *J. Halacha Contemp. Soc.*, **17**, 14–31.

Ruiz-Lopez, M.J., Martinez de Azagra, A., Serrano, A. & Casado-Flores, J. (1999). Brain death and evoked potentials in pediatric patients. *Crit. Care Med.*, **27**, 412–16.

Saposnik, G., Bueri, J.A., Maurino, J., Saizar, R. & Garetto, N.S. (2000). Spontaneous and reflex movements in brain death. *Neurology*, **54**, 221–3.

Schafer, J.A. & Caronna, J.J. (1978). Duration of apnea needed to confirm brain death. *Neurology*, **28**, 661–6.

Schroder, R. (1983). Later changes in brain death: signs of partial recirculation. *Acta Neuropathol. (Berl.)*, **62**, 15–23.

Shewmon, D.A. (1998a). 'Brainstem death, ' 'brain death' and death: a critical re-evaluation of the purported equivalence. *Issues Law Med.*, **14**, 125–45.

Shewmon, D.A. (1998b). Chronic 'brain death': meta-analysis and conceptual consequences. *Neurology*, **51**, 1538–45.

Shewmon, D.A. (1999). Spinal shock and 'brain death': somatic pathophysiological equivalence and implications for the integrative-unity rationale. *Spinal Cord*, **37**, 313–24.

Shivalkar, B., Van Loon, J., Wieland, W. et al. (1993). Variable effects of explosive or gradual increase of intracranial pressure on myocardial structure and function. *Circulation*, **87**, 230–9.

Simon, R.P. (1999). Hypoxia versus ischemia. *Neurology*, **52**, 7–8.

Singer, P.A., Siegler, M., Wittington, P.F. et al. (1989). Ethics of liver transplantation with living donors. *N. Engl. J. Med.*, **321**, 620–2.

Soifer, B. & Gelb, A. (1989). The multiple organ donor: identification and management. *Ann. Intern. Med.*, **110**, 814–23.

Soloveichik, A. (1979). The Halakhic definition of death. In *Jewish Bioethics*, ed. F. Rosner & J.D. Bleich, pp. 296–302. New York: Sanhedrin Press.

Sonoo, M., Tsai-Shozawa, Y., Aoki, M. et al. (1999). N18 in median somatosensory evoked potentials: a new indicator of medullary function useful for the diagnosis of brain death. *J. Neurol. Neurosurg. Psychiatry*, **67**, 374–8.

Spike, J. (1999). Brain death, pregnancy, and posthumous motherhood. *J. Clin. Ethics*, **10**, 57–65.

Starr, A. (1976). Auditory brain stem responses in brain death. *Brain*, **99**, 543–54.

Staworn, D., Lewison, L., Marks, J., Turner, G. & Levin, D. (1994). Brain death in pediatric intensive care unit patients: incidence, primary diagnosis, and the clinical occurrence of Turner's triad. *Crit. Care Med.*, **22**, 1301–5.

Stohr, M., Riffel, B., Trost, E. & Ulrich, A. (1987). Short-latency somatosensory evoked potentials in brain death. *J. Neurol.*, **234**, 211–14.

Task Force for the Determination of Brain Death in Children. (1987). Guidelines for the determination of brain death in children. *Arch. Neurol.*, **44**, 587–8.

Taylor, R.M. (1997). Reexamining the definition and criterion of death. *Semin. Neurol.*, **17**, 265–70.

Tendler, M.D. (1978). Cessation of brain function: ethical implications in terminal care and organ transplants. *Ann. NY Acad. Sci.*, **315**, 394–407.

Tolle, S.W., Bennett, W.M., Hickham, D.H. et al. (1987). Responsibilities of primary physicians in organ donation. *Ann. Intern. Med.*, **106**, 740–5.

Truog, R.D. (1997). Is it time to abandon brain death? *Hastings Cent. Rep.*, **27**(1), 29–37.

Turmel, A., Roux, A. & Bojanowski, M.W. (1991). Spinal man after declaration of brain death. *Neurosurgery*, **28**, 298–301.

Veatch, R.M. (1993). The impending collapse of the whole-brain definition of death. *Hastings Cent. Rep.*, **23** (4), 18–24.

Veatch, R.M. (1999). The conscience clause: how much individual choice in defining death can our society tolerate? In *The Definition of Death: Contemporary Controversies*, ed. S.J. Youngner, R.M. Arnold & R. Schapiro, pp. 137–60. Baltimore: John Hopkins University Press.

Veith, F.J., Fein, J.M., Tendler, M.D. et al. (1977). Brain death: a status report of medical and ethical considerations. *J. Am. Med. Assoc.*, **238**, 1651–5.

Wagner, W. (1996). Scalp, earlobe, and nasopharyngeal recordings of the median nerve somatosensory evoked P14 potential in coma and brain death. Detailed latency and amplitude analysis in 181 patients. *Brain*, **119**, 1507–21.

Walker, A.E., Diamond, E.L. & Moseley, J. (1975). The neuropathological findings in irreversible coma: a critique of the 'respirator brain.' *J. Neuropathol. Exp. Neurol.*, **34**, 295–323.

Wetzel, R.C., Setzer, N., Stiff, J.L. & Rogers, M.C. (1985). Hemodynamic responses in brain dead organ donor patients. *Anesth. Analg.*, **64**, 125–8.

White, R.J., Angstwurm, H. & Carrasco de Paula, I. (eds). (1992). Working Group on the Determination of Brain Death and its Relationship to Human Death. *Scripta Varia* 83. Vatican City: Pontifical Academy of Sciences.

Wijdicks, E.F. (1995). Determining brain death in adults. *Neurology*, **45**, 1003–11.

Wijdicks, E.F.M. & Bernat, J.L. (1999). Chronic 'brain death': meta-analysis and conceptual consequences (letter). *Neurology*, **53**, 1369–70.

Wilson, K., Gordon, L. & Selby, J.B., Jr. (1993). The diagnosis of brain death with Tc-99m HMPAO. *Clin. Nucl. Med.*, **18**, 428–34.

Yaqub, B.A. & Al-Deeb, S.M. (1996). Brain death: current status in Saudi Arabia. *Saudi Med. J.*, **17**, 5–10.

Yoshikai, T., Tahara, T., Kuroiwa, T. et al. (1997). Plain CT findings of brain death confirmed by hollow skull sign in brain perfusion SPECT. *Radiat. Med.*, **15**, 419–24.

Yoshioka, T., Sugimoto, H., Uenishi, M. et al. (1986). Prolonged hemodynamic maintenance by the combined administration of vasopressin and epinephrine in brain death: a clinical study. *Neurosurgery*, **18**, 565–7.

Youngner, S.J. & Arnold, R.M. (1993). Ethical, psychosocial, and public policy implications of procuring organs from non-heartbeating cadaver donors. *J. Am. Med. Assoc.*, **269**, 2769–74.

Youngner, S.J., Landefeld, C.S., Coulton, C.J., Juknialis, B.W. & Leary, M. (1989). 'Brain death' and organ retrieval. A cross-sectional survey of knowledge and concepts among health professionals. *J. Am. Med. Assoc.*, **261**, 2205–10.

25

Disorders of mood

Dean F. MacKinnon and J. Raymond DePaulo

Department of Psychiatry, Johns Hopkins University School of Medicine, Baltimore, MD, USA

Depression refers in the medical setting to clinically significant but transient emotional states which are called adjustment disorders and also to a clinical syndrome called major depression which occurs in unipolar depressive disorder and bipolar disorders. Confusion of adjustment disorders with depressive syndromes plagues both medical care and reasoning about mechanisms. Once identified, mood disorders (unipolar and bipolar disorders) are treated quite successfully with any of several medications and/or psychotherapy. The pathophysiology of mood disorders remains obscure, but clues are emerging as to the neuroanatomic components, molecular systems and genes involved in the vulnerability to mood disorder. The cumulative effect of these developments on a number of scientific fronts will be to unravel the complex knot of etiologic factors, leading to the refinement of current empirical treatment and the development of rational treatment. When we can identify the mechanisms of mood disorder, we will also gain an improved perspective from which to understand the role of environmental factors in the development of depressive and manic disorders.

In the official diagnostic nomenclature of American psychiatry a transition from the term 'affective disorders' to 'mood disorders' was made in 1987, though the diagnostic criteria for major depression and mania did not change appreciably. We use the term mood to denote a persistent emotional state, and affect or affective to refer to a constellation of phenomena generally associated with and including mood. We will use the term depression, hereafter, only to denote the syndrome of depressive illness.

Epidemiology

Mood disorders are among the most common illnesses in the community and in the medical clinic. Depression, in a variety of community samples worldwide, affects as many as one in six individuals in the course of a lifetime (Doris et al., 1999). Mania occurs in 1–2% of the population. Ten to twenty per cent of patients screened in a primary care clinic have a major depressive disorder (Zung et al., 1993); depression was found in over one-quarter of patients in a neurology practice (Carson et al., 2000). Mania is less often a presenting problem for non-psychiatric physicians, but can occur as an iatrogenic complication from the use of antidepressants (Benazzi, 1997), corticosteroids (Sharfstein et al., 1982), or psychostimulants (Masand et al., 1995). Moreover, a number of medical conditions are associated with the syndromes of mania and depression, as will be described below.

Mood disorders are extremely painful for families as well as patients, and are costly to society. Suicide is the cause of death in at least 5% of individuals with a mood disorder, as found in community samples (Inskip et al., 1998), and the rate of suicide among patients requiring hospitalization is three- to fourfold greater than that. Psychological autopsy studies reveal consistently that at least two-thirds of completed suicides had strong evidence for a mood disorder prior to death, even though many were never diagnosed or treated for it (Barraclough et al., 1974). Depression carries high direct costs from absenteeism and occupational disability (Druss et al., 2000; Greenberg et al., 1993) and medical expenditure (Simon et al., 1995), as well as high indirect costs via other highly destructive behaviours like those related to substance abuse.

Clinical facts

Central features

The depressive syndrome consists of a persistent and pervasive disturbance of affective state. The mood itself, however, is described as sad or depressed in only 50% of patients with major depression. The mood may be constantly dysphoric, or cycling through different dysphoric states, ranging from despair to apathy, anxiety, numbness, or irritability. The mood in the manic syndrome may be pleasantly euphoric, though often the accompanying excitement gives way to anxiety or irritability. A depressive or manic syndrome, as opposed to a normal lowering or elevation of mood, is concomitant with changes in self-attitude, vitality and neurovegetative functioning. The change in self-attitude manifests itself in depression with pathological guilt, self-loathing, feelings of worthlessness and failure. In mania, patients express expansive confidence and grandiosity, and with mixed or irritable manic states, there is often a combative self-righteousness. Vitality, or the physical sense of energy, capability, and stamina tend to be diminished in the depressed patient and elevated in the manic. Neurovegetative appetites for sex, sleep, food and stimulation are almost universally disturbed in some way in patients with mood disorder.

Mood disorder generally causes functional impairment, but impairment is neither necessary nor sufficient to differentiate mood disorder from normal emotional variation. Perturbations of energy and cognition tend to interfere with the conduct of work. Depressed patients tend to take longer to perform tasks, or think their way through problems. Manic patients can be so restless or distracted that they fail to complete tasks properly. However, the degree to which impairment is noticeable depends heavily on contextual factors, such as the difficulty of the work being performed, the stability of the patient's basic temperament (e.g. stoic vs. neurotic), and the depth of social resources on which the patient may draw. From similar reasoning, it is easy to see that many patients can exhibit severe functional decompensation in the absence of ongoing symptoms of mood disorder, if their discouragement leads to markedly altered behaviour.

Depressive and manic syndromes can be suspected based on chronic behavioural changes. However, behavioural changes alone do not make the diagnosis. The clinician must elicit the symptoms as described above to make the diagnosis. Depression, for example, should be suspected in patients exhibiting suicidal or self-mutilatory behaviour and in patients who withdraw socially and uncharacteristically fail to follow through with family and occupational obligations. Mania should be suspected when patients spend lavishly, engage in uncharacteristic sexual promiscuity, or exhibit other disinhibited behaviour. Because these behaviours may all arise under a variety of circumstances, it is important not only to elicit a history of any accompanying symptoms but also to know how the patient behaves at other times. In many cases, the diagnosis cannot be made without information from the patient's family about changes from prior behaviour.

A patient's resistance to or ignorance of the concept of mood disorder often obstructs diagnosis and treatment. Patients often do not recognize mood disorder as the primary source of their suffering. Mood disorder from the patient's perspective can be so insidious and pervasive that patients see their symptoms (however exaggerated compared to the normal range of human response) as an understandable reaction to adverse life events or to their own insufficient (or inflated) value as persons. Patients with depression may come to feel they deserve their despair; the belief that others would be better off without them all too often leads to suicide attempts. Manic patients, on the other hand, can evince an impenetrable arrogance, which thwarts efforts at management.

Classification

Patients with episodes of mania or hypomania are designated bipolar (synonymous with manic depressive illness) regardless of whether they have had documented depressive episodes. Patients with depressive episodes but no mania are called unipolar in the scholarly literature, and are given the diagnosis major depressive disorder in the official nomenclature of the American Psychiatric Association, the *Diagnostic and Statistical Manual (DSM)* (American Psychiatric Association, 1994). In many cases it is not easy to differentiate mild bipolar from unipolar depressive disorders, as patients and their families may not have recognized the milder manifestations of hypomania.

While most patients with bipolar or unipolar disorders have an episodic course, with substantial periods of remission, variations in the course of illness are accounted for in the classification scheme. Dysthymia refers to a mild-to-moderate depressive disorder, lasting years. Patients with four or more episodes of mania or depression per year are described as having 'rapid cycling'. Such patients can experience an episode once per season or can even cycle on a daily basis. Patients with the distinctive symptoms of mania and depression simultaneously are in what are called 'mixed states', first described by Kraepelin at the turn of the twentieth century (Kraepelin, 1921). Patients in mixed states often experience low and very irritable moods, but are physically and mentally hyperactive to the point of restlessness and distraction. Patients in these states are prone to violent and self-injurious rages.

The official operational definitions used in DSM diagnostic categories and based on clinical criteria sets ensure reliability, but not a valid nosology of mood disorders.

There is strong evidence for the validity of four or five of the subtypes listed in the manual. There may be meaningful biological distinctions between melancholic depression (blunted affect, insomnia, loss of appetite) and atypical depression (reactive mood, hypersomnia, hyperphagia) (Asnis et al., 1995) and between mood disorders with and without psychotic symptoms (Coryell, 1996). Other means of subtyping patients based on family history, comorbidity, and symptom severity remain a focus of research. Panic disorder, an anxiety disorder characterized by paroxysmal acute, severe anxiety, a feeling of impending death, derealization, and physical symptoms such as palpitations, shortness of breath, chest tightness and dizziness, occurs in 20% or more of individuals with bipolar and unipolar depressive disorders. Panic disorder comorbidity with bipolar disorder clusters in a subset of families containing multiple bipolar relatives and may be a marker of genetic heterogeneity in bipolar disorder (MacKinnon et al., 1998).

Somatic diseases and mood disorder

Patients with an unrecognized mood disorder often present with non-psychiatric complaints. Suspicion of an underlying mood disorder should be raised when patients present with uncontrollable pain, fatigue, requests for sleeping pills, and when there is uncharacteristic or unusually severe non-compliance with treatment or failure to rehabilitate after a medical illness. In the elderly, depression may manifest as an abrupt cognitive decline, though the diagnosis should be made only after delirium and dementia have been ruled out.

Depression is one of the most common comorbidities of medical illness (Coulehan et al., 1990). The interrelationship of depression and medical disorders underscores the significance of the task of identifying and treating depression. Depression is a major risk factor for the development of and morbidity from cardiovascular disease (Musselman et al., 1998). Mood disorders complicate the treatment and course of many neurological disorders, including seizure disorders (Wiegartz et al., 1999), cerebrovascular disease (Morris et al., 1993), Parkinson's Disease (Cummings & Masterman, 1999; Starkstein et al., 1990), Huntington's Disease (Peyser & Folstein, 1990), and multiple sclerosis (Patten & Metz, 1997). Mood disorders occur commonly with cancer (Spiegel, 1996) and AIDS, which produces both depressive and manic syndromes (Treisman et al., 1998). In some medical disorders with obscure pathology, like fibromyalgia (Ackenheil, 1998) and chronic fatigue syndrome (Lane et al., 1991) depression commonly coexists with the somatic symptoms and exacerbates the pain and fatigue.

In medically comorbid depression, however, the task of differentiating discouragement, which is also a common complication of illness, from depression is critical. The undertreatment of depression or overmedication of discouragement can have severe medical consequences in medically ill patients (Cassem, 1995). Medical illness often raises the risk for suicide in either case (Harris & Barraclough, 1994). Medically ill patients with depression have higher mortality rates (Covinsky et al., 1999; Herrmann et al., 1998). On the other hand, caution in prescribing is dictated by the significant risks of adverse side effects from medications (e.g. cardiac conduction delays with tricyclic antidepressants, delirium with any psychotropic medications), or unforeseen pharmacologic interactions (e.g. fluoxetine's inhibition of a cytochrome P-450 enzyme, lithium toxicity from concomitant use with thiazide diuretics or ibuprofen).

Therapeutic issues

Prior to the development of effective biological treatment for mood disorders, treatment focused on the containment of dangerous behaviour: suicide in melancholics, and violent agitation in manics, through institutionalization, sedation, and 'rest' (Goodwin & Jamison, 1990). In the middle third of the twentieth century, patients with milder forms of mood disorder often pursued psychoanalytically informed psychotherapy which, because it took place over a longer period than the expected natural duration of an episode of illness, was seen as probably effective in many cases. In the latter half of the twentieth century, an increasing array of effective pharmacologic and other biological treatments have supplanted the psychoanalytic and supplemented the pragmatic approach with empiric remedies and prophylaxis. The empiric means used to treat and forestall illness promise to inform our understanding of mechanisms of illness.

The first issue often confronting the physician treating depression is that patients can at the same time have major depression and be discouraged about having depression. Discouragement is an understandable emotional response to a state in which a mental disorder has caused one's enjoyment of life to be lost, one's bodily functions (sleep, appetite, libido) to be awry, and one's energy and cognitive fluency to be sapped. Biological treatments for depression all take weeks to months to have a full therapeutic effect, but patients tend to begin to feel better quickly when they are provided with hope for recovery. The amelioration of discouragement accounts for the rapid partial response seen both in placebo and treatment groups in many studies of antidepressant efficacy; however, after a week the continued progress towards recovery tends to occur only in the treatment groups.

All biological treatments in use for the treatment of mood disorders were discovered either serendipitously or from analogy with treatments discovered serendipitously. The older antidepressant classes, tricyclics (TCA) and monoamine oxidase inhibitors (MAOI) were observed incidentally to relieve depression in patients treated for psychosis and tuberculosis, respectively (Pletscher, 1991; Potter et al., 1991). Lithium, though it was known to be a component of mineral waters and even soft drinks early in the twentieth century, was found to be an effective antimanic agent only after its sedative properties were observed, incidentally, in guinea pigs being studied for the toxic effects of uric acid. Electroconvulsive therapy (ECT) arose from the observation (false, as it turns out) that epileptics are somehow protected from depression. Carbamazepine was observed, again incidentally, to improve mood symptoms in patients treated for epilepsy, and was applied to the treatment of bipolar disorder based on speculation about shared pathophysiologic mechanisms (Post et al., 1982).

Investigation of putative mechanisms of action of these treatments has led to newer generations of treatment either in use or under investigation for use against mood disorders. Serotonin selective reuptake inhibitors (SSRI) arose from insights derived from research on the binding properties of TCAs that showed, for example, high affinity of TCAs for serotonin receptors (Paul et al., 1981). Valproic acid was applied to mania because of its overlapping specificity with benzodiazepines for GABA receptors (Emrich et al., 1980). While the mechanism of action of ECT remains obscure, the concept of ECT has led to investigation into transcranial magnetic stimulation (TCMS) as a means to deliver a highly focused magnetic field across the skull without inducing the significant cognitive side effects often seen with ECT (George et al., 1995b).

Efficacy of many antidepressant and antimanic treatments has been established; however, efficacy of treatment with the aim of preventing relapse has been established only for the use of lithium in bipolar disorder. Antidepressant agents, when given in an adequate dose over 6 to 8 weeks tend to bring recovery in two-thirds to three-quarters of patients, across different antidepressant types (Nelson, 1999). ECT is more effective still in treating acute depression and mania (Mukherjee et al., 1994). Efficacy in alleviating mania has been established for lithium, several anticonvulsants, and an atypical neuroleptic (olanzapine). Long-term efficacy of antidepressant maintenance for recurrent depression is not well established, as effective dosages of medications tend not to be maintained in the long run (Mueller et al., 1999). In bipolar disorder long-term efficacy is established for lithium (Davis et al., 1999), while the evidence is less strong or non-existent for other agents currently in wide use (Bowden et al., 2000). Aside from medication, the advice offered by Kraepelin remains salient today:

That a very even tenor of life in *protected circumstances*, especially also with *avoidance of alcohol*, may have a certain prophylactic effect with individuals who are liable to attacks, may be regarded as probable considering the frequently indubitable influence of external injuries [Kraepelin, p. 202, emphasis his].

Patients with mood disorder are well advised to avoid alcohol and drugs and to sleep, work and exercise regularly.

Pathophysiology and etiology

Development of rational treatments to enhance the specificity of action in order to target patient subgroups, minimize side effects, and possibly accelerate treatment response, hinges on the elucidation of pathophysiologic mechanisms. Explorations of the biology of human emotional distress, pharmacologic mechanisms of action of antidepressant and antimanic agents, and variation in brain structure and function have opened windows to these mechanisms. Pathophysiologic investigation informs and is informed by the discovery of genetic markers linked to mood disorder vulnerability.

Depression and the stress response

Many patients and their physicians accept at face value the intuition that stress causes depression. A biochemical correlate of this intuition is the hypothesis that depression arises from an abnormality in the stress response mechanism, i.e. the hypothalamic–pituitary–adrenal (HPA) axis. There is some support for a relationship of HPA axis dysfunction and mood disorder, however the nature of the relationship remains uncertain. Depressive and manic syndromes occur with considerable frequency in Cushing's syndrome and with the use of corticosteroids. Patients with depression sometimes abnormally manifest nonsuppression of morning cortisol levels after an evening dose of dexamethasone (Carroll et al., 1968), however, without sufficient predictive power to aid in diagnosis (Arana et al., 1985). Consistent evidence of elevated cortisol levels in depressed patients has been difficult to establish (Posener et al., 2000; Steckler et al., 1999). Nevertheless, evidence continues to accumulate regarding the association of stress and HPA axis perturbations with altered emotional state. Corticotropin releasing factor (CRF) and its receptors have been implicated in the modulation of the stress response; mice bred to be lacking a CRF receptor show abnormally low anxiety in response to stress (Timpl et al., 1998), and human subjects with depression, panic disorder, or alcoholism all show a blunted corticotropin (ACTH) response to CRF (Holsboer et al., 1987). However, it is less clear that HPA axis dysfunction can be seen as a cause, rather than a cofactor or a result of mood disorder. Abnormal regulation of cortisol is seen with a variety of conditions that produce chronic stress, including non-depressed individuals who had experienced significant childhood trauma (Heim et al., 2000). Implication of chronic elevated stress and glucocorticoid levels as a cause of atrophy of hippocampal neurons (Magarinos et al., 1997; Sapolsky, 1996), which would predict diminished hippocampal volume in depressed patients, has found only mixed empirical support (Brown et al., 1999; Vakili et al., 2000).

Monoaminergic hypotheses

The noradrenergic hypothesis, derived in part from the emergence of depressive symptomatology in hypertensive patients taking reserpine, explains the mechanism of action of TCA medications and continues to gain empirical support (Lambert et al., 2000), but serotonergic dysfunction has been implicated more consistently as a possible pathophysiologic factor in depression. One line of empirical support for the serotonergic hypothesis is evidence of diminished serotonin function in the brains of depressed suicidal patients. The levels of serotonin metabolites have been found persistently to be decreased in the cerebrospinal fluid of patients with depression and suicidal intent (Traskman et al., 1981) and evidence for diminished functioning in the brain can be inferred from an increase in the number of serotonin receptors in the brains of suicide victims (Arango et al., 1990). The degree of serotonin deficiency correlates with the violence of the suicidal intention (Mann & Malone, 1997). Diminished levels of serotonin metabolites also have been discovered in the cerebrospinal fluid of violent and impulsive subjects in general (Stanley et al., 2000), so altered serotonin function is not necessarily specific to depression. The serotonin hypothesis is supported by the observation that correction of an apparent deficiency in serotonin neurotransmission correlates with alleviation of depressive symptoms. When depressed patients treated to at least partial remission with SSRI agents, which selectively block serotonin reuptake, are depleted of tryptophan, an amino acid precursor for serotonin, symptoms of depression return (Delgado et al.,

1990); however, recurrence of depressive symptoms under tryptophan depletion is not observed in patients in full remission (Moore et al., 2000). Continued elucidation of the mechanisms of regulation of serotonin activity at the synapse may lead to improvement in the focus of pharmacotherapy (Blier & de Montigny, 1994).

Mood instability and the mechanisms of action of lithium

Lithium exerts a variety of effects on neurons. One or some combination of these effects might be the key to the therapeutic mechanism of action of lithium, thus to the pathophysiologic mechanisms of mood disorder (Manji et al., 2000b). A general hypothesis is that lithium's modulating effects on signal transduction and thus gene expression may be salient for understanding affective psychopathology (Lachman & Papolos, 1995; Manji et al., 1995). Chronic lithium administration interferes with receptor-G protein coupling (Wang & Friedman, 1999), reduces levels of inositol triphosphate precursors (Huang et al., 2000), and inhibits phosphorylation of cyclic AMP (Wang et al., 1999) in rat brains. There is not, as yet, evidence of dysfunction in any of these pathways to explain why lithium's modulating effect is required in bipolar patients. There is evidence, however, to suggest that chronic administration of lithium and valproate may protect neurons by stimulating expression of a cytoprotective protein bcl-2 (Manji et al., 2000a). Whether mood instability is the result of a primary pathological process in structures related to affective modulation, or the effect on brain of manic hyperarousal is focal neurotoxicity, demonstration of the salutary effect of chronic lithium on brain corresponds nicely with the long-term efficacy of lithium in bipolar disorder.

Anatomy of mania and depression

A key challenge for neuroanatomic hypotheses of mood disorder is to explain both the state of illness and the episodic course of affective disorder. Epilepsies notwithstanding, the complete resolution of symptoms between mood disorder episodes appears inconsistent with an illness model involving a static brain lesion. Studies of depressive illness following stroke suggest that lesion location, the time since the stroke, and the extent of functional impairment independently predict depressive illness. Functional neuroimaging of actively depressed and remitted patients and of healthy subjects under emotional activation paradigms point to the limbic–cortical systems as important structures in the genesis and resolution of depressive states. Integration of structural and functional anatomy with hormonal, neurotransmitter and gene transcription hypotheses remains to be done.

Postmortem brain studies of patients with mood disorder, including suicide victims, have revealed no consistent histopathological differences in the brains of affected individuals, or gross evidence for pathology related to mood disorder (Goodwin & Jamison, 1990). Association of poststroke lesions and depressive symptomatology became feasible with the advent of clinical neuroimaging. Depression in the immediate poststroke period has been associated with left anterior stroke location (Astrom et al., 1993; Robinson & Szetela, 1981). These depressions were comparable phenomenologically to idiopathic major depressions. They also responded similarly to treatment with a tricyclic antidepressant (Lipsey et al., 1984). Depression following months or years behind a stroke tends to correlate more with the degree of residual functional impairment than with specific location of injury; however there is some association of delayed post-stroke depressive states and right occipital location (Robinson, 2000; Shimoda & Robinson, 1999).

Expanding on these lesion studies, volumetric and functional analysis of depressed patients without brain injury tends to implicate frontal and limbic structures in affective pathophysiology. One illustrative volumetric analysis revealed diminished frontal lobe volume relative to controls (Coffey et al., 1993); however, no particular portion of the frontal lobe was consistently affected, and other studies investigating structural changes with mood disorder have been inconsistent (Steffens & Krishnan, 1998). PET scanning of patients with depression has confirmed diminished metabolic activity in the left prefrontal cortex (Martinot et al., 1990), which correlates specifically with degree of mood disturbance and psychomotor retardation (Bench et al., 1993). Emotional activation paradigms involving the elicitation of sad emotions typically implicate frontal cortex as well as limbic structures, however laterality varies across studies (Beauregard et al., 1998; George et al., 1995a). Evidence for limbic–frontal reciprocity has emerged from PET studies of both depressed patients before and after successful pharmacologic treatment and healthy subjects induced to experience sad emotions, suggesting that mood regulation is a function of the relationship of cortical and limbic structures rather than the function of a single structure (Mayberg et al., 1999). Thus, a left frontal lobe diminished structurally and functionally by ischemic injury or other pathogenic processes may contribute to core symptoms of low mood and psychomotor disturbance, but may not be a necessary factor in pathophysiology.

Structures associated with the limbic system have a role to play in mood regulation, and probably do so as well in the pathophysiology of affective disorders. The amygdala, in particular, has been established through animal studies to be a centre for integration of the fear response (LeDoux, 2000) and has been found in one report to be activated (on the left side) with induction of sad mood in normal humans (Schneider et al., 1997). A contribution of the amygdala to affective psychopathology might explain mania seen in patients with temporal lobe epilepsy (Lyketsos et al., 1993) and could provide some anatomic support for the kindling model in idiopathic affective disorders (Post et al., 1982). The amygdala has extensive connections with prefrontal cortex (PFC), in particular with the subgenual prefrontal cortex, a structure implicated in the neuroanatomy of depression that also has connections with the lateral hypothalamus, nucleus accumbens, locus ceruleus, substantia nigra, and other deep brain and brainstem nuclei (Drevets, 1999). Functional and structural lesions in the subgenual PFC have been associated with mood disorder; patients with depression show diminished size and local cerebral blood flow in this region (Drevets et al., 1997); histopathological analysis finds a diminution principally in glia cells (Ongur et al., 1998). Lesions in this area do not duplicate a classic depressive syndrome; however, the amotivational syndrome arising from subgenual PFC certainly resembles a core feature of depressive states.

Linkages of brain dysfunction to depressive and manic psychopathology in the context of dementia and delirious states are not easily interpreted. Delirious states can present with depressive affect, withdrawal, and nihilistic or even suicidal statements; alternatively, delirious patients may appear as agitated, combative, or with manic features (e.g. denial of impairment from an obvious illness). Such symptomatology emerges routinely in the hospital setting in the context of delirium, whether due to systemic illness or intoxication. While the pathophysiology of manic or depressive-like symptoms in these contexts may in time prove informative to the understanding of idiopathic mood disorder, one must be alert to dissimilarities (not highlighted in many reports) between these known pathologic states and bipolar or depressive disorders. For example, late onset mood disorders have been associated with diffuse periventricular white matter ischemia, but also are independently correlated with generalized cognitive deficits (Steffens & Krishnan, 1998). Diffuse white matter hyperintensities have often been reported in bipolar disorder (Altshuler et al., 1995; Dupont et al., 1990) and in vascular and demyelinating disorders without affective syndromes. However, they have not been observed in first-episode manic patients (Strakowski et al., 1993), suggesting that diffuse white matter lesions are likely a contributing but not a primary causative factor in some cases of bipolar disorder.

Genetic risk

Familial risk for mood disorders is well established from family, twin, and adoption studies. Specific genetic risk factors for bipolar and unipolar disorders have not yet been discovered; however, it is possible from the evidence available to predict a complex genetic contribution to etiology. Genetic analysis promises to play a critical role in validating pathophysiologic mechanisms suggested by research in neuroanatomy and neuroendocrinology, and in suggesting further research into molecular mechanisms of illness.

Elevated familial risk for mood disorder is well established from family, twin and adoption studies (Bertelsen et al., 1977; MacKinnon et al., 1997; Mendlewicz & Rainer, 1977). Siblings of patients with bipolar disorder have about a fivefold elevated risk for bipolar disorder, and siblings of patients with unipolar disorder have about a twofold elevated risk (Tsuang & Faraone, 1990). Family study evidence also supports the conclusion that mood disorders do not elevate familial risk for schizophrenia, and vice versa (Gershon et al., 1982), so that these disorders may be seen as separate phenotypes, with probable separate pathophysiology. Analyses of patterns of inheritance of mood disorders have not consistently supported a dominant vs. recessive vs. X-linked mode of inheritance. Numerous explorations of the genome in families ascertained for bipolar disorder linkage study (genomic studies of unipolar disorder are, as of this writing, few in number) have yielded inconsistent support for linkage at a variety of genetic loci (Berrettini, 2000). While any one of these loci may or may not contain a gene coding for a protein involved in a mechanism salient to mood disorder, the fact that no one genetic locus is found to be linked to bipolar disorder in even a large minority of families suggests that bipolar disorder (and most likely unipolar disorder as well) is complex genetically as it is clinically.

The pattern of findings and non-findings in studies of genetic risk factors for mood disorder is consistent with a model in which vulnerability to mood disorder derives from the interaction of several proteins, neither of which is necessary or sufficient to produce symptoms individually. In other words, individual No. 1 may have an elevated risk for developing a first episode of mania or depression because of inheriting genetic variants A, B, and C, while individual No. 2 may have a similar risk because of C, D, and E, while No. 3's risk derives from F, G, and H. It can be seen that risk factors like C may be present in most, but not all individuals, while other risk factors may overlap not at all across individuals. Each genetic factor may elevate the risk by a factor of 2 or less, making detection even more difficult since a large proportion of individuals with a possible genetic risk factor will show no evidence of the phenotype. Multigenic etiology also may account for intrafamilial heterogeneity, a phenomenon that would severely limit the power to detect genetic risk using the methodologies available.

Progress in understanding the pathophysiology and etiology of mood disorders, therefore, is likely to hinge on cross-fertilization of scientific exploration across disciplines. This occurs already, in the form of candidate gene approaches in which known genetic loci coding for proteins involved in the function of neurotransmitter systems are tested for the association of polymorphisms (preferably with functional significance) with the phenotype under investigation. As the genome becomes completely mapped, and functions are assigned to the tens of thousands of genes as yet undiscovered as of this writing, it will be possible to evaluate using genetic analysis additional hypotheses to account for signal transduction defects, focal cytotoxicity in brain regions subserving affective modulation, impaired neuroendocrine regulation, and so on.

Conclusions and predictions

One of the most challenging and labour-intensive puzzles to be resolved in coming years is to differentiate mood disorders into clinically and pathophysiologically meaningful phenotypic subtypes. One can begin with the insight that unipolar depression responds differently than bipolar depression to antidepressants, sometimes. Increasingly, it will be possible to test hypotheses of clinical heterogeneity genetically, by linkage studies that show a common genetic variation in the affected individuals in some families, but not in others. Association of particular disease-related alleles with disease across families may yield additional pathophysiological insight, as molecular variations are related to physiologic dysfunction. While a presentation of current knowledge underscores the enormity of the gaps in our understanding of mood disorders, over the past generation the evidence has strengthened that mood disorders involve specific sorts of dysfunction in the brain and neuroendocrine systems. The means may now exist to begin to untangle the complexity of mental illness.

The intersecting study of neuroendocrine dysfunction, neuroanatomical pathology, cellular signal transduction and the genome will merge in time to provide the basis for a full description of the biological vulnerability to mood disorder. As soon as a single gene can be definitively linked to mood disorder, it will be possible to begin to dissect the genetic and biochemical complexities, and to investigate the brain functions underlying mood disorders. Once the biological mechanisms are understood, the environmental risk factors for depression will stand in stark relief, and may be approached with full knowledge of the potentials and limitations of interpersonal, behavioural, or social intervention in alleviating or preventing mood disorder. In time, cross-disciplinary correlations of genomic markers and specific biochemical or neuroanatomic markers of vulnerability traits and disease states will aid in the development of comprehensive theories of mood and mood disorder and the development of rational therapeutics.

References

Ackenheil, M. (1998). Genetics and pathophysiology of affective disorders: relationship to fibromyalgia. *Z. Rheumatol.* 57, Suppl. 2, 5–7.

Altshuler, L.L., Curran, J.G., Hauser, P., Mintz, J., Denicoff, K. & Post, R. (1995). T2 hyperintensities in bipolar disorder: magnetic resonance imaging comparison and literature meta-analysis. *Am. J. Psychiatry*, 152, 1139–44.

American Psychiatric Association (1994). *Diagnostic and Statistical Manual of Mental Disorders*, 4th edn. Washington, DC: APA Press.

Arana, G.W., Baldessarini, R.J. & Ornsteen, M. (1985). The dexamethasone suppression test for diagnosis and prognosis in psychiatry. Commentary and review. *Arch. Gen. Psychiatry*, 42, 1193–204.

Arango, V., Ernsberger, P., Marzuk, P.M. et al. (1990). Autoradiographic demonstration of increased serotonin 5-HT2 and beta-adrenergic receptor binding sites in the brain of suicide victims. *Arch. Gen. Psychiatry*, 47, 1038–47.

Asnis, G.M., McGinn, L.K. & Sanderson, W.C. (1995). Atypical depression: clinical aspects and noradrenergic function. *Am. J. Psychiatry*, 152, 31–6.

Astrom, M., Adolfsson, R. & Asplund, K. (1993). Major depression in stroke patients. A 3-year longitudinal study. *Stroke*, 24, 976–82.

Barraclough, B., Bunch, J., Nelson, B. & Sainsbury, P. (1974). A hundred cases of suicide: clinical aspects. *Br. J. Psychiatry*, 125, 355–73.

Beauregard, M., Leroux, J.M., Bergman, S. et al. (1998). The functional neuroanatomy of major depression: an fMRI study using an emotional activation paradigm. *Neuroreport*, 9, 3253–8.

Benazzi, F. (1997). Antidepressant-associated hypomania in outpatient depression: a 203-case study in private practice. *J. Affect. Disord.*, 46, 73–7.

Bench, C.J., Friston, K.J., Brown, R.G., Frackowiak, R.S. & Dolan, R.J. (1993). Regional cerebral blood flow in depression measured by positron emission tomography: the relationship with clinical dimensions. *Psychol. Med.*, 23, 579–90.

Berrettini, W.H. (2000). Genetics of psychiatric disease. *Annu. Rev. Med.*, 51, 465–79.

Bertelsen, A., Harvald, B. & Hauge, M. (1977). A Danish twin study of manic-depressive disorders. *Br. J. Psychiatry*, 130, 330–51.

Blier, P. & de Montigny, C. (1994). Current advances and trends in the treatment of depression. *Trends Pharmacol. Sci.*, 15, 220–6.

Bowden, C.L., Calabrese, J.R., McElroy, S.L. et al. (2000). A randomized, placebo-controlled 12-month trial of divalproex and lithium in treatment of outpatients with bipolar I disorder. Divalproex Maintenance Study Group. *Arch. Gen. Psychiatry*, 57, 481–9.

Brown, E.S., Rush, A.J. & McEwen, B.S. (1999). Hippocampal remodeling and damage by corticosteroids: implications for mood disorders. *Neuropsychopharmacology*, 21, 474–84.

Carroll, B.J., Martin, F.I. & Davies, B. (1968). Resistance to suppression by dexamethasone of plasma 11–O.H.C.S. levels in severe depressive illness. *Br. Med. J.*, 3, 285–7.

Carson, A.J., Ringbauer, B., MacKenzie, L., Warlow, C. & Sharpe, M. (2000). Neurological disease, emotional disorder, and disability: they are related: a study of 300 consecutive new referrals to a neurology outpatient department. *J. Neurol. Neurosurg. Psychiatry*, 68, 202–6.

Cassem, E.H. (1995). Depressive disorders in the medically ill. An overview. *Psychosomatics*, 36, S2–10.

Coffey, C.E., Wilkinson, W.E., Weiner, R.D., Ritchie, J.C. & Aque, M. (1993). The dexamethasone suppression test and quantitative cerebral anatomy in depression. *Biol. Psychiatry*, 33, 442–9.

Coryell, W. (1996). Psychotic depression. *J. Clin. Psychiatry*, 57, Suppl. 3, 27–31.

Coulehan, J.L., Schulberg, H.C., Block, M.R., Janosky, J.E. & Arena, V.C. (1990). Medical comorbidity of major depressive disorder in a primary medical practice. *Arch. Intern. Med.*, 150, 2363–7.

Covinsky, K.E., Kahana, E., Chin, M.H., Palmer, R.M., Fortinsky, R.H. & Landefeld, C.S. (1999). Depressive symptoms and 3-year mortality in older hospitalized medical patients. *Ann. Intern. Med.*, 130, 563–9.

Cummings, J.L. & Masterman, D.L. (1999). Depression in patients with Parkinson's disease. *Int. J. Geriatr. Psychiatry*, 14, 711–18.

Davis, J.M., Janicak, P.G. & Hogan, D.M. (1999). Mood stabilizers in the prevention of recurrent affective disorders: a meta-analysis. *Acta Psychiatr. Scand.*, 100, 406–17.

Delgado, P.L., Charney, D.S., Price, L.H., Aghajanian, G.K., Landis, H. & Heninger, G.R. (1990). Serotonin function and the mechanism of antidepressant action. Reversal of antidepressant-induced remission by rapid depletion of plasma tryptophan. *Arch. Gen. Psychiatry*, 47, 411–18.

Doris, A., Ebmeier, K. & Shajahan, P. (1999). Depressive illness. *Lancet*, 354, 1369–75.

Drevets, W.C. (1999). Prefrontal cortical–amygdalar metabolism in major depression. *Ann. NY Acad. Sci.*, 877, 614–37.

Drevets, W.C., Price, J.L., Simpson, J.R.J. et al. (1997). Subgenual prefrontal cortex abnormalities in mood disorders. *Nature*, 386, 824–7.

Druss, B.G., Rosenheck, R.A. & Sledge, W.H. (2000). Health and disability costs of depressive illness in a major U.S. corporation. *Am. J. Psychiatry*, **157**, 1274–8.

Dupont, R.M., Jernigan, T.L., Butters, N. et al. (1990). Subcortical abnormalities detected in bipolar affective disorder using magnetic resonance imaging. Clinical and neuropsychological significance. *Arch. Gen. Psychiatry*, **47**, 55–9.

Emrich, H.M., von Zerssen, D., Kissling, W., Moller, H.J. & Windorfer, A. (1980). Effect of sodium valproate on mania. The GABA-hypothesis of affective disorders. *Arch. Psychiatr. Nervenkr.*, **229**, 1–16.

George, M.S., Ketter, T.A., Parekh, P.I., Horwitz, B., Herscovitch, P. & Post, R.M. (1995a). Brain activity during transient sadness and happiness in healthy women. *Am. J. Psychiatry*, **152**, 341–51.

George, M.S., Wassermann, E.M., Williams, W.A. et al. (1995b). Daily repetitive transcranial magnetic stimulation (rTMS) improves mood in depression. *Neuroreport*, **6**, 1853–6.

Gershon, E.S., Hamovit, J., Guroff, J.J. et al. (1982). A family study of schizoaffective, bipolar I, bipolar II, unipolar, and normal control probands. *Arch. Gen. Psychiatry*, **39**, 1157–67.

Goodwin, F.K. & Jamison, K.R. (1990). *Manic Depressive Illness*, New York: Oxford University Press.

Greenberg, P.E., Stiglin, L.E., Finkelstein, S.N. & Berndt, E.R. (1993). The economic burden of depression in 1990. *J. Clin. Psychiatry*, **54**, 405–18.

Harris, E.C. & Barraclough, B.M. (1994). Suicide as an outcome for medical disorders. *Medicine*, **73**, 281–96.

Heim, C., Newport, D.J., Heit, S. et al. (2000). Pituitary-adrenal and autonomic responses to stress in women after sexual and physical abuse in childhood. *J. Am. Med. Assoc.*, **284**, 592–7.

Herrmann, C., Brand-Driehorst, S., Kaminsky, B., Leibing, E., Staats, H. & Ruger, U. (1998). Diagnostic groups and depressed mood as predictors of 22-month mortality in medical inpatients. *Psychosom. Med.*, **60**, 570–7.

Holsboer, F., von Bardeleben, U., Buller, R., Heuser, I. & Steiger, A. (1987). Stimulation response to corticotropin-releasing hormone (CRH) in patients with depression, alcoholism and panic disorder. *Horm. Metab. Res. Suppl.*, **16**, 80–8.

Huang, W., Galdzicki, Z., van Gelderen, P. et al. (2000). Brain myoinositol level is elevated in Ts65Dn mouse and reduced after lithium treatment. *Neuroreport*, **11**, 445–8.

Inskip, H.M., Harris, E.C. & Barraclough, B. (1998). Lifetime risk of suicide for affective disorder, alcoholism and schizophrenia. *Br. J. Psychiatry*, **172**, 35–7.

Kraepelin, E. (1921). *Manic Depressive Insanity and Paranoia*, Transl. R.M. Barclay, 1921, Edinburgh: E&S Livingstone, reprinted 1990, Salem, NH: Ayer Co.

Lachman, H.M. & Papolos, D.F. (1995). A molecular model for bipolar affective disorder. *Med. Hypotheses*, **45**, 255–64.

Lambert, G., Johansson, M., Agren, H. & Friberg, P. (2000). Reduced brain norepinephrine and dopamine release in treatment-refractory depressive illness: evidence in support of the catecholamine hypothesis of mood disorders. *Arch. Gen. Psychiatry*, **57**, 787–93.

Lane, T.J., Manu, P. & Matthews, D.A. (1991). Depression and somatization in the chronic fatigue syndrome. *Am. J. Med.*, **91**, 335–44.

LeDoux, J.E. (2000). Emotion circuits in the brain. *Annu. Rev. Neurosci.*, **23**, 155–84.

Lipsey, J.R., Robinson, R.G., Pearlson, G.D., Rao, K. & Price, T.R. (1984). Nortriptyline treatment of post-stroke depression: a double-blind study. *Lancet*, **i**, 297–300.

Lyketsos, C.G., Stoline, A.M., Longstreet, P. et al. (1993). Mania in Temporal Lobe Epilepsy. *Neuropsychiatry, Neuropsychol. Behav. Neurol.*, **6**, 19–25.

MacKinnon, D.F., Jamison, K.R. & DePaulo, J.R. (1997). Genetics of manic depressive illness. *Annu. Rev. Neurosci.*, **20**, 355–73.

MacKinnon, D.F., Xu, J., McMahon, F.J. et al. (1998). Bipolar disorder and panic disorder in families: an analysis of chromosome 18 data. *Am. J. Psychiatry*, **155**, 829–31.

Magarinos, A.M., Verdugo, J.M. & McEwen, B.S. (1997). Chronic stress alters synaptic terminal structure in hippocampus. *Proc. Natl. Acad. Sci., USA*, **94**, 14002–8.

Manji, H.K., Potter, W.Z. & Lenox, R.H. (1995). Signal transduction pathways. Molecular targets for lithium's actions. *Arch. Gen. Psychiatry*, **52**, 531–43.

Manji, H.K., Bowden, C.L. & Belmaker, R.H. (2000b). *Bipolar Medications: Mechanisms of Action.* Washington, DC: American Psychiatric Press.

Manji, H.K., Moore, G.J. & Chen, G. (2000a). Clinical and preclinical evidence for the neurotrophic effects of mood stabilizers: implications for the pathophysiology and treatment of manic-depressive illness. *Biol. Psychiatry*, **48**, 740–54.

Mann, J.J. & Malone, K.M. (1997). Cerebrospinal fluid amines and higher-lethality suicide attempts in depressed inpatients. *Biol. Psychiatry*, **41**, 162–71.

Martinot, J.L., Hardy, P., Feline, A. et al. (1990). Left prefrontal glucose hypometabolism in the depressed state: a confirmation. *Am. J. Psychiatry*, **147**, 1313–17.

Masand, P.S., Pickett, P. & Murray, G.B. (1995). Hypomania precipitated by psychostimulant use in depressed medically ill patients. *Psychosomatics*, **36**, 145–7.

Mayberg, H.S., Liotti, M., Brannan, S.K. et al. (1999). Reciprocal limbic-cortical function and negative mood: converging PET findings in depression and normal sadness. *Am. J. Psychiatry*, **156**, 675–82.

Mendlewicz, J. & Rainer, J.D. (1977). Adoption study supporting genetic transmission in manic – depressive illness. *Nature*, **268**, 327–9.

Moore, P., Landolt, H., Seifritz, E. et al. (2000). Clinical and physiological consequences of rapid tryptophan depletion. *Neuropsychopharmacology*, **23**, 601–22.

Morris, P.L., Robinson, R.G., Andrzejewski, P., Samuels, J. & Price, T.R. (1993). Association of depression with 10-year poststroke mortality. *Am. J. Psychiatry*, **150**, 124–9.

Mueller, T.I., Leon, A.C., Keller, M.B. et al. (1999). Recurrence after recovery from major depressive disorder during 15 years of observational follow-up. *Am. J. Psychiatry*, **156**, 1000–6.

Mukherjee, S., Sackeim, H.A. & Schnur, D.B. (1994). Electro-convulsive therapy of acute manic episodes: a review of 50 years' experience. *Am. J. Psychiatry*, **151**, 169–76.

Musselman, D.L., Evans, D.L. & Nemeroff, C.B. (1998). The relation-ship of depression to cardiovascular disease: epidemiology, biology, and treatment. *Arch. Gen. Psychiatry*, **55**, 580–92.

Nelson, J.C. (1999). A review of the efficacy of serotonergic and noradrenergic reuptake inhibitors for treatment of major depression. *Biol. Psychiatry*, **46**, 1301–8.

Ongur, D., Drevets, W.C. & Price, J.L. (1998). Glial reduction in the subgenual prefrontal cortex in mood disorders. *Proc. Natl. Acad. Sci., USA*, **95**, 13290–5.

Patten, S.B. & Metz, L.M. (1997). Depression in multiple sclerosis. *Psychother. Psychosom.*, **66**, 286–92.

Paul, S.M., Rehavi, M., Skolnick, P., Ballenger, J.C. & Goodwin, F.K. (1981). Depressed patients have decreased binding of tritiated imipramine to platelet serotonin 'transporter'. *Arch. Gen. Psychiatry*, **38**, 1315–17.

Peyser, C.E. & Folstein, S.E. (1990). Huntington's disease as a model for mood disorders. Clues from neuropathology and neuro-chemistry. *Mol. Chem. Neuropathol.*, **12**, 99–119.

Pletscher, A. (1991). The discovery of antidepressants: a winding path. *Experientia*, **47**, 4–8.

Posener, J.A., DeBattista, C., Williams, G.H., Kraemer, H.C., Kalehzan, B.M. & Schatzberg, A.F. (2000). 24-hour monitoring of cortisol and corticotropin secretion in psychotic and nonpsy-chotic major depression. *Arch. Gen. Psychiatry*, **57**, 755–60.

Post, R.M., Uhde, T.W., Putnam, F.W., Ballenger, J.C. & Berrettini, W.H. (1982). Kindling and carbamazepine in affective illness. *J. Nerv. Ment. Dis.*, **170**, 717–31.

Potter, W.Z., Rudorfer, M.V. & Manji, H. (1991). The pharmacologic treatment of depression. *N. Engl. J. Med.*, **325**, 633–42.

Robinson, R.G. (2000). An 82-year-old woman with mood changes following a stroke. *J. Am. Med. Assoc.*, **283**, 1607–14.

Robinson, R.G. & Szetela, B. (1981). Mood change following left hemispheric brain injury. *Ann. Neurol.*, **9**, 447–53.

Sapolsky, R.M. (1996). Why stress is bad for your brain. *Science*, **273**, 749–50.

Schneider, F., Grodd, W., Weiss, U. et al. (1997). Functional MRI reveals left amygdala activation during emotion. *Psychiatry Res.*, **76**, 75–82.

Sharfstein, S.S., Sack, D.S. & Fauci, A.S. (1982). Relationship between alternate-day corticosteroid therapy and behavioral abnormalities. *J. Am. Med. Assoc.*, **248**, 2987–9.

Shimoda, K. & Robinson, R.G. (1999). The relationship between poststroke depression and lesion location in long-term follow-up. *Biol. Psychiatry*, **45**, 187–92.

Simon, G.E., VonKorff, M. & Barlow, W. (1995). Health care costs of primary care patients with recognized depression. *Arch. Gen. Psychiatry*, **52**, 850–6.

Spiegel, D. (1996). Cancer and depression. *Br. J. Psychiatry. Suppl.*, 109–16.

Stanley, B., Molcho, A., Stanley, M. et al. (2000). Association of aggressive behavior with altered serotonergic function in patients who are not suicidal. *Am. J. Psychiatry*, **157**, 609–14.

Starkstein, S.E., Preziosi, T.J., Forrester, A.W. & Robinson, R.G. (1990). Specificity of affective and autonomic symptoms of depression in Parkinson's disease. *J. Neurol. Neurosurg. Psychiatry*, **53**, 869–73.

Steckler, T., Holsboer, F. & Reul, J.M. (1999). Glucocorticoids and depression. *Baillières Best Pract. Res. Clin. Endocrinol. Metab.*, **13**, 597–614.

Steffens, D.C. & Krishnan, K.R. (1998). Structural neuroimaging and mood disorders: recent findings, implications for classifica-tion, and future directions. *Biol. Psychiatry*, **43**, 705–12.

Strakowski, S.M., Wilson, D.R., Tohen, M., Woods, B.T., Douglass, A.W. & Stoll, A.L. (1993). Structural brain abnormalities in first-episode mania. *Biol. Psychiatry*, **33**, 602–9.

Timpl, P., Spanagel, R., Sillaber, I. et al. (1998). Impaired stress response and reduced anxiety in mice lacking a functional corticotropin-releasing hormone receptor 11. *Nat. Genet.*, **19**, 162–6.

Traskman, L., Asberg, M., Bertilsson, L. & Sjostrand, L. (1981). Monoamine metabolites in CSF and suicidal behavior. *Arch. Gen. Psychiatry*, **38**, 631–6.

Treisman, G., Fishman, M., Schwartz, J., Hutton, H. & Lyketsos, C. (1998). Mood disorders in HIV infection. *Depress. Anxiety*, **7**, 178–87.

Tsuang, M.T. & Faraone, S.V. (1990). *The Genetics of Mood Disorders*, Baltimore, MD: The Johns Hopkins University Press.

Vakili, K., Pillay, S.S., Lafer, B. et al. (2000). Hippocampal volume in primary unipolar major depression: a magnetic resonance imaging study. *Biol. Psychiatry*, **47**, 1087–90.

Wang, H.Y. & Friedman, E. (1999). Effects of lithium on receptor-mediated activation of G proteins in rat brain cortical mem-branes. *Neuropharmacology*, **38**, 403–14.

Wang, J.F., Asghari, V., Rockel, C. & Young, L.T. (1999). Cyclic AMP responsive element binding protein phosphorylation and DNA binding is decreased by chronic lithium but not valproate treatment of SH-SY5Y neuroblastoma cells. *Neuroscience*, **91**, 771–6.

Wiegartz, P., Seidenberg, M., Woodard, A., Gidal, B. & Hermann, B. (1999). Co-morbid psychiatric disorder in chronic epilepsy: rec-ognition and etiology of depression. *Neurology*, **53**, S3–8.

Zung, W.W., Broadhead, W.E. & Roth, M.E. (1993). Prevalence of depressive symptoms in primary care. *J. Fam. Pract.*, **37**, 337–44.

26

Schizophrenia

Paul J. Harrison

University Departments of Psychiatry and Clinical Neurology (Neuropathology), Oxford, UK

Although not the commonest psychiatric disorder, schizophrenia is at the heart of psychiatry. It is also the disorder which has caused most controversy in terms of its nature, its treatment, even its very existence. One particular debate has concerned its organic basis and, indirectly, the extent to which it is a disorder of brain or of mind. As such, schizophrenia, like epilepsy, has exemplified both the bridge and the gulf between neurology and psychiatry. When Kraepelin described the syndrome at the end of the nineteenth century, he persuaded his young colleague Alzheimer to investigate its neuropathology. However, no substantive progress was made and by the middle of the twentieth century the pendulum had swung almost entirely to psychological and sociological views of schizophrenia. The pendulum has swung back over the past 25 years, with convincing evidence of differences in the structure and function of the brain of patients with schizophrenia finally emerging.

Clinical features and epidemiology

Schizophrenia remains a clinical diagnosis, based upon the presence of certain types of delusions and hallucinations (sometimes grouped together as 'first rank symptoms') and thought disorder (Andreasen, 1995). These 'positive' symptoms are often complemented by the 'negative' symptoms of avolition, alogia and affective flattening. The criteria of the *Diagnostic and Statistical Manual of Mental Disorders* (4th edition) (DSM-IV; American Psychiatric Association, 1994) are used for most research studies (Table 26.1); the World Health Organization ICD-10 criteria are similar but require only a 1-month duration. Depending on the balance of symptoms, different subsyndromes are classically recognized: paranoid, hebephrenic (disorganized), catatonic, undifferentiated and simple subtypes. A final clinical domain, neglected until recently, is that there are neuropsychological deficits, with impaired performance across a wide range of memory and language tasks apparent in first episode patients (Bilder et al., 2000) as well as in most long-standing cases (Palmer et al., 1997). Interest in this aspect of schizophrenia has increased with recognition that the cognitive impairments may be a major contributor to poor outcome (Green, 1996).

Schizophrenia can begin at any time from early childhood onwards, with a peak age of onset in the third decade, occurring a few years earlier in men than women. The course and outcome are remarkably variable and unpredictable, but the prognosis is better than sometimes believed. Only a minority have a chronic, deteriorating course, though many others have recurrent or enduring functional deficits, including persistent negative symptoms and the cognitive deficits mentioned. There is a significant excess mortality from suicide and natural causes (Brown, 1997).

The diagnosis of schizophrenia is reliable, but as with any other syndromal diagnosis there are problems establishing its validity, deciding where its boundaries should be drawn, and debate as to whether it is a categorical or dimensional construct. In clinical practice, there are three main differential diagnostic issues. The first is to exclude a neurological or medical disorder producing a schizophrenia-like syndrome; there are many examples, including temporal lobe epilepsy, metachromatic leukodystrophy, Wilson's disease, Huntington's chorea, thyroid disease, and cerebral vasculitis (Lishman, 1998). The second is to identify a drug-induced psychosis; NMDA glutamate receptor antagonists such as phencyclidine (PCP) produce the most schizophrenia-like picture, although psychosis is also associated with amphetamine, cocaine, hallucinogen, and alcohol abuse. In one large study, an organic cause was identifiable in ~6% of people presenting with schizophrenia (Johnstone et al., 1987). Having excluded an organic

Table 26.1. Abbreviated DSM-IV diagnostic criteria for schizophrenia

A. Characteristic symptoms. Two or more of the following, each present for a significant part of a 1-month period:
1) Delusions
2) Hallucinations
3) Disorganized speech (e.g. derailment)
4) Disorganized or catatonic behaviour
5) Negative symptoms (i.e. affective flattening, alogia, avolition)

NB: Only one symptom needed if delusions are bizarre, or if the hallucinations consist of a voice keeping up a running commentary on the person's actions or thoughts, or two or more voices conversing with each other.

B. Functioning. Significant decline in one or more functional areas (work, relationships, self-care)

C. Duration. Continuous signs of disturbance for at least 6 months. (This may include prodromal or residual phases.)

D. Exclusion criteria.
1) Mood disorders or schizoaffective disorder
2) The disturbance is not due to the direct physiological effects of a substance
3) The disturbance is not due to a general medical condition
4) Autism or other pervasive developmental disorder

disorder, schizophrenia must be distinguished from other psychiatric disorders, especially bipolar disorder (manic depression), delusional disorder, schizoaffective disorder and certain personality disorders.

The lifetime risk of schizophrenia is about 0.8%, and is broadly similar across all cultures and countries (Cannon & Jones, 1996). There is an increased risk amongst relatives (e.g. 10% in the child of a schizophrenic parent, and about 40% in a monozygotic cotwin). Twin (Cardno & Gottesman, 2000) and adoption (Ingraham & Kety, 2000) studies show that the familial clustering is largely (if not entirely) due to shared genes not shared environment. Heritability is estimated at 60–90%, with most evidence implicating multiple genes and non-Mendelian inheritance. Several suggestive but small-effect loci have been identified, notably on chromosomes 1p, 5q, 6p, 8p, 13q and 18p (Owen et al., 2000); there is also an association with microdeletions of 22q11 (Bassett & Chow, 1999). Epigenetic factors may also be important (Petronis et al., 1999). There are few established environmental risk factors (McDonald & Murray, 2000), although prenatal events, especially birth complications, confer a small excess risk (Geddes et al., 1999).

Neuropathology

Structural imaging

Key findings

There have now been a large number of CT and MRI studies of the brain in schizophrenia. The cardinal find-

Table 26.2. Macroscopic brain changes in schizophrenia

Established by systematic reviews[1]
- Enlargement of lateral and third ventricles (+25–40%)
- Smaller brain volume (−3%)
- Smaller cortical volume (−4%)
- Smaller cortical grey matter volume (−6%)
- Relatively smaller medial temporal lobe volume (−5%)
- Relatively smaller thalamic volume (−4%)
- Larger basal ganglia (esp. globus pallidus)[2]

Other replicated (though still controversial) findings
- Greater cortical involvement of heteromodal association areas (esp. superior temporal gyrus)
- Decrease (or loss) of cerebral asymmetries

Notes:
[1] Summarized from Ward et al., 1996; Lawrie & Abukmeil, 1998; Nelson et al., 1998; Wright et al., 2000.
[2] Due to antipsychotic medication.

ings are summarised in Table 26.2 (see also Hopkins & Lewis, 2000). There is enlargement of the cerebral ventricles, accompanied by a loss of cortical volume (Ward et al., 1996; Lawrie & Abukmeil, 1998; Wright et al., 2000). Greater reductions occur in temporal lobe, especially medial structures (hippocampus, parahippocampal gyrus and amygdala; Nelson et al., 1998). Cerebral asymmetries may be reduced (Petty, 1999). Subcortical structures have not been well characterized, though there is good evidence for basal ganglia enlargement, especially of the globus pallidus; unlike all the other volume changes, this is due to antipsychotic medication (Harrison, 1999b;

Wright et al., 2000). There is some evidence for smaller thalamic size.

Characteristics of the findings

Monozygotic twins discordant for schizophrenia have provided valuable information. In virtually all pairs, the affected twin has the larger ventricles and smaller cortical and hippocampal size (Suddath et al., 1990). The discordant monozygotic twin study design allows two conclusions to be drawn. First, that structural abnormalities are a consistent finding in schizophrenia, their identification being aided by controlling for other genetic and environmental influences on neuroanatomy. Secondly, that the alterations are associated with expression of the schizophrenia phenotype rather than merely with the underlying shared genotype. Family studies support this interpretation, in that schizophrenics have bigger ventricles and smaller brains than their unaffected relatives. However, relatives who are obligate carriers (i.e. unaffected by schizophrenia but who seem to be transmitting the gene(s)) have larger ventricles than other relatives; moreover, both groups of relatives have larger ventricles and smaller brain structures than control subjects from families without schizophrenia (Harrison, 1999d). These data indicate that a proportion of the structural pathology of schizophrenia may be a marker of genetic liability to the disorder.

Ventricle–brain ratio (VBR) in schizophrenia follows a unimodal distribution, indicating that ventricular enlargement is not restricted to a subgroup but is present to a degree in all cases (Daniel et al., 1991). Conversely, it is important to emphasize that despite the mean group differences there is a significant overlap between subjects with schizophrenia and controls for every structural parameter. Furthermore, none of the established changes are known to be diagnostically specific. Hence the importance of the imaging data is in demonstrating the existence and location of brain pathology in schizophrenia, rather than for clinical purposes.

The structural abnormalities are present in first episode cases, excluding the possibility that they are a consequence of the illness or its treatment. Furthermore, cross-sectional studies show no correlation with duration of illness, suggesting that the alterations are largely static after onset. However, as longitudinal data emerge, the picture is becoming more complicated. First, there is increasing evidence that medial temporal lobe volumes selectively decrease in size during the prodrome and first episode of psychosis. Secondly, some longitudinal studies, spanning up to 10 years, find continuing divergence from controls (DeLisi, 1997) Overall the timing, progression and possible heterogeneity of brain changes in schizophrenia remain controversial, and are important as they bears upon the hypothesised nature of the disease process (see below).

There are few established correlations between brain structure and the symptoms or course of schizophrenia. For example, the expectation that enlarged ventricles might be a correlate of poor outcome has not been consistently demonstrated.

Microscopic and molecular neuropathology

Spurred on by the in vivo imaging evidence that there is a pathology of schizophrenia to be found, contemporary histological studies have addressed two main areas. First, to clarify the frequency and nature of neurodegenerative abnormalities in schizophrenia. Secondly, to investigate the cellular organization (cytoarchitecture) of the cerebral cortex and limbic system.

Gliosis

The issue of gliosis (reactive astrocytosis) has been extensively investigated since a report that gliosis was common in schizophrenia, especially in the diencephalon around the third ventricle (Stevens, 1982) . As gliosis is a sign of past inflammation, this implicated etiopathogenic scenarios for schizophrenia involving infective, ischemic, autoimmune, or neurodegenerative processes. However, over a dozen subsequent investigations have not found gliosis, and the consensus is now that gliosis is not a feature of schizophrenia (Roberts & Harrison, 2000). The issue has considerable implications. The gliotic response is said not to begin until the end of the second trimester in utero, and hence an absence of gliosis is taken as *prima facie* evidence of a disease process occurring before this time. Unfortunately, both the absence of gliosis, and its interpretation, are less clear than often assumed. Firstly, detecting gliosis is surprisingly difficult, and it can be argued that the data do not wholly rule out its occurrence. Secondly, despite the widely cited time point at which the glial response is said to begin, the matter has not been well investigated and it is prudent not to use this to time the pathology of schizophrenia with spurious accuracy. Furthermore, it is a moot point whether the subtle kinds of morphometric disturbance described in schizophrenia, whenever and however they occurred, would be sufficient to trigger detectable gliosis.

Alzheimer's disease in schizophrenia

It is sometimes claimed that Alzheimer's disease is commoner than expected in schizophrenia (perhaps on the assumption that it explains the high prevalence of cognitive impairment in elderly patients). However, a meta-analysis shows that this is false (Baldessarini et al., 1997), a conclusion which even applies in elderly schizophrenics with severe dementia, who show no evidence of any other neurodegenerative disorder either (Arnold et al., 1998). As such, the cognitive impairment of schizophrenia is unexplained. It may be a more severe manifestation of whatever substrate underlies schizophrenia, or it may be that the brain in schizophrenia is more vulnerable to cognitive impairment in response to a normal age-related amount of neurodegeneration.

Neural cytoarchitecture in schizophrenia

If neurodegenerative abnormalities are uncommon in, or epiphenomenal to, schizophrenia, it begs the question as to what *is* the pathology and how the macroscopic findings are explained microscopically. The answer has been sought in the cytoarchitecture of the cerebral cortex, with measurements of parameters such as the size, location, distribution and packing density of neurons and their synaptic connections (Table 26.3).

Three cytoarchitectural alterations have generated particular interest: abnormal neuronal organization (dysplasia) in the entorhinal cortex, disarray of hippocampal neurons, and an altered distribution of neurons in the subcortical white matter. These findings are important because they support the hypothesis of an early neurodevelopmental anomaly underlying schizophrenia. However, none have been unequivocally and independently replicated, and for each there is at least one non-replication (for references see Harrison, 1999a).

A less well-known yet seemingly more robust cytoarchitectural feature of schizophrenia is that many neurons are smaller (i.e. have a reduced cell body area or volume). This has been shown in three studies of pyramidal neurons in the hippocampus, and has also been reported in dorsolateral prefrontal cortex and for cerebellar Purkinje cells. Some studies find that neurons are also more closely packed. Outside the cerebral cortex, extensive cytoarchitectural data are limited to the thalamus, for which there are reports of a loss of neurons from the dorsomedial and anterior nuclei, though the matter remains controversial.

In summary, a range of differences in neuronal structure and organization have been reported to occur in schizophrenia (Table 26.3). The abnormalities sometimes taken to be characteristic of the disorder, V12 disarray, displacement and paucity of hippocampal and cortical neurons, are features which in fact have not been well demonstrated. This undermines attempts to date the pathology of schizophrenia to the second trimester in utero based on their presence (see below).

Table 26.3. Histological findings in schizophrenia

	Weight of evidence
Lack of neurodegenerative lesions (e.g. Alzheimer changes)	+++++
Lack of gliosis	++++
Smaller cortical and hippocampal pyramidal neurons	+++
Decreased cortical and hippocampal synaptic markers	+++
Decreased dendritic spine density	+++
Loss of neurons from dorsal thalamus	++
Abnormalities of white matter neurons	+
Entorhinal cortex dysplasia	+
Disarray of hippocampal neuron orientation	(±)
Loss of hippocampal or cortical neurons	0

Notes:

0: no good evidence. ±: equivocal data. + to +++++: increasing amount of supportive data.

Source: For detailed review and citations, see Harrison (1999a).

Studies of synapses and dendrites

Synapses and dendrites represent a potential site for pathology undetectable using standard approaches. Because they are hard to visualise directly, proteins localised to these parts of the neuron are used as markers for them (Honer et al., 2000).

Markers of presynaptic terminals are generally reduced in the hippocampus in schizophrenia. The magnitude of the loss varies according to the individual synaptic proteins (and hippocampal subfields) studied, implying that the synaptic pathology is not uniform. There is some evidence for preferential decrements in excitatory connections, in keeping with the indications of glutamatergic involvement mentioned above. Presynaptic markers are also reduced in prefrontal cortex, though in this region a subset of inhibitory neurons and terminals appears most affected (Lewis, 1997). Complementing these changes, a decreased density of dendritic spines has been seen in three studies (Glantz & Lewis, 2000). Although unproven, the usual and simplest interpretation is that these changes reflect fewer (or otherwise aberrant) synaptic contacts being formed and received.

Integrating the neuronal and synaptic findings

There is an encouraging convergence between neuronal and synaptic findings in schizophrenia. In particular, the decreases in presynaptic and dendritic markers are in keeping with the smaller neuronal cell bodies, since the size of the latter is proportional to the dendritic and axonal

Table 26.4. Major transmitter systems implicated in schizophrenia

Transmitter	Main supporting evidence
Dopamine (DA)	DA-releasing agents produce psychosis
	All antipsychotic drugs are DA (D_2 receptor) antagonists
	Postmortem: Increased levels of D_2 receptors and loss of cortical DA innervation
	In vivo: Increased basal and amphetamine-stimulated striatal DA levels
Glutamate	NMDA receptor antagonists produce a schizophrenia-like psychosis
	Postmortem: altered presynaptic glutamate, NMDA and non-NMDA receptors
	Partial NMDA receptor agonists (e.g. cycloserine) have some therapeutic benefit
	Roles of NMDA receptors in development and neurotoxicity
5-HT (Serotonin)	5-HT_2 agonists (e.g. LSD) are psychotomimetic
	Postmortem: Altered cortical 5-HT_{1A} and 5-HT_{2A} receptors
	5-HT_2 receptor polymorphisms associated with schizophrenia and clozapine response
	Atypical antipsychotics have high affinity for several 5-HT receptors
	Developmental and trophic roles of 5-HT
GABA	Postmortem: loss of cortical GABAergic cells, receptors, and synaptic markers

spread of the neuron. It is also consistent with the findings of increased neuronal density, in that dendrites and synapses are the major component of the neuropil and, if this is reduced, neurons will pack more closely together (Selemon & Goldman-Rakic, 1999). Moreover, it also corresponds with the results of proton magnetic resonance studies which have shown reductions of the neuronal marker *N*-acetyl-aspartate (NAA), as one would predict if the neurons are on average smaller and have less extensive projections (Bertolino et al., 1998).

Postmortem studies are limited to chronic schizophrenia, so it is impossible to prove that cytoarchitectural abnormalities are not the result of the illness or its treatment. However, several lines of evidence suggest that this is not the case. First, as the structural brain abnormalities and lower NAA signals occur in unmedicated and first-episode schizophrenia, it is reasonable to assume that the cytoarchitectural differences are also present then. Secondly, no correlations with duration of disease or medication exposure have been seen in postmortem studies. Thirdly, although antipsychotic treatment does have morphological consquences, the effects are largely restricted to the basal ganglia (Harrison, 1999b).

Where and what is the pathology?

Most of the positive findings reported in schizophrenia are in the hippocampal formation, dorsolateral prefrontal cortex and cingulate gyrus. However, this may be merely a sign that these areas have been the most intensively studied. Few studies have included a comparison region (e.g. striate cortex) and those which do not provide a clear picture as to the uniformity vs. selectivity of cerebral

involvement in schizophrenia. Neither are any of the individual histological abnormalities specific or pathological in the sense that a neurofibrillary tangle or Lewy body is. Rather, at present the favoured interpretation of the structural pathology as a whole is that it is a quantitative deviation of normal neuronal parameters, probably arising during development and putatively affecting functional connectivity between various brain regions. These hypotheses are elaborated below. However, it is important to remain critical of the empirical data, which could equally lead to the conclusion that, though brain structure is clearly altered in schizophrenia, its location, nature, origins, and consequences remain unknown.

Pathophysiology

Neurochemistry and neuropharmacology

A wide range of neurochemical parameters have been investigated in schizophrenia, both postmortem (Reynolds, 1995) and in vivo (Bigliani & Pilowsky, 1999; Soares & Inins, 1999), and a diverse collection of abnormalities reported. These especially affect monoamine and amino-acid neurotransmitter systems (Table 26.4).

Dopamine

The dopamine hypothesis of schizophrenia has been pre-eminent for over 30 years (Bennett, 1998). It proposes that the symptoms of schizophrenia result from dopaminergic overactivity, whether due to excess dopamine, or to an elevated sensitivity to it, e.g. because of increased numbers of dopamine receptors. The hypothesis originated with the discovery that effective antipsychotics were dopamine (D_2) receptor antagonists, and that dopamine-releasing agents such as amphetamine produce a paranoid psychosis. It received support from various postmortem findings of increased dopamine content and higher densities of D_2 receptors in schizophrenia. However, despite its longevity it has proven difficult to refine or refute the hypothesis, for two reasons. First, because antipsychotics have marked effects on the dopamine system, confounding all studies of medicated subjects, hence making postmortem studies problematic. Secondly, molecular biology has revealed a large and complex dopamine receptor family, increasing the potential sites and mechanisms of dysfunction.

Much attention has focused on D_2 receptors. Overall, the studies show an increased density in schizophrenia, but it has been difficult to distinguish what proportion of this is not attributable to antipsychotic medication (Zakzanis & Hansen, 1998). Most PET studies of unmedicated patients have not shown a change in D_2 receptors. However, recent evidence suggests that there may in fact be a genuine increase of D_2 receptors in schizophrenia, the uncertainty being due to methodological issues and perhaps an altered receptor conformation (Seeman & Kapur, 2000). Altered expression of D_1 and D_3 receptors has also been reported but this is either unconfirmed or contradicted by other studies. Particular controversy has surrounded the D_4 receptor, following a report that it was up-regulated several fold in schizophrenia; it has also been a candidate receptor to explain the unique therapeutic profile of the atypical antipsychotic drug clozapine. However the result appears to have been due to a 'D_4-like site' not the true D_4 receptor, and the status of the latter in schizophrenia is unknown (see Harrison, 1999c).

In contrast to the equivocal evidence about dopamine receptors, strong evidence for a functional abnormality of dopamine neurons in schizophrenia is emerging. Several PET and SPET studies have shown elevated striatal dopamine release in response to amphetamine, implying a dysregulation and hyper-responsiveness of dopamine neurons (Laruelle & Abi-Dargham, 1999). Importantly, the dopamine release abnormality is present in untreated patients, and is only present during an acute episode, suggesting that a hyperdopaminergic state may underlie the florid, positive symptoms – dopamine as the 'wind for the psychotic fire' (Laruelle & Abi-Dargham, 1999). Dopamine synthesis may also be increased (Lindström et al., 1999). Finally, a new study shows that dopamine levels and D_2 receptor occupancy are elevated in schizophrenia (Abi-Dargham et al., 2000), providing the best evidence yet for an underlying hyperdopaminergia in the disorder (Harrison, 2000). The position of dopaminergic abnormalities in the pathogenesis of schizophrenia is unknown, though one model envisages them as a consequence of a developmental pathophysiology affecting corticostriatal connections (Grace, 2000).

5-HT (Serotonin)

Suggestions of 5-HT involvement in schizophrenia arose because the hallucinogen lysergic acid diethylamide (LSD) is a 5-HT agonist. Recently, interest has focussed on the 5-HT_{2A} receptor (Harrison, 1999c). A high affinity for the receptor may explain the therapeutic advantages of atypical antipsychotics, and variants in the gene are a minor risk factor for schizophrenia and for non-response to the antipsychotic drug clozapine. Many studies have found lowered 5-HT_{2A} receptor expression in frontal cortex in schizophrenia, and there is a blunted neuroendocrine response to 5-HT_2 agonists. Elevated cortical 5-HT_{1A} receptors are also a replicated finding. Hypotheses to explain the role of 5-HT in schizophrenia include the trophic functions of the 5-HT system in neurodevelopment, interactions between 5-HT and dopamine neurons, and impaired 5-HT_{2A} receptor-mediated activation of prefrontal cortex (Kapur & Remington, 1996).

Glutamate

The observation that phencyclidine and other non-competitive antagonists of the NMDA subtype of glutamate receptor produce a psychosis resembling schizophrenia has driven hypotheses of glutamatergic dysfunction in the disorder. There is now some evidence in schizophrenia itself to support this proposal. For example, in medial temporal lobe, glutamatergic markers are decreased, with reduced expression of non-NMDA glutamate receptors (Meador-Woodruff & Healy, 2000). However, a different pattern is seen in other brain regions and affecting other glutamate receptor subtypes, precluding any simple conclusion. Mechanisms proposed to explain glutamatergic involvement in schizophrenia centre on its interactions with dopamine, and subtle forms of glutamate-mediated neurotoxicity (Tamminga, 1998).

Cerebral metabolic activity

Cerebral metabolism in schizophrenia has been extensively investigated using PET to measure regional cerebral blood flow (rCBF) and glucose utilization. SPET and fMRI have been applied as well (Du & McGuire, 1999).

Hypofrontality has been the most widely reported abnormality. Initially it was thought to be a reliable feature of schizophrenia, present in the resting state. However, whilst hypofrontality does occur in unmedicated subjects, it is not invariable, being seen most clearly when subjects are performing tasks which require activation of the frontal lobes (Andreasen et al., 1997; Spence et al., 1998). The interpretation of hypofrontality is still debated, notably the causality of its relationship to the undoubted impairment of schizophrenics on prefrontal working memory tasks (Weinberger & Berman, 1996).

The most comprehensive analysis correlating regional cerebral activity with clinical features is by Liddle and colleagues, who showed that the three subsyndromes of chronic schizophrenia which they had previously identified have characteristic patterns of rCBF (Liddle, 1996). For example, subjects with psychomotor poverty (a concept allied to negative symptoms) are hypofrontal whereas those with prominent positive symptoms have increased rCBF in the temporal lobe, especially in the hippocampus. Other studies show that the latter region does not activate normally during cognitive tasks, and that superior temporal gyrus activity has a relationship with auditory hallucinations.

Neurophysiology

Two aspects of sensorimotor functioning in schizophrenia are relevant to its neurobiology. First, sensory evoked potentials are altered. In particular, the P300 component is reduced and delayed in response to auditory stimuli, indicative of impaired sensory processing and further implicating the temporal lobes (Ford, 1999). The P300 alterations are also a trait marker of genetic vulnerability to schizophrenia (Blackwood, 2000). Secondly, there is a high rate of eye movement abnormalities in schizophrenia (Hutton & Kennard, 1998), especially affecting smooth pursuit tracking, suggesting impairment in the pathways subserving oculomotor control.

Together, the neurochemical, functional imaging and neurophysiological data illustrate the range and complexity of cerebral dysfunction which occurs in schizophrenia. Like the structural findings, they point to widespread abnormalities which cannot be reduced to a single locus or transmitter system. These uncertainties lead on to consideration of the two main pathogenic neurobiological theories of schizophrenia: as a disorder of neurodevelopment, and as a disorder of neural connectivity.

Pathogenic theories

Schizophrenia as a neurodevelopmental disorder

The neurodevelopmental model of schizophrenia in essence states that the disorder is due to abnormalities during maturation of the brain. It has become the prevail-

Table 26.5. Evidence for a neurodevelopmental origin of schizophrenia

- Structural brain changes present at or before onset of symptoms, and largely static thereafter
- No gliosis or other pathological signs of progressive or degenerative disease process
- Environmental risk factors are mostly pre- and perinatal
- Neurological, social and intellectual abnormalities seen in preschizophrenic children
- Increased prevalence of minor physical anomalies and abnormal fingerprint patterns, suggestive of intrauterine growth disturbance
- Increased prevalence of septum cavum pellucidum

ing pathogenic hypothesis (see Weinberger, 1995; Harrison, 1997; Waddington et al., 1999). A range of evidence is adduced in support of it (Table 26.5).

A 'strong' version of the theory is that the pathology of schizophrenia originates in the second trimester in utero. An earlier timing is excluded since overt brain abnormalities would be seen if neurogenesis were affected, whilst the lack of gliosis is taken to mean that the changes must have occurred prior to the third trimester. However, this form of the neurodevelopmental model is weak on two neuropathological grounds. First, because of the limitations of the absence-of-gliosis argument mentioned earlier. Secondly, the types of cytoarchitectural disturbance adduced in favour (neuronal disarray and malpositioning) are those suggestive of aberrant neuronal migration, a process which occurs at the appropriate gestational period. Yet, as mentioned (Table 26.3), these cytoarchitectural abnormalities have not been unequivocally shown to be present in schizophrenia. By comparison, the seemingly more robust cytoarchitectural findings (e.g. alterations in neuronal size, synapses and dendrites) could originate much later, such parameters being modifiable throughout life.

Other forms of the neurodevelopmental theory advocate a much wider and later time frame and include many maturational processes (e.g. cell adhesion, apoptosis, myelination and synaptic pruning), or suggest that it applies only to a subgroup of cases, or that neurotoxic processes are involved as well (DeLisi, 1997; Lieberman, 1999). Overall, a parsimonious view is that the data are indicative merely of an essentially developmental, as opposed to degenerative, disease process, rather than as pointing to a particular mechanism or timing. A simplified illustration of the neurodevelopmental model is shown in Figure 26.1.

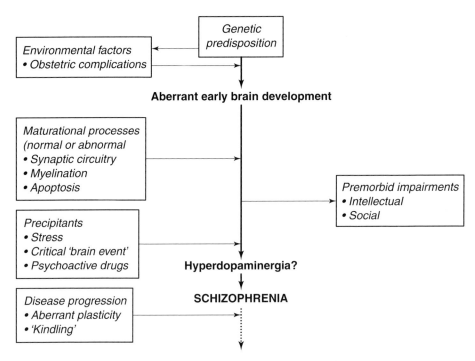

Fig. 26.1. Schematic representation of the neurodevelopmental model of schizoprenia.

Schizophrenia as a disorder of neural connectivity

Bleuler, who coined the term schizophrenia 90 years ago, proposed that the key symptoms are those of 'psychic splitting'. This view now has its counterpart in theories of aberrant functional connectivity between brain regions as the putative mechanism of psychosis (McGuire & Frith, 1996). One model advocates involvement of a circuit between frontal cortex, thalamus, striatum and cerebellum (Andreasen, 1999); another implicates fronto-temporal cortical connections. The conceptual and empirical basis for these proposals originated mainly in the functional imaging studies which show different patterns of activation and deactivation in schizophrenics. The cytoarchitectural features of schizophrenia described above may represent the neuroanatomical basis of this aberrant functional connectivity (Harrison, 1999a).

Treatment

The mainstay of schizophrenia treatment continues to be antipsychotic medication, which is effective in treating acute episodes in 60–70% of patients, and which markedly reduced relapse rates during maintenance therapy (Kane, 1999). However, the drugs cause many and severe side effects, and they have at most minimal efficacy against negative symptoms, depressive symptoms or cognitive deficits. The only drug which is unequivocally more effective than other antipsychotics is clozapine (Wahlbeck et al., 1999), and it is also free of extrapyramidal side effects. Unfortunately, its use is restricted because of the risk of agranulocytosis and the consequent need for regular blood tests.

Clozapine is the prototypical 'atypical' antipsychotic. The term was originally applied to drugs which in rodents were predictive of antipsychotic efficacy but which did not produce catalepsy; it is now often used just to refer to all recently introduced antipsychotics. The main controversy in schizophrenia therapy is whether these new drugs are, like clozapine, more effective and/or cause fewer side effects than conventional antipsychotics. A recent systematic review concluded that atypical antipsychotics as a group (other than clozapine) do cause less extrapyramidal side-effects, but their overall efficacy and tolerability is not clearly superior (Geddes et al., 2000). However, the trials have not adequately examined other outcomes, such as cognitive functioning, suicide rates, quality of life, and rates of tardive dyskinesia; it may well be in these domains that the atypical antipsychotics have their main advantages (e.g. Purdon et al., 2000).

Psychosocial treatments are an integral aspect of management (McGrath & Emmerson, 1999). Family interventions, cognitive therapy aimed at residual psychotic symptoms, and psychological therapy to increase medication compliance have all been shown to be effective (Huxley et al., 2000). In many countries, most patients are looked after by multidisciplinary mental health teams, which in addition to psychiatrists, psychologists and psychiatric nurses include social workers, occupational therapists and others. This range of skills and input is necessary given the range of difficulties and needs which many patients with schizophrenia have.

As yet, there have been few clear therapeutic improvements arising from the various advances in understanding schizophrenia, and the complexity of the disorder makes incremental progress more likely than fundamental advances in the near future. However, there are noteworthy efforts under way, such as trials to enhance glutamatergic functioning (Goff et al., 1999), early intervention to improve outcome (Birchwood et al., 1997) and even discussions about prevention (Tsuang et al., 2000).

In conclusion, considerable progress has been made in revealing the relationship between schizophrenia and the brain. Twenty-five years ago, even the existence of this relationship was doubted (Weinberger, 1995). Nevertheless, there has been no critical breakthrough in terms of identifying a specific biochemical or pathological marker for the disorder, nor a causative gene, and hence the understanding remains in many ways rudimentary. Equally, treatment continues to rely on dopamine-blocking antipsychotic drugs and complementary psychosocial interventions. Currently attention is focused on providing stronger evidence as to the origins and precise details of the molecular neurobiology which underlies this complex and heterogeneous syndrome.

References   * denotes key references

*Abi-Dargham, A., Rodenheiser, J., Printz, D. et al. (2000). Increased baseline occupancy of D_2 receptors by dopamine in schizophrenia. *Proc. Natl. Acad. Sci., USA*, **97**, 8104–9.

American Psychiatric Association (1994). *Diagnostic and Statistical Manual of Mental Disorders*, 4th edn. Washington, DC: American Psychiatric Association.

Andreasen, N.C. (1995). Symptoms, signs, and diagnosis of schizophrenia. *Lancet*, **346**, 477–81.

*Andreasen, N.C. (1999). A unitary model of schizophrenia – Bleuler's 'fragmented phrene' as schizencephaly. *Arch. Gen. Psychiatry*, **56**, 781–7.

Andreasen, N.C., O'Leary, D.S., Flaum, M. et al. (1997). Hypofrontality in schizophrenia: distributed dysfunctional circuits in neuroleptic-naive patients. *Lancet*, **349**, 1730–4.

Arnold, S.E., Trojanowski, J.Q., Gur, R.E., Blackwell, P., Han, L.Y. & Choi, C. (1998). Absence of neurodegeneration and neural injury in the cerebral cortex in a sample of elderly patients with schizophrenia. *Arch. Gen. Psychiat.*, **55**, 225–32.

Baldessarini, R.J., Hegarty, J.D., Bird, E.D. & Benes, F.M. (1997). Meta-analysis of postmortem studies of Alzheimer's disease-like neuropathology in schizophrenia. *Am. J. Psychiatry*, **154**, 861–3.

Bassett, A.S. & Chow, E.W.C. (1999). 22q11 deletion syndrome: A genetic subtype of schizophrenia. *Biol. Psychiatry*, **46**, 882–91.

Bennett, M.R. (1998). Monoaminergic synapses and schizophrenia: 45 years of neuroleptics. *J. Psychopharmacol.*, **12**, 289–304.

Bertolino, A., Callicott, J.H., Elman, I. et al. (1998). Regionally specific neuronal pathology in untreated patients with schizophrenia: A proton magnetic resonance spectroscopic imaging study. *Biol. Psychiatry*, **43**, 641–8.

Bigliani, V. & Pilowsky, L.S. (1999). *In vivo* neuropharmacology of schizophrenia. *Br. J. Psychiatry*, **174** (Suppl. 38), 23–33.

Bilder, R.M., Goldman, R.S., Robinson, D. et al. (2000). Neuropsychology of first-episode schizophrenia. Initial characterisation and clinical correlates. *Am. J. Psychiatry*, **157**, 549–59.

Birchwood, M., McGorry, P. & Jackson, H. (1997). Early intervention in schizophrenia. *Br. J. Psychiatry*, **170**, 2–5

Blackwood, D. (2000). P300, a state and a trait marker in schizophrenia. *Lancet*, **355**, 771–2.

Brown, S. (1997). Excess mortality of schizophrenia – a meta-analysis. *Br. J. Psychiatry*, **171**, 502–8.

*Cannon, M. & Jones, P. (1996). Schizophrenia. *J. Neurol., Neurosurg. Psychiatry*, **60**, 604–13.

Cardno, A.G. & Gottesman, I. (2000). Twin studies of schizophrenia: from bow-and-arrow concordances to Star Wars Mx and functional genomics. *Am. J. Med. Genet.*, **97**, 12–17.

Daniel, D.G., Goldberg, T.E., Gibbons, R.D. & Weinberger, D.R. (1991). Lack of a bimodal distribution of ventricular size in schizophrenia: a Gaussian mixture analysis of 1056 cases and controls. *Biol. Psychiatry*, **30**, 887–903.

DeLisi, L. (1997). Is schizophrenia a lifetime disorder of brain plasticity, growth and aging? *Schizophrenia Res.*, **23**, 119–29

Du, C.H.Y. & McGuire, P.K. (1999). Functional neuroimaging in psychiatry. *Phil. Trans. Roy. Soc. Lond. (Biol.)*, **354**, 1359–70.

Ford, J.M. (1999). Schizophrenia: the broken P300 and beyond. *Psychophysiology*, **36**, 667–82.

Geddes, J.R., Verdoux, H., Takei, N. et al. (1999). Schizophrenia and complications of pregnancy and labor: An individual patient data meta-analysis. *Schizophrenia Bull.*, **25**, 413–23.

Geddes, J., Freemantle, N., Harrison, P., Bebbington, P. for the National Schizophrenia Guideline Development Group. (2000). Atypical antipsychotics in the treatment of schizophrenia: systematic overview and meta-regression analysis. *Br. Med. J.*, **321**, 1371–6.

Glantz, L.A. & Lewis, D.A. (2000). Decreased dendritic spine density on prefrontal cortical pyramidal neurons in schizophrenia. *Arch. Gen. Psychiatry*, **57**, 65–73.

Goff, D.C., Tsai, G., Levitt, J. et al (1999). A placebo-controlled trial of D-cycloserine added to conventional neuroleptics in patients with schizophrenia. *Arch. Gen. Psychiatry*, **56**, 21–7.

Grace, A.A. (2000). Gating of information flow within the limbic system and the pathophysiology of schizophrenia. *Brain Res. Rev.*, **31**, 330–41.

Green, M.F. (1996). What are the functional consequences of neurocognitive deficits in schizophrenia? *Am. J. Psychiatry*, **153**, 321–30.

Harrison, P.J. (1997). Schizophrenia: a disorder of neurodevelopment? *Curr. Opin. Neurobiol.*, **7**, 285–9.

*Harrison, P.J. (1999a). The neuropathology of schizophrenia: a critical review of the data and their interpretation. *Brain*, **122**, 493–524.

Harrison, P.J. (1999b). The neuropathological effects of antipsychotic drugs. *Schizophrenia Res.*, **40**, 87–99.

Harrison, P.J. (1999c). Neurochemical alterations in schizophrenia affecting the putative receptor targets of atypical antipsychotics – focus on dopamine (D_1, D_3, D_4) and 5-HT_{2a} receptors. *Br. J. Psychiatry*, **174** (Suppl. 38), 12–22.

Harrison, P.J. (1999d). Brains at risk of schizophrenia. *Lancet*, **353**, 3–4.

Harrison, P.J. (2000). Dopamine and schizophrenia – proof at last? *Lancet*, **356**, 958–9.

Honer, W.G., Young, C. & Falkai, P. (2000). Synaptic pathology. In *The Neuropathology of Schizophrenia. Progress and Interpretation*, ed. P.J. Harrison & G.W. Roberts, pp. 105–36. Oxford: Oxford University Press.

Hopkins, R. & Lewis, S. (2000). Structural imaging findings and macroscopic pathology. In *The Neuropathology of Schizophrenia. Progress and Interpretation*, ed. P.J. Harrison & G.W. Roberts, pp. 5–55. Oxford: Oxford University Press.

Hutton, S. & Kennard, C. (1998). Oculomotor abnormalities in schizophrenia – a critical review. *Neurology*, **50**, 604–9.

Huxley, N.A., Rendall, M. & Sederer, L. (2000). Psychosocial treatments in schizophrenia – a review of the past 20 years. *J. Nervous Mental Dis.*, **188**, 187–201.

Ingraham, L.J. & Kety, S.S .(2000). Adoption studies of schizophrenia. *Am. J. Med. Genet.*, **97**, 18–22.

Johnstone, E.C., Macmillan, F. & Crow, T.J. (1987). The occurrence of organic disease of possible or probable aetiological significance in a population of 268 cases of first episode schizophrenia. *Psychol. Med.*,**17**, 371–9.

*Kane, J.M. (1999). Pharmacologic treatment of schizophrenia. *Biol. Psychiatry*, **46**, 1396–408.

Kapur, S. & Remington, G. (1996). Serotonin–dopamine interaction and its relevance to schizophrenia. *Am. J. Psychiatry*, **153**, 466–76.

*Laruelle, M. & Abi-Dargham, A. (1999). Dopamine as the wind of the psychotic fire: new evidence from brain imaging studies. *J. Psychopharmacol.*, **13**, 358–71.

Lawrie, S.M. & Abukmeil, S.S. (1998). Brain abnormality in schizophrenia – a systematic and quantitative review of volumetric magnetic resonance imaging studies. *Br. J. Psychiatry*, **172**, 110–20.

Lewis, D.A. (1997). Development of the prefrontal cortex during

adolescence: insights into vulnerable neural circuits in schizophrenia. *Neuropsychopharmacology*, **16**, 385–98.

Liddle, P.F. (1996). Functional imaging – schizophrenia. *Br. Med. Bull.*, **52**, 486–94.

Lieberman, J.A. (1999). Is schizophrenia a neurodegenerative disorder? A clinical and neurobiological perspective. *Biol. Psychiatry*, **46**, 729–39.

Lindström, L.H., Gefvert, O., Hagberg, G. et al. (1999). Increased dopamine synthesis rate in medial prefrontal cortex and striatum in schizophrenia indicated by L-(β-^{11}C)DOPA and PET. *Biol. Psychiatry*, **46**, 681–8.

Lishman, W.A. (1998). *Organic Psychiatry. The Psychological Consequences of Cerebral Disorder*, 3rd edn. Oxford: Blackwell Science, p. 922.

*McDonald, C. & Murray, R.M. (2000). Early and late developmental risk factors for schizophrenia. *Brain Res. Rev.*, **31**, 130–7.

McGrath, J. & Emmerson, W.B. (1999). Treatment of schizophrenia. *Br. Med. J.*, **319**, 1045–8.

*McGuire, P.K. & Frith, C.D. (1996). Disordered functional connectivity in schizophrenia. *Psychol. Med.*, **26**, 663–7.

Meador-Woodruff, J. & Healy, D. (2000). Glutamate receptor expression in schizophrenic brain. *Brain Res. Rev.*, **31**, 288–94.

Nelson, M.D., Saykin, A.J., Flashman, L.A. & Riordan, H.J. (1998). Hippocampal volume reduction in schizophrenia as assessed by magnetic resonance imaging – a meta-analytic study. *Arch. Gen. Psychiatry*, **55**, 433–40.

Owen, M.J., Cardno, A.G. & O'Donovan, M.C. (2000). Psychiatric genetics: back to the future. *Mol. Psychiatry*, **5**, 22–31.

Palmer, B.W., Heaton, R.K., Paulsen, J.S. et al. (1997). Is it possible to be schizophrenic and neuropsychologically normal? *Neuropsychology*, **11**, 437–47.

Petronis, A., Paterson, A.D. & Kennedy, J.L. (1999). Schizophrenia: An epigenetic puzzle? *Schizophrenia Bull.*, **25**, 639–55.

Petty, R.G. (1999). Structural asymmetries of the human brain and their disturbance in schizophrenia. *Schizophrenia Bull.*, **25**, 121–39.

Purdon, S.E., Jones, B.D.W., Stip, E., Labelle, A., Addington, D., David, S.R., Breier, A. & Tollefson, G.D. (2000). Neuropsychological change in early phase schizophrenia during 12 months of treatment with olanzapine, risperidone, or haloperidol. *Arch. Gen. Psychiatry*, **57**, 249–58.

Reynolds, G.P. (1995). Neurotransmitter systems in schizophrenia. *Int. Rev. Neurobiol.*, **38**, 305–39.

Roberts, G.W. & Harrison, P.J. (2000). Gliosis and its implications for the disease process. In *The Neuropathology of Schizophrenia. Progress and Interpretation*, ed. P.J. Harrison & G.W. Roberts, pp. 137–50. Oxford: Oxford University Press.

Seeman, P. & Kapur, S. (2000). Schizophrenia: more dopamine, more D2 receptors. *Proc. Natl. Acad. Sci., USA*, **97**, 7673–5.

*Selemon, L.D. & Goldman-Rakic, P.S. (1999). The reduced neuropil hypothesis: a circuit based model of schizophrenia. *Biol. Psychiatry*, **45**, 17–25.

*Soares, J.C. & Innis, R. (1999). Neurochemical brain imaging investigations of schizophrenia. *Biol. Psychiatry*, **46**, 600–16.

Spence, S.A., Hirsch, S.R., Brooks, D.J. & Grasby, P.M. (1998).

Prefrontal cortex activity in people with schizophrenia and control subjects. Evidence from positron emission tomography for remission of 'hypofrontality' with recovery from acute schizophrenia. *Br. J. Psychiatry*, 172, 316–23.

Stevens, J.R. (1982). Neuropathology of schizophrenia. *Arch. Gen. Psychiatry*, **39**, 1131–9.

Suddath, R.L., Christison, G.W., Torrey, E.F., Casanova, M.F. & Weinberger, D.R. (1990). Anatomical abnormalities in the brains of monozygotic twins discordant for schizophrenia. *N. Engl. J. Med.*, **322**, 789–94.

Tamminga, C.A. (1998). Schizophrenia and glutamatergic transmission. *Crit. Rev. Neurobiol.*, **12**, 21–36.

Tsuang, M.T., Stone, W.S. & Faraone, S.V. (2000). Towards the prevention of schizophrenia. *Biol. Psychiatry*, **48**, 349–56.

Waddington, J.L., Lane, A., Larkin, C. & O'Callaghan, E. (1999). The neurodevelopmental basis of schizophrenia: clinical clues from craniofacial dysmorphogenesis, and the roots of a lifetime trajectory of disease. *Biol. Psychiatry*, **46**, 31–9.

Wahlbeck, K., Cheine, M., Essali, A. & Adams, C. (1999). Evidence of clozapine's effectiveness in schizophrenia. A systematic review and meta-analysis of randomized trials. *Am. J. Psychiatry*, **156**, 990–9.

Ward, K.E., Friedman, L., Wise, A. & Schulz, S.C. (1996). Meta-analysis of brain and cranial size in schizophrenia. *Schizophrenia Res.*, **22**, 197–213.

*Weinberger, D.R. (1995). Schizophrenia. From neuropathology to neurodevelopment. *Lancet*, **346**, 552–7.

Weinberger, D.R. & Berman, K.F. (1996). Prefrontal function in schizophrenia: confounds and controversies. *Phil. Trans. Roy. Soc. Lond. (Biol.)*, **351**, 1495–503.

*Wright, I.C., Rabe-Hesketh, S., Woodruff, P.W.R., David, A.S., Murray, R.M. & Bullmore, E.T. (2000). Meta-analysis of regional brain volumes in schizophrenia. *Am. J. Psychiatry*, **157**, 16–24

Zakzanis, K.K. & Hansen, K.T. (1998). Dopamine D2 receptor densities and the schizophrenic brain. *Schizophrenia Res.*, **32**, 201–6.

27

Obsessive–compulsive disorder

Bavanisha Vythilingum,[1] Dan J. Stein[1] and Scott L. Rauch[2]

[1]MRC Anxiety Disorders Unit, Department of Psychiatry, University of Stellenbosch, Cape Town, South Africa
[2]Department of Psychiatry, Massachusetts General Hospital and Harvard University, Boston, MA, USA

Introduction

Obsessive–compulsive behaviour has long been described; religious scrupulosity is documented in medieval texts (Adams, 1973), repetitive hand washing as symbolic of guilt has been depicted by playwrights (Shakespeare: Macbeth) and 'obsessive–compulsive neurosis' generated by unconscious conflict was a cornerstone of psychodynamic theory (Freud, 1973). More recently, however, a new paradigm has emerged; obsessive–compulsive behaviour is now viewed as symptomatic of a highly prevalent medical disorder, characterized by specific psychobiological dysfunctions. Indeed, obsessive–compulsive disorder (OCD) is arguably one of the most incisive exemplars of a neuropsychiatric disorder, insofar as clear models now exist of how its characteristic psychopathology is mediated by specific neuroanatomical circuits and neurochemical systems. This chapter aims to provide a comprehensive review of the current state of knowledge on OCD, including epidemiology, clinical features, neurobiology and management.

Epidemiology

Prevalence

Until the 1980s OCD was viewed as a rare disorder, which only affected 0.005% of the population. These figures were based on a study by Rudin, which looked at the prevalence of OCD in a psychiatric in-patient population (Rudin, 1953). The Epidemiological Catchment Area (ECA) study of 1980–1984 radically changed views of the prevalence of OCD (Karno et al., 1988). Undertaken in five US commu-

nities, this study found lifetime prevalence rates for OCD to be 1.9–3.3%, making it the fourth most common psychiatric disorder, with a prevalence that was 25–60 times higher than previously believed. These figures were subsequently confirmed in similar studies in Canada (Kolada et al., 1994), Taiwan (Hwuh & Chang, 1989), and several other countries (Weismann et al., 1994), demonstrating that OCD is a disorder with a similar prevalence across nationalities.

The ECA figures, however, have been challenged. The ECA and cross-national study used the Diagnostic Interview Schedule (DIS); a structured interview designed for trained lay interviewers, to arrive at diagnoses. Several later studies have questioned the validity of DIS diagnoses. Nelson and Rice (1997) examined the 1-year temporal stability of the DIS and found it to be low, with only 19.2% of those who were originally diagnosed with OCD having this diagnosis confirmed on follow-up interview. Two follow-up studies of the ECA, using semistructured interviews conducted by psychiatrists (Antony et al., 1985; Helzer et al., 1985), supported these findings. However, these studies have been criticized in view of their small sample size and failure to use objective instruments to ascertain the diagnosis of OCD. More carefully designed studies, using standard rating scales followed by clinician rated diagnostic interviews have confirmed the ECA findings (Rasmussen & Eisen, 1998).

If OCD is so prevalent, why then has its prevalence been underestimated for so many years? In part this is perhaps due to reluctance on the part of sufferers to seek help, whether because of shame about symptoms or because of a lack of awareness of effective treatments. For example, survey of OCD patients found that the mean age of onset was 14.5 years and that professional help was only sought some 10 years later (Hollander et al., 1997a, b). The development of patient advocacy groups in the area of anxiety disorders and OCD, will hopefully contribute to increased awareness and earlier treatment.

Also important, however, is the problem of clinical misdiagnosis: in this study, the correct diagnosis was made only 6 years after professional help was sought (Hollander et al., 1997a, b). Patients with OCD may present to a range of different clinicians (e.g. to dermatologists for chapped hands following excessive washing, to primary medical practitioners for somatic obsessions, to internists for repeated concerns about AIDS, or to dentists for gum lesions from excessive tooth-brushing), and the diagnosis may be missed in these settings (Hollingsworth et al., 1980; Rapoport, 1989).

Demographic variables

Gender
In epidemiological samples of adults OCD appears to have equal prevalence between males and females (Karno et al., 1988; Valleni Basile et al., 1996; Zohar, 1999). Male gender may be associated with earlier age of onset, comorbid tics, and increased likelihood of perinatal trauma (Bogetto et al., 1999; Lensi et al., 1996).

Race
The ECA study found significantly fewer blacks presenting with OCD (Karno et al., 1988). However, this feature was observed in nine other mental disorders, and is probably a reflection of sociocultural issues, rather than representing a genetic difference in propensity to OCD. Similarly, although studies in Africa (Carothers, 1953; German, 1972) have found the prevalence of OCD to be lower than that described for the US, significant methodological problems exist with many of these studies (failure to use structured clinical interviews, lack of standardized diagnostic criteria). The Cross-National Epidemiological study (Weismann et al., 1994) found prevalence in Korea and Japan to be similar to the US, as did studies of OCD in India (Khanna et al., 1986) and Puerto Rico (Canino et al., 1987)

Socioeconomic status
In the ECA study (Karno et al., 1988) patients with OCD were more likely to be of lower socioeconomic status, and unemployed. However, in two epidemiological studies of children and adolescents, patients presenting with OCD were more likely to be of higher socioeconomic class (Thomsen, 1994; Valleni Basile et al., 1996). It is plausible that the lower socioeconomic status of adults with OCD reflects the impact their disease has on their ability to function in society.

Marital status
OCD sufferers are more likely to be single or divorced than the general population, a likely reflection of the degree of impairment associated with the disorder. Small clinical studies have suggested that the degree of impairment in sexual and marital functioning in OCD is not appreciably different from major depression (Staebler et al., 1993; Coryell, 1981) and panic disorder (Staebler et al., 1993).

Religion and culture
While the prevalence of OCD across different cultures appears to be similar, culture and religion may influence the content of obsessions and compulsions. Several studies in strictly religious communities (primarily Orthodox Jewish and Muslim), have found an increased prevalence of religious obsessions and scrupulosity (Greenberg & Witzum, 1994). Raphael et al. (1996) found more religious affiliation among patients with OCD than other psychiatric patients, but this was not specific to a single religion, and there is little evidence to suggest that increased religiousness is a predisposing factor to develop OCD (Greenberg & Witzum, 1994).

Quality of life and OCD

The enormous negative impact of OCD on patient's lives is reflected in the World Bank and WHO Global Burden of Disease study (Murray & Lopez, 1996), which found OCD to be among the ten most disabling conditions worldwide. The costs of OCD are enormous, reduced or lost productivity from OCD in the US alone has been estimated at $5.9 billion dollars a year (Dupont et al., 1995). Misdiagnosis may cost several billions of dollars a year in the USA (Hollander et al., 1997b).

Quality of life is a concept that is becoming increasingly important in health care and encompasses dimensions such as physical and social role functioning, interpersonal relationships, perceived health and mental well being. Studies of OCD show that it has significant impact on quality of life. Koran et al. (1996b) in a study of medication free patients, for example, found instrumental role performance (i.e. work, homemaking or student role functioning) and social functioning to be worse than that of the general population and of patients with type II diabetes.

These findings underscore the need for effective treatment of OCD. Both retrospective (Stein et al., 1996; Hollander et al., 1997b) and prospective (Bystritsky et al., 1999; Emmelkamp et al., 2000) studies have fortunately indicated that current treatments result in significant improvement in the quality of life in OCD patients.

Clinical features and diagnosis

Age of onset

The ECA study found a mean age of onset of OCD between 21 and 25 years, a figure that has been confirmed by several later studies (Kolada et al., 1994; Rasmussen & Eisen, 1998). However, a significant proportion of patients has onset of symptoms several years prior to the development of the full disorder. The Zurich cohort study (Degonda et al., 1993) reported that 70% of patients developed symptoms before the age of 20 and this has been confirmed in other studies. As noted earlier, there may be significant gender differences in the onset of OCD. Several studies have found males to have an earlier age of onset (17–19 years) than females (19–22 years) (Rasmussen & Eisen, 1990; Degonda et al., 1993).

Natural history and course of disease

OCD has typically been viewed as a chronic progressive unremitting disease. However, the picture may be more complex. Skoog and Skoog (1999) followed 144 patients over 40 years, with average length of follow-up from onset of 47 years. Eighty-three per cent of patients improved, with complete recovery in 20% and subclinical symptoms in 28%. Early age of onset, the presence of both obsessions and compulsions, magical obsessions and compulsive rituals, low baseline functioning and initial chronic course were associated with a worse course. What makes this study particularly interesting is that only 17 patients received medication and in 14 this was instituted after more than 30 years of OCD.

Studies in adolescents also suggest that OCD may improve over time. Flament et al. (1988) in a study of high school students, found that, of 12 students with OCD at baseline, only 5 still had clinical symptoms at 2 year follow-up; and Valleni Basile (Valleni Basile et al., 1996) found that in adolescents with OCD, the most common transition was from the more severe to the less severe category of OCD. While these studies paint a less gloomy picture of the course of OCD it must be emphasized that a significant proportion of patients continue to have disease after many years.

Symptomatology

The hallmark of OCD is the presence of obsessions and compulsion. While the spectrum of obsessions and compulsions is vast, the majority can be grouped into one of the following clusters (Rasmussen & Tsuang, 1986; Rettew et al., 1992).

Contamination fears

These are the most common of obsessions, and are often coupled with avoidance, checking and handwashing. Patients experience intense anxiety about being contaminated, often going to great lengths to avoid the feared object(s). It is interesting to note that, while the symptom structure has remained relatively constant, the actual feared object has changed over time, from the plague to syphilis and now AIDS (Rachman & Hodgson, 1980).

Checking

These patients experience intense worry that something terrible will happen because they failed to check something completely. Often they acknowledge that their fears are absurd, but experience intense anxiety if they do not perform their checking. They often experience a sense of 'incompleteness' (Janet, 1904) until their specified ritual is performed a certain number of times, when the anxiety stops. These patients show the experience of pathological doubt in its purest form. Leckman et al. (1997) found that checking was highly correlated with sexual, religious and somatic obsessions and that the strongest correlations were between aggressive impulses and checking rituals.

Sexual and aggressive obsessions

Some patients suffer from recurrent, unacceptable sexual thoughts or actions, which as Janet (1904) noted, are often the ones calculated to cause the most horror to the patient. For example, a deeply religious woman will have recurrent sexual thoughts of Jesus, or a mother will experience impulses to harm her children. Patients may experience severe guilt and anxiety, often coupled with the need for continual forgiveness or reassurance.

Symmetry and precision

Patients with obsessions about symmetry and precision may line objects up, straighten things, or perform ordering rituals. This may be accompanied by magical thinking; such patients worry that, unless things are ordered or symmetrical, a potential disaster may occur. Symmetry and ordering obsessions have been found to be associated with chronic tic disorders (Leckman et al., 1997).

Obsessional slowness may also occur as a result of symmetry and ordering concerns. Alternatively, however, obsessional slowness may reflect avoidance (for example, patients with contamination concerns may move slowly to avoid exposure to dirt). Patients with obsessional slowness tend to have more neurological soft signs (Hymas et al., 1991), and may represent a subgroup of patients with more severe illness (Veale, 1993).

Somatic obsessions

Somatic obsessions (for example, that a particular part of the body is misshapen or dysfunctional) occur in many disorders and differential diagnosis includes hypochondriasis, body dysmorphic disorder (BDD), and major depression with somatic features. Patients with OCD, however, tend to have multiple obsessions and compulsions.

Hoarding

Hoarding is defined as the acquisition of, and failure to discard possessions that are useless or have limited value (Frost & Gross, 1993). It may occur in response to several different kinds of obsessions e.g. fear of throwing something out by mistake, fear of misfortune occurring. It is a common symptom of OCD, present in up to 18% of patients (Rasmussen & Tsuang, 1986). It has been suggested that hoarding is associated with less insight (Greenberg, 1987; Frost & Gross, 1993), is found more frequently in patients with comorbid tic disorders, and is a predictor of worse response to SRIs (Black et al., 1998; Mataix-Cols et al., 1999).

OCD subtyping

Although advances in OCD demonstrate that it is a specific neuropsychiatric entity, the available data also indicate a degree of heterogeneity. Research interest has recently been directed at finding homogenous OCD subgroups with prognostic and therapeutic implications. Subtyping OCD by means of symptomatology (as above) provides a preliminary approach, to be supplemented by more sophisticated factor analytic techniques.

One of the first factor analyses (Hodgson & Rachman, 1977) used the Maudsley Obsessive Compulsive Inventory and yielded four factors 'checking', 'cleaning', 'slowness' and 'doubting'. However, the Maudsley is biased towards checking and cleaning items. Furthermore, over time patients' symptoms have been shown to evolve from one of these symptom clusters to another.

Rasmussen and Eisen (1991) have proposed three core subtypes of OCD: abnormal risk assessment, pathological doubt, and incompleteness. They argued that these subtypes cut across symptom clusters. In their work, symptoms involving incompleteness were more often associated with tics and compulsive personality features, whereas those without incompleteness were more likely to be associated with high levels of anxiety and comorbid anxiety disorders.

Baer (1994) in factor analysis of the Y-BOCS have provided data partially consistent with this hypothesis. Three factors best summarized the major symptoms: symmetry/hoarding, contamination/checking, and 'pure' obsessions, such as sexual, aggressive and religious obsessions. They noted similarities between symmetry/hoarding and incompleteness, a feature frequently found in Tourette's Syndrome. Symmetry/hoarding was significantly correlated with comorbid Tourette's Syndrome. Several later studies largely confirmed these findings but found symmetry and hoarding to be two different factors (Leckman et al., 1997).

Neuroimaging studies suggest that these factors may have different neuroanatomical correlations. Rauch and colleagues (Rauch et al., 1998a) found that pure obsessions correlated with bilateral striatal activity, symmetry and ordering negatively correlated with right caudate activity, and washing and cleaning symptoms correlated with orbitofrontal and anterior cingulate cortical activity.

These factors also appear to have clinical implications, for example cleaning/checking may respond best to behavioural treatment (Ball et al., 1996), while as we noted earlier, hoarding is associated with comorbid tic disorders and more likely to require the addition of neuroleptic medication (McDougle et al., 1993, 1994).

The relationship between OCD and tic disorders may provide particular insight into the subtyping of OCD. OCD is common in tic disorders and vice versa. Similarly, family studies have found higher rates of OCD in Tourette's syndrome probands, and higher rates of TS in OCD probands, suggesting a genetic link between the two disorders (Pauls et al., 1995).

Patients with and without tics may have phenotypic differences. For example, OCD patients with tics have male predominance, earlier age at onset, and higher frequency of tic-like compulsions such as the need to touch, tap, or rub items, blinking and staring rituals, as well as symmetry obsessions and feelings of incompleteness. Patients with tics are also more likely to experience sensory phenomena, such as bodily sensations, mental urges and a sense of inner tension (Miguel et al., 2000).

OCD patients with tics differ from those without tics in their response to treatment as well. A retrospective case controlled analysis found fluvoxamine to be less effective in patients with tics (McDougle et al., 1993). Furthermore, in one study patients with tics were more likely to respond to typical neuroleptic augmentation (McDougle et al., 1994). Such data suggests that patients with OCD and tics may represent a neurobiologically distinct subgroup. However, contrary to expectations, a recent controlled trial of risperidone (McDougle et al., 2000) found no significant difference in response between patients with and without tics.

Other aspects of the neurobiology of OCD may provide

an alternative basis for subtyping. Increased neurological soft signs have been found in OCD patients as compared to normal controls (Hollander et al., 1990), and in some but not all studies, this has been a predictor of poorer response to pharmacotherapy (Hollander et al., 1992; Thienemann & Koran, 1995). Similarly, the group of OCD patients with symptom onset in the context of streptococcal throat infection (see below) may represent a distinct subgroup. Thus, several possible ways of integrating data on symptoms, neurobiology and treatment into meaningful subgroups of OCD have been proposed, but further work is required to consolidate these approaches.

Diagnosis

DSM-IV (American Psychiatric Association, 1994) has provided diagnostic criteria for OCD. Like earlier versions, DSM-IV requires patients to experience either obsessions or compulsions which cause marked distress and significantly interfere with the person's social and/or occupational functioning. However, DSM-IV differs from earlier versions in two important ways: The need for insight and the presence of mental rituals.

The DSM-IV field trial (Foa et al., 1995) found that the large majority of patients were uncertain about whether or not their symptoms were unreasonable, and as result the need for insight was de-emphasized and a subcategory 'with poor insight' was added. Furthermore, the majority of patients were found to have mental rituals, and the definition of compulsions was changed to indicate that these are not necessarily physical actions.

Differential diagnosis

Other psychiatric disorders can present with phenomena similar to OCD. Patients with OCD spectrum disorders often experience recurrent, intrusive thoughts or behaviours but these are limited to a specific context (e.g. preoccupation with appearance in body dysmorphic disorder, hair pulling in trichotillomania, or excessive fears of having an illness as in hypochondriasis.) Similar distinctions occur with other anxiety disorders: social or specific phobia is characterized by preoccupations that are limited to a particular feared object or situation, while generalized anxiety disorder is characterized by excessive worry which involves real life situations.

Patients with dementia may display excessive list making, hoarding, counting and other behaviours that resemble compulsive rituals but are compensatory mechanisms. Patients with major depression may show somatic or paranoid ruminations, and patients with schizophrenia can display contamination concerns and hoarding behaviours. These patients however, typically have other symptoms as well, and the form of their symptoms may differ from the classical pattern of ego-dystonicity that characterizes OCD.

Tics and stereotyped movements must be distinguished from compulsions. The key differences are that they are not performed in response to an obsession and the patient does not attach meaning to these movements. However, it is important to bear in mind that the diagnosis of OCD and a tic disorder often coexist.

OCD must also be distinguished from obsessive compulsive personality disorder (OCPD). Unless they have a coexisting diagnosis of OCD, patients with OCPD do not have obsessions or compulsions, but rather their personality is characterized by a pervasive pattern of preoccupation with orderliness, perfectionism and control.

Superstitions and rituals are commonly encountered among a wide variety of people, but a diagnosis of OCD should only be considered if these behaviours are ego-dystonic, and cause significant distress or functional impairment.

Neurological disorders involving lesions of the frontal lobe, basal ganglia (particularly the caudate nucleus) or both, should be excluded. In a review of the relationship between frontal lobe degeneration and repetitive behaviours Ames et al. (1994) found 78% of patients showed some type of repetitive or compulsive behaviour. Similarly, many patients with lesions of the striatum develop behaviours that are consistent with a diagnosis of OCD. Case reports attest to a wide variety of etiologies for such lesion ranging from neurodegenerative disorders such as Huntington's disease, to infarction, to toxins like carbon monoxide or manganese (Cummings & Cunningham, 1992). There are also a few reports of temporal lobe lesions leading to OCD (Jenike & Brotman 1984; Zungu-Dirwayi et al., 1999).

Comorbid conditions

Comorbid conditions are frequent in OCD, with studies reporting that at least 50% of patients have a comorbid Axis I disorder and at least 40% of patients also meet criteria for personality disorder(s) (Piggot et al., 1994).

Axis I disorders

Major depressive disorder is the most common comorbid disorder in OCD, with at least 30% of patients meeting the criteria for a concurrent major depressive episode and lifetime prevalence as high as 70% (Piggot et al., 1994). Depression usually occurs secondary to OCD, with most patients reporting an onset of depressive symptoms after the onset of OCD. However, others report a separate course for their depressive symptoms vs. those of OCD, suggesting that in a subgroup of patients the disorders are unrelated or at least separate.

The relationship between OCD and mania has been less well studied, but recent evidence suggests that a significant number of patients have both disorders. Chen and Dilsaver (1995) found that 21% of subjects with bipolar disorder in the ECA survey had comorbid OCD while Kruger et al. (1995) found an incidence of 35%. Perugi et al. (1999) found that 16% of patients with OCD had comorbid bipolar disorder (mainly bipolar II). They found that these patients had a more gradual onset, more episodes of major depression and a higher rate of sexual and religious obsessions and fewer checking obsessions.

A substantial cohort of patients (40–60%) with OCD also have comorbid anxiety disorders, with the most common being panic disorder (12–15%), simple phobia (22–27%), and social phobia (11–18%). It has been suggested that the anxiety disorders represent states of altered risk assessment, and the high rates of comorbidity point to shared pathophysiological mechanisms (Piggot et al., 1994).

A substantial number of patients with OCD also have eating disorders, with lifetime rates of anorexia nervosa of 10–17% and rates for bulimia nervosa of 5–20% (Piggot et al., 1994). Similarly, patients with anorexia nervosa and bulimia nervosa have been reported to have a high incidence of obsessional features. This may have therapeutic implications with some studies suggesting that SSRI's may have preferential efficacy in these patients.

Axis II disorders

Due to changes in the conceptualization and diagnostic criteria of personality disorders, the co-morbidity of personality disorders with OCD has been difficult to elucidate. Nevertheless, in studies using DSM-III or IIIR criteria, personality disorders have been found to be very common in patients with OCD with some studies reporting that over 50% of patients meet the criteria for at least one personality disorder. Avoidant, dependent, histrionic or obsessive compulsive personality disorders appear to be the most common comorbid diagnoses (Piggot et al., 1994).

The relationship between OCD and OCPD has been an area of special interest. For many years the Freudian concept of the 'anal erotic character' dominated thinking about the relationship between OCD and OCPD. Here the disorders were viewed as existing along a continuum; with OCD being the final most severe form of the disorder. More recent evidence suggests that significant differences exist between the two disorders. OCD may be a predisposing factor for the development of OCPD. It has been suggested that patients may develop OCPD as an adaptive mecha-

nism to deal with disorder (Baer & Jenike, 1992), a possibility supported by the observation that OCD often predates the development of OCPD (Baer & Jenike, 1992). Obsessive–compulsive personality disorder occurs less frequently in OCD than previously thought but is still more common in OCD than in either the general population or in patients with major depression or panic disorder.

The role of personality disorders as predictors of outcome has received some study. Concomitant schizotypal personality disorder in particular has been consistently associated with poorer response to medication and behavioural therapy, and in some studies has been shown more likely to be associated with a response to typical neuroleptic augmentation (Ravizza et al., 1995). This is in keeping with studies reflecting dopamine dysfunction in schizotypal personality disorder (Siever, 1994). However, a trial of risperidone did not find a difference in response between those with and without schizotypal personality disorder (McDougle et al., 2000).

Etiology and pathophysiology

OCD is a complex disorder, in which several pathophysiological processes may be involved:

The genetics of OCD

Current data suggest that OCD has a substantial genetic component. Twin studies show concordance rates of approximately 80% in monozygotic twins and only 47–50% in dizygotic twins (Inyoue, 1965; Carey & Gottesman, 1981). Furthermore, several studies have found a greater prevalence of OCD and subsyndromal OCD in parents and first-degree relatives of OCD probands as compared to parents of psychiatrically normal controls (Black et al., 1992; Pauls et al., 1995).

Family studies have also borne out a link with Tourette's syndrome with greater prevalence of OCD in first-degree relatives of probands with Tourette's syndrome regardless of OCD comorbidity. Pauls et al. (Pauls & Leckman, 1986; Pauls et al., 1990) in two studies of Tourette's syndrome probands found familial patterns of Tourette's syndrome, chronic tics, and OCD that were consistent with an autosomal mode of transmission with incomplete penetrance. Two later studies replicated these findings (Van de Wetering, 1993; Eapen et al., 1993).

Taken together, these findings suggest that the risk for developing OCD is heritable and point to at least one form of OCD that is characterized by early onset and association with tic disorders.

Neuroanatomical models of OCD

The current neuroanatomical model of OCD emphasizes the role of cortico-striato-thalamo-cortical (CTSC) circuitry. Alexander et al. (1986, 1990) conceptualized this as being organized into multiple, parallel segregated circuits, which project from the cortex to corresponding striatal subterritories, from there to the basal ganglia, and via the thalamus back to the prefrontal regions from which they originated. Very briefly, these systems function to filter out extraneous input to the cortex, to ensure refined output and to mediate stereotyped rule-based processes without these reaching consciousness.

Modern imaging studies confirm the role of cortico-striato-thalamo-cortical circuitry in OCD.

Structural studies

Several volumetric studies of the caudate have shown structural abnormalities. The nature of the abnormalities described has been inconsistent, with some studies showing increased volume and others decreased volume; it is possible that caudate volume changes over time, with increased volume in the aftermath of streptococcal infection (Giedd et al., 2000), and later shrinkage.

Volumetric changes in the orbital frontal and anterior cingulate regions have been less well studied. Of three studies reported so far, only one (Szeszko et al., 1999) found structural abnormalities (reduced bilateral orbital frontal and amygdala volumes). Functional imaging studies, however, provide more robust evidence for involvement of these structures (see below).

White matter reductions in OCD have been reported and a subsequent replication study confirmed overall white matter reduction but increased opercular volume, which correlated with both severity of OCD and nonverbal immediate memory (Jenike et al., 1996). Finally, thalamic volumes normalize after treatment with paroxetine but not behaviour therapy, perhaps pointing to a different mechanism of action for the two modalities (Rosenberg et al., 2000a).

Studies using magnetic resonance spectroscopy (MRS) have also demonstrated striatal abnormalities. Two studies have found decreased N-acetyl-aspartate (NAA) levels in the striatum (Ebert et al., 1997; Bartha et al., 1998), suggesting decreased density of healthy neurons in this region. Furthermore, one of these studies failed to find significant differences in striatal volumes (Bartha et al., 1998), underscoring the purported greater sensitivity of MRS–NAA over current morphometric MRI methods.

Rosenberg's group has also demonstrated abnormalities in a pediatric population. Decreased NAA levels were found in right and left medial thalami, with the decreased levels in the left medial thalamus correlating with increased severity of disease (Fitzgerald et al., 2000). In addition caudate glutamatergic levels were found to be increased in children with OCD (Rosenberg et al., 2000b), but this was found to normalize after treatment with paroxetine, perhaps suggesting that paroxetine treatment is mediated by a serotonergically modulated reduction in fronto-striatal glutamatergic concentration.

Functional studies

Neutral state studies have implicated hyperactivity in the prefrontal cortex and less consistently striatal and cingulate involvement (Baxter et al., 1988; Nordahl et al., 1989; Swedo et al., 1989c; Benkelfat et al., 1990; Machlin et al., 1991; Rubin et al., 1992; Perani et al., 1995). Pre/posttreatment studies also point to involvement of these areas. Decreased activity after medication was found in the medial frontal cortex (Hoehn-Saric et al., 1991), and orbitofrontal cortex (Benkelfat et al., 1990; Swedo et al., 1992c), with one study correlating treatment response to activity in the right frontal cortex. Changes in the caudate and cingulum have also been reported (Benkelfat et al., 1990).

Baxter et al. (1992) found decreased right caudate activity in a group receiving medication as well as a different group receiving behaviour therapy. This was subsequently replicated in a second study of behaviour therapy, which also confirmed correlation between orbitofrontal and caudate activity pretreatment that disappeared posttreatment (Schwartz et al., 1996). These studies confirm that effective treatment of OCD, whether pharmacotherapeutic or psychotherapeutic in nature, is accompanied by specific changes in CTSC circuits.

Why should dysfunction in CTSC circuits lead to OCD symptoms? There is increasing evidence that striatal function is associated with the development, maintenance and selection of motoric cognitive and procedural strategies, this has been variously described as 'habit system' 'response set' and 'procedural mobilization'. Thus, it may be argued that striatal lesions can lead to the inappropriate release of genetically programmed sequences (such as hand-washing, hoarding, etc.).

An early heuristic model (Baxter et al., 1990) postulated that different circuits may be involved in the mediation of different kinds of OCD symptom. According to such a 'striatal topography model', the cognitive symptoms of OCD are mediated by the caudate, motoric symptoms by the putamen, and affective symptoms by paralimbic CTSC circuits. More recent evidence shows involvement of a range of CTSC circuits in OCD; nevertheless it may still be suggested that projections to specific fields or cells mediate different kinds of OCD symptoms.

Rauch et al. have suggested that the intrusive events that are the hallmark of OCD and related disorders represent failure of filtering at the level of the thalamus (Rauch et al., 1985). Information can be processed in two ways explicitly (i.e. consciously) and implicitly (i.e. unconsciously), with implicit operations being primarily processed via cortico-striatal systems. In OCD, pathology in the cortico-striatal pathways may allow this information to gain access to consciousness, presenting as intrusive phenomena. Rauch et al. has shown that the striatum is usually recruited during an implicit sequence learning task, but that in patients with OCD, this fails to occur and instead, medial temporal structures, usually associated with conscious information processing, are recruited (Rauch et al., 1985, 1997, 1998b).

In this model compulsions or tics may represent a compensatory mechanism. These repetitive behaviours may serve to recruit viable cortico-striatal-thalamic circuits, thereby facilitating filtering at the level of the thalamus. The repetitions required would reflect the inefficiency of such mechanisms. This is also consistent with clinical observation that patients often suddenly no longer experience the urge to perform a behaviour, 'as if a switch were turned off'. Presumably, once sufficient repetitions have been performed, a threshold level of filtering is reached and the intrusive stimuli no longer reach consciousness. Rauch et al. (1998a, b) have also demonstrated in functional imaging studies a characteristic pattern of thalamic deactivation with striatal recruitment.

Neuropsychology of OCD

Neuropsychological studies of OCD have demonstrated that the following domains of cognitive functioning are most consistently affected in patients with OCD: visuospatial skill, non-verbal memory, and executive abilities.

Visuospatial skills describe the patient's mental capacity to perceive and manipulate objects in two and three dimensional space (Lezak, 1995). Patients with OCD have been found to be impaired on a number of tests that purport to measure visuospatial memory (Flor-Henry et al., 1979; Insel et al., 1983; Behar et al., 1984; Head et al., 1989; Hollander et al., 1990, 1993; Boone et al., 1991; Christenson et al., 1992; Aronowitz et al., 1994, Savage et al., 1995).

Non-verbal memory refers to the ability to learn and recall new visual objects and images, preferably ones not easily described with words. Again, patients with OCD show impairment on several tests of nonverbal memory (Boone et al., 1991; Zielenski et al., 1991; Christenson et al., 1992; Savage et al., 1993, 1995; Aronowitz et al., 1994; Dirson et al., 1995; Cohen et al., 1996). In particular, their ability to encode new non-verbal information appears particularly affected (Boone et al., 1991; Zielenski et al., 1991; Savage et al., 1993, 1995; Aronowitz et al., 1994; Cohen et al., 1996). Deficits in the ability to retrieve previously stored non-verbal memories have also been described. To put it another way, patients with OCD have difficulty learning new non-verbal material, and once having learnt it, have problems in retrieving that memory.

Underlying both these deficits may be impairment of executive function. Executive function refers to the high-level control processes that modulate more elementary sensory, motor, cognitive, memory and affective functions. It requires the ability to take the overall context of the situation into account and use this knowledge to set priorities, implement strategic behaviour and shift behaviour appropriately as the situation changes (Lezak, 1995).

In general patients with OCD appear to have most difficulty in this last component of executive function, that is, they have trouble changing their behaviour appropriately as the situation changes (Malloy, 1987; Christenson et al., 1992).

This is reminiscent of the symptoms of OCD (Savage, 1998). Take as an example a compulsive checker. The excessive fear that something may happen if he fails to check may be linked to failure to appreciate the overall context of the situation. Checking may also be related to difficulty planning and implementing strategic actions. Continued checking in the face of its failure to reduce anxiety may be related to difficulty in flexibly modifying behaviour

This deficit in executive functioning may underlie the problems with non-verbal memory. If a person has poor executive function, and hence organizational problems, it is likely that they will not be able to break down visual structures into easily recognizable components, and hence find them more difficult to remember. Savage et al. demonstrated exactly this in a study that examined OCD patients' performance on the Rey–Osterreith complex figure test. Patients (and matched controls) were asked to copy a complex figure and then draw it immediately after the figure was removed and 30 minutes later. Patients with OCD showed impairment both in the organizational approach used to copy the figure as well as recall after the figure was removed (both immediate and delayed). Recent work also suggests impaired organizational strategies may mediate deficits in verbal memory as well (Savage et al., 2000).

These findings tie in well with evidence of fronto-striatal dysfunction demonstrated in imaging studies of patients with OCD. Studies of patients with Parkinson's disease and Huntington's disease, both disorders involving striatal degeneration, show evidence of executive dysfunction leading to memory and spatial deficits in these patients, with deficits in organizational approach similar to those found in OCD (Ogden et al., 1990; Grossman et al., 1993)

Autoimmune pathology in OCD

In a series of landmark studies (Swedo et al., 1989b, 1993), Swedo and colleagues confirmed earlier observations that OCD symptoms were common among children with Sydenham's chorea, and often preceded motor manifestations of the disease. Later work (Swedo et al., 1998) demonstrated that a subgroup had OCD symptoms of abrupt onset, and showed exacerbations that often were associated with demonstrable group A β-hemolytic streptococcus infection. In addition, a subset of children with OCD shows antineuronal antibodies.

Together, these finding have led to the designation of Pediatric Autoimmune Neuropsychiatric Disorders Associated with Streptococcal infections (PANDAS) (Swedo et al., 1998). Specific criteria include: (i) presence of OCD and/or a tic disorder, (ii) prepubertal onset, (iii) episodic course of symptom severity, (iv) association with group A β-hemolytic streptococcus infection (v) association with neurologic abnormalities.

Autoimmune basal ganglia damage has been identified as an important pathogenic mechanism in Sydenham's chorea (Husby et al., 1976). Furthermore, acute changes in striatal volume parallel the clinical course of PANDAS (Gibofsky et al., 1991). These findings therefore strengthen the case for striatal damage as a pathogenic mechanism for OCD.

Susceptibility to rheumatic fever and hence PANDAS (Gibofsky et al., 1991) may be inherited as an autosomal recessive trait. The B lymphocyte antigen d8/17 appears to serve as a marker for susceptibility to rheumatic fever, occurring in 100% of rheumatic fever sufferers (Khanna et al., 1989), with significantly higher expression in the rheumatic fever patients than in either unaffected first degree relatives or normal controls. As increased D8/17 has not been reported in poststreptococcal glomerulonephritis, it may indicate specific vulnerability to developing rheumatic fever and related complications. Elevated D8/17 expression has been described in patients with childhood onset OCD, Tourette's syndrome and autism, but not in trichotillomania (Swedo & Leonard, 1992; Niehaus et al., 1996; Murphy et al., 1997; Swedo et al., 1997; Chapman et al., 1998).

Neurochemistry and neuropharmacology

A number of neurotransmitter systems appear to play a role in mediating OCD symptoms.

Serotonin and OCD

The serotonergic hypothesis of OCD was first prompted by the observation that serotonergic reuptake inhibitors were more effective in alleviating the symptoms of OCD (Fernandez-Cordoba & Lopez-Ibor, 1967; Zohar & Insel, 1987; Greist et al., 1995b). Whether SSRI's work by correcting some fundamental abnormality on the serotonergic system or whether they modulate an intact system to compensate for underlying abnormalities in OCD is not yet known.

An interesting set of preclinical studies have found that, in order to desensitize the 5-HT1D autoreceptor in orbitofrontal cortex, the administration of relatively high doses of SSRI's for relatively long periods is required (low doses, short duration, and ECT does not have an effect) (Mansari et al., 1995). This work is reminiscent of clinical findings in OCD (see below), and suggests that this receptor may therefore have a particularly important role.

There is also work suggesting that 5-HT-2 receptors are important in OCD. Case reports suggest that certain hallucinogens (psilocybin and LSD), that are potent stimulators of the 5HT2A and 5HT2C receptors, can decrease OCD symptoms (Delgado & Morena, 1998). Conversely, ritanserin, a 5-HT-2 antagonist results in the exacerbation of OCD symptoms (Ergovesi et al., 1992). Arguably, enhancement of neurotransmission through 5HT2A or 5HT2C receptors may be a common pathway for drugs with therapeutic effect in OCD.

Studies of indirect measures of central serotonergic function (such as platelet receptor binding and CSF concentrations of 5HT metabolites) in OCD have been inconsistent. There is somewhat more consistency in studies of serotonergic agonists; OCD symptoms are exacerbated by mCPP (a 5HT1A and 5HTC agonist) (Zohar et al., 1987; Hollander et al., 1991; Piggot et al., 1993) and perhaps by sumatriptan (a 5HT-1D agonist) (Stein et al., 1999). Administration of sumatriptan during functional imaging demonstrated a significant association between symptom exacerbation and decreased frontal activity, arguably consistent with a role for the 5-HT1D receptor in OCD (Stein et al., 1999). Nevertheless, findings with both mCPP (Charney et al., 1988; Ho Pian et al., 1998; Goodman et al., 1996) and sumatriptan (Pian et al., 1998) have not always been consistent, and sumatriptan has poor blood–brain barrier penetration, so that additional work in this area remains necessary.

Dopaminergic systems and OCD

Preclinical studies demonstrate that stereotypic behaviour can be elicited by the administration of dopamine agonists, and decreased by dopamine blockers. Similarly, complex repetitive behaviours have been described in stimulant abusers (Ellinwood, 1967; Schiorring, 1975). Furthermore cocaine, which potentiates the effects of dopamine by blocking presynaptic uptake has been reported to exacerbate symptoms in patients with OCD and to induce such behaviour in subjects with a family but not personal history of OCD.

As noted earlier, there is also a strong association between OCD and Tourette's syndrome, a disorder for which a dopaminergic basis is well elucidated. For example, the principal dopamine metabolite homovanillic acid (HVA) is decreased in the CSF of patients with Tourette's syndrome (McDougle et al., 1989), and dopamine blockers are a standard form of treatment in TS. Recent imaging studies have demonstrated a significant increase in the number of striatal presynaptic dopamine carrier sites in the caudate and putamen in Tourette's patients (Singer et al., 1991; Malison et al., 1995; Wolf et al., 1996).

Pharmacologic studies in OCD support a potential role for the dopamine system. Only around 50–60% of patients respond to SSRIs, and patients with comorbid tics are particularly likely not to respond (McDougle et al., 1994). However, augmentation of SSRIs with dopamine blockers has been shown effective in both open (Jacobsen, 1995; Stein, 1997b) and controlled trials (McDougle et al., 2000). Typical neuroleptics are particularly effective in OCD patients with comorbid tics (McDougle et al., 1994), while the atypicals appear useful in OCD patients both with and without tics (Stein et al., 1997a, b; McDougle et al., 2000).

Neuropeptides and OCD

Preclinical evidence has linked neuropeptides to repetitive behaviour in animals and initial clinical investigations in OCD patients suggest that they may play a role in modulation of the disorder. Neuropeptides implicated in OCD include arginine vasopressin (AVP), oxytocin, adrenocorticotropic hormone (ACTH), corticotropin releasing factor (CRF), somatostatin, and the opioid system.

Preclinical studies have linked AVP with enhancement of memory acquisition and retrieval and with grooming behaviours. AVP may also inhibit extinction, decreasing the likelihood of changing a behavioural pattern once it has been established. Altemus et al. (1992) found OCD patients had significantly elevated basal levels of AVP and secreted more AVP into plasma in response to hypertonic saline. However, this was not found in a subsequent study (Leckman et al., 1994a). Nevertheless, in children and adolescents with OCD, a negative correlation between symptom severity and AVP levels was found (Swedo et al., 1992a).

Preclinical studies have shown that oxytocin administration markedly increases grooming behaviour. Further-more, oxytocin has been shown to induce maternal behaviour in female rats, but only in animals primed with estrogen (Insel, 1992). This may be relevant to explaining the increased risk for onset or exacerbation of OCD in pregnancy or the puerperium. Elevated levels of oxytocin (and estrogen) may induce OCD symptoms in a vulnerable subgroup of women. Higher CSF oxytocin levels have been found in adult patients with no family or personal history of tic disorders and oxytocin levels were significantly correlated with Y-BOCS scores (Leckman et al., 1994b). In children, the AVP/oxytocin ratio was negatively correlated with symptom severity (Swedo et al., 1992a). Administration of oxytocin to adults with OCD has, however, had no consistent therapeutic effect (Epperson et al., 1996).

ACTH and CRF are both noted to increase self-grooming in animals. In humans, both basal plasma ACTH and the increase following CRF administration was found to be less in adults with OCD than controls (Bailly et al., 1994). Studies of CRF levels have been inconsistent, with initial reports of elevated CRF in OCD patients not being confirmed in replication studies. In children, no correlation has been found between either CSF ACTH or CRF levels and symptoms severity (Swedo et al., 1992a). As both ACTH and CRF are released in response to stress, it is possible that any elevations found may be a non-specific response to the stress of a chronic illness.

In animals, somatostatin delays the extinction of active and passive avoidance behaviours (which may be similar to the persistent repetition of OCD) and can also produce stereotypic behaviours (Vecsei et al., 1986; Vecsei & Widerlov, 1988). Studies of both adults and children with OCD have found higher CSF somatostatin as compared to normals (adults) and conduct disordered children (Kruesi et al., 1990; Altemus et al., 1993).

Opioids mediate reward signals and it has been postulated that they may be involved in mechanisms that signal successful task completion. Deficiencies in these mechanisms may potentially explain the 'self-doubt' experienced by many patients with OCD. OCD patients have elevated serum antibodies for the dynorphin precursor prodynorphin (Roy et al., 1994). In Tourette's syndrome CSF dynorphin was found to correlate with OCD (but not tic) symptom severity (Leckman et al., 1988). However, no correlation was found between dynorphin levels and symptom severity in children with OCD. Furthermore, challenges with opioid antagonists in OCD have produced inconsistent results (Insel & Pickar, 1983; Keuler et al., 1996).

In summary, preclinical evidence suggests that various neuropeptides may play a role in the pathogenesis of OCD. Differences between results in adult and pediatric populations suggest developmental factors impact the functioning of the different neuropeptides. However, clinical studies so far have generally produced inconsistent results, and further studies are warranted to elucidate fully the role of these peptides.

OCD spectrum disorders

In recent years a group of disorders has been hypothesized to overlap phenomenologically and neurobiologically with OCD, the so-called OCD spectrum disorders (Hollander, 1993). These potentially include a broad range of conditions including disorders usually first diagnosed in childhood, infancy, or adolescence (Tourette's disorder, autistic disorder, stereotypic movement disorder), somatoform disorders (body dysmorphic disorder, hypochondriasis), and disorders of impulse control not otherwise specified (trichotillomania, pathological gambling). Nevertheless, the characterization of so varied a range of disorders as OCD related remains contentious, with some authors warning against premature and overinclusive classifications (Rasmussen, 1994).

Neurobiological data so far has pointed to several similarities between some of these disorders. Several of the OCD spectrum disorders have shown a selective response to serotonergic agents. Clomipramine has been shown to be superior to desipramine in a range of repetitive behaviours including hair-pulling (Swedo et al., 1989a), nail-biting (Leonard et al., 1991), stereotypic behaviours (Castellanos et al., 1996) and obsessive–compulsive symptoms in autistic disorder (Gordon et al., 1992). Data also indicates the selective efficacy of serotonin reuptake inhibitors (SRIs) for symptoms of body dysmorphic disorder (Hollander, 1993), obsessive–compulsive symptoms in Tourette's (Scahill et al., 1997), and self-injurious behaviour in mental retardation (Mikkelson et al., 1997). Augmentation of SRIs with dopamine blockers may also be useful in some of the disorders. Nevertheless, it should be remembered that SRIs may be selectively effective in disorders with markedly different phenomenology from OCD (such as premenstrual dysphoric disorder (Eriksson et al., 1995)).

There may also be neuroanatomical overlap between OCD and some of the putative OCD spectrum disorders. For example, in Tourette's disorder magnetic resonance imaging (MRI) studies have found abnormalities of the basal ganglia (including the putamen, Singer et al., 1993), and functional imaging studies have demonstrated abnormal activity in frontal-striatal regions. Findings are not precisely those found in OCD, but OCD symptoms in TD may correlate with increased metabolism in orbitofrontal cortex and putamen (Braun et al., 1995). Furthermore, in patients with obsessive–compulsive symptoms, regional cerebral blood flow patterns differed depending on whether a family history of TD was present, and patterns were similar to those seen in TD in patients from TD families (Moriarty et al., 1997).

In trichotillomania there is only limited brain imaging data. The data that does exist suggests that the caudate is not involved (O'Sullivan et al., 1997; Stein et al., 1997b), but that the left putamen may be smaller in trichotillomania than in controls (O'Sullivan et al., 1997). On functional imaging, however, patients with trichotillomania were found to have increased cerebellar and right superior parietal glucose metabolic rates compared to normal controls (Swedo et al., 1991). These authors also found that anterior cingulate and orbital-frontal metabolism correlated negatively with clomipramine response, a result they previously found in OCD. Increased orbital-frontal metabolism may conceivably comprise a compensatory response in both disorders.

Genetic overlap between OCD and TD has been of particular interest in the context of OCD spectrum disorders. Tics are more common than expected in the families of OCD probands, and OCD is more common in the families of TD patients than in those of controls. Furthermore, preliminary work on dopamine receptor polymorphisms suggests differences in OCD patients with and without tics (Nicolini et al., 1998). While trichotillomania and OCD may be more common in the families of trichotillomania probands than in the general population, this seems to be a relatively subtle finding (Lenane et al., 1992). Also, there was no increased prevalence of pathological gambling or eating disorders in families of OCD probands compared with controls (Black et al., 1994).

Neuroimmunological studies also point to the existence of a spectrum of disorders. Swedo et al. (1998) note that in the aftermath of β-hemolytic streptococcal infection, patients may present not only with OCD, but also with a range of other symptoms including tics and hair-pulling (Swedo et al., 1992b). Also, expression of the D8/17 lymphocyte marker appears increased in childhood-onset OCD and Tourette's (Murphy et al., 1997), and in autism (Hollander et al., 1997a), although not in trichotillomania (Niehaus et al., 1996).

Some authors (Stein & Hollander, 1993a, b) have suggested that one way of looking at the OCD spectrum may be in terms of the dimension of compulsivity and impulsivity. This perspective is based on the notion that compulsivity may reflect harm avoidance, whereas impulsivity reflects risk-seeking. Thus OCD falls on the compulsive end of an OCD spectrum, whereas impulsive disorders fall on the impulsive end, with disorders such as

Tourette's, trichotillomania, and obsessive–compulsive personality disorder demonstrating both compulsive and impulsive characteristics.

Serotonin receptor studies appear to provide some evidence in support of this. Whereas OCD appears to be characterized by hyperresponsivity of at least some serotonergic receptors, impulsivity has been strongly associated with serotonergic hypofunction. Similarly, whereas OCD is characterized by frontal hyperactivity on functional imaging, impulsivity is known to be associated with the loss of prefrontal function. Closer examination suggests, however, that such a distinction is overly simplistic. OCD patients may in fact demonstrate impulsive-aggressive symptoms and impulsive patients may have OCD symptoms. Furthermore, patients with OCD may demonstrate serotonergic hypofunction (Barr et al., 1992), and patients with frontal hypofunction may also demonstrate stereotypic symptoms.

One way of reconciling these data may be the presence or absence of compensatory responses. In OCD it is speculated that compensatory neurobiological changes such as upregulation of some serotonin receptors and frontal hyperfunction may occur. In contrast, in impulsive disorders, there is serotonin or frontal hypoactivity, with no compensatory response. Thus, whereas OCD patients characteristically demonstrate resistance to their symptoms, impulsive patients are able only to experience regret or shame after acting out their symptoms. Putative OCD spectrum disorders may involve both compulsive and impulsive features.

Further work is still needed to delineate fully the concept of an OCD spectrum of disorders. Currently, the most convincing evidence is for an overlap between Tourette's and OCD, with that for the other disorders remaining more speculative. In the interim, it may be useful to employ this construct as heuristic in both clinical and research settings.

Treatment of OCD

Treatment options for OCD fall into two main categories: behavioural therapy and medication.

Behavioural therapy

Behaviour therapy for OCD is not new, it was arguably described by Janet in the nineteenth century. The core features of behaviour therapy for OCD are exposure and response prevention, i.e. the subject is exposed to the feared stimulus and is then helped to resist the urge to carry out the compulsion.

The clustering of fears in OCD patients around certain themes (contamination, aggression etc) has been proposed by Seligman to represent 'prepared phobias' (Seligman, 1971) i.e. fears that we are highly prepared to acquire as they were probably linked to improved survival in earlier periods of human history. This ties in with findings suggesting that the basal ganglia are important in the development, maintenance and selection of cognitive and procedural strategies.

The theoretical basis from which exposure and response prevention operates was first proposed by Mowrer (Deese & Hulse, 1967), who stated that anxiety occurred in response to a specific event by classical conditioning. Rituals are engaged in to decrease the anxiety and if successful are reinforced and more likely to occur in the future (operant conditioning). Ritualistic behaviour preserves the fear response by preventing the person from remaining in contact with the anxiety provoking stimulus long enough to habituate. A vicious cycle of anxiety leading to rituals and back to anxiety is set up. As the disease evolves both the anxiety and the rituals becomes generalized to other stimuli.

Outcome studies of behavioural therapy have found it to be effective in the treatment of OCD. Meyer et al. (1974) in a study of 15 inpatients with OCD showed improvement in all, and of 12 followed up only 4 had experienced periods of relapse. Rachman et al. (Foa & Goldstein, 1978) in a crossover trial proved behavioural therapy to be superior to relaxation therapy. These findings have been replicated in USA, Greece and the Netherlands (Boulougaris, 1977; Emmelkamp, 1982; Baer & Minicheiello, 1988), suggesting cross cultural efficacy. Also, gains may be maintained over time. More recently, studies showing that behavioural therapy can be conducted using computer instruction have been undertaken. There is also a growing interest in more cognitive techniques.

Not all patients respond to behaviour therapy. Poor compliance is perhaps the most common predictor of failure; an unsurprising finding given that behavioural therapy demands a great deal of discipline from the patients. Other patients who are likely to have a poor response include those with pervasive checking rituals, overvalued ideation, obsessional slowness and schizotypal personality disorder. (Quality Assurance Project, 1985).

How does behaviour therapy compare to medication? The Quality Assurance Project meta-analysis looked at 71 trials conducted between 1961 and 1984. They found similar effect sizes for behavioural therapy and clomipramine. More recently Van Balkom et al. (1994) replicated and updated this meta-analysis and found equal efficacy for behavioural treatments and SSRIs (Chouinard, 1992).

Pharmacotherapy

Since the differential response of OCD to serotonergic agents was first noted, these have become the mainstay in the pharmacological management of OCD. Two main classes of agents have been found to be effective, clomipramine and the selective serotonin reuptake inhibitors.

Clomipramine is the most serotonergic of the tricyclic antidepressants and was in the fact the first agent shown to have differential efficacy in OCD. Clomipramine has been considered the standard therapy of OCD for years, and remains a useful agent. It is, however, associated with significant cholinergic and adrenergic side effects, which has limited its utility in clinical practice. Fluoxetine, fluvoxamine, sertraline, paroxetine and citalopram have all proven to be superior to placebo in controlled trials, and all are licensed in some parts of the world for use in patients with OCD (Chouinard, 1992; Montgomery et al., 1993; Wheadon et al., 1993; Tollefson et al., 1994; Greist et al., 1995a; Goodman et al., 1996).

Clinical experience suggests that the SRIs are needed in higher doses and for longer periods to produce an effect in OCD. However, in controlled trials the evidence for a dose–response relationship is only partial. Only paroxetine showed a significant dose–response relationship (Wheadon et al., 1993). Citalopram, fluoxetine and sertraline show a trend of better response at higher doses (Wheadon et al., 1993; Montgomery et al., 1993; Greist et al., 1995a), but this was not statistically significant and no dose response relationship was found for fluvoxamine.

The standard regimen is to treat for 10–12 weeks at the maximally tolerated dose. Initial response may take as long as 8 weeks, and maximal response as long as 20 weeks. Once a therapeutic response is achieved, therapy should be maintained for 6 months to a year. Medication should be tapered slowly and restarted should symptoms reoccur. There is some evidence that once a response is achieved patients can be maintained on somewhat lower doses (Pato et al., 1990; Ravizza et al., 1996; Mundo et al., 1997).

Relative efficacy

Meta-analytic studies have suggested that clomipramine is more effective than SSRIs in OCD (Bisserbee et al., 1995; Greist, 1995b; Piccinelli et al., 1995; Stein et al., 1995; Koran et al., 1996a). However, clomipramine was the first agent to be introduced for the treatment of OCD, and subsequent studies may have included more refractory patients, so resulting in a bias against the SSRIs in the meta-analyses. Indeed, direct head to head comparisons of fluoxetine, fluvoxamine, sertraline and paroxetine have shown equal efficacy of SSRIs with clomipramine, with the SSRIs being better tolerated (Piggot et al., 1990; Bisserbee et al., 1995; Koran et al., 1996a, Zohar & Judge, 1996).

Treatment resistance

Up to 60% of patients with OCD do not respond or experience only partial remission (Goodman et al., 1992). Treatment resistance can be defined as having failed an adequate 10–12 week trial of 2 different SSRIs or clomipramine at maximally tolerated doses. Several strategies have been proposed for the management of treatment resistant patients. Augmentation strategies, using tryptophan, lithium, clonazepam, buspirone and inositol, have all been used with varying degrees of success, but there are few positive controlled augmentation studies of these agents (Goodman et al., 1992; Fux et al., 1996).

Augmentation with neuroleptics has been proven effective in controlled studies. As noted earlier, augmentation of an SSRI with haloperidol produced a significant effect in treatment of refractory patients with co-morbid tic disorders and schizotypal personality predicting a response to neuroleptic augmentation (McDougle et al., 1994). The atypical neuroleptics may be effective also in patients without tics (McDougle et al., 2000), and in view of their superior side effect profile, are increasingly being used as augmenting agents.

Intravenous clomipramine has also been used as a strategy in treatment-resistant patients. Both open and controlled trials have shown benefit in patients previously refractory to oral clomipramine, with response being maintained after subsequent treatment with oral clomipramine (Fallon et al., 1992, 1998). Furthermore, intravenous pulse loading with clomipramine has been suggested to produce a faster response than either oral pulse loading or gradual intravenous dosing (Koran et al., 1997, 1998). However, further work is needed to determine the place of intravenous clomipramine in the treatment of OCD.

In pediatric patients, especially those who fulfill the criteria PANDAS, immunomodulatory treatment has been proposed. Several case reports (The Guillain Barré Study Group, 1985; Barron et al., 1992; Allen et al., 1995; Tucker et al., 1996) and a controlled trial (Perlmutter et al., 1999) have suggested that both plasmapheresis and intravenous immunoglobulin produce improvement in OCD symptoms. However, questions remain as to the generalizability of the results (the children studied are not representative of the pediatric population with OCD) and this treatment currently remains in the experimental phase.

Electroconvulsive therapy is generally not thought to be useful in OCD, but there are a few case reports of its efficacy in the elderly and in some treatment refractory patients (Casey & Davis, 1994; Maletzky et al., 1994; Rabheru &

Persad, 1997). Preliminary reports of the efficacy of transcranial magnetic stimulation (Greenberg et al., 1997) suggest that this modality may also have a place in the treatment of OCD, but at this stage it is still an experimental treatment.

Neurosurgery

Neurosurgery is generally limited to patients with severe, intractable OCD who have not responded to an exhaustive array of other available treatment. The four most common procedures used are: cingulotomy, capsulotomy, limbic leucotomy and subcaudate tractotomy (Jenike, 1998). In a review of the literature, Jenike (1998) found that at least partial relief can be obtained by surgery in some patients with malignant OCD. There is some evidence that right sided lesions are more effective. Lippitz et al. (1997, 1999) found that, in patients who had undergone capsulotomy, good outcome was associated with a lesion in small area within the middle of the right anterior limb of the internal capsule. There was no correlation between left sided lesions and outcome.

There is, however, a lack of controlled data about the efficacy of neurosurgery. This is due, in part to the ethical difficulties in finding an acceptable 'placebo' surgery. However, with the newer gamma knife techniques, which do not require craniotomy, such studies may now be feasible. Neurosurgery is not without risks, but these compare favourably with that of stereotactic operations for nonpsychiatric indications (Blaauw & Braakman, 1988). The risk of postoperative seizures is estimated at less than 1% (Ballantine, 1985; Jenike et al., 1991). In severely ill patients who have not benefited from any other intervention, neurosurgery should be considered as a treatment option.

Deep brain stimulation is another technique that may be useful in the treatment of severely ill patients with OCD. As with functional surgery for movement disorders, the use of deep brain stimulation is emerging as a possible alternative to ablative lesions for psychiatric indications as well (Nuttin et al., 1999)

Conclusion

OCD is a fascinating and complex disorder that has a markedly disruptive impact on the lives of those who suffer from it. It is comparatively recently that we have begun to unravel the mechanisms underlying this disorder, and much remains to be discovered. Nevertheless, we now know OCD to be a disorder mediated by particular neuroanatomical circuits, and to respond to specific interventions. Future work will undoubtedly extend and better integrate neuroanatomic, neurochemical, neurogenetic and neuroimmunological findings.

References

Adams, P.L. (1973). *Obsessive Children, A Sociopsychiatric Study*, pp. 235–6. New York: Brunner and Maze.

Alexander, G.E., DeLong, M.R. & Strick, P.L. (1986). Parallel organization of functionally segregated circuits linking basal ganglia and cortex. *Ann. Rev. Neurosci.*, **9**, 357–81.

Alexander, G.E., Crutcher, M.D. & Delong, M.R. (1990). Basal ganglia–thalamocortical circuits: parallel substrates for motor, oculomotor, 'prefrontal', and 'limbic' functions. *Progr. Brain Res.*, **85**, 119–46.

Allen, A.J., Leonard, H.L. & Swedo, S.E. (1995). Case study: a new infection-triggered autoimmune subtype of pediatric OCD and Tourette's syndrome. *J. Am. Acad. Child Adolesc. Psychiatry*, **34**, 307–11.

Altemus, M., Piggot, T., Kalogeras, K.T. et al. (1992). Abnormalities in the regulation of vasopressin and corticotropin releasing factor secretion in obsessive–compulsive disorder. *Arch. Gen. Psychiatry*, **49**, 9–20

Altemus, M., Piggot, T., L'Heureux, et al. (1993). CSF somatostatin in obsessive–compulsive disorder. *Am. J. Psychaitry*, **150**, 460–4.

American Psychiatric Association. (1994). *Diagnostic and Statistical Manual of Mental Disorders*, 4th edn. Washington, DC: APA.

Ames, D., Cummings, J.L., Wirshing, W.C. et al. (1994). Repetitive and compulsive behavior in frontal lobe lesions. *J. Neuropsychiat. Clin. Neurosci.*, **6**(2), 100–13.

Antony, J., Folstein, M. & Romanoski, A.J. (1985). Comparison of lay diagnostic interview schedule and a standardized psychiatric diagnosis. experience in eastern Baltimore. *Arch. Gen. Psychiatry*, **42**, 667–75.

Aronowitz, B.R., Hollander, E., DeCaria, C. et al. (1994). Neuropsychology of obsessive–compulsive disorder: preliminary findings. *Neuropsychiatr. Neuropsychol., Behav. Neurol.*, **7**, 81–6.

Baer, L. (1994). Factor analysis of symptoms subtypes of obsessive–compulsive disorder and their relation to personality and tic disorders. *J. Clin. Psychiatry*, Suppl. 55, 18–23.

Baer, L. & Jenike, M.A. (1992). Personality disorders in obsessive–compulsive disorder. *Psychiatr. Clin. North Am.*, **15**(4), 803–12.

Baer, L. & Minichiello, W.E. (1988). Behavior therapy for obsessive–compulsive disorder. In *Obsessive Compulsive Disorders: Practical Management*, 3rd edn, ed. M.A. Jenike, L. Baer & W.E. Minichiello. Mosby Inc.

Bailly, D., Servant, D., Dewailly, D. et al. (1994). Corticotropin releasing factor stimulation test in obsessive–compulsive disorder. *Biol. Psychiatry*, **35**, 143–6.

Ball, S.G., Baer, L. & Otto, M.W. (1996). Symptom subtypes of obsessive–compulsive disorder in behavioral treatment studies: a quantitative review. *Behav. Res. Ther.*, **34**(1), 47–51.

Ballantine, H.T., Jr. (1985). Neurosurgery for behavioral disorders. In *Neurosurgery*, ed. R.H. Wilkins & S.S. Rengachary, pp. 25–7. New York: Elsevier/North Holland Biomedical Press.

Barr, L.C., Goodman, W.K., Price, L.H., McDougle, C.J. & Charney, D.S. (1992). The serotonin hypothesis of obsessive–compulsive disorder: implications of pharmacologic challenge studies. *J. Clin. Psychiatry*, **53**, Suppl., 17–28.

Barron, K.S., Sher, M.R. & Silverman, E.D. (1992). Intravenous immunoglobulin therapy: magic or black magic. *J. Rheumatol.*, **19**, 94–7.

Bartha, R., Stein, M.B., Williamson, P.C. et al. (1998). A short echo ¹H spectroscopy and volumetric study MRI study of the corpus striatum in patients with obsessive–compulsive disorder and comparison subjects. *Am. J. Psychiatry*, **155** (11), 1584–91.

Baxter, L., Schwartz, J., Mazziotta, J. et al. (1988). Cerebral glucose metabolic rates in non-depressed patients with obsessive–compulsive disorder. *Am. J. Psychiatry*, **145**, 1560–3.

Baxter, L.R., Schwartz, J.M., Guze, B.H. et al. (1990). Neuroimaging in obsessive–compulsive disorder: seeking the mediating neuroanatomy. In *Obsessive Compulsive Disorder: Theory and Management*, ed. M.A. Jenike, L. Baer & W.E. Minichiello, 2nd edn, pp. 167–88. Chicago: Year Book Publishers.

Baxter, L.R., Jr, Schwartz, J.M., Bergman, K.S. et al. (1992). Caudate glucose metabolic rate changes with both drug and behavior therapy for obsessive–compulsive disorder. *Arch. Gen. Psychiatry*, **49**, 681–9.

Behar, D., Rapoport, J.L., Berg, C.J. et al. (1984). Computerized tomography and neuropsychological test measures in adolescents with obsessive–compulsive disorder. *Am. J. Psychiatry*, **141**, 363–8.

Benkelfat, C., Nordahl, T.E., Semple, W.E. et al. (1990). Local cerebral glucose metabolic rate in obsessive–compulsive disorder: patients treated with clomipramine. *Arch. Gen. Psychiatry*, **47**, 840–8.

Bisserbee, J., Wiseman, R. & Goldberg, M. (1995). Sertraline versus clomipramine in OCD, *American Psychiatric Association Annual Meeting, New Research Abstracts*, Miami, FL May 10–15.

Blaauw, G. & Braakman, R. (1988). Pitfalls in diagnostic stereotactic brain surgery. *Acta Neurochir.*, **42** (Suppl.), 161.

Black, D.W., Noyes, R., Goldstein, R.B. et al. (1992). A family study of obsessive–compulsive disorder. *Arch. Gen. Psychiatry*, **49**, 362–8.

Black, D.W., Goldstein, R.B., Noyes, R., Jr & Blum, N. (1994). Compulsive behaviors and obsessive–compulsive disorder (OCD): lack of a relationship between OCD, eating disorders, and gambling. *Comp. Psychiatry*, **35**, 145–8.

Black, D.W., Monahan, P., Gable, J., Blum, N., Clancy, G. & Baker, P. (1998). Hoarding and treatment response in 38 nondepressed subjects with obsessive–compulsive disorder. *J. Clin. Psychiatry*, **59**(8), 420–5.

Bogetto, F., Venturella, S., Albert, U., Maina, G. & Ravizza, L. (1999). Gender related clinical differences in obsessive–compulsive disorder. *Eur. Psychiatry*, **14**(8), 434–41.

Boone, K.B., Ananth, J., Philpott, L. et al. (1991). Neuropsychological characteristics of non-depressed adults with obsessive–compulsive disorder. *Neuropsychiatry Neuropsychol. Behav. Neurol.*, **4**, 96–109.

Boulougouris, J.C. (1977). Variables affecting the behavior modification of obsessive–compulsive patients treated by flooding. In *The Treatment of Phobic and Obsessive Compulsive Disorders*, ed. J.C. Boulougaris & A.D. Rabavilas. Oxford: Pergamon Press.

Braun, A.R., Randolph, C., Stoetter, B. et al. (1995). The functional neuroanatomy of Tourette's syndrome: an FDG-PET study. II Relationships between regional cerebral metabolism and associated behavioral and cognitive features of the illness. *Neuropsychopharmacology*, **13**, 151–68.

Bystritsky, A., Saxena, S., Maidment, K. et al. (1999). Quality of life changes among patients with obsessive–compulsive disorder in a partial hospitalization program. *Psychiat. Services*, **50**, 412–44.

Canino, G.J., Bird, H.R., Shrout, P.E. et al. (1987). The prevalence of specific psychiatric disorders in Puerto Rico. *Arch. Gen. Psychiatry*, **44**, 727–35.

Carey, G. & Gottesman, H. (1981). Twin and family studies of anxiety, phobic and obsessive–compulsive disorders. In *Anxiety: New Research and Changing Concepts*, ed. D.F. Klein & J.G. Rabkin, pp. 117–36. New York: Raven Press.

Carothers, J. (1953). *The African Mind in Health and Disease*. Geneva: World Health Organization.

Casey, D.A. & Davis, M.H. (1994). Obsessive compulsive disorder responsive to electroconvulsive therapy in an elderly woman. *South. Med. J.*, **87**(8), 862–4.

Castellanos, F.X., Ritchie, F.G., Marsh, W.L. & Rapoport, J.L. (1996). DSM IV stereotypic movement disorder: persistence of stereotypies of infancy in intellectually normal adolescents and adults. *J. Clin. Psychiatry*, **57**, 116–22.

Chapman, F., Visvanathan, K., Carreno-Manjarrez, R. & Zabriskie, J.B (1998). A flow cytometric assay for D8/17 B cell marker in patients with Tourette's syndrome and obsessive–compulsive disorder. *J. Immunol. Meth.*, **219**(1–2), 181–6.

Charney, D.S., Goodman, W.K., Price, L.H. et al. (1988). Serotonin function in obsessive–compulsive disorder. A comparison of the effects of tryptophan and *m*-chlorophenylpiperazine in patients and healthy subjects. *Arch. Gen. Psychiatry*, **45**(2), 177–85.

Chen, Y.W. & Dilsaver, S.C. (1995). Comorbidity for obsessive–compulsive disorder in bipolar and unipolar disorders. *Psychiatry Res.*, **59**(1–2), 57–64.

Chouinard, G. (1992). Sertraline in the treatment of obsessive–compulsive disorder: two double blind placebo controlled studies. *Int. Clin. Psychopharmacol.*, **7** (Suppl. 2), 37–41.

Christenson, K.J., Kim, S.W., Dysken, M.W. et al. (1992). Neuropsychological performance in obsessive–compulsive disorder. *Am. J. Psychiatry*, **31**, 4–18.

Cohen, L.J. et al. (1996). Specificity of neuropsychological impairment in obsessive–compulsive disorder: A comparison with social phobic and normal control subjects. *J. Neuropsychiatr. Clin. Neurosci.*, **8**, 82–5.

Coryell, W. (1981). Obsessive compulsive disorder and primary unipolar depression: comparisons of background, family history, course and mortality. *J. Nerv. Ment. Dis.*, **169**, 220–4.

Cummings, J.L. & Cunningham, K. (1992). Obsessive–compulsive disorder in Huntington's disease. *Biol. Psychiatry*, **31**(3), 263–70.

Deese, J. & Hulse, S.H. (1967). *The Psychology of Learning.* New York: McGraw Hill.

Degonda, M., Wyss, M. & Angst, J. (1993). The Zurich Study. XVIII Obsessive compulsive disorders and syndromes in the general population. *Eur. Arch. Psychiatr. Clin. Neurosci.*, **243**, 16–22.

Delgado, P.L. & Morena, F.A. (1998). Hallucinogens, serotonin and obsessive–compulsive disorder. *J. Psychoactive Drugs*, **30**(4), 359–66.

Dirson, S., Bouvard, M., Cottraux, J. & Martin, R. (1995). Visual memory impairment in patients with obsessive–compulsive disorder: a controlled study. *Psychother. Psychosom.*, **63**, 22–31.

Dupont, R.L., Rice, D.P., Shiraki, S. et al. (1995). Economic costs of obsessive–compulsive disorder. *Med. Interface*, 102–9.

Eapen, V., Pauls, D.L. & Robertson, M.M. (1993). Evidence for autosomal dominant transmission in Gilles de la Tourette syndrome. United Kingdom Cohort Study. *Br. J. Psychiatry*, **162**, 593–6.

Ebert, D., Speck, O., Konig, A. et al. (1997). ^{1}H-magnetic resonance spectroscopy in obsessive–compulsive disorder: evidence for neuronal loss in the cingulate gyrus and the right striatum. *Psychiatry Res.*, **74**(3), 173–6.

Ellinwood, E.H., Jr. (1967). Amphetamine psychosis I: description of the individuals and process. *J. Nerv. Ment. Dis.*, **144**, 273–83.

Emmelkamp, P.M.G. (1982). *Phobic and Obsessive Compulsive Disorders: Theory, Research and Practice.* New York: Plenum.

Emmelkamp, P.M.G., de Haan, E., Stout, R. & Goodman, W. (2000). A prospective study of psychosocial functioning and quality of life in obsessive–compulsive disorder. Presented at the Fourth International Obsessive Compulsive Disorder Conference, St Thomas USA.

Epperson, C.N., McDougle, C.J. & Price, L.H. (1996). Intranasal oxytocin in obsessive–compulsive disorder. *Biol. Psychiatry*, **40**, 547–9.

Ergovesi, S., Ronchi, P. & Smeraldi, E. (1992). 5HT2 receptor and fluvoxamine effect in obsessive–compulsive disorder. *Hum. Psychopharmacol.*, **7**, 287–89.

Fallon, B.A., Campeas, R., Schneier, F.R. et al. (1992). Open trial of intravenous clomipramine in five treatment-refractory patients with obsessive–compulsive disorder. *J. Neuropsychiatry Clin. Neurosci.*, **4**(1), 70–5.

Fallon, B.A., Liebowitz, M.R., Campeas, R. et al. (1998). Intravenous clomipramine for obsessive–compulsive disorder refractory to oral clomipramine: a placebo-controlled study. *Arch. Gen. Psychiatry*, **55**(10), 918–24.

Fernandez-Cordoba, E. & Lopez-Ibor, A.J. (1967). La monocloimipramina en enfermos psyquiatricos resistentes a otros tratamientos. *Acta Luso-Esp. Neurol. Psiquiatr. Ciene Afines*, **26**, 119–47.

Fitzgerald, K.D., Moore, G.J., Paulson, L.A. et al. (2000). Proton spectroscopic imaging of the thalamus in treatment-naïve pediatric obsessive–compulsive disorder. *Biol. Psychiatry*, **47**(3), 174–82.

Flament, M.F., Whitaker, A., Rapoport, J.L. et al. (1988). Obsessive–compulsive disorder in adolescence: an epidemiological study. *J. Am. Acad. Child Adolesc. Psychiatry*, **27**(6), 764–71.

Flor-Henry, P., Yeudall, L.T., Koles, Z.J. et al. (1979). Neuropsychological and power spectral EEG investigations of the obsessive–compulsive syndrome. *Biol. Psychiatry*, **14**, 119–30.

Foa, E.B. & Goldstein, A. (1978). Continuous exposure and complete response prevention in the treatment of obsessive–compulsive neurosis. *Behav. Res. Ther.*, **9**, 821–9.

Foa, E.B., Kozak, M.J., Goodman, W.K. et al. (1995). DSM IV field trial: obsessive–compulsive disorder. *Am. J. Psychiatry*, **152**(1), 90–6.

Freud, S. (1973). *Three Case Histories*, New York: Macmillan. (Translated by P Rieff; originally published in 1909.)

Frost, R.O. & Gross, R.C. (1993). The hoarding of possessions. *Behav. Res. Ther.*, **31**, 367–81.

Fux, M., Levine, J., Aviv, A. & Belmaker, R.H. (1996). Inositol treatment of obsessive–compulsive disorder. *Am. J. Psychiatry*, **153**(9), 1219–21.

German, G.A. (1972). Aspects of clinical psychiatry in sub-Saharan Africa. *Br. J. Psychiatry*, **121**, 461–79.

Gibofsky, A., Khanna, A., Suh, E. & Zabriskie, J.B. (1991). The genetics of rheumatic fever: relationship to streptococcal infection and autoimmune disease. *J. Rheumatol.*, Suppl. 30, 1–5.

Giedd, J.N., Rapoport, J.L., Garvey, M.A., Perlmutter, S. & Swedo, S.E. (2000). MRI assessment of children with obsessive–compulsive disorder or tics associated with streptococcal infection. *Am. J. Psychiatry*, **157**(2), 281–3.

Goodman, W.K., McDougle, C.J. & Price, L.H. (1992). Pharmacotherapy of obsessive–compulsive disorder. *J. Clin. Psychiatry*, **53** (Suppl. 4), 29–37.

Goodman, W.K., McDougle, C.J., Price, L.H. et al. (1995). *m*-Chlorophenylpiperazine in patients with obsessive–compulsive disorder: absence of symptom exacerbation. *Biol. Psychiatry*, **38**(3), 138–49.

Goodman, W.K., Kozak, M.J., Liebowitz, M. & White, K.L. (1996). Treatment of obsessive–compulsive disorder with fluvoxamine: a multicentre, double blind, placebo-controlled trial. *Int. Clin. Psychopharmacol.*, **11**, 21–9.

Gordon, C.T., Rapoport, J.L., Hamburger, S.D. et al. (1992). Differential response of seven subjects with autistic disorder to clomipramine and desipramine. *Am. J. Psychiatry*, **149**, 363–6.

Greenberg, B.D., George, M.S., Martin, J.D. et al. (1997). Effect of prefrontal repetitive transcranial magnetic stimulation in obsessive–compulsive disorder: a preliminary study. *Am. J. Psychiatry*, **154**(6), 867–9.

Greenberg, D. (1987). Compulsive hoarding. *Am. J. Psychother*, **41**, 409–16.

Greenberg, D. & Witztum, E. (1994). Cultural aspects of obsessive–compulsive disorder. In *Current Insights in Obsessive Compulsive Disorder*, ed. E Hollander, J. Zohar, D. Marazzati & B. Olivier. Chichester, UK: John Wiley.

Greist, J.H., Jefferson, J.W., Kobak, K.A. et al. (1995a). Efficacy and tolerability of serotonin transport inhibitors in obsessive–compulsive disorder: meta-analysis. *Arch. Gen. Psychiatry*, **52**, 53–60.

Greist, J., Chouinard, G., Duboff, E., Halaris, A., Kim, S.W. & Koran, L. (1995b). Double blind parallel comparison of three dosages of sertraline and placebo in outpatients with obsessive–compulsive disorder. *Arch. Gen. Psychiatry*, **52**, 289–95.

Grossman, M., Carvell, S., Peltzer, L. et al. (1993). Visual construction impairments in Parkinson's disease. *Neuropsychology*, **7**, 536–47.

The Guillain–Barré Syndrome Study Group. (1985). Plasmapheresis and acute Guillain–Barré syndrome. *Neurology*, **35**, 1096–104.

Head, D., Bolton, D. & Hymas, N. (1989). Deficit in cognitive shifting ability in patients with obsessive–compulsive disorders. *Biol. Psychiatry*, **25**, 929–37.

Helzer, J.E., Robins, L.N. & McEvoy, L.T. (1985). A comparison of clinical and diagnostic interview schedule diagnosis: physician reexamination of lay interview cases in general population. *Arch. Gen. Psychiatry*, **42**, 657–66.

Hodgson, R.J. & Rachman, S. (1977). Obsessional–compulsive complaints. *Behav. Res. Ther.*, **15**, 389–95.

Hoehn-Saric, R., Pearlson, G.D., Harris, G.J. et al. (1991). Effects of fluoxetine on regional cerebral blood flow in obsessive–compulsive patients. *Am. J. Psychiatry*, **148**, 1243–5.

Hollander, E. (1993). Obsessive–compulsive spectrum disorders: an overview. *Psychiat. Ann.*, **23**(7), 355–8.

Hollander, E., Schiffmann, E., Cohen, B. et al. (1990). Signs of central nervous system dysfunction in obsessive–compulsive disorder. *Arch. Gen. Psychiatry*, **47**, 27–32.

Hollander, E., De Caria, C., Gully, R. et al. (1991). Effects of chronic fluoxetine treatment on behavioral and neuroendrocrine responses to meta-chlorophenylpiperazine in obsessive–compulsive disorder. *Psychiatry Res.*, **36**(1), 1–17

Hollander, E., De Caria, C., Nitescu, A. et al. (1992). Serotonergic function in obsessive–compulsive disorder. Behavioural and neuroendocrine responses to oral *m*-CPP and fenfluramine in patients and healthy volunteers. *Arch. Gen. Psychiatry*, **49**, 21–8.

Hollander, E., Cohen, L., Richards, M. et al. (1993). A pilot study of the neuropsychology of obsessive–compulsive disorder and Parkinson's disease: basal ganglia disorders. *J. Neuropsychiatr. Clin. Neurosci.*, **5**, 104–6.

Hollander, E., Delgiudice-Asch, G., Simon, L. et al. (1997a). Repetitive behaviors and D8/17 positivity. *Am. J. Psychiatry*, **154**(11), 1630–1.

Hollander, E., Stein, D.J., Kwon, J.H. et al. (1997b). Psychosocial function and economic costs of obsessive compulsive disorder. *CNS Spectrums*, **2** (10), 16–20.

Hollingsworth, C., Tanguay, P., Grossman, L. et al. (1980). Long term outcome of obsessive–compulsive disorder in childhood. *J. Am. Acad. Child Psychiatry*, **9**, 134–44.

Ho Pian, K.L., Westenberg, H.G., den Boer, J.A. et al. (1998). Effects of meta-chlorophenylpiperazine on cerebral blood flow in obsessive–compulsive disorder and controls. *Biol. Psychiatry*, **44**(5), 367–70.

Husby, G., Van de Rijn, I., Zabriskie, J.B. et al. (1976). Antibodies reacting with cytoplasm of subthalamic and caudate nuclei neurons in chorea and rheumatic fever. *J. Exp. Med.*, **144**, 1094–110.

Hwuh, Y.E. & Chang, L. (1989). Prevalence of psychiatric disorders in Taiwan. *Acta Psychiatr. Scand.*, **79**, 136.

Hymas, N., Lees, A., Bolton, D. et al. (1991). The neurology of obsessional slowness. *Brain*, **114**, 2203–33.

Insel, T.R. (1992). Oxytocin – a neuropeptide for affiliation: evidence from behavioral, receptor sutoradiographic, and comparative studies. *Psychoneuroendocrinology*, **17**(1), 3–35.

Insel, T.R. & Pickar, D. (1983). Naloxone administration in obsessive–compulsive disorder: report of 2 cases. *Am. J. Psychiatry*, **140**, 1219–20.

Insel, T.R., Donnelly, E.F., Lalakea, M.L., Alterman, I.S. & Murphy, D.L. (1983). Neurological and neuropsychological studies of patients with obsessive–compulsive disorder. *Biol. Psychiatry*, **18**, 741–51.

Inyoue, E. (1965). Similar and dissimilar manifestations of obsessive–compulsive neurosis in monozygotic twins. *Am. J. Psychiatry*, **121**, 1171–5.

Jacobsen, F.M. (1995). Risperidone in the treatment of affective illness and obsessive–compulsive disorder. *J. Clin. Psychiatry*, **56**, 413–29.

Janet, P. (1904). *Les Obsessions et al psychasthenie*, ed 2. Paris 1904, Baillière.

Jenike, M.A. (1998). Neurosurgical treatment of obsessive–compulsive disorder. *Br. J. Psychiatry*, Suppl. **35**, 79–90.

Jenike, M.A. & Brotman, A.W. (1984). The EEG in obsessive–compulsive disorder. *J. Clin. Psychiatry*, **45**(3), 122–4.

Jenike, M.A., Baer, L., Ballantine, T. et al. (1991). Cingulotomy for refractory obsessive–compulsive disorder. A long-term follow-up of 33 patients. *Arch. Gen. Psychiatry*, **48**(6), 548–55.

Jenike, M.A., Breiter, H.C., Baer, L. et al. (1996). Cerebral structural abnormalities in obsessive–compulsive disorder. A quantitative morphometric magnetic resonance imaging study. *Arch. Gen. Psychiatry*, **53**(7), 625–32.

Karno, M., Goldin, J.M., Sorenson, S.B. & Burnom, A. (1988). The epidemiology of obsessive–compulsive disorder in five US communities. *Arch. Gen. Psychiatry*, **45**, 1094–9.

Keuler, D.J., Altemus, M., Michelson, D. et al. (1996). Behavioral effects of naloxone infusion in obsessive–compulsive disorder. *Biol. Psychiatry*, **40**, 154–6.

Khanna, A.K., Buskirk, D.R., Williams, R.C., Jr et al. (1989). Presence of a non-HLA B cell antigen in rheumatic fever patients and their families defined by a monoclonal antibody. *J. Clin. Invest.*, **83**(5), 1710–71.

Khanna, S., Rajendra, P.N. & Channabasavanna, S.M. (1986). Sociodemographic variables in obsessive–compulsive neurosis in India. *Int. J. Soc. Psychiatry*, **32**(3), 47–54.

Kolada, J.L., Bland, R.C. & Newman, S.C. (1994). Obsessive-compulsive disorder. *Acta Psychiatr. Scand.*, Suppl. **376**, 24–35

Koran, L.M., McElroy, S.L., Davidson, J.R.T., Rasmussen, S.A., Hollander, E. & Jenicke, M.A. (1996a). Fluvoxamine versus clomipramine for obsessive–compulsive disorder: a double-blind comparison. *J. Clin. Psychopharmacol.*, **16**, 121–9.

Koran, L.M., Thienemann, M.L. & Davenport, R. (1996b). Quality of life for patients with obsessive–compulsive disorder. *Am. J. Psychiatry*, **153**, 783–8.

Koran, L.M., Sallee, F.R., Pallanti, S. (1997). Rapid benefit of intravenous pulse loading of clomipramine in obsessive–compulsive disorder. *Am. J. Psychiatry*, **154** (3), 396–401.

Koran, L.M., Pallanti, S., Paiva, R.S. & Quercoli, L. (1998). Pulse loading versus gradual dosing of intravenous clomipramine in obsessive–compulsive disorder. *Eur. Neuropsychopharmacol.*, **8**(2), 121–6.

Kruesi, M.J.P., Swedo, S., Leonard, H. et al. (1990). CSF somatostatin in childhood psychiatric disorders: a preliminary investigation. *Psychiat. Res.*, **33**, 277–84.

Kruger, S., Cooke, R.G., Hasey, G.M., Jorna, T. & Persad, E. (1995). Comorbidity of obsessive–compulsive disorder in bipolar disorder. *J. Affect. Disord.*, **34**(2), 117–20.

Leckman, J.F., Riddle, M.A., Berrettini, W.H. et al. (1988). Elevated CSF dynorphin A[1–8] in Tourette's syndrome. *Life Sci.*, **43**, 2015–33.

Leckman, J.F., Goodman, W.K., North, W.G. et al. (1994a). Elevated cerebrospinal fluid levels of oxytocin in obsessive–compulsive-disorder. Comparison with Tourette's syndrome and healthy controls. *Arch. Gen. Psychiatry*, **51** (10), 782–92.

Leckman, J.F., North, W., Price, L.H. et al. (1994b). Elevated levels of CSF oxytocin in obsessive–compulsive disorder patients without a personal or family history of tics. *Arch. Gen. Psychiatry*, **51**, 782–92.

Leckman, J.F., Grice, D.E., Boardman, J. et al. (1997). Symptoms of obsessive–compulsive disorder. *Am. J. Psychiatry*, **154**, 911–17.

Lenane, M.C., Swedo, S.E., Rapoport, J.L. et al. (1992). Rates of obsessive–compulsive disorder in first degree relatives of patients with trichotillomania: a research note. *J. Child Psychol. Psychiatry*, **33**, 925–33.

Lensi, P., Cassano, G.B., Correddu, G., Ravagli, S., Kunovac, J.L. & Akiskal, H.S. (1996). Obsessive compulsive disorder. Familial – developmental history, symptomatology, comorbidity and course with special reference to gender related differences. *Br. J. Psychiatry*, **169**(1), 101–7.

Leonard, H.L., Lenane, M.C., Swedo, S.E. et al. (1991). A double blind comparison of clomipramine and desipramine treatment of severe onychophagia (nail biting). *Arch. Gen. Psychiatry*, **48**, 821–7

Lezak, M.D. (1995). *Neuropsychological Assessment*, 3rd edn. New York: Oxford University Press.

Lippitz, B., Mindus, P., Meyerson, B.A. et al. (1997). Obsessive compulsive disorder and the right hemisphere: topographic analysis of lesions after anterior capsulotomy performed with thermocoagulation. *Acta Neurochir. Suppl. (Wien)*, **68**, 61–3.

Lippitz, B.E., Mindus, P., Meyerson, B.A. et al. (1999). Lesion topography and outcome after thermocapsulotomy or gamma knife capsulotomy for obsessive–compulsive disorder: relevance of the right hemisphere. *Neurosurgery*, **44**(3), 452–8.

McDougle, C.J., Goodman, W.K., Delgado, P.L. et al. (1989). Pathophysiology of obsessive–compulsive disorder (letter). *Am. J. Psychiatry*, **146**, 1350–1.

McDougle, C.J., Goodman, W.K., Leckman, J.F., Barr, L.C., Heninger, G.R. & Price, L.H. (1993). The efficacy of fluvoxamine in obsessive–compulsive disorder: effects of comorbid chronic tic disorder. *J. Clin. Psychopharmacol.*, **13**(5), 354–8.

McDougle, C.J., Goodman, W.K., Leckman, J.K. et al. (1994). Haloperidol addition in fluvoxamine- refractory obsessive–com-pulsive disorder: A double placebo controlled study in patients with and without tics. *Arch. Gen. Psychiatry*, **51**, 302–8.

McDougle, C.J., Epperson, C.N., Pelton, G.H., Wasylink, S. & Price, L.H. (2000). A double-blind, placebo-controlled study of risperidone addition in serotonin reuptake inhibitor-refractory obsessive–compulsive disorder. *Arch. Gen. Psychiatry*, **57**(8), 794–801.

Machlin, S.R., Harris, G.J., Pearlson, G.D. et al. (1991). Elevated medial–frontal cerebral blood flow in obsessive–compulsive patients: a SPECT study. *Am. J. Psychiatry*, **148**, 1240–2.

Maletzky, B., McFarland, B., Burt, A. (1994). Refractory obsessive–compulsive disorder and ECT. *Convuls. Ther.*, **10**(1), 34–42.

Malison, R.T., McDougle, C.J., van Dyck, C.H. et al. (1995). [123I]B-CIT SPECT imaging of striatal dopamine binding in Tourette's disorder. *Am. J. Psychiatry*, **152**, 1359–61.

Malloy, P. (1987). Frontal lobe dysfunction in obsessive–compulsive disorder. In *The Frontal Lobes Revisited*, ed. E. Perecmam, pp. 207–23. IRBN Press.

Mataix-Cols, D., Rauch, S.L., Manzo, P.A., Jenike, M.A. & Baer, L. (1999). Use of factor-analyzed symptom dimensions to predict outcome with serotonin reuptake inhibitors and placebo in the treatment of obsessive–compulsive disorder. *Am. J. Psychiatry*, **156**(9), 1409–16.

Meyer, V., Levy, R. & Schnurer, A. (1974). The behavioral treatment of obsessive–compulsive disorders. In *Obsessional States*, ed. H.R. Beech. London: Methuen.

Miguel, E.C., do Rosario-Campos, M.C., Prado, H.S. et al. (2000). Sensory phenomena in obsessive–compulsive disorder and Tourette's disorder. *J. Clin. Psychiatry*, **61**(2), 150–6.

Mikkelson, E.J., Albert, L.G., Emens, M. et al. (1997). The efficacy of antidepressant medication for individuals with mental retardation. *Psych. Ann.*, **27**, 198–206.

Montgomery, S.A., McIntyre, A., Osterheider, M. et al. (1993). A double-blind, placebo-controlled study of fluoxetine in patients with DSM-III-R obsessive–compulsive disorder. *Europ. Neuropsychopharmacol.*, **3**, 143–52.

Moriarty, J., Eapen, V., Costa, D.C. et al. (1997). HMPAO SPECT does not distinguish obsessive–compulsive and tic syndromes in families multiply affected with Gilles de la Tourette's syndrome. *Psychol. Med.*, **27**, 737–40.

Mundo, E., Bianchi, L. & Bellodi, L. (1997). Efficacy of fluvoxamine, paroxetine, and citalopram in the treatment of obsessive–compulsive disorder: a single-blind study. *J. Clin. Psychopharmacol.*, **17**(4), 267–71.

Murphy, T.K., Goodman, W.K., Fudge, M.W. et al. (1997). B lymphocyte antigen D8/17: A peripheral marker for childhood-onset obsessive–compulsive disorder and Tourette's syndrome. *Am. J. Psychiatry*, **154**, 402–7.

Murray, C.J.L. & Lopez, A.D., eds. (1996). *Global Burden of Disease: A Comprehensive Assessment of Mortality and Disability from Diseases, Injuries and Risk Factors in 1990 and Projected to 2020.* Vol. 1, Harvard: World Health Organization.

Nelson, E. & Rice, J. (1997). Stability of diagnosis of obsessive–compulsive disorder in the epidemiologic catchment area study. *Am. J. Psychiatry*, **154**, 826–31.

Nicolini, H., Cruz, C., Paez, F. et al. (1998). Dopamine D2 and D4 receptor genes distinguish the clinical presence of tics in obsessive–compulsive disorder. *Gac. Med. Mex.*, **134**, 521–7.

Niehaus, D.J.H., Knowles, J.A., van Kradenburg, J. et al. (1996). D8/17 in obsessive–compulsive disorder and trichotillomania (let.). *S. Afr. Med. J.*, **89**, 755–6.

Nordahl, T.E., Benkelfat, C., Semple, W. et al. (1989). Cerebral glucose metabolic rates in obsessive–compulsive disorder. *Neuropsychopharmacology*, **2**, 23–8.

Nuttin, B., Cosyns, P., Demeulemeester, H. et al. (1999). Electrical stimulation in the anterior limbs of the internal capsules in patients with obsessive–compulsive disorder. *Lancet*, **354**(9189), 1526–7.

O'Sullivan, R.L., Rauch, S.L., Breiter, H.C. et al. (1997). Reduced basal ganglia volumes in trichotillomania measured via morphometric MRI. *Biol. Psychiatry*, **42**, 39–45.

Ogden, J.A., Growdon, J.H. & Corkin, S. (1990). Deficits in visuospatial tests involving forward planning in high-functioning parkinsonians. *Neuropsychiatr. Neuropsychol. Behav. Neurol.*, **3**, 125–39.

Pato, M., Hill, D.J. & Murphy, D.L. (1990). A clomipramine dosage reduction study in the course of long term treatment of OCD patients. *Psychopharmacol. Bull.*, **26**, 211–14.

Pauls, D.L. & Leckman, J.F. (1986). The inheritance of Gilles de la Tourette's syndrome and associated behaviors. *N. Engl. J. Med.*, **315**, 993–7.

Pauls, D.L., Pakstis, A.J., Kurlan, R. et al. (1990). Segregation and linkage analysis of Tourette's syndrome and related disorders. *J. Am. Acad. Child Adolesc. Psychiatry*, **29**, 195–203.

Pauls, D.L., Alsobrook, J.P. 2nd, Goodman, W., Rasmussen, S. & Leckman, J.F. (1995). A family study of obsessive–compulsive disorder. *Am. J. Psychiatry*, **152**(1), 76–84.

Perani, D., Colombo, C., Bressi, S. et al. (1995). FDG PET study in obsessive–compulsive disorder: a clinical metabolic correlation study after treatment. *Br. J. Psychiatry*, **166**, 244–50.

Perlmutter, S.J., Leitman, S.F., Garvey, M. et al. (1999). Therapeutic plasma exchange and intravenous immunoglobulin for obsessive–compulsive disorder and tic disorders in childhood. *Lancet*, **354**, 1153–8.

Perugi, G., Toni, C. & Akiskal, H.S. (1999). Anxious-bipolar comorbidity. Diagnostic and treatment challenges. *Psychiatr. Clin. North Am.*, **22**(3), 565–83. viii. Review.

Pian, K.L., Westenberg, H.G., van Megen, H.J. & den Boer, J.A. (1998). Sumatriptan (5-HT1D receptor agonist) does not exacerbate symptoms in obsessive–compulsive disorder. *Psychopharmacology (Berl.)*, **140**(3), 365–70.

Piccinelli, M., Pini, S., Bellantuono, C. & Wilkinson, G. (1995). Efficacy of drug treatment in obsessive–compulsive disorder: a meta-analytic review. *Br. J. Psychiatry*, **166**, 424–43.

Piggot, T.A., Pato, M.T., Bernstein, S.E. et al. (1990). Controlled comparisons of clomipramine and fluoxetine in the treatment of obsessive–compulsive disorder. *Arch. Gen. Psychiatry*, **47**, 1543–50.

Piggot, T.A., Hill, J.L., Grady, T.A. et al. (1993). A comparison of the behavioral effects of oral versus intravenous mCPP administration in OCD patients and the effect of metergoline prior to i.v. mCPP. *Biol Psychiatry*, **33**(1), 3–14

Piggot, T.A., L'Heureux, F., Dubbert, B. et al. (1994). Obsessive–compulsive disorder – comorbid conditions. *J. Clin. Psychiatry*, **55** (Suppl. 10), 15–27.

Quality Assurance Project. (1985). Treatment outlines for the management of obsessive–compulsive disorders. *Austr. NZ J. Psychiatry*, **19**, 240–53.

Rabheru, K. & Persad, E. (1997). A review of continuation and maintenance electroconvulsive therapy. *Can. J. Psychiatry*, **42**(5), 476–84.

Rachman, S.J. & Hodgson, R.J. (1980). *Obsessions and Compulsions*. Englewood Cliffs NJ: Prentice Hall.

Rapoport, J.L., ed. (1989). Obsessive Compulsive Disorder in Children and Adolescents. Washington: American Psychiatric Association.

Rasmussen, S.A. (1994). Obsessive compulsive spectrum disorders. *J. Clin. Psychiatry*, **55**, 89–91.

Rasmussen, S.A. & Eisen, J.L. (1990). Epidemiology of obsessive disorder. *J. Clin. Psychiatry*, **51**(Suppl.), 10–13.

Rasmussen, S.A. & Eisen, J.L. (1991). Phenomenology of OCD: clinical subtypes, heterogeneity and coexistence. In *Psychobiology of OCD*, ed. Y. Zohar, T.R. Insel & S.A. Rasmussen. New York: Springer Verlag.

Rasmussen, S.A. & Eisen, J.L. (1998). The epidemiology and clinical features of obsessive–compulsive disorder. In *Obsessive–Compulsive Disorders Practical Management*, 3rd edn, ed. M.A. Jenike, L. Baer & W.A. Minichiello. Mosby Inc.

Rasmussen, S.A. & Tsuang, M.T. (1986). Clinical characteristics and family history in DSM III obsessive–compulsive disorder. *Am. J. Psychiatry*, **143**, 317–22.

Rauch, S.L., Savage, C.R., Alpert, N.M. et al. (1985). A PET investigation of implicit and explicit sequence learning. *Hum. Brain Mapp.*, **3**, 271–86.

Rauch, S.L., Savage, C.R., Alpert, N.M. et al. (1997). Probing striatal function in obsessive–compulsive disorder: a PET study of implicit sequence learning. *J. Neuropsychiat.*, **9**, 568–73.

Rauch, S.L., Dougherty, D.D., Shin, L.M. et al. (1998a). Neural correlates of factor-analyzed OCD symptom dimensions: a PET study. *CNS Spectrums*, **3**, 37–43.

Rauch, S.L., Whalen, P.J., Curran, T. et al. (1998b). Thalamic deactivation during early implicit sequence learning: a functional MRI study. *Neuroreport*, **9**, 865–70.

Ravizza, L., Barzega, G., Bellino, S., Bogetto, F. & Maina, G. (1995). Predictors of drug treatment response in obsessive–compulsive disorder. *J. Clin. Psychiatry*, **56**(8), 368–73.

Ravizza, L., Barzega, G., Bellino, S., Bogetto, F. & Maina, G. (1996). Drug treatment of obsessive–compulsive disorder (OCD): long-term trial with clomipramine and selective serotonin reuptake inhibitors (SSRIs). *Psychopharmacol. Bull.*, **32**, 167–73.

Rettew, D.C., Swedo, S.E., Leonard, H.L. et al. (1992). Obsessions and compulsions across time in 79 children and adolescents with obsessive-compulsive disorder. *J. Am. Acad. Child Adolesc. Psychiatry*, **31**, 1050–6.

Rosenberg, D.R., Benazon, N.R., Gilbert, A. et al. (2000a). Thalamic volume in pediatric obsessive–compulsive disorder patients before and after behavioral therapy. *Biol. Psychiatry*, **48**(4), 294–300.

Rosenberg, D.R., MacMaster, F.P., Keshavan, M.S. et al. (2000b). Decrease in caudate glutamatergic concentrations in pediatric obsessive–compulsive disorder patients taking paroxetine. *J. Am. Acad. Child Adolesc. Psychiatry*, **39**(9), 1096–103.

Roy, B.F., Benkelfat, C., Hill, J.L. et al. (1994). Serum antibody for somatostatin-14 and prodynorphin in 209–240 in patients with obsessive–compulsive disorder, schizophrenia, Alzeheimer's disease, multiple sclerosis, and advanced HIV infection. *Biol. Psychiatry*, **35**, 335–44.

Rubin, R.T., Villaneuva-Myer, J., Ananth, J. et al. (1992). Regional xenon-133 cerebral blood flow and cerebral Technetium 99m HMPAO uptake in unmedicated patients with obsessive–compulsive disorder and matched normal control subjects. *Arch. Gen. Psychiatry*, **49**, 695–702.

Rudin, E. (1953). Ein Beitrag zur Frage der Zwangskrankheit insebesondere ihrere hereditaren Beziehungen. *Arch. Psychiatr. Nervenkr.*, **191**, 14–54.

Savage, C.R. (1998). Neuropsychology of obsessive–compulsive disorder: research findings and treatment implications. In *Obsessive–compulsive Disorders: Practical Management*, 3rd edn, ed. M.A. Jenike, L. Baer & W.E. Minichiello. Mosby Inc.

Savage, C.R., Keuthen, N.J., Jenike, M.A. et al. (1993). Recall and recognition memory in obsessive–compulsive disorder. *J. Neuropsychiatr. Clin. Neurosci.*, **8**, 99–103.

Savage, C.R., Baer, L., Keuthen, N.J. et al. (1995). Organizational strategies and nonverbal memory in obsessive–compulsive disorder. *Clin. Neuropsychol.*, **9**, 293–4.

Savage, C.R., Deckersbach, T., Wilhelm, S. et al. (2000). Strategic processing and episodic memory impairment in obsessive–compulsive disorder. *Neuropsychology*, **14**(1), 141–51.

Schahill, L., Riddle, M.A., King, R.A. et al. (1997). Fluoxetine has no marked effect on tic symptoms in patients with Tourettes: a double-blind placebo-controlled study. *J. Child Adolesc. Psychopharmacol.*, **7**, 75–85.

Schiorring, E. (1975). Changes in individual and social behavior induced by amphetamine and related compounds in monkeys and man. *Behavior*, **43**, 481–521.

Schwartz, J.M., Stoessel, P.W., Baxter, L.R. et al. (1996). Systematic changes in cerebral glucose metabolic rate after successful behavior modification. *Arch. Gen. Psychiatry*, **53**(2), 109–13.

Seligman, M.E.P. (1971). Phobias and preparedness. *Behav. Res. Ther.*, **2**, 307–20.

Shakespeare. *Macbeth*.

Siever, L.J. (1994). Biologic factors in schizotypal personal disorders. *Acta Psychiatr. Scand.*, **90** (Suppl. 384), 45–50.

Singer, H.S., Hahn, I.H. & Moran, T.H. (1991). Abnormal dopamine uptake sites in postmortem striatum from patients with Tourette's syndrome. *Ann. Neurol.*, **30**, 558–62.

Singer, H.S., Reiss, A.L., Brown, J.E. et al. (1993). Volumetric MRI changes in basal ganglia of children with Tourette's syndrome. *Neurology*, **43**(5), 950–6.

Skoog, G. & Skoog, I. (1999). A 40 year follow-up of patients with obsessive–compulsive disorder. *Arch. Gen. Psychiatry*, **56**, 121–7.

Staebler, C.R., Pollard, C.A. & Merkel, W.T. (1993). Sexual history and quality of current relationships in patients with obsessive–compulsive disorder: a comparison with two other psychiatric samples. *J. Sex. Marital Ther.*, **19**(2), 147–53.

Stein, D.J. & Hollander, E. (1993a). Impulsive aggression and obsessive–compulsive disorder. *Psychiatric Ann.*, **23**, 389–95.

Stein, D.J. & Hollander, E. (1993b). The spectrum of obsessive–compulsive related disorders. In *Obsessive–Compulsive Related Disorders*, ed. E. Hollander. Washington, DC: American Psychiatric Press.

Stein, D.J., Spadaccini, E. & Hollander, E. (1995). Meta-analysis of pharmacotherapy trials for obsessive–compulsive disorder. *Int. Clin. Psychopharmacol.*, **10**, 11–18.

Stein, D.J., Roberts, M., Hollander, E. et al. (1996). Quality of life and pharmaco-economic aspects of obsessive–compulsive disorder: a South African survey. *S. Afr. Med. J.*, **8**, 1579–85.

Stein, D.J., Bouwer, C. et al. (1997a). Risperidone augmentation of serotonin reuptake inhibitors in obsessive–compulsive and related disorders. *J. Clin. Psychiatry*, **58** (3), 119–22.

Stein, D.J., Coetzer, R., Lee, M. et al. (1997b). Magnetic resonance brain imaging in women with obsessive–compulsive disorder and trichotillomania. *Psychiatry Res.*, **74**, 177–82.

Stein, D.J., Van Heerden, B., Wessels, C.J. et al. (1999). Single photon emission computed tomography of the brain with Tc-99m HMPAO during sumatriptan challenge in obsessive–compulsive disorder: investigating the functional role of the serotonin autoreceptor. *Prog. Neuropsychopharmacol. Biol. Psychiatry*, **23** (6), 1079–99.

Swedo, S.E., Leonard, H.L., Rapoport, J.L. et al. (1989a). A double blind comparison of clomipramine and desipramine in the treatment of trichotillomania (hair pulling). *N. Engl. J. Med.*, **321**, 497–501.

Swedo, S.E., Rapoport, J.L., Cheslow, D.L. et al. (1989b). High prevalence of obsessive–compulsive symptoms in patients with Sydenham's chorea. *Am. J. Psychiatry*, **146**, 246–9.

Swedo, S.E., Shapiro, M.B., Grady, C.L. et al. (1989c). Cerebral glucose metabolism in childhood-onset obsessive–compulsive disorder. *Arch. Gen. Psychiatry*, **46**, 518–23.

Swedo, S.E., Rapoport, J.L., Leonard, H.L. et al. (1991). Regional cerebral glucose metabolism of women with trichotillomania. *Arch. Gen. Psychiatry*, **48**, 828–33.

Swedo, S.E., Leonard, H.L., Kruesi, M.J. et al. (1992a). Cerebrospinal fluid neurochemistry in children and adolescents with obsessive–compulsive disorder. *Arch. Gen. Psychiatry*, **49**, 29–36.

Swedo, S.E., Leonard, H.L., Lenane, M.C. & Rettew, D.C. (1992b). Trichotillomania: a profile of the disease from infancy through adulthood. *Int. Pediatrics*, **7**, 144–50.

Swedo, S.E., Pietrini, P., Leonard, H.L. et al. (1992c). Cerebral glucose metabolism in childhood onset obsessive–compulsive disorder: revisualization during pharmacotherapy. *Arch. Gen. Psychiatry*, **49**, 609–94.

Swedo, S.E., Leonard, H.L., Schapiro, M.B. et al. (1993). Sydenham's chorea: physical and psychological symptoms of St Vitus' dance. *Pediatrics*, **91**, 706–13.

Swedo, S.E., Leonard, H.L., Mittleman, B.B. et al. (1997). Identification of children with pediatric autoimmune neuropsychiatric disorders associated with streptococcal infections by a marker associated with rheumatic fever. *Am. J. Psychiatry*, **154**, 110–12.

Swedo, S.E., Leonard, H.L., Garvey, M. et al. (1998). Pediatric autoimmune neuropsychiatric disorders associated with streptococcal infections: clinical description of the first 50 cases. *Am. J. Psychiatry*, **155**, 264–71.

Szezsko, P.R., Robinson, D., Alvir, J.M.J. et al. (1999). Orbital frontal and amygdala volume reductions in obsessive–compulsive disorder. *Arch. Gen. Psychiatry*, **56**, 913–19.

The Guillain–Barré Syndrome Study Group. (1985). Plasmapheresis and acute Guillain–Barré syndrome. *Neurology*, **35**, 1096–104.

Thienemann, M. & Koran, L.M. (1995). Do soft signs predict treatment outcome in obsessive–compulsive disorder? *J. Neuropsychiatry Clin. Neurosci.*, **7**, 218–22.

Thomsen, P.H. (1994). Children and adolescents with obsessive–compulsive disorder: an analysis of sociodemographic background. A case-control study. *Psychopathology*, **27**(6), 303–11.

Tollefson, G.D., Rampey, A.H., Potvin, J.H. et al. (1994). A multicenter investigation of fixed-dose fluoxetine in the treatment of obsessive–compulsive disorder. *Arch. Gen. Psychiatry*, **51**, 559–67.

Tucker, D.M., Leckman, J.F., Schahill, L. et al. (1996). A putative poststreptococcal case of OCD with chronic tic disorder not otherwise specified. *J. Am. Acad. Child Adolesc. Psychiatry*, **35**, 1684–91.

Valleni Basile, L.A., Garrison, C.Z., Waller, J.L. et al. (1996). Incidence of obsessive-compulsive disorder in a community sample of young adolescents. *J. Am. Acad. Child Adolesc. Psychiatry*, **35**(7), 898–906.

Van Balkom, A.J., Van Oppen, P., Vermeulen, A.W.A. et al. (1994). A meta-analysis on the treatment of obsessive–compulsive disorder: a comparison of antidepressant, behavior therapy, and cognitive therapy. *Clin. Psychol. Rev.*, **14**, 359–81.

van de Wetering, B.J.M. (1993). The Gilles de la Tourette syndrome: a psychiatric genetic study. PhD Thesis, Erasmus University, Rotterdam, Netherlands.

Veale, D. (1993). Classification and treatment of obsessional slowness. *Br. J. Psychiatry*, **162**, 198–203.

Vecsei, L. & Widerlov, E. (1988). Effects of intracerebroventricularly administered somatostatin on passive avoidance, shuttlebox and openfield activity in rats. *Neuropeptides*, **12**, 237–42.

Vecsei, L., Bollok, L., Penke, B. et al. (1986). Somatostatin and (D-Trp8, D-Cys14) somastatin delay extinction and reverse electroconvulsive shock-induced amnesia in rats. *Psychoneuroendocrinology*, **11**, 111–15.

Weissman, M.M., Bland, R.C., Canino, G.J. et al. (1994). The cross national epidemiology of obsessive–compulsive disorder. The Cross National Collaborative Group. *J Clin. Psychiatry*, **55** (Suppl.), 5–10.

Wheadon, D.E., Bushnell., W.D. & Steiner, M. (1993). A fixed dose comparison of 20, 40, or 60mg paroxetine to placebo in the treatment of obsessive–compulsive disorder [poster]. Presented at the Annual Meeting of the American College of Neuropsychopharmacology (ACNP), December; San Juan, Puerto Rico.

Wolf, S.S., Jones, D.W., Knable, M.B. et al. (1996). Tourette syndrome: Prediction of phenotypic variation in monozygotic twins by caudate nucleus D2 receptor binding. *Science*, **273**, 1225–7.

Zielinski, C.M., Taylor, M.A. & Juzwin, K.R. (1991). Neuropsychological deficits in obsessive–compulsive disorder. *Neuropsychiatr. Neuropsychol. Behav. Neurol.*, **4**, 110–26.

Zohar, A.H. (1999). The epidemiology of obsessive–compulsive disorder in children and adolescents. *Child Adolesc. Psychiatr. Clin. N. Am.*, **8** (3), 445–60.

Zohar, J. & Insel, T.R. (1987). Obsessive–compulsive disorder: psychobiological approaches to diagnosis, treatment, and pathophysiology. *Biol. Psychiatry*, **22**, 667–87.

Zohar, J. & Judge, R. (1996). OCD Paroxetine Study Investigators. Paroxetine versus clomipramine in the treatment of obsessive–compulsive disorder. *Br. J. Psychiatry*, **169**, 468–74.

Zohar, J., Mueller, E.A., Insel, T.R., Zohar-Kadouch, R.C. & Murphy, D.L. (1987). Serotonergic responsivity in obsessive–compulsive disorder. Comparison of patients and healthy controls. *Arch. Gen. Psychiatry*, **44**(11), 946–51.

Zungu-Dirwayi, N., Hugo, F., van Heerden, B.B. & Stein, D.J. (1999). Are musical obsessions a temporal lobe phenomenon? *J. Neuropsychiatry Clin. Neurosci.*, **11**(3), 398–400.

28

Autism and autistic spectrum disorders

Barry Gordon

Division of Cognitive Neurology, Department of Neurology The Johns Hopkins University School of Medicine, Baltimore, MD, USA

Autism is a neurodevelopmental disorder characterized by the early (before 3 years of age, if not earlier) presentation of deficits in social abilities (and in all abilities that depend upon social abilities) and language (delays and/or inappropriate use) and by repetitive behaviours or apparent obsessions. Approximately 70% of individuals with autism are mentally retarded, and nearly 50% of cases never develop useful speech. These disturbances are lifelong, although they may be modified by education, by circumstances, and perhaps by maturation. Autism is surprisingly common, with an incidence of approximately 1/1000. Although first described in 1943 by Kanner (1943) and in 1944 by Asperger (1944), it came under far more intense scrutiny and saw greater public awareness beginning in the 1970s. Milder forms have been recognized, other conditions (such as the general categories of 'developmental language delays' and 'mental retardation') are now being appreciated as frequently harbouring the diagnosis of autism, and individuals with autism are being more publicly visible, and even in some cases speaking out on their own behalf (e.g. Grandin & Scariano, 1996).

Nevertheless, autism is a confusing condition to many health care professionals. The term 'autism' is confusing partly because its characteristic deficits, in social abilities, communication and language use, and in the flexibility and spontaneity of behaviour, are all domains that are often difficult to assess without a detailed history from good observers, and in which a wide range of normalcy (in development tempo or degree of achievement) is generally allowed. The diagnosis of autism is also confusing to many because the term does not really apply to a single condition or even to a spectrum of severity along a single dimension of disease features. Instead, it describes a set of multidimensional clinical entities that differ in both their specific pattern of features and in the severity of each feature. The term can be used to characterize an award-winning math-

ematician (Baron-Cohen et al., 1999) as well as a mute, severely retarded child who spins in a corner by himself all day long. Whether such cases have a unifying neurobiologic basis is not yet known. Therefore, the diagnosis of autism is still based on an imperfect phenomenology, not on neurobiology. Because diagnostic standards have also varied over time and across different researchers and clinicians, older data on 'autism' have to be interpreted with caution, whereas information about conditions such as 'childhood schizophrenia' and many examples of 'mental retardation' and 'idiot savants' must now be reinterpreted as possible examples of autistic disorders. Therefore, there is less certain knowledge than one would like about such a relatively common, and frequently devastating, lifelong condition. This chapter will summarize what is reasonably well known or can be reasonably inferred about this condition or conditions, leaving many aspects of the controversies underlying these summaries to the more primary literature. Filipek et al. (1999) review the status of different diagnostic entities and diagnostic criteria and processes. Cohen and Volkmar (1997), Wetherby and Prizant (2000), and Accardo et al. (2000) are recent book-length treatments. Recent general reviews include those by Rapin (1997), Happé and Frith (1996), Minshew et al. (1997), and Bailey et al. (1996), with Ciaranello and Ciaranello (1995) focusing on neurobiology. Piven (1997) and Ingram et al. (2000) review the current knowledge of the genetics of autism. Recent reviews of treatment options include, for behaviour, Heflin and Simpson (1998), Howlin (1998), and Koegel and Koegel (1995), with Zimmerman et al. (2000) reviewing pharmacologic options. Gordon (2000) gives a theoretical overview of the strategies for behavioural treatments and possibly for pharmacological ones as well. Outcome studies have been summarized by Nordin and Gillberg (1998). Sperry (2001) presents the illustrative stories of ten autistic children, followed from childhood through adulthood.

Table 28.1. Diagnostic Criteria for 299.00 autistic disorder

A. A total of six or more items from (1), (2), and (3), with at least two from (1) and one each from (2) and (3)	(1) Qualitative impairment in social interaction as manifested by at least two of the following:	(a) Marked impairment in the use of multiple non-verbal behaviours such as eye-to-eye gaze, facial expression, body postures, and gestures to regulate social interaction (b) Failure to develop peer relationships appropriate to developmental level (c) A lack of spontaneous seeking to share enjoyment, interests, or achievements with other people (e.g. by a lack of showing, bringing, or pointing out objects of interest) (d) Lack of social or emotional reciprocity
	(2) Qualitative impairments in communication as manifested by at least one of the following	(a) Delay in, or total lack of, the development of spoken language (not accompanied by an attempt to compensate through alternative modes of communication, such as gesture or mime) (b) In individuals with adequate speech, marked impairment in the ability to initiate or sustain a conversation with others (c) Stereotyped and repetitive use of language or idiosyncratic language (d) Lack of varied, spontaneous make-believe play or social imitative play appropriate to developmental level
	(3) Restricted repetitive and stereotyped patterns of behaviour, interests, and activities, as manifested by at least one of the following	(a) Encompassing preoccupation with one or more stereotyped and restricted patterns of interest that is abnormal either in intensity or focus (b) Apparently inflexible adherence to specific, nonfunctional routines or rituals (c) Stereotyped and repetitive motor mannerisms (e.g. hand or finger flapping or twisting, or complex whole-body movements) (d) Persistent preoccupation with parts of objects
B. Delays or abnormal functioning in at least one of the following areas prior to age three years C. The disturbance is not better accounted for by Rett's syndrome or Childhood Disintegrative Disorder	(1) Social interaction (2) Language as used in social communication, or (3) Symbolic or imaginative play	

Source: From DSM-IV TR (American Psychiatric Association and American Psychiatric Association: Task Force on DSM-IV, 2000). Copyright 2000, American Psychiatric Association. Reprinted with permission.

Defining symptomatology

Terminology is confusing for autism and for the many named conditions that fall under the same term or that have apparent similarities with aspects of autism (autistic spectrum disorder, pervasive developmental disorder, high-functioning autism, Asperger's syndrome, non-verbal learning disability, Rett's syndrome, childhood disintegrative disorder, childhood schizophrenia). Some confusion has arisen because prior classification schemes were often based upon relatively small samples and were also somewhat prescriptive rather than data driven. More recent approaches have emphasized larger-scale surveys and classifications emerging from data clusters and correlations (e.g. Rapin, 1996).

The DSM–IV–TR (American Psychiatric Association and American Psychiatric Association: Task Force on DSM-IV, 2000) currently provides the most accepted definition and classification of autistic conditions; those definitions are reproduced in Table 28.1. (The ICD-10 [World Health Organization, 1993] definitions are very similar, although there are differences that may be important for research classifications.)

The DSM–IV–TR criteria incorporate three key features that define the condition and its relatives.

A defect in social awareness and understanding

Individuals with autism do not respond to other people the way that normal individuals do. Other people may be ignored or treated as though they were objects, or these individuals may fail to appreciate other people's emotional states, feelings, wants, or desires. While they may show some warmth and friendliness, particularly towards family members, even this is markedly reduced compared to normal. For many reasons, the social deficit seems to be a core characteristic of the condition.

A defect in communication

Individuals with autism frequently have delayed or absent speech or, if they have speech capabilities, often do not use these capabilities to communicate effectively. They appear to be unaware of the social uses of speech.

Repetitive and stereotypical behaviours, or fixed and unusual interests

These three characteristics do have a strong tendency to co-occur; they do not seem to be just an arbitrary collection. Some of the behavioural manifestations of autism do occur in other conditions but, in many ways, as Rutter and Bailey (1993) have pointed out, often appear to be more intrinsic to the autistic condition in affected individuals. Studies of children and adults (Wing & Gould, 1978, 1979; Shah et al., 1982; Rutter et al., 1992) and family studies (Bolton et al., 1994; Bailey et al., 1998b; Piven, 2000) have shown that these types of abnormalities tend to co-occur in the same individuals and in milder form in relatives. Nonetheless, these abnormalities still span a wide variety of individual presentations. Several subtypes of the autistic spectrum have either been identified in the literature or seen to be of practical or perhaps research significance (Zimmerman & Gordon, 2000).

Subtypes

Asperger's syndrome

Individuals whose only real deficits are 'qualitative impairments in reciprocal social interaction' with 'restricted, repetitive, and stereotyped patterns of behaviour, interests and activities' (World Health Organization, 1993), without any delays or impairments in language or cognitive development, are given this label. Frequently, these individuals also have a history of delayed motor milestones and

motoric clumsiness. (In some classification schemes, these motor impairments are critical for the diagnosis, although it is not clear why they have to be.) In many ways, individuals with Asperger's syndrome can be considered almost the purest form of expression of an isolated defect in social awareness and interaction. As currently defined, the features of the syndrome of non-verbal learning disabilities have a high degree of overlap with those of Asperger's syndrome (Klin et al., 1995), probably representing a failure of precise differentiation. There are many reasons to believe that deficits in social awareness can exist in relatively pure form, apart from any deficits in other non-verbal domains, such as visuospatial functions.

High-functioning autism

Individuals with autistic features, but who have language capabilities and IQs>70 (sometimes, performance IQs>70), are in this category. The exact characterization of these individuals is controversial, and the upper boundary (with Asperger's syndrome) and lower boundary (with low-functioning autism) are not very distinct. High-functioning autism is now generally distinguished from Asperger's by a history of language delay, which individuals with Asperger's do not have. However, given that the pace of language development has a relatively wide range in normal individuals, the distinction between high-functioning autism and Asperger's may prove to be more of a quantitative difference in many cases than a qualitative one. Relative to individuals with Asperger's, individuals with high-functioning autism have lower verbal IQs and higher performance IQs (Klin et al., 1995).

Low-functioning autism

Generally, this category is reserved for individuals with autism who have low verbal IQs (<70). Fifty to 75% of individuals diagnosed as being autistic fall into this category. Approximately 50% of individuals with autism have not just low verbal IQs, but little or no speech. This category is also not precisely defined, partly because the spectrum of verbal abilities is relatively wide and often not easy to categorize in and of itself. For example, a fair percentage of individuals with autism demonstrate echolalia (Howlin, 1982; Roberts, 1989). Frequently, however, speech comprehension is impaired in such cases. IQ in autism is also not well defined (Lincoln et al., 1995), because these children do not necessarily cooperate on the tests, and because their pattern of disabilities prevents standard IQ tests from tapping more central functions.

Autism following regression

Approximately 20–25% of individuals with autism have a history of initially normal development followed by regression. Most often, the parent reports that the child had been developing words, then ceased to add new words and lost the words that he/she had acquired. This finding, most often reported between the age of 18 months and 3 years, has been difficult to study. To the extent that it has been (Rogers & DiLalla, 1990; Kurita et al., 1992; Tuchman & Rapin, 1997; Volkmar et al., 1997), evidence suggests that the actual phenomena may be more complex. Many, if not all, of these children were slower in word acquisition or had some other developmental abnormality or delay preceding the loss of words. In more than half of these children, the loss of words is accompanied by a change in social responsiveness. Regression does not necessarily predict autism, although the best clinical evidence suggests that the risk of autism with this pattern is quite high.

The reasons for this regression are even less clear than the existence of the phenomenon itself. However, a potentially significant possibility is that these cases represent secondary influences causing the autistic spectrum condition. As a result, this group of individuals is under intense scrutiny for possible immunologic and other exogenous etiologies for the autistic spectrum disorder. The best available current evidence has effectively ruled out an association between immunizations and autism in general (Afzal et al., 2000; DeStefano & Chen, 2000). However, the possibility remains that this group is enriched in secondary causes, for which the search continues.

It was once thought that children with regression otherwise followed the typical course of low-functioning individuals. However, there is now clinical evidence that at least some of these individuals can become higher functioning. Autism following regression is categorized here as a separate subtype not because its outcomes are not already categorized, but because its course may help to identify a different cause or causes than is true in other cases of autism.

Broader autism phenotype

The likelihood that autism does not have sharply defined boundaries and may have milder, fragmentary presentations is supported by the evidence for a broader autism phenotype in the relatives of autistic individuals (Bailey et al., 1998b; Piven, 2000). These relatives show a higher incidence of somewhat similar deficits in cognitive functions (relatively lower performance on verbal but not non-verbal IQ scores, poor performance on tests of reading comprehension, rapid automized naming, and executive function, and deficits in pragmatic language and speech), and problems with social cognition (difficulties in accurate interpretation of others' mental states). They suffer more frequently from affective disorders (major depression and anxiety). Relatives of autistic individuals also show a higher frequency of particular personality characteristics (aloofness, rigidity, hypersensitivity to criticism, and anxiety and a history of fewer close friendships) than do those from families without autism. This evidence suggests that there may be elements of autism that can occur in isolation and with less severity.

Autism likely to be secondary to other disorders

Autism has been reliably associated with several other conditions, such as tuberous sclerosis, and less reliably associated with many others (such as fetal alcohol syndrome) (see Table 28.2). Autism is a frequent consequence of tuberous sclerosis (Smalley, 1998). Sixty to 70% of mentally retarded individuals with tuberous sclerosis are autistic as well, and many of these individuals also have epilepsy (Curatolo et al., 1991; Smalley et al., 1992; Hunt & Shepherd, 1993; Gillberg et al., 1994). Particular involvement of the temporal lobes (Bolton & Griffiths, 1997) or of the cerebellum (Weber et al., 2000) has been claimed to be present in those individuals with autistic features. Autism or autistic-like features have also been reported to occur in 15–25% of individuals with Fragile X syndrome (Dykens & Volkmar, 1997; Bailey et al., 1998c). There are scattered reports of associations with other conditions, as noted in Table 28.2, although all have to be interpreted with extreme caution (Dykens & Volkmar, 1997). Severe physical and social deprivation has also been reported to cause autistic-like behaviours (Rutter et al., 1999).

What is also noteworthy about autism's associations is what it is not associated with. Autism has not been associated with focal lesions, even with perinatal focal lesions. Autism and autistic-like features are not seen in other neurodevelopmental conditions, even those with mental retardation. This relative rarity of autism as a secondary consequence of other conditions is part of the evidence for accepting it as an entity in its own right, as difficult as it may be to try to relate its various aspects.

Epidemiology

Prevalence

The prevalence of autism is approximately 1/1000 (Gillberg & Wing, 1999), although it may be as high as 1/500 or even greater, if relatively mild and more circumscribed deficits are included. The exact incidence and prevalence of

Table 28.2. Suspected etiologies or associations of autistic spectrum disorders

Presumed single gene deficit	*HOXA1, HOXB1* (Ingram et al., 2000)
Presumed polygenetic	(thought to be most common) (Szatmari et al., 1998; Piven, 2000)
In the context of otherwise known conditions	Fragile X syndrome (Bailey et al., 1998c)
	Tuberous sclerosis (Smalley, 1998)
	Phenylketonuria (?) (Dykens & Volkmar, 1997)
	Angelman syndrome
	Down's syndrome (rare; see Dykens & Volkmar, 1997)
	Turner's syndrome (Creswell & Skuse, 1999)
Structural brain anomalies (including those with known genetics)	Neural migration defects
	Moebius syndrome
	Joubert syndrome (Holroyd et al., 1991; Ozonoff et al., 1999)
	Duane syndrome
Toxins	Thalidomide (Stromland et al., 1994)
	Valproic acid (Williams & Hersh, 1997)
	Ethanol (Aronson et al., 1997)
Intrauterine infections	CMV (?) (Gillberg & Coleman, 1992)
	Rubella (?) (Gillberg & Coleman, 1992)
Perinatal cerebral injury	Anoxia–ischemia
	Hippocampal sclerosis
	Herpes simplex
Epileptic syndromes	Infantile spasms
	Lennox-Gastaut syndrome
Environmental (?)	Suspected, not established

Note:
For sources not otherwise referenced, see Dykens and Volkmar (1997), Ingram et al. (2000) and Rapin (2000).

autism are understandably not completely clear and are also controversial. Such estimates require both an appropriate set of screening criteria and a guarantee that all appropriate screening is performed to adequate standards in all of the potential population. Surveys coming closest to these ideals include those reported from Japan (Gillberg, 1995), Nova Scotia (Bryson et al., 1988), and Sweden (Gillberg & Wing, 1999).

In many school districts, the incidence of autism has given the appearance of rising, much to the concern of parents and school officials, probably not because of any change in the actual incidence of the condition (Fombonne, 2001), but instead because of greater awareness and, in some cases, to families moving into regions with allegedly better school systems.

Male predominance

Males are more commonly affected than females, by a ratio of approximately 4:1 overall (Gillberg & Coleman, 1992). This male predominance seems to be particularly true of Asperger's syndrome, where the male:female ratio has been reported to be as high as 10:1 (Gillberg, 1989). Skuse (Creswell & Skuse, 1999; Skuse, 2000) has suggested an explanation for the male predominance in autism; he has posited that a genetic factor that influences other genetic factors responsible for social behaviours is part of the X-chromosome. This factor is functional only on the paternally derived X-chromosome; it is imprinted on the maternal X-chromosome. The X-chromosome of boys can only come from the mother; hence, they become more susceptible to any other factors impairing the expression of genes related to social behaviour. Skuse and his colleagues (Creswell & Skuse, 1999; Skuse, 2000) have shown, in partial support of this hypothesis, that the individuals with Turner syndrome who show autistic features are those with maternal X-chromosomes.

Causative or risk factors

Genetics

The best available evidence is that most cases (if not all) of autism represent genetic disorders (or a genetic predisposition coupled with as-yet-unknown non-genetic factors) (Bailey et al., 1998a; Szatmari et al., 1998; Maestrini et al., 2000; Piven, 2000). In a comparison of monozygotic twins vs. dizygotic twins, autism was present by strict definition in 36–91% of monozygotic twins but in 0% of same-sex dizygotic twins (Bailey et al., 1995). Using a broader definition of cognitive or social abnormalities, 92% of monozygotic twins were concordant compared to 10% of dizygotic twins. It has been suggested that anywhere from 2–20 interacting genes may be involved in the pathogenesis of autism. The strongest evidence for the identity of any one of these genes (which is also evidence that suggests that only one need be at fault) comes from the recent demonstration that the HOXA1 gene, or perhaps the HOXB1 gene, is abnormal in a large percentage of individuals with autism (with the frequency of specific mutations in the autistic group ranging from 21–35% (Ingram et al., 2000)). The HOXA1 gene has been thought to be responsible for the developmental organization of the hindbrain. If this finding is confirmed, it would provide a clue as to why children with autism not infrequently appear to have motor abnormalities of the face and lower cranial nerves, and perhaps why the mental retardation and other defects associated with autism have a very different pattern from those occurring in most other conditions.

The risk to couples who already have one autistic child of having an additional autistic child has been estimated as anywhere from 1.5% to 10–20%, much greater than the general risk of approximately 0.1% (Piven et al., 1990; Jorde et al., 1990; Bolton et al., 1994). Families considering having more children obviously are interested in having a more precise estimate of risk within this almost tenfold estimated range, but it is difficult to refine the estimate more precisely, partly because of the different inclusion criteria used. Broader inclusion criteria are not necessarily incorrect, because of the existence of the broader autism phenotype referred to earlier. However, this broad autism phenotype does lead to an apparent overestimation of the chances of having a child with autism, because children with milder and/or less pervasive abnormalities are also included.

Non-genetic factors

These factors must exist, because the concordance rate even among identical twins is <100% (estimated at 60%, Bailey et al., 1998b). However, at the current time, there is no reliable understanding of what these non-genetic factors can be or how they may operate. Well-publicized cases of 'clusters' of autistic cases have not been proven to be due to any known environmental agent or combinations of agents. Immunization (Wakefield et al., 1998), and more recently, mercury exposure (Bernard et al., 2000)

from the carrier used for immunization has been suggested as the 'cause' or contributors to autism. However, not only have these not been proven, there is considerable negative evidence against them (DeStefano & Chen, 2000).

There have been some promising laboratory models of how autism might be acquired. Pletnikov and his colleagues (1999) have shown deficits in social behaviour in juvenile rats who had neonatal infection with Borna disease virus. Bachevalier and colleagues (1994) have shown that some autistic-like behaviours can be seen in monkeys with neonatal injuries to the medial temporal lobes.

As a precaution to researchers in this area, it is perhaps well to keep in mind that, although autism is now known to be the most genetically determined of all the developmental neurobehavioural syndromes, as recently as 1976, genetics were not thought to have a role (Hanson & Gottesman, 1976). The biases and methodologic flaws that led to this erroneous conclusion need to be kept in mind.

Clinical presentation

Initial clinical presentation

Absent or below-average language development is the most common symptom prompting evaluation of these children, but retrospective clinical reports and research studies have suggested that disorders are apparent much earlier in infancy, perhaps as early as 12 months or even earlier. In research studies, the earliest definable feature separating children who will later be diagnosed as autistic from those who would develop normally has been failure of eye contact (based on retrospective review of videotapes of home movies and tapes) (Werner et al., 2000). In retrospect, parents will often note that the infant did not make normal eye contact, did not follow the parent's gaze or pointing (did not seem to have joint attention), and did not point himself.

Clinically, infants with autism are often reported to be irritable, 'colicky', and poor sleepers. Infants may seem to resist being touched, arching the back on contact, or may be unexpectedly passive to touching or holding, even by complete strangers. Early babbling is not abnormal but may not progress, and first words may be delayed, develop at a slower pace than normal, or even seem to be lost by age 2–2½ (see above, 'Autism following regression'). Gross motor development (sitting, crawling, and walking) is not necessarily delayed, although a minority of autistic children will show delayed gross motor development and, later, clumsiness.

The presentation of autism is dependent upon the severity of the defining autistic deficits themselves and upon the severity of any other associated deficits in sensory function, motor function, or cognition. Many feel that autism can be reliably diagnosed before the age of 2 in most cases. However, it frequently takes much longer to recognize and to be actionable. In some cases, appreciation of autism is delayed until the child enters preschool or school, when more objective individuals can observe and compare behaviours. In fact, more recent awareness of the full diagnostic criteria has meant that some individuals have not been diagnosed until adulthood, when their pattern of social isolation, lack of social understanding, and inappropriate social behavioural responses are identified as being a manifestation of Asperger's syndrome. Social deficits might well be masked by achievement in other areas and by selective isolation and involvement that does not stress those areas of deficiencies.

Other associated findings or conditions

Although the defining symptoms of autism are behavioural, these individuals frequently have a number of other impairments or peculiarities. Many are listed in Table 28.3, although this is far from an exhaustive list; more complete tabulations and references can be found in the general reviews cited earlier and in Rapin (1996) and Leary and Hill (1996). One important limitation of such a list is that most of the available data cannot give individual correlations. Therefore, it is not known what features are related to other features and which are not. There may be clues to the neurobiology in those patterns, but these have not been studied systematically.

The seizures and EEG abnormalities noted in Table 28.3 deserve special mention. Two or more unprovoked seizures (epilepsy) occur in 20–40% of individuals with autism, particularly low-functioning, non-verbal individuals (Rapin, 1997). Seizures are most common in infancy and next most commonly occur in adolescence.

EEG abnormalities have been reported in even a larger proportion of individuals with autism, particularly when extended recordings are done (Tuchman, 2000). The clinical significance of these EEG abnormalities, in the absence of overt seizures, is unclear. Although aggressive antiepileptic treatment and even surgery have been used in such individuals, there is no compelling biological reason to believe that the EEG abnormalities are the primary cause of any of the symptomatology of autism, and there is no empirical evidence that treatment of these abnormalities *per se* actually results in improvement of autistic conditions. However, both of these possibilities are under continued investigation.

Neurobiology

A number of attempts have been made to identify a fundamental behavioural deficit that underlies the surface manifestations of autism. Suggestions include: 'mind-blindness', or a lack of awareness of other people (Baron-Cohen, 1995); executive disorders (Russell, 1997); failures of higher information processing (Minshew et al., 1997); and a failure of central coherence (Frith, 1989), the normal tendency to make consistent scripts for events and situations. Although each of these seems to explain large portions of the autistic disorder, no grand unified behavioural theory seems to be very plausible; the deficits in autism are too diverse and present at too many levels of the neuraxis (and perhaps somatically as well; see below).

Neuropathologic, structural imaging and functional imaging assessments of individuals with autism have been hampered by the relatively small numbers and, in some cases, atypical features of individuals who either are available for postmortem examination or are compliant with imaging studies. Several cooperating research efforts to collect the brains from individuals with autism and controls will undoubtedly help to correct this situation in the future. At the present time, available data have relatively little internal coherence or consistency. It does seem to be a reliable finding that the brains of autistic individuals are either normal sized or slightly larger than average. What elements of cerebral tissue are responsible for the increased size in these individuals is not known. Abnormalities have been reported by macroscopic and/or microscopic neuropathological studies and/or by imaging studies (structural or functional imaging) in the brainstem, cerebellar vermis, medial temporal lobes, and cortex and subcortical structures (e.g. Courchesne, 1997; Kemper & Bauman, 1998; Bailey et al., 1998a; Aylward et al., 1999; Ohnishi et al., 2000), although with considerable differences of opinion between investigators (see, for example, Courchesne, 1997 and Piven & Arndt, 1995). The variability and inconsistencies do suggest that either the reported abnormalities have nothing directly to do with autism itself or that autism may be a byproduct of damage or dysfunction of many different levels and sites in the nervous system. To the extent that autism is a neurogenetic condition, it is almost certain that the chain connecting expressed symptomatology with the underlying genetic defect or defects is likely to be extremely complex (Caviness, 2001).

What is clear about the neuropathology of autism is that no single focal lesion, or even currently used combination of lesions, can reproduce the symptomatology. Bachevalier et al. (1994) have created animal models for some aspects of autism in neonatal monkeys by bilateral ablation of the

Table 28.3. Autism and autistic spectrum disorders: other associated conditions/findings

Physical characteristics	Macrocephaly
	Mid-facial dysmorphic features (e.g. increased inter-pupillary distance) (Bailey et al., 1995)
	Other morphological abnormalities (Rodier et al., 1997; Walker, 1977)
Gastrointestinal disorders	Constipation and/or diarrhea
Sensory disorders	Apparent heightened sensitivity to sound (hyperacusis)
	Seemingly lowered sensitivity to pain
	Abnormal sensory response, increased to decreased (Rapin, 2000)
Motor disorders	Strabismus (Kaplan et al., 1999)
	Oromotor dyspraxia
	Hypotonia with increased joint mobility
	Dysmetria and intention tremor
	Awkward fine motor movements
	Limb apraxias
	Abnormal postures (hands, head, etc.)
	Toe walking
Other neurologic disorders	Sleep disorders with early night wakening (Hoshino et al., 1984)
	EEG abnormalities
	Seizures
	Impaired eye-blink conditioning
Cognitive/behavioural features	Smelling of food and people
	Gaze avoidance 'looking out of the corner of the eye'
	Spinning without dizziness
	Attentional disorders: difficulty holding attention, difficulty diverting attention (e.g. Courchesne et al., 1994)
	Apparent auditory processing deficits (Rapin et al., 1977)
	Apparent relative or absolute superiority (Happé & Frith, 1996) in:
	Visual perception
	WAIS Block design subtest
	Drawing
	Jigsaw puzzles
	Perfect pitch (Heaton et al., 1998)
	Music
	Rote memory
	Lightning calculations
	'Executive function' disorders: disorders of planning, strategy and attention (see above)
	Self-injurious behaviour
	Violence or aggression (goal-directed, or accidental)
	Repetitive, stereotypical behaviours

Notes:
For sources not otherwise referenced, see Happé and Frith (1996), Rapin (1997).

hippocampus, amygdala, or associated structures. This research is encouraging because it also begins to address the issue that lesions in early life may interrupt or redirect development, in addition to whatever deficits for which they may be directly responsible. Certainly, many individual components of the autistic condition can be seen behaviourally in focal brain lesions, even in adults, or seem to occur in other developmental disorders, such as atten-tion–deficit–hyperactivity disorder or Tourette's syndrome, and severe learning disabilities. However, despite these superficial similarities, it remains to be seen whether the seemingly identical overt behavioural abnormalities are caused by the same underlying behavioural impairments or malfunctions.

Although many biochemical and neurotransmitter systems have been considered as possible causes or contributors to the autistic deficit(s) (Cook, 1990), none have been reliably found to be abnormal, and no treatment of any putative transmitter system has yet been found to be of positive benefit.

Rett's syndrome (Bibat & Naidu, 2001), which has recently been identified as being caused by a mutation of a specific gene (Amir et al., 1999), the methyl-CpG-binding protein-2 gene (*MECP2*) on the X-chromosome, is an instructive example of the behavioural–neurobiologic correlations to be expected for autism. The condition primarily affects girls of all ethnic groups. Initially, there is stagnation of cognitive development, then profound motor and cognitive regression, then partial recovery and stability. Among the behavioural features that Rett's syndrome has in common with autism are loss of language functions, loss of fine motor functions, stereotypic hand movements, constipation, and seizures. (This list is selective; many somatic and neurologic features of Rett's syndrome are not typically seen in autism.)

The *MECP2* gene has been found to have 78 mutations so far in known Rett's syndrome cases (Shahbazian & Zoghbi, 2001). It is now appreciated that there are very mild cases as well as extremely severe cases (probably lethal in most hemizygous males) (Shahbazian & Zoghbi, 2001). Finally, even though the gene is widely expressed throughout the body, the bulk of pathology caused by the mutations seem to be confined to the central nervous system. Even more specifically, the neuropathologic abnormalities that have been described, selective vulnerability of the zona compacta of the substantia nigra, the nucleus basalis of Meynert, the caudate, frontal lobes, and cerebellum, and a distinctive pattern of cerebral cortical abnormalities (Bibat & Naidu, 2001), cannot be easily related to fairly prototypical signs of classic Rett's syndrome. Therefore, Rett's syndrome is further evidence that there must be a bidirectional perspective on these conditions, from the genes up to the neuropathology and behaviour, and from the behaviours and behavioural abnormalities down to the genes, if we are to hope to have a unified account of the neurobiology of these conditions (Caviness, 2001). The situation for autism is likely to be no less complex than that for Rett's syndrome.

Diagnosis

Guidelines for the diagnosis of autistic spectrum disorders have recently been accepted by a number of professional bodies (Filipek et al., 1999, 2000); guidelines are available on the Web (www.aan.com/public/practiceguidelines/autism.pdf). These guidelines divide the diagnosis into an initial screening phase, followed by more specific assessment for individuals identified as high risk for autism or related developmental disorders by the screen. The guidelines for screening reflect in part an increased awareness that developmental delays or idiosyncrasies need to be taken seriously in many cases; children do not necessarily 'grow out of them', as folklore may have taught. Moreover, earlier diagnosis needs to be encouraged because it is likely that, the earlier the intervention, the more positive the eventual outcome.

Several studies have demonstrated that, if a parent expresses concern about a child's development, they are almost always correct; such concerns need to be taken seriously. It is also the case, however, that many parents are not aware or concerned about even apparently obvious developmental delays. Therefore, the physician and health care provider need to have a high suspicion for such abnormalities, even in the absence of parental reports.

One practical problem in making a diagnosis is that the relevant information and assessments are not available at a single time but may be spread out over weeks to months. A related problem is that the relevant information is often in the possession of separate individuals and professions. A speech pathologist may note delayed speech. An occupational therapist may note clumsiness. Parents will realize that the child does not seem to play appropriately and does not have social contact, even with familiar family members. Often, these various observations are treated in isolation without realizing their common origin and interdependent significance.

One important diagnostic quandary is the child who has some features of autism or elements of autistic-like behaviour or dysfunction but does not meet full criteria for autism. Some such individuals seem to overcome these handicaps. Others will express them more persistently and more clearly, and will be more easily classified as autistic. However, regardless of the particular label, each of these elements or dysfunctions is itself a deficit that needs to be addressed by the child's medical and educational system.

Autism is a diagnosis that can be made with a fair amount of certainty, depending on the information base, the severity of the disorder and associated conditions, and the child's age. Moreover, in addition to the diagnosis itself, outcome predictions can be refined by observing the child's response to therapeutic intervention. Outcome itself is probably better, the earlier the intervention. Therefore, overall, it is better for a child to have suspicions aired and to have the appropriate medical and educational mechanisms engaged as early as possible.

Treatments

Autism cannot yet be 'cured' in the way that some other conditions can be cured and eliminated. Given the increasing evidence as to the fundamental nature of autism, it is unlikely that it will be possible to reverse the underlying neurobiologic deficits once they have had a pervasive influence on the developing brain. However, although features of the autistic spectrum disorders are essentially lifelong, this does not mean that they cannot be ameliorated in some way, either by treating the individual or by altering the individual's environment. Behavioural techniques and, to a lesser extent, pharmacological treatments, can improve some aspects of the functioning and adjustment of these individuals.

Behavioural treatments

Even though the basic neurobiologic deficit(s) in autism are not known, there are some basic principles that should guide behavioural treatment attempts (see also Gordon, 2000). Human beings normally have a variety of processes available to them for effecting change in the nervous system as a result of experience, existing at many different neural levels and time scales (Posner et al., 1997). One way of categorizing these processes of learning for behavioural purposes is as follows: at the most basic, least-demanding level, passive correlations can often extract considerable information from the environment, without the necessity for feedback, reward, punishment, or expectation. However, adding feedback, even in just basic rewards or punishments (e.g. food or the withholding of food) vastly increases the rate of learning. This reward/punishment feedback mechanism seems to be a fairly basic and pervasive one; it is evident in non-human animals, and in infants and young children. Some animals, and human children, also have the ability to learn through imitation. Finally, the most complex and subtle forms of learning are perhaps those which are accomplished by mental prediction, assessment of consequences, and selected actions, in essence, fast forwarding different scenarios and examining how they might turn out. The normally functioning human being has all of these mechanisms available to him or her, and all are typically used in almost every learned activity. For example, although learning to play video games involves conscious thought for tactics and strategy, winning or losing activates fundamental learning circuits, and basic perceptual and motor skills are more finely honed by practice, regardless of whether the game is won or lost.

From this perspective, individuals with autism may fail to learn for a large number of reasons: they may lack the perceptual, motoric, or conceptual abilities to understand basic functions and concepts; they may lack the executive abilities necessary to allocate their attention and their efforts; and they may lack the social awareness and needs that help motivate learning. To try to overcome these problems requires exactly the same types of strategies as are used for learning and teaching in general, except they have to be adapted to the narrower abilities of these children, the shorter conceptual leaps that they can take, and to their more constricted motivations. Behavioural treatments can, therefore, logically try to simplify the environment of the child on the one hand and increase the child's capabilities for dealing with that environment on the other.

Although these principles seem fairly straightforward, in the current educational environment, there have actually been a large number of different methods for teaching and training proposed, including Discrete Trial Training (the Lovaas method: Lovaas et al., 1971), the TEACCH method (Schopler et al., 1993; Schopler & Mesibov, 1994), pivotal behaviours (Koegel & Koegel, 1995), floor play (Greenspan, 1992; Greenspan & Wieder, 1998), the Eden method (Holmes, 1997), the Walden approach (McGee et al., 2001), and others (Handleman et al., 2001). There is evidence for the effectiveness of many if not all of these approaches (e.g. Helfin & Simpson, 1998; Howlin, 1998; Rogers, 1998; Sheinkopf & Siegel, 1998; Ozonoff & Cathcart, 1998). However, these various approaches do differ in a number of fundamental assumptions: in the level of functioning (or of functions) for which they are most appropriate; in their basic philosophies as to which are the core or fundamental deficits to be addressed first; and in their adopted methodologies for achieving behavioural changes in those particular functional deficits. Understanding these differences can help identify which approach is best for which child.

Assignment of fundamental deficits

As an example of philosophic differences, the explicit position espoused by Greenspan (1992) might be contrasted with the implicit positions of applied behavioural analysis and discrete trial training approaches (e.g. Lovaas & Taubman, 1981). For Greenspan, 'The primary goal of intervention is to enable children to form a sense of their own personhood, a sense of themselves as intentional, interactive individuals' (Greenspan, 1992). In the applied behavioural analysis tradition, these children have deficits in a number of specific skills. Training is, therefore, directed at improving the specific skills, presumably in the hope that they would coalesce into a better-functioning, complete human being. The evidence from neurobiology would seem to lend more weight to the implicit applied behavioural analysis position, in that it is generally assumed, with much evidence supporting this, that our mental abilities (including perhaps even our sense of self) are, in fact, a collection of much more specific, discrete, and relatively independent underlying mental functions. If not all of those discrete abilities are present, then normal complete 'personhood' cannot be expected to be achieved. (Autism itself provides examples of how some specific functions can be impaired, while others can be relatively spared.) However, despite this seeming contrast in starting positions, Greenspan's own approach seems to also be focused upon specific functions and abilities (Greenspan & Wieder, 1998), albeit those thought to underlie the development of personhood, and those whose learning can be capitalized upon through special situations and interests in each particular child. This partial convergence of methodologies is perhaps another reason why a comparison of these methods is so confusing for parents and teachers alike.

Methods for achieving behavioural change

Specific methods that have been endorsed range from teacher-imposed, single-trial-at-a-time learning, with rewards (or withholding of rewards) (e.g. Lovaas & Taubman, 1981), to using the child's own spontaneous interests and actions as the basis for instruction (e.g. Greenspan & Wieder, 1998).

From the general perspective on learning discussed above, the ideal learning situation for each individual with autism is not so much a matter of a particular philosophy, but instead, identifying the particular pattern of abilities and disabilities that each individual exhibits at any one point in time, and of choosing the best methods for overcoming those disabilities at that time. For some deficits, in some children, trial-by-trial guidance and rewarding will be necessary (the discrete trial and Lovaas approaches). Other children may have fewer deficits and be more spontaneous and more capable of learning through their own intrinsic devices, with the proper guidance. For these children, approaches that capitalize on these features (such as pivotal behaviours (Koegel & Koegel, 1995) and floor play (Greenspan & Wieder, 1998) may be more appropriate.

A similar approach applies to the question of environmental adaptation. There is an ongoing debate as to whether the environment of these individuals should be simplified or not, to foster learning. For lower-functioning children, environmental adaptations consist of a routinized school environment and a simplified, routinized home environment. Each step involved in, for example, tooth brushing, may be indicated by picture icons as a constant reminder for the child of what is necessary after what. The number of choices may be reduced; commands and comments may be simplified to avoid confusion. For example, a low-functioning child may not apparently recognize that 'sit' and 'sit down' are meant to refer to the same thing.

There is a valid concern that simplification may be counterproductive, especially with higher-functioning children, leading to decreased motivation and to a decreased exposure to the natural variation and richness of a normal environment. This may reduce the child's ability to generalize to new materials or to respond to new situations. Achieving an adequate balance between adequate simplification and productive complexity is an ongoing debate in the teaching of such children. However, it remains the case that many children cannot begin to learn, or learn how to learn, unless they are started in a simplified, structured environment. Even in regular education, the learning environment is made more structured than outside reality usually is. For other children, less simplification and more variety are probably desirable.

In practice, it is often hard to tell many of these methods apart, despite their strong theoretical contrasts. Their goals and methods often seem to overlap and even blend. The overriding principles that need to be kept in mind are that the educational process, and the strategies for education, of any particular individual with autism can and must change with the individual's circumstances. Furthermore, no matter how successful the reported intervention is reputed to be, all interventional strategies must be tested by examination of the actual data for each individual.

Pharmacological treatments

Drugs have not yet been shown to produce improvement in any functions in these individuals. However, there are reasonable expectations, and some data exist that appropriate drug therapy can reduce problem behaviours in at least some individuals (Cook, 1990; Minshew, 2000; Zimmerman et al., 2000). Such behaviours and suggested drug treatment regimens are given in Table 28.4.

Treatment coordination

Regardless of whether behavioural treatments, drug treatments, or both, are used, the treatment of autistic individuals is a constantly changing process that requires different types of expertise at different points in time. Treatment plans must be adapted at any point in time to a particular individual's pattern of abilities and disabilities and to their family and school circumstances. Plans must have goals that are appropriate for that individual's

Table 28.4. Possible pharmacologic treatments for selected disorders in autism

Hyperactivity Distractibility Impulsivity	Stimulant medications	Methylphenidate, 5–60 mg/day in 3–5 divided doses
		Dextroamphetamine 5–40 mg/day in 3–5 divided doses
		Adderall, 5–30 mg/kg/day in two divided doses
	Clonidine, 0.1–0.4 mg/day in 2–3 doses or via transdermal skin patch	
	Naltrexone, 0.5–2.0 mg/kg/day in two divided doses	
Rituals Compulsions	Antidepressants SSRIs	Fluoxetine, 5–80 mg/day in 1–2 divided doses or 10–20 mg every other day
		Paroxetine, 2.5–50 mg/day in 1–2 divided doses
		Sertraline, 25–200 mg/day in 1–2 divided doses
		Fluvoxamine, 25–300 mg/day in 1–3 divided doses
	Tricyclic antidepressants	Citalopram, 5–40 mg/day in 1–2 divided doses
		Clomipramine, 25–200 mg/day in 1–2 divided doses
Aggression Irritability	Sympatholytic agents	Propranolol, 20–320 mg/day in 3–4 divided doses
		Naldolol, 40–100 mg/day in daily dose
	Anticonvulsants	Carbamazepine to a blood level of 8–12 micrograms/ml
		Valproate to a blood level of 50–125 micrograms/ml
	Naltrexone, 0.5–2.0 mg/kg in 1–2 divided doses	
	Lithium to a serum level of 0.8–1.2 meq/litre	
	Neuroleptic agents	Risperidone, 0.5–4.0 mg/day in 1–3 divided doses
		Olanzapine, 2.5–20 mg/day in 1–3 divided doses

Source: Adapted from Minshew (2000). Used with permission.

required functions, current status, and expected trajectory of change. Physicians are not typically involved in this therapeutic process, although their input is critical for justifying it. More typically, the educational process is in the hands of a varying combination of parents, educators, speech pathologists, physical therapists, behavioural psychologists, occupational therapists, and others. For most individuals with autism, it is critical that there be some strong coordinating individual or group that can help to identify goals, prioritize methods, and monitor the progress of any particular program that the child has, eliminating inconsistencies and redundancies, solving unforeseen problems, and trying to capitalize on successes.

Prospects

Although individuals with autism face a lifelong condition, it can be ameliorated in many cases and in many ways. Higher-functioning individuals in particular have a good chance of a successful life; indeed, some of the signature behavioural characteristics of autism can be positives in the right career or career niche. Success in many areas of life is determined less by weaknesses than by strengths, and these individuals may have many strengths.

Meanwhile, autism has become an area of enormous interest, both in its own right and for what it can reveal about the mind and the brain and their pathologies and possible treatments.

Acknowledgements

Preparation of this chapter has been supported in part by an endowment and gifts from an anonymous family, by gifts from The Benjamin and Adith Miller Family Endowment on Aging, Alzheimer's and Autism Research, and by gifts in memory of Bernard Gordon.

The author's perspectives on autism have benefited from discussions with many individuals, including Drs Dana Boatman, Katharina Boser, Geraldine Dawson, Martha Denckla, Pauline A. Filipek, Rebecca Landa, Catherine Lord, O. Ivar Lovaas, William J. McIlvane, James L. McClelland, Ruth Nass, Isabel Rabin, Judith Rumsey, Tristram Smith, Paula Tallal, and Andrew Zimmerman. Most of all, the author has benefited from direct contact with individuals with autism and their schools, teachers, aides, and parents, including The Forum School (Wycoff, New Jersey; Dr Steven Krapes, Linda Edwards, and Brielle Boedart), the LEAP Program of the Kennedy Krieger School

(Baltimore, Maryland; Marilyn Cataldo, Keri Demos, and Melanie Wagner), the Mamaroneck Union Free School District (Mamaroneck, NY; Dr Sherry Parker King, Dr Fern Aefsky, and Jane Friedlander), and from teachers and therapists such as Maureen Boner, Anne Fetherston, and Jessica O'Grady, and many others. I particularly thank Nancy Cook, and also Maura Whelan and Renning Ji, for their help in the preparation of this chapter. None, of course, are responsible for any errors or omissions made here.

References

Accardo, P.J., Magnusen, C. & Capute, A.J. (2000). *Autism: Clinical and Research Issues*, Baltimore: York Press.

Afzal, M.A., Minor, P.D. & Schild, G.C. (2000). Clinical safety issues of measles, mumps and rubella vaccines. *Bull. World Health Org.*, 78, 199–204.

American Psychiatric Association and American Psychiatric Association: Task Force on DSM-IV (2000). *Diagnostic and Statistical Manual of Mental Disorders: DSM-IV-TR*, 4th edition revised, Washington, DC: American Psychiatric Association.

Amir, R.E., Van den Veyver, I.B., Wan, M., Tran, C.Q., Francke, U. & Zoghbi, H.Y. (1999). Rett syndrome is caused by mutations in X-linked MECP2, encoding methyl-CpG-binding protein 2. *Nat. Genet.*, 23, 185–8.

Aronson, M., Hagberg, B. & Gillberg, C. (1997). Attention deficits and autistic spectrum problems in children exposed to alcohol during gestation: a follow-up study. *Dev. Med. Child Neurol.*, 39, 583–7.

Asperger, H. (1944). Die 'Autistischen Psychopathen' im kindesalter. *Arch. Psychiatr. Nervenkr.*, 117, 76–136.

Aylward, E.H., Minshew, N.J., Goldstein, G. et al. (1999). MRI volumes of amygdala and hippocampus in non-mentally retarded autistic adolescents and adults. *Neurology*, 53, 2145–50.

Bachevalier, J. (1994). Medial temporal lobe structures and autism: a review of clinical and experimental findings. *Neuropsychologia*, 32, 627–48.

Bailey, A., Le Couteur, A., Gottesman, I. et al. (1995). Autism as a strongly genetic disorder: evidence from a British twin study. *Psychol. Med.*, 25, 63–77.

Bailey, A., Phillips, W. & Rutter, M. (1996). Autism: towards an integration of clinical, genetic, neuropsychological, and neurobiological perspectives. *J. Child Psychol. Psychiatry*, 37, 89–126.

Bailey, A., Luthert, P., Dean, A. et al. (1998a). A clinicopathological study of autism. *Brain*, 121, 889–906.

Bailey, A., Palferman, S., Heavey, L. & Le Couteur, A. (1998b). Autism: the phenotype in relatives. *J. Autism. Dev. Disord.*, 28, 369–92.

Bailey, D.B., Jr., Mesibov, G.B., Hatton, D.D., Clark, R.D., Roberts, J.E. & Mayhew, L. (1998c). Autistic behavior in young boys with fragile X syndrome. *J. Autism Dev. Disord.*, 28, 499–508.

Baron-Cohen, S. (1995). *Mindblindness, An Essay on Autism and Theory of Mind*. Cambridge: MIT Press.

Baron-Cohen, S., Wheelwright, S., Stone, V. & Rutherford, M. (1999). A mathematician, a physicist and a computer scientist with Asperger syndrome: performance on folk psychology and folk physics tests. *Neurocase*, 4, 475–83.

Bernard, S., Enayati, A., Roger, H., Binstock, T., Redwood, L. & McGinnis, W. (2000). *Autism: A Unique Type of Mercury Poisoning*. Cranford, NJ: ARC Research.

Bibat, G. & Naidu, S. (2001). Rett syndrome: an update. *Neurologist*, 7, 73–81.

Bolton, P., Macdonald, H., Pickles, A. (1994). A case-control family history study of autism. *J. Child Psychol. Psychiatry*, 35, 877–900.

Bolton, P.F. & Griffiths, P.D. (1997). Association of tuberous sclerosis of temporal lobes with autism and atypical autism. *Lancet*, 349, 392–5.

Bryson, S.E., Clark, B.S. & Smith, I.M. (1988). First report of a Canadian epidemiological study of autistic syndromes. *J. Child Psychol. Psychiatry*, 29, 433–45.

Caviness, V.S. (2001). Research strategies in autism: a story with two sides. *Curr. Opin. Neurol.*, 14, 141–3.

Ciaranello, A.L. & Ciaranello, R.D. (1995). The neurobiology of infantile autism. *Annu. Rev. Neurosci.*, 18, 101–28.

Cohen, D.J. & Volkmar, F.R. (1997). *Handbook of Autism and Pervasive Developmental Disorders*, 2nd edn. New York: John Wiley.

Cook, E.H. (1990). Autism: review of neurochemical investigation. *Synapse*, 6, 292–308.

Courchesne, E. (1997). Brainstem, cerebellar and limbic neuroanatomical abnormalities in autism. *Curr. Opin. Neurobiol.*, 7, 269–78.

Courchesne, E., Townsend, J., Akshoomoff, N.A. et al. (1994). Impairment in shifting attention in autistic and cerebellar patients. *Behav. Neurosci.*, 108, 848–65.

Creswell, C.S. & Skuse, D.H. (1999). Autism in association with Turner syndrome: genetic implications for male vulnerability to pervasive developmental disorders. *Neurocase*, 5, 511–18.

Curatolo, P., Cusmai, R., Cortesi, F., Chiron, C., Jambaque, I. & Dulac, O. (1991). Neuropsychiatric aspects of tuberous sclerosis. *Ann. NY Acad. Sci.*, 615, 8–16.

DeStefano, F. & Chen, R.T. (2000). Autism and measles, mumps, and rubella vaccine: No epidemiological evidence for a causal association. *J. Pediatr.*, 136, 125–6.

Dykens, E.M. & Volkmar, F.R. (1997). Medical conditions associated with autism. In *Handbook of Autism and Pervasive Developmental Disorders*, ed. D.J. Cohen, & F.R. Volkmar, pp. 388–410. New York: John Wiley.

Filipek, P.A., Accardo, P.J., Baranek, G.T. et al. (1999). The screening and diagnosis of autistic spectrum disorders. *J. Autism Dev. Disord.*, 29, 439–84.

Filipek, P.A., Accardo, P.J., Ashwal, S. et al. (2000). Practice parameter: screening and diagnosis of autism: report of the Quality Standards Subcommittee of the American Academy of Neurology and the Child Neurology Society. *Neurology*, 55, 468–79.

Fombonne, E. (2001). Is there an epidemic of autism? *Pediatrics*, **107**, 411–12.

Frith, U. (1989). *Autism: Explaining the Enigma*. Oxford: Blackwell.

Gillberg, C. (1989). Asperger syndrome in 23 Swedish children. *Dev. Med. Child Neurol.*, **31**, 520–31.

Gillberg, C. (1995). Autism and its spectrum disorders. Epidemiology and neurobiology. *Jpn J. Child Adolesc. Psychiatry*, **36**, 342–87.

Gillberg, C. & Coleman, M. (1992). *The Biology of the Autistic Syndromes*, 2nd edn, London: Mac Keith Press.

Gillberg, C. & Wing, L. (1999). Autism: not an extremely rare disorder. *Acta Psychiatr. Scand.*, **99**, 399–406.

Gillberg, I.C., Gillberg, C. & Ahlsen, G. (1994). Autistic behaviour and attention deficits in tuberous sclerosis: a population-based study. *Dev. Med. Child. Neurol.*, **36**, 50–6.

Gordon, B. (2000). Commentary: a neural systems perspective for improving behavioral treatments for autism. *J. Autism Dev. Disord.*, **30**, 503–8.

Grandin, T. & Scariano, M.M. (1996). *Emergence: Labeled Autistic*. New York: Warner Books.

Greenspan, S.I. (1992). Reconsidering the diagnosis and treatment of very young children with autistic spectrum or pervasive developmental disorders. *Zero to Three*, **13**, 1–9.

Greenspan, S.I. & Wieder, S. (1998). *The Child with Special Needs*. Reading, MA: Perseus.

Handleman, J.S. & Harris, S.L. (2001). *Preschool Education Programs for Children with Autism*, Pro-Ed, Austin, TX.

Hanson, D.R. & Gottesman, I. (1976). The genetics, if any, of infantile autism and childhood schizophrenia. *J. Autism Child Schizophr.*, **6**, 209–34.

Happé, F. & Frith, U. (1996). The neuropsychology of autism. *Brain*, **119**, 1377–400.

Heaton, P., Hermelin, B. & Pring, L. (1998). Autism and pitch processing: a precursor for savant musical ability? *Music Percept.*, **15**, 291–306.

Heflin, L.J. & Simpson, R.L. (1998). Interventions for children and youth with autism: prudent choices in a world of exaggerated claims and empty promises. Part 1: intervention and treatment option review. *Focus Autism Other Dev. Disabil.*, **13**, 194–211.

Holmes, D.L. (1997). *Autism Through the Lifespan: The Eden Model*. Bethesda, MD: Woodbine House.

Holroyd, S., Reiss, A.L. & Bryan, R.N. (1991). Autistic features in Joubert syndrome: a genetic disorder with agenesis of the cerebellar vermis. *Biol. Psychiatry*, **29**, 287–94.

Hoshino, Y., Watanabe, H., Yashima, Y., Kaneko, M. & Kumashiro, H. (1984). An investigation on sleep disturbance of autistic children. *Folia Psychiatr. Neurol. Jpn*, **38**, 45–51.

Howlin, P. (1982). Echolalic and spontaneous phrase speech in autistic children. *J. Child Psychol. Psychiatry*, **23**, 281–93.

Howlin, P. (1998). Practitioner review: psychological and educational treatments for autism. *J. Child Psychiatry*, **39**, 307–22.

Hunt, A. & Shepherd, C. (1993). A prevalence study of autism in tuberous sclerosis. *J. Autism Dev. Disord.*, **23**, 323–39.

Ingram, J.L., Stodgell, C.J., Hyman, S.L., Figlewicz, D.A., Weitkamp, L.R. & Rodier, P.M. (2000). Discovery of allelic variants of HOXA1 and HOXB1: genetic susceptibility to autism spectrum disorders. *Teratology*, **62**, 393–405.

Jorde, L.B., Mason-Brothers, A., Waldmann, R. et al. (1990). The UCLA-University of Utah epidemiologic survey of autism: genealogical analysis of familial aggregation. *Am. J. Med. Genet.*, **36**, 85–8.

Kanner, L. (1943). Autistic disturbances of affective contact. *Nerv. Child*, **2**, 217–50.

Kaplan, M., Rimland, B. & Edelson, S.M. (1999). Strabismus in autism spectrum disorder. *Focus Autism Other Dev. Disabil.*, **14**, 101–5.

Kemper, T.L. & Bauman, M. (1998). Neuropathology of infantile autism. *J. Neuropathol. Exp. Neurol.*, **57**, 645–52.

Klin, A., Volkmar, F.R., Sparrow, S.S., Cicchetti, D.V. & Rourke, B.P. (1995). Validity and neuropsychological characterization of Asperger syndrome: convergence with nonverbal learning disabilities syndrome. *J. Child Psychol. Psychiatry*, **36**, 1127–40.

Koegel, R. & Koegel, L. (1995). *Teaching Children with Autism*. Baltimore: Paul H. Brookes.

Kurita, H., Kita, M. & Miyake, Y. (1992). A comparative study of development and symptoms among disintegrative psychosis and infantile autism with and without speech loss. *J. Autism Dev. Disord.*, **22**, 175–88.

Leary, M.R. & Hill, D.A. (1996). Moving on: autism and movement disturbance. *Ment. Retard.*, **34**, 39–53.

Lincoln, A.J., Allen, M.E. & Piacentini, A. (1995). The assessment and interpretation of intellectual abilities in people with autism. In *Learning and Cognition in Autism*, eds. E. Schopler & G.B. Mesibov, pp. 89–117. New York: Plenum Press.

Lovaas, O.I. & Taubman, M.T. (1981). Language training and some mechanisms of social and internal control. *Analysis Intervent. Dev. Disabil.*, **1**, 363–72.

Lovaas, O.I., Scheibman, L., Koegel, R. & Rehm, R. (1971). Selective responding by autistic children to multiple sensory input. *J. Abnorm. Psychol.*, **77**, 211–22.

McGee, G.G., Morrier, M. & Daly, T. (2001). The Walden early childhood programs. In *Preschool Education Programs for Children with Autism*, ed. J.S. Handleman & S.L. Harris. Austin, TX: Pro-Ed.

Maestrini, E., Paul, A., Monaco, A.P. & Baily, A. (2000). Identifying autism susceptibility genes. *Neuron*, **28**, 19–24.

Minshew, N., Goldstein, G. & Siegel, D. (1997). Neuropsychologic functioning in autism: profile of a complex information processing disorder. *J. Int. Neuropsychol. Soc.*, **3**, 303–16.

Minshew, N.J. (2000). In *Autism: Neurologic Basis and Symptoms Across the Ages*, pp. 71–85. San Diego, CA: American Academy of Neurology.

Nordin, V. & Gillberg, C. (1998). The long-term course of autistic disorders: update on follow-up studies. *Acta Psychiatr Scand.*, **97**, 99–108.

Ohnishi, T., Matsuda, H., Hashimoto, T. et al. (2000). Abnormal regional cerebral blood flow in childhood autism. *Brain*, **123**, 1838–44.

Ozonoff, S. & Cathcart, K. (1998). Effectiveness of a home program intervention for young children with autism. *J. Autism Dev. Disord.*, **28**, 25–32.

Ozonoff, S., Williams, B.J., Gale, S. & Miller, J.N. (1999). Autism and autistic behavior in Joubert syndrome. *J. Child Neurol.*, **14**, 636–41.

Piven, J. (1997). The biological basis of autism. *Curr. Opin. Neurobiol.*, **7**, 708–12.

Piven, J. (2000). The broad autism phenotype. In *Autism: Clinical and Research Issues*, ed P.J. Accardo, C. Magnusen, & A.J. Capute, pp. 215–24. Baltimore: York Press.

Piven, J. & Arndt, S. (1995). The cerebellum and autism. *Neurology*, **45**, 398–402.

Piven, J., Gayle, J., Chase, G.A. et al. (1990). A family history study of neuropsychiatric disorders in the adult siblings of autistic individuals. *J. Am. Acad. Child Adolesc. Psychiatry*, **29**, 177–83.

Pletnikov, M.V., Rubin, S.A., Vasudevan, K., Moran, T.H. & Carbone, K.M. (1999). Developmental brain injury associated with abnormal play behavior in neonatally Borna disease virus-infected Lewis rats: a model of autism. *Behav. Brain Res.*, **100**, 43–50.

Posner, M.I., DiGirolamo, G.J. & Fernandez-Duque, D. (1997). Brain mechanisms of cognitive skills. *Conscious Cogn.*, **6**, 267–90.

Rapin, I. (1996). *Preschool Children with Inadequate Communication Developmental Language Disorder, Autism, Low IQ*. London: Cambridge University Press.

Rapin, I. (1997). Autism. *N. Engl. J. Med.*, **337**, 97–104.

Rapin, I. (2000). In *Autism: Neurologic Basis and Symptoms Across the Ages*. American Academy of Neurology, San Diego, CA, pp. 1–26.

Rapin, I., Mattis, S., Rowan, A.J. & Golden, G.G. (1977). Verbal auditory agnosia in children. *Dev. Med. Child. Neurol.*, **19**, 197–207.

Roberts, J.M.A. (1989). Echolalia and comprehension in autistic children. *J. Autism Dev. Disord.*, **19**, 271–81.

Rodier, P.M., Bryson, S.E. & Welch, J.P. (1997). Minor malformations and physical measurements in autism: data from Nova Scotia. *Teratology*, **55**, 319–25.

Rogers, S.J. (1998). Empirically supported comprehensive treatments for young children with autism. *J. Clin. Child Psychol.*, **27**, 168–79.

Rogers, S.J. & DiLalla, D.L. (1990). Age of symptom onset in young children with pervasive developmental disorders. *J. Am. Acad. Child Adolesc. Psychiatry*, **29**, 863–72.

Russell, J. (1997). *Autism as an Executive Disorder*. Oxford: Oxford University Press.

Rutter, M. & Bailey, A. (1993). Thinking and relationships: mind and brain – some reflections on 'theory of mind' and autism. In *Understanding Other Minds: Perspectives from Autism*, ed. S. Baron-Cohen & H. Tager-Flusberg, pp. 481–504. Oxford: Oxford University Press.

Rutter, M., Mawhood, L. & Howlin, P. (1992). Language delay and social development. In *Specific Speech and Language Disorders in Children: Correlates, Characteristics, and Outcomes*, ed. P. Fletcher, D.M.B. Hall & E. Auger. San Diego: Singular Publishing Group.

Rutter, M., Andersen-Wood, L., Beckett, C. et al. (1999). Quasi-autistic patterns following severe early global privation. English and Romanian Adoptees (ERA) Study Team. *J. Child Psychol. Psychiatry*, **40**, 537–49.

Schopler, E. & Mesibov, G.B. (1994). *Behavioral Issues in Autism*. New York: Plenum Press.

Schopler, E., Van Bourgondien, M.E. & Bristol, M.M. (1993). *Preschool Issues in Autism*. New York: Plenum Press.

Shah, A., Holmes, N. & Wing. L. (1982). Prevalence of autism and related conditions in adults in a mental handicap hospital. *Appl. Res. Ment. Retard.*, **3**, 303–17.

Shahbazian, M.D. & Zoghbi, H.Y. (2001). Molecular genetics of Rett syndrome and clinical spectrum of *MECP2* mutations. *Curr. Opin. Neurol.*, **14**, 171–6.

Sheinkopf, S.J. & Siegel, B. (1998). Home-based behavioral treatment of young children with autism. *J. Autism Dev. Disord.*, **28**, 15–24.

Skuse, D.H. (2000). Imprinting, the X-chromosome, and the male brain: explaining sex differences in the liability to autism. *Pediatr. Res.*, **47**, 9–16.

Smalley, S.L. (1998). Autism and tuberous sclerosis. *J. Autism Dev. Disord.*, **28**, 407–14.

Smalley, S.L., Tanguay, P.E., Smith, M. & Gutierrez, G. (1992). Autism and tuberous sclerosis. *J. Autism Dev. Disord.*, **22**, 339–55.

Sperry, V.W. (2001). *Fragile Success: Ten Autistic Children, Childhood to Adulthood*, Baltimore, MD: Paul H. Brookes.

Stromland, K., Nordin, V., Miller, M., Akerstrom, B. & Gillberg, C. (1994). Autism in thalidomide embryopathy: a population study. *Dev. Med. Child Neurol.*, **36**, 351–6.

Szatmari, P., Jones, M.B., Zwaigenbaum, L. & MacLean, J.E. (1998). Genetics of autism: overview and new directions. *J. Autism Dev. Disord.*, **28**, 351–68.

Tuchman, R. (2000). Treatment of seizure disorders and EEG abnormalities in children with autism spectrum disorders. *J. Autism Dev. Disord.*, **30**, 485–9.

Tuchman, R.F. & Rapin, I. (1997). Regression in pervasive developmental disorders: seizures and epileptiform electroencephalogram correlates. *Pediatrics*, **99**, 560–6.

Volkmar, F.R., Klin, A., Marans, W. & Cohen, D.J. (1997). Childhood disintegrative disorder. In *Handbook of Autism and Pervasive Developmental Disorders*, ed. D.J. Cohen & F.R. Volkmar, pp. 47–59. New York: John Wiley.

Wakefield, A.J., Murch, S.H., Anthony, A. et al. (1998). Ileal–lymphoid–nodular hyperplasia, non-specific colitis, and pervasive developmental disorder in children. *Lancet*, **351**, 637–41.

Walker, H.A. (1977). Incidence of minor physical anomaly in autism. *J. Autism Child Schizophr.*, **7**, 165–76.

Weber, A.M., Egelhoff, J.C., McKellop, J.M. & Franz, D.N. (2000). Autism and the cerebellum: evidence from tuberous sclerosis. *J. Autism Dev. Disord.*, **30**, 511–17.

Werner, E., Dawson, G., Osterling, J. & Dinno, N. (2000). Brief report: recognition of autism spectrum disorder before one year of age: a retrospective study based on home videotapes. *J. Autism Dev. Disord.*, **30**, 157–62.

Wetherby, A.M. & Prizant, B.M. (2000). *Autism Spectrum Disorders. A Transactional Developmental Perspective*. Baltimore: Paul H. Brookes.

Williams, P.G. & Hersh, J.H. (1997). A male with fetal valproate syndrome and autism. *Dev Med. Child Neurol.*, **39**, 632–4.

Wing, L. & Gould, J. (1978). Systematic recording of behaviors and skills of retarded and psychotic children. *J. Autism Child Schizophr.*, **8**, 79–97.

Wing, L. & Gould, J. (1979). Severe impairments of social interaction and associated abnormalities in children: epidemiology and classification. *J. Autism Dev. Disord.*, **9**, 11–29.

World Health Organization (1993). *The ICD-10. The ICD-10 Classification of Mental and Behavioural Disorders: Diagnostic Criteria for Research.* Geneva: World Health Organization.

Zimmerman, A.W. & Gordan, B. (2000). Neural mechanisms in autism. In *Autism: Clinical and Research Issues*, ed. P.J. Accardo, C. Magnusen, & A.J. Capute, pp. 1–24. Baltimore: York Press.

Zimmerman, A.W., Bonfardin, B. & Myers, S.M. (2000). Neuropharmacological therapy in autism. In *Autism: Clinical and Research Issues*, ed. P.J. Accardo, C. Magnusen, & A.J. Capute, pp. 241–302. Baltimore: York Press.

29

Attention deficit hyperactivity disorder: spectrum and mechanisms

Martha Bridge Denckla

Kennedy Krieger Institute, Baltimore, Maryland. MD, USA

Attention deficit hyperactivity disorder (ADHD) is among the most prevalent disorders (3 to 5% of school-age children) treated by physicians who manage children/adolescents, comprising as much as half of child psychiatric practice (Cantwell, 1996). Media attention has been inspired by the extension of the ADHD diagnosis to adults, acknowledgement of frequent comorbidity or antecedent status with respect to other conditions, and concern over the increase in stimulant prescriptions; it may appear that ADHD, or at least its importance, is a novelty. In truth, the essential description of the disorder has a 75-year-long history under a variety of names: 'incorrigibles', 'brain damaged', 'hyperkinetic', and 'Minimal Brain Dysfunction' (Barkley, 1990). Since 1980, the term 'attention' has been the initial and therefore most prominent feature of the names given to the syndrome, either 'attention deficit' alone or combined with 'hyperactivity' (and 'impulsivity') comprising the other central features defining the clinical category (American Psychiatric Association Diagnostic and Statistical Manual, 1994). The current *Diagnostic and Statistical Manual* (*DSM–IV*) lists three subtypes: a combined or full ADHD; a predominantly inattentive; and a predominantly hyperactive/impulsive subtype (*American Psychiatric Association Diagnostic and Statistical Manual*, 1994). Experts suspect that the predominantly hyperactive/impulsive subtype is most often seen in preschool children; there is more controversy about the predominantly inattentive subtype (except when it is only a residual form of the full syndrome, occurring in the adolescent and adult portions of the lifespan); controversial is whether those who present as children with the predominantly inattentive type have a disorder that is quite different. The heterogeneity of ADHD is one of the commonly documented but difficult characteristics of the disorder.

Diagnosis

Hyperactivity may be the first sign to be noticed, obvious in nursery school when not much sustained attention or independent self-control is expected. A small percentage of children diagnosed with ADHD are retrospectively described as difficult right from the moment of birth and as children who 'run rather than walk' as soon as they get up on their feet. Most children with the ADHD diagnosis are also impulsive, which can be in terms of 'on the mind, out the mouth' and is not necessarily gross physical activity or aggressivity. Impulsivity can take the form of not waiting one's turn or thinking before acting, interrupting, talking too much, talking too loud, blurting out whatever comes to mind. Impulsivity is more characteristic of ADHD than is true inattentiveness. Impulsive children may seem clumsy and accident prone because they are uninhibited when exploring the environment in a state of activation/excitation.

Time management, organization of possessions, and sustained on-task effort of any kind present difficulties at any age for people with ADHD. It is often stated that children with ADHD forget what they have for homework, forget to bring in what homework they have done, may bring their homework to school and forget to hand it in, fail to finish things, make careless mistakes, and appear to be in a kind of 'brownian motion' between activities, yet sustain attention on games/play of their own predilection.

Although they appear just 'immature for age' or 'exaggerated children', children with ADHD can make life difficult for everyone around them as well as for themselves, causing disruption and disorganization in homes and schools. Often, they experience social rejection by other children who find their behaviour somewhere between annoying and completely obnoxious, while teachers and parents may regard the children's deportment as belonging to 'moral turpitude' categories such as irresponsibility, lack of motivation, or laziness. Secondary emotional overlay comes in the wake of rejection and the experience of negative reactions from others, so that anger and frustration may distort the psychosocial adjustment of children with ADHD; they can easily become oppositional, argumentative, and, while denying their own mistakes, attribute the causes of their actions to others. Because children with ADHD do not perform academically up to expectations based on their intellects or talents, because often and repeatedly they are subjected to negative comments, scolding, and punishments, they frequently suffer from poor self-esteem, generating still further disorders like depression and anxiety.

Adolescents and adults with ADHD are more likely to look like the 'predominantly inattentive type' even though, fulfilling full criteria for development of the full syndrome before the age of seven years, they have previously been hyperactive. What persists is a picture of fidgety restlessness, disorganization, forgetfulness, poor boredom tolerance, impatience and a generally 'immature'/disheveled lifestyle. As teenagers, they misplace their possessions, mismanage their time, neglect their homework, and do not achieve the level of self-control considered appropriate for the level of independence craved by most teenagers. Persisting in the adult picture is difficulty setting priorities, managing time, keeping track of possessions, and remembering an agenda. Adult 'hyperactivity' in a sense is persistent in the more time-stretched-out sense of moving frequently, changing primary relationships frequently and changing jobs more frequently than do others of their age.

ADHD is diagnosed at least three times more often in boys than in girls; and this difference, more boys than girls, is even more pronounced among those who are seen in psychiatric rather than pediatric settings. Boys appear more likely to be disruptive, hyperactive, overtly impulsive, and express the comorbidity of oppositional-defiant disorder. Girls are often diagnosed at a later age, and more often with the predominantly inattentive type; close clinical inspection of such girls, however, reveals considerable impulsivity in their leisure behaviours outside of school and a greater degree (than is obvious to the observer) of inhibitory insufficiency in the extent to which they are able to control their mental activities.

Diagnosis of ADHD is complicated by symptoms/signs suggestive of other psychiatric diagnoses and must be distinguished from these or declared comorbid with these. Common comorbidities in childhood are academic learning disabilities and developmental motor coordination disorder. The term minimal brain dysfunction was popular between 1968 and 1980 and was used to describe a mixture

of attention deficit hyperactivity disorder symptoms, learning disabilities, and developmental motor coordination disorder (Barkley, 1990). More than 20% of children with ADHD have depressive or anxiety disorders; up to one-third of children with ADHD are aggressive and may receive a formal diagnosis of oppositional-defiant disorder. Some experts believe that the 'externalizing' or acting-out behaviours comprising so-called disruptive 'comorbidity' result from the same underlying failure of behavioural inhibition or impulse control that is fundamental to ADHD. Those whose profiles are complicated by the aggressive, oppositional-defiant, or misconduct symptomatology also have a high rate of alcoholism and drug abuse, sometimes because of antisocial personality, sometimes because of attempts towards self-medication for mood issues (Biederman et al., 1993; Mannuzza et al., 1993). Comorbidity with Tourette's syndrome is discussed in the chapter by Singer, this volume.

There are times when a 'secondary' ADHD gives clues as to the biological basis of the disorder in general; for example, the hyperactive/impulsive group called the 'incorrigibles' were children who suffered brain damage in the wake of the encephalitis lethargica epidemic in the 1920s after World War I. ADHD also occurs secondary to several genetic disorders, head injuries and toxic exposures such as lead poisoning and fetal alcohol syndrome (The Harvard Mental Health Letter, 2000). It is now widely accepted that the core of the disorder is a failure of self-control, most prominently in the sense of behavioural inhibition, inability to respond adequately to routine reward and punishment, and/or deficiencies in what is called 'executive function' (see below). So far, ADHD cannot be diagnosed by any form of neuroimaging, neuropsychological tests, or blood tests.

Differential diagnosis is complicated by the fact that circumstances and situations have to be taken into account in order to rule out that signs/symptoms resembling ADHD result from improper schooling/child rearing, or stress in the form of abuse or neglect. It is sometimes difficult to make a differential diagnosis between bipolar disorder and ADHD (The Harvard Mental Health Letter, 2000). The way in which the child is handled may make the child behave so markedly differently in one situation from another, contemporaneously, that it may be difficult to sort out whether or not the child has the fundamental biological disorder of ADHD; sometimes a child will be perfectly well behaved with a kind but firm teacher, but then be completely out of control in a daycare setting where there is a less structured approach to managing the room. In general, children with ADHD behave better one-to-one, in small groups, or in situations in which the adult management is kind but firm, and the expectations are clear, as are the consequences of either positive or negative behaviours.

Diagnosis should require a thorough medical/psychiatric history and examination, a neuropsychological/psychoeducational evaluation, and use of questionnaires and rating scales in the context of careful clinical interviews with parents, teachers, and the children themselves. (Unfortunately, this is exceedingly time consuming, so that ideal diagnostic procedures are rarely feasible in today's medical care environment.) Information about family history and about the fine-grained details of home and school life are also important. There may need to be involvement beyond neurologists, psychiatrists, and teachers in the form of information from school counsellors and clinical child psychologists, as well. If there are learning disabilities or language disorders, special educators and language therapists will become participants in the process.

Much of the neurobiological thinking about the disorder has arisen from the fact that certain stimulant drugs in a majority of cases provide striking immediate improvement in the most troublesome and most disruptive symptoms of ADHD; however, response to stimulants is *not* diagnostic of ADHD.

A valid diagnosis of ADHD requires that the problems as quantified on rating scales must be a sufficient number of standard deviations from the mean for the behaviours exhibited by children at that age/level of development. The problems must have begun before the age of seven and must be persistent across time. The requirement that they be pervasive across situations runs into some of the difficulties noted above, but at least in settings similarly structured there should be pervasive problems. It is not that a high level of activity is considered intolerable as long as activity and impulse control are regulated; it is that the child cannot get along with others, obey reasonable requests from parents and teachers, and cannot progress academically because of impersistence. When clinicians follow established guidelines, the diagnosis of ADHD is reliable (NIH Consensus Statement, 1998).

Prognosis

Even the staunchest advocates of a biological interpretation of the basis for attention deficit hyperactivity disorder have been aware of the fact that there are major environmental interactions in the appearance and in the severity of the disorder. The increased demands for sustained attention, and self-control (at an earlier age than decades ago) due to patterns of parental employment, and even the burden of 'virtual reality' distractions may have profoundly influenced attentional and inhibitory capacities and accentuated the perception that a child is inadequate developmentally. Negative parenting practices predict more of the non-compliant and the externalizing behaviours, particularly those that go beyond the age inappropriate and are antisocial (Hinshaw et al., 1997). A persistent misconception is that a biological interpretation of ADHD leads to the conclusion that parenting and schooling do not matter; this prevails even among highly educated persons thinking about the controversies surrounding ADHD. Experience of clinicians is that the child's environment may powerfully influence the prognosis even when there are strong indicators of a biological set of predispositions of ADHD. How the family and the school react to the child, adolescent, and even young adult across the lifespan and how they cope with the problems, seek help and modify the environment for the person with ADHD may be crucial in shaping development; and for all we know, this may be in a very literal brain-development sense as well as the total adaptive sense. Underlying tendencies may be worsened by overly lenient, difficult, inconsistent, or hostile teaching and parenting. The most important complications of ADHD seem to emerge under the worst of circumstances, while optimal parenting and teaching promote strengths in children with ADHD, including positive peer relations (Tannock, 1998).

Neurobiology

Neuropsychology

Since 1980, contemporaneous with the emphasis upon the word 'attention' in the name of the disorder and also a general consensus that psychological processes should guide our understanding of the disorder, neuropsychologists have been struck by analogies between test/assessment behaviours seen in patients with 'frontal lobe' lesions and similar ones in children with ADHD. From this has come a large body of literature focused upon the frontal-lobe-associated construct of 'executive dysfunction' in children with attention deficit hyperactivity disorder, which has itself been the inspiration for a great deal more in the way of study of the normal development of the executive system in childhood. By 1991, a very influential textbook on learning disabilities was constructing a framework in which ADHD was affiliated with frontal lobe, particularly dorsolateral, dysfunction (Pennington, 1991). Executive functions are historically linked to prefrontal, especially dorsolateral, regions and their subcortical, 'domain-general' interconnected regions. The parallel circuits connecting corresponding subdivisions of the frontal lobes and various subdivisions of the basal ganglia have been scrutinized; there is now a general conceptual model to the effect that children with attention deficit hyperactivity disorder, particularly those with the frequent comorbidity of developmental motor coordination disorder, are deficient in one (or more) sectors of the frontal striatal circuitry involving control; there are seen various clinical combinations of motor control, cognitive control, and emotional control deviating from normal developmental attainments. Although there have been both positive and negative findings with respect to each of several tests of executive function in sampled populations with attention deficit hyperactivity disorder, examination of executive functions constitutes a major clinical advance and also inspires the focus of the anatomic imaging work, hypothesis-driven because it measures those structures that are reasonable frontal or basal ganglia 'candidates' implicated in the types of controlled processes on which ADHD-related failures are found (Tannock, 1998; Barkley, 2000).

The executive deficits found have largely been those that involve response inhibition and working memory. As for the adjacent 'motor' domain, there have been many publications on response inhibition in the context of behavioural neurology (Voeller et al., 1991). More recently, eye movements have been studied and a variety of different findings have been forthcoming with respect to antisaccades and remembered saccades (Mostofsky et al., 2000). Clinicians frequently see that tests of executive function, particularly in children, adolescents, and adults with the predominantly inattentive type of ADHD, successfully characterize young patients in a way that is instantaneously recognizable to their parents; however, it has not proven possible to turn around the diagnostic algorithm in such a way that one could classify persons as qualifying for the diagnosis of ADHD on the basis of their executive dysfunctions (Grodzinsky & Barkley, 1999). In his book on ADHD, which is subtitled *The Nature Of Self-Control* (Barkley, 1997), Barkley attempts a linear model explanation of executive function, whereby inhibition is the fundamental and driving precursor of all subsequent developmental executive difficulties, however multiple the manifestations. (Motor control enters into Barkley's thinking as he takes note of the disinhibition on motor examination in the form of overflow movements.) On the other hand, other researchers have suggested that a more pervasive cognitive dysfunction with more proactive organization of components, rather than a precursor deficit restricted to response inhibition, is characteristic of children with attention deficit hyperactivity disorder

(Oosterlaan & Sergeant, 1998). Even tests previously thought of as completely within the linguistic domain, such as rapid automatized naming (considered to be one of the best predictors of reading disability) have been shown to be impaired in children with ADHD (Tannock et al., 2000). Furthermore, narrative language skills are not always normal in an ADHD group that is not clinically considered to have language deficits of a more basic nature, because higher order executive function deficits operating upon the domain of language emerge when important pre-writing formulation skills are tested (Purvis & Tannock, 1997). Many professionals who specialize in evaluating school problems are now of the opinion, as is the writer of this contribution, that ADHD implies cognitive control issues that do constitute 'true learning disabilities'. The separation between 'learning disabilities' and 'ADHD' is increasingly untenable (Fischer et al., 1990; Cox et al., 1997; Denckla & Cutting, 1999).

On continuous performance tests, particularly of the go/no-go type, most patients with ADHD show prolonged reaction times and a high degree of variability (inconsistency) of their reaction times (Reader et al., 1994). Paradoxically, most patients with ADHD are slow on response preparation, so timed tasks are the most useful ones in corroborating the diagnosis of ADHD. Output under timed conditions with rule-governed control demands brings out deficits in ADHD, as on the letter-word fluency task aptly called Controlled Word Association. Clinicians have found it useful to look at the organizational scores, particularly in a developmental context, from the copying of the Rey Osterrieth complex figure. The California Verbal Learning Test for children also provides a useful opportunity to contrast the level of recall with the learning characteristics and error types. Children with ADHD, who have mainly proactive executive deficits, tend to be poor in strategy (clustering) and also respond less well under free recall conditions than they do when they are given by the examiner the explicit structure of category cues. Those with severe impulsivity make enormous numbers of intrusion errors. The occurrence of repetition errors may indicate poor working memory (Denckla, 1994, 1996).

Neurophysiology of ADHD

Although for many years de-emphasized, recently there has been reborn interest in the epileptiform EEG associated with attention deficit hyperactivity disorder. Epileptiform discharges were reported in a rather large study of children with ADHD, even after all patients with a history of clinical seizures were excluded from the study.

'Definite noncontroversial epileptiform activity' was present in 30%, with epileptiform spike discharges of a focal nature in 24% (temporal/occipital) and generalized spike/waves in 6%. Normal records were found in 47%, but only 28% were completely normal (Hughes et al., 2000). Transcranial magnetic stimulation, when used to study patients with ADHD, indicates immaturity (relative to age-matched peers) in the development of cortical inhibitory pathways; children with ADHD showed reduced intracortical inhibition relative to other children of their age (Moll et al., 2000). Functional magnetic resonance imaging has been used in order to demonstrate altered neuronal activity accompanying relevant response preparation/inhibition tasks; when tested without medication, boys with ADHD showed greater-than-normal activity in the frontal lobe during the more difficult of two tasks requiring response inhibition. Also, the ADHD group showed impaired inhibitory control on both 'easy' and 'hard' go/no-go tasks associated with reduced striatal activation; but they showed improved striatal function when given methylphenidate (Vaidya et al., 1998).

Neuroimaging

Over the past decade, there have been a dozen papers indicating significant regional brain differences in ADHD as determined by quantitative volumetric brain magnetic resonance imaging (MRI). Findings (smaller volumes) have always been more prominent in boys than in girls, but consistently across all studies from all groups is that boys with ADHD have reduced total cerebral volumes compared with controls (boys matched for age and intelligence). Girls with ADHD have not been shown to differ from controls in their total cerebral volume; however, as previously reported in boys with ADHD, girls with ADHD showed similar subtotal volume reductions in bilateral posterior prefrontal brain, bilateral caudate nucleus, left globus pallidus, and posterior inferior cerebellar vermis (F.X. Castellanos, personal communication, 1998). See also MRI volumetrics of Tourette/comorbid ADHD, reviewed by Singer, this volume.

Considerable consensus across studies from different centres reveals the following structures to be smaller in boys with ADHD: frontal regions, caudate, globus pallidus (Aylward et al., 1996; Castellanos et al., 1996; Filipek et al., 1997; Giedd et al., 1994), and posterior inferior cerebellar vermis (Berquin et al., 1998; Mostofsky et al., 1998b). Only one study differed from the majority's emphasis on the anterior structures, reporting additional parietal volume reductions in a group of 15 boys, one-third of whom were said to be stimulant non-responders (Filipek et al., 1997;

Semrud-Clikeman et al., 1994). The symptom/sign of disinhibition in children with ADHD correlates with reversed asymmetry of the caudate; measures of attention correlate with right hemisphere white matter volumes (Semrud-Clikeman et al., 2000).

Neurotransmitters implicated in ADHD

Although most research has focused upon dopaminergic mechanisms, recent reviews related to the mechanisms underlying attention deficit hyperactivity disorder provide considerable evidence supporting a noradrenergic hypothesis of ADHD (Biederman & Spencer, 2000). Response to drugs with mixed noradrenergic and dopaminergic pharmacological loci of action have long been the starting point for this hypothesis, albeit the dopamine focus has been dominant. In addition (see genetics section below), although new and controversial, several research publications, with some degree of replication, have found associations between ADHD and two genes, the dopamine transporter and one particular dopamine receptor, D4 subtype (Swanson et al., 2000a). A recent PET study of children with ADHD using the tracer [18F] DOPA indicates unusually high accumulation of that neurochemical in the dopamine-rich region of the high midbrain, while no other dopamine-rich regions significantly differed between groups with and without ADHD (Ernst et al., 1999); this recent PET study was considered to be suggestive of dysfunction at the level of the dopaminergic nuclei in children with ADHD. Noradrenergic activation is documented as essential to the normal operation of attention, especially the arousal infrastructure; the noradrenergic system is well known to be necessary for the modulation of higher cortical functions that include selective attention, vigilance, and executive function in general. Research based upon animal (including primate) models suggests that either too much $\mathscr{L}_1$ receptor or too little $\mathscr{L}_2$ receptor stimulation can impair prefrontal cortex (Arnsten, 2000). Epinephrine itself, linked to adrenomedullary functioning during cognitive testing in boys with diagnosed ADHD, has been reported to be correlated with both parent- and teacher-rated behaviours categorized under 'inattention'. Lower adrenomedullary epinephrine status in individuals with ADHD while they are performing the cognitive 'stress' of schoolwork appears to be associated with the inattentive subtype but not so much with the full syndrome (Anderson et al., 2000).

Serotonin is another neurotransmitter that may play a role, particularly among those children who are prominently aggressive from an early age. Serotonin activity has also been implicated in working memory performance in some studies of children with ADHD (Gainetdinov et al., 1999; Spivak et al., 1999; Oades, 2000).

Providing transition to the subject of genetics, comparison of the effect of 20 genes that involve dopamine, serotonin, and neuroadrenergic metabolism on quantitative scores in a multivariate linear regression analysis predicting ADHD in a large population indicated that adrenergic genes accounted for more of the variance in ADHD than either the dopaminergic or serotonergic genes combined; but it must be noted that even the six adrenergic genes contributed only 6.9% of the variance, while all genes combined accounted for 11.6% of the variance (Comings et al., 2000).

Genetic basis of ADHD

Genes related to neurotransmitters and neurotransmitter receptors

Molecular genetic studies of ADHD have suggested the possible involvement of one or more dopaminergically relevant genes, either a dopamine transporter gene (associated with a mechanism of excess dopamine reuptake) or the 7-repeat allele of DRD4 (associated with a reduced sensitivity of the receptor at the postsynaptic level) (Thapar et al., 1999; Swanson et al., 2000a). Neuropsychological tests of attention in those with the 7-repeat allele of DRD4 gene contradicted the primary hypothesis of this study; those with the candidate abnormal gene (7-repeat allele DRD4) seemed to be free of difficulties on the neuropsychological tests, exhibiting average reaction times and consistent responses (Swanson et al., 2000a, b).

The DRD4 gene and its relationship with ADHD remain controversial. Two negative studies from Israel concern the exon 3 repeat polymorphism (Eisenberg et al., 2000; Kotler et al., 2000) and a study from Ireland concerning the 7-repeat allele was similarly negative (Hawi et al., 2000). On the other hand, there have been several studies documenting DRD4 variants conferring ADHD risk (McCracken et al., 2000; Barr et al., 2000; Muglia et al., 2000).

The human dopamine transporter gene was further analysed; gene variants that alter levels of DAT expression survive as excellent candidate mechanisms for underlying ADHD as well as, in a less specific fashion, other frequently comorbid associated neuropsychiatric disorders (Vandenbergh et al., 2000). Some evidence for the serotonin HTR 2 A receptor gene as relevant to ADHD opens an entirely new avenue of molecular genetics research on ADHD, leading to speculation that there is a complex interplay in ADHD among neurotransmitter systems rather than strictly emphasis upon the dopamine system (Quist et al., 2000).

Clarifying the genetic architecture of ADHD

Using a sophisticated statistical analysis called latent class analysis in a twin study of school-age children, only two subtypes emerged, one inattentive and the other combined, each of which is a dimensional domain (Neuman et al., 1999). Another twin study suggested that extreme hyperactivity/impulsivity might be genetically and etiologically separable from the usual moderate full syndrome and extrapolated without reservation to families with girls as ADHD probands (Faraone et al., 2000). A common genetic factor (revealed in a large twin pair study) underlies maternally reported and concordant maternal/teacher-reported ADHD; when teacher-only-ADHD is reported, weaker genetic influence is supported and environmental factors loom larger (Thapar et al., 2000).

In multiplex families with ADHD, the gender ratio appeared to be consistent with a genetic model in which a greater loading of familial influences was necessary for the girls to develop ADHD (Smalley et al., 2000).

Treatment

Most of the controversy about the diagnosis of ADHD has emanated from its almost complete identification (in the public mind) with treatment involving stimulant medication. In what is probably the most widely replicated body of literature on psychopharmacology dealing with the pediatric age group it has been shown that methylphenidate (Ritalin) and dextroamphetamine (Dexedrine) provide improvement for between 75 and 90% of children and adults with ADHD. Side effects are few and rarely serious, all being confined to observable effects upon the central nervous system (eating, sleeping, mood, tics). In 1998, the Council on Scientific Affairs of the American Medical Association conducted a 20-year review of the scientific literature and concluded that stimulant drugs were not being prescribed excessively or being misused (The Harvard Mental Health Letter, 2000). Stimulant treatment of ADHD in public schools in Maryland (mainly methylphenidate) is variably prescribed to students for school purposes, being fourfold greater for males than for females, twice as often for white as for minority students, and three times as often for elementary as opposed to high school students. The majority of the children taking stimulant medication had their medical supervision and prescriptions undertaken by pediatricians (63%); when medications other than methylphenidate (Ritalin) were prescribed, the prescribing physician was a psychiatrist in 29% of such cases (Safer & Malove, 2000). Recent studies on the long-term risk of drug abuse and alcoholism among those who as children were treated with prescription stimulants reaches a conclusion opposite to that of increased risk; rather, the risk for drug abuse in adolescents is lessened by successful childhood stimulant medication treatment of ADHD (Degrandpre & Hinshaw, 2000).

A recent major clinical trial sponsored by the National Institute of Mental Health was conducted at several medical centres and universities for, so far, a 14-month period (MTA Cooperative Group, 1999a). Clear benefits of stimulant medication were documented for carefully diagnosed children with ADHD (who had their medication optimally managed by initial dosage adjustment, monthly family visits to the doctors, and mandatory contact with school personnel). Medication management of this high quality was superior in outcome, in terms of reducing signs/symptoms, to medication-free intensive psychosocial intervention (involving long-term parent training, school consultation, and summer programmes of contingency management/behaviour modification). The careful medication regimen was clearly superior to 'community' standards of stimulant medication treatment lacking the close monitoring and titrating. A lower dose of medication was effective in the group receiving the combined medical and behavioural treatment (MTA Cooperative Group, 1999b).

Medication alone is not even initially effective, when there are comorbid conditions, like learning disabilities, which require remediation. Cognitive interventions for non-academic behaviours are not as useful as contingency management techniques. Schools, following Federal law, must accommodate ADHD as a disability under the Section 504 of the American with Disabilities Act. This is a different law from the one that governs learning disabilities (P.L. 94–142). A 504 Plan for ADHD should feature the following: extended time on tests, frequent breaks on tests, close monitoring, predictable schedules, constant feedback, tangible rewards and response costs; and those with ADHD should be positioned in the classroom close to the teacher and as far as possible from sources of distraction. It appears that the main reason that non-pharmacological treatments do not receive as much focus as pharmacological ones is that they are very demanding of adult time, expertise and effort; and given that the ADHD is chronic, it appears likely that the psychosocial treatments need to be chronic, whatever the modality (Pelham & Gnagy, 1999).

In conclusion, despite fears that 'drugging children' into compliance is the motivation for making the diagnosis of ADHD, there is considerable clinical and research evidence supporting the view that ADHD represents a group of real neurological, mainly neurodevelopmental, disorders involving control processes (motor, cognitive, and emotional). This point of view acknowledges that 'the brain both shapes and is shaped by the environment; underlying psychobiological risk factors can be treated environmentally and some conditions resulting from stressful life events could be dealt with by biological intervention . . .' (Degrandpre & Hinshaw, 2000).

References

American Psychiatric Association. (1994). *Diagnostic and Statistical Manual of Mental Disorders*, 4th edn. Washington, DC: American Psychiatric Association.

Anderson, G.M., Dover, M.A., Yang, B.P. et al. (2000). Adrenomedullary function during cognitive testing in attention deficit hyperactivity disorder. *J. Acad. Child Adolesc. Psychiatry*, **39** (5), 635–43.

Arnsten, A.F. (2000). Genetics of childhood disorders: XVIII. ADHD, part 2: norepinephrine has a critical modulatory influence on prefrontal cortical function. *J. Acad. Child Adolesc. Psychiatry*, **39** (9), 1201–3.

Aylward, E.H., Reiss, A.L., Reader, M.J. Singer, H.S., Brown, J.E. & Denckla, M.B. (1996). Basal ganglia volumes in children with attention deficit hyperactivity disorder. *J. Child Neurol.*, **11**, 112–15.

Barkley, R.A. (1997). *ADHD and the Nature of Self-Control*. New York: Guilford Press.

Barkley, R.A. (1990). *Attention Deficit Hyperactivity Disorder: A Handbook for Diagnosis and Treatment*. New York: Guilford Press.

Barkley, R.A. (2000). Genetics of childhood disorders XVII ADHD, part I: the executive functions and ADHD. *Am. Acad. Child Adolesc. Psychiatry*, **39**, 1064–7.

Barr, C.L., Wigg, K.G., Bloom, S. et al. (2000). Further evidence from haplotype analysis for linkage of the dopamine D4 receptor gene and attention deficit hyperactivity disorder. *Am. J. Med. Genet.*, **96** (3), 262–7.

Berquin, P.C., Giedd, J.N., Jacobsen, L.K. et al. (1998). Cerebellum in attention-deficit hyperactivity disorder: a morphometric MRI study. *Neurology*, **50**, 1087–93.

Biederman, J. & Spencer, T.J. (2000). Is ADHD a noradrenergic disorder. *J. Am. Acad. Child Adolesc. Psychiatry*, **39**, 1330.

Biederman, J., Faraone, S., Spencer, T. et al. (1993). Patterns of psychiatric comorbidity cognition and psychosocial functioning in adults with attention deficit hyperactivity disorder. *Am. J. Psychiatry*, **150**, 1792–8.

Cantwell, D.P. (1996). Attention deficit disorder: a review of the past ten years. *J. Am. Acad. Child Adolesc. Psychiatry.*, **35**, 978–87.

Castellanos, F.X., Giedd, J.N., Marsh, W.L. et al. (1996). Quantitative brain magnetic resonance imaging in attention deficit hyperactivity disorder. *Arch. Gen. Psychiatry*, **53** (7), 607–16.

Comings, D.E., Gade-Andavolu, R., Gonzalez, N. et al. (2000). Comparison of the role of dopamine, serotonin, and noradrenaline genes in ADHD, odd and conduct disorder: multivariate regression analysis of 20 genes. *Clin. Genet.*, **57** (3), 178–96.

Cox, C.S., Chee, E., Chase, G.A. et al. (1997). Reading proficiency affects the construct validity of the Stroop test interference score. *Clin. Neuropsychol.*, **11**, 105–10.

Degrandpre, R.J. & Hinshaw, S.P. (2000). ADHD: serious psychiatric problem or all-American cop-out? *Cerebrum: The Dana Forum on Brain Science.*, **2**(3), 12–38.

Denckla, M.B. (1994). Measurement of Executive Function. In *Frames of Reference for the Assessment of Learning Disabilities: New Views on Measurement Issues*, ed. G.R. Lyon, pp. 117–42. Baltimore: Brooks Publishing Co.

Denckla, M.B. (1996). Research on executive function in a neurodevelopmental context: application of clinical measures. *Devel. Neuropsychol.*, **12**, 5–15.

Denckla, M.B. & Cutting, L.E. (1999). History and significance of rapid automatized naming. *Ann. Dyslexia*, **49**, 29–41.

Eisenberg, J., Zohar, A., Mei-Tal, G. et al. (2000). A haplotype relative risk study of the dopamine D4 receptor (DRD4) exon III repeat polymorphism and attention deficit hyperactivity disorder (ADHD). *Am. J. Med. Genet.*, **96** (3), 258–61.

Ernst, M., Zametkin, A.J., Matochik, J.A., Pascualvaca, D., Jons, P.H. & Cohen, R.M. (1999). High midbrain [^{18}F]DOPA accumulation in children with attention deficit hyperactivity disorder. *Am. J. Psychiatry*, **156** (8), 1209–15.

Faraone, S.V., Biederman, J., Mick, E. et al. (2000). Family study of girls with attention deficit hyperactivity disorder. *Am. J. Psychiatry*, **157** (7), 1077–83.

Filipek, P.A., Semrud-Clikeman, M., Steingard, R.J., Renshaw, P.F., Kennedy, D.N. & Biederman, J. (1997). Volumetric MRI analysis comparing attention deficit hyperactivity disorder and normal controls. *Neurology*, **48**, 589–601.

Fischer, M., Barkley, R.A., Edelrock, C.S. & Smallish, L. (1990). The adolescent outcome of hyperactive children diagnosed by research criteria, II: academic, attentional, and neuropsychological status. *J. Cons. Clin. Psychology*, **58**, 580–8.

Gainetdinov, R.R., Wetsel, W.C., Jones, S.R., Levin, E.D., Jaber, M. & Caron, M.G. (1999). Role of serotonin in the paradoxical calming effect of psychostimulants on hyperactivity. *Science*, **283** (5400), 397–401.

Giedd, J.N., Castellanos, F.X., Casey, B.J. et al. (1994). Quantitative morphometry of the corpus callosum in attention deficit hyperactivity disorder. *Am. J. Psychiatry*, **151**, 665–9.

Grodzinsky, G.M. & Barkley, R.A. (1999). Predictive power of frontal lobe tests in the diagnosis of attention-deficit hyperactivity disorder. *Clin. Neuropsychol.*, **13** (1), 12–21.

Hawi, Z., McCarron, M., Kirley, A., Daly, G., Fitzgerald, M. & Gill, M. (2000). No association of the dopamine DRD4 receptor (DRD4) gene polymorphism with attention deficit hyperactivity disorder (ADHD) in the Irish population. *Am. J. Med. Genet.*, **96** (3), 268–72.

Hinshaw, S.P., Zupan, B.A., Simmel, C., Nigg, J.T & Melnick, S. (1997). Peer status in boys with and without attention deficit hyperactivity disorder: predictions from overt and covert antisocial behavior, social isolation, and authoritative parenting beliefs. *Child Devel.*, **68** (5), 880–96.

Hughes, J.R., DeLeo, A.J. & Melyn, M.A. (2000). The electroencephalogram in attention deficit hyperactivity disorder: emphasis on epileptiform discharges. *Epilepsy Behav.*, **1**, 271–7.

Kotler, M., Manor, I., Sever, Y. et al. (2000). Failure to replicate an excess of the long dopamine D4 exon III repeat polymorphism in ADHD in a family-based study. *Am. J. Med. Genet.*, **96** (3), 278–81.

McCracken, J.T., Smalley, S.L., McGough, J.J. et al. (2000). Evidence for linkage of a tandem duplication polymorphism upstream of the dopamine D4 receptor gene (DRD4) with attention deficit hyperactivity disorder. *Mol. Psychiatry*, **5** (5), 531–6.

Mannuzza, S., Klein, R.G., Bessler, A., Malloy, P. & LaPadula, M. (1993). Adult outcome of hyperactive boys: educational achievement, educational rank and psychiatric status. *Arch. Gen. Psychiatry*, **50**, 565–76.

Moll, G.H., Heinrich, H., Trott, D.E., Wirth, S. & Rothenberger, A. (2000). Deficient intracortical inhibition in drug naïve children with attention deficit hyperactivity disorder. *Neurosci. Lett.*, **284**, 121–5.

Mostofsky, S.H., Reiss, A.L., Lockhart, P. & Denckla, M.B. (1998). Evaluation of cerebellar size in attention deficit hyperactivity disorder. *J. Child Neurol.*, **13**, 434–9.

Mostofsky, S.H., Lasker, A.G., Denckla, M.B., Cutting, L.E. & Zee, D.S. (2000). Oculomotor findings in attention deficit hyperactivity disorder (ADHD): evidence for deficits in frontal lobe functioning and importance of gender differences. *Neurology*, **54** (7) Suppl. 3, A243.

MTA Cooperative Group (1999a). Fourteen month randomized clinical trial of treatment strategies for attention deficit hyperactivity disorder. *Arch. Gen. Psychiatry*, **56**, 1073–86.

MTA Cooperative Group (1999b). Moderators and mediators of treatment response for children with ADHD: the MTA study. *Arch. Gen. Psychiatry*, **56**, 1088–96.

Muglia, P., Jain, U., Macciardi, F. & Kennedy, J.L. (2000). Adult attention deficit hyperactivity disorder and the dopamine D4 receptor gene. *Am. J. Med. Genet.*, **96** (3), 273–7.

Neuman, R.J., Todd, R.D., Heath, A.C. et al. (1999). Evaluation of ADHD typology in three contrasting samples: a latent class approach. *J. Am. Acad. Child Adolesc. Psychiatry*, **38** (1), 25–33.

NIH Consensus Statement (1998).

Oades, R.D. (2000). Differential measures of 'sustained attention' in children with attention deficit hyperactivity or tic disorders: relations to monoamine metabolism. *J. Psychiatr. Res.*, **93**, 165–78.

Oosterlann, J. & Sergeant, J.A. (1998). Response inhibition and response re-engagement in attention-deficit/hyperactivity disorder, disruptive, anxious and normal children. *Behav. Brain Res.*, **94** (1), 33–43.

Pelham, W.E. & Gnagy, E.M. (1999). Psychosocial and combined treatments for ADHD. *Ment. Retard. Dev. Disabil. Res. Rev.*, **5**, 225–36.

Pennington, B.F. (1991). *Diagnosing Learning Disabilities: A Neuropsychological Framework*. New York: Guilford Press.

Purvis, K.L. & Tannock, R. (1997). Language abilities in children with attention deficit hyperactivity disorder, reading disabilities, and normal controls. *J. Abnorm. Child Psychol.*, **25** (2), 133–4.

Quist, J.F., Barr, C.L., Schachar, R. et al. (2000). Evidence for the serotonin HTR2A receptor gene as a susceptibility factor in attention deficit hyperactivity disorder. *Mol. Psychiatry*, **5**(5), 537–41.

Reader, M.J., Harris, E.L., Schuerholz, L.J. & Denckla, M.B. (1994). Attention deficit hyperactivity disorder and executive dysfunction. *Devel. Neuropsychol.*, **10** (4), 493–512.

Safer, D.J. & Malove, M. (2000). Stimulant treatment in Maryland public schools. *Pediatrics*, **106**, 533–9.

Semrud-Clikeman, M., Filipek, P.A. & Biederman, J. (1994). Attention deficit hyperactivity disorder: differences in the corpus callosum by MRI morphometric analysis. *J. Am. Acad. Child Adolesc. Psychiatry*, **33**, 875–81.

Semrud-Clikeman, M., Steingard, R.J., Filipek, P., Biederman, J., Bekken, K. & Renshaw, P.F. (2000). Using MRI to examine brain–behavior relationships in males with attention deficit disorder with hyperactivity. *J. Am. Acad. Child Adolesc. Psychiatry*, **39**, 477–84.

Smalley, S.L., McGough, J.J., De l'Homme, M. et al. (2000). Familial clustering of symptoms and disruptive behaviors in multiplex families with attention deficit hyperactivity disorder. *J. Am. Acad. Child Adolesc. Psychiatry*, **39** (9), 1135–43.

Spivak, B., Vered, Y., Yoran-Hegesh, R. et al. (1999). Circulatory levels of catecholamines, serotonin and lipids in attention deficit hyperactivity disorder. *Acta Psychiatr. Scand.*, **99**(4), 300–4.

Swanson, J.M., McBurnett, K., Wigal, T. et al. (1993). Effect of stimulant medication on children with attention deficit hyperactivity disorder: a 'review of reviews'. *Except. Child.*, **60**(2), 154–61.

Swanson, J., Oosterlaan, J., Murias, M. et al. (2000a). Attention deficit hyperactivity disorder children with a 7-repeat allele of the dopamine receptor D4 gene have extreme behavior but normal performance on critical neuropsychological tests of attention. *Proc. Natl. Acad. Sci., USA.*, **97**(9), 4754–9.

Swanson, J.M., Flodman, P., Kennedy, J. et al. (2000b). Dopamine genes and ADHD. *Neurosci. Biobehav. Rev.*, **24**(1), 21–5.

Tannock, R. (1998). Attention deficit hyperactivity disorder: advances in cognitive, neurobiological, and genetic research. *J Child Psychol. Psychiatry.* **39**, 69–99.

Tannock, R., Martinussen, R. & Frijters, J. (2000). Naming speed performance and stimulant effects indicate effortful, semantic processing deficits in attention deficit hyperactivity disorder. *J. Abnorm. Child Psychol.*, **28** (3), 237–52.

Thapar, A., Holmes, J., Poulton, K. & Harrington, R. (1999). Genetic basis of attention deficit and hyperactivity. *Br. J. Psychiatry*, **174**, 105–111.

Thapar, A., Harrington, R., Ross, K. & McGuffin, P. (2000). Does the definition of ADHD affect heritability. *J. Am. Acad. Child Adolesc. Psychiatry*, **39**, 1528–36.

The Harvard Mental Health Letter (August and September 2000). **17**, 2–3.

Vaidya, C.J., Austin, G. & Kirkorian, G. (1998). Selective effects of methylphenidate in attention deficit hyperactivity disorder: a functional magnetic resonance study. *Proc. Natl. Acad. Sci., USA*, **95**, 14494–9.

Vandenbergh, D.J., Thompson, M.D., Cook, E.H. et al. (2000). Human dopamine transporter gene: coding region conservation among normal, Tourette's disorder, alcohol dependence and attention deficit hyperactivity disorder populations. *Mol. Psychiatry*, **5** (3), 283–92.

Voeller, K.K.S. (1991). What can neurologic models of attention, intention and arousal tell us about ADHD. *J. Child Neurol.*, **3**, 209–16.

30

The neurobiology of drug addiction

Charles A. Dackis and Charles P. O'Brien

Treatment and Research Center, Department of Psychiatry, University of Pennsylvania, Philadelphia, PA, USA

Although neuroscientists have made considerable progress investigating and characterizing the brain regions that are involved in addiction, the integration of this information with clinical practice is still in its infancy. The neurobiology of addiction addresses the dynamic interaction between addictive drugs and the brain, ranging from drug intoxication to chronic neuroadaptations such as withdrawal, tolerance and craving. While psychological, psychosocial and environmental factors play important roles, addiction is primarily a brain disease (Leshner & Koob, 1999), and a greater understanding of its neurobiology should uncover new and effective treatments. Currently, there is an urgent need for medications capable of reducing craving and recidivism, perhaps by reversing brain disruptions associated with chronic substance abuse. Aside from refining treatment, addiction research has also shed light on the brain's reward centres that so dominate our lives. These centres have evolved over millions of years to reinforce feeding, mating, and other survival-related activities. Tampering with brain reward circuitry, through the process of addiction, produces many of the dangerous and lethal consequences that are associated with addictive illness.

Through the development of technological advances, scientists have developed sophisticated probes into the brain regions that are involved in drug reward. Addictive agents affect different neurotransmitter systems at various anatomical sites, creating distinct 'fingerprints' on the reward circuitry. However, the administration of all addictive substances increases extracellular dopamine (DA) levels in the nucleus accumbens (NAc), a location that has been named the 'universal addiction site'. This remarkable fact will be our starting point in a discussion of pathways that interconnect the midbrain, limbic system, and medial prefrontal cortex (PFC). Repeated administration of addictive drugs often produces opposite brain effects, and evidence of impaired DA neurotransmission has been reported with chronic cocaine, opiate, alcohol and marijuana exposure. Other neuroadaptations have also been identified and will be reviewed, by substance, in an attempt to integrate brain mechanisms with clinical phenomena such as drug withdrawal, craving and progression.

The nature of addiction

The hallmark of addiction is a progressive loss of control over drug intake, regardless of negative consequences. The willingness of drug addicts to risk death, disease, incarceration, job loss, financial ruin and family strife may seem counterintuitive. However, when the dynamics of addiction are understood, the lack of control exhibited by drug addicts becomes more comprehensible. A useful framework for conceptualizing addiction has been proposed by Wikler (Wikler & Pescor, 1967), based on classical and operant conditioning theory. In this construct, initial drug use may occur for a number of reasons, including boredom, curiosity, recreation and peer pressure. Drug euphoria, resulting from physiological effects on endogenous reward centres, 'positively' reinforces repeated drug use in the pursuit of pleasure. Over time, neuroadaptations affecting brain reward centres lead to phenomena such as drug withdrawal, craving and dysphoria. These unpleasant states, temporarily alleviated by drugs, 'negatively' reinforce repeated drug use. Craving and withdrawal symptoms can also be triggered by conditioned cues that are associated with drug procurement and drug use. Alternating negative and positive reinforcement drives a viscous cycle of addiction that becomes increasingly entrenched and uncontrollable. Since the cycle of addiction is essentially etched onto the brain's reward substrate, the compulsive drive to use drugs takes on the strength and characteristics of a primary survival drive.

Anatomy and circuitry of endogenous reward centres

Since 'pleasure centres' in the lateral hypothalamus were first discovered by Olds in the 1950s, brain regions supporting electrical and drug self-stimulation have been intensively researched (Bardo, 1998). However, much of what is known about these reward centres is based on animal experiments that may not be easily generalized to humans. Aside from cross-species differences in anatomical, neurotransmitter and molecular systems, it is a wide leap from animal behaviour to human subjective experience. With these caveats in mind, it is apparent that a number of structures with synaptic connections to the medial forebrain bundle are intrinsically involved in drug reward and natural reward states (Wise, 1996). These structures include the DA-rich ventral tegmentum (VTA), PFC, NAc, and elements of the limbic system.

Drugs as diverse as psychostimulants, opiates, alcohol, marijuana, nicotine and phencyclidine (PCP) acutely increase levels of extracellular DA in the NAc (Koob et al., 1998). The shell of the NAc shares embryological and cytoarchitectural similarities with the central nucleus of the amygdala and the bed nucleus of the stria terminalis, comprising what has been termed the extended amygdala (Heimer & Alheid, 1991). The extended amygdala has reciprocal connections with the forebrain, hippocampus, midbrain, ventral pallidum, mediodorsal thalamus and the lateral hypothalamus (Koob et al., 1998). The NAc can be functionally divided into its ventromedial shell, essentially a limbic structure, and its core that is associated with the ventral striatum. The shell is implicated in reward function and the core projects motor-related information to the substantia nigra. The proximity of predominately reward and motor structures within the NAc provides a direct anatomical interface between motivational and behavioural function (Pennartz et al., 1994).

The NAc shell region is composed primarily of medium-sized spiny cells. These neurons utilize GABA as their primary neurotransmitter but may also contain endogenous opioid peptide (EOP) neurotransmitters. EOP neurotransmitters such as dynorphin and enkephalin are contained primarily in output neurons within the NAc. All three classes of opiate receptors are found in the NAc. Agonists for the mu and delta receptors are rewarding in this region, whereas kappa agonists are aversive (Akil et al., 1998). In addition, the activation of mu and delta receptors releases DA, while kappa agonists inhibit DA release. There is evidence that separate populations of NAc neurons in the striatum contain either enkephalin or dynorphin, with enkephalin-containing neurons usually expressing D_2

receptors and dynorphin-containing neurons typically expressing D_1 receptors (Akil et al., 1998). Dynorphin and enkephalin projections are thought to be involved in compensatory actions in response to excessive DA neurotransmission, and alterations in these systems may underlie neuroadaptations associated with opiates, stimulants, and other addictive agents. The presence of opioids and opiate receptors in this universal addiction site is noteworthy.

The NAc receives 'reward circuit' DA projections from the VTA and returns inhibitory reciprocal fibres to this DA-rich centre. DA projections of the reward circuit have complicated actions on medium-sized spiny cells. D_2-mediated effects are inhibitory and reduce the formation of cAMP within NAc target cells (Self et al., 1998). D_1 receptors, on the other hand, stimulate cAMP formation and have a modulatory role that involves either inhibition or excitation, depending on the resting state of NAc target cells. Medium-sized spiny cells tend to be in either an active or inactive state, and D_1 activation causes a prolongation of the pre-existing state (Hernandez-Lopez et al., 1997). Therefore, while D_2 receptor activation inhibits medium-sized spiny cells, D_1 activation can either inhibit or stimulate the firing rates of these output neurons.

The NAc is stimulated by glutamate-containing axons that originate in the PFC, amygdala, hippocampus, and thalamus (Pennartz et al., 1994). The PFC sends massive descending fibres that actually join DA terminals of the reward circuit to form 'dual-synapses' on medium-sized spiny cells (Sesack & Pickel, 1992). Similar convergent DA and glutamate terminals in the NAc have been demonstrated with excitatory inputs from the hippocampus (CA3 area), amygdala and thalamus. Also, the NAc sends reciprocal fibres to each of these glutamatergic areas. Dense glutamate-containing fibres from the amygdala travel via the stria terminalis before converging on the spines and distal dendrites of NAc neurons. Hippocampal projections, possibly involved in reward memory, originate in the subiculum and pass through the fimbria-fornix to target cells in the NAc. Convergent synaptic input from glutamate and DA projections allows for the simultaneous processing of cortical and midbrain reward information by GABA\EOP-containing cells of the NAc.

Aside from glutamate and DA, the NAc is also influenced by other neurotransmitter systems. It receives serotonin terminals from the dorsal and median raphe, and norepinephrine projections from the locus coeruleus and the nucleus tractus solitarius. Cholinergic neurons intrinsic to the NAc synapse on the dendritic shafts of a population of medium-sized spiny cells that do not receive DA projections (Pickel & Chan, 1990). This finding provides evidence that discrete populations of medium-sized spiny cells in the NAc have different functions. The convergence of DA, GABA, glutamate, EOP, serotonin, norepinephrine and acetylcholine-containing neurons in the NAc allows for complex interactions involving these critical neurotransmitter systems.

The NAc shell sends GABA and opioid-containing projections throughout the reward circuitry. NAc projections extend directly to the lateral hypothalamic and preoptic areas that are involved in the consummatory functions of feeding, drinking, and sexual activity. Morphine is self-administered directly into the lateral hypothalamus, suggesting a role for EOP systems in consummatory reward. Indirect outflow from the NAc passes through the ventral pallidum, a structure intrinsically involved in motivation and drug seeking behaviour (Bardo, 1998). In addition to serving as a relay point to other anatomical regions, the ventral pallidum processes reward information through opioid modulation (Napier & Mitrovic, 1999). The ventral pallidum conveys NAc projections to the pedunculopontine tegmental nucleus, a region composed of large cholinergic cells and smaller glutamate neurons. Cholinergic neurons of the pedunculopontine tegmentum project to the VTA and stimulate nicotinic receptors that are located on DA cell bodies. Implicated in the acquisition of drug-rewarded behaviour, the pedunculopontine nucleus also projects to the amygdala and lateral hypothalamus.

Another important NAc pathway traverses through the ventral pallidum to the mediodorsal thalamic nucleus, an area associated with feelings of fear and anxiety. The mediodorsal thalamus is generally viewed as limbic and has extensive connections to the PFC and anterior cingulate. The anterior cingulate, which also receives direct VTA projections, has numerous functions that include pain perception and the assignment of emotional valence to perceived stimuli. The pallidal–thalamocortical circuit has been termed the 'motive circuit' and is thought to initiate adaptive responses to reward information received from the NAc (Kalivas et al., 1999). The PFC (Grant et al., 1996) and cingulate area (Childress et al., 1999) are hypermetabolic in humans during cocaine cue craving, suggesting that the multisynaptic circuit connecting the NAc, ventral pallidum, mediodorsal thalamus, and cortical regions has an important role in the addictive process. As the neurobiology of craving is further unravelled by additional imaging studies, new treatments for this tenacious negative reinforcer may result.

The amygdala plays a role in reward and reward-related memory. The basolateral nucleus of the amygdala consists largely of glutamatergic pyramidal cells while the central nucleus is mainly populated by GABA-containing projection neurons. As with the NAc, the amygdala is rich in endogenous opioids. The central nucleus of the amygdala, NAc, and bed nucleus of the stria terminalis (extended amygdala) share many characteristics (Heimer & Alheid, 1991). The amygdala sends excitatory glutamatergic axons to the NAc and receives reciprocals from this important reward centre. Preclinical and imaging studies demonstrate that the amygdala is involved in the recognition of emotionally relevant stimuli. Imaging studies in humans have reported hypermetabolism in the amygdala during cocaine cue craving (Grant et al., 1996; Childress et al., 1999), and amygdaloid suppression during cocaine administration (Breiter et al., 1997). Animal studies report that lesions of the basolateral amygdala interfere with the process by which neutral stimuli become secondary reinforcers of cocaine administration and motivate drug-seeking behaviour and cue-induced relapse (Whitelaw et al., 1996). While the basolateral amygdala is involved in the acquisition of cocaine-seeking behaviour, the central nucleus of the amygdala is implicated in alcohol reward and withdrawal. This GABA/EOP-rich region may also be affected by CRF abnormalities that are associated with addiction. CRF is a centrally acting neuropeptide that, aside from its ability to activate the hypothalamic–pituitary–adrenal axis, also mediates behavioural responses to stress. Elevations in CRF are found during withdrawal from many substances (cocaine, opiates, THC, and alcohol) and CRF antagonists reverse aversive affects of alcohol and opiate withdrawal when administered into the central nucleus of the amygdala (Koob et al., 1998).

The VTA is the source of all mesocorticolimbic DA and serves a crucial role in drug reward and in natural drive states, including the procurement of food, fluid, and sex. DA neurons comprise about 85% of the cell bodies in the VTA and display either baseline pacemaker activity, or episodic burst firing when activated. Burst firing occurs during consummatory activity (such as feeding) and later upon exposure to cues associated with these behaviours, suggesting an interesting learning capability of mesocorticolimbic DA neurons (Schultz et al., 1997). The major projection bundles from the VTA extend to the NAc, the frontal lobe (prefrontal and anterior cingulate cortex), and the amygdala. It is not clear how these three important projections and their target sites interrelate on a functional basis through their extensive interconnections.

DA neurons in the VTA are under intensive local and distal regulation, receiving input from GABA, glutamate, acetylcholine, EOP, and serotonergic-containing neurons. Local inhibition is mediated through somato-dendritic D_2 autoreceptors and local GABA interneurons. Inhibitory fibres also project from the NAc (directly and via the ventral pallidum), amygdala and other limbic structures. Glutamatergic projections and cholinergic axons from the laterodorsal

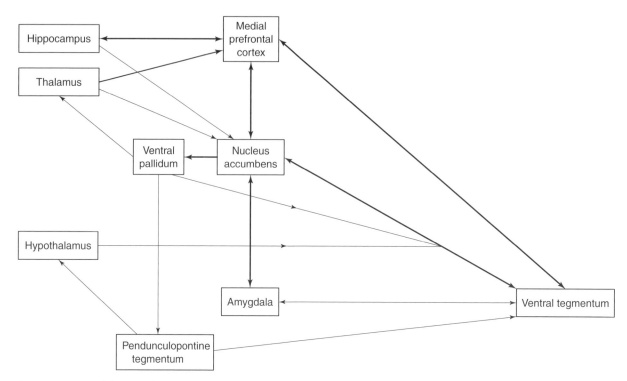

Fig. 30.1. Circuits of the reward centres are schematically represented. Attention is directed to the 'reward circuit' involving DA projections from the VTA to the NAc. The NAc, termed the 'universal reward site' contains GABA\EOP projection neurons and is implicated in all drug reward states. The 'motive circuit' connects the NAc and ventral pallidum with glutamatergic neurons of the thalamus and PFC. Cholinergic projections from the pedunculopontine tegmentum terminate on nicotinic receptors.

tegmental and pedunculopontine nuclei provide excitatory input to the VTA. The activation of inhibitory mu opioid receptors on GABA interneurons of the VTA (and GABA cells projecting to the VTA) releases DA neurons from tonic GABA inhibition (Leshner & Koob, 1999). DA neurons in the VTA also receive direct synaptic input from EOP-containing terminals, and are modulated by the raphe nuclei and the hypothalamus.

Glutamate-containing pyramidal cells in the PFC tonically stimulate VTA neurons, and thereby regulate the basal outflow of DA throughout the limbic system. Glutamatergic terminals synapse directly on DA neurons at the cell body level and activate NMDA and AMPA receptors. These cortical projections and reciprocal DA axons run through the medial forebrain bundle, a tract that has been intensely studied in reward, working memory, and schizophrenia research. DA projections to the PFC form synapses on the dendritic spines and shafts of cortical glutamatergic neurons, modulating their activity (Carr et al., 1999) and completing an interactive loop that is undoubtedly central to reward function. DA projections also modulate local inhibitory circuitry through synaptic connections on cortical GABA neurons. In addition to enhancing working memory, DA projections to the PFC appear to be involved in memory-guided goal-directed behaviour (Durstewitz et al., 2000). PFC pyramidal neurons that receive DA input are also innervated by glutamatergic projections from the hippocampus, a structure that is implicated in memory. The role of memory in the perpetuation of repeated drug use is an essential component of addiction.

The reward circuitry outlined in this discussion is summarized in Fig. 30.1. It is useful to note that there are three major VTA bundles projecting to the NAc, PFC, and amygdala. These structures are extensively interconnected and send reciprocal fibres back to the VTA to form a series of loops within the reward circuitry. The major neurotransmitter systems that comprise these circuits include DA, glutamate, GABA and EOP-containing neurons. Since these neurotransmitters are intimately involved in the acute and chronic actions of addictive substances, researchers have focused on therapeutic agents that directly or indirectly affect their associated neuronal pathways. Given the central modulatory role of mesocortico-limbic DA neurons, intact VTA function is probably crucial in the normal orchestration of reward circuits. The dysregulation of DA neurons with chronic addiction, combined with target cell neuroadaptations, will be reviewed in the following sections, and may explain many of the clinical aspects of addiction. The next sections will focus on the major classes of addictive drugs with regard to their neurobiology and clinical characteristics.

Central stimulants: cocaine and amphetamine

Historically, central stimulants have caused a number of drug epidemics, especially when perceived to be safe. Stimulants are associated with intense euphoria, well outside the normal range of human experience, and their repeated use leads to rapidly progressive addiction in many individuals. The power of stimulant reward is illustrated by the fact that cocaine and amphetamine are readily self-administered by animals to the point of death, and preferred over sex, food and water (Dackis & Gold, 1985). Aside from producing euphoria, stimulants suppress hunger and food intake, reverse fatigue and increase psychomotor activity. Cocaine is often administered through the intrapulmonary route (as crack), which is the most rapid means of delivery to the brain. The relatively mild withdrawal seen with stimulants, characterized by depressed mood, hypersomnia, hyperphagia, anergia and psychomotor retardation, illustrates that severe physical withdrawal is not crucial in the perpetuation of drug addiction. There is significant evidence that repeated stimulant exposure disrupts the functional integrity of the brain's reward centres.

The rewarding effect of cocaine and amphetamine results from increased DA neurotransmission in reward circuits. Amphetamine promotes the presynaptic release of DA (through reverse transport) while cocaine blocks the dopamine transporter (DAT), a membrane-bound protein that regulates synaptic DA levels (see Fig. 30.2). There is a strong correlation between euphoria and the rate at which cocaine enters the brain and blocks the DAT (Volkow et al., 1999). Cocaine also blocks serotonin and norepinephrine reuptake, and has local anesthetic action on neurons. The acute administration of cocaine and amphetamine dramatically reduces DA neuronal firing in the VTA by activating D_2 autoreceptors. This finding demonstrates that increased DA neurotransmission, not increased DA burst firing, is an essential feature of stimulant euphoria. Also consistent with increased DA neurotransmission during stimulant reward are the findings that DA antagonists block self-administration and reduce euphoric effects (Koob et al., 1998).

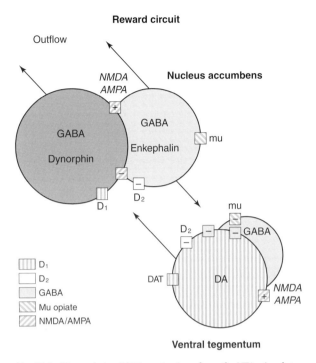

Fig. 30.2. 'Reward circuit' DA projections from the VTA stimulate D_1 and D_2 receptors on dynorphin and enkephalin-containing GABA neurons. Receptor effects (+ or −) are noted, and D_1 effects are modulatory. NMDA/AMPA receptors are excitatory, receiving glutamatergic projections from numerous cortical regions. Heroin acts on mu receptors, releasing DA from tonic inhibition. Cocaine acts on the DAT, increasing DA neurotransmission.

It has been suggested that increased DA neurotransmission cannot entirely explain stimulant reward because DAT knockout mice (lacking the DAT) self-administer cocaine, leading to the speculation that serotonin or norepinephrine systems are involved in stimulant reward. However, DAT knockout animals have high resting levels of extra-neuronal DA and may have developed specific brain mechanisms to overcome their genetic deficit. For instance, the norepinephrine reuptake transporter has a high affinity for DA and may play a role in the self-administration of cocaine by these mice. Thus, the balance of evidence continues to support DA as the key neurotransmitter associated with stimulant reward.

Given the importance of DA neurotransmission in stimulant reward, attention is directed toward postsynaptic DA receptors. At least five distinct DA receptors (D_{1-5}) have been identified, although D_1 and D_5 receptors (often termed D_1) share many structural similarities, and D_{2-4} receptors (often termed D_2) also have homologous residue sequences. Second messenger systems linked to DA receptors are intimately involved in the reinforcing action of stimulants. D_2 receptor stimulation inhibits cAMP formation by activating the inhibitory guanine nucleotide binding protein (G_i-protein). If G_i-proteins in the NAc are inactivated with pertussis toxin, stimulant reinforcement is greatly reduced (Self et al., 1998). Therefore, stimulant reward is associated with D_2 inhibition of cAMP within medium-sized spiny cells in the NAc. Opiates also acutely inhibit cAMP in these neurons through mu and delta receptors coupled to G_i-proteins.

Opposing the action of G_i-proteins are G_s-proteins that increase cAMP levels and activate cAMP-dependent protein kinase. Activation of this pathway affects ion channels, neuronal enzymes and even nuclear transcription factors that can change long-term gene expression. It has been theorized that genetic changes are involved in the transformation from drug use to drug abuse. D_1 receptors are coupled to G_s-proteins and their stimulation increases cAMP levels. Therefore, D_1 and D_2 receptors have opposite effects on cAMP formation. Furthermore, cAMP inhibition enhances stimulant reward, while cAMP stimulation has the opposite effect (Self et al., 1998). Repeated cocaine administration increases cAMP levels in the NAc and upregulates D_1 receptors, resulting in a reduced capacity of DA to lower cAMP levels that could underlie tolerance (Self et al., 1998). Reduced D_2 receptors (associated with decreased metabolism in cingulate gyrus and orbitofrontal cortex) have been reported in human cocaine addicts although it is unclear whether these abnormalities are cocaine induced, or represent a pre-existing abnormality that may predispose certain individuals to cocaine dependence (Volkow et al., 1993). Anecdotal evidence from cocaine users suggests acute tolerance within a session and chronic tolerance to subjective effects over time. In a PET study of methylphenidate, another DAT inhibitor, less DA release was observed in cocaine abusers than in normal controls (Volkow et al., 1999). These findings indicate that repeated stimulant administration may render GABA\EOP neurons in the NAc less responsive to D_2-mediated inhibition and more responsive to D_1 effects.

In addition to changes in signal transduction, repeated cocaine exposure has been reported to produce DA depletion. DA depletion has been theorized to underlie the craving and dysphoria associated with cocaine dependence, and may result from the synaptic metabolism of DA during DAT blockade (Dackis & Gold, 1985). Consistent with DA depletion are reports of hyperprolactinemia (a marker for diminished DA tone) (Mendelson et al., 1989), reduced DA release (Volkow et al., 1999) and persistent reductions in DA activity in cocaine addicts (Wu et al., 1997). In addition, preclinical studies show low DA titres in the NAc (Robertson et al., 1991) and reductions in spontaneous VTA neuronal firing (Peoples et al., 1999) after chronic cocaine exposure. DA depletion, in combination with reduced D_2 receptor transduction, could explain the increases in reward thresholds that have been measured after repeated exposure to cocaine (Koob et al., 1998). If DA dysregulation contributes to the craving and dysphoria seen in stimulant addicts, its reversal could improve the recidivism that characterizes stimulant dependence (Dackis & Gold, 1985).

Cocaine craving, a major factor contributing to relapse, can be vigorously triggered by conditioned cues. While rehabilitative approaches advocate the avoidance of 'people, places and things' associated with drug use, this practice is seldom practical for patients immersed in the drug environments of our inner cities. Cue-induced craving has been reported to produce robust limbic activation in cocaine addicts (Grant et al., 1996; Childress et al., 1999), but not in cocaine naïve individuals (Childress et al., 1999), providing a graphic illustration of an acquired brain abnormality. Interestingly, preclinical studies have identified select NAc cells that actually fire in anticipation of cocaine, and this finding may have bearing on cue-induced craving mechanisms (Carelli, 2000). Also, the fact that specific NAc cells fire in anticipation of food and water (Miyazaki et al., 1998) suggests that cocaine has the capacity to recruit brain mechanisms that are normally activated in the presence of survival-related opportunities.

After repeated administration, sensitization develops to a number of toxic and behavioural effects of stimulants. This 'reverse tolerance' is exemplified by kindling in animals (sensitization to the convulsant effects of cocaine) and appears to involve glutamatergic mechanisms. In humans, clear evidence of sensitization is elusive although it has also been proposed to explain the clinical phenomenon of progressively worsening stimulant craving. Amphetamine and cocaine vigorously release glutamate into the PFC, NAc, and several other limbic regions (Reid et al., 1997) through the stimulation of D_1 receptors and, with repeated stimulant use, there develops an increased capacity of the D_1 receptor to release glutamate (Kalivas & Duffy, 1998) (see Fig. 30.3). Sensitization is also associated with D_2 autoreceptor downregulation in the VTA (Li et al., 1999) and supersensitivity of glutamate NMDA receptors (Itzhak, 1995). Stimulant sensitization can be prevented with NMDA antagonists and ablation of the PFC (Li et al., 1999), suggesting an important role for glutamate in this phenomenon. Glutamate depletion has been reported with chronic cocaine administration (Keys et al., 1998), and may result from the overstimulation of glutamatergic neurons.

Excessive brain levels of glutamate can produce neurotoxicity and cell death as a result of Ca^{2+} inflow through

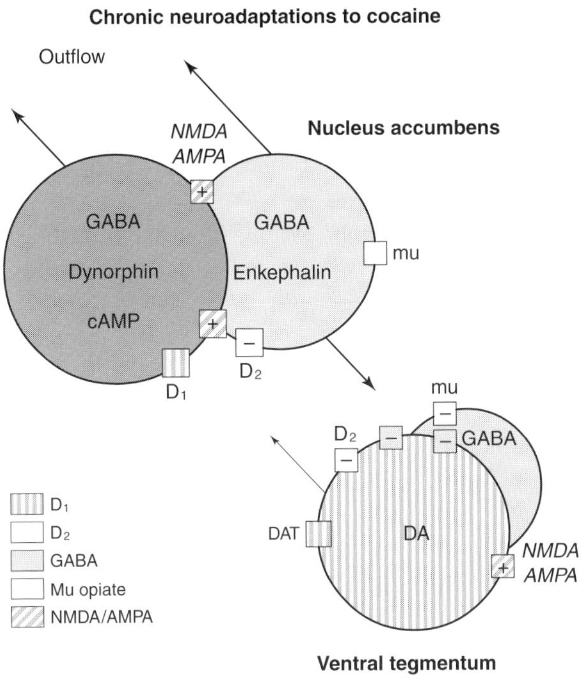

Chronic neuroadaptations to cocaine

Fig. 30.3. Chronic cocaine exposure results in DA depletion and reduced outflow from the VTA. This effect is compounded by reduced D_2 and increased D_1 receptor transduction, increasing cAMP with NAc neurons. Up-regulation of NMDA/AMPA receptors in the NAc and down-regulation of D_2 autoreceptors contribute to sensitization. The NAc becomes increasingly resistant to VTA inhibition as levels of cAMP rise within GABA\EOP neurons. Over time, these changes may reduce hedonic function and contribute to clinical features of cocaine dependence.

NMDA-gated ion channels. Glutamate toxicity, in combination with focal defects of cerebral perfusion attributed to vasoconstriction (Holman et al., 1991), may account for longstanding neuropsychological impairment reported in some stimulant addicts. Reduced metabolism in the glutamate-rich orbitofrontal cortex has actually been reported during stimulant withdrawal (Volkow & Fowler, 2000). Alterations in glutamate-containing PFC neurons could adversely affect frontal lobe processing, including executive function and the ability to suppress limbic impulses.

Cocaine also affects serotonin, norepinephrine, and GABA-containing neurons. Repeated cocaine administration depletes norepinephrine and serotonin, possibly through increased synaptic metabolism during the blockade of associated membrane transporters. In addition, the stimulation of serotonin (5-HT_{1b}) receptors increases cocaine reward (Parsons et al., 1998). These and other findings may justify research of serotonergic agents in

cocaine patients. Cocaine addicts also have benzodiazepine receptor upregulation, strengthening of GABA neurotransmission and enhanced sensitivity to benzodiazepine treatment (Volkow et al., 1998), suggesting likely research opportunities with GABA agents.

Unfortunately, there are no proven pharmacological treatments for stimulant dependence. Cocaine overdose can only be treated by supportive measures and prolonged elimination from the body can result from cocaine's nonlinear pharmacokinetics. The blockade of stimulant reward through neutralizing antibodies to cocaine has been demonstrated in animals and a cocaine vaccine study in humans is under investigation. DA antagonists reduce cocaine euphoria in humans but cause a number of side effects, may worsen craving (Dackis & Gold, 1985), and are unlikely to be acceptable to cocaine addicts. Also, reward blockade would not be expected to ameliorate neuroadaptations of chronic stimulant exposure. Effective detoxification and relapse prevention agents have yet to be identified for psychostimulants, although this is an area of intensive, government-sponsored research. As discussed, GABA/EOP-containing neurons in the NAc receive DA terminals from the VTA and convey reward-related signals to other structures, including regions of the thalamus, PFC, and hypothalamus. Disruption in DA neurotransmission, either through presynaptic DA depletion or postsynaptic transduction changes could drastically affect the orchestration of reward flow in the brain. Current research is being directed toward agents that might reverse DA, GABA, EOP and glutamatergic imbalances that are associated with stimulant addiction.

Opiates

Opiates produce their intensely rewarding effects by activating endogenous opioid receptors, the natural targets of endogenous endorphins, enkephalins, and dynorphins. The genes of mu, delta, and kappa receptors have been cloned, and the former two are involved in opiate reward while kappa receptors may contribute to aversion (Wise, 1996). Mu receptor agonists hyperpolarize medium-sized spiny cells, and this action contributes to their rewarding effect. GABA inhibition also results in DA burst firing with DA release into the NAc. Drug addicts frequently use heroin in conjunction with cocaine (speedballing), a combination that increases NAc extracellular DA by over 1000% (Gerasimov et al., 1999). Although GABA-mediated DA burst firing has been proposed as a mechanism of opiate reward, selective lesions of DA terminals within the NAc do not attenuate IV heroin self-administration (Pettit et al.,

Table 30.1. Intoxication and withdrawal signs and symptoms are listed for several classes of drugs

	Stimulants	PCP	Marijuana	Alcohol/Sedatives	Opiates
Intoxication	Tachycardia	Tachycardia	Tachycardia	Bradycardia	Bradycardia
	Hypertension	Hypertension	Hypertension	Hypotension	Hypotension
	Hyperthermia	Hyperthermia	Hyperthermia	Hypothermia	Hypothermia
	Arousal	Arousal	Paranoia	Sedation	Sedation
	Diaphoresis	Aggression	Diaphoresis	Hypokinesis	Hypokinesis
	Mydriasis	Psychosis	Mydriasis	Ataxia	Pinned pupils
	Hyperkinesis	Ataxia	Ataxia	Slurred speech	Slurred speech
	Euphoria	Salivation	Paranoia	Decreased respirations	Analgesia
	Psychosis	Rigidity	Dry mouth		Head Nodding
	Myoclonus	Red eyes			
	Nystagmus	Nystagmus			
Withdrawal	Bradycardia	Prolonged	Depression	Tachycardia	Tachycardia
	Hypersomnia	Psychosis	Insomnia	Insomnia	Insomnia
	Hyperphagia		Anxiety	Nausea	Nausea
	Depression		Irritability	Anxiety	Anxiety
	Hypokinesis		Anorexia	Hypertension	Hypertension
			Tachycardia	Tachycardia	
				Hyperreflexia	Hyperreflexia
				Diaphoresis	Diaphoresis

Notes:
Note the similarity among alcohol, sedatives, and opiates with regard to intoxication and withdrawal symptoms

1984). This finding demonstrates that opiate reward is not dependent on DA activation, and appears to include two separate (DA-dependent and DA-independent) components. Also consistent with DA-independent opiate reward is the fact that opiates are directly self-administered into a number of brain regions, including the NAc, lateral hypothalamus, amygdala, and the CA3 region of the hippocampus.

Opiates hyperpolarize neurons by increasing the outflow of K^+ through receptor-gated ion channels, and by closing Na^+ channels. As with stimulants, opiates also have the ability to acutely inhibit cAMP through mu and delta receptors coupled to G_i-proteins. Repeated opiate administration has the opposite effect of elevating cAMP levels within NAc cells, and increased cAMP has also been reported in the locus coeruleus, amygdala and thalamus after repeated opiate administration (Terwilliger et al., 1991). The activation of the cAMP pathway renders noradrenergic neurons less sensitive to opiate inhibition, resulting in rebound noradrenergic hyperactivity that has been hypothesized to underlie opiate withdrawal. Increased noradrenergic cAMP has also been reported with chronic stress, and there is an established relationship between stress and recidivism. In addition to noradrenergic effects, chronic exposure to opiates produces DA inhi-

bition. During opiate withdrawal, extracellular DA is reduced in the NAc (Rossetti et al., 1992), and chronic opiate exposure leads to dramatically reduced DA firing rates that persist well beyond physical withdrawal (Diana et al., 1999). DA depletion may contribute to the reward inhibition and dysphoria that has been reported in opiate dependence (Dackis & Gold, 1992; Rossetti et al., 1992).

Opiate addiction has been a significant health problem in this country for many years, especially since the invention of the hypodermic syringe in the nineteenth century. Its poor prognosis is undoubtedly affected by the lure of opiate euphoria, a subjective and physiological state that differs greatly from psychostimulant intoxication (see Table 30.1). These drug states have opposite effects on vital signs, general arousal, libido, aggression, and vigilance. In addition, opiate use typically leads to a state of contentedness that lasts several hours, whereas cocaine use rapidly engenders additional cocaine craving (O'Brien et al., 1992).

A number of treatments are currently available for opiate dependence. Overdose is potentially lethal, usually due to respiratory inhibition, and can be reversed with naloxone, a mu receptor antagonist. Opiate withdrawal offers a classic example of how an understanding of brain mechanisms can uncover new treatments. A large body of clinical and preclinical research predicted the efficacy of clonidine, an alpha-$_2$ adrenergic agonist, based on its ability to reverse noradrenergic hyperactivity associated with opiate withdrawal. Although alpha$_2$- agonists are effective for opiate withdrawal, patients usually prefer methadone. Heroin detoxification with methadone can be achieved with descending doses in about three days (Dackis & Gold, 1992) and dosing should be guided by clinical signs of withdrawal rather than patient-reported symptoms. Detoxification alone is seldom sufficient treatment and should be provided in concert with drug rehabilitation.

Even after detoxification and rehabilitative treatment, the majority of heroin addicts tend to relapse. Methadone maintenance, the transfer from intravenous heroin to a long-acting oral agonist, can achieve greater retention, reduced heroin use, and lower rates of HIV infection (Sees et al., 2000), viral hepatitis, and bacterial endocarditis. When combined with psychosocial treatment, an adequate dose of methadone can effectively stabilize many otherwise treatment refractory individuals. Two additional replacement agents are available to treat opiate addicts. Levo-alpha-acetylmethadol (LAAM), FDA approved since 1993, is a longer acting opioid that can be administered three times per week. Buprenorphine is a partial mu opiate agonist, an attribute that provides a 'ceiling' effect and diminishes lethality with overdose. Buprenorphine also attenuates the subjective effects of heroin. The availability of methadone, LAAM and buprenorphine provides the clinician with several options in treating these difficult patients.

A final treatment strategy for heroin dependence involves blocking heroin euphoria with naltrexone. Naltrexone has a high affinity for the mu and kappa receptors, and antagonizes neurotransmission by displacing opiate agonists such as morphine, heroin, and methadone. Since opiate receptor blockade produces acute withdrawal in dependent individuals, naltrexone should not be administered prior to the completion of detoxification. Special populations that may benefit from naltrexone are professionals with regular workplace exposure to drugs and probationers who are mandated to treatment (Cornish et al., 1997). Unfortunately, there has been little practitioner interest in this treatment, perhaps due to compliance issues. A long-acting depot form of naltrexone that provides clinically effective blood levels for 30–60 days is currently in clinical trials. It is hoped that this advance will improve medication adherence and reduce impulsive relapses.

THC and PCP

Marijuana is a widely abused substance, particularly by young people. Along with nicotine, another early exposure drug, marijuana has the potential to serve as a gateway to other drugs of abuse, perhaps due to its ability to activate reward circuitry and release DA into the NAc. Also, the persistence of marijuana's metabolites in the urine, combined with the widespread practice of pre-employment drug testing, can prohibitively affect the careers of both habitual and casual users. Marijuana produces drug seeking behaviour and addictive patterns, and its chronic use has been associated with withdrawal symptoms. As with alcohol, opiates, and stimulants, elevations in CRF occur during THC withdrawal (Rodriguez de Fonseca et al., 1997) and chronic exposure to marijuana reduces the firing rates of mesocorticolimbic DA cells (Diana et al., 1998). THC binds the cannabinoid receptor for which an endogenous ligand, anandamide, has been recently isolated (Devane & Axelrod, 1994). Cannabinoid receptors are found in the hippocampus, thalamus, cortex, and striatum, are coupled to G-proteins, and acutely inhibit cAMP levels. THC administration also reduces GABA output and releases DA into the NAc through a Ca^{2+}-dependent mechanism that can be blocked by naloxone (Chen et al., 1990). Therefore, THC appears to activate reward circuitry by stimulating DA and opiate systems. These actions of THC provide a neurochemical rationale for the well-established clinical prohibition of smoking marijuana when attempting recovery from other drugs of abuse.

Phencyclidine (PCP) exerts its rewarding effect through the blockade of NMDA receptors. Originally developed as an intravenous anesthetic, PCP ('angel dust') use was discontinued in humans due to the untoward effects of agitation, delusions, impaired judgment, and violent behaviour. PCP and other NMDA receptor antagonists have been proposed to have potential value in stroke models. The NMDA receptor is a complicated macromolecule that depolarizes neurons by opening gated Ca^{2+} channels, generally in the presence of both glutamate and glycine. This receptor is distinguished from two other glutamate receptor types, AMPA and KA, by its voltage-dependent characteristics, high permeability to Ca^{2+}, and activation of a nitric oxide cascade. PCP rewarding action may result, to some extent, from its ability to directly inhibit NAc medium spiny neurons. As previously discussed, these cells are normally activated by glutamatergic pyramidal neurons of the prefrontal cortex, and modulated by DA projections from the VTA. As a result of GABA inhibition, PCP has been reported to cause neurotoxicity through the release of excessive amounts of acetylcholine in the brain (Kim et al., 1999). Although PCP is not widely used at this time, a reduction in perceived risk could potentially lead to increased use of this dangerous agent. For example, MDMA ('ecstasy') has neurotoxic effects on serotonin neurons (Kosten, 1990) but is currently popular and has low risk perception. The addictiveness of PCP, a specific NMDA antagonist, demonstrates the importance of glutamate pathways in the neurobiology of addiction.

Nicotine

Nicotine differs from previously discussed substances by its legality and the lack of functional impairment associated with its use. However, the tenacious quality of nicotine, combined with its extensive and serious medical complications, makes it arguably the most lethal of all addictive substances. Nicotine directly accounts for an estimated 400 000 deaths per year (Epping-Jordan et al., 1998). Nicotine dependence involves reinforcement, tolerance, and withdrawal, and smokers often cite craving as the greatest impediment to quitting. Substitution therapy with a nicotine patch or nicotine gum has limited effectiveness, perhaps because these routes of administration do not provide the rapid delivery of nicotine seen with the intrapulmonary route. Encouraging results have been found with buproprion, an antidepressant that inhibits the DAT (O'Brien & McKay, 1998).

Nicotine stimulates nicotinic receptors that are located on DA cell bodies in the VTA and on DA terminals in the NAc (Dani & Heinemann, 1996), causing a release of DA into the shell of the NAc. In animal models, nicotine self-administration is reduced by destruction of mesocortico-limbic DA neurons (Corrigall et al., 1992) and by the administration of DA antagonists (Corrigall et al., 1994). Opiate antagonists also reduce nicotine self-administration, suggesting the involvement of both DA and EOP mechanisms. Nicotine withdrawal has been associated with changes in the distribution of nicotine receptors in the brain and with markedly reduced measurements of brain reward (Epping-Jordan et al., 1998). It is possible that a reduction in brain reward contributes to the intense craving characteristic of nicotine dependence. Since nicotine stimulates reward circuits it stands to reason that patients seeking recovery from other drugs might have more success if they quit smoking. Interestingly, 12-step self-help based approaches do not generally advocate nicotine avoidance and research is clearly needed to determine whether nicotine abstinence can improve recovery rates from other addictive agents.

Alcohol and sedative hypnotics

Alcohol has numerous actions on GABA, opiate, glutamate, DA, and serotonin neurotransmitter systems. Unlike other addictive agents with high affinity for membrane-bound proteins, alcohol mediates its effects on ion channels by disrupting the membrane lipid matrix. Alcohol facilitates GABA-mediated neurotransmission by promoting Cl^- influx through $GABA_A$-gated ion channels. This effect on Cl^- influx decreases with repeated alcohol administration, and may contribute to the development of alcohol tolerance (Koob & Weiss, 1992). A number of studies report that GABA neurotransmission is increased during alcohol intoxication and decreased during alcohol withdrawal. Consistent with these findings is the fact that alcohol withdrawal can be reversed with GABA agonists (such as benzodiazepines) and alcohol withdrawal seizures respond to GABAergic anticonvulsants.

The importance of opiate mechanisms in alcohol reward is illustrated by the fact that mu antagonists reduce alcohol consumption, especially when administered directly into the central nucleus of the amygdala (Koob & Weiss, 1992). Also, alcohol administration increases endorphin levels while alcoholics in withdrawal have reduced levels of beta-endorphin (CSF) (Koob & Weiss, 1992). Alcohol-induced DA release into the NAc is blocked by opiate antagonists (Acquas et al., 1993), suggesting an opiate mechanism of this phenomenon. Although the precise mechanism of alcohol's effect on opiate systems in the brain is not known, the appreciation of EOP involvement led to the landmark development of naltrexone as a treatment for alcoholism (Volpicelli et al., 1992).

DA mechanisms are also involved in alcoholism. Rats selectively bred for alcohol preference have an exaggerated DA response to alcohol, whereas D_2 receptor deficient (D_2 knockout) rats show a marked aversion to alcohol (Koob & Weiss, 1992). Alcohol directly and robustly excites DA neurons of the VTA (Brodie et al., 1999), increases DA synthesis and turnover, and releases DA into the NAc (Koob & Weiss, 1992). In addition, DA antagonists applied to the NAc reduce alcohol self-administration (Koob et al., 1998). These findings suggest an important role for DA in alcohol reward. However, the selective destruction of DA terminals in the NAc does not reduce alcohol self-administration (Koob et al., 1998), suggesting an additional DA-independent mechanism in alcohol reward.

Alcohol has chronic actions on DA neurons that are similar to those seen with cocaine and opiates. With chronic alcohol exposure, there is a reduction in DA release (Weiss et al., 1996) and a sustained inhibition of DA firing that persists well beyond the withdrawal state (Diana et al., 1996). This has led to the hypothesis that alcohol-induced DA depletion leads to hedonic inhibition, craving and relapse tendencies of alcoholics (Wise, 1996), as has been proposed with individuals addicted to opiates (Rossetti et al., 1992), cocaine (Dackis & Gold, 1985), and marijuana (Diana et al., 1998). The high prevalence of depression and suicide in alcoholics and other substance abusers could also result, to some degree, from impaired hedonic function.

Alcohol has additional actions on serotonin, glutamate, and noradrenergic systems. Alcohol preferring rats have reduced levels of brain serotonin, and pharmacological enhancement of serotonin reduces alcohol intake (Koob & Weiss, 1992). However, serotonin depletion also reduces alcohol intake, and serotonergic agents have not been found effective in treating alcoholism (O'Brien & McKay, 1998). Additionally, alcohol reduces NMDA neurotransmission through allosteric blockade of Ca^{2+} and Na^+ channels, resulting in a reduction of ion current that is linearly related to alcohol intoxication (Lovinger et al., 1989). Conversely, alcohol withdrawal is associated with increased NMDA neurotransmission (Fitzgerald & Nestler, 1995). Alcohol withdrawal may also involve noradrenergic hyperactivity as evidenced by the presence of hypertension, tachycardia, hyperreflexia, diaphoresis, insomnia, tremor, and anxiety (Koob & Weiss, 1992). Detoxification from alcohol is seldom a sufficient treatment for alcoholics and does not eliminate the protracted craving and recidivism that is characteristic of alcoholism. Rehabilitation through professional and self-help approaches should be strongly encouraged with these patients.

Medications currently available for treating alcoholism include detoxification agents, disulfiram, and naltrexone. Detoxification has been reviewed elsewhere (Dackis & Gold, 1992) and generally involves prescribing descending doses of benzodiazepines (or barbiturates) over 3–5 days. Disulfiram inactivates aldehyde dehydrogenase, resulting in high levels of the toxic metabolite, acetaldehyde, when alcohol is consumed. This results in aversive subjective effects that should theoretically discourage drinking. However, double-blind trials have not shown disulfiram to be better than placebo (O'Brien & McKay, 1998) and alcoholics tend to simply discontinue disulfiram and resume drinking. Also, disulfiram does not reverse chronic neuroadaptive changes caused by alcohol and is ineffective against alcohol craving.

Promising results in the treatment of alcoholism have been demonstrated with naltrexone. Naltrexone reduces alcohol consumption and ameliorates craving for alcohol, and its effectiveness may continue beyond the period in which the drug is taken (O'Brien & McKay, 1998). Naltrexone also reduces the rewarding effects of alcohol, presumably by blocking opiate-mediated reward. In spite of numerous studies confirming the efficacy of naltrexone in the treatment of alcoholism, its clinical use is not widespread. Acamprosate, a GABA receptor agonist, is currently under investigation and has been shown to be effective in five studies in Europe (O'Brien & McKay, 1998).

Sedative hypnotics, particularly benzodiazepines, are widely prescribed for anxiety, muscle tension, insomnia, and convulsions. Benzodiazepines, barbiturates, and alcohol produce a similar and characteristic state of reduced anxiety, disinhibition, euphoria, sedation, and hypnosis (Koob & Nestler, 1997). Sedatives facilitate GABA-mediated neurotransmission through allosteric actions on the GABA receptor complex, opening GABA-gated chloride channels. This action serves to inhibit target neurons and, in this regard, sedatives share effects and cross-tolerance with alcohol (Koob & Nestler, 1997). Unlike alcohol, sedatives have no effect on the NMDA receptor. Clinically, it is imperative to maintain a high degree of suspicion for sedative dependence since it is often covert, and withdrawal can be protracted. Successful detoxification from sedatives can be achieved by instituting a descending dose schedule of either phenobarbital (for barbiturates) or long-acting benzodiazepines like chlordiazepoxide (for benzodiazepines), and detoxification may require several weeks duration (Dackis & Gold, 1992). With the exception of treating withdrawal, sedatives should not normally be prescribed to alcoholics due to their addiction potential, similarity in brain action, and ability to reinstate alcohol intake.

In conclusion, extensive research into the neurobiology of addiction has yielded a number of interesting findings and some new treatments. It is evident that addictive drugs with diverse pharmacological and subjective effects activate common reward pathways (see Table 30.2). Increased DA neurotransmission is universally found during drug intoxication, while DA depletion and reduced DA neurotransmission appears to be a feature of chronic addiction. The NAc, thought to be a crucial target of DA projections, is largely composed of GABA/EOP-containing projection neurons. These medium-sized spiny cells convey reward-related information to a number of brain regions known to be associated with motivation and feeling states, including the thalamus, cingulate and frontal cortex, and the hypothalamus. The inhibition of GABA/EOP medium-sized spiny cells occurs in all intoxication states. While GABA/EOP neurons in the NAc are inhibited during drug intoxication, suppression may become increasingly difficult with repeated drug exposure due to molecular changes associated with the cAMP second messenger pathway. Neuroadaptations such as this may contribute to clinical phenomena associated with addictive illness, including tolerance, withdrawal, and hedonic inhibition

Table 30.2. Acute mechanisms of action of major addictive drugs

Alcohol	Facilitates GABA-mediated neurotransmission
	Antagonizes NMDA-mediated neurotransmission
Amphetamine	Releases DA through reverse transport
	Releases 5-HT, norepinephrine
Cocaine	Antagonist at DAT, local anesthetic action
	Antagonist at 5-HT and norepinephrine transporters
Heroin and opiates	Agonist at opiate receptors
Marijuana	Agonist at cannabinoid receptors
Nicotine	Agonist at nicotinic cholinergic receptors
Phencyclidine	Antagonist at NMDA receptors

(see Table 30.3). Since inhibition of medium-sized spiny neurons within the reward centres appears to be an important feature of drug reward, medications capable of altering GABA/EOP function should be high on the list of potential therapeutic agents to be investigated. Although pharmacological treatments for addiction are currently limited, additional treatments may result from a refined understanding of the neuronal and molecular aspects of addiction.

Several lines of evidence support the existence of two separate reward systems in the brain that are activated by different classes of addictive agents. Alcohol and opiates are self-administered even after the chemical ablation of DA terminals (Koob et al., 1998), strongly suggesting the existence of DA-independent reward mechanisms. Also, the intoxication produced by opiates, alcohol, and sedatives differs markedly from that of stimulants, also suggesting the activation of different brain mechanisms. Stimulants and opiates may act on different brain systems that have evolved to reward the procurement and consumption, respectively, of survival needs. Stimulants

Table 30.3. Acute and chronic neurotransmitter effects of addictive substances are indicated. Chronic neuroadaptations are often opposite to acute effects

	Acute actions	Chronic neuroadaptations
Stimulants	Increase DA levels in the NAc	Deplete DA
	Reduce cAMP in the NAc	Increase cAMP in the NAc
	Reduce DA and NE firing rates	Increase CRF
	Decrease GABA firing rates	Increase NMDA receptor sensitivity
		Reduce D_2 autoreceptor sensitivity
		Decrease orbitofrontal metabolism
		Reduce brain reward
Opiates	Release DA into the NAc	Deplete DA
	Reduce cAMP in the NAc	Increase cAMP in the NAc
	DA burst firing	NE hyperactivity
	Inhibit GABA neurons	Increase cAMP in the locus coeruleus
		Increase CRF
Alcohol	Releases DA into the NAc	Depletes DA
	Decreases NMDA neurotransmission	Reduces DA firing rates
	Increases GABA neurotransmission	Increasees NMDA neurotransmission
	Increases EOP levels	Decreases GABA neurotransmission
	Produces DA burst firing	Reduces EOP levels
		Increases CRF
		Reduces brain reward
Nicotine	Release DA into the NAc	Reduces brain reward
	DA burst firing	
Marijuana	Releases DA into the NAc	Depletes DA
	Reduces cAMP in the NAc	Increases cAMP in the NAc
	Blocks GABA output	Increases CRF

promote vigilance, psychomotor and autonomic activation, environmental interaction, and intensification of craving. These activating effects would be desirable in the pursuit of survival goals. Opiates, on the other hand, produce euphoria, behavioural suppression, relaxation, and satiation, and may act on a system designed to punctuate consumption and provide consummatory reward.

Basic science research supports many clinical practices that are currently used in the treatment of addiction. Since all addictive drugs activate reward circuits, and appear to produce similar neuroadaptations with chronic use, reinstatement of addiction is a risk when any addictive agent is used. This notion supports the clinical principle that recovery from one class of addictive drugs is best achieved when all addictive drugs are avoided. The avoidance of cues associated with drug use, a central theme of drug rehabilitation, is strongly supported by PET studies showing limbic activation during cue-induced craving. Reliance on peers and professional caretakers during early recovery may be especially important to counter powerful limbic craving, and compensate for the lack of internal resolve that may result from impaired frontal lobe executive function. Genetic variations affecting the reward circuitry could explain why certain individuals are more likely to develop addiction. The possibility that nicotine use could undermine recovery, through its ability to stimulate the VTA–NAc pleasure circuit, warrants research. Given the biological underpinnings of addiction, clinicians should view addiction as a disease rather than a weakness, and maintain a compassionate and non-judgmental approach to their patients. In addition to being seriously afflicted with a brain disease, drug addicts and alcoholics are often victimized by prejudice and misunderstanding. Hopefully, further elucidation of the neurobiology of addiction will change perceptions, diminish prejudice, and reduce obstacles faced by afflicted individuals who are seeking acceptance and access to medical care.

References

Acquas, E., Meloni, M. & Di Chiara, G. (1993). Blockade of delta-opioid receptors in the nucleus accumbens prevents ethanol-induced stimulation of dopamine release. *Eur. J. Pharmacol.*, **230**, 239–41.

Akil, H., Owens, C., Gutstein, H., Taylor, L., Curran, E. & Watson, S. (1998). Endogenous opioids: overview and current issues. *Drug Alcohol Depend.*, **51**, 127–40.

Bardo, M.T. (1998). Neuropharmacological mechanisms of drug reward: beyond dopamine in the nucleus accumbens. *Crit. Rev. Neurobiol.*, **12**, 37–67.

Breiter, H.C., Gollub, R.L., Weisskoff, R.M. et al. (1997). Acute effects of cocaine on human brain activity and emotion. *Neuron*, **19**, 591–611.

Brodie, M.S., Pesold, C. & Appel, S.B. (1999). Ethanol directly excites dopaminergic ventral tegmental area reward neurons. *Alcohol Clin. Exp. Res.*, **23**, 1848–52.

Carelli, R.M. (2000). Activation of accumbens cell firing by stimuli associated with cocaine delivery during self-administration [In Process Citation]. *Synapse*, **35**, 238–42.

Carr, D.B., O'Donnell, P., Card, J.P. & Sesack, S.R. (1999). Dopamine terminals in the rat prefrontal cortex synapse on pyramidal cells that project to the nucleus accumbens. *J. Neurosci.*, **19**, 11049–60.

Chen, J.P., Paredes, W., Li, J., Smith, D., Lowinson, J. & Gardner, E. L. (1990). Delta 9-tetrahydrocannabinol produces naloxone-blockable enhancement of presynaptic basal dopamine efflux in nucleus accumbens of conscious, freely-moving rats as measured by intracerebral microdialysis. *Psychopharmacology*, **102**, 156–62.

Childress, A.R., Mozley, P.D., McElgin, W., Fitzgerald, J., Reivich, M. & O'Brien, C.P. (1999). Limbic activation during cue-induced cocaine craving. *Am. J. Psychiatry*, **156**, 11–18.

Cornish, J.W., Metzger, D., Woody, G.E. et al. (1997). Naltrexone pharmacotherapy for opioid dependent federal probationers. *J. Subst. Abuse Treat.*, **14**, 529–34.

Corrigall, W.A., Franklin, K.B., Coen, K.M. & Clarke, P.B. (1992). The mesolimbic dopaminergic system is implicated in the reinforcing effects of nicotine. *Psychopharmacology*, **107**, 285–9.

Corrigall, W.A., Coen, K.M. & Adamson, K.L. (1994). Self-administered nicotine activates the mesolimbic dopamine system through the ventral tegmental area. *Brain Res.*, **653**, 278–84.

Dackis, C.A. & Gold, M.S. (1985). New concepts in cocaine addiction: the dopamine depletion hypothesis. *Neurosci. Biobehav. Rev.*, **9**, 469–77.

Dackis, C.A. & Gold, M.S. (1992). Psychiatric hospitals for treatment of dual diagnosis. In *Substance Abuse, A Comprehensive Textbook*, ed. J.H. Lowinson, pp. 467–85. Baltimore: Williams & Wilkins.

Dani, J.A. & Heinemann, S. (1996). Molecular and cellular aspects of nicotine abuse. *Neuron*, **16**, 905–8.

Devane, W.A. & Axelrod, J. (1994). Enzymatic synthesis of anandamide, an endogenous ligand for the cannabinoid receptor, by brain membranes. *Proc. Natl. Acad. Sci., USA*, **91**, 6698–701.

Diana, M., Pistis, M., Muntoni, A. & Gessa, G. (1996). Mesolimbic dopaminergic reduction outlasts ethanol withdrawal syndrome: evidence of protracted abstinence. *Neuroscience*, **71**, 411–15.

Diana, M., Melis, M., Muntoni, A.L. & Gessa, G.L. (1998). Mesolimbic dopaminergic decline after cannabinoid withdrawal. *Proc. Natl. Acad. Sci., USA*, **95**, 10269–73.

Diana, M., Muntoni, A.L., Pistis, M., Melis, M. & Gessa, G.L. (1999). Lasting reduction in mesolimbic dopamine neuronal activity after morphine withdrawal. *Eur. J. Neurosci.*, **11**, 1037–41.

Durstewitz, D., Seamans, J.K. & Sejnowski, T.J. (2000). Dopamine-mediated stabilization of delay-period activity in a network model of prefrontal cortex. *J. Neurophysiol.*, **83**, 1733–50.

Epping-Jordan, M.P., Watkins, S.S., Koob, G.F. & Markou, A. (1998). Dramatic decreases in brain reward function during nicotine withdrawal. *Nature*, **393**, 76–9.

Fitzgerald, L.W. & Nestler, E.J. (1995). Molecular and cellular adaptations in signal transduction pathways following ethanol exposure. *Clin. Neurosci.*, **3**, 165–73.

Gerasimov, M R., Ashby, C.R., Jr., Gardner, E.L., Mills, M.J., Brodie, J.D. & Dewey, S.L. (1999). Gamma-vinyl GABA inhibits methamphetamine, heroin, or ethanol-induced increases in nucleus accumbens dopamine. *Synapse*, **34**, 11–19.

Grant, S., London, E.D., Newlin, D.B. et al. (1996). Activation of memory circuits during cue-elicited cocaine craving. *Proc. Natl. Acad. Sci., USA*, **93**, 12040–5.

Heimer, L. & Alheid, G.F. (1991). Piecing together the puzzle of basal forebrain anatomy. *Adv. Exp. Med. Biol.*, **295**, 1–42.

Hernandez-Lopez, S., Bargas, J., Surmeier, D.J., Reyes, A. & Galarraga, E. (1997). D1 receptor activation enhances evoked discharge in neostriatal medium spiny neurons by modulating an L-type Ca^{2+} conductance. *J. Neurosci.*, **17**, 3334–42.

Holman, B.L., Carvalho, P.A., Mendelson, J. et al. (1991). Brain perfusion is abnormal in cocaine-dependent polydrug users: a study using technetium-99m-HMPAO and ASPECT. *J. Nucl. Med.*, **32**, 1206–10.

Itzhak, Y. (1995). Cocaine kindling in mice. Responses to *N*-methyl-D,L-aspartate (NMDLA) and L-arginine. *Mol. Neurobiol.*, **11**, 217–22.

Kalivas, P.W. & Duffy, P. (1998). Repeated cocaine administration alters extracellular glutamate in the ventral tegmental area. *J. Neurochem.*, **70**, 1497–502.

Kalivas, P.W., Churchill, L. & Romanides, A. (1999). Involvement of the pallidal-thalamocortical circuit in adaptive behavior. *Ann. NY Acad. Sci.*, **877**, 64–70.

Keys, A.S., Mark, G.P., Emre, N. & Meshul, C.K. (1998). Reduced glutamate immunolabeling in the nucleus accumbens following extended withdrawal from self-administered cocaine. *Synapse*, **30**, 393–401.

Kim, S.H., Price, M.T., Olney, J.W. & Farber, N.B. (1999). Excessive cerebrocortical release of acetylcholine induced by NMDA antagonists is reduced by GABAergic and alpha2-adrenergic agonists. *Mol. Psychiatry*, **4**, 344–52.

Koob, G.F. & Nestler, E.J. (1997). The neurobiology of drug addiction. *J. Neuropsychiatry Clin. Neurosci.*, **9**, 482–97.

Koob, G.F. & Weiss, F. (1992). Neuropharmacology of cocaine and ethanol dependence. *Recent Dev. Alcohol*, **10**, 201–33.

Koob, G.F., Sanna, P.P. & Bloom, F.E. (1998). Neuroscience of addiction. *Neuron*, **21**, 467–76.

Kosten, T.R. (1990). Neurobiology of abused drugs. Opioids and stimulants. *J. Nerv. Ment. Dis.*, **178**, 217–27.

Leshner, A I. & Koob, G.F. (1999). Drugs of abuse and the brain. *Proc. Assoc. Am. Physicians*, **111**, 99–108.

Li, Y., Hu, X.T., Berney, T.G. et al. (1999). Both glutamate receptor antagonists and prefrontal cortex lesions prevent induction of cocaine sensitization and associated neuroadaptations. *Synapse*, **34**, 169–80.

Lovinger, D.M., White, G. & Weight, F.F. (1989). Ethanol inhibits NMDA-activated ion current in hippocampal neurons. *Science*, **243**, 1721–4.

Mendelson, J.H., Mello, N.K., Teoh, S.K., Ellingboe, J. & Cochin, J. (1989). Cocaine effects on pulsatile secretion of anterior pituitary, gonadal, and adrenal hormones. *J. Clin. Endocrinol. Metab.*, **69**, 1256–60.

Miyazaki, K., Mogi, E., Araki, N. & Matsumoto, G. (1998). Reward-quality dependent anticipation in rat nucleus accumbens. *Neuroreport*, **9**, 3943–8.

Napier, T.C. & Mitrovic, I. (1999). Opioid modulation of ventral pallidal inputs. *Ann. NY Acad. Sci.*, **877**, 176–201.

O'Brien, C.P. & McKay, J.R. (1998). Pharmacological treatments of substance use disorders. In *A Guide to Treatments That Work*, ed. P.E. Nathan & J.M. Gorman, pp. 127–55. New York: Oxford University Press.

O'Brien, C.P., Childress, A.R., McLellan, A.T. & Ehrman, R. (1992). Classical conditioning in drug-dependent humans. *Ann. NY Acad. Sci.*, **654**, 400–15.

Parsons, L.H., Weiss, F. & Koob, G.F. (1998). Serotonin1B receptor stimulation enhances cocaine reinforcement. *J. Neurosci.*, **18**, 10078–89.

Pennartz, C.M., Groenewegen, H.J. & Lopes da Silva, F.H. (1994). The nucleus accumbens as a complex of functionally distinct neuronal ensembles: an integration of behavioural, electrophysiological and anatomical data. *Prog. Neurobiol.*, **42**, 719–61.

Peoples, L.L., Uzwiak, A.J., Gee, F. & West, M.O. (1999). Tonic firing of rat nucleus accumbens neurons: changes during the first 2 weeks of daily cocaine self-administration sessions. *Brain Res.*, **822**, 231–6.

Pettit, H.O., Ettenberg, A., Bloom, F.E. & Koob, G.F. (1984). Destruction of dopamine in the nucleus accumbens selectively attenuates cocaine but not heroin self-administration in rats. *Psychopharmacology*, **84**, 167–73.

Pickel, V.M. & Chan, J. (1990). Spiny neurons lacking choline acetyltransferase immunoreactivity are major targets of cholinergic and catecholaminergic terminals in rat striatum. *J. Neurosci. Res.*, **25**, 263–80.

Reid, M.S., Hsu, K., Jr. & Berger, S.P. (1997). Cocaine and amphetamine preferentially stimulate glutamate release in the limbic system: studies on the involvement of dopamine. *Synapse*, **27**, 95–105.

Robertson, M.W., Leslie, C.A. & Bennett, J.P., Jr. (1991). Apparent synaptic dopamine deficiency induced by withdrawal from chronic cocaine treatment. *Brain Res.*, **538**, 337–9.

Rodriguez de Fonseca, F., Carrera, M.R.A., Navarro, M., Koob, G.F. & Weiss, F. (1997). Activation of corticotropin-releasing factor in the limbic system during cannabinoid withdrawal [see comments]. *Science*, **276**, 2050–4.

Rossetti, Z.L., Hmaidan, Y. & Gessa, G.L. (1992). Marked inhibition of mesolimbic dopamine release: a common feature of ethanol, morphine, cocaine and amphetamine abstinence in rats. *Eur. J. Pharmacol.*, **221**, 227–34.

Schultz, W., Dayan, P. & Montague, P.R. (1997). A neural substrate of prediction and reward. *Science*, **275**, 1593–9.

Sees, K.L., Delucchi, K.L., Masson, C. et al. (2000). Methadone maintenance vs 180-day psychosocially enriched detoxification for treatment of opioid dependence: a randomized controlled trial [see comments]. *J. Am. Med. Assoc.*, **283**, 1303–10.

Self, D.W., Genova, L.M., Hope, B.T., Barnhart, W.J., Spencer, J.J. & Nestler, E.J. (1998). Involvement of cAMP-dependent protein kinase in the nucleus accumbens in cocaine self-administration and relapse of cocaine-seeking behavior. *J. Neurosci.*, **18**, 1848–59.

Sesack, S.R. & Pickel, V.M. (1992). Prefrontal cortical efferents in the rat synapse on unlabeled neuronal targets of catecholamine terminals in the nucleus accumbens septi and on dopamine neurons in the ventral tegmental area. *J. Comp. Neurol.*, **320**, 145–60.

Terwilliger, R.Z., Beitner-Johnson, D., Sevarino, K.A., Crain, S.M. & Nestler, E.J. (1991). A general role for adaptations in G-proteins and the cyclic AMP system in mediating the chronic actions of morphine and cocaine on neuronal function. *Brain Res.*, **548**, 100–10.

Volkow, N.D. & Fowler, J.S. (2000). Addiction, a disease of compulsion and drive: involvement of the orbitofrontal cortex [In Process Citation]. *Cereb. Cortex*, **10**, 318–25.

Volkow, N.D., Fowler, J.S., Wang, G.J. et al. (1993). Decreased dopamine D2 receptor availability is associated with reduced frontal metabolism in cocaine abusers. *Synapse*, **14**, 169–77.

Volkow, N.D., Wang, G.J., Fowler, J.S. et al. (1998). Enhanced sensitivity to benzodiazepines in active cocaine-abusing subjects: a PET study. *Am. J. Psychiatry*, **155**, 200–6.

Volkow, N.D., Fowler, J.S. & Wang, G.J. (1999). Imaging studies on the role of dopamine in cocaine reinforcement and addiction in humans. *J. Psychopharmacol.*, **13**, 337–45.

Volpicelli, J.R., Alterman, A.I., Hayashida, M. & O'Brien, C.P. (1992). Naltrexone in the treatment of alcohol dependence [see comments]. *Arch. Gen. Psychiatry*, **49**, 876–80.

Weiss, F., Parsons, L.H., Schulteis, G. et al. (1996). Ethanol self-administration restores withdrawal-associated deficiencies in accumbal dopamine and 5-hydroxytryptamine release in dependent rats. *J. Neurosci.*, **16**, 3474–85.

Whitelaw, R.B., Markou, A., Robbins, T.W. & Everitt, B.J. (1996). Excitotoxic lesions of the basolateral amygdala impair the acquisition of cocaine-seeking behaviour under a second-order schedule of reinforcement. *Psychopharmacology (Berl.)*, **127**, 213–24.

Wikler, A. & Pescor, F.T. (1967). Classical conditioning of a morphine abstinence phenomenon, reinforcement of opioid-drinking behavior and 'relapse' in morphine-addicted rats. *Psychopharmacologia*, **10**, 255–84.

Wise, R.A. (1996). Neurobiology of addiction. *Curr. Opin. Neurobiol.*, **6**, 243–51.

Wu, J.C., Bell, K., Najafi, A. et al. (1997). Decreasing striatal 6–FDOPA uptake with increasing duration of cocaine withdrawal [see comments]. *Neuropsychopharmacology*, **17**, 402–9.

Part III

Disorders of motor control

31

Mechanisms of motor control

James Ashe[1] and Apostolos P. Georgopoulos[2]

[1] Brain Sciences Center, VAMC, and Department of Neurology and Neuroscience, University of Minnesota, MN, USA
[2] Brain Sciences Center, VAMC, and Department of Neurology, Neuroscience, and Psychiatry, University of Minnesota, MN, USA

Historical overview

The idea that the cortex of the brain could be responsible for the control of movement or indeed that any function could be localized to the cortex is a relatively new one. Until the middle of the nineteenth century it was generally thought that the cerebral cortex was the repository of thoughts and ideas. Nevertheless, Robert Boyle, one of the founders of the Royal Society and originator of the eponymous Boyle's Law, had suggested in 1691 that some aspects of motor function could be localized within the cerebral cortex. Franz Joseph Gall, the father of phrenology, had been a strong advocate of localized function within the cortex, and had suggested that the frontal lobes contained centres for speech some decades before Broca. Observations made by the British neurologist John Hughlins Jackson on patients with focal seizures convinced him that motor activity was localized within the surface of the brain. However, the first experimental demonstration of such localization came with the electrical stimulation experiments of Fritsch and Hitzig in 1870 (Fig. 31.1). They applied galvanic current to the brain of a dog and were able to elicit movements on the opposite side of the body. In 1875 David Ferrier (Ferrier, 1875) did similar experiments on the cortex of the monkey using faradic stimulation. Given the relatively crude methodology employed, the movements elicited by Ferrier through stimulation of different areas conform well to the somatotopic map currently accepted. Sherrington and his colleagues (Leyton & Sherrington, 1917) did a series of detailed experiments, using more refined stimulation methods, on the brains of anthropoid apes to more precisely define the motor and sensory areas of the cortex. Their findings were more detailed than those of Ferrier and not much different from the current standard maps of somatotopic distribution (Fig. 31.2).

Stimulation experiments were also done on the human brain. One of the most dramatic and earliest descriptions

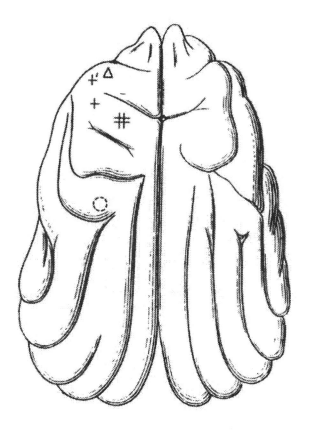

Fig. 31.1. Figure from the classic experiment of Fritsch and Hitzig in 1870. Shows the exposed cortical surface of the dog viewed from above. The symbols denote parts of the surface to which galvanic current was applied and the type of movement elicited in different groups of muscles on the opposite side of the body: # (hindlimb), + (forelimb), +' (forelimb), △ (neck), ○ (facial). (From Fritsch and Hitzig, 1870, figure 2.)

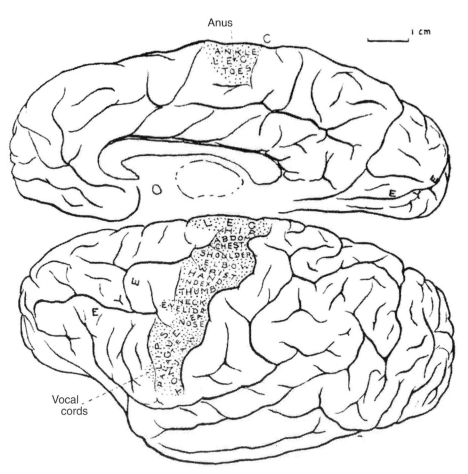

Fig. 31.2. Medial (above) and lateral view of the cortical surface of the brain of the gorilla. Points along the precentral gyrus where stimulation was applied are indicated by dots. The body parts in which movements were elicited following localized stimulation are also shown. (From Leyton and Sherrington, 1917, figure 10.)

of cortical stimulation in a human is to be found in an account by a Dr Bartholow of the Medical College of Ohio (Bartholow, 1874). He describes inserting a needle electrode into the parietal lobe of a patient through a defect in the skull. When current was passed through the electrode, movements were elicited on the opposite side of the body as well as pain and other sensations. Since these pioneering studies, we have gained a much clearer concept as to how the frontal lobes relate to the control of voluntary movement through the use of a variety of investigational techniques.

Investigating the functional properties of motor areas

The are a wide variety of methods that can be used to examine the functional properties of the different motor areas. As already mentioned, most of the earlier data came from electrical stimulation and lesion studies in animals, and from the observation of human subjects with brain lesions following trauma or stroke. After the introduction of extracellular neuronal recording in awake monkeys by Jasper (Ricci et al., 1957) it became possible to more precisely relate dynamic neural activity to aspects of motor behaviour. More recently, the use of functional imaging techniques (Ugurbil et al., 1999), such as positron emission tomography (PET) and functional magnetic resonance imaging (fMRI), and other approaches such as transcranial magnetic stimulation (Hallett, 2000) has made it possible to study motor areas in the normal human brain in a relatively non-invasive way and at high spatial resolution. The techniques that may be used in the investigation of motor function differ as regards spatial resolution, temporal resolution, and invasiveness and

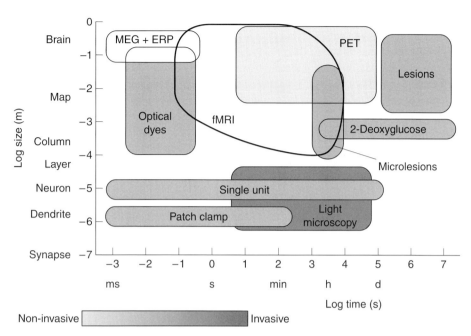

Fig. 31.3. The spatial resolution, temporal resolution, and invasiveness of different experimental techniques used to study the brain. Abbreviations: MEG, magnetoencephalography; ERP, event related potentials; fMRI, functional magnetic resonance imaging; and PET, positron emission tomography. (From Cohen and Bookheimer, 1994, figure 4.)

consequently provide very different types of information (see Fig. 31.3).

Motor cortex and other cortical motor areas

The results of early stimulation studies suggested that the motor portion of the frontal lobe was coextensive with the precentral gyrus, defined cytoarchitectonically as Brodmann area (BA) 4. However with the passage of time it became clear that this narrow view of what constituted 'motor cortex' was not consistent with data from lesion studies (Fulton, 1935) or stimulation experiments in both humans (Penfield & Welch, 1949) and monkeys (Woolsey et al., 1952). We now recognize that the cortical motor areas include both BA 4 and 6. The motor cortex proper or primary motor cortex is in area 4, while several distinct premotor areas, both functionally and anatomically, are located in area 6 (Geyer et al., 2000).

Motor cortex

The motor cortex in BA 4 is designated 'primary' because (i) historically it had been regarded as the only motor area, (ii) its neurons have the most direct and prominent connection to motor neurons in the spinal cord via the corti-cospinal tract, (iii) it is particularly important for the control of hand and finger movement, and (iv) lesions of this area or its projections frequently result in the most severe motor deficits.

A central question in motor physiology has been whether the motor cortex controls movement by specifying the activation of individual muscles or is primarily involved at a 'higher' level such as the control of whole movements or movement parameters like direction, force, velocity, acceleration etc? This issue of the 'representation' of movement within the motor cortex has been addressed using a variety of different approaches.

Clinical observation

Before the experimental studies of cortical stimulation of Frisch and Hitzig in the dog and Ferrier in the monkey, the neurologist John Hughlings Jackson in 1864 put forward an hypothesis about the cortical representation of movements based on his clinical observations in patients with stroke or convulsions (Jackson, 1864). He noted that, in patients with stroke, or other lesions of the cortex, the main deficit was an inability to perform certain movements rather than weakness in specific muscles and that, even with large lesions, many movements remained intact. There were several components to his hypothesis. He believed that the neural mechanisms of sensorimotor processes, rather than muscles were represented in the motor cortex: 'The nervous centres represent movements not muscles; cords not notes'. He also believed that all the movements of which an individual is capable are represented in the motor cortex. A direct extension of this is that the hand, for example, a body part capable of a great variety of movements will be more widely 'represented' within the motor cortex, than the leg or the trunk. Jackson conceived of a pattern of overlapping representations of body parts within the motor cortex, the extent of any representation being determined by the repertoire of movements a particular body part possessed.

Cortical stimulation

The first direct approach to the issue of representation as conceived by Jackson was through experiments using cortical stimulation, in which electrical stimulation was applied to the cerebral cortex and movements of limbs, joints, and muscles were observed (Penfield & Rasmussen, 1950). These studies showed that the principal body parts were represented separately though not equally, and that the order of this arrangement conformed in a general way to the body surface (somatotopy). However, these studies did not show how movements were represented, merely, that body parts were organized in an orderly way on the cortical surface and that there were direct excitatory connections between the motor cortex and motoneurons in the spinal cord.

Neural recording

The most detailed information to date about the representation of movement has come from neural recording from cells in the motor cortex of subhuman primates during the performance of movement under controlled conditions. Particular attention has been paid to whether the motor cortex plans and codes for movement in spatial terms such as direction and amplitude. In one experiment monkeys were trained to make arm movements from a central starting point to one of eight targets evenly spaced on a circle. During this task a large proportion of cells in the motor cortex were 'tuned' to the direction of movement (Fig. 31.4). Such cells had a preferred direction of movement in which the activity of the cell was highest and the activity decreased progressively as one deviated further from this direction. The interesting question is how cells in the motor cortex with these properties indicate or 'code' the direction of limb movement. Georgopoulos and colleagues (Georgopoulos et al., 1983) proposed, and subsequently demonstrated, that the coding of direction is actually done by a population of cells though the construction of a population vector which predicts the direction of an upcoming arm movement. The concept of the population vector is that for any movement each cell in the motor cortex which is directionally tuned, makes a contribution in its preferred direction, and the magnitude of this contribution is proportional to the angle between its preferred direction and the actual direction of movement. Figure 31.5 (see colour plate section) illustrates this concept for movement in one direction.

These and similar experiments (Alexander & Crutcher, 1990; Ashe & Georgopoulos, 1994; Kakei et al., 1999) suggest that the motor cortex represents movement in terms of the direction of the limb in space rather than on the basis of the activation of individual muscles. This raises the issue of how and at what level the activation of specific muscles, essential for goal directed movement, is achieved. It is likely that during infancy we learn the mapping between the spatial aspects of limb movements and the muscles that need to be activated for those movements to occur. Thereafter, spatial instructions from the motor cortex will automatically activate the appropriate muscles to execute the movement. Recent data which supports this intuitive conclusion comes from experiments in human subjects who were asked to make movements to targets in the presence of a complicated force field opposing the movement (Shadmehr & Mussa-Ivaldi, 1994). At first the movement trajectories were quite disrupted by the force field (Fig. 31.6(a)). However, over time, the movement trajectories reverted to those before the force field was imposed (Fig. 31.6(b)). The fact that the subjects adapted to the force field and produced smooth straight trajectories although they had received little instruction as to what movements to make suggests that movement is planned in terms of trajectory. To probe exactly how this adaptation was achieved, the force field was suddenly withdrawn (Fig. 31.6(c)). Subjects now produced movements with abnormal trajectories (almost the mirror image of the original perturbation) as if they were compensating for the forces they expected to experience. Therefore it is likely that the subjects built an 'internal model' of the forces which mapped the signals being produced by the motor cortex onto the forces being generated by the muscles. Whether one sees a reflection of this internal model in the activity of cells in the motor cortex during motor learning is currently being investigated in a number of laboratories (Gandolfo et al., 2000; Li et al., 2001). What is clear is that one does not see such activity once behaviours have been mastered.

If there is little evidence of a translation of a spatial signal to one indicating muscle activation in the motor cortex then where does this necessary transformation occur? Bizzi and colleagues (Bizzi et al., 1991; Gistzer et al., 1993; Tresch & Bizzi, 1999) have shown in experiments in the frog and rat

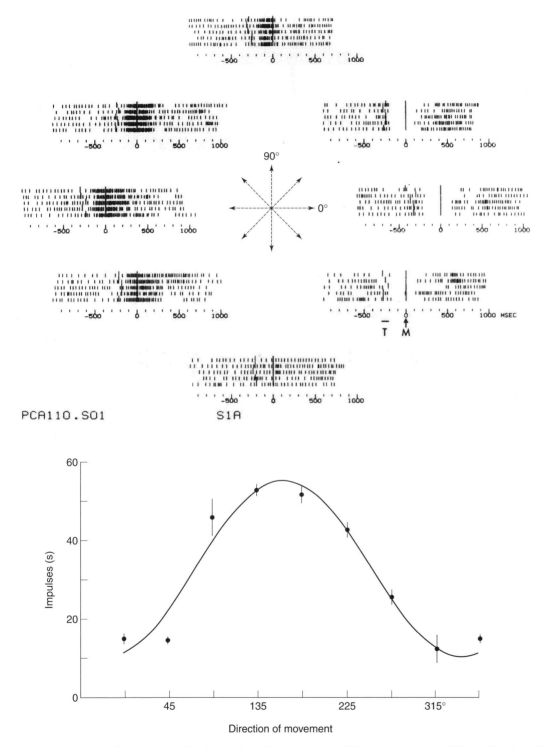

PCA110.SO1   S1A

Fig. 31.4. Variation in the frequency of discharge of a single motor cortex cell during movement in different directions. *Upper half,* Each small tick indicates an action potential; the display shows impulse activity during five repetitions (trials) of movements made in each of the eight directions indicated in the centre diagram. Trials are oriented to the onset of movement *M. Lower half,* Direction tuning curve of the same cell; the average frequency of cell activity during the response time and movement time is plotted for each of the eight directions. (From Georgopoulos et al., 1982, figure 4.)

(a)

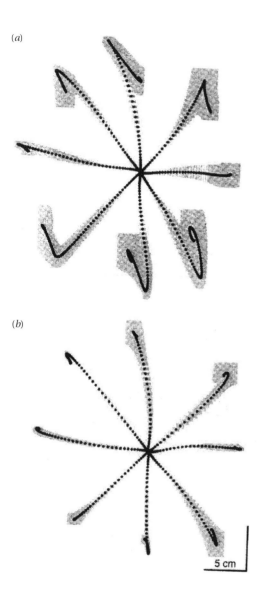

(b)

(c)

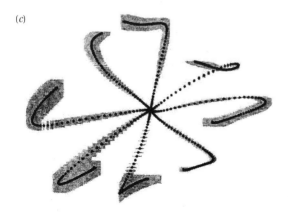

Fig. 31.6. Averages ± SD of hand trajectories during (a) the initial exposure to the force field, (b) following adaptation to the field and (c) after the force field was abruptly withdrawn toward the end of the training period. (From Shadmehr and Mussa-Ivaldi, 1994, modified from figures 9 and 13.)

that a set of 'motor primitives', which could form the basis of activating specific sets of muscles during multijoint movement, can be elicited through microsimulation of the spinal grey matter. These primitives may form the building blocks for voluntary movement by translating spatial signals from the motor cortex into appropriate muscle output. In addition, other spinal interneuronal systems such as the propriospinal system in the cat (Lundberg, 1979) have been shown to be important in the patterned activation of the different muscles required for reaching. Propriospinal neurons at the C3–C4 level in the cat have monosynaptic connections to motoneurons supplying proximal muscles. These propriospinal neurons, in turn, have monosynaptic connections to several supraspinal systems, including the corticospinal tract. Interruption of the projections from the interneurons results in abnormal reaching movements (Alstermark et al., 1981). These propriospinal interneurons may participate in the integration of reaching movements at a spinal level, and effectively translate signals from cells in the motor cortex that relate to the direction of force output of the whole limb (Georgopoulos et al., 1982) into appropriate patterns of muscle activation.

The premotor cortex

If the motor cortex is the most important area for the control of voluntary movement this inevitably raises the issue of the function of the other motor areas in the frontal lobe: the premotor areas (see Fig. 31.7). The functional division between the motor cortex and the other frontal motor areas is not strict nor is there the rigid hierarchy among them that had been previously thought (see Geyer et al., 2000). The motor cortex and premotor areas operate in parallel in the production of movement. Differences in the functional properties among these areas are relative rather than absolute.

Lateral premotor cortex

There are at least two distinct subareas within the lateral premotor cortex in humans: the dorsal (PMD) and ventral (PMV) premotor cortex, and there may be even more based on evidence from subhuman primates (Geyer et al., 2000). There has been a great deal of controversy about the consequences of lesions of the human lateral premotor area. Earlier workers noted a loss of skilled movements, forced grasping, and spasticity, similar to those deficits seen with motor cortex lesions (Fulton, 1935); while others documented few if any adverse effects of lesions (Walshe, 1935). One consistent finding in humans has been prominent weakness in proximal muscles which led to the suggestion that an important function of the lateral premotor cortex was to place the limb in a position appropriate for action. More detailed work from neural recording in non human primates has pinpointed some clear functional divisions between the two major portions of lateral premotor cortex.

Neurons in the PMV can have both tactile and visual receptive fields (Rizzolatti et al., 1988; Graziano & Gross, 1998). The interesting feature, however, is that the visual receptive fields move with the arm and not with the eyes (Graziano & Gross, 1998). This feature enables the integration of somatosensory, visual and motor information and provides the substrate for the online visual guidance of movement which is now thought to be a prominent function of the PMV. Cells in the PMD show many of the same features as those in the motor cortex such as directional properties (Caminiti et al., 1990). This area may also be the site of the final step in the transformation of visual signals, which are initially coded in retinal coordinates, to a coordinate framework based on the arm (Johnson et al., 1996). The most compelling theory of PMD function is that it is involved in stimulus–response mapping. Neurons in this area integrate information about the properties of the stimulus, including its spatial location, with the attentional state of the subject, and the action or response required, so that we can more effectively interact with our environment.

Medial premotor areas

The medial premotor region contains both the supplementary motor area (SMA) and the cingulate motor areas. The SMA is further subdivided into two regions which are functionally and anatomically distinct, the SMA proper and the pre-SMA which is just anterior to it (Tanji, 1994). The cingulate motor areas in the human may contain up to three separate functional regions (Picard & Strick, 1996).

SMA

Data from subjects with lesions involving the SMA or medial premotor cortex have suggested that an important function of the SMA is in the temporal organization of sequences of movements, particularly when these sequences are produced from memory (Goldberg & Bruce, 1985; Halsband et al., 1993). For example, following a stroke in the medial premotor cortex a concert pianist was no longer able to make transitions smoothly from one note to the next or maintain the relative timing values of the notes although the actual spatial sequence was correct (Foerster,

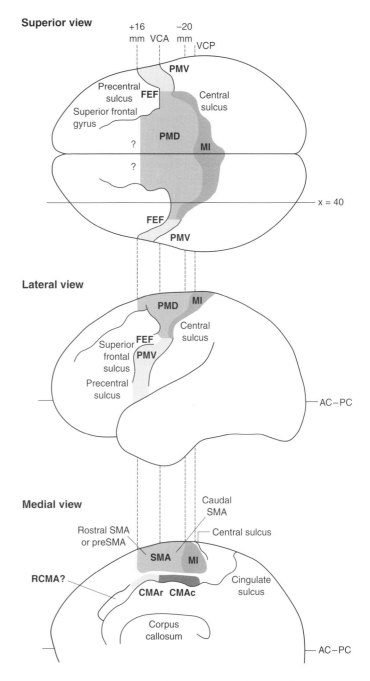

Fig. 31.7. Schematic diagrams of the proposed subdivisions of the cortical motor areas in humans from three different perspectives. AC-PC, anterior commisure–posterior commisure plane; CMAc, caudal cingulate motor area; CMAr, rostral cingulate motor area; FEF, frontal eye fields; M1, primary motor cortex; PMD, dorsal premotor cortex; PMV, ventral premotor cortex; RCMA, rostral anterior cingulate motor area; SMA, supplementary motor areas; VCA and VCP, coronal plane through the anterior and posterior commisure, respectively; *x* = 40, 40 mm from midline. (Adapted from Roland and Zilles, 1996, figure 1.)

1936). The Russian psychologist Luria noted that, although the ability to perform simple movements was preserved following lesions of the medial premotor cortex, there were impairments in complex sequences of movements, particularly when such movements had to be learned (Luria, 1966). In addition, the medial motor areas are involved in the control of bimanual movements; there is strong evidence for this, both from neural recording in monkeys and imaging in humans. The SMA has been subdivided on functional and anatomical grounds into the SMA proper, which has prominent connections to the motor cortex and projections to the spinal cord, and the preSMA which is more closely connected to the prefrontal cortex (Tanji, 1994). PreSMA is more active while learning novel motor behaviours, whereas SMA is prominently involved during the performance of previously learned sequential behaviours. The reports of akinetic mutism following medial premotor lesions in humans are almost certainly due to the involvement of the far anterior portions of the cingulate gyrus which do not have a prominent motor function.

Cingulate motor areas

Three distinct subregions have been defined within the cingulate motor area; all of which are buried in the cingulate sulcus (Picard & Strick, 1996). These comprise a rostral anterior cingulate motor area (RCMA) and two more posterior areas (see Fig. 31.7) divided into cingulate motor area rostral (CMAr) and caudal (CMAc). The RCMA has functions which appear little related to the control of action but is engaged in such operations as spatial attention, working memory, semantic and episodic memory (see Cabeza & Nyberg, 1997) and the online monitoring of performance (Carter et al., 1998). Nevertheless, there are direct projections from the cingulate motor areas to the spinal cord (Dum & Strick, 1991) and in the case of the more posterior areas a substantial number of the neurons project to motoneurons supplying the distal muscles of the upper limb (Dum & Strick, 1991; He et al., 1995). Therefore, these areas, like the motor cortex, may be involved in the control of distal movements. However, the specific function of the cingulate motor area is unclear. In imaging studies of the whole brain, activity within the most posterior cingulate motor areas seems to parallel that within the SMA. There have been few lesion studies restricted to this region, and comprehensive neural recordings have not been performed.

Motor deficits following stroke in humans

The constellation of motor symptoms resulting from stroke in humans seem to be primarily related to damage to the motor cortex or to its subcortical projection fibres (see Rondot, 1969; Rascol et al., 1982; Foix & Levy, 1927; Mohr et al., 1993). Given that vascular lesions generally do not respect cytoarchitectonic boundaries in the brain such statements are approximate at best. While it is not our purpose to treat the various stoke syndromes in any great depth, we can recognise two general types which primarily affect the motor system. The first is the result of infarction of the middle cerebral artery (MCA) or one of its principal branches, the second, the typical lacune, due to small vessel disease in or around the internal capsule.

MCA

Infarction of the main trunk of the MCA often leads to quite a profound deficit with contralateral hemiplegia, hemianesthesia and hemianopia in addition to deviation of the eyes and head toward the lesion. Lesser degrees of infarction such as from occlusion of the upper division of the MCA lead primarily to contralateral motor and sensory deficits which are less severe. There is some controversy as to the expected distribution of weakness in these cases. It has been generally held that the most severe weakness was in the distal arm and lower face and leg in keeping with the principles outlined by Broadbent in the nineteenth century (Broadbent, 1872) and consistent with the areal somatotopic distribution of these body parts on the precentral gyrus. However, this view has been recently challenged particularly by Mohr (Mohr et al., 1993) who maintains that usually proximal and distal movements are equally affected. Monoplegias are extremely rare and when present almost invariably indicate a cortical lesion.

Lacunes

Stroke due to small vessel ischemia in and around the internal capsule is perhaps the most common form of stroke seen clinically. The deficits associated with up to 70% of lacunar strokes are predominantly motor in character and have often been described as representing a form of pure motor stroke (Fisher & Curry, 1965; Rascol et al., 1982). However, it is pure only to the extent that there are not significant deficits in sensation, behaviour, language or vision. Although sensory symptoms may be frequent objective signs are rare. Face, arm and leg are generally equally affected. It has been commonly held that there was a fairly strict somatotopic distribution within the internal capsule. The results of studies correlating radiological lesions with deficits in humans would suggest that this is not the case.

Clinical–physiological interpretation

One of the more striking aspects of the deficits in patients following stroke is that, even in cases in which there is not profound weakness, there is poverty of movement. This seems to fit well with the concept of Jackson that the motor cortex is primarily concerned with movements rather than with muscles; when this representation is disrupted it is the movements rather than the muscles which are affected. The relative lack of correlation between weakness and the general impairment of motor function in patients with stroke has led neurologists to search for other causes. The standard explanation for this lack of correlation is that the motor impairment is primarily related to spasticity (Mizrahi & Angel, 1979; Dietz et al., 1991). Nevertheless, the weight of clinical evidence (Sahrmann & Norton, 1977), in addition to what we currently know about the physiology of motor control, would seem to go against this thesis. Obviously, extreme spasticity can further disrupt the ability to move but numerous studies have failed to find a quantitative relation between the extent of spasticity and the motor deficits.

Recovery of motor function following stroke

Some recovery of motor function is the rule after stroke. The extent and time course of recovery is quite variable and dependent on a host of factors which are not well understood (Twitchell, 1951; Bard & Hirschberg, 1965; Seitz, 1997). The natural history of the recovery from stroke has received less attention than it might have given the social and economic cost of the disorder. Recovery when it does occur generally begins early and is evident first in the proximal muscles (Twitchell, 1951). Patients who make a full recovery do so within the first month and it is not usual to find much additional improvement more than six months after the original stroke. There is controversy as to what constitute reliable prognostic indicators for motor recovery following stroke but prominent spasticity and a long interval from the onset of deficit to the first sign of recovery are not good signs. When recovery does occur, it is invariably associated with cortical reorganization.

Cortical reorganization is a well-described phenomenon following injury. It has been documented in animals following damage to, or disruption of, sensory input (Merzenich et al., 1983) and has been shown to occur in motor cortical areas of non-human primates after amputation, section of motor nerves (Donoghue & Sanes, 1988), or as a result of micro-infarction to adjacent areas of cortex (Nudo et al., 1996; Nudo & Milliken, 1996). Glees and Cole

(1950, 1952) were the first to study reorganization in the motor system under controlled conditions. Following experimentally induced lesions of the motor cortex in the monkey, they found, on the basis of cortical stimulation, evidence of reorganization both in areas surrounding the cortical lesion (1950) and also in homologous regions in the other hemisphere (1952). The issue was re-examined more recently by Nudo and colleagues (Nudo et al., 1996; Nudo & Milliken, 1996) who showed that loss of hand and wrist representation after micro-infarcts in the motor cortex of the monkey was restored through reorganization following rehabilitation (Nudo et al., 1996, Fig. 31.8, see colour plate section). Without rehabilitation, although there was reorganization in the motor cortex, the representations in the areas damaged by infarction were not restored. Clearly, restoration of function is not dependent on motor cortex reorganization *per se* and presumably can be mediated by other cortical areas.

Functional imaging studies in humans following stroke have confirmed the suggestion of Glees and Cole (1952) that recovery of function is associated with a re-organization involving lateral premotor areas ipsilateral to the infarct and the motor cortex contralateral to the infarct (Chollet et al., 1991; Weiller et al., 1992; Cramer et al., 1997). Whereas there appears to be abundant data (Brodal, 1972; Kim et al., 1993) to support a role for the motor cortex (contralateral to the lesion) ipsilateral to the motor deficit in the control of movement and consequently its involvement in recovery of function, the evidence for significant reorganization in lateral premotor areas contributing to recovery is not nearly as strong. Recent data (Lewis et al., 1999) suggest that the medial premotor areas, which have prominent corticospinal projections, may make the largest contribution to recovery of function.

Effects of rehabilitation

Studies in normal subjects have shown that cortical motor areas can undergo reorganization on the basis of different patterns of limb or finger use. For example, there is an increased representation of left-hand digits in the motor cortex of string players and the extent of this increase is correlated with the age at which the subjects began to play the instrument (Elbert et al., 1995). The potential for use-dependent changes in cortical representation within the sensory motor system has obvious implications for rehabilitation in patients following stroke. Although spontaneous reorganization of the cortex does occur after experimentally induced cortical stroke in primates (Nudo & Milliken, 1996), this reorganization does not result in restored movement capacity unless accompanied by specific rehabilitation (Nudo et al., 1996). The technique of constraint-induced movement therapy (or 'forced use'), in which the unaffected limb is restrained in a sling and the impaired one is trained in a series of motor tasks over a two week period, has been shown to lead to long-lasting improvement in function in patients with chronic stroke (Taub et al., 1993; Miltner et al., 1999), and is associated with concomitant changes in cortical excitability (Liepert et al., 2000). The encouraging preliminary results with the technique in both humans and subhuman primates offer hope that it will provide an efficacious form of rehabilitation of motor function in stroke patients when used on a larger scale.

The future: neural signals to control prosthetic devices

One of the more exciting developments for the future is that it may be possible to apply what has been learned about the neural control of movement to enable the use of signals from the intact motor cortex to control prosthetic devices. An even more ambitious project would be the use of neural signals to directly drive muscles, which would clearly be beneficial in patients with spinal cord injury and in a subgroup of patients following stroke.

The idea behind such a development is a relatively simple one and is based on a concept already discussed above: that many cells in the motor cortex are directionally tuned (Georgopoulos et al., 1982) and that a population of such cells can be used to predict the upcoming motor output under a variety of conditions (Georgopoulos et al., 1983, 1986). The issue is how one transforms such neural signals into a coordinated contraction of limb muscles to generate an appropriate motor output (Lukashin et al., 1996; Amirikian & Georgopoulos, 1999). This transformation can be carried out by an artificial neural network, using actual neural signals as an input, which it then recoded as graded muscle activation. For example, Fig. 31.9 shows neural data which were recorded while a monkey exerted force in a particular direction; these data were then used to instruct a model arm to produce the same behaviour.

Other recent experiments suggest that the goal of a neurally driven device is a realistic goal for the future. Chapin and colleagues have sampled neural signals in the cortex and thalamus of the rat and used them to control a relatively simple one-dimensional robot arm (Chapin et al., 1999). While the behaviour used in the experiment was relatively trivial compared to what might be required in real life, the authors also demonstrated that the animal could learn different strategies to control the neurons responsible for the movement of the robot arm. Such plasticity between neural activity in motor cortex and behaviour makes it more likely that patients could eventually learn to control prosthetic devices or even their own muscles. More recently, this work was expanded and extended to the monkey (Wessberg et al., 2000). Neural signals obtained from chronically implanted microwire electrodes in several cortical motor areas were used to predict hand trajectories in three dimensions, and more importantly, could be employed to control a robotic arm in real time. These approaches needs further modification and refinement so that they can be useful for application in humans. The work cited is best regarded as a promising start rather than a final solution.

Acknowledgements

This work was supported in part by a Merit Review Award from the Department of Veterans Affairs, the Brain Sciences chair, and by NIH grants NS32437 and NS17413.

References

Alexander, G.E. & Crutcher, M.D. (1990). Preparation for movement: neural representations of intended direction in three motor areas of the monkey. *J. Neurophysiol.*, **64**, 133–49.

Alstermark, B., Lundberg, A., Norrsell, U. & Sybirska, E. (1981). Integration in descending motor pathways controlling the forelimb in the cat. Differential behavioral defects after spinal cord lesions interrupting defined pathways from higher centers to motoneurons. *Exp. Brain Res.*, **42**, 290–318.

Amirikian, B. & Georgopoulos, A.P. (1999). Cortical populations and behaviour: Hebb's thread. *Can. J. Exp. Psychol.*, **53**, 21–34.

Ashe, J. & Georgopoulos, A.P. (1994). Movement parameters and neuronal activity in motor cortex and area 5. *Cereb. Cortex*, **6**, 590–600.

Bard, G. & Hirschberg, G. (1965). Recovery of voluntary motion in upper extremity following hemiplegia. *Arch. Phys. Med. Rehabil.*, **46**, 567–72.

Bartholow, R. (1874). Experimental investigations into the functions of the human brain. *Am. J. Med. Sci.*, **CXXXIV**, 305–13.

Bizzi, E., Mussa-Ivaldi, F.A. & Giszter, S. (1991). Computations underlying the execution of movement: a biological perspective. *Science*, **253**, 287–91.

Broadbent, W. (1872). On the cerebral mechanism of speech and thought. *Trans. R. Med. Chir. Soc. (Lond.)*, 145.

Brodal, A. (1972). Cerebrocerebellar pathways anatomical data and some functional implications. *Acta Neurol. Scand.*, **48**, 153–95.

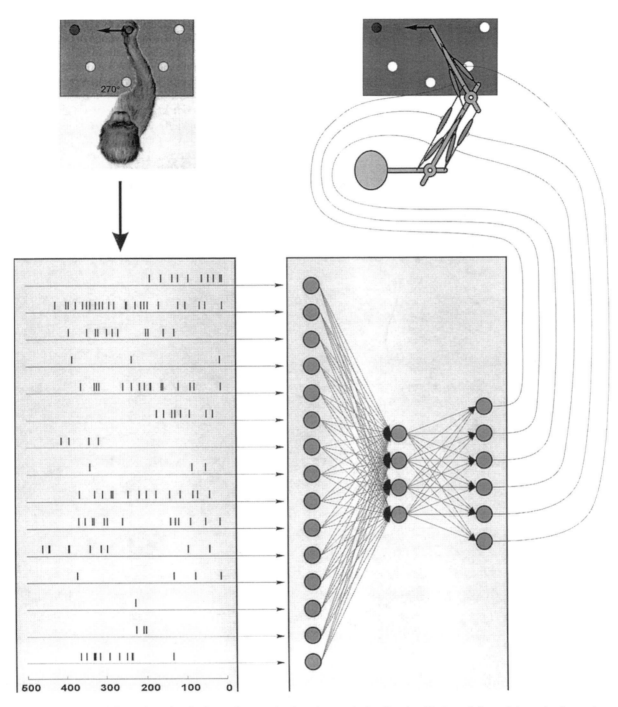

Fig. 31.9. The upper left panel is a sketch of a monkey exerting force in a particular direction. The lower left panel shows the time series of action potentials in 15 separate cells in the motor cortex during the task. The lower right illustrates the three-layered feed forward neural network used to transform the signal and the upper right shows the performance of a model of the arm on the basis of the transformed signals. (From Amirikian and Georgopoulos, 1999, figure 8.)

Cabeza, R. & Nyberg, L. (1997). Imaging cognition – an empiral review of PET studies with normal subjects. *J. Cogn. Neurosci.*, **9**, 1–26.

Caminiti, R., Johnson, P.B. & Urbano, A. (1990). Making arm movements within different parts of space: dynamic aspects in the primate motor cortex. *J. Neurosci.*, **10**, 2039–58.

Carter, C.S., Braver, T.S., Barch, D.M., Botvinick, M.M., Noll, D. & Cohen, J.D. (1998). Anterior cingulate cortex, error detection, and the online monitoring of performance. *Science*, **280**, 747–9.

Chapin, J.K., Moxon, K.A., Markowitz, R.S. & Nicolelis, M.A. (1999). Real-time control of a robot arm using simultaneously recorded neurons in the motor cortex. *Nat. Neurosci.*, **2**, 664–70.

Chollet, F., DiPiero, V., Wise, R.J.S., Brooks, D.J., Dolan, R.J. & Frackowiak, R.S.J. (1991). The functional anatomy of motor recovery after stroke in humans: a study with positron emission tomography. *Ann. Neurol.*, **29**, 63–71.

Cohen, M.S. & Bookheimer, S.Y. (1994). Localization of brain function using magnetic resonance imaging. *Trends Neurosci.*, **17**, 268–77.

Cramer, S.C., Nelles, G., Benson, R.R. et al. (1997). A functional MRI study of subjects recovered from hemiparetic stroke. *Stroke*, **28**, 2518–27.

Dietz, V., Trippel, M. & Berger, W. (1991). Reflex activity and muscle tone during elbow movements in patients with spastic paresis. *Ann. Neurol.*, **30**, 767–79.

Donoghue, J.P. & Sanes, J.N. (1988). Organization of adult motor cortex representation patterns following neonatal forelimb nerve injury in rats. *J. Neurosci.*, **8**, 3221–32.

Dum, R.P. & Strick, P.L. (1991). The origin of corticospinal projections from the premotor areas in the frontal lobe. *J. Neurosci.*, **11**, 667–89.

Elbert, T., Pantev, C., Wienbruch, C., Rockstroh, B. & Taub, E. (1995). Increased cortical representation of the fingers of the left hand in string players. *Science*, **270**, 305–7.

Ferrier, D. (1875). Experiments in the brain of monkeys. *Proc. R. Soc. Lond. (Biol.)*, **23**, 409–30.

Fisher, C. & Curry, H. (1965). Pure motor hemiplegia of vascular origin. *Arch. Neurol.*, **13**, 30–44.

Flor, H., Elbert, T., Knecht, S. et al. (1995). Phantom-limb pain as a perceptual correlate of cortical reorganization following arm amputation. *Nature*, **375**, 482–4.

Foerster, O. (1936). Motorische felder und bahnen. In *Handbuch der Neurologie*, ed. O. Bumke & O. Foerster, pp. 1–357. Berlin: Springer.

Foix, C. & Levy, M. (1927). Les ramollissements sylviens. *Rev. Neurol. (Paris)*, 11–51.

Fritsch, G. & Hitzig, E. (1870). Ueber die elektrische Erregbarkeit des Grosshirns. *Arch. Anat. Physiol. Wis. Med.*, **37**, 300–32.

Fulton, J.F. (1935). A note on the definition of 'motor' and 'premotor' areas. *Brain*, **58**, 311–16.

Gandolfo, C., Li, R., Benda, B., Schioppa, C. & Bizzi, E. (2000). Cortical correlates of learning in monkeys adapting to a new dynamical environment. *Neurobiology*, **97**, 2259–63.

Georgopoulos, A.P., Kalaska, J.F., Caminiti, R. & Massey, J.T. (1982). On the relations between the direction of two-dimensional arm movements and cell discharge in primate motor cortex. *J. Neurosci.*, **2**, 1527–37.

Georgopoulos, A.P., Caminiti, R., Kalaska, J.F. & Massey, J.T. (1983). Spatial coding of movement: a hypothesis concerning the coding of movement direction by motor cortical populations. *Exp. Brain Res.*, Suppl. **7**, 327–36.

Georgopoulos, A.P., Schwartz, A.B. & Kettner, R.E. (1986). Neuronal population coding of movement direction. *Science*, **233**, 1416–19.

Geyer, S., Schormann, T., Mohlberg, H. & Zilles, K. (2000). Areas 3a, 3b, and 1 of human primary somatosensory cortex. Part 2. Spatial normalization to standard anatomical space. *Neuroimage*, **11**, 684–96.

Giszter, S.F., Mussa-Ivaldi, F.A. & Bizzi, E. (1993). Convergent force fields organized in the frog's spinal cord. *J. Neurosci.*, **13**, 467–91.

Glees, P. & Cole, J. (1950). Recovery of skilled motor functions after small repeated lesions of motor cortex in macaque. *J. Neurophysiol.*, **13**, 137–48.

Glees, P. & Cole, J. (1952). Ipsilateral representation in the motor cortex: its significance in relation to motor function. *Lancet*, **i**, 1191–2.

Goldberg, M.E. & Bruce, C.J. (1985). Cerebral cortical activity associated with the orientation of visual attention in the rhesus monkey. *Vision Res.*, **25**, 471–81

Graziano, M.S. & Gross, C.G. (1998). Spatial maps for the control of movement. *Curr. Opin. Neurobiol.*, **8**, 195–201.

Hallett, M. (2000). Transcranial magnetic stimulation and the human brain. *Nature*, **406**, 147–50.

Halsband, U., Ito, N., Tanji, J. & Freund, H.J. (1993). The role of premotor cortex and the supplementary motor area in the temporal control of movement in man. *Brain*, **116**, 243–66.

He, S.Q., Dum, R.P. & Strick, P.L. (1995). Topographic organization of corticospinal projections from the frontal lobe: motor areas on the medial surface of the hemisphere. *J. Neurosci.*, **15**, 3284–306.

Jackson, J.H. (1864). Loss of Speech. In *Clinical Lectures and Reports of the London Hospital*, vol. 1, p. 459.

Johnson, P.B., Ferraina, S., Bianchi, L. & Caminiti, R. (1996). Cortical networks for visual reaching: physiological and anatomical organization of frontal and parietal lobe arm regions. *Cereb. Cortex*, **6**, 102–19.

Kakei, S., Hoffman, D.S. & Strick, P.L. (1999). Muscle and movement representations in the primary motor cortex. *Science*, **285**, 2136–9.

Kim, S.G. & Ugurbil, K. (1997). Functional magnetic resonance imaging of the human brain. *J. Neurosci. Meth.*, **74**, 229–43.

Kim, S-G., Ashe, J., Hendrich, K. et al. (1993). Motor cortex, hemispheric asymmetry, and handedness. *Science*, **261**, 615–17.

Lewis, S., Dassonville, P., Zhu, X-H., Kim, S-G., Ugurbil, K. & Ashe, J. (1999). Functional reorganization within cortical motor areas associated with recovery of motor function following stroke. *Soc. Neurosci. Abstr.*, **25**, 384.

Leyton, A.S.F. & Sherrington, C.S. (1917). Observations on the excitable cortex of the chimpanzee, orang-utan and gorilla. *Q. J. Exp. Physiol.*, **11**, 135–222.

Li, C-S.R., Padoa-Schioppa, C. & Bizzi, E. (2001). Neuronal correlates of motor performance and motor learning in the primary motor cortex of monkeys adapting to an external force field. *Neuron*, **30**, 593–607.

Liepert, J., Bauder, H., Wolfgang, H.R., Miltner, W.H., Taub, E. & Weiller, C. (2000). Treatment-induced cortical reorganization after stroke in humans. *Stroke*, **31**, 1210–16.

Lukashin, A.V., Amirikian, B.R. & Georgopoulos, A.P. (1996). A simulated actuator driven by motor cortical signals. *Neuroreport*, **7**, 2597–601.

Lundberg, A. (1979). Integration in a propriospinal motor centre controlling the forelimb in the cat. *Igaku Shoin, Tokyo*, 47–64.

Luria, A. (1966). *Higher Cortical Functions in Man*. New York: Basic Books .

Merzenich, M.M., Kaas, J.H., Wall, J., Nelson, R.J., Sur, M. & Felleman, D. (1983). Topographic reorganization of somatosensory cortical areas 3b and 1 in adult monkeys following restricted deafferentation. *Neuroscience*, **8**, 33–55.

Miltner, W.H., Braun, C., Arnold, M., Witte, H. & Taub, E. (1999). Coherence of gamma-band EEG activity as a basis for associative learning. *Nature*, **397**, 434–6.

Mizrahi, E.M. & Angel, R.W. (1979). Impairment of voluntary movement by spasticity. *Ann. Neurol.*, **5**, 594–5.

Mohr, J.P., Foulkes, M.A., Polis, A.T. et al. (1993). Infarct topography and hemiparesis profiles with cerebral convexity infarction: the Stroke Data Bank. *J. Neurol. Neurosurg. Psychiatry*, **56**, 344–51.

Nudo, R.J. & Milliken, G.W. (1996). Reorganization of movement representations in primary motor cortex following focal ischemic infarcts in adult squirrel monkeys. *J. Neurophysiol.*, **75**, 2144–9.

Nudo, R.J., Wise, B.M., SiFuentes, F. & Milliken, G.W. (1996). Neural substrates for the effects of rehabilitative training on motor recovery after ischemic infarct. *Science*, **272**, 1791–4.

Penfield, W. & Rasmussen, T. (1950). *The Cerebral Cortex of Man*. New York: MacMillan.

Penfield, W. & Welch, K. (1949). The supplementary motor area in the cerebral cortex of man. *Trans. Am. Neurol. Assoc.*, **74**, 179–84.

Picard, N. & Strick. P.L. (1996). Motor areas of the medial wall: a review of their location and functional activation. *Cereb. Cortex*, **6**, 342–53.

Randot, P. (1969). Syndromes of central motor disorder. *Handbook of Clinical Neurology*, vol. **1**, p. 169.

Rascol, A., Montastruc, J.L., Guiraud-Chaumeil, B. & Clanet, M. (1982). Bromocriptine as the 1st treatment of Parkinson's disease. Long term results. *Rev. Neurol.*, **138**, 401–8.

Ricci, G., Doane, B. & Jasper, H. (1957). Microelectrode studies of conditioning. In *Premier Congres International des Science Neurologiques*. Bruxelles: Snoeck-Ducaju.

Rizzolatti, G., Camarda, R., Fogassi, L., Gentilucci, M., Luppino, G. & Matelli, M. (1988). Functional organization of inferior area 6 in the macaque monkey. II. Area F5 and the control of distal movements. *Exp. Brain Res.*, **71**, 491–507.

Rondot, P. (1969). Syndromes of central motor disorder. In *Handbook of Clinical Neurology*, ed. P.J. Vinken & G.W. Bruyn, pp. 169–217. Amsterdam: North-Holland.

Sahrmann, S.A. & Norton, B.J. (1977). The relationship of voluntary movement to spasticity in the upper motor neuron syndrome. *Ann. Neurol.*, **2**, 460–5.

Seitz, R.J. (1997). Recovery of executive motor functions. In *Handbook of Neuropsychology*, ed. F. Boller & J. Grafman, pp. 185–207. New York: Elsevier.

Shadmehr, R. & Mussa-Ivaldi, F.A. (1994). Adaptive representation of dynamics during learning of a motor task. *J. Neurosci.*, **14**, 3208–24.

Tanji, J. (1994). The supplementary motor area in the cerebral cortex. *Neurosci. Res.*, **19**, 251–68.

Taub, E., Miller, N.E., Novack, T.A. et al. (1993). Technique to improve chronic motor deficit after stroke. *Arch. Phys. Med. Rehabil.*, **74**, 347–54.

Tresch, M.C. & Bizzi, E. (1999). Responses to spinal microstimulation in the chronically spinalized rat and their relationship to spinal systems activated by low threshold cutaneous stimulation. *Exp. Brain Res.*, **129**, 401–16.

Twitchell, T. (1951). The restoration of motor function following hemiplegia in man. *Brain*, **74**, 443–80.

Ugurbil, K., Hu, X., Chen, W., Zhu, X.H., Kim, S.G. & Georgopoulos, A. (1999). Functional mapping in the human brain using high magnetic fields. *Phil. Trans. R. Soc. Lond. B Biol. Sci.*, **354**, 1195–213.

Walshe, F. (1935). On the 'syndrome of the premotor cortex' (Fulton) and the definition of the terms "premotor" and "motor": with a consideration of Jackson's views on the cortical representation of movements. *Brain*, **58**, 49–80.

Weiller, C., Chollet, F., Friston, K.J., Wise, R.J. & Frackowiak, R.S. (1992). Functional reorganization of the brain in recovery from striatocapsular infarction in man. *Ann. Neurol.*, **31**, 463–72.

Wessberg, J., Stambaugh, C.R., Kralik, J.D. et al. (2000). Real-time prediction of hand trajectory by ensembles of cortical neurons in primates. *Nature*, **408**, 361–5.

Woolsey, C.N. (1952). *Patterns of Localization in Sensory and Motor Areas of the Cerebral Cortex*, pp. 193–206. New York: Hoeber.

32

The apraxias

Ramón C. Leiguarda

Raúl Carrea Institute of Neurological Research, FLENI, Buenos Aires, Argentina

Apraxia is a term used to denote a wide spectrum of higher-order motor disorders owing to acquired brain disease affecting the performance of skilled, learned movements with or without preservation of the ability to perform the same movement outside the clinical setting in the appropriate situation or environment. The disturbance of purposive movements cannot be termed apraxia, however, if it results from a language comprehension disorder or from dementia, or if the patient suffers from any elementary motor or sensory deficit (i.e. paresis, dystonia, ataxia) which could fully explain the abnormal motor behaviour (Heilman & Rothi, 1985; Roy & Square, 1985; De Renzi, 1989). The praxic disorder may affect various body parts such as the eyes, face, trunk, or limbs, and may involve both sides of the body (i.e. ideational and ideomotor apraxias), preferentially one side (i.e. limb-kinetic apraxia), or, alternatively, interlimb coordination, as in the case of apraxia of gait.

Apraxias are poorly recognized but common disorders that can result from a wide variety of focal (i.e. stroke, trauma) or diffuse brain damage (i.e. corticobasal degeneration, Alzheimer's disease) (Heilman & Rothi, 1985; Freund, 1992). There are two main reasons why apraxia may go unrecognized. Firstly, many patients with apraxia, particularly ideomotor apraxia, show a voluntary–automatic dissociation, which means that the patient does not complain about the deficit because the execution of the movement in the natural context is relatively well preserved, and the deficit appears mainly in the clinical setting when the patient is required to represent explicitly the content of the action outside the situational props. Secondly, although in apraxic and aphasic patients specific functions are selectively affected, language and praxic disturbances frequently coexist and the former may interfere with the proper evaluation of the latter (Freund, 1992).

Limb apraxias

Liepmann (1920) posited that the idea of the action, or movement formula, containing the space–time form picture of the movement, was stored in the left parietal lobe. In order to carry out a skilled movement, the space–time plan has to be retrieved and associated via cortical connections with the innervatory pattern stored in the left sensorimotorium that conveys the information to the left primary motor area. When the left limb performs the movement, the information has to be transmitted from the left to the right sensorimotorium through the corpus callosum to activate, thereafter, the right motor cortex. Liepmann conceived ideational apraxia as a disruption of the space–time plan or its proper activation, so that it was impossible to construct the idea of the movement; the patient does not know what to do. In contrast, in ideomotor apraxia, the space–time plan is intact but it can no longer guide the innervatory engrams which implement the movement because it is disconnected from them; the patient knows what to do but not how to do it. Finally, limb-kinetic apraxia appears when the disruption of the innervatory engrams interferes with the selection of the required muscle synergies to perform the skilled movement.

Heilman and Rothi (1985) and Rothi et al. (1991) proposed that the 'movement formulae' or 'visuokinesthetic motor engrams' were stored in the left inferior parietal lobule (IPL), and translated into an innervatory pattern in the supplementary motor area (SMA) rather than in the convexity of the premotor cortex (PM). A neuropsychological model was advanced involving specific dissociation of verbal, visual or tactile inputs into an action lexicon (represented in the parietal lobe) in which visuokinesthetic motor engrams programme skilled movements (Rothi et al., 1991).

Table 32.1. *Assessment of limb praxis*

Intransitive movements:	non-representational (e.g. touch your nose, wriggle your fingers)
	representational (e.g. wave good-bye, hitch-hike)
Transitive movements:	(e.g. use a hammer, use a screwdriver) under verbal, visual and tactile modalities
Imitation of meaningful and meaningless movements, postures and sequences.	
Multiple step tasks:	(e.g. prepare a letter for mailing)
Tool[a] selection tasks:	to select the appropriate tool to complete a task, such as a hammer for a partially driven nail
Alternative tool selection tasks:	to select an alternative tool such as pliers to complete a task such as pounding a nail, when the appropriate tool (i.e. hammer) is not available
Gesture recognition tasks:	to assess the capacity to comprehend gestures, either verbally (to name gestures performed by the examiner), as well as non-verbally (to match a gesture performed by the examiner with cards depicting the tool / object[b] corresponding to the pantomime)

Notes:

[a] Tool: implement with which an action is performed (e.g. hammer, screwdriver).

[b] Object: the recipient of the action (e.g. nail, screw).

Source: De Renzi (1989); Rothi et al. (1997).

In 1985, Roy and Square refined a praxis model into a conceptual system and a production system. The conceptual system was conceived to contain knowledge of object and tool use and organization of single actions into a sequence. On the other hand, the production system incorporates a sensori motor component of knowledge, as well as encompassing the perceptual motor processes for organizing and executing action. Dysfunction of the praxis conceptual system would give rise to conceptual or ideational apraxia, whereas impairment of the praxis production system would induce ideomotor and limb-kinetic apraxias. At present, however, it is possible to interpret the different types of limb apraxias, particularly ideomotor and limb kinetic apraxias, on the basis of our current knowledge of the modular organization of the brain (Leiguarda & Marsden, 2000).

Evaluation of limb praxis

A systematic evaluation of limb praxis is critical in order: (i) to identify the presence of apraxia; (ii) to classify correctly the nature of limb praxis deficit according to the errors committed by the patient; and (iii) to gain an insight into the underlying mechanism of the patient's abnormal motor behaviour (Table 32.1).

Several types of transitive movements are used in the evaluation of praxis and it is not an uncommon finding that apraxic patients perform some but not all movements in a particularly abnormal fashion and/or that individual differences appear in some but not all components of a

given movement. Therefore, the dissimilar complexity and features of transitive movements should be considered in order to analyse and interpret praxic errors accurately. For instance: (i) movements may or may not be repetitive in nature (e.g. hammering versus using a bottle opener to remove the cap); (ii) an action may be composed of sequential movements (e.g. to reach for a glass and take it to the lips in drinking); (iii) a movement may primarily reflect proximal limb control (transport) such as transporting the wrist when carving a turkey, proximal and distal limb control such as reaching and grasping a glass of water, or primarily distal control as when the patient is asked to manipulate a pair of scissors; and (iv) movements may be performed in the peripersonal space (e.g. carving a turkey), in body-centred space (e.g. tooth-brushing), or require the integration of both, such as the drinking action.

Analysis of a patient's performance is based on both accuracy and error patterns (Table 32.2). Three-dimensional motion analysis of the spatio-temporal characteristics of gestural movements has provided an accurate method to capture objectively the nature of the praxis errors observed in clinical examination. Patients with ideomotor apraxia, due to focal left hemisphere lesions (Clark et al., 1994; Poizner et al., 1995), and different asymmetric cortical degenerative syndromes (Leiguarda & Starkstein, 1998), have shown slow and hesitant build-up of hand velocity, irregular and non-sinusoidal velocity profiles, abnormal amplitudes, alterations in the plane of motion and in the direction and shapes of wrist trajectories, decou-

Table 32.2. Types of praxis errors

I. Temporal

S = sequencing: some pantomimes require multiple positionings that are performed in a characteristic sequence. Sequencing errors involve any perturbation of this sequence including addition, deletion, or transposition of movement elements as long as the overall movemen structure remains recognizable.

T = timing: this error reflects any alterations from the typical timing or speed of a pantomime and may include abnormally increased, decreased, or irregular rate of production or searching or groping behaviour.

O = occurrence: pantomimes may involve either single (i.e. unlocking a door with a key) or repetitive (i.e. screwing in a screw with a screwdriver) movement cycles. This error type reflects any multiplication of single cycles or reduction of a repetitive cycle to a single event.

II. Spatial

A = amplitude: any amplification, reduction, or irregularity of the characteristic amplitude of a target pantomime.

IC = internal configuration: when pantomiming, the fingers and hand must be in specific spatial relation to one another to reflect recognition and respect for the imagined tool. This error type reflects any abnormality of the required finger/hand posture and its relationship to the target tool. For example, when asked to pretend to brush teeth, the subject's hand may close tightly into a fist with no space allowed for the imagined toothbrush handle.

BPO = body-part-as-object: the subject uses his/her finger, hand, or arm as the imagined tool of the pantomime. For example, when asked to smoke a cigarette, the subject might puff on his or her index finger.

ECO = external configuration orientation: when pantomiming, the fingers/ hand/arm and the imagined tool must be in a specific relationship to the 'object' receiving the action. Errors of this type involve difficulties orienting to the 'object' or in placing the 'object' in space. For example, the subject might pantomime brushing teeth by holding his hand next to his mouth without reflecting the distance necessary to accommodate an imagined toothbrush. Another example would be when asked to hammer a nail, the subject might hammer in differing locations in space reflecting difficulty in placing the imagined nail in a stable orientation or in a proper plane of motion (abnormal planar orientation of the movement).

M = movement: when acting on an object with a tool, a movement characteristic of the action and necessary to accomplish the goal is required. Any disturbance of the characteristic movement reflects a movement error. For example, a subject, when asked to pantomime using a screwdriver, may orient the imagined screwdriver correctly to the imagined screw but instead of stabilizing the shoulder and wrist and twisting at the elbow, the subject stabilizes the elbow and twists at the wrist or shoulder.

III. Content

P = perseverative: the subject produces a response that includes all or part of a previously produced pantomime.

R = related: the pantomime is an accurately produced pantomime associated in content with the target. For example, the subject might pantomime playing a trombone for a target of a bugle.

N = non-related: the pantomime is an accurately produced pantomime not associated in content with the target. For example, the subject might pantomime playing a trombone for a target of shaving.

H = the patient performs the action without benefit of a real or imagined tool. For example, when asked to cut a piece of paper with scissors, he or she pretends to rip the paper.

IV. Other

C = concretization. The patient performs a transitive pantomime not on an imagined object but instead on a real object not normally used in the task. For example, when asked to pantomime sawing wood, the patient pantomimes sawing on his or her leg.

NR = no response.

UR = unrecognizable response: the response shares no temporal or spatial features of the target.

Source: Rothi et al. (1997).

pling of hand speed and trajectory curvature, and loss of interjoint coordination (Figs. 32.1–32.3). All these studies have evaluated gestures, such as carving a turkey or slicing a loaf of bread, which mainly explore the transport or reaching phase of the movement. However, the majority of transitive gestures included in most apraxia batteries are prehension (reaching and grasping) movements which reflect proximal (transport) as well as distal limb control (grasping). The kinematic analysis of aiming movements in apraxic patients has demonstrated spatial deficits, in particular when visual feedback is unavailable, whereas the analysis of prehension movements has shown disruption of both the transport and grasp phases of the movements as well as transport-grasping uncoupling (Caselli et al., 1999;

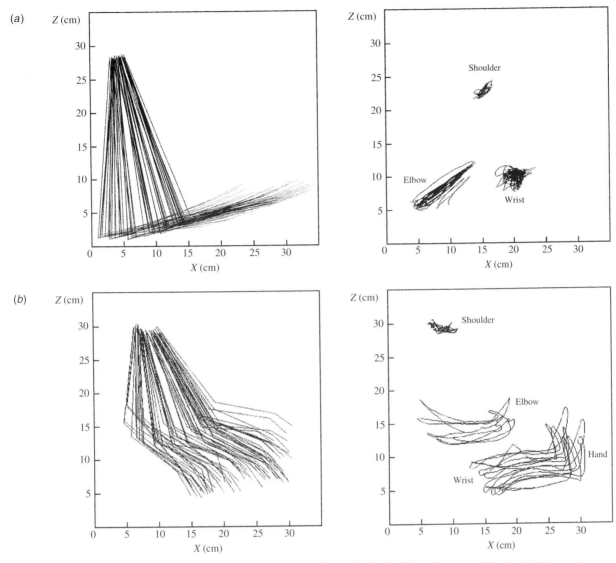

Fig. 32.1. Left: Lateral view of successive arm, forearm, wrist and hand positions during the performance of the bread-slicing gesture. Right: Frontal view of successive cycles of shoulder, elbow, wrist and hand trajectories. (*a*) Control subject. (*b*) Patient with ideomotor apraxia. Wrist trajectories in the control subject are located perpendicular to the goal object and aligned in the sagittal plane with slight vertical and horizontal displacement. The patient's wrist path showed abnormal horizontal displacement. Note also the incorrect orientation of movement axis.

Haaland et al., 1999; Leiguarda et al., 2000). Furthermore, the study of manipulating finger movements has disclosed abnormal workspace and breakdown of the temporal profiles of the scanning movements in patients with limb-kinetic apraxia (Leiguarda et al., 2000). Thus, exploration into the kinematics of reaching, grasping and manipulating provides information regarding the specific neural subsystems involved in patients with different types of limb praxic disorders.

Interhemispheric differences in the control of praxic skills

Apraxia as tested by the imitation of gestures and object use pantomime has been found in about 50% of patients with left hemisphere damage and in less than 10% of those with right hemisphere damage (De Renzi, 1989). Most of the errors exhibited by ideomotor apraxia patients are equally seen in left or right hemisphere-damaged patients

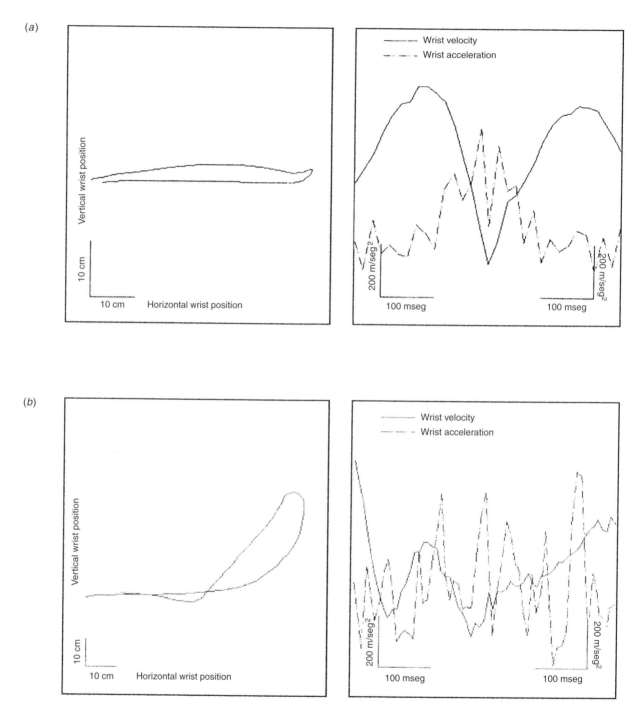

Fig. 32.2. Phase reversal in a control subject (*a*) and in a patient with ideomotor apraxia (*b*). The patient showed an abnormal widening of the wrist path during the reversal phase with a resulting spatial separation of irregular onward and outward path. The spatial distortion corresponds with a grossly disrupted relationship between wrist velocity and wrist acceleration.

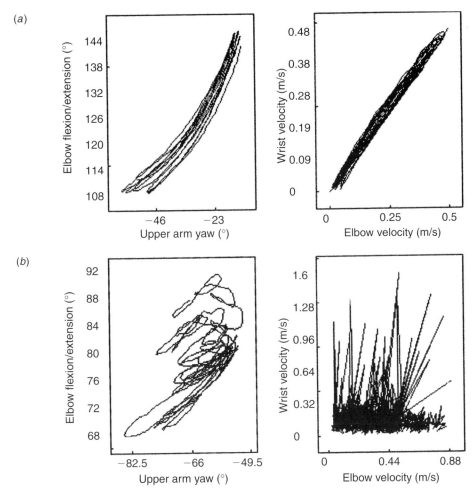

Fig. 32.3. Interjoint coordination (*a*) in a control subject and (*b*) in a patient with ideomotor apraxia. The control subject showed a smooth and linear relationship between elbow flexion–extension and upper arm yaw. As the elbow extended, the upper arm moved laterally across the body in a well-coordinated pattern. In contrast, the patient showed distorted angle–angle relationships owing to poor coordination between elbow flexion–extension and upper arm yaw as well as asynchronous intersegmental joint velocities.

when they pantomime non-representative and representative/intransitive gestures, but are observed predominantly in left hemisphere-damaged patients when they pantomime transitive movements, because it is this action which is performed outside the natural context (Haaland & Flaherty, 1984). Schnider et al. (1997) also emphasized that the left hemisphere motor dominance reflected by ideomotor apraxia refers to spatially and temporally complex movements carried out in an artificial context. Moreover, it has been suggested that, whereas either hemisphere would be able to process intransitive movements as well as transitive movements using tools/objects, the left hemisphere would be dominant not only for the 'abstract' performance (pantomiming to verbal command) of transitive movements but also for learning and reproducing novel move-

ments such as meaningless movements and sequences (Rapcsak et al., 1993). Impairment in sequencing is apparent in left hemisphere-damaged patients when the tasks place demands on memory, but also when the temporal aspects of sequencing, reflecting response preparation and programming, are considered (Harrington & Haaland, 1992). Rushworth et al. (1998) have further proposed that the left hemisphere is not only dominant for learning to select movements in a sequence but also for learning to select a limb movement that is appropriate for the use of an object. Thus, is seems likely that the interhemispheric differences in the control of praxic skills would largely depend on the context in which the movement is performed and on the cognitive requirements of the task; that is, when a single and/or sequence of object-oriented movements are performed outside the usual context and depend on higher-level cognitive abilities for planning and self-monitoring the action, the left hemisphere emerges as more dominant than the right (Haaland & Harrington, 1996).

Types of limb apraxia

Ideational or conceptual apraxia

In 1905 Pick described a patient who was unable to carry out a series of acts involving the utilization of several objects leading to an action goal (e.g. prepare a letter for mailing), although he was also able to use properly single tools and objects. Liepmann (1908) defined ideational apraxia as an impairment of tasks requiring a sequence of several acts with tools and objects. However, other authors use the term to denote a failure to use single tools appropriately (De Renzi, 1989). To overcome this confusion, Ochipa et al. (1992) have suggested restricting the term ideational apraxia to a failure to conceive a series of acts leading to an action goal, and introduced the term conceptual apraxia to denote deficits in the different types of tool-action knowledge as proposed by Roy and Square (1985). However, a strict difference between ideational and conceptual apraxia is not always feasible, since patients with ideational apraxia not only fail on tests of multiple object use, but may also perform abnormally when using a single object (De Renzi & Lucchelli, 1988).

Patients with ideational or conceptual apraxia exhibit primarily content errors in the performance of transitive movements (see Table 32.2), because they are unable to associate tools and objects with their corresponding action. They may also lose the ability to associate tools with the objects that receive their action; thus, when a partially driven nail is shown, the patient may select a pair of scissors rather than a hammer from an array of tools to perform the action. Not only are patients unable to select the appropriate tool to complete an action, but they may also fail to describe a function of a tool or point to a tool when the function is described by the examiner, even when the patient names the tool properly when shown to him/her. Patients with conceptual apraxia lose the mechanical advantage afforded by tools (mechanical knowledge). For example, when asked to complete an action and the appropriate tool is not available (e.g. a hammer to drive a nail), they may not select the most adequate tool for that action (e.g. a wrench) but rather one which is inadequate (e.g. a screwdriver) (Ochipa et al., 1992). These patients may also be impaired in the sequencing of tool/object use (Pick, 1905; Liepmann, 1920; Poeck,

1983). Patients with ideational or conceptual apraxia are disabled in everyday life, because they use tools/objects improperly, they misselect tools/objects for an intended activity, perform a complex sequential activity (e.g. make express coffee) in a mistaken order or do not complete the task at all (Foundas et al., 1995). Ideational apraxia has been traditionally allocated to the left parieto-occipital and parieto-temporal regions (Liepmann, 1920), although frontal and frontotemporal lesions may also cause ideational (De Renzi & Luchelli, 1988) or conceptual apraxia (Heilman et al., 1997).

Ideomotor apraxia

Ideomotor apraxia has been defined as 'a disturbance in programming the timing, sequencing and spatial organization of gestural movements' (Rothi et al., 1991). Patients with ideomotor apraxia exhibit mainly temporal and spatial errors (see Table 32.2). The movements are incorrectly produced but the goal of the action can usually be recognized. Occasionally, however, the performance is so severely deranged that the examiner cannot recognize the movement. Transitive movements are more affected than intransitive ones on pantomiming to commands and patients usually improve on imitation when performance is compared to responses to verbal commands (Heilman & Rothi, 1985). Acting with tools/objects is carried out better than pantomiming their use, but even so, movements may not be entirely normal. The improvement in performance observed when the patient actually uses the tool/object is due to the advantage provided by visual and tactile-kinesthetic cues emanating from the tool/object and by the fact that in this condition, the patient is performing the movement in a more natural context and therefore less dependent on the left hemisphere. Ideomotor apraxia is commonly associated with damage to the parietal association areas, less frequently with lesions of the PM cortex and SMA and usually with disruption of the intrahemispheric white matter bundles which interconnect them (Leiguarda & Marsden, 2000). Although small lesions of the basal ganglia and thalamus may cause ideomotor apraxia, in the majority of patients the pathology extends to the internal capsule and periventricular and peristriatal white matter (Pramstaller & Marsden, 1996). Most studies examining possible clinico-anatomical correlation for ideomotor apraxia have found a strong association of apraxia with large cortico-subcortical lesions in the suprasylvian, perirolandic region of the left dominant hemisphere, but no specific lesion site which correlated with apraxia. Disruption of cortico-cortical and cortico-subcortical connection due to white matter damage seems essential for the occurrence of apraxia (Kertesz & Ferro, 1984; Alexander et al., 1992; Schnider et al., 1997; Leiguarda & Marsden, 2000).

Limb-kinetic apraxia

This type of apraxia was originally described by Kleist (1907), who called it 'innervatory apraxia' to stress the loss of hand and finger dexterity due to inability to connect and to isolate individual innervation. The deficit is mainly confined to finger and hand movements contralateral to the lesion, regardless of its hemispheric side, with preservation of power and sensation. Manipulatory finger movements are predominantly affected, but in most cases all movements, either complex or routine, independently of the modality to evoke them, are coarse, awkward, mutilated and 'amorphous' (Liepmann, 1908). Fruitless attempts usually precede wrong movements, which in turn are frequently contaminated by extraneous movements. Imitation of finger postures is also abnormal and some patients use the less affected or normal hand to reproduce the requested posture. The severity of the deficit is consistent, exhibiting the same degree in everyday activities as in the clinical setting; thus, there is no voluntary-automatic dissociation (Liepmann, 1908; Faglioni & Basso, 1985).

Limb-kinetic apraxia has been scantily reported with focal lesions (Faglioni & Basso, 1985); there are two potential explanations: first, most PM lesions also involve the precentral cortex, and, therefore, the contralateral paresis or paralysis precludes the expression of the praxic deficit; and, secondly, bilateral activation of the PM cortex and SMA are often observed with unilateral movements; thus, a unilateral lesion would not be enough for an overt deficit, since bilateral involvement would be most likely necessary. As a matter of fact, all recently pathologically confirmed cases of limb-kinetic apraxia suffered a degenerative process such as corticobasal degeneration and Pick's disease, involving frontal and parietal cortices or, predominantly, the PM cortex (Leiguarda & Marsden, 2000).

Callosal apraxia

Patients with damage to the body of the corpus callosum with or without genu involvement (Liepmann & Maas, 1907; Watson & Heilman, 1983; Graff-Radford et al., 1987; Leiguarda et al., 1989) may develop unilateral apraxia of the non-dominant limb whose characteristics vary according to the type of test given and the lateralization pattern of praxic skills in each patient. Some patients could not correctly pantomime to verbal commands with their left hand, but performed normally on imitation and object use (Geschwind & Kaplan, 1962), whereas others could not use their left hand on command, by imitation or while holding the object (Watson & Heilman, 1983; Leiguarda et al., 1989). Moreover,

a few patients could not pantomime to verbal commands and while holding the object, but performed fairly well on imitation (Graff-Radford et al., 1987), or improved over time on imitation and object use (Watson & Heilman, 1983). Thus, the most enduring callosal type of praxic defect is demonstrated when verbal-motor tasks, such as pantomiming to command, are used (Graff-Radford et al., 1987).

Modality-specific or disassociation apraxias

The modality-specific (De Renzi et al., 1982) or disassociation apraxias (Rothi et al., 1991) refer to those types of praxic deficits exhibited by patients who commit errors only, or predominantly, when the movement is evoked by one but not all modalities. Thus, the impairment of patients who performed abnormally only under verbal commands has been attributed to a left hemispheric lesion most likely affecting the audio-verbal inputs to the parietal lobe (De Renzi et al., 1982) or a callosal lesion (Geschwind & Kaplan, 1962). Patients who performed poorly to seen objects, but were able to pantomime gestures normally to verbal command, have also been reported as having lesions interrupting the flow of visual information toward the parietal lobe. On occasion, praxic deficits may be confined to the tactile modality. Finally, patients have been reported who, unlike those with ideomotor apraxia improving on imitation, were more impaired when imitating than when pantomiming to command, or could not imitate but performed flawlessly under other modalities. Deficits may be restricted solely to the imitation of meaningless gestures with preserved imitation to meaningful gestures (De Renzi et al., 1982; Rothi et al., 1991; Ochipa et al., 1994; Goldenberg & Hagmann, 1997).

The anatomofunctional substrates of limb praxis

The fact that most studies exploring possible clinico-anatomical correlations for different types of limb apraxia have failed to unveil a consistent and specific lesion site for the disorder, strongly suggests that praxic functions are distributed across several distinct anatomofunctional neural systems, working in concert but with each one controlling specific processes (i.e. parieto-frontal systems and reaching/grasping, fronto-striatal system and sequential motor events). Damage to these systems would produce selective praxic-related deficits depending on the movement context and cognitive demand of the action.

Parallel parieto-frontal circuits for sensorimotor integration

Recent anatomical and functional studies have identified in primates a series of segregated parieto-frontal circuits, working in parallel and each one involved in a specific sensorimotor transformation process; that is, their function is to transform the sensory information encoded in the coordinates of sensory epithelia (e.g. retina, skin) into information for movements (Rizzolatti et al., 1998). The transformation process involves parallel mechanisms that simultaneously engage functionally related parietal and frontal areas linked by reciprocal cortico-cortical connections. The posterior parietal cortex comprises a multiplicity of areas, each involved in the analysis of particular aspects of sensory information (i.e. somatosensory, visual, auditory, vestibular). The coordinate system may vary in different parts of the parietal cortex according to the nature of the actions evoked by sensory input. The motor cortex, in turn, is also made up by many areas, each containing an independent body movement representation, and playing a specific role in motor control, according to its afferent and efferent connections. The proposed functions of the main circuits originating from the superior parietal lobule (SPL) include: visual and somatosensory transformation for reaching (MIP-F_2), somatosensory transformation for reaching (PEc/PEip-F_2), somatosensory transformation for posture (PEci-F_3), and transformation of body part location data into information necessary for the control of body part movements (PE-F_1). The circuits originating in the IPL are devoted to visuomotor transformation for grasping and manipulation (AIP-F_5), the internal representation of actions (PF-F_5), coding peripersonal space for limb and neck movements (VIP-F_4), and visual transformation for eye movements (LIP-FEF) (Fig. 32.4) (Rizzolatti et al., 1998).

Selective apraxia-related deficits resulting from damage to the parieto-frontal circuits

Patients with lesions of the postero-superior parietal cortex develop a disorder of visually guided reaching called optic ataxia (Balint, 1909). Some of the patients not only misreach the target but also misshape the hand before grasping and on occasion commit errors in hand orientation (Jeannerod et al., 1994). Freund (1992) has suggested using the term 'visuomotor apraxia' rather than optic ataxia because inaccuracy of the movement (ataxia) is not the sole feature of the disorder, as performance is also misdirected, decomposed and faulty in the execution of its parts. Visuomotor apraxia most likely results from disruption of the parieto-frontal circuit devoted to visual and somatosensory transformation for reaching.

Lesions in the SPL involving circuits that subserve somatosensory transformation for reaching, somatosensory transformation for posture and transformation of body part location data into information for the control of

body part movements would explain the external configuration and movement types of praxic errors such as faulty orientation and abnormal limb configuration. Heilman et al. (1986) described a right-handed patient with an apraxia due to a right superior parietal lesion; her performance with the left hand was characterized by minor temporal but gross spatial errors, particularly with the eyes closed; she erroneously moved the arm in space and abnormally oriented the limb in relation to the object. She failed to display visuomotor ataxia, and grasping appeared to be preserved. Selective deficits limited to the grasping phase of the movement that can mirror some of the internal configuration types of praxic errors have also been described in humans with damage to parieto-frontal circuits in the IPL. Jeannerod et al. (1994) reported a patient who, following a bilateral parieto-occipital infarction, showed a severe and bilateral grasping impairment; the hand was widely open, without correlation between grip and object size, and the grasp was awkward and inaccurate. Binkofski et al. (1998) studied patients with lesions involving the anterior bank of the intraparietal sulcus (IPs), possibly the human homologue of the anterior intraparietal area (AIP), who had selective temporal and spatial kinematic deficits in the coordination of finger movements required for grasping a switch with minor disturbances of the reaching phase of the movement. The report of Sirigu et al. (1995) clearly demonstrated the relationship between grasping and praxis. Their patient, with bilateral hypometabolism in the posterior parietal regions, showed a selective praxic deficit for hand postures during grasping objects in the context of utilization gestures, with apparently normal movement trajectories and accurate manual grasp scaling during simple reaching movements. Thus, object attributes are likely to be processed differently according to the task in which subjects are involved. When a subject is requested only to grasp an object but not to use it, the brain extracts the structural attributes of objects (i.e. form, size, orientation) relevant to action to generate the appropriate movement. However, during utilization gestures, in addition to data about object characteristics, prior knowledge about functional properties of objects needs to be integrated into the grasping subsystem to produce an accurate manual grasp (Jeannerod et al., 1995; Sirigu et al., 1995).

Lesions in animals and humans involving areas of the motor cortex making up the parieto-frontal circuits also cause distinct types of praxic-like deficits, though less selectively than those observed with damage to the parietal component of the circuits. Persistent impairment of skilled movement has been observed with damage to the PM cortex. Luria (1980) stressed the 'loss of the kinetic melody',

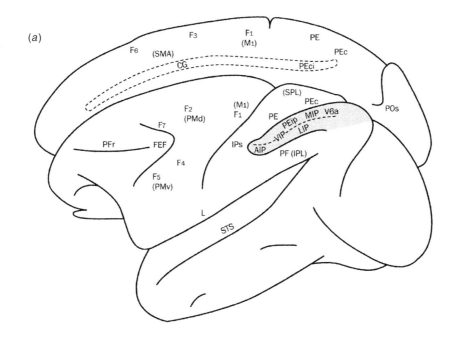

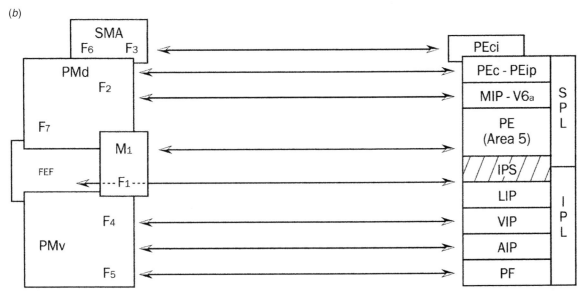

Fig. 32.4. (a) Lateral and medial views of the cerebral hemisphere of macaque monkey. The intraparietal sulcus has been opened (shaded grey) to show areas located in its medial and lateral bank. (b) Simplified diagram of the organization of the parallel parieto-frontal circuits for sensory-motor integration. The parcellation of the agranular frontal cortex is defined according to Matelli et al. (1985, 1991) studies in monkeys. F1 corresponds to primary motor cortex, F2 and F7 correspond to the dorsal premotor cortex (PMd) and F4 and F5 to the ventral premotor cortex (PMv). F6 and F3 correspond to the pre-supplementary motor area (SMA) and SMA proper, respectively. The arm is represented in F1, F2, F3, F4 and F5 whereas the leg only in F1, F2 and F3. F6 and F7 are almost devoid of corticospinal neurons. In the posterior parietal lobe there are also multiple representations of the arm, leg and face. All parietal areas are defined according to Pandya and Seltzer (1982), except those buried within the intraparietal sulcus (IPs) which are defined according to physiological data (Rizzolatti et al., 1998); AIP, anterior intraparietal area; CG, cingulate gyrus; FEF, frontal eye-field; L, lateral fissure; LIP, lateral intraparietal area; MIP, medial intraparietal area; PE, dorsal part of area 5; PEc, posterior part of PE; PEci, posterior part of cingulate sulcus; PEip, rostral part of the medial bank of IPs; PF, anterior part of the convexity of IPL; POs, parieto-occipital sulcus; PFr, prefrontal cortex; STS, superior temporal sulcus; VIP, ventral intraparietal area; V6a, visual area 6 in the rostral bank of the POs. Monkey IPL is not homologous to human IPL, since it is devoid of Brodmann areas 39 and 40. (Source: Leiguarda & Marsden, 2000.)

resulting in a disintegration of the dynamics of the motor act and of complex skilled movements in patients with PM lesions, which is mainly apparent when the task requires the learning of a new skilled movement. Patients with frontal lobe lesions may exhibit deficits in visually steering the arm accurately, particularly during rapid movements (catch a thrown ball) due to abnormal temporal sequencing of muscular activation (Freund & Hummelsheim, 1985). On the other hand, the cingulate and SMA seem to play a leading role in bimanual interaction since patients with damage to these areas show difficulties whenever the two hands must act simultaneously (i.e. buttoning, tying shoelaces) but experience no trouble with unimanual dexterity (Stephan et al., 1999). In addition, patients with PM lesions exhibit a deficit in conditional motor learning (Halsband & Freund, 1990) which may underlie the inappropriate selection of actions in relation to the context exhibited by apraxic patients (Passingham, 1993).

Fronto-striatal and fronto-parietal systems: sequencing of movements

Patients with apraxia exhibit several types of sequential errors, such as deletions, transpositions, additions, perseverations and non-related types of substitutions (Roy & Square, 1985; Rothi et al., 1997). Functional brain imaging studies have shown that different neural systems are actively engaged in the preparation and generation of a sequential action, depending on whether a sequence has been prelearned or is a new one, and contingent to the complexity of the attentional demands of the task (Grafton et al., 1995; Catalan et al., 1998).

The SMA, primary sensorimotor cortex, basal ganglia (mid-posterior putamen) and cerebellum would be mainly involved in the execution of automatic, overlearned, sequential movements, whereas the prefrontal, PM and posterior parietal cortices and the anterior part of the caudate/putamen would be particularly recruited, in addition to such areas engaged in the execution of simple movement sequences, when a complex or newly learned sequence, which requires attention, integration of multimodal information and working memory processes for its appropriate selection and monitoring, has to be performed (Grafton et al., 1995; Catalan et al., 1998.

Thus, different neural systems would be engaged depending on the type of movement sequence requested to be executed during praxis evaluation. When the sequence is well known or automated, or else performed from memory, the SMA-basal ganglion system would be preferentially recruited. However, most of the sequences used to test praxis are new (e.g. sequencing of movement

in the movement imitation test for ideomotor apraxia); or, the content of an otherwise well learned goal-directed action (e.g. multiple sequential use of objects test for ideational apraxia) has to be explicitly represented. In any case, the system made up by the prefrontal, PM and parietal cortices, the striatum and white matter fascicles would be specifically engaged. In addition, it might be possible that within this system there are many different subsystems subserving functionally separate cognitive computations involved in motor sequencing (i.e. timing, motor attention, selection of limb movements and object-oriented responses) which may be selectively damaged by the pathological process and thus produce different types of sequencing impairment in apraxic patients (Harrington & Haaland, 1992; Rushworth et al., 1998).

The temporo-parieto-frontal system: recognition and imitation of actions

Action recognition deficits have been observed in patients with parietal, temporal, frontal and basal ganglion lesions predominantly in the left hemisphere (Ferro et al., 1983; Varney & Damasio, 1987). On the other hand, abnormal performance on imitation has been found in patients with parietal, frontal, temporal, subcortical and basal ganglion lesions (Hermsdöfer et al., 1996). Thus, recognition and imitation of actions seem to be subserved through distributed neural systems preferentially though not exclusively dependent on the left dominant hemisphere. These systems would be made up by several interconnected nodes mainly in the parietal and frontal cortices, but also in the temporal cortex and perhaps subcortical structures, each devoted to preferential functions within each system. Single-unit studies in monkeys and functional neuroimaging studies tend to support these assumptions.

Di Pellegrino et al. (1992) discovered a particular subset of neurones in F5 which discharge during the time a monkey observes meaningful hand movements made by the experimenter, in particular when interacting with objects; they called them 'mirror neurons' and speculated that they belonged to an observation/execution matching system involved in understanding the meaning of motor events as well as in action imitation (Rizzolatti et al., 1998). Neurons with properties similar to those of mirror neurons in F5 are also found in the superior temporal sulcus (STS) in monkeys (Carey et al., 1997). Two other types of neurons, which may contribute to the recognition and imitation of postures and actions, have also been found in the STS. One type encodes the visual appearance of particular parts of the body (i.e. fingers, hands, arms), which combine in such a way that the collection of components can specify a particular meaningful posture or action. The second type encodes specific body movements, such as walking and turning (Carey et al., 1997). Cells responding to hand–object interaction might also be present in area 7b, located in the rostral part of the IPL, which sends its cortical output to the F5; in turn, area 7b receives projection from the STS region, and the latter is interconnected with the frontal lobe, thus closing a cortical circuit involved in the perception of hand–object interaction. The crucial cognitive role of the STS-7b-F5 network would be the internal representation of actions which, when evoked by an action made by others, would be involved in two related functions, namely, action recognition and action imitation (Rizzolatti et al., 1998).

PET studies in humans support neurophysiological findings in monkeys. Grasping observation markedly increased cerebral blood flow in the cortex of the STS, in the rostral part of Broca's area and in the rostral part of the left IPs on the left hemisphere of right-handed subjects (Rizzolatti et al., 1996; Grafton et al., 1996). Furthermore, the imitation of meaningful actions seems to be mediated by the implicit knowledge about the form as well as the meaning of the gesture, which is processed by regions involved in the planning and generation of actions plus the temporal cortex, whereas imitation of meaningless actions would depend on the decoding of their spatiotemporal layout in the occipito-parietal-PM cortex pathway (Decety et al., 1997), or on the analysis of arbitrary body movements or components (i.e. hand open, finger extended) by cells in the temporal cortex and their corresponding parietal and/or premotor connections (Carey et al., 1997).

Limb apraxias due to dysfunction of the parieto-frontal circuits: higher-order defects of sensorimotor integration

Disruption of parieto-frontal circuits and their subcortical connections, subserving the transformation of sensory information into action, would give rise to most of the praxic errors observed in ideomotor apraxia. Damage to circuits devoted to sensorimotor transformation for grasping, reaching and posture, as well as for transformation of body part location into information necessary for the control of body part movements, would produce incorrect finger and hand posture and abnormal orientation of the tool/object, inappropriate configuration of the arm and faulty orientation of the movement (both with respect to the body and the target of the movement in extrapersonal space), as well as movement trajectory abnormalities. These errors may be similarly observed in the limb contralateral to a left or right parietal lesion, if an associated elemental motor or sensory deficit does not preclude their proper interpretation. However, they would be particularly reflective of ideomotor apraxia, and then also observed in the limb ipsilateral to a left hemisphere lesion, when the patient pantomimes a transitive movement under verbal command. Thus, the praxic quality of the errors in ideomotor apraxia would be determined by the context in which the movement is performed and the cognitive requirements of the task.

Selective praxic deficits may be observed when specific circuits are involved in the parietal or frontal lobes. Damage to the SPL in circuits subserving somatosensory transformation for reaching, posture and movements would produce praxic errors, such as abnormal limb orientation and configuration, resembling those observed in patients with apraxia secondary to superior parietal lesions (Heilman et al., 1986). When the circuits subserving grasping mechanisms are damaged in the IPL, a praxic deficit characterized by a mismatch between finger and hand postures and the object to be grasped will be observed (Sirigu et al., 1995).

Lesions in the PM dorsal cortex and SMA involving the corresponding parieto-frontal circuits will most likely cause milder errors in limb position, configuration, orientation and trajectory than those observed with parietal lesions. These deficits will be more evident in the contralateral limb due to close interrelation between both premotor cortices during movements, although subtle abnormalities may be observed in the limb ipsilateral to a damaged left hemisphere, particularly when the subject pantomimes transitive movements to verbal command. Involvement of the circuits subserving sensorimotor transformation for grasping in the PM ventral cortex may produce some of the ideomotor type of praxis errors confined to hand movements. However, it seems possible that damage to this region of the premotor cortex, particularly when bilateral, would primarily disrupt particular segments of the action and the specificity for different hand and finger movements and configurations. The 'motor vocabulary' necessary for the proper selection of finger and hand movements (Jeannerod et al., 1995) would be impaired and a limb-kinetic type of praxis deficit would appear in the hand contralateral to the more affected hemisphere, regardless of the pattern of cerebral dominance (Leiguarda & Marsden, 2000).

Treatment of limb apraxia

Limb apraxia has a definitive ecological impact on patients' lives, since it interferes with activities of daily living. Patients may use and select tools/objects improperly and may be unable to perform a routine sequential action. In addition, the presence of limb apraxia may negatively affect the acquisition and use of gestural communication in aphasic patients (Foundas et al., 1995). Furthermore, although the natural evolution of limb apraxia is still unknown, it seems that some aspects of the disorder improve over time, but others are persistent. Therefore, the praxic disorder should be correctly identified and treated together with associated neurological deficits.

Maher and Ochipa have suggested two strategies to manage patients' disability. One is to modify the environment in order to facilitate activities of daily living and to reduce the risk of injuries. The other would be to directly treat specific praxic deficits based on their functional relevance and patients' needs. Although still not well established, preliminary studies indicate that therapeutic gains are restricted to the specific defect or trained activity, and treatment is more effective when implanted into patients' natural environment (Maher & Ochipa, 1997; Goldenberg & Hagmann, 1998).

Distribution of the apraxias in other body parts

Spatial and temporal errors committed by patients with limb (ideomotor) apraxia are remarkably similar to those observed in patients with oral verbal (speech) and oral non-verbal (buccofacial) apraxias which may reflect some common disruption of motor control (Roy & Square-Storer, 1990). Apraxia of speech or verbal apraxia is defined as an articulatory prosodic speech disorder due to 'an impaired ability to program the positioning of the speech musculature . . . and the sequencing of muscle movements' (Darley et al., 1975). The disorder is distinct from aphasia and dysarthria, but often coexists with them, in particular with Broca's aphasia. Apraxic speech is characterized by articulatory errors of different types, slow rate and prosodic deviation or abnormalities of speech rhythm and stress patterns, becoming more evident on longer and phonetically more complex utterances. Frontal (PM), insula, anterior limb of the internal capsule, basal ganglion and parietal damage in the left hemisphere may cause apraxia of speech; the presentation of the motor speech disorder may differ according to lesion location. Both deficits of postural shaping and disruption for sequencing muscle contractions during speech seem to respond to therapy (Square-Storer & Apeldoorn, 1991). Buccofacial or oral non-verbal apraxia is a disturbance of voluntary facial acts; patients exhibit spatial and temporal errors of similar quality to those observed in limb and speech apraxia when performing movements such as sticking out the tongue,

blowing out a match or sucking on a straw. Buccofacial apraxia often coexists with Broca's aphasia, but they can be completely dissociated. The disorder is more frequently observed with damage to the frontal and central operculum, insula, centrum semiovale and basal ganglia (Raade et al., 1991).

Apraxia of eyelid opening can be defined as a nonparalytic inability to open the eyes at will in the absence of visible contraction of the orbicularis oculi muscle. Many patients show a forceful contraction of the frontalis muscle and/or a backward thrusting of the head on attempting eyelid opening and use different types of manoeuvres to help open the eyes including opening the mouth, massaging the lids and manual elevation of the lids. Apraxia of eyelid opening can occur in isolation or associated with blepharospasm. Treatment with botulin toxin may be effective in patients with associated blepharospasm and when the disorder is due to a continuation of orbicularis oculi activity following voluntary closure of the eyes (pretarsal motor persistence) but not when it is only the result of involuntary palpebral levator inhibition (Goldstein & Cogan, 1965; Boghen, 1997).

Gerstmann and Schilder (1926) described apraxia of gait as a genuine disturbance of walking due to frontal lesions. However, it remains controversial whether it is a specific disorder or rather it represents a spectrum of higher-order walking syndromes (see Chapter 41). Apraxia of gait is defined as the loss of ability to use the lower limbs properly in the act of walking, which cannot be accounted for by demonstrable sensory impairment or motor weakness (Meyer & Barron, 1960). Gait is characterized by slowness of initiation, loss of balance, 'magnetic attraction of the foot to the ground', and inability to pedal, to kick or to trace a circle with the foot, as well as increased tone (Gegenhalten) and brisk reflexes in the lower limbs with grasping foot responses. The disorder is caused by bilateral damage to the frontal lobes or by white matter lesions interrupting the connections between premotor cortex, supplementary motor area and cerebellum and basal ganglia.

References   * denotes key references

Alexander, M.P., Baker, E., Naeser, M.A., Kaplan, E. & Palumbo, C. (1992). Neuropsychological and neuroanatomical dimensions of ideomotor apraxia. *Brain*, **115**, 87–107.

Balint, R. (1909). Seelenlähmung des Schavens, optische Ataxie, raum-liche Störung der Aufmerksamkeit. *Monatsschr. Psychiatr. Neurol.*, **250**, 51–81.

Binkofski, F., Phil, M., Posse, S., Stephan, K.M., Hefter, H., Seitz, R.J. & Freund, H.J. (1998). Human anterior intraparietal area subserves prehension: a combined lesion and functional MRI activation study. *Neurology*, **50**, 1253–9.

*Boghen, D. (1997). Apraxia of lid opening: a review. *Neurology*, **48**, 1491–4.

*Carey, D.P., Perrett, D. & Oram, M. (1997). Recognizing, understanding and reproducing action. In *Handbook of Neuropsychology*, ed. F. Boller & J. Grafman Jr., vol. 11 pp. 111–29. Amsterdam: Elsevier Science Publishers.

Caselli, R.J., Stelmach, G.E., Caviness, J.V. et al. (1999). A kinematic study of progressive apraxia with and without dementia. *Mov. Disorders*, **14**, 276–87.

Catalan, M.J., Honda, M., Weeks, R., Cohen, L. & Hallett, M. (1998). The functional neuroanatomy of simple and complex sequential finger movements: a PET study. *Brain*, **121**, 253–64.

*Clark, M.A., Merians, A.S., Kothari, A. et al. (1994). Spatial planning deficits in limb apraxia. *Brain*, **117**, 1093–106.

Darley, F.L., Aronson, A.E. & Brown, J.R. (1975). *Motor Speech Disorders–Audiotapes*. Philadelphia: W.B. Saunders.

*De Renzi, E. (1989). Apraxia. In *Handbook of Neuropsychology*, ed. F. Boller and J. Grafman, vol. 2 pp. 245–63. Amsterdam: Elsevier Science Publishers.

De Renzi, E. & Lucchelli, F. (1988). Ideational Apraxia. *Brain*, **113**, 1173–88.

De Renzi, E., Faglioni, P. & Sorgato, P. (1982). Modality-specific and supramodal mechanisms of apraxia. *Brain*, **105**, 301–12.

*Decety, J., Grèzes, J., Costes, N. et al. (1997). Brain activity during observation of actions: influence of action content and subject's strategy. *Brain*, **120**, 1763–77.

di Pellegrino, G., Fadiga, L., Fogassi, L., Gallese, V. & Rizzolatti, G. (1992). Understanding motor events: a neurophysiological study. *Exp. Brain Res.*, **91**, 176–80.

*Faglioni, P. & Basso, A. (1985). Historical perspectives on neuroanatomical correlates of limb apraxia. In *Neuropsychological Studies of Apraxia and Related Disorders*, ed. E.A. Roy, pp. 3–44. Amsterdam: North-Holland.

Ferro, J., Martins, I., Mariano, G. & Castro Caldas, A. (1983). CT scan correlates of gesture recognition. *J. Neurol., Neurosurg., Psychiatry*, **46**, 943–52.

Foundas, A., Macauley, B.L., Raymer, A.M., Maher, L.M., Heilman, K.M. & Rothi, L.J.G. (1995). Ecological implications of limb apraxia: evidence from mealtime behavior. *J. Int. Neuropsychol. Soc.*, **1**, 62–6.

*Freund, H.J. (1992). The apraxias. In *Diseases of the Nervous System. Clinical Neurobiology*, ed. A.K. Asbury, G.M. McKhann & W.J. McDonald, 2nd edn, pp. 751–67. Philadelphia: W.B. Saunders.

Freund, H.J. & Hummelsheim, H. (1985). Lesions of premotor cortex in man. *Brain*, **108**, 697–733.

Gerstmann, J. & Schilder, P. (1926). Über eine besondere Gangstörung bei Stirnhirner krankung. *Wien. Med. Wochenschr*, **76**, 97–102.

Geschwind, N. & Kaplan, E. (1962). A human cerebral disconnection syndrome. *Neurology*, **12**, 675–85.

Goldenberg, G. & Hagmann, S. (1997). The meaning of meaningless gestures: a study of visuo-imitative apraxia. *Neuropsychologia*, **35**, 333–41.

Goldenberg, G. & Hagmann, S. (1998). Therapy of activities of daily living in patients with apraxia. *Neuropsychol. Rehab.*, **8**, 123–42.

Goldstein, J.E. & Cogan, D.G. (1965). Apraxia of lid opening. *Arch. Ophthalmol.*, **73**, 155–9.

Graff-Radford, N.R., Welsh, K. & Godersky, J. (1987). Callosal apraxia. *Neurology*, **37**, 100–5.

Grafton, S.T., Hazeltine, E. & Ivry, R. (1995). Functional mapping of sequence learning in normal humans. *J. Cog. Neurosci.*, **7**, 497–510.

*Grafton, S.T., Arbid, M.A., Fadiga, L. & Rizzolatti, G. (1996). Localization of grasp representations in humans by positron emission tomography 2. Observation compared with imagination. *Exp. Brain Res.*, **112**, 103–11.

Haaland, K.Y. & Flaherty, D. (1984). The different types of limb apraxia errors made by patients with left vs. right hemisphere damage. *Brain Cognit.*, **3**, 370–84.

Haaland, K.Y. & Harrington, D.L. (1996). Hemispheric asymmetry of movement (Review). *Curr. Opin. Neurobiol.*, **6**, 796–800.

Haaland, K.Y., Harrington, D.L. & Knight, R.T. (1999). Spatial deficits in ideomotor limb apraxia: a kinematic analysis of aiming movements. *Brain*, **122**, 1169–82.

Halsband, U. & Freund, H.J. (1990). Premotor cortex and conditional motor learning in man. *Brain*, **113**, 207–22.

Harrington, D.L., Haaland, K.Y. & Knight, R.T. (1998). Cortical networks underlying mechanisms of time perception. *J Neurosci*, **18**, 1085–95.

*Heilman, K.M. & Rothi, L.J.G. (1985). Apraxia. In *Clinical Neuropsychology*, ed. K.M. Heilman & E. Valenstein, pp. 131–50. New York: Oxford University Press.

Heilman, K.M., Rothi, L.J.G., Mack, L., Feinberg, T. & Watson, R. (1986). Apraxia after superior parietal lesion. *Cortex*, **22**, 141–50.

*Heilman, K.M., Maher, L.H., Greenwald, L. & Rothi, L.J. (1997). Conceptual apraxia from lateralized lesions. *Neurology*, **49**, 457–64.

Hermsdörfer, J., Mai, N., Spatt, J., Marquardt, C., Veltkamp, R. & Goldenberg, G. (1996). Kinematic analysis of movement imitation in apraxia. *Brain*, **119**, 1575–86.

Jeannerod, M., Decety, J. & Michel, F. (1994). Impairment of grasping movements following a bilateral posterior parietal lesion. *Neuropsychologia*, **32**, 369–80.

Jeannerod, M., Arbid, M.A., Rizzolatti, G. & Sakata, H. (1995). Grasping objects: the cortical mechanisms of visuomotor transformation. *Trends Neurosci*, **18**, 314–20.

Kertesz, A. & Ferro, J.M. (1984). Lesion size and location in ideomotor apraxia. *Brain*, **107**, 921–33.

Kleist, K. (1907). Kortikale (innervatorische) Apraxie. *Jahrbuch für Psychiatrie und Neurologie*, **28**, 46–112.

*Leiguarda, R. & Marsden, D. (2000). Limb apraxias: higher-order disorders of sensorimotor integration (Review). *Brain*, **123**, 860–79.

Leiguarda, R. & Starkstein, S. (1998). Apraxia in the syndromes of Pick complex. In *Pick's Disease and Pick Complex*, ed. A. Kertesz & D.G. Muñoz, pp. 129–43. New York: Wiley-Liss.

Leiguarda, R., Starkstein, S. & Berthier, M. (1989). Anterior callosal haemorrhage. A partial interhemispheric disconnection syndrome. *Brain*, **112**, 1019–37.

Leiguarda, R., Merello, M. & Balej, J. (2000). Apraxia in corticobasal degeneration. *Adv Neurol*, **82**, 103–21.

Liepmann, H., (1908). *Drei Aufsätze aus dem Apraxiegebiet*. Berlin: Karger.

Liepmann, H. (1920). Apraxie. *Ergeb Gesamten Medizin*, **1**, 516–43.

Liepmann, H. & Maas, O. (1907). Eie Fall von linksseitiger Agraphie und Apraxie bei rechtsseitiger Lähmung. *Monatsschr. Psychiatrie Neurol.*, **10**, 214–27.

Luria, A.R. (ed.) (1980). In *Higher Cortical Function in Man*, ed. 2nd edn. New York: Basic Books.

Maher, L.M. & Ochipa, C. (1997). Management and treatment of limb apraxia. In *Apraxia: the Neuropsychology of Action*, ed. L.J.G. Rothi & K.M. Heilman, pp. 75–92. Hove, UK: Psychology.

Matelli, M., Luppino G. & Rizzolatti, G. (1985). Patterns of cytochrome oxidase activity in the frontal agranular cortex of the macaque monkey. *Behav. Brain Res.*, **18**, 125–36.

Matelli, M., Luppino, G. & Rizzolatti, G. (1991). Architecture of superior and mesial area 6 and the adjacent cingulated cortex in the macaque monkey. *J. Comp. Neurol.*, **311**, 445–62.

*Meyer, J.S. & Barron, D.W. (1960). Apraxia of gait: a clinico-physiological study. *Brain*, **83**, 261–84.

Ochipa, C., Rothi, L.J.G. & Heilman, K.M. (1992). Conceptual apraxia in Alzheimer's disease. *Brain*, **115**, 1061–71.

Ochipa, C., Rothi, L.J.G. & Heilman, K.M. (1994). Conduction apraxia. *J. Neurol., Neurosurg. Psychiatry*, **57**, 1241–4.

Pandya, D.N. & Seltzer, B. (1982). Intrinsic connections and architectonics of posterior parietal cortex in the rhesus monkey. *J. Comp. Neurol.*, **204**, 196–210.

Passingham, R. (1993). The frontal lobes and voluntary action. In *Oxford Psychology Series 21*. Oxford: Oxford: University Press.

Pick, A. (1905). *Studien über Motorische Apraxie und ihre Mahestenhende Erscheinungen: ihre Bedeutung in der Symptomatologie Psychopathologischer Symptomenkomplexe*. Leipzig: Deuticke.

Poeck, K. (1983). Ideational apraxia. *J. Neurol.*, **230**, 1–5.

Poizner, H., Clark, M.A., Merians, A.S., Macauley, B., Rothi, L.J.G. & Heilman, K.M. (1995). Joint coordination deficits in limb apraxia. *Brain*, **118**, 227–42.

Pramstaller, P. & Marsden, C.D. (1996). The basal ganglia and apraxia (Review). *Brain*, **119**, 319–41.

Raade, A.S., Rothi, L.J.G. & Heilman, K.M. (1991). The relationship between buccofacial and limb apraxia. *Brain Cognit.*, **16**, 130–46.

Rapcsak, S.Z., Ochipa, C., Beeson, P. & Rubens, A. (1993). Praxis and the right hemisphere. *Brain Cognit.*, **23**, 181–202.

Rizzolatti, G., Fadiga, L., Matelli, M., Bettinardi, V., Paulesu, E. & Perani, D. (1996). Localization of grasp representations in humans by positron emission tomography. 1. Observation versus execution. *Exp. Brain Res.*, **111**, 246–52.

*Rizzolatti, G., Luppino, G. & Matelli, M. (1998). The organization of the cortical motor system: new concepts (Review). *Electroencephalogr. Clin. Neurophysiol.*, **106**, 283–96.

*Rothi, L.J.G., Ochipa, C. & Heilman, K.M. (1991). A cognitive neuropsychological model of limb praxis. *Cogn. Neuropsychol.*, **8**, 443–58.

Rothi, L.J.G., Raymer, A.M. & Heilman, K.M. (1997). Limb praxis assessment. In *Apraxia: the Neuropsychology of Action*, ed. L.J.G. Rothi & K.M. Heilman, pp. 61–74. Hove, UK: Psychology.

*Roy, E.A. & Square, P.A. (1985). Common considerations in the study of limb, verbal, and oral apraxia. In *Neuropsychological Studies of Apraxia and Related Disorders*, ed. E.A. Roy, pp. 111–61. North-Holland: Amsterdam.

Roy, E.A. & Square-Storer, P.A. (1990). The apraxis-correlative studies of fine motor control and action sequencing. In *Cerebral Control of Speech and Limb Movements: Advances in Psychology*, ed. G. Hammond, pp. 477–502. Amsterdam: Elsevier Science.

Rushworth, M.F.S., Nixon, P.D., Wade, D.T., Renowden, S. & Passingham, R.E. (1998). The left hemisphere and the selection of learned actions. *Neuropsychologia*, **36**, 11–24.

Schnider, A., Hanlon, R.E., Alexander, D.N. & Benson, F. (1997). Ideomotor apraxia: behavioural dimensions and neuroanatomical basis. *Brain Lang.*, **58**, 125–36.

Sirigu, A., Cohen, L., Duhamel, J., Pillon, B., Dubois, B. & Agid, Y. (1995). A selective impairment of hand posture for object utilization in apraxia. *Cortex*, **31**, 41–5.

Square-Storer, P.A. & Apeldoorn, S. (1991). An acoustic study of apraxia of speech in patients with different lesion loci. In *Dysarthria and Apraxia of Speech: Perspectives on Managements*, ed. C.A. Moore, K.M. Yorbeton & D.R. Benkelman, pp. 271–86. Baltimore: ML Paul H. Brooks.

Stephan, K.M., Binkofski, F., Halsband, J. et al. (1999). The role of the ventral medial wall motor areas in bimanual co-ordination: a combined lesion and activation study. *Brain*, **122**, 351–68.

Varney, N. & Damasio, H. (1987). Locus of lesion in impaired pantomime recognition. *Cortex*, **23**, 699–703.

Watson, R.T. & Heilman, K.M. (1983). Callosal apraxia. *Brain*, **106**, 391–403.

33

Parkinson's disease

Marian L. Evatt, Mahlon R. DeLong and Jerry L. Vitek

Department of Neurology, Emory University School of Medicine, Atlanta, Georgia, GA, USA

Clinical neuroscience

Movement disorders may be classified as hyperkinetic, characterized by excessive, involuntary movement or hypokinetic, characterized by decreased and slowed movement. First described by James Parkinson in 1817, Parkinson's disease (PD) is the archetypal hypokinetic disorder and the second most common neurodegenerative disorder after Alzheimer's disease. Though incidence and prevalence increase with age, the total estimated incidence is 20/100000 and prevalence is 150/100000 (Schapira, 1999). In the United States, approximately one million patients have PD. The estimated societal cost tops $25 billion (Scheife et al., 2000) and is expected to rise as the population ages.

Parkinsonism: classification/clinical symptoms

'Parkinsonism' is a term describing syndromes combining bradykinesia, tremor, muscle rigidity, gait and balance disturbances. The term 'idiopathic PD' traditionally referred to patients exhibiting two or more of the cardinal signs (rest tremor, rigidity and bradykinesia) who responded to levodopa replacement therapy and did not show evidence of other neurologic disease. Given the discovery of inherited dopa-responsive PD, parkinsonian syndromes with good, sustained clinical response to dopaminergic therapy are best termed 'primary PD' (PPD). Infection, drugs, metabolic abnormalities, or other disease states may cause symptomatic parkinsonism. 'Parkinson-plus' (PD-plus) or atypical parkinsonism includes such syndromes as multiple system atrophy (MSA), progressive supranuclear palsy (PSP), Lewy body disease (LBD), the tauopathies (corticobasalganglionic degeneration and frontotemporal dementias), as well as the amyloidopathies (Alzheimer's

disease with parkinsonism). These conditions typically exhibit little or no response to levodopa therapy, prominent and early gait and balance disturbance, autonomic and cognitive symptoms (Table 33.1). Table 33.2 lists signs and symptoms occuring in PPD and parkinsonian syndromes. See Chapter 34 for further discussion of the atypical syndromes.

Diagnostic criteria and clinical features for primary Parkinson's disease (PPD)

Although James Parkinson published the first description of the 'shaking palsy' almost 200 years ago, we still have no standardized diagnostic test for PPD. Clinical criteria for PPD vary, but most movement disorders experts agree a patient must demonstrate at least two of the three cardinal signs and experience significant, long lasting (>5 years) improvement with dopaminergic therapy (Gelb et al., 1999). With these clinical criteria and experience, neurologists' diagnostic accuracy can approach 92% (Jankovic et al., 2000). Single photon emission tomography (SPECT) or ^{18}Fluoro-dopa scans may support the diagnosis, but these techniques are currently used largely in research studies and require clinical correlation for an accurate diagnosis (Staffen et al., 2000). Thus, history and clinical exam remain the primary determinants of diagnosis.

PD begins insidiously, often with non-specific complaints of malaise, fatigue or weakness. Since most patients manifest symptoms between ages 55 and 65, these symptoms are often attributed to aging or other disorders, particularly if the typical rest tremor is absent. The asymmetric 'pill-rolling' tremor typical of PPD appears at rest and/or with sustained posture, has a frequency of 4–7 hertz (Hz) and improves with movement of the affected limb. The tremor usually begins in the fingers or hand and spreads

Table 33.1. Classification of parkinsonism

Primary parkinsonism
Idiopathic ('sporadic') PD
Genetic primary PD
Identified mutations (rare)
    PARK1 (α-synuclein)
      – 2 mutations
    PARK2 (Parkin gene mutation)
      – multiple polymorphisms
    PARK3

Symptomatic parkinsonism
Drugs
    Antiemetics (e.g. compazine, metoclopramide)
    Neuroleptics
    Dopamine depleting agents (reserpine, tetrabenazine)
    α-methyldopa
    Lithium carbonate
    Valproic acid
    Fluoxetine

Vascular parkinsonism
Parkinson-plus sydromes
    'Alpha-synucleopathies': Multiple systems atrophies and Lewy body dementia
    'Tauopathies' (disorders with primary tau pathology): Progressive supranuclear palsy, Corticobasal degeneration, Fronto-temporal
      dementia
    'Amyloidopathies' (disorders with primary amyloid pathology, secondary tau pathology and dementia): Alzheimer's disease with
      parkinsonism, (Sporadic, APP, PS1 and PS2 related)

Toxins
    1-methyl-1, 2, 4, 6-tetrahydropyridine (MPTP)
    Manganese
    Cyanide
    Methanol
    Carbon monoxide
    Carbon disulfide

Metabolic conditions
    Hypoparathyroidism or pseudo-hypoparathyroidism with basal ganglia calcifications

Miscellaneous acquired conditions
    Normal pressure hydrocephalus
    Catatonia
    Cerebral palsy
    Repeated head trauma ('dementia pugilistica')

Genetic disorders with parkinsonian features
    Wilson's disease
    Hallervorden–Spatz disease
    Chediack Hagashi disease
    SCA-3 spinocerebellar ataxia
    X-linked dystonia–parkinsonism (DYT3)
    Huntington's disease (Westphalt variant)
    Prion disease

Infectious and post-infectious diseases
    Postencephalitic PD
    Neurosyphilis

Table 33.2. Neurologic signs in selected neurodegenerative disorders

Frequency and intensity of neurologic signs in selected neurodegenerative disorders

| | MSA | | | | | | | |
	SND	SDS	OPCA	PSP	PD	DLBD	AD	CBGD
Parkinsonism	++++	+++	++	++++	++++	++++	++	++++
Cerebellar signs	++	+	++++	+	0	0	+	+
Pyramidal signs	++	++++	++	+	++	++	+	+
Autonomic failure	++	++++	++	++	++	+	+	++
Cognitive dysfunction	++	+	++	+++	++	++++	++++	++
Oculomotor impairment	+	+	+++	++++	++	++	+	++
Dysarthria	+++	+	+++	+++	++	++	++	+++
Dysphagia	++	+	++	+++	++	++	++	+
Peripheral neuropathy	+	+	++	+	0	0	+	++
Involuntary movements	+	+	++	+	+++	+++	+	++
Prominent gait problem	++++	++++	++++	++++	++	+++	+	+++

Notes:

0 = none; + = uncommon; ++ = common or moderate; +++ = frequent or marked; ++++ = present in nearly all cases or severe.
SND striatal nigral degeneration; SDS = Shy-Drager Syndrome; OPCA = olivopontocerebellar atrophy; PSP = progressive supranuclear palsy; DLBD = diffuse Lewy body disease; AD = Alzheimer's disease; CBGD = corticobasal ganglionic degeneration.
Source: (From Shulman and Wiener, Multiple System Atrophy. In Watts RL, Koller, WC. Movement Disorders 1997, with permission.)

proximally, usually involving the opposite side within 1–2 years. Parkinsonian tremor may appear in the tongue, jaw or facial muscles, but titubation or voice tremor suggests essential tremor. However, in one familial form of PPD essential tremor may occur as an alternate phenotype (Farrer et al., 1999). Such observations have generated comment about the possible relationship between essential and parkinsonian tremor (Deuschl, 2000).

Patients may appear bradykinetic during both 'automatic' (e.g. walking) and 'commanded' tasks (e.g. rapidly alternating hand pronation/supination) as well as activities of daily living and fine motor tasks. Hypophonic speech is a particularly disabling manifestation of bradykinesia.

The rigidity seen in PPD presents as a uniform resistance to passive limb movement. Although subclinical tremor often imparts a 'cogwheel' quality to parkinsonian rigidity, the rigidity does not vary with velocity, thus differentiating it from spasticity. Patients may report 'heaviness' or 'weakness', but rarely complain of 'rigidity'.

Parkinsonian gait is narrow-based and slow, with short shuffling steps, diminished armswing, and *en-bloc* turning. With advancing disease, patients experience increased problems with initiating gait and 'freezing'. Predominant gait symptoms, ataxic gait and significant postural instability early in the course of the illness suggest atypical PD (Table 33.2).

Although PPD is considered a movement disorder, patients experience multiple associated non-motor signs, symptoms and syndromes (Table 33.3). Cognitive, behavioural and mood changes may reflect disruption of the non-motor circuits that parallel the motor circuits of the basal ganglia or involvement of other biogenic amine systems (Alexander et al., 1990).

Symptomatic PD

At one time, postencephalitic parkinsonism accounted for many of the symptomatic parkinsonian cases seen in clinics. However, after the 1918–1930 epidemic, encephalitis lethargica virtually disappeared. Drug-induced, dementia-associated and vascular parkinsonism are now the most common forms of symptomatic parkinsonism (Rajput et al., 1984; Baldereschi et al., 2000).

Dopamine(DA)-blocking and DA-depleting drugs are commonly associated with symptomatic parkinsonism. These include traditional neuroleptics, antiemetic medications (metoclopramide, promethazine, and prochorperazine) and some antihypertensive agents (reserpine and calcium channel blockers cinnarizine and flunarizine). The motor signs of drug-induced parkinsonism are generally symmetric. Rest tremor occurs less commonly than in PPD. The severity of drug-induced parkinsonism correlates with D2 receptor blocking in the basal ganglia. Newer, 'atypical' antipsychotic drugs differ from the traditional neuroleptics in their receptor binding characteristics. Though the

Table 33.3. Common signs and symptoms in Parkinson's disease

Motor
Dystonia
Hypomimia ('masked faces')
Stooped posture
Propulsive/retropulsive gait
Micrographia
'Freezing' or start hesitation
Difficulty arising from a seated position

Autonomic
Constipation
Urinary dysfunction
Erectile dysfunction
Excessive sweating
Orthostatic hypotension
Drooling
Dry mouth (treated patients)

Sensory
Pain/dysesthesia syndromes

Cognitive/psychiatric
Frontal lobe dysfunction
Depression
Anxiety

Sleep
Restless legs syndrome (RLS)
REM-behaviour sleep disorder (RBD)
Excessive daytime somnolence (EDS)

mechanism of reduced extrapyramidal side effects (EPS) associated with atypical antipsychotics is uncertain, it seems related to a higher serotonin to DA blockade ratio and a relatively higher affinity for D3 receptors. Using 'atypical' neuroleptics (clozapine, quetiapine, olanzepine) reduces the risk of drug-induced parkinsonism, but even these atypical agents have been reported to cause parkinsonism (Glazer, 2000; Modestin et al., 2000). Multiple other drugs, including valproate, have been reported to induce parkinsonism, but the mechanism is unclear (Armon et al., 1996; Onofrj et al., 1998).

Although experts agree vascular parkinsonism exists, its precise phenotype is less clear. In general, affected patients have akinetic-rigid 'lower body' symptoms with prominent gait and balance problems. Action tremor is seen more commonly than in PPD. Associated findings include vascular risk factors, atherosclerotic disease, upper motor neuron signs, pseudobulbar palsy, and dementia. Dopaminergic therapy offers little benefit and anticholin-

ergics and amantadine frequently induce hallucinosis or delerium. These clinical signs and evidence of diffuse white matter disease on imaging studies suggest vascular parkinsonism, but postmortem examination is necessary to exclude other causes of parkinsonism.

Etiology: pathology, genetics and pathogenic theories

Gross examination of the brainstem of a patient with PPD reveals the classic loss of pigmentation in the substantia nigra (SN). The basal ganglia (caudate, putamen, globus pallidus) appear normal. On microscopic examination, one sees loss of neuromelanin-containing neurons and gliosis in the substantia nigra pars compacta (SNc). This loss causes DA deficiency in the striatum and in extrastriatal nigral projections to the motor and limbic basal ganglia circuits (Braak & Braak, 2000). The motor portion of the striatum (the putamen) is the earliest and most severely depleted, most likely accounting for the early development of skeletal signs and symptoms.

Large, round, intracellular eosinophilic inclusions, named Lewy bodies (LB) after the neuropathologist who first described them in 1912, are seen in the nigral pigmented neurons as well as multiple other cortical and subcortical locations. These inclusions contain abnormally phosphorylated neurofilaments and have a halo surrounding a core that stains with antibodies to both ubiquitin and α-synuclein. Lewy bodies are found in the SN in about 75% of clinically diagnosed PPD cases and are considered a pathological hallmark for Parkinson's disease. However, LB have also been described in other neurodegenerative diseases including Alzheimer's disease, some prion diseases and diffuse Lewy Body disease (DLBD). They are not present in autosomal recessive juvenile parkinsonism (ARJP) and thus are sensitive, but not specific for PPD.

At least four different mutations (Park1, Park2, Park3, Park4, Table 33.4) have been described in families whose clinical course is consistent with PPD. Two of these mutations (Park1 and Park3) are in genes coding for α-synuclein and an enzyme involved in ubiquitin metabolism. Both ubiquitin and α-synuclein are major components of LB. Mutant proteins may self-aggregate and form the cores of LB or contribute to the selective vunerability of dopaminergic neurons to oxidant stress (Riess et al., 2000; Polymeropoulos et al., 1997). A third mutation, (Park2) (Matsumine et al., 1998) is found in ARJP patients who have not demonstrated LB when autopsied. This lack of LB in ARJP and the finding of DLBD pathology in a Park4

Table 33.4. Genetically mediated dopa-responsive parkinsonism

Gene	Chromosome	Inheritance	Gene product	Phenotype
Park1	4q21–23	AD	missense mutation in α-synuclein	onset <50 years old, rapid progressive, +Lewy bodies
Park2	6q25–27	AR	point mutation or deletion of parkin gene	onset <40 years, dopa-responsive; early motor fluctuations
Park3	2p	AD	?	40% penetrance
Park 4	4p15	AD	missense mutation of ubiqutin carboxy terminal hydrolase L1	PPD and essential tremor phenotypes

affected patient illustrates the difficulty of classifying parkinsonism solely on clinical or pathologic criteria.

Uncertainty surrounding genetic and environmental factors in PPD has been the rule. A small percentage of cases are familial, but the role of heredity in sporadic cases has been questioned. Early twin studies revealed conflicting concordance results and argued against heredity playing a significant role in PPD. However, monozygotic twins in these studies were prematurely classified discordant (Piccini et al., 1999), suggesting genetics may factor in development of some forms of parkinsonism. The 40% penetrance of the Park3 mutation makes it a target of investigation as a 'risk factor' for sporadic PPD.

Though it is not yet clear how mutations in these genes are related to the selective SN cell death seen in PD, other genetic polymorphisms or mutations may also play a role. Kruger et al., reported apolipoprotein E4 combined with a certain α-synuclein allele increases the risk of a person developing PD (Kruger et al., 1999). Furthermore, apoE genotype may modulate the age of PPD onset (Zareparsi et al., 1997).

Oxidative stress, along with mitochondrial dysfunction, excess nitric oxide formation, and inflammatory processes are all considered contributors to accelerated dopaminergic neuronal apoptosis and development of PPD. Increased glutamatergic output from the subthalamic nucleus (STN) may contribute to degeneration of SN_c neurons via excitotoxic mechanisms (Marsden & Olanow, 1998). Inflammatory responses have also been implicated as glial cells may accelerate DA cell loss via release of cytokines (Hirsch et al., 1998). The 30% decrease in mitochondrial complex I activity found in SN neurons in PPD may contribute to a lowered threshold for apoptosis or susceptiblity to environmental toxins (Schapira et al., 1998).

Langston's description of parkinsonism induced by 1-methyl-4-phenyl-1, 2, 3, 6-tetrahydropyridine (MPTP, a neurotoxic contaminant of synthetic heroin), suggested environmental toxins could precipitate PPD and lead to the development of the primate MPTP model of PD (Langston et al., 1983). MPTP is converted to MPP+ by monoaminoxidase-B (MAO-B). MPP+, a mitochondrial complex I inhibitor, is concentrated in dopaminergic cells by the DA re-uptake system. Thus, MPP+ is selectively toxic to the striatal-nigral system, producing motor deficits in humans, non-human primates and a few other species that closely mimic the clinical signs of PPD. These motor symptoms respond to antiparkinson medications. In addition, MPTP-treated animals may develop dyskinesias and dystonic postures, though MPTP-induced tremor is usually seen with posture rather than at rest. As with motor symptoms, MPTP pathology varies from PPD pathology. Notably, LB are not seen (though older primates may show LB-like inclusions) and MPTP damage is selective for the SN_C. The first model to nearly replicate PPD motor signs, MPTP-parkinsonism is currently the standard to which other models are compared and by which new PPD treatments are tested.

Recently, Greenamyre et al. (1999) and Betarbet and Greenamyre (2000) described a new model of PPD based on chronic, low-level exposure of rats to rotenone, a mitochondrial respiratory chain inhibitor, an 'organic' pesticide used in gardening and aquamanagement. This model appears to more closely mimic the time course and neurobiology of PPD than the MPTP model, but its development in primates and confirmation of its validity awaits further study.

Pathophysiology circuit

The basal ganglia are viewed as components of multiple segregated circuits, including motor, oculomotor, associative, and limbic circuits (Alexander et al., 1990). The motor circuit is implicated in the pathophysiology of both hypo- and hyperkinetic movement disorders (DeLong, 1990). It originates from pre- and postcentral sensorimotor fields and includes specific portions of the putamen, the external

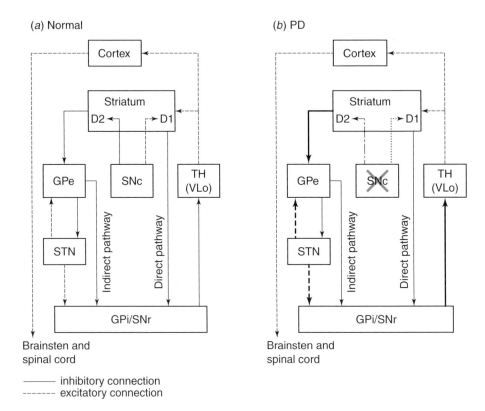

Fig. 33.1. Physiology model of PD. GPe = globus pallidus, external segment; SN$_C$ = substantia nigra, pars compacta; TH = thalamus; VLo = ventrolateral nucleus; STN = subthalamic nucleus; GPi = globus pallidus, internal segment; SNr = substantia nigra, pars reticulata.

(GPe) and internal (GPi) segments of the globus pallidus, the substantia nigra pars reticulata (SNr), the subthalamic nucleus (STN) and portions of the motor thalamus (ventralis lateralis pars oralis, (VLo) and ventralis anterior, (VA)), and returns to the same precentral motor fields from which it originates (Alexander et al., 1990). The striatum (the major input structure of the basal ganglia), influences GPi and SNr (the major output structures), via two routes: a 'direct' pathway from striatum to GPi/SNr and an 'indirect' pathway from the striatum via the GPe and STN (Fig. 33.1).

All the intrinsic connections of the basal ganglia are inhibitory, except for the STN→GPi/SNr pathway, which is excitatory. The dopaminergic nigrostriatal pathway appears to modulate the activity of the two striato-pallidal pathways by activating different DA receptor subtypes (D1 and D2). Thus, DA appears to facilitate transmission in the 'direct' pathway via D$_1$ receptors and to inhibit transmission in the 'indirect' pathway via D$_2$ receptors (Albin et al., 1989; Gerfen et al., 1990). Output from GPi/SNr exerts a tonic inhibition on thalamocortical neurons (Yoshida et al., 1972).

Based on this model of intrinsic basal ganglia circuitry, putamenal DA depletion leads to increased mean dis-

charge rates of GPi neurons, excessive inhibition of the thalamic pallidal receiving areas, and correspondingly reduced thalamocortical activity. Consistent with model predictions, single neuron recording studies in parkinsonian animals demonstrated increased tonic discharge rates of GPi neurons and reduced discharge rates in VLo (the pallidal receiving area) (Miller & DeLong, 1988; Filion et al., 1991; Vitek et al., 1994). The observed increases in tonic activity in GPi neurons indicate increased activity in the 'indirect' pathway and decreased activity in the 'direct' pathway in parkinsonian conditions. Increasing striatal inhibition leads to decreased GPe activity, which increases STN activity (Filion et al., 1989, 1991; Bergman et al., 1990). It is proposed that increased STN activity increases GPi output, which, in turn, suppresses thalamocortical activity and leads to dyskinesia and bradykinesia (DeLong, 1990). Consistent with these predictions, temporary or permanent inactivation of the GPi or STN, (in both animal PD models and patients with PPD) is associated with significant improvement in parkinsonian motor signs (Bergman et al., 1990; Wichmann et al., 1994; Lozano et al., 1995; Baron et al., 1996; Gross et al., 1997; Lang et al., 1997; Kumar et al., 1998; Vitek et al., 1998a, b; Volkmann et al.,

1998). Furthermore, this improvement in parkinsonian motor signs coincides with increased cortical metabolic activity (supplementary motor area and dorsolateral prefrontal cortex) (Grafton et al., 1995; Eidelberg et al., 1996; Davis et al., 1997; Samuel et al., 1997; Limousin et al., 1997).

However, this scheme of basal ganglia function (based solely on changes in discharge rate) has several problems. The model predicts that thalamotomy should worsen parkinsonian motor signs by further reducing thalamocortical activity. Contrary to these predictions, most studies report that thalamotomy causes little or no change in bradykinesia, but is highly effective in alleviating parkinsonian tremor and rigidity (Narabayashi, 1986; Montastruc et al., 1994). The model also predicts that pallidotomy should induce excessive involuntary movement (dyskinesias), by disinhibiting the thalamus and increasing thalamocortical activity. However pallidotomy is very effective in alleviating levodopa-induced dyskinesias in addition to improving rigidity, bradykinesia and tremor. These observations are difficult to reconcile with the hypothesis that rate changes alone account for the development of PPD. Many investigators have suggested the observed changes in the pattern of discharge and increased synchronization of neuronal activity reported in animal models and humans with PD play an important role in PPD motor symptoms (Hutchison et al., 1994; Nina et al., 1995; Wichmann & DeLong, 1996; Raz et al., 1997; Vitek, 1997; Vitek et al., 1998).

Changes in pallidal and thalamic receptive field characteristics and neuronal activity patterns (in addition to (or as well as) the levels of neuronal activity) likely provide a significant contribution to the development of parkinsonian motor signs. Disruption of the normal spatio-temporal pattern of cortical neuronal activity may disrupt thalamocortical signal transmission. In the MPTP rodent PD model, improvement of parkinsonian motor signs follows lesioning of the STN. The resulting normalization of pallidal and thalamic neuronal activity (Ryan & Sanders, 1993) coincides with normalization of cortical metabolic activity patterns and improvement in motor signs after stereotactic surgeries in humans with PPD (Grafton et al., 1995; Eidelberg et al., 1996; Davis et al., 1997; Limousin et al., 1997; Samuel et al., 1997). Thus, thalamotomy and pallidotomy are effective in alleviating parkinsonian motor signs because each removes or reduces abnormal neuronal activity that disrupts function in the motor circuit.

Therapeutic principles

The main treatment goals are controlling secondary disability and minimizing associated complications (decon-

ditioning, joint contractures, fractures, etc.) with symptomatic therapy. For all patients, adjunctive therapies including daily stretching and regular physical activity are strongly recommended. Stretching helps maintain flexibility, decreasing the risk of injury from falls, and exercise training may decrease parkinsonian signs (Schenkman et al., 1998; Reuter et al., 1999). Several detailed algorithms for managing early and late PD have recently been published (Olanow & Koller, 1998; Silver & Ruggieri, 1998). The treatment options outlined below fall into three categories: symptom relief, prevention of l-dopa side effects and neuroprotective strategies.

Still considered the most potent symptomatic antiparkinson agent, l-dopa first became widely available in the early 1970s. Although initially administered in high doses without regard to long-term complications, dyskinesias and motor fluctuations were soon observed with chronic l-dopa treatment. Fifty percent of patients with PPD develop dyskinesias after 5 years of l-dopa therapy (Friedman, 1985; Blanchet et al., 1996; Denny & Behari, 1999) and current evidence suggests that the emergence and severity of dyskinesias depend on damaged nigrostriatum exposed to supraphysiologic pulsatile dopaminergic stimulation (Schuh & Bennett, 1993; Chase et al., 1994; Bedard et al., 1999). Younger patients appear more susceptible to motor fluctuations (Quinn et al., 1987; Gibb & Lees, 1988; Giovannini et al., 1991; Pantelatos & Fornadi, 1993; Friedman, 1994; Schrag et al., 1998), and it may be particularly important in younger patients to avoid l-dopa therapy as long as possible. Concerns over such l-dopa-induced side effects and neurotoxicity have led to an ever-increasing emphasis on l-dopa sparing and the early use of DA agonists (Montastruc et al., 1994; Rinne et al., 1998; Rascol et al., 2000; Shulman, 2000).

In addition to priming the basal ganglia for development of dyskinesias, l-dopa neurotoxicity could occur through oxidative stress. L-dopa metabolism generates free radicals, hydrogen peroxide and quinones, all of which can create oxidative stress in dopaminergic neurons. Administering supplemental l-dopa could accelerate or promote apoptotic death of dopaminergic cells. However, evidence from several studies suggests l-dopa delays death in elderly parkinsonian patients about 5 years (Clarke, 1995). Review of the l-dopa toxicity literature (including autopsy cases) found no evidence of l-dopa neurotoxicity in doses comparable to those used clinically (Agid et al., 1999; Weiner, 1999). More recently, Datla et al., provided evidence chronic l-dopa may be protective in 6-hydroxydopamine-lesioned rats (Datla et al., 2001).

The most common side effects of l-dopa are nausea, vomiting, orthostatic hypotension, and hallucinosis. L-dopa is converted to DA in both the periphery and the brain; while l-dopa crosses the blood–brain barrier, DA does not. Combining l-dopa with a peripheral decarboxylase inhibitor (carbidopa) increases the amount of available l-dopa for conversion to DA in the brain. Levodopa conversion to DA in the area postrema is decreased, thereby decreasing nausea and vomiting. Domperidone, a peripheral DA receptor antagonist, may be used as an antiemetic.

Several other agents commonly used for symptomatic management of PPD include DA agonists, anti-cholinergics, amantadine and catechol-*o*-methyl transferase (COMT) inhibitors. Dopamine agonists offer the advantage of directly stimulating postsynaptic DA receptors, thus bypassing the degenerating nigrostriatal nerve terminals. Other advantages include lack of competition with dietary amino acids for absorption and transport into the brain (Rabey, 1995), longer duration of action than standard carbidopa/l-dopa (thus providing more sustained DA receptor stimulation) and lack of auto-oxidation (thus reducing free radical generation and reducing oxidative stress) (Olanow, 1992).

The DA agonists currently used in the United States include ergotamine derivatives (bromocriptine and pergolide) and non-ergolines (pramipexole and ropinirole). Dopamine agonists vary in their affinity for dopamine receptor subtypes and 5-hydroxytryptiline (5-HT) receptors, but none of these compounds has shown clinical superiority in alleviating symptoms. Cabergoline is a long-acting agonist that is clinically available in Europe, but its use in the United States is limited to the treatment of hyperprolactinemia. Apomorphine and lisuride, also available in Europe, have the advantage of parenteral administration. Apomorphine, with its short half-life may be particularly helpful for patients with severe motor fluctuations. The nonergoline structure of ropinerole and pramipexole potentially could limit such side effects as orthostatic hypotension and should decrease the occurrence of pulmonary and retroperitoneal fibrosis associated with ergoline compounds.

Anticholinergic drugs, the first drugs shown to improve parkinsonian symptoms (Duvoisin, 1967), help balance the relative cholinergic excess caused by DA depletion. Though mildly beneficial for rigidity and bradykinesia, anticholinergics are now largely added to target tremor symptoms. Currently used anticholinergics include trihexyphenidyl (Artane), benztropine (Cogentin), and biperiden (Akineton). Ethopropazine (Parsitan) is no longer manufactured in the United States, but can be obtained from Canada and some compounding pharma-

cies in the United States. Neuropsychiatric and cognitive side effects limit anticholinergic usefulness.

Amantadine, an antiviral agent serendipitously discovered to have anti-parkinson activity, is thought to act by blocking the reuptake of DA into presynaptic neurons, directly stimulating postsynaptic DA receptors, and possibly inhibiting cholinergic activity (Bailey & Stone, 1975; Calne, 1993). More recently, Stoof, et al., recognized that amantadine may act as an NMDA receptor antagonist (Stoof et al., 1992). Amantadine can provide effective monotherapy in early PD, but more importantly provides significant (up to 60%) reduction in dyskinesias (Metman et al., 1999).

As PPD progresses, intracellular DA storage capacity declines and the DA availability becomes more closely tied to circulating blood levels. The COMT inhibitors entacapone and tolcapone have been studied as adjunctive therapy in PD and can extend the duration of l-dopa action by reducing the peripheral degradation of l-dopa. COMT catalyses the breakdown of l-dopa to 3-*o*-methyldopa (3-OMD). Tolcapone and entacapone both inhibit COMT peripherally, and tolcapone also inhibits COMT centrally. Both increase the fraction of l-dopa available to enter the brain. Thus, concomitant l-dopa and COMT inhibitor administration may provide more stable concentrations than can be achieved by fractionating the carbidopa/l-dopa dose or by using controlled release l-dopa formulations.

In addition to symptomatic treatment, neuroprotective strategies are receiving increasing interest. Several clinical trials are in progress to investigate whether DA agonists and such other medications as riluzole could slow PD progression (Dunnett & Bjorklund, 1999). Selegeline was one of the first drugs clinically studied for potential neuroprotection. In the DATATOP study, vitamin E (dosed at 400 IU/day) did not significantly delay the need for l-dopa initiation. Selegeline did delay initiation of l-dopa therapy, but its symptomatic benefit and long washout period confounded this endpoint. Whether seleginine slows the progression of PD remains an unanswered question.

The search for neuroprotection continues with DA agonists and other agents (Marsden & Olanow, 1998; Olanow et al., 1998; Schapira, 1999) Multiple lines of evidence suggest DA agonists may be neuroprotective. Dopamine agonists diminish the need for l-dopa and may therefore minimize the formation of toxic metabolites. In addition, recent evidence suggests that DA agonists have direct antioxidant effects possibly by acting as free radical scavengers (Yoshikawa et al., 1994).

Associated management issues

Coexisting illnesses (e.g. depression, dementia and manic-depressive disorder) can make patients more susceptible to medication side effects and may require the treating neurologist to manage more than the motor manifestations of PPD. Depression, occuring in up to 40% of PPD patients (Cummings & Masterman, 1999), may exacerbate parkinsonian signs and symptoms. Depressed PD patients may be managed similarly to other depressed geriatric patients. Many pharmacists are reluctant to dispense antidepressants to patients who are also taking selegeline, but concern regarding a potential 'serotonin syndrome' interaction is not generally warranted (Heinonen & Myllyla, 1998; Ahlskog, 1999). Patients should also be screened for other medical causes of depression (e.g. hypothyroidism, B12 deficiency).

Patients with cognitive impairment are particularly susceptible to delusions, frank hallucinosis and thought disruption from overstimulation of DA receptors. With a higher ratio of serotonin $5HT_{2a}$ to DA D_2 blockage, the newer atypical antipsychotics clozapine and quetiapine are particularly useful in managing such complications (Juncos, 1999). Electroconvulsive therapy may benefit both depression and parkinsonian symptoms (Anderson et al., 1987).

Along with neuropsychiatric issues, PD patients commonly suffer sleep disruption (Clarenbach, 2000; Larsen et al., 2000; Razmy & Shapiro, 2000). Restless legs syndrome (RLS), a common disorder, responds to DA agents but may be exacerbated by some of the antidepressants used to control depressive symptoms. REM behaviour disorder is a parasomnia commonly seen in PPD. Finally, excessive daytime somnolence and sleep attacks related to dopaminergic therapy are also common in PPD and can be extremely disabling and dangerous (Clarenbach, 2000).

Surgical therapy

Patients with PPD whose motor symptoms can no longer be adequately controlled by medical therapy or who develop intractable drug-induced side effects are candidates for surgical therapy (Fine et al., 2000). Surgical procedures for PD include restorative measures (transplantation using fetal, porcine or retinal tissue), ablative procedures (thalamotomy, pallidotomy and subthalamotomy) and chronic stimulation procedures (thalamic, pallidal, subthalamic).

Although the initial efforts to replace dying dopaminergic neurons with autologous adrenal transplants benefited some patients, such transplants do not offer enough benefit to justify such treatment routinely. Fetal cell transplants seem to offer the best results in animal models and have been tried in humans. Although patients have shown improved bradykinesia and rigidity, freezing and tremor was unaffected and some patients developed severe 'runaway' dyskinesias, even off medications (Fahn, 2000; Freed et al., 2001). Transplant clinical trials thus far have included only patients with advanced PPD, but these patients may not be the ideal candidates for a such a procedure. In the future, transplantation may be a standard therapy, but currently many issues limit it to experimental status.

Thalamotomy is effective for the treatment of Parkinsonian tremor (Tasker, 1998a, b; Linhares & Tasker, 2000). Lesions are generally placed in the cerebellar receiving area, (the ventralis intermedius (V_{im}) nucleus). If extended more anteriorly into the basal ganglia receiving areas (ventralis oralis posterior and ventralis oralis anterior), thalamotomy may also improve rigidity and drug-induced dyskinesias. Thalamotomy is not effective for bradykinesia, freezing, postural instability or the gait disorder associated with PD. Due to an unacceptably high incidence (30–50%) of aphasia, dysarthria or dysphonia, bilateral thalamotomy is not recommended.

A number of studies have demonstrated that pallidotomy is effective for PPD. Lesions within the posteroventral 'sensorimotor' portion of the GPi improve all the cardinal motor signs of PD including tremor, rigidity, bradykinesia, as well as motor fluctuations, drug-induced dyskinesias and dystonia. Although pallidotomy may also improve axial symptoms including gait, balance and freezing, such benefit following unilateral pallidotomy is less consistent than that for appendicular symptoms and many patients lose their benefit 6 months to 2 years postpallidotomy. Bilateral pallidotomy reportedly benefits axial symptoms, but is associated with an unacceptably high incidence of hypophonia. Urinary incontinence and cognitive decline have also been reported following bilateral pallidotomy, though these complications occur less commonly and may result from lesions that encroach on non-motor areas of GPi and/or the internal capsule. Lack of postpallidotomy improvement suggests the patient does not have idiopathic PD or was lesioned outside of the sensorimotor portion of the GPi (Vitek et al., 1998; Eskander et al., 2000).

In recent years, deep brain stimulation (DBS) via implanted electrodes has been employed in place of stereotactic ablation. An implantable programmable pulse generator activates the electrodes. Chronic DBS may reversibly suppress or normalize neuronal activity in neurons by activating an inhibitory interneurons, depolarization block, interupting or normalizing irregular and abnormally bursting activity patterns.

Widely used in Europe, thalamic DBS is now FDA approved for tremor in the United States. Thalamic DBS is effective in the treatment of parkinsonian and other forms of tremor. However, since additional motor symptoms inevitably develop in PPD, pallidotomy or pallidal or sub-thalamic DBS, should be recommended for PPD patients. Bilateral DBS in the STN or GPi can be performed as a staged procedure or simultaneously. Although some centres support using STN DBS for midline symptoms and GPi DBS for dyskinesias, both procedures are effective in treating the cardinal motor signs of PD and may allow reduced dosing of antiparkinson medications (Burchiel et al., 1999; Krause et al., 2001). Kumar and others have reported benefit lasting 6 to 12 months though the long-term effect of DBS remains ill-defined (Krause et al., 2001).

Future directions: prevention and/or restoration

In the future, treatment strategies will likely provide neuroprotection and neurorescue in PPD (Schapira, 1999). Strategies which decrease iron, lipid peroxidation products and reactive oxygen species accumulation, increase antioxidant concentrations, and improve mitochondrial dysfunction may help accomplish these goals. Such anti-apoptotic agents as the neuroimmunophylins offer another potential avenue of rescue and protection and anti-glutaminergic drugs are being investigated as disease modifying agents. Lastly, transplant studies are currently under way with DA-producing human and pig mesencephalic tissue, genetically engineered dopaminergic cells, and cells expressing trophic factors (GDNF and BDNF). Recently, Kordower et al., successfully delivered glial cell line derived nerve growth factor (GDNF) via a lentiviral injection into the striatum and substantia nigra (Kordower et al., 2000) of rhesus monkeys. The implants successfully expressed GDNF, improved markers of dopaminergic function in MPTP-treated monkeys. Most importantly, the monkeys improved clinically and in quantitative motor testing.

References

Agid, Y., Ahlskog, E., Albanese, A. et al. (1999). Levodopa in the treatment of Parkinson's disease: a consensus meeting. *Mov. Disord.*, **14**(6), 911–13.

Ahlskog, J.E. (1999). Medical treatment of later-stage motor problems of Parkinson disease. *Mayo Clin. Proc.*, **74**(12), 1239–54.

Albin, R.L., Young, A.B. & Penney, J.B. (1989). The functional anatomy of basal ganglia disorders. [see comments]. *Trends Neurosci.* **12**(10), 366–75.

Alexander, G.E., Crutcher, M.D. & DeLong, M.R. (1990). Basal ganglia-thalamocortical circuits: parallel substrates for motor, oculomotor, 'prefrontal' and 'limbic' functions. In *Progress in Brain Research*, ed. H.B.M. Uylings. New York: Elsevier Science Publishers.

Andersen, K., Balldin, J., Gottifres, C.G. et al. (1987). A double-blind evaluation of electroconvulsive therapy in Parkinson's disease with 'on–off' phenomena. *Acta Neurol. Scand.*, **76**(3), 191–9.

Armon, C., Shin, C., Miller, P. et al. (1996). Reversible parkinsonism and cognitive impairment with chronic valproate use. *Neurology*, **47**(3), 626–35.

Bailey, E.V. & Stone, T.W. (1975). The mechanism of action of amantadine in Parkinsonism: a review. *Arch. Int. Pharmacodyn. Ther.*, **216**(2), pp. 246–62.

Baldereschi, M., Di Carlo, A., Rocca, W.A. et al. (2000). Parkinson's disease and parkinsonism in a longitudinal study: two-fold higher incidence in men. ILSA Working Group. Italian Longitudinal Study on Aging. *Neurology*, **55**(9), 1358–63.

Baron, M.S., Vitek, J.L., Bakay, R.A. et al. (1996). Treatment of advanced Parkinson's disease by posterior GPi pallidotomy: 1-year results of a pilot study [see comments]. *Ann. Neurol.*, **40**(3), 355–66.

Bedard, P.J., Blanchet, P.J., Levesque, D. et al. (1999). Pathophysiology of L-dopa-induced dyskinesias. *Mov. Disord.*, **14**(Suppl. 1), 4–8.

Bergman, H., Wichmann, T. & DeLong, M.R. (1990). Reversal of experimental parkinsonism by lesions of the subthalamic nucleus. *Science*, **249**(4975), 1436–8.

Blanchet, P.J., Allard, P., Gregoire, L., Tardif, F. & Bedard, P.J. (1996). Risk factors for peak dose dyskinesia in 100 levodopa-treated parkinsonian patients. *Can. J. Neurol. Sci.*, **23**(3), 189–93.

Braak, H. & Braak, E. (2000). Pathoanatomy of Parkinson's disease. *J. Neurol.*, **247**(Suppl. 2), II3–10.

Burchiel, K.J., Anderson, V.C., Favre, J. & Hammerstad, J.P. (1999). Comparison of pallidal and subthalamic nucleus deep brain stimulation for advanced Parkinson's disease: results of a randomized, blinded pilot study. *Neurosurgery*, **45**(6), 1375–84.

Calne, D.B. (1993). Treatment of Parkinson's disease [see comments]. *N. Engl. J. Med.*, **329**(14), 1021–7.

Chase, T.N., Engber, T.M. & Mouradian, M.M. (1994). Palliative and prophylactic benefits of continuously administered dopaminomimetics in Parkinson's disease. *Neurology*, **44**(7 Suppl. 6), S15–18.

Clarenbach, P. (2000). Parkinson's disease and sleep. *J. Neurol.*, **247**(Suppl. 4), IV/20–3.

Clarke, C.E. (1995). Does levodopa therapy delay death in Parkinson's disease? A review of the evidence [see comments]. *Mov. Disord.*, **10**(3), 250–6.

Cummings, J.L. & Masterman, D.L. (1999). Depression in patients with Parkinson's disease. *Int. J. Geriat. Psychiatry*, **14**(9), 711–18.

Datla, K.P., Blunt, S.B. & Dexter, D.T. (2001). Chronic L-DOPA administration is not toxic to the remaining dopaminergic nigrostriatal neurons, but instead may promote their functional recovery, in rats with partial 6–OHDA or FeCl(3) nigrostriatal lesions. *Mov. Disord.*, **16**(3), 424–34.

Davis, K.D., Taub, E., Houle, S. et al. (1997). Globus pallidus stimulation activates the cortical motor system during alleviation of parkinsonian symptoms [see comments]. *Nat. Med.*, **3**(6), 671–4.

DeLong, M.R. (1990). Primate models of movement disorders of basal ganglia origin. *Trends Neurosci.*, **13**(7), 281–5.

Denny, A.P. & Behari, M. (1999). Motor fluctuations in Parkinson's disease. *J. Neurol. Sci.*, **165**(1), 18–23.

Deuschl, (2000). The pathophysiology of parkinsonian tremor: a review. *J. Neurol.*, **247**(Suppl. 5), V33–48.

Dunnett, S.B. & Bjorklund, P.A. (1999). Prospects for new restorative and neuroprotective treatments in Parkinson's disease. *Nature*, **399**(6738 Suppl.), A32–9.

Duvoisin, R.C. (1967). Cholinergic–anticholinergic antagonism in parkinsonism. *Arch. Neurol.*, **17**(2), 124–36.

Eidelberg, D., Moeller, J.R., Ishakawa, T. et al. (1996). Regional metabolic correlates of surgical outcome following unilateral pallidotomy for Parkinson's disease. *Ann. Neurol.*, **39**(4), 450–9.

Eskandar, E.N., Shinobu, L.A., Penney, J.B., Jr, Cosgrove, G.R. & Connihan, T.J. (2000). Stereotactic pallidotomy performed without using microelectrode guidance in patients with Parkinson's disease: surgical technique and 2-year results. *J. Neurosurg.*, **92**(3), 375–83.

Fahn, S. (2000). Double-blind controlled trial of embryonic dopaminergic tissue transplants in advanced Parkinson's disease. In 6th International Congress of Parkinson's Disease and Movement Disorders, Barcelona, Spain.

Farrer, M., Gwinn-Hardy, K., Muenter, M. et al. (1999). A chromosome 4p haplotype segregating with Parkinson's disease and postural tremor. *Hum. Mol. Genet.*, **8**(1), 81–5.

Filion, M., Tremblay, L. & Bedard, P.J. (1989). *Excessive and Unselective Responses of Medial Pallidal Neurons to both Passive Movements and Striatal Stitmulation in Monkeys with MPTP-induced Parkinsonism*, pp. 157–64. London: John Libbey.

Filion, M., Tremblay, L. & Bedard, P.J. (1991). Effects of dopamine agonists on the spontaneous activity of globus pallidus neurons in monkeys with MPTP-induced parkinsonism. *Brain Res.*, **547**(1), 152–61.

Fine, J., Duff, J., Chen, R. et al. (2000). Long-term follow-up of unilateral pallidotomy in advanced Parkinson's disease. *N. Engl. J. Med.*, **342**(23), 1708–14.

Freed, C.R., Grerene, P.E., Breeze, R.E. et al. (2001). Transplantation of embryonic dopamine neurons for severe Parkinson's disease. *N. Engl. J. Med.*, **344**(10), 710–19.

Friedman, A. (1985). Levodopa-induced dyskinesia: clinical observations. *J. Neurol.*, **232**(1), 29–31.

Friedman, A. (1994). Old-onset Parkinson's disease compared with young-onset disease: clinical differences and similarities. *Acta Neurol. Scand.*, **89**(4), 258–61.

Gelb, D.J., Oliver, E. & Gilman, S. (1999). Diagnostic criteria for Parkinson disease. *Arch. Neurol.*, **56**(1), 33–9.

Gerfen, C.R., Engber, T.M., Mahan, L.C. et al. (1990). D1 and D2 dopamine receptor-regulated gene expression of striatonigral and striatopallidal neurons [see comments]. *Science*, **250**(4986), 1429–32.

Gibb, W.R. & Lees, A.J. (1988). *A* comparison of clinical and pathological features of young- and old-onset Parkinson's disease. *Neurology*, **38**(9), 1402–6.

Giovannini, P., Piccolo, I., Genitrini, S. et al. (1991). Early-onset Parkinson's disease. *Mov. Disord.*, **6**(1), 36–42.

Glazer, W.M. (2000). Extrapyramidal side effects, tardive dyskinesia, and the concept of atypicality. *J. Clin. Psychiatry*, **61**(3), 16–21.

Grafton, S.T., Waters, C., Sutton, J., Lew, M.F. & Couldwell, W. (1995). Pallidotomy increases activity of motor association cortex in Parkinson's disease: a positron emission tomographic study. *Ann. Neurol.*, **37**(6), 776–83.

Greenamyre, J.T., Mackenzie, G., Peng, T.I. & Stephens, S.E. (1999). Mitochondrial dysfunction in Parkinson's disease. *Biochem. Soc. Symp.*, **66**, 85–97.

Gross, C., Rougier, A., Guehl, D. et al. (1997). High-frequency stimulation of the globus pallidus internalis in Parkinson's disease: a study of seven cases. *J. Neurosurg.*, **87**(4), 491–8.

Heinonen, E.H. & Myllyla, V. (1998). Safety of selegiline (deprenyl) in the treatment of Parkinson's disease. *Drug Safety*, **19**(1), 11–22.

Hirsch, E.C.P., Hunot, S.P., Damier, P.M.D.P. & Faucheux, B.P. (1998). Glial Cells and inflammation in parkinson's disease: a role in neurodegeneration? [Miscellaneous article]. *Ann. Neurol. Cell Death, Neuroprotection in Parkinson's Dis.*, **44**(3)(Suppl. 1), S115–20.

Hutchison, W.D., Lozano, A.M., Davis, K.D. et al. (1994). Differential neuronal activity in segments of globus pallidus in Parkinson's disease patients. *Neuroreport*, **5**(12), 1533–7.

Jankovic, J., Rajput, A.H., McDermott, M.P. & Perl, D.P. (2000). The evolution of diagnosis in early Parkinson disease. Parkinson Study Group. *Arch. Neurol.*, **57**(3), 369–72.

Juncos, J.L. (1999). Management of psychotic aspects of Parkinson's disease. *J. Clin. Psychiatry*, **60**(Suppl. 8), 42–53.

Kordower, J.H., Emborg, M.E., Bloch, J. et al. (2000). Neurodegeneration prevented by lentiviral vector delivery of GDNF in primate models of Parkinson's disease. *Science*, **290**(5492), 767–73.

Krause, M., Fogel, W., Heck, A. et al. (2001). Deep brain stimulation for the treatment of Parkinson's disease: subthalamic nucleus versus globus pallidus internus. *J. Neurol., Neurosurg. Psychiatry*, **70**(4), 464–70.

Kruger, R., Vieira-Saecher, A.M., Kuhn, W. et al. (1999). Increased susceptibility to sporadic Parkinson's disease by a certain combined alpha-synuclein/apolipoprotein E genotype. *Ann. Neurol.*, **45**(5), 611–17.

Kumar, R., Lozano, A.M., Montgomery, E. & Lang, A.E. (1998). Pallidotomy and deep brain stimulation of the pallidum and subthalamic nucleus in advanced Parkinson's disease. *Mov. Disord.*, **13**(Suppl. 1), 73–82.

Kumar, R., Lang, A., Rodriguez-Oroz, M.C. et al. (2000). Deep brain stimulation of the globus pallidus pars interna in advanced Parkinson's disease. *Neurology*, **55**(12) (Suppl. 6), S34–9.

Lang, A.E., Lozano, A., Duff, J. et al. (1997). Medial pallidotomy in late-stage Parkinson's disease and striatonigral degeneration. *Adv. Neurol.*, **74**, 199–211.

Langston, J.W., Ballard, P., Tetrud, J.W. & Irwin, I. (1983). Chronic Parkinsonism in humans due to a product of meperidine-analog synthesis. *Science*, **219**(4587), 979–80.

Larsen, J.P., Karlsen, K. & Tandberg, E. (2000). Clinical problems in non-fluctuating patients with Parkinson's disease: a community-based study. *Mov. Disord.*, **15**(5), 826–9.

Limousin, P., Greene, J., Pollak, P. et al. (1997). Changes in cerebral activity pattern due to subthalamic nucleus or internal pallidum stimulation in Parkinson's disease. *Ann. Neurol.*, **42**(3), 283–91.

Linhares, M.N. & Tasker, R.R. (2000). Microelectrode-guided thalamotomy for Parkinson's disease. *Neurosurgery*, **46**(2), 390–5; discussion 395–8.

Lozano, A.M., Lang, A.E., Galvez-Jimenez, N. et al. (1995). Effect of GPi pallidotomy on motor function in Parkinson's disease [see comments]. [Erratum appears in *Lancet*, 1996, Oct 19;348(9034):1108]. *Lancet*, **346**(8987), 1383–7.

Marsden, C.D. & Olanow, C.W. (1998). The causes of Parkinson's disease are being unraveled and rational neuroprotective therapy is close to reality. *Ann. Neurol.*, **44**(3 Suppl. 1), S189–96.

Matsumine, H., Yamamura, Y., Hattori, N. et al. (1998). A microdeletion of D6S305 in a family of autosomal recessive juvenile parkinsonism (PARK2). *Genomics*, **49**(1), 143–6.

Metman, L.V., Del Dotto, P., Le Poole, K. et al. (1999). Amantadine for levodopa-induced dyskinesias: a 1-year follow-up study. *Arch. Neurol.*, **56**(11), 1383–6.

Miller, W.C. & DeLong, M.R. (1988). Parkinsonian symptomatology. An anatomical and physiological analysis. *Ann. NY Acad. Sci.*, **515**, 287–302.

Modestin, J., Stephan, P.L., Erni, T. & Umari, T. (2000). Prevalence of extrapyramidal syndromes in psychiatric inpatients and the relationship of clozapine treatment to tardive dyskinesia. *Schizophrenia Res.*, **42**(3), 223–30.

Montastruc, J.L., Rascol, O., Senard, J.M. & Rascol, A. (1994). A randomised controlled study comparing bromocriptine to which levodopa was later added, with levodopa alone in previously untreated patients with Parkinson's disease: a five-year follow up. *J. Neurol., Neurosurg. Psychiatry*, **57**(9), 1034–8.

Narabayashi, H. (1986). Tremor: its generation mechanism and treatment. In *Handbook of Clinical Neurology*, pp. 597–607.

Nini, A., Feingold, A., Slovin, H. & Bergman, H. (1995). Neurons in the globus pallidus do not show correlated activity in the normal monkey, but phase-locked oscillations appear in the MPTP model of parkinsonism. *J. Neurophysiol.*, **74**(4), 1800–5.

Olanow, C.W. (1992). A rationale for dopamine agonists as primary therapy for Parkinson's disease. *Can. J. Neurol. Sci.*, **19**(1 Suppl.), 108–12.

Olanow, C.W. & Koller, W.C. (1998). An algorithm (decision tree) for the management of Parkinson's disease: treatment guidelines. *Am. Acad. Neurol., Neurology*, **50**(3 Suppl. 3), S1–57.

Olanow, C.W., Jenner, P. & Brooks, D. (1998). Dopamine agonists and neuroprotection in Parkinson's disease. *Ann. Neurol.*, **44**(3 Suppl. 1), S167–74.

Onofrj, M., Thomas, A. & Paci, C. (1998). Reversible parkinsonism induced by prolonged treatment with valproate. *J. Neurol.*, **245**(12), 794–6.

Pantelatos, A. & Fornadi, F. (1993). Clinical features and medical treatment of Parkinson's disease in patient groups selected in accordance with age at onset. *Adv. Neurol.*, **60**, 690–7.

Piccini, P., Burn, D.J., Ceravalo, R., Maraganore, D. & Brooks, D.J. (1999). The role of inheritance in sporadic Parkinson's disease: evidence from a longitudinal study of dopaminergic function in twins [see comments]. *Ann. Neurol.*, **45**(5), 577–82.

Polymeropoulos, M.H., Lavedan, C., Leroy, E. et al. (1997). Mutation in the alpha-synuclein gene identified in families with Parkinson's disease [see comments]. *Science*, **276**(5321), 2045–7.

Quinn, N., Critchley, P. & Marsden, C.D. (1987). Young onset Parkinson's disease. *Mov. Disord.*, **2**(2), 73–91.

Rabey, J.M. (1995). Second generation of dopamine agonists: pros and cons. *J. Neur. Transm., Suppl.*, **45**, 213–24.

Rajput, A.H., Offord, K.P., Beard, C.M. & Kurland, L.T. (1984). Epidemiology of parkinsonism: incidence, classification, and mortality. *Ann. Neurol.*, **16**(3), 278–82.

Rascol, O., Brooks, D.J., Korczyn, A.D. et al. (2000). A five-year study of the incidence of dyskinesia in patients with early Parkinson's disease who were treated with ropinirole or levodopa. 056 Study Group. *N. Engl. J. Med.*, **342**(20), 1484–91.

Raz, A., Fiengold, A., Vaadia, E., Abeles, M. & Bergman, H. (1997). In phase neuronal oscillations in the basal ganglia of tremulous MPTP-treated vermet monkeys. In *Society for Neuroscience Abstracts*.

Razmy, A. & Shapiro, C.M. (2000). Interactions of sleep and Parkinson's disease. *Semin. Clin. Neuropsychiatry*, **5**(1), 20–32.

Reuter, I., Engelhardt, M., Stecker, K. & Baas, H. (1999). Therapeutic value of exercise training in Parkinson's disease. *Med. Sci. Sports Exercise*, **31**(11), 1544–9.

Riess, O., Kuhn, W. & Kruger, R. (2000). Genetic influence on the development of Parkinson's disease. *J. Neurol.*, **247**(Suppl. 2), II69–74.

Rinne, U.K., Bracco, F., Chouza, C. et al. (1998). Early treatment of Parkinson's disease with cabergoline delays the onset of motor complications. Results of a double-blind levodopa controlled trial. The PKDS009 Study Group. *Drugs*, **55**(Suppl. 1), 23–30.

Ryan, L.J. & Sanders, D.J. (1993). Subthalamic nucleus lesion regularizes firing patterns in globus pallidus and substantia nigra pars reticulata neurons in rats. *Brain Res.*, **626**(1–2), 327–31.

Samuel, M., Ceballos-Baumann, A.O., Turjanski, N. et al. (1997). Pallidotomy in Parkinson's disease increases supplementary motor area and prefrontal activation during performance of volitional movements an H2(15)O PET study. *Brain*, **120**(8), 1301–13.

Schapira, A.H. (1999). Science, medicine, and the future: Parkinson's disease. *Br. Med. J.*, **318**(7179), 311–14.

Schapira, A.H., Gu, M., Taanman, J.W. et al. (1998). Mitochondria in the etiology and pathogenesis of Parkinson's disease. *Ann. Neurol.*, **44**(3 Suppl. 1), S89–98.

Scheife, R.T., Shumock, G.T., Burskin, A., Gottwald, M.D. & Luer, M.S. (2000). Impact of Parkinson's disease and its pharmacologic treatment on quality of life and economic outcomes. *Am. J. Health-Syst. Pharmacy*, **57**(10), 953–62.

Schenkman, M., Cutson, T.M., Kuchibhatla, M. et al. (1998). Exercise to improve spinal flexibility and function for people with Parkinson's disease: a randomized, controlled trial. *J. Am. Geriat. Soc.*, **46**(10), 1207–16.

Schrag, A., Ben-Shlomo, Y., Brown, R., Marsden, C.D. & Quinn, N. (1998). Young-onset Parkinson's disease revisited – clinical features, natural history, and mortality. *Mov. Disord.*, **13**(6), 885–94.

Schuh, L.A. & Bennett, J.P., Jr. (1993). Suppression of dyskinesias in advanced Parkinson's disease. I. Continuous intravenous levodopa shifts dose response for production of dyskinesias but not for relief of parkinsonism in patients with advanced Parkinson's disease [see comments]. *Neurology*, **43**(8), 1545–50.

Shulman (2000). Levodopa toxicity in Parkinson disease: reality or myth?: reality – practice patterns should change. *Arch. Neurol.*, **57**(3), 406–7.

Silver, D.E. & Ruggieri, S. (1998). Initiating therapy for Parkinson's disease. *Neurology*, **50**(6 Suppl. 6), S18–22; discussion S44–8.

Staffen, W., Mair, A., Unterrainer, J. et al. (2000). [123I] beta-CIT binding and SPET compared with clinical diagnosis in parkinsonism. *Nucl. Med. Commun.*, **21**(5), 417–24.

Stoof, J.C., Booij, J. & Drukarch, B. (1992). Amantadine as N-methyl-D-aspartic acid receptor antagonist: new possibilities for therapeutic applications? *Clin. Neurol. Neurosurg.*, **94 Suppl.**, S4–6.

Tasker, R.R. (1998a). Ablative therapy for movement disorders. Does thalamotomy alter the course of Parkinson's disease? *Neurosurg. Clin. N. Am.*, **9**(2), 375–80.

Tasker, R.R. (1998b). Deep brain stimulation is preferable to thalamotomy for tremor suppression. *Surg. Neurol.*, **49**(2), 145–53; discussion 153–4.

Vitek, J. (1997). Stereotaxic surgery and deep brain stimulation for movement disorders. In *Movement Disorders in Neurologic Principles and Practice*, ed. R.W. & W. Koller, pp. 237–55. New York: McGraw-Hill, Inc.

Vitek, J.L., Ashe, J. & Kaneoke, Y. (1994). Spontaneous neuronal activity in the motor thalamus: alteration in pattern and rate in parkinsonism. *Neuroscience*, 561.

Vitek, J.L., Bakay, R.A., Hashimoto, T. et al. (1998). Microelectrode-guided pallidotomy: technical approach and its application in medically intractable Parkinson's disease [see comments]. *J. Neurosurg.*, **88**(6), 1027–43.

Volkmann, J., Sturm, V., Weiss, P. et al. (1998). Bilateral high-frequency stimulation of the internal globus pallidus in advanced Parkinson's disease. *Ann. Neurol.*, **44**(6), 953–61.

Weiner, W.J. (1999). The initial treatment of Parkinson's disease should begin with levodopa [In Process Citation]. *Mov. Disord.*, **14**(5), 716–24.

Wichmann, T. & DeLong, M.R. (1996). Functional and pathophysiological models of the basal ganglia. *Curr. Opin. Neurobiol.*, **6**(6), 751–8.

Wichmann, T., Bergman, H. & DeLong, M.R. (1994). The primate subthalamic nucleus. III. Changes in motor behavior and neuronal activity in the internal pallidum induced by subthalamic inactivation in the MPTP model of parkinsonism. *J. Neurophysiol.*, **72**(2), 521–30.

Yoshida, M., Rabin, A. & Anderson, M. (1972). Monosynaptic inhibition of pallidal neurons by axon collaterals of caudato-nigral fibers. *Exp. Brain Res.*, **15**(4), 333–47.

Yoshikawa, T., Minamiyama, Y., Naito, Y., & Kondo, M. (1994). Antioxidant properties of bromocriptine, a dopamine agonist. *J. Neurochem.*, **62**(3), 1034–8.

Zareparsi, S., Kaye, J., Camicoli, R. et al. (1997). Modulation of the age at onset of Parkinson's disease by apolipoprotein E genotypes [see comments]. *Ann. Neurol.*, **42**(4), 655–8.

34

Other extrapyramidal syndromes: parkinsonism-plus and other forms of secondary parkinsonism

Kailash P. Bhatia

Department of Clinical Neurology, Institute of Neurology, London, UK

There are numerous other causes of an extrapyramidal syndrome manifesting as parkinsonism apart from Parkinson's disease (see previous chapter). Traditionally, these are listed etiologically as shown in Table 34.1. In this list three broad groups emerge namely that referred to as the parkinsonism-plus syndromes (also called atypical parkinsonian syndromes), the symptomatic or secondary parkinsonian conditions and the hereditary/heredodegenerative disorders (Table 34.1). The parkinsonism-plus syndromes are so called because they are multisystem degenerations and have other features in addition to parkinsonism. This older classification, although useful, has its limitations because the divisions drawn are somewhat artificial and there is a fair amount of overlap in the disorders listed under the different subheadings. For example, additional clinical features can also be present in disorders in the two groups apart from the parkinson-plus disorders and it is being realized that a genetic basis may even underlie parkinsonian disorders thought to be sporadic like progressive supranuclear palsy (PSP). Great advances at the molecular, ultrastructural and genetic level are leading to a newer way of classifying many of these degenerative diseases affecting the basal ganglia causing extrapyramidal syndromes (Dickson, 1997; Spillantini, 1999). Many parkinsonian syndromes can now be viewed as being caused by the genetic or sporadic occurrence of diseases characterized on the basis of cytoskeletal pathology and staining of particular proteins, for example, alpha-synucleinopathies where alpha-synuclein is present (Spillantini, 1999; Goedert, 2001) or taupathies wherein there is deposition of tau protein (Morris et al., 1999a). This way, many of the disorders listed in Table 34.1 can now be reclassified as shown in Tables 34.2 and 34.3 on a molecular basis. Thus PSP and corticobasal degeneration and the inherited condition of frontotemporal dementia parkinsonism as well as dementia pugilistica or encephalitis

lethargica from the secondary parkinsonism division are all grouped together as 'taupathies', while multiple system atrophy (MSA) and Parkinson's disease and dementia with Lewy bodies go together as 'alpha-synucleinopathies' (Spillantini et al., 1998a).

It is beyond the scope of this chapter to detail each of the conditions causing parkinsonism listed in Table 34.1, hence this chapter will focus on some of the conditions most likely to be confused with Parkinson's disease, namely progressive supranuclear palsy (PSP), corticobasal degeneration (CBD) and multiple system atrophy (MSA) among the parkinsonism-plus syndromes with a brief mention of other related conditions as well as some secondary or symptomatic parkinsonian disorders. The UK brain bank series study looking at a 100 cases diagnosed as having Parkinson's disease in life found that 25 of these had other diagnosis at pathology (Hughes et al., 1992). The most commonly misdiagnosed conditions were atypical parkinsonian disorders, namely progressive supranuclear palsy (PSP), multiple system atrophy (MSA), and vascular parkinsonism (CBD). It is important too for the clinician to recognize the parkinsonism-plus conditions as they usually have a poor response to levodopa replacement treatment and have a bleak prognosis with regard to survival.

Progressive supranuclear palsy (PSP)

Background

PSP is a progressive neurodegenerative condition with the anatomical pathology centred around the basal ganglia and brainstem accounting for its distinctive clinical features. PSP was first recognized as a distinct syndrome by Steele, Richardson and Olszewski in 1963 and their initial

Table 34.1. Classification of parkinsonism

Idiopathic (primary)
Parkinson's disease

Parkinsonism-plus
Progressive supranuclear palsy (PSP)
  PSP of the French West Indies (Guadelope)
Multiple system atrophy (MSA)
  Striatonigral degeneration (SND/MSA-P)
  Shy–Drager syndrome (SDS)
  Olivopontocerebellar degeneration (MSA-C)
Corticobasal ganglionic degeneration (CBD)
Dementia syndromes
  Parkinsonism–dementia–ALS complex of Guam
  Frontotemporal dementia parkinsonism–chromosome
    17 (FTDP-17)
  Dementia with Lewy Bodies (Diffuse Lewy body disease)
  Creutzfeldt–Jakob disease
  Alzheimer's disease

Hereditary/heredodegenerative disorders
Wilson's disease
Hallervorden-Spatz disease
Huntington's disease
Neuroacanthocytosis
SCA-3 (Machado–Joseph) and other spinocerebellar ataxias
Lubag (X-linked dystonia–parkinsonism)
Ceroid lipofuscinosis
Hereditary hemochromatosis
Hereditary ceruloplasmin deficiency (Apoceruloplasminemia)
Familial basal ganglia calcification (Fahr's syndrome)

Symptomatic (secondary)
Infectious and postinfectious
  Postencephalitic (encephalitis lethargica)
  Other encephalitides
Toxins – manganese, cobalt, MPTP, cyanide, CO, methanol,
  ethanol
Drugs
  Dopamine receptor blockers (antipsychotics/antiemetics),
    dopamine storage depletors, α-methylparatyrosine, α-
    methyldopa, calcium channel blockers, SSRI's
Vascular–multi-infarct, Binswanger
Brain tumours
Head trauma – including dementia pugilistica
Vascular
Metabolic–hypoparathyroidism, hepatocerebral degeneration
Other – hemiparkinsonism/hemiatrophy, normal pressure
  hydrocephalus, paraneoplastic

Table 34.2. Conditions characterized by the deposition of tau containing neurofibrillary tangles (taupathies)

Progressive supranuclear palsy (PSP)
Corticobasal degeneration (CBD)
Frontotemporal dementia parkinsonism-chromosome 17
  (FTDP-17)
Pick's disease
Post-encephalitic parkinsonism (encephalitis lethargica)
Post-traumatic parkinsonism
Parkinson dementia complex of Guam
Alzheimer's disease
Niemann–Pick type C
Subacute sclerosing panencephalitis

Source: From Morris et al. (1999b).

Table 34.3. Parkinsonian syndromes with alpha-synuclein accumulation (alpha-synucleinopathies)

Lewy body diseases
Idiopathic Parkinson's disease
Inherited Lewy body diseases (mutations of the alpha-synuclein
  gene, PARK3, PARK4)
Dementia with Lewy Bodies
Halloverden Spatz disease

Multiple system atrophy (MSA)
Striatonigral degeneration
Shy–Drager syndrome
Olivopontocerebellar atrophy

Source: From Goedert & Spillantini (2001).

description has proven to be remarkably accurate (Steele et al., 1964). Despite the distinctive clinical presentation, however, the condition is probably underdiagnosed (Nath et al., 2001).

Clinical aspects

PSP typically occurs late in life usually in the sixth decade with the median age at disease onset between 60 and 66 years (Nath & Burn, 2000). Onset below age 40 years is virtually unknown. A prevalence of 1.4/100000 had been reported from New Jersey (Golbe et al., 1988) and 1 per 100000 as per a more national survey from the UK (Nath et al., 2001). A recent cross-sectional study from the UK has shown that the age-adjusted prevalence for PSP was 6.4 per 100000 (Schrag et al., 1999). There have been only two reported case control studies of PSP both by the same group. The first study suggested that PSP patients were more likely to live in areas of relatively sparse population (Davis et al., 1988). However, a follow-up study failed to identify any particular risk factor except for the likelihood of having completed 12 years of education or more that differentiated PSP patients from matched controls (Golbe et al., 1996). Recently, one study reported a higher prevalence of presymptomatic high blood pressure in PSP patients (81%) compared to Parkinson's disease patients (15%) (Ghika & Bogousslavsky, 1997); however, another subsequent series could not replicate these figures and found this in a much smaller number (24%) of patients with PSP (Fabbrini et al., 1998). PSP has been considered to be a sporadic condition and in one study of 104 patients, Jankovic et al. (1990) failed to find another affected person among 400 first-degree relatives. However, some reports of familial clustering have appeared in the literature from time to time (Brown et al., 1993; de Yebenes et al., 1995; Tetrud et al., 1996). Recently, 12 families were put together, 8 of whom with probable autosomal dominant inheritance with pathological confirmation in 4 probands (Rojo et al., 1999).

Most patients present with a gait disturbance with a tendency to fall backwards. Indeed 70% of PSP cases would have falls in the first year of the illness. Some may present with a complaint of visual disturbance, particularly when reading or walking downstairs due to lack of control of saccadic eye movements (see below). A growling gruff dysarthria and swallowing difficulty may be associated with presenting symptoms. Despite these disabling presenting features, surprisingly the mean interval from symptom onset to diagnosis of PSP is usually delayed even up to 3–4 years (Maher & Lees, 1986; Golbe et al., 1988). Thus, the average patient with PSP remains undiagnosed for approximately half of the natural history of their disease.

Clinically, most patients have an erect posture in contrast to the flexed posture of Parkinson's disease. Also, unlike Parkinson's disease most signs of parkinsonism in PSP are axial that is involving postural balance, gait and speech with less pronounced distal limb involvement. In contrast to PD, PSP patients have a stiff somewhat broad-based gait quite often marked by start hesitation, freezing and disequilibrium leading to a tendency to fall. There is early loss of postural reflexes as compared to PD (Litvan et al., 1997a). PSP patients, when asked to stand up from sitting, tend to jump up abruptly from the seated position, only to fall back immediately into the chair which has been called the 'rocket sign' and probably results from a combination of postural instability and frontal–subcortical disturbance (Litvan, 1997). Sitting 'en bloc', in which the patient's feet come high off the floor as they sit down, also tends to occur in 30% of cases (Collins et al., 1995). An increase of axial tone with rigidity of

the trunk and neck rather than of the limbs is typical and rest tremor is uncommon or does not occur. Bradykinesia is common and affects nearly half the patients by the time of diagnosis and up to 95% of patients during the course of their illness (Verny et al., 1996). Striking frontalis overactivity with markedly reduced blink frequency and hypomimia produce the so-called 'reptilian' stare with regard to facial appearance (Verny et al., 1996). The characteristic feature from which the term 'progressive supranuclear palsy' is derived is the supranuclear gaze problem (Troost & Daroff, 1977). Typically, voluntary down-gaze is slow and incomplete but, when the oculo-cephalic manoeuvre is engaged, full down-gaze is possible. Because up-gaze may be restricted with ageing, and restriction in this direction can also occur with other disorders, downward gaze palsy is more specific for the diagnosis of PSP (Lees, 1987). Some other causes of vertical supranuclear gaze palsy include Whipple's disease (Averbuch-Heller et al., 1999), Niemann Pick type C (Shulman et al., 1995), and other conditions including CBD, prion disease (Brown et al., 1994) and spino-cerebellar ataxia (SCA) including SCA2 and SCA3. Square wave jerks, saccadic intrusions when fixing gaze on a stationary object, can also be seen in PSP (Rascol et al., 1991). Unlike corticobasal degeneration, involvement of horizontal saccades occurs only later in PSP (Vidhailhet et al., 1994), a useful differentiating feature. In the late stages, complete supranuclear restriction of eye movements may be seen (Rivaud-Pechoux et al., 2000). Difficulty in eyelid opening may caused by blepharospasm and/or apraxia of eyelid opening. A pseudobulbar palsy occurs in 85–90% of cases, and a frontal lobe-like syndrome sometimes with marked emotional lability is present in 80% of cases with 52% developing this in the first year (Brusa et al., 1980; Verny et al., 1996). Speech and swallowing can be affected early and may be presenting features (Daniel et al., 1995). PSP patients may have stuttering, stammering hypophonic speech. Echolalia, pallilalia and pallilogia can be present. A poor or unsustained response to levodopa is characteristic of PSP (Litvan et al., 1997a). The condition is unfortunately relentlessly progressive with death from disease onset in about 5–6 years (Maher & Lees, 1986; Brusa et al., 1980). An early onset, presence of falls and early down-gaze palsy seems to be associated with a more rapid progression (Santacruz et al., 1998).

Pathology, clinicopathological correlation, tau ultrastructure and genetics of PSP

PSP is characterized pathologically by abundant neurofibrillary tangles (NFTs) which consist of hyperphosphorylated tau and neuropil threads in select basal ganglia and brainstem regions (Fig. 34.1, see colour plate section). Thus PSP is one of group of tau neurofibrillary disorders (Table 34.2) (Dickson, 1997; Morris et al., 1999a). Tau is a microtubule binding protein which serves to promote and stabilize the polymerization of monomeric tubulin into microtubules. Tau is present mainly in axons and expressed also in glial cells, especially in pathological conditions. In PSP, for example, tau deposition is seen as tufted astrocytes (Fig. 34.2, see colour plate section). The tau protein itself is alternatively spliced from the tau gene with six different types of proteins (isoforms) appearing in normal adult human brain (Morris et al., 1999a). These isoforms differ in the presence of three or four repeated microtubule binding domains (three or four repeat tau) and the extra microtubule binding domain is determined by the inclusion of exon 10 of the tau gene. Tau deposition or dysfunction in these disorders is not thought to be an incidental finding but appears to be the pathogenic cause of neurodegeneration (Hutton et al., 1998; Goedert & Spillantini, 2001).

The main lesions in PSP are in the substantia nigra pars compacta, and reticulata, internal segment of the globus pallidus, subthalamic nucleus, midbrain and pontine reticular formation. Cortical damage and glial pathology is more variable and allows distinction between this disorder from CBD and Pick's disease which have distinctive cortical involvement. The most striking neurochemical abnormality is marked reduction in striatal dopamine, dopamine receptor density, choline acetyl transferase activity and loss of nicotinic cholinergic receptors in the basal forebrain (Young, 1985; Ruberg et al., 1985; Juncos et al., 1991). However, in contrast to the striatum the mesolimbic structures are relatively spared with normal dopamine levels in the nucleus accumbens.

There is a good correlation for PSP between the pathological anatomical substrate and the predominant clinical features. Postural instability is probably due to involvement of the dentate and pedunculopontine nucleus as well as bilateral globus pallidus. Involvement of the substantia nigra, medial pallidum and subthalamic nucleus (Feany & Dickson, 1996) may result in the bradykinesia and limb rigidity. The superior colliculus involvement may account for the increased axial tone. Impairment of vertical saccades is probably due to involvement of rostral interstitial nucleus of Cajal and nucleus of Darkshewitsch and the rostral interstitial nucleus of the medial longitudinal fasciculus (Juncos et al., 1991). Echolalia, pallilalia, grasping and groping behaviour arises from frontal lobe or frontal basal ganglia connections. PSP pathology may affect the spinal cord, and Onuf's nucleus in the sacral spinal cord has been shown to be affected and can result in loss of bladder control and abnormal sphincter elec-

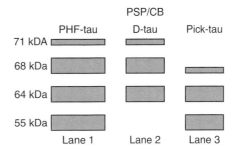

Fig. 34.3. Electrophoretic migration patterns in different taupathies. Lane 1 represents paired helical filament-tau (PHF-tau) characteristic of certain taupathies like Alzheimer's disease and certain forms of frontotemporal dementia linked to chromosome 17 (FTD-17). All six isoforms of tau contribute and a triplet pattern migrating at 68, 64 and 55 kilodaltons is observed. Lane 2 with a doublet pattern migrating at 68 and 64 kilodaltons is observed in conditions such as PSP and CBD. Abnormal tau in both these conditions is composed of four repeat isoforms. Lane 3 shows two bands migrating at 64 and 55 kilodaltons characteristic of conditions like Pick's disease. The tau in this condition is composed of three repeat isoforms. (Courtesy Dr Tamas Revesz, Dept. of Neuropathology, Institute of Neurology, London.)

tromyogram changes (Scaravilli et al., 2000; Valldeoriola et al., 1995)

These changes are associated with nerve cell loss, gliosis, and occasional granulovacuolar or ballooned argyrophilic neuronal degeneration (Jellinger et al., 1995). Ultrastructural and protein chemistry of neurofibrillary tangles allows subdivision of the different taupathies. In contrast to other neurodegenerative disorders with tau pathology like AD, Pick's disease and CBD which are characterized by flame-shaped NFTs, the NFTs of PSP are mainly of the globose type (Fig. 34.1, see colour plate section). They are made up of clusters of straight filaments arranged in circling and interlacing bundles, and have a diameter of 12 to 15 nm (Roy et al., 1974). This filamentous phenotype therefore differs from the paired helical filaments typically found in Alzheimer's disease (Dickson, 1997). Also, on electrophoresis the paired helical filaments of Azheimer's disease are made up of three distinct bands of 55, 64 and 68 kDa and they are composed of all six isoforms of the tau gene, containing both four and three repeat isoforms. In PSP the straight filaments are composed of only two bands at 64 and 68 kDa (Fig. 34.3) and the tau protein is made up only of a subset of tau isoforms consisting only of four repeat tau (Conrad et al., 1997; Morris et al., 1999a). Thus taupathies can be classified according to tau repeat isoforms deposited.

Most cases of PSP are isolated with no family history and it is considered to be a sporadic condition. However, a number of families have been described with autosomal dominant PSP (Rojo et al., 1999), although neither a linked chromosomal locus nor a causative gene have been identified in any of these (Morris et al., 1999a). As a rare exception recently there has been report of a family with PSP pathology with a novel mutation of exon 10 of the tau gene (Stanford et al., 2000). However, no mutations were identified on sequencing exons 9–13 of the tau gene in over 60 patients with PSP (Baker et al., 1999). This is the area where most of the mutations causing frontotemporal dementia with parkinsonism linked to chromosome 17 had been detected. In fact, no mutations were found on sequencing the entire coding region of the tau gene in any of these PSP patients in whom this was carried out (Baker et al., 1999). Also there appears to be no effect of alpha-synuclein, synphilin, or APOE genotypic variability for the development of PSP (Morris et al., 2000). However, analysis of sporadic PSP cases has led to a suggestion of an association between a polymorphic dinucleotide marker within the tau gene and PSP (Conrad et al., 1997; Higgins et al., 1998, 1999, 2000; Baker et al., 1999; Morris et al., 1999b). In PSP there appears to be an over-representation of the more common allele A0 and the genotype A0/A0 which is not found in PD, MSA or CBD. This may be a predisposing factor to PSP in the same way as as apolipoprotein E e4 allele is in Alzheimer's disease.

Diagnostic tests, diagnostic criteria and differential diagnosis

CT or MRI brain scans of patienst with PSP may show generalized and/or brainstem atrophy mainly of the dorsal midbrain. The degeneration of the superior colliculus gives a flattened appearance of the third ventricle on MRI scans; aqueductal dilatation and increased olivary signal have also been noted (Savoiarda et al., 1994, Schrag et al., 2000). If midbrain atrophy is seen on MRI, differentiation of PSP from PD is possible as MRI is normal but not from other akinetic-rigid syndromes, for example MSA, where similar changes may be present. MR spectroscopy has shown reductions in N-acetylaspartate in the lentiform nucleus of PSP patients but not so in PD patients (Federico et al., 1997). Metabolic studies using PET have demonstrated global reduction in cerebral metabolism with particular affectation of the frontal and striatal regions using labelled oxygen or glucose markers (Brooks, 1994). ^{18}F-dopa PET uptake is reduced in the caudate and putamen thus discriminating from PD but not other akinetic-rigid syndromes like MSA which can have a similar picture. Ten to 25% reduction of uptake in caudate and putamen using

^{11}C-raclopride, a D2 receptor ligand, and also for ^{11}C-diprenorphine, an opoid receptor ligand, has been shown in PSP (Brooks, 1994).

Ideal diagnostic criteria for PSP would reliably separate the condition from other akinetic-rigid syndromes, notably Parkinson's disease and also other neurodegenerative disorders with parkinsonism and dementia (Lopez et al., 1999). Many different diagnostic criteria have been proposed to assist the clinician in making an accurate diagnosis of PSP (Lees, 1987; Collins et al., 1995; Tolosa et al., 1994; Litvan et al., 1996a). Of these the National Institute of Neurological Disorders and Stroke and Society for Progressive Supranuclear Palsy, Inc. (NINDS–SPSP) diagnostic criteria are shown in Table 34.4 (Litvan et al., 1996b) which have been validated and also evaluated and found to have good specificity (Lopez et al., 1999). A difficult problem can be with an early case of PSP, before the characteristic clinical features have emerged. The patient may not yet have the typical vertical supranuclear gaze paresis and it is clear that sometimes the development of 'core' diagnostic features may be delayed, or may not occur at all. Thus, in one series comprising 17 pathologically confirmed cases of PSP, 10 of the cases did not have a vertical supranuclear gaze paresis documented antemortem and all 10 of these were misdiagnosed (Daniel et al., 1995). Phenotypic variants for PSP can also cause diagnostic confusion. There have been unusual phenotypes of pathologically confirmed cases, for example, early and severe dementia or that with pure akinesia and unilateral limb dystonia or apraxia leading to a mistaken diagnosis of CBD (Matsuo et al., 1991; Davis et al., 1985; Pharr et al., 1999). PSP is most often clinically misdiagnosed as PD or as cerebrovascular disease (false-negative clinical diagnosis) (Litvan et al., 1996c). In the clinicopathological series of Hughes et al. (1992), mentioned earlier, 25% of the 24 cases clinically diagnosed as having PD, but without Lewy bodies at postmortem, were actually found to have PSP. Conversely, there are pathologically confirmed cases of corticobasal degeneration, multiple system atrophy, dementia with Lewy bodies, prion disease and Whipple's disease, that were clinically misdiagnosed as having PSP (false-positive clinical diagnosis) (Litvan et al., 1996c; Fearnley et al., 1991; Averbuch-Heller et al., 1999). Overall, looking at which factors best differentiate PSP from other related disorders, according to one study, postural instability, leading to falls (typically backwards) within the first year of disease onset, coupled with a vertical supranuclear gaze paresis have been shown to have good discriminatory diagnostic value when comparing PSP with other akinetic-rigid syndromes (Litvan et al., 1997a, b).

Table 34.4. NINDS–SPSP Clinical criteria for the diagnosis of PSP

PSP	Mandatory inclusion criteria	Mandatory exclusion criteria	Supportive criteria
Possible	Gradually progressive disorder Onset age 40 or later Either vertical supranuclear palsy or both slowing of vertical saccades and postural instability with falls <1 year disease onset No evidence of other diseases that could explain the foregoing features, as indicated by exclusion criteria	Recent history of encephalitis Alien limb syndrome, cortical sensory deficits, focal frontal or temporoparietal atrophy Hallucinations or delusions unrelated to dopaminergic therapy Cortical dementia of Alzheimer type Prominent, early cerebellar symptoms or unexplained autonomic dysautonomia	Symmetric akinesia or rigidity, proximal more than distal Abnormal neck posture, especially retrocollis Poor or absent response of parkinsonism to levodopa Early dysphagia & dysarthria Early onset of cognitive impairment including >2 of: apathy, impairment in abstract thought, decreased verbal fluency, utilization or imitation behaviour, or frontal release signs
Probable	Gradually progressive disorder Onset age 40 or later Vertical supranuclear palsy and prominent postural instability with falls <1 year disease onset No evidence of other diseases that could explain the foregoing features, as indicated by exclusion criteria		
Definite	Clinically probable or possible PSP and histopathological evidence of typical PSP		

Source: Adapted from Litvan et al. (1997a).

Management

PSP patients usually do not have significant benefit from dopaminergic medication. In some there may be some initial improvement but this is not sustained. There have been some suggestions that amantadine may be useful with the motor features of PSP but this has not been formally tested in a randomized trial. Cholinergic drugs such as physostigmine have been said to be useful for certain aspects. Following physostigmine administration in PSP patients, a significant reduction in errors of performance was found in four out of seven on neuropsychological tests; however, motor disability was not significantly altered (Blin et al., 1995). Alpha-2 antagonist drugs like idaxozan and efaroxon have been mooted for motor symptoms; however, there is no clear evidence that these are useful (Ghika et al., 1991; Rascol et al., 1998). Botulinum toxin is useful for blepharospasm and less so for levator inhibition or apraxia of eyelid opening. Supportive therapy is the mainstay rather than drug treatment. Physiotherapy and occupational therapy are important to help balance with aids and avoid falls. Early speech therapy and assessment of swallowing function may be helpful in avoiding aspiration and its complications. In some instances feeding may have to be done by means of a percutaneous gastrostomy tube, but such an intervention should take into account the patients and the relatives' wishes with regard to quality of life and how advanced the disease process may be.

PSP in the French West Indies

Clues to the etiology of PSP may come from the recent observation of a large cohort of PSP patients in the small island of Guadelope in the French West Indies (Caparros-Lefebvre et al., 1999). Out of 87 consecutive patients with parkinsonism referred to a single neurological department, 31 had PSP which was a gross over-representation. A case control study established that a higher proportion of the PSP patients, but not the PD patients, consumed herbal teas and tropical fruits. As these are known to contain benzyltetrahydroisoquinolines, this is being considered as the possible exogenous environmental toxin in addition to a possible genetic susceptibility.

Corticobasal degeneration (CBD)

Background

Corticobasal degeneration (CBD), is a rare sporadic neurodegenerative disorder recognized relatively recently with the first description of three patients by Rebeiz, Kolodny and Richardson in 1967. These patients had an asymmetric onset of slow, awkward voluntary limb movement, tremor, dystonic posturing, stiffness, lack of dexterity, and 'numbness or deadness' of the affected limb. The gradual progression of symptoms included gait disorder, limb rigidity, impairment of position sense, and other sensory modalities (Rebeiz et al., 1967, 1968). Cognitive function was said to remain relatively intact (Rebeiz et al., 1967, 1968). A fairly characteristic clinical picture thus emerged. Pathology also was thought to be quite typical with asymmetric frontoparietal cortical atrophy, neuronal loss with associated gliosis, and swollen neuronal cell bodies which were devoid of Nissl substance, thus prompting the descriptive term 'achromatic'. There was considerable loss of pigmented neurons in the substantia nigra in all three patients, variable subcortical neuronal involvement, and secondary corticospinal tract degeneration. Different terms reflecting the cortical and subcortical pathology and the characteristic achromasia appeared in the literature describing clinically similar cases including corticonigral degeneration with neuronal achromasia (Rebeiz et al., 1967, 1968; Lippa et al., 1990), corticobasal ganglionic degeneration (Watts et al., 1985; Riley and Lang, 1988; Greene et al., 1990), corticobasal ganglionic degeneration with neuronal achromasia (Watts et al., 1989), syndrome of progressive rigidity with apraxia (LeWitt et al., 1989) and corticobasal degeneration (CBD) (Gibb et al., 1989; Thompson & Marsden, 1992; Rinne et al., 1994; Wenning et al., 1998), which is the term commonly used now for this condition.

Clinical features

CBD presents in mid to late adult life, with a mean onset of symptoms at 63 years (Wenning et al., 1998). However, cases of CBD have been reported as early as 40 years old and the youngest case with pathologic confirmation was 45 years old. Population prevalence is not known and although both sexes are affected, some have wondered about a slight preponderance of women (Rinne et al., 1994; Schneider et al., 1994; Watts et al., 1997). The clinical phenotype of CBD is well described most recently in three large series of patients (Rinne et al., 1994; Wenning et al., 1998; Kompoliti et al., 1998) one of them with post-

mortem confirmation (Wenning et al., 1998). The typical presentation is that of an asymmetric progressive akinetic-rigid syndrome poorly responsive to levodopa treatment. The most common initial symptom reported, limb clumsiness, has been observed in 50% of the patients at the first visit in some studies. Rinne et al. (1994) describing a large series of 36 patients with CBD outlined five common types of clinical presentation. The most common presentation was with a 'useless' arm which could be due to combined rigidity, dystonia, akinesia or apraxia, with or without myoclonus. A similar presentation but affecting a leg and presenting as a gait disorder was next most common. Other presentations included a sensory disturbance with pain, or 'clumsiness', or a speech disturbance. Only one patient in this series presented with behavioural changes, and cognitive problems were described as an uncommon presenting feature, being noted only later in the illness. However, of late it is becoming clear that many patients with pathologic findings of CBD may have dementia as the presenting and predominant feature (Grimes et al., 1999).

On examination, limb rigidity or dystonia and focal reflex myoclonus manifesting as an irregular action/postural tremor are the prominent clinical features. Asymmetric limb dystonia is observed in a vast majority of patients (Wenning et al., 1998; Vanek & Jankovic, 2000; Litvan et al., 1997b). The arm is the most frequently affected region and typically is held adducted at the shoulder with flexion of the forearm at the elbow. The fingers are flexed at the metacarpophalangeal joints, often digging into the palms of the hand, sometimes with associated contractures causing fixed posturing (Watts et al., 1997; Vanek & Jankovic, 2000). Akinesia, rigidity and apraxia are the most common findings during the course of CBD (Kumar et al., 1998; Riley & Lang, 2000). Typically, ideomotor and limb kinetic apraxia are seen in patients with CBD with ideational apraxia being less common (Leiguarda et al., 1994). Ideomotor apraxia is manifested by impairment of timing, sequencing, spatial organization, and in copying gestures made by the examiner. In limb kinetic apraxia there is a decrease in dexterity and fine movements. Ideomotor apraxia is usually bilateral and can be tested on the less affected side in advanced cases, as often the severe rigidity and dystonia of the more affected side make apraxia testing virtually impossible (Leiguarda et al., 1994). Orofacial apraxia with impairment of tongue and lip movements is also not infrequent in CBD (Ozsancak et al., 2000). Apart from apraxia, other cortical signs including cortical sensory loss or alien limb phenomenon are often present. The alien limb phenomenon is a failure to recognize ownership of a limb in the absence of visual cues. It is

Table 34.5. Clinical manifestations of CBD

Basal ganglia signs	Cerebral cortical signs	Other manifestations
Akinesia, rigidity	Cortical sensory loss	Postural-action tremor
Limb dystonia	Alien limb phenomenon	Hyperreflexia
Athetosis	Dementia	Impaired ocular motility
Postural instability, falls	Apraxia	Dysarthria
Orolingual dyskinesias	Frontal release reflexes	Focal reflex myoclonus
	Dysphasia	Impaired eyelid motion
		Dysphagia

Source: From Riley et al. (1990).

associated with autonomous activity of the extremity including posturing and levitation. About 40% or so of patients with CBD develop the alien limb phenomenon during the course of the illness, although it is rare on initial presentation (Kumar et al., 1998).

Eye movement abnormalities are also common in CBD and the extraocular movements appear slow and hypometric. Horizontal saccadic latencies are significantly increased in patients with CBD whereas vertical saccades are usually normal at least initially helping to differentiate CBD from PSP (Vidhailet et al., 1994; Litvan et al., 1997b). Slowness of speech production, and dysphonia, echolalia, and palilalia can be present as in PSP and also, like the latter, swallowing disorders are very common, especially in advanced stages.

Riley and colleagues suggested a set of diagnostic criteria for CBD (Table 34.5) (Riley et al., 1990; Riley & Lang, 1993). These consisted of unilateral onset and asymmetric course of an insidious and progressive disorder with the following clinical manifestations which were divided into three main groups: (i) those suggestive of dysfunction of the cerebral cortex namely cortical sensory loss, apraxia, alien limb, frontal release signs; (ii) those attributed to involvement of the basal ganglia namely akinesia, rigidity, limb dystonia, and postural instability and (iii) additional findings which did not localize to either cortex or basal ganglia such as action tremor, hyperreflexia, Babinski signs, oculomotor impairment, dysarthria and dysphagia.

Prognosis

The symptoms are progressive and death usually ensues 5 to 10 years after disease onset. Early onset of bilateral parkinsonism and the presence of a frontal lobe syndrome are associated with shorter survival in CBD patients (Wenning et al., 1998).

Pathology

Superior frontoparietal cortical atrophy in CBD is often asymmetrical and involves perirolandic cortex (Schneider et al., 1994). Microscopic examination reveals neuronal loss and gliosis in cortical and subcortical regions. Superficial spongiosis in atrophic cortical regions is common. Ballooned and achromatic neurons lacking Nissl substance, eosinophilic on H & E staining, and often vacuolar, observed in cortical and subcortical regions are a characteristic feature of CBD (Rebeiz et al., 1968; Watts et al., 1985; Smith et al., 1992). By immunochemistry ballooned neurons do not stain for alpha-synuclein and are sometimes positive for ubiquitin (Smith et al., 1992). However, focal tau immunoreactivity is detected in ballooned neurons as well as in neurofibrillary tangles, neuropil threads, grains, glial, and neuronal inclusions seen in this condition (Dickson, 1999; Feany & Dickson, 1996). They are frequently identified on silver stain preparations and on tau immunohistochemistry within cortical neurons, and subcortical structures including the basal ganglia, and brainstem nuclei. The locus ceruleus, raphe nuclei, tegmental grey matter, and substantia nigra have frequent neurofibrillary lesions that are tau immunoreactive (Feany & Dickson, 1996). Tau pathology in glial cells is also expressed in CBD (Dickson, 1999; Feany & Dickson, 1996). Tau-positive astrocytic plaques are argyrophilic structures identified in many cases of CBD. They are thought to be characteristic of CBD although they have also been observed in PSP (Dickson, 1999).

There appears to be considerable neuropathological overlap between Pick's disease, progressive supranuclear palsy (PSP), and CBD (Dickson, 1999; Gearing et al., 1994). All three conditions may have ballooned neurons along with variable degeneration of the substantia nigra, basal ganglia, and tau-positive inclusions (Gearing et al., 1994; Schneider et al., 1994). However, the temporal cortex as well as the hippocampus that are usually involved in Pick's disease are spared in CBD and Pick bodies, which are characteristic of Pick's disease, are rarely observed in CBD. Also in CBD astrocytic tau plaques are seen, while in PSP there are tufted astrocytes (Fig. 34.2, see colour plate section) with tau within the distal and proximal processes (Dickson, 1999). Electrophoretic pattern of tau can separate Pick's disease from CBD, PSP (and frontotemporal dementia). Only Pick's disease has two bands migrating at 64 and 55 kdalton while in the others there are 60 and 64 kdalton bands (Fig. 34.3) (Dickson, 1999; Dickson et al., 2000). Both CBD and PSP have four repeat tau (Dickson et al., 2000).

It appears to be a sporadic condition, although rare familial cases have been reported and there is a suggestion that like PSP those with the specific tau haplotypes may be at risk factor for CBD (Di Maria et al., 2000; Houlden et al., 2001). Tau sequencing in 57 neuropathologically confirmed cases failed to reveal the presence of pathogenic mutations; however, analysing tau polymorphisms in CBD cases vs. controls the frequency of H1, H1/H1 was significantly increased. CBD and PSP thus seem to share a common genetic risk factor (Houlden et al., 2001).

Differential diagnosis

The characteristic features of CBD are so distinctive that it is often possible to make a confident clinical diagnosis (Feifel et al., 1994; Litvan, 1997). However, prototypic phenotypes may have atypical (non-CBD) pathology (Boeve et al., 1999; Bhatia et al., 2000). Examples of these CBD look-alikes include vascular lesions, leukodystrophies, Pick's and Alzheimer's disease, PSP and other etiologies (Bhatia et al., 2000). On the other hand, there are also examples of atypical phenotypes, for example presenting with early dementia, who have classic CBD pathology (Bergeron et al., 1996). CBD appears to be underdiagnosed, particularly in the early stages of presentation (Wenning et al., 1998; Litvan et al., 1997b). When it presents with the motor disorder phenotype, PSP is the commonest misdiagnosis (Litvan et al., 1997b). Differentiating the two can be difficult; however, CBD patients presented with lateralized motor (e.g. parkinsonism, dystonia or myoclonus) and cognitive signs (e.g. ideomotor apraxia, aphasia or alien limb), while PSP patients often had severe postural instability at onset, symmetric parkinsonism, vertical supranuclear gaze palsy, speech and frontal lobe-type features. Litvan et al. (1997b) have suggested that limb dystonia, ideomotor apraxia, myoclonus, and asymmetric akinetic-rigid syndrome with late onset of gait or balance disturbances were the best predictors for the diagnosis of CBD.

However, as mentioned recently, it has become clear that a fair proportion of patients with pathological proven CBD may have dementia as their presenting and/or as the main feature (Grimes et al., 1999). Thus conditions like Pick's disease, Alzheimer's disease and frontotemporal dementia which can have some extrapyramidal manifestations also come into the differential (Boeve et al., 1999; Litvan et al., 1997b).

Radiographic studies may help but are not by themselves diagnostic. Cortical asymmetry with fronto-parietal atrophy on CT or MRI may suggest CBD. Compared with CBD, MRI in patients with PSP shows atrophy in the midbrain (Schrag et al., 2000). AD, on the other hand, may be differentiated from CBD by recognizing diffuse temporal and hippocampal atrophy. CBD patients show a global reduction of oxygen and glucose metabolism demonstrated by FDG positron emission tomography (PET) scans most prominent in the cerebral hemisphere contralateral to the most affected limb (Brooks, 2000). There is a corresponding reduction of CBF most evident in the frontoparietal, medial frontal, and temporal cortical regions (Okuda et al., 1999; Laureys et al., 1999; Sawle et al., 1991). Dysfunction of the nigrostriatal dopaminergic system has been demonstrated by decreased ^{18}fluorodopa (F-Dopa) uptake in the striatum with PET, and reduced postsynaptic striatal D2 receptor binding of $[^{123m}I]$-iodobenzamide (IBZM) on SPECT scanning. Caudate and putamen are similarly affected in CBD, whereas in PD F-Dopa uptake is selectively reduced in the putamen (Brooks, 2000). The characteristic pattern of asymmetrically reduced frontoparietal cerebral cortical metabolism and/or CBF coupled with bilateral reduction of F-Dopa uptake in the caudate and putamen provides strong supportive evidence in a patient with a clinical diagnosis of possible CBD (Brooks, 2000).

Therapy

Pharmacotherapy for CBD has generally been of limited benefit. CBD patients show limited or no beneficial response to carbidopa/levodopa and other dopaminergic agents. However, these drugs are worth trying as some improvement in clinically diagnosed CBD occurred in 24% of patients receiving carbidopa/levodopa in one report (Kompoliti et al., 1998). Dopamine agonists provide less clinical improvement than carbidopa/levodopa and are more likely to produce side effects. Clonazepam can be beneficial for treatment of the action tremor and myoclonus. Baclofen and tizanidine may improve rigidity and tremor, but they have only a modest effect. Anticholinergics have been reported to yield benefit in a small number of patients but their benefit wanes quickly and they are poorly tolerated (Kompoliti et al., 1998). Likewise, amantadine is of little or no benefit and may produce side effects. Botulinum toxin injections may be useful in the treatment of painful focal upper limb dystonia and blepharospasm (Vanek & Jankovic, 2000).

As for PSP, other aspects of patient care, not involving pharmacotherapy, are important for these CBD patients and their carers. Physiotherapy is useful for maintenance of mobility and may help prevent contractures. Speech therapy may help optimize speech function and guard against aspiration secondary to swallowing difficulty. Unfortunately, the disease is relentlessly progressive to a state of bilateral rigid immobility, and the patients usually die from aspiration pneumonia or urinary tract infection.

Frontotemporal dementia parkinsonism-chromosome 17

Frontotemporal dementia is a condition characterized by a behavioural disorder of insidious onset and variable progression. Clinically, its early features reflect frontal lobe dysfunction characterized by personality change, worsening memory and executive functions, and stereotypical and perseverative behaviour. Parkinsonism, postural instability and supranuclear gaze palsy are other characteristics showing similarities to other taupathies like PSP and CBD. Progressive dysphasia is prominent in some kindreds and signs of anterior horn disease may also be distinctive features. The condition can be rapidly progressive with the parkinsonism being unresponsive to levodopa therapy.

Pathologically, there is degeneration of the neocortex with marked frontal and temporal lobe atrophy and involvement of the subcortical basal ganglia and brainstem nuclei which led to the use of the term pallido-ponto-nigral degeneration (PPND) to describe some of these families (Wzolek et al., 1992). In cases where family aggregation is observed, it is inherited as an autosomal dominant, age-dependent disorder. Other terms for such families had included familial Pick's disease and disinhibition–dementia–parkinsonism–amyotrophy complex (Wilhelmsen–Lynch disease). However, there was linkage to chromosome 17q21 in many of the different kindreds (Lynch et al., 1994, Wilhelmsen et al., 1994; Wijker et al., 1996; Reed et al., 1998) described above, which led to the search of primary genetic etiology of these conditions. It became clear that, in all such families there was significant tau deposition in those where there was pathology, and they were all related disorders now called

frontotemporal dementia parkinsonism-17 (FTDP-17). The link with tau was further established, as the tau gene was known to be located on chromosome 17q and it is clear tau gene mutations cause FTDP-17 (Poorkaj et al., 1998). Hutton et al. (1998) described three missense mutations and three mutations in the 5' splice site of exon 10. Subsequently, many more different mutations have been found associated with FTDP (Dumanchin et al., 1998; Spillantini et al., 1998a, b; D'Souza et al., 1999). The location of most mutations in the microtubule binding region of the tau gene (Dumanchin et al., 1998) suggests that disruption of this process is likely to be central to the neurodegenerative process. It has also confirmed that abnormal tau deposition in this disorder leads to neurodegeneration (Spillantini et al., 2000). An other possibility is a proapoptotic effect by the tau mutations (Furukawa et al., 2000). Bird et al. (1999) in a clinical pathological comparison of three families with frontotemporal dementia and with an identical mutation in the tau gene (P301L) found marked clinical and pathological variabity in these families. This suggested that unidentified environmental and/or genetic factors were producing phenotypic variability on the background of an identical mutation. PET scanning in kindreds said to have pallido-ponto-nigral degeneration type of FTDP-17 showed a reduction of Fluoro-dopa uptake, which affected both caudate and putamen (Pal et al., 2001). 11C-Raclopride scans showed normal to elevated striatal D2-receptor binding and cerebral glucose metabolism globally reduced but with maximal involvement of frontal regions (Pal et al., 1999). The fact that there was severe presynaptic dopaminergic dysfunction with intact striatal D2 receptors in these patients suggested that the dopa unresponsiveness is probably a result of pathology downstream to the striatum. The pattern of presynaptic dysfunction contrasts with that seen in idiopathic parkinsonism, where the putamen is affected more than the caudate nucleus, but is similar to that in other atypical Parkinsonian conditions such as PSP. The differential diagnosis is from other conditions presenting with dementia and parkinsonism like Pick's disease, PSP, CBD and rarely Alzheimer's. A family history is usually lacking in these disorders compared to FTDP-17. However, rarely familial CJD or prion disease can present with a phenotype of FTDP-17. Recently, a family with CJD associated with a point mutation at codon 183 of the prion protein gene presented at median age of 44 years with behavioural disturbances as the predominant presenting symptom. Eight of the nine patients manifested parkinsonian signs and dementia thus resembling FTDP-17 (Nitrini et al., 2001).

Multiple system atrophy (MSA)

Background

Multiple system atrophy (MSA) is a sporadic progressive degenerative neurological disorder characterized clinically by the combination of varying degrees of parkinsonism, autonomic dysfunction and impaired cerebellar function (Quinn, 1989). Early descriptions focused on the most conspicuous clinical manifestation, so that it was variously described as striatonigral degeneration (SND), (predominant parkinsonism with a poor response to levodopa), Shy–Drager syndrome (SDS) (parkinsonism and/or cerebellar syndrome with predominant autonomic dysfunction) and sporadic olivopontocerebellar atrophy (sOPCA) (predominant cerebellar dysfunction). Although sOPCA was described in 1900 by Dejerine and Thomas, it was not until the 1960s that other presentations of MSA were documented by Shy and Drager (1960), Adams et al. (striatonigral degeneration, 1961) and Graham and Oppenheimer (1969). The term MSA thus describes a syndrome with features overlapping with SDS, SND and sOPCA (Quinn, 1989). The discovery of the characteristic histology marked by the glial cytoplasmic inclusions by Papp and Lantos in 1989 which are present in all these three types defined MSA as a clinico-pathological entity. MSA seems to be greatly under-recognized and, in one series of 35 pathologically proven cases of MSA, 30% had an incorrect diagnosis of Parkinson's disease (PD) at the time of death (Wenning et al., 1995).

The population prevalence of MSA has been estimated at 4.4 per 100 000, thus representing 2.4% of cases of parkinsonism (Schrag et al., 1999). The disease affects both men and women usually starting in the sixth decade, the median age at onset being 54 years. Onset before age 30 years has not been described and the incidence of the disease appears to decline after peaking in the early 50s. Median survival from first symptom to death was 9.5 years in one large clinical series (Wenning et al., 1994) but only 6.2 years in a large retrospective meta-analysis of pathologically proven cases from the literature (Ben Shlomo et al., 1997).

Clinical features

The clinical features and their frequency are listed, from a report of 203 pathologically verified cases of MSA, in Table 34.6 (Wenning et al., 1997). Bradykinesia, rigidity, and postural and rest tremor as well as dysequilibrium and gait unsteadiness characterize the parkinsonism associated with MSA. Although 67% of patients have resting tremor, a

Table 34.6. Clinical features in 203 cases of MSA

Features	Frequency (%)	CI (95%)
Autonomic symptoms		
Urinary incontinence	55	(48–62)
Postural faintness	51	(44–58)
Impotence	47	(37–56)
Recurrent syncope (>2)	18	(12–23)
Urinary retention	18	(13–24)
Fecal incontinence	12	(8–17)
Parkinsonism		
Akinesia	83	(77–88)
Tremor*	67	(60–73)
Present at rest	39	(32–46)
Pill-rolling	8	(5–12)
Jerky	3	(1–6)
Not specified	25	(18–32)
Rigidity	63	(56–70)
L-Dopa response		
Best Poor	72	(62–83)
Good	28	(17–38)
Last Poor	95	(75–92)
Good	5	(1–12)
Dyskinesias	27	(17–38)
Orofacial	15	(8–25)
Limbs	10	(4–19)
Fluctuations	24	(15–35)
Cerebellar signs		
Gait ataxia	49	(42–56)
Limb ataxia	47	(40–54)
Intention tremor	24	(18–30)
Nystagmus	23	(18–30)
Pyramidal signs		
Hyperreflexia	46	(39–53)
Extensor plantar response	41	(34–48)
Spasticity	10	(6–15)
Other features		
Intellectual deterioration		
Mild	22	(17–29)
Moderate	2	(1–5)
Severe	0.5	(0–3)
Stridor	13	(9–18)
Dystonia	12	(8–17)
Anisocoria	8	(5–12)
Contractures	7	(4–11)

Notes:

* Some patients had more than one type of tremor.

CI, confidence interval.

Source: From Wenning et al. (2001).

classic pill rolling rest tremor typical of PD is almost never or very rarely (8%) present in MSA patients. Up to 90% of patients with the parkinsonian presentation (MSA-P) treated with levodopa do not have a sustained response over the long term although there may be some initial benefit. Also unusual levodopa-induced dyskinesia often involving the orofacial region, as a dystonic grimacing of one side of the face, occur in MSA (Wenning et al., 1994). The cerebellar disorder consists of gait ataxia commonly leading to early falls when associated with the extrapyramidal loss of postural reflexes. Limb kinetic ataxia, scanning dysarthria and cerebellar oculomotor disturbances are other features of cerebellar dysfunction. Autonomic failure in MSA is manifested predominantly as symptomatic orthostatic hypotension which is defined as a 20 mm Hg fall of systolic or 10 mm Hg fall of diastolic blood pressure. Erectile disturbance is common and may be the earliest feature of MSA in males. Other features include increased constipation, hypohidrosis or anhidrosis. Urinary bladder disturbances are also common including urinary urgency, frequency, nocturia and urge incontinence.

Mild cognitive problems occur in about 22% of cases but moderate to severe dementia rules against the diagnosis of MSA. Apart from the main features mentioned above, softer signs or 'red flags' as they are called by Quinn (1995) often indicate the diagnosis. These include REM sleep behaviour disorder, inspiratory sighs, snoring, stridor, myoclonus, contractures and the so-called disproportionate anterocollis where the head is severely flexed forward with a fairly upright stance or/and the 'Pisa' syndrome where the patient leans to one side. Diagnostic criteria for MSA (Gilman et al., 1998) are shown in Tables 34.7, 34.8 and 34.9, which have to be used together.

Differential diagnosis

The difficulty most commonly faced is to differentiate MSA from PD or PSP. Colosimo et al., in 1995 attempted to identify factors that could assist in the early differentiation of MSA-P from PD and PSP and suggested that, in patients with symmetric onset, rapid progression, lack of tremor, orthostasis and little benefit from levodopa the diagnosis of MSA should be very carefully considered (Colosimo et al., 1996). Wenning et al. (2000) posing the same question developed a model based on the emergence of features within the first five years of the illness. The four features selected included: presence of autonomic features (2), poor initial response to levodopa (2), early fluctuations (2) and initial rigidity (2). Of note, 23% of PD subjects' initial response to levodopa was poor,

while 58% of MSA cases had a poor response. Dementia and psychiatric symptoms were more common in PD than MSA. Speech impairment and axial instability were almost universal in the MSA cases. Autonomic failure occurred in 84% of the MSA cases but also in 26% of the PD cases. These findings should be considered when making the diagnosis in a given patient.

Diagnostic investigations

The diagnosis of MSA is thus largely clinical, based on the history and examination. No investigation is diagnostic by itself but diagnostic tests may help in supporting the clinical impression and help with excluding the differential diagnosis. In patients with urogenital complaints, external sphincter electromyography frequently shows prolonged and polyphasic muscle potentials consistent with deinervation and reinervation of voluntary sphincter muscles. However, sphincter EMG is a sophisticated technique that is not widely available. Also, because interpretation of the results requires great caution, since it may be affected by previous traumatic childbirth, abdominal, rectal, or retropubic prostatic surgery, and also since it is often abnormal in PSP (Valldeoriola et al., 1995) it is not particularly helpful in distinguishing between MSA and PSP. Nonetheless, if correctly undertaken and interpreted, the presence of an abnormal sphincter EMG can still be a useful ancillary investigation pointing away from idiopathic PD (Palace et al., 1997; Tison et al., 2000).

CT brain scans may show infratentorial atrophy in MSA patients. In almost 90% of patients with MSA brain, MRI shows characteristic changes in the striatum, brainstem and cerebellum (Schrag et al., 1998, 2000; Schultz et al., 1999). In T_2-weighted images there is frequently a hyperintense signal seen adjacent to the posterolateral putamen which itself displays a hypointense signal due to atrophic changes. What is the morphological basis of the hyperintense band is not entirely certain but it may be due to activated microglia seen adjacent to atrophic putamenal tissue. This appearance is a useful diagnostic marker with an estimated sensitivity of 93% and specifity of 88%. Another characteristic appearance is the so called 'hot cross bun' sign of MSA (Fig. 34.4); on T_2-weighted images of the brainstem, a hyperintense signal in the shape of a cross seen in the pons (Schrag et al., 1998). MR spectroscopy has shown reduced N-acetylcysteine as a metabolic correlate of neuronal cell loss in MSA (Davie et al., 1995) but, as yet, this has limited diagnostic value in a given patient. Functional imaging may be a useful adjuvant in support of the diagnosis but the changes are not specific

Table 34.7. Diagnostic categories of MSA

I. Possible MSA
One criterion plus two features from separate other domains. When the criterion is parkinsonism, a poor levodopa response qualifies as one feature (hence only one additional feature is required)

II. Probable MSA
Criterion for: autonomic failure/urinary dysfunction plus poorly levodopa responsive parkinsonsim or cerebellar dysfunction

III. Definite MSA
Pathologically confirmed by the presence of a high density of glial cytoplasmic inclusions in association with a combination of degenerative changes in the nigrostriatal and olivopontocerebellar pathways

Table 34.8. Exclusion criteria for the diagnosis of MSA

I. History
Symptomatic onset under 30 years of age
Family history of a similar disorder
Systemic disease or other identifiable causes for features listed in Table 34.7
Hallucinations unrelated to medication

II. Physical examination
DSM criteria for dementia
Prominent slowing of vertical saccades or vertical supranuclear gaze palsy
Evidence of local cortical dysfunction such as aphasia, alien limb syndrome, and parietal dysfunction

III. Laboratory investigation
Metabolic, molecular genetic, and imaging evidence of an alternative cause of features listed in Table 34.3

Source: From Gilman et al. (1998).

Table 34.9. Clinical domains, features and criteria used in the diagnosis of MSA

I. Autonomic and urinary dysfunction
A. Autonomic and urinary features
    1. Orthostatic hypotension by (20 mm Hg systolic or 10 mm Hg diastolic)
    2. Urinary incontinence or incomplete bladder emptying
B. Criterion for autonomic failure or urinary dysfunction in MSA
Orthostatic falls in blood pressure by (30 mm Hg systolic or 15 mm Hg diastolic) or urinary incontinence (persistent, involuntary partial or total bladder emptying, accompanied by erectile dysfunction in men) or both

II. Parkinsonism
A. Parkinsonian features
    1. Bradykinesia (slowness of voluntary movement with progressive reduction in speed and amplitude during repetitive actions)
    2. Rigidity
    3. Postural instability (not caused by primary visual, vestibular, cerebellar, or proprioceptive dysfunction)
    4. Tremor (postural, resting or both)
B. Criterion for parkinsonism in MSA
    Bradykinesia plus at least one of items 2 to 4

III. Cerebellar dysfunction
A. Cerebellar features
    1. Gait ataxia (wide based stance with steps in irregular length and direction)
    2. Ataxic dysarthria
    3. Limb ataxia
    4. Sustained gaze-evoked nystagmus
Criterion for cerebellar dysfunction in MSA
Gait ataxia plus at least one of items 2 to 4

IV. Corticospinal tract dysfunction
A. Corticospinal tract features
    1. Extensor plantar responses with hyperreflexia
B. Corticospinal tract dysfunction in MSA: no corticospinal tract features are used in defining the diagnosis of MSA

Notes:
A feature (A) is characteristic of the disease and a criterion (B) is a defining feature or composite of features required for diagnosis.

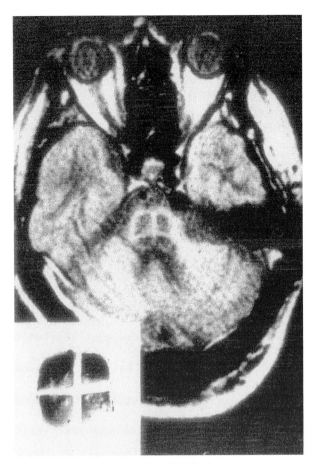

Fig. 34.4. MRI T$_2$-weighted image of the brainstem in a patient with multiple system atrophy showing infratentorial atrophy and typical signal change in the pons in the form of a cross resembling that seen on hotcross buns (inset) which are baked typically over Easter. (Courtesy Prof. Niall Quinn, Institute of Neurology, Queen Square, with permission from Journal of Neurology, Neurosurgery and Psychiatry.)

for MSA. IBZM SPECT shows reduced striatal dopamine D2 receptor binding in MSA and may predict l-dopa unresponsiveness with these patients turning out to have either MSA-P or PSP (Schulz et al., 1994; Schwarz et al., 1998). However, dopamine transporter ligands such as beta CIT so far are not particularly useful for the differential diagnosis (Brucke et al., 1997; Pirker et al., 2000). Fluorodopa PET scanning shows reduced uptake both in the putamen and caudate, a pattern different from PD but which may be seen with other atypical parkinsonian conditions like PSP or CBD. Increased striatal binding of both D2 and D1 receptor ligands (11C-SCH 23390) has been noted (Brooks et al., 1992; Momose et al., 1997; Shinotoh et al., 1993). On the other hand, there is decreased uptake in the putamen

and caudate with opiod receptor ligand ^{11}C-diprenorphine (Burn et al., 1995). Specialized imaging can thus suggest that the patient has an atypical parkinsonian condition and not Parkinson's disease but cannot definitely differentiate between the different atypical parkinsonian disorders.

Pathology

Pathologically, there is neuronal loss and gliosis in substantia nigra, striatum (mainly posterior putamen), inferior olives, cerebellar Purkinje cells and pontine nuclei, and the intermediolateral cell columns and Onuf's nucleus of the spinal cord, to varying degrees according to clinical emphasis (Terao et al., 1994; Daniel, 1992). The current nomenclature is MSA-P, in which parkinsonism is more prominent, and MSA-C, in which cerebellar dysfunction is more prominent. The identification of a common pathology, the presence of glial cytoplasmic inclusions (GCIs) in oligodendrocytes (Papp et al., 1989), in these syndromes confirmed the suspicion that these disorders are manifestations of the same process. Glial inclusion formation which is thus characteristic of MSA has been added to the consensus diagnostic criteria of definite MSA (Gilman et al., 1998). GCIs are argyrophilic and half-moon, oval or conical in shape (Fig. 34.5, see colour plate section). They are distributed selectively in the basal ganglia, supplementary and primary motor cortex, reticular formation, bases pontis, the middle cerebellar peduncle and the cerebellar white matter (Lantos, 1998; Papp & Lantos, 1994). The origin of the GCIs is not known, but they are known to consist of filaments 20–30 nm in diameter and are antigenic for ubiquitin and tau (Lantos, 1998). The tau in MSA, however, resembles nomal adult tau (Cairns et al., 1997; Spillantini et al., 1998a, b; Takeda et al., 1997). Recently, alpha-synuclein has been observed in both neuronal and glial cytoplasmic inclusions in MSA brains (Fig. 34.3) (Wakabayashi et al., 1998; Arima et al., 1998; Tu et al., 1998). This has led to the notion that MSA belongs to the group of synucleinopathies like PD and DLB (Spillantini, 1999). What the role of alpha-synuclein is in the pathogenesis of MSA is not clear. Usually, this protein is found in the soluble fraction of neuronal cytoplasm, however in pathological states for example MSA, alpha-synuclein forms insoluble aggregates. Whether this is a primary event or a secondary epiphenomenon of MSA pathology remains to be discovered.

MSA is known to be a sporadic condition and abnormalities of alpha-synuclein gene causing autosomal dominant Parkinson's disease (A53T and A30P) have not been found in confirmed cases of MSA (Ozawa et al., 1999; Kruger et al.,

1998) suggesting that these mutations are not the pathogenic cause of MSA.

Therapy

Although MSA patients have a poor or unsustained response to levodopa almost 30% do have some benefit initially and hence it is worth trying (Wenning et al., 1994). In fact as per one report about 5% of cases still responded to levodopa after 5 years of treatment (Wenning et al., 1994). Patients with MSA also develop dyskinesias but unlike PD these are dystonic and often involve the face (Wenning et al., 1994). Dopamine agonists are generally not beneficial and poorly tolerated. Amantidine has not been found to be useful (Colosimo et al., 1996). The parkinsonian features of MSA are not helped by stereotactic surgery including pallidotomy and subthalamic nucleus stimulation and, in fact, the suspicion of MSA is a contraindication for these procedures. Management of orthostatic hypotension can be difficult. Increased salt intake, elastic stockings and head-up tilt of about 30 degrees are useful physical measures. Drugs like fludrocortisone, ephedrine and octreotide may be useful. For bladder urgency and urge incontinence, oxybutinin can be helpful. Physical therapy including use of walking aids and speech as well as occupational therapy can be very useful in these cases usually more so than drug treatments.

Dementia with Lewy bodies (DLB)

This condition which used to be called diffuse Lewy body disease has recently been defined as a clinical pathological entity (McKeith et al., 1996) in a consensus report of an international consortium. The syndrome is characterized by cognitive deficit and parkinsonism. Onset age is between 50 and 85 years. Cognitive impairment in DLB resembles that seen in Alzheimer's disease (AD), but memory loss is less marked early on; however, differentiation on clinical grounds alone may be difficult. Fluctuations in cognitive state often present as confusional states. Pathologically there are Lewy bodies, alpha-synuclein immunoreactive Lewy neuritis and neuronal loss in the neocortex and subcortical nuclei. Thus dementia with Lewy bodies is a synucleinopathy (Spillantini, 1999). Diffuse and neuritic amyloid plaques and neocortical neurofibrillary tangles can also be seen in about a quarter of cases. What is the relationship between Lewy bodies and the Alzheimer's type of change is still unresolved. However, it is clear that the clinical syndrome of dementia, psychosis and autonomic failure can occur with the presence of Lewy bodies alone (without significant Alzheimer's changes). Compared to Alzheimer's disease on formal neurospsychometry, attention and working memory appears to be disproportionately impaired in DLB, and these patients are worse off in visuospatial and constructional tasks and perception (Gnanlingham et al., 1997; Calderon et al., 2001). About 80% with DLB will develop extrapyramidal features in the course of the disease (McKeith et al., 1996). The parkinsonism in DLB may differ somewhat from PD, with symmetrical signs, uncommon resting tremor, frequent myoclonic jerks and an unpredictable response to levodopa. Recurrent visual hallucinations, depression and delusions are common, as is a REM sleep disorder which may precede the other features (Boeve et al., 1999). Autonomic dysfunction can be present leading to syncope and falls. The clinical criteria for the diagnosis of DLB have been suggested (McKeith et al., 1996). In addition to the progressive cognitive decline, two of the following are required for the diagnosis of 'probable' DLB (one for possible DLB): (i) Fluctuating course with pronounced variations in attention and alertness; (ii) recurrent, well-formed visual hallucinations and (ii) motor features of parkinsonism. Supportive features (not required for the diagnosis) include repeated falls, syncope, transient loss of consciousness, neuroleptic sensitivity, systematized delusions and hallucinations in other modalities. Clinically, differentiation from other Parkinsonian-plus syndromes can be difficult. Both MSA, if the autonomic features are present, and PSP, if there is dementia and supranuclear gaze palsy which can sometimes be seen in DLB (Lewis & Gawel, 1990), can come into the differential as can different dementing disorders including Alzheimer's and Pick's disease and corticobasal degeneration to name a few. However, as yet there are no specific antemortem biological markers for DLB and the clinical differentiation between these disorders remains a diagnostic challenge. Recent advances in structural and functional imaging can be useful but not definitive in making the diagnosis. Structural brain imaging shows generalized atrophy in DLB and in 50% or so the medial temporal lobe appears to be relatively preserved unlike Alzheimer's disease (Barber et al., 1999). Dopaminergic dysfunction in DLB can be shown by SPECT studies using dopamine transporter and this may help differentiate it from AD (Walker et al., 1999) but not from other parkinsonian syndromes.

Secondary/symptomatic parkinsonism

These are listed in Table 34.1 and some of them will be discussed in the section below.

Postencephalitic parkinsonism (PEP) and other infections

Encephalitis lethargica or postencephalitic parkinsonism (PEP) occurring after the pandemics of influenza beween 1918 and 1926 is well recognized (Calne & Lees, 1988). The parkinsonism in these cases usually occurred after a latent period, sometimes of many years. The presence of associated features such as oculogyric crises, blepharospasm and rarely, chorea, tic, and dystonia helped differentiate this disorder from PD. However, there appear to be many similarities between PEP and PSP and the Parkinson–dementia complex of Guam both clinically and pathologically (Geddes et al., 1993). Neuropathologists have great difficulty differentiating PSP and PEP on postmortem brains (Geddes et al., 1993). However, when clinical data is available, the sensitivity and reliability of diagnosis of PEP improves significantly (Litvan et al., 1996a, b). All three conditions display neurofibrillary tangles in subcortical and cortical areas and therefore a common etiology has been suspected but seems unlikely. New sporadic cases of PEP still occur rarely (Howard & Lees, 1987). However, other types of encephalitis such as Japanese B encephalitis in south east Asia, Western Equine encephalitis and others can also cause parkinsonism. Unlike encephalitis lethargica where there was a long latency period, in Japanese B and others, mentioned earlier the parkinsonism appears as the acute phase is resolving. Creutzfeldt–Jacob disease can present as a rapidly progressive parkinsonian syndrome with dementia and myoclonus associated (Brown et al., 1993). Parkinsonian signs and dementia resembling FTDP-17 have been described in a familial CJD with prion gene mutation (Nitrini et al., 2001).

Drug-induced parkinsonism

Perhaps the commonest secondary cause of parkinsonism is due to drugs. Neuroleptic drugs or dopamine receptor blockers are the usual culprit. Mostly, these drugs have been used to treat psychosis or other psychiatric disorders but it is important to remember that these drugs can be used for other indications, for example metoclopromide which is used to treat gastrointestinal symptoms and is a powerful D2 receptor blocking agent. The prevalence of neuroleptic-induced parkinsonism is estimated variably from 5% to 60% in those treated with these drugs. Female more than male, age, and possible genetic tendency are possible risk factors. Neuroleptic drug may be unmasking latent Parkinson's disease. One study by Rajput et al. (1982) showed that some patients who recovered from neuroleptic-induced parkinsonism had pathological changes of PD on postmortem.

Also, apart from neuroleptics, calcium channel blockers like cinnarazine and flunnarazine and even serotonin reuptake inhibitors (SSRIs) can induce parkinsonism.

Vascular parkinsonism

The clinical features here are fairly characteristic with gait difficulty freezing being the prominent feature as well as postural reflex impairment. Apart from that urinary and cognitive symptoms may be present. As there is no true bradykinesia involving the upper limbs some refer to this condition as a form of pseudo-parkinsonism (Quinn, 1995). There is usually no tremor and the response to levodopa is poor. Imaging will show multiple lacunes involving the basal ganglia. Rarely, a frontal tumour like a meningioma or other mass lesion may present with a similar clinical picture. Removal of the tumour can lead to resolution of the parkinsonian features, which must be caused by indirect pressure effects on the dopaminergic nigrostriatal pathway.

Toxins

A variety of toxins and heavy metals can cause parkinsonism. Exposure to manganese causing toxicity in miners without proper protective gear produces an atypical parkinsonian syndrome manifested as akinesia, postural reflex loss usually without tremor (Pal et al., 1999). There are dystonic features affecting the feet and legs and causing a peculiar gait with the patients walking on their toes, referred to as 'cock-walk'. The early phase of the intoxication may be characterized by psychic, non-motor signs. The neurological syndrome does not respond to levodopa. If these extrapyramidal findings are present, they are likely to be irreversible and even progress after termination of the exposure to manganese (Pal et al., 1999). Imaging of the brain may reveal MRI signal changes in the globus pallidus, striatum, and midbrain. Positron emission tomography reveals normal presynaptic and postsynaptic nigrostriatal dopaminergic function (Pal et al., 1999). Gliosis in the pallidal segments underlies the well-established phase of the intoxication. The mechanism of toxicity is not clear and oxidative stress is considered as a possibility.

Carbon monoxide, cyanide, MPTP, n-hexane and organophosphates (Bhatt et al., 1999) all can produce a parkinsonian syndrome. Bhatt et al. (1999) described five patients with exposure to organophosphates who acutely developed an atypical parkinsonian syndrome poorly responsive to levodopa which reversed in four patients completely after withdrawal from exposure and one patient experienced repeated episodes of parkinsonism with inadvertent re-exposure.

Trauma

A direct link between trauma and parkinsonism has been long debated (Stern, 1991; Jankovic, 1994). However, it is widely accepted that repeated head injury for example in boxers leads to what is described as the chronic traumatic brain injury (CTBI) syndrome (Jordan, 2000). This presents with varying degrees of motor, cognitive, and/or behavioural impairments. Parkinsonism is a feature of the motor syndrome, along with gait imbalance and loss of postural reflexes. The severe form of CTBI is referred to as 'dementia pugilistica'. The diagnosis of CTBI is dependent upon documenting a progressive neurological condition that is consistent with the clinical symptomatology of CTBI attributable to brain trauma and unexplainable by an alternative pathophysiological process (Jordan, 2000). Pathologically, CTBI shares many characteristics with Alzheimer's disease (i.e. neurofibrillary triangles, diffuse amyloid plaques, acetylcholine deficiency, and/or tau immunoreactivity) (Jordan, 2000). The mainstay of treatment of CTBI is prevention; however, medications used in the treatment of Alzheimer's disease and/or parkinsonism could be tried, although no controlled trials have been done.

More contentious is the notion that head injury can cause or precipitate Parkinson's disease. Although trauma is mentioned in epidemiological studies, there is only a weak causal relationship between trauma and PD as a result of recall bias, time between injury and onset of the condition and other factors. Long-term prospective data fail to corroborate an increased incidence of PD among a cohort of head injury patients (Williams et al., 1991). There are some exceptions. Recently, Bhatt et al. (2000) reported three patients who developed a rapidly evolving post-traumatic akinetic-rigid syndrome following head injury, the clinical manifestations of which were similar to parkinson's disease, including response to levodopa. In all three cases imaging studies showing traumatic damage to the substantia nigra; however, the parkinsonian syndrome appeared only after a delay of 1–5 months after the injury. However trauma remains a rare cause of parkinsonism. Cardoso & Jankovic (1995), have proposed that even peripheral injury can result in movement disorders including parkinsonism. However, not all agree with this assumption. For example, recently there was a report of parkinsonism following electric injury to the hand (Morris et al., 1998) but this claim was refuted by Quinn and Marganore (2000), who suggested that this was a coincidence.

Hereditary/heredodegenerative disorders

These have been listed in Table 34.1 and many of these disorders are detailed elsewhere in other chapters. A few conditions will be mentioned briefly here. About 10% or 50 of patients with Huntington's disease present with an akinetic rigid syndrome rather than chorea and this is often referred to as the Westphal's variant. This presentation is more common in the juvenile onset cases who are more likely to have inherited the CAG triplet repeat disorder from their fathers.

Wilson's disease usually presents with dystonia, imbalance, dysartria, and psychiatric or cognitive disturbances. Sometimes they may manifest with parkinsonism and all juvenile onset parkinsonian patients must have serum copper and ceruloplasmin assay and a slit-lamp examination for presence of Kayser–Fleischer rings. It is important not to miss this potentially treatable disorder. Copper chelating agents like D-penicillamine can be very effective.

Neuroacanthocytosis mostly occurs as a neurological syndrome with chorea, personality change, orofacial dyskinesias or dystonia causing feeding difficulty and self-mutilation, and often absent tendon reflexes due to an axonal peripheral neuropathy (Hardie et al., 1991). Rarely, parkinsonism may be the predominant feature rather than the chorea (Peppard et al., 1990) and sometimes there can be progression from an earlier hyperkinetic disorder to a later parkinsonian state (Stevenson & Hardie, 2001). Diagnosis requires the demonstration of acanthocytes in a peripheral blood smear and serum creatine kinase is frequently elevated.

Hallervorden–Spatz syndrome usually presents in childhood predominantly as a dystonic syndrome often with associated dementia, psychiatric disturbances and retinal pigmentary changes. Rarely, onset in adolescence or adulthood may be with predominant parkinsonism. Pathologically there are spheroids seen and there is deposition of iron in the globus pallidus and zona reticulata of the substantia nigra. The diagnosis may be indicated by MRI changes due to the iron deposition producing the typical 'eye of the tiger' sign with a zone of decreased intensity (due to iron) with hyperintensity on T_2-weighted images. Treatment is only symptomatic and not usually beneficial.

References

Adams, R.D., van Bogaert, L. & van der Eecken, H. (1961). Dégénérescences nigrostriées et cérébello-nigro-striées. *Psychiat. Neurolog.*, **142**, 219–59.

Arima, K., Ueda, K., Sunohara, N. et al. (1998). NACP/alpha-synuclein immunoreactivity in fibrillary components of neuronal and oligodendroglial cytoplasmic inclusions in the pontine nuclei in multiple system atrophy. *Acta Neuropathol. (Berl.)*, **96**, 439–44.

Averbuch-Heller, L., Paulson, G.W., Daroff, R.B. & Leigh, R.J. (1999). Whipple's disease mimicking progressive supranuclear palsy: the diagnostic value of eye movement recording. *J. Neurol., Neurosurg. Psychiatry*, **66**, 532–5.

Baker, M., Litvan, I., Houlden, H. et al. (1999). Association of an extended haplotype in the tau gene with progressive supranuclear palsy. *Hum. Mol. Genet.*, **8**, 711–15.

Barber, R., Gholkar, A., Ballard, C., Scheltens, P., McKeith, I. & O'Brien, J.T. (1999). Medial temporal lobe atrophy on MRI in dementia with Lewy bodies: a comparison with Alzheimer's disease, vascular dementia and normal ageing. *Neurology*, **52**, 1153–8.

Barclay, C.L., Bergeron, C. & Lang, A.E. (1999). Arm levitation in progressive supranuclear palsy. *Neurology*, **52**, 879–82.

Ben-Shlomo, Y., Wenning, G.K., Tison, F. & Quinn, N.P. (1997). Survival of patients with pathologically proven multiple system atrophy: a meta-analysis. *Neurology*, **48**, 384–93.

Bergeron, C., Pollanen, M.S., Weyer, L., Black, S.E. & Lang, A.E. (1996). Unusual clinical presentations of cortico–basal ganglionic degeneration. *Ann. Neurol.*, **40**, 893–900.

Bhatia, K.P., Lee, M.S., Rinne, J.O. et al. (2000). Corticobasal degeneration look-alikes. *Adv. Neurol.*, **82**, 169–82.

Bhatt, M.H., Elias, M.A. & Mankodi, A.K. (1999). Acute and reversible parkinsonism due to organophosphate pesticide intoxication: five cases. *Neurology*, **52**(7), 1467–71.

Bhatt, M., Desai, J., Mankodi, A., Elias, M. & Wadia, N. (2000). Posttraumatic akinetic-rigid syndrome resembling Parkinson's disease: a report on three patients. *Mov. Disord.*, **15**(2), 313–17.

Bird, T.D., Nochlin, D., Poorkaj, P. et al. (1999). A clinical pathological comparison of three families with frontotemporal dementia and identical mutations in the tau gene (P301L). *Brain*, **122**, 741–56.

Blin, J., Baron, J.C., Dubois, B. et al. (1990). Positron emission tomography study in progressive supranuclear palsy. Brain hypometabolic pattern and clinicometabolic correlations. *Arch. Neurol.*, **47**, 747–52.

Blin, J., Mazetti, P., Mazoyer, B. et al. (1995). Does the enhancement of cholinergic neurotransmission influence brain glucose kinetics and clinical symptomatology in progressive supranuclear palsy? *Brain*, **118**, 1485–95.

Boeve, B.F., Maraganore, D.M., Parisi, J.E. et al. (1999). Pathologic heterogeneity in clinically diagnosed corticobasal degeneration. *Neurology*, **53**, 795–800.

Brooks, D.J. (1994). PET studies in progressive supranuclear palsy. *J. Neural. Transm. Suppl.*, **42**, 119–34.

Brooks, D.J. (2000). Corticobasal degeneration. Functional imaging studies in corticobasal degeneration. *Adv. Neurol.*, **82**, 209–15.

Brooks, D.J., Ibanez, V., Sawle, G.V. et al. (1992). Striatal D2 receptor status in patients with Parkinson's disease, striatonigral degeneration, and progressive supranuclear palsy, measured with ^{11}C-raclopride and positron emission tomography. *Ann. Neurol.*, **31**, 184–92.

Brown, J., Lantos, P., Stratton, M. et al. (1993). Familial progressive supranuclear palsy. *J. Neurol., Neurosurg. Psychiatry*, **56**, 473–6.

Brown, P., Gibbs, C.J. Jr, Rodgers-Johnson, P. et al. (1994). Human spongiform encephalopathy: the National Institutes of Health series of 300 cases of experimentally transmitted disease. *Ann. Neurol.*, **35**, 513–29.

Brucke, T., Assenbaum, S., Pirker, W. et al. (1997). Measurement of the dopaminergic degeneration in Parkinson's disease with [^{123}I] beta-CIT and SPECT: correlation with clinical findings and comparison with multiple system atrophy and progressive supranuclear palsy. *J. Neural. Transm. Suppl.*, **50**, 9–24.

Burn, D.J., Rinne, J.O., Quinn, N.P., Lees, A.J., Marsden, C.D. & Brooks, D.J. (1995). Striatal opioid receptor binding in Parkinson's disease, striatonigral degeneration and Steele–Richardson–Olszewski syndrome, a [^{11}C]diprenorphine PET study. *Brain*, **118**, 951–8.

Cairns, N.J., Atkinson, P.F., Hanger, D.P., Anderton, B.H., Daniel, S.E. & Lantos, P.L. (1997). Tau protein in the glial cytoplasmic inclusions of multiple system atrophy can be distinguished from abnormal tau in Alzheimer's disease. *Neurosci. Lett.*, **230**, 49–52.

Calderon, J., Perry, R.J., Erzincliglu, S.W., Berrios, G.E., Dening, T.R. & Hodges, J.R. Perception, attention and working memory are disproportionately impaired in dementia with Lewy bodies compared with Alzheimer's disease. *J. Neurol., Neurosurg. Psychiatry*, **70**, 154–61.

Calric, D.B. & Lees, A.J. (1988). Late progression of postencephalic Parkinson's syndrome. *Can. J. Neurol. Sci.*, **15**, 135–8.

Caparros-Lefebvre, D., Elbaz, A. and the Caribbean parkinsonism study group. (1999). Possible relation of atypical parkinsonism in the French West Indies with consumption of tropical plants: a case control study. *Lancet*, **354**, 281–6.

Cardosa, F. & Jankovic, J. (1995). Peripherally induced tremor and parkinsonism. *Arch. Neurol.*, **52**, 263–70.

Collins, S.J., Ahlskog, J.E., Parisi, J.E. & Maraganore, D.M. (1995). Progressive supranuclear palsy: neuropathologically based diagnostic clinical criteria. *J. Neurol., Neurosurg. Psychiatry*, **58**, 167–73.

Colosimo, C., Merello, M. & Pontieri, F.E. (1996). Amantadine in parkinsonian patients unresponsive to levodopa: a pilot study [letter]. *J. Neurol.*, **243**, 422–5.

Conrad, C., Andreadis, A., Trojanowski, J.Q. et al. (1997). Genetic evidence for the involvement of tau in progressive supranuclear palsy. *Ann. Neurol.*, **41**, 277–81.

Daniel, S.E. (1992). The neuropathology and neurochemistry of multiple system atrophy. In *A Textbook of Clinical Disorders of Autonomic Nervous System*, ed. R. Bannister & C. Mathias, 3rd edn, pp. 564–85. Oxford: Oxford University Press.

Daniel, S.E., de Bruin, V.M. & Lees, A.J. (1995). The clinical and pathological spectrum of Steele–Richardson–Olszewski syndrome (progressive supranuclear palsy): a reappraisal. *Brain*, **118**, 759–70.

Davie, C.A., Wenning, G.K., Barker, G.J. et al. (1995). Differentiation of multiple system atrophy from idiopathic Parkinson's disease using proton magnetic resonance spectroscopy. *Ann. Neurol.*, **37**, 204–10.

Davis, P.H., Bergeron, C. & McLachlan, D.R. (1985). Atypical presentation of progressive supranuclear palsy. *Ann. Neurol.*, **17**, 337–43.

Davis, P.H., Golbe, L.I., Duvoisin, R.C. & Schonberg, B.S. (1988). Risk factors for progressive supranuclear palsy. *Neurology*, **38**, 1546–52.

Dejerine, J. & Thomas, A.A. (1900). L'atrophie olivo-ponto-cérébelleuse. *Nouvelle Iconographie de le Salpêtrière*, **13**, 330–70.

De Yebenes, J.G., Sarasa, J.L., Daniel, S.E. & Lees, A.J. (1995). Familial progressive supranuclear palsy. Description of a pedigree and review of the literature. *Brain*, **118**, 1095–104.

Dickson, D.W. (1997). Neurodegenerative disorders with cytoskeletal pathology: a biological classification. *Ann. Neurol.*, **42**, 541–4.

Dickson, D.W. (1999). Neuropathologic differentiation of progressive supranuclear palsy and corticobasal degeneration. *J. Neurol.*, **246**(2), 116.

Dickson, D.W., Liu, W-K., Ksiezak-Redig, H. & Yen, S-H. (2000). Neuropathology and molecular consideration. *Adv. Neurol.*, **82**, 9–28.

Di Maria, E., Tabaton, M., Vigo, T. et al. (2000). Corticobasal degeneration shares a common genetic background with progressive supranuclear palsy. *Ann. Neurol.*, **47**, 374–7.

D'Souza, I., Poorkaj, P., Hong, M. et al. (1999). Missense and silent tau gene mutations cause frontotemporal dementia with parkinsonism-chromosome 17 type, by affecting multiple alternative RNA splicing regulatory elements. *Proc. Natl. Acad. Sci., USA*, **11**(96), 5598–603.

Dumanchin, C., Camuzat, A., Campion, D. et al. (1998). Segregation of a missense mutation in the microtubule-associated protein in tau gene with familial frontotemporal dementia and parkinsonisms. *Hum. Mol. Genet.*, **7**, 1825–9.

Fabbrini, G., Vanacore, N., Bonifati, V. et al. (1998). Presymptomatic hypertension in progressive supranuclear palsy. *Arch. Neurol.*, **55**, 1153–4

Feany, M.B. & Dickson, D. (1996). Neurodegenerative disorders with extensive tau pathology: a comparative study and review. *Ann. Neurol.*, **40**(2), 139–48.

Fearnley, J.M., Revesz, T., Brooks, D.J., Frackowiak, R.S. & Lees, A.J. (1991). Diffuse Lewy body disease presenting with a supranuclear gaze palsy. *J. Neurol., Neurosurg. Psychiatry*, **54**, 159–61.

Federico, F., Simone, I.L., Lucivero, V. et al. (1997). Proton magnetic resonance spectroscopy in parkinson's disease and progressive supranuclear palsy. *J. Neurol., Neurosurg. Psychiatry*, **62**, 239–342.

Feifel, E., Brenner, M., Teiwes, R., Lucking, C.H. & Deuschl, G. (1994). Corticobasal degeneration. The significance of clinical criteria for establishing the diagnosis. *Nervenarzt.*, **65**, 653–9.

Furukawa, K., D'Souza, I., Crudder, C.H. et al. (2000). Pro-apoptotic effects of tau mutations in chromosome 17 frontotemporal dementia and parkinsonism. *Neuroreport*, **11**, 57–60.

Gearing, M., Olson, D.A., Watts, R.L. & Mirra, S.S. (1994). Progressive supranuclear palsy: neuropathologic and clinical heterogeneity. *Neurology*, **44**, 1015–24.

Geddes, J.F., Hughes, A.J., Lees, A.J. & Daniel, S.E. (1993). Pathological overlap in cases of parkinsonism associated with neurofibrillary tangles. A study of recent cases of postencephalitic parkinsonism and comparison with progressive supranuclear palsy and Guamanian parkinsonism–dementia complex. *Brain*, **116**, 281–302.

Ghika, J., Tennis, M., Hoffman, E., Schoenfeld, D. & Growdon, J. (1991). Idazoxan treatment in progressive supranuclear palsy. *Neurology*, **41**, 986–91.

Ghika, J. & Bogousslavsky, J. (1997). Presymptomatic hypertension is a major feature in progressive supranuclear palsy. *Arch. Neurol.*, **54**, 1104–8.

Gibb, W.R.G., Luthert, P.J. & Marsden, C.D. (1989). Corticobasal degeneration. *Brain*, **112**, 1171–92.

Gilman, S., Low, P.A., Quinn, N. et al. (1998). Consensus statement on the diagnosis of multiple system atrophy. *J. Auton. Nerv. Syst.*, **74**, 189–92.

Gnanlingham, K.K., Byrne, E.J., Thornton, A., Sambrook, M.A. & Bannister, P. (1997). Motor and cognitive function in Lewy body dementia: comparison with Alzheimer's and Parkinson's disease. *J. Neurol., Neurosurg. Psychiatry*, **62**, 243–52.

Goedert, M. (2001). Alpha-synuclein and neurodegenerative diseases. *Nat. Rev. Neurosci.*, **2**, 492–501.

Goedert, M. & Spillantini, M.G. (2001). Tau gene mutations and neurodegeneration. *Biochem. Soc. Symp.*, **67**, 59–71.

Golbe, L.I., Davis, P.H., Schoenberg, B.S. & Duvoisin, R.C. (1988). Prevalence and natural history of progressive supranuclear palsy. *Neurology*, **38**, 1031–4.

Golbe, L.I., Rubin, R.S., Cody, R.P. et al. (1996). Follow up study of the risk factors in progressive supranuclear palsy. *Neurology*, **47**, 148–54.

Graham, J.G. & Oppenheimer, D.R. (1969). Orthostatic hypotension and nicotine sensitivity in a case of multiple system atrophy. *J. Neurol., Neurosurg. Psychiatry*, **32**, 28–34.

Greene, P.E., Fahn, S., Lang, A.E., Watts, R.L., Eidelberg, D. & Powers, J.M. (1990). Case 1, 1990: Progressive unilateral rigidity, bradykinesia, tremulousness, and apraxia, leading to fixed postural deformity of the involved limb. *Mov. Disord.*, **5**, 341–51.

Grimes, D.A., Lang, A.E. & Bergeron, C.B. (1999). Dementia as the most common presentation of cortical-basal ganglionic degeneration. *Neurology*, **53**, 1969–74.

Hardie, R.J., Pullon, H.W., Harding, A.E. et al. (1991). Neuroacanthocytosis. A clinical haematological and pathological study of 19 cases. *Brain*, **114**, 13–49.

Higgins, J.J., Litvan, I., Pho, L.T., Li, W. & Neem, L.E. (1998). Progressive supranuclear gaze palsy is in linkage disequilibrium with the tau and not the alpha-synuclein gene. *Neurology*, **50**, 270–3.

Higgins, J.J., Adler, R.L. & Loveless, J.M. (1999). Mutational analysis of the tau gene in progressive supranuclear palsy. *Neurology*, **53**, 1421–4.

Higgins, J.J., Golbe, L.I., De Biase, A., Jankovic, J., Factor, S.A. & Adler, R.L. (2000). An extended 5′-tau susceptibility haplotype in progressive supranuclear palsy. *Neurology*, **14**, 55, 1364–7.

Houlden, H., Baker, M., Morris, H.R. et al. (2001). Corticobasal degeneration and progressive supranuclear palsy share a common tau haplotype. *Neurology*, **56**(12), 1702–6.

Hughes, A.J., Daniel, S.E., Kilford, L. & Lees, A.J. (1992). Accuracy of clinical diagnosis of idiopathic Parkinson's disease: a clinico-pathological study of 100 cases. *J. Neurol., Neurosurg. Psychiatry*, **55**, 181–4.

Howard, R.S. & Lees, A.J. (1987). Encephalitis lethargica. A report of recent cases. *Brain*, **110**, 19–33.

Hutton, M., Lendon, C.L., Rizzu, P. et al. (1998). Association of missense and 5-splice-site mutations in tau with the inherited dementia FTDP-17. *Nature*, **393**, 702–5.

Jankovic, J. (1994). Posttraumatic movement disorders. Central and peripheral mechanisms. *Neurology*, **44**, 2008–14.

Jankovic, J., Friedman, D.I., Pirozzolo, F.J. & McCrary, J.A. (1990). Progressive supranuclear palsy: motor, neurobehavioural and neuroophthalmological findings. *Adv. Neurol.*, **53**, 293–304.

Jellinger, K.A., Bancher, C., Hauw, J.J. & Verny, M. (1995). Progressive supranuclear palsy: neuropathologically based diagnostic clinical criteria. *J. Neurol., Neurosurg. Psychiatry*, **59**, 106.

Jordan, B.D. (2000). Chronic traumatic brain injury associated with boxing. *Semin. Neurol.*, **20**(2), 179–85.

Juncos, J.L., Hirsch, E.C., Malessa, S., Duyckaerts, C., Hersh, L.B. & Agid, Y. (1991). Mesencephalic cholinergic nuclei in progressive supranuclear palsy. *Neurology*, **41**, 25–30.

Kompoliti, K., Goetz, C.G., Boeve, B.F. et al. (1998). Clinical presentation and pharmacological therapy in corticobasal degeneration. *Arch. Neurol.*, **55**(7), 957–61

Kumar, R., Bergeron, C., Pollanen, M.S. & Lang, A.E. (1998). Cortical basal ganglionic degeneration. In *Parkinson's Disease and Movement Disorders*, ed. J. Jankovic & E. Tolosa, pp. 297–316. Baltimore: Williams & Wilkins.

Kruger, R., Kuhn, W., Muller, T. et al. (1998). Ala30Pro mutation in the gene coding alpha-synuclein in Parkinson's disease. *Nat. Genet.*, **18**, 106–108.

Lantos, P.L. (1998). The definition of multiple system atrophy: a review of the recent developments. *J. Neuropathol. Exp. Neurol.*, **57**, 1099–111.

Laureys, S., Salmon, E., Garraux, G. et al. (1999). Fluorodopa uptake and glucose metabolism in early stages of corticobasal degeneration. *J. Neurol.*, **246**(12), 1151–8.

Leiguarda, R., Lees, A.J., Merello, M., Starkstein, S. & Marsden, C.D. (1994). The nature of apraxia in corticobasal degeneration. *J. Neurol., Neurosurg. Psychiatry*, **57**, 455–9.

Lees, A.J. (1987). The Steele–Richardson–Olszewski syndrome (progressive supranuclear palsy). In *Movement Disorders 2*, ed. C.D. Marsden & S. Fahn, pp. 272–87. London: Butterworths.

Lewis, A.J. & Gawel, M.J. (1990). Diffuse Lewy body disease with dementia and oculomotor dysfunction. *Mov. Disord.*, **5**, 143–7.

LeWitt, P., Friedman, J., Nutt, J., Korczyn, A., Brogna, C. & Truong,

D. (1989). Progressive rigidity with apraxia: the variety of clinical and pathological features. *Neurology*, **39**(Suppl. 1), 140.

Lippa, C.F., Smith, T.W. & Fontneau, N. (1990). Corticonigral degeneration with neuronal achromasia. A clinicopathological study of two cases. *J. Neurol. Sci.*, **98**, 301–10.

Litvan, I. (1997). Progressive supranuclear palsy and corticobasal degeneration. In *Baillières Clinical Neurology*, ed. N.P. Quinn, pp. 167–85. London: Ballière Tindall.

Litvan, I., Agid, Y., Calne, D. et al. (1996a). Clinical research criteria for the diagnosis of progressive supranuclear palsy (Steele–Richardson–Olszewski syndrome): report of the NINDS–SPSP international workshop. *Neurology*, **47**, 1–9

Litvan, I., Mangone, C.A., McKee, A. et al. (1996b). Natural history of progressive supranuclear palsy (Steele–Richardson–Olszewski syndrome) and clinical predictors of survival: a clinicopathological study. *J. Neurol., Neurosurg. Psychiatry*, **60**, 615–20.

Litvan, I., Agid, Y., Jankovic, J. et al. (1996c). Accuracy of clinical criteria for the diagnosis of progressive supranuclear palsy (Steele–Richardson–Olszewski syndrome). *Neurology*, **46**, 922–30.

Litvan, I., Hauw, J.J., Bartko, J.J. et al. (1996d). Validity and reliability of the preliminary NINDS neuropathologic criteria for progressive supranuclear palsy and related disorders. *J. Neuropathol. Exp. Neurol.*, **55**, 97–105.

Litvan, I., Campbell, G., Mangone, C.A. et al. (1997a). Which clinical features differentiate progressive supranuclear palsy (Steele–Richardson–Olszewski syndrome) from related disorders? A clinicopathological study. *Brain*, **12**, 65–74.

Litvan, I., Agid, Y. & Goetz, C. (1997b). Accuracy of the clinical diagnosis of corticobasal degeneration: a clinicopathologic study. *Neurology*, **48**(1), 119–25.

Lopez, O.L., Litvan, I., Catt, K.E. et al. (1999). Accuracy of four clinical diagnostic criteria for the diagnosis of neurodegenerative dementias. *Neurology*, **53**, 1292–9.

Lynch, T., Sano, M., Marder, K.S. et al. (1994). Clinical characteristics of a family with chromosome 17-linked disinhibition–dementia–parkinsonism–amyotrophy complex. *Neurology*, **44**, 1878–84.

McKeith, I.G., Galasko, D., Kosaka, K. et al. (1996). Consensus guidelines for the clinical and pathologic diagnosis of dementia with Lewy bodies (DLB): report of the consortium on DLB international workshop. *Neurology*, **47**, 1113–24.

Maher, E.R. & Lees, A.J. (1986). The clinical features and natural history of the Steele–Richardson–Olszewski syndrome (progressive supranuclear palsy). *Neurology*, **36**, 1005–8.

Matsuo, H., Takashima, H., Kishikawa, M. et al. (1991). Pure akinesia: an atypical manifestation of progressive supranuclear palsy. *J. Neurol., Neurosurg. Psychiatry*, **54**, 397–400.

Momose, T. & Sasaki, Y. (1997). Striatal dopamine D2 receptor in Parkinson disease and its related disorders assessed by C-11 NMSP and PET. *Nippon Rinsho*, **55**, 227–32.

Morris, H.R., Moriabadi, N.F., Lees, A.J., Dick, D.J. & Turjanski, D. (1998). Parkinsonism following electrical injury to the hand. *Mov. Disord.*, **13**(3), 600–2

Morris, H.R., Lees, A.J. & Wood, N.W. (1999a). Neurofibrillary tangle parkinsonian disorders – tau pathology and tau genetics. *Mov. Disord.*, **14**(5), 731–6.

Morris, H.R., Janssen, J.C., Bandmann, O. et al. (1999b). The tau gene A0 polymorphism in progressive supranuclear palsy and related neurodegenerative diseases. *J. Neurol., Neurosurg. Psychiatry*, **66**, 665–7.

Morris, H.R., Vaughan, J.R., Datta, S.R. et al. (2000). Multiple system atrophy/progressive supranuclear palsy: alpha-synuclein, synphilin, tau, and APOE. *Neurology*, **55**, 1918–20.

Nath, U. & Burn, D.J. (2000). The epidemiology of progressive supranuclear palsy. *Parkinsonism Rel. Disord.*, **6**, 145–53.

Nath, U., Ben-Shlomo, Y., Thomson, R.G. et al. (2001). The prevalence of progressive supranuclear palsy (Steele–Richardson–Olszewski syndrome) in the UK. *Brain*, **124**, 1438–49.

Nitrini, R., Silva, L.S., Rosemberg, S. et al. (2001). Prion disease resembling frontotemporal dementia and parkinsonism linked to chromosome 17. *Arq. Neuropsiquiatr.*, **59**(2–A), 161–4.

Okuda, B., Tachibana, H., Kawabata, K., Takeda, M. & Sugita, M. (1999). Cerebral blood flow correlates of higher brain dysfunctions in corticobasal degeneration. *J. Geriat. Psychiatry, Neurology*, **12**(4), 189–93.

Ozawa, T., Takano, H., Onodera, O. et al. (1999). No mutation in the entire coding region of the alpha-synuclein gene in pathologically confirmed cases of multiple system atrophy. *Neurosci. Lett.*, **270**, 110–12.

Ozsancak, C., Auzou, P. & Hannequin, D. (2000). Dysarthria and orofacial apraxia in cortcobasal degeneration. *Mov. Disord.*, **15**, 905–10.

Pal, P.K,. Samii, A. & Calne, D.B. (1999). Manganese neurotoxicity: a review of clinical features, imaging and pathology. *Neurotoxicology*, **20**, 227–38.

Pal, P.K., Wszolek, Z.K., Kishore, A. et al. (2001). Positron emission tomography in pallido-ponto-nigral degeneration (PPND) family (frontotemporal dementia with parkinsonism linked to chromosome 17 and point mutation in tau gene). *Parkinsonism Relat. Disord.*, **7**, 81–8.

Palace, J., Chandiramani, V.A. & Fowler, C.J. (1997). Value of sphincter electromyography in the diagnosis of multiple system atrophy. *Muscle Nerve*, **20**, 1396–403.

Papp, M.I. & Lantos, P.L. (1994). The distribution of oligodendroglial inclusions in multiple system atrophy and its relevance to clinical symptomatology. *Brain*, **117**, 235–43.

Papp, M.I., Kahn, J.E. & Lantos, P.L. (1989). Glial cytoplasmic inclusions in the CNS of patients with multiple system atrophy (striatonigral degeneration, olivopontocerebellar atrophy and Shy–Drager syndrome). *J. Neurol. Sci.*, **94**, 79–100.

Peppard, R.F., Lu, C.S., Chu, N.S., Teal, P., Martin, W.R. & Calne, D.B. (1990). Parkinsonism with neuroacanthocytosis. *Can. J. Neurol. Sci.*, **17**, 298–301.

Pharr, V., Litvan, I., Brat, D.J., Troncoso, J., Reich, S.G. & Stark, M. (1999). Ideomotor apraxia in progressive supranuclear palsy: a case study. *Mov. Disord.*, **14**, 162–6.

Pirker, W., Asenbaum, S., Bencsits, G. et al. (2000). [123I]beta-CIT-SPECT in multiple system atrophy, progressive supranuclear palsy, and corticobasal degeneration. *Mov. Disord.*, **15**, 1158–67.

Poorkaj, P., Bird, T.D., Wijsman, E. et al. (1998). Tau is a candidate gene for chromosome 17 frontotemporal dementia. *Ann. Neurol.*, **43**(6), 815–25.

Quinn, N. (1989). Multiple system atrophy – the nature of the beast. *J. Neurol., Neurosurg, Psychiatry*, Suppl., 78–89.

Quinn, N. (1995). Parkinsonism – recognition and differential diagnosis. *Br. Med. J.*, **310**, 447–52.

Quinn, N. & Maraganore, D. (2000). Parkinsonism following electrical injury to the hand. *Mov. Disord.*, **15**(3), 587–8.

Rajput, A.H., Rozdilsky, B., Hornykiewicz, O., Shannak, K., Lee, T. & Seeman, P. (1982). Reversible drug-induced parkinsonism. Clinicopathologic study of two cases. *Arch. Neurol.*, **39**, 644–6.

Rascol, O., Sabatini, U., Simonetta-Moreau, M. et al. (1991). Square wave jerks in parkinsonian syndromes. *J. Neurol., Neurosurg. Psychiatry*, **54**, 599–602.

Rascol, O., Sieradzan, K., Peyro-Saint-Paul, H. et al. (1998). Efaroxan, an alpha-2 antagonist, in the treatment of progressive supranuclear palsy. *Mov. Disord.*, **13**, 673–6.

Rebeiz, J.J., Kolodny, E.H. & Richardson, E.P. (1967). Cortico-dentatonigral degeneration with neuronal achromasia: a progressive disorder of late adult life. *Trans. Am. Neurol. Assoc.*, **92**, 23–6.

Rebeiz, J.J., Kolodny, E.H. & Richardson, E.P. (1968). Cortico-dentatonigral degeneration with neuronal achromasia. *Arch. Neurol.*, **18**, 20–33.

Reed, L.A., Schmidt, M.L., Wszolek, Z.K. et al. (1988). The neuropathology of a chromosome 17-linked autosomal dominant parkinsonism and dementia ('pallido-ponto-nigral degeneration'). *J. Neuropathol. Exp. Neurol.*, **57**, 588–601.

Riley, D.E. & Lang, A.E. (1988). Corticobasal ganglionic degeneration (CBGD): Further observations in six additional cases. *Neurology*, **38**(Suppl. 1), 360.

Riley, D.E. & Lang, A.E. (1993). Cortico-basal ganglionic degeneration. In *Parkinsonian Syndromes*, ed. M.B. Stern & W.C. Koller, pp. 379–92. New York: Marcel Dekker.

Riley, D.E. & Lang, A.E. (2000). Clinical diagnostic criteria. *Adv. Neurol.*, **82**, 29–34.

Riley, D.E., Lang, A.E., Lewis, A. et al. (1990). Cortico-basal ganglionic degeneration. *Neurology*, **40**, 1203–12.

Rinne, J.O., Lee, M.S., Thompson, P.D. & Marsden, C.D. (1994). Corticobasal degeneration: a clinical study of 36 cases. *Brain*, **117**, 1183–96.

Rivaud-Pechoux, S., Vidailhet, M., Gallouedec, G., Litvan, I., Gaymard, B. & Pierrot-Deseilligny, C. (2000). Longitudinal ocular motor study in corticobasal degeneration and progressive supranuclear palsy. *Neurology*, **54**, 1029–32.

Rojo, A., Pernaute, R.S., Fontan, A. et al. (1999). Clinical genetics of familial progressive supranuclear palsy. *Brain*, **122**, 1233–45.

Roy, S., Datta, C.K., Hirano, A., Ghatak, N.R. & Zimmerman, H.M. (1974). Electron microscopic study of neurofibrillary tangles in Steele–Richardson–Olszewski syndrome. *Acta Neuropathol. (Berl.)*, **29**, 175–9

Ruberg, M., Javoy-Agid, F., Hirsch, E. et al. (1985). Dopaminergic and cholinergic lesions in progressive supranuclear palsy. *Ann. Neurol.*, **18**, 523–9.

Santacruz, P., Uttl, B., Litvan, I. & Grafman, J. (1998). Progressive supranuclear palsy. A survey of the disease course. *Neurology*, **50**, 1637–47.

Savoiardo, M., Girotti, F., Strada, L. & Ciceri, E. (1994). Magnetic resonance imaging in progressive supranuclear palsy and other parkinsonian disorders. *J. Neural. Transm. Suppl.*, **42**, 93–110.

Sawle, G.V., Brooks, D.J., Marsden, C.D. & Frackowiak, R.S. (1991). Corticobasal degeneration. A unique pattern of regional cortical oxygen hypometabolism and striatal fluorodopa uptake demonstrated by positron emission tomography. *Brain*, **114**, 541–56.

Scaravilli, T., Pramstaller, P.P., Salerno, A. et al. (2000). Neuronal loss in Onuf's nucleus in three patients with progressive supranuclear palsy. *Ann. Neurol.*, **48**, 97–101.

Schneider, J.A., Watts, R.L., Gearing, M., Brewer, R.P. & Mirra, S.S. (1994). Corticobasal degeneration: neuropathological and clinical heterogeneity. *Neurology*, **48**, 959–89.

Schrag, A., Kingsley, D., Phatouros, C. et al. (1998). Clinical usefulness of magnetic resonance imaging in multiple system atrophy. *J. Neurol., Neurosurg., Psychiatry*, **65**, 65–71.

Schrag, A., Ben-Shlomo, Y. & Quinn, N.P. (1999). Prevalence of progressive supranuclear palsy and multiple system atrophy: a cross-sectional study. *Lancet*, **354**, 1771–5.

Schrag, A., Good, C.D., Miszkiel, K. et al. (2000). Differentiation of atypical parkinsonian syndromes with routine MRI. *Neurology*, **54**(3), 697–702.

Schulman, L.M., Lang, A.E., Jankovic, J. et al. (1995). Case 1, 1995: psychosis, dementia, chorea, ataxia, and supranuclear gaze dysfunction. *Mov. Disord.*, **10**, 257–62.

Schulz, J.B., Klockgether, T., Petersen, D. et al. (1994). Multiple system atrophy: natural history, MRI morphology, and dopamine receptor imaging with 123IBZM-SPECT. *J. Neurol., Neurosurg., Psychiatry*, **57**, 1047–56.

Schulz, J.B., Skalej, M., Wedekind, D. et al. (1999). Magnetic resonance imaging-based volumetry differentiates idiopathic Parkinson's syndrome from multiple system atrophy and progressive supranuclear palsy. *Ann. Neurol.*, **45**, 65–74.

Schwarz, J., Tatsch, K., Gasser, T. et al. (1998). 123I-IBZM binding compared with long-term clinical follow up in patients with de novo parkinsonism. *Mov. Disord.*, **13**, 16–19.

Shinotoh, H., Inoue, O., Hirayama, K. et al. (1993). Dopamine D1 receptors in Parkinson's disease and striatonigral degeneration: a positron emission tomography study. *J. Neurol., Neurosurg., Psychiatry*, **56**, 467–72.

Shy, G.M. & Drager, G.A. (1960). A neurologic syndrome associated with orthostatic hypotension. *Arch. Neurol.*, **2**, 511–27.

Simpson, D.A., Wishnow, R., Gargulinski, R.B. & Pawlak, A.M. (1995). Oculofacial-skeletal myorhythmia in central nervous system Whipple's disease: additional case and review of the literature. *Mov. Disord.*, **10**, 195–200

Smith, T.W., Lippa, C.F. & de Girolama, U. (1992). Immunocytochemical study of ballooned neurons in cortical degeneration with neuronal achromasia. *Clin. Neuropathol.*, **11**, 28–35.

Spadoni, F., Stefani, A., Morello, M., Lavaroni, F., Giacomini, P. & Sancesario, G. (2000). Selective vulnerability of pallidal neurons in the early phases of manganese intoxication. *Exp. Brain Res.*, **135**(4), 544–51.

Spillantini, M.G. (1999). Parkinson's disease, dementia with Lewy bodies and multiple system atrophy are alpha-synuleinopathies. *Parkinsonism and Related Disorders*, **5**, 157–62.

Spillantini, M.G., Crowther, R.A., Jakes, R., Cairns, N.J., Lantos, P.L. & Goedert, M. (1998a). Filamentous alpha-synuclein inclusions link multiple system atrophy with Parkinson's disease and dementia with Lewy bodies. *Neurosci. Lett.*, **251**, 205–8.

Spillantini, M.G., Murrell, J.R., Goedert, M., Farlow, M.R., Klug, A. & Ghetti, B. (1998b). Mutation in the tau gene in familial multiple system tauopathy with presenile dementia. *Proc. Natl. Acad. Sci., USA*, **95**(13), 7737–41.

Spillantini, M.G., Van Swieten, J.C. & Goedert, M. (2000). Tau gene mutations in frontotemporal dementia and parkinsonism linked to chromosome 17 (FTDP-17). *Neurogenetics*, **2**, 193–205.

Stanford, P.M., Halliday, G.M., Brooks, W.S. et al. (2000). Progressive supranuclear palsy pathology caused by a novel silent mutation in exon 10 of the tau gene: expansion of the disease phenotype caused by tau gene mutations. *Brain*, **123**, 880–93.

Steele, J.C., Richardson, J.C. & Olszewski, J. (1964). Progressive supranuclear palsy: a heterogenous degeneration involving the brainstem, basal ganglia and cerebellum with vertical gaze and pseudobulbar palsy, nuchal dystonia and dementia. *Arch. Neurol.*, **10**, 333–59.

Stern, M.B. (1991). Head trauma as a risk for Parkinson's disease. *Mov. Disord.*, **6**, 95–7.

Stevenson, V.L. & Hardie, R.J. (2001). Acanthocytosis and neurological disorders. *J. Neurol.*, **248**, 87–94.

Takeda, A., Arai, N., Komori, T., Iseki, E., Kato, S. & Oda, M. (1997). Tau immunoreactivity in glial cytoplasmic inclusions in multiple system atrophy. *Neurosci. Lett.*, **234**, 63–6.

Terao, S., Sobue, G., Hashizume, Y., Mitsuma, T. & Takahashi, A. (1994). Disease-specific patterns of neuronal loss in the spinal ventral horn in amyotrophic lateral sclerosis, multiple system atrophy and X-linked recessive bulbospinal neuronopathy, with special reference to the loss of small neurons in the intermediate zone. *J. Neurol.*, **241**, 196–203.

Tetrud, J.W., Golbe, L.I., Forno, L.S. & Farmer, P.M. (1996). Autopsy proven progressive supranuclear palsy in two siblings. *Neurology*, **46**, 931–4.

Thompson, P.D. & Marsden, C.D. (1992). Corticobasal degeneration. In *Clinical Neurology, Unusual Dementias*, ed. M.N. Rosser, Vol. 1(3), pp. 677–86. London: Baillière Tindall.

Tison, F., Arne, P., Sourgen, C., Chrysostome, V. & Yeklef, F. (2000). The value of external anal sphincter electromyography for the diagnosis of multiple system atrophy. *Mov. Disord.*, **15**, 1148–57.

Tolosa, E., Valldeoriola, F. & Marti, M.J. (1994). Clinical diagnosis and diagnostic criteria of progressive supranuclear palsy (Steele–Richardson–Olszewski syndrome). *J. Neural. Transm. Suppl.*, **42**, 15–31.

Troost, B.T. & Daroff, R.B. (1977). The ocular motor defects in progressive supranuclear palsy. *Ann. Neurol.*, **2**, 397–403.

Tu, P., Galvin, J.E., Baba, M. et al. (1998). Glial cytoplasmic inclusions in white matter oligodendrocytes of multiple system atrophy brains contain insoluble α-synuclein. *Ann. Neurol.*, **44**, 415–422.

Vanek, Z.F. & Jankovic, J. (2000). Corticobasal degeneration. Dystonia in corticobasal degeneration. *Adv. Neurol.*, **82**, 61–7.

Valldeoriola, F., Valls-Sole, J., Tolosa, E.S. & Marti, M.J. (1995). Striated anal sphincter denervation in patients with progressive supranuclear palsy. *Mov. Disord.*, **10**, 550–5.

Verny, M., Jellinger, K.A., Hauw, J.J., Bancher, C., Litvan, I. & Agid, Y. (1996). Progressive supranuclear palsy: a clinicopathological study of 21 cases. *Acta Neuropathol.*, **91**, 427–31.

Vidailhet, M., Rivaud, S., Gouider-Khouja, N. et al. (1994). Eye movements in parkinsonian syndromes. *Ann. Neurol.*, **35**, 420–6.

Wakabayashi, K., Yoshimoto, M., Tsuji, S. & Takahashi, H. (1998). α-Synuclein immunoreactivity in glial cytoplasmic inclusions in multiple system atrophy. *Neurosci. Lett.*, **249**, 180–2.

Walker, Z., Costa, D.C., Ince, P., McKeith, I.G. & Katona, C. (1999). In-vivo demonstration of dopaminergic degeneration in dementia with Lewy Bodies. *Lancet*, **354**, 646–7.

Watts, R.L., Williams, R.S., Young, R.R. & Haley, E.C. (1985). Corticobasal ganglionic degeneration. *Neurology*, **35**(Suppl. 1), 178.

Watts, R.L., Mirra, S.S., Young, R.R., Burger, P.C., Villier, J.A. & Heyman, A. (1989). Cortico-basal ganglionic degeneration (CBGD) with neuronal achromasia: clinical–pathological study of two cases. *Neurology*, **39**(Suppl. 1), 140.

Watts, R.L., Mirra, S.S. & Richardson, E.P. (1994). Corticobasal ganglionic degeneration. In *Movement Disorders 3*, ed. C.D. Marsden & S. Fahn, pp. 282–99. London: Butterworth Heinneman.

Watts, R., Brewer, R.P., Schneider, J.A. & Mirra, S.S. (1997). Corticobasal degeneration In *Movement Disorders: Neurologic Principles and Practice*, ed. R.L. Watts & W.C. Kollen, pp. 611–21. McGraw Hill, Inc.

Wenning, G.K., Ben-Shlomo, Y., Magalhaes, M., Daniel, S.E. & Quinn, N.P. (1994). Clinical features and natural history of multiple system atrophy: an analysis of 100 cases. *Brain*, **117**, 835–45.

Wenning, G.K., Ben-Shlomo, Y., Magalhães, M., Daniel, S.E. & Quinn, N.P. (1995). A clinicopathological study of 35 cases of multiple system atrophy. *J. Neurol., Neurosurg. Psychiatry*, **58**, 160–6.

Wenning, G.K., Tison, F., Ben-Shlomo, Y., Daniel, S.E. & Quinn, N.P. (1997). Multiple system atrophy: a review of 203 pathologically proven cases. *Mov. Disord.*, **12**, 133–47.

Wenning, G.K., Litvan, I., Jankovic, J. et al. (1998). Natural history and survival of 14 patients with corticobasal degeneration confirmed at postmortem examination. *J. Neurol., Neurosurg. Psychiatry*, **64**, 184–9.

Wenning, G.K., Seppi, K., Scherfler, C., Stefanova, N. & Puschban, Z. (2001). Multiple system atrophy. *Sem. Neurol.*, **21**, 33–40.

Wijker, M., Wszolek, Z.K., Wolters, E.C. et al. (1996). Localization of the gene for rapidly progressive autosomal dominant parkinsonism and dementia and pallido-ponto-nigral degeneration to chromosome 17q21. *Hum. Mol. Genet.*, **5**, 151–4.

Wilhelmsen, K.C., Lynch, T., Pavlou, E., Higgins, M. & Nygaard, T.G. (1994). Localization of disinhibition–dementia–parkinsonism–amyotrophy complex to 17q21–22. *Am. J. Hum. Genet.*, **55**, 1159–65.

Williams, D.B., Annegers, J.F., Kokmen, F., O'Brien, P.C. & Kurland, L.T. (1991). Brain injury and neurologic sequelae: a cohort study of dementia, parkinsonism and amyotrophic lateral sclerosis. *Neurology*, **41**, 1154–7.

Wszolek, Z.K., Pfeiffer, R.F., Bhatt, M.H. et al. (1992).Rapidly progressive autosomal dominant parkinsonism and dementia with pallido-ponto-nigral degeneration. *Ann. Neurol.*, **32**(3), 312–20.

Yasuda, M., Takamatsu, J., D'Souza, I. et al. (2000). A novel mutation at position +12 in the intron following exon 10 of the tau gene in familial frontotemporal dementia (FTD-Kumamoto) *Ann. Neurol.*, **47**, 422–9.

Young, A.B. (1985). Progressive supranuclear palsy: postmortem chemical analysis. *Ann. Neurol.*, **18**(5), 521–2.

35

Tremors

Jyh-Gong Hou and Joseph Jankovic

Parkinson's Disease Center and Movement Disorders Clinic, Department of Neurology,
Baylor College of Medicine, Houston, Texas, USA

Tremor, the most common movement disorder, is defined as a rhythmic, oscillatory movement of a body part produced by alternating or synchronous contractions of agonist and antagonist muscles. It ranges from a normal, barely noticeable, physiologic phenomenon to a severe, disabling movement disorder. Tremors can be classified according to their phenomenology, distribution, frequency, amplitude or etiology (Deuschl et al., 1998). Phenomenologically, tremors are subdivided into two major categories: rest tremors and action tremors. Rest tremors occur when the body part is fully supported against gravity and not actively contracting. In contrast, action tremors manifest during voluntary muscle contraction on an antigravity posture (postural tremor) or a goal-directed movement (kinetic tremor) (Table 35.1). This phenomenologic classification is far from ideal since there are many overlapping features among different tremors, but it remains the most widely accepted classification.

Rest tremor is present predominantly in Parkinson's disease (PD). It may also occur in other conditions such as different forms of parkinsonism, severe essential tremor (ET) and midbrain lesions. Postural tremors are typical of physiologic tremor, enhanced physiologic tremor, and ET. Task- or position-specific tremors are action tremors that occur only during specific motor activities, such as writing ('primary writing tremor') or maintaining at a certain posture. Kinetic tremors exist in cerebellar or midbrain disorders. Isometric tremor is seen during a voluntary isometric contraction, such as making a tight fist or contracting abdominal muscles. Tremors associated with dystonia, myoclonus, tardive dyskinesia, and other movement disorders may exhibit mixed phenomenology. Other disorders that produce rhythmic, but not necessarily oscillatory movements include segmental myoclonus, myorhythmia, asterixis, fasciculations, clonus, epilepsia partialis continua, shivering, head bobbing, and tituba-tion. In this chapter we will first review the current notions of the tremor pathophysiology and then discuss the clinical features and treatment of the different types of tremors.

Pathophysiologic mechanisms of tremors

The broad clinical spectra of tremors suggest that different pathophysiologic mechanisms underlie various forms of tremors. Based on a large body of evidence from experimental and clinical physiologic studies, tremors originate from two types of mechanisms: (i) central and (ii) peripheral. The central oscillators consist of neuronal networks with auto-rhythmic properties and spontaneous bursting propagated through central nervous system (CNS) motor pathways. The peripheral components of tremors are influenced by mechanical characteristics of the affected body parts (muscles, tendons, and joints) and sensorimotor reflex mechanisms (Hallett, 1998). With the development of novel electrophysiologic and functional imaging techniques, the knowledge of mechanisms of tremors has been significantly advanced in recent years.

Intracellular recordings of certain neurons reveal autorhythmic (pacemaker) properties. Studying neurons of the inferior olive, Llinas and colleagues (Llinas, 1988) demonstrated that, as a result of low-threshold Ca^{2+} conductance, these neurons generate action potentials (low-threshold spike or LTS) at subthreshold depolarization. A fast action potential, generated by Na^+ current into the cell body, is followed by a slow, high-threshold Ca^{2+} spike that activates prolonged (80–100 ms) K^+-mediated hyperpolarization. This is followed by an abrupt rebound response mediated by a low-threshold Ca^{2+} conductance large enough to generate a second Na^+-dependent action potential. The cycle then repeats, resulting in rhythmical bursting. Other CNS regions besides inferior olivary also

Table 35.1. Classification and differential diagnosis of tremors

Rest tremors (Typical 3 to 6 Hz)	Action tremors
Parkinson's disease	*Postural tremor*
Other parkinsonian syndromes	*Physiologic tremor*
Multiple system atrophies (SND, SDS, OPCA)	*Enhanced physiologic tremor*
Progressive supranuclear palsy	(Typical 8–12 Hz)
Cortical–basal–ganglionic degeneration	(a) Stress-induced: emotion, exercise, fatigue, anxiety, fever
Parkinsonism–dementia–ALS of Guam	(b) Endocrine: hypoglycemia, thyrotoxicosis, pheochromocytoma,
Diffuse Lewy body disease	adrenocorticosteroids
Progressive pallidal atrophy	(c) Drugs: beta agonists (theophylline, terbutaline, epinephrine, etc),
	dopaminergic drugs (levodopa, dopamine agonists), stimulants
Heredodegenerative disorders	(amphetamines), psychiatric drugs (lithium, neuroleptics, tricyclics)
Huntington's disease	methylxanthines (coffee, tea), valproic acid, cyclosporin, interferon
Wilson's disease	(d) Toxins: Hg, Pb, As, Bi, Br, alcohol withdrawal
Neuroacanthocytosis	
Hallervorden–Spatz disease	*Essential tremor*
Gerstmann–Strausler–Scheinker disease	(Typical 4–8 Hz)
Ceroid lipofuscinosis	(a) Autosomal dominant
	(b) Sporadic
Secondary parkinsonism	
Toxic: MPTP, CO, Mn, methanol, cyanide, CS_2	*Postural tremor associated with*
Drug-induced: dopamine receptor blocking drugs	(a) Dystonia
(neuroleptics, the 'rabbit syndrome'), dopamine	(b) Parkinsonism
depleting drugs (reserpine, tetrabenazine), lithium,	(c) Myoclonus
flunarizine, cinnarizine	(d) Hereditary motor–sensory neuropathy (Roussy–Levy)
Vascular: multi-infarct, Binswanger's, 'lower body	(e) Kennedy's syndrome (X-linked spino–bulbar atrophy)
parkinsonism'	
Trauma: pugilistic encephalopathy, midbrain injury	*Task- or position-specific tremors*
Tumour and paraneoplastic	(a) Handwriting
Infectious: postencephalitic, fungal, AIDS, SSPE,	(b) Orthostatic
Creutzfeldt-Jakob disease	(c) Other (e.g. occupational) task-specific tremors
Metabolic: hypoparathyroidism, mitochondrial	
Cytopathies, chronic hepatic degeneration	*Kinetic (intention, terminal) tremors*
Normal pressure hydrocephalus	(Typical 2.5–4 Hz)
	(a) Cerebellar disorders (cerebellar outflow): multiple sclerosis, trauma,
Spasmus nutans	stroke, Wilson's disease, drugs, toxins
	(b) Midbrain lesions
	Isometric tremor
	Muscular contraction during sustained exertion
Tremors with mixed phenomenology	*Miscellaneous tremors and other rhythmic movements*
A Parkinson's disease and other parkinsonian	A Myoclonus: rhythmical segmental myclonus (e.g. palatal), oscillatory
syndromes (rest and postural)	myoclonus, asterixis, mini-polymyoclonus
B Essential tremor (postural and kinetic)	B Dystonic tremors
Severe essential tremor (postural and rest)	C Cortical tremors
C Midbrain (rubral) tremor (postural, kinetic and rest)	D Epilepsia partialis continua
D Tardive tremor (rest, postural and kinetic)	E Nystagmus
E Myorhythmia (rest and kinetic)	F Clonus
F Neuropathic tremor (postural or rest)	G Fasciculations
G Psychogenic tremor (rest, postural or kinetic)	H Shivering
	I Shuddering attacks
	J Head bobbing (3rd ventricular cysts)
	K Aortic insufficiency with head titubation

contain neuronal networks with self-generating bursts of activities. For example, high-frequency oscillations are induced in local cortical circuits from cortex-striatum-mesencephalon organotypic cultures (Plenz & Kitai, 1996). Neurons from the subthalamic nucleus and external globus pallidus generate synchronized oscillating bursts at 0.4, 0.8 and 1.8 Hz in cell cultures.

Different types of tremors originate from different central oscillators. By studying awake decerebrate monkeys, Lamarre (1984) found two different types of rhythmic discharges from two different regions: 3 to 6 Hz spontaneous rhythmic discharges in the ventral thalamus and 7 to 12 Hz discharges in the olivo-cerebellar system. The 3 to 6 Hz thalamic neuron discharges were facilitated by a lesion in the ventromedial tegmentum of the midbrain. Such thalamic deafferentiation was thought to express parkinsonian rest tremor.

Central mechanisms

Central oscillators are thought to play a major role in the generation of rest tremor in PD, with only minimal contribution from the peripheral mechanical-reflex mechanisms. Rest tremor can be produced in a monkey treated with the neurotoxin 1-methyl-4-phenyl-1, 2, 3, 6- tetrahydropyridine (MPTP) which damages dopaminergic neurons in SN pars compacta (SNpc) (Bergman et al., 1994). The investigators demonstrated that subthalamic nucleus (STN) and globus pallidus interna (GPi), the outflow nucleus from the basal ganglia, were overactive in the monkeys with MPTP-induced parkinsonism (Blandini et al., 2000). According to a model of the basal ganglia circuitry, the degeneration of SNpc and reduced striatal dopamine (DA) result in excessive inhibition from striatal neurons that project to globus pallidus externa (GPe) and consequent disinhibition of the subthalamic nucleus (STN) via indirect pathway (Obeso et al., 2000). The nigrostriatal denervation decreases inhibition of globus pallidus interna (GPi) via the direct pathway. The combined effects of increased activity of the indirect pathway and decreased activity of the direct pathway result in increased activity of the STN and GPi. Since the outflow pathway from the GPi to the thalamus is mediated by the inhibitory neurotransmitter gamma-amino-butyric acid (GABA), the increased GPi activity in PD results in overinhibition of the thalamo-cortical-spinal pathway, clinically expressed as bradykinesia and tremor. The latter is presumably due to an inhibition of those thalamic neurons that normally suppress the oscillators in the ventral thalamus 'unmasking' the normally suppressed pacemakers. The 3 to 6 Hz spontaneous bursts from ventral thalamus are transmitted via the thalamo-cortical-spinal circuitry to the spinal motor neurons leading to synchronization of motor unit discharges, manifested as tremor. This model is used to explain the physiologic basis of surgical treatment of PD by thalamotomy, pallidotomy and deep brain stimulation (DBS).

Unlike PD, there are no morphologic or biochemical abnormalities found in autopsied brains of patients with ET (Rajput et al., 1991). Clinical physiologic studies demonstrate that the frequency of ET is not affected by mass loading to the studied limb. This indicates that central oscillators but not stretch reflex or limb mechanics play a major role in ET (Hallett, 1998). Tremorgenic oscillators in the CNS, possibly in those brainstem nuclei projecting to the cerebellum, are believed to be responsible for the tremor of ET. This is supported by the finding that harmaline, a monoamine oxidase inhibitor that causes tremor similar to human ET in animal models, induces rhythmic activities in the olivo-cerebellar system (Wilms et al., 1999). Metabolic PET studies (Wills et al., 1994) and functional MRI (Bucher et al., 1997), however, suggest that the tremor generators for ET reside in bilateral cerebellum and red nucleus. Cerebellar involvement in ET is also supported by subtle signs of cerebellar dysfunctions, impaired tandem gait, postural instability, kinetic tremor in advanced stage of ET, and disappearance of ipsilateral ET after cerebellar infarct (Deuschl et al., 2000). Alcohol reduces the amplitude of ET possibly by inhibiting cerebellar hyperactivity, as demonstrated by PET studies during tremor (Boecker et al., 1996). However, some argue that cerebellar dysfunction is not specific for ET since other forms of tremors such as PD, neuropathic tremor, and orthostatic tremor (see below) are associated with an increase in cerebellar blood flow on PET (Boeker & Brooks, 1998). Thalamus has been also postulated to play a role in ET either because it contains populations of pacemaker neurons or because it simply relays rhythmic discharges from the cerebello-olivary pathway to the motor cortex and then to the spinal cord, synchronizing the motor neuron pool and thus producing the oscillatory movement (Hua et al., 1998). The involvement of thalamus in ET is supported by the observation that thalamotomy and thalamic stimulation improve ET (Ondo et al., 1998).

Ever since the classic descriptions by Holmes (1917) that cerebellar injuries cause hypotonia, ataxia, and kinetic tremor, this form of tremor has been related with dysfunctions of cerebellum and its outflow pathways. Lesions in the midbrain (red nucleus) are associated with a slow, 2 to 3 Hz frequency tremor, sometimes referred to as myorhythmia. Higher brain stem (midbrain, pons) lesions lead to tremor at 5–7 Hz, and lower brainstem lesions produce a faster frequency at 8–11 Hz. Several anatomic–

physiologic studies have demonstrated that disruptions of the dentatorubrothalamic outflow pathway induce kinetic tremor. Such lesions result in error timing on contractions of the agonist and antagonist muscle groups.

Peripheral mechanisms

The limb muscle coupled with bones, tendons and joints is virtually a mechanical spring system that resonates and vibrates at its natural frequency. The resonant frequency varies from different joints and is inversely related to the mass of the body part. Walsh (1992) formulated an equation to calculate this frequency of vibration (f_0): $f_0 = 1/(2\pi)(K/J)^{1/2}$, where K is the stiffness exerted on a structure and J is the moment of inertia. Several factors may modify the resonance. Ballistocardiac effect influences the frequency and amplitude of peripherally generated tremors. Loading the extremity with weight mass reduces the resonant frequency. This oscillation of the muscle–joint coupling is the major contributor to physiologic tremor with typical frequency at 8 to 12 Hz. Muscle spindle primary afferent ending receptors are very sensitive, particularly in contracting muscles with α-γ co-activation, sending signals to the spinal cord and eliciting a stretch reflex. With appropriate timing, the stretch reflex produces synchronization of spinal motor neurons and generation of muscle contraction. The contraction induces another stretch reflex, and the cycle repeats itself, resulting in an oscillatory movement (McAuley & Marsden, 2000). The stretch reflex–muscle spindle feedback is controlled and modified by central oscillators and other supraspinal influences. The presence of stretch reflex loop is essential for enhanced physiologic tremor; tremors of PD and ET are much less dependent on the peripheral stretch reflex.

Clinical features and treatments of tremors

Rest tremors

Rest tremor is an oscillatory movement of a body part when that part is supported against gravity. By definition, rest tremor disappears or diminishes during voluntary muscle contraction or movement. It is difficult, however, to apply this definition to certain body parts such as lips, chin and face that are often involved in rest tremor. It should also be emphasized that all tremors, including rest tremors, disappear when the body part is at a complete rest state or during sleep and hand rest tremor is typically exacerbated when a patient with PD walks. The classical clinical picture of PD rest tremor is an asymmetric onset of 3 to 6 Hz supinating-pronating (pill-rolling) hand oscillation.

Other body parts frequently involved by PD tremor include individual fingers, lips, jaw, tongue, legs and feet. Head tremor, which is typical for ET, however, is rarely seen in PD. About 70% of PD patients present with rest tremor and nearly all patients with PD manifest tremor some time during the course of their illness (Hughes et al., 1993). Patients with tremor-dominant form of PD generally have a younger age at onset, relative sparing of cognition, slower progression and more favourable prognosis than PD patients with postural instability and gait difficulty, or PIGD (Jankovic et al., 1990). The amplitude varies between different patients and may vary from minute to minute in the same patient. When PD patients hold their arms outstretched horizontally in front of their body, the rest tremor usually disappears. In some patients the tremor reappears after a latency of several seconds (up to a minute). Although this tremor occurs during maintenance of a posture, this 're-emergent tremor' shares the same mechanisms with rest tremor because its amplitude and frequency are both similar to those of rest tremor (Jankovic et al., 1999).

While PD is the most common cause, there are many other etiologies including secondary parkinsonism and parkinsonism-plus syndromes presenting with rest tremor (Table 35.1). Advanced ET can also cause rest tremor. Although some authors argued that the coexistence of PD and ET simply represents a chance of occurrence of two common diseases (Pahwa & Koller, 1993), there is a growing body of evidence that the presence of ET is a risk factor for later development of PD (Jankovic, 2000). Several autosomal dominant families have been described in which some members have ET and others have PD (Jankovic et al., 1995; Findley, 2000).

Treatment

The discussion of treatment of rest tremors is beyond the intended scope of this chapter, but it is essentially the same as treatment of PD (Jankovic & Marsden, 1998). For a summary of treatment options on different types of tremors, please refer to Table 35.2. The choices of medical treatment of PD rest tremor include dopamine replacement with levodopa, dopamine receptor agonists, amantadine, and anticholinergic agents. Clozapine, an atypical neuroleptic (Ceravolo et al., 1999) and mirtazapine, an antidepressant with both noradrenergic and serotoninergic properties (Pact & Giduz, 1999) have been also found effective. Local injections of botulinum toxin (BTX) into the affected muscles reduce the tremor amplitude (Jankovic et al., 1996). The antitremor action of BTX is not well understood, but has been attributed to the action of BTX on the extrafusal and intrafusal motor fibres, reducing

Table 35.2. Medical treatment of tremor variants

Variant	Treatment		
Rest tremor	T, L, PH	BTX	DBS
Postural hand/arm tremor	P, PRI, A, PH	BTX	DBS
Head tremor	C, PRI, P	BTX	
Voice tremor	P	BTX	
Facial/tongue tremor	P, PRI, L	BTX	
Task-specific tremor	T, P, PRI	BTX	
Orthostatic tremor	G, C, PRI, PH, L		
Kinetic hand/arm tremor	C, P, PRI, BU, PH	BTX	DBS

Notes:

A = Alprazolam.
BTX = Botulinum toxin.
BU = Buspirone.
C = Clonazepam.
DBS = Deep brain stimulation.
G = Gabapentin.

L = Levodopa.
P = Propranolol.
PH = Phenobarbital.
PRI = Primidone.
T = Trihexyphenidyl.

spindle afferent input to the spinal cord. This restores presynaptic inhibition between antagonist muscles and reduces tremor (Modugno et al., 1998). While BTX injections may be quite effective in the treatment of parkinsonian rest tremor, it is particularly useful in ET and in dystonic tremor (see below).

For drug-resistant and disabling tremors, several surgical treatment options include thalamotomy, pallidotomy and high frequency deep brain stimulation (DBS) of the STN or GPi (Jankovic, 1999; Lang, 2000). Ventral lateral thalamotomy involving the nucleus ventralis intermedius (VIM) used to be the most popular choice of surgical options, but now VIM DBS (in ET), GPi DBS and STN DBS (in PD) are far more common. Patients can turn the pulse generator (stimulator) on or off by applying a magnet over the area where the stimulator is subcutaneously implanted, usually in the upper chest. These procedures have the advantage over the ablative procedures because the stimulating parameters can be customized to each patient and they are safer and more effective than the traditional thalamotomy (Schuurman et al., 2000). While VIM DBS reduces contralateral tremor in about 46–92% of patients (Ondo et al., 1998; Koller et al., 1999), GPi or STN DBS offers the possibility of improvement on tremor and other parkinsonian features as well, including levodopa-induced motor complications (Krack et al., 1998; Krauss et al., 2001). Rare complications of DBS are hemorrhage, seizures, contralateral hemiparesis, dysequilibrium, and infection due to foreign bodies (stimulating electrode, the pulse generator and their connections).

Action tremors

Physiologic tremor

Physiologic tremor is universally present in all people, but it is not considered pathological, until it interferes with social or occupational (fine motor) activities. Many factors may exacerbate the amplitude of physiologic tremor, including endogenous factors such as emotional stress, anxiety, fatigue, hypoglycemia, endocrine effects (e.g. hyperthyroidism, hyperadrenergic states in response to hypoglycemia); exogenous CNS stimulants such as caffeine, amphetamines, beta-agonists, lithium, neuroleptics, anticonvulsants, and tricyclic antidepressants (Diederich & Goetz, 1998). Delirium tremens, the tremor induced by acute alcohol withdrawal, is a variant of enhanced physiological tremor. Enhanced physiologic tremor is usually reversible after causative agents are removed. Chronic use of certain drugs, such as the neuroleptics, however, can produce persistent parkinsonian or tardive tremor. Tardive tremor is manifested by a mixture of rest, postural and kinetic tremor with a frequency of 3 to 5 Hz (Stacy & Jankovic, 1992). In contrast to parkinsonian tremor, tardive tremor improves rather than worsens with anti-dopaminergic agents such as tetrabenazine, a dopamine depleting and dopamine receptor blocking drug.

Several studies have demonstrated an overlap in physiologic characteristics between physiologic and isometric tremors. Isometric tremors usually do not require treatment with the exception of orthostatic tremor (Deuschl et al., 1998) (see below).

Treatment

In most cases, enhanced physiologic tremors are reversible and the treatment strategies should focus on elimination of the triggering factors such as anxiety, caffeine, drugs (e.g. lithium), hyperthyroidism, pheochromocytoma, and hypoglycemia. If tremor is embarrassing or troublesome, beta adrenergic blockers (propranolol or nadolol) and benzodiazepines may be useful (Wasielewski et al., 1998).

Essential tremor

ET is characterized by postural or kinetic tremor with frequency usually at 4 to 8 Hz, but sometimes may be as high as 12 Hz (Jankovic, 2000b). Head tremor has a slower frequency at 2 to 8 Hz. The amplitude and frequency of ET are less dependent on position of the limb or mass loading, different from those of physiologic tremor. Although the term 'benign essential tremor' is still used in the literature, it is important to recognize that ET can be very disabling. The tremor may interfere with eating, speaking, writing, daily activities and cause social embarrassment leading to social withdrawal.

Various epidemiologic studies show prevalence rates ranging from 0.4 to 5.6%, depending on different methodologies, diagnostic criteria and study populations (Louis et al., 1998). The age at onset appears to be a bimodal distribution, with peaks at the second and sixth decades (Lou & Jankovic, 1991). Since there are no physiologic, genetic or biological markers for ET, the diagnosis is based on clinical criteria. According to one set of criteria, definite ET is a bilateral postural tremor, with or without kinetic component, involving hands or forearms persistent for more than 5 years (Jankovic, 2000b). The tremor may be asymmetrical and other body parts may be affected. Other causes of tremor must be excluded. Probable ET includes the same criteria as of definite ET, but tremor may be confined to one body part and the duration is greater than 3 years. Primary orthostatic tremor, isolated voice, tongue, chin tremors, position- and task-specific tremors must be excluded. There are two types of possible ET. Criteria for type 1 possible ET are the same as of probable ET, but patients may exhibit other neurologic disorders (parkinsonism, dystonia, myoclonus, peripheral neuropathy, restless legs syndrome, or mild extrapyramidal signs). Type 2 possible ET consists of a monosymptomatic and isolated tremor of uncertain relationship to ET. It includes position- and task-specific tremors such as occupational tremors (primary writing tremors), primary orthostatic tremor, isolated voice, chin, tongue, leg tremor and unilateral postural hand tremor. Core and secondary criteria were proposed to facilitate a practical approach to the diagnosis of ET (Elble, 2000). Core criteria include bilateral action tremor of the hands and forearms (but not rest tremor), absence of other neurologic signs (except for the Froment's sign), and isolated head tremor without signs of dystonia. Secondary criteria include long duration (>3 years), positive family history, and beneficial response to alcohol. There are diagnostic red flags which indicate diagnoses other than ET, such as unilateral tremor, leg tremor, rigidity, bradykinesia, rest tremor, gait disturbance, focal tremor, isolated head tremor with abnormal posture (head tilt or turning), sudden or rapid onset, and on drug treatment that may cause or exacerbate tremor.

Upper extremities are involved most frequently in ET, typically manifesting a 4 to 8 Hz symmetrical hand tremor. Similar to enhanced physiologic tremor, emotion, stress and fatigue make ET worse. Head is another body part frequently affected, either in a form of anterior–posterior oscillation (yes–yes nodding) or lateral, side-to-side (no–no

shaking) oscillation at 2–8 Hz. Body parts also affected by ET include larynx (voice), jaw, lips, face and tongue. The lower extremities are rarely involved (Lou & Jankovic, 1991; Elble, 2000). ET often develops insidiously and progresses slowly, becoming more severe over years. The prevalence increases with age, affecting 5% to 14% of people above 65 years old (Brin & Koller, 1998). Older patients tend to have lower frequency (4–12 Hz) than younger patients (8–12 Hz) (Elble, 2000). Because the frequency of physiologic tremor is similar to ET, it may be difficult to differentiate mild ET from enhanced physiologic tremor. The way to differentiate is that mass loading of the limb decreases the frequency of physiologic tremor, but not ET.

ET is a genetic disorder inherited as an autosomal dominant pattern. The frequency of positive family history among first-degree relatives ranges from 17% to 100%. These wide variations in reported family histories are mostly due to different methodologies used to ascertain ET among family members and different characteristics of study populations (Findley, 2000). Based on studies of large ET families, Higgins et al. (1998) found a marker on chromosome 2p22–p25, termed *ETM*. The ET gene locus, *FET1*, on chromosome 3q13 (Gulcher et al., 1997), was mapped in other families with ET. Although classic ET is a monosymptomatic disorder without other neurologic signs and symptoms, in some patients and families ET is associated with parkinsonism, dystonia and other neurologic disorders. In one such family, the disorders (ET, parkinsonism, or both) were linked to chromosome 4p14–16.3 (Farrer et al., 1999). It is anticipated that there will be more gene loci and mutations identified in tremor families which will eventually lead to a genetic classification of ET.

Task- or position-specific tremors represent either variants (forme fruste) of ET or dystonia (Jankovic, 2000). The patients experience tremor when performing fine-coordinated motor activities, such as writing, playing a musical instrument, golfing or holding objects in certain positions (Bain et al., 1995). The pathophysiology of these tremors is not clear. One possibility is an abnormal CNS response to muscle spindle input from forearm muscles. Isolated voice, tongue and chin tremors also have features that seem to overlap with focal dystonia (Deuschl et al., 2000). Although many patients with dystonia have a postural tremor that is phenomenologically identical to ET, this tremor does not appear to be associated with the known GAG deletion in the *DYT1* gene (Dürr et al., 1993). Orthostatic tremor, another position-specific tremor, is characterized by a rapid (14–16 Hz) frequency tremor present in the legs while standing or during isometric contraction of trunk muscles. It is associated with 'vibration' in the legs, calf cramps and a feeling of unsteadiness after standing for a few minutes (Heilman, 1984). Jaw and other cranial muscles may occasionally be involved. Electrophysiologic recordings from the legs show bilateral coherence supporting the notion that this type of tremor is generated from a single central oscillator (McAuley et al., 2000).

Treatment

The choice of treatment for ET largely depends on the severity of the tremor and how it interferes with patient's daily activities. The antitremor medications decrease tremor amplitude but not frequency. In addition to medical treatment, factors affecting tremor such as drugs, alcohol, caffeine, anxiety, or temperature should be eliminated or minimized whenever possible. The main therapeutic options for ET include beta-adrenergic blockers and primidone (Koller et al., 2000). The beta-adrenergic blockers, especially propranolol, have been considered the treatment choice since the early 1970s. The other beta-blockers (metoprolol, nadolol and timolol) seem to be less effective than propranolol. The pharmacological mechanism of beta-blockers in the treatment of ET is not clear. Since there is no direct correlation between lipid solubility (and consequent ability to cross the blood brain barrier) and their efficacy, peripheral mechanisms seem to play a key role in reducing tremor (Guan & Peroutka, 1990). Beta-blockers are generally well tolerated, but may cause excessive daytime drowsiness, fatigue, erectile dysfunction and depression. They should not be prescribed in patients with diabetes, asthma or congestive heart failure. The efficacy of primidone in reducing tremor amplitude is about 40–50%, similar to that of propranolol. The drug is metabolized into phenylethylmalonamide (PEMA) and phenobarbital. Neither PEMA nor phenobarbital seem to have an independent antitremor activity, suggesting that the parent compound is the active drug (Sasso et al., 1991). The most common side effect is excessive daytime drowsiness, and up to 25% of patients, particularly the elderly patients, experience an acute reaction that is manifested by nausea, vomiting, sedation, confusion and ataxia. This idiosyncratic reaction may be prevented by initiating the drug with a very low dose (e.g. 25 mg at bedtime) followed by a slow and gradual titration over several weeks (up to 750 mg per day in 3 divided doses).

Many patients with ET report transient improvement of tremor after alcohol ingestion. Some use alcohol (often not judiciously) at social events to ameliorate tremor (Koller et al., 2000). Benzodiazepines, especially clonazepam, are also used to reduce ET. Other drugs with antitremor effect include the antiepileptic drugs gabapentin and topiramate (Ondo et al., 2000). Orthostatic tremor responds well to clonazepam, gabapentin and perhaps levodopa (Wills et

al., 1999). BTX injections into the muscles involved in the generation of tremor have been found to be beneficial (Jankovic et al., 1996). BTX is particularly useful in controlling head tremor, which usually does not respond well to other medical therapies. Vocal and palatal tremors are also effectively treated with BTX injections. Kaji et al. (1995) showed that local injection of lidocaine into the target muscle produced peripheral deafferentiation and transient reduction in the amplitude of postural tremor (as well as focal dystonia, such as writer's cramp).

Neurosurgical intervention should be reserved only for those patients with severe ET who are disabled or functionally impaired despite optimal medical therapies. While thalamotomy was the surgical treatment of choice in the past, in recent decades DBS of the ventral intermediate (VIM) nucleus of the thalamus has become the surgical treatment of choice because it is safer and more effective (Schuurman et al., 2000). Besides VIM, chronic cortical stimulation may improve contralateral action tremor, but this is not a practical treatment modality (Nguyen et al., 1998). Subthalamic nucleus is currently being investigated as a target for refractory proximal ET (Kitagawa et al., 2000).

Kinetic tremor

Kinetic tremor, formerly named 'intention' tremor, is a form of action tremor in which the oscillation occurs when voluntary contraction of muscles produces a goal-directed movement (e.g. finger-to-nose). This tremor has been referred as 'midbrain' or 'rubral' tremor although CNS areas, especially thalamic lesions, may present a similar clinical picture (Vidailhet et al., 1998). Diseases affecting the cerebellum or the cerebellar outflow pathways cause not only kinetic tremor, but also ataxia, dysmetria and other cerebellar signs (Deuschl et al., 2000). 'Titubation', which is a slow rhythmic oscillation of whole body or head with increasing amplitude on movement, is associated with cerebellar dysfunction (San Pedro et al., 1998). Kinetic tremor is often unilateral, present on the side ipsilateral to the cerebellar lesion, with a slow frequency raging between 2 and 5 Hz. Amplitude is medium to coarse, and is more robust when approaching the target (terminal tremor). Disorders commonly causing kinetic tremor include multiple sclerosis (MS), Friedreich's ataxia, stroke, trauma, and Wilson's disease. Alcohol abuse and toxicity due to various anticonvulsants (phenytoin and valproic acid) may also induce kinetic tremor.

Myorhythmia is a special type of tremor that is characterized by a slow 1 to 3 Hz frequency, continuous or intermittent rhythmic movement existing at rest and persisting during activity. It has irregular presentations mixed with rest, kinetic and postural tremors and is not as rhythmic as other tremors (Deuschl et al., 1998). It is often accompanied by ataxia and ipsilateral 3rd nerve palsy. This slow tremor arises from lesions in the red nucleus, midbrain, cerebellum or thalamus with secondary interruption of various pathways. It is also associated with palatal myoclonus due to an interruption of the dentato-rubro-olivary pathway (Yanagisawa et al., 1999). Etiologies of myorhythmia include cerebellar degeneration, ischemic or hemorrhagic lesions, Whipple's disease and Wilson's disease. Autopsy and PET studies suggest that the combination of rest and kinetic tremors is typically associated with disruptions in both cerebello-thalamic and nigrostriatal systems (Remy et al., 1995).

Treatment

Before selecting a symptomatic therapy for the kinetic tremor, it is important to thoroughly evaluate the patient in search of an etiology-specific treatment. Of all different tremors, kinetic tremor is the most resistant to symptomatic pharmacologic therapy. No drug has been found to provide a reliable benefit (Wasielewski et al., 1998). Clonazepam, which works on both serotoninergic and GABA systems, is used frequently for symptomatic relief. Buspirone, a 5-HT1A agonist and odansetron, a 5-HT3 antagonist were reported effective in improving cerebellar tremor (Lou et al., 1995; Rice et al., 1997). Tetrahydrocannabinol and cannabinoids may improve spasticity and tremor in patients with multiple sclerosis (Baker et al., 2000). Surgical treatment is less effective in kinetic tremor, but for some incapacitating kinetic tremors, surgical intervention, such as VIM DBS, may be the only option (Schulder et al., 1999; Taha et al., 1999).

Miscellaneous tremors

Tremors associated with peripheral neuropathy

Tremors often accompany peripheral neuropathies, particularly the dysgammaglobulinemic neuropathies, and hereditary motor–sensory neuropathies (Cardoso & Jankovic, 1993). Since the amplitude of tremor in patients with hereditary motor–sensory neuropathy does not directly correlate with the severity of motor weakness, sensory loss, or slowing of nerve conduction, the mechanism of the tremor may be pathophysiologically independent of the neuropathy. Peripheral injuries induce tremor, whether or not associated with reflex sympathetic dystrophy or the complex regional pain syndrome (Cardoso & Jankovic, 1995). There is growing evidence of central reor-ganization in response to altered peripheral input that may underlie peripherally induced tremors (Jankovic, 2001).

Psychogenic tremor

Psychogenic tremor sometimes can be difficult to differentiate from neurologic ('organic') tremor, but several series have provided useful diagnostic criteria (Deuschl et al., 1998). These include: (i) sudden onset, (ii) spontaneous remission, (iii) various combinations of different types of tremors, (iv) changing amplitude and frequency, (v) tremor increases with attention and decreases with distraction, (vi) poor response to antitremor drugs, (vii) selective disability, (viii) entrainment of the tremor with voluntary repetitive movement, (ix) absent finger tremor, and (x) remission with psychotherapy. Many patients with psychogenic tremor not only have abrupt onset but also present with maximal disability at onset (Kim et al., 1999). Some additional or associated features may help diagnose psychogenic tremor, such as false weakness, false sensory symptoms, multiple somatizations, self-inflicted injuries, bizarre movements or pseudoseizures, and subtle or obvious psychiatric illness. The management of patients with psychogenic tremor is often challenging and should include careful exploration of psychological as well as physical factors that may be contributing to the tremor. By helping the patient provide insight into the psychodynamics of the tremor, the physician may successfully treat not only the tremor, but also the underlying psychological disturbance. Antidepressant medications often play an ancillary role. Prognosis varies from poor to complete remission, largely depending on the insight of the patient and the family.

References   * denotes key references

Bain, P.G., Findley, L.J., Britton, T.C. et al. (1995). Primary writing tremor. *Brain*, **118**, 1461–72.

Baker, D., Pryce, G., Croxford, J.L. et al. (2000). Cannabinoids control spasticity and tremor in a multiple sclerosis model. *Nature*, **404**, 84–7.

Bergman, H., Wichmann, T., Karmon, B. & DeLong, M.R. (1994). The primate subthalamic nucleus: 2. Neuronal activity in the MPTP model of parkinsonism. *J. Neurophysiol.*, **72**, 507–20.

Blandini, F., Nappi, G., Tassorelli, C. & Martignoni, E. (2000). Functional changes of the basal ganglia circuitry in Parkinson's disease. *Prog. Neurobiol.*, **62**, 63–88.

Boecker, H. & Brooks, D.J. (1998). Functional imaging of tremor. *Mov. Disord.*, **13**(Suppl. 3), 64–72.

Boecker, H., Wills, A.J., Ceballos-Baumann, A. et al. (1996). The effect of ethanol on alcohol-responsive essential tremor: a position emission tomography study. *Ann. Neurol.*, **39**, 650–8.

Brin, M.F. & Koller, W.C. (1998). Epidemiology and genetics of essential tremor. *Mov. Disord.*, **13**(Suppl. 3), 55–63.

Bucher, S.F., Seelos, K.C., Dodel, R.C. et al. (1997). Activation mapping in essential tremor with functional magnetic resonance imaging. *Ann. Neurol.*, **41**, 32–40.

Cardoso, F.C. & Jankovic, J. (1993). Hereditary motor–sensory neuropathy and movement disorders. *Muscle Nerve*, **16**, 904–10.

Cardoso, F. & Jankovic, J. (1995). Peripherally-induced tremor and parkinsonism. *Arch. Neurol.*, **52**, 263–70.

Ceravolo, R., Salvetti, S., Piccini, P. et al. (1999). Acute and chronic effects of clozapine in essential tremor. *Mov. Disord.*, **14**, 468–72.

*Deuschl, G., Bain, P., Brin, M. and an Ad Hoc Scientific Committee. (1998). Consensus statement of the Movement Disorder Society on Tremor. *Mov. Disord.*, **13**(Suppl. 3), 2–23.

Deuschl, G., Wenzelburger, R., Loffler, K., Raethjen, J. & Stolze, H. (2000). Essential tremor and cerebellar dysfunction: clinical and kinematic analysis of intention tremor. *Brain*, **123**, 1568–80.

Diederich, N.J. & Goetz, C.G. (1998). Drug-induced movement disorders. *Neurol. Clin.*, **16**, 125–39.

Dürr, A., Stevanin, G., Jedynak, C.P. et al. (1993). Familial essential tremor and idiopathic torsion dystonia are different genetic entities. *Neurology*, **43**, 2212–14.

*Elble, R.J. (2000). Diagnostic criteria for essential tremor and differential diagnosis. *Neurology*, **54**(Suppl. 4), S2–6.

Farrer, M., Gwinn-Hardy, K., Muenter, M. et al. (1999). A chromosome 4p haplotype segregating with Parkinson's disease and postural tremor. *Hum. Mol. Genet.*, **8**, 81–5.

*Findley, L.J. (2000). Epidemiology and genetics of essential tremor. *Neurology*, **54**(Suppl. 4), S8–13.

Guan, X-M. & Peroutka, S.J. (1990). Basic mechanisms of action of drugs used in the treatment of essential tremor. *Clin. Neuropharmacol.*, **13**, 210–23.

Gulcher, J.R., Jónsson, P., Kong, A. et al. (1997). Mapping of a familial essential tremor gene, *FET1*, to chromosome 3q13. *Nat. Genet.*, **17**, 84–7.

*Hallett, M. (1998). Overview of human tremor physiology. *Mov. Disord.*, **13**(Suppl. 3), 43–8.

Heilman, K.M. (1984). Orthostatic tremor. *Arch. Neurol.*, **412**, 880–1.

Higgins, J.J., Loveless, J.M., Jankovic, J. & Patel, P. (1998). Evidence that a gene for essential tremor maps to chromosome 2p in four families. *Mov. Disord.*, **13**, 972–7.

Holmes, G. (1917). The symptoms of acute cerebellar injuries due to gunshot injuries. *Brain*, **40**, 461–535.

Hua, S.E., Lenz, F.A., Zirh, T.A. et al. (1998). Thalamic neuronal activity correlated with essential tremor. *J. Neurol., Neurosurg. Psychiatry*, **64**, 273–6.

Hughes, A.J., Daniel, S.E., Blankson, S. & Lees, A.J. (1993). A clinicopathologic study of 100 cases of Parkinson's disease. *Arch. Neurol.*, **50**, 140–8.

Jankovic, J. (1999). New and emerging therapies for Parkinson disease. *Arch. Neurol.*, **56**, 785–90.

*Jankovic, J. (2000). Essential tremor: clinical characteristics. *Neurology*, **54**(Suppl. 4), S21–5.

Jankovic, J. (2001). Can peripheral trauma induce dystonia and other movement disorders? Yes! *Mov. Disord.*, **16**, 7–12.

Jankovic, J. (2002). Therapeutic strategies in Parkinson's disease. In *Parkinson's Disease and Movement Disorders*, 3rd edn, ed. J. Jankovic & E. Tolosa, pp. 191–220. Philadelphia, PA: Lippincott.

Jankovic, J., McDermott, M., Carter, J. et al. (1990). Variable expression of Parkinson's disease: a base-line analysis of the DATATOP cohort. The Parkinson Study Group. *Neurology*, **40**, 1529–34.

Jankovic, J., Beach, J., Schwartz, K. & Contant, C. (1995). Tremor and longevity in relatives of patients with Parkinson's disease, essential tremor and control subjects. *Neurology*, **45**, 645–8.

Jankovic, J., Schwartz, K., Clemence, W., Aswad, A. & Mordaunt, J. (1996). A randomized, double-blind, placebo-controlled study to evaluate botulinum toxin type A in essential hand tremor. *Mov. Disord.*, **11**, 250–6.

Jankovic, J., Schwartz, K.S. & Ondo, W. (1999). Re-emergent tremor of Parkinson's disease. *J. Neurol., Neurosurg. Psychiatry*, **67**, 646–50.

Kaji, R., Kohara, N., Katayama, M. et al. (1995). Muscle afferent block by intramuscular injection of lidocaine for the treatment of writer's cramp. *Muscle Nerve*, **18**, 234–5.

Kim, Y.J., Pakiam, A.S.I. & Lang, A.E. (1999). Historical and clinical features of psychogenic tremor: a review of 70 cases. *Can. J. Neurol. Sci.*, **26**, 190–5.

Kitagawa, M., Murata, J., Kikuchi, S. et al. (2000). Deep brain stimulation of subthalamic area for severe proximal tremor. *Neurology*, **55**, 114–16.

Koller, W.C., Lyons, K.E., Wilkins, S.B. & Pahwa, R. (1999). Efficacy of unilateral deep brain stimulation of the VIM nucleus of the thalamus for essential head tremor. *Mov. Disord.*, **14**, 847–50.

Koller, W.C., Hristova, A. & Brin, M. (2000). Pharmacologic treatment of essential tremor. *Neurology*, **54**(Suppl. 4), S30–8.

Krack, P., Pollak, P., Limousin, P. et al. (1998). Subthalamic nucleus or internal pallidal stimulation in young onset Parkinson's disease. *Brain*, **121**, 451–7.

Krauss, J.K., Jankovic, J. & Grossman, R.G., eds. (2001). *Surgery for Movement Disorders*, pp. 1–449. Philadelphia, PA: Lippincott Williams & Wilkins.

Lamarre, Y. (1984). Animal models of physiological, essential and parkinsonian-like tremors. In *Movement Disorders: Tremor*, ed. L.J. Findley & R. Capildeo, pp. 183–94. New York: Oxford University Press.

*Lang, A.E. (2000). Surgery for Parkinson disease. *Arch. Neurol.*, **57**, 1118–25.

Llinas, R.R. (1988). The intrinsic electrophysiological properties of mammalian neurons: insights into central nervous system function. *Science*, **242**, 1654–64.

Lou, J.S. & Jankovic, J. (1991). Essential tremor: clinical correlates in 350 patients. *Neurology*, **41**, 234–8.

Lou, J.S., Goldfarb, L., McShane, L. et al. (1995). Use of buspirone for treatment of cerebellar ataxia. An open-label study. *Arch. Neurol.*, **52**, 982–8.

*Louis, E.D., Ottman, R. & Hauser, W.A. (1998). How common is the most common adult movement disorder? Estimates of the prevalence of essential tremor throughout the world. *Mov. Disord.*, **13**, 5–10.

*McAuley, J.H. & Marsden, C.D. (2000). Physiological and pathological tremors and rhythmic central motor control. *Brain*, **123**, 1545–67.

McAuley, J.H., Britton, T.C., Rothwell, J.C., Findley, L.J. & Marsden, C.D. (2000). The timing of primary orthostatic tremor bursts has a task-specific plasticity. *Brain*, **123**, 254–66.

Modugno, N., Priori, A., Berardelli, A., Vacca, L., Mercuri, B. & Manfredi, M. (1998). Botulinum toxin restores presynaptic inhibition of group Ia afferents in patients with essential tremor. *Muscle Nerve*, **21**, 1701–5.

Montigny, C. de & Lamarre, Y. (1973). Rhythmic activity induced by harmaline in the olivo–cerebello–bulbar system of the cat. *Brain Res.*, **53**, 81–95.

Nguyen, J.-P., Pollin, B., Feve, A. et al. (1998). Improvement of action tremor by chronic cortical stimulation. *Mov. Disord.*, **13**, 84–8.

Obeso, J.A., Rodriguez-Oroz, M.C., Rodriguez, M. et al. (2000). Pathophysiology of the basal ganglia in Parkinson's disease. *TINS*, **23**(Suppl.), S8–19.

Ondo, W., Jankovic, J., Lai, E. et al. (1998). Assessment of motor function following stereotactic pallidotomy. *Neurology*, **50**, 266–70.

Ondo, W., Hunter, C., Vuong, K.D., Schwartz, K. & Jankovic, J. (2000). Gabapentin for essential tremor: a multiple-dose, double-blind, placebo-controlled trial. *Mov. Disord.*, **15**, 678–82.

Pact, V. & Giduz, T. (1999). Mirtazapine treats resting tremor, essential tremor, and levodopa-induced dyskinesias. *Neurology*, **53**, 1154.

Pahwa, R. & Koller, W.C. (1993). Is there a relationship between Parkinson's disease and essential tremor? *Clin. Neuropharmacol.*, **16**, 30–5.

Plenz, D. & Kitai, S. (1996). Generation of high-frequency oscillations in local circuits of rat somatosensory cortex cultures. *J. Neurophysiol.*, **76**, 4180–4.

Plenz, D. & Kitai, S. (1999). A basal ganglia pacemaker formed by the subthalamic nucleus and external globus pallidus. *Nature*, **400**, 677–81.

Rajput, A.H., Rozdilsky, B., Ang, L. & Rajput, A. (1991). Cinicopathologic observations in essential tremor: report of six cases. *Neurology*, **41**, 1422–4.

Remy, P., de Recondo, A., Defer, G. et al. (1995). Peduncular rubral

tremor and dopaminergic denervation: a PET study. *Neurology*, **45**, 472–7.

Rice, G.P.A., Lesaux, J., Vandervoort, P., Macewan, L. & Ebers, G.C. (1997). Odansetron, a 5-HT3 antagonist, improves cerebellar tremor. *J. Neurol., Neurosurg. Psychiatry*, **62**, 282–4.

San Pedro, E.C., Mountz, J.M., Liu, H.G. & Deutsch, G. (1998). Postinfectious cerebellitis: clinical significance of Tc-99m HMPAO brain SPECT compared with MRI. *Clin. Nucl. Med.*, **23**, 212–16.

Sasso, E., Perucca, E., Fava, R. & Calzetti, S. (1991). Quantitative comparison of barbiturates in essential hand and head tremor. *Mov. Disord.*, **6**, 65–8.

Schulder, M., Sernas, T., Mahalick, D., Adler, R. & Cook, S. (1999). Thalamic stimulation in patients with multiple sclerosis. *Stereotact. Funct. Neurosurg.*, **72**, 196–201.

*Schuurman, P.R., Bosch, A., Bossuyt, P.M. et al. (2000). A comparison of continuous thalamic stimulation and thalamotomy for suppression of severe tremor. *N. Engl. J. Med.*, **342**, 461–8.

Stacy, M. & Jankovic, J. (1992). Tardive tremor. *Mov. Disord.*, **7**, 53–7.

Taha, J.M., Janszen, M.A. & Favre, J. (1999). Thalamic deep brain stimulation for the treatment of head, voice, and bilateral limb tremor. *J. Neurosurg.*, **91**, 68–72.

Vidailhet, M., Jedynak, C.P., Pollak, P. & Agid, Y. (1998). Pathology of symptomatic tremors. *Mov. Disord.*, **13**(Suppl. 3), 49–54.

Volkmann, J., Joliot, M., Mogilner, A. et al. (1996). Central motor loop oscillations in parkinsonian resting tremor revealed by magnetoencephalography. *Neurology*, **46**, 1359–70.

Walsh, E.G. (1992). *Muscles, Masses and Motion*, pp. 67–77. London: MacKeith Press.

*Wasielewski, P.G., Burns, J.M. & Koller, W.C. (1998). Pharmacologic treatment of tremor. *Mov. Disord.*, **13**(Suppl. 3), 90–100.

*Wills, A.J., Jenkins, I.H. & Thompson, P.D. (1994). Red nuclear and cerebellar but no olivary activation associated with essential tremor: a positron emission tomographic study. *Ann. Neurol.*, **36**, 636.

Wills, A.J., Brusa, L., Wang, H.C., Brown, P. & Marsden, C.D. (1999). Levodopa may improve orthostatic tremor: case report and trial of treatment. *J. Neurol., Neurosurg. Psychiatry*, **66**, 681–4.

Wilms, H., Sievers, J. & Deuschl, G. (1999). Animal models of tremor. *Mov. Disord.*, **14**, 557–71.

Yanagisawa, T., Sugihara, H., Shibahara, K., Kamo, T., Fujisawa, K. & Murayama, M. (1999). Natural course of combined limb and palatal tremor caused by cerebellar-brain stem infarction. *Mov Disord.*, **14**, 851–4.

36

Myoclonus

Peter Brown

Sobell Department of Motor Neuroscience, Institute of Neurology and
National Hospital for Neurology and Neurosurgery, London, UK

Myoclonus is defined as shock-like involuntary movements. Most often these are due to brief bursts of muscle activity, resulting in positive myoclonus. Jerks, however, may also result from sudden short inhibitions of ongoing tonic muscle activity, termed negative myoclonus or asterixis. Myoclonus may be physiological, such as hiccups, or due to a variety of hereditary or acquired conditions. In particular, it may be seen in primary generalized epilepsy, but as this syndrome is dominated by epilepsy rather than myoclonus, it will not be considered further here.

Clinical overview of physiologically based classification

Although etiological classifications have not proven very useful in predicting the response to drugs, electrophysiological investigations have been able to distinguish several different pathophysiological mechanisms with therapeutic implications. To a large degree, the pathophysiological type of myoclonus can be suspected on clinical grounds. The most useful clinical distinction is between generalized, multifocal and focal/segmental jerks. Generalized myoclonus involves the majority of the body in a synchronous jerk. It may spare the face and be predominantly axial, as in propriospinal myoclonus, or include the face, as in brainstem myoclonus. The latter may only consist of reflex jerks, as in exaggerated startle/hyperekplexia, or may also involve prominent spontaneous jerks as in brainstem reticular reflex myoclonus. A useful confirmatory sign of a brainstem origin is the presence of jerks in response to auditory stimulation, particularly unexpected sounds. Multifocal myoclonus involves different parts of the body at different times. There may also be the occasional generalized jerk, but the clinical picture is dominated by multifocal jerks. Such patients may be divided into those in whom the distal limbs are especially involved, and are likely to have cortical myoclonus, and those in whom the jerks are most noticeable proximally, particularly round the shoulders. These are likely to have essential myoclonus. Helpful confirmatory signs of cortical and essential myoclonus are an exacerbation of jerking upon voluntary action and the presence of dystonic posturing, respectively. Focal/segmental jerks are the most obscure as they may arise at virtually any level of the nervous system, including the spinal cord.

Clinical suspicion of particular pathophysiological types of myoclonus can be supported by simple investigation. Epileptic EEG abnormalities are suggestive of a cortical origin, as are giant cortical SEPs following median or tibial nerve stimulation. EMG studies are useful in focal myoclonus as signs of segmental denervation often accompany spinal segmental myoclonus. Similarly, imaging of brain and spinal cord can be very helpful in demonstrating the structural lesion that often accompanies generalized or focal myoclonus.

Cortical myoclonus

Pathophysiology

Cortical myoclonus is the result of an abnormal discharge in the sensorimotor cortex, and rapidly conducting corticospinal pathways. It may consist of reflex myoclonus, spontaneous jerks or myoclonus elicited by voluntary action, and tends to be focal or multifocal. It is characterized by brief bursts of electromyographic activity (EMG), usually less than 70 ms in duration. EMG bursts are preceded by pathological enlargement of the cortical components of the sensory evoked potential in reflex jerks, or a time-locked cortical correlate in the electroencephalographic activity (EEG) in action or spontaneous myoclonus

(Fig. 36.1). In each case the relevant EEG wave precedes the EMG burst by an interval more or less appropriate for conduction in the fastest corticospinal pathways. For the intrinsic muscles of the hand, this interval is about 20 ms. Although the EEG waves prior to the jerks are often several tens of microvolts in amplitude, averaging techniques, such as backaveraging, are usually necessary to identify their morphology and distribution.

Some patients may also have cortical negative myoclonus, either action induced or reflex. In this a brief silencing of muscle activity occurs preceded by a cortical wave. Sudden lapses in posture result, particularly noticeable during gait, and tend to be more resistant to drug treatment than positive reflex or action myoclonus. In addition, in some patients with multifocal myoclonus, myoclonic activity spreads within and between the sensorimotor cortices, so that bilateral or generalized jerks also occur. Spread is somatotopic, and cranial nerve innervated muscles are activated rostro-caudally, unlike the caudo-rostral activation seen in hyperekplexia.

The cortical inhibitory processes, which would normally keep spread in check, are deficient in cortical myoclonus. This can be shown in vivo using the technique of transcutaneous stimulation of the motor cortex (Brown et al., 1996). A conditioning magnetic shock to either the ipsilateral or contralateral motor cortex normally inhibits the response to a succeeding test shock, demonstrating the presence of both cortico-cortical and transcallosal inhibition in healthy subjects. Both types of inhibition are severely impaired in patients with cortical myoclonus and evidence of cortical spread of myoclonic activity.

Etiology and clinical features

Cortical myoclonus is most marked in the distal limb, and in focal forms is usually confined to this site. If widespread, myoclonus is multifocal, with or without additional bilateral or generalized jerks. The latter are associated with more marked disability. Reflex jerks may be elicited by touch and tap, or visual stimuli. Marked sensitivity to photic stimulation suggests Unverricht–Lundborg disease. Sensitivity to auditory stimuli suggests a startle syndrome, although some patients may have a combination of cortical myoclonus and pathological startle. Multifocal jerks occurring with voluntary action are very suggestive of a cortical origin for the myoclonus. As well as involving arm function, jerks may affect speech and gait. Extraocular muscles are spared.

Focal cortical myoclonus is usually due to vascular or neoplastic lesions of the sensorimotor cortex. When spontaneous jerks are frequent, focal cortical myoclonus is

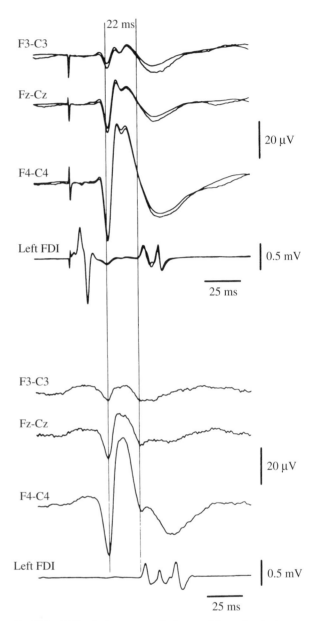

Fig. 36.1. (*a*) Cortical sensory evoked potentials to electrical stimulation of the left ulnar nerve at the wrist. (*b*) Backaveraged EEG activity preceding voluntary action jerks in a patient with coeliac disease and cortical myoclonus. A giant EEG wave is recorded, largest contralateral to the stimulated or moved hand. The positive (downgoing) component of the wave precedes the reflex response (*a*) or action jerk (*b*) by 22 ms, an interval appropriate for conduction from motor cortex to hand via the fastest pyramidal pathways. (Reprinted from Bhatia et al., 1995, with permission.)

often called epilepsia partialis continua. Multifocal myoclonus may occur in posthypoxic encephalopathy, as first described by Lance and Adams (1963), or as part of a progressive illness, as in the syndromes of progressive myoclonic ataxia and progressive myoclonic epilepsy. Causes with a genetic basis usually have an onset before the age of 20. Progressive myoclonic ataxia describes those patients with prominent myoclonus and ataxia, but little in the way of epilepsy or progressive dementia. The term encompasses the Ramsay Hunt syndrome. Progressive myoclonic ataxia is most commonly due to Unverricht–Lundborg disease, mitochondrial encephalopathy or coeliac related encephalopathy. The latter usually comes on in middle-age or later and enteric coeliac disease may be asymptomatic (Bhatia et al., 1995). The diagnosis is confirmed by small bowel biopsy. Unverricht-Lundborg disease is due to mutations in the gene on chromosome 21q that codes for cystatin B, an inhibitor of cysteine protease. The mitochondrial encephalopathy associated with myoclonus is usually the MERRF syndrome of myoclonus, epilepsy and ragged red fibres. This is typically due to point mutations in the mitochondrial gene that codes for tRNA (Lys). An elevated CSF lactate level is suggestive of the diagnosis, which can often be confirmed by mitochondrial DNA analysis of blood.

Progressive myoclonic epilepsy describes those patients with myoclonus, severe epilepsy and relentless cognitive decline. The commonest causes are sialidosis, Lafora's disease, lipidosis, neuronal ceroid lipofuscinosis, dentato-rubro-pallido-luysian atrophy and Huntington's disease, although mitochondrial encephalopathy can also be responsible. Dentato-rubro-pallido-luysian atrophy and Huntington's disease are due to CAG triplet repeat expansions on chromosome 12p and 4, respectively. Sialidosis is due to mutations in the sialidase gene and confirmatory tests include assays for urine oligosaccharides and fibroblast α-neuraminidase. Juvenile neuronal ceroid lipofuscinosis is caused by mutations in the CLN3 gene, a gene of unknown function that encodes a 438-amino acid protein of possible mitochondrial location. The remaining forms of neuronal ceroid lipofuscinosis and Lafora disease have been mapped by linkage analysis but the corresponding gene defects are still unknown. Lafora disease is an autosomal recessive storage disease characterized by polyglucosan acid-Schiff positive inclusions (Lafora bodies) in cells of brain, liver, muscle and skin, in sweat gland ducts.

Cortical myoclonus may also be a relatively minor aspect of several degenerative diseases, where the clinical picture is dominated by other features. Examples are multiple system atrophy and Alzheimer's disease. Multifocal myoclonus, particularly of the hands, may be present in corticobasal degeneration, but it seems likely that the myoclonus in this condition is subserved by different pathways to classical cortical myoclonus. In particular, cortical sensory evoked potentials are not giant, and the latency of reflex responses is very short, raising the possibility of a direct relay of somatosensory afferent input to the motor cortex without involvement of the sensory cortex. Patients with Creutzfeldt–Jacob disease usually have myoclonus, which at least in some cases has a cortical origin.

Pharmacology and treatment

Drug treatment is primarily aimed at bolstering deficient inhibitory processes. In particular, a reduction of 25 to 50% of GABA levels has been reported in the cerebrospinal fluid of patients with posthypoxic myoclonus and progressive myoclonic epilepsy, and GABAergic drugs form the cornerstone of treatment. Of these sodium valproate is the most effective, and increases cortical GABA levels as well as potentiating GABA postsynaptic inhibitory activity. The drug is introduced slowly, with most patients needing doses of 1200 to 2000 mg/day. Transient gastrointestinal upset may occur during initial treatment, usually with nausea and vomiting, but sometimes with abdominal pain and diarrhea. Hair loss, tremor, hepatotoxicity and drowsiness may also occur.

Benzodiazepines and barbiturates facilitate GABAergic transmission by effects on the GABA receptor–ionophore complex. Clonazepam is the most useful antimyoclonic agent. Large doses of clonazepam are often necessary (as much as 15 mg/day). Undue drowsiness and ataxia are the only major side effects and can be largely overcome by gradually increasing the dosage. Abrupt reductions and withdrawls can result in a marked deterioration in myoclonus and withdrawal fits. Tolerance may develop over a period of several months in some patients. Primidone and phenobarbital are occasionally useful.

Piracetam is structurally similar to GABA, but it does not elicit specific GABAergic effects nor modify GABA levels in the brain, and its mechanism of action remains unclear. The drug's effectiveness is largely limited to cortical myoclonus, regardless of aetiology. This suggests that, where possible, electrophysiological assessment of the physiological type of myoclonus should be undertaken before considering treatment with the drug. Piracetam is well tolerated and does not alter blood levels of other anticonvulsants. In particular, it is non-sedating. It is usually prescribed as add-on therapy, but can be effective when given alone. Therapeutic dosages range between 2.4 g and 21.6 g. Abrupt withdrawal of piracetam has been associated with a severe worsening of myoclonus and seizures in a minority of patients.

Disturbances of serotoninergic function have also been incriminated in cortical myoclonus. CSF concentrations of the principal metabolite of serotonin, 5-hydroxyindoleacetic acid, are reduced in these patients. However, treatment with serotonin precursors like 5-hydroxytryptophan, is poorly tolerated and, nowadays, only used as a last resort.

Phenytoin and carbamazepine are rarely helpful. In some patients, particularly those with Unverricht–Lundborg disease, phenytoin may exacerbate myoclonus. Carbamazepine may worsen myoclonic seizures. Vigabatrin, an irreversible inhibitor of GABA transaminase, surprisingly does not seem very useful. It may lead to a paradoxical increase in myoclonus in some patients, or, occasionally, myoclonus in its own right.

In summary, the treatments of first choice in cortical myoclonus are sodium valproate and clonazepam. However, most patients only gain adequate relief from their myoclonus when drugs are used in combination (Obeso et al., 1988). Gait disturbance tends to be the most resistant feature and a bouncy unsteady gait with frequent falls may persist despite control of action and reflex myoclonus in the upper limbs. The combination of clonazepam, primidone and either sodium valproate, piracetam or both may be necessary to provide substantial relief of myoclonus. Polytherapy is generally well tolerated, but doses may be limited by ataxia and drowsiness. Piracetam has particular advantages in these circumstances, as its addition to existing treatments is rarely accompanied by sedation.

Prognosis

Prognosis is dictated by the underlying condition. However, two conditions merit particular comment. The progressive myoclonic ataxia associated with coeliac disease often starts in the foot, slowly spreading to the other foot and upper limbs. Most patients become wheelchair bound or die within 2 years, regardless of dietary restriction (Bhatia et al., 1995). In posthypoxic myoclonus the disability following the hypoxic event is often severe, but it has recently been realized that late improvement in the myoclonic syndrome and the level of disability can occur years after onset (Werhahn et al., 1997). Some patients are eventually able to discontinue antimyoclonic medication and to walk unaided. Cognitive deficits are found in about half, but are usually mild. Epilepsy may be a problem in the first year, particularly during the initial

Table 36.1. Diagnostic criteria for hereditary essential myoclonus

Onset under 20 years old
Males and females equally affected
Myoclonus with a benign course, compatible with a life of normal span
Dominant mode of inheritance, but with variable severity
Absence of seizures, dementia, gross ataxia and other neurological deficits
Normal EEG

period of posthypoxic coma, but thereafter only persists in the minority of cases. Other neurological deficits are rare.

Myoclonus in association with dystonia

Essential myoclonus

Essential myoclonus is commonly inherited as an autosomal dominant trait with variable penetrance and expression, when it is termed hereditary essential myoclonus (the terms essential familial myoclonus, familial myoclonia, ballistic overflow myoclonus and benign essential myoclonus have also been used). The diagnostic criteria for this condition have been set out by Mahloudji and Pikielny (1967), and are summarized in Table 36.1. The jerks are present at rest, but become more marked with action. They are worst around the neck and proximal arms, and may dramatically improve with alcohol. In many cases there is also evidence of dystonic posturing or a family history of dystonia. Sporadic cases are very similar and may be examples of hereditary essential myoclonus with incomplete penetrance, new mutations or truly sporadic phenocopies.

Myoclonic jerks arise from a distortion of the normal reciprocal activation pattern of ballistic movements, so that muscle activity is no longer restricted to appropriate muscles. EMG activity may also be prolonged, with conspicuous cocontraction. Stimulus sensitivity is not a prominent feature, although jerks can sometimes be provoked by unexpected loud noises. Cortical somatosensory evoked potentials are normal. Back-averaging of the EEG activity preceding jerks reveals no cortical correlate or an unusual generalized wave preceding the jerks by a longer interval than seen in cortical myoclonus.

The available but limited pharmacological evidence suggests a cholinergic–serotoninergic imbalance. Therapeutic trials have shown moderate benefit from benztropine mesylate and 5-HTP, although the latter is poorly tolerated. The deterioration of the myoclonus following parenteral physostigmine also supports a relative cholinergic overactivity. Antiepileptic treatments are not helpful, with the possible exception of clonazepam. Drug treatments generally fail to match the amelioration seen with alcohol, and as a result there is a real danger of alcoholism in this condition. Deep brain stimulation of the globus pallidus interna may be considered in intractable cases.

Myoclonic dystonia

Some families with idiopathic dystonia may have family members with jerks (termed myoclonic dystonia), but myoclonus is not found in the absence of dystonia and does not show a dramatic response to alcohol, distinguishing these families from those with hereditary essential myoclonus (Quinn, 1996).

Brainstem myoclonus and the startle syndrome: segmental

Brainstem myoclonus usually leads to generalized myoclonic jerks, as in brainstem reticular reflex myoclonus and hyperekplexia. Focal forms are rare, although diaphragmatic myoclonus may arise in the rostral medulla. Palatal myoclonus is best considered as a form of tremor.

Hyperekplexia/startle syndrome

The most striking clinical characteristic of the generalized forms of brainstem myoclonus is the exaggerated motor response to unexpected auditory and, sometimes, somesthetic and visual stimuli. Hyperekplexia is the commonest cause of the startle syndrome. It may be idiopathic, inherited as an autosommal dominant condition, or symptomatic. There is now general agreement that the response in hereditary and symptomatic hyperekplexia is a pathological exaggeration of the normal startle reflex (Brown et al., 1991b; Matsumoto et al., 1992). Both types of response are the result of activity in a common reflex centre in the lower brainstem. Thus (when allowance is made for the blink reflex which is usually elicited concurrently) the first EMG activity in the startle is recorded in sternocleidomastoid, with other cranial, trunk and limb muscles following in an orderly fashion, as myoclonic activity spreads up the brainstem and down the spinal cord (Fig. 36.2). Caudal muscles are recruited relatively slowly, and involvement of the

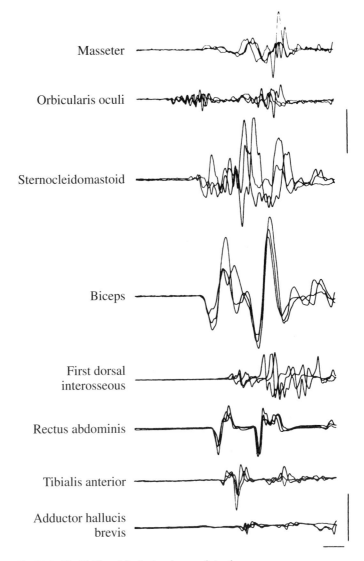

Fig. 36.2. The EMG activity in the abnormal startle response elicited by auditory stimulation in a patient with symptomatic hyperekplexia. The unrectified EMG activity in three single trials is superimposed. Each trial was started at the point of presentation of a 124 dB tone. Following the normal auditory blink reflex, EMG activity was recorded first in sternocleidomastoid, and then later in masseter and trunk limb muscles. The latencies to the intrinsic hand muscles of the hand and foot were disproportionately long. The horizontal calibration line represents 20 ms. The vertical calibration line represents 0.5 and 4.0 mV for the upper three channels, and the lower five channels, respectively. (Reprinted from Brown et al., 1991a, with permission.)

intrinsic hand and foot muscles is disproportionately delayed.

The reflex jerks to auditory, somesthetic or visual stimuli involve many muscles, both proximal and distal, bilaterally and synchronously to produce a sudden shock-like movement usually involving a grimace, abduction of the arms, and flexion of the neck, trunk, elbows, hips and knees. Thus the reflex jerks resemble the normal startle reaction in general character, although, clinically, they are greatly exaggerated in amplitude, more extensive in distribution and habituate poorly. Somesthetic stimuli are most effective when applied to the mantle area; that is the head, face and upper chest.

Many patients also exhibit generalized tonic spasms with unexpected stimuli, and it is these that lead to frequent injury and which are the most disabling feature of the condition. The pathophysiology of these tonic spasms is not known. They may be a brainstem phenomenon or the result of activity in the motor and supplementary motor cortex, as in startle epilepsy. Tonic spasms consist of generalized stiffening, lasting a few seconds, usually in response to unexpected somesthetic or acoustic stimuli. During these tonic spasms patients are unable to take any protective action and, if erect, fall stiffly to the ground, without losing consciousness. When present, tonic spasms tend to dominate the clinical picture. The tonic episodes are quite different to the brief, generalized startle reflexes seen in these patients and occur less frequently than the latter. They are also distinct from the tonic spasms of multiple sclerosis, which are usually painful, unilateral and rarely stimulus sensitive.

In addition, patients may experience excessive jerking, particularly during or going off to sleep. These paroxysms of jerking involve repetitive flexion of all four limbs, especially the legs. They are usually spontaneous. Consciousness is preserved in diurnal attacks, although jerking may be severe enough to cause incontinence of urine. The pathophysiology of the episodes of jerking, like that of the tonic spasms, is unclear.

Carbamazepine, phenytoin and the benzodiazepines, particularly clonazepam, form the mainstay of treatment, which is directed at the disabling tonic spasms rather than the exaggerated startle responses.

Hereditary hyperekplexia

Hereditary hyperekplexia is due to a mutation in the $alpha_1$ subunit of the glycine receptor, which may lead to altered ligand binding or disturbance of the chloride ion-channel part of the receptor (Shiang et al., 1993). Gycine receptors are widely distributed within the central nervous system, and this change in the $alpha_1$ subunit may account for the range of abnormalities which can be present in this condition. Stiffness and apneic attacks as a baby, hyperreflexia, a hesitant wide-based gait, epilepsy, and low intelligence may occur in addition to an exaggerated startle, tonic spasms and paroxysms of jerking.

The clinical and electrophysiological findings vary between members of the same family, and many relatives may only have an excessive startle reaction, without other neurological abnormalities. The mutation in the glycine receptor is rarely found in these minor forms, despite its presence in more affected relatives and it is possible that these minor forms represent a normal variant or 'copied' behaviour.

Acquired hyperekplexia

Clinically, idiopathic and symptomatic hyperekplexia are usually only distinguished from hereditary hyperekplexia by the absence of a family history and the presence of any signs attributable to the underlying disease in symptomatic forms. Patients have an exaggerated startle reflex, with or without tonic spasms and paroxysms of jerking. Tonic spasms are occasionally complicated by laryngeal spasm, with the risk of respiratory arrest. So far, sporadic cases have not been found to have mutations in the glycine receptor. Symptomatic hyperekplexia is usually due to brainstem disease, such as infarct, hemorrhage or encephalitis.

Startle epilepsy

Startle epilepsy can readily be distinguished from hyperekplexia, although similar pathophysiological mechanisms may operate in the tonic episodes of each condition. Startle epilepsy is seen in the setting of early brain damage, usually perinatal anoxia (Chauvel et al., 1992). Most patients have a hemiparesis, and mental retardation is common. Seizures begin in childhood or adolescence, and tend to be frequent. They consist of tonic spasms, lasting up to 30s, with preservation of consciousness. The spasms are typically asymmetrical and predominatly involve the paretic limbs. They may be elicited by unexpected auditory, visual or somesthetic stimulation, or occur spontaneously. Other seizure types occur in about a quarter of patients. Cranial imaging is abnormal in the majority of cases, usually showing unilateral atrophy involving the lateral central and pericentral cortex. The interictal EEG is generally abnormal with localized or diffuse slow waves and spikes. Ictal scalp-recorded EEG shows a fast low amplitude discharge often preceded by a high voltage spike at the vertex. Using depth electrodes the tonic seizures have been shown to originate in the motor or supplementary motor cortex.

Brainstem reticular reflex myoclonus

This rare form of generalized myoclonus may occur in posthypoxic encephalopathy, brainstem encephalitis and uremia. It responds to anticonvulsant drugs, particularly clonazepam and sodium valproate. Clinically, it is distinguished from hyperekplexia by the frequent occurrence of spontaneous, as well as reflex jerks to auditory and somesthetic stimulation. The latter is most effective over the distal limbs, rather than the mantle area typical of hyperekplexia. The basic pattern of muscle recruitment in the jerks is similar to that recorded in hyperekplexia in so far as activity seems to spread from the caudal brainstem (Hallett et al., 1977). EMG activity is recorded first in trapezius and sternocleidomastoid, and later in other cranial, trunk and limb muscles. The relative latencies to onset of reflex EMG activity in these muscles increases with the distance of their respective segmental innervations from the lower brainstem.

These generalized jerks are therefore believed to arise in the reticular formation of the caudal brainstem. Despite this, several important electrophysiological distinctions exist between brainstem reticular reflex myoclonus and hyperekplexia, making it likely that their origins within the bulbopontine reticular formation are different. The difference between the relative latencies of trunk and limb muscles is small in the jerks of brainstem reticular reflex myoclonus, indicating that the spinal motor pathways are rapidly conducting, with velocities comparable to those of rapidly conducting pyramidal pathways. This is in contrast to the findings in hyperekplexia. Also, in reticular reflex myoclonus the relative latencies of the intrinsic hand and foot muscles are not disproportionately prolonged, as in hyperekplexia.

Startle responses with unknown physiology

There remain several other conditions in which an exaggerated startle is a prominent feature, but the physiology of the motor response is unclear. Infantile GM2 gangliosidosis (Tay–Sachs and Sandhoff's diseases) is characterized by hypotonia, irritability and abnormal startle responses in infancy. Developmental regression, progressive blindness with a cherry red macular spot, deafness, seizures and spasticity ensue. Death usually occurs before the third year. The physiology of the abnormal startle is unknown in this condition, but a relationship to the normal startle or Moro response seems unlikely as the motor response consists of a sudden extension of the arms, head and trunk.

Tics in Gilles de la Tourette's syndrome usually are spontaneous, but sometimes may be triggered by external stimuli and may have the appearance of an exaggerated startle response. They rarely represent a diagnostic problem as the other clinical features of Gilles de la Tourette's syndrome are distinctive. In jumping, latah and myriachit unexpected sensory stimulation leads to an initial violent start followed by automatic speech or behaviour, such as echolalia, echopraxia or the assumption of a defensive posture.

Spinal myoclonus

The spinal cord possesses both local segmental organization and long propriospinal pathways linking activity across many segments. Pathological activity in either system can lead to myoclonus. Very rarely, focal myoclonus may be due to a lesion of the spinal root, plexus or peripheral nerve.

Propriospinal myoclonus

In this form of myoclonus a spinal myoclonic generator recruits axial muscles up and down the spinal cord via long propriospinal pathways (Brown et al., 1991a; Schulz-Bonhage et al., 1996). The disorder generally develops in middle age, and follows cervical trauma, albeit mild, in about half of cases. Its course is relatively benign, with a history of involuntary jerking stretching back up to 25 years. Spontaneous remission is unusual. Myoclonus usually takes the form of axial flexion jerks involving the neck, trunk, and hips, although a minority of patients may have truncal extension jerks. It may occur spontaneously, particularly on lying flat, or be precipitated by somesthetic stimuli. Myoclonic EMG activity usually consists of repetitive bursts with a frequency of 1–7Hz. EMG bursts can be quite long, lasting several hundred milliseconds. The jerks may be stimulus sensitive, particularly to taps to the abdomen, biceps or patella tendons. The orderly recruitment of rostral and caudal segments from a given spinal focus often confirms a spinal origin for the myoclonus (Fig. 36.3), although it is not always possible to distinguish such a pattern of activation. Clonazepam has proven the most effective treatment for propriospinal myoclonus, and leads to partial improvement in over half of patients. Other anticonvulsants have been largely unhelpful.

Segmental spinal myoclonus

Segmental spinal myoclonus is often symptomatic of an underlying structural lesion, such as an intrinsic or extrinsic

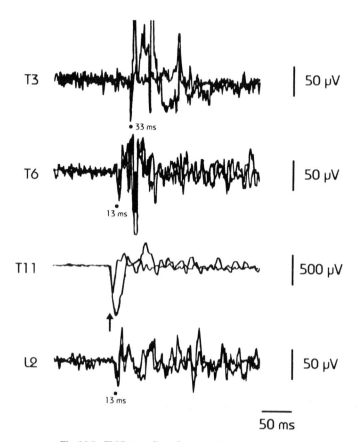

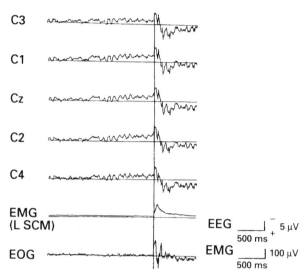

Fig. 36.4. Records from a patient with psychogenic myoclonus. EEG activity has been realigned to the onset of the jerk recorded in left sternocleidomastoid (L SCM) and then averaged to give the 'backaveraged EEG'. This shows a slow negative wave (the Bereitschaftspotential) starting 1.3 seconds before the EMG onset. Compare this wave to the brief, giant wave, which precedes cortial myoclonus by 20 or so milliseconds in Fig. 36.1. (Reprinted from Terada et al., 1995, with permission.)

Fig. 36.3. EMG recordings from erector spinae at various vertebral levels from the second lumbar vertebra (L2) to the third thoracic vertebra (T3) in a patient with stimulus-sensitive propriospinal myoclonus. Two recordings are superimposed. Jerks were elicited by tapping the electrode overlying T11 (arrowed). Latencies are given with respect to the stimulus artefact at T11. Propagation occurs away from the lower thoracic level. (Reprinted from Schulze-Bonhage et al., 1996, with permission.)

malignancy or syringomyelia, or of viral or paraneoplastic myelitis (Brown, 1994). It is confined to one or a few contiguous myotomes, and is most often rhythmic, the frequency of the jerks varying between 1 and 2 per minute to 240 per minute. EMG bursts may be up to 1000 ms in duration. Clues to a spinal origin are the independence from supraspinal influences and persistence of myoclonus in sleep. The condition may or may not be stimulus sensitive.

Segmental spinal myoclonus is believed to result from the isolation of spinal motoneurones from inhibitory influences or from direct cellular injury. Treatment is that of the underlying cause, where this is possible. Symptomatic treatment is only moderately effective. Clonazepam is the drug of first choice and, in dosages of up to 6 mg daily, may diminish or abolish myoclonus.

Diazepam, carbamazepine and tetrabenazine have been useful in occasional cases.

Psychogenic myoclonus

Clinical features suggestive, but not diagnostic, of a psychogenic origin are the sudden onset of an inconsistent and variable movement disorder, which does not overly trouble the subject. Additional clues are the lessening of movements when distracted and, conversely, a dramatic increase in severity and complexity of movements during direct observation, settling again when no longer under direct observation. The absence of signs of organic neurological disease and the unusual nature of the movements are also suggestive, but not necessarily diagnostic of a psychogenic etiology. More convincing is the disappearance of the movement disorder when supposedly unobserved or following suggestion and placebo. The typical indicators of a conversion disorder, such as psychological precipitants, multiple somatizations and secondary gain may or may not be present.

The electrophysiological pattern of psychogenic jerks is indistinguishable from that of voluntary movements. In particular, EMG burst duration is almost always longer than 70ms (unlike cortical myoclonus) and may involve a triphasic activation of agonist and antagonist muscles. The pattern of recruitment of muscles with different segmental origins is variable, and the latencies of reflex jerks are long. In patients with spontaneous jerks good electrophysiological evidence in favour of psychogenic myoclonus is the presence of a slow negative wave (Terada et al., 1995), the Bereitschaftspotential, in the EEG backaveraged from the jerks (Fig. 36.4).

References

Bhatia, K.P., Brown, P., Gregory, R. et al. (1995). Progressive myoclonic ataxia associated with coeliac disease: the myoclonus is of cortical origin, but the pathology is in the cerebellum. *Brain*, 118, 1087–93.

Brown, P.(1994). Spinal myoclonus. In *Movement Disorders 3*, ed. C.D. Marsden & S. Fahn, pp. 459–76. London: Butterworth.

Brown, P., Thompson, P.D., Rothwell, J.C. et al. (1991a). Axial myoclonus of propriospinal origin. *Brain*, 114, 197–214.

Brown, P., Rothwell, J.C., Thompson, P.D. et al. (1991b). The hyperekplexias and their relationship to the normal startle reflex. *Brain*, 114, 1903–28.

Brown, P., Ridding, M.C., Werhahn, K.J., Rothwell, J.C. & Marsden, C.D. (1996). Abnormalities of the balance between inhibition and excitation in the motor cortex of patients with cortical myoclonus. *Brain*, 119, 309–18.

Chauvel, P., Trottier, S., Vignal, J.P. & Bancaud, J. (1992). Somatomotor seizures of frontal lobe origin. *Adv. Neurolol.*, 57, 185–232.

Hallet, M., Chadwick, D., Adam, J. et al. (1977). Reticular reflex myoclonus: a physiological type of human post-hypoxic myoclonus. *J. Neurol., Neurosurg. Psychiatry*, 40, 253–64.

Lance, J.W. & Adams, R.D. (1963). The syndrome of intention or action myoclonus as a sequel to hypoxic encephalopathy. *Brain*, 86, 111–36.

Mahloudji, M. & Pikeilny, R.T. (1967). Hereditary essential myoclonus. *Brain*, 90, 669–74.

Matsumoto, J., Fuhr, P., Nigro, M. & Hallett, M. (1992). Physiological abnormalities in hereditary hyperekplexia. *Ann. Neurol.*, 32, 41–50.

Obeso, J.A., Artieda, J., Rothwell, J.C. et al. (1988). The treatment of severe action myoclonus. *Brain*, 112, 765–77.

Quinn, N.P. (1996). Essential myoclonus and myoclonic dystonia. *Mov. Disord.*, 11, 119–24.

Schulz-Bonhage, A., Knott, H. & Ferbert, A. (1996). Pure stimulus-sensitive truncal myoclonus of propriospinal origin. *Mov. Disord.*, 11, 87–90.

Shiang, R., Ryan, S.G., Zhu, Y., Hahn, A.F., O'Connell, P. & Wasmuth, J.J. (1993). Mutations in the alpha$_1$ subunit of the inhibitory glycine receptor cause the dominant neurologic disorder, hyperekplexia. *Nat. Genet.*, 5, 351–7.

Terada, K., Ikeda, A., Van Ness, P.C. et al. (1995). Presence of Bereitschaftspotential preceding psychogenic myoclonus: clinical application of jerk-locked averaging. *J. Neurol., Neurosurg. Psychiatry*, 58, 745–7.

Werhahn, K.J., Brown, P., Thompson, P.D. & Marsden, C.D. (1997). The clinical features and prognosis of chronic post-hypoxic myoclonus. *Mov. Disord.*, 12, 216–20.

37

Dystonia

Barbara Illowsky Karp, Susanne Goldstein and Mark Hallett

Office of the Clinical Director and Human Motor Control Section NINDS, NIH, Bethesda, Maryland, USA

Dystonia is a movement disorder characterized by sustained involuntary muscle contraction causing abnormal twisting, repetitive movements or posturing that tend to have a directional predominance. Descriptions of dystonic patients, who were often believed to be hysterical, first appeared at the beginning of the twentieth century (Zeman & Dyken, 1968). In 1908, Schwalbe ascertained the hereditary nature of the illness and its variable expression (Schwalbe, 1908). The term 'dystonia musculorum deformans' was first used by Oppenheim (1911), while Mendel and Flateau, emphasizing the twisted posture, called the disease 'torsion dystonia' or 'torsion spasm' (Flateau & Sterling, 1911; Zeman & Dyken, 1968).

After a period of relative inattention, interest in dystonia revived in the 1970s with a fuller delineation of the symptomatology allowing the recognition of focal forms. More recent technological developments have culminated in the identification of genetic mutations underlying generalized torsion dystonia, dopa-responsive dystonia, and some focal dystonias. New therapies have been developed including botulinum toxin injections, stereotactic surgery, and deep brain stimulation.

Classification

Dystonia can be classified by etiology, by the body area involved, and by the age of onset. The division by etiology into primary (idiopathic) and secondary (symptomatic) dystonia provides a schema for evaluating the patient. The classification by affected region is especially useful for the primary dystonias, where the epidemiology, prognosis, treatment and genetics differ by dystonia type. Classifying dystonia by age of onset is also most applicable to primary dystonia, where it serves to separate idio-

pathic generalized torsion dystonia of childhood onset from the focal dystonias which typically present in adulthood.

A classification suggested by Fahn et al., divides dystonias into primary dystonia, 'dystonia-plus' syndromes in which dystonia combines with other neurological symptomatology, secondary dystonia where an underlying pathological process causing dystonia can be identified, and heredofamilial dystonia in which there is an underlying neurodegenerative disorder (Fahn et al., 1998).

Signs and symptoms

Idiopathic dystonia often first manifests as a feeling of discomfort or stiffness in the affected body part. Abnormal movement ensues and initially may only be apparent when performing specific acts, interfering with smooth and accurate performance. As it progresses, dystonia occurs with other voluntary movements and may eventually be present even at rest. Dystonic muscles may hypertrophy; fixed contractures and deformity occur in severe cases. Dystonia disappears during sleep. Prolonged muscle spasm can lead to aching, but severe pain is generally absent except in cervical dystonia.

Dystonia may be the sole movement disorder present or it may be accompanied by postural or action tremor (Cohen et al., 1987; Jedynak et al., 1991; Lou & Jankovic, 1991; Dubinsky et al., 1993). As shown in the Fig. 37.1, some patients have 'gestes antagonistes' or tricks whereby a simple touch or movement temporarily relieves the dystonia. Primary sensory function assessed by routine neurologic examination, strength, muscle tone, and reflexes are normal in idiopathic dystonia. The presence of such neurologic signs should therefore suggest another diagnosis.

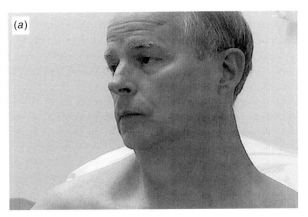 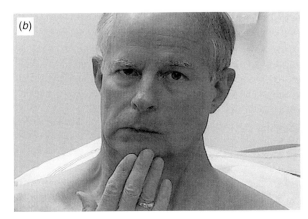

Fig 37.1. (*a*) Resting position of the head in a patient with torticollis. (*b*) Resting position of the head during the geste antagoniste. A light touch to the chin allows the head to return to a forward position.

Primary dystonias

The generalized dystonias include idiopathic torsion dystonia (formerly called 'dystonia musculorum deformans') and 'dystonia-plus' syndromes such as dopa-responsive dystonia, paroxysmal choreoathetosis/dystonia, rapid onset dystonia/parkinsonism and myoclonic dystonia.

Idiopathic generalized torsion dystonia (early-onset torsion dystonia) typically presents between ages 6 and 12, almost always before age 24 (Marsden & Harrison, 1974; Bressman et al., 2000). The first sign in many patients is limb involvement (Bressman et al., 2000), such as gait impairment due to foot flexion and inversion. When dystonia presents with early onset and limb involvement, it is especially likely to progress and become generalized, but affects the cranial muscles in only 11% of patients. Symptoms usually stabilize after 5–10 years. While patients often become wheelchair bound, lifespan is nearly normal. Remissions lasting hours to years occur in up to 20% of patients.

Early-onset generalized torsion dystonia is most frequently an autosomal dominant disease with a reduced penetrance. In the most common form, DYT1, the clinical expression is highly variable and members of the same family may have focal rather than generalized symptoms. The gene underlying this disorder has been identified and will be discussed below.

Dopa-responsive dystonia (DRD) is a less common form of generalized dystonia characterized by childhood-onset, diurnal variation and exquisite sensitivity to low doses of l-dopa (Segawa et al., 1976; Nygaard et al., 1990). In this disorder, dystonic symptoms progressively worsen during the day and improve with sleep. The presence of spasticity and mild hyperreflexia in some patients may lead to the mistaken diagnosis of cerebral palsy. Parkinsonism may develop later in the course. Genetic mutations underlying both autosomal dominant and autosomal recessive forms of DRD have been identified and will be discussed below.

In paroxysmal dystonic choreoathetosis (PDC), attacks of generalized dystonia sometimes accompanied by choreoathetosis begin in infancy or childhood. In kinesigenic dyskinesia, brief attacks follow exercise or movement. In the rarer non-kinesigenic PDC, episodes are precipitated by alcohol, stress or caffeine and last minutes to hours (Bhatia, 1999). Patients are asymptomatic between attacks.

Myoclonic dystonia is an autosomal dominant disease with myoclonus and dystonia beginning in adolescence (Quinn et al., 1988; Klein et al., 1999). Both symptoms may respond dramatically to alcohol ingestion. Unlike early-onset idiopathic generalized torsion dystonia, it typically spares the legs.

Focal dystonias

Focal dystonias are named by the predominant site of involvement. The extent to which the various forms of focal dystonia share genetic or physiological underpinnings is unknown. Focal dystonia can be the presenting feature of generalized dystonia, but especially in later-onset cases, tends to remain focal.

Cervical dystonia (spasmodic torticollis) is the most common focal dystonia with approximately 9 cases/100 000 population (Nutt et al., 1988). Women are more often affected than men and the usual age of onset is 40–60 years (Jankovic et al., 1991). Cervical dystonia is named by the direction of head movement. The most common pattern is torticollis, where the head turns to one side due in part to overactivity of the opposite sternocleidomastoid muscle. In retrocollis, the head tilts backward due to over-contraction of neck extensors such as splenius capitus. In anterocollis the neck is flexed due to hyperactivity of the anterior scalenes and sternocleidomastoids. Laterocollis, head tilt, and other patterns are less common. Cervical dystonia is often accompanied by tremor and shoulder elevation. Unlike other focal dystonias, cervical dystonia is often painful.

Patients with blepharospasm often first complain of uncomfortable sensations in or around the eyes. Bilateral involuntary eye closure ensues leading to visual impairment, and, at worst, functional blindness. In Meige syndrome, blepharospasm combines with oromandibular dystonia where the abnormal movements encompass the jaw, face, and neck.

Dystonia of the vocal cords is called spasmodic dysphonia. The most common form is adductor spasm, in which dystonia of the thyroarytenoid muscles produces a hoarse, choked voice. The less common abductor spasm is due largely to cricoarytenoid dystonia and leads to an intermittent soft, whispery voice.

Focal hand dystonia often arises in those whose work entails repetitive small hand movements or following a period of particularly excessive hand use. The initial sign may be a feeling of tightness or stiffness in the affected limb. As the dystonia develops, abnormal hand posture may become apparent accompanied by loss of speed, impaired movement fluency, and inaccurate motor control. At its onset, limb dystonia may be task-specific, i.e. present only during a particular action such as writing or playing a musical instrument. Other movements, even those utilizing the same muscles, can be performed normally. In some patients, the dystonia progresses to include other activities and at times, may become obvious even at rest. When limb dystonia involves the contiguous proximal limb girdle musculature, it is called segmental dystonia.

Hemidystonia, in which only half of the body is affected, is often secondary to structural brain damage (Marsden et al., 1985).

Secondary dystonia

Dystonia can be part of the symptomatology of a wide range of metabolic and degenerative diseases, can accompany or follow brain damage, or be caused by medications (Table 37.1). When identifiable brain lesions are present in patients with symptomatic dystonia, the basal ganglia, especially the putamen, are likely to be involved (Marsden et al., 1985; Bhatia & Marsden, 1994; Kostic et al., 1996;

Table 37.1. Dystonia in association with other disorders and causes of secondary dystonia

Degenerative and metabolic diseases
Parkinson's disease
Parkinsonian syndromes
Lubag
Machado-Joseph
Corticobasalganglionic degeneration
Dentato-rubro-pallido-luysian atrophy
Huntington's disease
Hallervorden Spatz disease
Wilson's disease
Gangliosidoses
Lipidoses
Amino acidurias
Leigh's disease

Injury or toxicity
Perinatal birth injury/ cerebral palsy
Head trauma
Peripheral trauma
Cervical cord injury
Post-encephalitis
Post-hypoxia
Poisoning (manganese, cyanide, methanol, carbon monoxide)
Pontine and extrapontine myelinolysis
Brain tumour
Multiple Sclerosis
Psychogenic
Medications
Neuroleptics,
Anticonvulsants
Antidepressants
L-dopa

Lehericy et al., 1996). Conversely, dystonia is the most common movement disorder associated with basal ganglia damage (Bhatia & Marsden, 1994). Dystonia can occasionally arise from damage in the thalamus, subthalamic area, brainstem, or with posterior fossa or cervical lesions (Jankovic & Patel, 1983; Lee & Marsden, 1994; Cammarota et al., 1995; Jho & Janetta, 1995; Krauss et al., 1997).

Dystonia is part of the symptomatology of several known basal ganglia diseases. It is seen with Parkinson's disease and other parkinsonian and degenerative disorders such as X-linked dystonia/parkinsonism (Lubag), rapid-onset dystonia–parkinsonism, and corticobasal ganglionic degeneration. In Wilson's disease, dystonia may arise before tremor or cerebellar signs. Neuroleptic medications are a common cause of both acute dystonic reactions and tardive dystonia, especially in the psychiatric population.

Table 37.2. Genetics of dystonia

Genotype	Location	Mutation	Phenotype
DYT1	9q34	GAG deletion in Torsin A	Early-onset generalized dystonia
DYT2	Unknown	Unknown	Autosomal recessive dystonia in Gypsies(Gimenez-Roldan et al., 1988)
DYT3	Xq13.1	Unknown	X-linked dystonia/parkinsonism (Lubag)
DYT4	Unknown	Unknown	Hereditary whispering dystonia in an Australian family (Parker, 1985)
DYT5	14q22.1-22.2	GTP cyclohydrolase I	Dopa-responsive dystonia-autosomal dominant
	11p15.5	Tyrosine hydroxylase	Dopa-responsive dystonia-autosomal recessive
DYT6	8p21-q22	Unknown	Phenotype intermediate to early- and late-onset dystonia in Mennonites
DYT7	18p	Unknown	Adult-onset torticollis and spasmodic dysphonia
DYT8	2q33-35	?channelopathy	Paroxysmal non-kinesigenic dystonic choreoathetosis
DYT9	1p	Unknown	Paroxysmal choreoathetosis with episodic ataxia
DYT10	16p11.2-q12.1	Unknown	Paroxysmal kinesigenic dystonic choreoathetosis
DYT11	11q23	Dopamine receptor D2	Myoclonic dystonia
DYT12	19q13	Unknown	Rapid onset dystonia-parkinsonism

Post-hemiplegic dystonia follows ischemic brain damage or trauma and is probably due to aberrant cerebral reorganization. Extrapontine myelinolysis, a neurologic disorder caused by rapid correction of hyponatremia, frequently affects the basal ganglia and dystonia often develops weeks to months after the initial brain insult (Wu & Lu, 1992; Seiser et al., 1998).

Dystonia, especially hemidystonia, can follow head trauma with a latency of months to years (Krauss et al., 1992, 1996). The contralateral basal ganglia and thalamus are the most frequent lesion sites in post-traumatic dystonia (Lee et al., 1994).

There is also an association between peripheral trauma and the development of dystonia (Schott, 1985; Jankovic & Van Der Linden, 1988). Bhatia et al. reported a history of trauma to the dystonic body part within 3 months preceding the onset of dystonia in 39% of patients with primary axial dystonia (Bhatia et al., 1997). Similarly, peripheral trauma appeared to trigger the onset in up to 20% of cases with idiopathic generalized torsion dystonia reported by Fletcher et al. (1991). Tarsy identified differences in cervical dystonia developing immediately after trauma from that developing later and from idiopathic torticollis (Tarsy, 1998). Acute onset torticollis reached maximal intensity within days of the injury, had a more fixed posture, no relief with sensory tricks, and poorer response to botulinum toxin injection.

Dental procedures and facial trauma can trigger oromandibular dystonia, even in areas of the face and oropharynx not directly traumatized. These patients often have pain and dysesthesia as well as dystonia (Sankhla et al., 1998; Schrag et al., 1999).

Dystonia is no longer considered a hysterical disorder, but can be psychogenic in some patients. Psychogenic dystonia should be suspected when there is no identified underlying cause, abrupt onset, rapid progression to fixed posture, prominent pain, other psychogenic neurologic signs, and multiple somatizations (Lang, 1995).

Secondary dystonias can be recognized by the clinical setting and by the presence of neurological signs other than dystonia. Evaluation for treatable form of dystonia, such as Wilson's disease, should be undertaken in all patients in whom an etiology is not apparent.

Epidemiology

Nutt et al. (1988) found a prevalence of generalized dystonia of 3.4/100000 and focal dystonia of 29.5/100000 in Rochester, Minnesota in 1980. The European Dystonia Study Group found that, except for writer's cramp, segmental and focal dystonias are more common in women, but that men tend to have an earlier age of onset (Epidemiologic Study of Dystonia in Europe Collaborative Group, 1999).

Genetics

Table 37.2 summarizes the identified dystonia genes.

Idiopathic torsion dystonia

Early-onset idiopathic torsion dystonia is most often an autosomal dominant disorder with 30–40% penetrance.

Ozelius et al., first reported the localization of the gene (DYT1) for this disorder to chromosome 9q34 in 1989 (Ozelius et al., 1989). In 1997, the same group identified the gene itself (Ozelius et al., 1997). Early-onset torsion dystonia is caused by a GAG deletion in the DYT1 gene resulting in the loss of a glutamine residue from a conserved region of an ATP binding protein, Torsin A. Although the function of Torsin A is not known, it is structurally related to heat shock proteins. Torsin A is expressed in the substantia nigra pars compacta, the major source of dopaminergic neurons projecting to the basal ganglia (Augood et al., 1999).

The DYT1 mutation is present in 2.7/100 000 Ashkenazi Jews but only in 0.5/100 000 of the general population. Early-onset idiopathic torsion dystonia in Ashkenazi Jews appears to have arisen from a single founder mutation (Risch et al., 1995). The GAG deletion in the Torsin A gene is responsible for 60–75% of cases of early-onset idiopathic dystonia. The DYT1 mutation can be associated with atypical phenotypes in different members of the same family, such as postural hand tremor or stuttering (Slominsky et al., 1999).

Less is known about the genetics of adult-onset idiopathic dystonias. Up to 25% of patients with focal dystonias have other affected family members and these disorders may also be autosomal dominant with incomplete penetrance and variable phenotypic expression (Waddy et al., 1991; Stojanovic et al., 1995; Leube et al., 1997). The DYT1 mutation is not involved (Valente et al., 1998). There is similarly no evidence that the DYT1 founder mutation plays a role in the development of secondary dystonia (Bressman et al., 1997).

Dopa-responsive dystonia

Dopa-responsive dystonia (DRD) can be an autosomal dominant or recessive disorder. Autosomal dominant DRD is caused by mutations on chromosome 14q22.1–22.2 in the gene for the tetrahydrobiopterin (BH4) biosynthetic enzyme, GTP cyclohydrolase I (GCH1). BH4 is a required cofactor for tyrosine hydroxylase, the first enzyme in the synthesis of dopamine from tyrosine. These patients therefore have low basal ganglia neopterin and biopterin levels. Putaminal tyrosine hydroxylase levels may also be low (Furukawa & Kish, 1999; Furukawa et al., 1999; Ichinose & Nagatsu, 1999). More than 30 mutations have been reported in the GCH1 gene, but the specific mutation does not predict the clinical picture. As with idiopathic early-onset dystonia, there is marked phenotypic variation even in the same family. Mutations in the tyrosine hydroxylase gene itself have been found in patients with autosomal recessive DRD (Nygaard et al., 1990; Ichinose & Nagatsu, 1999).

Other dystonias

Almasy et al. (1997) identified DYT 6 in the pericentromeric region of chromosome 8 in 2 Mennonite families with a phenotype intermediate to that of early and late-onset dystonia. Leube et al. (1996) identified DYT7 on chromosome 18p in a single pedigree from northwest Germany with adult-onset spasmodic torticollis and spasmodic dysphonia.

Autosomal dominant paroxysmal non-kinesigenic dystonic choreoathetosis has been mapped to chromosome 2q31–36 and, similar to other paroxysmal movement disorders, may be a channelopathy (Fink et al., 1997; Jarman et al., 1997; Matsuo et al., 1999). Paroxysmal kinesigenic dystonic choreoathetosis appears to localize to chromosome 16 (Bennett et al., 2000). Myoclonic dystonia is associated with a mutation in the dopamine D2 receptor on chromosome 11 (Klein et al., 1999). The area of the X-chromosome linked to the DYT3 gene associated with X-linked dystonia/parkinsonism is being narrowed (Nemeth et al., 1999). Rapid onset dystonia-parkinsonism is a rare autosomal dominant disease in which dystonia and parkinsonism evolve over hours or days. This disorder has been linked to chromosome 19q13 (Brashear et al., 1998; Kramer et al., 1999). Despite the progress made to date, idiopathic dystonias appear to have wide genetic heterogeneity and the presently identified genes cannot account for most cases (Jarman et al., 1999).

Pathology

While isolated cases of neuronal loss and gliosis have been reported (Zeman & Dyken, 1968; Zweig et al., 1988), routine pathological examination is generally unrevealing in idiopathic dystonia (Zeman, 1970; Hornykiewicz et al., 1986; Gibb et al., 1988; Furukawa et al., 2000). X-linked dystonia–parkinsonism, however, has been associated with a mosaic pattern of striatal gliosis (Altrocchi & Forno, 1983; Gibb et al., 1992; Waters et al., 1993), and hypopigmentation of dopaminergic cells in the substantia nigra may be seen in dopa-responsive dystonia (Rajput et al., 1994).

Becker et al. (1999) recently reported increased copper and a trend towards increased manganese in the globus pallidus and putamen in idiopathic adult-onset dystonia. These changes in metal deposition may explain the increased basal ganglia echogenicity on transcranial sonography in patients with idiopathic dystonia reported by Naumann and Becker (Naumann et al., 1996; Becker et al., 1997). Naumann et al. (1998c) failed to find changes in *N*-acetyl aspartate/creatine-lactate/creatine ratio in focal hand dystonia, suggesting no neuronal loss or change in aerobic metabolism.

Neurochemistry

Although a unifying neurochemical abnormality has not been identified in dystonia, dopamine is likely to be involved. Dystonia is part of the symptomatology of other disorders with dopaminergic dysfunction such as Parkinson's disease, myoclonus-dystonia, dopa-responsive dystonia, rapid-onset dystonia parkinsonism, and X-linked dystonia–parkinsonism. Dystonia also arises with l-dopa treatment in Parkinson's disease patients. Neuroleptic medications, which are dopamine antagonists, can cause both acute and tardive dystonia.

Direct measurement of neurotransmitters and their metabolites in cerebrospinal fluid (CSF) or pathological specimens have given inconsistent results. Low CSF levels of homovanillic acid (HVA), the major metabolite of dopamine, have been found in isolated cases of idiopathic dystonia (Tabaddor et al., 1978; Ashizawa et al., 1980), but are usually normal (Marsden & Harrison, 1974). CSF HVA is low in dopa-responsive dystonia, and rapid-onset dystonia–parkinsonism (Nygaard et al., 1990; Brashear et al., 1998). Hornykeiwicz also found decreased striatal dopamine in a single patient with idiopathic dystonia (Hornykiewicz et al., 1986). In contrast, striatal dopamine and HVA concentrations were normal in a single patient with the DYT1 mutation reported by Furukawa et al. (2000).

In vivo positron emission tomography (PET) and single photon emission tomography (SPECT) studies have similarly given inconsistent results. Kishore et al., found elevated D2 receptor binding in the striatum in both patients and asymptomatic gene carriers of dopa-responsive dystonia (Kischore, 1998), and Leenders et al. (1993) found increased striatal uptake of C11-methyl-spiperone contralateral to dystonia in 6 focal dystonia patients. Perlmutter et al. (1997a), however, found decreased F18-spiperone binding in the putamen in idiopathic blepharospasm and oromandibular dystonia, and Naumann et al. (1998a) found decreased D2 receptor binding in the striatum of patients with torticollis. In the same study, Naumann found normal presynaptic tracer uptake; however, Playford et al. (1993) reported decreased F18-dopa uptake in the putamen in idiopathic

dystonia. Vidailhet et al. (1999) found decreased F-dopa uptake in the striatum of patients with dystonia secondary to midbrain strokes that paralleled the severity of the dystonia.

Animal studies have also implicated dopamine. In MPTP-poisoned animals, dystonia appears before the onset of parkinsonian symptoms. In these animals, Perlmutter et al. (1997b) found that the dystonic phase was associated with a 98% decrease in dopamine in the ipsilateral caudate and putamen and decreased D2 receptor number bilaterally, which increased as the dystonia improved. In the spontaneously dystonic hamster, D1 and D2 binding are decreased in the dorsomedial striatum as well as in limbic structures (Nobrega et al., 1999).

Although the strongest evidence is for dopaminergic dysfunction, other neurotransmitters may be involved. Jankovic and Patel (1983) and Hornykiewicz et al. (1986) found abnormalities of several neurotransmitters, especially norepinephrine, in patients with idiopathic dystonia. The dystonic dt rat has more marked changes in norepinephrine than dopamine (Richter & Loscher, 1998). The response of some dystonia patients to anticholinergic medications raises the possibility of an abnormality in acetylcholine function or in interactions between dopaminergic and cholinergic pathways.

Both decreased activity in the D2-mediated indirect pathway (Perlmutter et al., 1997a; Todd & Perlmutter, 1998) and increases in the D1-direct pathway (Eidelberg et al., 1995; Karp et al., 1999) in the basal ganglia have been proposed as underlying dystonia. Either condition would lead to impaired thalamic inhibition by the globus pallidus and thus to excess thalamic stimulation of the cerebral cortex. Rather than being due to an absolute underactivity or overactivity in either pathway, dystonia may arise from an imbalance between the two.

Animal models

There are two animal lines with spontaneously-arising dystonia. The dt rat develops generalized dystonia after a period of normal motor development which worsens with stress and disappears during rest (Richter & Loscher, 1998). Similar to human idiopathic dystonia, cerebral gross and microscopic pathology are normal. Studies in these rats have suggested cerebellar and noradrenergic dysfunction. In the dystonic hamster (dt^{SZ}), dystonia is precipitated by stress and worsened by selective dopamine uptake inhibitors and intrastriatal injection of dopamine agonists (Rehders et al., 2000). During dystonic attacks, dopamine transporter binding is decreased in the nucleus accumbens and ventral tegmental area (Norbrega, 1999).

Dystonia can be induced in otherwise normal animals. Matsumura et al. (1991) showed that local application of bicuculline, a GABA antagonist, onto motor cortex caused disordered movement and changed the EMG pattern from reciprocal activity of antagonist muscles to co-contraction. At the cellular level, there was a loss of cell directionality and conversion of silent cells into active ones (Matsumura et al., 1992). Guehl et al., used bicuculline injections into the ventrolateral (VL) thalamus to produce dystonia (Guehl et al., 2000). In these animals, injections into the rostral VL thalamus caused severe dystonic posturing, difficulty performing a sequential motor task, and, by EMG, prolonged muscle bursts with co-contraction of antagonist muscles. Injection into the caudal VL thalamus led to dystonia with myoclonus. Byl et al. (1996) showed that repetitive hand movements in monkeys could induce a motor dysfunction similar to dystonia associated with enlargement and overlap of somatosensory neuron receptive fields for the fingers in primary sensory cortex (Topp & Byl, 1999). A role for aberrant plasticity in the development of dystonia is also supported by studies in rats, where facial palsy coupled with mild dopamine deficiency induced by unilateral injection of 6–OH-dopamine caused blepharospasm with increased excitability of the blink reflex (Schicatano et al., 1997).

Physiology

Dystonic movements have been studied electromyographically since the mid-twentieth century (Herz, 1944; Tournay & Paillard, 1955). They are characterized by cocontraction of agonist/antagonist muscles with loss of normal alternation, prolonged duration of muscle bursts with superimposed shorter, repeated bursts of activity, lack of selectivity for individual movements, overflow of contraction to muscles not normally activated by the task being performed, and failure of some muscles to activate voluntarily (Cohen & Hallett, 1988; Berardelli et al., 1998). The time needed to switch between components of a voluntary complex motor task is increased (Agostino et al., 1992). Using cross-correlational analysis, Farmer et al. (1998) showed that dystonic cocontraction is distinct from voluntary cocontraction and is due to abnormal presynaptic synchronization of antagonistic motor pools.

Reciprocal inhibition is a process by which activation of a muscle suppresses activity in its antagonist. Deficient reciprocal inhibition, which could result in co-contraction of antagonist muscles, has been demonstrated in patients with generalized dystonia, writer's cramp, spasmodic torticollis, and blepharospasm (Rothwell et al., 1983; Nakashima et al., 1989a; Panizza et al., 1989, 1990; Deuschl

et al., 1992; Chen et al., 1995; Valls-Sole & Hallett, 1995). Deficient inhibition can also be demonstrated in the blink reflex in blepharospasm, generalized dystonia, spasmodic torticollis, and spasmodic dysphonia, in some cases even in the absence of clinical eyelid involvement (Berardelli et al., 1985; Cohen et al., 1989). Similar abnormalities are seen in perioral reflexes (Topka & Hallett, 1992) and exteroceptive silent periods (Nakashima et al., 1989b). Although reduction of spinal cord and brainstem inhibition are present in dystonia, the fundamental physiological disturbance is more likely to be in supraspinal commands.

Several lines of evidence point to dysfunction of the cortical motor system in dystonia. Movement-related cortical potentials with self-paced finger movements in patients with arm dystonia show a diminished amplitude of the NS component, thought to be generated in the motor cortex (van der Kamp et al., 1995; Deutschl, 1995). Changes both in premotor potential peak amplitude and in localization were found by Feve et al. (1994) in more severely affected secondary and idiopathic dystonia patients. Yazawa et al. (1999) found that the premotor potential preceding voluntary wrist relaxation was also decreased in amplitude. The contingent negative variation, an EEG potential generated in a warned, reaction time task, is similarly deficient with head turning in patients with torticollis (Kaji et al., 1995b) and with hand movement in patients with writer's cramp (Ikeda et al., 1996; Hamano et al., 1999). A localized deficiency of event-related desynchronization in the beta frequency range of the EEG before unilateral movement in patients with writer's cramp confirmed a focal abnormality of the contralateral sensorimotor regions (Toro, 1993). These studies demonstrate abnormalities in cerebral preparation for movement in dystonia (Berardelli et al., 1998).

Other evidence of cerebral dysfunction in dystonia comes from cerebral blood flow studies. Ceballos-Baumann et al. (1995) found depressed activity of the caudal SMA and bilateral sensorimotor cortex, with overactivity of the contralateral lateral premotor cortex, cingulate, dorsolateral prefrontal cortex, and lentiform nucleus with self-paced movements and handwriting in patients with dystonia (Ceballos-Baumann et al., 1997). Magyar-Lehmann et al. (1997) found increased glucose metabolism bilaterally in the lentiform nucleus in patients with torticollis. Ibanez et al. (1999) found deficient activation of somatosensory cortex, premotor cortex, cingulate, and SMA during writing and with sustained hand muscle contraction in patients with writer's cramp. Eidelberg et al. (1995) found increased metabolic activity of contralateral lentiform nucleus, pons, and midbrain which was dissociated from thalamic activity and correlated with symptom severity in patients with unilateral dystonia.

Hyperexcitability of motor cortex can be demonstrated by transcranial magnetic stimulation (TMS). Ikoma et al., showed that motor threshold and motor evoked potential (MEP) amplitude were normal; with increases in the level of background contraction, however, there was an abnormal increase in MEP size with increasing stimulus intensity in writer's cramp (Ikoma et al., 1996). They and Byrnes et al. (1998) also found enlarged motor maps for dystonic muscles suggesting cortical reorganization. Hyperexcitability of the motor cortex may arise from deficient intracortical inhibition. Ridding et al. (1995) and Siebner et al. (1999) demonstrated less inhibition of MEPs elicited by dual stimulus and repetitive TMS in patients with focal hand dystonia. Chen et al. (1997) found similar defective inhibition at long interstimulus intervals with sustained background contraction only in the symptomatic hand in writer's cramp. A shortening of the silent period elicited by TMS in dystonia patients also indicated defective inhibition (Ikoma et al., 1996; Chen et al., 1997; Filipovic et al., 1997; Rona et al., 1998; Curra et al., 2000). Taken together, these results suggest relative overactivation of prefrontal motor planning areas and underactivation of inhibitory sensorimotor areas in dystonia (Berardelli et al., 1998).

Although dystonia is a movement disorder, abnormalities of sensory systems may contribute (Hallett, 1995). While the routine sensory examination is normal, subtly abnormal kinesthesia may be present (Grunewald et al., 1997). In some cases, ill-defined abnormal sensations may elicit or accompany dystonic movements, as in patients with blepharospasm who have photophobia or eye irritation (Ghika et al., 1993). Sensory gestes can temporarily relieve dystonia. Aberrant sensory feedback may contribute to the development of dystonia following peripheral trauma. Sensory dysfunction in dystonia may arise at the level of the processing of muscle spindle input. Kaji et al. (1995b) found that vibration induced dystonia in patients with hand cramp, which could be reversed by cutaneous stimulation similar to the sensory geste or by lidocaine block. PET and evoked potential studies have detected abnormal brain responses to somatosensory input in dystonia (Tempel & Perlmutter, 1990; Reilly et al., 1992; Tempel & Perlmutter, 1993; Tinazzi et al., 1999, 2000). Cortical sensory maps for individual fingers may be distorted and temporal discrimination impaired (Bara-Jimenez et al., 1998, 2000). Intracerebral recordings have shown expanded thalamic sensory receptive fields (Lenz et al., 1999).

Basal ganglia dysfunction may underlie the cortical abnormalities. Direct recording from neurons in patients with primary dystonia undergoing neurosurgical procedures have found lowered firing rates, enlarged sensory receptive fields, and irregular discharge patterns in the basal ganglia (Vitek et al., 1998a). Defects in the TMS-elicited silent period have been found in diseases known to involve the basal ganglia, such as Parkinson's disease and Huntington's chorea (Roick et al., 1992; Priori et al., 1994). Bromocriptine can increase intracortical inhibition in normal subjects, demonstrating dopaminergic influences on cortical function (Ziemann et al., 1997).

Although most evidence points to the basal ganglia as the fundamental site of dysfunction in dystonia, abnormalities can also be found the thalamus, an area where sensory and motor functions converge. As noted above, bicuculline injections into the thalamus can produce dystonia (Guehl et al., 2000). Recordings made during thalamic surgery in patients with secondary dystonia show sensory reorganization (Lenz & Byl, 1999; Lenz et al., 1999). Thalamotomy lesions in the Vim or Vop nuclei can treat dystonia in some patients.

Treatment

Since the etiology of dystonia is not yet known, its treatment remains symptomatic. Current therapeutic options include oral medications, chemodenervation, peripheral nerve or muscle surgery, and brain neurosurgical procedures. Often despite optimal management, there are residual dystonic symptoms. Oral medications are most useful in generalized, hemi-, segmental, and severe cervical dystonia. Focal dystonias are often well controlled with botulinum toxin injections. This approach is less successful in the treatment of widespread dystonic symptoms because toxic doses would be required. Surgery is reserved for medication-refractory dystonia. Physical therapy, occupational therapy and alternative treatments can be combined with pharmacotherapy or surgery. The management of secondary dystonias is similar to that of primary dystonias, except where specific treatment is available for an underlying disorder such as Wilson's disease.

Pharmacotherapy

Dopaminergic agents

Although dopamine dysfunction likely plays a role in the etiology of dystonia, neither dopaminergic agonists nor antagonists are generally effective treatments. An important exception is dopa-responsive dystonia (DRD), in which symptoms are well-controlled with low doses of l-dopa. The response of DRD is also remarkable in that it can be sustained for years without the medication side effects common in Parkinson's disease patients. Although DRD usually presents in childhood with lower limb involvement, atypical presentations during adulthood have also been described (Steinberger et al., 1998, 1999). Patients with idiopathic dystonia should therefore have a trial of L-dopa treatment (Bandmann et al., 1998; Jankovic, 1998).

Antidopaminergic medications

While dopamine receptor antagonist medications, such as the conventional neuroleptics may be particularly useful in suppressing tardive dystonia (Kang et al., 1986), they may also benefit patients with idiopathic generalized or focal dystonia (Fahn, 1987; Lang, 1988). Their use, however, is often complicated by significant side effects such as parkinsonism, which may require the concomitant use of anticholinergic drugs. Sedation and depression are also common. More seriously, typical neuroleptics can cause neuroleptic malignant syndrome or permanent tardive dyskinesia. The efficacy of newer neuroleptics, such as risperidone, has not yet been fully evaluated. Clozapine, an atypical neuroleptic agent, is useful in treating tardive dystonia (Trugman et al., 1994; Wolf & Mosnaim, 1994; Adityanjee & Estrera, 1996; Raja et al., 1996) and, in a small open-label trial, also helped patients with idiopathic generalized and focal dystonia (Karp et al., 1999).

Approximately 25% of dystonia patients benefit from dopamine depleting agents such as reserpine or tetrabenazine (Greene et al., 1988; Jankovic & Beach, 1997). These drugs, however, can cause intolerable sedation and depression, limiting their use.

Anticholinergic agents

Although their mechanism of action in treating dystonia is not known, anticholinergic medications are often the most effective oral drugs. Approximately 50% of children and 40% of adults with idiopathic dystonia benefit from trihexiphenidyl, although high doses may be required (Fahn, 1983). The use of anticholinergic medication is limited by side effects, many of which are dose-related. Systemic side effects include blurred vision, dry mouth and constipation. The elderly are particularly susceptible to central side effects such as sedation, confusion and short-term memory loss.

Muscle relaxants and antispasmodics

Clonazepam and other benzodiazepines are rarely adequate to treat dystonia when used as sole agents (Greene et al., 1988), however they are often used as adjunctive therapy. There have been no controlled trials of clonazepam as an antidystonic agent, but some anecdotal evidence supports its efficacy in dystonic tremor (Davis et al., 1995). Side effects of benzodiazepines include sedation, depression, and drug dependence.

Muscle relaxants and antispasmodics such as baclofen or possibly tizanidine may also help patients with severe or generalized dystonia. Similar to benzodiazepines, they are not very effective when used alone, but may contribute to dystonia relief when combined with other medications (Greene et al., 1988). Side effects of oral baclofen and tizanidine include sedation, dizziness, weakness, and fatigue.

Baclofen can also be administered as a continuous intrathecal infusion via an implanted pump, which delivers a high dose directly into the spinal fluid, thereby limiting systemic adverse effects. This approach improves spasticity and there is some evidence of efficacy in dystonia, although higher doses may be required (Penn et al., 1995; Albright et al., 1996; Ford et al., 1996, 1998a; Siebner et al., 1998). Ford et al. (1996) retrospectively reviewed 13 patients undergoing baclofen pump implantation. After a mean of 21 months, 55% patients had continued benefit, but only 27% had sustained improved function. Thirty-eight per cent had severe, treatment-related complications. Penn et al. (1995) tried intrathecal baclofen in five patients who had failed oral baclofen. Three patients with generalized or secondary dystonia had mild or brief improvement, while two with focal leg dystonia had marked improvement. Unfortunately, some patients who initially respond become tolerant to intrathecal baclofen and lose benefit over time. Because pump implantation is associated with significant morbidity, including infection, CSF leaks, baclofen over-infusion, meningitis, lethargy and skin erosion, it should only be undertaken if there is a good response to a test drug infusion before pump insertion and after carefully weighing the risks and benefit (Ford et al., 1998a).

Botulinum toxin

Dr Alan Scott pioneered the use of intramuscular injection of small doses of botulinum toxin to treat strabismus (Scott, 1981). Its success in treating ocular disorders associated with muscular overcontraction led to successful trials in dystonia. Botulinum toxin has become the first line of treatment for focal dystonia.

Botulinum toxin is the most potent biological toxin known. It acts presynaptically, blocking the release of acetylcholine at the neuromuscular junction, thereby chemically denervating the muscle. There are seven distinct botulinum toxin serotypes which cleave SNAP-25, a protein needed for acetylcholine vesicle fusion with the presynaptic membrane, synaptobrevin-2/VAMP, a compo-

Table 37.3. Botulinum toxin serotype sites of action

Serotype	Site of Action
Type A	SNAP-25
Type B	VAMP/ synaptobrevin
Type C	Syntaxin 1A, 1B
Type D	SNAP-25; VAMP/synaptobrevin
Type E	SNAP-25
Type F	VAMP/ synaptobrevin
Type G	VAMP/ synaptobrevin

nent of the synaptic vesicle membrane or syntaxin, a plasma membrane-associated protein (Table 37.3) (Tsui, 1996). Since type A has been the only form commercially available until recently, the discussion below centres on clinical experience with this serotype. Type B toxin, recently marketed, differs in dosage and possibly duration of action and frequency of adverse effects. Although type F has been studied in limited clinical trials, it will not be commercially developed.

During preparation for clinical use, botulinum toxin is precipitated with hemaglutinin and other proteins. The weight of the drug therefore does not correlate well with clinical potency. Botulinum toxin dose is, rather, quantified in terms of the mouse unit (MU) defined as the LD50 for 18–20 gram female Swiss-Webster mice injected intraperitoneally. Extrapolating from data on intramuscular injection in monkeys, the human LD50 is estimated to be 40 MU/kg for type A toxin (Scott & Suzuki, 1988). When used to treat dystonia, benefit from botulinum toxin becomes apparent within 2 weeks, peaks between 2 and 6 weeks, and wears off about 10–12 weeks after injection, although the time course varies widely. Regardless of the response duration, repeated injections are needed to maintain benefit. There are presently two commercially available preparations of botulinum toxin type A, Botox®(Allergan, Inc, USA), and Dysport® (Speywood Pharmaceuticals, England). The doses of these two products are not equivalent. Due to differences in preparation, Botox® is approximately 3–5 times as potent as Dysport® (Tsui, 1996). Botulinum toxin can effectively treat all forms of focal dystonia including blepharospasm (Scott et al., 1985), cervical dystonia (Jankovic & Schwartz, 1990), oromandibular dystonia (Hermanowicz & Truong, 1991), and limb dystonia (Karp et al., 1994), but is less successful if large muscles or many body areas are involved.

Up to 10% of patients receiving the original type A botulinum toxin preparations develop clinical resistance due to the formation of blocking antibodies. The incidence of antibody formation in patients receiving the newer toxin preparations is not yet known. Sensitization is especially likely in patients who receive large doses and frequent injections. Patients who lose response to repeated injections should be tested for the presence of antibodies. The currently available immunoassay has high specificity, but variable sensitivity; a rabbit bioassay correlates better with clinical resistance (Borodic et al., 1996). The absence of weakness following a trial injection into a non-dystonic muscle, such as the frontalis, can also be used to demonstrate loss of toxin efficacy (Hanna & Jankovic, 1998).

There is little immune cross-reactivity between botulinum toxin types. Therefore, in the face of antibody development, patients may be switched to another serotype. Resumption of clinical benefit has been demonstrated in patients with antibodies to type A toxin who are switched to type F or type B (Tsui et al., 1995; Borodic et al., 1996; Chen et al., 1998; Sankhla et al., 1998a). Plasmapharesis was used in a single patient with botulinum toxin resistance to decrease antibody burden (Naumann et al., 1998c). The patient was able to benefit from a subsequent injection. Duane et al. (2000) used mycophenolate, an immunosuppressant, to maintain non-detectable antibody titers and botulinum toxin responsivity in three patients with cervical dystonia and previous loss of response. It is not yet known if either of these latter approaches to botulinum-toxin resistant patients will be practical for long-term management.

The most common side effect of botulinum toxin injections is greater weakness than intended in the injected or contiguous muscles. To help avoid spread, small volume injections into multiple sites are preferable to a single large injection. Weakness is always transient, typically resolving in a matter of weeks. Dysfunction due to excessive weakness depends on the location of injection. For example, injection of the anterior neck muscles may lead to dysphagia. Ptosis and diplopia may result from injections around the eyes. Weakness is rarely a problem with lower limb injections. Although electrophysiological changes in neuromuscular junction function in muscles remote to the injection site can be demonstrated (Girlanda et al., 1992), there are few clinically significant systemic side effects. Transient low-grade fever, malaise, fatigability and flu-like symptoms have been noted (Tsui et al., 1986). Other rare adverse reactions to botulinum toxin include allergic reactions and a Guillain–Barré-like syndrome (Haug et al., 1990; LeWitt & Trosch, 1997). Neuromuscular disorders, such as myasthenia gravis, Eaton–Lambert syndrome, amyotrophic lateral sclerosis and the concomitant use of aminoglycosides are relative contraindications to using botulinum toxin. The safety of botulinum toxin in pregnancy and during nursing has not been evaluated.

Neuroablative drugs

Intramuscular injection of phenol permanently destroys the surrounding peripheral nerve and muscle tissue (Gracies et al., 1997). Although phenol is less expensive than botulinum toxin, its use requires additional precautions. Phenol injection is painful. It can only be used on motor nerves, as destruction of sensory nerves can lead to severe, persistent dysesthesia. Two pilot studies showed benefit in three of five patients with torticollis (Massey, 1995; Garcia Ruiz & Sanchez Bernardos, 2000). Although effects were longer lasting than those of botulinum toxin, repeated phenol injections were sometimes necessary.

Doxorubicin is an antimitotic drug that destroys muscle. Wirtschafter et al., injected this medication to treat 18 patients with blepharospasm (Wirtschafter, 1991; Wirtschafter & McLoon, 1998). Of ten patients able to complete a series of up to ten injections, nine had remission lasting longer than one year. Caution is warranted, however, because of significant adverse effects including skin ulceration, pigmentary changes, urticaria and diplopia.

Local anesthesia

Noting the possible sensory contributions to dystonia discussed above, Kaji et al. (1995b) injected lidocaine at doses that blocked muscle spindle afferents. Thirteen of 15 patients had clinical improvement lasting up to 24 hours. Benefit was prolonged up to 21 days if 10% ethanol was injected at the same time. The utility of oral mexiletine for the treatment of dystonia is currently being explored (Ohara et al., 1997, 1998).

Peripheral surgery

Dystonia surgery is usually reserved for those patients who are refractory to medical management, develop antibodies to botulinum toxin, or desire a more permanent solution.

Several techniques have been employed to treat cervical dystonia, including rhizotomy, peripheral denervation of the spinal accessory nerve, ramisectomy and myectomy (Lang, 1998). An early surgical approach combined anterior cervical rhizotomy with selective resection of the spinal accessory nerve (Hamby & Schiffer, 1969; Gauthier et al., 1988). Hernesniemi et al. reported 23 patients with spasmodic torticollis, 11 of whom underwent SCM myotomy and 12 of whom had cervical rhizotomy (Hernesniemi & Keranen, 1990). Only two of the myotomy patients reported subjective improvement lasting up to 4 years after surgery. The remainder of the patients had poor response. Complications of both procedures were significant, including neck and shoulder weakness, neck instability, pain and dysphagia (Horner et al., 1992; Lang,

1998). Myectomy or myotomy of the trapezius muscle similarly achieved only moderate improvement (Hernesniemi & Keranen, 1990; Krauss et al., 1999).

Peripheral denervation and selective sectioning of the spinal accessory nerve are more successful in treating cervical dystonia, but also entail significant complications including sensory loss or hyperesthesia, weakness of the trapezius, and dysphagia (Bertrand et al., 1987; Bertrand, 1993). Ford et al. (1998b) conducted a retrospective study of selective ramisectomy in botulinum toxin-resistant cervical dystonia patients. One-third of 16 patients had at least moderate benefit, but all except one remained unable to work. Given the limited benefit and the high frequency of adverse effects and dystonia recurrence, such procedures should be reserved for patients with severe, refractory cervical dystonia.

Peripheral nerve surgery, such as carpal tunnel release, is generally not helpful in limb dystonia. Ulnar nerve transposition, however, may benefit the occasional patient whose hand dystonia may be secondary to an occult ulnar neuropathy (Ross et al., 1995; Charness et al., 1996). Tendonotomy or even limb amputation have been performed for severe, disabling limb dystonia (Moberg-Wolff, 1998).

Myectomy of the orbicularis oculi and neurectomy of the facial nerve have been used for blepharospasm. Up to 90% of patients initially have improved visual function with such procedures, but blepharospasm recurrence is common. Forty-six per cent of the patients reported by Chapman et al. (1999) who benefited from myectomy required botulinum toxin injections within 5 years of surgery. Side effects of myectomy include forehead numbness, chronic periorbital lymphedema, keratitis, ptosis, and lid retraction (Lang, 1998).

Sectioning of the recurrent laryngeal nerve benefits many patients with adductor spasmodic dysphonia (Schiratzki & Fritzell, 1988; Fritzell et al., 1993). Symptom recurrence, often attributed to nerve fibre regeneration, is common after surgery, and may require an additional procedure or botulinum toxin injections (Ludlow et al., 1990).

Thalamotomy, pallidotomy and deep brain stimulation

Stereotactic neurosurgery was used to treat dystonia as early as the 1950s. In 1979, Cooper reviewed his 20-year experience with thalamotomy for primary and secondary generalized dystonia (Cooper, 1979). Most patients had bilateral procedures. Seventy per cent had subjective improvement. In the series reported by Andrew et al. (1983), 64% of 55 patients with focal or generalized dystonia improved after thalamotomy, but benefit persisted longer than a year in only 25%. Lesioning the contralateral thalamus was especially helpful in hemidystonia. Bilateral thalamotomy was more successful than unilateral in patients with torticollis. In Tasker's review of 56 patients with lesions in either the ventral intermediate or posterior ventral oral nucleus of the thalamus operated on between 1961 and 1985, 34% of those with secondary dystonia and 32% with primary generalized dystonia had at least 50% improvement in their symptoms (Tasker et al., 1988). Unfortunately, symptoms recurred in most patients following surgery; the longest remission was six years. Thalamotomy complications were frequent and included hemiparesis, numbness, dysarthria and dysphagia. Adverse effects were more common with bilateral procedures. Overall lack of uniformity in technique, target and patient selection led to a wide range of outcomes and the procedures were largely abandoned.

Recent stereotactic advances have led to a revival in neurosurgical approaches to treating dystonia. Surgical targets for dystonia are largely the thalamus and internal globus pallidus (GPi), components of the fronto-basal ganglionic-thalamo-cortical circuit that appears to be involved in the generation of dystonia (Lenz et al., 1998; Vitek, 1998; Vitek et al., 1998a, b).

Initially shown beneficial in Parkinson's disease, pallidotomy has more recently been applied to the treatment of dystonia. Ondo et al. (1998) reported improvement lasting up to 9 months in 8 patients with primary and secondary generalized dystonia. The patients with idiopathic dystonia had greater benefit than those with secondary dystonia. Lozano et al. reported improvement in single cases of patients with idiopathic or symptomatic childhood-onset dystonia with bilateral GPi procedures (Lozano et al., 1997; Lin et al., 1998, 1999; Lai et al., 1999). Complications from pallidotomy including hemiparesis, hemianopsia, dysarthria, dysphagia, cognitive and mood disorders were more common with bilateral procedures.

Ablative techniques such as pallidotomy and thalamotomy leave permanent lesions in the target structure. Many physicians therefore now prefer deep brain stimulation (DBS), which entails the implantation of electrodes in the same brain targets. Activation of the electrodes suppresses neuronal firing. The electrodes are controlled by a stimulator implanted under the skin which can be turned on or off at will. Stimulus parameters can be adjusted to those providing maximal relief of symptoms with minimal adverse effects. If needed, the electrodes and stimulator can be repositioned or removed.

Kumar et al., used bilateral GPi DBS to treat generalized dystonia and found significant improvement that was sustained for at least one year (Kumar et al., 1999). Interestingly,

PET scanning 1 year after surgery showed a decrease in previously hyperactive motor cortex activity. Tronnier et al., reported GPi DBS in three patients with generalized dystonia, two with idiopathic and one with secondary dystonia (Tronnier & Fogel, 2000). Both patients with idiopathic dystonia had marked improvement, while the patient with secondary dystonia had only moderate improvement. Symptomatic dystonia may however also respond to DBS. Loher reported a single patient with post-traumatic hemidystonia who had improvement in dystonic symptoms sustained for at least four years (Loher et al., 2000).

Deep brain stimulation can also target the thalamus. A case study of hemidystonia secondary to a thalamic lesion reported marked benefit from ventroposterolateral nucleus stimulation (Sellal et al., 1993). Benabid et al., however, found only mild improvement with nucleus ventralis intermedius stimulation in two patients with idiopathic dystonia (Benabid et al., 1996).

There is more limited experience with stereotactic procedures for focal dystonia. Individual case reports have shown mixed results in treating limb dystonia and blepharospasm with thalamotomy (Goto et al., 1997; Iacono et al., 1998).

Ancillary therapies

Ancillary non-pharmacological, non-surgical therapies such as physical and occupational therapy help many dystonic patients maintain as much function and mobility as possible. Splints and neck braces in patients with limb or cervical involvement may be helpful. Biofeedback benefited a single patient with writer's cramp reported by O'Neill et al. (1997). Specific large muscle EMG biofeedback eased writing in 10 of 13 writer's cramp patients with proximal muscle involvement reported by Deepak et al. (Deepak & Behari, 1999). Biofeedback, acupuncture, massage and other alternative therapies may increase patient comfort, but their use in dystonia has not been studied systematically. Our patients have had mild relief of dystonia-associated pain, but no sustained benefit from acupuncture. Since these therapies may offer some relief to individual patients and since they can be safely combined with medical or surgical treatment, physicians should consider their use.

Conclusions

Dystonia is a hyperkinetic movement disorder characterized by sustained or tremulous twisting or turning postures. Physiologic and pharmacologic data suggest dopaminergic dysfunction of the basal ganglia and defective cerebral inhibition at several levels. Optimal management takes advantage of oral medications, chemodenervation, and ancillary, non-pharmacologic therapies. Surgery and deep brain stimulation are currently reserved for medically refractory dystonia. As our understanding of the genetic, physiologic, and biochemical bases of dystonia grows, more specific, curative therapies may well become available.

References

Adityanjee & Estrera, A.B. (1996). Successful treatment of tardive dystonia with clozapine. *Biol. Psychiatry*, **39**, 1064–5.

Agostino, R., Berardelli, A., Formica, A., Accornero, N. & Manfredi, M. (1992). Sequential arm movements in patients with Parkinson's disease, Huntington's disease, and dystonia. *Brain*, **115**, 1481–95.

Albright, A.L., Barry, M.J., Fasick, P., Barron, W. & Shultz, B. (1996). Continuous intrathecal baclofen infusion for symptomatic generalized dystonia. *Neurosurgery*, **38**(5), 934–8.

Almasy, L., Bressman, S.B., Raymond, D. et al. (1997). Idiopathic torsion dystonia linked to chromosome 8 in two Mennonite families. *Ann. Neurol.*, **42**, 670–3.

Altrocchi, P.H. & Forno, L.S. (1983). Spontaneous oral–facial dyskinesia: neuropathology of a case. *Neurology*, **33**, 802–5.

Andrew, J., Fowler, C.J. & Harrison, M.J. (1983). Stereotaxic thalamotomy in 55 cases of dystonia. *Brain*, **106**(4), 981–1000.

Ashizawa, T., Patten, B.M. & Jankovic, J. (1980). Meige's syndrome. *South. Med. J.*, **73**(7), 863–6.

Augood, S.J., Martin, D.M., Ozelius, L.J. et al. (1999). Distribution of the mRNAs encoding TorsinA and TorsinB in the normal adult human brain. *Ann. Neurol.*, **46**, 761–9.

Bandmann, O, Marsden, CD & Wood, NW. (1998). Atypical presentations of dopa-responsive dystonia. *Adv. Neurol.*, **78**, 283–90.

Bara-Jimenez, W., Catalan, M.J., Hallett, M. & Gerloff, C. (1998). Abnormal somatosensory homunculus in dystonia of the hand. *Neurology*, **44**, 828–31.

Bara-Jimenez, W., Shelton, P., Sanger, T.D. & Hallett, M. (2000). Sensory discrimination capabilities in patients with focal hand dystonia. *Ann. Neurol.*, **47**(3), 377–80.

Becker, G., Naumann, M., Schubeck, M. et al. (1997). Comparison of transcranial sonography, magnetic resonance imaging and single photon emission computed tomography findings in idiopathic spasmodic torticollis. *Mov. Disord.*, **12**(1), 79–88.

Becker, G., Berg, D., Rausch, W.D. et al. (1999). Increased tissue copper and manganese in the lentiform nucleus in primary adult-onset dystonia. *Ann. Neurol.*, **46**, 260–3.

Benabid, A.L., Pollak, P., Gao, D. et al. (1996). Chronic electrical stimulation of the ventralis intermedius nucleus of the thalamus as a treatment of movement disorders. *J. Neurosurg.*, **84**(2), 203–14.

Bennett, L.B., Roach, E.S. & Bowcock, A.M. (2000). A locus for paroxysmal kinesigenic dyskinesia maps to human chromosome 16. *Neurology*, **54**, 125–30.

Berardelli, A., Rothwell, J.C., Day, B.L. & Marsden, C.D. (1985). Pathophysiology of blepharospasm and oromandibular dystonia. *Brain*, **108**, 593–608.

Berardelli, A., Rothwell, J.C., Hallett, M. et al. (1998). The pathophysiology of primary dystonia. *Brain*, **121**, 1195–212.

Bertrand, C.M. (1993). Selective peripheral denervation for spasmodic torticollis: surgical technique, results, and observations in 260 cases. *Surg. Neurol.*, **40**(2), 96–103.

Bertrand, C., Molina-Negro, P., Bouvier, G. & Gorczyca, W. (1987). Observations and analysis of results in 131 cases of spasmodic torticollis after selective denervation. *Appl. Neurophysiol.*, **50**(1–6), 319–23.

Bhatia, K.P. (1999). The paroxysmal dyskinesias. *J. Neurol.*, **246**, 149–55.

Bhatia, K.P. & Marsden, C.D. (1994). The behavioural and motor consequences of focal lesions of the basal ganglia in man. *Brain*, **117**(4), 859–76.

Bhatia, K.P., Quinn, N.P. & Marsden, C.D. (1997). Clinical features and natural history of axial predominant adult onset primary dystonia. *J. Neurol., Neurosurg. Psychiatry*, **63**, 788–91.

Borodic, G., Johnson, E., Goodnough, M. & Schantz, E. (1996). Botulinum toxin therapy, immunologic resistance, and problems with available materials. *Neurology*, **46**(1), 26–9.

Brashear, A., Butler, I.J., Hyland, K., Farlow, M.R. & Dobyns, W.B. (1998). Cerebrospinal fluid homovanillic acid levels in rapid-onset dystonia–parkinsonism. *Ann. Neurol.*, **43**, 521–6.

Bressman, S.B., de Leon, D., Raymond, D. et al. (1997). Secondary dystonia and the DYT1 gene. *Neurology*, **48**(6), 1571–7.

Bressman, S.B., Sabatti, C., Raymond, D. et al. (2000). The DYT1 phenotype and guidelines for diagnostic testing. *Neurology*, **54**, 1746–52.

Byl, N.N., Merzenich, M.M. & Jenkins, W.M. (1996). A primate genesis model of focal dystonia and repetitive strain injury. *Neurology*, **47**, 508–20.

Byrnes, M.L., Thickbroom, G.W., Wilson, S.A. et al. (1998). The corticomotor representation of upper limb muscles in writer's cramp and changes following botulinum toxin injection. *Brain*, **121**, 977–88.

Cammarota, A., Gershanik, O.S., Garcia, S. & Lera, G. (1995). Cervical dystonia due to spinal cord ependymoma: involvement of cervical cord segments in the pathogenesis of dystonia. *Mov. Disord.*, **10**(4), 500–3.

Ceballos-Baumann, A.O., Passingham, R.E., Warner, T. et al. (1995). Overactive prefrontal and underactive motor cortical areas in idiopathic dystonia. *Ann. Neurol.*, **37**, 363–72.

Ceballos-Baumann, A.O., Sheean, G., Passingham, R.E., Marsden, C.D. & Brooks, D.J. (1997). Botulinum toxin does not reverse the cortical dysfunction associated with writer's cramp. A PET study. *Brain*, **120**, 571–82.

Chapman, K.L., Bartley, G.B., Waller, R.R. & Hodge, D.O. (1999). Follow-up of patients with essential blepharospasm who underwent eyelid protractor myectomy at the Mayo Clinic from 1980 through 1995. *Ophthal. Plast. Reconstr. Surg.*, **15**(2), 106–10.

Charness, M.E., Ross, M.H. & Shefner, J.M. (1996). Ulnar neuropathy and dystonic flexion of the fourth and fifth digits: clinical correlation in musicians. *Muscle Nerve*, **19**(4), 431–7.

Chen, R.S., Tsai, C.H. & Lu, C.S. (1995). Reciprocal inhibition in writer's cramp. *Mov.Disord.*, **10**(5), 556–61.

Chen, R., Wassermann, E.M., Canos, M. & Hallett, M. (1997). Impaired inhibition in writer's cramp during voluntary muscle activation. *Neurology*, **49**, 1054–9.

Chen, R., Karp, B.I. & Hallett, M. (1998). Botulinum toxin type F for treatment of dystonia: long-term experience. *Neurology*, **51**(5), 1494–6.

Cohen, L.G. & Hallett, M. (1988). Hand cramps: clinical features and electromyographic patterns in a focal dystonia. *Neurology*, **38**, 1005–12.

Cohen, L.G., Hallett, M. & Sudarskyt, L. (1987). A single family with writer's cramp, essential tremor, and primary writing tremor. *Mov. Disord.*, **2**(2), 109–16.

Cohen, L.G., Ludlow, C.L., Warden, M. et al. (1989). Blink reflex excitability recovery curves in patients with spasmodic dysphonia. *Neurology*, **39**, 572–7.

Cooper, I.S. (1979). 20-year followup study of the neurosurgical treatment of dystonia musculorum deformans. *Adv. Neurol.*, **14**, 423–52.

Curra, A., Romaniello, A., Berardelli, A., Cruccu, G. & Manfredi, M. (2000). Shortened cortical silent period in facial muscles of patients with cranial dystonia. *Neurology*, **54**, 130–5.

Davis, T.L., Charles, P.D. & Burns, R.S. (1995). Clonazepam-sensitive intermittent dystonic tremor. *South. Med. J.*, **88**(10), 1069–71.

Deepak, K.K. & Behari, M. (1999). Specific muscle EMG biofeedback for hand dystonia. *Appl. Psychophysiol. Biofeedback*, **24**(4), 267–80.

Deuschl, G., Heinen, F., Kleedorfer, B. et al. (1992). Clinical and polymyographic investigation of spasmodic torticollis. *J. Neurol.*, **239**, 9–15.

Deuschl, G, Toro, C, Matsumoto, J. & Hallett, M. (1995). Movement-related cortical potentials in writer's cramp. *Ann. Neurol.*, **38**, 838–8.

Duane, D.D., Monroe, J. & Morris, R.E. (2000). Mycophenolate in the prevention of recurrent neutralizing botulinum toxin A antibodies in cervical dystonia. *Mov. Disord.*, **15**(2), 365–6.

Dubinsky, R.M., Gray, C.S., Koller, W.C. (1993). Essential tremor and dystonia. *Neurology*, **43**: 2382–4.

Eidelberg, D., Moeller, J.R., Ishikawa, T. et al. (1995). The metabolic topography of idiopathic torsion dystonia. *Brain*, **118**, 1473–4.

Epidemiologic Study of Dystonia in Europe Collaborative Group (1999). Sex-related influences on the frequency and age of onset of primary dystonia. *Neurology*, **53**, 1871–3.

Fahn, S. (1983). High dosage anticholinergic therapy in dystonia. *Neurology*, **33**(10), 1255–61.

Fahn, S. (1987). Systemic therapy of dystonia. *Can. J. Neurol. Sci.*, **14**(3 Suppl.), 528–32.

Fahn, S., Bressman, S. & Marsden, C.D. (1998). Classification of dystonia. In *Dystonia 3. Advances in Neurology*, ed. S. Fahn, M. DeLong & C.D. Marsden, pp. 1–10. Philadelphia: Lippincott-Raven.

Farmer, S.F., Sheehan, G.L., Mayston, M.J. et al. (1998). Abnormal motor unit synchronization of antagonist muscles underlies pathological co-contraction in upper limb dystonia. *Brain*, **121**, 801–14.

Feve, A., Bathien, N. & Rondot, P. (1994). Abnormal movement related potentials in patients with lesions of basal ganglia and anterior thalamus. *J. Neurol., Neurosurg. Psychiatry*, **57**, 100–4.

Filipovic, S.R., Ljubisavljevic, M., Svetel, M. et al. (1997). Impairment of cortical inhibition in writer's cramp as revealed by changes in electromyographic silent period after transcranial magnetic stimulation. *Neurosci. Lett.*, **222**, 167–70.

Fink, J.K., Hedera, P., Mathay, J.G. & Albin, R.L. (1997). Paroxysmal dystonic choreoathetosis linked to chromosome 2q: clinical analysis and proposed pathophysiology. *Neurology*, **49**(1), 177–83.

Flateau, E. & Sterling, W. (1911). Progressiver Torsionspasms bei Kindren. *Z. Gasamte Neurol. Psychiatr.*, **7**, 586–612.

Fletcher, N.A., Harding, A.E. & Marsden, C.D. (1991). The relationship between trauma and idiopathic torsion dystonia. *J. Neurol., Neurosurg. Psychiatry*, **54**, 713–17.

Ford, B., Greene, P., Louis, E.D. et al. (1996). Use of intrathecal baclofen in the treatment of patients with dystonia. *Arch. Neurol.*, **53**(12), 1241–6.

Ford, B., Greene, P.E., Louis, E.D. et al. (1998a). Intrathecal baclofen in the treatment of dystonia. *Adv. Neurol.*, **78**, 199–210.

Ford, B., Louis, E.D., Greene, P. & Fahn, S. (1998b). Outcome of selective ramisectomy for botulinum toxin resistant torticollis. *J. Neurol., Neurosurg. Psychiatry*, **65**(4), 472–8.

Fritzell, B., Hammarberg, B., Schiratzki, H. et al. (1993). Long-term results of recurrent laryngeal nerve resection for adductor spasmodic dysphonia. *J. Voice*, **7**(2), 172–8.

Furukawa, Y. & Kish, S.J. (1999). Dopa-responsive dystonia: recent advances and remaining issues to be addressed. *Mov. Disord.*, **14**(5), 709–15.

Furukawa, Y., Nygaard, T.G., Gutlich, M. et al. (1999). Striatal biopterin and tyrosine hydroxylase protein reduction in dopa-responsive dystonia. *Neurology*, **53**, 1032–41.

Furukawa, Y., Hornykiewicz, O., Fahn, S. & Kish, S.J. (2000). Striatal dopamine in early-onset primary torsion dystonia with the DYT1 mutation. *Neurology*, **54**(5), 1193–5.

Garcia Ruiz, P.J. & Sanchez Bernardos, V. (2000). Intramuscular phenol injection for severe cervical dystonia. *J. Neurol.*, **247**(2), 146–7.

Gauthier, S., Perot, P. & Bertrand, G. (1988). Role of surgical anterior rhizotomies in the management of spasmodic torticollis. *Adv. Neurol.*, **50**, 633–5.

Ghika, J., Regli, F. & Growdon, J.H. (1993). Sensory symptoms in cranial dystonia: a potential role in etiology? *J. Neurol. Sci.*, **116**, 142–7.

Gibb, W.R.G., Lees, A.J. & Marsden, C.D. (1988). Pathological report of four patients presenting with cranial dystonias. *Mov. Disord.*, **3**(3), 211–21.

Gibb, W.R.G., Kilford, L. & Marsden, C.D. (1992). Severe generalised dystonia associated with a mosaic pattern of striatal gliosis. *Mov. Disord.*, **7**(3), 217–23.

Gimenez-Roldan, S., Delgado, G., Marin, M., Villanueva, J.A. & Mateo, D. (1988). Hereditary torsion dystonia in Gypsies. *Adv. Neurol.*, **50**, 73–81.

Girlanda, P., Vita, G., Nicolosi, C., Milone, S. & Messina, C. (1992). Botulinum toxin therapy: distant effects on neuromuscular transmission and autonomic nervous system. *J. Neurol., Neurosurg. Psychiatry*, **55**, 844–5.

Goto, S., Tsuiki, H., Soyama, N. et al. (1997). Stereotactic selective Vo-complex thalamotomy in a patient with dystonic writer's cramp. *Neurology*, **49**(4), 1173–4.

Gracies, J.M., Elovic, E., McGuire, J. & Simpson, D.M. (1997). Traditional pharmacological treatments for spasticity. Part I: Local treatments. *Muscle Nerve Suppl.*, **6**(91), S61–91.

Greene, P., Shale, H. & Fahn, S. (1988). Experience with high dosages of anticholinergic and other drugs in the treatment of torsion dystonia. *Adv. Neurol.*, **50**, 547–56.

Grunewald, R.A., Yoneda, Y., Shipman, J.M. & Sagara, H.J. (1997). Idiopathic focal dystonia: a disorder of muscle spindle afferent processing? *Brain*, **120**, 2179–85.

Guehl, D., Burbaud, P., Boraud, T. & Bioulac, B. (2000). Bicuculline injections into the rostral and caudal motor thalamus of the monkey induce different types of dystonia. *Eur. J. Neurosci.*, **12**(3), 1033–7.

Hallett, M. (1995). Is dystonia a sensory disorder?' *Ann. Neurol.*, **38**, 139–40.

Hamano, T., Kaji, R., Katayama, M. et al. (1999). Abnormal contingent negative variation in writer's cramp. *Clin. Neurophysiol.*, **110**(3), 508–15.

Hamby, W.B. & Schiffer, S. (1969). Spasmodic torticollis: results after cervical rhizotomy in 50 cases. *J. Neurosurg.*, **31**(3), 323–6.

Hanna, P.A. & Jankovic, J. (1998). Mouse bioassay versus Western blot assay for botulinum toxin antibodies: correlation with clinical response. *Neurology*, **50**(6), 1624–9.

Haug, B.A., Dressler, D. & Prange, H.W. (1990). Polyradiculoneuritis following botulinum toxin therapy. *J. Neurol.*, **237**, 62–3.

Hermanowicz, N. & Truong, D.D. (1991). Treatment of oromandibular dystonia with botulinum toxin. *Laryngoscope*, **101**(11), 1216–18.

Hernesniemi, J. & Keranen, T. (1990). Long-term outcome after surgery for spasmodic torticollis. *Acta Neurochir.*, **103**(3–4), 128–30.

Herz, E. (1944). Dystonia. 1. Historical review: analysis of dystonic symptoms and physiologic mechanisms involved. *Arch. Neurol. Psychiatry*, **51**(4), 305–18.

Horner, J., Riski, J.E., Ovelmen-Levitt, J. & Nashold, B.S. Jr. (1992). Swallowing in torticollis before and after rhizotomy. *Dysphagia*, **7**(3), 117–25.

Hornykiewicz, O., Kish, S.J., Becker, L.E., Farley, I. & Shannak, K. (1986). Brain neurotransmitters in dystonia musculorum deformans. *N. Engl. J. Med.*, **315**, 347–53.

Iacono, R.P., Kuniyoshi, S.M. & Schoonenberg, T. (1998). Experience with stereotactics for dystonia: case examples. *Adv. Neurol.*, **78**, 221–6.

Ibanez, V., Sadato, N., Karp, B., Dieber, M-P. & Hallett, M. (1999). Deficient activation of the premotor cortical network in patients with writer's cramp. *Neurology*, **53**, 96–105.

Ichinose, H. & Nagatsu, T. (1999). Molecular genetics of Dopa-responsive dystonia. *Adv. Neurol.*, **80**, 195–8.

Ikeda, A., Shibasaki, H., Kaji, R. et al. (1996). Abnormal sensorimotor integration in writer's cramp: study of contingent negative variation. *Mov. Disord.*, **11**, 683–90.

Jankovic, J. (1998). Medical therapy and botulinum toxin in dystonia. *Adv. Neurol.*, **78**, 169–83.

Ikoma, K., Samii, A., Mercuri, B., Wassermann, E.M. & Hallett, M. (1996). Abnormal cortical motor excitability in dystonia. *Neurology*, **46**(5), 1371–6.

Jankovic, J. & Beach, J. (1997). Long-term effects of tetrabenazine in hyperkinetic movement disorders. *Neurology*, **48**(2), 358–62.

Jankovic, J. & Patel, S.C. (1983). Blepharospasm associated with brainstem lesions. *Neurology*, **33**(9), 1237–40.

Jankovic, J. & Schwartz, K. (1990). Botulinum toxin injections for cervical dystonia. *Neurology*, **40**, 277–80.

Jankovic, J. & Van Der Linden, C. (1988). Dystonia and tremor induced by peripheral trauma: predisposing factors. *J.Neurol., Neurosurg. Psychiatry*, **51**, 1512–19.

Jankovic, J., Leder, S., Warner, D. & Schwartz, K. (1991). Cervical dystonia: clinical findings and associated movement disorders. *Neurology*, **41**, 1088–91.

Jarman, P.R., Davis, M.B., Hodgson, S.V., Marsden, C.D. & Wood, N.W. (1997). Paroxysmal dystonic choreoathetosis. Genetic linkage studies in British family. *Brain*, **120**(12), 2125–30.

Jarman, P.R., del Grosso, N., Valente, E.M. et al. (1999). Primary torsion dystonia: the search for genes is not over. *J. Neurol., Neurosurg., Psychiatry*, **67**, 395–7.

Jedynak, C.P., Bonnet, A.M. & Agid, Y. (1991). Tremor and idiopathic dystonia. *Mov. Disord.*, **6**(3), 230–6.

Jho, H.D. & Janetta, P. (1995). Microvascular decompression for spasmodic torticollis. *Acta Neurochir. (Wien)*, **134**(1–2), 21–6.

Kaji, R., Ikeda, A., Ikeda, T. et al. (1995a). Physiological study of cervical dystonia. Task-specific abnormality in contingent negative variation. *Brain*, **118**, 511–22.

Kaji, R., Kohara, N., Katayama, M. et al. (1995b). Muscle afferent block by intramuscular injection of lidocaine for the treatment of writer's cramp. *Muscle Nerve*, **18**, 234–5.

Kang, U.J., Burke, R.E. & Fahn, S. (1986). Natural history and treatment of tardive dystonia. *Mov. Disord.*, **1**(3), 193–208.

Karp, B.I., Cohen, L.G., Cole, R. et al. (1994). Long-term botulinum toxin treatment of focal hand dystonia. *Neurology*, **44**, 70–6.

Karp, B., Goldstein, S.R., Chen, R. et al. (1999). An open trial of clozapine for dystonia. *Mov. Disord.*, **14**(4), 652–7.

Kishore, A, Nygaard, T.G., del la Fuente-Fernandez, R. et al. (1998). Striatal D2 receptors in symptomatic and asymptomatic carriers of dopa-responsive dystonia measured with [^{11}C]-raclopride and positron-emission tomography, *Neurology*, **50**, 1028–32.

Klein, C., Brin, M.F., Kramer, P. et al. (1999). Association of a missense change in the D2 dopamine receptor with myoclonus dystonia. *Proc. Natl. Acad. Sci., USA*, **96**(9), 5173–6.

Kostic, V.S., Stojanovic-Svetel, M. & Kacar, A. (1996). Symptomatic dystonias associated with structural brain lesions: report of 16 cases. *Can. J. Neurol. Sci.*, **23**(1), 53–6.

Kramer, P.L., Mineta, M., Klein, C. et al. (1999). Rapid-onset dystonia-parkinsonism: linkage to chromosome 19q13. *Ann. Neurol.*, **6**, 176–82.

Krauss, J.K., Mohadjer, M., Braus, D.F. et al. (1992). Dystonia following head trauma: a report of nine patients and review of the literature. *Mov. Disord.*, **7**(3), 263–72.

Krauss, J.K., Trankle, R. & Kopp, K.H. (1996). Post-traumatic movement disorders in survivors of severe head injury. *Neurology*, **47**(6), 1488–92.

Krauss, J.K., Seeger, W. & Jankovic, J. (1997). Cervical dystonia associated with tumors of the posterior fossa. *Mov. Disord.*, **12**(3), 443–7.

Krauss, J.K., Koller, R. & Burgunder, J.M. (1999). Partial myotomy/myectomy of the trapezius muscle with an asleep–awake–asleep anesthetic technique for treatment of cervical dystonia. Technical note. *J. Neurosurg.*, **91**(5), 889–91.

Kumar, R., Dagher, A., Hutchison, W.D., Lang, A.E. & Lozano, A.M. (1999). Globus pallidus deep brain stimulation for generalized dystonia: clinical and PET investigation. *Neurology*, **53**(4), 871–4.

Lai, T., Lai, J.M. & Grossman, R.G. (1999). Functional recovery after bilateral pallidotomy for the treatment of early-onset primary generalized dystonia. *Arch. Phys. Med. Rehabil.*, **80**(10), 1340–2.

Lang, A.E. (1988). Dopamine agonists and antagonists in the treatment of idiopathic dystonia. *Adv. Neurol.*, **50**, 561–70.

Lang, A.E. (1995). Psychogenic dystonia: a review of 18 cases. *Can. J. Neurol. Sci.*, **22**(2), 136–43.

Lang, A.E. (1998). Surgical treatment of dystonia. *Adv. Neurol.*, **78**, 185–98.

Lee, M.S. & Marsden, C.D. (1994). Movement disorders following lesions of the thalamus or subthalamic region. *Mov. Disord.*, **9**, 493–507.

Lee, M.S., Rinne, J.O., Ceballos-Baumann, A., Thompson, P.D. & Marsden, C.D. (1994). Dystonia after head trauma. *Neurology*, **44**(8), 1374–8.

Leenders, K., Hartvig, P., Forsgren, L. et al. (1993). Striatal [11C]-*N*-methyl-spiperone binding in patients with focal dystonia (torticollis) using positron emission tomography. *J. Neural. Trans. [P-D Sect.]*, **5**, 79–87.

Lehericy, S., Vidailhet, M., Dormont, D. et al. (1996). Striatopallidal and thalamic dystonia. A magnetic resonance imaging anatomoclinical study. *Arch. Neurol.*, **53**(3), 241–50.

Lenz, F.A. & Byl, N.N. (1999). Reorganization in the cutaneous core of the human thalamic principal somatic sensory nucleus (ventral caudal) in patients with dystonia. *J. Neurophysiol.*, **82**(6), 3204–12.

Lenz, F.A., Suarez, J.I., Metman, L.V. et al. (1998). Pallidal activity during dystonia: somatosensory reorganisation and changes with severity. *Jr. Neurol., Neurosurg. Psychiatry*, **65**(5), 767–70.

Lenz, F.A., Jaeger, C.J., Seike, M.S. et al. (1999). Thalamic single neuron activity in patients with dystonia: dystonia-related activity and somatic sensory reorganization. *J. Neurophysiol.*, **82**(5), 2372–92.

Leube, B., Rudnicki, D., Ratzlaff, T. et al. (1996). Idiopathic torsion dystonia: assignment of a gene to chromosome 18p in a German family with adult onset, autosomal dominant inheritance and purely focal distribution. *Hum. Mol. Genet.*, **5**(10), 1673–7.

Leube, B., Kessler, K.R., Goecke, T., Auburger, G. & Benecke, R. (1997). Frequency of familial inheritance among 488 index patients with idiopathic focal dystonia and clinical variability in a large family. *Mov. Disord.*, **12**(6), 1000–6.

LeWitt, P.A. & Trosch, R.M. (1997). Idiosyncratic adverse reactions to intramuscular botulinum toxin type A injection. *Mov. Disord.*, **12**(6), 1064–7.

Lin, J.J., Lin, S.Z., Lin, G.Y., Chang, D.C. & Lee, C.C. (1998). Application of bilateral sequential pallidotomy to treat a patient with generalized dystonia. *Eur. Neurol.*, **40**(2), 108–10.

Lin, J.J., Lin, G.Y., Shih, C. et al. (1999). Benefit of bilateral pallidotomy in the treatment of generalized dystonia. Case report. *J. Neurosurg.*, **90**(5), 974–6.

Loher, T.J., Hasdemir, M.G., Burgunder, J.M. & Krauss, J.K. (2000). Long-term follow-up study of chronic globus pallidus internus stimulation for posttraumatic hemidystonia. *J. Neurosurg.*, **92**(3), 457–60.

Lou, J.S. & Jankovic, J. (1991). Essential tremor: clinical correlates in 350 patients. *Neurology*, **41**, 234–8.

Lozano, A.M., Kumar, R., Gross, R.E. et al. (1997). Globus pallidus internus pallidotomy for generalized dystonia. *Mov. Disord.*, **12**(6), 865–70.

Ludlow, C.L., Naunton, R.F., Fujita, M. & Sedory, S.E. (1990). Spasmodic dysphonia: botulinum toxin injection after recurrent nerve surgery. *Otolaryngol. Head Neck Surg.*, **102**(2), 122–31.

Magyar-Lehmann, S., Antonini, A., Roelcke, U. et al. (1997). Cerebral glucose metabolism in patients with spasmodic torticollis. *Mov. Disord.*, **12**(5), 704–8.

Marsden, C.D. & Harrison, M.J.G. (1974). Idiopathic torsion dystonia (dystonia musculorum deformans). A review of forty-two patients. *Brain*, **97**, 793–810.

Marsden, C.D., Obeso, J.A., Zarranz, J.J. & Lang, A.E. (1985). The anatomical basis of symptomatic hemidystonia. *Brain*, **108**, 463–83.

Massey, J.M. (1995). Treatment of spasmodic torticollis with intramuscular phenol injection. *J. Neurol., Neurosurg. Psychiatry*, **58**(2), 258–9.

Matsumura, M., Sawaguchi, T., Oishi, T., Ueki, K. & Kubota, K. (1991). Behavioral deficits induced by local injection of bicuculline and muscimol into the primate motor and premotor cortex. *J. Neurophysiol.*, **65**, 1542–53.

Matsumura, M., Sawaguchi, T. & Kubota, K. (1992). GABAergic inhibition of neuronal activity in the primate motor and premotor cortex during voluntary movement. *J. Neurophysiol.*, **68**, 692–702.

Matsuo, H., Kamakura, K., Saito, M. et al. (1999). Familial paroxysmal dystonic choreoathetosis. Clinical findings in a large Japanese family and genetic linkage to 2q. *Arch. Neurol.*, **56**, 721–6.

Moberg-Wolff, E.A. (1998). An aggressive approach to limb dystonia: a case report. *Arch. Phys. Med. Rehabil.*, **79**, 589–90.

Nakashima, K., Rothwell, J., Day, B. et al. (1989a). Reciprocal inhibition between forearm muscles in patients with writer's cramp and other occupational cramps, symptomatic hemidystonia and hemiparesis due to stroke. *Brain*, 112, 681–97.

Nakashima, K., Thompson, P.D., Rothwell, J.C. et al. (1989b). An exteroceptive reflex in the sternocleidomastoid muscle produced by electrical stimulation of the supraorbital nerve in normal subjects and patients with spasmodic torticollis. *Neurology*, 39, 1354–8.

Naumann, M., Becker, G., Toyka, K.V., Supprian, T. & Reiners, K. (1996). Lenticular nucleus lesion in idiopathic dystonia detected by transcranial sonography. *Neurology*, 47, 1284–90.

Naumann, M., Pirker, W., Reiners, K. et al. (1998a). Imaging the pre- and postsynaptic side of striatal dopaminergic synapses in idiopathic cervical dystonia: a SPECT study using 123I epidepride and 123I beta CIT. *Mov. Disord.*, 13(2), 319–23.

Naumann, M., Toyka, K.V., Mansouri Taleghani, B. et al. (1998b). Depletion of neutralising antibodies resensitises a secondary non-responder to botulinum A neurotoxin. *J. Neurol., Neurosurg. Psychiatry*, 65(6), 924–7.

Naumann, M., Warmuth-Metz, M., Hillerer, C., Solymosi, L. & Reiners, K. (1998c). H1 Magnetic resonance spectroscopy of the lentiform nucleus in primary focal hand dystonia. *Mov. Disord.*, 13(6), 929–33.

Nemeth, A.H., Nolte, D., Dunne, E. et al. (1999). Refined linkage disequilibrium and physical mapping of the gene locus for x-linked dystonia-parkinsonism (DYT3). *Genomics*, 60, 320–9.

Nobrega, J.N., Gernert, M., Loscher, W. et al. (1999). Tyrosine hydroxylase immunoreactivity and [H3]win 35, 428 binding to the dopamine transporter in a hamster model of idiopathic paroxysmal dystonia. *Neuroscience*, 92, 211–17.

Nutt, J.G., Muenter, M.D., Aronson, A., Kurland, L.T. & Melton, L.J. (1988). Epidemiology of focal and generalized dystonia in Rochester, Minn. *Mov. Disord.*, 3(3), 188–94.

Nygaard, T., Trugman, J., Yebenes, J. & Fahn, S. (1990). Dopa-responsive dystonia: the spectrum of clinical manifestations in a large North American family. *Neurology*, 40, 66–9.

Ohara, S., Hayashi, R., Momoi, H., Miki, J. & Yanagisawa, N. (1998). Mexiletine in the treatment of spasmodic torticollis. *Mov. Disord.*, 13(6), 934–40.

Ohara, S., Miki, J., Momoi, H. et al. (1997). Treatment of spasmodic torticollis with mexiletine: a case report. *Mov. Disord.*, 12(3), 466–9.

Ondo, W.G., Desaloms, J.M., Jankovic, J. & Grossman, R.G. (1998). Pallidotomy for generalized dystonia. *Mov. Disord.*, 13(4), 693–8.

O'Neill, M.A., Gwinn, K.A., & Adler, C.H. (1997). Biofeedback for writer's cramp. *Am. J. Occup. Ther.*, 51; 605–7.

Oppenheim, H. (1911). Uber eine eigenartige Kramfkrankheit des kindlichen und jugendlichen Alters (Dysbasia lordotica progressiva, Dystonia musculorum deformans). *Neurol. Centrabl.*, 30, 1090–107.

Ozelius, L., Kramer, P.L., Moskowitz, C.B. et al. (1989). Human gene for torsion dystonia located on chromosome 9q32–34. *Neuron*, 2, 1427–34.

Ozelius, L., Hewett, J.W., Page, C.E. et al. (1997). The early onset torsion dystonia gene (DYT1) encodes an ATP-binding protein. *Nat. Genet.*, 17, 40–8.

Panizza, M., Hallett, M. & Nilsson, J. (1989). Reciprocal inhibition in patients with hand cramps. *Neurology*, 39, 85–9.

Panizza, M., Lelli, S., Nilsson, J. & Hallett, M. (1990). H-reflex recovery curve and reciprocal inhibition of H-reflex in different kinds of dystonia. *Neurology*, 40, 824–8.

Parker, N. (1985). Hereditary whispering dysphonia. *J. Neurol., Neurosurg. Psychiatry*, 48(3), 218–24.

Penn, R.D., Gianino, J.M. & York, M.M. (1995). Intrathecal baclofen for motor disorders. *Mov. Disord.*, 10(5), 675–7.

Perlmutter, J.S., Stambuk, M.K., Markham, J. et al. (1997a). Decreased 18F-Spiperone binding in putamen in idiopathic focal dystonia. *J. Neurosci.*, 17(2), 843–50.

Perlmutter, J.S., Tempel, L.W., Black, K.J., Parkinson, D. & Todd, R.D. (1997b). MPTP induces dystonia and parkinsonism. Clues to the pathophysiology of dystonia. *Neurology*, 49(5), 1432–8.

Playford, E.D., Fletcher, N.A., Sawle, G.V., Marsden, C.D. & Brooks, D.J. (1993). Striatal F18-dopa uptake in familial idiopathic dystonia. *Brain*, 116, 1191–9.

Priori, A., Berardelli, A., Inghilleri, M., Accornero, N. & Manfredi, M. (1994). Motor cortical inhibition and the dopaminergic system. Pharmacological changes in the silent period after transcranial brain stimulation in normal subjects, patients with Parkinson's disease and drug-induced parkinsonism. *Brain*, 117, 317–23.

Quinn, N.P., Rothwell, J.C., Thompson, P.D. & Marsden, C.D. (1988). Hereditary myoclonic dystonia, hereditary torsion dystonia and hereditary essential myoclonus: an area of confusion. *Adv. Neurol.*, 50, 391–401.

Raja, M., Maisto, G., Altavista, M.C. & Albanese, A. (1996). Tardive lingual dystonia treated with clozapine. *Mov. Disord.*, 11(5), 585–6.

Rajput, A.H., Gibb, W.R., Zhong, X.H. et al. (1994). Dopa-responsive dystonia: pathological and biochemical observations in a case. *Ann. Neurol.*, 35(4), 396–402.

Rehders, J.H., Loscher, W. & Richter, A. (2000). Evidence for striatal dopaminergic overactivity in paroxysmal dystonia indicated by microinjections in a genetic rodent model. *Neuroscience*, 97(2), 267–77.

Reilly, J.A., Hallett, M., Cohen, L.G., Tarkka, I.M. & Dang, N. (1992). The N30 component of somatosensory evoked potentials in patients with dystonia. *Electroenceph. Clin. Neurophysiol.*, 84, 243–7.

Richter, A. & Loscher, W. (1998). Pathology of idiopathic dystonia: findings from genetic animal models. *Progr. Neurobiol.*, 54, 633–77.

Ridding, M.C., Sheean, G., Rothwell, J.C., Inzelberg, R. & Kujiraj, T. (1995). Changes in the balance between motor cortical excitation and inhibition in focal, task specific dystonia. *J. Neurol., Neurosurg. Psychiatry*, 59(5), 493–8.

Risch, N., de Leon, D., Ozelius, L. et al. (1995). Genetic analysis of idiopathic torsion dystonia in Ashkenazi Jews and their recent descent from a small founder population. *Nat. Genet.*, 9, 152–9.

Roick, H., Giesen, H.J., Lange, H.W. & Benecke, R. (1992). Postexcitatory inhibition in Huntington's disease. *Mov. Disord.*, 7, 27.

Rona, S., Berardelli, A., Vacca, L., Inghilleri, M. & Manfredi, M.

(1998). Alterations of motor cortical inhibition in patients with dystonia. *Mov. Disord.*, **13**, 118–24.

Ross, M.H., Charness, M.E., Lee, D. & Logigian, E.L. (1995). Does ulnar neuropathy predispose to focal dystonia? *Muscle Nerve*, **18**, 606–11.

Rothwell, J.C., Obeso, J.A., Day, B.L. & Marsden, C.D. (1983). Pathophysiology of dystonias. *Adv. Neurol.*, **39**, 851–63.

Sankhla, C., Jankovic, J. & Duane, D. (1998a). Variability of the immunologic and clinical response in dystonic patients immunoresistant to botulinum toxin injections. *Mov. Disord.*, **13**(1), 150–4.

Sankhla, C., Lai, E.C. & Jankovic, J. (1998b). Peripherally induced oromandibular dystonia. *J. Neurol., Neurosurg., Psychiatry*, **65**, 722–8.

Schicatano, E.J., Basso, M.A. & Evinger, C. (1997). Animal model explains the origins of cranial dystonia benign essential blepharospasm. *J. Neurophysiol.*, **77**, 2842–6.

Schiratzki, H. & Fritzell, B. (1988). Treatment of spasmodic dysphonia by means of resection of the recurrent laryngeal nerve. *Acta Otolaryngol. Suppl.*, **449**, 115–17.

Schott, G.D. (1985). The relationship of peripheral trauma and pain to dystonia. *J. Neurol., Neurosurg. Psychiatry*, **48**, 698–701.

Schrag, A., Bhatia, K.P., Quinn, N.P. & Marsden, C.D. (1999). Atypical and typical cranial dystonia following dental procedures. *Mov. Disord.*, **14**(3), 492–6.

Schwalbe, W. (1908). *Eine eigentumliche tonische Krampfform mit hysterischen Symptomen.* Berlin.

Scott, A.B. (1981). Botulinum toxin injection of eye muscles to correct strabismus. *Trans. Am. Ophthalmol. Soc.*, **79**, 734–70.

Scott, A.B. & Suzuki, D. (1988). Systemic toxicity of botulinum toxin by intramuscular injection in the monkey. *Mov. Disord.*, **3**, 333–5.

Scott, A.B., Kennedy, R.A. & Stubbs, H.A. (1985). Botulinum A toxin injection as a treatment for blepharospasm. *Arch. Ophthalmol.*, **103**(3), 347–50.

Segawa, M., Hosaka, A., Miyagawa, F., Nomura, Y. & Imai, H. (1976). Hereditary progressive dystonia with marked diurnal fluctuation. In *Advances in Neurology*, ed. R. Eldridge & S. Fahn, pp. 215–33. New York: Raven Press.

Seiser, A., Schwarz, S., Aichinger-Steiner, M.M. et al. (1998). Parkinsonism and dystonia in central pontine myelinolysis. *J. Neurol., Neurosurg. Psychiatry*, **65**, 119–21.

Sellal, F., Hirsch, E., Barth, P., Blond, S. & Marescaux, C. (1993). A case of symptomatic hemidystonia improved by ventroposterolateral thalamic electrostimulation. *Mov. Disord.*, **8**(4), 515–18.

Siebner, H.R., Dressnandt, J., Auer, C. & Conrad, B. (1998). Continuous intrathecal baclofen infusion induced a marked increase of the transcranially evoked silent period in a patient with generalized dystonia. *Muscle Nerve*, **21**(9), 1209–12.

Siebner, H.R., Auer, C. & Conrad, B. (1999). Abnormal increase in the corticomotor output to the affected hand during repetitive transcranial magnetic stimulation of the primary motor cortex in patients with writer's cramp. *Neurosci. Lett.*, **262**, 133–6.

Slominsky, P.A., Markova, E.D., Shadrina, M.I. et al. (1999). A common 3bp deletion in the DYT1q gene in Russian families with early-onset torsion dystonia (abstract). *Hum. Mutat.*, **14**, 269.

Steinberger, D., Weber, Y., Korinthenberg, R. et al. (1998). High penetrance and pronounced variation in expressivity of GCH1 mutations in five families with dopa-responsive dystonia. *Ann. Neurol.*, **43**(5), 634–9.

Steinberger, D., Topka, H., Fischer, D. & Muller, U. (1999). GCH1 mutation in a patient with adult-onset oromandibular dystonia. *Neurology*, **52**(4), 877–9.

Stojanovic, M., Cvetkovic, D. & Kostic, V.S. (1995). A genetic study of idiopathic focal dystonias. *J. Neurol.*, **242**, 508–11.

Tabaddor, K., Wolfson, L.I. & Sharpless, N.S. (1978). Ventricular fluid homovanillic acid and 5-hydroxyindoleacetic acid concentrations in patients with movement disorders. *Neurology*, **28**, 1249–53.

Tarsy, D. (1998). Comparison of acute- and delayed-onset posttraumatic cervical dystonia. *Mov. Disord.*, **13**(3), 481–5.

Tasker, R.R., Doorly, T. & Yamashiro, K. (1988). Thalamotomy in generalized dystonia. *Adv. Neurol.*, **50**, 615–31.

Tempel, L.W. & Perlmutter, J.S. (1990). Abnormal vibration-induced cerebral blood flow responses in idiopathic dystonia. *Brain*, **113**(3), 691–707.

Tempel, L.W. & Perlmutter, J.S. (1993). Abnormal cortical responses in patients with writer's cramp. *Neurology*, **43**, 2252–7.

Tinazzi, M., Frasson, E., Polo, A. et al. (1999). Evidence for an abnormal cortical sensory processing in dystonia: selective enhancement of lower limb P37–N50 somatosensory evoked potential. *Mov. Disord.*, **14**(3), 473–80.

Tinazzi, M., Priori, A., Bertolasi, L. et al. (2000). Abnormal central integration of a dual somatosensory input in dystonia: evidence for sensory overflow. *Brain*, **123**(1), 42–50.

Todd, R.D. & Perlmutter, J.S. (1998). Mutational and biochemical analysis of dopamine in dystonia: evidence for decreased dopamine D2 receptor inhibition. *Mol. Neurobiol.*, **16**(2), 135–47.

Topka, H. & Hallett, M. (1992). Perioral reflexes in orofacial dyskinesia and spasmodic dysphonia. *Muscle Nerve*, **15**, 1016–22.

Topp, K.S. & Byl, N.N. (1999). Movement dysfunction following repetitive hand opening and closing: anatomical analysis in Owl monkeys. *Mov. Disord.*, **14**(2), 295–306.

Tournay, K.A. & Paillard, J. (1955). Torticolis spasmodique et electromyographie. *Rev. Neurol. (Paris)*, **93**, 347–55.

Tronnier, V.M. & Fogel, W. (2000). Pallidal stimulation for generalized dystonia. Report of three cases. *J. Neurosurg.*, **92**(3), 453–6.

Trugman, J.M., Leadbetter, R., Zalis, M.E., Burgdorf, O. & Wooten, G.F. (1994). Treatment of severe axial tardive dystonia with clozapine: case report and hypothesis. *Mov. Disord.*, **9**, 441–6.

Tsui, J.K. (1996). Botulinum toxin as a therapeutic agent. *Pharmacol. Ther.*, **72**(1), 13–24.

Tsui, J.K.C., Eisen, A., Stoessl, A.J., Calne, S. & Calne, D.B. (1986). Double-blind study of botulinum toxin in spasmodic torticollis. *Lancet*, **ii**, 245–7.

Tsui, J.K., Hayward, M., Mak, E.K. & Schulzer, M. (1995). Botulinum toxin type B in the treatment of cervical dystonia: a pilot study. *Neurology*, **45**(11), 2109–10.

Valente, E.M., Warner, T.T., Jarman, P.R. et al. (1998). The role of DYT1 in primary torsion dystonia in Europe. *Brain*, **121**, 2335–9.

Valls-Sole, J. & Hallett, M. (1995). Modulation of electromyographic activity of wrist flexor and extensor muscles in patients with writer's cramp. *Mov. Disord.*, **10**(6), 741–8.

van der Kamp, W., Rothwell, J.C., Thompson, P.D., Day, B.L. & Marsden, C.D. (1995). The movement related cortical potential is abnormal in patients with idiopathic torsion dystonia. *Mov. Disord.*, **5**, 630–3.

Vidailhet, M., Dupel, C., Leheriya, S. et al. (1999). Dopaminergic dysfunction in midbrain dystonia. *Arch. Neurol.*, **56**, 982–9.

Vitek, J.L. (1998). Surgery for dystonia. *Neurosurg. Clin. N. Am.*, **9**(2), 345–66.

Vitek, J.L., Zhang, J., DeLong, M.R., Mewes, K. & Bakay, R.A.E. (1998a). Neuronal activity in the pallidum in patients with medially intractable dystonia. In *Dystonia 3. Advances in Neurology*, ed. S. Fahn, M. DeLong & C.D. Marsden. Philadelphia: Lippincott-Raven.

Vitek, J.L., Zhang, J., Evatt, M. et al. (1998b). GPi pallidotomy for dystonia: clinical outcome and neuronal activity. *Adv. Neurol.*, **78**, 211–19.

Waddy, H.M., Fletcher, N.A., Harding, A.E. & Marsden, C.D. (1991). A genetic study of idiopathic focal dystonias. *Ann. Neurol.*, **29**, 320–4.

Waters, C.H., Faust, P.L., Powers, J. et al. (1993). Neuropathology of Lubag (x-linked dystonia parkinsonism). *Mov. Disord.*, **8**(6), 387–90.

Wirtschafter, J.D. (1991). Clinical doxorubicin chemomyectomy. An experimental treatment for benign essential blepharospasm and hemifacial spasm. *Ophthalmology*, **98**(3), 357–66.

Wirtschafter, J.D. & McLoon, L.K. (1998). Long-term efficacy of local doxorubicin chemomyectomy in patients with blepharospasm and hemifacial spasm. *Ophthalmology*, **105**(2), 342–6.

Wolf, M.E. & Mosnaim, A.D. (1994). Improvement of axial dystonia with the administration of clozapine. *Int. J. Clin. Pharmacol. Ther.*, **32**(6), 282–3.

Wu, C.L. & Lu, C.S. (1992). Delayed-onset dystonia following recovery from central pontine myelinolysis. *J. Formos. Med. Assoc.*, **91**(10), 1013–16.

Yazawa, S., Ikeda, A., Kaji, R. et al. (1999). Abnormal cortical processing of voluntary muscle relaxation in patients with focal hand dystonia studied by movement-related potentials. *Brain*, **122**(7), 1357–66.

Zeman, W. (1970). Pathology of torsion dystonias. *Neurology*, **20**, 79–88.

Zeman, W. & Dyken, P. (1968). Dystonia musculorum deformans. In *Diseases of the Basal Ganglia. Handbook of Clinical Neurology*, ed. P.J. Vinker & G.W. Bruyn, pp. 517–43. Amsterdam: North-Holland Publishing Co.

Ziemann, U., Tergau, F., Bruns, D., Baudewig, J. & Paulus, W. (1997). Changes in human motor cortex excitability induced by dopaminergic and anti-dopaminergic drugs. *Electroenceph. Clin. Neurophysiol.*, **105**, 430–7.

Zweig, R.M., Hedreen, J.C., Jankel, W.R. et al. (1988). Pathology in brainstem regions of individuals with primary dystonia. *Neurology*, **38**, 702–6.

38

Tourette syndrome

Donna J. Stephenson and Harvey S. Singer

Department of Neurology, Johns Hopkins University, Baltimore, Maryland, USA

In 1885 George Gilles de la Tourette, a Parisian neuropsychiatrist, described nine patients with a chronic disorder characterized by the presence of multiple motor and vocal tics. He recognized many of the salient clinical features of the syndrome that today bears his name, including its onset in childhood, the tendency of tics to wax and wane, and the presence of a variety of comorbid neurobehavioural problems such as obsessive–compulsive symptoms, anxieties, and phobias. Nevertheless, Gilles de la Tourette (1885) and his mentor Charcot attributed this disorder to a form of 'hereditary insanity' and felt it was a degenerative disorder with 'no hope of a complete cure'. Today, Tourette syndrome (TS) is considered a complex neuropsychiatric disorder with a wide spectrum of behavioural manifestations and psychological comorbidities.

Clinical features

Tics are the cardinal feature of TS. They encompass a wide variety of involuntary movements and sounds and are formally defined as involuntary, sudden, rapid, brief, repetitive, non-rhythmic stereotyped movements or vocalizations. Motor tics consist of involuntary movements and are subdivided into simple and complex subtypes. Simple motor tics are movements of single muscle groups. Examples include eye blinking, head jerking, and facial twitching. Complex motor tics consist of a coordinated pattern of movements that may be non-purposeful (facial or body contortions) or appear to be more purposeful but actually serve no purpose (touching, smelling, jumping, obscene gestures). Copropraxia describes the presence of obscene gestures, whereas echopraxia is the imitation of the gestures of others as a tic manifestation. Phonic (vocal) tics involve the production of sound. Simple phonic tics include sniffing, grunting, and throat clearing. Complex phonic tics involve the production of partial or complete words, phrases, or sentences. Palilalia is the repetition of one's own words and echolalia is the repetition of words of another person. Coprolalia is a dramatic type of tic that consists of the involuntary utterance of obscene words and phrases. Although once considered necessary for the diagnosis of TS, coprolalia occurs in only a small minority of patients with TS (Goldenberg et al., 1994). Tics are commonly misdiagnosed as other problems such as chronic respiratory symptoms, visual problems, asthma, allergies and anxiety.

Several features differentiate tics from other movements, including their variability, duration, exacerbating factors, supressibility, diminution during sleep, subjective perceptions and associated disturbances. Tics typically wax and wane in severity and may not be apparent during a routine office visit. As one tic fades, another may take its place. Several tics may occur at one time, or there may be a quiescent period with no tics noticed. A videotape of the movements is often helpful when the diagnosis is in question. Tics evolve over time and vary in their temporal pattern. Often exacerbated by fatigue, anxiety, and stress, tics may lessen during periods of relaxation. Although they are not usually evident on casual observation during sleep, they are present on polysomnograms. Most individuals are able briefly to suppress their tics. During the period of voluntary suppression, patients frequently describe a build-up of 'inner tension' that is relieved when the tic occurs or the effort to suppress the tics is discontinued. Tics are often preceded by a 'feeling' or sensory phenomenon, labeled a premonitory urge or sensory tic.

Infrequently tics can be mistaken for other movements or disorders. Stereotypies are involuntary, patterned, purposeless, repetitive, rhythmic movements that can be simple or complex. They often occur in the setting of mental retardation, pervasive developmental disorders, and other syndromes of brain dysfunction, but can also occur as a normal developmental feature of childhood. Mannerisms are an individual's embellishments of otherwise intentional normal movement patterns (e.g. baseball player at bat). Compulsions are behaviours that are experienced as alien but necessary to fulfil an inner 'need.' There is significant comorbidity of obsessive–compulsive disorder with TS, and sometimes it may be difficult to distinguish between compulsive movements and tics (Miguel et al., 1995). Seizures are occasionally confused with complex motor tics, but are distinguished from them by non-suppressible prolonged movements, loss of awareness, postictal state, and abnormal electroencephalogram. Myoclonus, tremor, dystonia, and chorea are usually clearly distinguishable from tics by observation. Sydenham's chorea (SC), which occurs in the same age group as TS, can have tics as part of the presenting motor disorder. A wide range of conditions, drugs and toxins have been associated with tics (Table 38.1). A spectrum of movements that are not tics may also occur in patients with TS. For example, it is possible that some movements may be drug-induced (akathisia, dystonia, chorea, parkinsonism) or associated with comorbid conditions such as obsessive–compulsive disorder (OCD), attention deficit hyperactivity disorder (ADHD), or antisocial behaviour (Kompoliti & Goetz, 1998).

Although the diagnosis of a tic disorder typically requires an age of onset before 18 to 21 years, the mean age of onset for tics in TS is between 6 and 7 years (Shapiro & Shapiro, 1982). Seventy-five per cent of patients have symptoms by 11 years. Infrequent cases of adult-onset tics have been reported (Chovinard & Ford, 2000). Often tics come to attention gradually, but on occasion there is an apparently explosive onset (Singer et al., 2000). Boys are three times as likely as girls to be diagnosed with TS. The most common presenting tics are those classified as simple motor tics, e.g. eye blinking, facial and head movements. Vocal tics are uncommon as a presenting symptom (Shapiro & Shapiro, 1982). Tics are usually most severe during late childhood and early adolescence (8 to 12 years). More complex tics, including coprolalia, may develop several years after the initial tic appeared (Shapiro & Shapiro, 1982). About one-third of patients with TS will have complete remission of their tics during late adolescence, and a significant improvement in tic severity is seen in an additional third of patients (Erenberg et al., 1987; Bruun, 1988; Bruun & Budman, 1993). The remaining one-third will continue to have significant tics into adulthood. Childhood tic severity is not a good predictor of tic severity later in life.

Table 38.1. Conditions in which tics may be seen

Chromosomal abnormalities	9p mosaicism
	XXX
	Fragile X
	XXY
	XYY
Developmental disorders	Static encephalopathies
	Cerebral palsy
	Autistic spectrum disorders
Neurodegenerative disorders	Huntington's chorea
	Lesch–Nyhan syndrome
	Hallovorden–Spatz
	Neuroacanthocytosis
	Subacute sclerosing panencephalitis
	Wilson's disease
	Primary dystonia
Drugs	Tardive dyskinesia (tardive Tourette)
	Dopaminergic drugs
	CNS stimulants
	Carbamazepine
	Phenobarbital
	Phenytoin
	Lamotrigine
	Clomipramine
	Wellbutrin
	Cocaine
Infections	Encephalitis (para or post)
	Lyme infection
	Sydenham's chorea
	Creutzfedt–Jakob disease
	HIV
	Neurosyphilis
Trauma	Head trauma
	Stroke
	Cardiopulmonary bypass with hypothermia
Toxins	CO poisoning
	Wasp-venom encephalopathy
	Lead poisoning
	Gasoline inhalation
Metabolic disorders	Citrullinemia
Other conditions reported to have tics	Duchenne muscular dystrophy
	Tuberous sclerosis
	Anorexia nervosa
	Type 1 neurofibromatosis

Source: From Fahn & Ehrenberg (1988).

Table 38.2. Diagnostic criteria for Tourette syndrome (TS Classification Group)

(i)   The presence of multiple motor and at least one vocal (phonic) tics
(ii) A waxing and waning course with tics evolving in a progressive manner
(iii) The presence of tic symptoms for at least 1 year
(iv) Onset before age 21
(v)   Absence of a precipitating illness, e.g. encephalitis, stroke or degenerative disease
(vi) Observation of tics by a knowledgeable individual

Diagnostic criteria

Tic disorders are classified into transient and chronic forms. Transient tic disorder is quite common, affecting 5–24% of school children. By definition, the disorder lasts less than 1 year and typically involves only a few motor or vocal tics. Chronic tic disorders (CTD) are diagnosed after a duration of at least 1 year and include chronic motor tic disorder, chronic vocal tic disorder, Tourette syndrome, and Tourette disorder. To meet the diagnosis of chronic motor (or phonic) tic disorder an individual must have either several motor (or several phonic tics), but not both. Chronic motor/phonic tic disorder is a heritable trait (often occurring in families with TS) and responds similarly to TS therapies. Non-specific tic disorder is a category in the DSM IV that encompasses chronic tic disorders that do not meet criteria for CTD or TS (APA, 1994). Terms often used for this category include Tourettism, Tourette-like, or secondary tic disorder.

Criteria for *Tourette syndrome* have been developed by the Tourette Syndrome Classification Group and are set out in Table 38.2 (1993). The DSM IV criteria for Tourette disorder (TD) are similar to those for TS, with several additions including an 'impairment' criterion requiring that 'marked distress or significant impairment in social, occupational, or other important areas of functioning' be present (APA, 1994). Furthermore, the DSM IV requires an age of onset before 18 years and a tic-free interval that is not longer than 3 months. Coprolalia, echolalia, and copropraxia are not inclusion criteria in either TS or TD, nor is there a requirement for coexisting comorbid features. Since the duration of tics is an essential criterion for tic disorder diagnosis, individuals presenting with a brief history of tics are called 'tic disorder-diagnosis deferred' while awaiting further temporal observation. Accurate distinction of a chronic tic disorder into CTD, TS, or non-specific tic disorder is important for research investigations, but has little relevance for discussion of outcome or treatment.

Rating scales

Although the diagnosis of tics is generally straightforward, it is challenging to rank tics objectively in terms of symptom severity and their impact on quality of life. Several questionnaires and rating scales have been developed for this purpose. Self-report checklists such as the Tourette Syndrome Questionnaire (TSQ) (Jagger et al., 1982) and the Tourette Syndrome Symptom List (TSSL) (Cohen et al., 1980) are easy to administer. The Tourette Syndrome Severity Scale (TSSS) (Shapiro & Shapiro, 1984; Shapiro et al., 1988), the Hopkins Motor and Vocal Tic Scale (Walkup et al., 1992), and the Yale Global Tic Severity Scale (YGTSS) (Lechman et al., 1989) are three different scales that are based on patient observation and historical information. The TSSS and YGTSS take into account not only the phenomenology of tics but also their impact on quality of life. Video-based rating systems offer the advantage of video replay for reliable tic assessment, but may be difficult to obtain in a busy office setting. The Rush Video-based Tic Rating Scale is a 10-minute film protocol that includes near and far body views obtained with the patient relaxed with and without the examiner present. It has recently been suggested that videos obtained in the home environment, rather than the physician's office, may be more accurate indicators of tic severity (Goetz et al., 1999). Other common questionnaires used to assess neuropsychiatric comorbidities include the Child Behaviour Checklist (Achenbach, 1991), Parent Symptom Questionnaire for ADHD (Conners, 1970), and the Child Yale-Brown Obsessive Compulsive Scale (CY-BOCS) (Goodman et al., 1989a, b).

Associated behaviours and psychopathology

Individuals with TS frequently manifest other behavioural and psychiatric problems. The most common comorbidities are attention deficit hyperactivity disorder (ADHD) and obsessive–compulsive disorder (OCD) and this diagnosis is often referred to as the 'TS triad.' In addition to these typical findings, the scope of comorbidity includes anxiety disorders, bipolar and non-bipolar mood disorders, and episodic behaviour disorder (Table 38.3). In several studies, severely ill patients with tic disorders have been shown to be more impaired by their non-tic

Table 38.3. Frequency of comorbid conditions in TS

OCD	30–70%
ADHD	50–75%
Anxiety disorders	20–80%
Mood disorders	20–80%
Episodic control disorders	25%
Sleep problems	12–62%
Academic difficulties	50%

symptoms than by their tics (Coffey et al., 2000; Robertson, 2000). Rates of comorbidity vary depending on the clinical setting in which individuals are seen, i.e. patients seen in a psychiatry clinic are more likely to be diagnosed with comorbid psychiatric conditions than if they are seen in a neurologist's office.

Obsessive–compulsive disorder

Obsessions are defined as recurrent ideas, thoughts, images, or impulses that intrude upon conscious thought and are persistent and unwelcome (ego-dystonic). Compulsions are repetitive, seemingly purposeful, behaviours usually performed in response to an obsession, or in accord with certain rules, or in a stereotyped fashion. Obsessive–compulsive behaviours (OCB) become a disorder (OCD) when activities are sufficiently severe to cause marked distress, take up more than 1 hour of the day, or have a significant impact on normal routine, function, social activities, or relationships. The incidence of OCB in TS is typically reported to be from 30–70% (Frankel et al., 1986; Comings & Comings, 1987d; Kano et al., 1997; King et al., 1999). Obsessive behaviours generally emerge several years after the onset of tics, usually during early adolescence. Comorbidity with OCD is associated with a more severe tic phenotype (de Groot et al., 1997). In one study, subjects with more severe tics, notably coprolalia, were more likely to have OCB (Kano et al., 1997). Studies comparing OCB in persons with and without TS have suggested clinical differences. In patients with TS, obsessions may have sexual, violent, religious, and/or aggressive themes, and compulsions include a need for order or routine and a requirement for things to be symmetrical or 'just right.' Hence, compulsions typically involve arranging, ordering, hoarding, touching, tapping, rubbing, counting, checking for errors, and 'evening-up' rituals. In contrast, in pure OCD, obsessions are predominantly concerned with contamination, dirt, germs, being neat and clean, fear of errors, bad happenings, or illness, and compulsions tend to

involve cleaning and washing (Robertson, 2000). Biological differences have reported between pure OCD and TS–OCD groups based on levels of CSF oxytocin (Leckman et al., 1994). Patients from both groups, however, have premonitory sensations and urges. Obsessive–compulsive behaviours are associated with a preceding trigger of anxiety or fear rather than a true sensation (itch, tightening, tingling) or a feeling of tension before a tic. After the action is performed, there is a brief relief from the trigger. Despite these differences, it may be difficult to distinguish whether actions such as touching, tapping, and picking represent tics or compulsions. Because of similarities in features, many investigators believe complex tics and compulsions represent a clinical spectrum of symptoms with many overlapping features. The concept that tics and obsessive–compulsive symptoms represent a continuum is supported by evidence that there is a genetic association between OCD and TS. Nevertheless, OCD is etiologically heterogeneous and not all cases are associated with a chronic tic disorder. The pharmacologic treatment of tics and OCD is distinctly different.

Attention deficit hyperactivity disorder (ADHD)

ADHD (see also Chapter 29) is characterized by impulsivity, hyperactivity, and a decreased ability to maintain attention. The disorder is common in TS probands and is reported to affect about 50–75% of referred TS cases (Golden, 1984; Comings & Comings, 1987a; Matthews, 1988; Comings, 1990; Walkup et al., 1999). Often children are diagnosed with ADHD before the onset of tics. ADHD typically begins about age 4–5 years and in TS patients, usually precedes the onset of tics by 2 to 3 years. Its appearance is not associated with the concurrent severity of tics, although ADHD is common in patients with more severe tic symptoms. Associated ADHD appears to be the most important contributing factor to poor school performance in a child with TS (Park et al., 1993; Abwender et al., 1996). Comparisons between children with ADHD-only and TS+ADHD have suggested that mood and anxiety problems were associated with ADHD and not the presence of tics (Spencer et al., 1998). Investigators have also suggested that some of the apparent increases in personality disorders in adults with TS are secondary to the presence of childhood ADHD (Robertson, 2000). Impairments in TS patients with ADHD appear to differ quantitatively and qualitatively from those observed in patients with primary ADHD without tics: those with primary ADHD have significantly more impairment on tests that measure visual search and mental flexibility, have slower reaction times, and make fewer correct responses on both simple and choice reaction time tasks (Silverstein et al., 1995). Whether a genetic relationship exists between TS and ADHD remains controversial. Pauls and colleagues have suggested that there may be two distinct populations of TS patients with comorbid ADHD: (i) those with onset of ADHD before the onset of tics; and (ii) those, possibly genetically associated, with onset after, or in concert with, the onset of tics (Pauls et al., 1993).

Other psychopathologies

Several studies have shown an increased incidence of anxiety and depression in patients with TS (Comings & Comings, 1987a, b; Robertson, 1989; Coffey et al., 1992; Robertson et al., 1993). Although the incidence of generalized anxiety disorder in TS subjects (range 19 to 80%) exceeds that in controls, some investigators believe that symptoms, especially separation anxiety, may be secondary to moderate or severe TS (Coffey et al., 1992; Robertson, 2000). TS patients also have a higher prevalence of depression than do controls. Some investigators believe that depression correlates positively with earlier onset and longer duration of tics, whereas others find no correlations between depression and the number of tics. Genetic studies show that major depressive disorder is genetic but that TS and this disorder are unrelated (Pauls et al., 1994). Personality disorders are more common in TS, but this increase has been attributed to long-term outcome of childhood ADHD (Robertson et al., 1997). Sudden, unpredictable, explosive outbursts of anger, irritability, temper, and aggression have been reported in about 25% of clinically referred patients with tic disorders (Comings et al., 1989; Wand et al., 1993; Budman et al., 2000). These explosive outbursts occur more frequently in children and resemble intermittent explosive disorder. Their presence appears to correlate highly with the combined comorbidity of ADHD and OCD (Santangelo et al., 1994; Park et al., 1996). A variety of other behavioural/emotional problems have been identified, including aggressiveness, immaturity, withdrawal, conduct disorder, oppositional defiant disorder, and somatic complaints (Singer & Rosenberg, 1989; Walkup et al., 1992, 1995). Whether these disorders are related to tic severity, are secondary to the presence of ADHD, or are the result of having a stigmatizing disorder is unclear.

Sleep problems

Sleep disturbances, including somnambulism (sleep walking), night terrors, nightmares, talking in sleep, rest-lessness, and difficulty falling asleep, have been reported in 12 to 62% of patients with TS (Comings & Comings, 1987f; Allen et al., 1992). Studies with polysomnographs have revealed decreased rapid eye movement sleep, but have not shown consistent abnormalities in delta sleep (Mendelson et al., 1980; Glaze et al., 1983). The use of sleep behaviour questionnaires has confirmed that patients with TS have an increased incidence of insomnia, dreams, required bedtime rituals, and parasomnias (Allen et al., 1992). This study found that the incidence of sleep problems was significantly increased in patients with comorbid ADHD, however, suggesting that ADHD may be a significant determinant for sleep problems in TS. Overlapping clinical and pathologic features have been proposed to exist between individuals with TS and the restless legs syndrome. Both groups have excess periodic leg and arm movements during sleep (Voderholzer et al., 1997).

Academic difficulties

Several studies have shown that learning problems are common in children with TS (Hagin & Kugler, 1988; Burd et al., 1992) and that TS is more prevalent in children in special education classes (Comings et al., 1990; Kurlan et al., 1994b). Individuals with TS typically have normal levels of intellectual functioning, although there may be a discrepancy between performance and verbal IQ, an impairment of visual perceptual achievement, or a decrease in visual–motor skills. Learning difficulties have been reported in up to 51% of children with TS, but are most common in those with both TS and ADHD. Several studies have identified differences in neuropsychological and neuromotor capabilities between children with TS only and those with TS + ADHD. For example, children with TS only had higher full scale IQ scores than did children with TS + ADHD (Faraone et al., 1993; Schuerholz et al., 1996). In a study designed to determine whether a discrepancy-based learning disability was associated with a specific subset of TS patients, results showed that comorbid ADHD accounted for the increased incidence of learning disabilities (Schuerholz et al., 1996). Children without ADHD also performed better on tests of executive function. Nevertheless, individuals with TS, irrespective of the presence of ADHD, often require extra time to complete their assignments. This difficulty has been associated, in part, with a linguistic executive dysfunction that affects the speed and efficiency of memory search. For example, a group of bright children with TS only and no learning disabilities had slowed responses on measures of executive function, especially those that were timed. Most notable was slowing on the Letter Word Fluency Task, which requires the ability to search memory efficiently. TS boys, compared to age-matched controls, had slowed reaction time during a continuous performance test (Shucard et al., 1997), but the effect of comorbid variables was not measured. In patients with TS without ADHD, school difficulties may be related to tic severity, the use of tic-suppressing medicine, executive dysfunction, a direct consequence of having a stigmatizing disorder, or other psychopathologies (Singer et al., 1995).

Epidemiology

Tourette syndrome occurs worldwide, with increasing evidence of common features in all cultures and races. The true incidence and prevalence of TS have yet to be accurately determined. Among the multiple factors accounting for inconclusive estimates are the following: mildly affected individuals do not seek medical care; the diagnostic criteria have evolved over time; TS symptoms vary in their intensity and severity; misdiagnosis of TS by practitioners; and estimates are influenced by selection and attribution bias. In a retrospective review of medical records in Rochester, Minnesota over 12 years, the calculated incidence from identified cases was 0.46 per 100 000 or 1000 new cases annually in the United States (Lucas et al., 1982). The estimated prevalence of TS has varied greatly in individual studies; estimates of 49.5 (65), 23 (72), 5.2 (73), 2.9 (9), and 0.7 (10) per 10 000 in school age children and adolescents. More recent studies, however, have suggested a prevalence rate of approximately 1% of school-age children. A study of 13- to 14-year-old mainstream British students revealed a prevalence of 299 per 10 000 children with mild to severe tics. The validity of this study has been questioned, however, because this population was not reassessed or formally diagnosed by an expert (Shapiro & Shapiro, 1982). In Houston, Texas, investigators found a prevalence rate of definite TS or TS by history in 0.7% of students (Kadesjö & Gillberg, 2000), in Sweden the prevalence was estimated at up to 1.1% of school-aged children (Hanna et al., 1999) and in Rochester NY up to 3.5% of school-aged children (Kinlan et al., 2001). All authors suggest that mild TS is more common than was previously recognized. In adult populations, prevalence estimates have been much lower (Coffey et al., 1992), presumably because the natural history is that tics become less severe after adolescence. Investigators have also shown that children in special school populations have an increased prevalence of tic disorders (Comings et al., 1990), as do children with autism, Asperger syndrome, and autistic spectrum disorders (Baron-Cohen et al., 1999).

Genetics

Although Georges Gilles de la Tourette suggested that TS is an inherited disorder, the precise pattern of transmission and the identification of the gene remain elusive. Strong support for a genetic disorder is provided by studies of monozygotic twins, which show an 86% concordance rate with TS as compared to 20% in dizygotic twins (Price et al., 1985; Hyde et al., 1992). Earlier proposals suggesting a sex-influenced autosomal dominant role of inheritance with variable expressivity as either TS, chronic tic disorder, or OCD (Pauls & Leckman, 1986) have been seriously questioned. Other investigators have proposed hypotheses of a single major locus in combination with a multifactorial background, i.e. either additional genes or environmental factors (Walkup et al., 1996). The search for a genetic site is being actively pursued, but to date no reproducible locus has been identified. In a systematic genome scan of 76 affected sib-pair families with a total of 110 sib pairs, the multipoint maximum likelihood scores for two regions (4q and 8p) showed a trend, but did not reach acceptable statistical significance (The Tourette Syndrome Association, 1999). Linkage analysis in a large French Canadian family showed a LOD score of 3.24 for chromosome 11 (11q23), which replicated findings described in a South African population (Simonic et al., 1998; Merette et al., 2000). A region on chromosome 19p has also been implicated in a genome scan of multigenerational families and three of five patients with a fragile site at 16q22–23.37 had TS. Linkage studies to candidate genes associated with specific synaptic markers, including dopamine D1–5 receptors, have not found a consistent linkage to a large variety of factors (Barr et al., 1997, 1999a; Brett et al., 1997; Hebebrand et al., 1997; Devor et al., 1998; Thompson et al., 1998; Stober et al., 1999). Several variables have been proposed to explain the unsuccessful genome search, including problems defining the phenotype, inaccurate diagnostic assessment, improper ascertainment methods, and problems with genetic modelling and data analysis. Nevertheless, some investigators have suggested that TS is not genetic, but rather represents a common disorder in the general population (Kurlan, 1994). Further complicating our understanding of TS genetics is the controversial issue of genomic imprinting (sex of the transmitting parent may affect the clinical phenotype) (Furtado & Suchowersky, 1994; Lichter et al., 1995; Eapen et al., 1997) and bilineal transmission (genetic contribution from both sides of the family (Comings et al., 1989; Kurlan et al., 1994a; McMahon et al., 1996; Hanna et al., 1999; Lichter et al., 1999). For example, it has been shown that paternal transmission of the affected gene leads to increased vocal

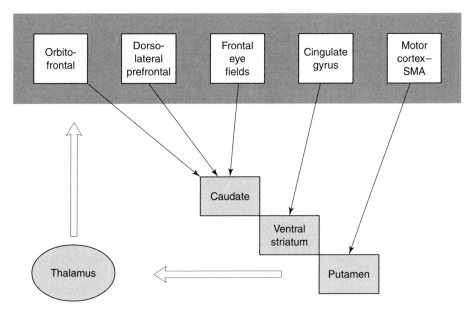

Fig. 38.1. Postulated frontal–subcortical pathways involved in Tourette syndrome.

tics and ADHD, whereas maternal transmission is linked to greater motor tic complexity and obsessive compulsive symptoms (Lichter et al., 1995). Additionally, one study estimates bilineality for tics, OCD, and ADHD to be 26% in TS families, further complicating interpretation of genetic data (Hanna et al., 1999). Studies also emphasize that factors other than genetic dose effects, such as genetic heterogeneity, epigenetic factors, and gene-environment interactions, may play an important role in determining tic severity in TS. A hypothesized role for environmental factors, especially infections, in the presentation or exacerbation of tics and OCD (Swedo et al., 1998) remains a controversial issue awaiting more definitive evidence (Kurlan, 1998).

Pathophysiology

Neuroanatomy

The exact neuroanatomic localization of TS remains unknown. Published postmortem studies are limited to seven cases; one suggested arrested development of the striatum and four showed a reduction in dynorphin-like immunoreactivity in the striatal projections to the globus pallidus and ventral pallidum (Richardson, 1982; Haber & Wolfer, 1992). Routine non-invasive neuroradiographic studies (CT and MRI) have identified only isolated defects that are considered to be incidental non-specific findings,

unrelated to the basic pathology. Nevertheless, several publications have described localized lesions in the striatum, globus pallidus, and gyrus rectus of the left frontal lobe associated with clinical tics (Singer & Walkup, 1991). Neuropathologic and radiographic investigations have shown abnormalities in persons with secondary tics (Tourettism). For example, in a postmortem study of encephalitis lethargica, subjects with acquired tics had an array of small focal lesions in the central grey matter that extended into the midbrain tegmentum (Wohlfart et al., 1961; Sacks, 1982). Tourette-like symptoms also appear in association with a variety of acute and chronic neurologic disorders (see Table 38.1).

Although the exact neuroanatomic localization for tics has yet to be established, a series of parallel frontal subcortical circuits that link specific regions of the frontal cortex to subcortical structures (Alexander et al., 1986; Alexander & Crutcher, 1990; Cummings, 1993) provide a unifying framework for understanding the interconnected neurobiologic relationships that exist between ADHD and movement disorders (see Fig. 38.1). In brief, the striatum is distinguished by the presence of several structurally and functionally distinct subcortical and cortical circuits that are shared by the frontal lobe, striatum, globus pallidus, and thalamus. Each of these circuits has been associated with a behavioural abnormality seen in TS. The motor circuit, a potential site for generation of tics, originates primarily from the supplementary motor cortex and projects to the putamen in a somatotopic distribution. The oculomotor circuit, a potential site of origin for ocular tics, begins primarily in the frontal eye fields and connects to the central region of the caudate. The dorsolateral prefrontal circuit links Brodmann's areas 9 and 10 with the dorsolateral head of the caudate and appears to be involved with executive function and motor planning. Dysfunction of this pathway could lead to attentional difficulties such as ADHD. The lateral orbitofrontal circuit originates in the inferolateral prefrontal cortex and projects to the ventromedial caudate. Orbitofrontal injury is associated with OCD, personality changes, disinhibition, irritability and mania. Lastly, the anterior cingulate circuit arises in the anterior cingulate gyrus and projects to the ventral striatum (olfactory tubercle, nucleus accumbens, and ventral medial aspect of the caudate and putamen) which receives additional input from the amygdala, hippocampus, and entorhinal and perirhinal cortex. Mutism, apathy and OCD are associated with this circuit. An important aspect of a circuit hypothesis is that lesions in one part (e.g. globus pallidus) of the circuit could produce signs and symptoms similar to those caused by a lesion in another region of the circuit (e.g. prefrontal cortex).

Direct evidence for pathophysiologic involvement of frontal subcortical circuits, especially the basal ganglia, in TS is derived from volumetric MRI studies (Peterson et al., 1993; Singer et al., 1993), area measurements of the corpus callosum (Peterson et al., 1993; Baumgartner et al., 1996), functional imaging of glucose metabolism and blood flow (Riddle et al., 1992; Baxter & Guse, 1993), oculomotor paradigms (Farber et al., 1999; Dursun et al., 2000; Mastofsky et al., 2001), and neuroimaging studies in subjects with ADHD and OCD (Aylward et al., 1996; Trivedi, 1996). For example, volumetric MRI studies in TS have shown significant differences in the symmetry of the putamen and lenticular region in boys (Singer et al., 1993) and a reduction in the size of these structures in adults (Peterson et al., 1993). On the basis of a quantitative MRI study of monozygotic twins, other investigators have suggested that, rather than an abnormality of the lenticular region, the caudate may be the important site (Hyde et al., 1995). A recent study in girls, however, showed no significant differences in basal ganglia or corpus callosum size between those with and without TS, suggesting that there may be gender differences in the neurobiologic manifestations of TS (Mostofsky et al., 1999; Zimmerman et al., 2000). Functional imaging studies have identified abnormalities in glucose metabolism and perfusion of the basal ganglia, especially on the left (Riddle et al., 1992; Stoetter et al., 1992; Baxter & Guse, 1993). In the HMPAO SPECT study of Riddle et al. (1992), TS was associated with

a 4% reduction of blood flow to the left putamen and globus pallidus. In a small number of TS patients, event-related $[^{15}O]H_2O$ PET combined with time-synchronized audio and videotaping, identified aberrant activity in interrelated sensorimotor, language, executive, and paralimbic circuits (Stern et al., 2000). Transcranial magnetic stimulation (TMS) in children with tic disorders identified a shortened cortical silent period (Ziemann et al., 1997), suggesting a reduced motor inhibition believed to be at the level of the basal ganglia. In preliminary functional MRI studies, Peterson et al. (1998) compared images acquired during periods of voluntary tic suppression with those acquired when subjects were allowed spontaneous expression of their tics. Significant changes in signal intensity were seen in the basal ganglia and thalamus, as well as in connected cortical regions. Lastly, functional MRI imaging of five patients with TS during finger tapping showed an increased area of cerebral activation in both sensorimotor cortex and supplementary motor area as compared to these areas in healthy subjects (Biswal et al., 1990).

Neurochemistry

The distribution of classical neurotransmitters within the basal ganglia's frontal–subcortical circuits raises the possibility that a variety of transmitters are involved in the pathobiology of TS (Graybiel, 1990; Graybiel et al., 1994). In general, current hypotheses are based on extrapolations from clinical trials evaluating the response to specific medications; from studies of CSF, blood, and urine in relatively small numbers of patients; from SPECT and PET investigations; and from neurochemical assays on a limited number of postmortem brain tissues (Singer, 1997; Singer & Wendlandt, 2001). Genetic linkage analyses have also been performed in an attempt to identify specific candidate genes that are associated with components of neurotransmission. To date, the dopaminergic, GABAergic, cholinergic, serotoninergic, noradrenergic, and opioid systems have all been implicated. Which, if any, of these systems is the primary pathologic factor remains to be determined. Since many transmitter systems are interrelated in the production of complex actions, it is indeed possible, if not probable, that imbalances exist among several transmitter systems. Moreover, investigators must vigorously pursue mechanisms that could unify findings of alterations within multiple transmitter systems, i.e. such possibilities as second-messenger pathways, vesicle release proteins, channel abnormalities, or synaptic membrane dysfunction. Furthermore, any hypotheses about specific neurotransmitter deficiencies must account for variability in tic manifestations, fluctuating symptoms, and potential resolution in adulthood.

Neurochemical studies on postmortem tissues are limited to four TS cases. Singer et al. (1991) found a significant elevation of striatal [^{3}H]mazindol binding suggesting an elevation of dopamine transporter sites. Additionally a reduction in cyclic AMP was observed in cerebral cortex (Singer et al., 1990), but subsequent investigations identified no specific abnormality within several second messenger pathways (Singer et al., 1995a). Anderson et al. (1992) evaluating the same cases, compared levels of catecholamines, serotonin (5-HT), amino acids, and metabolites in 13 brain regions. Results showed reductions of 5-HT, tryptophan, and 5-hydroxyindoleacetic acid in subcortical structures, decreased glutamate levels in the globus pallidus and substantia nigra pars reticulata, and diminished glycine levels in substantia nigra pars reticulata. These data would suggest the possibility of altered serotoninergic transmission in the striatum and a reduced influence of glutamate in subthalamic efferent pathways. Because of the small number of available postmortem samples, emphasis has shifted to studies by in vivo neurochemical imaging. Dopaminergic hypotheses, including abnormalities of both pre- and postsynaptic function (supersensitive postsynaptic dopamine receptors, dopamine hyperinnervation, abnormal presynaptic function, or excessive release of dopamine) have been studied by PET and SPECT techniques. Overall, studies of D2 dopamine receptors have not consistently shown significant differences between TS patients and controls. Nevertheless, several investigations have supported the hypothesis that the dopamine receptor is involved in the neurobiology of TS (Wolf et al., 1996; Wong et al., 1997; Muller-Vahl et al., 2000). Similarly, attempts to provide support for a postulated dopamine hyperinnervation hypothesis by PET or SPECT binding have resulted in contradictory reports (Maison et al., 1995; Heinz et al., 1998). Studies evaluating dorsal striatal dopaminergic innervation by use of in vivo measures of vesicular monoamine transporter type 2 (VMAT2) binding, however, do not support the concept of increased striatal innervation. The possibility that deficits in a variety of presynaptic dopamine functional elements play a role has been supported by higher accumulations of [^{18}F]fluorodopa in the left caudate nucleus and right midbrain compared with levels in control subjects (Ernst et al., 1999). Lastly, increased intrasynaptic dopamine release from the putamen has been proposed, based on kinetic modelling of [^{11}C]raclopride binding after pretreatment with a central stimulant (Singer et al., in press). A [^{125}I]-CIT SPECT binding study has reported a negative correlation between overall tic severity and binding in the midbrain (serotoninergic) and thalamus (serotonin or noradrenergic) (Heinz et al., 1998). The authors suggest that serotoninergic transmission is a modifying, but not causal, factor in the pathogenesis of tics. In summary, available data have not confirmed a definite consistent abnormality of synaptic neurotransmission.

Neuroimmunology

Recently it has been proposed that TS, like Sydenham's chorea (SC), may be part of an immune-mediated neurologic response to a Group AB-hemolytic streptococcus infection (GABHS). SC is a major manifestation of rheumatic fever, along with carditis, migratory polyarthritis, erythema marginatum, and subcutaneous nodules. Typically, systemic manifestations of rheumatic fever occur 1–5 weeks after a GABHS pharyngitis, whereas chorea, which may be the sole manifestation, occurs from 2–6 months after antecedent infection. The pathophysiology responsible for the chorea has been speculated to be autoimmune, probably due to 'molecular mimicry,' i.e. shared antigens by the bacteria and host organs (Cairns, 1988; Stollerman, 1991).

The proposed spectrum of neurobehavioural disorders associated with GABHS infection has been expanded to include some children with TS and/or OCD termed 'pediatric autoimmune neuropsychiatric disorders associated with streptococcal infection' (PANDAS) (Swedo et al., 1997, 1998). A possible association between GABHS and tics was initially proposed in case reports describing the explosive onset of tics after a preceding streptococcal infection (Kondo & Kabasawa, 1978; Matarazzo, 1992; Kiessling et al., 1993). More recently, Swedo and colleagues proposed diagnostic criteria that include: the presence of OCD and/or tic disorder; prepubertal age at onset; sudden, 'explosive' onset of symptoms and/or a course of sudden exacerbations and remissions; a temporal relationship between symptoms and GABHS; and the presence of neurologic abnormalities, including hyperactivity and choreiform movements. Volumetric MRI analysis in 34 children with PANDAS showed that the average size of the caudate, putamen, and globus pallidus, but not thalamus or total cerebrum, was significantly greater in the affected group than in 82 healthy children (Gredd et al., 2000). In a study of first degree relatives of children with PANDAS, the rates of tic disorders and OCD were similar to those published for tic disorders and OCD (Lougee et al., 2000). The authors suggest that this supports the hypothesis of an environmental trigger in a genetically vulnerable population. An immune-mediated mechanism involving molecular mimicry has been proposed for PANDAS (i.e. antibodies produced against GABHS cross-react with neuronal tissue in specific brain regions), similar to the Sydenham's chorea model. Indirect support for this hypothesis is derived from the response of a small number of patients with PANDAS to two forms of immunotherapy, intravenous immunoglobulin (IVIG) and plasmapheresis (PEX) (Perlmutter et al., 1999); the documentation of antineuronal antibodies in patients with TS (Singer et al., 1998); and the development of dyskinesias (paw- and floor-licking, head- and paw-shaking) and phonic utterances in rodents after the microinfusion of dilute IgG from TS subjects into their striatum (Hallett et al., 2000).

The existence of PANDAS, however, remains controversial (Kurlan, 1998). For example, no prospective epidemiologic study has confirmed that an antecedent GABHS infection is specifically associated with either the onset or exacerbation of tic disorders or OCD. Subjects with PANDAS lack other stigmata of streptococcal infection, such as rash, arthritis, or valve disease. Diagnostic criteria established for PANDAS are also potentially confounded by the phenotypic variability commonly associated with tic disorders: a normal fluctuation in the frequency and severity of symptoms; exacerbation of tics by stress, anxiety, fatigue, and illness; the occurrence of 'sudden, abrupt' onset and/or recurrence of tics in non-PANDAS subjects (Singer et al., 2000); a variable response to pharmacotherapy; and the lack of a precise definition for choreiform movements. Additionally, longitudinal laboratory data, rather than studies that utilize only a throat culture or only a single antistreptolysin O (ASO) or antideoxyribonuclease B titre, are necessary to confirm the presence of a prior GABHS infection.

Evidence to support an immune-mediated hypothesis for PANDAS also remains largely circumstantial. For example, although plasmapheresis was claimed be beneficial, the therapeutic response did not parallel to the rate of antibody removal, it is unclear how peripheral changes affect events across the blood–brain barrier, and the mechanism for the beneficial response remains undetermined. Additionally, despite reported higher antineuronal antibody values in children with neurobehavioural problems and/or movement disorders including tics (Husby et al., 1976; Kiessling et al., 1992; Singer et al., 1998), the sensitivity and specificity of these studies remain a major issue. Antineuronal antibodies are present in control groups and Western blot analyses suggest that there are

Table 38.4. Tic-suppressing medications

Non-neuroleptics
  Clonidine
  Guanfacine
  Baclofen
  Clonazepam
Neuroleptics
  Pimozide
  Fluphenazine
  Haloperidol
  Trifluphenazine
Atypical neuroleptics
  Risperidone
  Olanzapine
  Ziprasidone
Alternatives
  Botulinum toxin
  Tetrabenazine
  Pergolide
  Nicotine
  THC

multiple differences in antibody repertoires in children with TS (Wendlaudt et al., 2001). Longitudinal studies will be required to clarify the current controversies.

Treatment

Treatment of TS must take into account not only the severity of tics but the significance of comorbid academic, social, and neuropsychiatric problems. The symptom causing the most difficulty for the patient must be targeted first. The mere presence of tics does not in itself justify initiation of pharmacotherapy (Table 38.4). Medications should be targeted and reserved only for those problems that are functionally disabling and not remediable by non-drug interventions.

Patients with tics that are not causing any psychosocial or physical problems (i.e. no loss of self-esteem, no peer problems, no difficulty participating in academic, social, and after-school activities, no disruption of classroom setting, and no musculoskeletal problems) should be counseled and observed for the progression of symptoms. A variety of behavioural treatments including conditioning techniques, relaxation training, biofeedback, and hypnosis have been utilized as alternative therapeutic approaches for tics with variable short- and long-term success (Turpin, 1983; Bergin et al., 1998).

Tic-suppressing medications can be broadly divided into a 'mild' (non-neuroleptic) group and the neuroleptics (typical or atypical). Initial treatment of tics generally begins with non-neuroleptics. This category includes clonidine, guanfacine, baclofen and clonazepam. Clonidine can be especially effective in individuals with relatively mild tics who also have ADHD with aggressive features or poor impulse control. There is some suggestion that motor tics are more effectively suppressed with clonidine than are vocal tics (Leckman et al., 1985, 1991; Goetz et al., 1987). For tics alone, a BID dosing schedule is often adequate. For patients with comorbid ADHD, a QID schedule is often necessary for a consistent therapeutic effect. Common side effects include drowsiness, dry mouth, itchy eyes, postural hypotension, bradycardia and headaches. Clonidine should be tapered gradually to avoid rebound tic exacerbation and hypertension.

Individuals who fail initial therapy or who present with severe tics may benefit from neuroleptic or atypical neuroleptic medications. Neuroleptics, D2 dopamine receptor antagonists, are the most effective tic-suppressing agents (about 70–80% effective), but side effects may limit their usefulness. Side effects include weight gain, dysphoria, movement abnormalities (acute dystonic reactions, bradykinesia, akathisia, tardive and withdrawal dyskinesias), depression, and poor school performance. Haloperidol has historically been the most frequently used neuroleptic in this class, but more recently it has been replaced by pimozide because of greater tolerability (Shapiro et al., 1989; Sallee et al., 1997). Before initiating treatment with pimozide, an ECG should be obtained in order to identify a prolonged Q–T_c interval, a contraindicating factor. Other neuroleptics used in TS include fluphenazine and trifluoperazine.

The atypical neuroleptics were designed to decrease the extrapyramidal side effects common to most D2 receptor antagonists. As a group, risperidone, olanzapine, ziprasidone, clozapine, and quetiapine all have greater affinity for 5-HT2 (serotonin) receptors than for D2 receptors. Of these, risperidone and olanzapine have been used most extensively in TS. Risperidone may be most beneficial when tics occur with comorbid OCD (Robertson et al., 1996). A recent study has identified equal efficacy in the suppression of tics with use of either risperidone or pimozide (Beuggeman et al., 2001). In several studies olanzapine has been shown to be generally well tolerated and beneficial for tics (Bengi & Semerci, 2000; Onofrj et al., 2000; Stamenkovic et al., 2000).

Several additional pharmacotherapies have been proposed as tic-suppressing agents. Tetrabenazine, a dopamine antagonist that depletes presynaptic storage of dopamine and blocks postsynaptic dopamine receptors, has effectively suppressed tics (Jankovic et al., 1984; Jankovic & Beach, 1997). Dopamine agonists, such as pergolide, somewhat unexpectedly improved tics at approximately one-tenth the dose used for treatment of Parkinson's disease (Lipinski et al., 1997). Nicotine, in gum or patch form, has been shown to have brief beneficial effects when used in conjunction with neuroleptics (Dursun & Reveley, 1997; Sanberg et al., 1988, 1989, 1997). In uncontrolled trials, marijuana and delta-9-tetrahydrocannabinol, the major psychoactive component of marijuana, have been reported to be beneficial (Muller-Vahl et al., 1999, 2000). Botulinum toxin, which reduces muscle activity by inhibiting acetylcholine release at neuromuscular junctions, has been shown not to only reduce tics but also the premonitory urge associated with the tics (Kwak et al., 2000). Suggestions that Botox® produces a universal improvement in simple tics (Trimble et al., 1998; Awaad, 1999) have not been supported in all studies (Marras et al., 2000). Several patients with coprolalia have been successfully treated with injections either into a single vocal cord or both thyroarytenoid muscles (Scott et al., 1996; Trimble et al., 1998). Penicillin and immune therapies including IVIG and plasmapheresis for PANDAS are currently under investigation. Neurosurgical interventions for severe intractable tics are rarely indicated. Procedures used have included focal lesions of frontal, cingulate, thalamic, and cerebellar areas (Rauch et al., 1995). Thalamic deep brain stimulation, a modern stereotactic treatment proposed for use in other movement disorders, has been suggested as a potential therapy for the control of tics.

ADHD

Although psychostimulant medications are generally regarded as the treatment of choice for ADHD, their use in children with TS was controversial because of their proposed potential to provoke or intensify tics in a substantial minority. Several new reports providing additional information on the question of the role of stimulants in worsening tic disorders can be summarized as follows: there is strong evidence that stimulants have a beneficial effect on ADHD and, in most children receiving low-moderate doses of methylphenidate, there appears to be no clinically significant effect on tics (Lowe et al., 1982; Castellanos et al., 1997; Gadow et al., 1999; Nolan et al., 1999; Law & Schachar, 1999). Tics may fluctuate but usually do not require pharmacologic adjustments. Other medications suggested for the treatment of ADHD symptoms in children with TS include clonidine, guanfacine, desipramine, deprenyl, and nortriptyline. In the occasional situation where a stimulant is required for attendance in school or performance at work and tics remain constant, stimulants and tic-suppressing medications are given simultaneously.

OCD

Over the past decade the treatment of OCD has expanded, with the addition of a variety of serotonin reuptake inhibitor antidepressants including fluoxetine, fluvoxamine, clomipramine, paroxetine, and sertraline. These medications, also effective in anxiety disorders, can sometimes be helpful in addressing the stress associated with the stigma of a chronic tic disorder.

In conclusion, although much is known about TS and related disorders, much remains to be done. Tourette syndrome is a chronic neuropsychiatric disorder that has been recognized for well over a century. Although defined by the presence of vocal and motor tics, comorbidities, such as OCD and ADHD, often cause more significant impairment than the tics. TS is considered to be an inherited disorder, although the precise pattern of transmission and the identification of the gene remains elusive. Genetic heterogeneity, epigenetic factors and gene–environmental interactions may play an important role in phenotypic expression. Evidence supports involvement of frontal–subcortical circuits and synaptic neurotransmission. Nevertheless, the precise localization and specific subcellular mechanism have yet to be determined. Pharmacotherapy is available for tic suppression, but is strictly symptomatic, not universally effective, and often limited by side effects.

References

Abwender, D.A., Como, P.G., Kurlan, R. et al. (1996). School problems in Tourette's syndrome. *Arch. Neurol.*, **53**, 509–11.

Achenbach, T.M. (1991). *Manual for the Child Behavior Checklist/4–18 and 1991 Profile.* Burlington: University of Vermont Department of Psychiatry.

Alexander, G.E. & Crutcher, M.D. (1990). Functional architecture of basal ganglia circuits: neuronal substrates of parallel processing. *Trends. Neurosci.*, **13**, 266–71.

Alexander, G.E., Delong, M.R. & Strick, P.L. (1986). Parallel organization of functionally segregated circuits linking basal ganglia and cortex. *Annu. Rev. Neurosci.*, **9**, 357–81.

Allen, R.P., Singer, H.S., Brown, J.E. et al. (1992). Sleep disorders in Tourette syndrome: a primary or unrelated problem? *Pediatr. Neurol.*, **8**, 275–80.

American Psychiatric Association (APA) (1994). *Diagnostic Manual and Statistical Manual of Mental Disorders,* 4th edn. Wahington DC: American Psychiatric Association.

Anderson, G.M., Pollak, E.S., Chatterjee, D. et al. (1992). Postmortem analysis of subcortical monoamines and amino acids in Tourette's syndrom. In *Advances in Neurology*, ed. T.N. Chase, A.J. Friedhoff & D. Cohen, Vol. 58. New York: Raven Press.

Awaad, Y. (1999). Tics in Tourette syndrome: new treatment options. *J. Child. Neurol.*, **14**, 316–19.

Aylward, E.H., Reiss, A.L., Reader, M.J. et al. (1996). Basal ganglia volumes in children with attention-deficit hyperactivity disorder. *J. Child. Neurol.*, **11**, 112–15.

Baron-Cohen, S., Scahill, V.L., Izaguirre, J., Hornsey, I.I. & Robertson, M.M. (1999). The prevalence of Gilles de la Tourette syndrome in children and adolescents with autism: a large scale study. *Psychol. Med.*, **29**, 1151–9.

Barr, C.L., Wigg, K.G., Zovko, E., Sandor, P. & Tsui, L.C. (1997). Linkage analysis of the dopamine D5 receptor gene and Gilles de la Tourette syndrome. *Am. J. Med. Genet.*, **74**, 58–61.

Barr, C.L., Wigg, K.G., Pakstis, A. et al. (1999a). Genome scan for linkage to Gilles de la Tourette syndrome. *Am. J. Med. Genet.*, **88**, 437–45.

Barr, C.L., Wigg, K.G. & Sandor, P. (1999b). Catechol-*o*-methyltranferase and Gilles de la Tourette syndrome. *Mol. Psychiatry*, **4**, 492–5.

Baumgartner, T.L., Singer, H.S., Denckla, M.B. et al. (1996). Corpus callosum morphology in children with Tourette syndrome and attention deficit hyperactivity disorder. *Neurology*, **47**, 277–482.

Baxter, L.R., Jr & Guze, B.J. (1993). Neuroimaging. In *Handbook of Tourette's Syndrome and Related Tic and Behavioral Disorders*, ed. R. Kurlan, pp. 289–304. New York: Marcel Dekker.

Bengi Semerci, Z. (2000). Olanzapine in Tourette's disorder. *J. Am. Acad. Child Adolesc. Psychiatry*, **39**, 140.

Bergin, A., Waranch, H.R., Brown, J., Carson, K. & Singer, H.S. (1998). Relaxation therapy in Tourette syndrome: a pilot study. *Pediatr. Neurol.*, **18**, 136–42.

Biswal, B., Ulmer, J.L., Krippendorf, R.L. et al. (1998). Abnormal cerebral activation associated with a motor task in Tourette syndrome. *Am. J. Neuroradiol.*, **19**, 1509–12.

Brett, P.M., Curtis, D., Robertson, M.M. & Gurlin, H.M. (1997). Neuroreceptor subunit genes and the genetic susceptibility to Gilles de la Tourette syndrome. *Biol. Psychiatry*, **42**, 941–7.

Bruggeman, R. & van der Linden, C. Group Study (2001). Risperidone versus pimozide in Tourette's disorder: a comparative double-blind parallel-group study. *J. Clin Psychiatry*, **62**, 50–6.

Bruun, R.D. (1988). The natural history of Tourette's syndrome. In *Tourette's Syndrome and Tic Disorders: Clinical Understanding and Treatment*, ed. D.J. Cohen, R.D. Bruun & J.F. Leckman. New York: John Wiley.

Bruun, R.D. & Budman, C.L. (1993). The natural history of Gilles de la Tourette's syndrome. In *Handbook on Tourette's Syndrome and Related Tic Diosorders*, ed. R. Kurlan. New York: Marcel Dekker.

Budman, C.L., Bruun, R.D., Park, K.S., Lesser, M. & Olson, M. (2000). Explosive outbursts in children with Tourette's disorder. *J. Am. Acad. Child Adolesc. Psychiatry*, **39**, 1270–6.

Burd, L., Kerbeshian, J., Wikenheiser, M. & Fisher, W. (1986). A prevalence study of Gilles de la Tourette syndrome in North

Dakota school-age children. *J. Am. Acad. Child Psych.*, **25**, 552–3.

Burd, L., Kauffman, D.W. & Kerbeshian, J. (1992). Tourette syndrome and learning disabilities. *J. Learn. Disabil.*, **25**, 598–604.

Cairns, L.M. (1988). Immunologic studies in acute rheumatic fever. *NZ Med. J.*, **101**, 388–91.

Castellanos, F.X., Giedd, J.N., Elia, J. et al. (1997). Controlled stimulant treatment of ADHD and comorbid Tourette's syndrome: effects of stimulant and dose. *J. Am. Acad. Child Adolesc. Psychiatry*, **35**, 589–96.

Chouinard, S. & Ford, B. (2000). Adult onset tic disorders. *J. Neurol., Neurosurg. Psychiatry*, **68**, 738– 43.

Coffey, B., Frazier, J. & Chen, S. (1992). Comorbidity, Tourette syndrome, and anxiety disorders [review]. *Adv. Neurol.*, **58**, 95–104.

Coffey, B.J., Biederman, J., Smoller, J.W. et al. (2000). Anxiety disorders and tic severity in juveniles with Tourette's disorder. *J. Am. Acad. Child Adolesc. Psychiatry*, **39**, 562–8.

Cohen, D.J., Detlor, J., Young, G. et al. (1980). Clonidine ameliorates Gilles de la Tourette syndrome. *Arch. Gen. Psychiatry*, **37**, 1350–7.

Comings, D. (1990). ADHD in Tourette syndrome. In *Tourette Syndrome and Human Behavior*, ed. D. Comings, pp. 99. Duarte, CA: Hope Press.

Comings, D.E. & Comings, B.G. (1987a). A controlled study of Tourette syndrome. I. Attention-deficit disorder, learning disorders, and school problems. *Am. J. Hum. Genet.*, **41**, 701–41.

Comings, D.E. & Comings, B.G. (1987b). A controlled study of Tourette syndrome. II. Conduct. *Am. J. Hum. Genet.*, **41**, 742–60.

Comings, D.E. & Comings, B.G (1987c). A controlled study of Tourette syndrome. III. Phobias and panic attacks. *Am. J. Hum. Genet.*, **41**, 761–81.

Comings, D.E. & Comings, B.G (1987d). A controlled study of Tourette syndrome. IV. Obsessions, compulsions and schizoid behaviors. *Am. J. Hum. Genet.*, **41**, 782–803.

Comings, B.G. & Comings, D.E. (1987e). A controlled study of Tourette syndrome. V. Depression and mania. *Am. J. Hum. Genet.*, **41**, 804–21.

Comings, D.E. & Comings, B.G. (1987f). A controlled study of Tourette syndrome: VI. Early development, sleep problems, allergies, and handedness. *Am. J. Hum. Genet.*, **41**, 822–38.

Comings, D.E., Comings, B.G. & Knell, E. (1989). Hypothesis: homozygosity in Tourette syndrome. *Am. J. Med. Genet.*, **34**, 413–21.

Comings, D.E., Himes, J.A. & Comings, B.G. (1990). An epidemiologic study of Tourette's syndrome in a single school district. *J. Clin. Psychiatry*, **51**, 463–9.

Conners, C.K. (1970). Symptom patterns in hyperkinetic, neurotic, and normal children. *Child Dev.*, **41**, 667–82.

Cummings, J. (1993). Frontal–subcortical circuits and human behavior. *Arch. Neurol.*, **50**, 873–980.

Debray-Ritzen, P. & Dubois, H. (1980). Maladies des tics de l'enfant. *Rev. Neurol.*, **136**, 15.

de Groot, C.M., Yeates, K.O., Baker, G.B. & Bornstein, R.A. (1997). Impaired neuropsychological functioning in Tourette's syndrome subjects with co-occuring obsessive–compulsive and attention deficit symptoms. *J. Neuropsych. Clin. Neurosci.*, **9**, 267–72.

Devor, E.J., Dill-Devor, R.M. & Magee, H.J. (1998). The Bal I and Msp I polymorphisms in the dopamine D3 receptor gene display linkage disequilibrium with each other but no association with Tourette syndrome. *Psychiatr. Genet.*, **8**, 49–52.

Dursun, S.M. & Reveley, M.A. (1997). Differential effects of transdermal nicotine on microstructured analyses of tics in Tourette's syndrome: an open study. *Psychol. Med.*, **27**, 483–7.

Dursun, S.M., Burke, J.G. & Reveley, M.A. (2000). Antisaccade eye movement abnormalities in Tourette Syndrome: evidence for cortico-striatal network dysfunction? *J. Psychopharmacol.*, **14**, 37–9.

Eapen, V., O'Neill, J., Gurling, H. & Robertson, M.M. (1997). Sex of parent transmission effect in Tourette's syndrome: evidence for earlier age at onset in maternally transmitted cases suggests a genomic imprinting effect. *Neurology*, **48**, 934–7.

Erenberg, G., Cruse, R.P. & Rothner, A.D. (1987). The natural history of Tourette syndrome: a follow-up study. *Ann. Neurol.*, **22**, 383–5.

Ernst, M., Zamekin, A.J., Jons, P.H., Matochik, J.A., Pascualvaca, D. & Cohen, R.M. (1999). High presynaptic dopaminergic activiety in children with Tourette's disorder. *J. Am. Acad. Child Adolesc. Psychiatry*, **38**, 86–94.

Fahn, S. & Erenberg, G. (1988). Differential diagnosis of tic phenomena: a neurologic perspective. In *Tourette Syndrome and Tic Disorders*, ed. D.J. Cohen, R. Bruun & J.E. Leckman, pp. 41–54. New York, NY: John Wiley.

Faraone, S.V., Biederman, J., Lehman, B.K. et al. (1993). Intellectual performance and school failure in children with attention deficit hyperactivity disorder and in their siblings. *J. Abnorm. Psychol.*, **102**, 616–23.

Farber, R.H., Swerdlow, N.R. & Clementz, B.A. (1999). Saccadic performance characteristics and the behavioural neurology of Tourette's syndrome. *J. Neurol., Neruosurg. Psychiatry*, **66**, 305–12.

Frankel, M., Cummings, J.L., Robertson, M.M. et al. (1986). Obsessions and compulsions in Gilles de la Tourette's syndrome. *Neurology*, **36**, 378–82.

Furtado, S. & Suchowersky, O. (1994). Investigation of the potential role of genetic imprinting in Gilles de la Tourette syndrome. *Am. J. Med. Genet.* **51**, 51–4.

Gadow, K.D., Sverd, J., Sprafkin, J., Nolan, E.E. & Grossman, S. (1999). Long-term methylphenidate therapy in children with comorbid attention-deficit hyperactivity disorder and chronic multiple tic disorder. *Arch. Gen. Psychiatry*, **56**, 330–6.

Giedd, J.N., Rapoport, J.L., Garvey, M.A., Perlmutter, S. & Swedo, S.E. (2000). MRI assessment of children with obsessive–compulsive disorders of tics associated with streptococcal infection. *Am. J. Psychiatry*, **157**, 281–3.

Gilles de la Tourette, G. (1885). Etude sur une affection nerveuse caracterisee par de l'incoordination motrice accompagnee d'echolalie et de copralalie. *Arch. Neurol.*, **9**, 19–42; 158–200.

Glaze, D.G., Frost, J.D. & Jankovic, J. (1983). Sleep in Gilles de la Tourette's syndrome: disorder of arousal. *Neurology*, **33**, 586–92.

Goetz, C.G., Tanner, C.M., Wilson, R.S., Carroll, V.S., Garron, P.G. & Shannon, K.M. (1987). Clonidine and Gilles de la Tourette's syndrome: double-blind study using objective rating methods. *Ann. Neurol.*, **21**, 307–10.

Goetz, C.G., Pappert, E.J., Louis, E.D., Raman, R. & Leugans, S. (1999). Advantages of a modified scoring method for the Rush Video-Based Tic Rating Scale. *Mov. Disord.*, **14**, 502–6.

Golden, G.S. (1984). Psychologic and neuropsychologic aspects of Tourette's syndrome. *Neurol. Clin.*, **2**, 91–102.

Goldenberg, J.N., Brown, S.B. & Weiner, W.J. (1994). Coprolalia in younger patients with Gilles de la Tourette syndrome. *Mov. Disord.*, **9**, 622–5.

Goodman, W.K., Price, L.H., Rasmussen, S.A. et al. (1989a). The Yale–Brown obsessive compulsive scale. II. Validity. *Arch. Gen. Psychiatry*, **46**, 1012–16.

Goodman, W.K., Price, L.H., Rasmussen, S.A. et al. (1989b). The Yale–Brown obsessive compulsive scale. I. Development, use and reliability. *Arch. Gen. Psychiatry*, **46**, 1006–11.

Graybiel, A.M. (1990). Neurotransmitters and neuromodulators in the basal ganglia. *Trends Neurosci.*, **13**, 244–51.

Graybiel, A.M., Aosake, T., Flaherty, A.W. et al. (1994). The basal ganglia and adaptive motor control. *Science*, **265**, 1826–31

Haber, S.N. & Wolfer, D. (1992). Basal ganglia peptidergic staining in Tourette syndrome: a follow-up study. In *Advances in Neurology*, ed. T.N. Chase, A.J. Friedhoff & D.J. Cohen, Vol. 58, pp. 145–50. New York: Raven Press.

Hagin, R.A. & Kugler, J. (1988). School problems associated with Tourette's syndrome. In *Tourette's Syndrome and Tic Disorder*, ed. D.J. Cohen, R.D. Bruun & J.F. Leckman. New York: Wiley.

Hallett, J.J., Harling-Berg, C.J., Knopf, P.M., Stopa, E.G. & Kiessling, L.S. (2000). Anti-striatal antibodies in Tourette syndrome cause neuronal dysfunction. *J. Neuroimmunol.*, **111**, 195–202.

Hanna, P.A., Janjua, P.N., Contant, C.F. & Jankovic, J. (1999). Bilineal transmission in Tourette syndrome. *Neurology*, **53**, 813–38.

Hebebrand, J.H., Nothen, M.M., Ziegler, A. et al. (1997). Nonreplication of linkage disequilibrium between the dopamine D4 receptor locus and Tourette syndrome. *Am. J. Hum. Genet.*, **61**, 238–9.

Heinz, A., Knable, M.B., Wolf, S.S. et al. (1998). Tourette's syndrome: [I-123] beta-CIT SPECT correlates of vocal tic severity. *Neurology*, **51**, 1069–74.

Husby, G., van de Rijn, I., Zabriskie, J.B. et al. (1976). Antibodies reacting with cytoplasm of subthalamic and caudate nuclei neurons in chorea and acute rheumatic fever. *J. Exp. Med.*, **144**, 1094–110.

Hyde, T.M., Aronson, B.A., Randolph, C., Rickler, K.C. & Weinberger, D.R. (1992). Relationship of birth weight to the phenotypic expression of Gilles de la Tourette's syndrome. *Neurology*, **42**, 652–58.

Hyde, T.M., Stacey, M.E., Coppola, R.C. et al. (1995). Cerebral morphometric abnormalities in Tourette's syndrome: a quantitative MRI study in monozygotic twins. *Neurology*, **45**, 1176–82.

Jagger, J., Prusoff, B.A., Cohen, D.J. et al. (1982). The epidemiology of Tourette's syndrome: a pilot study. *Schizopr. Bull.*, **8**, 267–78.

Jankovic, J. & Beach, J. (1997). Long-term effects of tetrabenazine in hyperkinetic movement disorders. *Neurology*, **48**, 358–62.

Jankovic, J., Glaze, D.G. & Frost, J.D.J.R. (1984). Effect of tetrabenazine on tics and sleep of Gilles de la Tourette's syndrome. *Neurology*, **34**, 688–92.

Kadesjö, B. & Gillberg, C. (2000). Tourette's disorder: epidemiology and comorbidity in primary school children. *J. Am. Acad. Child Adolesc. Psychiatry*, **39**, 548–55

Kano, Y., Ohta, M. & Nagai, Y. (1997). Differences in clinical characteristics between Tourette syndrome coprolalia. *Psych. Clin. Neurosci.*, **51**, 331–7.

Kiessling, L.S. (1989). Tic disorders associated with evidence of invasive group A beta hemolytic streptococcal disease [Abstract]. *Devel. Med. Child Neurol.*, **31**(Suppl. 59), 48.

King, R.A., Leckman, J.F., Scahill, L. & Cohen, D.J. (1999). Obsessive–compulsive disorder, anxiety and depression. In *Tourette's Syndrome – Tics, Obsessions, Compulsions: Developmental Psychopathology and Clinical Care*, ed. J.F. Leckman & D.J. Cohen, pp. 63–78. New York, NY: Wiley.

Kompoliti, K. & Goetz, C.G. (1998). Hyperkinetic movement disorders misdiagnosed as tics in Gilles de la Tourette syndrome. *Mov. Disord.*, **13**, 477–80.

Kondo, K. & Kabasawa, T. (1978). Improvement in Gilles de la Tourette syndrome after corticosteroid therapy. *Ann. Neurol.*, **4**, 387.

Kurlan, R. (1994). Hypothesis II: Tourette's syndrome is part of a clinical spectrum that includes normal brain development. *Arch. Neurol.*, **51**, 1145–50.

Kurlan, R. (1998). Tourette's syndrome and 'PANDAS': will the relation bear out? *Neurology*, **50**, 1530–4.

Kurlan, R., Eaper, V., Stern, J., McDermott, M.P. & Robertson, M.M. (1994a). Bilineal transmission in Tourette's syndrome families. *Neurology*, **44**, 2336–42.

Kurlan, R., Whitmore, D., Irvine, C., McDermott, M.P. & Como, P.G. (1994b). Tourette's syndrome in a special education population: a pilot study involving a single school district. *Neurology*, **44**, 699–702.

Kurlan, R., McDermott, M.P., Deeley, C. et al. (2001). Prevalence of tics in schoolchildren and association with placement in special education. *Neurology*, **57**, 1383–8.

Kwak, C.H., Hanna, P.A. & Jankovic, J. (2000). Botulinum toxin in the treatment of tics. *Arch. Neurol*, **57**, 1190–3.

Law, S.F. & Schachar, R.J. (1999). Do typical clinical doses of methylphenidate cause tics in children treated for attention–deficit hyperactivity disorder? *J. Am. Acad. Child Adolesc. Psychiatry*, **38**, 944–51.

Leckman, J.F., Detlor, J., Harcherik, D.F., Ort, S., Shaywitz, B.A. & Cohen, D.J. (1985). Short- and long- term treatment of Tourette's syndrome with clonidine: a clinical perspective. *Neurology*, **35**, 343–51.

Leckman, J.F., Riddle, M.A. & Hardin, M.T. (1989). The Yale Global Tic Severity Scale: initial testing of a clinician-rated scale of tic severity. *J. Am. Acad. Child Adolesc. Psychiatry*, **28**, 566–73.

Leckman, J.F., Hardin, M.T., Riddle, M.A., Stevenson, J., Ort, S.I. & Cohen, D.J. (1991). Clonidine treatment of Gilles de la Tourette's syndrome. *Arch. Gen. Psychiatry*, **48**, 324–8.

Leckman, J.F., Goodman, W.K., North, W.G. et al. (1994). Elevated cerebrospinal fluid levels of oxytocin in obsessive–compulsive disorder. Comparison with Tourette's syndrome and healthy controls. *Arch. Gen. Psychiatry*, **51**, 782–92.

Lichter, D.G., Jackson, L.A. & Schachter, M. (1995). Clinical evidence of genomic imprinting in Tourette's syndrome. *Neurology*, **45**, 924–8.

Lichter, D.G., Dmochowski, J., Jackson, L.A. & Trinidad, K.S. (1999). Influence of family history on clinical expression of Tourette's syndrome. *Neurology*, **52**, 308–19.

Lipinski, J.F., Sallee, F.R., Jackson, C. & Sethuraman, G. (1997). Dopamine agonist treatment of Tourette disorder in children: results of an open-lable trial of pergolide. *Mov. Disord.*, **12**, 402–7.

Lougee, L., Perlmutter, S.J., Nicolson, R., Garvey, M.A. & Swedo, S.E. (2000). Psychiatric disorders in first-degree relatives of children with pediatric autoimmune neuropsychiatric disorders associated with streptococcal infections (PANDAS). *J. Am. Acad. Child Adolesc. Psychiatry*, **39**, 1120–6.

Lowe, T.L., Cohen, D.J., Detlor, J., Kremenitzer, M.W. & Shaywitz, B.A. (1982). Stimulant medications precipitate Tourette's syndrome. *J. Am. Med. Assoc.*, **247**, 1729–31.

Lucas, A.R., Beard, C.M., Rajput, A.H. et al. (1982). Tourette syndrome in Rochester, Minnesota, 1968–1979. In *Gilles de la Tourette Syndrome*, ed. T.N. Chase & A.J. Friedhoff, p. 267. New York: Raven Press.

McMahon, W.M., van de Wetering, B.J.M., Filloux, F., Betit, K., Coon, H. & Leppert, M. (1996). Bilineal transmission and phenotypic variation of Tourette's disorder in a large pedigree. *J. Am. Acad. Child Adolesc. Psychiatry*, **35**, 672–80.

Maison, R.T., McDougle, C.J., van Dycke, et al. (1995). [*125*]Beta-CIT SPECT imaging demonstrates increased striatal dopamine binding in Tourette's syndrome. *Am. J. Psychiatry*, **152**, 1359–61.

Marras, C., Sime, E.A., Andrews, D.J. & Lang, A.E. (2000). Botulinum toxin injections for simple motor tics: a randomized, placebo-controlled trial. *Neurology*, **54**(Suppl. 3), A49.

Matarazzo, E.B. (1992). Tourette's syndrome treated with ACTH and prednisone: report of two cases. *J. Child. Adolesc. Psychopharmacol.*, **2**, 215–26.

Matthews, W.S. (1988). Attention deficits and learning disabilities in children with Tourette's syndrome. *Pediatr. Ann.*, **17**, 410–16.

Mendelson, W.B., Caine, E.D., Goyer, P. et al. (1980). Sleep in Gilles de la Tourette syndrome. *Biol. Psychiatry*, **15**, 339–43.

Merette, C., Brassard, A., Potvin, A. et al. (2000). Significant linkage for Tourette syndrome in a large French Canadian family. *Am. J. Hum. Genet.*, **67**, 1008–13.

Miguel, E.C., Coffey, B.J., Baer, L., Savage, C.R., Rauch, S.L. & Jenike, M.A. (1995). Phenomenology of intentional repetitive behaviors in obsessive–compulsive disorder and Tourette's syndrome. *J. Clin. Psychiatry*, **56**, 246–55.

Mostofsky, S.H., Wendlandt, J., Cutting, L., Denckla, M.B. & Singer, H.S. (1999). Corpus callosum measurements in girls with Tourette syndrome. *Neurology*, **53**, 1345–7.

Mostofsky, S.H., Lasker, A.G., Singer, H.S. et al. (2001). Oculomotor abnormalities in boys with Tourette syndrome with and without ADHD. *J. Am. Acad. Child Adolesc. Psychiatry*, **403**, 1464–72.

Muller-Vahl, K.R., Kolbe, H., Schneider, U. & Emrich, H.M. (1998). Cannabinoids: possible role in pathophysiology and therapy of Gilles de la Tourette syndrome. *Acta Psychiatr. Scand.*, **98**, 502–6.

Muller-Vahl, K.R., Schneider, U., Kolbe, J. & Emrich, H.M. (1999). Treatment of Tourette's syndrome with delta-9-tetrahydrocannabinol. *Am. J. Psychiatry*, **156**, 495.

Muller-Vahl, K.R., Berding, G., Kolbe, I.I. et al. (2000). Dopamine D2 receptor imaging in Gilles de la Tourette syndrome. *Acta Neurol. Scand.*, **101**, 165–71.

Nolan, E.E., Gadow, K.D. & Sprafkin, J. (1999). Stimulant medication withdrawn during long-term therapy in children with comorbid attention-deficit hyperactivity disorder and chronic multiple tic disorder. *Pediatrics*, **103**, 730–7.

Onofrj, M., Paci, C., D'Andreamatteo, G. & Toma, L. (2000). Olanzapine in severe Gilles de la Tourette syndrome: a 52-week double-blind cross-over study vs. low dose pimozide. *J. Neurol.*, **247**, 443–6.

Park, S., Como, P.G., Cui, L. et al. (1993). The early course of the Tourette's syndrome clinical spectrum. *Neurology*, **43**, 1712–15.

Park, K.N., Budman, C.L., Bruun, R.D. et al. (1996). Rage attacks in children and adolescents with Tourette's disorder. *Sci. Proc. Am. Acad. Child Adolesc. Psychiatr.*, **12**, 110.

Pauls, D.L. & Leckman, J.F. (1986). The inheritance of Gilles de la Tourette syndrome and associated behaviors: evidence for autosomal dominant transmission. *N. Eng. J. Med.*, **315**, 993–7.

Pauls, D.L., Leckman, J.F. & Cohen, D.J. (1993). Familial relationship between Gilles de la Tourette's syndrome, attention deficit disorder, learning disabilities, speech disorders, and stuttering. *J. Am. Acad. Child Adolesc. Psychiatr.*, **32**, 1044–50.

Pauls, D.L., Leckman, J.F. & Cohen, D.J. (1994). Evidence against a genetic relationship between Tourette's syndrome and anxiety, depression, panic and phobic disorders. *Br. J. Psychiatry*, **164**, 215–21.

Perlmutter, S.J., Leitman, S.F., Garvey, M.A. et al. (1999). Therapeutic plasma exchange and intravenous immunoglobulin for obsessive–compulsive disorder and tic disorders in childhood. *Lancet*, **354**, 1153–8.

Peterson, B.S., Riddle, M.A., Cohen, D.J. et al. (1993). Reduced basal ganglia volumes in Tourette's syndrome using three-dimensional reconstruction techniques from magnetic resonance images. *Neurology*, **43**, 941–9.

Peterson, B.S., Leckman, J.F., Cuncan, J. et al. (1994). Corpus callosum morphology from MR images in Tourette's syndrome. *Psychiatry Res.*, **55**, 85–99.

Peterson, B.S., Skudlarski, P., Anderson, A.W. et al. (1998). A functional magnetic resonance imaging study of tic suppression in Tourette syndrome. *Arch. Gen. Psychiatry*, **55**, 326–33.

Price, R.A., Kidd, K.K., Cohen, D.J. et al. (1985). A twin study of Tourette syndrome. *Arch. Gen. Psychiatry*, **42**, 815–20.

Rauch, S.L., Baer, L., Cosgrove, G.R. & Jenike, M.A. (1995). Neurosurgical treatment of Tourette's syndrome: a critical review [Review] *Compr. Psychiatry*, **36**, 141–56.

Richardson, E.P. (1982). Neuropathological studies of Tourette syndrome. In *Advances in Neurology*, ed. A.J. Friedhoff & T.N. Chase, Vol. 35, pp. 83–7. New York: Raven Press.

Riddle, M.A., Rasmusson, A.M., Woods, S.W. et al. (1992). SPECT imaging of cerebral blood flow in Tourette syndrome. In

Advances in Neurology, ed. T.N. Chase, A.J. Friedhoff & D.J. Cohen, Vol. 58, pp. 207–11. New York: Raven Press.

Robertson, M.M. (1989). Gilles de la Tourette syndrome: the current status. *Br. J. Psychiatry*, **154**, 147–69.

Robertson, M.M. (2000). Tourette syndrome, associated conditions and the complexities of treatment. *Brain*, **123**, 425–62.

Robertson, M.M., Channon, S., Baker, J. et al. (1993). The psychopathology of Gilles de la Tourette's syndrome: a controlled study. *Br. J. Psychiatry*, **162**, 114–17.

Robertson, M.M., Scull, D.A., Eapen, V. & Trimble, M.R. (1996). Risperidone in the treatment of Tourette syndrome: a retrospective case note study. *J. Psychopharmacol.*, **10**, 317–20.

Robertson, M.M., Banerjee, S., Hiley, P.J. & Tannock, C. (1997). Personality disorder and psychopathology in Tourette's syndrome: a controlled study. *Br. J. Psychiatry*, **171**, 283–6.

Sacks, O.W. (1982). Acquired tourettism in adult life. In *Advances in Neurology*, Vol. 35, ed. A.J. Friedhoff & T.N. Chase, pp. 89–92. New York: Raven Press.

Sallee, F.R., Nesbitt, L., Jackson, C., Sine, L. & Sethuraman, G. (1997). Relative efficacy of haloperidol and pimozide in children and adolescents with Tourette disorder. *Am. J. Psychiatry*, **8**, 1057–62.

Sanberg, P.R., Fogelson, H.M., Manderscheid, P.Z., Parder, K.W., Norman, A.B. & McConville, B.J. (1988). Nicotine gum and haloperidol in Tourette syndrome [letter]. *Lancet*, **i**, 592.

Sanberg, P.R., McConville, B.J., Fogelson, H.M. et al. (1989). Nicotine potentiates the effects of haloperidol in animals and in patients with Tourette syndrome. *Biomed. Pharmacother.*, **34**, 19–23.

Sanberg, P.R., Silver, A.A., Shyle, R.D. et al. (1997). Nicotine for the treatment of Tourette's syndrome. *Pharmacol. Ther.*, **74**, 21–5.

Santangelo, S.L., Pauls, D.L., Goldstein, J.M. et al. (1994). Tourette's syndrome: what are the influences of gender and comorbid obsessive compulsive disorder? *J. Am. Acad. Child Psychiatry*, **33**: 795–804.

Schuerholz, L.J., Baumgardner, T.L., Singer, H.S., Reiss, A.L. & Denckla, M.B. (1996). Neuropsychological status of children with Tourette's syndrome with and without attention deficit hyperactivity disorder. *Neurology*, **46**, 958–65.

Scott, B.L., Jankovic, J. & Conovan, D.T. (1996). Botulinum toxin infection into vocal cord in the treatment of malignant coprolalia associated with Tourette's syndrome. *Mov. Disord.*, **11**, 431–3.

Shapiro, A.K & Shapiro, E.S. (1982). An update of Tourette syndrome. *Am. J. Psychother.*, **36**, 379–90.

Shapiro, A.D. & Shapiro, E. (1984). Controlled study of pimozide vs. placebo in Tourette's syndrome. *J. Am. Acad. Child Psychiatry*, **23**, 161–73.

Shapiro, A.K., Shapiro, E.R., Young, J.G. et al. (1988). Measurement in tic disorders. In *Gilles de la Tourette Syndrome*, ed. A.K. Shapiro, E.S. Shapiro & J.G. Young, 2nd edn, pp. 451–80. New York: Raven Press.

Shapiro, E., Shapiro, A.K., Fulop, G. et al. (1989). Controlled study of haloperidol, pimozide, and placebo for the treatment of Gilles de la Tourette's syndrome. *Arch. Gen. Psychiatry.*, **46**, 722–30.

Shucard, D.W., Benedict, R.H., Tekok-Kilic, A. & Lichter, D.G. (1997). Slowed reaction time during a continous performance test in children with Tourette's syndrome. *Neuropsychology*, **11**, 147–55.

Silverstein, S.M., Como, P.G., Palumbo, D.R. et al. (1995). Multiple scores of attentional dysfunction in adults with Tourette's syndrome: comparison with attention deficit-hyperactivity disorder. *Neuropsychology*, **9**, 157–64.

Simonic, I., Gericke, G.S., Ott, J. & Weber, J.L. (1998). Identification of genetic markers associated with Gilles de la Tourette syndrome in an Afrikaner population. *Am. J. Hum. Genet.*, **63**, 839–46.

Singer, H.S. (1997). Neurobiology of Tourette syndrome. *Neurologic Clinics of North America*, **15**(2), 357–79.

Singer, H.S. & Rosenberg, L.A. (1989). Development of behavioral and emotional problems in Tourette syndrome. *Pediatr. Neurol.*, **43**, 950.

Singer, H.S. & Walkup, J.T. (1991). Tourette syndrome and other tic disorders: diagnosis, pathophysiology, and treatment. *Medicine*, **70**, 15–32.

Singer, H.S. & Wendlandt, J.T. (2001). Neurochemistry and synaptic neurotransmission in Tourette syndrome. In *Advances in Neurology*, ed. D.J. Cohen, C.G. Goetz & J. Jankovic, pp. 163–78. Philadelphia: Lippincott Williams and Wilkins.

Singer, H.S., Hahn, I-H., Krowiak, E. et al. (1990). Tourette syndrome: a neurochemical analysis of postmortem cortical brain tissue. *Ann. Neurol.*, **27**, 443–6.

Singer, H.S., Hahn, I-H. & Moran, T.H. (1991). Abnormal dopamine uptake sites in postmortem striatum from patients with Tourette syndrome. *Ann. Neurol.*, **30**, 558–62.

Singer, H.S., Reiss, A.L., Brown, J.E. et al. (1993). Volumetric MRI changes in basal ganglia of children with Tourette's syndrome. *Neurology*, **43**, 950–6.

Singer, H.S., Dickson, J., Martinie, D. et al. (1995a). Second messenger systems in Tourette's syndrome. *J. Neurol. Sci.*, **128**, 78–83.

Singer, H.S., Schuerholz, L.J. & Denckla, M.B. (1995b). Learning difficulties in children with Tourette syndrome. *J. Child Neurol.*, **10**(Suppl. 1), S58–61.

Singer, H.S., Guiliano, J.D., Hansen, B.H. et al. (1998). Antibodies against human putamen in children with Tourette Syndrome. *Neurology*, **50**, 1618–24.

Singer, H.S., Giuliano, J.D., Hansen, B.H. et al. (1999). Antibodies against a neuron-like (HTB-10 neuroblastoma) cell in children with Tourette syndrome. *Biol Psychiatry*, **46**, 775–80.

Singer, H.S., Giuliano, J.D., Zimmerman, A. & Walkup, J.T. (2000). Infection as an environmental stimuli in children with tic disorders. *Pediatr. Neurol.*, **22**, 380–3.

Spencer, T., Biederman, J., Hardin, M. et al. (1998). Disentangling the overlap between Tourette's disorder and ADHD. *J. Child Psychol. Psychiatr*y, **39**, 1037–44.

Stamenkovic, M., Schnidler, S.D., Aschauer, H.N. et al. (2000). Effective open-label treatment of Tourette' disorder with olanzapine. *Int. Clin. Psychopharmacol.*, **15**, 23–8.

Stern, E., Silbersweig, D.A., Chee, K.Y. et al. (2000). A functional neuroanatomy of tics in Tourette syndrome. *Arch. Gen. Psychiatry*, **57**, 741–8.

Stober, G., Hebebrand, J., Cichon, S. et al. (1999). Tourette syndrome and the norepinephrine transporter gene: results of a systematic mutation screening. *Am. J. Med. Genet.*, **88**, 158–63.

Stoetter, B., Blesa, R. & Chase, T.N. (1992). Regional abnormalities in cerebral glucose metabolism in Tourette's syndrome [abstract]. *Neurology*, **42**, 396.

Stollerman, G.H. (1991). Rheumatogenic streptococci and autoimmunity. *Clin. Immunol. Immunopathol.*, **61**, 131–42.

Swedo, S.E., Leonard, H.L., Mittleman, B.B. et al. (1997). Identification of children with pediatric autoimmune neuropsychiatric disorders associated with streptococcal infections by a marker associated with rheumatic fever. *Am. J. Psychiatry*, **154**, 110–12.

Swedo, S.E., Leonard, H.L., Garvey, M. et al. (1998). Pediatric autoimmune neuropsychiatric disorders associated with streptococcal infections: clinical description of the first 50 cases. *Am. J. Psychiatry*, **155**, 264–71.

The Tourette Syndrome Association International Consortium for Genetics. (1999). A complete genome screen in sib pairs affected by Gilles de la Tourette syndrome. *Am. J. Hum. Genet.*, **65**, 1428–36.

The Tourette Syndrome Classification Group. (1993). Definition and classification of tic disorders. *Arch. Neurol.*, **50**, 1013–16.

Thompson, M., Comings, D.E., Feder, L., George, S.R. & O'Dowd, B.F. (1998). Mutation screening of the dopamine D1 receptor gene in Tourette's syndrome and alcohol dependent patients. *Am. J. Med. Genet.*, **81**, 241–4.

Trimble, M.R., Whurr, R., Brookes, G., Robertson, M.M. & Traverse, L. (1998). Vocal tics in Gilles de la Tourette syndrome treated with botulinum toxin injections. *Mov. Disord.*, **13**, 617–19.

Trivedi, M.H. (1996). Functional neuroanatomy of obsessive compulsive disorder. *J. Clin. Psychiatr.* (Suppl.), 26.

Turpin, G. (1983). The behavioral management of tic disorders: a critical review. *Adv. Behav. Res. Therapy*, **5**, 203–45.

Voderholzer, U., Muller, N., Haag, C., Riemann, D. & Straube, A. (1997). Periodic limb movements during sleep are a frequent finding in patients with Gilles de la Tourette's syndrome. *J. Neurology*, **244**, 521–6.

Walkup, J.T., Rosenberg, L.A., Brown, J. & Singer, H.S. (1992). The validity of instruments measuring tic severity in Tourette's syndrome. *J. Am. Acad. Child Adolesc. Psychiatr.*, **31**, 472–7.

Walkup, J.T., Scahill, J.D. & Riddle, M.A. (1995). Disruptive behavior, hyperactivity, and learning disabilities in children with Tourette's syndrome. *Adv. Neurol.*, **65**, 259–72.

Walkup, J.T., LaBuda, M.C., Singer, H.S., Brown, J., Riddle, M.A. & Herko, O. (1996). Family study and segregation analysis of Tourette syndrome: evidence for a mixed model of inheritance. *Am. J. Hum. Genet.*, **59**, 684–93.

Walkup, J.T., Khan, S., Schuerholz, L., Paik, Y.S., Leckman, J.F. & Schultz, R.T. (1999). Phenomenology and natural history of tic-related ADHD and learning disabilities. In *Tourette's Syndrome–Tics, Obsessions, Compulsions: Developmental Psychopathology and Clinical Care*, ed. J.F. Leckman & D.J. Cohen, pp. 63–78. New York, NY: John Wiley.

Wand, R.R., Matazow, G.S., Shady, G.A., Furer, P. & Staley, D. (1993). Tourette syndrome: associated symptoms and most disabling features. *Neurosci. Biobehav. Rev.*, **17**, 271–5.

Wendlandt, J.T., Grus, F.H., Hansen, B.H. & Singer, H.S. (2001). Striatal antibodies in children with Tourette's syndrome: multivariate discriminant analysis of IgG repertoires. *J. Neuroimmunol.*, **119**, 106–13.

Wohlfart, G., Ingvar, D.H. & Hellberg, A.M. (1961). Compulsory shouting (Benedek's klazomania) associated with oculogyric spasms in chronic epidemic encephalitis. *Acta Psychiatr. Scand.*, **36**, 369–77.

Wolf, S.S., Jones, D.W., Knable, M.B. et al. (1996). Tourette syndrome: prediction of phenotypic variation in monozygotic twins by caudate nucleus D2 receptor binding. *Science*, **273**, 1225–7.

Wong, D.F., Singer, H.S., Brandt, J. et al. (1997). D2-like dopamine receptor density in Tourette syndrome measured by PET. *J. Nucl. Med.*, **38**, 1243–7.

Ziemann, U., Paulus, W. & Rosenberger, A. (1997). Decreased motor inhibition in Tourette's disorder: evidence from transcranial magnetic stimulation. *Am. J. Psychiatry*, **154**, 1277–84.

Zimmerman, A.M., Abrams, M.T., Giuliano, J.D., Denckla, M.B. & Singer, H.S. (2000). Subcortical volumes in female children with Tourette syndrome: support for a gender effect. *Neurology*, **54**, 224–9.

39

Cerebral palsy

Alexander H. Hoon, Jr[1] and Michael V. Johnston[2]

[1] Department of Pediatrics, Johns Hopkins University School of Medicine and Kennedy Krieger Institute, Baltimore, MD, USA
[2] Departments of Neurology and of Pediatrics, Johns Hopkins University School of Medicine and Kennedy Krieger Institute, Baltimore, MD, USA

Cerebral palsy (CP) is a clinical diagnostic term referring to a group of upper motor neuron syndromes secondary to disorders of early brain development (Johnston, 1998a). In addition to primary impairments in motor function, there may be associated problems with speech, cognition, epilepsy, visual impairment seizures and orthopedic deformities. Although CP is considered non-progressive, neurological findings may change or progress over time (Saint Hilaire et al., 1991; Scott & Jankovic, 1996).

CP is the most prevalent and costly form of chronic motor disability that begins in childhood. Although comprehensive longitudinal studies are limited, the majority of affected children live into adulthood (Crichton et al., 1995). In the United States, financial costs of care are estimated to be in the billions of dollars (Kuban & Leviton, 1994). The non-economic impact on affected individuals and their families is substantial (Murphy et al., 2000).

At the end of the nineteenth century, William Osler published his lectures on *The Cerebral Palsies of Children*, with a CP classification based on neuroanatomy, etiology and extremity involvement. 'Dividing the motor path into an upper corticospinal segment, extending from the cells of the cortex to the grey matter of the cord, and a lower spinomuscular, extending from the ganglia of the anterior horns to the motorial end plates, the palsies which I propose to consider have their anatomical seat in the former, and may result from a destructive lesion of the motor centres, or of the pyramidal tract, in hemisphere, internal capsule, crus or pons' (Osler, 1987). The current concept of CP is built on Osler's description, using imaging techniques, molecular genetic probes and measurement tools to further etiological understanding, improve classification and refine treatment options (Hoon & Melhem, 2000; Brunstrom et al., 2000).

Several strongly conflicting theories of causation have been proposed. In the mid-1800s, Sir William Little suggested that most CP was related to difficulties with delivery, a view which has had legal ramifications extending to the present time (Little, 1861). Approximately 50 years later, Sigmund Freud offered an alternative hypothesis that cerebral palsy reflected 'symptoms of deeper underlying influences which have dominated the development of the fetus' (Freud, 1968). Recent epidemiological studies indicate that most cases are related to prenatal disorders of genetic and environmental origin (Hagberg et al., 1996; Palmer et al., 1995). A small but distinguishable group results from perinatal hypoxic–ischemic insults, and a third group from injury in early childhood.

Modern neuroimaging techniques, including cranial ultrasound, computerized tomography (CT) and magnetic resonance (MR) imaging, provide clues to the timing and pathogenesis in 70–90% of patients (Truwit et al., 1992; Hoon, 1995). The ongoing development of advanced nuclear magnetic resonance methods, including diffusion-weighted imaging (Inder et al., 1999a; Johnson et al., 1999), diffusion tensor imaging (Mori et al., 1999) and MR spectroscopy (Shu et al., 1997; Novotny et al., 1998), hold promise to further etiological understanding.

Neuroimaging studies, including brain MR imaging, have demonstrated links between specific CP syndromes and patterns of selective vulnerability of specific components of developing motor systems (Dammann & Leviton, 1997; Nelson et al., 1998). These patterns are related to age-dependent changes in cellular metabolism, neuronal connectivity and circulation (Johnston, 1998b). Important examples readily seen with MR imaging include white matter vulnerability between 24 and 34 weeks, termed periventricular leukomalacia (PVL), as well as neuronal vulnerability at term (Okumura et al., 1997; Menkes & Curran, 1994).

Effective management of patients with CP requires the participation of a team of physicians, clinicians and therapists that provides careful, continuing neurodiagnostic evaluation along with therapeutic intervention to manage tone and other rehabilitative needs. Coordination of services with community based clinicians is also required to ensure that affected individuals have full opportunities to learn in school and participate in society.

Epidemiology

The overall prevalence of CP in developed countries is 2–3/1000 (Murphy et al., 1993; Hagberg et al., 1996). This figure has remained relatively constant over the last two decades, despite dramatic improvements in obstetrical and neonatal intensive care. This suggests that obstetrical interventions such as tocolysis (medication to slow or stop labour, eg, ritodrine, magnesium), the increased rate of Caesarean section and fetal heart rate monitoring have had little impact in reducing the incidence of CP (Canadian Preterm Labor Investigators Group, 1992; Scheller & Nelson, 1994; Parer & King, 2000).

Prematurity is strongly associated with CP (Surveillance of Cerebral Palsy in Europe, 2000). The improved survival of very low birthweight infants has led to an absolute increase in the number of children with the disorder. A second related factor is the recent increase in multiple births; there is a tendency for these infants to be low in birthweight, with a consequent increased risk of developing CP (Grether et al., 1993). Overall, while most premature infants develop normally, concerns have been expressed that one undesirable result of the success of neonatal medicine is the increased survival of children with severe neurodevelopmental handicaps, including CP (Hack & Fanaroff, 1999; Colver et al., 2000).

However, births at term are far more numerous than premature births and the majority of children with CP are born full term. Studies based on the NIH Perinatal Collaborative Project indicate that in more than 80% of cases, CP is associated with disorders of prenatal origin (Nelson & Ellenberg, 1986). Major risk factors for CP, in addition to low birthweight and prematurity, include maternal infections and/or fever at term, endocrine disturbances such as hypothyroidism and other factors listed in Table 39.1.

Cerebral palsy syndromes

CP can be classified into four broad groups based on differences in tone and limb involvement: bilateral spasticity, unilateral spasticity, extrapyramidal (dyskinetic) and

Table 39.1. Epidemiological factors associated with cerebral palsy

Maternal	Fetal/neonatal
History of fetal loss	Congenital malformations
Long interval between	Fetal growth retardation
menstrual cycles	Twin gestation
Low socioeconomic group	Abnormal fetal presentation
Mental retardation	Nuchal cord
Fever in labour	Prematurity
Chorioamnionitis	Premature separation of
Febrile urinary tract infections	placenta
Thrombophilic disorders	Newborn encephalopathy
Thyroid disorders	

Table 39.2. Common cerebral palsy syndromes

Bilateral spasticity	Extrapyramidal (dyskinetic)
Spastic diplegia	Bradykinesia
Spastic quadriplegia	Dystonia
Unilateral spasticity	Choreoathetosis
Spastic hemiplegia	Hemiballismus

hypotonia/ataxia, and further subcategorized into clinically recognizable syndromes such as spastic diplegia (Table 39.2). These syndromes often have differing etiological antecedents (Table 39.3) and relatively distinct clinical features (Table 39.4).

The majority of patients with CP have relatively symmetric upper motor neuron involvement, with spasticity being the primary neurologic abnormality. Most of these individuals have either spastic diplegia or spastic quadriplegia depending on whether the lower limbs are preferentially involved (diplegia) or whether all four extremities are heavily involved (quadriplegia). A smaller group with unilateral spasticity is referred to as hemiplegic CP.

Patients with abnormalities of tone and posture associated with basal ganglia involvement are classified as extrapyramidal (dyskinetic) CP. They usually have rigidity rather than spasticity, variability in truncal and appendicular tone, and additional manifestations of basal ganglia involvement including bradykinesia, dystonia, choreoathetosis or hemiballismus.

A small group of patients with atypical features such as hypotonia and or ataxia are classified with hypotonic/ataxic CP. Many patients with this type of congenital motor disorder, along with a substantial portion of the extrapyramidal

Table 39.3. *Common causes of cerebral palsy by syndrome*

Spastic diplegia	Spastic quadriplegia	Hemiplegia	Extrapyramidal
PVL[a]	PVL[a] (Severe)	Stroke[d]	Near-total asphyxia
Hereditary spastic paraparesis	Multicystic encephalomalacia[b]	Periventricular hemorrhagic infarction[e]	Kernicterus
HIV	Genetic-developmental[c]	Genetic-developmental[f]	Genetic-metabolic[g]
	Hydrocephalus		Hypothermic circulatory arrest (heart surgery)

Notes:

[a] Secondary to hypoxia–ischemia, maternal infection, fetal/neonatal infection and endocrine/metabolic disorders in the mother or fetus (e.g, thyroid disorder); [b] secondary to partial prolonged asphyxia, intrauterine infection, bacterial meningitis, non-accidental trauma; [c] holoprosencephaly, neuronal migration disorders, agenesis of the corpus callosum; [d] secondary to thrombophilic disorders, embolic disorders, trauma, infection; [e] (Grade 4 IVH); [f] unilateral schizencephaly; [g] mitochondrial disorders, methylmalonic aciduria, glutaric aciduria, type I Huntington disease, Hallervorden–Spatz.

Table 39.4. *Clinical features of cerebral palsy*

	Spastic diplegia	Spastic quadriplegia	Hemiplegia	Extrapyramidal	Hypotonia/ataxia
Tone	Spasticity	Spasticity	Spasticity	Rigidity	Hypotonia
Extremity involvement	LE>UE	LE=UE	Unilateral	UE>LE	UE=LE
Movement disorders	Clonus, spasms, toe walking	Clonus, spasms	Clonus, spasms	Dystonia, chorea, athetosis	Ataxia
Speech/swallowing	Mild impairment	Impaired	Intact	Impaired or absent speech	Variable
Cognitive impairment	Mild–moderate, learning disorders	Moderate–severe	Intact to mild	Intact to moderate	Variable
Associated problems	Strabismus, orthopedic deformities	Orthopedic deformities, epilepsy	Epilepsy	Orthopedic deformities Genetic–metabolic disorders	Undiagnosed genetic–metabolic disorders

group, have undiagnosed genetic/metabolic disorders including disorders of mitochondrial energy metabolism.

Spastic diplegia

Spastic diplegia is the clinical syndrome with spasticity greater in the legs than the arms, seen most commonly in children born prematurely. As premature infants usually receive careful developmental follow-up after discharge from the NICU, those with spastic diplegia are often identified during the first 6–12 months of life with signs of delayed motor development.

Spastic diplegia is primarily a disorder of developing white matter and is nearly always associated with neuropathological and neuroimaging findings of PVL. PVL is characterized by destruction of cerebral white matter in regions near the lateral ventricles. It consists of areas of focal necrosis with complete cellular loss, and surrounding regions with selective glial cell injury. PVL is easily demonstrated on MR imaging either as characteristic 'squared off', enlarged ventricles or as moderate ventricular enlargement with periventricular gliotic scarring, as seen on T_2-weighted sequences (Fig. 39.1). PVL is typically more prominent in the posterior ventricular system, particularly in the periatrial area, and is associated with thinning of the corpus callosum.

PVL is strongly associated with premature birth, with the highest incidence at 28 weeks gestation; later in gestation the incidence markedly declines, becoming far less frequent after 32 weeks gestation. While most children with PVL are born prematurely, a few are born at term. It is very likely that most of these children acquired PVL earlier

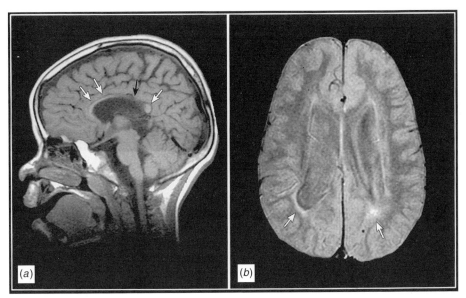

Fig. 39.1. These MR images obtained in childhood show the MR imaging findings of PVL. (*a*) Marked thinning of the corpus callosum (white arrows) with area of complete loss (black arrow); (*b*) Ventriculomegaly with scalloped irregular borders and periventricular gliosis (white arrows). Clinically the child had severe motor and cognitive impairments. (These images were previously published in Hoon & Melhem, 2000.)

during gestation (Miller et al., 2000). Preferential involvement of myelinating corticospinal fibres closest to the ventricles, which control the lower extremities, explains the greater involvement of the legs than the arms in spastic diplegia.

Considerable clinical and experimental evidence indicates that PVL and associated spastic diplegia reflect the selective vulnerability of immature oligodendroglia to stressors such as hypoxia–ischemia or infection at a critical period in their development (Dammann & Leviton, 1997). In many premature infants, PVL is probably produced by reductions in blood flow to marginally perfused periventricular regions as a result of dysfunctional vascular regulatory mechanisms related to prematurity and other contributing factors, including respiratory distress syndrome/prolonged mechanical ventilation, sepsis and necrotizing enterocolitis (Volpe, 1997). Experimental evidence suggests that glutamate released during ischemic episodes may trigger excitotoxic injury in immature oligodendroglia, in part because these cells are less protected from oxygen free radical damage than more mature oligodendroglia (Oka et al., 1993).

Infection, especially gram-negative infection, in either the mother or infant has also been associated with PVL based on clinical and experimental evidence. PVL has been reported to be more frequent in infants whose mothers had febrile urinary tract infections during pregnancy and in infants with sepsis related to necrotizing entercolitis. PVL may also be associated with thyroid or other endocrine metabolic disturbances.

In contrast, low grade (I–II) intraventricular bleeding does not appear to be a strong predictor of motor disability or PVL (Paneth, 1999). However, periventricular hemorrhagic infarction associated with grade IV hemorrhage is often associated with unilateral white matter destruction and asymmetric spasticity (Volpe, 1995).

MR imaging is quite sensitive and specific for PVL associated with spastic diplegia, and is useful for ruling out other causes of motor dysfunction. MR imaging is useful even in older patients with PVL since the changes appear to be permanent. Evidence from quantitative brain MR studies suggests that ventricular enlargement with PVL correlates with greater motor and cognitive impairment related to loss of white matter connections among different regions of the cerebral cortex (Melhem et al., 2000). Quantitative MR imaging is also useful for detecting neuronal abnormalities that may coexist with PVL (Inder et al., 1999b). By contrast, CT scanning is relatively insensitive to PVL, showing only the most severe involvement as enlargement of the ventricles with the characteristic 'squared-off' ventricular profile.

Cranial ultrasound is often informative in the newborn period when the anterior fontanel remains open. Cranial ultrasound can often detect the progression from

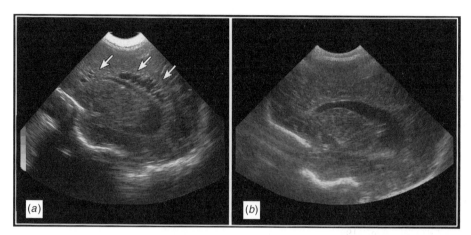

Fig. 39.2. These images show the evolution of cystic PVL on sagittal cranial ultrasound images in a 27 week infant. (*a*) Hypoechoic areas corresponding to cystic degeneration in periventricular white matter at 2 months of age (white arrows); (*b*) Resolution of the cysts with compensatory ventriuculomegaly at 6 months of age. The findings in Panel A carry a risk for CP which approaches 100%. (These images were previously published in Hoon & Melhem, 2000.)

periventricular enhanced signal intensity to cyst formation to ventricular enlargement that can occur during the postnatal period in premature infants (Fig. 39.2). Persistent ventriculomegaly seen on ultrasound in premature infants is a strong risk factor for CP, probably because it reflects loss of periventricular white matter (Paneth et al., 1994).

Spastic quadriplegia

Spastic quadriplegia is the pattern of bilateral spasticity affecting all four extremities. It is the result of a broader range of pathological insults than spastic diplegia, including severe PVL, multicystic encephalomalacia, genetic/developmental brain malformations and hydrocephalus. As with other forms of CP, low birthweight, prematurity and complicated neonatal course are important risk factors. Delayed motor development in the first year is usually more prominent than in spastic diplegia.

In the subgroup with severe PVL, extensive white matter involvement leads to disruption of arm as well as leg fibres as they descend from the motor cortex. These children are often born very prematurely. Some may have also sustained posthemorrhagic hydrocephalus with pressure-related disruption of white matter.

Patients in a second major subgroup have relatively symmetric destructive lesions of the cerebral cortex. One important type of destructive lesion is multicystic encephalomalacia, which refers to multiple cystic cavities in the cortex separated by glial septations. It results from diffuse insults occurring from late gestation through infancy (Barkovich, 2000). It can be produced by intrauter-

ine infections, partial prolonged hypoxia–ischemia, perinatal herpes simplex, bacterial meningitis, or non-accidental trauma during infancy. Parasagittal watershed infarctions associated with hypotension in sick term infants may present as quadriplegia with more weakness in the shoulders and upper extremities (Pasternak, 1987).

A third subgroup includes patients with genetic/developmental brain malformations, such as holoprosencephaly, lissencephaly, pachygyria and agenesis of the corpus callosum which commonly lead to microcephaly and spastic quadriplegia. TORCH infections (toxoplasmosis, rubella, cytomegalovirus, herpes, and other bacterial and viral) can also result in pachygryria, with similar clinical findings. Brain MR imaging is very useful for distinguishing these disorders, some of which have specific recurrence risks (Hoon & Melhem, 2000). CT is still useful for detecting intracranial calcifications.

A final common subgroup includes those with fetal or neonatal hydrocephalus, reflecting a variety of pathologies affecting the development and maintenance of CSF pathways, including aqueductal stenosis and Dandy Walker syndrome. Outcome is related to the presence and severity of associated anomalies (Pretorius et al., 1985) as well as the need for multiple shunt revisions.

Hemiplegic cerebral palsy

One-third of patients with CP have unilateral spasticity, termed hemiplegic CP, which usually affects the arms more than the legs. A higher proportion of these infants are born at term than in groups of patients with diplegia or quadri-

Table 39.5. Thrombophilic disorders associated with vascular occlusions in CP

Factor V Leiden
N-Methylene-tetrahydrofolate reductase deficiency
Prothrombin mutation
Deficiency of Protein S, Protein C, or Antithrombin III
Anticardiolipin antibodies

plegia. Several studies indicate that most term infants with hemiplegic CP sustained cerebral infarctions or strokes prior to birth (Scher et al., 1991; Nelson, 1991). Neuropathological and neuroimaging studies demonstrate the presence of wedge-shaped lesions suggesting vascular infarctions or irregularities in the periventricular white matter (Taudorf et al., 1984). In a large postmortem study of cerebral infarctions in neonates, arterial vascular occlusions were found to be the most common lesion, and the most common associated cause was sepsis with or without disseminated intravascular coagulation (Barmada et al., 1979). Venous sinus thrombosis is probably also a significant cause of hemiparesis, though it has been difficult to identify until the era of modern neuroimaging.

In a study of focal white matter necrosis in infants, markers for infection are prominent risk factors as are congenital malformations, placental vascular malformations, multiple births and maternal and intra-amniotic infections (Leviton & Paneth, 1990). Prenatal white matter necroses and hemipareses have also been found to be associated with polyhydramnios, and the in utero death of one twin. In premature infants, hemiparetic CP can be produced by Grade IV intraventricular hemorrhages with periventricular white matter infarction due to venous infarction. Overall, hemiparetic CP is far more likely than other syndromes to be caused by infarctions secondary to vascular occlusions.

Recently, inherited thrombophilic disorders such as Factor V Leiden have been recognized to be a significant cause of vascular occlusions in fetuses and infants, and may be nearly as frequent as infection as a precipitating cause of hemiparetic CP (Thorarensen et al., 1997) (Table 39.5). Recent studies suggest that Factor V leiden may be responsible for obstetrical complications in mothers such as pre-eclampsia, as well as for bleeding disorders and strokes in infants (Harum et al., 1999). In one study of mothers with complicated pregnancies, acquired or inherited thrombophilic disorders were diagnosed in more than half of these women (Kupferminc et al., 1999). These studies suggest that patients with hemiparetic CP should be evaluated carefully for possible thrombophilic disorders, which may carry a recurrence risk in subsequent pregnancies.

A third group of disorders which may cause hemiplegia is schizencephaly, some forms of which may have a genetic etiology (Brunelli et al., 1996). Unilateral schizencephaly is associated with hemiplegic CP, while bilateral schizencephaly results in spastic quadriplegia.

Brain MR imaging is the most useful diagnostic modality in patients with hemiplegia. It provides clear distinction between vascular insults which are lined with gliotic white matter and the grey matter lining seen in schizencephaly (Candy et al., 1993).

Extrapyramidal cerebral palsy

Approximately 20% of patients with CP have a prominent extrapyramidal syndrome with rigidity more than spasticity and involvement of the upper extremities more than lower extremities. It is usually associated with a marked reduction in speech production but relatively preserved intelligence. Most of these individuals have an overall reduction and slowing of movement (bradykinesia), but some have hyperkinetic disorders including chorea, athetosis, dystonia and hemiballismus. (An additional group of children have spastic diplegia or quadriplegia associated with extrapyramidal signs, and are referred to as having a 'mixed' CP.)

The entire group of patients with extrapyramidal CP is quite heterogeneous because of the wide spectrum of acquired and inherited disorders of the basal ganglia responsible for the syndrome (Hoon et al., 1997). In some patients the motor disability remains stable over time, while in others there is progressive neurological decline. This important distinction may require careful, repeated neurological examinations to establish.

One important subgroup of extrapyramidal CP patients results from selective injury to the basal ganglia, especially the putamen and thalamus, occurring in acute near-total asphyxia in the last few weeks of a term gestation (Johnston & Hoon, 1998). Several authors have reported the neuroimaging picture of basal ganglia injury in these patients, with MR imaging proving to be particularly helpful (Menkes & Curran, 1994; Pasternak & Gorey, 1998). Early MR imaging, within a few weeks of injury, often shows increased signal on T_1-weighted images in the caudate, putamen and thalami while follow-up is more likely to show enhanced T_2-weighted signal in the posterior portion of the putamen and lateral thalami. The peri-rolandic cerebral cortex is sometimes involved as well. The selective vulnerability of these regions may reflect hyperactivity of prominent excitatory glutamate-containing neurons that

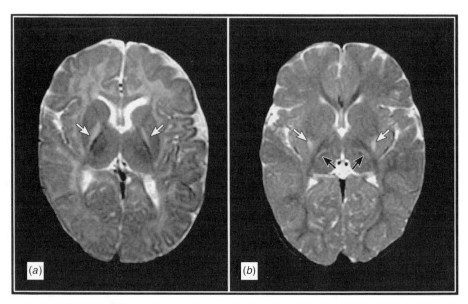

Fig. 39.3. MR images from two infants with clinically similar neonatal encephalopathies, including seizures and ventilatory failure. (*a*) Globus pallidus hyperintensities (white arrows) seen in bilirubin encephalopathy; (*b*) Putaminal (white arrows) and thalamic (black arrows) hyperintensities seen in perinatal hypoxic–ischemic encephalopathy. Both result in extrapyramidal CP.

connect these regions with the cerebral cortex in reciprocal circuits. This pattern of selective vulnerability has also been reproduced in animal models of hypoxia–ischemia. MR imaging can provide strong evidence that hypoxic–ischemic injury to the basal ganglia from asphyxia is responsible for extrapyramidal CP in some patients.

Other patients with extrapyramidal CP may have heterogeneous disorders that require careful diagnostic evaluation. This subgroup of patients is most likely to contain undiagnosed metabolic–genetic disorders, where careful follow-up is important to detect changes that may reflect a progressive disorder. MR imaging can readily distinguish patients with extrapyramidal CP associated with lesions in the globus pallidus from those with putaminal injury in asphyxia. Pallidal injuries are common in kernicterus from hyperbilirubinemia (Fig. 39.3), but may also be caused by mitochondrial disorders with or without lactic acidosis. Some patients with extrapyramidal CP may have pallidal injury after heart surgery as infants (Kupsky et al., 1995). These patients are more likely than others to have hyperkinetic disorders such as chorea or hemiballismus.

Patients with degenerative disorders that affect the globus pallidus, such as Hallervorden–Spatz disease, may progress at such a slow rate initially that they appear to have idiopathic extrapyramidal CP. Other disorders that can present as undiagnosed CP include glutaric aciduria Type I and juvenile Huntington disease, both of which have prominent basal ganglia lesions on MR imaging (Morton et al., 1991;

Lenti & Bianchini, 1993). Methylmalonic aciduria can also present with prominent lesions of the globus pallidi after metabolic 'strokes' (Heidenreich et al., 1988). Patients with other, more obscure disorders of intermediary or neurotransmitter metabolism, or of idiopathic or genetic dystonia, may present initially as extrapyramidal CP. Rarely, patients with a defect in GTP cyclohydrolase (Segawa's disease or dopa-responsive dystonia) may present with severe idiopathic extrapyramidal CP early in life (Korf, 1998).

Because of the diverse nature of disorders that can present as extrapyramidal CP, this group of patients requires careful diagnostic evaluation. The etiological evaluation should include brain MR imaging, urine organic acids, plasma amino acids, lactate and chromosomes. Evaluation of CSF biopterin, neurotransmitter and amino acid metabolism is often indicated, especially in patients with idiopathic extrapyramidal CP with normal MR scans. Careful follow-up is important as many of these patients progress or change over time. Furthermore, patients with extrapyramidal CP secondary to acquired lesions such as asphyxia may progress or display new movement disorders including dystonia in teenage or adult years, probably due to continuing reorganization of the nervous system.

Hypotonic/ataxic cerebral palsy

A few patients with congenital motor disorders present predominantly with hypotonic truncal tone, delayed

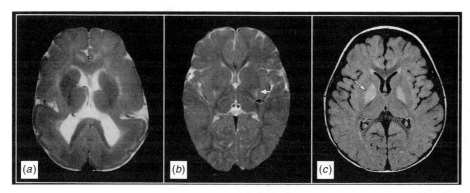

Fig. 39.4. MR images from three children presenting with severe CP. (*a*) Lissencephaly in Miller–Dieker syndrome; (*b*) perinatal hypoxic–ischemic encephalopathy (from Fig. 39.3), and (*c*) methymalonic acidemia with globus pallidus hyperintensities (white arrows).

motor milestones and an abnormal gait with an ataxic appearance (Dubowitz, 1980). These patients are distinguished by the lack of lower motor neuron signs, suggesting a disorder of upper motor neurons. Like extrapyramidal CP, this is a very heterogeneous group, which probably contains many patients with undiagnosed genetic-metabolic disorders. This group is probably the least likely of all the cerebral palsy syndromes to be caused by an acquired condition such as asphyxia. Careful neurodiagnostic evaluation of these patients is also indicated with MR as well as metabolic testing. Recognized disorders include congenital malformations of the cerebellar vermis with mega-cisterna magna, mitochondrial disorders, carbohydrate-deficient glycoprotein disorder, disorders of neurotransmitter metabolism, and Joubert's syndrome. Periodic re-evaluation of these children is indicated.

Diagnostic evaluation

The evaluation of patients with motor delay should begin with a careful history, including details of the prenatal, perinatal and postnatal course. Maternal perception of decreased fetal movement is an important sign of prenatal onset. If there is no history of an acute neonatal encephalopathy, then the etiology is not related to perinatal events. Family history is important to identify those with potential genetic disorders. The review of systems should include questions about vision, hearing, snoring, feeding, bowel and bladder function as well as any cardiac and pulmonary problems. The neurological examination should be comprehensive, including careful observation for adventitious movements, including chorea, athetosis, hemiballismus and dystonia.

An assessment of functional abilities should be obtained, and measures of cognitive function whenever possible. The functional assessment of children with CP is best done in conjunction with skilled physical and occupational therapists. Children may be classified both by the extent of mobility aids required (from point canes to wheelchairs), as well as by their ability to ambulate independently in various settings (from home to gymnasium to community). Physical therapists can be of great benefit here, recommending appropriate aids to mobility as well as setting functional goals for the child, which will foster independence. The cognitive evaluation should be done by a neuropsychologist experienced in the assessment of intelligence in motor impaired patients to provide an accurate reflection of abilities.

The diagnostic evaluation should commence with an MR imaging study (Fig. 39.4). Findings from this study can often be used to determine the need for additional testing. For example, in a child with extrapyramidal CP and imaging abnormalities in the globus pallidus, a comprehensive evaluation for genetic–metabolic disorders should be completed. In those with developmental brain malformations including neuronal migration disorders such as lissencephaly and schizencephaly, specific molecular testing may be important to identify an etiology and to determine recurrence risk (Gleeson et al., 2000).

Depending on the clinical setting, there are a number of other diagnostic modalities. All children with CP should have an ophthalmological evaluation by a specialist experienced in CP. This is important both because of the large number who have refractive errors as well as the potential diagnostic clues which can be identified from a dilated examination of the optic nerve and retina.

Based on clinical examination, if there is evidence to suggest a genetic etiology, a karyotype as well as specific molecular probes should be obtained. If there is evidence of rigidity on examination, a disorder of energy production involving mitochondrial function should be considered, with a lactate, plasma amino acid and urinary organic acid profile obtained. If there is significant ataxia, the cerebellum should be carefully assessed on MR imaging, with testing to include various forms of SCA as well as carbohydrate deficient glycoprotein disorders; Angelman syndrome should also be considered.

If the initial diagnostic work-up is unrevealing, ongoing clinical follow-up may reveal further information that will assist in diagnosis and clinical care. While many parents seek 'closure' of the search for cause so that they can proceed with rehabilitation, most nevertheless remain interested in establishing the cause, and will continue with a carefully orchestrated ongoing diagnostic search.

Associated impairments

While CP refers primarily to the motor involvement, affected individuals frequently have a range of associated impairments (Table 39.3). Up to half of children with CP have mental retardation. A third have seizure disorders. Learning disabilities are also linked with CP. Impairments in hearing and vision should also be considered, as well as disorders of speech, swallowing and feeding.

Furthermore, for the affected child, there may be social and emotional limitations. These children often have a difficult time once they become aware of differences from their peers. It is important for families to encourage them to develop skills in other areas, which may include horseback riding, and in other forms of therapeutic recreation. This will promote a sense of confidence and self-esteem.

While educational opportunities are often available until age 21 under the provisions of the Individuals with Disabilities Education Act (IDEA), rehabilitative and supportive services are less well organized in adulthood. Despite the American with Disabilities Act, barriers to employment continue to exist.

Rehabilitation

There are a number of rehabilitative motor interventions for individuals with CP. Depending on the clinical situation, the rehabilitative goals may be ease of care, preventing orthopedic deformities or facilitating function. The specific goals of affected individuals and their families should be carefully considered in formulating rehabilitation plans.

In young children, the mainstays of rehabilitation are occupational and physical therapy (Bartlett & Palisano, 2000). These techniques serve to lessen the effects of inhibitory reflexes and to facilitate the acquisition of gross and fine motor skills. They may also have benefit in other areas of development including language, and the promotion of confidence and self esteem.

In children with spasticity, there may be progressive orthopedic deformities. In the past, surgeries were done in a sequential fashion, one at a time. However, more recently, multiple soft tissue and/or bone procedures have been conducted simultaneously (Fabry et al., 1999). Initially, soft tissue releases are usually employed for those with contractures. Bony procedures to the leg, hip and spine may also be required. Whether pharmacological interventions will lessen the need for orthopedic surgery is unclear at this time.

For patients with localized spasticity, botulinum toxin has been effectively utilized to improve gross and fine motor abilities (Wissel et al., 1999; Koman et al., 2000). Beneficial effects are related to the temporary weakening of specific muscle groups interfering with function. Botulinum injections are extremely safe, with effects lasting up to three to four months.

A range of oral pharmacological agents has been effectively utilized to diminish spasticity (Pranzatelli, 1996). Diazepam has been employed in the past, although concerns over cognitive side effects limited its use. More recently, baclofen has been preferentially used, recognizing that there are less cognitive side effects from this drug. However, patients should be cautioned against abruptly discontinuing baclofen, which can precipitate hallucinations or seizures. Depending on the clinical situation, other antispasticity agents such as dantrolene and tiazadine can be used.

For patients with extrapyramidal CP, pharmacological agents modulating dopamine action in the striatum have been effectively utilized. For those with chorea, drugs to deplete dopamine such as reserpine, tetrabenazine, clonzapam and carbamazepine have been used. For patients with dystonia, athetosis or bradykinesia, drugs to increase dopamine flux including trihexyphenidyl and levodopa (usually administered with carbidopa) have been effectively employed.

Recently, intrathecal baclofen, delivered by a programmable pump placed in the abdomen connected to a catheter ending in the intrathecal space, has been employed for patients with spasticity of spinal as well as cerebral origin (Penn & Kroin, 1985; Albright et al., 1993). Studies have indicated that intrathecal baclofen effectively reduces spasticity (Gilmartin et al., 2000), and may be of benefit in improving function (Latash & Penn, 1996). Intrathecal baclofen has also been reported to be of benefit in dystonic CP (Albright et al., 1996). Complications of this therapy include catheter kinking as well as infection, possibly requiring replacement of the catheter or pump.

Selective dorsal rhizotomy, a neurosurgical procedure in which a percentage of sensory rootlets in the LS spine are cut, is felt by some groups to be an effective intervention for spastic diplegia (Park & Owen, 1992). In carefully chosen patients with relatively pure forms of spastic diplegia, this procedure reduces spasticity and improves function (Steinbok et al., 1997). However, other groups have reported no benefit from this procedure over intensive physical therapy (Graubert et al., 2000). Furthermore, there may be both short- and long-term complications from this procedure (Abbott, 1992; Tuir & Kalen, 2000).

Recently, there has been interest in stereotactic neurosurgical procedures similar to those performed for Parkinson disease (De Salles, 1996). Preliminary work indicates that in carefully selected patients, the severity of dystonia and hemiballismus may be decreased. Depending on the clinical setting, both ablative as well as neural stimulation procedures may be done.

Because therapies have not achieved all the goals that families want for their children or for themselves, parents and those affected may seek alternative therapies. Such therapies are wide ranging, from herbal remedies to hyperbaric oxygen. While some may be beneficial, each should be carefully considered. Care should be taken as some herbs may have significant toxicities, and with regard to hyperbaric oxygen tanks, there have been concerns that high oxygen tension may damage developing white matter pathways (Huang et al., 2000).

Prognosis

Families as well as affected individuals often seek information about long-term prognosis so that appropriate medical, financial and life care plans can be made. They may also worry about whether other family members are at risk. The key step to providing information in these matters is to conduct a comprehensive etiological evaluation at the time that the diagnosis of CP is made. Such a work-up can provide specifics of prognosis and recurrence risk when a recognized genetic or metabolic disorder is identified, as well as reassurance when a sporadic cause is identified.

Given the progressive nature of some CP syndromes, ongoing medical follow-up is required both for the individual patient, as well as to establish guidelines for groups of patients. For example, some adults with extrapyramidal CP are at risk for progressive cervical spine disease, which if untreated can lead to sudden quadriplegia (Harada et al. 1996) (Fig. 39.5). Others may develop progressive neuro-

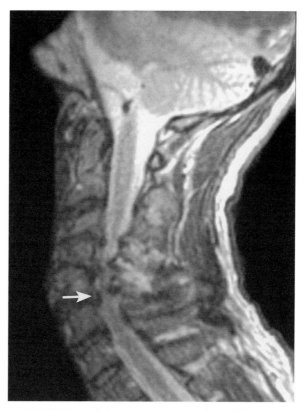

Fig. 39.5. MR image from an adult with extrapyramidal CP, who sustained cord compression (white arrow) from repetitive head movements used to control a communication system.

logical symptoms necessitating new treatment modalities (Scott & Jankovic, 1996).

In conclusion, advances in neurobiology, as well as brain imaging, have expanded the understanding of the pathogenesis of CP. Combining imaging techniques with clinical examination can refine classification and establish homogeneous groups so that rehabilitative interventions can be more effectively assessed.

References

Abbott, R. (1992). Complications with selective posterior rhizotomy. *Pediatr. Neurosurg.*, **18**, 43–7.

Albright, A.L., Barron, W.B., Fasick, M.P., Polinko, P. & Janosky, J. (1993). Continuous intrathecal baclofen infusion for spasticity of cerebral origin. *J. Am. Med. Assoc*, **270**, 2475–7.

Albright, A.L., Barry, M.J., Fasick, P., Barron, W. & Shultz, B. (1996). Continuous intrathecal baclofen infusion for symptomatic generalized dystonia. *Neurosurgery*, **38**, 934–8.

Barkovich, J.A. (2000). *Pediatric Neuroimaging*, 3rd edn, pp. 157–209. Philadelphia: Lippincott Williams & Wilkins.

Barmada, M.A., Moossy, J. & Shuman, R.M. (1979). Cerebral infarcts with arterial occlusion in neonates. *Ann. Neurol.*, **6**, 495–502.

Bartlett, D.J. & Palisano, R.J. (2000). A multivariate model of determinants of motor change for children with cerebral palsy. *Phys. Ther.*, **80**, 598–614.

Brunelli, S., Faiella, A., Capra, V. et al. (1996). Germline mutations in the homeobox gene EMX2 in patients with severe schizencephaly. *Nat. Genet.*, **12**, 94–6.

Brunstrom, J.E., Bastian, A.J., Wong, M. & Mink, J.W. (2000). Motor benefit from levodopa in spastic quadriplegic cerebral palsy. *Ann. Neurol.*, **47**, 662–5.

Canadian Preterm Labor Investigators Group (1992). Treatment of preterm labor with the beta-adrenergic agonist ritodrine. *N. Engl. J. Med.* **327**, 308–12.

Candy, E.J., Hoon, A.H., Capute, A.J. & Bryan, R.N. (1993). MRI in motor delay: important adjunct to classification of cerebral palsy. *Pediatr. Neurol.*, **9**, 421–9.

Colver, A.F., Gibson, M., Hey, E.N., Jarvis, S.N., Mackie, P.C. & Richmond, S. (2000). Increasing rates of cerebral palsy across the severity spectrum in north-east England 1964–1993. The North of England Collaborative Cerebral Palsy Survey. *Arch. Dis. Child Fetal Neonatal Ed.*, **83**, F7–12.

Crichton, J.U., Mackinnon, M. & White, C.P. (1995). The life-expectancy of persons with cerebral palsy. *Dev. Med. Child Neurol.*, **37**, 567–76.

Dammann, O. & Leviton, A. (1997). Maternal intrauterine infection, cytokines, and brain damage in the preterm newborn. *Ped. Res.*, **42**, 1–8.

De Salles, A.A.F. (1996). Role of stereotaxis in the treatment of cerebral palsy. *J. Child Neurol.*, **11**(Suppl. 1), S43–50.

Dubowitz, V. (1980). *The Floppy Infant*, 2nd edn. Philadelphia: J.B. Lippincott Co.

Fabry, G., Liu, X.C. & Moleraers, G. (1999). Gait pattern in patients with spastic diplegic cerebral palsy who underwent staged operations. *J. Pediatr. Orthop.*, **8**, 33–8.

Freud, S. (1968). *Infantile Cerebral Paralysis*. Coral Gables: University of Miami Press.

Gilmartin, R., Bruce, D., Storrs, B.B. et al. (2000). Intrathecal baclofen for management of spastic cerebral palsy: multicenter trial. *J. Child Neurol.*, **15**, 71–7.

Gleeson, J.G., Minnerath, S., Kuzniecky, R.I. et al. (2000). Somatic and germline mosaic mutations in the doublecortin gene are associated with variable phenotypes. *Am. J. Hum. Genet.*, **67**, 574–81.

Graubert, C., Song, K.M., McLaughlin, J.F. & Bjornson, K.F. (2000). Changes in gait at 1 year post-selective dorsal rhizotomy: results of a prospective randomized study. *J. Pediatr. Orthop.*, **20**, 496–500.

Grether, J.K., Nelson, K.B. & Cummins, S.K. (1993). Twinning and cerebral palsy: experience in four northern California counties, births 1983 through 1985. *Pediatrics*, **92**, 854–8.

Hack, M. & Fanaroff, A.A. (1999). Outcomes of children of extremely low birthweight and gestational age in the 1990's. *Early Hum. Dev.*, **53**, 193–218.

Hagberg, B., Hagberg, G., Olow, I. & van Wendt, L. (1996). The changing panorama of cerebral palsy in Sweden. VII. Prevalence and origin in the birth year period 1987–90. *Acta Paediatr.*, **85**, 954–60.

Harada, T., Ebara, S., Anwar, M.M. et al. (1996). The cervical spine in athetoid cerebral palsy: a radiological study of 180 patients. *J. Bone Joint Surg. Br.*, **78**, 613–19.

Harum, K.H., Hoon, A.H. & Casella, J.F. (1999). Factor V Leiden: a risk factor for cerebral palsy. *Dev. Med. Child Neurol.*, **41**, 781–5.

Heidenreich, R., Natowicz, M., Hainline, B.E. et al. (1988). Acute extrapyramidal syndrome in methylmalonic acidemia: 'metabolic stroke' involving the globus pallidus. *J. Pediatr.*, **113**, 1022–7.

Hoon, A.H. (1995). Neuroimaging in the high risk infant: relationship to outcome. *J. Perinatol.*, **15**, 389–94.

Hoon, A.H. & Melhem, E.R. (2000). Neuroimaging: applications in disorders of early brain development. *J. Dev. Behav. Pediatr.*, **21**, 291–302.

Hoon, A.H., Reinhardt, E.M., Kelley, R.I. et al. (1997). Brain MR imaging in suspected extrapyramidal cerebral palsy: observations in distinguishing genetic-metabolic from acquired etiologies. *J. Pediatr.*, **131**, 240–5.

Huang, F., Wu, J., Lin, H., Mao, S., Kang, B. & Wan, F. (2000). Prolonged exposure to hyperbaric oxygen induces neuronal damage in primary rat cortical cultures. *Neurosci. Lett.*, **293**, 159–62.

Inder, T., Huppi, P.S., Zientara, G.P et al. (1999a). Early detection of periventricular leukomalacia by diffusion-weighted magnetic resonance imaging techniques. *J. Pediatr.*, **134**, 631–4.

Inder, T.E., Huppi, P.S., Warfield, S. et al. (1999b). Periventricular white matter injury in the premature infant is followed by reduced cerebral cortical gray matter volume at term. *Ann. Neurol.*, **46**, 755–60.

Johnson, A.J., Lee, B.C.P. & Lin, W. (1999). Echoplanar diffusion-weighted imaging in neonates and infants with suspected hypoxic–ischemic injury: correlation with patient outcome. *Am. J. Radiol.*, **172**, 219–26.

Johnston, M.V. (1998a). Can a mother's infection damage her baby's brain? *Neurology Network Commentary*, **2**, 305–11.

Johnston, M.V. (1998b). Selective vulnerability of the neonatal brain. *Ann. Neurol. (Editorial)*, **44**, 155–6.

Johnston, M.V. & Hoon, A.H. (1998). Excitotoxicity and patterns of brain injury from fetal or perinatal asphyxia. In *Asphyxia and Fetal Brain Damage*, ed. D. Maulik, pp. 113–25. Wiley-Liss, Inc.

Koman, L.A., Mooney, J.F. Smith, B.P., Walker, F. & Leon, J.M. (2000). Botulinum toxin type A neuromuscular blockade in the treatment of lower extremity spasticity in cerebral palsy: a randomized, double-blind, placebo-controlled trial. *J. Pediatr. Orthop.*, **20**, 108–15.

Korf, B.R. (1998). The hereditary dystonias: an emerging story with a twist. *Ann. Neurol.*, **44**, 4–5.

Kuban, K.C.K. & Leviton, A. (1994). Cerebral palsy. *N. Engl. J. Med.*, **330**, 188–95.

Kupferminc, M.J., Eldor, A., Steinman, N. et al. (1999). Increased frequency of genetic thrombophilia in women with complications of pregnancy. *N. Engl. J. Med.*, **340**, 9–13.

Kupsky, W.J., Drozd, M.A. & Barlow, C.F. (1995). Selective injury of the globus pallidus in children with post-cardiac surgery choreic syndrome. *Dev. Med. Child Neurol.*, **37**, 135–44.

Latash, M.L. & Penn, R.D. (1996). Changes in voluntary motor control induced by intrathecal baclofen in patients with spasticity of different etiology. *Physiother Res. Int.*, **1**, 229–46.

Lenti, C. & Bianchini, E. (1993). Neuropsychological and neuroradiological study of a case of early-onset Huntington's chorea. *Dev. Med. Child Neurol.*, **35**, 1007–14.

Leviton, A. & Paneth, N. (1990). White matter damage in preterm newborns – an epidemiologic perspective. *Early Hum. Dev.*, **24**, 1–22.

Little, W.J. (1861). On the influence of abnormal parturition, difficult labors, premature birth and asphyxia neonatorum, on the mental and physical condition of the child, especially in relation to deformities. *Trans. Obstet. Soc. Lond.*, **3**, 293–344.

Melhem, E.R., Hoon, A.H., Ferrucci, J.T. et al. (2000). Periventricular leukomalacia: relationship between lateral ventricular volume on brain MR images and severity of cognitive and motor impairment. *Radiology*, **214**, 199–204.

Menkes, J.H. & Curran, J. (1994). Clinical and MR correlates in children with extrapyramidal cerebral palsy. *Am. J. Neuroradiol.*, **15**, 451–7.

Miller, S.P., Shevell, M.I., Patenaude, Y. & Gorman, A.M. (2000). Neuromotor spectrum of periventricular leukomalacia in children born at term. *Ped. Neurol.*, **23**, 155–9.

Mori, S., Crain, B.J., Chacko, V.P. & van Zijl, P.C.M. (1999). Three-dimensional tracking of axonal projections in the brain by magnetic imaging. *Ann. Neurol.*, **45**, 265–9.

Morton, D.H., Bennett, M.J., Seargeant, L.E., Nichter, C.A. & Kelley, R.I. (1991). Glutaric aciduria type I: a common cause of episodic encephalopathy and spastic paralysis in the Amish of Lancaster County, Pennsylvania. *Am. J. Med. Genet.*, **41**, 89–95.

Murphy, C.C., Yeargin-Allsopp, M., Decoufle, P. & Drews, C.D. (1993). Prevalence of cerebral palsy among ten-year-old children in metropolitan Atlanta, 1985 through 1987. *J. Pediatr.*, **123**, S13–20.

Murphy, K.P., Molnar, G.E. & Lankasky, K. (2000). Employment and social issues in adults with cerebral palsy. *Arch. Phys. Med. Rehabil.*, **81**, 807–11.

Nelson, K.B. (1991). Prenatal origin of hemiparetic cerebral: how often and why? *Pediatrics*, **88**, 1059–61.

Nelson, K.B. & Ellenberg, J.H. (1986). Antecedents of cerebral palsy: multivariate analysis of risk. *N. Engl. J. Med.*, **315**, 81–6.

Nelson, K.B., Dambrosia, J.M., Grether, J.K. & Phillips, T.M. (1998). Neonatal cytokines and coagulation factors in children with cerebral palsy. *Ann. Neurol.*, **44**, 665–75.

Novotny, E., Ashwal, S. & Shevell, M. (1998). Proton magnetic resonance spectroscopy: an emerging technology in pediatric neurology research. *Ped. Res.*, **44**, 1–10.

Oka, A., Belliveau, M.J., Rosenberg, P.A. & Volpe, J.J. (1993). Vulnerability of oligodendroglia to glutamate: pharmacology, mechanisms, and prevention. *J. Neurosci.*, **13**, 1441–53.

Okumura, A., Hayakawa, F., Kato, T., Kuno, K. & Watanabe, K. E. (1997). MRI findings in patients with spastic cerebral palsy. I: correlation with gestational age at birth. *Dev. Med. Child Neurol.*, **39**, 363–8.

Osler, W. (1987). *The Cerebral Palsies of Children*. London: Mac Keith Press.

Palmer, L., Blair, E., Petterson, B. & Burton, P. (1995). Antenatal antecedents of moderate and severe cerebral palsy. *Paediatr. Perinat. Epidemiol.*, **9**, 171–84.

Paneth, N. (1999). Classifying brain damage in preterm infants. *J. Pediatr.*, **134**, 527–9.

Paneth, N., Rudelli, R., Kazam, E. & Monte, W. (1994). *Brain Damage in the Preterm Infant*, pp. 171–85. London: MacKeith Press.

Parer, J.T. & King, T. (2000). Fetal heart rate monitoring: is it salvageable? *Am. J. Obstet. Gynecol.*, **182**, 982–7.

Park, T.S. & Owen, J.H. (1992). Surgical management of spastic diplegia in cerebral palsy. *N. Engl. J. Med.*, **326**, 745–9.

Pasternak, J.F. (1987). Parasagittal infarction in neonatal asphyxia? *Ann. Neurol.*, **21**, 202–3.

Pasternak, J.F. & Gorey, M.T. (1998). The syndrome of acute near-total intrauterine asphyxia in the term infant. *Pediatr. Neurol.*, **18**, 391–8.

Penn, R.D. & Kroin, J.S. (1985). Continuous intrathecal baclofen for severe spasticity. *Lancet,* **ii** (8447), 125–7.

Pranzatelli, M.R. (1996). Oral pharmacotherapy for the movement disorders of cerebral palsy. *J. Child Neurol.*, **11**(Suppl. 1), S13–22.

Pretorius, D.H., Davis, K., Manco-Johnson, M.L., Manchester, D., Meier, P.R. & Clewell, W. (1985). Clinical course of fetal hydrocephalus: 40 cases. *Am. J. Roentgenol.*, **144**, 827–31.

Saint Hilaire, M-H., Burke, R.E., Bressman, S.B., Brin, M.F. & Fahn, S. (1991). Delayed-onset dystonia due to perinatal or early childhood asphyxia. *Neurology*, **41**, 216–22.

Scheller, J.M. & Nelson, K.B. (1994). Does cesarean delivery prevent cerebral palsy or other neurologic problems of childhood? *Obstet. Gynecol.*, **83**, 624–30.

Scher, M.S., Belfar, H., Martin, J. & Painter, M.J. (1991). Destructive brain lesions of presumed fetal onset: antepartum causes of cerebral palsy. *Pediatrics*, **88**, 898–906.

Scott, B.L. & Jankovic, J. (1996). Delayed-onset progressive movement disorders after static brain lesions. *Neurology*, **46**, 68–74.

Shu, S.K., Ashwal, S., Holshouser, B.A., Nystrom, G. & Hinshaw, D.B. (1997). Prognostic value of ^{1}H-MRS in perinatal CNS insults. *Pediat. Neurol.*, **17**, 301–18.

Steinbok, P., Reiner, A.M., Beauchamp, R., Armstrong, R.W. & Cochrane, D.D. (1997). A randomized clinical trial to compare selective posterior rhizotomy plus physiotherapy with physiotherapy alone in children with spastic diplegic cerebral palsy. *Dev. Med. Child Neurol.*, **39**, 178–84.

Surveillance of Cerebral Palsy in Europe (2000). Surveillance of cerebral palsy in Europe: a collaboration of cerebral palsy surveys and registers. *Dev. Med. Child Neurol.*, **42**, 816–24.

Taudorf, K., Melchior, J.C. & Pedersen, H. (1984). CT findings in spastic cerebral palsy, clinical, aetiological and prognostic aspects. *Neuropediatrics*, **15**, 120–4.

Thorarensen, O., Ryan, S., Hunter, J. & Younkin, D.P. (1997). Factor V Leiden mutation: an unrecognized cause of hemiplegic cerebral palsy, neonatal stroke, and placental thrombosis. *Ann. Neurol.*, **42**, 372–5.

Truwit, C.L., Barkovich, A.J., Koch, T.K. & Ferriero, D.M. (1992). Cerebral palsy: MR findings in 40 patients. *Am. J. Neuroradiol.*, **13**, 67–78.

Tuir, M. & Kalen, V. (2000). The risk of spinal deformity after selective dorsal rhizotomy. *J. Pediatr. Orthop.*, **20**, 104–7.

Volpe, J.J. (1995). Intracranial hemorrhage: germinal matrix-intraventricular hemorrhage of the premature infant. In *Neurology of the Newborn*, 3rd edn. Philadelphia: W.B. Saunders Co.

Volpe, J.J. (1997). Brain injury in the premature infant: neuropathology, clinical aspects, pathogenesis, and prevention. In *Neurologic Disorders of the Newborn*, ed. A.J. du Plessis, pp. 562–87. Philadelphia: W.B. Saunders Co.

Wissel, J., Heinen, F., Schenkel, A. et al. (1999). Botulinum toxin A in the management of spastic gait disorders in children and young adults with cerebral palsy: a randomized, double-blind study of 'high-dose' versus 'low-dose' treatment. *Neuropediatrics*, **30**, 120–4.

40

Gait and balance disorders

John G. Nutt[1] and Fay B. Horak[2]

[1] Department of Neurology and Department of Pharmacology and Physiology, Oregon Health Sciences University, USA
[2] Neurological Sciences Institute and Department of Pharmacology and Physiology, Oregon Health Sciences University, USA

Walking requires two capabilities: maintenance of balance (protection of upright stance via anticipatory and reactive postural mechanisms) and movement through the environment via locomotion. Postural responses and locomotion are dependent upon all levels of the nervous and musculoskeletal systems. Consequently, gait and balance disorders are common manifestations of many diseases.

The clinician commonly thinks of gait disorders in terms of walking pattern, emphasizing the movements of the legs. And literally this is correct; 'gait' is defined by Webster's *Third International Dictionary* as the 'manner of walking' or 'sequence of foot movements.' Accordingly, the neurological exam emphasizes evaluation of strength, tone, coordination, sensation and reflexes of the limbs. The result is that clinical neurology focuses on locomotion.

The importance of balance or equilibrium to walking is not recognized or explicitly acknowledged. Yet balance is the key and critical element in safe ambulation. Many so-called gait disorders are in reality balance disorders, not disorders in the sequence of foot movements. For example, Bruns' 'frontal ataxia' (Bruns, 1892) and van Bogart and Martins' 'apraxia of gait' (1929) are descriptions of patients who could not even stand independently. Although impairments of gait or locomotion can sometimes be separated from impairments of balance or postural equilibrium, locomotion and balance are more often inextricably intertwined (Mori, 1987). Thus, classifications need to consider disorders of both gait and balance.

The aim of this chapter is to present a classification scheme for gait and balance disorders. We first consider a classification based on neurological functions required for purposeful ambulation using Hughlings Jackson's hierarchical scheme of lower, middle and higher functions. This classification suggests the range of neurological impairments that can disrupt ambulation and the relationships among various gait and balance disorders.

Patients' walking and balance patterns do not necessarily reflect impairments in neural functioning but rather the patient's compensatory strategies for coping with the impairments. Different impairments may elicit common compensatory strategies. For this reason, classification by impairments is inadequate for clinical diagnosis. The second portion of our classification scheme considers the common compensatory strategies as clinical patterns or syndromes for which there are differential diagnoses. Problems with ambulation are separated into clinical patterns or syndromes that are predominantly disorders of balance and those that are predominantly disorders of locomotion, recognizing that in most diseases, both postural control and locomotion are affected to some extent. Because falls are a common presenting complaint, we offer a separate classification for fall patterns.

Physiology of locomotion and postural control

The temporal and spatial sequence of contractions of leg muscles for locomotion are programmed at the spinal cord level by central pattern generators (CPGs) (Grillner & Wallen, 1985). Well-patterned hind leg stepping responses can be elicited by treadmill stimulation in cats with total thoracic cord transection (Grillner & Wallen, 1985) and in the legs of humans with paraplegia and quadriplegia (Dietz et al., 1994). This spinal stepping can be activated by sensory stimulation resulting from treadmill motion and by non-specific dorsal root sensory stimulation. The CPGs are normally activated by descending pathways arising in brainstem locomotor centres (Orlovsky & Shik, 1976). Electrical stimulation of the brainstem locomotor centres will produce stepping and, at higher intensity, trotting and running movements of the legs of cats and monkeys (Eidelberg et al., 1981). Cerebellum, basal ganglia and primary motor areas refine and adapt locomotion to varying conditions such as for precision walking on the rungs of a horizontal ladder (Armstrong, 1988). Other cortical areas coordinate locomotion with the individual's voluntary or purposeful actions.

The neuroanatomical control of posture is less well understood than is locomotion. The isolated spinal cord does not have postural responses. The hindlimbs of paraplegic cats can support the weight of the trunk with background muscle tone but do not respond to postural perturbation to prevent a fall (Macpherson & Fung, 1999). Postural support must be provided for the spinal cats walking on a treadmill (Grillner & Wallen, 1985) indicating that postural responses must be mediated through centres above the spinal cord. Coordinated postural responses can be elicited from brainstem. Evidence for brainstem programming of postural control comes from the studies in intact cats with implanted electrodes in dorsal and ventral tegmental regions of the pons. Stimulation of the ventral tegmental region would make a lying cat stand up and then begin walking. Stimulation of the dorsal tegmental region reversed this effect; a walking cat would first stop and then would lie down (Mori, 1987). Thus, at least some postural responses appear to arise from the brainstem.

Higher centres are presumed to adapt postural control to the environment and to the individual's needs. For example, frontal cortical areas coordinate anticipatory postural adjustments that precede and accompany any voluntary movement to protect postural stability. These adaptations require accurate neural maps of the body in relation to the earth's gravitational field, the support surface and the immediate environment as well as the relation of various body segments to each other. These maps are synthesized from information obtained from a variety of sensory modalities (Horak & Macpherson, 1996). Somatosensory information from proprioceptors in muscles and joints is the most important for coordination of posture and gait, including triggering rapid postural responses. Cutaneous information provides information about the contour and characteristics of surfaces, the pressure under the feet in contact with support surfaces, and a stable reference for posture. Vestibular information helps control trunk and head orientation in space, as well as stable gaze during locomotion. Vision is primarily used in a predictive manner to avoid obstacles and plan trajectories and step placement during gait. In addition to online sensory information, postural responses are modified and adapted to behaviour goals by context, previous experience and expectation.

Systems classification of gait and balance syndromes

A hierarchical classification, modelled after Hughlings Jackson's approach, considers three levels of neural function controlling gait and balance; lower, middle and higher levels (Table 40.1). 'Lower' to 'higher' correlates with 'simpler' to 'more complex' neural processing. It will be apparent that clinicians are most comfortable diagnosing disorders caused by neurological dysfunction arising at lower levels and motor dysfunction at the middle level of this classification. The effects of sensory disorganization and higher neurological dysfunction on balance and gait are less well defined clinically. We emphasize these less recognized and problematic disorders in the text and references. It is important to note that a given disorder may produce balance and gait dysfunction by effects at several levels. For example, mild to moderate parkinsonism is envisioned as causing mid-level dysfunction by reducing the force generation for balance and locomotor synergies. More severe parkinsonism may also affect higher level functions such as adaptation of balance synergies to environmental conditions and coordination of synergies.

Lower level

The lower level has three components. The first component consists of the intrinsic locomotor synergies (CPGs) programmed in the spinal grey matter and the postural responses programmed in the brainstem. These locomotor and postural synergies are the building blocks of successful ambulation. A patient with complete spinal cord section may have no behavioural evidence of locomotor synergies because they lack the necessary facilitation to elicit them. Spinal lesions may also injure CPGs disrupting spinal locomotor synergies and thereby timing of muscle contractions required for locomotion although frequently other neurological dysfunctions from higher spinal and brainstem lesions complicate interpretation. Lower level synergies may be disinhibited by higher lesions so that spinal stepping (Dietz et al., 1994) and decerebrate, tonic neck and perhaps grasp responses may emerge. Another possible abnormal postural response in humans resulting from disinhibition is the involuntary hyperextension or pushing the centre of mass behind the base of support seen in some patients upon standing.

The second component of the lower level is the primary sensory modalities with which the person locates themselves with respect to the support surface, the gravitational field, and the immediate environment and also senses the relative

Table 40.1. Neural systems/anatomical classification

I. LOWER LEVEL

A. *Spinal locomotor and brainstem postural synergies*

1. Absence of synergies
2. Abnormal spatial–temporal organization of synergies
   a. Spinal cord lesions disrupting CPGs
3. Disinhibition of synergies with higher lesions
   a. Spinal stepping
   b. Decerebrate posturing, tonic neck responses
   c. Hyperextension, pushing backwards

B. *Primary Sensory Input* (vestibular, visual, somatosensory)

1. Absent or distorted input
   a. Veering ataxia of acute vestibular lesions
   b. Sensory ataxia with loss of proprioception from peripheral nerve or posterior column lesions
   c. Veering, careful gait of newly blind

C. *Force Production* (muscle and nerve)

1. Weakness
   a. Steppage gait (foot drop) of peripheral nerve lesions
   b. Waddling gait of muscular dystrophies and polymyositis with involvement of proximal muscle
   c. Hyperextended knees with quadriceps weakness

II. MIDDLE LEVEL

A. *Perception/Orientation* (organization of primary sensation into spatial maps of body in gravitational field by parietal cortex, putamen, premotor cortex and their subcortical connections)

1. Distorted spatial maps
   a. Central vestibular lesions of brainstem and thalamus
   b. Parietal lesions and 'pusher syndrome'
2. Distorted maps or neglect of spatial information
   a. Thalamic astasia
   b. Putaminal astasia
   c. Progressive supranuclear palsy?
   d. Non-dominant parietal lesions?

B. *Force Scaling* (modulation of force for optimization of postural and locomotor synergies by basal ganglia, cerebellum and primary motor cortex)

1. Movement disorders
   a. Hypo- and hyperkinetic disorders of basal ganglia origin
   b. Hypermetric and dysmetric disorders of cerebellar origin
   c. Spasticity and clumsiness from corticospinal system damage

III. HIGHER LEVEL

A. *Synergy selection, coordination and adaptation* of locomotor and postural responses (less conscious functions) mediated by frontal lobe and subcortical connections.

1. Dyscoordination of voluntary movement and postural responses
   a. Reduction or loss of anticipatory responses with frontal lobe lesions
2. Altered inhibition or excitation of lower postural and gait synergies
   a. Hyperextension and pushing centre of mass behind support
   b. Freezing with frontal, subcortical and basal ganglia lesions
3. Adaptation of postural synergies to conditions
   a. Postural inflexibility of advanced parkinsonism
   b. Inability to use experience to anticipate appropriate magnitude of postural responses in cerebellar disease
   c. Appropriate slowing, shortening of stride and en bloc turns with perceived postural instability
4. Inappropriate sequencing of postural synergies
   a. 'Apraxia' of postural shifts as from lying to sitting and sitting to standing

Table 40.1 (*cont.*)

B. Cognitive (attention and insight for adaptation to person's goals and limitations (more conscious functions) mediated by all cortical regions

1. Impaired attention
    a. Falls related to centrally active medications, delirium and dementia
2. Imparied insight
    a. Falls related to inappropriate behaviour in dementia
    b. Psychogenic gait disturbances

positions of various limb segments, trunk and head. Under most conditions, the information from the visual, vestibular and proprioceptive sensory systems is redundant so that an accurate spatial sense is possible with input from just one or two of the sensory systems. The disequilibrium of acute and chronic vestibular dysfunction and the sensory ataxia associated with proprioceptive dysfunction are examples of gait and balance disorders associated with reduced, unbalanced and disordered sensory input.

The third component of the lower system is the musculoskeletal system and peripheral motor nerves connecting it to the CNS. These tissues are responsible for generating forces to preserve balance and to move in space. Damage or disease affecting these structures, the effectors of postural and locomotor strategies, will obviously alter the execution of the strategies. Skeletal deformities, arthritis, muscle disease and peripheral motor neuropathies will affect gait and postural responses. For the neurologist, the waddling gait and locked knees of muscular dystrophies and polymyositis and the steppage gait of peripheral neuropathies such as Charcot Marie Tooth disease are prime examples of this type of dysfunction.

Middle level

At the middle level there are two components. The first component is composed of the neural structures that integrate sensory information into spatial maps. This function probably takes place in many areas of the brain. Spatial maps concerned with motor function have been identified in the putamen and premotor cortex. Maps concerned with visual function exist in frontal eye fields and the superior colliculus. Surprisingly, the parietal lobes appear to be more important in creating the spatial maps which may actually reside elsewhere in the brain (Gross & Graziano, 1995). Distorted maps can result in body tilt or lean or inappropriately asymmetrical postural responses. Examples of this type of disorientation are the altered perception of visual and postural verticality that may accom-

pany lesions of central vestibular connections (Dieterich & Brandt, 1993; Bisdorff et al., 1996) and parietal lesions (Karnath, 1994; Karnath et al., 2000). Other candidates for this type of dysfunction in orienting in space are progressive supranuclear palsy, thalamic astasia (Marsden & Gorelick, 1988) and putaminal astasia (Labadie et al., 1989) syndromes in which patients appear to be either unaware of postural vertical or indifferent to this information. As patients with these clinical syndromes have not been studied carefully, it is not known if these syndromes are attributable to lack of synthesizing information into maps or to sensory neglect, motor neglect, or other types of dysfunction.

The second component of the middle level function is the precise modulation of force for optimal locomotor and postural control. The central motor system has this role. Basal ganglia, cerebellum and cortical motor areas sharpen and adapt locomotor and postural coordination but do not create the synergies. The clinical manifestations of dysfunction at this level are parkinsonism (slow/bradykinetic and stiff/rigid postural and locomotor synergies), hyperkinetic movement disorders (involuntary movements superimposed on normal strategies), ataxia (hypermetric and dysmetric synergies) and spasticity (slowed, stiff and imprecise synergies). These clinical syndromes are a distortion, not loss, of appropriate postural and locomotor synergies caused by the imprecise execution of appropriate synergies. Skilled and precise voluntary stepping are impaired; walking a line or performing a dance step become challenging.

Higher level

At the higher level, two components are hypothesized. The first largely operates at an unconscious level. It is responsible for selecting, accessing and coordinating the appropriate brainstem and spinal synergies for balance and walking. The selection of synergies is based on the information about the body, its location in space and the goals of the individual. Sensitivity to context is an important component of this function. For example, balance and locomotor synergies should be different for walking on a slick versus a non-slippery surface and for responding to a postural perturbation when holding onto a support versus when standing without a handhold. Anticipatory postural responses that accompany voluntary movements to prevent postural perturbations caused by the voluntary movements may be impaired by lesions of premotor or supplementary regions (Massion, 1992).

A second group of higher level problems is with disinhibition of inappropriate postural responses and inability to elicit appropriate locomotor synergies. The tendency for some patients to push their centre of mass behind their support base may be an example of disinhibition of an inappropriate postural tone. It may be seen with frontal lesions, deep white matter lesions and severe parkinsonism (which may induce frontal dysfunction). Freezing appears to be disturbed access to locomotor synergies and is associated with the same array of frontal, subcortical white matter and basal ganglia lesions (Yanagisawa et al., 1991; Achiron et al., 1993; Giladi et al., 1997).

A third group of higher level problems relates to the ability to adapt to changes in environmental conditions and to predict appropriate responses. Subjects with basal ganglia disease have difficulty adapting postural synergies to changes in support surfaces (Horak et al., 1992) and subjects with cerebellar disease have difficulty adapting postural synergies based on prior experience (Horak & Diener, 1994). A gait that is often considered as abnormal and variously termed senile, elderly or cautious gait, is the slowed, short stepped gait with *en bloc* turns. However, this gait pattern is an appropriate response to perceived instability and shows that at least some of the higher level function is intact.

A fourth group of higher level problems is totally deranged synergies that may fit the concept of apraxia. Although the term 'apraxia of gait' is in common use, its appropriateness and clinical definition are problematic (Nutt et al., 1993). However, the term 'apraxia of balance' may be justified for righting responses that are entirely disrupted and ineffective. Inappropriate righting responses such as trying to arise from a chair without bringing the feet underneath the seated body, and bizarre postural responses upon standing may be associated with frontal lobe lesions and deep white matter lesions (Bruns, 1892; van Bogart & Martin, 1929; Meyer & Barron, 1960; Petrovici, 1968; Thompson & Marsden, 1987; Nutt et al., 1993). What is commonly termed apraxia of gait is subsumed under freezing and apraxia of balance in our classification.

A second component of the highest system operates at a more conscious level to modify locomotor synergies. It is responsible for precision stepping such as on stepping stones or performing unfamiliar dance steps. If there are lower and middle level postural and locomotor difficulties, this higher level compensates as best it can to allow ambulation within the constraints imposed by the lower level dysfunction. Under these circumstances, walking and balance are elevated from operation at the largely unconscious level to operation at a conscious level. The more balance and gait are under conscious control, the more attention is required. In this situation, balance and gait deteriorate when attempting a simultaneous, cognitive task such as conversation, searching for keys in a pocket or carrying a fragile object (Wright & Kemp, 1992). Falls occur in older patients who do not direct sufficient attention to walking and balance or who do not have the insight to avoid posturally challenging situations. This may be the reason that dementia and centrally active drug use in the elderly emerge in epidemiological studies as predisposing factors to falls (Tinetti et al., 1988; Salgado et al., 1994).

Psychogenic gait disorders would also be seen as representative of dysfunction at this higher level (Keane, 1989; Lempert et al., 1991).

Classification of balance and gait disorders by clinical patterns

The postural responses and locomotor patterns that the clinician observes are not the direct consequence of the neurological impairments but instead reflect the compensatory strategies the patient uses to cope with the impairments. Impairments at different levels may invoke clinically similar compensatory postural and gait patterns. For example, a hyperextended, locked knee to prevent knee buckling in stance may be a compensatory strategy for weak quadriceps muscles, hypermetric synergies from a cerebellar disorder or lack of proprioceptive feedback in an individual with profound somatosensory loss.

The pattern classification assumes that there are gait and balance features that define different strategies for which there is a limited differential. The patterns or syndromes are not exclusive; a patient may demonstrate more than one abnormal pattern.

The classification is based on the history and observation of gait and postural responses. History is particularly important for patients with falls, as they are generally not directly observed. Gait and balance features are observed not only during stance and gait, but also during transitions from sit to stand and turning, when balance is challenged by walking in tandem with a narrow base of support, and responding to postural perturbations such as the 'pull test.'

Table 40.2. Fall patterns

1. Collapsing (akinetic seizures, syncope, orthostatic hypotension)
2. Toppling
    a. Drifting into a fall while standing
    b. While changing position/posture
    c. Weaving from side to side or in all directions until falling
3. Tripping
4. Freezing
5. Falling in specific situations or with concurrent sensory symptoms
6. Non-patterned

The perceived limits of stability can also be evaluated by examining how far the subject can lean forward and backwards in standing and laterally in sitting. Ability to maintain orientation with limited somatosensory information can be evaluated by standing on compliant foam with eyes open and closed. These features will describe gait and balance patterns. Each pattern will have a differential. Other clinical features derived from the neurological exam, imaging and laboratory testing will help differentiate between causes of a given pattern but are not used to define the pattern. The proposed pattern classification has three categories; fall patterns, disequilibrium patterns and gait patterns.

Fall patterns

Fall patterns (Table 40.2) are based on history. The first distinction is between falling because of loss of postural tone and falls with retained tone. 'Collapsing in a heap' is a common description of falls from loss of postural tone. Akinetic seizures, negative myoclonus, syncope, otolithic crises and orthostatic hypotension cause collapsing falls. The recognition of the collapsing fall syndrome is an important distinction as the differential, diagnostic tests and treatments are very different from the other falls to be considered below.

In falls with retained muscle tone, the patient falls in some direction and does not just collapse. It may be helpful to distinguish whether the patient actually falls to the ground or has 'near-falls.' 'Near-falls' suggest that the patient recognizes when they are out of equilibrium and performs a late or inadequate postural response. In contrast, patients who consistently fall to the ground clearly have grossly inadequate postural control or are unaware, until too late, that equilibrium has been compromised. Patients and their caregivers can often provide helpful information regarding the environmental situation, task attempted and type of fall pattern. It is also useful to re-enact the circumstances that led to a fall during the clinical exam.

Toppling falls are falls where the patient 'topples like a falling tree.' They may occur when the subject is just standing as seen in progressive supranuclear palsy or thalamic and putaminal astasia (Masdeu & Gorelick, 1988; Labadie et al., 1989) or when the subject is changing position as is characteristic of parkinsonism. In these disorders there is often inadequate or no effort to arrest the fall. Patients with cerebellar disease may weave about when standing and fall in any direction but have protective responses.

Tripping falls occur because the feet do not clear the support surface adequately. The falls are generally forward. Foot drop, spasticity and parkinsonism are common causes of tripping falls.

Freezing falls occur when the feet do not move quickly enough to stay under the falling forward centre of mass. The patients typically fall forward on to their knees and outstretched arms.

Falls that occur only when the patient is experiencing vertigo, in the dark, or in sensory conflict situations such as when surrounded by moving objects, suggest a peripheral or central vestibular deficit. Falls when walking on uneven surfaces suggest inadequate sensory information for control of balance, especially somatosensory loss as occurs with peripheral neuropathy and dorsal column disease. In these sensory type falls, patients generally recognize their spatial disorientation and attempt to use their arms to grab onto stable objects or voluntarily sit down to prevent injury.

Finally, non-patterned falls, falls that do not seem to fit a consistent pattern, may represent failure of attention and insight producing carelessness as can occur in dementia.

Disequilibrium syndromes

Disequilibrium syndromes (Table 40.3) are characterized by impairments of balance that markedly impede or preclude locomotion. They are identified by inspection of arising, standing with eyes open and closed, standing on foam, walking, tandem walking, turning, response to postural perturbation and limits of stability while standing and sitting.

Disequilibrium can result from dyscoordination within postural synergies; the relative timing of postural muscle contractions is inappropriate. The clinical consequence is buckling and excessive motion of joints. Cortical lesions and partial spinal cord lesions can produce abnormal timing of postural responses. An example of a dyscoordi-

Table 40.3. Disequilibrium patterns

1. Dyscoordination: excessive motion, buckling, etc. of limb segments caused by disordered timing affecting temporal patterns of body segment movements
2. Dysmetric (hypermetric): excessive sway and over-reaction to postural disturbance caused by correct timing but inappropriately large movements
3. Hypometric: postural responses are too small because force develops slowly
4. Sensory deprivation: situation-dependent disequilibrium related to circumstances that limit sensory input
5. Sensory disorganization: apparent disregard for postural vertical leading to drifting off balance or distorted perception of verticality causing active moving into unstable postures
6. Apraxic: completely abnormal or inappropriate postural responses

nated pattern is the delayed onset of postural responses in gastrocnemius such that the hamstrings muscle activation that normally follows gastrocnemius, comes earlier than it, resulting in knee buckling (Nashner et al., 1983).

In dysmetric disequilibrium, there is increased postural sway while standing still. The postural responses are appropriately organized but improperly scaled and often are hypermetric (Horak & Diener, 1994). Postural pertubation often elicits a response that is too large and causes the body to be thrown into another unstable position. Dysmetric, often hypermetric, postural responses are characteristic of cerebellar disorders, the prototype for dysmetric disequilibrium. However, the involuntary movements of chorea can also produce the dysmetric disequilibrium syndrome. High anxiety, fear of falling and suggestibility can also produce hypermetric postural responses. Distraction by another task, such as testing stereognosis, will often reduce sway in patients with anxiety and suggestibility.

Hypokinetic or bradykinetic postural responses are frequent in parkinsonism. The development of force is slow so that the execution of postural responses is slow and may not be sufficiently timely or forceful to maintain upright balance. Recovery from the pull test is noticeably slow, the upper body moving back over the centre of support over a few seconds or longer. Sometimes the patients fall without an apparent effort to resist the perturbation. Despite responses that clinically appear delayed, weak or even absent, the latency of postural responses measured by surface EMG electrodes are not prolonged, but amplitude is reduced (Horak et al., 1992).

Disequilibrium resulting from sensory deprivation is characteristic of vestibular disorders, severe peripheral neu-

ropathies and posterior column disease. Disequilibrium occurs because there is inadequate sensory information to trigger and modify postural responses. These disorders are revealed by situations that deprive the patients of other sensory input such as standing with eyes closed or standing on foam (Horak et al., 1990).

Disequilibrium from sensory disorganization appears to be the cause of falls with thalamic, putaminal, and cortical, particularly parietal and possibly frontal lesions. Primary sensory input is intact but the synthesis of the information into spatial maps is disturbed or there is inattention to the spatial information. Falls are characterized by drifting off balance with no apparent effort to correct balance in thalamic (Masden & Gorelick, 1988) and putaminal astasia (Labadie et al., 1989) progressive supranuclear palsy and advanced parkinsonism. Parietal lesions may be associated with actively pushing the centre of mass toward the lesioned side secondary to a distorted sense of body vertical (Karnath et al., 2000).

Apraxic disequilibrium is the disorganization of arising and standing because the righting and standing synergies are completely inappropriate. The most common example is patients who try to arise from sitting without bringing the feet under the chair but other mechanically impossible strategies for righting and standing may be seen. These types of disequilibrium disorders are commonly associated with frontal lobe dysfunction (Nutt et al., 1993) but may also be seen with advanced parkinsonism.

Gait syndromes

Gait syndromes are based on abnormalities that are apparent while the patient is walking. Waddling and foot drop gait patterns identify weakness. The distance between the feet (base) may be widened or, less commonly, narrowed while standing or walking. Gait speed and stride length are reduced with any gait disorder or perceived risk to upright balance and are therefore of no diagnostic assistance. The cadence or regularity of steps, both length and base, may vary during walking. Deviation or veering from intended direction of travel may be observed. Stiffness or rigidity of the legs or trunk may be apparent by the loss of the normal fluidity of gait. Difficulty initiating or maintaining gait (freezing) is one of the more striking abnormalities of gait. Adaptability may be estimated by the patient's ability to modify walking speed, avoid obstacles, perform precision walking or turn about.

Eight gait patterns are proposed (Table 40.4). The proposed gait patterns are not exclusive; patients may show elements of more than one pattern. Also, gait patterns are not fixed but may change or progress across time in conjunction

Table 40.4. Gait patterns

1. Ataxic: irregular cadence and progression
a. Cerebellar ataxia
b. Sensory ataxia
c. Chorea
2. Stiff/rigid: loss of fluidity, stiffness of legs and trunk
a. Spasticity
b. Parkinsonism
c. Dystonia
d. Diffuse cortical and subcortical diseases, such as multi-infarct state
3. Weakness: waddling and foot drop
a. Muscle disorders
b. Peripheral neuropathies
c. Corticospinal tract lesions
4. Veering: deviation of gait to one side
a. Vestibular disorders
b. Cerebellar disorders
5. Freezing: start and turn hesitation
a. Parkinsonism
b. Multi-infarct state
c. Normal pressure hydrocephalus
6. Wide-based: widened base with standing and walking
a. Midline cerebellar disorders
b. Multi-infarct state
c. In conjunction with ataxic syndromes
7. Cautious: slowing, short steps and *en bloc* turns
a. Non-specific, multifactorial
8. Psychogenic: bizarre, inconsistent, distractible

with the evolution of the neurological problems. Many gait syndromes begin as a cautious gait and evolve into other syndromes. Finally, gait pattern classification is not to say that the patients have no balance disorders; most do, and the abnormal gait pattern may be a compensatory response to the balance difficulties.

Ataxic gaits are a result of uncertainty when and where the feet will make contact with the support surface with each step. This can be a consequence of dysmetric control of the centre of mass and leg movements as in cerebellar disorders, superimposed involuntary movements as in chorea, impaired proprioception in the feet and legs as in sensory ataxia and a moving support surface as on a ship deck. Ataxic gaits are characterized by irregular, excessive centre of mass motion and disorderly progression (locomotion). Typically, these abnormalities are associated with a widened base and shorter stride. Cadence is also irregular.

Stiff/rigid gaits are gaits in which the usual fluidity of walking is lost. Rotation of trunk is reduced or absent. The range of motion at the knees and hips is reduced, as is arm swing. Base may be abnormally narrow or wide; stride is shortened. Examples are spasticity, parkinsonism, dystonia, multi-infarct states (vascular parkinsonism) and musculoskeletal disorders. The stiffness may be unilateral as in spastic hemiparesis or hemidystonia.

Gaits disturbed by proximal or distal weakness are well recognized. Proximal weakness prevents fixation of the pelvis during single support portions of gait. Myopathies and dystrophies that typically affect proximal muscles commonly produce waddling gaits although occasionally multiple root and peripheral nerve lesions are responsible. Hyperextension of the knee may also occur with proximal weakness. Distal weakness generally affects dorsiflexors of the ankle, requiring the leg to be lifted higher for the toe to clear the ground. Peripheral neuropathies are the common cause of this problem. Corticospinal tract lesions affect the distal leg muscles more than proximal muscles but stiffness and circumduction of the leg differentiate this from weakness caused by peripheral nerve lesions.

Veering gaits are those in which the patient tends to lean, fall or deviate in one direction while walking. Peripheral and central vestibular disorders are the common cause but other brainstem and thalamic lesions may cause similar patterns.

Freezing gaits are those characterized by difficulty initiating (start hesitation and 'slipping clutch' phenomena) and maintaining locomotion while maneuvering in tight quarters, passing through doorways and turning (turn hesitation). There appear to be at least two distinguishable patterns of the freezing gait. Most commonly freezing is associated with a stiff/rigid gait and a narrow base. These patients may have no or reduced lateral sway when trying to initiate walking. Idiopathic parkinsonism, parkinsonism plus syndromes, normal pressure hydrocephalus and vascular parkinsonism are common diagnoses (Giladi et al., 1997). A less common form of freezing is associated with widened base and often exaggerated truncal sway and arm swing to initiate gait. It is this pattern to which 'slipping clutch' is an apt description. It has been associated with multi-infarct state.

Wide based gaits indicate problems with lateral stability. In isolation, that is without dysmetria of the legs and with normal cadence, wide based gaits are seen in midline cerebellar syndromes such as alcoholic cerebellar atrophy and in multi-infarct states.

Cautious gait is marked by mild to moderate slowing, shortening of stride and *en bloc* turns with only minimal widening of the base. Other gait abnormalities are absent. It is termed cautious because it is the gait pattern assumed by a normal person who is concerned about their balance such as when walking on a slippery surface. Cautious gait is an appropriate response to perceived threats to postural balance. As such, cautious gait is non-specific and may be associated with a variety of problems that impact a person's ability to walk safely. Cautious gait may also be of multifactorial etiology.

A final category is psychogenic gait disorders. Although balance may be disturbed in patients with a psychogenic origin for the problem, most can ambulate as well and therefore are considered as gait disorders. A variety of bizarre patterns that fit none of the above descriptions are possible. Distractibility, inconsistencies and other non-physiological signs are common tip-offs to the diagnosis Keane, 1989; Lampert et al., 1991). Because some of the apraxic disequilibrium syndromes and dystonic gaits may be very bizarre, they can be easily confused with psychogenic gaits.

An 'over cautious' pattern sometimes termed space phobia or fear of falling occurs in some older people with mild, multisystem impairments, generally in response to a fall or some other event arousing their anxiety about falling. Gait is slow, often wide-based, staggering and with prolonged double stance duration. The person must hold on to another person, furniture or the wall to walk (Murphy & Isaacs, 1982). The clinician needs to be 'cautious' about this syndrome and not make the diagnosis without thorough evaluation, including a MRI to look for silent infarcts.

Diagnosis of balance and gait disorders

The remainder of the neurological exam will direct the workup of fall, balance and gait disorders. For unexplained balance and gait disorders, a MRI is indicated and may reveal unexpected infarcts, hydrocephalus, atrophy and particularly subcortical white matter ischemic lesions (Baloh et al., 1995). Vitamin B12 deficiency is another rare cause of unexplained balance and gait disorders.

Treatment of balance and gait disorders

If a treatable lesion is discovered as a cause of imbalance or gait disorders, this is obviously the target of therapy. In many cases there is no single abnormality that is responsible for gait and balance abnormalities and a multifactorial etiology is likely. This is particularly true in the elderly where mild sensory and motor deficits may produce a cautious or pathological gait syndrome. Attempts to improve as many of these factors as possible, even seemingly inconsequential factors, may improve gait and reduce falls (Tinetti et al., 1994). Assessment of home safety to remove

hazards, optimize lighting and instal hand-holds is an important method of reducing falls. Strengthening and balance exercises, even in the elderly, reduce risks for falls (Province et al., 1995).

Rehabilitation of balance and gait disorders

The goal of rehabilitation is to eliminate impairments if possible and, if not, to facilitate the most optimal compensatory strategies given the constraints imposed by the impairments. Some impairments, such as weakness and poor range of motion can be readily improved. The extent to which higher level neurological problems affecting balance and gait can be remediated is less clear. However, even if the specific impairments, such as sensory loss, dysmetria, and distorted internal body maps may not be readily improved with exercise and experience, studies have shown that functional balance and gait can be successfully trained (Woollacott & Moore, 1992). Not only can sway area and gait speed improve with training, the use of sensory information for postural orientation can improve and the incidence of falls can be significantly reduced.

The particular therapeutic goal and approach to treatment of balance and gait disorders must be specific to the underlying physiological constraints or impairments. Thus, balance and gait problems due to abnormal timing and scaling of postural synergies would be treated differently from problems due to loss of sensory information and from adaptation and cognitive problems. For example, abnormal synergies for controlling postural sway could be retrained using kinematic biofeedback and functional electrical stimulation during postural sway activities. In contrast, balance and gait in an individual without vestibular information for postural orientation should be retrained by focusing on sensory substitution and increase sensitivity of the remaining visual and somatosensory senses. Patients who compensate poorly for lack of joint coordination by co-contracting the neck or increasing limb spasticity, can be exposed to alternative, less energy inefficient movement patterns, with or without prosthetic or assistive devices. Patients with Parkinson's disease who have difficulty initiating a step, can be shown how to use external cues or imagined cues to trigger a step. In general, rehabilitation of balance and gait should involve exposing subjects to particular tasks and environments that allow the nervous system to discover the most optimal and effective strategies available for their specific functional goals.

In conclusion, this chapter proposes two new classifications that would serve different purposes. The systems oriented balance and gait disorders classification is intended to provide a logical hierarchy and indicate inter-relations of balance and gait disorders. It is partially hypothetical because higher level disorders have received less attention in clinical and laboratory investigations and the proper places for some disorders in the classification are unproven. The pattern or syndrome classification is intended to help the clinician consider the diagnostic possibilities for falls, abnormal postural responses and abnormal gait patterns.

Safe, efficient ambulation is a wonderful attribute of health. Understanding the many ways in which it may be disturbed by neurological disease should lead to better methods to treat or cope with dysfunction.

References   * denotes key references

Achiron, A., Ziv, I., Goren, M. et al. (1993). Primary progressive freezing gait. *Mov. Disord.*, **8**, 293–7.

Armstrong, D.M. (1988). Supraspinal control of locomotion. *J. Physiol.*, **405**, 1–37.

Baloh, R.W., Yue, Q., Socotch, T.M. & Jacobson, K.M. (1995). White matter lesions and disequilibrium in older people: I. case-control comparison. *Arch. Neurol.*, **52**, 970–4.

Bisdorff, A.R., Wolsley, C.J., Anastasopoulos, D., Bronstein, A.M. & Gresty, M.A. (1996). The perception of body verticality (subjective postural vertical) in peripheral and central vestibular disorders. *Brain*, **119**, 1523–34.

Bruns, L.. (1892). Uber storugen des gleichgewichtes bei stirnhirntumoren. *Dtsch. Med. Wochensch.*, **18**, 138–40.

Dieterich, M. & Brandt, T. (1993). Thalamic infarctions: differential effects on vestibular function in the roll plane (35 patients). *Neurology*, **43**, 1732–40.

Dietz, V., Colombo, G. & Jensen, L. (1994). Locomotor activity in spinal man. *Lancet*, **344**, 1260–3.

Eidelberg, E., Walden, J.G. & Nguyen, L.H. (1981). Locomotor control in Macaque monkeys. *Brain*, **104**, 647–63.

Giladi, N., Kao, R. & Fahn, S. (1997). Freezing phenomenon in patients with parkinsonian syndromes. *Mov. Disord.*, **12**, 302–5.

Grillner, S. & Wallen, P. (1985). Central pattern generators for locomotion with special reference to vertebrates. *Ann. Rev. Neurosci.*, **8**, 233–61.

Gross, C.G. & Graziano, M.S.A. (1995). Multiple representations of space in the brain. *Neuroscientist*, **1**, 43–50.

Horak, F.C. & Diener, H.C. (1994). Cerebellar control of postural scaling and central set in stance. *J. Neurophysiol.*, **72**, 479–93.

Horak, F.B. & Macpherson, J.M. (1996). Postural orientation and equilibrium: interaction and coordination. *Handbook of Physiology*, pp. 255–92. New York: Oxford University Press.

Horak, F.B., Nashner, L.M. & Diener, H.C. (1990). Postural strategies associated with somatosensory and vestibular loss. *Exp. Brain Res.*, **82**, 167–77.

Horak, F.B., Nutt, J.G. & Nashner, L.M. (1992). Postural inflexibility in parkinsonian subjects. *J. Neurol. Sci.*, **111**, 46–58.

Karnath, H-O. (1994). Subjective body orientation in neglect and the interactive contribution of neck muscle proprioception and vestibular stimulation. *Brain*, **117**, 1001–12.

Karnath, H-O., Ferber, S. & Dichgans, J. (2000). The origin of contraversive pushing: evidence for a second graviceptive system in humans. *Neurology*, **55**, 1298–304.

Keane, J.R. (1989). Hysterical gait disorders: 60 cases. *Neurology*, **39**, 586–9.

Labadie, E.L., Awerbuch, G.I., Hamilton, R.H. & Rapesak, S.Z. (1989). Falling and postural deficits due to acute unilateral basal ganglia lesions. *Arch. Neurol.*, **45**, 492–6.

Lempert, T., Brandt, T., Dieterich, M. & Huppert, D. (1991). How to identify psychogenic disorders of stance and gait. *J. Neurol.*, **238**, 140–6.

Macpherson, J.M. & Fung, J.R. (1999). Weight support and balance in stance in the chronic spinal cat. *J. Neurophysiol.*, **82**, 3066–81.

Masdeu, J.C. & Gorelick, P.B. (1988). Thalamic astasia: inability to stand after unilateral thalamic lesions. *Ann. Neurol.*, **23**, 596–603.

Massion, J. (1992). Movement, posture, and equilibrium: interaction and coordination. *Prog. Neurobiol.*, **38**, 35–56.

Meyer, J.S. & Barron, D.W. (1960). Apraxia of gait: a clinicophysiological study. *Brain*, **83**, 261–84.

Mori, S. (1987). Intergration of posture and locomotion in acute decerebrate cats and in awake freely moving cats. *Prog. Neurobiol.*, **28**, 161–95.

Murphy, J. & Isaacs, B. (1982). The post-fall syndrome: a study of 36 elderly patients. *Gerontology*, **82**, 265–70.

Nashner, L.M., Shumway-Cook, A. & Marin, O. (1983). Stance posture in selected groups of children with cerebral palsy: deficits in sensory organization and muscular coordination. *Exp. Brain Res.*, **49**, 393–409.

*Nutt, J.G., Marsden, C.D. & Thompson, P.D. (1993). Human walking and higher level gait disorders, particularly in the elderly. *Neurology*, **43**, 268–79.

Orlovsky, G.N. & Shik, M.L. (1976). Control of locomotion: a neurophysiological analysis of the cat locomotor system. *Int. Rev. Physiol.*, **10**, 281–317.

Petrovici, I. (1968). Apraxia of gait and of trunk movements. *J. Neurol. Sci.*, **7**, 229–43.

*Province, M.A., Hadley, E.C., Hornbrook, M.C. et al. (1995). The effects of exercise on falls in elderly patients: a preplanned meta-analysis of the FICSIT trials. *J. Am. Med. Assoc.*, **273**, 1341–7.

Salgado, R., Lord, S.R., Packer, J. & Ehrlich, F. (1994). Factors associated with falling in elderly hospital patients. *Gerontology*, **40**, 325–31.

Thompson, P.D. & Marsden, C.D. (1987). Gait disorder of subcortical arteriosclerotic encephalopathy: Binswanger's disease. *Mov. Disord.*, **2**, 1–8.

*Tinetti, M.E., Speechley, M. & Ginter, S.F. (1988). Risk factors for falls among elderly persons living in the community. *N. Engl. J. Med.*, **319**, 1701–7.

*Tinetti, M.E., Baker, D.I., McAvay, G. et al. (1994). A multifactorial intervention to reduce the risk of falling among elderly people living in the community. *N. Engl. J. Med.*, **331**, 821–7.

van Bogart, L. & Martin, P. (1929). Sur deux signes du syndrome de desequilibration frontale: l'apraxie de la marche et l'antonie statique. *Encephale*, **24**, 11–18.

Woollacott, M.H. & Moore, S. (1992). Improvements in balance in the elderly through training in sensory organization abilities. In *Sensorimotor Impairments in the Elderly*, ed. G.E. Stelmach & V. Homberg, pp. 377–92. Kluwer Academic Publishers.

Wright, D.L. & Kemp, T.L. (1992). The dual-task methodology and assessing the attentional demands of ambulation with walking devices. *Phys. Ther.*, **72**, 306–15.

Yanagisawa, N., Ueno, E. & Takami, M. (1991). Frozen gait of Parkinson's disease and vascular parkinsonism – a study with floor reaction forces and EMG. In *Neurobiological Basis of Human Locomotion*, ed. M. Shimamura, S. Grillner & V.R. Edgerton, pp. 291–304. Tokyo: Japan Scientific Societies Press.

Part IV

Disorders of the special senses

41

Smell

Richard L. Doty[1] and Steven M. Bromley[1,2]

[1] Smell and Taste Center, University of Pennsylvania Medical Center, Philadelphia, PA, USA
[2] Neurological Institute of New York, Columbia-Presbyterian Medical Center, New York, NY, USA

Possibly owing to the fact that, historically, most disorders of smell function have been difficult to diagnose and treat, physicians often downplay this sense in the routine neurological examination. This is unfortunate when one considers that olfactory disorders are relatively common and profoundly effect a patient's quality of life. Along with its sister sense of taste (see Chapter 42), olfaction determines, among other things, the flavour of foods and beverages, and provides an early warning system for detecting leaking natural gas, spoiled food, fire and other adverse environmental situations. Importantly, olfactory disturbances can be an early sign of such serious diseases or anomalies as Alzheimer's disease, idiopathic Parkinson's disease, epilepsy, multiple sclerosis, and schizophrenia. Although some patients initially present with a frank complaint of a smell disturbance, others are unaware of their dysfunction, pointing out the need for routine quantitative olfactory assessment, which is now easily performed in the office.

In this chapter, we (a) summarize key aspects of olfactory anatomy and physiology, (b) present up-to-date practical techniques for the management and quantitative evaluation of the olfactory system, and (c) describe basic olfactory disorders commonly encountered in the neurological setting.

Anatomy and physiology

Olfactory neuroepithelium: a portal to the central nervous system

The olfactory receptors are located within a ~ 2 cm² neuroepithelium lining the cribriform plate and regions of the superior turbinate, middle turbinate, and septum. The neurologist should be aware of the fact that, in addition to the main olfactory system (CN I), other specialized neural systems are present in the nose. These include (a) trigemi-nal (CN V) afferents responsible, for example, for the coolness of menthol vapours (Doty, 1995a), (b) a rudimentary and non-functional vomeronasal organ (VNO) near the base of the septum (Bhatnagar & Meisami, 1998; Smith & Bhatnagar, 2000), and (c) the poorly understood nervus terminalis or terminal nerve (CN O). CN O, a highly conserved neural plexus that ramifies throughout the nasal epithelium, is distinguished by ganglia at nodal points and a high gonadotropin content, and presumably plays no role in human odour perception (Schwanzel-Fukuda & Pfaff, 1995). Throughout life, islands of respiratory-like epithelial metaplasia appear within the epithelium, presumably as a result of cumulative viral, bacterial, and other insults Among the cells within the neuroepithelium (see Fig. 41.1) are (a) the *bipolar sensory receptor neurons* which harbour the seven domain transmembrane odorant receptors on multiple cilia extending from each dendritic knob, (b) the *supporting or sustentacular cells*, which have microvillae and serve structural and metabolic functions, (c) the poorly understood *microvillar cells* located at the surface of the epithelium, (d) the *cells that line the Bowman's glands and ducts*, and (e) the *globose (light)* and *horizontal (dark) basal cells* – cells located near the basement membrane from which most of the other cell types arise (Huard et al., 1998).

Olfactory nerve cells, as well as the proximal extraneural spaces, are well-established conduits for the movement of viruses and exogenous agents from the nasal cavity into the brain. In the case of viruses, transit times occur at rates usually intermediate between slow and fast axonal transport, e.g. around 3 mm/day for rabies virus, 8–16 mm/day for herpes simplex virus, and 14 mm/day for retrovirus (Stroop, 1995). This pathway has been recognized for some time (e.g. Clark, 1929; Hurst, 1936), as has the knowledge that chemical cauterization of the olfactory mucosa protects against viral-related CNS infection (Armstrong & Harrison, 1935; Burnet & Lush, 1938). Such knowledge led to

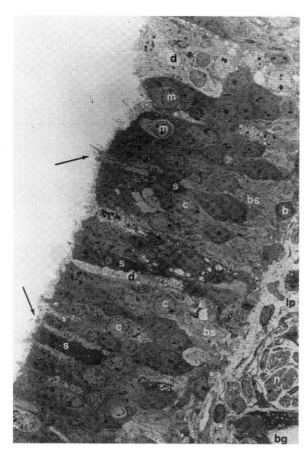

Fig. 41.1. Low-power electron micrograph (×670) of a longitudinal section through a biopsy specimen of human olfactory mucosa taken from the nasal septum. Four cell types are indicated: ciliated olfactory receptors (c), microvillar cells (m), supporting cells (s), and basal cells (b). The arrows point to ciliated olfactory knobs of the bipolar receptor cells. d = degenerating cells; bs = base of the supporting cells; lp = lamina propria; n = nerve bundle; bg = Bowman's gland. (Photo courtesy of David T. Moran.)

a prophylaxis movement in the late 1930s to spray noses of school children with zinc sulfate during poliomyelitis outbreaks (Peet et al., 1937; Schultz & Gebhardt, 1937; Tisdall et al., 1937). More recently, the 'olfactory vector hypothesis' has been proposed to explain both the olfactory loss and the etiology of several common neurodegenerative diseases (Doty, 1991; Doty et al., 1992a; Ferreyra-Moyano & Barragan, 1989; Roberts, 1986; Hawkes et al., 1999).

Olfactory neural transduction

Once odorants traverse the olfactory mucus and reach the cilia, they contact and bind to receptors which initiate the transduction cascades that ultimately result in action potentials. Around 1000 olfactory receptor types are believed to exist, and a given receptor cell contains only one type of receptor (Buck & Axel, 1991). Neurons expressing the same gene seem to be randomly distributed, at least in the mouse, within one of four segregated strip-like 'spatial zones' of the neuroepithelium, and olfactory neurons expressing a given gene seem to project to the same glomeruli within the olfactory bulb (Ngai et al., 1993). A given odorant activates an idiosyncratic pattern of activity across the population of receptors: a pattern that serves as the initial basis for odour perception and discrimination (Shepherd & Firestein, 1991).

Despite the fact that, under normal circumstances, there is continuous neurogenesis within basal segments of the epithelium, many receptor cells are long-lived and become replaced only after damage (Hinds et al., 1984). Both endogenous and exogenous factors promote receptor cell death and replenishment from the basal progenitor stem cells (Mackay-Sim & Kittel, 1990).

The olfactory bulb

The neural components of the olfactory bulb, the first neural processing station in the olfactory pathway, are arranged in six concentric layers: the olfactory nerve layer, the glomerular layer, the external plexiform layer, the mitral cell layer, the internal plexiform layer, and the granule cell layer (Fig. 41.2). The axons of the olfactory nerve cells synapse, within the glomeruli of the glomerular layer, with the dendrites of mitral and tufted cells, the major second order neurons of the olfactory system. The latter cells, in turn, send collaterals that synapse within the periglomerular and external plexiform layers, resulting in 'reverberating' circuits in which negative and positive feedback occur. For example, mitral cells modulate their own output by activating granule cells (which are inhibitory to them). Reciprocal inhibition between neighbouring mitral or tufted cells presumably sharpens the contrast between adjacent channels, perhaps analogous to what occurs among visual receptors within the retina.

The mitral and tufted axons project ipsilaterally to the primary olfactory cortex via the lateral olfactory tract without synapsing in the thalamus. However, some projections from primary to secondary (e.g. orbitofrontal) cortex do relay through the thalamus (see Fig. 41.3). Furthermore, contralateral projections also occur via the anterior commissure, largely from pyramidal cells of the anterior olfactory nucleus (AON).

The primary olfactory cortex

In addition to the AON, the mitral and tufted cells target (from rostral to caudal) (a) the piriform cortex, (b) the olfactory tubercle, (c) the entorhinal area, (d) the peri-amygdaloid cortex, and (e) the corticomedial amygdala (Fig. 41.3). Most of the olfactory cortical structures have three distinct layers. The superficial segment of layer 1 contains synapses between (a) the incoming mitral and tufted cell axons and (b) the apical dendrites of the pyramidal cells, the principal olfactory cortical neurons. The deeper segments of layer 1 contain connections among intracortical association areas. Layers 2 and 3 are made up of cell bodies and processes of the pyramidal cells. Small populations of intrinsic short axon cells are present within all three layers. The axons of the pyramidal neurons project reciprocally, via layer 2 and 3 connections, to numerous regions, including the anterior commissure, the mediodorsal thalamus, the posterior hypothalamus, and the medial hypothalamus and hippocampus. Centrifugal fibres richly project from sectors of the olfactory cortex and other central structures to the olfactory bulb, presumably modulating the incoming flow of olfactory sensory signals (Kratskin, 1995) (Fig. 41.4).

Olfactory cortical regions: functional anatomy

While lesions of the olfactory neuroepithelium, the olfactory fila, or the olfactory bulbs and tracts rostral to the olfactory trigone can produce *total anosmia* on the affected side, lesions within olfactory structures more posterior to the olfactory trigone do not typically cause *complete* loss (Gloor, 1997). Orbitofrontal cortex lesions produce difficulties in discriminating or identifying odours, and odour discrimination is reportedly impaired following amygdalotomy (Zatorre and Jones-Gotman, 1991; Jones-Gotman et al., 1997a). In multiple sclerosis, the number of plaques within the inferior medial temporal and inferior frontal lobes correlates strongly ($r = -0.94$) with odour identification test scores (Doty et al., 1997a, 1998). Recent functional imaging studies have reported greater right than left orbitofrontal cortex activation by odorants, suggesting some hemispheric specialization (Malaspina et al., 1998; Yousem et al., 1997a; Zatorre et al., 1992). Olfactory stimulation reliably and significantly activates posterior lateral cerebellar areas, whereas sniffing alone activates mainly anterior central cerebellar regions (Sobel et al., 1998a, b; Yousem et al., 1997).

Classification of olfactory disorders

Olfactory disorders can be reliably classified as follows: *anosmia*: inability to detect qualitative olfactory sensations (i.e. absence of smell function); *partial anosmia*: ability to perceive some, but not all, odorants; *hyposmia* or

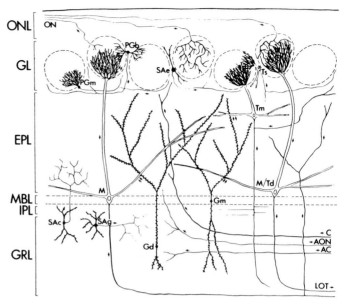

Fig. 41.2. Diagram of major layers and types of neurons in the mammalian olfactory bulb, as based on stained Golgi material. Main layers are indicated on the left as follows: ONL = olfactory nerve layer; GL = glomerular layer; EPL = external plexiform layer; MBL = mitral cell body layer; IPL = internal plexiform layer; GRL = granule cell layer; ON = olfactory nerves; PGb = periglomerular cells with biglomerular dendrites; PGm = periglomerular cell with monoglomerular dendrites; SAe = short-axon cell with extraglomerular dendrites; M = mitral cell; M/Td = displaced mitral or deep tufted cell; Tm = middle tufted cell; Ts = superficial tufted cell; Gm = granule cell with cell body in mitral body layer; Gd = granule cell with cell body in deep layers; SAc = short-axon cell of Cajal; SAg = short-axon cell of Golgi; C = centrifugal fibres; AON = fibres from anterior olfactory nucleus; AC = fibres from anterior commissure; LOT = lateral olfactory tract. (From Shepherd, 1972; Copyright © 1972 American Physiological Society.)

microsmia: decreased sensitivity to odorants; *hyperosmia*: abnormally acute smell function; *dysosmia* (sometimes termed cacosmia or parosmia): distorted or perverted smell perception to odorant stimulation; *phantosmia*: a dysosmic sensation perceived in the absence of an odour stimulus (a.k.a. olfactory hallucination); and *olfactory agnosia*: inability to recognize an odour sensation, even though olfactory processing, language, and general intellectual functions are essentially intact, as in some stroke patients. Presbyosmia is sometimes used to describe smell loss due to ageing, but this term is less specific than those noted above (e.g. it does not distinguish between anosmia and hyposmia) and is laden, by definition, with the notion that it is age per se that is causing the age-related deficit.

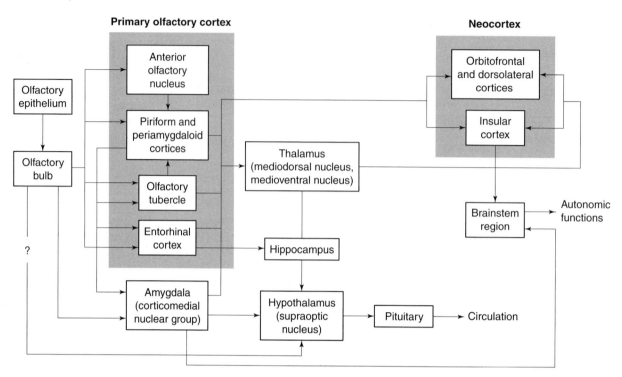

Fig. 41.3. Major afferent neural connections of the olfactory system. Structures common to both the olfactory and limbic systems include the olfactory tubercle, the entorhinal cortex, the amygdala, the hippocampus, and the hypothalamus. Although it is well established that the olfactory fibres project from the amygdala to the 'feeding centre' of the hypothalamus (especially the ventromedial and ventrolateral nuclei), it is unclear whether direct olfactohypothalamic routes exist in humans, as may be the case in some other vertebrates. (Copyright © 2001, Richard L. Doty.)

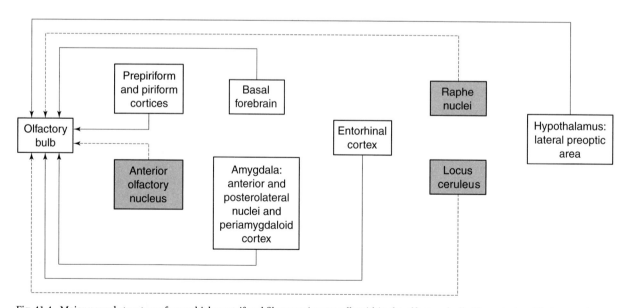

Fig. 41.4. Major neural structures from which centrifugal fibres project to cells within the olfactory bulb. The anterior olfactory nucleus, locus ceruleus, and raphae nuclei are known to have projections to both olfactory bulbs. The other depicted structures are presumed to have primarily, if not solely, ipsilateral projections to the bulbs. (Copyright © 2001, Richard L. Doty.)

Clinical evaluation of olfactory function

History

Details concerning the nature, timing of onset, duration and pattern of fluctuations, if any, of the patient's chemosensory problem are all very important. Discovery of precipitating antecedent events, such as head trauma, viral upper respiratory infections, toxic exposures, and nasal surgeries is critical. A history of allergy should be sought. The use of drugs (e.g. intranasal cocaine), alcohol (e.g. chronic alcoholism in the context of Wernicke and Korsakoff syndromes), and smoking tobacco are also important given the association between smell loss and such factors. A determination of the medications that the patient is or was taking is needed, as some drugs, such as angiotensin-converting enzyme (ACE) inhibitors, often have distinct influences on olfaction. It is critical to be aware that while patients often complain of problems with smell and taste, quantitative testing usually reveals only an olfactory problem, reflecting decreased retronasal stimulation of the olfactory receptors during deglutition (Burdach & Doty, 1987).

The examiner should ascertain whether the patient has any other medical conditions potentially associated with smell impairment (e.g. renal failure, liver disease, hypothyroidism, diabetes, or dementia). Questions regarding epistaxis, discharge (clear, purulent or bloody), nasal obstruction, allergies and somatic symptoms, including headache or irritation may have localizing value. A family history of smell dysfunction may suggest a genetic etiology. Subtle symptoms of central tumours, dementia, parkinsonism, and seizure activity (e.g. automatisms, occurrence of black-outs, auras, and *déjà vu*) should be sought. Delayed puberty in association with anosmia (with or without midline craniofacial abnormalities, deafness, and renal anomalies) suggests the possibility of Kallmann's syndrome or some variant thereof.

Physical examination and laboratory tests

The neurological component of the evaluation should focus on cranial nerve function, with particular attention to possible skull base and intracranial lesions. Visual acuity, visual field, and optic disc examinations aid in the detection of possible intracranial mass lesions and in the detection of the Foster Kennedy syndrome (ipsilateral anosmia, ipsilateral optic atrophy, and contralateral papilledema secondary to raised intracranial pressure) (Watnick & Trobe, 1989). The otolaryngological examination should employ nasal endoscopy, both flexible and rigid, to ensure thorough assessment of the olfactory meatal area. Appropriate medical imaging should be employed to assess sinonasal tract inflammation (e.g. computerized tomography), as well as brain lesions and the integrity of the olfactory bulbs, tracts, and cortical parenchyma (e.g. magnetic resonance imaging). Some laboratory tests (e.g. blood serum tests) may be helpful in detecting underlying medical conditions suggested by history and physical examinations, such as infection, nutritional deficiencies (e.g. B6, B12), allergy, diabetes mellitus, and thyroid, liver, and kidney disease (Bromley, 2000).

Quantitative olfactory testing

A number of practical standardized clinical smell tests are now commercially available (for review, see Doty, 2001a), providing the neurologist with the ability to (a) determine of the validity of patients' complaints (including the detection of malingering), (b) characterize the exact nature of the problem, (c) reliably monitor changes in function over time (including those of iatrogenic etiology), and (d) accurately establish compensation for permanent disability. The most widely used of these tests are self-administered 'scratch and sniff' tests, ranging from the 3-item Pocket Smell Test™ to the 40-item University of Pennsylvania Smell Identification Test (UPSIT; commercially termed the Smell Identification Test™ or SIT) (Doty, 1995b; Doty et al., 1996). Available in English, Spanish, French, and German language versions, the latter test can be self-administered in 10 to 15 minutes by most patients in the waiting room, and scored in less than a minute by non-medical personnel. Results are expressed in terms of a percentile score of a patient's performance relative to age- and sex-matched controls, as well in categories of function: normosmia, mild microsmia, moderate microsmia, severe microsmia, anosmia, and probable malingering. Malingering is inferred from improbable responses in the forced-choice setting.

Although olfactory event-related potentials (OERPs) are available in some specialized medical centers, including our own, their general practicality is limited. They require expensive equipment capable of delivering well-delineated 'square wave' odorant pulses to the olfactory receptors within a background of continuously flowing warmed and humidified air (Doty & Kobal, 1995). Unlike their visual and auditory counterparts, OERPs are unable to discern where in the pathway the anomaly exists.

Causes of olfactory dysfunction

In general, olfactory dysfunction is due to one of three causes: (a) conductive or transport impairments from obstruction of the nasal passages (e.g. by chronic nasal inflammation, polyposis, etc.); (b) sensorineural impairment from damage to the olfactory neuroepithelium (e.g. by viruses, airborne toxins, etc.); and (c) central olfactory neural impairment from CNS damage (e.g. tumours, masses impacting on olfactory tract, etc.). These categories are not necessarily mutually exclusive. For example, both damage and blockage of airflow to the receptors can occur from chronic rhinosinusitis.

As seen in Table 41.1, there are a number of known etiologies for olfactory disturbance. Nearly two-thirds of cases of chronic anosmia or hyposmia (i.e. those which are presumably permanent) are due to prior upper respiratory infections, head trauma, and nasal and paranasal sinus disease, and most reflect permanent damage to the olfactory neuroepithelium (Deems et al., 1991). Other causes include iatrogenic interventions (e.g. septoplasty, rhinoplasty, turbinectomy, radiation therapy, medications), intranasal neoplasms (e.g. inverting papilloma, hemangioma, and esthesioneuroblastoma), intracranial tumours or lesions (e.g. Foster Kennedy Syndrome, olfactory groove meningiomas, frontal lobe gliomas), neurodegenerative diseases, toxic exposures (which includes smoking), epilepsy, psychiatric disorders, and various endocrine and metabolic disorders. Details regarding some of the more common entities associated with smell loss are discussed below.

Ageing

In later life, decreased smell function is the rule, rather than the exception, and is largely responsible for the well-documented age-related increases in accidental gas poisonings and explosions, as well as weight loss, malnutrition, impaired immunity, and worsening of some medical illnesses (Doty et al., 1984a, Miletic et al., 1996; Mattes & Cowart, 1994). In contrast to the ~ 1% of persons under the age of 65 years with major smell loss, about half of the population between 65 and 80 years of age has such loss (Fig. 41.5). Over the age of 80, this figure rises to nearly 75% (Doty et al., 1984a). Often an accumulation of damage over the years is the culprit and a single event, such as a bad cold, can be the precipitating factor. In some cases, the olfactory loss may reflect, as a result of age-related appositional bone growth, the pinching off of the olfactory fila as they traverse the ethmoid bone (Kalmey et al., 1998). In general, the number olfactory receptors and olfactory bulb glomeruli decrease markedly with age (Smith, 1942; Meisami et al., 1998).

Post-upper respiratory infections

The most common cause of *permanent* smell loss in the adult human is that induced by upper respiratory infections

Table 41.1. Reported agents, diseases, drugs, interventions and other etiologic categories associated in the medical or toxicological literature with olfactory dysfunction. Note that categories are not mutually exclusive

Industrial dusts, metals, volatiles
Acetone
Acids (e.g. sulfuric)
Ashes
Benzene
Benzol
Butyl acetate
Cadmium
Carbon disulfide
Cement
Chalk
Chlorine
Chromium
Coke/coal
Cotton
Cresol
Ethyl acetate
Ethyl & methyl acrylate
Flour
Formaldehyde
Grain
Hydrazine
Hydrogen selenide
Hydrogen sulfide
Iron carboxyl
Lead
Mercury
Nickel
Nitrous gases
Paint solvents
Paper
Pepper
Peppermint oil
Phosphorus oxychloride
Potash
Silicone dioxide
Spices
Trichloroethylene

Drugs
Adrenal steroids (chronic use)
Amino acids (excess)
   Cysteine
   Histidine
Analgesics
   Antipyrine
Anesthetics, local
   Cocaine HCl
   Procaine HCl
   Tetracaine HCl

Table 41.1. (*cont.*)

Anticancer agents (e.g. methotrexate)
Antihistamines (e.g. chlorpheniramine malate) *See also* Table 41.2.
Antimicrobials
   Griseofulvin
   Lincomycin
   Macrolides
   Neomycin
   Penicillins
   Streptomycin
   Tetracyclines
   Tyrothricin
Antirheumatics
   Mercury/gold salts
   D-Penicillamine
Antithyroids
   Methimazole
   Propylthiouracil
   Thiouracil
Antivirals
Cardiovascular/hypertensives
Gastric medications
   Cimetidine
Hyperlipoproteinemia medications
   Artovastatin calcium (Lipitor)
Cholestyramine
Clofibrate
Intranasal saline solutions with:
   Acetylcholine
   Acetyl, β-methylcholine
   Menthol
   Strychnine
   Zinc sulfate
Local vasoconstrictors
Opiates
Codeine
   Hydromorphone HCl
   Morphine
Psychopharmaceuticals (e.g. LSD, psilocybin)
Sympathomimetics
   Amphetamine sulfate
   Fenbutrazate HCl
Phenmetrazine theoclate

Endocrine/metabolic
Addison's disease
Congenital adrenal hyperplasia
Cushing's syndrome
Diabetes mellitus
Froelich's syndrome
Gigantism
Hypergonadotropic hypogonadism
Hypothyroidism
Kallmann's syndrome
Pregnancy

Table 41.1. (*cont.*)

Panhypopituitarism
Pseudohypoparathyroidism
Sjögren's syndrome
Turner's syndrome

Infections – viral/bacterial
Acquired immunodeficiency syndrome (AIDS)
Acute viral rhinitis
Bacterial rhinosinusitis
Bronchiectasis
Fungal
Influenza
Rickettsial
Microfilarial

Lesions of the nose/airway blockage
Adenoid hypertrophy
Allergic rhinitis
   Perennial
   Seasonal
Atrophic rhinitis
Chronic inflammatory rhinitis
Hypertrophic rhinitis
Nasal polyposis
Rhinitis medicamentosa
Structural abnormality
   Deviated septum
   Weakness of alae nasi
Vasomotor rhinitis

Medical interventions
Adrenalectomy
Anesthesia
Anterior craniotomy
Arteriography
Chemotherapy
Frontal lobe resection
Gastrectomy
Hemodialysis
Hypophysectomy
Influenza vaccination
Laryngectomy
Oophorectomy
Paranasal sinus exenteration
Radiation therapy
Rhinoplasty
Temporal lobe resection
Thyroidectomy

Neoplasms – intracranial
Frontal lobe gliomas and other tumours
Midline cranial tumours
   Parasagital meningiomas
   Tumours of the corpus callosum

Table 41.1. (*cont.*)

Olfactory groove/cribriform plate meningiomas
Osteomas
Paraoptic chiasma tumours
  Aneurysms
  Craniopharyngioma
  Pituitary tumours (esp. adenomas)
  Suprasellar cholesteatoma
  Suprasellar meningioma
Temporal lobe tumours

Neoplasms – Intranasal
Neuro-olfactory tumours
  Esthesioepithelioma
  Esthesioneuroblastoma
  Esthesioneurocytoma
  Esthesioneuroepithelioma
Other benign or malignant nasal tumours
  Adenocarcinoma
  Leukemic infiltration
  Nasopharyngeal tumours with extension
  Neurofibroma
  Paranasal tumours with extension
  Schwannoma

Neoplasms – extranasal and extracranial
Breast
Gastrointestinal tract
Laryngeal
Lung
Ovary
Testicular

Neurologic
Amyotrophic lateral sclerosis
Alzheimer's disease
Cerebral abscess (esp. frontal or ethmoidal regions)
Down's syndrome
Familial dysautonomia
Guam ALS/PD/dementia
Head trauma
Huntington's disease
Hydrocephalus
Korsakoff's psychosis
Migraine
Meningitis
Multiple sclerosis
Myesthenia gravis
Paget's disease
Parkinson's disease
Refsum's syndrome
Restless leg syndrome
Syphilis
Syringomyelia

Table 41.1. (*cont.*)

Temporal lobe epilepsy
  Hamartomas
  Mesial temporal sclerosis
  Scars/previous infarcts
  Vascular insufficiency/anoxia
  Small multiple cerebrovascular accidents
  Subclavian steal syndrome
  Transient ischemic attacks

Nutritional/metabolic
Abetalipoproteinemia
Chronic alcoholism
Chronic renal failure
Cirrhosis of liver
Gout
Protein calorie malnutition
Total parenteral nutrition w/o adequate replacement
Trace metal deficiencies
  Copper
  Zinc
Whipple's disease
Vitamin deficiency
  Vitamin A
  Vitamin B6
  Vitamin B12

Pulmonary
Chronic obstructive pulmonary disease

Psychiatric
Anorexia nervosa (severe stage)
Attention deficit disorder
Depressive disorders
Hysteria
Malingering
Olfactory reference syndrome
Schizophrenia
Schizotypy
Seasonal affective disorder

(URIs), such as those associated with the common cold, influenza, and pneumonia. Often the respiratory illness is described as being more severe than usual. Exactly what predisposes someone to viral- or bacterial-induced smell dysfunction or the mechanisms underlying it remains unclear. Direct insult to the olfactory neuroepithelium is likely, but central structures may also be affected. In general, patients with URI-related anosmia have markedly reduced numbers of receptors and when receptors are present, they appear abnormal compared to those patients with hyposmia (Jafek et al., 1990). Although spontaneous recovery in

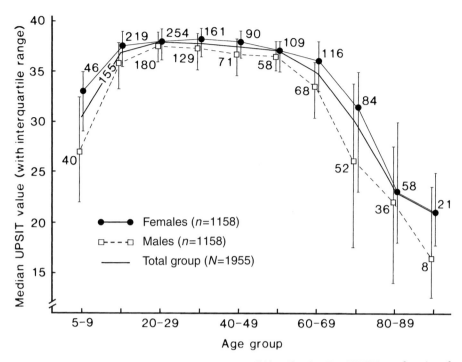

Fig. 41.5. Scores on the University of Pennsylvania Smell Identification Test (UPSIT) as a function of age and gender in a large heterogeneous group of subjects. Numbers by data points indicate sample sizes. (From Doty et al., 1984b; Copyright © 1984, American Association for the Advancement of Science.)

these patients is theoretically possible given the propensity of olfactory neurons to regenerate, meaningful recovery is unlikely when marked loss has been present for a period of time.

Head trauma

Smell disturbance following head trauma is common, particularly where rapid acceleration/deceleration of the brain occurs (i.e. coup contra coup injury). On average, blows to the occiput have been found to produce greater olfactory loss than blows to the front of the head (Doty et al., 1997b). The most common mechanisms include disruption of the sinonasal tract from shearing forces, and direct contusion and ischemia to the olfactory bulb and frontal and temporal poles (Fig. 41.6). The prevalence of olfactory dysfunction in patients with head trauma is typically below 15% (Yousem et al., 1999), and is proportional to the severity of the injury (Doty et al., 1997b). Dysosmia, when present, typically decreases significantly over the post-trauma period (Doty et al., 1997b). In severe cases, MRI images reveal damage to the olfactory bulbs, tracts, and areas of the temporal and frontal lobes (Yousem et al., 1996). Animal studies show that intracranial hemorrhage and ischemia can lead to degeneration of the olfactory epi-

thelium without transection of the olfactory nerves (Nakashima et al., 1983).

Nasal and sinus disease

Unlike the sensorineural dysfunction that can follow a viral syndrome or head trauma, olfactory impairment that accompanies nasal or sinus disease has been traditionally viewed as being solely conductive. However, empirical data suggest that surgical (e.g. excision of polyps) or medical (e.g. administration of topical or systemic steroids) treatment rarely returns function to normal levels, implying that blockage alone cannot explain the olfactory loss (Doty & Mishra, 2001). Recently it has been shown that the severity of histopathological changes within the olfactory mucosa of patients with chronic rhinosinusitis is positively related to the magnitude of olfactory loss (Kern, 2000). Furthermore, biopsies from the neuroepithelial region of patients with nasal disease are less likely to yield olfactory-related tissue than biopsies from controls (Feron et al., 1998). The same is true for anosmic vs. non-anosmic rhinosinusitis patients, the former of whom exhibit a generally more pathological epithelium (e.g. disordered arrangement of cells, more islands of respiratory-like epithelium) (Lee et al., 2000).

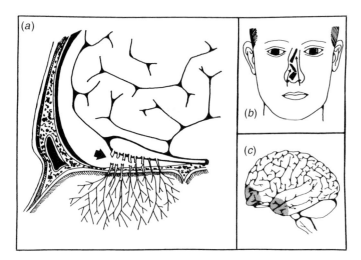

Fig. 41.6. Mechanisms of post-traumatic olfactory dysfunction. (*a*) Shearing or tearing of the olfactory fila. (*b*) Injury to the sinonasal tract (*c*) Cortical contusions and brain hemorrhage. (From Costanzo & Zasler, 1991; Copyright © 1991, Raven Press, Ltd.)

CNS neoplasms

According to Finelli and Mair (1991), the single most egregious error of neurologists is failure to recognize the symptom of anosmia as the principal or sole feature of an olfactory groove neoplasm. Tumours impinging on the olfactory bulbs or tracts, such as olfactory groove meningiomas, frontal lobe gliomas, and suprasellar ridge meningiomas arising from the dura of the cribriform plate, have been associated with olfactory disturbance, as have tumours on the floor of the third ventricle, pituitary tumours that extend above the sella turcica, and tumours in the temporal lobe or uncinate convolution.

Neurodegenerative and other neurological diseases

Olfactory deficits have been described in such neurological disorders as Alzheimer's disease, idiopathic Parkinson's disease, Huntington's disease, alcoholic Korsakoff's syndrome, Pick's disease, the parkinson dementia complex of Guam, amyotrophic lateral sclerosis, schizophrenia, and multiple sclerosis (Mesholam et al., 1998; Doty, 1991; Doty et al., 1998; Moberg et al., 1997a; b). Importantly, olfactory dysfunction may be the first clinical sign of Alzheimer's disease (AD) and idiopathic Parkinson's disease (PD) (Doty et al., 1987, 1988b). Although not classically considered a neurodegenerative disease, schizophrenia also is associated with smell loss that appears to be correlated with disease duration, suggesting a possible progressive or degenerative component to this disorder in olfaction-related pathways (Moberg et al., 1997b). The olfactory

bulbs and tracts of patients with schizophrenia are markedly smaller than those of controls (Turetsky et al., 2000).

Two studies have recently demonstrated that smell testing is useful in identifying persons at risk for later significant cognitive decline or AD. Graves et al. (1999) tested 1985 Japanese–American people around the age of 60 with cognitive tests and an abbreviated version of the UPSIT, and then rescreened 1604 of these people after two years. They also genotyped 69% of the follow-up participants for apolipoprotein E (apoE). Overall, olfactory dysfunction in the presence of one or more APOE-e4 alleles was associated with a very high risk of subsequent cognitive decline, and smell testing identified persons who came to exhibit later cognitive decline better than did a global cognitive test. More recently, Devanand et al. (2000) administered the UPSIT to 90 outpatients with mild cognitive impairment at 6-month intervals, along with matched healthy controls. Patients with mild cognitive impairment scored lower on the UPSIT than did the controls. Most importantly, patients with low UPSIT scores (<34) were more likely to develop AD than the other patients. Low UPSIT scores, combined with lack of awareness of olfactory deficits on the part of the patients, predicted the time to development of AD. UPSIT scores from 30–35 showed moderate to strong sensitivity and specificity for diagnosis of AD at follow-up.

The underlying physiological basis of the olfactory loss in patients with AD is not yet clear, although this disorder is associated with a profound loss of neurons in the anterior olfactory nucleus, olfactory bulb, and layer II of the entorhinal cortex (Doty, 1991; Gomez-Isla et al., 1996). Limbic brain regions which receive olfactory bulb mitral and tufted cell projections are disproportionately laden with neurofibrillary tangles and neuritic plaques (Delacourte et al., 1999). Deficits in the neurotransmitter acetylcholine may somehow relate to this problem, as it is well established that (a) individuals with no history of cognitive loss that are in the early histopathologic stages of AD exhibit a cholinergic deficit within the inferior temporal lobe and (b) drugs that alter cholinergic function alter the ability to smell. For example, scopolamine, a muscarinic cholinergic antagonist, reportedly decreases olfactory sensitivity (Serby et al., 1990), whereas physostigmine, a cholinesterase inhibitor, improves odour discrimination performance, at least in rats (Doty et al., 1999a).

In idiopathic PD, bilateral olfactory deficits occur before the onset of most of the classical neurological signs and symptoms (Doty et al., 1988b). The PD-related olfactory impairment is unrelated to disease stage, use of antiparkinson medications, duration of the illness, and severity of the symptoms, such as tremor, rigidity, bradykinesia or gait disturbance (Doty et al., 1992b). Since olfactory loss is pervasive and marked in PD, as well as in AD, and is absent or not present to the same degree in a number of other neurological disorders, it can be used to distinguish among disorders that share many symptoms and signs with PD (Doty, 1991). For example, while patients with essential tremor, progressive supranuclear palsy, multiple system atrophy and parkinsonism induced by the proneurotoxin 1-methyl-4-phenyl-1, 2, 3, 6-tetrahydropyridine (MPTP) share a number of motor symptoms with idiopathic PD, they have little or no olfactory dysfunction (Doty, 1991). Like idiopathic PD, familial PD is also associated with olfactory impairment, and this heritable defect occurs independently of the parkinsonian phenotype (Markopoulou et al., 1997).

In multiple sclerosis, olfactory loss is directly proportional to the number of MS-related plaques in central brain regions associated with olfactory processing (e.g. inferior middle temporal lobe and periorbital frontal cortex) (Doty et al., 1997b, 1998). A 1:1 longitudinal association is present between UPSIT scores and changes in plaque load over time (Doty et al., 1999b), implying that olfactory function increases and decreases as the plaque numbers increase and decrease. In effect, knowledge of a patient's UPSIT score largely predicts the plaque load in the olfaction-related regions.

Other causes

A number of environmental and industrial chemicals have been linked to olfactory dysfunction, including acrylates, cadmium, benzene, formaldehyde, solvents, and nickel dust, although few well-controlled studies exist in this area and most reports are largely anecdotal (Doty & Hastings, 2001). With regard to cigarette smoking, olfactory ability decreases as a function of cumulative smoking dose and cessation of smoking can result in improvement in olfactory function over time (Frye et al., 1990). Medications commonly affect smell function and should be considered early in an evaluation, especially in the context of a new drug therapy (Table 41.2). Olfactory hallucinations occur in mesial temporal lobe seizures and migraine. Hyperosmia is classically associated with pregnancy and hyperemesis gravidarum, although objective evidence of true hypersensitivity, rather than hyperreactivity, is still lacking. Despite the fact that some patients with apparent multiple chemical hypersensitivity syndrome (MCS) report heightened ability to smell, olfactory thresholds are not meaningfully altered (Doty et al., 1988a). Hyperosmia reportedly occurs in some cases of epilepsy during the interictal period, although, as noted above, most patients with long-term epilepsy and intractable seizure activity,

such as candidates for temporal lobe resection, are hyposmic.

Treatment of olfactory disorders

As alluded to earlier, meaningful treatments are available for some, but not all, patients whose olfactory dysfunction is conductive; i.e. resulting from blockage of airflow to the olfactory neuroepithelium. Such therapies include allergy management, topical and systemic corticosteroid therapies, and surgical procedures to reduce inflammation or obstructions (e.g. polyps). A brief course of systemic steroid therapy can be useful in distinguishing between conductive and sensorineural olfactory loss, as patients with the former will often respond positively to some extent to the treatment, although longer term systemic steroid therapy is not advised. Topical nasal steroids are often ineffectual in returning smell function because the steroid fails to reach the affected regions in the upper nasal passages. Increased efficacy presumably occurs when the nasal drops or spray are administered in the head-down Moffett position.

Patients with sensorineural causes of olfactory disturbance are difficult to manage, and the prognosis for patients suffering from long-standing total loss due to upper respiratory illness or head trauma is poor. Most patients who recover smell function subsequent to trauma do so within 12 weeks of injury (Costanzo et al., 1995). Although there are no verified treatments for trauma-related olfactory loss, anti-inflammatory agents may minimize post-traumatic sequelae in some cases. Recent rat research suggests that application of nerve growth factor onto the olfactory epithelium may alleviate axotomy-induced degenerative changes in the olfactory receptor neurons, although it is not known whether this has any functional consequence or if such a procedure in humans would be efficacious (Yasuno et al., 2000).

Tobacco smoking by itself rarely causes complete loss of the sense of smell, although patients who quit smoking typically have dose-related improvement in olfactory function and flavour sensation over time (Frye et al., 1990). Central lesions, such as CNS tumours that impinge on olfactory bulbs and tracts and epileptogenic foci within the medial temporal lobe that result in olfactory seizures, can often be resected in a manner that allows for some restoration of olfactory function. Medications that induce distortions of olfaction can often be discontinued and replaced with other types of medications or modes of therapy. Importantly, dopaminergic and cholinergic therapies do not improve the olfactory dysfunction seen in Parkinson's disease, and there is no evidence that neuroleptics alter the

Table 41.2. Selected medications that reportedly alter smell and/or taste. Most of these agents are noted in the Physician's Desk Reference (PDR) as having adverse effects on the olfactory system

Antianxiety agents
Alprazolam (Xanax)
Buspirone (BuSpar)

Antibiotics
Ampicillin
Azithromycin (Zithromax)
Ciprofloxacin (Cipro)
Clarithromycin (Biaxin)
Enalapril (Vaseretic)
Griseofulvin (Grisactin)
Metronidazole (Flagyl)
Ofloxacin (Floxin)
Terbinafine (Lamisil)
Ticarcillan (Timentin)
Tetracycline

Anticonvulsants
Carbamazepine (Tegretol)
Phenytoin (Dilantin)

Antidepressants
Amitriptyline (Elavil)
Clomipramine (Anafranil)
Desipramine (Norpramin)
Doxepin (Sinequan)
Imipramine (Tofranil)
Nortriptyline (Pamelor)

Antihistamines and decongestants
Chlorpheniramine
Loratadine (Claritin)
Pseudoephedrine

Antihypertensives and cardiac medications
Acetazolamide (Diamox)
Amiodarone (Pacerone)
Amiloride (Midamor)
Amiodarone (Cordarone)

Betaxolol (Betoptic)
Captopril (Capoten)
Diltiazem (Cardizem)
Enalapril (Lexxel, Vasotec, Vaseretic)
Hydrochlorothiazide (Esidix)
Nifedipine (Procardia)
Nitroglycerin
Propafenone (Rythmol)
Propranolol (Inderal)
Spironolactone (Aldactone)
Tocainide (Tonocard)

Anti-inflammatory agents
Auranofin (Ridaura)
Beclomethasone (Beclovent, Beconase)
Budesonide (Rhinocort)
Colchicine
Dexamethasone (Decadron)
Flunisolide (Nasalide, Aerobid)
Fluticasone (Flonase)
Gold (Myochrysine)
Hydrocortisone
Penicillamine (Cuprimine)

Antimanic drugs
Lithium

Antimigrane agents
Dihydroergotamine (Migranal)
Naratriptan (Amerge)
Rizatriptan (Maxalt)
Sumatriptan (Imitrex)

Antineoplastics
Cisplatin (Platinol)
Doxorubicin (Adriamycin)
Levamisole (Ergamisol)
Methotrexate (Rheumatrex)
Vincristine (Oncovin)

Antiparkinsonian agents
Levodopa (Larodopa; with carbidopa: Sinemet)

Antipsychotics
Clozapine (Clozaril)
Trifluoperazine (Stelazine)

Antithyroid agents
Methimazole (Tapazole)
Propylthiouracil

Antiviral agents
Ganciclovir (Cytovene)
Interferon (Ruferon-A)
Zalcitabine (HIVID)

Bronchodilators
Biotolterol (Tornalate)
Pirbuterol (Maxair)

Lipid-lowering agents
Atorvastatin (Lipitor)
Fluvastatin (Lescol)
Lovastatin (Mevacor)
Pravastatin (Pravachol)

Muscle relaxants
Baclofen (Lioresal)
Dantrolene (Dantrium)

Pancreatic enzyme preparations
Pancrelipase (Cotazym)

Smoking cessation aids
Nicotine (Nicotrol)

olfactory loss of patients with schizophrenia. Despite the fact there are advocates for zinc and vitamin therapies, there is no compelling evidence that these therapies work except in cases where frank zinc or vitamin deficiencies exist.

Prognosis for recovery seems to be better for patients with not too severe microsmia (e.g. UPSIT scores above 25) than for those with anosmia or severe microsmia. In some etiologies, this reflects the less extensive damage into the basal cell layer of the epithelia and possibly less fibrosis around the foramina of the cribriform plate through which the olfactory nerve axons pass. An important component to therapy for many patients is the quantitative establishment of the true degree of olfactory loss. This places the patient's problem into overall perspective; thus, it can be therapeutic for an older person to learn that, while his or her smell function is not what it used to be, it still falls above the average of his or her peer group.

Acknowledgement

This paper was supported, in part, by Grants PO1 DC 00161, RO1 DC 04278, RO1 DC 02974, and RO1 AG 27496 from the National Institutes of Health, Bethesda, MD, USA (R.L. Doty, Principal Investigator).

References

Armstrong, C. & Harrison, W.T. (1935). Prevention of intranasally-inoculated poliomyelitis of monkeys by instillation of alum into the nostrils. *Pub. Health Rep., 22*, 725–30.

Bhatnagar, K.P. & Meisami, E. (1998). Vomeronasal organ in bats and primates: extremes of structural variability and its phylogenetic implications. *Microsc. Res. Tech., 43*, 465–75.

Bromley, S.M. (2000). Smell and taste disorders: a primary care approach. *Am. Fam. Phys., 61*, 427–36.

Buck, L. & Axel, R. (1991). A novel multigene family may encode odorant receptors: a molecular basis for odor recognition. *Cell, 65*, 175–87.

Burdach, K.J. & Doty, R.L. (1987). The effects of mouth movements, swallowing, and spitting on retronasal odor perception. *Physiol. Behav., 41*, 353–6.

Burnet, F.M. & Lush, D. (1938). Infection of the central nervous system by louping ill virus. *Aust. J. Exp. Biol. Med. Sci., 16*, 233–40.

Clark, W.E.L. (1929). Anatomical investigation into the routes by which infections may pass from the nasal cavities into the brain. *Rep. Pub. Health Med. Sub., 54*, 1–27.

Costanzo, R.M. & Zasler, N.D. (1991). Head trauma. In *Smell and Taste in Health and Disease*, ed. T.V. Getchell, R.L. Doty, L.M. Bartoshuk, & J.B. Snow, Jr. pp. 711–30. New York: Raven Press.

Costanzo, R.M., DiNardo, L.J. & Zasler, N.D. (1995). Head injury and olfaction. In *Handbook of Olfaction and Gustation*, ed. R.L. Doty, pp. 493–502. New York: Marcel Dekker.

Deems, D.A., Doty, R.L., Settle, R.G. et al. (1991). Smell and taste disorders, a study of 750 patients from the University of Pennsylvania Smell and Taste Center. *Arch. Otolaryngol. Head Neck Surg., 117*, 519–28.

Delacourte, A., David, J.P., Sergeant, N. et al. (1999). The biochemical pathway of neurofibrillary degeneration in aging and Alzheimer's disease. *Neurology, 52*, 1158–65.

Devanand, D.P., Michaels-Marston, K.S., Liu, X. et al. (2000). Olfactory deficits in patients with mild cognitive impairment predict Alzheimer's disease at follow-up. *Am. J Psychiatry, 157*, 1399–1405.

Doty, R.L. (1991). Olfactory dysfunction in neurogenerative disorders. In *Smell and Taste in Health and Disease*, ed. T.V. Getchell, R.L. Doty, L.M. Bartoshuk & J.B. Snow, Jr. pp. 735–51. NY: Raven Press.

Doty, R.L. (1995a). Intranasal trigeminal chemoreception. In *Handbook of Olfaction and Gustation*, ed. R.L. Doty, pp. 821–33. New York: Marcel Dekker.

Doty, R.L. (1995b). *The Smell Identification Test™ Administration Manual, 3rd edn*, pp. 1–57. Haddon Hts., NJ: Sensonics, Inc.

Doty, R.L. (2001a). Olfaction. *Ann. Rev. Psychol. 52*, 423–52.

Doty, R.L. (2001b). Olfaction and gustation in normal aging and Alzheimer's disease. In *Functional Neurobiology of Aging*, ed. P.R. Hof, & C.V. Mobbs, pp. 647–58. San Diego: Academic Press.

Doty, R.L. & Hastings, L. (2001). Neurotoxic exposure and olfactory impairment. *Clin. Occupat. Environ. Med., 1*, 547–75.

Doty, R.L. & Kobal, G. (1995). Current trends in the measurement of olfactory function. In *Handbook of Olfaction and Gustation*, ed. R.L. Doty, pp. 191–225. New York: Marcel Dekker.

Doty, R.L. & Mishra, A. (2001). Influences of nasal obstruction, rhinitis, and rhinosinusitis on the ability to smell. *Laryngoscope, 111*, 409–23.

Doty, R.L., Shaman, P., Applebaum, S.L. et al. (1984a). Smell identification ability: changes with age. *Science, 226*, 1441–3.

Doty, R.L., Shaman, P. & Dann, M. (1984b). Development of the University of Pennsylvania Smell Identification Test: a standardized microencapsulated test of olfactory function. *Physiol. Behav., 32*, 489–502.

Doty, R.L., Reyes, P.F. & Gregor, T. (1987). Presence of both odor identification and detection deficits in Alzheimer's disease. *Brain Res. Bull., 18*, 597–600.

Doty, R.L., Deems, D.A., Frye, R.E., Pelberg, R. & Shapiro, A. (1988a). Olfactory sensitivity, nasal resistance, and autonomic function in patients with multiple chemical sensitivities. *Arch. Otolaryngol. Head Neck Surg., 114*, 1422–7.

Doty, R.L., Deems, D.A. & Stellar, S. (1988b). Olfactory dysfunction in parkinsonism: a general deficit unrelated to neurologic signs, disease stage, or disease duration. *Neurology, 38*, 1237–44.

Doty, R.L., Singh, A., Tetrude, J. & Langston, J.W. (1992a). Lack of olfactory dysfunction in MPTP-induced parkinsonism. *Ann. Neurol., 32*, 97–100.

Doty, R.L., Stern, M.B., Pfeiffer, C., Gollomp, S.M. & Hurtig, H.I. (1992b). Bilateral olfactory dysfunction in early stage treated and untreated idiopathic Parkinson's disease. *J. Neurol. Neurosurg. Psychiatry, 55*, 138–42.

Doty, R.L., Marcus, A. & Lee, W.W. (1996). Development of the 12-item cross-cultural smell identification test (CC-SIT). *Laryngoscope, 106*, 353–6.

Doty, R.L., Li, C., Mannon, L.J. & Yousem, D.M. (1997a). Olfactory dysfunction in multiple sclerosis. *N. Engl. J. Med., 336*, 1918–19.

Doty, R.L., Yousem, D.M., Pham, L.T., Kreshak, A.A., Geckle, R. & Lee, W.W. (1997b). Olfactory dysfunction in patients with head trauma. *Arch. Neurol., 54*, 1131–40.

Doty, R.L., Li, C., Mannon, L.J. & Yousem, D.M. (1998). Olfactory dysfunction in multiple sclerosis: Relation to plaque load in inferior frontal and temporal lobes. *Ann. NY Acad. Sci., 855*, 781–86.

Doty, R.L., Bagla, R. & Kim, N. (1999a). Physostigmine enhances performance on an odor mixture discrimination test. *Physiol. Behav., 65*, 801–4.

Doty, R.L., Li, C., Mannon, L.J. & Yousem, D.M. (1999b). Olfactory dysfunction in multiple sclerosis: relation to longitudinal changes in plaque numbers in central olfactory structures. *Neurology, 53*, 880–2.

Feron, F., Perry, C., McGrath, J.J. & Mackay, S. (1998). New techniques for biopsy and culture of human olfactory epithelial neurons. *Arch. Otolaryngol. Head Neck Surg.*, **124**, 861–6.

Ferreyra-Moyano, H. & Barragan, E. (1989). The olfactory system and Alzheimer's disease. *Internat. J. Neurosci.*, **49**, 157–97.

Finelli, P.F. & Mair, R.G. (1991). Disturbances of taste and smell. In *Neurology in Clinical Practice*, ed. G.M. Fenichel, & C.D. Marsden, pp. 209–16. Boston: Butterworth-Heinemann.

Frye, R.E., Schwartz, B.S. & Doty, R.L. (1990). Dose-related effects of cigarette smoking on olfactory function. *J. Am. Med. Assoc.*, **263**, 1233–6.

Gloor, P. (1997). *The Temporal Lobe and the Limbic System*, pp. 273–323. New York: Oxford University Press.

Gomez-Isla, T., Price, J.L., McKeel, D.W. Jr, Morris, J.C., Growdon, J.H. & Hyman, B.T. (1996). Profound loss of layer II entorhinal cortex neurons occurs in very mild Alzheimer's disease. *J. Neurosci.*, **16**, 4491–500.

Graves, A.B., Bowen, J.D., Rajaram, L. et al. (1999). Impaired olfaction as a marker for cognitive decline: interaction with apolipoprotein E epsilon4 status. *Neurology*, **53**, 1480–7.

Hawkes, C.H., Shephard, B.C. & Daniel, S.E. (1999). Is Parkinson's disease a primary olfactory disorder? *Quart. J. Med.*, **92**, 473–80.

Hinds, J.W., Hinds, P.L. & McNelly, N.A. (1984). An autoradiographic study of the mouse olfactory epithelium: evidence for long-lived receptors. *Anat. Rec.*, **210**, 375–83.

Huard, J.M., Youngentob, S.L., Goldstein, B.L., Luskin, M.B. & Schwob, J.E. (1998). Adult olfactory epithelium contains multipotent progenitors that give rise to neurons and non-neural cells. *J. Comp. Neurol.*, **400**, 469–86.

Hurst, E.W. (1936). Newer knowledge of virus diseases of nervous system: review and interpretation. *Brain*, **59**, 1–34.

Jafek, B.W., Hartman, D., Eller, P.M., Johnson, E.W., Strahan, R.C. & Moran, D.T. (1990). Postviral olfactory dysfunction. *Am. J. Rhinol.*, **4**, 91–100.

Jones-Gotman, M., Zatorre, R.J., Cendes, F. et al. (1997). Contribution of medial versus lateral temporal-lobe structures to human odour identification. *Brain*, **120**, 1845–56.

Kalmey, J.K., Thewissen, J.G. & Dluzen, D.E. (1998). Age-related size reduction of foramina in the cribriform plate. *Anat. Rec.*, **251**, 326–9.

Kern, R.C. (2000). Chronic sinusitis and anosmia: pathologic changes in the olfactory mucosa. *Laryngoscope*, 110, 1071–7.

Kratskin, I. (1995). Functional anatomy, central connections, and neurochemistry of the mammalian olfactory bulb. In *Handbook of Olfaction and Gustation*, ed. R.L. Doty, pp. 103–26. New York: Marcel Dekker.

Lee, S.H., Lim, H.H., Lee, H.M., Park, H.J. & Choi, J.O. (2000). Olfactory mucosal findings in patients with persistent anosmia after endoscopic sinus surgery. *Ann. Otol. Rhinol. Laryngol.*, **109**, 720–5.

Mackay-Sim, A. & Kittel, P.W. (1990). On the life span of olfactory receptor neurons. *Eur. J. Neurosci.*, **3**, 209–15.

Malaspina, D., Perera, G.M., Lignelli, A. et al. (1998). SPECT imaging of odor identification in schizophrenia. *Psychiat. Res.*, **82**, 53–61.

Markopoulou, K., Larsen, K.W., Wszolek, E.K. et al. (1997). Olfactory dysfunction in familial parkinsonism. *Neurology*, **49**, 1262–7.

Mattes, R.D. & Cowart, B.J. (1994). Dietary assessment of patients with chemosensory disorders. *J. Am. Diet. Assoc.*, **94**, 50–6.

Meisami, E., Mikhail, L., Baim, D. & Bhatnagar, K.P. (1998). Human olfactory bulb: aging of glomeruli and mitral cells and a search for the accessory olfactory bulb. *Ann. NY. Acad. Sci.*, **855**, 708–15.

Mesholam, R.I., Moberg, P.J., Mahr, R.N. & Doty, R.L. (1998). Olfaction in neurodegenerative disease: a meta-analysis of olfactory functioning in Alzheimer's and Parkinson's diseases. *Arch. Neurol.*, **55**, 84–90.

Miletic, I.D., Schiffman, S.S., Miletic, V.D. & Sattely-Miller, E.A. (1996). Salivary IgA secretion rate in young and elderly persons. *Physiol. Behav.*, **60**, 243–8.

Moberg, P.J., Doty, R.L., Mahr, R.N. et al. (1997a). Olfactory identification in elderly schizophrenia and Alzheimer's disease. *Neurobiol. Aging*, **18**, 163–7.

Moberg, P.J., Doty, R.L., Turetsky, B.I. et al. (1997b). Olfactory identification deficits in schizophrenia: correlation with duration of illness. *Am. J. Psychiatry*, **154**, 1016–18.

Moran, D.T., Rowley, J.C., III, Jafek, B.W. & Lovell, M.A. (1982). The fine structure of the olfactory mucosa in man. *J. Neurocytol.*, **11**, 721–46.

Nakashima, T., Kimmelman, C.P. & Snow, B.J. (1983). Progressive olfactory degeneration due to ischemia. *Surg. Forum*, **34**, 566–8.

Ngai, J., Chess, A., Dowling, M.M., Necles, N., Macagno, E.R. & Axel, R. (1993). Coding of olfactory information: topography of odorant receptor expression in the catfish olfactory epithelium. *Cell*, **72**, 667–80.

Peet, M.D., Echols, D.H. & Richter, H.J. (1937). The chemical prophylaxis for poliomyelitis: the technique of applying zinc sulfate intranasally. *J. Am. Med. Assoc.*, **108**, 2184–7.

Roberts, E. (1986). Alzheimer's disease may begin in the nose and may be caused by aluminosilicates. *Neurobiol. Aging*, **7**, 561–7.

Roper, S & Glimore, R.L. (1995). Orbitofrontal resections for intractable partial seziures. *J. Epilepsy*, **8**, 186.

Schultz, E.W. & Gebhardt, L.P. (1937). Zinc sulfate prophylaxis in poliomyelitis. *J. Am. Med. Assoc.*, **108**, 2182–4.

Schwanzel-Fukuda, M. & Pfaff, D.W. (1995). Structure and function of the nervus terminalis. In *Handbook of Olfaction and Gustation*, ed. R.L. Doty, pp. 835–64. New York: Marcel Dekker.

Serby, M., Flicker, C., Rypma, B., Weber, S., Rotrosen, J.P. & Ferris, S.H. (1990). Scopolamine and olfactory function. *Biol. Psychiat.*, **28**, 79–82.

Shepherd, G.M. (1972). Synaptic organization of the mammalian olfactory bulb. *Physiol. Rev.*, **52**, 864–917.

Shepherd, G.M. & Firestein, S. (1991). Toward a pharmacology of odor receptors and the processing of odor images. *J. Ster. Biochem. Mol. Biol.*, **39**, 583–92.

Smith, C.G. (1942). Age incident of atrophy of olfactory nerves in man. *J. Comp. Neurol.*, **77**, 589–94.

Smith, T.D. & Bhatnagar, K.P. (2000). The human vomeronasal organ. Part II. prenatal development. *J. Anat.*, **197**, 421–36.

Sobel, N., Prabhakaran, V., Desmond, J.E. et al. (1998a). Sniffing and smelling: separate subsystems in the human olfactory cortex. *Nature*, **392**, 282–6.

Sobel, N., Prabhakaran, V., Hartley, C.A. et al. (1998b). Odorant-induced and sniff-induced activation in the cerebellum of the human. *J. Neurosci.*, **18**, 8990–9001.

Stroop, W.G. (1995). Viruses and the olfactory system. In *Handbook of Olfaction and Gustation*, ed. R.L. Doty, pp. 367–93. New York: Marcel Dekker.

Tisdall, F.F., Brown, A., Defries, R.D., Ross, M.A. & Sellers, A.H. (1937). Nasal spraying as preventive of poliomylitis. *Can. Pub. Health J.*, **28**, 431–4.

Turetsky, B.I., Moberg, P.J., Yousem, D.M., Doty, R.L., Arnold, S.E. & Gur, R.I. (2000). Olfactory bulb volume is reduced in patients with schizophrenia. *Am. J. Psychiatry*, **157**, 828–30.

Watnick, R.L. & Trobe, J.D. (1989). Bilateral optic nerve compression as a mechanism for the Forster-Kennedy sydrome. *Ophthalmology*, **96**, 1793–8.

West, S.E. & Doty, R.L. (1995). Influence of epilepsy and temporal lobe resection on olfactory function. *Epilepsia*, **36**, 531–42.

Yasuno, H., Fukazawa, K., Fukuoka, I., Kondo, E., Sakagami, M. & Noguchi, K. (2000). Nerve growth factor applied onto the olfactory epithelium alleviates degenerative changes of the olfactory receptor neurons following axotomy. *Brain Res.*, **887**, 53–62.

Yousem, D.M., Geckle, R.J., Bilker, W.B., McKeown, D.A. & Doty, R.L. (1996). Posttraumatic olfactory dysfunction: MR and clinical evaluation. *Am. J. Neuroradiol.*, **17**, 1171–9.

Yousem, D.M., Williams, S.C., Howard, R.O. et al. (1997). Functional MR imaging during odor stimulation: preliminary data. *Radiology*, **204**, 833–8.

Yousem, D.M., Geckle, R.J., Bilker, W.B., Kroger, H. & Doty, R.L. (1999). Posttraumatic smell loss: relationship of psychophysical tests and volumes of the olfactory bulbs and tracts and the temporal lobes. *Acad. Radiol.*, **6**, 264–72.

Zatorre, R.J. & Jones-Gotman, M. (1991). Human olfactory discrimination after unilateral frontal or temporal lobectomy. *Brain*, **114**, 71–84.

Zatorre, R.J., Jones-Gotman, M., Evans, A.C. & Meyer, E. (1992). Functional localization and lateralization of human olfactory cortex. *Nature*, **360**, 339–40.

42

Taste

Steven M. Bromley[1, 2] and Richard L. Doty[1]

[1] Smell & Taste Center, University of Pennsylvania Medical Center, Philadelphia, PA, USA
[2] Neurological Institute of New York, Columbia-Presbyterian Medical Center, New York, NY, USA

Taste modifies the act of eating, and subsequently has a tremendous impact on one's behaviour and well-being. The physiologic role of the gustatory system is multifold and includes: (a) triggering ingestive and digestive reflex systems that alter the secretion of oral, gastric, pancreatic, and intestinal juices (Schiffman, 1997; Giduck et al., 1987), (b) reinforcing the ingestive process by enhancing the feelings of pleasure and satiety (Warwick et al., 1993), and (c) enabling the individual to determine the quality of sampled foodstuffs and distinguish nutrients (which usually taste 'good') from potential toxins (which usually taste 'bad') (McLaughlin & Margolskee, 1994; Scott & Giza, 1995). Although rarely appreciated, gustatory dysfunction can alter food choices and patterns of consumption, resulting in weight loss, malnutrition, and possibly impaired immunity (Schiffman & Wedral, 1996; Mattes & Cowart, 1994). Increased sensitivity and aversion to bitter-tasting substances on the part of the pregnant mother during the first trimester presumably reflects the need to detect and avoid bitter tasting poisons and teratogens during this critical phase of fetal development. Similarly, increased preferences for salty and bitter tasting substances during the remainder of pregnancy likely encourage the eating of a varied diet and the ingestion of much needed electrolytes to expand fluid volume (Duffy et al., 1998). In someone who is hypertensive or diabetic, taste loss can lead to a dangerous tendency to over-compensate for the loss by adding additional salt or sugar to the food.

In this chapter, we review clinically important aspects of the anatomy and physiology of the gustatory system, describe approaches for quantitatively evaluating this system, and present examples of common types of gustatory dysfunction, along with means for their management or treatment.

Anatomy and physiology

Taste buds, papillae, and initiation of taste transduction

The ~4600 goblet-shaped taste buds are located on the tongue's dorsal surface, the tongue–cheek margin, the base of the tongue, the soft palate, the pharynx, the larynx, the epiglottis, the uvula, and the first third of the esophagus (Miller, 1995). Most are found on the surface of the tongue within the protruding papillae. The fungiform, foliate and vallate (also called circumvallate) papillae harbor most of the taste buds; filiform papillae do not (Fig. 42.1).

Each taste bud contains between 50 and 150 slender epithelial cells arranged in a manner similar to the segments of a grapefruit. The taste pore opens into the centre of the bud, the taste pit, into which microvillae of sensory cells project. Each bud contains not only sensory and supporting cells, but progenitor cells from which the other cell types arise. Light, dark, and intermediate cells can be identified on the basis of their ultrastructural appearance and the presence or lack of dense granules in their apical portion (Farbman, 1980). Taste bud cells have the propensity to replace themselves ('turn over') periodically, with a time course of around two weeks (Beidler & Smallman, 1965).

A tastant initiates gustatory transduction and ultimately action potentials in one of two ways: by directly gating apical ion channels on microvillae of taste bud cells (a process that probably occurs with sour- and salty-tasting substances) or by activating receptors coupled to G-proteins that, in turn, are coupled to various second messenger systems (a process that probably occurs for sweet- and bitter-tasting agents; for review, see Margolskee, 1995). The

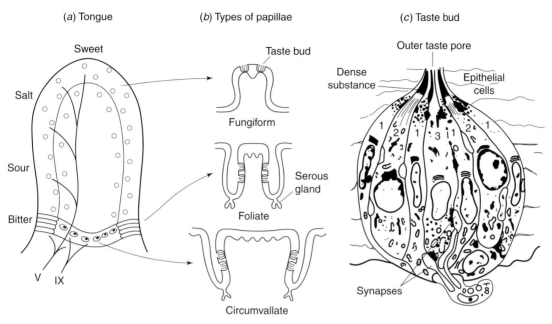

(a) Tongue   *(b)* Types of papillae   *(c)* Taste bud

Fig. 42.1. (*a*) Lingual distribution of (*b*) types of papillae that harbour (*c*) taste buds. In (*c*), 1 and 2 are presumably supporting cells, which secrete materials into the lumen of the taste buds; 3 is a sensory receptor cell; and 4 is a basal cell from which the other types of cells arise. (Modified from Shepherd, 1994.)

full range of primary taste sensations may be broader than simply sweet, sour, salty, and bitter, including 'metallic' (iron salts), 'umami' (monosodium glutamate, disodium gluanylate, disodium inosinate), and 'chalky' (calcium salts) (Schiffman, 1997; Kurihara & Kasiwayangi, 2000). The olfactory and trigeminal systems contribute to overall flavour perception by providing aroma, texture, temperature and spiciness.

Saliva and its role in taste function

Saliva contains dozens of different proteins and peptides (Table 42.1) and is secreted into the oral cavity by numerous glands, most importantly the paired parotid, submandibular, and sublingual salivary glands. Saliva is involved in the taste process, *per se*, in at least four ways. First, before tastants can enter the taste buds, they must be solubilized, and tastants dissolve or mix with saliva before entering the taste pore. Secondly, saliva serves as a filter to influence the concentration of tastants that enter the taste buds. For example, when bitter-tasting tannin-containing foods are ingested, there is an increase in the amount of proline-rich salivary proteins that bind tannins (Beidler, 1995). Such binding decreases the amount of tannins available to the taste buds, thereby increasing the taste threshold to the tannins. Third, saliva rinses away tastants and other mate-

rials that are introduced into the mouth, decreasing their tendency to linger in the oral cavity. Finally, saliva appears to play a role in taste bud maintenance. For example, taste buds within the fungiform papillae of rats disappear following removal of the submandibular and sublingual salivary glands: disappearance that can be reversed by adding epidermal growth factor to their drinking water (Morris-Witman et al., 2000).

Multiple peripheral pathways to the gustatory nucleus

The taste buds are innervated by branches of several cranial nerves which, unlike CN I, are mixed motor and sensory nerves transmitting multiple forms of information. The facial nerve (CN VII) supplies the taste buds within the fungiform and filiform papillae on the anterior two-thirds of the tongue (via the chorda tympani) and those on the soft palate (via the lesser palatine nerve branch of the greater petrosal nerve). The cell bodies of these afferent gustatory fibres are located in the geniculate ganglion. A short distance of the CN VII taste fibres is shared with the lingual nerve (CN V3) proximal to the tongue. The glossopharyngeal nerve (CN IX) supplies the circumvallate and most foliate taste buds within the posterior third of the tongue via its lingual–tonsillar branch. The

Table 42.1. *Proteins and peptides in mammalian whole saliva*

N-Acetyl-D-glucosaminidase	IgA
Agglutinagen A	IgG
Agglutinagen B	IgM
Agglutinagen C	Kallikrein
Albumin	Lactoferrin
Aldolase	Lactoperoxidase
Amylase family	Lethal factor
Angiotensin II	Lingual lipase
Anticomplimentary factor	Lipoproteins
Antileukoprotease	Lysozyme
Antitrypsin	Mesodermal growth factor
Aproerytherin	Metalloprotease
Biopterin	Monopterin
Bone marrow colony-	Mucins
stimulating factor	Neopterin
Calmodulin	Nerve growth factor
Carbonic anhydrase	Neural tube growth factor
Cathespin	Parotid glycoprotein family
Collagenase	Peroxidase
Cystatin family	Plasminogen activator
Elastase	Platelet-activating factor
Endothelial growth-	Proline-rich proteins
stimulating factor	Prostaglandins
Esterase	Pterin
Esterase B	Renin
Esteropeptidase	Sialomucin
Ferritin	Sialotonin
Fibronectin	Somatostatin
Fucosyltransferase	Statherin
Gastrin	Tissue plasminogen activator
Glucagon	Tonin
Glutamine-glutamic acid	Transferrin
protein family	VEG protein
Granulocytosis-inducing	Vitamin B-binding proteins
factor	Wound contraction factor
5-Hydroxymethylpterin	Xanthopterin

Notes:
If individual protein family members and isoenzymes are included separately, the total number approaches 200.
Source: Reprinted with permission from Beidler, (1995). Copyright © 1995, Marcel Dekker, Inc.

pharyngeal branch of this nerve innervates taste buds in the nasopharynx. The nerve cell bodies of these visceral gustatory afferent fibres are located immediately outside the jugular foramen in the petrosal ganglion. The vagus nerve (CN X) innervates the taste buds on the epiglottis, aryepiglottal folds, and esophagus (via the internal portion of the superior laryngeal branch).

Table 42.2. *Relative potency, in terms of taste thresholds, among different chemical compounds that have primarily sweet, sour, salty, or bitter tastes*

Salty-tasting substances	Index	Sour-tasting substances	Index
Sodium chloride	1	Hydrochloric acid	1
Ammonium chloride	2.5	Formic acid	1.1
Sodium fluoride	2	Chloracetic acid	0.9
Calcium chloride	1	Lactic acid	0.85
Potassium chloride	0.6	Tartaric acid	0.7
Sodium bromide	0.4	Malic acid	0.6
Lithium chloride	0.4	Acetic acid	0.55
Sodium iodide	0.35	Citric acid	0.46

Sweet-tasting substances	Index	Bitter-tasting substances	Index
Sucrose	1	Quinine	1
Sucrononic acid	200,000	Denatonium	1000
Saccharin	675	Strychnine	3.1
Aspartame	150	Nicotine	1.3
Chloroform	40	Brucine	1.1
Fructose	1.7	Phenylthiourea	0.9
Alanine	1.3	Caffeine	0.4
Glucose	0.8	Morphine	0.02

Notes:
The thresholds can vary as much as several thousand-fold from one compound to another, even within the same class.
Reprinted with permission from McLaughlin & Margolskee (1994).
Source: Copyright © 1994, Sigma Xi, The Scientific Research Society.

Gustatory cortical regions: functional anatomy

All the peripheral gustatory fibres enter the brainstem and project to the nucleus of the tractus solitarius (NTS), which begins in the rosterolateral medulla and extends caudally along the ventral border of the vestibular nuclei. From this structure, connections are made to higher processing centres described below. The cells of the NTS also make reflexive connections, via the interneurons of the reticular formation, with cranial nuclei that control (a) muscles of facial expression, (b) taste-mediated behaviours such as chewing, licking, salivation and swallowing, and (c) pre-absorptive insulin release (Smith & Shipley, 1992).

In primates, the projections from the NTS to higher centres likely ascend ipsilaterally within the central tegmental tract, to synapse ultimately within the parvicellular division of the ventroposteromedial thalamic nucleus

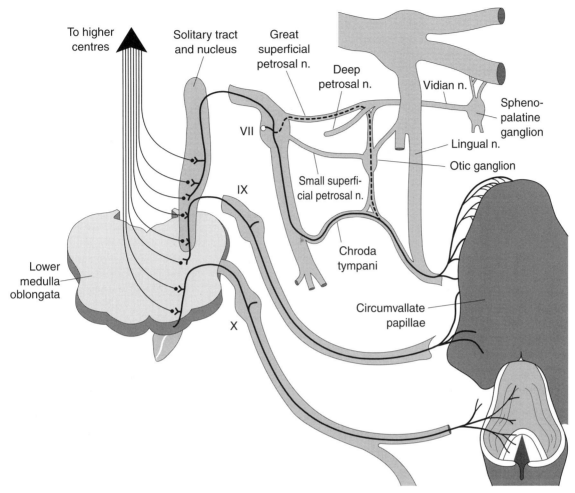

Fig. 42.2. Distribution of cranial nerves to gustatory regions. CN VIII fibres from the geniculate ganglion innervate taste buds on the anterior portion of the tongue and on the soft palate. CN IX fibres from cell bodies within the petrosal ganglion innervate taste buds on foliate and vallate papillae of the tongue, as well as pharyngeal taste buds. CN X fibres from cell bodies in the nodose ganglion innervate taste buds on the epiglottis, larynx and esophagus. (Modified and adapted from Netter, F.H. The CIBA Collection of Medical Illustrations, Vol. 1. Nervous System. Ciba Pharmaceutical Corporation, New York, 1964.)

(termed the thalamic taste nucleus or TTN) (Beckstead et al., 1980; Onoda & Ikeda, 1999). From the TTN, fibres then project to the primary taste cortex, which is located deep in the parietal operculum and adjacent parainsular cortex near somatosensory centres for oral sensation and motor centres for the control of jaw and tongue movement (Pritchard et al., 1986). Functional imaging studies suggest tastants activate insular and perisylvian regions, including the frontal operculum, superior temporal gyrus (opercular part), and inferior parts of the pre- and postcentral gyrus (Gloor, 1997; Faurion et al., 1998). A secondary cortical taste region is located in the caudomedial/caudolateral orbitofrontal cortex, extending several millimetres in front of the primary taste cortex (Rolls, 1995).

Little is known about the role the gustatory cortical regions in the processing of taste information, although none are purely gustatory, as they also contain neurons responsive to touch and temperature (Pritchard, 1991). The orbitofrontal cortex processes information from several sensory pathways (including olfactory, gustatory, and visual), and has been linked to emotion, feeding and social behaviour (Rolls & Baylis, 1994; Rolls et al., 1998). The degree to which taste function is represented on each side of the brain is also poorly understood. In an fMRI study, Cerf et al. (1998) found the superior part of the insula is likely bilaterally innervated; however, significant lateralization of taste function was present in the inferior insula, such that in right-handed subjects there was relatively more left inferior insula activation, whereas in left-handed subjects the reverse was true.

Classification of gustatory disorders

The classification of gustatory disorders follows a schemata similar to that of olfactory disorders: ageusia: inability to detect qualitative gustatory sensations; i.e. absence of taste; hypogeusia: decreased sensitivity to tastants; dysgeusia: distortion in the perception of a normal taste (e.g. the presence of an unpleasant taste when a normally pleasant tastant is presented); gustatory agnosia: inability to recognize a taste sensation, even though gustatory processing, language, and general intellectual functions are essentially intact.

Clinical evaluation of gustatory function

History

The clinical history for taste dysfunction largely overlaps that described in Chapter 41 for olfactory dysfunction. It is especially important to distinguish alterations in sweet, sour, bitter, and salty perception from changes in the perception of such sensations as chocolate, lemon, chicken, spaghetti, etc., since most 'taste' complaints reflect loss or distortions of the latter sensations which depend upon retronasal stimulation of CN I. Problems with speech articulation, salivation, chewing, swallowing, oral pain or burning, dryness of the mouth, periodontal disease, bruxism and foul breath odour should be noted, along with hearing and balance problems (since previous ear infections and surgery can alter chorda tympani function and produce taste loss or distortions). A determination of recent dental procedures and the patient's history of radiation exposure should also be made. Stomach problems may also be relevant, since acid reflux can damage or irritate taste buds. A careful assessment of medication usage is critical since, as described in detail later in this chapter, a number of drugs, including lipid-lowering agents, antibiotics and antihypertensives, produce significant taste disturbances.

Physical examination and imaging

In the evaluation of the oral cavity, particular attention should be directed towards the teeth and gums, since dysgeusia may result from exudates commonly found in gingivitis or pyorrhea. Inspection of fillings, bridges and other dental work should be made along with inspection of the mucosal surfaces, which may show signs of scarring, inflammation, or atrophy. A whitish lingual plaque can reflect candidiasis, lichen planus, leukoplakia, or food products. Local causes of glossitis include (a) mechanical trauma (e.g. tongue biting, jagged teeth, ill-fitting dentures), (b) irritation (e.g. that due to excessive use of alcohol, tobacco, O_2-liberating mouthwashes or peroxides), and (c) burns. Systemic causes of glossitis include (a) vitamin deficiencies (e.g. B vitamins, C, zinc), (b) anemia (e.g. pernicious, iron-deficiency), and (c) dermatologic syndromes (e.g. Behcet's syndrome, lichen planus, erythema multiforme, aphthous lesions, and pemphigus). Palpation should be performed to detect masses, neoplastic lesions or collections deep in the tongue's musculature. Neurologically, the integrity of CN VII, IX, and X can be evaluated by screening for deficits in non-gustatory functions of these nerves (e.g. facial musculature, swallow, salivation, gag, voice production).

Quantitative gustatory testing

Regional taste testing is needed to establish the function of each of the nerves innervating specific taste bud fields, as whole-mouth tests are insensitive to even complete dysfunction of one or several of the nerves that innervate the tongue. Two general stimulus presentation approaches can be employed. In *chemical testing*, liquid stimuli are presented to target regions of the tongue or oral cavity via pipettes, Q-tips, or filter paper disks. In *electrical testing* (also termed electrogustometry), low levels of electrical current are presented to taste bud fields via small electrodes (Frank & Smith, 1991).

Accurate quantitative taste testing can be quite time consuming, more so for chemical than for electrical testing because of rinsing and stimulus delivery (e.g. intertrial interval) issues. In chemical testing, for example, stimuli representing each of the four basic tastes are typically administered to each side of the anterior (CN VII) and posterior (CN IX) tongue, with rinsing and expectoration following. Thus, a minimum of 16 trials (4 tastants × 4 tongue regions), as well as 16 rinses and expectorations, are needed to provide a single trial of each taste quality stimulus within the back and front hemilingual surfaces. If a paired blank in a forced-choice trial (e.g. water) is to be presented, then an additional 16 trials are needed. Since multiple stimuli are required to produce reliable responses, a typical taste test requires a considerable number of trials. The regional test used by us employs a micropipette to present 15μl aliquots of suprathreshold tastants (sucrose, citric acid, sodium chloride, and caffeine) that are equated in viscosity to left and right anterior and posterior tongue regions. A single concentration of each stimulus is presented to each of the four target tongue regions six times, in counterbalanced order, along with a subsequent water rinse. Thus, 96 stimuli and 96 rinses are presented.

Gustatory dysfunction: causes and treatments

Although total loss or markedly diminished whole-mouth gustation exists, such changes are rarely produced by non-metabolic diseases or disorders unassociated with central ischemic or other damage, since regeneration of taste buds can occur and peripheral damage would have to involve multiple pathways to induce taste loss. Thus, while 433 of 585 patients (74%) studied at the University of Pennsylvania with verifiable olfactory loss complained of both smell and taste disturbance, less than 4% had verifiable whole-mouth gustatory dysfunction, and even that dysfunction was limited (Deems et al., 1991).

Regional deficits in taste dysfunction are much more common. For example, in one study sensitivity to three relatively low concentrations of NaCl was measured on the tongue tip and 3 cm posterior to the tongue tip in 12 young (20–29 years of age) and 12 elderly (70–79 years of age) subjects. On average, the young subjects were more sensitive to NaCl on the tongue tip than on the more posterior stimulation site and exhibited, at both tongue loci, an increase in detection performance as the stimulus concentration increased. The elderly subjects, who would be expected to exhibit, at worse, moderate deficits on whole-mouth testing, typically performed at chance level (Matsuda & Doty, 1995).

Most people, including older persons, are unaware of regional taste deficits, despite their wide prevalence. Patients rarely recognize their loss of taste sensation on half of the anterior tongue following unilateral sectioning of the chorda tympani in middle ear surgery. This lack of awareness reflects, in part, the redundancy of the multiple taste nerves, as well as possibly compensatory mechanisms. Anesthetizing or lesioning the chorda tympani (CN VII) unilaterally reportedly enhances taste perception on the rear of the tongue (CN IX), particularly on the side contralateral to that of the anesthesia or lesion (Kveton & Bartoshuk, 1994). The latter phenomenon, which has been interpreted as release of inhibition, probably occurs centrally, since the taste pathways are generally believed not to be crossed until the level of the thalamus.

A wide range of disorders and interventions have been associated with at least some loss of taste function. Mechanisms can include: (a) the release of bad-tasting materials from oral medical conditions (e.g. gingivitis, sialadenitis, oral infections), (b) transport problems of taste chemicals to the taste buds (e.g. caused by excessive chronic dryness of the oral cavity or damage to taste pores from a burn), (c) destruction or loss of taste buds themselves (e.g. from radiotherapy of the oral cavity), (d) damage to one or more neural pathways innervating the taste buds (e.g. Bell's palsy, trauma, dental or surgical procedures), and (e) involvement of central neural structures (e.g. tumour, stroke, multiple sclerosis, epilepsy).

Damage to brainstem structures that subserve taste may produce dysgeusia, although usually not without significant impairment of other cranial nerves or long tracts. Notable brainstem areas involved in taste that are susceptible to injury include the tractus solitarius and its nucleus (where injury produces ipsilateral ageusia) and the pontine tegmentum which involves both gustatory lemnisci (where injury produces bilateral ageusia). Bilateral injury to the thalamus can result in ageusia, although unilateral lesions above the brainstem do not usually cause complete loss of function (likely due to the multiple areas involved in processing taste information). Gustatory disturbance as a result of stroke (either ischemic or hemorrhagic) or demyelination (as seen in multiple sclerosis) (Catalanotto et al., 1984) commonly involve lesions in the gustatory pathway that can be discerned by MRI (Onoda & Ikeda, 1999; Yabe et al., 1995). An example of a stroke-related ischemia in a region of the upper medulla near the right nucleus tractus solitarius that produced altered taste ability is shown in Fig. 42.3 (note that, in this image, the left and right sides are reversed). Taste identification scores and a localized complaint of dysgeusia was greater in the right than in the left CN VII and CN IX lingual fields.

It is noteworthy that gustation may also be affected by injury to cortical association areas outside of the primary gustatory pathways. The concept of left unilateral neglect, typically resulting from contralateral injury to the right hemisphere (e.g. parietal lobe, thalamus, basal ganglia), appears to exist for taste in a manner similar to the visual, auditory, tactile, and olfactory sensory systems (Bellas et al., 1988). A specific syndrome of buccal hemineglect may exist in which patients neglect mouth and food products in the left half of the mouth and are unable to initiate chewing and swallowing when food is in this location (Andre et al., 2000). This syndrome can result in choking or a socially-embarrassing tendency to drool and regurgitate unnoticed food.

Bell's palsy

Although Bell's palsy is frequently associated with ipsilateral loss of taste over the anterior two-thirds of the tongue,

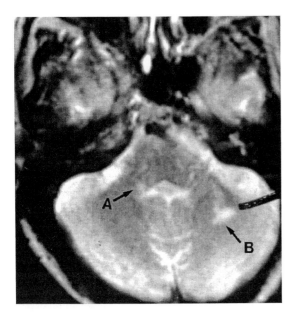

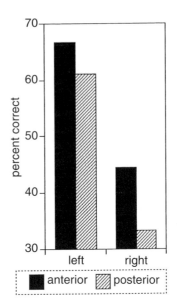

Fig. 42.3. L: Axial T2 (2500/90) MR scan through the upper brain stem reveals a hyperintensive infarct lesion (4×3 mm) in the right medulla (Arrow A). Note also large infarct (15×8 mm) inside the white matter of the left cerebellum (Arrow B). R: Identification scores on the University of Pennsylvania Taste Assessment Test (UPTAT) showing relative decrement on right side of tongue. From a 65-year-old woman with a history of ministrokes who developed a persistent salty/metallic dysgeusia and soreness on the right side of the tongue following a severe 2-day bout of emesis accompanied by marked dehydration and increased blood pressure but unaccompanied by fever. (Copyright © 2001, Richard L. Doty.)

the patient may not recognize this loss. Taste loss in Bell's palsy reflects a lesion somewhere in the neural pathway extending from the pons, along the nervus intermedius portion of the facial nerve (CN VII), through the geniculate ganglion, to the point where the chorda tympani joins the facial nerve in the facial canal. In addition to ipsilateral taste loss and commonly recognized facial weakness, hyperacusis (due to weakness of the stapedius muscle) and impairment of the taste-salivary reflex are present in many cases.

Trauma

Post-traumatic ageusia, as a result of peripheral or central injury, is much less common than post-traumatic anosmia, with solitary ageusia of one or more primary taste modalities occurring in less than 1% of persons with major head injury (Sumner, 1967; Deems et al., 1991). However, the prognosis for post-traumatic ageusia is far better than for post-traumatic anosmia, and recovery from ageusia, when present, usually occurs over a period of a few weeks to months. The etiology of post-traumatic taste dysfunction varies. Head trauma that results in injury to the middle ear, a finding encountered with basilar temporal bone fractures, can potentially result in both ipsilateral

impairment of taste and salivary function (by damaging the chorda tympani nerve *and* preganglionic parasympathetic fibres). Trauma to the jaw (e.g. from a punch with a fist) or to the mouth (e.g. from difficult orotracheal intubation, aggressive dental procedures) can result in numbness and taste loss over the anterior two-thirds of the ispilateral tongue, since the chorda tympani-lingual nerve carries both taste and touch information. Compression injury to this nerve may have a greater effect on taste than on fine-touch sensory components, since the chorda tympani fibres of the conjoined nerve are more superficial and posterolateral, and therefore more susceptible to partial transection or pressure on the side of the nerve (Wantanabe et al., 1995). Although presently there are no well-validated treatments for trauma-induced gustatory dysfunction, early steroidal intervention may minimize damage due to inflammatory sequelae in some cases.

Surgical iatrogenesis

A number of surgical procedures have been associated with taste dysfunction. Ear surgery, including tympanoplasty, mastoidectomy, and stapedectomy can damage CN VII (Bull, 1965; Moon & Pullen, 1963; Kveton & Bartoshuk,

1994). The chorda tympani nerve fibres are often stretched or sectioned during surgery for otosclerosis, resulting in taste loss or dygeusia. Such aberrations can last long after the operation (Bull, 1965). Damage to the glossopharyngeal nerve is not uncommon as a result of tonsillectomy, bronchoscopy, or laryngoscopy (Ohtuka et al., 1994; Donati et al., 1991; Arnhold-Schneider & Bernemann, 1987), reflecting the close proximity of the muscle layer of the palatine tonsillar bed to the lingual branch of CN IX (Ohtsuka et al., 1994). Third molar extraction, a very common dental procedure, can damage the lingual nerve and its coexisting chorda tympani fibres, as they lie in close proximity to the mandibular third molars. Such damage is very common; recently the taste function of 17 patients was quantitatively evaluated before third molar extraction, and at 1 month and 6 months thereafter (Shafer et al., 1999). Measurable taste deficits were found in most of these patients that persisted for at least 6 months after surgery, even though complaints of the deficits were rare. Patients with the most deeply impacted teeth exhibited the most severe loss. The chorda tympani nerve may also be injured by the injection of local anesthesia, either by direct contact with the needle or as a result of neurotoxic effects of the anesthetic compound (typically lidocaine and epinephrine) (Shafer et al., 1999; Nickel, 1993). While it is generally assumed that most cases of iatrogenic damage to nerves subserving gustatory function resolve spontaneously over time (reflecting the ability of nerves to regenerate), the limited data available suggest that complete recovery is, in fact, the exception (Bull, 1965; Shafer et al., 1999).

Infections

Local infections have the potential to disturb or impair taste. Important anatomical regions include (a) the teeth and periodontal tissue, (b) the salivary glands, (c) surfaces of the tongue, mouth, and oropharynx, and (d) the middle ear. Importantly, the use of appropriate doses of antibiotic medications may, in and of themselves, have detrimental consequences on taste function (Morris & Kelly, 1993; Schwartz et al., 1996; Adelglass et al., 1998; Magnasco & Magnasco, 1985). Proper oral hygiene and routine dental care should be emphasized to patients as a way of protecting themselves against oral infections.

Medications

Pharmacological agents appear to result in taste disturbances much more frequently than olfactory disturbances. Over 250 medications have been noted in the literature to alter the sense of taste, including antiproliferative drugs, antirheumatic drugs, antibiotic drugs, psychotropic drugs and drugs with sulfhydryl groups, such as penicillamine and captopril (Ackerman & Kasbekar, 1997; Doty et al., 1991; Deems et al., 1991; Bromley, 2000; Schiffman et al., 1998; Schiffman, 1997). Angiotensin-converting enzyme inhibitors are commonly associated with taste disturbance, such as hypogeusia, or excessive metallic, bitter, or sour dysgeusic tastes (Ackerman & Kasbekar, 1997). Such psychotropic medications as amytriptyline, clomipramine, desipramine, imipramine, doxepin, and trifluoperazine as well as protease inhibitors used in the treatment of HIV and AIDS, not only have a taste of their own, but can significantly alter the intensity of other tastants, such as salt and sugar (Schiffman et al., 1998, 1999). Drug-induced taste disorders can, in some instances, be reversed by discontinuance of the offending drug, by employing alternative medications, or by changing drug dosage. However, many pharmacological agents appear to induce long-term alterations in taste that may take months to disappear even after discontinuance of the drug. In situations where xerostomia and excessive dryness occurs as a result of a drug (e.g. an anticholinergic agent), a physician can offer artificial saliva (e.g. Xerolube) to improve comfort, particularly if alternative medications are not available and drug dose cannot be decreased. However, if specific salivary proteins are needed for taste bud maintenance, saliva substitutes may not completely alleviate the chronic effects of lack of saliva on the taste buds.

Although various carcinomas apparently can alter taste function, it is important to recognize that conditioned taste aversions commonly occur among cancer patients undergoing chemo- or radiation therapy. In effect, malaise from the therapy becomes conditioned to the taste of foodstuffs, even if the malaise occurs hours after the intake of the food. In some cases, such conditioned aversions are transient, but in other cases they can be relatively long lasting and can lead to generalized anorexia and cachexia. A strategy for minimizing such aversions is to have the patient consume a novel food immediately before the initiation of therapy. Somehow subsequent conditioned aversions become focused primarily on the novel food, protecting against the formation of conditioned aversions to preferred food items (Chambers & Bernstein, 1995).

Epilepsy

Taste function can be altered by seizure activity, and on occasion gustatory auras appear. Like olfactory auras, gustatory auras usually represent seizure activity predominately within the temporal lobes, although on rare occasion such activity arises from the orbitofrontal region (Hausser-Hauw & Bancaud, 1987; Acharya et al., 1998; Roper & Gilmore, 1995). Sensations have been reported to include 'peculiar', 'rotten', 'sweet', 'like a cigarette', 'like rotten apples', and 'like vomitus' (for review, see West & Doty, 1995), although many of these 'tastes' likely represent smell sensations miscategorized as tastes by both the patients and their physicians. Usually, taste auras produced by simple partial seizures disappear after the use of antiseizure medications, although this may not be the case with intractable epilepsy. Surgery, e.g. temporal lobe resection, successfully halts most gustatory auras (Acharya et al., 1998).

Other medical causes

There are a number of other causes of gustatory disturbance, including diabetes (where there can be a progressive loss of taste beginning with glucose and extending to other sweeteners, salty stimuli, and then all stimuli), familial dysautonomia (a genetic disorder with lack of taste buds and papillae), hypothyroidism, myasthenia gravis, and Guillain-Barré syndrome. In cases of taste loss secondary to hypothyroidism, thyroxin replacement can normalize taste sensitivity (Mattes & Kare, 1986). In newly diagnosed non-insulin dependent diabetics (based on plasma glucose concentration and glycosolated hemoglobin percentage), quantifiable taste impairment not only exists, but may be somewhat reversible with correction of the hyperglycemia (Perros et al., 1996). Both chronic renal failure and end-stage liver disease have been associated with alterations in taste function, and in some circumstances, transplantation may improve detection thresholds (Bloomfield et al., 1999). It is not clear whether the prodrome or acute headache phase associated with migraine involves definable gustatory phenomena as seen with olfaction. Certain tastes may, however, induce a migraine (Blau and Solomon, 1985). A distinct entity from glossopharyngeal neuralgia, Burning Mouth syndrome (BMS), often referred to as glossalgia or glossodynia, is the subjective sensation of intense burning in the mouth without obvious physical cause that may respond to tricyclic antidepressants (for review, see Tourne & Fricton, 1992). BMS is sometimes associated with dysgeusia.

Fortunately, most cases of idiopathic dysgeusias spontaneously resolve within 2 years (Deems et al., 1996). In some cases, antifungal and antibiotic treatments have been reported to be useful in resolving dysgeusias, although double blind studies of the efficacy of such treatments are lacking. Chlorhexidine, which has a strong positive charge, has been suggested as having possible efficacy for mitigating some salty or bitter dysgeusias when used as mouthwash (Helms et al., 1995).

Acknowledgements

This paper was supported, in part, by Grants PO1 DC 00161, RO1 DC 04278, RO1 DC 02974, and RO1 AG 27496 from the National Institutes of Health, Bethesda, MD, USA (R.L. Doty, Principal Investigator).

References

Acharya, V., Acharya, J. & Luders, H. (1998). Olfactory epileptic auras. *Neurology*, **51**, 56–61.

Ackerman, B.H. & Kasbekar, N. (1997). Disturbances of taste and smell induced by drugs. *Pharmacotherapy*, **17**, 482–96.

Adelglass, J., Jones, T.M., Ruoff, G. et al. (1998). A multicenter, investigator-blinded, randomized comparison of oral levofloxacin and oral clarithromycin in the treatment of acute bacterial sinusitis. *Pharmacotherapy*, **18**, 1255–63.

Andre, J.M., Beis, J.M., Morin, N. & Paysant, J. (2000). Buccal hemineglect. *Arch. Neurol.*, **57**, 1734–41.

Arnhold-Schneider, M. & Bernemann, D. (1987). Uber die Haufigkeit von Geschmacksstorungen nach Tonsillektomie. *HNO*, **35**, 195–198.

Beckstead, R.M., Morse, J.R. & Norgren, R. (1980). The nucleus of the solitary tract in the monkey: projections to the thalamus and brain stem nuclei. *J. Comp. Neurol.*, **190**, 259–82.

Beidler, L.M. (1995). Saliva: Its functions and disorders. In *Handbook of Olfaction and Gustation*, ed. R.L. Doty, pp. 503–19. New York: Marcel Dekker.

Beidler, L.M. & Smallman, R.L. (1965). Renewal of cells within taste buds. *J. Cell Biol.*, **27**, 263–72.

Bellas, D.N., Novelly, R.A., Eskenazi, B. & Wasserstein, J. (1988). The nature of unilateral neglect in the olfactory sensory system. *Neuropsychologia*, **26**, 45–52.

Blau, J.N. & Solomon, F. (1985). Smell and other sensory disturbances in migraine. *J. Neurol.*, **232**, 275–6.

Bloomfield, R.S., Graham, B.G., Schiffman, S.S. & Killenberg, P.G. (1999). Alterations of chemosensory function in end-stage liver disease. *Physiol. Behav.*, **66**, 203–7.

Bromley, S.M. (2000). Smell and taste disorders: a primary care approach. *Am. Fam. Phys.*, **61**, 427–36.

Bull, T.R. (1965). Taste and the chorda tympani. *J. Laryngol. Otol.* **79**, 479–93.

Catalanotto, F.A., Dore-Duffy, P., Donaldson, J.O., Testa, M., Peterson, M. & Ostrom, K.M. (1984). Quality-specific taste changes in multiple sclerosis. *Ann. Neurol.*, **16**, 611–15.

Cerf, B., Lebihan, D., Van De Moortele PF, Mac, L.P. & Faurion, A.

(1998). Functional lateralization of human gustatory cortex related to handedness disclosed by fMRI study. *Ann. NY. Acad. Sci.*, **855**, 575–8.

Chambers, K.C. & Bernstein, I.L. (1995). Conditioned flavor aversions. In *Handbook of Olfaction and Gustation*, ed. R.L. Doty, pp. 745–73. New York: Marcel Dekker.

Deems, D.A., Doty, R.L., Settle, R.G. et al. (1991). Smell and taste disorders, a study of 750 patients from the University of Pennsylvania Smell and Taste Center. *Arch. Otolaryngol. Head Neck Surg.*, **117**, 519–28.

Deems, D.A., Yen, D.M., Kreshak, A. & Doty, R.L. (1996). Spontaneous resolution of dysgeusia. *Arch. Otolaryngol. Head Neck Surg.*, **122**, 961–3.

Donati, F., Pfammatter, J.P., Mauderli, M. & Vassella, F. (1991). Neurologische Komplikationen nach Tonsillektomie. *Schweiz. Med. Wochenschr.*, **121**, 1612–17.

Doty, R.L., Bartoshuk, L.M. & Snow, J.B., Jr. (1991). Causes of olfactory and gustatory disorders. In *Smell and Taste in Health and Disease*, ed. T.V. Getchell, R.L. Doty, L.M. Bartoshuk, & J.B. Snow, Jr., 449–61. New York: Raven Press.

Duffy, V.B., Bartoshuk, L.M., Striegel-Moore, R. & Rodin, J. (1998). Taste changes across pregnancy. *Ann. NY. Acad. Sci.*, **855**, 805–9.

Farbman, A.I. (1980). Renewal of taste bud cells in rat circumvallate papillae. *Cell Tissue Kinet.*, **13**, 349–57.

Faurion, A., Cerf, B., Le, B.D. & Pillias, A.M. (1998). fMRI study of taste cortical areas in humans. *Ann. NY. Acad. Sci.*, **855**, 535–45.

Frank, M.E. & Smith, D.V. (1991). Electrogustometry: a simple way to test taste. In *Smell and Taste in Health and Disease*, ed. T.V. Getchell, R.L. Doty, L.M. Bartoshuk, & J.B. Snow, Jr., pp. 503–14. New York: Raven Press.

Frey, L. (1923). Le syndrome du nerf auriculo-temporal. *Rev. Neurol.*, **2**, 97–104.

Giduck, S.A., Threatte, R.M. & Kare, M.R. (1987). Cephalic reflexes: their role in digestion and possible roles in absorption and metabolism. [Review]. *J. Nutrit.*, **117**, 1191–6.

Gloor, P. (1997). *The Temporal Lobe and the Limbic System*, pp. 273–323. New York: Oxford University Press.

Hausser-Hauw, C. & Bancaud, J. (1987). Gustatory hallucinations in epileptic seizures. Electrophysiological, clinical and anatomical correlates. *Brain*, **110**, 339–59.

Helms, J.A., Della-Fera, M.A., Mott, A.E. & Frank, M.E. (1995). Effects of chlorhexidine on human taste perception. *Arch. Oral. Biol.*, **40**, 913–20.

Kurihara K. & Kashiwayanagi M. (2000). Physiological studies on umami taste. *J. Nutrit.*, **130**, 931S–4S.

Kveton, J.F. & Bartoshuk, L.M. (1994). The effect of unilateral chorda tympani damage on taste. *Laryngoscope*, **104**, 25–9.

Magnasco, L.D. & Magnasco, A.J. (1985). Metallic taste associated with tetracycline therapy. *Clin. Pharm.*, **4**, 455–6.

Margolskee, R.F. (1995). Receptor mechanisms in gustation. In *Handbook of Olfaction and Gustation*, ed. R.L. Doty, pp. 575–95. New York: Marcel Dekker.

Matsuda, T. & Doty, R.L. (1995). Regional taste sensitivity to NaCl: relationship to subject age, tongue locus and area of stimulation. *Chem. Senses*, **20**, 283–90.

Mattes, R.D. & Cowart, B.J. (1994). Dietary assessment of patients with chemosensory disorders. *J. Amer. Diet. Assoc.*, **94**, 50–6.

Mattes, R.D. & Kare, M.R. (1986). Gustatory sequelae of alimentary disorders. *Digest. Dis.*, **4**, 129–38.

McLaughlin, S. & Margolskee, R.F. (1994). The sense of taste. *Am. Scientist*, **82**, 538–45.

Miller, I.J. (1995). Anatomy of the peripheral taste system. In *Handbook of Olfaction and Gustation*, ed. R.L. Doty, pp. 521–47. New York: Marcel Dekker.

Moon, C.N. & Pullen, E.W. (1963). Effects of chorda tympani section during middle ear surgery. *Laryngoscope*, **73**, 392–405.

Morris-Witman, J., Sego, R., Brinkley, L. & Dolce, C. (2000). The effects of sialoadenectomy and exogenous EGF on taste bud morphology and maintenance. *Chem. Senses*, **25**, 9–19.

Morris, J.T. & Kelly, J.W. (1993). Rifabutin-induced ageusia [letter]. *Ann. Intern. Med.*, **119**, 171–2.

Netter, F.H. (1964). *The CIBA Collection of Medical Illustrations, Vol. 1. Nervous System.*, New York: Ciba Pharmaceutical Corporation.

Nickel, A.A. (1993). Regional anesthesia. *Oral Maxil. Surg. Clin. N. Amer.*, **5**, 17–24.

Ohtsuka, K., Tomita, H. & Murakami, G. (1994). [Anatomical study of the tonsillar bed: the topographical relationship between the palatine tonsil and the lingual branch of the glossopharyngeal nerve]. [Japanese]. *Nippon Jibiinkoka Gakkai Kaiho [J. Oto-Rhino-Laryngol. Soc.Japan*, **97**, 1481–93.

Ohtuka, K., Tomita, H., Yamauchi, Y. & Kitagoh, H. (1994). [Taste disturbance after tonsillectomy]. [Japanese]. *Nippon Jibiinkoka Gakkai Kaiho [J. Oto-Rhino-Laryngol. Soc. Japan*, **97**, 1079–88.

Onoda, K. & Ikeda, M. (1999). Gustatory disturbance due to cerebrovascular disorder. *Laryngoscope*, **109**, 123–8.

Perros, P., MacFarlane, T.W., Counsell, C. & Frier, B.M. (1996). Altered taste sensation in newly-diagnosed NIDDM. *Diabetes Care*, **19**, 768–70.

Pritchard, T.C. (1991). The primate gustatory system. In *Smell and Taste in Health and Disease*, ed. T.V. Getchell, R.L. Doty, L.M. Bartoshuk, & J.B. Snow, Jr. pp. 109–125. New York: Raven Press.

Pritchard, T.C., Hamilton, R.B., Morse, J.R. & Norgren, R. (1986). Projections of thalamic gustatory and lingual areas in the monkey, Macaca fascicularis. *J. Comp. Neurol.*, **244**, 213–28.

Rolls, E.T. (1995). Central taste anatomy and neurophysiology. In *Handbook of Olfaction and Gustation*, ed. R.L. Doty, pp. 549–73. New York: Marcel Dekker.

Rolls, E.T. & Baylis, L.L. (1994). Gustatory, olfactory, and visual convergence within the primate orbitofrontal cortex. *J. Neurosci.* **14**, 5437–52.

Rolls, E.T., Critchley, H.D., Browning, A. & Hernadi, I. (1998). The neurophysiology of taste and olfaction in primates, and umami flavor. *Ann. NY. Acad. Sci.*, **855**, 426–37.

Schiffman, S.S. (1997). Taste and smell losses in normal aging and disease. *J. Am. Med. Assoc.*, **278**, 1357–62.

Schiffman, S.S., Graham, B.G., Suggs, M.S. & Sattely-Miller, E.A.

(1998). Effect of psychotropic drugs on taste responses in young and elderly persons. *Ann. NY. Acad. Sci.,* **855**, 732–737, 1998.

Schiffman, S.S. & Wedral, E. (1996). Contribution of taste and smell losses to the wasting syndrome. *Aging Nutrit.,* **7**, 106–20.

Schiffman, S.S., Zervakis, J., Heffron, S. & Heald, A.E. (1999). Effect of protease inhibitors on the sense of taste. *Nutrition,* **15**, 767–72.

Schwartz, H., Krause, R., Siepman, N. et al. (1996). Seven-day triple therapy with lansoprazole, clarithromycin, and metronidazole for the cure of *Helicobacter pylori* infection: a short report. *Helicobacter,* **1**, 251–5.

Scott, T.R. & Giza, B.K. (1995). Theories of gustatory neural coding. In *Handbook of Olfaction and Gustation*, ed. R.L. Doty, pp. 611–33. New York: Marcel Dekker.

Scrivani, S.J., Keith, D.A., Kulich, R., Mehta, N. & Maciewicz, R.J. (1998). Posttraumatic gustatory neuralgia: a clinical model of trigeminal neuropathic pain. *J. Orofacial Pain,* **12**, 287–92.

Shafer, D.M., Frank, M.E., Gent, J.F. & Fischer, M.E. (1999). Gustatory function after third molar extraction. *Oral Surg. Oral. Med. Oral Pathol. Oral Radiol. Endodont.,* **87**, 419–28.

Sharav, Y., Benoliel, R., Schnarch, A. & Greenberg, L. (1991). Idiopathic trigeminal pain associated with gustatory stimuli. *Pain,* **44**, 171–2.

Shepherd, G.M. (1994). *Neurobiology,* p. 248 New York: Oxford University Press.

Smith, D.V. & Shipley, M.T. (1992). Anatomy and physiology of taste and smell. *J. Head Trauma. Rehabil.,* **7**, 1–14.

Soria, E.D., Candaras, M.M. & Truax, B.T. (1990). Impairment of taste in the Guillain–Barré syndrome. [Review]. *Clin. Neurol. Neurosurgery,* **92**, 75–9.

Sumner, D. (1967). Post-traumatic ageusia. *Brain,* **90**, 187–202.

Tourne L.P. & Fricton, J.R. (1992). Burning Mouth syndrome. Critical review and proposed clinical management. *Oral Surg., Oral Med., Oral Pathology,* **74**, 158–67.

Wantanabe, K., Tomita, H. & Murkami, G. (1995). Morphometric study of chorda tympani-derived fibers along their course in the lingual nerve. *J. ORL Soc. Jap.,* **98**, 80–9.

Warwick, Z.S., Hall, W.G., Pappas, T.N. & Schiffman, S.S. (1993). Taste and smell sensations enhance the satiating effect of both a high-carbohydrate and a high-fat meal in humans. *Physiol. Behav.,* **53**, 553–63.

West, S.E. & Doty, R.L. (1995). Influence of epilepsy and temporal lobe resection on olfactory function. *Epilepsia,* **36**, 531–42.

Yabe, I., Andoh, S., Mito, Y., Saski, H. & Tashiro, K. (1995). Multiple sclerosis presenting with taste disturbance [in Japanese]. *Neurol. Med.,* **43**, 383–5.

Yanagisawa, K., Bartoshuk, L.M., Catalanotto, F.A., Karrer, T.A. & Kveton, J.F. (1998). Anesthesia of the chorda tympani nerve and taste phantoms. *Physiol. Behav.,* **63**, 329–35.

43

Disorders of vision

Antony Morland[1] and Christopher Kennard[2]

[1] Department of Psychology, Royal Holloway College, Egham, Surrey, UK
[2] Division of Neuroscience and Psychological Medicine, Imperial College School of Medicine, Charing Cross Campus, London, UK

Vision is the primary sensory input to the brain in terms both of the number of sensory fibres and in the amount of cortical processing area devoted to its analysis. As a consequence there is a protean number of disorders, which range in their pathophysiological mechanisms from disturbed axon conduction, as in optic neuritis, to the abnormal cortical sensory processing apparent in the generation of visual hallucinations. The localization of visual disturbances is often assisted by appropriate analysis and interpretation of visual field defects (Fig 43.1).

Anterior visual pathway

Disorders of the optic nerve

Optic neuritis

Optic neuritis (ON) is a term used to describe an idiopathic optic neuropathy or one resulting from inflammatory, infectious or most commonly demyelinating etiology. In the majority of cases the optic disc is normal on ophthalmoscopy and the term retrobulbar neuritis is used. In those cases in which the optic disc is swollen then the terms papillitis or anterior ON are used.

Clinical features

In typical ON there is usually acute unilateral loss of visual acuity and visual field, which may progress over hours or a few days, reaching its maximal impairment within 1 week. Ninety per cent of cases complain of ocular pain which is noted especially with eye movement, and which may precede the visual impairment by a few days (Lepore, 1991). The visual loss may range from contrast defects with maintained acuity to no light perception. A defect of colour vision is almost universal. Although ON is generally asso-

ciated with a central scotoma a wide variety of field defects may be found ranging from a central scotoma to altitudinal and nerve fibre layer defects (Keltner et al., 1993). An afferent pupillary defect is present in over 90% of patients with acute ON. The patient is usually aged under 40 years, although ON may occur at any age, and improvement takes place in most patients (90%) to normal or near normal visual acuity over several weeks. There may be persistent subtle residual defects of colour vision, depth perception and contrast sensitivity, which may continue for several months. Subsequent disc pallor may occur but does not correlate closely with the level of visual recovery (McDonald & Barnes, 1992).

ON exemplifies a number of the pathophysiological consequences of axonal demyelination, which may be partial or complete. These include slowed conduction (indicated by the delay in the P100 of the visual evoked potential), and susceptibility of partially demyelinated axons to small increases in local temperature (Uhtoff's phenomenon in which patients with ON become aware of increased visual impairment during exercise), and to mechanical distortion (visual phosphenes on eye movement).

Atypical ON may be unilateral or involve bilateral simultaneous onset of ON in an adult patient. There is often lack of pain and there may be other ocular findings suggestive of an inflammatory process, such as an anterior uveitis. Other features include a worsening of visual function beyond 14 days of onset, in a patient outside the 20–50-year age span. They may also have evidence of other systemic conditions, particularly inflammatory or infectious diseases.

A number of disorders may be associated with typical or atypical ON (Table 43.1).

The evaluation of patients with ON rather depends on whether or not it is a typical or atypical case. Typical ON probably does not necessitate any additional laboratory

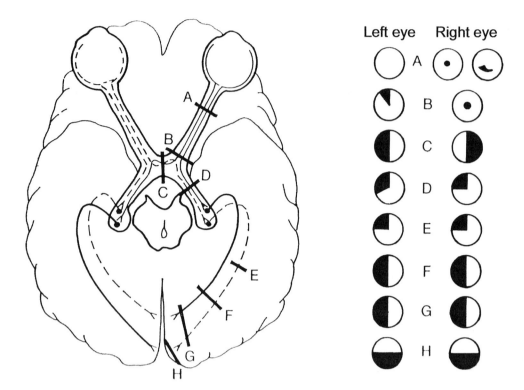

Fig. 43.1. Patterns of visual field loss: (*a*) Optic nerve lesions result in a central scotoma or arcuate defect. (*b*) Optic nerve lesions just prior to the chiasm produce junctional scotoma due to ipsilateral optic nerve involvement with the inferior contralateral crossing fibres (dotted line). (*c*) chiasm lesions produce a bitemporal hemianopia. (*d*) Optic tract lesions result in an incongruous hemianopic field defect. (*e*), (*f*) Lesions of the optic radiation result in either homonymous quadrantanopia or hemianopia depending on the extent and location of the lesion (upper quadrant, temporal lobe; lower quadrant, parietal lobe). (*g*) Lesions of the striate cortex produce a homonymous hemianopia, sometimes with macular sparing, particularly with vascular disturbances. (*h*) Partial lesions of the superior or inferior bank of the striate cortex cause inferior or superior altitudinal field defects, respectively.

investigations, although an abnormal MRI brain scan significantly increases the likelihood of developing multiple sclerosis (Morrisey et al., 1993).

Those patients with atypical ON should have a chest X-ray, laboratory tests including a blood count, biochemistry, and tests for collagen and vascular disease and syphilis serology. Examination of the spinal fluid (CSF) is probably justified in this group of patients.

Management
Although IV methylprednisolone leads to a more rapid visual recovery, at the end of 6 months the visual acuity is no better than without the treatment (Beck et al., 1992). Therefore, steroid treatment of patients with typical ON is unnecessary, unless there is severe ocular pain which cannot be managed with analgesics, or if there is already poor vision in the fellow eye due to some other disease process. The role of beta interferon in preventing the development of multiple sclerosis after a single attack of

ON in a patient with an abnormal MRI scan is still unclear.

Ischemic optic neuropathy
Ischaemic optic neuropathy is due to infarction of the optic nerve head, and can be either the more common non-arteritic (idiopathic ischemic neuropathy, anterior ischemic optic neuropathy, AOIN) or arteritic type, when it is usually associated with giant cell arteritis.

Non-arteritic ischemic optic neuropathy
This is characterized by abrupt, painless and generally non-progressive visual loss, associated with an arcuate or altitudinal visual field loss, and tends to occur in patients aged between 45 and 80 years. In nearly all cases, there is optic disc edema, often associated with one or more splinter hemorrhages at the disc margin. Optic atrophy rapidly ensues after the ischemic event. Although previously considered irreversible, as many as 40% of patients may show

Table 43.1. Causes of typical and atypical optic neuritis

Unknown etiology
Multiple sclerosis
Cerebral angiography
CO poisoning
Meningitis
Air embolism
Neoplasm
Tentorial herniation
Cardiac arrest
Systemic lupus erythematosis
Dialysis equilibrium

Table 43.2. Causes of optic atrophy

Deficiency states
Thiamine ('tobacco–alcohol amblyopia')
B12 (pernicious anemia, 'tobacco amblyopia')
Drugs/toxins
Ethambutol
Chlormycetin
Streptomycin
Isoniazid
Chlorpropamide
Digitalis
Chloroquine
Placidyl
Antabuse
Heavy metals
Hereditary optic atrophies
Dominant (juvenile)
Leber's
Associated heredodegenerative neurologic syndromes
Recessive, associated with juvenile diabetes
Demyelination
Grave's disease
Atypical glaucoma
Macular dystrophies

some improvement, and there is a 40% chance of involvement of the fellow eye within 5 years (Ischemic optic neuropathy decompression trial research group, 1995).

The cause of AION remains obscure, although it has been associated with small optic discs (Burde, 1993). The most important aspect of management, since there is no treatment of proven benefit, is to exclude the possibility of the arteritic form, when the fellow eye is particularly vulnerable to similar involvement.

Arteritic ION
The arteritic form of ION usually occurs in giant cell (cranial, temporal) arteritis (GCA), but also rarely occurs in lupus and polyarteritis nodosa. Anyone with AION over the age of 50 should be suspected of having GCA. This often occurs in the context of headache, malaise, weight loss, anorexia, anemia, proximal muscle ache or stiffness, temporal artery tenderness, jaw claudication and fever. These symptoms and signs usually precede the visual loss. The disc infarction is similar to that seen in non-arteritic AION.

A high index of suspicion is required for GCA, and if suspected an urgent erythrocyte sedimentation rate (ESR) and temporal artery biopsy should be arranged. At the same time as the blood for the ESR is taken, the patient should be immediately started on systemic steroids (prednisolone 80 mg daily, plus 200 mg i.v. hydrocortisone immediately). In most patients the ESR is markedly elevated, as is the C-reactive protein. Occasionally the ESR may be normal. A biopsy of the superficial temporal artery should be obtained as soon as possible after the diagnosis has been considered. The biopsy will not be affected by the use of corticosteroids for at least 48 hours. A positive temporal artery biopsy confirms the diagnosis of giant cell arteritis, but in 25% of patients skip areas are found in biopsy specimens, and therefore a negative biopsy may sometimes be obtained.

Steroid treatment should not be tapered or withdrawn

too early, since a relapse of symptoms is common. The dose of prednisolone can be gradually tapered after 2–3 weeks to maintain a normal ESR and the patient asymptomatic. Treatment should be continued for at least 6–12 months.

Optic atrophy
Optic atrophy is the final result of a variety of disturbances to the optic nerve or retina. The disc appears pale, which is due to death of the retinal ganglion cells with a dying back of their nerve fibres. This can, therefore, result from diseases which directly involve the ganglion cells themselves or from damage to the axons in the pregeniculate visual pathway, resulting in retrograde atrophy. The development of optic atrophy is usually slow, dependent on its cause. In most instances the optic atrophy is bilateral, the disc appearing chalky-white in colour with clearly defined margins and an absence of disc vasculature and retinal nerve fibres. The differential diagnosis of optic atrophy is considered in Table 43.2.

Heredo-familial optic neuropathies
The hereditary optic neuropathies can either be those which are autosomal dominant or recessive, or those which are due to point mutations in mitochondrial DNA.

The autosomal conditions usually present in childhood with impaired vision and pale optic discs, and due to space restrictions will not be considered further.

Leber's hereditary optic neuropathy (LHON)

This mitochondrial disorder develops primarily in males (approximately 14% women) in the second to third decade of life. It is characterized by an abrupt loss of central vision in one eye usually followed by a loss of vision in the remaining eye which may occur weeks, months or sometimes years later. Occasionally visual loss may occur simultaneously in the two eyes. There is no associated pain on eye movement in contrast to acute ON, and the visual loss is usually permanent with optic atrophy and large absolute central scotomas. However, the fundoscopic picture in the acute phase often shows swelling of the papillary nerve fibre layer, circumpapillary telangiectatic microangiopathy and tortuosity of the retinal vessels (Riorden-Eva et al., 1995).

There is a maternal pattern of inheritance and a number of point mutations in mitochondrial DNA have been identified, particularly at the 11778 location and less frequently at 3460 and 14484 (Mackey, 1994). Patients with the point mutation at 14484 are more likely to show some visual recovery when compared with patients who have a defect at the 11778 (37% as opposed to 4%). It is appropriate, therefore, to carry out genetic testing in those individuals presenting with atypical ON of the appropriate sex and age, even if a positive family history is not available. There is no effective treatment for this condition.

Nutritional and toxic optic neuropathies

Bilateral, slowly progressive central visual loss with centro-caecal scotomas, and usually normal or mild temporally atrophic optic discs characterizes optic nerve failure due to either nutritional deficiency or a toxic cause. Once a family history of one of the hereditary familial diseases has been excluded, this condition should be considered, and is usually due to a combination of alcohol abuse, deficiencies within the B vitamin complex and a frequently high tobacco consumption. With treatment by abstinence of the likely toxic agents and vitamin supplementation, recovery of vision usually occurs, unless the condition is so long standing that optic atrophy has intervened. Recent epidemics of optic neuropathy in Cuba (Sadun et al., 1994), and in West Africa have probably been related to multiple dietary deficiencies.

A wide variety of instances have been cited as causing toxic optic neuropathy which include ethambutol, chloramphenicol, halogenated hyroxyquinolones, lead, isoniazid and vincristine.

Tumours of the optic nerve

Optic nerve sheath meningiomas

Primary optic nerve sheath meningiomas, most frequently found in middle-aged women, are usually unilateral but if bilateral raise the possibility of central neurofibromatosis (NF2). Although most patients will have mild (2–4 mm) proptosis at the time of their initial consultation, patients complain of dimming of vision and decreased colour vision. Visual loss progresses over years with optic disc swelling gradually being supplanted by optic atrophy, with or without the evolution of optociliary venous (retinochoroidal anastamoses) shunt vessels (Dutton, 1992).

The CT picture in patients with these tumours is most often one of diffuse narrow enlargement of the optic nerve, with bulbous swellings of the nerve in the region of the globe and orbital apex. 'Railroad-track' calcification of the optic nerve sheath in the orbit is a characteristic feature. Use of MRI has enabled optic nerve sheath meningiomas to be distinguished from optic nerve gliomas, where the former but not the latter shows that the nerve is readily distinguished from the optic nerve sheath (Lindblom et al., 1992).

Management of patients with optic nerve sheath meningiomas is controversial. While there is general agreement that nerve sheath tumours are most aggressive in children and become progressively more indolent with advancing age, there is no consensus as to the best way to treat these lesions. Clinical resection, particularly when there is intracranial spread, is usually incomplete. These patients rarely die from the meningioma and it is probably best to observe. In some instances radiotherapy has been shown to result in some visual improvement.

Optic nerve gliomas

Optic nerve gliomas, which may also involve the chiasm, are of two distinct types. By far the commonest is the benign glioma of childhood, and the other the malignant glioblastoma in adults (Dutton, 1994). Approximately a quarter of cases occur in the setting of NF-1.

Benign optic nerve gliomas usually present within the first two decades of life, with a peak incidence at 1–6 years of age. The usual presenting manifestations are proptosis and visual loss. The fundus may show either papilledema or optic atrophy. The clinical course of childhood optic nerve gliomas is highly variable. In some tumours enlargement proceeds slowly for a time but then reaches a plateau, while in others the enlargement proceeds unabated (Hoyt & Bagdassarian, 1969). Necropsy has suggested that these tumours are in fact hamartomas rather than true neoplasms. Optic nerve gliomas are generally managed conservatively, although some favour radiation therapy for lesions with chiasmal involvement and surgery for at least those tumours restricted to the orbit.

Optic nerve gliomas of adulthood are malignant gliomas which usually arise in males aged 40–60 years. These patients often present with a rapid onset of visual failure, which on some occasions may mimic acute ON. The tumour rapidly progresses and the patient usually dies within a short period.

Disorders of the optic chiasm

Approximately 25% of all brain tumours occur in the chiasmal region and since half of these cases initially present with visual loss, an appreciation of the various field abnormalities is important. Although there are a number of other causes for the chiasmal syndrome, eg trauma and demyelination, these are rare. The neuro-ophthalmological signs of a compressive optic chiasm lesion are primarily a field defect and deterioration of visual acuity, which depend on the relationship of the chiasm to the pituitary. The classical field defect of a chiasmal lesion is a bitemporal hemianopia, since pituitary tumours first affect the medial aspect of the chiasm (Holder, 1991). Damage to the lateral aspects of the chiasm due to aneurysm result in nasal field defects. These two observations indicate that the human chiasm is organized in an orderly fashion with medial and lateral aspects of the chiasm comprising fibres originating from the nasal and temporal retinal fibres respectively, which was first anatomically observed by Hoyt and Luis (1963). Hemianopic field defects associated with a compressive optic chiasm lesion may be complete or incomplete and may or may not be symmetrical. Due to the optic nerve being compromised in addition to the chiasm it is unusual to have a bitemporal hemianopia without some reduction in central visual acuity in at least one eye.

The main symptom resulting from the chiasmal syndrome is usually a progressive deterioration of vision, often with associated dimming of the visual field, particularly temporally. A fairly frequent symptom in patients with the chiasmal syndrome is diplopia. This may be a vertical or horizontal separation of images, which usually occurs in the absence of a demonstrable ocular motor paresis. An explanation for this hemifield slide phenomenon is the absence of the temporal field in each eye, which normally acts as a physiological linkage for the two nasal fields. Minor ocular motor imbalance, which does not normally affect binocular fusion, now results in an inability to maintain the two fields in juxtaposition. Some patients will also complain of a disturbance of depth deception, experiencing problems with such tasks as sewing, threading needles or using precision tools. This phenomenon, called chiasmic postfixation blindness, is due to the presence of a blind area beyond the fixation point. The image of objects located in this area falls on the nasal retina which is blind (Kirkham, 1972).

Abnormalities in decussation at the chiasm can also result from congenital disorders. In albinism, in addition to nasal fibres, some temporal fibres also cross at the optic chiasm. The additional crossed fibres result in a systematic shift of the line of decussation into the extra foveal temporal retina. Albinism has many phenotypes and is expressed as a hypopigmentation of the skin, hair and eyes in oculocutaneous albinism (OC) and of the eyes only in ocular albinism (OA). Oculocutaneous albinos can be either tyrosinase positive or negative and further phenotypic subdivisions have been documented (Abadi & Pascal, 1989). There is considerable variability in the visual disorders suffered by albinos. All patients suffer loss of visual acuity, which is invariably associated with foveal hypoplasia. Albinos can also suffer photophobia and nystagmus, the latter contributing to reduced acuity (Abadi & Pascal, 1991). It should be noted, however, that acuity is also reduced in the rare cases where patients are able to fixate, showing that nystagmus alone does not underlie the acuity loss (Abadi & Pascal, 1991). Usually, albinism can be readily diagnosed with fundoscopy and iris transillumination, but some cases can be more difficult to detect. The most reliable measurement that detects the albino aberrant visual projections is the VEP, which has been shown to diagnose patients in 97/98 cases. As nystagmus is often present, however, pattern-onset VEP has revealed the most reliable results in adults (Apkarian, 1992). Appropriate stimulus selection has also proved effective in detecting albino pathway 'misrouting' in infants, so early detection is possible with VEPs (Apkarian et al., 1991). Visual stimulation during fMRI has also proved effective in documenting the albino visual projections (Morland et al., 2001).

Stereopsis was thought to be absent in all patients with congenital chiasmatic abnormalities because fibres representing the central visual field from both eyes project to different hemispheres. There has been one report, however, that documents stereopsis in approximately 10% of albinos, who also had reasonably stable fixation and ocular alignment. This interesting observation implies that adaptive mechanisms involving interhemispheric communication must develop to mediate this aspect of binocular vision (Apkarian, 1996; Zeki & Fries, 1980).

Disorders of the optic tract, radiation and occipital lobe

Optic tract lesions

Lesions of the optic tract, although rare (less than 3% of visual field defects in a series of 100 homonymous hemianopias), often produce specific signs and visual field abnormalities which allow definitive diagnosis (Newman & Miller, 1983). The optic tract is the first point in the visual pathways where the ipsilateral temporal and contralateral nasal retinal nerve fibres come together, and so the field defect is usually a partial or complete homonymous hemianopia. When partial there is often gross incongruity between the visual field defects found in each eye, which may also be found with lesions of the lateral geniculate nucleus and more rarely the optic radiations. Ophthalmoscopically optic pallor due to retrograde degeneration may be observed. This takes a characteristic form with band or 'bow tie' atrophy in the eye opposite to the lesion due to loss of nasal retinal fibres. Ipsilateral to the lesion, temporal pallor is observed.

Occipital lobe

On reaching the occipital lobe there is a high degree of order in the fibres of the optic radiation and lesions, which are usually due to infarction, trauma or tumour, produce congruent field defects which are homonymous. The only features of the field defect which help localize the lesion to the occipital lobe, rather than the anterior optic radiation, is the presence of macula sparing or a temporal crescent in a homonymous hemianopia.

In macula sparing there is preservation of the visual field within a region of 1–2° up to 10° around the fixation point in the hemianopic field. In the more usual situation the hemianopic field is split along the vertical meridian through the fixation point (macula splitting). Although it has been argued that macula sparing is a result of poor fixation during visual field testing, this would only account for about 1–2° of sparing (Bishoff et al., 1995). Despite the continued controversy concerning the cause of macula sparing there appear to be two main anatomical factors which may explain this phenomenon. Firstly, there is evidence that there is a vertically orientated median strip centred on the fovea in which retinal ganglion cells project either ipsilaterally or contralaterally (Fukuda et al., 1989). The macula, therefore, is bilaterally represented but since this strip is at most responsible for 2° of the central field this is insufficient to explain many cases of macula sparing. The second more probable explanation is the rich anastomotic network between terminal branches of the middle cerebral artery and the posterior cerebral artery which supply the area of the striate cortex containing the macula representation in the occipital pole (Sugishita et al., 1993).

Lesions at the pole of the occipital lobe result in small homonymous central scotomas, which may lead the patient to present with reading difficulties and may be missed if only the peripheral field is examined to confrontation. The central 10° of the primary visual cortex (Horton & Hoyt, 1991). More anterior lesions of the occipital lobe involving the more anterior part of the calcarine fissure, which contains the representation of the unpaired peripheral nasal retina, results in a monocular defect in the peripheral temporal field, called the 'temporal crescent', 60–90° from the fixation point. However, it should be remembered that the most common cause for such unilateral peripheral visual field defects is a retinal lesion rather than an intracranial one. The converse of this defect may be found in which there is sparing of the temporal crescent in a homonymous hemianopia. This usually occurs with a vascular lesion affecting the more posterior striate cortex (Benton et al., 1980).

Bilateral lesions of the occipital lobes may result in varying degrees of homonymous hemianopia, ranging from small bilateral central homonymous scotomas to complete blindness. The extent of the abnormality may vary between the two halves, being partial or complete, hemianopic or quadrantic. Sometimes restricted bilateral lesions of the occipital lobes may result in small bilateral homonymous central scotomas. Altitudinal field defects usually occur as a result of trauma (rarely tumours or vascular events) involving upper or lower occipital poles bilaterally (Holmes, 1918).

fMRI, which can spatially localize brain blood oxygenation accurately, can be used to investigate the effect of lesions of the radiation on cortical activity. It is possible, therefore, to use fMRI during visual stimulation to determine the reason for visual field loss, when damage to the cortical grey matter is absent. Retinotopic mapping fMRI methods, that have become commonplace in the research of normal visual function (DeYoe et al., 1996), may become increasingly useful in investigating visual field defects resulting from occipital damage (Baseler et al., 1999).

Cortical blindness

Cortical blindness usually indicates selective involvement of the occipital visual cortex. The essential features are (i) complete loss of all visual sensation, (ii) loss of reflex lid closure to threat, (iii) normal pupillary light reactions, (iv) normal retina and full extraocular eye movements. The commonest etiology is hypoxia of the striate cortex. Patients with cortical blindness may sometimes be unaware of their visual defect (anosognosia) and vigorously deny it, known as Anton's syndrome. This may occur with lesions elsewhere causing total blindness. There is no satisfactory explanation for this syndrome and the various hypotheses are discussed by Lessell (1975). Several hypotheses have been proposed to explain this syndrome including an alteration in emotional reactivity, 'psychiatric' denial as an accentuation of a common response to illness, a memory disorder for example in Korsokoff's syndrome, and associated lesions elsewhere in areas of the brain responsible for the recognition and interpretation of visual images.

Disorders of higher visual processing

Residual visual function in hemianopias

In his classic work Holmes (1918) showed that the striate cortex damage results in a complete hemianopia. However, incomplete damage to the occipital lobe may result in retention of some aspects of visual perception, the most commonly observed being the ability to perceive small moving objects in the homonymous hemianopia (Riddoch, 1917; Zeki & ffytche, 1998). Riddoch's phenomenon may be the first evidence of recovery of a homonymous hemianopia. This is then usually followed by perception of static targets and finally colour perception returns. Unfortunately, the Riddoch phenomenon is not only found in occipital lesions, but has been reported in patients with lesions in the anterior visual pathways (Safran & Glaser, 1980).

The retention of the ability to localize objects in space and limited pattern discrimination in monkeys in whom both striate cortices had been removed, led to interest in the possible visual functions in the hemianopic field of human patients (Weiskrantz, 1986). Since these patients are unaware of any residual visual capacity and appear blind by standard clinical perimetric methods this visual capacity has been termed 'blindsight' (Weiskrantz et al., 1974; Weiskrantz, 1986). Using forced-choice discrimination methods such patients have revealed their ability to locate stimuli both by saccadic eye movements and by pointing (Cowey & Stoerig, 1991). The extent of the residual visual capacity is varied amongst the patients so far reported, and as yet there is poor correlation with the precise location of lesions in the occipital lobe.

Residual visual function also extends the ability to discriminate between stimuli on the basis of their motion (Barbur et al., 1980; Blythe et al., 1986a, 1987; Morland et al., 1999; Zeki and ffytche, 1998), orientation (Morland et al., 1996; Weiskrantz, 1986), spatial periodicity (Weiskrantz, 1986), and spectral content (Blythe et al., 1987; Morland et al., 1999; Stoerig & Cowey, 1989, 1992). The extent to which different patients have conscious experience of such visual abilities is variable (Weiskrantz, 1986; Weiskrantz et al., 1974) and in individual patients is dependent on the characteristics of the visual stimulus (Morland et al., 1999; Zeki & ffytche, 1998). In one patient

with damage to striate cortex, stimulation with visual motion activates extrastriate cortical areas (Barbur et al., 1993; Zeki and ffytche, 1998). However, a general consistency between activity in extrastriate cortex and residual motion processing in hemianopes has yet to be revealed in studies of more than one patient (Barton & Sharpe, 1997).

Reports have documented a reduction in the size of scotomata in patients with cortical lesion following training (Zihl & von Cramon, 1979). Patients were trained to detect targets present within, but near, the boundary of their scotomata. This resulted in an increased visual sensitivity within the trained region that transferred interocularly and to different stimulus attributes such as colour (Zihl & von Cramon, 1979). Further studies also revealed that scotomata could be reduced when patients are trained to saccade to targets in their blind visual fields (Zihl, 1981; Zihl & von Cramon, 1985). Recent work has revealed that hemianopic patients visually scan natural images differently from normal (Pambakian et al., 2000). The degree of abnormality in the scan paths was greatest for patients with the longest period between the lesion onset and time of testing, which suggests development of coping strategies. In addition to the training implemented by Zihl's group (Zihl, 1981; Zihl & von Cramon, 1979, 1985) it may also be possible to train patients to scan scenes so the effects of the visual field defects may be minimized and adaptive strategies may be enhanced (Zihl, 2000; Pambakian et al., 2000).

Functional visual loss in prestriate lesions

There is increasing evidence from electrophysiological studies in primates that once initial processing of visual information has occurred in the striate cortex, segregation of different properties of the visual stimulus occurs in the prestriate cortex (Zeki & Shipp, 1988; Zeki, 1993). This cortical region contains a number of individual representations of the contralateral hemifield, each containing neurons with a particular response characteristic. For example, some areas contain neurons which are selective for colour (V4), and another for motion (V5, middle temporal gyrus, MT). There appears, therefore, to be parallel processing of different aspects of visual information in these various cortical areas before an organized synthesis of the visual scene can be generated. Specific lesions in one or other of these areas might be expected to give rise to an appropriate specific loss of a visual modality. In this section such specific losses are described for colour (achromatopsia), movement (akinetopsia) and faces (prosopagnosia).

Colour

Acquired disorders of colour vision due to lesions of the central nervous system are of two types. In one the colour sense is normal but the naming and recognition of colour is impaired. This can occur as part of an aphasia e.g. Wernicke's or anomic, in the syndrome of alexia without agraphia or as one feature of visual agnosia (see below). In the second type there is an inability to see colours (dyschromatopsia or achromatopsia) (Zeki, 1990).

Patients with lesions in the region of the lingual and fusiform gyri, which lies in the anterior inferior region of the occipital lobe and is considered to be the human homologue of the monkey visual area V4, complain that they cannot see colours and that everything looks grey or in varying shades of black and white (Meadows, 1974a). They are unable to identify the figures on pseudoisochromatic test plates, although able to correctly name the colours of brightly coloured objects. In addition they are unable to perform normally on the Farnsell–Munsworth 100-hue test. Patients with cerebral dyschromatopsia may or may not realize that their colour sense is impaired. Other functions such as visual acuity, object recognition and depth perception are all normal, but there is often an associated visual field defect, usually a bilateral superior homonymous quadrantanopia sometimes also associated with prosopagnosia.

There is good evidence that cortical lesions disrupt selective aspects of colour processing. One patient with reduced colour discrimination appeared to have colour naming responses that were consistent with a lack of colour constancy (Kennard et al., 1995). Colour constancy describes the ability to perceive an object colour as constant when illumination changes to cause a change in the spectral distribution of light reflected from that object. Neurons in the macaque visual area V4 exhibit colour-constant responses, whereas those in V1 do not (Zeki, 1980). This evidence suggests that the lesions of the lingual and fusiform gyri in the patient documented by Kennard et al. (1995) included the human homologue of V4. Functional imaging experiments on normal observers have also implicated the same cortical regions as colour selective (McKeefry & Zeki, 1997; Zeki et al., 1991). Other patients have also been shown to lack colour constancy, some of them with lesions to putative V4 (Clarke et al., 1998), while in other patients lesions appeared exclusive of this cortical area (Ruttiger et al., 1999).

Movement

A case has been reported of a woman who exhibited a selective deficit of movement perception (Zihl et al., 1983). She had no impression of movement in depth and could only discriminate between a stationary and a moving target in the periphery of her otherwise intact visual fields.

The patient had bilateral lesions involving the lateral occipito-parieto-temporal junction, which PET has revealed is specifically activated during motion perception and, therefore, appears to be the human homologue of the monkey visual area V5 (Zeki, 1991).

Moving boundaries that are defined by second order features (as opposed to luminance boundaries) are not discriminated normally in patients with lesions in lateral occipital regions (Plant & Nakayama, 1993). A more recent study, however, appears to indicate a considerable overlap in the cortical areas responsible for processing first and second order motion (Greenlee & Smith, 1997).

Visual associated agnosia

The term visual agnosia refers to a rare condition in which there is an inability to recognize and name or demonstrate the use of an object presented visually, in the absence of a language deficit, general intellectual dysfunction or attentional disturbances. The patient is, however, able to name the object when using other sensory modalities such as touch or sound. Teuber (1965) described visual agnosia as a 'percept stripped of its meaning'.

Visual agnosia has been classified in a number of different ways. One classification depends on the specific category of visual material which cannot be recognized, for example a disturbance of recognition of objects (object agnosia), faces (prosopagnosia) and colour (colour agnosia) which may occur in isolation or in various combinations. Lissauer's (1890) classic dichotomous classification of visual agnosia is, however, still relevant today. When a patient is able to copy and match-to-sample objects that he fails to name or recognize visually, his agnosia is termed associative; if he fails on all these tasks or demonstrates perceptual abnormalities his agnosia is termed apperceptive (Tranel & Damasio, 1996).

Apperceptive visual agnosia

Well documented cases of apperceptive visual agnosia are rare (Warrington & James, 1988). They show an inability to copy or match-to-sample drawings which they cannot recognize, and recognition and matching of all other stimuli which demand shape or pattern perception is also affected. Most cases have been associated with cerebral damage due to cardiac arrest, carbon monoxide poisoning or bilateral cerebrovascular infarction. Less severe apperceptive disorders are associated with unilateral and generally right cerebral damage.

Associative visual agnosia

Unlike apperceptive agnosia there is no doubting the existence of associative agnosia as a definite neuropsychological syndrome since a number of well-documented cases have been reported (Humphreys & Riddoch, 1993).

These cases exhibit the ability to copy and/or match-to-sample items which they fail to identify visually, without any evidence of primary sensory or sensory motor disturbance. The syndrome is commonly associated with colour agnosia, prosopagnosia and alexia in various combinations. This may reflect task and processing similarities between recognition of faces and objects, resulting in defects of both. Alternatively, lesions giving rise to object agnosia may involve adjacent areas specific for colour or face processing.

Patients with associative visual agnosia show an increasing difficulty in identifying an object when presented as the object itself, as a picture or a line drawing. Auditory and tactile recognition is usually intact. There is no uniformity about the field defects which are often present. A further commonly found feature is the strong tendency these patients have to perseverate either previously viewed objects or, more commonly, the verbal response to them.

A number of hypotheses to explain visual agnosia have been proposed. Geschwind (1965) suggested that agnosia was not a defect of a unitary process of recognition, but rather a special form of a modality-specific naming defect. Using a disconnection explanation similar to that given for dyslexia without dysgraphia and colour agnosia, he suggested that the confabulatory verbal responses are due to a pathological disconnection of the intact speech area from the intact sensory area. Ratcliff and Newcome (1982) have argued, however, that since object recognition, as opposed to naming, is mediated by the semantic system, disconnection must be a visual-semantic one and not merely visual–verbal. However, patients with surgically sectioned cerebral commisures are able to extract meaning from words and pictures when visual input is restricted to the right hemisphere, making it unlikely that this disconnection of an intact right hemisphere would be sufficient to cause agnosia.

A second hypothesis, proposed by Warrington (1975), suggests that the disorder is due to a disturbance of access to visual semantic information itself, since in her patient 'all links of associations were lost, not just verbal' and hence a visual–verbal disconnection was not a sufficient explanation. She regarded preservation of the ability to make same/different judgements with respect to photographs of objects taken from different angles as evidence of preserved 'perceptual classification'. However, other authors have suggested a defect of visual categorization in their patients (Albert et al., 1975). It has to be concluded that both the anatomical basis and clinical criteria for associative visual agnosia are still uncertain, but excellent reviews are available by Farah (1990) and Tranel and Damasio (1996).

Prosopagnosia

Prosopagnosia is a specific inability to recognize familiar faces despite a normal ability to recognize everyday objects, and is therefore, different from visual agnosia (Meadows, 1974b). Although facial recognition is a visual pattern discrimination of great complexity patients with prosopagnosia have no difficulty in discriminating unfamiliar faces and matching faces correctly. Indeed there appears to be no disturbance of visual perception, patients being able to accurately recognize many stimuli which are visually more complex than human faces. It appears that the disorder is not specific to faces but to complex non verbal visual stimuli that belong to a group where individual members are visually similar and yet individually different. For example, prosopagnosics cannot recognize their own car and do not recognize different makes of car; however, they can distinguish different classes of vehicle, e.g. ambulance or fire engine. Similarly a case has been reported of a farmer suddenly becoming unable to distinguish individual animals within his herd and of a bird watcher developing an inability to recognize different species of birds.

Prosopagnosics appear, therefore, to be unable to match a current visual stimulus within a class such as faces, with the memory traces of other members of this specific class which have been built up from past experience (De Renzi, 1997). Pathophysiologically there is disorder of visually triggered contextual memory. Under normal circumstances after multiple exposures to a stimulus, a template of the stimulus is stored, perhaps at several levels, but in prosopagnosics there is a defect in activating this template. Recent brain imaging studies have suggested that these processes involve the inferior temporal lobe and also the ventrolateral frontal cortex (Haxby et al., 1996). Electrophysiological recordings from superior temporal sulcus in monkeys have identified neurones which are specifically responsive to faces, cells which may well be involved in the facial recognition process (Perrett et al., 1984).

Most cases of prosopagnosia are due to infarction, head injury or hypoxia resulting in bilateral lesions in the ventromedial aspects of the occipitotemporal region (Damasio et al., 1982).

Visual illusions

Visual illusions occur when the visually perceived target appears altered in size, shape, colour, position in space and in number of images (Kölmel, 1993). The illusory type of defects may occur in the entire field of vision, or may effect only the object or the background. The term 'dysmetropsia' indicates the apparent smallness (micropsia), largeness (macropsia) or irregularity of shape (metamorphopsia) of objects. Dysmetropsia usually occurs as a result of retinal disease due to distortion of the relative distance between rods and cones. However, these distortions can also occur as a result of cortical dysfunction, for example in the aura of migraine or epilepsy, chiasmic compression or focal cerebral lesions. Visual allesthesia is a transfer of visual images from one half field to the other (Jacobs, 1980). There may also rarely be an inversion of the visual scene or tilting of the environment in patients with the lateral medullary syndrome (Wallenberg's syndrome) (Hornstein, 1974). This relates to a disturbance of the vestibular inputs required for normal visual perception.

Visual hallucinations

Visual hallucinations occur under many circumstances, eg drug withdrawal, anoxia, migraine, infection and schizophrenia in addition to those related to focal neurological disease. Those in the latter category may be unformed, consisting of flashes of light (coloured or white), lines, simple shapes or they may be complex highly organized hallucinations of people, objects, etc. (Kölmel, 1993).

Although it is considered that simple visual hallucinations signify involvement of the occipital lobe and complex ones involvement of the temporal lobe this is not always the case, for example complex hallucinations have been observed by patients with hemianopias due to occipital lobe lesions (Kölmel, 1985).

It has long been considered that visual hallucinations could result from irritative foci analogous to epileptic discharges, and certainly electrical stimulation of the occipital and temporal lobes (Penfield and Perot, 1963) supports this suggestion. Other mechanisms in some cases may be a release phenomenon to be found in the context of sensory deprivation (Charles Bonnet syndrome), in which visual cortical areas are deprived of normal visual impulses so releasing cortical activity which normal visual inputs keep suppressed (ffytche et al., 1998) This is the explanation usually given to hallucinations occurring in elderly patients who have impaired vision (Teunisse et al., 1995). However, the term 'peduncular hallucinations' was first described by L'Hermitte (1922) to describe visual hallucinations which appear animated, slow moving, cartoon-like and are usually frightening for the patient. This type of hallucination is usually associated with inversion of the sleep–wake cycle, with diurnal somnolence and nocturnal insomnia, and occurs with lesions in the upper brainstem (McKee et al., 1990).

Palinopsia

Palinopsia is a rare disorder in which there is persistence (perseveration) or recurrence of visual images after the exciting stimulus has been removed (Bender et al., 1968). Although in the literature both perseveration and recurrence of visual images have been lumped together under the term palinopsia it has been argued that they may be distinct (Blythe et al., 1986b). It most commonly occurs during the progressive evolution or resolution of a homonymous hemianopic field defect, usually resulting from a posterior cerebral hemisphere lesion due to neoplasia (Bender et at, 1968), vascular disease or trauma.

Bender et al. (1968) suggested four possible mechanisms for this phenomenon: sensory seizures, psychogenic elaboration or fantasies, visual after-images or hallucinations. Although some patients with palinopsia have had seizures, most have no evidence of seizure activity on the electroencephalogram and the palinopsia does not respond to treatment with anticonvulsants. Patients with palinopsia show no signs of psychopathology and, therefore, it is unlikely that they are due to psychogenic collaborations. Similarly, there is no evidence that visual after-effects in patients with palinopsia are enhanced and such an explanation would not explain the late recurrence of the image (by some several minutes) which occurs in some patients. However, palinopsia may be a type of release phenomenon as described for visual hallucinations. In favour of this possibility is a fact that formed release hallucinations can occur in patients with palinopsia and that in both conditions there is evidence of an interruption of cortical visual processing.

Specific types of palinoptic phenomena are illusory visual spread and polyopia. In illusory visual spread (Critchley, 1951) there is an extension of visual perception over an area greater than that excited by the object presented to the observer. In the time domain visual perseveration of moving objects has also been reported and one patient experienced accelerated movement of a perseverated image.

In instances of usually right-sided occipital lesions patients may experience monocular diplopia or more commonly polyopia (the seeing of multiple images) which persist whichever eye is closed. Rare cases of cerebral induced monocular diplopia emphasize the importance of ensuring that this phenomenon is not present in patients complaining of diplopia. Other causes for monocular diplopia include ocular causes such as corneal irregularities, iris lesions and retinal detachment.

Certain cases of polyopia may be due to epileptic phenomena (Bender & Sobein, 1963) but Bender (1945) in a description of four cases tried to explain the phenomenon as a result of impaired fixation.

References   *denotes key references

Abadi, R.V. & Pascal, E. (1989). The recognition and management of albinism. *Ophthal. Physiol. Opt.*, **9**, 3–15.

Abadi, R.V. & Pascal, E. (1991). Visual resolution limits in human albanism. *Vis. Res.* **31**, 1445–7.

Albert, M.L., Reches, A.. & Silverberg, R. (1975). Associative visual agnosia without alexia. *Neurology*, **25**, 322–6.

Apkarian, P. (1992). A practical approach to albino diagnosis. VEP misrouting across the age span. *Ophthal. Paediatr. Genet*, **13**, 77–88.

Apkarian, P. (1996). Chiasmal crossing defects in disorders of binocular vision. *Eye*, **10**, 222–32.

Apkarian, P., Eckhardt, P.G. & van Schooneveld, M.J. (1991). Detection of optic pathway misrouting in the human albino neonate. *Neuropediatrics*, **22**, 211–15.

Barbur, J.L., Ruddock, K.H. & Waterfield, V.A. (1980). Human visual responses in the absence of the geniculo-calcarine projection. *Brain*, **103**, 905–28.

Barbur, J.L., Watson, J.D., Frackowiak, R.S. & Zeki, S. (1993). Conscious visual perception without V1. *Brain*, **116**, 1293–302.

Barton, J.J.S. & Sharpe, J.A. (1997). Motion direction discrimination in blind hemifields. *Ann. Neurology*, **41**, 255–64.

Baseler, H.A., Morland, A.B. & Wandell, B.A. (1999). Topographic organization of human visual areas in the absence of input from primary cortex. *J. Neurosci.*, **19**, 2619–27.

*Beck, R.W. & ONTT Study Group (1992). A randomised, controlled trial of corticosteriods in the treatment of acute optic neuritis. *N. Engl. J. Med.*, **326**, 581–8.

Bender, M.B. (1945). Polyopsia and monocular diplopia of cerebral origin. *Arch. Neurol. Psych.*, **54**, 323–38.

Bender, M.B. & Sobein, A.J. (1963). Polyopia and palinopia in homonymous fields of vision. *Trans. Am. Neurol. Assoc.*, **88**, 56–7.

Bender, M.B., Feldman, M. & Sobein, A.J. (1968). Palinopsia. *Brain*, **91**, 321–38.

Benton, S., Levy, I. & Swash, M. (1980). Vision in the temporal crescent in occipital infarction. *Brain*, **103**, 83–95.

Bishoff, P., Lang, J. & Huber, A. (1995). Macular sparing as a perimetric artifact. *Am. J. Ophthalmol.*, **119**, 72–80.

Blythe, I.M., Bromley, J.M. & Kennard, C. et al. (1986a). A study of systemic visual perseveration involving central mechanisms. *Brain*, **109**, 661–75.

Blythe, I.M., Bromley, J.M., Kennard, C. & Ruddock, K.H. (1986b). Visual discrimination of target displacement remains after damage to the striate cortex in humans. *Nature*, **320**, 619–21.

Blythe, I.M., Kennard, C. & Ruddock, K.H. (1987). Residual vision in patients with retrogeniculate lesions of the visual pathways. *Brain*, **110**, 887–905.

Burde, R.M. (1993). Optic disc risk factors for nonarteritic anterior ischaemic optic neuropathy. *Am. J. Ophthalmol.*, **115**, 759–63.

Clarke, S., Walsh, V., Schoppig, A., Assal, G. & Cowey, A. (1998). Colour constancy impairments in patients with lesions of the prestriate cortex. *Exp. Brain Res.*, **123**, 154–8.

Cowey, A. & Stoerig, P. (1991). The neurobiology of blindsight. *Trends Neurosci.*, **14**, 140–5.

Critchley, M. (1951). Types of visual perseveration, palinopsia and illusory visual spread. *Brain*, 74, 267–99.

*Damasio, A.R., Damasio, H. & Van Hoesen, G.W. (1982). Prosopagnosia: anatomic basis and behavioural mechanisms. *Neurology*, **32**, 331–41.

De Renzi, E. (1997). Prosopagnosia. In *Behavioural Neurology and Neuropsychology*, ed. T.E. Finberg, M.J. Farah, pp. 245–55. New York: McGraw-Hill.

DeYoe, E.A., Carman, G.J., Bandettini, P. et al. (1996). Mapping striate and extrastriate visual areas in human cerebral cortex. *Proc. Natl Acad. Sci., USA*, **93**, 2382–6.

Dutton, J.J. (1992). Optic nerve sheath meningiomas. *Surv. Ophthalmol.*, **37**, 167–83.

Dutton, J.J. (1994). Gliomas of the anterior visual pathway. *Surv. Ophthalmol.*, **38**, 427–52.

Farah, M.J. (1990). *Visual Agnosia: Disorders of Optic Recognition and What They Tell Us About Normal Vision*. Cambridge, MA: MIT Press.

ffytche, D.H., Howard, R.J., Brammer, M.J. et al. (1998). The anatomy of conscious vision: an fMRI study of visual hallucinations. *Nature Neurosci.*, **1**, 738–42.

Fukuda, Y., Sawai, H., Watanbe, M. et al. (1989). Nasotemporal overlap of crossed and uncrossed retinal ganglion cell projection in the Japanese monkey (*Macaca fuscata*). *J. Neurosci.*, **9**, 2353–73.

Geschwind, N. (1965). Disconnection syndromes in animal and man. *Brain*, **88**, 237–94, 585–644.

Greenlee, M.W. & Smith, A.T. (1997). Detection and discrimination of first- and second-order motion in patients with unilateral brain damage. *J. Neurosci.*, **17**, 804–18.

Haxby, J.V., Ungerleider, L.G., Horwitz, B. et al. (1996). Face encoding and recognition in the human brain. *Proc. Natl Acad. Sci. USA*, **93**, 922–7.

Holder, G. (1991). Chiasmal and retrochiasmal lesions. In *Principals and Practice of Clinical Electrophysiology. Mosby Year Book*, ed. J. R. Heckenlively & G. A. Arden. St Louis.: Mosby.

Holmes, G. (1918). Disturbances of vision by cerebral lesions. *Br. J. Ophthalmol.*, **2**, 353–84.

Hornstein, G. (1974). Wallenberg's syndrome. Part I: General symptomatology, with special reference to visual disturbances and imbalance. *Acta Neurol. Scand.*, **50**, 434–46.

*Horton, J.C. & Hoyt, W.F. (1991). The representation of the visual field in human striate cortex: a revision of the classic Holme's map. *Arch. Ophthalmol.*, **109**, 816–24.

Hoyt, W.F. & Bagdassarian, S.A. (1969). Optic glioma of childhood: natural history and rationale for conservative management. *Br. J. Ophthalmol.*, **53**: 793–8.

Hoyt, W.F. & Luis, A. (1963). The primate optic chiasm. Details of visual fibre organisation studied by silver impregnation techniques. *Arch. Ophthalmol.*, **70**, 69–85.

Humphreys, G.W. & Riddoch. M.J. (1993). Object agnosias. In *Visual Perceptual Visual Defects*, ed. C. Kennard, pp. 339–59. London: Baillière Tindall.

Ischemic optic neuropathy decompression trial research group (1995). Optic nerve decompression surgery for nonarteritic anterior ischemic optic neuropathy (NAION). is not effective and may be harmful. *J. Am. Med. Assoc.*, **273**, 625–32.

Jacobs, I. (1980). Visual allesthesia. *Neurology*, **30**, 1059–63.

Keltner, J.L., Johnson, C.A., Spurr, J.O. et al. (1993). Baseline visual field profile of optic neuritis: the experience of the Optic Neuritis Treatment Trial. *Arch. Ophthalmol.*, **111**, 231–4.

Kennard, C., Lawden, M., Morland, A.B. & Ruddock, K.H. (1995). Colour identification and colour constancy are impaired in a patient with incomplete achromatopsia associated with prestriate cortical lesions. *Proc. R. Soc. Lond. B. Biol. Sci.*, **260**, 169–75.

Kirkham, T.H. (1972). The ocular symptomatology of pituitary tumours. *Proc. Roy. Soc. Med.*, **65**, 517–18.

Kölmel, H.W. (1985). Complex visual hallucinations in the hemianopic field. *J. Neurol. Neurosurg. Psych.*, **48**, 29–38.

*Kölmel, H.W. (1993). Visual illusions and hallucinations. In *Visual Perceptual Defects*, ed. C. Kennard, pp. 243–64. London: Baillière-Tindell.

Lepore, F.E. (1991). The origin of pain in optic neuritis. Determinants of pain in 101 eyes with optic neuritis. *Arch. Neurol.*, **48**, 748–9.

Lessell, S. (1975). Higher disorders of visual function: negative phenomena. In *Neuro-ophthalmology*, vol 8, ed. J.S. Glaser & J.L. Smith, pp. 1–26. St Louis: C.V. Mosby.

L'Hermitte, J. (1992). Syndrome de la calotte du pedonche cerebral: les troubles psycho-sensoriels dans les lesians du mescephale. *Rev. Neurol.*, **38**, 1359–65.

Lindblom, B., Truit, C.L. & Hoyt, W.F. (1992). Optic nerve sheath meningioma: definition of intraorbital, intracanalicular and intracranial components with magnetic resonance imaging. *Ophthalmology*, **99**, 560–6.

Lissauer, H. (1890). Ein Fall von Seelenblindheit nebst einem Beitrage zur Theorie derselben. *Arch. Psychiatr. Nervenkr.*, **21**, 22–70.

Mackey, D.A. (1994). Three subgroups of patients from the United Kingdom with Leber's hereditary optic neuropathy. *Eye*, **8**, 431–6.

McDonald, W.I. & Barnes, D. (1992). The ocular manifestations of multiple sclerosis. I. Abnormalities of the afferent visual system. *J. Neurol. Neurosurg. Psych.*, **55**, 747–52.

McKee, A.C., Lavine, D.N., Kowll, N.W. et al. (1990). Peduncular hallucinosis associated with isolated infarction of the substantia nigra, pars reticulata. *Ann. Neurol.*, **27**, 500–4.

McKeefry, D.J. & Zeki, S. (1997). The position and topography of the human colour centre as revealed by functional magnetic resonance imaging. *Brain*, **120**, 2229–42.

Meadows, J.C. (1974a). Disturbed perception of colours associated with localised cerebral lesions. *Brain*, **97**, 615–32.

Meadows, J.C. (1974b). The anatomical basis of prosopagnosia. *J. Neurol. Neurosurg. Psych.*, **37**, 489–501.

Morland, A.B., Ogilvie, J.A., Ruddock, K.H. & Wright, J.R. (1996). Orientation discrimination is impaired in the absence of the striate cortical contribution to human vision. *Proc. R. Soc. Lond. B. Biol. Sci.*, **263**, 633–40.

Morland, A.B., Jones, S.R., Finlay, A.L., Deyzac, E., Le, S. & Kemp, S. (1999). Visual perception of motion, luminance and colour in a human hemianope. *Brain*, **122**, 1183–98.

Morland, A.B., Baseler, H.A., Hoffmann, M.B. Sharpe & L.T. Wandell, B.A. (2001). Abnormal retinotopic representations in human visual cortex revealed by fMRI. *Acta Psychol.*, **107**, 229–47.

*Morrisey, S.P., Miller, D.H., Kendall, B.E. et al. (1993). The significance of brain magnetic resonance imaging abnormalities at presentation with clinically isolated syndromes suggestive of multiple sclerosis. *Brain*, **116**, 135–46.

Newman, S.A. & Miller, N.R. (1983). Optic tract syndrome: Neuroophthalmic considerations. *Arch. Ophthalmol.*, **101**, 1241–50.

Pambakian, A.L., Wooding, D.S., Patel, N., Morland, A.B., Kennard C. & Mannan, S.K. (2000). Scanning the visual world: a study of patients with homonymous hemianopia. *J. Neurol. Neurosurg. Psychiatry*, **69**, 751–9.

Penfield, W. & Perot, P. (1963). The brain's record of auditory and visual experience. *Brain*, **86**, 596–696.

Perrett, D.I., Smith, P.A.J., Potter, D.D. et al. (1984). Neurones responsive to faces in the temporal cortex: studies of functional organisation, sensitivity to identity and relation to perception. *Hum. Neurobiol.*, **3**, 197–208.

Plant, G.T. & Nakayama, K. (1993). The characteristics of residual motion perception in the hemifield contralateral to lateral occipital lesions in humans. *Brain*, **116**, 1337–53.

Ratcliff, G. & Newcombe, F. (1982). Object recognition: some deductions from the clinical evidence. In *Normality and Pathology of Cognitive Function*, ed. A. Ellis, pp. 147–71. New York: Academic Press.

Riddoch, G. (1917). Dissociation in visual perceptions due to occipital injuries, with special reference to appreciation of movement. *Brain*, **40**, 15–57.

*Riordan-Eva, P., Sanders, M.D., Govan, C.G. et al. (1995). The clinical features of Leber's hereditary optic neuropathy defined by the presence of a pathogenic mitochondrial DNA mutation. *Brain*, **118**, 319–37.

Ruttiger, L., Braun, D.I., Gegenfurtner, K.R., Petersen, D., Schonle, P. & Sharpe, L.T. (1999). Selective color constancy deficits after circumscribed unilateral brain lesions. *J. Neurosci.*, **19**, 3094–106.

Sadun, A.A., Martone, J.F., Muci-Mendoza, R. et al. (1994). Epidemic optic neuropathy in Cuba: eye findings. *Arch. Ophthalmol.*, **112**, 691–9.

Safran, A.B. & Glaser, J.S. (1980). Statokinetic dissociation in lesions of the anterior visual pathways. *Arch. Ophthalmol.*, **98**, 291–5.

Stoerig, P. & Cowey, A. (1989). Wavelength sensitivity in blindsight. *Nature*, **342**, 916–18.

Stoerig, P. & Cowey, A. (1992). Wavelength discrimination in blindsight. *Brain*, **115**, 425–44.

Sugishita, M., Hemmi, I., Sakuma, I. et al. (1993). The problem of macular sparing after unilateral occipital lesions. *J. Neurol.*, **241**, 1–9.

Teuber, H.L. (1965). Somatosensory disorders due to cortical lesions. *Neuropsychologia*, **3**, 287–94.

Teunisse, R.J., Cruysberg, J.R.M., Verbeek, A. et al. (1995). The Charles Bonnet Syndrome. A large prospective study in The Netherlands. *Br. J. Psych.*, **166**, 254–7.

Tranel, D. & Damasio, A.R. (1996). Agnosias and apraxias. In *Neurology in Clinical Practice*. ed. W.G. Bradley, T.C.B. Daroff, G.H. Fenichel et al., pp. 119–29. Boston: Butterworth, Heinemann.

Warrington, E.K. (1975). The selective impairment of semantic memory. *Qtr. J. Expl. Psychol.*, **27**, 635–58.

Warrington, E.K. & James, M. (1988). Visual aperceptive agnosia: a clinco-anatomical study of three cases. *Cortex*, **24**, 13–32.

Weiskrantz, L. (1986). *Blindsight – A Case Study and Implications*, Oxford Psychology Series No. 12. Oxford: Clarendon Press.

Weiskrantz, L., Warrington, E.K., Sanders, M.D. & Marshall, J. (1974). Visual capacity in hemianopic field following a restricted occipital ablation. *Brain*, **97**, 709–28.

Zeki, S. (1980). The representation of colours in the cerebral cortex. *Nature*, **284**, 412–8.

Zeki, S. (1990). A century of cerebral achromatopsia. *Brain*, **113**, 1727–77.

Zeki, S. (1991). Cerebral akinetopsia (visual motion blindness). A review. *Brain*, **114**, 811–24.

*Zeki, S. (1993). *A Vision of the Brain*. London: Blackwell.

Zeki, S. & ffytche, D.H. (1998). The Riddoch syndrome: insights into the neurobiology of conscious vision. *Brain*, **121**, 25–45.

Zeki, S. & Fries, W. (1980). A function of the corpus collosum in the Siamese cat. *Proc. Roy. Soc. Lond. B. Biol. Sci.*, **207**, 249–58.

Zeki, S. & Shipp, S. (1988). The functional logic of cortical connections. *Nature*, **335**, 311–17.

*Zeki, S., Watson, J.D., Lueck, C.J., Friston, K.J., Kennard, C. & Frackowiak, R.S. (1991). A direct demonstration of functional specialization in human visual cortex. *J. Neurosci.*, **11**, 641–9.

Zihl, J. (1981). Recovery of visual functions in patients with cerebral blindness. Effect of specific practice with saccadic localization. *Exp. Brain Res.*, **44**, 159–69.

Zihl, J. (2000). *Rehabilitation of Visual Disorders after Brain Injury*. UK: Psychology Press, Hove.

Zihl, J. & von Cramon, D. (1979). Restitution of visual function in patients with cerebral blindness. *J. Neurol. Neurosurg. Psychiatry*, **42**, 312–22.

Zihl, J. & von Cramon, D. (1985). Visual field recovery from scotoma in patients with postgeniculate damage. A review of 55 cases. *Brain*, **108**, 335–65.

Zihl, J, von Cramon, D. & Mai, N. (1983). Selective disturbance of movement vision after bilateral brain damage. *Brain*, **106**, 313–40.

44

Oculomotor control: normal and abnormal

David S. Zee[1] and R. John Leigh[2]

[1]Department of Neurology, Johns Hopkins Hospital, Baltimore, MD, USA
[2]Department of Neurology, University Hospitals of Cleveland, OH, USA

An approach to understanding eye movements best begins by considering how they serve vision (Leigh & Zee, 1999). One class of eye movements brings objects of interest onto the fovea and includes saccades and quick phases of nystagmus, which are the fastest of eye movements and allow us to rapidly change our line of sight. A second class of eye movements holds images steady on the fovea and includes pursuit, which allows us to track small objects moving across our visual environment, and vestibular slow phases, which hold images steady on the fovea during head motion. Optokinetic slow phases (OKN, full-field visual following) also help stabilize gaze during head rotation. Vergence eye movements rotate the eyes in opposite directions; they bring the images of an object of interest onto both foveae at once, and then keep them there.

Head motion is of two types: angular (rotations), sensed by the semicircular canals, and linear (translations) sensed by the otoliths. For head rotations, horizontal (yaw), vertical (pitch) and, roll (ear to shoulder), compensatory slow phases in the orbit must be equal and opposite to the angular motion of the head. For head translations, fore–aft, up–down or side-to-side, slow phases must be scaled to the location of the point of regard; the closer the target the greater the amplitude of the compensatory slow-phase for a given amount of translational motion. During natural movements of the head, rotational and translational vestibular reflexes work together with the visual-following reflexes, OKN, pursuit and vergence, so that subjects can maintain their line of sight on the particular location of interest in three-dimensional space.

Oculo-motor control signals

To interpret abnormal ocular motility it is helpful to understand the way the central nervous system controls eye movements under normal circumstances (Leigh & Zee, 1999). Here, we review the normal patterns of innervation for moving the eyes to change gaze accurately, and for holding the eyes steady to maintain gaze on a stationary object of interest. The major hindrance to rotation of the globe is orbital viscosity because the moment of inertia of the globe is relatively small. For rapid eye movements (saccades and quick phases of nystagmus), a powerful contraction of the extraocular muscles is necessary to overcome viscous drag. This is accomplished by a phasic increase in the frequency of neural discharge called the pulse of innervation. Once the eyes are brought to their new position they must be held there against elastic-restoring forces of the orbital tissues, which would return the globe to the primary position. Preventing this centripetal drift requires a sustained contraction of the extraocular muscles. This is produced by a tonic level of neural activity called the step of innervation. The oculomotor control signal for saccadic eye movements is this pulse-step of innervation (Fig. 44.1). This pattern of activity is reflected in the discharge of both ocular motoneurons and the eye muscles themselves.

The immediate premotor command for the saccadic pulse is generated by burst neurons, which for horizontal saccades lie within the pontine paramedian reticular formation (PPRF) and for vertical saccades lie in the prerubral fields of the mesencephalon in the rostral interstitial nucleus of the medial longitudinal fasciculus (riMLF). Burst neurons discharge at high frequencies beginning just before and time locked to the saccade itself. Otherwise they are silent because of inhibitory inputs from omnipause neurons, which are located between the rootlets of the abducens nerve in the nucleus raphe interpositus. Omnipause neurons discharge tonically except during saccades in any direction, when they pause and allow burst neurons to generate a saccade. A separate class of saccade-related neurons, inhibitory burst cells, are located in the

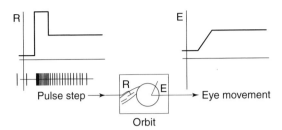

Fig. 44.1. Neural signal for a saccade. (Right) Eye movement; E is eye position in the orbit, and the abscissa scale represents time. (Left) Neural signal sent to the extraocular muscles to produce the saccade. The vertical lines indicate the occurrence of action potentials of an ocular motoneuron. The graph above is a plot of the neuron's discharge rate (R) against time. It shows the neurally encoded pulse (velocity command) and step (position command). (From Leigh & Zee, 1999.)

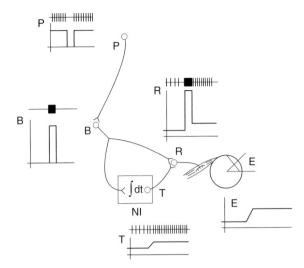

Fig. 44.2. Relationship between pause cells (P) and burst cells (B) during saccades. Pause cells cause discharging just before each saccade, allowing the burst cells to generate the pulse. The pulse is integrated by the neural integrator (NI) to produce the step. The pulse and step combine to produce the innervational change on the ocular motor neurons (OMN) that produces the saccadic eye movement (E). Vertical lines represent individual discharges of neurons. Underneath the schematized neural (spike) discharge is a plot of discharge rate versus time. (From Leigh & Zee, 1999.)

medulla, they act as a brake, and help stop saccades so that they do not overshoot the target.

The step of innervation is created by a neural gaze-holding network or neural integrator that integrates, in the mathematical sense, the saccadic eye velocity command to produce the appropriate position-coded information for the ocular motoneurons. The medial vestibular nucleus and the adjacent nucleus prepositus hypoglossi are important for the neural integration of horizontal oculomotor signals (Arnold et al., 1999). For integration of vertical oculomotor signals the interstitial nucleus of Cajal, coupled with activity in the vestibular and prepositus nuclei (Helmchen et al., 1998) are important. The flocculus of the cerebellum also contributes to the integration of both vertical and horizontal eye movements (Zee et al., 1981); its input is in part from cell groups that lie in the paramedian tracts (PMT) adjacent to the MLF along its extent from the rostral medulla to the caudal midbrain (Büttner-Ennever & Horn, 1996; Nakamagoe et al., 2000). All types of versional eye movements require a step component of innervation to hold gaze at the end of a movement; they share a common neural integrator. Fig. 44.2 shows the relationship between burst neurons, pause neurons, and the neural integrator for the generation of saccadic commands.

Control of horizontal conjugate gaze

The abducens nucleus itself is the site of assembly of the premotor commands for horizontal conjugate eye movements (Büttner-Ennever & Büttner, 1988). The nucleus contains two main types of neurons: abducens motor neurons, with axons that innervate the lateral rectus muscle; and abducens internuclear neurons, with axons

that project, via the contralateral medial longitudinal fasciculus (MLF), to the medial rectus subdivision of the contralateral oculomotor nucleus (Fig. 44.3). Lesions of the abducens nucleus, therefore, cause a conjugate gaze palsy, an inability to move the eyes beyond the midline with any type of ipsilaterally-directed versional eye movement (saccadic, pursuit, optokinetic or vestibular). There may also be some horizontal gaze-evoked nystagmus on looking contralateral to the side of the lesion, probably due to involvement of fibres of passage crossing to the contralateral abducens nucleus from the ipsilateral medial vestibular nucleus, or the involvement of the PMT cell group (Müri et al., 1996). Lesions of the MLF, on the other hand, deprive the ipsilateral medial rectus of its innervation during versional eye movements. This leads to paresis of adduction during conjugate gaze but with intact adduction during convergence: internuclear ophthalmoplegia (INO) (Gamlin et al., 1989). There is often a nystagmus in the abducting eye, which may reflect involvement of the PMT cell group adjacent to the MLF, or commissural pathways connecting the two neural integrators on either side of the brain stem. In some cases of INO the abducting nystagmus reflects an adaptive response to the patient habitually fixing with the paretic eye. If a 'conjugate' gaze palsy is not perfectly conjugate, a coexisting abducens nerve lesion

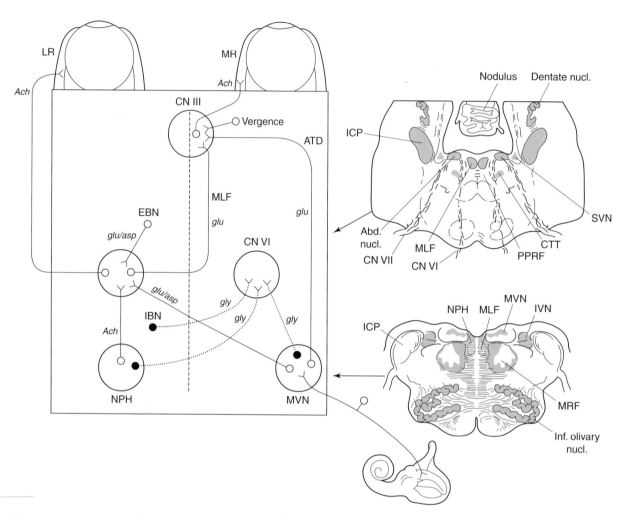

Fig. 44.3. Anatomic scheme for the synthesis of signals for horizontal eye movements. The abducens nucleus (CN VI) contains abducens motoneurons that innervate the ipsilateral lateral rectus muscle (LR) and abducens internuclear neurons that send an ascending projection in the contralateral medial longitudinal fasciculus (MLF) to contact medial rectus (MR) motoneurons in the contralateral third nerve nucleus (CN III). From the horizontal semicircular canal, primary afferents on the vestibular nerve project mainly to the medial vestibular nucleus (MVN), where they synapse and then send an excitatory connection to the contralateral abducens nucleus and an inhibitory projection to the ipsilateral abducens nucleus. Saccadic inputs reach the abducens nucleus from ipsilateral excitatory burst neurons (EBN) and contralateral inhibitory burst neurons (IBN). Eye position information (the output of the neural integrator) reaches the abducens nucleus from neurons within the nucleus prepositus hypoglossi (NPH) and adjacent MVN. The medial rectus motoneurons in CN III also receive a command for vergence eye movements. Putative neurotransmitters for each pathway are shown: Ach, acetylcholine; asp, aspartate; glu, glutamate; gly, glycine. The anatomic sections on the right correspond to the level of the arrowheads on the schematic on the left. Abd. nucl., abducens nucleus; ATD: ascending trait of Deiters; CN VI, abducens nerve; CN VII, facial nerve; CTT, central tegmental tract; ICP, inferior cerebellar peduncle; IVN, inferior vestibular nucleus; Inf. olivary nucl., inferior olivary nucleus; MRF, medullary reticular formation; SVN, superior vestibular nucleus. (From Leigh & Zee, 1999.)

(abduction affected more than adduction) is suggested. A brainstem lesion affecting one abducens nucleus and the adjacent MLF causes paralysis of both ipsilateral conjugate gaze and adduction of the ipsilateral eye. The only remaining movement during attempted conjugate gaze is abduction of the contralateral eye. This is the 'one-and-a-half' syndrome (Wall & Wray, 1983).

How do saccadic, pursuit, and vestibular commands reach the abducens nucleus? The velocity commands for horizontal saccades come from the burst cells located in the pontine paramedian reticular formation (PPRF) adjacent to the abducens nucleus. Lesions here impair ipsilateral saccades, but vestibular slow phases and smooth pursuit may be spared (Johnston & Sharpe, 1989; Kommerell et al., 1987; Horn et al., 1997). This is because vestibular inputs and pursuit commands reach the abducens nucleus by direct projections from the vestibular nuclei; only if these pathways are involved will vestibular or pursuit movements also be affected. The output of the neural integrator (the step (tonic) component for versional eye movements) appears to reach the abducens nucleus via projections from the nucleus prepositus hypoglossi and the medial vestibular nucleus (see Fig. 44.3). Mesencephalic lesions, too, may affect horizontal eye movements, presumably by interrupting descending pathways carrying higher-level commands. A deficit in contralateral saccades and ipsilateral pursuit is the usual finding (Zackon & Sharpe, 1984).

The excitatory command for the horizontal vestibulo-ocular reflex comes from the contralateral vestibular nuclear complex. When the head is still, neurons in the right and left vestibular nuclei discharge tonically at the same rate. During horizontal head rotation the lateral semicircular canal in one labyrinth is stimulated and the lateral canal in the other is inhibited. This creates an imbalance between the discharge rates of the right and left vestibular nuclei; activity increases on one side and decreases on the other. The difference encodes head velocity and provides the command that generates the slow phase of vestibular nystagmus.

Control of vertical conjugate gaze

The midbrain is important for vertical eye movements (Fig. 44.4) (Horn & Büttner-Ennever, 1998; Bhidayasiri et al., 2000). The vertical premotor saccadic command arises in burst cells located in the riMLF. This structure lies ventral to the sylvian aqueduct in the prerubral fields at the junction of the midbrain and thalamus. Each burst neuron projects to motoneurons in a manner such that the eyes are tightly coordinated (yoked) during vertical saccades.

Saccadic innervation from riMLF is unilateral to depressor muscles but bilateral to elevator muscles, with axons crossing within the oculomotor nucleus. Thus, riMLF lesions may cause conjugate saccadic palsies that are either complete or selectively downwards (but not upwards). The riMLF on each side of the midbrain contains burst neurons for both up and down saccades, but only for ipsilateral torsional saccades. Therefore, unilateral riMLF lesions can be detected at the bedside if torsional quick phases are absent during ipsidirectional head rotations in roll (ear to shoulder). There also may be a spontaneous torsional nystagmus with quick phases directed with the top poles beating toward the side opposite to the lesion (Helmchen et al., 1996). Bilateral lesions of the riMLF in monkeys and in humans produce a predominantly downward deficit for saccades or paralyse all vertical saccades. Bilateral experimental lesions of the riMLF in monkeys abolish vertical and torsional saccades (Suzuki et al., 1995) but vertical gaze-holding, vestibular eye movements, and pursuit are preserved, as are horizontal saccades.

The interstitial nucleus of Cajal (INC) is important for holding the eye in eccentric gaze after a vertical saccade, and coordinating eye-head movements in roll. Bilateral INC lesions limit the range of vertical gaze, but vertical saccades are not slowed (Helmchen et al., 1998). The posterior commissure (PC) is the route by which INC projects to ocular motoneurons. Inactivation of the PC causes vertical gaze-evoked nystagmus, but destructive lesions cause a more profound defect of vertical gaze, probably due to involvement of the nucleus of the PC.

Unilateral lesions of the INC cause a spontaneous torsional nystagmus with quick phases directed such that the top poles of the eyes beat toward the side of the lesion. There may be a 'see-saw' component to this nystagmus. There also is an ocular tilt reaction (OTR) with contralateral head tilt, skew deviation with hypertropia of the ipsilateral eye, and ocular counterroll with extorsion of the contralateral eye, and intorsion of the ipsilateral eye. This pattern of ocular tilt reaction is similar to that produced by a lesion of the contralateral utricular nerve (Riordan-Eva et al., 1997) and is encountered clinically with a variety of brain stem lesions that involve central otolithic pathways (Brandt & Dieterich, 1994). Lesions in the vestibular periphery or vestibular nuclei (as occurs with Wallenberg's syndrome) usually produce an ipsilateral pattern of ocular tilt reaction, with an ipsilateral head tilt, skew deviation with hypertropia of the contralateral eye, and extorsion of the ipsilateral and intorsion of the contralateral eye. Lesions in the MLF produce a contralateral pattern of ocular tilt reaction similar to that produced with lesions in the INC. Lesions in the MLF also produce an asymmetry in the vertical

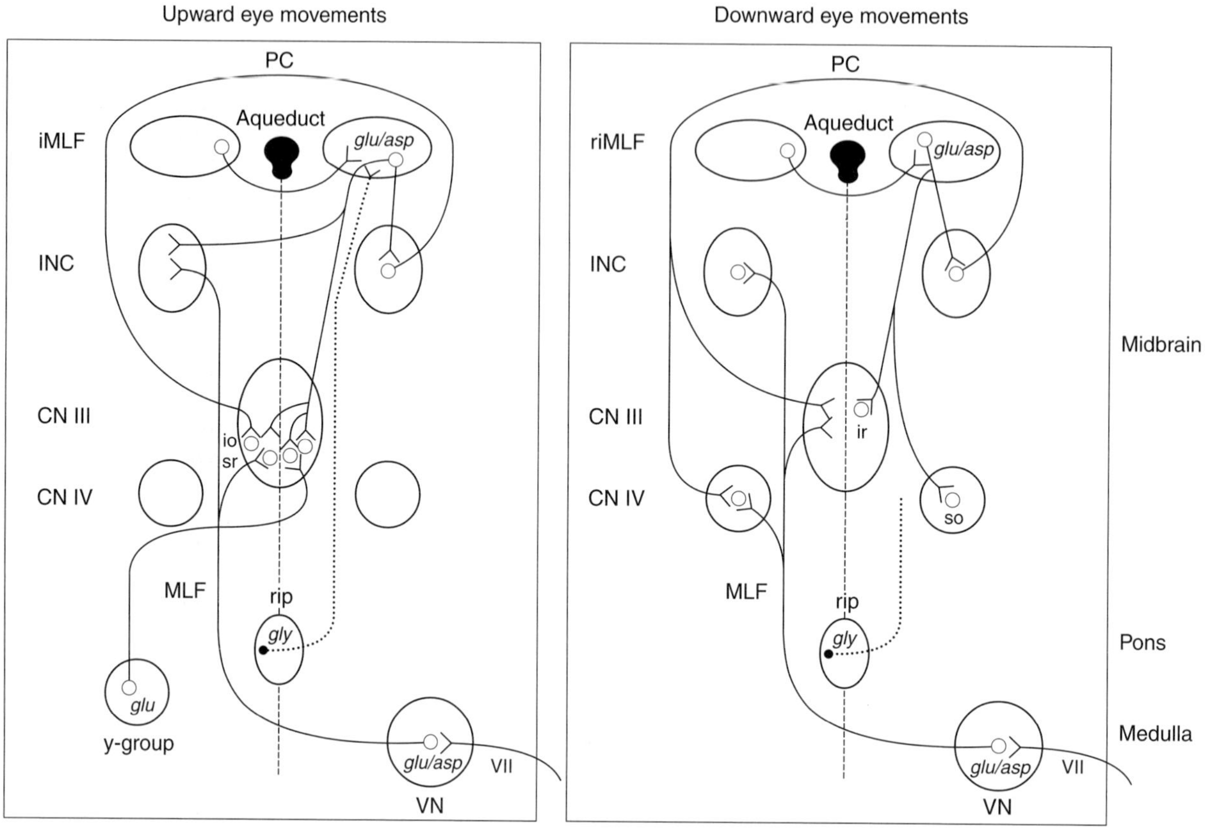

Fig. 44.4. Anatomic schemes for the synthesis of upward, downward, and torsional eye movements. From the vertical semicircular canals, primary afferents on the vestibular nerve (VN) synapse in the vestibular nuclei (VN) and ascend into the medial longitudinal fasciculus (MLF) and brachium conjunctivum (not shown) to contact neurons in the trochlear nucleus (CN IV), oculomotor nucleus (CN III), and the interstitial nucleus of Cajal (INC). (For clarity, only excitatory vestibular projections are shown.) The rostral interstitial nucleus of the medial longitudinal fasciculus (riMLF), which lies in the prerubral fields, contains saccadic burst neurons. It receives an inhibitory input from omnipause neurons of the nucleus raphe interpositus (rip), which lie in the pons (for clarity, this projection is only shown for upward movements). Excitatory burst neurons in riMLF project to the motoneurons of CN III and CN IV and send an axon collateral to INC. Each riMLF neuron sends axon collaterals to yoke-pair muscles (Hering's law). Projections to the elevator subnuclei (innervating the superior rectus and inferior oblique muscles) may be bilateral because of axon collaterals crossing at the level of the CN III nucleus. Projections of inhibitory burst neurons are less well understood, and are not shown here. The INC provides a gaze-holding signal, and projects to vertical motoneurons via the posterior commissure. Signals contributing to vertical smooth pursuit and eye-head tracking reach CN III from the y-group via the brachium conjunctivum and a crossing ventral tegmental tract. Neurotransmitters: asp, aspartate; glu, glutamate; gly, glycine. (From Leigh & Zee, 1999.)

vestibulo-ocular reflex (better response with slow phases upwards) due to the sparing of fibres mediating anterior semicircular canal reflexes, which run in part outside the MLF (Cremer et al., 1999).

Higher-level control of saccades

The brainstem circuits that generate the premotor commands for saccades are triggered by inputs both directly

from the cerebral hemispheres, and indirectly from the cerebral cortex and the basal ganglia via the superior colliculus (SC). The cerebellum is also an important circuit for generating saccades and receives inputs from the cerebral hemispheres via the pontine relay nuclei. Recent research has emphasized the role of the SC in saccade generation. Although pharmacological inactivation of the SC in experimental animals severely disrupts normal saccadic programming (Lee et al., 1988), destructive lesions in the SC do not permanently abolish voluntary saccades (Albano et al., 1982). So the cerebral projections to the brainstem, and to the cerebellum via the nucleus reticularis tegmenti pontis (NRTP) also seem important. Lesions restricted to the superior colliculus in humans are rare and are reported to cause relatively minor changes in the triggering of saccades (Pierrot-Deseilligny et al., 1991). A crucial finding is that bilateral lesions of the frontal eye fields and the superior colliculus cause an enduring, severe deficit of voluntary saccades (Schiller et al., 1987). A similar defect occurs with combined bilateral lesions of the frontal and parietal eye fields (Lynch, 1992). Thus, parallel descending pathways are involved in generating voluntary saccades, and it appears that each is capable of triggering saccades.

The frontal lobes contain three major areas that contribute to the control of saccadic eye movements: frontal eye fields (FEF), supplementary eye fields (SEF), and dorsolateral prefrontal cortex. The cingulate cortex and the intralaminar thalamic nuclei, with which the frontal and supplementary eye fields have reciprocal connections, are also important in the control of saccades. Recent studies in normal humans using functional imaging and transcranial magnetic stimulation, combined with studies in patients with focal cerebral lesions, have allowed a more precise understanding of the contribution of the different cerebral areas to the control of saccades (e.g. Gaymard et al., 1998; O'Driscoll et al., 2000; Connolly et al., 2000).

In humans, the FEF is located around the lateral part of the precentral sulcus, involving adjacent areas of the precentral gyrus, the middle frontal gyrus, and the superior frontal gyrus, and corresponding to confluent portions of Brodmann areas 6 and 4, but not area 8 (Blanke et al., 2000). The supplementary eye field (SEF) lies on the dorsomedial surface of the hemisphere, in the posterior–medial portion of the superior frontal gyrus. The dorsolateral prefrontal cortex occupies the middle frontal gyrus and adjacent cortex, corresponding to Brodmann areas 46 and 9.

Acute inactivation of the frontal eye fields in monkey (and presumably in humans), causes an 'ocular motor scotoma', so that all voluntary contralateral saccades with sizes and directions corresponding to the injected site are abolished. Such animals also have a pronounced gaze preference towards the side of the lesion, which is also the case for humans with acute frontal lobe lesions. In humans with chronic frontal eye field lesions there are increases in the reaction time of saccades, especially to remembered target locations, and to imagined targets during the 'antisaccade' task in which patients are required to look in the direction opposite to that of a suddenly-appearing target (Ploner et al., 1999). Other findings include hypometria of saccades made to visual or remembered targets located contralaterally to the side of the lesion, a reduced ability to make sac-

cades in anticipation of predictable stepping movement of a target, when the target moves away from the side of the lesion, and an impaired ability to inhibit inappropriate saccades to a novel visual stimulus. Patients with lesions in the supplementary eye fields have an impaired ability to make a remembered sequence of saccades to an array of visible targets and also have some difficulty with memory-guided saccades. Patients with lesions in the dorsolateral prefrontal cortex show defects in predictive saccades, memory-guided saccades and antisaccades.

The parietal lobe also plays an important role in the control of saccades. Its influence is largely through projections to the superior colliculus, though there are also reciprocal projections between the frontal eye fields and more posterior structures. The parietal eye field (PEF), which in humans lies close to the horizontal portion of the intraparietal sulcus, projects directly to the superior colliculus. The PEF seems important for triggering visually-guided saccades to explore reflexively the visual environment. Patients with unilateral and especially right-sided parietal lesions may show contralateral inattention, ipsilateral gaze deviation or preference, and increased latency for visually- and memory-guided saccades. Bilateral parietal lobe lesions can lead to Balint's syndrome: peripheral visual inattention (simultanagnosia), inaccurate arm pointing ('optic ataxia'), and difficulty in making visually-guided saccades. If all voluntary eye movements are affected, involvement of both frontal and parietal lobes is likely, and the term 'ocular motor apraxia' has been used.

All three frontal areas project to brain stem structures important in saccadic programming via parallel descending pathways. Although direct projections from frontal cortex to the pontine reticular formation do exist, at least in monkeys, the indirect projections via the superior colliculus seem more important.

The frontal eye fields send a direct projection to the superior colliculus but also an indirect projection to the superior colliculus via the caudate nucleus and the pars reticulata of the substantia nigra. The latter, indirect pathway is composed of two serial inhibitory links: a phasically active caudate-nigral inhibition and a tonically active nigrocollicular inhibition (Hikosaka & Wurtz, 1989). If the frontal eye fields cause caudate neurons to discharge, the nigrocollicular inhibition is removed and the superior colliculus is able to activate a saccade. Thus, disease affecting the caudate could impair the ability to make saccades in complex tasks, often related to memory, expectation and reward (Vermersch et al., 1999). Conversely, disease affecting the pars reticulata of the substantia nigra might disinhibit the superior colliculus and so cause excessive, inappropriate saccades. Such a combination of deficits is encountered in patients with disease of the basal ganglia, such as Huntington's disease (Lasker & Zee, 1997). The subthalamic nucleus, too, has a role for the generation of saccades. Stimulation here in patients with Parkinson's disease leads to an improvement in the generation of memory-guided saccades (Rivaud-Pechoux et al., 2000a).

To summarize, the influence of frontal and parietal cortex on the control of saccades appears to be via two parallel descending pathways. One pathway is via the frontal eye field to the superior colliculus (directly, and indirectly via the basal ganglia). This pathway appears to be more concerned with self-generated changes in gaze, related to remembered, anticipated, or learned behaviour and potential reward. The other pathway is directly from posterior parietal cortex to the superior colliculus. This pathway is more concerned with reorienting gaze to novel visual stimuli and in particular with shifting visual attention to the location of new targets appearing in extrapersonal space. There are, however, strong interconnections between, and common projection sites of, the parietal and the frontal lobes, which precludes a strict separation of function between the two pathways (Chafee & Goldman-Rakic, 2000).

Control of smooth pursuit

In monkeys, a subdivision of the visual system is concerned with the perception of motion. It starts with retinal ganglion cells that project to the magnocellular layers of the lateral geniculate nucleus. Some striate cortex neurons respond to moving visual stimuli, but most information processing occurs in the middle temporal visual area (MT), to which striate cortex projects (Komatsu & Wurtz, 1988). Discrete lesions of the middle temporal area in monkeys produce a scotoma for motion in the affected visual field (Dürsteler & Wurtz, 1988). The consequences are that saccades can still be made accurately to stationary targets in the affected visual field, but moving stimuli cannot be tracked accurately by saccades or smooth pursuit.

The middle temporal visual area projects to the adjacent medial superior temporal visual area (MST); neurons here not only encode moving visual stimuli but also carry an eye movement signal (Newsome et al., 1988). Lesions of the medial superior temporal area cause a deficit of horizontal smooth pursuit for targets moving toward the side of the lesion. Human homologues of the MT and MST are in the occipito-temporo-parietal junction, where Brodmann areas 19, 37, and 39 meet.

Signals about target motion are also passed from posterior structures to frontal areas, which also have neurons that discharge in relation to pursuit and in which areas lesions create abnormalities of pursuit tracking (Shi et al., 1998). Functional imaging studies, too, implicate both posterior and anterior cerebral regions in control of pursuit eye movements (Berman et al., 1999; Petit & Haxby, 1999). Both the frontal and extrastriate visual areas project to the pontine nuclei, especially the dorsolateral pontine nuclei (DLPN) with further relay onto the paraflocculus, flocculus, and dorsal vermis of the cerebellum (Fig. 44.5). The nucleus of the optic tract (NOT) within the midbrain, which receives inputs from areas MT and MST, may be important in the initiation of pursuit by virtue of its projections to the pontine nuclei (Yakushin et al., 2000). The cerebellum plays a critical role in synthesizing the pursuit signal. The dorsal vermis and fastigial nucleus may contribute mainly to the onset of pursuit, whereas the paraflocculus and flocculus mainly sustain the pursuit response. The output of the flocculus and paraflocculus is primarily through the vestibular nuclei and y-group (for vertical responses), but it remains unclear how the fastigial nucleus effects its control of pursuit.

Like the control of saccades there may be a dichotomy between the frontal and parietal contributions to smooth pursuit, the former being associated with more voluntary, internally generated aspects and the latter with more reflexive, externally triggered tracking (Petit & Haxby, 1999; Berman et al., 1999). Similar considerations apply to vergence and changing our line of sight in depth; frontal areas may be more important for generating volitional changes, posterior structures for more reflexive responses (Gamlin & Yoon, 2000).

Cerebellar influences on eye movements

The cerebellum plays an important role in both immediate on-line and long-term adaptive oculomotor control (Walker & Zee, 2000; Dieterich et al., 2000; Demurget et al., 2000). The latter refers to the mechanisms that ensure that eye movements remain appropriate to their stimulus in normal development and aging as well as disease. Three distinct cerebellar syndromes have been identified as the result of studies of discrete lesions.

First, lesions of the flocculus and paraflocculus impair smooth visual tracking – both smooth pursuit with the head still and steady fixation of a target rotating with the head (Zee et al., 1981). The latter, called cancellation of the vestibulo-ocular reflex, is comparable to fixation suppression of caloric nystagmus. Floccular lesions also cause horizontal gaze-evoked nystagmus, which implicates the vestibulocerebellum in the normal function of the neural

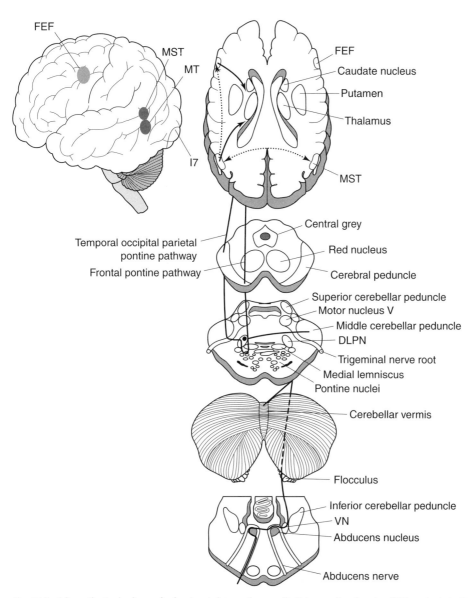

Fig. 44.5. A hypothetical scheme for horizontal smooth pursuit. Primary visual cortex (V1) projects to the homologue of the middle temporal visual area (MT) that in humans lies at the temporal–occipital–parietal junction. MT projects to the homologue of the medial superior temporal visual area (MST) and also to the frontal eye field (FEF). MST also receives inputs from its contralateral counterpart. MST projects through the retrolenticular portion of the internal capsule and the posterior portion of the cerebral peduncle to the dorsolateral pontine nucleus (DLPN). The DLPN also receives inputs important for pursuit from the frontal eye field; these inputs descend in the medial portion of the cerebral peduncle. The DLPN projects, mainly contralaterally, to the flocculus, paraflocculus, and ventral uvula of the cerebellum; projections also pass to the dorsal vermis. The flocculus projects to the ipsilateral vestibular nuclei (VN), which in turn project to the contralateral abducens nucleus. Note that the sections of brain stem are in different planes from those of the cerebral hemispheres. (From Leigh & Zee, 1999.)

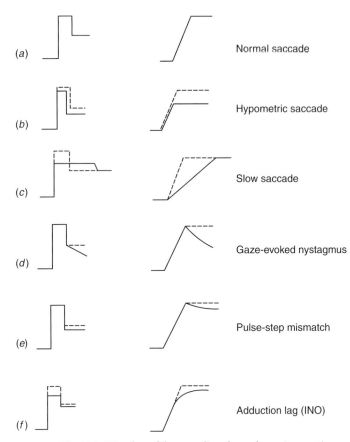

Fig. 44.6. Disorders of the saccadic pulse and step. Innervation patterns are shown on the left, eye movements on the right. Dashed lines indicate the normal response. (*a*) Normal saccade. (*b*) Hypometric saccade: pulse amplitude (width × height) is too small but pulse and step are matched appropriately. (*c*) Slow saccade: decreased pulse height with normal pulse amplitude and normal pulse-step match. (*d*) Gaze-evoked nystagmus: normal pulse, poorly sustained step. (*e*) Pulse-step mismatch (glissade): step is relatively smaller than pulse. (*f*) Pulse-step mismatch due to internuclear ophthalmoplegia (INO): the step is larger than the pulse, and so the eye drifts onward after the initial rapid movement. (From Leigh & Zee, 1999.)

gaze-holding integrator. Other signs of flocculectomy are downbeat nystagmus, rebound nystagmus, and postsaccadic drift or glissades (see under 'Disorders of saccadic eye movements').

Secondly, lesions of the nodulus and adjacent uvula cause a prolongation of vestibular responses as well as periodic alternating nystagmus (Waespe et al., 1985). There also is a failure of tilt-suppression of post-rotary nystagmus (Wiest et al., 1999).

Thirdly, lesions of the dorsal vermis (lobules V–VII) and the underlying fastigial nuclei cause both pursuit abnor-

malities and saccadic dysmetria. Vermal lesions produce hypometric saccades and impaired pursuit, especially when the eyes initiate their smooth tracking response. Fastigial nuclei lesions produce predominantly hypermetric saccades with relative preservation of pursuit.

The cerebellum also plays an important role in mediating the adaptive capabilities of the oculomotor system. Floccular lesions interfere with the adaptive capability of maintaining the accuracy of vestibular eye movements as well as preventing postsaccadic drift (Yagi et al., 1981; Lisberger et al., 1984; Optican et al., 1986). Lesions in the dorsal vermis produce abnormalities of adaptation for saccades and pursuit (Takagi et al., 1998, 2000).

Disorders of saccadic eye movements

Abnormalities of saccades can be divided into disorders of accuracy, velocity, latency, and stability. Furthermore, they can be analysed as disorders of the saccadic innervational commands: the pulse, the step, and the match between the pulse and the step (Fig. 44.6). For optimal performance the saccadic pulse must be the appropriate amplitude (approximately height × width) to ensure that the saccade is accurate, and of the appropriate height to ensure that the saccade is of high velocity. The saccadic pulse and step must be perfectly matched to prevent drift of the eyes after the saccade. A change in amplitude of the pulse creates saccadic overshoot, saccadic dysmetria. This sign is characteristic of disorders of the dorsal vermis or the fastigial nuclei of the cerebellum, although it appears with lesions in other parts of the nervous system. In Wallenberg's syndrome, for example, a specific pattern of saccadic dysmetria occurs. Saccades overshoot to the side of the lesion and undershoot away from the side of the lesion, and with attempted purely vertical saccades there is an inappropriate horizontal component toward the side of the lesion; this is called 'ipsipulsion' of saccades. With lesions of the superior cerebellar peduncle, the opposite pattern, 'contrapulsion', occurs: saccades overshoot opposite to the side of the lesion (Ranalli & Sharpe, 1986).

A decrease in the height of the saccadic pulse causes slow saccades. Normally, saccades follow a relatively invariant relationship between peak velocity and amplitude, called the 'main sequence'. Slow horizontal saccades usually imply disease affecting the horizontal burst cells in the pons, such as olivopontocerebellar atrophy (e.g. spinocerebellar ataxia types 1 and 2 (SCA1 and 2)). Slow vertical saccades usually imply disease affecting the vertical burst cells of the midbrain, such as progressive supranuclear palsy (Rivaud-Pechoux et al., 2000b) or Neimann–Pick disease (Rottach et al., 1997). A mismatch in size between the pulse and the step produces brief (several hundred millisecond) postsaccadic drift or glissades. Postsaccadic drift occurs with disease of the vestibulocerebellum. The combination of slow, hypometric saccades and postsaccadic drift also occurs with internuclear ophthalmoplegia (INO), ocular motor nerve palsies, myasthenia gravis and ocular myopathies.

Disorders of saccadic initiation lead to an increase in saccadic latency (the normal saccadic latency is 200 ms). Often an associated head movement or a blink is needed to help initiate the saccade. Impaired saccadic initiation has been reported in patients with a variety of conditions including frontal or parietal lobe lesions, congenital or acquired 'oculomotor apraxia', Huntington's disease, Parkinson's disease and Alzheimer's disease. In patients with Parkinson's disease the saccade initiation deficit is often most obvious when they are instructed to voluntarily make repetitive saccades back and forth between two stationary targets.

Inappropriate saccades disrupt steady fixation, so called saccadic intrusions (Fig. 44.7). They include square-wave jerks, small-amplitude (up to 5°) saccades that take the eyes off target and are followed within 200 ms by a corrective saccade. Square-wave jerks may occur in normal, elderly subjects or in patients with cerebral hemisphere lesions, but they are especially prominent in progressive supranuclear palsy and in cerebellar disease. Square-wave jerks may be an exaggeration of the microsaccades that occur in normal individuals during fixation and can be most easily detected by ophthalmoscopy when the patient is instructed to fixate a target seen with the other eye. Macro-square-wave jerks (10–40° in amplitude) have been observed in multiple sclerosis and olivopontocerebellar atrophy. Macrosaccadic oscillations consist of sequences of markedly hypermetric saccades, separated by a normal intersaccadic interval (several hundred milliseconds), that continually overshoot the target. This causes a prominent back-and-forth oscillation about the point of fixation. Macrosaccadic oscillations reflect an increase in saccadic system gain (the saccade amplitude-target displacement relationship). They are typically found in patients with lesions in the midline deep cerebellar nuclei (Selhorst et al., 1976) but may be found with lesions in the pons (Averbuch-Heller et al., 1996).

Saccadic intrusions should be differentiated from excessive distractibility, in which novel visual targets that are behaviourally irrelevant evoke inappropriate saccades. Excessive distractibility can be demonstrated in the antisaccade task. When instructed to make a saccade in the direction opposite that of a visual stimulus (antisaccade

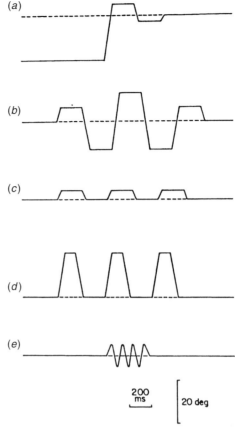

Fig. 44.7. Schematic of saccadic intrusions and oscillations. (*a*) Dysmetria: inaccurate saccades. (*b*) Macrosaccadic oscillations: hypermetric saccades about the position of the target; (*c*) Square-wave jerks: small, uncalled-for saccades away from and back to the position of the target; (*d*) Macrosquare-wave jerks: large, uncalled-for saccades away from and back to the position of the target; (*e*) Ocular flutter: to-and-fro, back-to-back saccades without an intersaccadic interval. (From Leigh & Zee, 1999.)

paradigm), patients with Huntington's disease, Alzheimer's disease, schizophrenia, and frontal lobe lesions make an inappropriate saccade to the visual target.

Saccadic oscillations without an intersaccadic interval (back-to-back, to-and-fro saccades) are called ocular flutter when they are limited to the horizontal plane and opsoclonus when they are multidirectional (horizontal, vertical, and torsional). Either type of oscillation may occur in patients with various types of encephalitis, as a remote effect of neuroblastoma or other tumours, and in association with toxins. An immunological basis is suggested (Connolly et al. 1997). Such oscillations are typically brought out by a change in gaze, eye closure, an associated blink, or combined saccadic-vergence eye movements (Bhidayasiri et al., 2001). Flutter and opsoclonus may reflect a disorder of saccadic omnipause neurons (Zee & Robinson, 1979), although other explanations are possible (Leigh & Zee, 1999; Ridley et al., 1987). Voluntary nystagmus is another example of saccadic oscillations without an intersaccadic interval.

Disorders of smooth pursuit

Smooth pursuit eye movements that cannot keep up with the moving target, and require 'catch-up' saccades to keep the fovea on target are a common clinical finding. Impaired pursuit is often a side effect of medications such as sedatives and anticonvulsants. It also occurs with disease of the cerebellum or of the brainstem in, for example, progressive supranuclear palsy. Smooth pursuit capability also decreases with age. With lesions of the cerebral hemispheres typically pursuit is impaired for tracking directed toward the side of the lesion.

'Reversal' of smooth pursuit may be seen in some patients with congenital nystagmus: the smooth eye movements are directed opposite to the motion of the target.

Abnormalities of smooth pursuit are usually accompanied by commensurate disturbance of tracking of smoothly moving targets with combined movements of eye and head. This is tested by asking the patient to fixate a target rotating with the head. If cancellation (fixation suppression) of the vestibulo-ocular reflex is intact, no nystagmus is seen and the eyes remain stationary in orbit. When pursuit is defective, cancellation is also impaired and a nystagmus appears. Only when the vestibulo-ocular reflex is abnormal will noticeable discrepancies between smooth pursuit and eye–head tracking be evident.

Mechanisms of nystagmus

Nystagmus is a repetitive, to-and-fro movement of the eyes. When pathologic, it reflects abnormalities in the mechanisms that hold images steady on the retina: visually mediated eye movements (fixation), the vestibulo-ocular reflex, and the neural integrator which makes it possible to hold eccentric gaze (Stahl & Leigh, 2001). A disturbance of any of these mechanisms may cause drifts of the eyes (the slow phases of nystagmus) during attempted steady fixation. Corrective quick phases of saccades then rest the eyes.

Constant-velocity drifts of the eyes (Fig. 44.8(a)) with corrective quick phases produce jerk nystagmus, which is

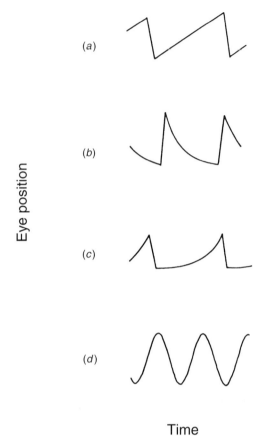

Fig. 44.8. Four common slow-phase waveforms of nystagmus. (a) Constant velocity drift of the eyes. This occurs in nystagmus caused by peripheral or central vestibular disease and also with lesions of the cerebral hemispheres. The added quick phases give a 'sawtooth' appearance. (b) Drift of the eyes back from an eccentric orbital position toward the midline (gaze-evoked nystagmus). The drift shows a negative exponential time course, with decreasing velocity. This waveform reflects an unsustained eye position signal caused by an impaired neural integrator. (c) Drift of the eyes away from the central position with a positive exponential time course (increasing velocity). This waveform suggests an unstable neural integrator and is encountered in the horizontal plane in congenital nystagmus and in the vertical plane in cerebellar disease. (d) Pendular nystagmus, which is encountered as a type of congenital nystagmus and with acquired disease. (From Leigh & Zee, 1999.)

usually caused by an imbalance of vestibular or possibly optokinetic or pursuit drives. Lesions of the peripheral vestibular apparatus (labyrinth or nerve VIII) usually cause a mixed horizontal–torsional nystagmus with slow phases directed toward the side of the lesion. Because visually mediated movements are preserved, peripheral vestibular nystagmus is suppressed during fixation. This visual suppression of vestibular nystagmus may be evaluated at the bedside by using the ophthalmoscope; when the fixing eye is transiently covered, drifts of the optic disc and retinal vessels may appear or increase in velocity if there is an underlying vestibular imbalance. Frenzel goggles can also be used to remove fixation and bring out nystagmus. Nystagmus induced by a change in head position is frequently due to free-floating otoconia that have become trapped in one of the semicircular canals, benign positional vertigo, but may also be due to central disease. In particular, purely vertical positional nystagmus is suggestive of a posterior fossa lesion.

Nystagmus caused by disease of central vestibular connections may be purely torsional, purely vertical (downbeat or upbeat), or purely horizontal (i.e. without the torsional component that is usually seen with peripheral lesions). Smooth pursuit is usually also affected, so the velocity of slow-phase drift of central vestibular nystagmus does not diminish with fixation. Downbeat nystagmus in primary position usually reflects disease at the craniocervical junction, such as the Arnold–Chiari malformation or degenerative lesions of the cerebellum. Downbeat nystagmus is usually increased by convergence or lateral gaze. Patients with episodic ataxia (EA1) often have interictal downbeat nystagmus; they can be treated with diamox (Brandt & Strupp, 1997). Upbeat nystagmus in primary position occurs with lesions at the pontomedullary or pontomesencephalic junction or in the fourth ventricle. In the medulla it often involves the nucleus intercalatus, one of the perihypoglossal nuclei. Purely torsional nystagmus usually reflects intrinsic brain stem involvement in the vestibular nuclei or lesions in the vestibulocerebellum. Periodic alternating nystagmus (horizontal jerk nystagmus that changes direction every 2 minutes) is a form of central vestibular nystagmus (Leigh et al., 1981) and can be created experimentally by removing the cerebellar nodulus (Waespe et al., 1985). It can be successfully treated with Baclofen (Halmagyi et al., 1980).

Nystagmus on attempted eccentric gaze and with slow phases that show a declining exponential time course (see Fig. 44.8(b)) is due to an unsustained eye position command. This is gaze-evoked nystagmus, and it commonly occurs as a side effect of certain medications, especially anticonvulsants, hypnotics, and tranquillizers; with disease of the cerebellar flocculus; or, in the brainstem, with lesions in the paramedian tracts, the nucleus prepositus hypoglossi, and the medial vestibular nuclei. These last structures are frequently involved in Wernicke's encephalopathy and account for the gaze-evoked nystagmus and vestibular paresis in this condition. With prolonged eccentric gaze, gaze-evoked nystagmus may damp and actually change direction, so-called centripetal nystagmus. Following eccentric gaze, a rebound nystagmus occurs when the eyes return to the primary position; slow phases are directed toward the prior position of eccentric gaze. Rebound nystagmus usually coexists with other cerebellar eye signs.

Latent nystagmus also has slow phases with exponentially decreasing velocity (Abadi & Scallan, 2000). Latent nystagmus appears when one eye is occluded; then both eyes drift conjugately with slow phases of the viewing eye directed toward the nose. Latent nystagmus is commonly associated with strabismus (usually an esotropia) and dissociated vertical deviations (DVD) in which the eye under cover is higher. Latent nystagmus is acquired early in life but does not imply any underlying neurologic disease.

Nystagmus with slow phases that show an increasing exponential time course (see Fig. 44.8(c)) are typical of congenital nystagmus and may be due to instability of smooth pursuit or gaze-holding mechanisms. Congenital nystagmus is usually horizontal, accentuated by attempted fixation, diminished by convergence or active eyelid closure, associated with a head turn, and sometimes accompanied by 'reversed' smooth pursuit in which slow phases are directed oppositely to that of the target. Occasionally, acquired lesions of the cerebellum produce nystagmus with slow phases that have increasing exponential waveforms; this is usually vertical.

Pendular nystagmus consists of a slow phase that is a sinusoidal oscillation (see Fig. 44.8(d)) rather than a unidirectional drift. Quick phases may be superimposed. Congenital nystagmus often appears pendular, although the slow-phase waveform of the nystagmus is usually not a true sinusoid and the nystagmus becomes jerk at extremes of horizontal gaze. Acquired pendular nystagmus may be a manifestation of multiple sclerosis or a sequel to brainstem infarction with inferior olivary hypertrophy (the syndrome of palatal tremor) (Deuschl et al., 1994). It has recently been proposed that pendular nystagmus in patients with multiple sclerosis may be caused by an instability in the neural integrator that normally guarantees steady gaze (Das et al., 2000). Acquired pendular nystagmus may have both horizontal and vertical components, and the amplitude and phase relationships of the two sine waves determine the trajectory taken by the eyes. For example, the trajectory is oblique if the sine waves are in phase and, more commonly elliptical (or circular) if they are 90° out of phase. Acquired pendular nystagmus is frequently disconjugate and may even be horizontal in one eye and vertical in the other. Gabapentin and memantine often diminish the intensity of acquired pendular nystagmus (Starck et al., 1997; Averbuch-Heller et al., 1997).

Convergence-retraction nystagmus, which occurs with midbrain lesions and usually coexists with upgaze paralysis

Table 44.1. *Pulling actions of the extraocular muscles with the eye in primary position*

Muscle	Primary action	Secondary action	Tertiary action
Lateral rectus	Abduction	–	–
Medial rectus	Adduction	–	–
Superior rectus	Elevation	Intorsion	Adduction
Inferior rectus	Depression	Extorsion	Adduction
Superior oblique	Intorsion	Depression	Abduction
Inferior oblique	Extorsion	Elevation	Abduction

(Parinaud's syndrome), actually consists of asynchronous adducting saccades (Keane, 1990). Cocontraction may also occur, causing the eyes to retract into the orbit. See–saw nystagmus (one eye goes up, the other down, with variable torsion) may be related to an imbalance in activity in structures that receive projections from the otolith organs (Kanter et al., 1987). The lesions are usually in the midbrain though see–saw nystagmus may accompany lesions in more caudal parts of the brainstem or cerebellum (Pieh and Gottlob, 2000). Humans with developmental disorders of the optic chiasm may have see–saw nystagmus (Dell'Osso et al., 1999a).

Ocular alignment: anatomic and physiologic principles

The primary pulling directions of the six extraocular muscles, when the eye is in primary position, are summarized in Table 44.1. The lateral rectus always abducts and the medial rectus always adducts the eye, but the actions of the vertical muscles depend on the starting position of the eye. The vertical recti and the oblique muscles pull the globe in both vertical and torsional directions. It is important to test the vertical recti and oblique muscles with the eye in a position that will cause the muscle in question to have its greatest vertical action. Thus, to test the vertical recti, bring the eye first into the abducted position; to test the oblique muscle, bring the eye first into the adducted position.

The fibres of the extraocular muscles show histological and histochemical differences from those of limb muscles (Spencer & Porter, 1988; Demer et al., 1995, 1997). As each muscle is traced anteriorly, two parallel layers are formed. The more central or 'global' portion of extraocular muscle contains fibre types that are specialized for developing transient, high tensions, to move the eyes quickly. This global layer of extraocular muscle contains about 60% of

total muscle fibre and inserts via a tendon on the sclera of the globe. The more peripheral or 'orbital' layer of extraocular muscle is composed of fibre types that are specialized for sustaining tonic tension. An important recent discovery is that the orbital fibre layer of each muscle does not insert on the globe but, instead, attaches to a pulley of connective tissue (Demer et al., 2000). The pulley for each muscle lies contiguous with the orbital wall or its fascia, between the globe equator and the posterior pole of the eye. Thus, the functional point of origin of the extraocular muscles is not, as previously thought, at the orbital apex, but corresponds to the current position of the pulleys (Clarke et al., 2000). In this sense, all the extraocular muscles are similar to the superior oblique muscle, which has its functional origin at the trochlea (the only pulley that does not move). This scheme is consistent with older electromyographic studies of human extraocular muscles, which demonstrated a 'division of labour' between the global and orbital layers (Scott & Collins, 1973). Furthermore, the geometric rules that govern the axes of rotation of the eyes (such as Listing's law, which limits rotational axes during saccades and pursuit to an approximately frontoparallel plane, and so specifies eye torsion in eccentric gaze positions) may be imposed by the properties of the pulleys.

Extraocular muscle contains pallisade proprioceptors, which lie at the junction of the multiply-innervated extraocular muscle fibres and its tendon of insertion into the globe (Ruskell, 1999). These multiply innervated fibres receive their input from a discrete set of moto neurons, which ring the periphery of the classic borders of the oculomotor, trochlear, and abducens nuclei (Büttner-Ennever, 2000). Thus, it seems possible that the multiply-innervated fibres and pallisade proprioceptors could function similarly to muscle spindles in skeletal muscle though they may also influence dynamic properties of eye movements (Knox et al., 2000; Dell'Osso et al., 1999b). There is, however, no stretch reflex, in the classical sense, associated with the extraocular muscles (Keller & Robinson, 1971). These ocular proprioceptors also seem concerned with localization of objects for limb movements, or long-term adaptation to injury (Lewis et al., 1994, 1999; Ruskell, 1999; Weir et al., 2000).

The courses of the oculomotor nerves

The anatomy of the oculomotor, trochlear, and abducens nerves is reviewed in detail by Leigh and Zee (1999). The oculomotor nucleus sends fibres to extraocular muscles, to the levator palpebrae superioris, pupillary constrictor, and ciliary body. The oculomotor nucleus is a paired structure; its anatomy is summarized in Fig. 44.9. The classic scheme

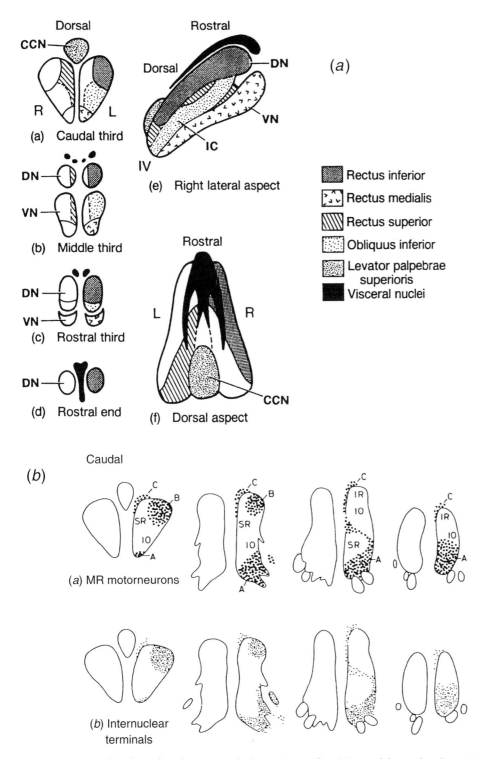

Fig. 44.9. (*a*) Warwick's scheme, based on retrograde denervation studies. CCN, caudal central nucleus; DN, dorsal nucleus; IC, intermediate nucleus; IV, trochlear nucleus; VN, ventral nucleus; R, right; L, left. (*b*) Scheme of Büttner-Ennever and Akert, based on radioactive tracer techniques. Top: The medial rectus (MR) motoneurons, identified by injecting isotope into medial rectus muscle, lie in three groups, A, B, and C. IO, inferior oblique; IR, inferior rectus; SR, superior rectus. Bottom: These same three areas also receive inputs from abducens internuclear neurons as demonstrated by injecting isotope into the contralateral sixth nerve nucleus. (From Leigh & Zee, 1999.)

of Warwick (1953), shown in Fig. 44.9(*a*), has been modified by Büttner-Ennever and Akert (1981) on the basis of studies with tracer techniques. The latter authors demonstrated that the medial rectus neurons (see Fig. 44.9(*b*), top) are distributed in three areas, A, B, and C. Neurons from area C receive pretectal inputs, and their axons mainly innervate the orbital layers of the medial rectus muscle. Neurons in all three locations receive inputs from the internuclear neurons of the contralateral abducens nucleus via the MLF (see Fig. 44.9(*b*), bottom). Projections from the oculomotor nucleus are ipsilateral except those to the superior rectus, which are totally crossed, and those to the levator palpebrae superioris, which are both crossed and uncrossed.

Clinical testing of diplopia: symptoms

Misalignment of the visual axes, strabismus, causes the two images of a seen object to fall on non-corresponding areas of the two retinas. This usually causes diplopia – the sensation of seeing an object at two different locations in space. In addition, the two foveae are simultaneously presented different images, so occasionally two different objects are perceived at the same point in space. This is called visual confusion.

If diplopia is monocular the cause is usually astigmatism or spherical refractive errors, incipient cataract, corneal irregularity, lens dislocation, or eye trauma. Such patients may report that the two images differ in brightness or that there are more than two images. Monocular diplopia caused by lens or corneal abnormality can be overcome by pinhole vision. Rarely, monocular diplopia is due to retinal detachment or to cerebral disorders.

Patients who complain of little or no visual disturbance despite an obvious ocular misalignment usually have had their strabismus from early in life. Thus, it is important to inquire about any history of strabismus, eye patching, eye surgery or abnormal head posture; old photographs may be of help.

Clinical testing of diplopia: physiologic principles

A clinical scheme for diplopia is summarized in Table 44.2. After looking for head tilts or turns, visual acuity, visual fields, pupils, and eyelids should be checked as preliminaries to testing ocular motility. Establishing the range of movement of each eye while the other is covered (ductions) and with both eyes viewing (versions) may reveal

Table 44.2. *A summary scheme for diplopia testing*

Preliminary examinations
    Look for head tilts and turns
    Check visual acuity and visual fields
    Examine pupils and eyelids
Determine range of movement
    First, with one eye viewing (ductions)
    Second, with both eyes viewing (versions)
Use objective tests to estimate amount of diplopia in the nine cardinal positions of gaze
    Red glass test
    Maddox rod
    Lancaster red–green test
Use the cover test to examine the tropia in the nine cardinal positions of gaze (prisms can be used to measure the deviation; For vertical deviations, use the Bielschowsky head-tilt test (Fig. 44.11).

limitation of movement caused by extraocular muscle palsy. The direction of any limitation of movement can be correlated with the pulling action of a muscle (see Table 44.1). It is often useful to ask the patient to follow a penlight and to note the relative positions of the two corneal reflections with the eyes in each field of gaze. Subjective tests of diplopia depend on the patient's report of the subjective visual direction of images from one test object for each eye. If both images lie on corresponding retinal elements, for example, both foveae, the object will be reported to lie in the same visual direction. If the two images lie on non-corresponding retinal elements the object may appear to lie in two visual directions and the patient will report diplopia. Two further principles are important in this type of testing: (i) the images are maximally separated when the patient looks into the direction of action of the paretic muscle and (ii) the target seen by the paretic eye is projected more peripherally. The red glass and the Maddox rod (which takes a point source of light and makes it appear as a straight line) help the patient identify which image corresponds to the paretic eye.

Cover tests demand less cooperation by the patient than does the red glass or the Maddox rod. Cover tests depend on the principle that when one eye is required to fix on an object, it preferentially does so with the fovea. (Certain exceptions to this rule, caused by anomalous retinal correspondence, occur in congenital strabismus.) If the principal visual axis is not directed toward the object, an eye movement (saccade) will be necessary to move the image of the object, toward the fovea. The detection and estimated size of this corrective saccade ('movement of

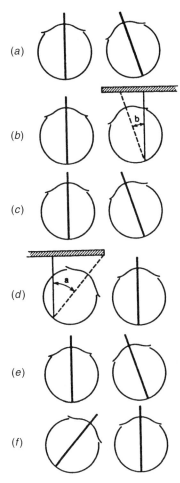

Fig. 44.10. The cover test. (*a*) Initially, with both eyes viewing, there is an esotropia (right eye turned in). (*b*) When the cover is placed before the nonfixating right eye, no movement occurs; nor does it occur when (*c*) the cover is removed. (*d*) When the left eye is covered, the right eye must fixate the target and a movement of redress occurs. Note that the deviation of the sound eye under cover (the secondary deviation-a) is greater than that of the paretic eye under cover (primary deviation-b). When the cover is removed, either (*e*) the left eye again takes up fixation, or (*f*) the paretic eye continues to fixate, if the patient is an 'alternate fixator'. (From Leigh & Zee, 1999.)

redress') provide an indication of misalignment of the visual axes.

The cover test (Fig. 44.10) reveals a tropia, a misalignment of the visual axes when both eyes are viewing. The patient is instructed to fix on a target that requires a visual discrimination (e.g. a letter) and ensures a fixed accommodative state. First, with the eyes in primary position, cover the right eye and look for a movement of the uncovered left eye (movement of redress). If no movement of the left eye

is seen when the right eye is covered, remove the cover and then cover the left eye, looking for a movement of redress of the right eye. For horizontal deviations, exotropia (outward deviation) points to medial rectus weakness and esotropia (inward deviation) to lateral rectus weakness. Repeat this test with the eyes brought into the nine cardinal positions of gaze by rotating the head while the eyes fixate on the same target. In this way, the field of gaze in which the deviation is maximal can be determined.

Testing for vertical strabismus with the Bielschowsky head-tilt test

After a paralytic strabismus has been present for some months, changes in the innervation and mechanical properties of the muscles occur so that the deviation may no longer increase when the eyes look into the direction of action of the paretic muscle. This so-called spread of comitance can be particularly troublesome in the diagnosis of vertical muscle palsies. In this situation, noting any change of vertical deviation as the patient tilts the head (ear to shoulder) to the right or to the left can often be helpful (Bielschowsky, 1940). Classically, with a superior oblique palsy, the deviation is increased when the patient's head is tilted to the side of the palsy and reduced with a head tilt to the opposite side (Fig. 44.11). In a patient who has a third nerve palsy and who is unable to adduct the eye, the action of the superior oblique muscle can be best evaluated by looking for intorsion of the abducted eye on attempted downward gaze.

Topologic diagnosis of oculomotor nerve palsies

Causes of palsies of cranial nerves III, IV and VI are summarized in Tables 44.3–44.5.

Etiology of abducens nerve palsy

Disease affecting the abducens nucleus causes an ipsilateral conjugate gaze palsy. This is because the abducens nucleus contains not only abducens motor neurons (bound for the sixth nerve) but also abducens internuclear neurons that pass into the contralateral MLF and so reach the contralateral medial rectus subnucleus (see Fig. 44.3). Hereditary gaze palsies and Möbius' syndrome (horizontal gaze palsy, facial diplegia, and associated developmental anomalies) are probably due to failure of development of the abducens nucleus (Carr et al., 1997). Duane's retraction syndrome is characterized by narrowing of the palpebral fissure on

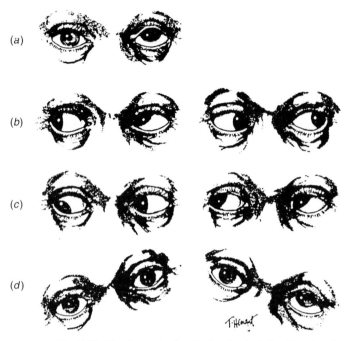

Fig. 44.11. The diagnosis of vertical ocular deviation. The steps in the diagnosis of a left superior oblique palsy are shown. (*a*) In primary position there is a left hypertropia. This could be due to weakness of elevators of the right eye or depressors of the left eye. (*b*) The deviation becomes worse on gaze to the right. This implies weakness of the right superior rectus or the left superior oblique. (*c*) With the eyes in right gaze, the deviation is more marked on looking down. This implies weakness of the left superior oblique muscle. (*d*) The Bielschowsky head-tilt test. With a rightward head tilt, there is no detectable vertical deviation of the eyes. (This would be the patient's preferred head position.) With the head tilted to the left, there is an exaggeration of the left hypertropia. (From Leigh & Zee, 1999.)

adduction (retraction) and (i) limitation of abduction but full adduction (type I), (ii) limitation of adduction but full abduction (type II) or (iii) limitation of both abduction and adduction (type III). Rare cases of Duane's syndrome are acquired, for example, through orbital injury, but in most patients the syndrome is due to abnormal development of the abducens nucleus and aberrant innervation of the lateral rectus muscle by axons from the oculomotor nucleus. Patients with Duane's syndrome seldom complain of diplopia. The syndrome occurs more frequently in females and affects the left eye more than the right.

Lesions of the fascicles of the abducens nerve usually also involve structures through which the nerve passes. For example, sixth nerve palsy may be accompanied by ipsilateral facial weakness and contralateral hemiplegia (Millard–Gubler syndrome). Within its subarachnoid

Table 44.3. Causes of abducens nerve palsy

Nucleus
    Congenital gaze palsy and Mobius syndrome
    Duane's syndrome (some cases)
    Infarction
    Tumour
    Wernicke's encephalopathy
Fascicular
    Infarction
    Demyelination
    Tumour
Subarachnoid
    Meningitis (infectious and neoplastic)
    Trauma
    Subarachnoid hemorrhage
    Cerebellopontine angle and clivus tumour
    Aneurysm including an ectatic basilar artery
Petrous
    Infection of petrous tip or mastoid
    Trauma
    Expanding supratentorial lesion
    After lumbar puncture
Cavernous sinus and superior orbital fissure
    Tumour (e.g. nasopharyngeal carcinoma, pituitary adenoma, meningioma)
    Aneurysm
    Cavernous sinus thrombosis
    Carotid – cavernous sinus thrombosis
    Dural arteriovenous fistula
    Infectious, including herpes zoster
Localization uncertain
    Infarction (often in association with diabetes or hypertension)

Table 44.4. Causes of trochlear nerve palsy

Nuclear and fascicular
    Trauma
    Hemorrhage or infection
    Demyelination
Subarachnoid
    Trauma
    Tumour
    Meningitis
Cavernous sinus and superior orbital fissure
    Tumour
    Aneurysm
    Herpes zoster
    Tolosa-Hunt syndrome
Localization uncertain
    Infarction (often in association with diabetes or hypertension)

Table 44.5. Causes of oculomotor nerve palsy

Nuclear
  Congenital hypoplasia
  Infarction
  Tumour
Fascicular
  Infarction
  Tumour
Subarachnoid
  Aneurysm of posterior communicating or basilar arteries
  Meningitis – infectious or neoplastic
  Nerve infarction (often in association with diabetes or hypertension)
  Tumour
At the tentorial edge
  Uncal herniation
  Trauma
Cavernous sinus and superior orbital fissure
  Aneurysm
  Tumour (pituitary adenoma, meningioma, nasopharyngeal carcinoma)
  Pituitary infarction
  Cavernous sinus thrombosis
  Carotid cavernous fistula
  Infections, including herpes zoster
  Tolosa–Hunt syndrome
Orbit
  Trauma
  Tumour
Localizing uncertain
  Migraine

course, the sixth nerve may be involved along with other cranial nerves by infective or neoplastic meningitis, chordoma, or enlarged ectatic basilar aneurysm (Table 44.3). Both abnormally increased and decreased intracranial pressure may be associated with abducens nerve palsies (Mokri et al., 1997).

As the abducens nerve rises and passes over the petrous bone, it lies close to the fifth nerve. These adjacent nerves may be involved by infection of the petrous bone causing diplopia and facial pain, Gradenigo's syndrome; deafness commonly coexists.

Within the cavernous sinus the sixth nerve may be involved with carotid aneurysm, carotid-cavernous fistula, dural arteriovenous shunts, or tumours, and may occasionally be recurrent (Blumenthal et al., 1997). Abducens palsy may be accompanied by Horner's syndrome (caused by involvement of adjacent oculosympathetic fibres) or involvement of other cranial nerves in the cavernous sinus.

Abducens nerve palsy should always be differentiated from myasthenia gravis, divergence paresis, convergence spasm (spasm of the near triad) and diseases within the orbit (see Table 44.7).

Etiology of trochlear nerve palsy

Involvement of the trochlear nucleus is rare; when it does occur there is often an associated Horner's syndrome due to involvement of the adjacent descending sympathetic pathways. The most common site of involvement is the subarachnoid course of the nerve. Here the fourth nerves emerge together from the anterior medullary velum. Thus, bilateral fourth nerve palsy after blunt head trauma is most likely due to contrecoup forces transmitted to the emerging nerves by the free edge of the tentorium. It may be associated with cerebellar gait ataxia if the superior vermis is also damaged. The nerves may also be involved in their subarachnoid course by tumour or as a consequence of neurosurgical procedure (Table 44.4).

Within the cavernous sinus, involvement of the trochlear nerve by tumour or aneurysm is usually accompanied by involvement of adjacent cranial nerves. In many cases of trochlear nerve palsy, no cause can be found, although sometimes diabetes or hypertension is associated, and the presumed etiology is ischemic.

Superior oblique palsy should be differentiated from involvement of other vertical extraocular muscles, skew deviation, or restrictive disease of the orbit, especially due to thyroid ophthalmopathy. The Bielschowsky head-tilt test, forced duction tests, and imaging of the orbit, help in making the diagnosis.

Another syndrome peculiar to the superior oblique muscle is superior oblique myokymia. Affected patients typically complain of brief, recurrent episodes of monocular blurring of vision, or tremulous sensations in one eye (Brazis et al., 1994). Some also report vertical or torsional diplopia or oscillopsia. Attacks usually last less than 10 seconds, but they may occur many times per day. The attacks may be brought on by looking downward, by tilting the head toward the side of the affected eye, or by blinking. Most patients with superior oblique myokymia have no underlying disease, though cases have been reported following trochlear nerve palsy, head injury, possible demyelination or brainstem stroke, and with cerebellar tumour. The mechanism for superior oblique myokymia is uncertain but some degree of damage to the trochlear nerve is probably a common predisposing factor.

The eye movements of superior oblique myokymia are often difficult to appreciate on gross examination, but the spasms of torsional–vertical rotations can sometimes be detected by looking for the movement of a conjunctival vessel as the patient announces the onset of symptoms. They are more easily detected during examination with an ophthalmoscope or slit lamp.

No treatments for superior oblique myokymia are consistently effective, but individual patients may respond to carbamazepine, baclofen, and systemically or topically administered beta blockers. In some patients, superior oblique myokymia spontaneously resolves (Brazis et al., 1994) but in others the symptoms are so troublesome that surgical treatment is considered.

Etiology of oculomotor nerve palsy

Lesions of the nucleus of the third nerve are rare. When they occur, they usually involve structures important for vertical conjugate gaze. Based on current knowledge of the anatomic organization of the oculomotor nucleus it is possible to set certain criteria for diagnosis of nuclear third nerve palsy; unilateral third nerve palsy with contralateral superior rectus paresis and bilateral partial ptosis, and bilateral third nerve palsy associated with spared levator function (internal ophthalmoplegia may be present or absent) almost invariably reflect a lesion in the oculomotor nucleus. However, it is important to recognize that in this small area of the midbrain, the nuclei and fascicles of the oculomotor nerve lie in close proximity, and both may be affected to varying degrees (Umapathi et al., 2000).

Fascicular third nerve lesions usually also involve adjacent structures. Claude's syndrome consists of third nerve palsy, contralateral cerebellar ataxia, and tremor; it is due to involvement of the red nucleus and its cerebellar connections. Weber's syndrome consists of a third nerve palsy and contralateral hemiplegia, the latter caused by involvement of one cerebral peduncle. Benedikt's syndrome combines third nerve palsy, contralateral ataxia, and contralateral hemiplegia; if vertical gaze impairment is also present, it is referred to as Nothnagel's syndrome. Fascicular lesions may lead to a pattern of weakness that mimics effects of more distal lesions.

After its exit from the brainstem, the third nerve runs in the subarachnoid space and is susceptible to meningeal processes (infection, tumour, blood). The third nerve may be compressed by aneurysm, usually from the posterior communicating artery and sometimes from the basilar artery (Table 44.5). In such cases only rarely is the pupil affected alone. A common clinical challenge is to differentiate third nerve compression due to aneurysm from nerve infarction in association with diabetes or hypertension, in which cerebral arteriography is not indicated. The presence of pupillary involvement can be relied on to identify

those patients that harbour an aneurysm. Initially, however, the pupil may be spared, so pupil-sparing third nerve palsy requires careful observation for a week before a decision can be made about arteriography. After a week, third nerve palsy with complete pupillary sparing is rarely due to aneurysm. Cases of complete extraocular palsy with normal pupils due to aneurysm are rare. Partial pupillary involvement may be grounds for an arteriogram, although mild involvement of the pupil may occur with noncompressive processes. Spontaneous resolution of an oculomotor paresis does not necessarily mean that aneurysm is excluded. In patients with an acute oculomotor palsy individuals between 20 and 50 years of age are more likely to have an aneurysm (Trobe, 1998) whereas children younger than 11 years almost never do. MRI and angiography often help to differentiate nerve infarction from compressive or brainstem lesions, and gadolinium enhancement of the cisternal portion of the oculomotor nerve is a sensitive index of neoplastic or inflammatory processes, including migraine.

At least some cases of third nerve infarction, usually in association with diabetes, hypertension, or collagen-vascular disease, involve the subarachnoid portion of the nerve. Another site is within the cavernous sinus. Such 'medical third nerve palsies' usually are acute in onset, preceded by facial or orbital pains, and characterized by total or relative sparing of the pupil.

At the tentorial edge the third nerve may be compressed by the uncus of the temporal lobe during cerebral herniation. Pupillary dilatation may be the first warning of such herniation.

Within the cavernous sinus the oculomotor nerve may be compressed by aneurysm or tumour. With carotid aneurysm, about half of all patients suffer pain in the face; abducens and trochlear palsies may coexist. Sparing of the pupils is more common with cavernous sinus than with posterior communicating aneurysms. Tumours in the region of the cavernous sinus often grow slowly and pain is not a usual feature. Often multiple cranial nerves are involved. A relatively common finding with such slowly progressive processes is aberrant regeneration of the oculomotor nerve (Boghen et al., 1979). This is characterized by anomalous synkinetic movements; most commonly the lid elevates during adduction or depression of the eye. Aberrant regeneration of the third nerve also occurs after trauma, intracavernous aneurysms and congenital third nerve palsy. Tumours arising near the cavernous sinus, including meningioma, pituitary adenomas, and lymphomas, may cause third nerve palsy; usually other nerves in the cavernous sinus are also affected. Typically, the tumours grow slowly without producing any pain.

Table 44.6. Causes of multiple oculomotor nerve palsies

Brainstem
    Tumour
    Infarction
Subarachnoid
    Meningitis (infective and neoplastic)
    Trauma
    Clivus tumour
    Aneurysm – ectatic basilar artery
    Sarcoidosis
Cavernous sinus and superior orbital fissure
    Aneurysm
    Tumour (pituitary adenoma, meningioma, nasopharyngeal
        carcinoma)
    Cavernous sinus thrombosis
    Pituitary infarction
    Carotid-cavernous fistula
    Sphenoid sinus mucocele
    Infections (herpes zoster)
    Tolosa–Hunt syndrome
Orbital
    Trauma
    Tumour
    Mucormycosis
Localization uncertain
    Post-inflammatory neuropathy (Guillain–Barré and Miller
        Fisher syndrome)

Table 44.7. Differential diagnosis of ocular motor nerve palsies

Concomitant strabismus
Disorders of vergence, especially spasm of the near triad
Brainstem disorders causing abnormal prenuclear inputs
    (e.g. skew deviation)
Myasthenia gravis
Restrictive ophthalmopathy (e.g. Brown's superior oblique
    tendon sheath syndrome)
Trauma (e.g. blow-out fracture of the orbit)
Ophthalmic Graves' disease
Orbital metastases
Orbital pseudotumour
Orbital infections (e.g. trichinosis)
Disease affecting extraocular muscle
    Oculopharyngeal dystrophy
    Myotubular myopathy
    Myotonic dystrophy
Kearns–Sayre syndrome (mitochondrial cytopathies)

Sometimes, the diagnosis only becomes evident with serial MRI scans. Occasionally, hemorrhage occurs into a pituitary tumour, causing the syndrome of pituitary apoplexy.

As the oculomotor nerve passes through the superior orbital fissure it divides into superior and inferior branches; isolated involvement of either ramus has been reported.

Etiology of multiple oculomotor nerve palsies

The main causes of multiple oculomotor nerve palsies are trauma, basal arachnoiditis and tumour infiltrations, lesions within the cavernous sinus (where the three nerves are adjacent), and generalized neuropathies (Table 44.6).

A low-grade inflammatory disorder of the cavernous sinus produces the Tolosa–Hunt syndrome (Campbell & Okazaki, 1987). It is a disease of middle or later life, and the presenting complaints are retro-orbital pain and diplopia. The third or sixth nerve or combinations of oculomotor nerves may be involved. Sensation over the first two divisions of the trigeminal nerve may be impaired. Slight proptosis and impairment of visual acuity may occur. Diagnosis

is by imaging, which demonstrates soft-tissue infiltration in the cavernous sinus, sometimes with extension into the orbit apex, but without erosion of bone (Goto et al., 1990). Corticosteroid medications usually produce a prompt improvement.

The third, fourth, and sixth cranial nerves may be involved as part of a generalized neuropathy associated with toxins or the Guillain–Barré syndrome. The Miller–Fisher variant of the latter condition consists of ophthalmoplegia, areflexia, and ataxia. The pattern of ophthalmoparesis may sometimes suggest central involvement, mimicking gaze palsies or internuclear ophthalmoplegia. Evidence suggests that anti-GQ1b antibodies play a key role in producing the disturbance of eye movements in Miller–Fisher syndrome, Guillain–Barré syndrome, and Bickerstaff's encephalitis (Newsome-Davis, 1997; Ohtsuka et al., 1998). As in Guillain–Barré syndrome, *C. jejuni* may be the responsible trigger, since anti-GQ1b antibodies bind to surface epitopes on this organism (Jacobs et al., 1995). Testing for anti-GQ1b antibodies may be positive in patients presenting with unexplained ophthalmoparesis (Yuki, 1996).

Disorders of ocular alignment not related to disease of the oculomotor nerves

Table 44.7 summarizes the various central and peripheral disorders that may mimic oculomotor palsies. Concomitant strabismus, in which the deviation is constant for all fields of gaze, is most commonly encountered in children but may occasionally present in adulthood, for example, after one eye has been patched for ophthalmic reasons. Spasm of the near triad (convergence spasm) occurs in hysterical patients and can usually be detected by careful observation of the pupils and by demonstration of a full range of eye movements with one eye viewing or in response to rapid, passive head turns (Griffin et al., 1976). The skew deviation associated with the ocular tilt reaction (OTR) may be difficult to distinguish from peripheral muscle palsies (Donahue et al., 1999).

When diplopia is due to myasthenia gravis, characteristics findings are fatigue brought on by sustained upward or lateral gaze and involvement of extraocular muscles supplied by more than one nerve. Ptosis is common. Such patients may have characteristic 'quiver' eye movements, in which saccades begin at a high speed but fatigue in mid-flight. Intramuscular administration of neostigmine, looking for a change in saccade accuracy, may be useful in documenting a response to anticholinesterase inhibitors in ocular myasthenia gravis. Improvement in eye or lid movements following application of an ice pack or after a brief nap is also diagnostically helpful.

Restrictive ophthalmopathy includes congenital conditions such as Brown's syndrome, in which the adducted eye cannot be elevated (Wilson et al., 1989), sequelae of orbital trauma, and inflammatory conditions. Thyroid ophthalmopathy characteristically causes impaired elevation, and extortion of the eye on abduction (Dresner & Kennerdell, 1985). Thyroid function tests may be abnormal and MRI or computed scanning of the orbit, or orbital ultrasonography may demonstrate enlarged extraocular muscles. Progressive limitation of ocular motility, accompanied by ptosis, is a feature of mitochondrial disorders as well as a number of dystrophic processes. Diplopia is an uncommon complaint in these conditions.

References * denotes key references

Abadi, R.V. & Scallan, C.J. (2000). Waveform characteristics of manifest latent nystagmus. *Invest. Ophthalmol. Vis. Sci.*, **41**, 3805–17.

Albano, J.F., Mishkin, M., Westbrook, L.E. et al. (1982). Visuomotor deficits following ablation of monkey superior colliculus. *J. Neurophysiol.*, **48**, 338–51.

*Arnold, D.B., Robinson, D.A. & Leigh, R.J. (1999). Nystagmus induced by pharmacological inactivation of the brainstem ocular motor integrator in monkey. *Vision Res.*, **39**, 4286–95.

Averbuch-Heller, L., Kori, A.A., Rottach, K. et al. (1996). Dysfunction of pontine omnipause neurons causes impaired

fixation: macrosaccadic oscillations with a unilateral pontine lesion. *Neuro-Ophthalmology*, **16**, 99–106.

Averbuch-Heller, L., Tusa, R.J., Fuhry, L. et al. (1997). A double-blind controlled study of Gabapentin and Baclofen as treatment for acquired nystagmus. *Ann. Neurol.*, **41**, 818–25.

Berman, R.A., Colby, C.L., Genovese, C.R. et al. (1999). Cortical networks subserving pursuit and saccadic eye movements in humans: an fMRI study. *Hum. Brain Mapp.*, **8**, 209–25.

*Bhidayasiri, R., Plant, G.T. & Leigh, R.J. (2000). A hypothetical scheme for the brainstem control of vertical gaze. *Neurology*, **54**, 1985–93.

Bhidayasiri, R., Somers, J.T., Kim, J-I. et al. (2001). Ocular oscillations induced by shifts of the direction and depth of fixation. *Ann. Neurol.*, **41**, 24–8.

Bielschowsky, A. (1940). *Lectures on Motor Anomalies.* Hanover, NH: Darmouth College Publications.

Blanke, O., Spinelli, L., Thut, G. et al. (2000). Location of the human frontal eye field as defined by electrical cortical stimulation: anatomical, functional and electrophysiological characteristics. *NeuroReport*, **11**, 1907–13.

Blumenthal, E.Z., Gomori, J.M. & Dotan, S. (1997). Recurrent abducens nerve palsy caused by dolichoectasia of the cavernous internal carotid artery. *Am. J. Ophthalmol.*, **124**, 255–7.

Boghen, D., Chartrand, J.P., LaFlammer, J.P. et al. (1979). Primary aberrant third nerve regeneration. *Ann. Neurol.*, **6**, 415–18.

Brandt, T. & Dieterich, M. (1994). Vestibular syndromes in the roll plane: topographic diagnosis from brain stem to cortex. *Ann. Neurol.*, **36**, 337–47.

Brandt, T. & Strupp, M. (1997). Episodic ataxia type 1 and 2 (familial periodic ataxia/vertigo). *Audiol. Neurootol.*, **2**, 373–83.

Brazis, P.W., Miller, N.R., Henderer, J.D. et al. (1994). The natural history and results of treatment of superior oblique myokymia. *Neuro-Ophthalmology*, **106**, 1169–70.

Büttner-Ennever, J.A. (2000). A dual motor control of extraocular muscles. *Neuro-Ophthalmology*, **23**, 147–9.

Büttner-Ennever, J.A. & Akert, K. (1981). Medial rectus subgroups of the oculomotor nucleus and their abducens internuclear input in the monkey. *J. Comp. Neurol.*, **107**, 17–27.

Büttner-Ennever, J.A. & Büttner, U. (1988). The reticular formation. In *Reviews of Oculomotor Research. Vol. 2. Neuroanatomy of the Oculomotor System*, ed. J.A. Büttner-Ennever, pp. 119–76. Amsterdam: Elsevier.

Büttner-Ennever, J.A. & Horn, A.K. (1996). Pathways from cell groups of the paramedian tracts to the floccular region. *Ann. NY Acad. Sci.*, **781**, 532–40.

Campbell, R.J. & Okazaki, H. (1987). Painful ophthalmoplegia (Tolosa–Hunt variant): autopsy findings in a patient with necrotizing intracavernous carotid vasculitis and inflammatory disease of the orbit. *Mayo Clin. Proc.*, **62**, 520–6.

Carr, M., Ross, D., Zuker, R. (1997). Cranial nerve defects in congenital facial palsy. *J. Otolaryngol.*, **26**, 80–7.

Chafee, M.V. & Goldman-Rakic P.S. (2000). Inactivation of parietal and prefrontal cortex reveals interdependence of neural activity during memory-guided saccades. *J. Neurophysiol.*, **83**, 1550–66.

Clarke, R.A., Miller, J.M. & Demer, J.L. (2000). Three-dimensional location of human rectus pulleys by path inflections in secondary gaze positions. *Invest. Ophthalmol. Vis. Sci.*, **41**, 3787–97.

Connolly, A.M., Pestronk, A., Mehta, S. et al. (1997). Serum autoantibodies in childhood opsoclonus-myoclonus syndrome: an analysis of antigenic targets in neural tissues. *J. Pediatr.*, **130**, 974–88.

Connolly, J.D., Goodale, M.A., DeSouza, J.F. et al. (2000). A comparison of frontoparietal fMRI activation during anti-saccades and anti-pointing. *J. Neurophysiol.*, **84**, 1645–55.

Cremer, P.D., Migliaccio, A.A., Halmagyi, G.M. et al. (1999). Vestibulo-ocular reflex pathways in internuclear ophthalmoplegia. *Ann. Neurol.*, **45**, 529–33.

*Das, V.E., Oruganti, P., Kramer, P.D. & Leigh, R.J. (2000). Experimental tests of a neural-network model for ocular oscillations caused by disease of central myelin. *Exp. Brain Res.*, **133**, 189–97.

Dell'Osso, L.F., Hogan, D., Jacobs, J.B. et al. (1999a). Eye movements in canine hemichiasma: does human hemichiasma exist? *Neuro-Ophthalmol.*, **22**, 47–58.

Dell'Osso, L.F., Hertle, R.W., Williams, R.W. et al. (1999b). A new surgery for congenital nystagmus: effects of tenotomy on an achiastmatic canine and the role of extraocular proprioception. *J. AAPOS*, **3**, 166–82.

Demer, J.L., Miller, J.M., Poukens, V. et al. (1995). Evidence for fibromuscular pulleys of the recti extraocular muscles. *Invest. Ophthalmol. Vis. Sci.*, **36**, 1125–36.

Demer, J.L., Poukens, V., Miller, J.M. et al. (1997). Innervation of extraocular pulley smooth muscle in monkeys and humans. *Invest. Ophthalmol. Vis. Sci.*, **38**, 1774–85.

Demer, J.L., Oh, S.Y. & Poukens, V. (2000). Evidence for active control of rectus extraocular muscle pulleys. *Invest. Ophthalmol. Vis. Sci.*, **41**, 1280–90.

Demurget, M., Pélisson, D., Grethe, J.S. et al. (2000). Functional adaptation of reactive saccades in humans: a PET study. *Exp. Brain Res.*, **132**, 243–59.

Deuschl, G., Toro, C., Valls-Solo, J. et al. (1994). Symptomatic and essential tremor. I. Clinical, physiological and MRI analysis. *Brain*, **117**, 773–88.

Dieterich, M., Bucher, S.F., Seelos, K.C. et al. (2000). Cerebellar activation during optokinetic stimulation and saccades. *Neurology*, **54**, 148–55.

Donahue, S.P., Lavin, P.J. & Hamed, L.M. (1999). Tonic ocular tilt reaction stimulating a superior oblique palsy: diagnostic confusion with the 3-step test. *Arch. Ophthalmol.*, **117**, 347–52.

Dresner, S.C. & Kennerdell, J.S. (1985). Dysthyroid orbitopathy. *Neurology*, **35**, 1628–34.

Dürsteler, M.S. & Wurtz, R.H. (1988). Pursuit and optokinetic deficits following chemical lesions of cortical areas MT and MST. *J. Neurophysiol.*, **60**, 940–65.

Fukushima, K., Fukushima, J., Harada, C. et al. (1990). Neuronal activity related to vertical eye movement in the region of the interstitial nucleus of Cajal in alert cats. *Exp. Brain Res.*, **79**, 43–64.

Gamlin, P.D. & Yoon, K. (2000). An area for vergence eye movement in primate frontal cortex. *Nature*, **407**, 1003–7.

Gamlin, P.D.R., Gnadt, J.W. & Mays, L.E. (1989). Lidocaine-induced

unilateral internuclear ophthalmoplegia: effects on convergence and conjugate eye movements. *J. Neurophysiol.*, **62**, 82–95.

*Gaymard, B., Ploner, C.J., Rivaud, S., Vermersch, A.I. & Pierrot-Deseilligny, C. (1998). Cortical control of saccades. *Exp. Brain Res.*, **123**, 159–63.

Goto, Y., Hosokawa, S., Goto, I. et al. (1990). Abnormality in the cavernous sinus in three patients with Tolosa-Hunt syndrome: MRI and CT findings. *J. Neurol. Neurosurg. Psychiatry*, **53**, 231–4.

Griffin, J.F., Wray, S.H. & Anderson, D.P. (1976). Misdiagnosis of spasm of the near reflex. *Neurology*, **26**, 1018–20.

Halmagyi, G.M., Rudge, P., Gresty, M.A. et al. (1980). Treatment of periodic alternating nystagmus. *Ann. Neurol.*, **8**, 609–11.

Helmchen, C., Glasauer, S., Bartl, K. et al. (1996). Contralesionally beating torsional nystagmus in a unilateral rostral midbrain lesion. *Neurology*, **47**, 482–6.

Helmchen, C., Rambold, H., Fuhry, L. & Büttner, U. (1998). Deficits in vertical and torsional eye movements after uni- bilateral muscimol inactivation of the interstitial nucleus of Cajal of the alert monkey. *Exp. Brain Res.*, **119**, 436–52.

Hikosaka, O. & Wurtz, R.H. (1989). The basal ganglia. In *Review of Oculomotor Research. Vol. 3 The Neurobiology of Saccadic Eye Movements*, ed. R.E. Wurtz & M.E. Goldberg, pp. 257–81. Amsterdam: Elsevier.

Horn, A.K.E., & Büttner-Ennever, J.A. (1998). Premotoneurons for vertical eye-movements in the rostral mesencephalon of monkey and man: the histological identification by paravalbumin immunostaining. *J. Comp. Neurol.*, **392**, 413–27.

Horn, A.K.E., Büttner-Ennever, J.A., Suzuki, Y. et al. (1997). Histological identification of premotoneurons for horizontal saccades in monkey and man by parvalbumin immunostaining. *J. Comp. Neurol.*, **359**, 350–63.

Jacobs, B.C., Endtz, H.P., van der Meché, F.G.A. et al. (1995). Serum antiGQ1b IgG antibodies recognize surface epitopes on *Campylobactor jejuni* from patients with Miller Fisher syndrome. *Ann. Neurol.*, **37**, 260–4.

Johnston, J.L. & Sharpe, J.A. (1989). Sparing of the vestibulo-ocular reflex with lesions of the paramedian pontine reticular formation. *Neurology*, **39**, 876.

Kantner, D.S., Ruff, R.L., Leigh, R.J. et al. (1987). See-saw nystagmus and brainstem infarction. MRI findings. *Neuro-Ophthalmology*, **7**, 279–83.

Keane, J.R. (1990). The pretectal syndrome: 206 patients. *Neurology*, **40**, 684–90.

Keller, E.L. & Robinson, D.A. (1971). Absence of a stretch reflex in extraocular muscles of the monkey. *J. Neurophysiol.*, **34**, 908–19.

Knox, P.C., Weir, C.R. & Murphy, P.J. (2000). Modification of visually-guided saccades by a nonvisual afferent feedback signal. *Invest. Ophthalmol. Vis. Sci.*, **41**, 2561–5.

Komatsu, H. & Wurtz, R.H. (1988). Relation of cortical area MT and MST to pursuit eye movements. I. Localization and visual properties of neurons. *J. Neurophysiol.*, **60**, 580–603.

Kommerell, G., Henn, V., Bach, M. et al. (1987). Unilateral lesion of the paramedian pontine reticular formation. Loss of rapid eye movements with preservation of vestibulo-ocular reflex and pursuit. *Neuro-Ophthalmology*, **7**, 93–8.

*Lasker, A.G. & Zee, D.S. (1997). Ocular motor abnormalities in Huntington's disease. *Vision Res.*, **37**, 3639–45.

Lee, C., Rohrer, W.H. & Sparks, D.H. (1988). Population coding of saccadic eye movements by neurons in the superior colliculus. *Nature*, **332**, 357–60.

*Leigh, R.J. & Zee, D.S. (1999). *The Neurology of Eye Movements*, New York, NY: Oxford University Press.

Leigh, R.J., Robinson, D.A. & Zee, D.A. (1981). A hypothetical explanation for periodic alternating nystagmus: instability in the optokinetic–vestibular system. *Ann. NY Acad. Sci.*, **374**, 619–35.

Lewis, R.F., Zee, D.S., Gaymard, B. et al. (1994). Extraocular muscle proprioception functions in the control of ocular alignment and eye movement conjugacy. *J. Neurophysiol.*, **71**, 1028–31.

Lewis, R.F., Zee, D.S., Goldstein, H.P. & Guthrie, B.L. (1999). Proprioceptive and retinal afference modify post-saccadic drift. *J. Neurophysiol.*, **82**, 551–63.

Lisberger, S.G., Miles, F.A. & Zee, D.S. (1984). Signals used to compute errors in the monkey vestibulo-ocular reflex: possible role of the flocculus. *J. Neurophysiol.*, **52**, 1140–53.

Lynch, J.C. (1992). Saccade initiation and latency deficits after combined lesions of the frontal and posterior eye fields in monkey. *J. Neurophysiol.*, **68**, 1913–16.

Mokri, B., Piepgras, D.G. & Miller, G.M. (1997). Syndrome of orthostatic headaches and diffuse pachymeningeal gadolinium enhancement. *Mayo Clin. Proc.*, **72**, 400–13.

Müri, R.M., Chermann, J.F., Cohen, L. et al. (1996). Ocular motor consequences of damage to the abducens nucleus area in humans. *J. Neuro-ophthalmol.*, **65**, 374–7.

Nakamogoe, K., Iwamomto, Y. & Yoshida, K. (2000). Evidence for brainstem structures participating in oculomotor integration. *Science*, **228**, 857–9.

Newsome, W.T., Wurtz, R.H. & Komatsu, H. (1988). Relation of cortical areas MT and MST to pursuit eye movements. II. Differentiation of retinal from extraretinal inputs. *J. Neurophysiol.*, **60**, 604–20.

Newsome-Davis, J. (1997). Myasthenia gravis and the Miller–Fisher variant of Guillaire–Barré syndrome. *Curr. Opin. Neurol.*, **10**, 18–21.

O'Driscoll, G.A., Wolff, A-L.V., Benkelfat, C. et al. (2000). Functional anatomy of smooth pursuit and predictive saccades. *NeuroReport*, **11**, 1335–40.

Ohtsuka, K., Nakamura, Y., Hashimoto, M. et al. (1998). Fisher syndrome associated with IgG anti GQ1b antibody following infection by a specific serotype of *Camplyobacter jejuni*. *Ophthalmology*, **105**, 1281–5.

Optican, L.M., Zee, D.S. & Miles, F.A. (1986). Floccular lesions abolish adaptive control of post-saccadic ocular drift in primates. *Exp. Brain. Res.*, **64**, 596–8.

Petit, L. & Haxby, J.V. (1999). Functional anatomy of pursuit eye movements in humans as revealed by fMRI. *J. Neurophysiol.*, **82**, 463–71.

Pieh, C. & Gottlob, I. (2000). Arnold–Chiari malformation and nystagmus of skew. *J. Neurol. Neurosurg. Psychiatry*, **69**, 124–6.

Pierrot-Deseilligny, C., Rosa, A., Masmoudi, K. et al. (1991).

Saccade deficits after a unilateral lesion affecting the superior colliculus. *J. Neurol. Neurosurg., Psychiatry*, **54**, 1106–9.

Ploner, C.J., Rivaud-Pechoux, S., Gaymard, B.M., Agid, Y. & Pierrot-Deseilligny, C. (1999). Errors of memory-guided saccades in humans with lesions of the frontal eye field and the dorsolateral prefrontal cortex. *J. Neurophysiol.*, **82**, 1086–90.

Ranalli, P.J. & Sharpe, J.A. (1986). Contrapulsion of saccades and ipsilateral ataxia: a unilateral disorder of the rostral cerebellum. *Ann. Neurol.*, **20**, 311–16.

Ridley, A., Kennard, C., Schlotz, C.L. et al. (1987). Omnipause neurons in two cases of opsoclonus associated with oat cell carcinoma of the lung. *Brain*, **110**, 1699–709.

Riordan-Eva, P., Harcourt, J.P., Faldon, M. (1997). Skew deviation following vestibular nerve surgery. *Ann. Neurol.*, **41**, 94–9.

Rivaud-Pechoux, S., Vermersch, A.I., Gaymard, B. et al. (2000a). Improvement of memory guided saccades in parkinsonian patients by high frequency subthalamic nucleus stimulation. *J. Neurol. Neurosurg. Psychiatry*, **68**, 381–4.

Rivaud-Pechoux, S., Vidailhet, M., Gallouedec, G., Litvan, I., Gaymard, B. & Pierrot-Deseilligny, C. (2000b). Longitudinal ocular motor study in corticobasal degeneration and progressive supranuclear palsy. *Neurology*, **54**, 1029–32.

Rottach, K.G., von Maydell, R.D., Das, V.E. et al. (1997). Evidence for independent feedback control of horizontal and vertical saccades from Niemann–Pick type C disease. *Vision Res.*, **37**, 3627–38.

Ruskell, G.L. (1999). Extraocular muscle proprioceptors and proprioception. *Prog. Retinal Eye Res.*, **18**, 269–91.

Schiller, P.H., Sandell, J.H. & Maunsell, J.H.R. (1987). The effect of frontal eye field and superior colliculus lesions on saccadic latencies in the rhesus monkey. *J. Neurophysiol.*, **57**, 1033–49.

Scott, A.B. & Collins, C.C. (1973). Division of labor in human extraocular muscle. *Arch. Ophthalmol.*, **90**, 319–22.

Selhorst, J.B., Stark, L., Ochs, A.L. et al. (1976). Disorders in cerebellar ocular motor control. II. Macrosaccadic oscillations: an oculographic control system, and clinico-anatomical analysis. *Brain*, **99**, 509–22.

Shi, D., Friedman, H.R. & Bruce, C.J. (1998). Deficits in smooth-pursuit eye movements after muscimol inactivation within the primate's frontal eye field. *J. Neurophysiol.*, **80**, 458–64.

Spencer, R.F. & Porter, J.D. (1988). Structural organization of the extraocular muscles. In *Reviews of Oculomotor Research*, Vol. 2. *Neuroanatomy of the Oculomotor System*, ed. J.A. Büttner-Ennever, pp. 33–79. Amsterdam: Elsevier.

*Stahl, J.S. & Leigh, R.J. (2001). Nystagmus. Current Neurology and Neuroscience Report.

Starck, M., Albrecht, H., Pollmann, W. et al. (1997). Drug therapy for acquired pendular nystagmus in multiple sclerosis. *J. Neurol.*, **244**, 9–16.

Suziki, Y., Büttner-Ennever, J.A., Straumann, D. et al. (1995). Deficits in torsional and vertical rapid eye movements and shift of Listing's plane after uni- and bilateral lesions of the rostral interstitial nucleus of the medial longitudinal fasciculus. *Exp. Brain Res.*, **106**, 215–32.

Takagi, M., Zee, D.S. & Tamargo, R. (1998). Effects of lesions of the oculomotor vermis on eye movements in primate: saccades. *J. Neurophysiol.*, **80**, 1911–31.

Takagi, M., Zee, D.S. & Tamargo, R. (2000). Effects of lesions of the oculomotor vermis on eye movements in primate: pursuit. *J. Neurophysiol.*, **83**, 2047–62.

Trobe, J.D. (1998). Managing oculomotor nerve palsy. *Arch. Ophthalmol.*, **116**, 798.

Umapathi, T., Koon, S.W., Mukkam, R.P. et al. (2000). Insights into the three-dimensional structure of the oculomotor nuclear complex and fascicles. *J. Neuroophthalmol.*, **20**, 138–44.

Vermersch, A.I., Gaymard, B.M., Rivaud-Pechoux, S., Ploner, C.J., Agid, Y. & Pierrot-Deseilligny, C. (1999). Memory guided saccade deficit after caudate nucleus lesion. *J. Neurol. Neurosurg. Psychiatry*, **66**, 524–7.

Waespe, W., Cohen, B. & Raphan, T. (1985). Dynamic modification of the vestibulo-ocular reflex by nodulus and uvula. *Science*, **228**, 199–202.

*Walker, M.F. & Zee, D.S. (2000). Cerebellar control of gaze. In *Proceedings of the INOS 2000 meeting*, in press.

Wall, M. & Wray, S.H. (1983). The one-and-a-half syndrome: a study of 20 cases and review of the literature. *Neurology*, **33**, 971–80.

Warwick, R. (1953). Representation of the extra-ocular muscles in the oculomotor nuclei of the monkey. *J. Comp. Neurol.*, **98**, 449–503.

Weir, C.R., Knox, P.C. & Dutton, G.N. (2000). Does extraocular muscle proprioception influence oculomotor control? *Br. J. Ophthalmol.*, **84**, 1071–7.

Wiest, G., Deecke, L., Trattnig, S. et al. (1999). Abolished tilt suppression of the vestibulo-ocular reflex caused by a selective uvulo-nodular lesion. *Neurology*, **52**, 417–19.

Wilson, M.E., Eustis, H.S., Jr. & Parks, M.M. (1989). Brown's syndrome. *Surv. Ophthalmol.*, **34**, 153–72.

Yagi, T., Shimizu, M., Sekine, S. et al. (1981). New neurotological test for detecting cerebellar dysfunction. Vestibulo-ocular reflex changes with horizontal vision-reversal prisms. *Ann. Otol. Rhinol. Laryngol.*, **90**, 276–80.

Yakushin, S.B., Gizzi, M., Reisine, H. et al. (2000). Functions of the nucleus of the optic tract (NOT). II. Control of ocular pursuit. *Exp. Brain Res.*, **131**, 433–47.

Yuki, N. (1996). Acute paresis of extraocular muscles associated with IgG anti GQ1b antibody. *Ann. Neurol.*, **39**, 668–72.

Zackon, D.H. & Sharpe, J.A. (1984). Midbrain paresis of horizontal gaze, *Ann. Neurol.*, **16**, 495–504.

Zee, D.S. & Robinson, D.A. (1979). A hypothetical explanation of saccadic oscillations. *Ann. Neurol.*, **5**, 405–14.

Zee, D.S., Yamazaki, A., Butler, P.H. et al. (1981). Effects of the ablation of flocculus and paraflocculus on eye movements in primate. *J. Neurophysiol.*, **46**, 878–99.

45

Disorders of the auditory system

Borka Ceranic and Linda M. Luxon

Neuro-otology Department, The National Hospital for Neurology and Neurosurgery, Queen Square, London, UK

The human auditory system possesses a remarkable ability to evaluate the acoustic environment and to provide the information necessary for normal function and survival. The process of evaluation begins at the periphery, in the ear. In the cochlea, auditory information is frequency analysed, amplified or attenuated, sharply tuned and transformed into electrical neural impulses, which are transmitted and processed in the auditory nerve. In the central auditory system, complex processing of acoustic signals, such as binaural fusion and sound localization, takes place, as well as various perceptual and cognitive processes. The efferent system plays a role in modulation of the auditory information, by balancing the processes of excitation and inhibition. Tonotopic organization, i.e. the anatomical arrangement according to sound frequencies, exists throughout the entire auditory system, and facilitates the maintenance and enhancement of frequency discrimination. The integral parts of the auditory system interact through complex, mainly feedback mechanisms, creating a highly dynamic system, in which abnormal functioning at one level may have functional consequences at other level(s). This functional plasticity in the auditory system is, for instance, reflected in the phenomenon of tonotopic reorganization in the cortex as a result of cochlear damage, and, in the opposite direction, an abnormality in the central auditory system may lead to disinhibition phenomena at the cochlear level. There is a myriad of functional disorders, resulting from pathology in the auditory system, with the loss of hearing sensitivity being the most important. From a neurological point of view, the understanding of auditory dysfunction has considerable importance, as neurological lesions may be associated with damage of auditory pathways. The identification of auditory dysfunction, its relationship to particular anatomical structure(s), and localization of the underlying pathological process, are

subjects of continuing interest to both clinicians and scientists. With advances in science and technology, there has been significant progress in gaining better insight into this fascinating system.

Functional anatomy of the auditory system

Outer and middle ear

The outer ear assists in localizing a sound source and serves to reinforce the resonance of the tympanic membrane.

The middle ear (Fig. 45.1) contains the three interarticulated auditory ossicles, which form an elastic spring, the stiffness of which is controlled by the two middle ear muscles, the stapedius and the tensor tympani. Acoustic stimulation leads to contraction, mainly of the stapedius, reducing the middle ear transmission of sound. The neural network of the stapedial reflex is integrated in the lower brainstem and consists of both ipsilateral and contralateral routes, with the efferent pathway in the facial nerve.

The inner ear – cochlea

The inner ear (Fig. 45.1) consists of the organs of balance and the cochlea. The cochlea is divided longitudinally by the basilar and Reissner's membranes into three chambers: the scala vestibuli, tympani and media. The scala vestibuli and tympani contain perilymph. Via the Sylvian aqueduct, the perilymphatic system communicates with the subarachnoid space of the posterior cranial fossa. The scala media is continuous with the vestibular membranous labyrinth, which contains endolymph. The organ of Corti (Fig. 45.2) contains the auditory sensory receptor, located on the basilar membrane and includes both outer (OHC) and

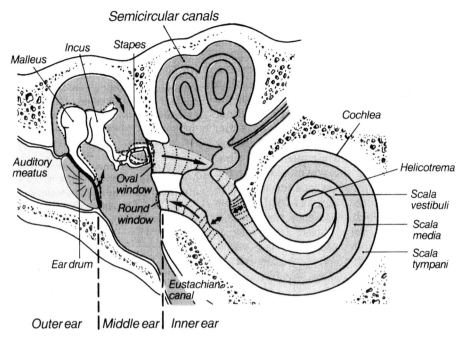

Fig. 45.1. A cross-section of the middle and inner ear. The dotted lines in the middle ear (together with arrows) indicate vibratory movements of the ossicular chain, and the perilymph of the inner ear is driven by sound pressure waves; in the inner ear, longitudinal arrows show the direction of the travelling wave propagation and transverse arrows the site of maximal displacement and vibrations of the scala media. (Adapted from Despopulous & Silbernagl, 1991.)

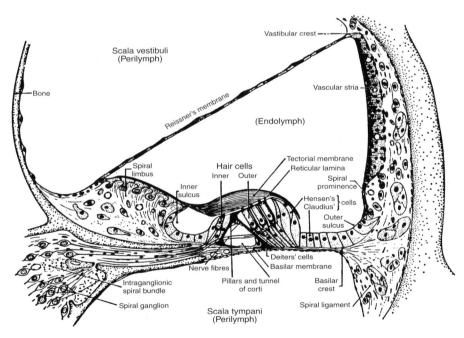

Fig. 45.2. A cross-section of the organ of Corti. (Davis and Associates, 1953.)

Organ of Corti

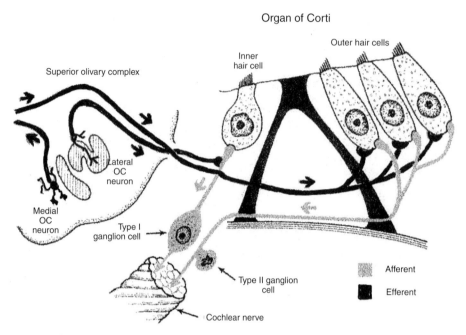

Fig. 45.3. The afferent and efferent innervation of the cochlea. (Schuknecht, 1993.)

inner hair cells (IHC). The OHCs are characterized by the presence of contractile elements, actin–myosin complexes, which are responsible for active mechanical responses in the cochlea.

The vibrations of the stapes footplate in the oval window, induced by sound pressure, cause a passive dynamic displacement of the cochlear partition in the shape of a travelling wave (von Békésy, 1960). As the walls of the endolymphatic duct (scala media) are flexible, the travelling waves are transmitted to the scala tympani, and the wave-like distortion of the endolymphatic duct causes Reissner's membrane and the basilar membrane to swing from one side to the other alternately.

However, the cochlea is not just a passive mechanical signal analyser, but plays an active role in the mechanical processing of sound. The source of active behaviour, as mentioned above, is the OHCs, with their motor capacity for fast oscillating and slow tonic contractions. The fast contractions (Brownell et al., 1985) are phase-locked to the stimulating sound and follow sound-driven passive vibrations of the cochlear partition. They stimulate the actinomyosin network of OHCs, acting to oppose viscous damping in the cochlea and to enhance the oscillations of the cochlear partition. These active oscillations of the OHCs are responsible for the generation of otoacoustic emissions (described below). The slow tonic contractions of OHCs (Zenner, 1986) can alter the stiffness of the cochlear partition in a sharply restricted area, thus modifying

the envelope of the travelling wave. These slow contractions result from the activity of the efferent system.

The OHC fast (a.c.) motility, which amplifies sound (by ≈40 dB, near hearing threshold), is linearly correlated to the intensity of sound. However, with an increase in sound pressure level, the cochlea is capable of correcting undesirable (high) shifts of the basilar membrane by the slow OHC (d.c.) movements, leading to reduction of the passive displacement, and non-linear compression of cochlear dynamics (attenuation). Thus, OHCs act as controlled mechano-amplifiers, and feed mechanical oscillations to the IHCs, which are directly involved in the transformation of mechanical energy into neural activity.

Cochlear innervation

The organ of Corti has efferent and afferent innervation (Fig. 45.3). Efferent fibres (see below Efferent system) originate in the superior olivary complex. The lateral olivocochlear (OC) fibres project to afferent fibres of the IHCs, while the medial OC fibres project directly onto the OHCs. About 90–95% (Spoendlin, 1979) of the afferents originate from the IHCs, while approximately 5–10% of them originate from the OHCs. This means that the acoustic information transferred from the cochlea almost exclusively comes from the IHCs.

In contrast, about 95% of all efferent fibres have direct and wide synaptic contact with the OHC bodies, whilst an almost negligible number of the efferent neurons have indirect postsynaptic contact with IHCs. The afferent fibres form the cochlear nerve, and efferent fibres form the olivo-cochlear bundle, which travels within the vestibular nerve bundle.

Glutamate is the main neurotransmitter of the afferent fibres. Beside its potent excitatory effect, glutamate also displays a highly neurotoxic effect, observed in various pathological conditions, e.g. acoustic trauma (Puel, 1995).

The efferent olivocochlear innervation to the OHCs provides control of the OHCs via predominantly cholinergic fibres (basal OHCs, for high frequencies) and γ-amino-butyric acid (GABA)-ergic fibres (apical OHCs, for low-frequencies).

The distinctly different innervation pattern of the IHCs and OHCs implies specific physiological roles of the dual sensory system in the cochlea: IHCs as the primary sensory cells that generate action potentials in the auditory nerve, and OHCs as the active mechanoreceptors, which are controlled and modulated by the central nervous system.

Retrocochlear afferent auditory system

The auditory nerve

The auditory nerve, together with the vestibular nerve, passes through the internal acoustic meatus. The high frequency fibres lie on the periphery, while mid–low frequency fibres lie more medially in the nerve. This may explain why the high frequencies are often affected initially by an acoustic neuroma. The auditory nerve enters the brainstem at the cerebellopontine angle, behind the cerebellar peduncle. It branches into three major divisions, to the cochlear nuclei (CN) (Fig. 45.4). These three divisions are located on the posterolateral surface of the ponto-medullary junction, so an extra-axial expanding lesion (e.g. from the cerebellopontine angle) may affect the branches or the nuclei causing, respectively, peripheral and central auditory deficits. As the CN receive only ipsilateral input, pathology at this site produces unilateral hearing deficit. The afferents are arranged in the CN according to frequency (tonotopic organization) and various cell types in the CN analyse different aspects of sound. The CN play a fundamental role in the extraction of temporal auditory information (amplitude modulation) from auditory nerve responses and, within these nuclei, lateral inhibition enhances auditory contrast.

The fibres from the CN project ipsi- and contralaterally to the superior olivary complex (SOC), lateral lemniscus (LL) and the nuclei along the LL, and to the reticular formation. Some of the fibres from the CN bypass the SOC and the nuclei of the LL and project directly to the inferior col-

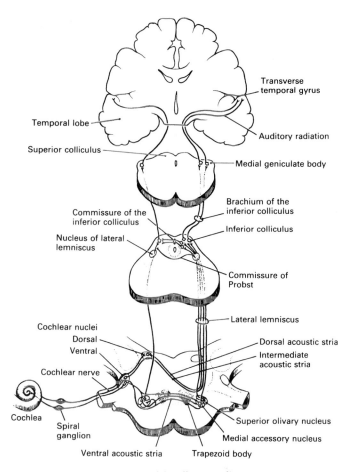

Fig. 45.4. Schematic illustration of the afferent auditory system. (Benjamin & Todd Troust, 1988.)

liculus. Bilateral projections from the CNs to the higher auditory pathways enable the comparison of intensity and travelling time of sound (lateralization).

The superior olivary complex (SOC)

The SOC is composed of several nuclei, including the lateral (LSO) and medial (MSO) nuclei. Both of these structures receive bilateral innervation, and, therefore, provide the anatomical basis for binaural representation and integration of binaurally presented signals (interaural time, phase and intensity difference). A lesion in the SOC may lead to abnormal binaural interaction. However, unilateral disruption of auditory pathways at this level and above, would not lead to a significant hearing loss, due to the crossed, bilateral ascending auditory input.

The lateral lemniscus (LL)

The LL is a major auditory tract containing afferent and efferent fibres. The LL on both sides communicate through the commissure of Probst, or via the pontine reticular formation.

The inferior colliculus (IC)

The IC receives the auditory fibres predominantly crossing from the opposite side. The IC is highly tonotopically organized and is characterized by extremely sharp tuning curves, suggesting a high degree of frequency resolution. Some of the neurons in the IC are time and spatially sensitive, suggesting a role in temporal and spatial resolution, and ultimately, in sound localization coding.

The medial geniculate body (MGB)

The MGB has ventral, dorsal and medial divisions, of which the ventral contains mainly acoustically responsive cells, while the other divisions are sensitive to both sensory and acoustic stimulation. The MGB is also tonotopically organized and is thought to play a role in the analysis of both binaural stimuli and inter-aural intensity differences. At this level, the processing of natural speech is thought to begin.

From the MGB, there are multiple and complex thalamocortical projections upon the tonotopically organized cortical fields. The major thalamo-cortical pathway, consisting mainly of auditory fibres, originates from the ventral MGB and projects to the primary auditory cortical area in Heschl's gyrus. Another thalamo-cortical pathway, containing in addition to auditory, somatic and, possibly, visual fibres, runs towards the external capsule, and from there to the insula.

The auditory cortical area

The auditory cortical area encompasses the posterior three-quarters of the Sylvian fissure, including the superior temporal lobe, the inferior–posterior frontal lobe and the inferior parietal lobe. Heschl's gyrus is considered the primary auditory cortical area, which receives most of the thalamocortical projections and is tonotopically organized, suggesting that most of the auditory information is processed initially in this area. The secondary auditory cortical areas include the planum temporale, which is significantly longer on the left than on the right side and is located approximately in Wernicke's area, suggesting involvement in receptive language function (left hemisphere is dominant for speech) (Musiek, 1986). Other acoustically responsive areas are the supramarginal gyrus and the insula. The inferior part of the parietal and frontal lobes and the claustrum are also responsive to acoustic stimulation.

The primary auditory area has intra- and interhemispheric connections to different parts of the brain. The auditory cortical areas also have connections to the frontal lobe, including the arcuate fasciculus, which connects Wernicke's and Broca's areas. These connections enable activation of different specialized secondary areas, depending on the complexity of the auditory signals. The secondary, association, areas for hearing are responsible for a variety of complex auditory processing, including the analysis of complex sounds (e.g. noise, music or speech decoding); short-term memory for comparison of tones; inhibition of unwanted motor responses and for intent listening. Lesions of these areas in the dominant hemisphere may lead to a specific loss of function (e.g. sensory aphasia in a lesion of the left hemisphere).

The corpus callosum (CC) contains inter-hemispheric auditory fibres, which connect the cortices of each hemisphere, predominantly homolaterally. The auditory segment of the CC is confined to the posterior half. This is supported by the findings on central auditory tests in patients with section of the posterior part of the CC (Musiek, 1986). The results of animal research indicate the presence of excitatory and inhibitory fibres, suggesting a role of the CC in modulating the activity in both hemispheres, allowing optimal integration of cortical responses. This may be of particular importance for those processes, in which one hemisphere may be dominant, e.g. left hemisphere is dominant for language and sequencing of auditory stimuli, while the right is dominant for spatial auditory perception and the perception of music.

Efferent system

The efferent system runs in parallel to the afferent system, from the cortex to the cochlea, but it is less well defined than the afferent auditory system. It is thought that there is a pathway from the cortex to the MGB and another from the cortex to the various nuclei in the brainstem. The IC receives input from both the cortex and the MGB. From the IC, there are efferent connections to the SOC system and the CN, and to the nuclei of the LL.

The best known part of the efferent system is the olivo-cochlear (OC) system (Fig. 45.3), arising from the SOC. Fibres from the lateral SO nucleus are arranged in the predominantly uncrossed, lateral olivo-cochlear bundle (LOCB) which projects to afferent fibres of the IHC (see above). The fibres from the medial nucleus are arranged in the mainly crossed, medial olivo-cochlear bundle (MOCB) and project directly onto the OHC. During this course, the MOCB runs in the floor of the fourth ventricle.

The medial efferent olivo-cochlear (MOC) system is considered to be inhibitory (Wiederhold, 1986) and responsible for the control of the OHC motility. It also appears to be responsible for automatic gain control, adaptation and homeostasis of the cochlea. Anatomical and physiological studies of the IC connections with the SOC system strongly suggest that the IC plays a role in the activity of the OC system.

However, very little is known about the lateral olivo-cochlear system. It is believed that it modulates sensitivity of the afferent receptors and may have a protective role against excessive noise and/or excitotoxicity (Pujol, 1994; Sahly et al., 1999).

The efferent auditory system with its multisynaptic connections from the cortex to the cochlea suggests the presence of an efficient feedback mechanism, providing a balance between excitatory and inhibitory stimuli. Its assumed role is to facilitate and enhance the targeted acoustic signal and to inhibit unwanted signal, such as noise. It also mediates frequency-selective auditory attention.

Extra-auditory neural connections

The auditory pathways have connections with other parts of the central nervous system.

The reticular formation

A serotoninergic input to the lower brainstem area may provide a basis for modulation of the olivocochlear and middle ear (stapedial and tensor tympani) reflexes (Thompson & Thompson, 1995).

The somatosensory system

The medial division of the MGB (a multisensory thalamic area) probably plays the most important role in the phylogenetically 'old' connection between the auditory and somatosensory systems. Connections with the somatosensory system are also possible via the *extralemniscal system*, which branches off from the classical ascending lemniscal auditory system at the level of the IC and projects to the association cortices (prefrontal area, limbic portions, temporal, parietal and occipital areas) rather than to the primary auditory cortex (Graybiel, 1972). Neurons of the extralemniscal system respond much less specifically to sound stimulation than neurons in the lemniscal system and receive input, not only from the auditory, but also from the somatosensory system. Therefore, somatosensory stimulation, in addition to auditory stimulation, may lead to the perception of sound (e.g. electrical stimulation of the median nerve in some individuals may lead to the perception of tinnitus: Møller et al., 1992).

Another important relay in the polysensory system is the superior colliculus, which includes maps of visual and tactile receptive fields, aligned with the auditory map, and which, in part, therefore, coordinates auditory, visual and somatic information (Huffman & Henson, 1990).

The hypothalamus
The hypothalamus provides input to the auditory pathway via the IC (Adams, 1980).

The limbic system
The limbic system receives projections from the MGB and this link is hypothesized to serve in the attachment of emotional significance to acoustic stimuli (LeDoux et al., 1983).

The cerebellum
The cerebellum is linked to the auditory system probably via the cochlear nuclei (Gacek, 1973), allowing adjustment in the position of the body and the head to the location of sound. The descending acousticomotor system (Huffman & Henson, 1990) involves acousticomotor centres in the cerebellum, the superior colliculus and the medial nucleus of the MGB, which receive projections from the external nucleus (multisensory nucleus) of the inferior colliculus, allowing multisensory integration.

Functional correlates of the pathology in the auditory system

Abnormalities at different levels of the auditory system may have different functional consequences. The most important is hearing loss, which may be associated with other dysfunctions, including loudness recruitment, abnormal auditory adaptation, tinnitus and/or hyperacusis. Other auditory attributes, such as those related to frequency selectivity, temporal resolution (detection of a gap between two stimuli), pitch perception, sound localization, auditory pattern perception, speech perception, or those related to other complex processing of the auditory information are beyond the scope of this brief description.

Hearing loss

Peripheral hearing loss results from abnormalities of the external/ middle ear, cochlea and auditory nerve, up to the entry into the brainstem, beyond which, central hearing impairment occurs. Hearing loss may be divided into two types: conductive and sensorineural. Conductive hearing loss is consequent upon occlusion of the external ear canal, or secondary to pathology of the middle ear and indicates inadequate transmission of sound from the environment to the inner ear. Sensorineural hearing impairment results

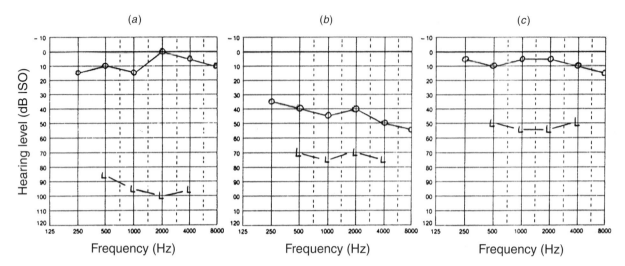

Fig. 45.5. Examples of cochlear dynamic range: in normal subjects (*a*), in cochlear lesion with loudness recruitment (*b*) and narrow dynamic range in hyperacusis (*c*).

most commonly from pathology in the cochlea, less commonly from the auditory nerve, and rarely from a central auditory abnormality.

It is of clinical importance to distinguish conductive from sensorineural hearing loss; sensorineural hearing loss of cochlear origin from that of retrocochlear origin; sensorineural hearing loss resulting from pathology of the VIIIth nerve, from that due to brainstem pathology and higher auditory pathways. The distinction may be extremely difficult if pathology involves both sensory and neural structures.

Loudness recruitment

Loudness recruitment can be defined as an abnormal growth of loudness as a function of suprathreshold sound intensity. This phenomenon is associated with cochlear lesions, in particular OHC damage, although it has been reported in patients with brainstem lesions (Dix & Hood, 1973). One of possible explanations of loudness recruitment is the loss of non-linearity in response to sound as a function of the intensity. In the cochlea, the source of non-linearity are the OHC (as explained in the section on Functional anatomy), which are responsible for the enhancement of sensitivity of signals at low intensity, while responses at high sound levels display saturation. Therefore, patients with extensive OHC lesion, have reduced hearing sensitivity at low sound levels, while with increasing sound intensity, the growth of loudness is passive and linear. An analogous explanation for the presence of loudness recruitment in brainstem lesions could be offered, which may arise due to

the damage of neural fibres/nuclei, which are responsible for non-linear intensity coding.

Patients with this type of abnormality complain that loud sounds (e.g. >70 dB) are uncomfortable and even painful. Loudness discomfort levels (LDL) represent the lowest intensity of sound which the individual finds uncomfortably loud, and in normal subjects is in the range 95–115 dB hearing level (Fig. 45.5(a)). In cochlear pathology, the dynamic range is reduced (Fig, 45.5(b)).

Tone decay (or abnormal auditory adaptation)

This phenomenon refers to a very rapid decrease in neuronal responses, while the response to the onset of a sound may be normal or near normal. A reduction of the number of normally functioning auditory nerve fibres has been proposed as one explanation of this phenomenon. It manifests by the loss of sensitivity to a continuous tone (but normal sensitivity to an interrupted tone) in the affected ear, while hearing sensitivity in the unaffected ear persists as long as the stimulation.

Hyperacusis

Hyperacusis can be defined as an abnormal growth in loudness but, unlike loudness recruitment, patients complain of loud perception of ordinary environmental sounds. In the majority of cases it is associated with normal hearing. It is assumed that hyperacusis results from raised spontaneous auditory activity and is considered by some authors to be a condition preceding tinnitus. One of the hypotheses for the underlying mechanism is disinhibition of efferent feedback auditory control, leading to an increased gain in auditory function. This hypothesis may explain hyperacusis which has been reported in facial/Bell's palsy and in the Ramsay–Hunt syndrome. In these cases, the stapedial reflex, which normally reduces acoustic input, is affected. Hyperacusis is judged clinically by measuring loudness discomfort levels (LDL) which are considerably lower in patients with hyperacusis than in normal subjects (Fig. 45.5(c)).

Tinnitus

Tinnitus is an auditory perception in the absence of external stimulation and it has been assumed that it results from an altered state of excitation and/or inhibition within the auditory system. Aberrant activity, which may be caused by different pathologies and at different levels of the auditory system, may interact with psychological factors, such as stress or depression.

Tinnitus is a subjective phenomenon and so far there has been no convincing objective evidence for tinnitus-related activity. However, the recent emergence of functional imaging techniques has provided new insight into the generation of this symptom. Single-proton emission computed tomography (SPECT), positron-emission tomogaphy (PET) and functional magnetic resonance imaging (fMRI) have demonstrated that more auditory cortical areas are activated in patients with tinnitus than in controls subjects, including the medial temporal lobe and the limbic areas (Shulman et al., 1995; Lockwood et al., 1998, 1999; Levine, 1999). The extent of the neuronal network involved is thought to influence the quality and attributes of tinnitus (e.g. a link to the limbic system may explain the emotional response to tinnitus).

Undoubtedly, functional imaging techniques have pushed forward the frontiers in research on tinnitus, supporting some of the hypotheses and providing new information on spatial aspects of tinnitus-related processing. However, temporal aspects of neural activity which may underlie tinnitus generation remain poorly understood.

Several pathophysiological mechanisms for the generation of tinnitus may be considered:

Abnormal afferent excitation at the cochlear level

- Spontaneous cochlear (OHC) activity, identified by the recording of spontaneous otoacoustic emissions, could be a cause of tinnitus in a small number ($\approx$4%) of patients (for review see Ceranic et al., 1995).
- Glutamate neuro-excito-otoxicity, e.g. in exposure to excessive noise (Pujol, 1994).
- Modulation (enhanced sensitivity) of NMDA and non-

NMDA receptors by endogenous opioid peptides dynorphins, released onto the IHC synaptic region by the lateral olivocochlear fibres, as a part of the response to stress (Sahly et al., 1999).

Efferent dysfunction/reduction of GABA effect

Several studies have suggested dysfunction (a reduction in the suppressive effect) of the medial olivocochlear system, and furthermore, a global efferent dysfunction (Attias & Bresloff, 1998), as the underlying mechanisms to tinnitus.

It has also been suggested that general age-related reduction of GABA may contribute to the development of tinnitus in the elderly.

Abnormal auditory activation

- Irritative lesions (e.g. tumours, Espir et al., 1997; Milicic & Alçada, 1999)
- Activation of the auditory system through the activation of other motor/sensory systems, e.g. visual, such as that occurring in a gaze-evoked tinnitus, or tinnitus provoked by jaw clenching (Lockwood et al., 1999); tinnitus evoked by electrical stimulation of the median nerve (Møller et al., 1992). There are also patients who have developed gaze-evoked tinnitus after surgical removal of an acoustic neuroma (Cacace et al., 1994).

Alteration of spontaneous activity due to tonotopic reorganization

Peripheral lesions/dysfunctions, with sound deprivation or overstimulation, result in plastic transformations within the brain (Møller, 2000). The findings from electrophysiological studies and functional imaging (PET, fMRI) of expansion of the brain regions responsive to tones, provide strong evidence for plastic transformation of the brain in these patients. Similar observations have been made in experimental animals after damage to the cochlea (Recanzone et al., 1993). The area in the auditory cortex deprived of its characteristic frequency acquires a new characteristic frequency, which corresponds to that at the edge of the region of cochlear damage, leading to an expansion of cortical representation of a restricted frequency band adjacent to the region of cochlear loss (Robertson & Irvine, 1989). These data suggest that tinnitus may be due to altered spontaneous activity in the CNS due to aberrant neural pathways formed during plastic transformation of the brain.

Stress-related neuro-humoral activity

Circumstantial evidence exists that stress is of relevance in the generation of tinnitus, particularly in individuals with negative psychological conditions, or individuals with psychiatric disturbances. Stress may activate various

biological functions, including the sympathetic adrenal medullary system, with secretion of catecholamines, and the hypothalamic pituitary–adrenocortical system, with the secretion of glucocorticoids (e.g. Cortisol). Failure in homeostasis may lead to abnormal functioning of the auditory system, including the emergence of tinnitus.

Investigation

In addition to the assessment of auditory function, it is important to test vestibular function, in view of the common pathology which may occur at the labyrinthine (Fig. 45.1) and vestibulocochlear nerve levels. There is also the possibility of an abnormality in the acoustico-motor centres in the cerebellum, which reflects in concurrent central auditory and vestibular manifestations (Shulman & Strashun, 1999).

A detailed otoscopic examination is essential in the investigation of hearing disorder and the most relevant tests which serve to define auditory dysfunction are described.

Tuning fork tests

These are simple tests to differentiate conductive from sensorineural hearing loss: the Rinne test identifies a conductive component to hearing loss and the Weber test may detect asymmetrical sensorineural hearing loss, or lateralize a conductive loss.

Pure-tone audiometry

This is a routine clinical technique to determine hearing threshold levels for pure-tone stimuli. In conductive hearing loss the audiogram indicates an air–bone gap, as bone conduction is normal, while cochlear/retrocochlear lesions produce sensorineural hearing impairment, with similar deficits in both air and bone conduction (Fig. 45.6).

Tympanometry

Tympanometry assesses the mechanical properties of the middle ear: the ear drum compliance and the pressure in the middle ear. This test complements the identification of middle ear disorders.

Stapedial reflex

Unilateral acoustic stimulation leads to contraction of the stapedial muscle bilaterally (Fig. 45.7), thus increasing the resistance to the sound transmission through the middle ear, by up to 15 dB.

Acoustic reflex thresholds are measured in response to ipsi- and contralateral tones. They are elevated/absent in conductive and retrocochlear hearing loss. Depending on the site of a lesion and the part of the reflex arc involved, different, characteristic patterns of ipsi- and contra-lateral reflexes can be observed (Fig. 45.8).

Decay of the stapedial reflex reflects abnormal transmission of acoustic signal through the auditory nerve, by the inability to sustain the reflex over a certain period of time. Decay is, therefore, indicative of a neural (e.g. in acoustic neuroma), or a brainstem lesion.

Speech audiometry

The speech discrimination score is affected by the site of a lesion. In the case of cochlear hearing loss, the discrimination score parallels to the hearing loss and can be restored by increasing the intensity of sound. However, in the case of neural hearing loss, there is disproportionally worse speech discrimination than would be expected considering the pure-tone audiometric thresholds.

Otoacoustic emissions

Otoacoustic emissions (OAEs) are weak signals that can be recorded in the sealed ear canal and are considered to reflect cochlear, OHC activity (Kemp, 1978).

All OAEs can be divided in two classes: spontaneous and evoked. Spontaneous otoacoustic emissions are continuous narrow-band signals emitted by the cochlea in the absence of any stimulation. Evoked otoacoustic emissions are recorded following stimulation by different stimuli: transient evoked otoacoustic emissions (TEOAEs), evoked by transient impulses, or distortion product otoacoustic emissions (DPOAEs), evoked by two continuous tones at closely spaced frequencies. TEOAEs can be recorded in almost all normal subjects (Fig. 45.9). DPOAEs have similar characteristics as TEOAEs, however, they provide more frequency specific responses.

OAEs are applied in the evaluation of cochlear function and are particularly valuable in difficult-to-test subjects (e.g. children, or mentally retarded patients). They can also be used in the differential diagnosis of cochlear and retrocochlear lesions: if TEOAEs are recorded in subjects with a moderate or severe sensorineural hearing loss, this would strongly suggest a retrocochlear lesion.

It is important to note that OAE application is limited to those subjects with normal middle ear function, as a middle ear abnormality may alter the transfer of acoustic signals to the cochlea.

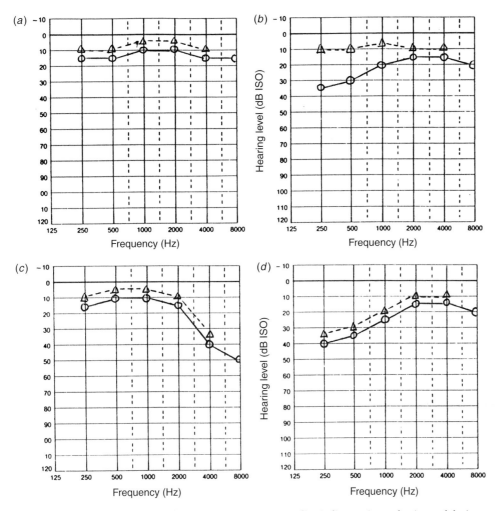

Fig. 45.6. Standard pure-tone audiogram, where the continuous line indicates air-conduction and the interrupted line indicates bone-conduction hearing threshold levels: (*a*) normal, (*b*) conductive, (*c*) sensorineural high-frequency sloping and (*d*) sensorineural low-frequency hearing loss.

Olivocochlear suppression test

This is an emerging technique for exploring the medial olivo-cochlear system, or so-called phenomenon of 'reciprocal cochlear interaction', in which acoustic stimulation of one ear suppresses TEOAEs in the opposite ear. The MOC suppression test provides general information on the structural integrity of the medial olivo-cochlear reflex arc, and a glimpse into the modulation of cochlear mechanics by efferent stimulation.

Electrophysiological testing

Electrocochleography (ECochG)

Three groups of ECochG potentials can be recorded: the cochlear microphonic, the summating potential, both thought to derive from mainly OHC activity, and the compound action potential, the synchronized activity of the auditory fibres, in response to stimulus onset.

ECochG is mainly used for the evaluation of cochlear function, e.g. in Menière's disease (the pathophysiological rationale is that deflection of the cochlear basilar membrane, consequent upon hydrops, creates an enlarged negative summation potential).

The auditory brainstem response (ABR)

The ABR is thought to be generated within the auditory pathway up to the inferior colliculus (Fig. 45.10). The ABR is particularly useful for the detection of acoustic neurinoma (typically prolonged wave V latency on the affected side) and is very sensitive in intra-axial brainstem lesions. The ABR is also used for objective threshold estimation,

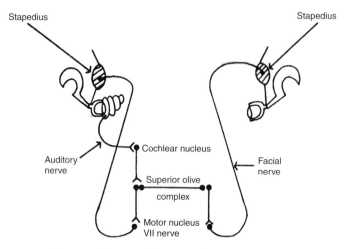

Fig. 45.7. Schematic illustration of main components of the ipsilateral and contralateral acoustic reflex. (Luxon & Cohen, 1997.)

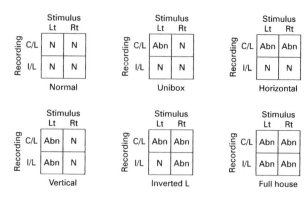

Fig. 45.8. Patterns of acoustic reflex thresholds and common interpretations (Lt-left, Rt-right, C/L-contralateral, I/L-ipsilateral): Unibox = small unilateral brain lesion medial to the cochlear nucleus; Horizontal = midline brainstem lesion; Vertical = left VIIIth nerve lesion; Inverted L = intra-axial brainstem lesion plus extension to the cochlear nucleus or VIIIth nerve on the affected side (a conductive lesion may present in this way); Full house = a midline brainstem lesion with extension to involve the cochlear nuclei and/or VIIIth nerves (N.B. bilateral conductive lesion needs exclusion); Abn = abnormal; N = normal. (Luxon & Cohen, 1997.)

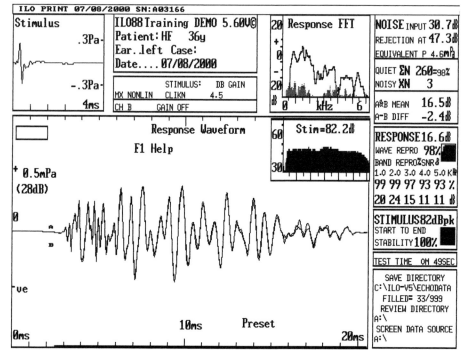

Fig. 45.9. Transient evoked otoacoustic emissions recorded following non-linear click stimulation (82.2 dBSPL) from a normal subject; in the response window (the largest box, denoted as Response Waveform), the waveforms (A and B), resulting from the signals averaged in two separate buffers, show a very high (98%) correlation (A and B almost completely overlap), suggesting a very good cochlear response; response signals are also analysed in frequency domain (Fast Fourier Transforms – FFT), shown above right; the overall response amplitude is automatically displayed, in this case 16.6 dBSPL, shown in the middle right box.

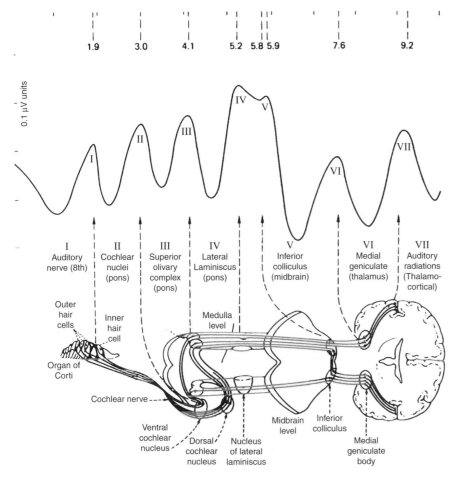

Fig. 45.10. Diagram of the anatomical correlates of the waves observed in the brainstem responses. (Duane, 1977.)

and the resistance to drug effects and general anesthesia make this technique suitable for objective evaluation of hearing thresholds in children.

Middle latency response (MLR)

The temporal lobe or thalamocortical projections are important for generation of the MLR, although it is most likely that multiple generators exist. Evaluation of the MLR is used for assessing the integrity of the central nervous system beyond the brainstem and for threshold estimation of low-frequency hearing sensitivity, as it is less dependent on neural synchrony than ABR. However, it is sensitive to the state of consciousness.

Auditory cortical responses (ACRs)

The ACRs originate mainly from the auditory cortical areas in the temporal lobe. They are generally elicited with a tone burst and, therefore, provide frequency specific responses, which are well correlated with subjective pure-tone thresh-olds. The ACRs are mainly used for objective threshold estimation, particularly in medico-legal cases, and are only applicable in alert subjects.

Event-related potentials (ERPs)

Unlike other auditory evoked responses, the ERPs are considered to be endogenous potentials, resulting from cognitive processing of sensory information. The temporal lobe and limbic structures, including hippocampus and amygdala, have been implicated as the major sources for the ERP.

The Mismatch negativity (MMN) is a component of the ERPs, generated by a change-discrimination process that mainly occurs in the auditory cortex. The MMN is attention-independent and can be obtained even from uncooperative individuals. In auditory pathology, the MMN might be useful in objective evaluation of cochlear implant function and for objective diagnosis of aphasic patients, dysphasic children and of children with auditory-based learning disabilities (Näätänen, 1995).

Central behavioural testing

Central behavioural tests (CBT) are applied in conjunction with electrophysiological tests and imaging techniques to define and localize an abnormality within the central auditory pathways. One of the limitations of these tests is that the assessment of central structures may be affected by peripheral abnormalities. In addition, due to the parallel organization within the central nervous system and involvement of several structures in a particular function, results may not provide information on the localization of a lesion. Another important consideration in CBT is the availability of adequate normative data.

CBT can be classified according to a common parameter, such as mode of presentation (e.g. monaural or binaural), or type of stimuli used (e.g. tones or speech), as outlined in Table 45.1 (Luxon & Cohen, 1997).

In the construction of the test battery, specific auditory tasks are used to assess specific auditory functions of a particular anatomical structure. For example, in the brainstem, binaural acoustic integration, the extraction of signals from background noise and sound localization occur, and, therefore, assessment of these functions is targeted. Cortical and hemispheric pathology produces subtle auditory dysfunctions which may not be correlated to a specific anatomical location. The classic findings of CBT are functional deficits in the ear contralateral to cortical and hemispheric pathology on dichotic testing.

Functional imaging techniques

Functional magnetic resonance imaging (fMRI) of auditory cortical activity

It has been observed that passive and active speech listening generate greater activation of the left than the right hemispheres and this is thought to be related to the left hemisphere specialization for processing spectral changes (Hall et al., 2000) (Fig. 45.11, see colour plate section).

Positron emission tomography (PET)

Studies on functional organization within the auditory cortex support the view of the existence of a hierarchy in functioning of the cortical areas. For example, simple auditory stimuli activate predominantly the contralateral primary cortical area 41, stimuli with interrupted pattern activate bilateral area 42, and stimuli with complex spectral, intensity and temporal structure, such as speech or music, activate more extensive association auditory areas (Mirz et al., 1999).

Table 45.1. Behavioural tests of central auditory processing

A. Monoaural tests
- Degraded speech (filtered speech, interrupted speech, or compressed speech)
- Masked speech (speech-in-noise)
- Synthetic sentence identification with ipsilateral competing message (SSI–ICM)

B. Binaural interaction tests
- Congruent
    Dichotic digit
    Dichotic word
    Dichotic sentence identification
    Nonsense syllables
- Non-congruent
    Binaural fusion
    Rapid alternating speech
    Interaural intensity difference
    Masking level difference (MLD)
    Interaural timing

C. Binaural separation
- Competing sentences
- Threshold of interference

D. Sequencing tasks
- Pitch pattern
- Duration pattern
- Intensity pattern
- Psychoacoustic pattern discrimination

Etio-pathogenesis of hearing disorders

External/middle ear

The pathology at this level may sometimes affect the more proximal auditory pathway. A severe form of otitis externa (*Pseudomonas aeruginosa*), may spread through the adjacent structures and affect the auditory nerve. The middle ear disease can expand towards the apex of petrous bone (petrositis), affecting the abducens nerve and trigeminal ganglion, with the presentation of Gradenigo's syndrome: otitis media, VIth nerve palsy and trigeminal neuralgia. Involvement of the auditory nerve may lead to hearing loss on that side.

Inner ear (cochlea)

Cochlear lesions can be acquired due to various noxious factors, such as ischemia, hypoxia, trauma, excessive

Table 45.2. Causes of auditory disorders

Congenital and hereditary lesions associated with hearing loss
May be a part of many syndromes (Table 45.3)
- *Failure in normal development*
  Michel defect – complete inner ear aplasia
  Mondini defect – incomplete development of the labyrinth
  Scheibe defect – membranous cochleosaccular dyplasia
- *Secondary degeneration* – isolated auditory defect or in
  association with other abnormalities (e.g. Arnold–Chiari);
  Syndromes of inherited spinal degenerations, ataxia and
  neuropathies (e.g. Friedreich's ataxia)

Trauma and toxicity
- mechanical (transverse fracture of the temporal bone,
  concussion of the inner ear with secondary degeneration)
- barotrauma
- surgical intervention
- radiotherapy
- ototoxicity (salicylates, aminoglycosides, thalidomide,
  vincristine)
- acoustic trauma

Infection:
- microbial (syphilis, Lyme disease, meningitis, postchronic
  suppurative otitis media)
- viral (AIDS, Ramsay–Hunt syndrome)
- mycotic

Ischemia:
- vertebrobasilar ischemia
- arterial occlusion (subclavian steal syndrome)
- aneurysm (anterior inferior cerebellar artery)
- stroke
- vasculitis
- polycythemia (emboli)
- coagulopathies (hereditary coagulation disorders, sickle cells)
Risk factors: cardiovascular disease, hypertension,
cardiopulmonary bypass surgery

Neoplasia:
- vestibular schwannoma (syn. acoustic neuroma)
- primary and secondary lesions

Metabolic and endocrine disorders:
- diabetes mellitus
- uremic polyneuropathy
- thyroid dysfunctions

Autoimmune disorders/vasculitis
rheumatoid arthritis, Cogan syndrome, systemic lupus
erythematosus, Takayasu disease, Behçet syndrome,
polyarteritis nodosa

Table 45.3. Genetic syndromes associated with hearing
loss

I. Chromosomal: Down syndrome (trisomy 21), Turner syndrome
(X Ch)

II. Autosomal:

Autosomal dominant	*Autosomal recessive*
– Waardenburg	– Usher progressive hearing loss
Type 1 (Ch 2q)	Type 1 (Ch 14q)
Type 2 (Ch 3q)	Type 2 (Ch 1q)
– Neurofibromatosis	Type 3 (Ch 3q)
Type 1 (Ch 17q)	– Pendred (Ch 7q)
Type 2 (Ch 22q)	– Albinism
– BOR syndrome (Ch 8q)	
– Klippel–Feil	
– Wildervanks	
– Treacher-Collins (Ch 5q)	
– Jervell Lange Neilsen syndrome (Ch 7q 11p)	
– Stickler syndrome (Ch 12q)	
– Crouzon syndrome (Ch 10q25–26)	
– Otosclerosis (multifactorial)	

III. X-linked:	*IV. Mitochondrial*
– Alport syndrome (Xq21–22)	– Kearns–Sayre
– Norrie syndrome (Xp11–3)	– Myoclonic epilepsy
– Perilymph gusher syndrome (Xq13)	– Maternally inherited diabetes
– Encephalopathy-hearing loss (Xq22)	– Maternally inherited susceptibility to aminoglycosides
– Large vestibular aqueduct syndrome	
– X-linked non-syndromic deafness	– MELAS

noise, ototoxic drugs (salicylates, aminoglycosides, thalidomide *cis*-platinum, or vincristine), due to age-related degeneration (presbyacusis), autoimmune disorders, or may result from a number congenital/ hereditary abnormalities (Tables 45.2, 45.3 and 45.4).

The molecular and biological mechanisms of ototoxic effects and other forms of cochlear damage, have been the subject of extensive scientific investigation over recent years. Formation of reactive oxygen metabolites (ROM), including free oxygen radicals and other metabolites, are thought to be central to damage of cochlear tissue, as these highly reactive compounds can oxidize a wide variety of targets, such as proteins, mitochondrial DNA (mtDNA), or lipids. Better understanding of these mechanisms has led to a series of experimental studies with coadministration of antioxidants, or ROM scavengers. For example, use of iron chelators was found to reduce gentamicin ototoxicity (Schacht, 1998), and calorie restriction, vitamin C and E

Table 45.4. Causes of hearing loss arising from dysfunctional neurological tissue

Inner ear:	Degeneration of the spiral ganglion cells (inherited – in Roussy–Levy syndrome)
	Neurinoma of the spiral ganglion
Auditory nerve:	Hereditary neuropathies
	Friedreich's ataxia, Charcot–Marie–Tooth and other hereditary motor-sensory neuropathies, Leber's optic neuropathy
	Auditory neuropathies associated with DIDMOAD, MELAS and other mitochondrial disorders
	Idiopathic auditory neuropathy
	Tumours: Acoustic neurinoma (incl. NF1 and NF2)
	Cerebello-pontine angle lesions
	Metastatic tumours
	Paraneoplastic syndromes
	Infections: Ramsay–Hunt syndrome
	Basal meningitis (bacterial, TB)
	Vascular: Loop, aneurysm
	Malformations: Arnold–Chiari
	Multiple sclerosis (n. root entry zone)
	Trauma (including radiation therapy)
Central nervous system:	
	Tumours: primary and metastatic
	Vascular: Infarct, hemorrhage
	Infections: Encephalitis
	Neurosyphilis
	Lyme disease
	Multiple sclerosis
	Syringo-bulbia
	Neuro-sarcoid
	Neuro-Behçet
	Trauma

supplementation, and melatonin treatment, attenuated age-related hearing loss (Seidman, 2000). These findings herald an exciting future, with potential identification of pharmacological and nutritional strategies for prevention of ototoxicity and different forms of cochlear degeneration.

Cochlear damage is reflected in degeneration and abnormal function of the proximal auditory structures. Loss of hair cells leads to degeneration of the auditory fibres, while efferent fibres remain intact. Neuronal and transneuronal degeneration of auditory axons in the brainstem of an adult mammal, resulting from cochlear damage, has been observed (Morest et al., 1997). Recordings of the spontaneous activity of the auditory nerve have shown a reduction in rate (Liberman & Kiang, 1978) and single fibre recordings have indicated that auditory sensitivity is lost and fre-

quency resolution reduced (Pickles, 1988). However, cochlear lesions lead to an increased excitability of the cochlear nucleus, inferior colliculus (Salvi & Ahroon, 1983) and medial geniculate body (Gerken, 1979). Studies of the auditory cortical neurons have indicated changes in frequency selectivity and a sequence of changes in the relative levels of excitatory and inhibitory inputs to the primary cortical neurons. This leads to an expansion of the receptive field of the cortical neurons (Rajan et al., 1992), which in turn raises the threshold sensitivity and broadens frequency selectivity.

Menière's disease, a condition with both cochlear and vestibular manifestations, deserves special mention. It is considered that endolymphatic hydrops is the underlying pathophysiological abnormality, although it has been suspected that some other mechanisms may be involved, with endolymphatic hydrops being an epiphenomenon. In the absence of known etiology, the diagnosis of Menière's disease is based on the characteristic clinical history, with the classical triad of episodic symptoms of tinnitus, diminished hearing and vertigo, a documented sensorineural shift on pure-tone audiometry and/or reduced speech discrimination score test, as defined by the Committee on Hearing and Equilibrium, American Academy of Ophthalmology and Otolaryngology (1995). Fluctuating sensorineural hearing loss in Menière's disease, typically affects predominantly low frequencies, as in Fig. 45.6(*d*).

Auditory nerve

Different lesions of the auditory nerve, such as trauma, infection (microbial, viral and mycotic), neoplasia (acoustic neuroma, primary and metastatic tumours in the internal acoustic meatus), autoimmune, or congenital/ hereditary disorders (Tables 45.2, 45.3 and 45.4), lead to unilateral neural loss. An example of mononeuritis of the eight nerve is the Ramsay–Hunt syndrome (Herpes zoster oticus), with a deep burning pain in the affected ear, followed by a vesicular eruption in the external auditory canal and concha, and subsequent hearing loss and vertigo. The auditory nerve can also be damaged due to pathological processes in the temporal bone, such as otosclerosis, Paget disease, fibrous displasia, or osteopetroses. With regard to congenital abnormalities, in addition to primary abnormalities (i.e. failure in normal development), secondary lesions may occur. Secondary degeneration of the auditory nerve has been reported in association with other defects in many syndromes (e.g. neurofibromatosis, Treacher-Collins, Wildervank, Usher, Kearns-Sayre, Waardenburg, Pendred, Alport) (Yeoh, 1997). In Arnold–Chiari malformation, it is thought that invagination of the brainstem leads to the stretching of the auditory nerve and to auditory symptoms, which could be caused by cochlear anoxia, while associated increased intracranial pressure may be responsible for pulsatile tinnitus. Degeneration of the auditory nerve is also associated with various inherited spinal degenerations, ataxia and neuropathies (Friedreich's ataxia, hereditary sensory neuropathy) and as an isolated phenomenon (Booth, 1997).

Acoustic neuroma (AN) has been reported to represent 10% of intracranial tumours and over 95% of cerebellopontine lesions (Gonzalez-Revilla, 1948). In addition to the effect on the auditory nerve, AN may cause cochlear degeneration due to chronic partial obstruction of the blood supply by the tumour, biochemical alterations in the inner ear fluids, loss of efferent control of active mechanical tuning and degeneration due to neuronal loss (Prasher et al., 1995). Analysis of 500 patients who underwent AN resection, revealed that unilateral auditory symptoms occur in 83% of patients and that tinnitus was the initial symptom in 11% of patients (Ramsden, 1987), while in a study on 1000 patients, it was found that acoustic disturbances occur in 95% of patients (Matthies & Samii, 1997). The prevalence of tinnitus is higher in patients with a partial hearing loss than in deaf patients, however, postoperative deafness does not mean relief from tinnitus: this symptom may exist in 46% of postoperatively deaf patients (Matthies & Samii, 1997), suggesting that, although the onset of tinnitus may be due to the peripheral effect, its maintenance is mediated through the more proximal, central mechanisms.

Multiple sclerosis may occasionally affect the central auditory system, and even less commonly the auditory nerve. Auditory symptoms have been reported in less than 4% of patients, they are usually unilateral and, in most cases, are of transient character (Booth, 1997).

Auditory neuropathy is a recently recognized clinical entity (Starr et al., 1996) without apparent pathology, with normal cochlear function (normal otoacoustic emissions and cochlear microphonics), but abnormal auditory brainstem evoked responses and poor speech discrimination. Patients present typically with a mild or moderate hearing loss and are characterized by poor response to traditional hearing aids. One of the hypothetical explanations of this disorder is an altered temporal synchrony in firing of the auditory nerve, which could be an early sign of demyelination (Starr et al., 1996), but there is also a possibility of selective damage to the inner hair cells, which may reduce neural input (Salvi et al., 1999).

Central auditory pathways

With the increase in complexity of auditory pathways from the cochlea to the cortex, together with multiple representations of each ear, on each side of the brain, auditory function becomes more complex and multifaceted. Central lesions (Table 45.4) may cause varying degrees of hearing impairment and other auditory dysfunctions, such as disproportionately impaired speech discrimination (relative to hearing sensitivity), tinnitus, hyperacusis, hallucinations, and various abnormalities in sound processing, including derangements of binaural acoustic integration, sound localization, signal sequencing, or auditory pattern recognition.

Lesions of the brainstem can be caused by a variety of lesions, including neoplastic and vascular abnormalities, such as vertebrobasilar disease, mini strokes, vascular spasms, or vascular loops. Intra- and extra-axial lesions of the brainstem may affect auditory function in different ways (Musiek & Baran, 1986). An intra-axial lesion of the brainstem, especially in the pons, is likely to cause a bilateral auditory disorder, as it may disrupt the majority of crossing fibres from the cochlear nuclei and the superior olivary complex. Intra-axial lesions, for example, secondary to central pontine haemorrhage, have given rise to bilateral low-frequency hearing loss, reflecting the tonotopic organisation of the auditory pathways, with the lowest frequencies being encoded centrally (Cohen et al., 1996). An extra-axial lesion of the mid to low lateral pons may directly affect the cochlear nuclei, the only superficially located auditory structure, leading to ipsilateral deficits. An extra-axial or intra-axial lesion at the level of the inferior colliculus (midbrain) and MGB (thalamus) is more likely to cause a contralateral deficit on behavioural central tests. In general, lesions of the brainstem appear to affect dichotic integration tasks rather than dichotic separation tasks. Large space-occupying lesions in the brainstem or cerebellum may cause multiple deficits, with additional secondary effects due to compression, displacement, vascular disruption, or hydrocephalus.

Subcortical and cortical auditory pathways

The pathology of the auditory cortex (grey matter) and hemispheres (grey and white matter) results mainly from ischemic, neoplastic or demyelinating lesions. Hearing deficit at this level is very rare and is most likely to be caused by vascular disease of both temporal lobes.

Management

Hearing loss

It is important to ensure all preventive measures are undertaken to avoid permanent hearing loss, e.g. regulations regarding occupational noise exposure and serum monitoring of known ototoxic drugs, e.g. gentamicin. In the majority of cases, hearing loss is permanent, but in some patients hearing loss can be treated surgically or pharmacologically. In those with irreversible hearing loss, the management is directed towards reduction of the effect of any auditory disability or handicap, by the application of different types of amplification devices and implants.

Surgical treatment

In a small proportion of cases, limited to those with middle ear disorders, surgical intervention may improve or restore hearing, for example, following myringotomy, with or without grommet insertion, in otitis media with effusion, stapedectomy for otosclerosis, or in osteogenesis imperfecta. Surgical procedures for acoustic neuroma, may preserve hearing, but usually lead to an increased, if not total, hearing loss. Surgical treatment is also used in Ménière's disease, primarily for management of vestibular symptoms, although the evidence for conservative procedures, such as endolymphatic sac decompression, remain controversial. Destructive procedures, e.g. labyrinthectomy and vestibular nerve section, should be undertaken with great care in the light of the significant prevalence of bilateral Ménière's disease.

Pharmacological treatment

This form of treatment is more orientated towards preservation, rather than towards an improvement of hearing, and is determined by the etiology of hearing loss. In hearing loss, such as Ménière's disease, treatment is directed towards the assumed underlying pathophysiological mechanism (endolymphatic hydrops), and consists of diuretic treatment and/or dietary restriction of sodium intake, which has been reported to improve symptoms in 60–70% of patient (Gates, 1999). Autoimmune hearing disorders are treated with steroids (glucocorticoids), and their application in some cases of idiopathic hearing loss has also been recommended, although with questionable effect, as spontaneous remission may occur (McKee, 1997).

Rehabilitation

This is the management option for most patients with hearing loss (Stephens, 1997).

I. Instrumentational rehabilitation consists of the application of personal and environmental devices.

Personal instrumentation is the most important component of rehabilitation and includes:

1. Hearing aid systems (hearing aid and ear mould). There is a wide range of devices, from low- to high-powered, from simple linear to sophisticated programmable digital hearing aids, whose application depends on many factors, including configuration and severity of hearing loss.

2. Bone anchored hearing aids, are applied in patients with significant conductive hearing loss and consist of a surgically implanted (mastoid) titanium base to which is attached an electronic amplification system, allowing bone-transmission of sound.

3. Vibrotactile hearing aids are applied in individuals with profound hearing impairment in whom is not possible to deliver acoustic signal above the threshold. Vibrotactile information is delivered via a vibration transducer, often worn on the forearm.

4. Cochlear implants bypass the transduction mechanisms of the cochlea by electrically stimulating the auditory nerve directly, and they are used in profoundly hearing-impaired individuals.

5. Brainstem implants are applied in patients who have no remaining auditory nerve, e.g. subsequent to surgical removal of vestibular neuroma. The cochlear nucleus, as the termination site for all auditory fibres, and therefore, most peripheral of the central structures, is the target of stimulation.

II. Non-instrumental rehabilitation includes the application of environmental aids, those using sound to enhance loudness and clarity (e.g. additional speaker/receiver, or induction coil systems), or those using visual information (e.g. text telephones, subtitle TV/videos, or video telephones) and alerting and warning systems (e.g. flashing doorbell or the telephone bell, also include use of trained dogs).

Tinnitus

There are several lines in the management of this complex symptom.

Treatment of underlying disorders

Medical evaluation may indicate conditions which could be of relevance for the emergence of tinnitus (cardiovascular, renal, metabolic and autoimmune disease, or the effects of medications and drugs). Auditory assessment may identify the presence and site of a lesion, which could be treatable.

Pharmacological treatment

There have been attempts, with varying success, to base pharmacological treatment on hypothetical underlying mechanisms, as highlighted above in the section on tinnitus. Ca^{2+}-antagonists (nimodipine), $GABA_A$ and $GABA_B$ agonists (benzodiazepines and baclofen, respectively), and drugs for depression of neuronal response to excitatory stimuli and hyperpolarization of neuronal membranes (phenytoin, carbamazepine) have all been tried.

In patients with significant associated anxiety, or depression, treatment with tranquillizers and antidepressants (e.g. tricyclic nortriptyline) may be of value. More recently, selective serotonin reuptake inhibitors, as modulators of tonic inhibition of auditory pathways, were found to be effective in some patients with tinnitus, particularly in those with associated depression.

The quality of evidence for the efficacy of pharmacological treatment of tinnitus is poor. This is largely due to the difficulty in undertaking adequate studies, as tinnitus is a symptom of different pathologies and different underlying mechanisms may be involved. Therefore, it is of importance to identify any audiological, or relevant abnormality in order to provide 'tailored' treatment for each individual.

Tinnitus retraining therapy (TRT)

TRT includes counselling and sound therapy (see below Instrumentation), based on neurophysiological model of tinnitus (Jastreboff & Hazell, 1993). Directive counselling is aimed at providing the patient with clear information about the possible mechanism(s) of tinnitus and how it can be influenced adversely or beneficially; person-centred counselling deals with the stress and needs and ways of dealing with problems; cognitive counselling is aimed at identifying and dispelling patients' false beliefs, attitudes, or fears.

Instrumentation

Hearing aids are the first line in management for patients with associated hearing loss, as they reduce awareness of tinnitus by amplification of external sounds. Tinnitus maskers and low-level noise generators may mask or at least reduce the effect of tinnitus. Other devices, as a part of a masking strategy, include pillow speakers or a tape recorder, which may alleviate tinnitus at night, while walkmans can be used during the day.

Surgical treatment

In addition to evidence-based surgical treatment of specific underlying lesions, other surgical procedures, for the treatment of tinnitus *per se*, such as auditory nerve section, or cochlear destruction, have provided little evidence of effectiveness and may even make tinnitus worse.

References   * denotes key references

Adams, J.C. (1980). Crossed and descending projections to the inferior colliculus. *Neurosci. Lett.*, **19**, 1–5.

Attias, J. & Bresloff, J. (1998). Neurophysiology of tinnitus. In *Advances in Noise Research*, Vol. 1, *Biological Effects of Noise*, ed. D. Prasher & L. Luxon, pp. 226–35. London: Whurr Publishers.

Benjamin, E., Todd Troost, B. (1988). Central auditory disorders. In *Otolaryngology* 1, ed. G.M. English, pp. 1–33. Philadelphia: J.B.Lippincott Co.

*Booth, J.B. (1997). Sudden, and fluctuant sensorineural hearing loss. In *Scott-Brown's Otolaryngology: Otology*, ed. A.G. Kerr, Chapter 17. Oxford: Butterworth-Heinemann.

*Brownell, W.E., Bader, C.R., Bertrand, D. & de Ribaupierre, Y. (1985). Evoked mechanical responses of isolated cochlear outer hair cells. *Science*, **227**, 194–6.

Cacace, A.T., Lovely, T.J., McFarland, D.J., Parnes, S.M. & Winter, D.F. (1994). Anomalous cross-modal plasticity following posterior fossa surgery: some speculations on gaze-evoked tinnitus. *Hear. Res.*, **81**, 22–32.

Ceranic, J.B., Prasher, D.K. & Luxon L.M. (1995). Tinnitus and otoacoustic emissions. *Clin. Otolaryngol.*, **20**, 192–200.

Cohen, M., Luxon, L. & Rudge, P. (1996). Auditory deficits and hearing loss associated with focal brainstem haemorrhage. *Scand. Audiol.*, **25**, 133–41.

Committee on Hearing and Equilibrium, the American Academy of Ophthalmology and Otolaryngology (1995). Committee on Hearing and Equilibrium guidelines for diagnosis and evaluation of therapy in Menière's disease. *Otolaryngol. Head Neck Surg.*, **113**, 181–5.

Davis, H. and Associates. (1953). Acoustic trauma in the guinea pig. *J. Acoust. Soc. Am.*, **25**, 1180–9.

Despopulous, A. & Silbernagl, S. (1991). Physiology of the ear. In *Color Atlas of Physiology*, p. 319. New York: Thieme Medical Publishers Inc.

Dix, M.R. & Hood, J.D. (1973). Symmetrical hearing loss in brainstem lesions. *Acta Otolaryngol. (Stockh.)*, **75**, 165–77.

Duane, D.D. (1977). A neurological perspective of central audiatory dysfunction. In *Central Auditory Dysfunction*, ed. R.W. Keith, Orlando: FI: Grune & Stratton.

Espir, M., Illingworth, R., Ceranic, B. & Luxon, L.M. (1997). Paroxysmal tinnitus due to meningeoma in the cerebellopontine angle. *J. Neurol. Neurosurg. Psych.*, **62**, 401–3.

Gacek, R. (1973). A cerebellocochlear nucleus pathway in the cats. *Exp. Neurol.*, **41**, 101–12.

Gates, G. (1999). Menière's disease: medical therapy. In *Menière's Disease*, ed. J.P. Harris, pp. 329–40. The Hague: Kugler Publications.

Gerken, G.M. (1979). Central denervation hypersensitivity in the auditory system of the cat. *J. Acoust. Soc. Am.*, **66**, 721–7.

Gonzalez-Ravilla, A. (1948). Differential diagnosis of tumours at the cerebellar recess. *Bull. Johns Hopkins Hosp.*, **83**, 187–212.

Graybiel, A.M. (1972). Some fiber pathways related to the posterior thalamic region in the cat. *Brain Beh. Evol.*, **6**, 363–93.

Hall, D.A., Haggard, M.P., Akeroyd, M.A. et al. (2000). Modulation and tasks effects in auditory processing measured using fMRI. *Hum. Brain Mapp.*, **10**, 107–19.

*Huffman, R.F. & Henson, O.W. Jr. (1990). The descending auditory pathway and acousticomotor system: connections with the inferior colliculus. *Brain Res. Rev.*, 15, 295–323.

Jastreboff, P.J. & Hazell, W.P. (1993). A neurophysiological approach to tinnitus: clinical implications. *Br. J. Audiol.*, **27**, 7–17.

*Kemp, D.T. (1978). Stimulated acoustic emissions from within the human auditory system. *J. Acoust. Soc. Am.*, **64**, 1386–91.

LeDoux, J.E., Sakaguchi, A. & Reis, D.J. (1983). Subcortical efferent projections of the medial geniculate nucleus mediate emotional responses conditioned to acoustic stimuli. *J. Neurosci.*, **4**, 683–98.

Levine, R.A. (1999). Somatic (craniocervical) tinnitus: a pivotal role for dorsal cochlear nucleus ? *ARO*, Abs **22**, 6.

Liberman, N.C. & Kiang, N.Y. (1978). Acoustic trauma in cats. *Acta Otolaryngol.*, Suppl 358, 1–63.

Lockwood, A.H., Salvvi, R.J., Coad, M.L., Towsley, M.L., Wack, D.S. & Murphy, B.W. (1998). The functional neuroanatomy of tinnitus: evidence from limbic system links and neuronal plasticity. *Neurology*, **50**, 114–20.

Lockwood, A.H., Salvi, R.J., Burkard, R.F., Galantowicz, P.J., Coad, M.L. & Wack, D.S. (1999). Neuroanatomy of tinnitus. *Scand. Audiol.*, Suppl 51, 47–52.

*Luxon, L.M. & Cohen, M. (1997). Central auditory dysfunction. In *Scott-Brown's Otolaryngology: Adult Audiology*, ed. D. Stephens, Chapter 17. Oxford: Butterworth-Heinemann.

*McKee, G.J. (1997). Pharmacological treatment of hearing and balance disorders. In *Scott-Brown's Otolaryngology: Adult Audiology*, ed. D. Stephens, Chapter 6. Oxford: Butterworth-Heinemann.

Matthies, C. & Samii, M. (1997). Management of 1000 vestibular schwannomas (acoustic neuromas): clinical presentation. *Neurosurgery*, **40**, 1–9.

Milicic, D. & Alçada, M. (1999). A tinnitus objectivization: how we do it. *Int. Tinnitus J.*, **5**, 5–15.

Mirz, F., Ovesen, T., Ishizu, K. et al. (1999). Stimulus-dependent central processing of auditori stimuli. *Scand. Audiol.*, **28**, 161–9.

Møller, A.R. (2000). Similarities between severe tinnitus and chronic pain. *J. Am. Ac. Audiol.*, **11**, 115–24.

Møller, A.R., Møller, M.B. & Yokota, M. (1992). Some forms of tinnitus may involve the extralemniscal auditory pathway. *Laryngoscope*, **109**, 1165–71.

Morest, K.D., Kim, J. & Bohne, B.A. (1997). Neuronal and transneuronal degeneration of auditory axons in the brainstem after cochlear lesion in the chinchilla: cochleotopic and non-cochleotopic patterns. *Hear. Res.*, **103**, 151–68.

Musiek, F.E. (1986). Neuroanatomy, neurophysiology and central auditory assessment. Part II: the cerebrum. *Ear Hear.*, **7**, 283–94.

*Musiek, F.E. & Baran, J.A. (1986). Neuroanatomy, neurophysiology and central auditory assessment. Part I: brain stem. *Ear Hear.*, **7**, 207–19.

Musiek, F.E. & Lamb, L. (1994). Central auditory assessment: an overview. In *Handbook of Clinical Audiology*, ed. J. Katz, pp. 197–211. Baltimore: Williams & Wilkins.

Näätänen, R. (1995). The mismatch negativity: a powerful tool for cognitive neuroscience. *Ear Hear.*, **16**, 6–15.

Pickles, J.O. (1988). The auditory nerve. In *Introduction to the Physiology of Hearing*, ed. J.O. Pickles, pp. 78–111. London: Academic Press.

Prasher, D.K., Tun, T., Brooks, G.B. & Luxon, L.M. (1995). Mechanisms of hearing loss in acoustic neuroma: an otoacoustic emission study. *Acta Otolaryngol.*, **115**, 375–81.

*Puel, J.L. (1995). Chemical synaptic transmission in the cochlea. *Prog. Neurobiol.*, **47**, 449–76.

Pujol, R. (1994). Lateral and medial efferents: a double neurochemical mechanism to protect and regulate inner and outer hair cell function in the cochlea. *Br. J. Audiol.*, **28**, 185–91.

Rajan, R., Irvine, D.R.F., Calford, M.B. & Wise, L.Z. (1992). Effects of frequency-specific losses in cochlear neural activity on the processing and representation of frequency in primary auditory cortex. In *Noise Induced Hearing Loss*, ed. A.L. Dancer, D. Henderson, R.J. Salvi & R.P. Hamernik, pp. 119–29. St. Louis: Mosby Year Book.

Ramsden, R.T. (1987). Acoustic tumours. In *Scott-Brown's Otolaryngology: Otology*, ed. A.G. Kerr, Chapter 21. London: Butterworths.

Recanzone, G.H., Schreiner, C.E. & Merzenich, M.M. (1993). Plasticity in the frequency representation of primary auditory cortex following discrimination training in adult owl monkeys. *J. Neurosci.*, **13**, 87–103.

Robertson, D. & Irvine, R.F. (1989). Plasticity of frequency organisation in auditory cortex of Guinea pigs with partial unilateral deafness. *J. Comp. Neurol.*, **282**(82), 456–71.

*Sahley, T.L., Nodar, R.H. & Musiek, F.E. (1999). Endogenous dynorphins: possible role in peripheral tinnitus. *Int. Tinnitus J.*, **5**, 76–91.

Salvi, R.J., Wang, J., Ding, D., Stecker, N. & Arnold, S. (1999). Auditory deprivation of the central auditory system resulting from selective inner hair cell loss: animal model of auditory neuropathy. *Scand. Audiol.*, **28**, Suppl. 51, 1–12.

Salvi, R.J. & Ahroon, W.A. (1983). Tinnitus and neural activity. *J. Speech Hear. Res.*, **26**, 629–32.

Seidman, M.D. (2000). Effects of dietary restrictions and antioxidants on presbyacusis. *Laryngoscope*, **110**, 727–38.

Schacht, J. (1998). Aminoglycoside ototoxicity: prevention in sight? *Otolaryngol. Head Neck Surg.*, **118**, 674–77.

Schuknecht, H.F. (1993). *Pathology of the Ear*, p. 67. Philadelphia: Lea & Febiger.

Shulman, A. & Strashun, A. (1999). Descending auditory system/cerebellum/tinnitus. *Int. Tinnitus J.*, **5**, 92–106.

Shulman, A., Strashun, A.M., Afriyie, M., Aronson, F., Abel, W. & Goldstein, B. (1995). SPECT imaging of brain and tinnitus – neurotologic/neurologic implications. *Int. Tinnitus J.*, **1**, 13–29.

Spoendlin, H. (1979). Neural connections of the outer hair cell system. *Acta Otolaryngol.*, **87**, 381–7.

Starr, A., Picton, T.W., Sininger, Y., Hood, L.J. & Berlin, C.I. (1996). Auditory neuropathy. *Brain*, **119**, 741–53.

*Stephens, D. (1997). Audiological rehabilitation. In *Scott-Brown's Otolaryngology: Adult Audiology*, ed. D. Stephens, Chapter 13. Oxford: Butterworth-Heinemann.

Thompson, A.M. & Thompson, G.C. (1995). Light microscopic evidence of serotoninergic projections to olivocochlear neurones in the bush baby otolemur garnetti. *Brain Res.*, **695**, 263–66.

von Békésy, G. (1960). *Experiments on Hearing.* New York: McGraw-Hill.

Wiederhold, M.L. (1986). Physiology of the olivocochlear system. In *Neurobiology of Hearing, The Cochlea*, ed. R. Altschuler, R. Bobin & D. Hoffman, pp. 349–70. New York: Raven Press.

Yeoh, L.H. (1997). Causes of hearing loss. In *Scott-Brown's Otolaryngology: Adult Audiology*, ed. D. Stephens, Chapter 10. Oxford: Butterworth-Heinemann.

Zenner, H.P. (1986). Motile responses in outer hair cells. *Hear. Res.*, **22**, 83–90.

46

Vertigo and vestibular disorders

Thomas Brandt

Department of Neurology, Klinikum Grosshadern, University of Munich, Germany

Vertigo is an unpleasant distortion of static gravitational orientation, or an erroneous perception of motion of either the sufferer or the environment. It is not a disease entity, but rather the outcome of many pathological or physiological processes. Vertigo is best described as a multisensory and sensorimotor syndrome with perceptual, postural, ocular motor and autonomic manifestations induced by either

- unusual and therefore unadapted (motion) stimulation of the intact sensory systems, or
- pathological (lesional) dysfunction.

Vertigo, dizziness, and disequilibrium are common complaints of patients of all ages, particularly the elderly. As presenting symptoms, they occur in 5–10% of all patients seen by general practitioners and 10–20% of all patients seen by neurologists and otolaryngologists. The clinical spectrum of vertigo is broad, extending from vestibular rotatory vertigo with nausea and vomiting to presyncope light-headedness, from drug intoxication to hypoglycemic dizziness, from visual vertigo to phobias and panic attacks, and from motion sickness to height vertigo. Appropriate preventions and treatments differ for different types of dizziness and vertigo; they include drug therapy, physical therapy, psychotherapy and surgery.

The 'vestibular' vertigo syndromes

Vertigo usually implies a mismatch between the vestibular, visual, and somatosensory systems. These three sensory systems subserve both static and dynamic spatial orientation, locomotion, and control of posture by constantly providing reafferent cues. The sensory information is partially redundant in that two or three senses may simultaneously provide similar information about the same action. Thanks to this overlapping of their functional ranges, it is possible for one sense to substitute, at least in part, for deficiencies in the others. When information from two sensory sources conflicts, the intensity of the vertigo is a function of the degree of mismatch; it is increased if information from an intact sensory system is lost, as for example in a patient with pathological vestibular vertigo who closes his eyes. The distressing sensorimotor consequences of the mismatch are frequently based on our earlier experiences with orientation, balance, and locomotion, i.e. there is a mismatch between the expected and the actually perceived pattern of multisensory input.

Vertigo may thus be induced by physiological stimulation of the intact sensorimotor systems (height vertigo; motion sickness) or by pathological dysfunction of any of the stabilizing sensory systems, especially the vestibular system (Table 46.1). The symptoms of vertigo include sensory qualities identified as arising from vestibular, visual, and somatosensory sources. As distinct from one's perception of self-motion during natural locomotion, the experience of vertigo is linked to impaired perception of a stationary environment; this perception is mediated by central nervous system processes known as 'space constancy mechanisms'. Loss of the external stationary reference system required for orientation and postural regulation contributes to the distressing mixture of self-motion and surround motion (Brandt & Daroff, 1980b).

Signs and symptoms

Physiological and clinical vertigo syndromes (Table 46.2) are commonly characterized by a combination of phenomena involving perceptual, ocular motor, postural and autonomic manifestations: vertigo, nystagmus, ataxia, and nausea (Fig. 46.1; Brandt & Daroff 1980b). These four manifestations correlate with different aspects of vestibular function and emanate from different sites within the central nervous system.

Table 46.1. Physiological or pathological vertigo

Physiological stimulation	Height vertigo
	Motion sickness
Pathological dysfunction	Labyrinthine and vestibular nerve disorders
	Central vestibular disorders

Table 46.2. Syndromal manifestations of vertigo

Syndrome	Manifestation
Perceptual	Vertigo, disorientation
Ocular motor	Nystagmus, ocular deviation
Postural	Ataxia, falls
Autonomic	Nausea, vomiting, anxiety

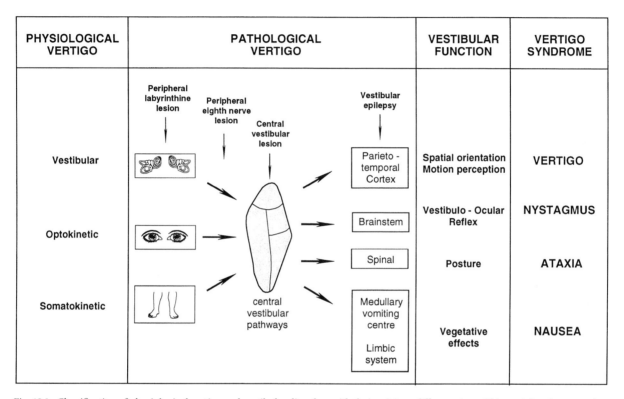

Fig. 46.1. Classification of physiological vertigo and vestibular disorders with their origin at different sites within peripheral or central vestibular structures. Vestibular disorders are not clinical entities but different sensorimotor syndromes arising from unusual stimulation or lesional dysfunction. (From Brandt & Daroff, 1980b.)

1. The vertigo itself results from a disturbance of cortical spatial orientation.
2. Nystagmus is secondary to a direction-specific imbalance in the vestibulo-ocular reflex, which activates brainstem neuronal circuitry.
3. Vestibular ataxia and postural imbalance are caused by inappropriate or abnormal activation of monosynaptic and polysynaptic vestibulospinal pathways.
4. The unpleasant autonomic responses with nausea, vomiting, and anxiety travel along ascending and descending vestibulo-autonomic pathways to activate the medullary vomiting center.

Under certain conditions, distressing symptoms and malaise may be preceded by a pleasurable autonomic sensation, which is presumably mediated through the limbic system and accounts for the popularity of amusement park rides and the like.

The mismatch concept

Physiological vertigo (motion sickness) and pathological vertigo (peripheral or central vestibular dysfunction) are thought to be generated by an acute sensorimotor conflict (mismatch) between the converging sensory inputs and

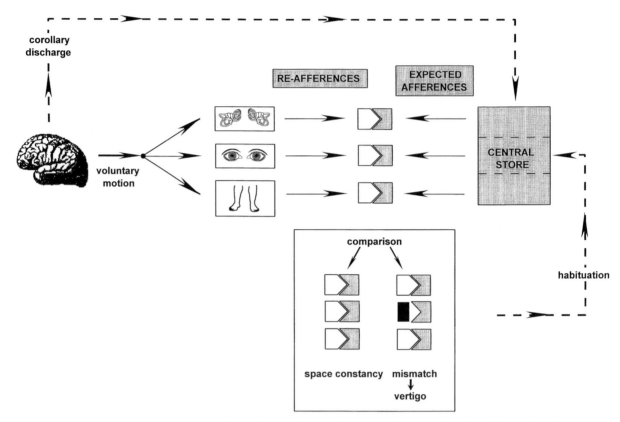

Fig. 46.2. Schematic diagram of the sensory conflict or the neural mismatch concept of vertigo and motion sickness. An active movement leads to stimulation of the sensory organs whose messages are compared with a multisensory pattern of expectation calibrated by earlier experience of motions (central store). The pattern of expectation is prepared either by the efference copy signal which is emitted parallel to and simultaneously with the motion impulse, or by vestibular excitation during passive transportation in vehicles. If concurrent sensory stimulation and the pattern of expectation are in agreement, self-motion is perceived while 'space constancy' is maintained. If, for example, there is no appropriate visual report of motion, as a result of the field of view being filled with stationary environmental contrasts (reading in the car), a sensory mismatch occurs. With repeated stimulation, motion sickness is induced through summation; the repeated stimulation leads to a rearrangement of the stored pattern of expectation, however, so that a habituation to the initially challenging stimulation is attained within a few days. An acute unilateral labyrinthine loss causes vertigo, because the self-motion sensation induced by the vestibular tone imbalance is contradicted by vision and the somatosensors.

the expected sensory patterns (Fig. 46.2) or a vestibular tone imbalance. A mismatch arises, for example, when the multisensory consequences of being a passenger in a moving vehicle or of moving actively do not match the expected patterns which have been calibrated by prior experience of active locomotion. Thus, it is the sensory mismatch (e.g. visual–vestibular or between right and left vestibular input) rather than the sensory loss which causes vertigo. The absence of one channel of the redundant sensory input, important as it is for demanding balancing tasks in sports, rarely manifests as vertigo. Inappropriate information from one or multiple sensory systems produces an illusion of body motion and causes vertigo. An acute unilateral labyrinthine dysfunction (see vestibular

neuritis) causes vertigo because the sensation of self-motion induced by the vestibular tone imbalance is contradicted by vision and the somatosensors.

Approaching the patient

Dizziness is a vexing symptom, difficult to assess because of its purely subjective character and its variety of sensations. The sensation of spinning or rotatory vertigo is much more specific; if it persists, it undoubtedly indicates acute pathology of the labyrinth, the vestibular nerve, or the caudal brainstem, which contains the vestibular nuclei.

History taking allows the early differentiation of vertigo

and disequilibrium disorders into seven categories that serve as a practical guide for differential diagnosis:

(i)   dizziness and light-headedness (e.g. hyperventilation, intoxication)

(ii)   single or recurrent attacks of (rotatory) vertigo (e.g. Menière's disease, basilar migraine)

(iii)   sustained (rotatory) vertigo (e.g. Wallenberg's syndrome)

(iv)   positional/positioning vertigo (e.g. benign paroxysmal positional vertigo, central positional vertigo)

(v)   oscillopsia, the apparent motion of the visual scene (e.g. bilateral vestibular failure, downbeat nystagmus)

(vi)   vertigo associated with auditory dysfunction (e.g. Menière's disease, Cogan's syndrome)

(vii)   dizziness or to-and-fro vertigo with postural imbalance (e.g. somatoform phobic postural vertigo, central vestibular disorders, episodic ataxia)

Management of vestibular disorders

The prevailing good prognosis of vertigo should be emphasized, because

–   many forms of vertigo have a benign cause and are characterized by spontaneous recovery of vestibular function or central compensation of a peripheral vestibular tone imbalance, and

–   most forms of vertigo can be effectively relieved by pharmacological treatment (Table 46.3), physical therapy (Table 46.4), surgery (Table 46.5), or psychotherapy [7].

There is, however, no common treatment, and vestibular suppressants (Table 46.6) provide only symptomatic relief of vertigo and nausea. A specific therapeutic approach thus requires recognition of the numerous particular pathomechanisms involved (Baloh & Halmagyi, 1996; Brandt, 1999; Bronstein et al., 1996). Such therapy can include causative, symptomatic, or preventive approaches.

Antivertiginous and antiemetic drugs

A variety of drugs used for symptomatic relief of vertigo and nausea (Table 46.4) have the major side effect of general sedation (Foster & Baloh, 1996). Vestibular suppressants, including anticholinergics, antihistamines, and benzodiazepines, provide symptomatic relief of distressing symptoms by down-regulating vestibular excitability. Antiemetics preferably control nausea and vomiting by acting on the medullary vomiting center, the chemoreceptor trigger zone, or the gastrointestinal tract itself. Vestibular suppressants are often acetylcholine and hista-

Table 46.3. Pharmacologic therapies for vertigo

Therapy	Vertigo
Vestibular suppressants	Symptomatic relief of nausea (in acute peripheral and vestibular nuclei lesions), prevention of motion sickness
Antiepileptic drugs	Vestibular epilepsy, vestibular paroxysmia (disabling positional vertigo), paroxysmal dysarthria and ataxia in MS, other central vestibular paroxysms, superior oblique myokymia
Beta-receptor blockers	Basilar migraine (vestibular migraine; benign recurrent vertigo)
Betahistine	Menière's disease
Antibiotics	Infections of the ear and temporal bone
Ototoxic antibiotics	Menière's disease (Menière's drop attacks)
Corticosteroids	Vestibular neuritis, autoimmune inner ear disease
Baclofen	Downbeat or upbeat nystagmus or vertigo
Acetazolamide	Familial periodic ataxia or vertigo

Source: From Brandt (1999).

Table 46.4. Physical therapies for vertigo

Therapy	Vertigo
Deliberate manoeuvres	Benign paroxysmal positioning vertigo
Vestibular exercises	Vestibular rehabilitation, central compensation of acute vestibular loss, habituation for prevention of motion sickness, improvement of balance skills (e.g. in the elderly)
Physical therapy (neck collar)	Cervical vertigo (fiction or reality?)

Source: From Brandt (1999).

mine antagonists, which act as acetylcholine antagonists by competitive inhibition at muscarinic receptors in the vestibular nuclei, their most likely site of action. Vestibular suppression by benzodiazepines is best explained by their $GABA_A$ agonistic effect, because GABA is the major neuroinhibitory transmitter for vestibular neurons. Antiemetics are effective mainly due to their dopamine (D_2) antagonist

Table 46.5. *Surgical interventions for vertigo*

Surgery	Vertigo
Surgical decompression of eighth nerve	Tumour (acoustic neurinoma) or cyst
Surgical decompression of vertebral artery	Rotational vertebral artery occlusion
Ampullary nerve section or canal plugging	Benign paroxysmal positioning vertigo
Endolymphatic shunt	Menière's disease
Vestibular nerve section or labyrinthectomy	Intractable Menière's disease
Surgical patching	Perilymph fistula

Source: From Brandt (1999).

properties, but some antiemetics also have muscarinergic or antihistaminic (H₁) properties that may assist in vestibular suppression as well. Primary vestibular suppressants such as scopolamine also effectively suppress vomiting by virtue of their muscarinergic action. Antiemetics are more selective in action. They are primarily used to control nausea and vomiting; for treatment of severe vertigo with nausea, they are often combined with antivertiginous drugs (Foster & Baloh, 1996).

There are only four clear indications for the use of antivertiginous (vestibular suppressants) and antiemetic drugs to control vertigo, nausea, and vomiting (Brandt, 1999):

(i)   to prevent nausea due to acute peripheral vestibulopathy (for the first 1–3 days or as long as nausea lasts),

(ii) to prevent severe vertigo and nausea due to acute brainstem or archicerebellar lesions near the vestibular nuclei,

(iii) to prevent severe vertigo attacks that frequently recur, and

(iv) to prevent motion sickness.

For conditions 1 and 2, fast-acting compounds with vestibular and general sedation should be preferably administered, e.g. diazepam or promethazine combined with dimenhydrinate if nausea and vomiting are exceptionally severe. These drugs should not be given after nausea has disappeared, because they prolong the time course of central compensation of an acute vestibular tone imbalance.

Mobility and vestibular excitability are major requirements for recovery and vestibular rehabilitation. Antivertiginous and antiemetic drugs are not indicated for patients suffering from chronic dizziness. A prophylactic treatment with vestibular suppressants, e.g. scopolamine or dimenhydrinate, is justified only in exceptional situations of rare patients who have frequent and severe vertigo attacks. In severe cases of benign paroxysmal positioning vertigo it may become necessary to control nausea and vomiting when performing physical liberatory manoeuvres. It is our own experience that severe central positioning vomiting is best controlled by benzodiazepines rather than antiemetics or typical vestibular suppressants (Arbusow et al., 1998). Scopolamine administered transdermally as Transderm Scop provides a continuous blood level over a 3-day period and effectively prevents motion sickness. The selection of vestibular suppressants and antiemetic drugs should take into account that those that reach a peak effect 7–9 hours after ingestion (Manning et al., 1992) are ineffective for treating short vertigo attacks.

Vestibular compensation

Central compensation of a unilateral peripheral vestibular loss is considered the prototype of brain plasticity. Readjustment of the vestibular reflexes, which act on eye and body muscles, requires sensory feedback from the sensory mismatch elicited by voluntary movements. Therefore, on the basis of our current knowledge of vestibular physiology, continued management should consist of vestibular exercises that promote central compensation (Strupp et al., 1998).

Postural normalization in frogs after a complete unilateral labyrinthectomy occurs within about 60 days (Flohr et al., 1981). Recovery from vestibular lesions is neither a simple nor a single process; multiple processes are involved. Analysis of the mechanisms of recovery requires a careful comparison of normalization between parallel phenomena at the behavioural level, on the one hand, and the neuronal level, on the other. Incongruences in the time course and the magnitude of the changes in behaviour and neuronal activity clearly indicate that multiple processes of compensation occur in distributed neuronal networks for vestibulo-ocular, vestibulo-spinal and perceptual disturbances at different locations and at different times (Dieringer, 1995; Curthoys & Halmagyi, 1994).

Substitution of vestibular function

Vestibular compensation is less perfect than generally believed. For instance, after acute unilateral vestibular

Table 46.6. Commonly used antivertiginous and antiemetic drugs

Drug	Dosage	Action
Anticholinergics		Muscarine antagonist
Scopolamine (Transderm Scop)	0.6 mg po q 4–6 h or	
	Transdermal patch: 1 q 3 days	
Antihistamines		
Dimenhydrinate (Dramamine)	50 mg po q 4–6 h or im q 4–6 h or	Histamine (H$_1$) antagonist
	100 mg suppository q 8–10 h	Muscarine antagonist
Meclizine (Antivert, Bonine)	25 mg po q 4–6 h	Histamine (H$_1$) antagonist
		Muscarine antagonist
Promethazine (Phenergan)	15 or 50 mg po q 4–6 h or im q 4–6 h or	Histamine (H$_1$) antagonist
	suppository q 4–6 h	Muscarine antagonist
		Dopamine (D$_2$) antagonist
Phenothiazine		
Prochlorperazine (Compazine)	5 or 10 mg po q 4–6 h or	Muscarine antagonist
	im q 6 h or 25 mg suppository q 12 h	Dopamine (D$_2$) antagonist
Butyrophenone		
Droperidol (Inapsine)	2.5 or 5 mg im q 12 h	Muscarine antagonist
		Dopamine (D$_2$) antagonist
Benzodiazepines		
Diazepam (Valium)	5 or 10 mg po bid–qid im q 4–6 h or iv q 4–6 h	GABA$_A$ agonist
Clonazepam (Klonopin)	0.5 mg po tid	GABA$_A$ agonist

Source: From Brandt 1999.

deafferentation, which occurs in vestibular neuritis, the process of normalization is impressive for *static* conditions in the absence of head motion: the initial rotatory vertigo, spontaneous nystagmus, and postural imbalance subside. Compensation is, however, less impressive for *dynamic* conditions, especially when the vestibular system is exposed to high-frequency head accelerations (Curthoys & Halmagyi, 1994). The dynamic disequilibrium, i.e. VOR asymmetry, causes oscillopsia, the illusory movement of the environment due to excessive slip of images upon the retina during fast head movements or walking, because after uni- and bilateral peripheral vestibular lesions the VOR cannot generate fast compensatory eye rotations during high-frequency head rotations. The dynamic vestibular tone imbalance can be detected clinically by provoking a directional head-shaking nystagmus (Hain et al., 1987) or by bedside testing of the VOR with rapid head rotation (Halmagyi & Curthoys, 1988).

Vestibular compensation is usually considered a central 'repair mechanism' for a vestibular tone imbalance secondary to a peripheral vestibular loss. However, central compensation is also possible for central vestibular tone imbalances, which is best demonstrated by the cessation of nystagmus and lateropulsion in Wallenberg's syndrome.

It is still poorly understood which central vestibular syndromes can be compensated and which cannot. Upbeat and downbeat nystagmus may serve as an example. Acquired upbeat nystagmus is rarely permanent, whereas acquired downbeat nystagmus may be permanent.

Three types of vestibular dysfunction

Basically there are three types of vestibular dysfunction.

Congenital or acquired bilateral vestibular failure = vestibular loss

Key symptoms are oscillopsia associated with head movements (due to the defective vestibulo-ocular reflex) and unsteadiness of gait, particularly in the dark or on unlevel ground (when visual and somatosensory input cannot substitute for the missing vestibulo-spinal control).

These patients have no complaints when standing still without head movement.

Diagnosis is made by a bedside test for defective vestibulo-ocular reflex and the absence of nystagmic reaction to both caloric and rotatory pendular testing.

Acute unilateral lesions of the labyrinth, vestibular nerve, or central vestibular pathways = vestibular tone imbalance

Key symptoms are rotatory vertigo or perceived body tilt with spontaneous nystagmus, ocular torsion, or skew deviation associated with a direction-specific deviation of gait and body falls (due to the lesion-induced vestibular tone imbalance).

Typically a lesion-induced vestibular tone imbalance manifests as an acute syndrome with slow gradual restitution within days to weeks by either central compensation, sensory substitution, or resolution of the lesion.

Diagnosis is made by the combination of perceptual, ocular motor, and postural signs and symptoms. The direction of nystagmus or deviation of posture and gait allows one to determine the particular tone imbalance in one of the three major planes of action of the vestibular system (yaw, pitch, or roll).

Inadequate paroxysmal stimulation of the vestibular system = vestibular attacks

Key symptoms are attacks of vertigo, ocular motor dysfunction, and postural imbalance which may occur spontaneously (basilar migraine, paroxysmal vertigo of childhood, episodic ataxia type I or II, vestibular epilepsy) or may be elicited by changes in head position (benign paroxysmal positional vertigo, vestibular paroxysmia).

Diagnosis of the different etiologies for these attacks is based on careful taking of patient history, clinical examination, and testing of the vestibular function.

Table 46.7 shows the frequency of vertigo syndromes diagnosed in our Neurological Dizziness Unit and gives relevant examples that will be described in the following.

Bilateral vestibular failure

Bilateral vestibular failure (BVF) is a disorder of the peripheral labyrinth or the eighth nerve which has various etiologies. It is either acquired or congenital, or familial or sporadic. BVF occurs simultaneously or sequentially in both ears, and takes either an abrupt or slowly progressive course. A chronic bilateral loss of vestibular function is surprisingly well tolerated. Moreover, there is no continuing distressing vertigo, spontaneous nystagmus, or postural falls, which are typical signs of a vestibular tone imbalance caused by acute unilateral lesions. The key symptoms are oscillopsia during locomotion or head movements and unsteadiness, particularly in the dark. The entity was first

Table 46.7. Frequency of different vertigo syndromes in 3038 patients seen in a neurological dizziness unit (1989–1999)

Diagnosis	Frequency	
	n	%
1. Benign paroxysmal positional vertigo	533	17.6
2. Somatoform phobic postural vertigo	434	14.3
3. Central vestibular syndromes with vertigo	364	12.0
4. Peripheral vestibulopathy (vestibular neuritis)	263	8.7
5. Basilar migraine, vestibular migraine	241	7.9
6. Menière's disease	200	6.6
7. Bilateral vestibular failure	89	2.9
8. Psychogenic vertigo (without 2)	89	2.9
9. Vestibular paroxysmia (neurovascular cross-compression)	63	2.1
10. Perilymph fistula	7	0.3
Various rare vertigo syndromes	112	3.7
Unknown etiology	132	4.3
Other central vestibular syndromes (without vertigo)	396	13.0
Other disorders	115	3.8

described by Dandy (1941) in patients who had undergone bilateral vestibular neurectomies. Generally patients with BVF are first referred not only for assessment of dizziness and dysequilibrium, but also for examination of ocular motor disorders, ataxia, or hearing loss, conditions in which BVF is often not suspected prior to investigation (Rinne et al., 1995).

The diagnosis is made with the simple bedside test for defective vestibulo-ocular reflex during rapid, passive head turns (Halmagyi & Curthoys, 1988). It is confirmed by the absence of nystagmic reaction to both caloric and rotatory pendular testing while the patient sits in a rotary chair. The most frequent etiologies include ototoxicity, autoimmune disorders, meningitis, neuropathies, sequential vestibular neuritis, cerebellar degeneration, tumours, and miscellaneous otological diseases. So-called idiopathic BVF is found in more than 20% of patients (Baloh et al., 1989; Vibert et al., 1995; Rinne et al., 1995). Subjective symptoms in the acute stage tend to improve with time by processes of somatosensory and visual 'substitution' of vestibular function. Vestibular rehabilitation is supportive of this improvement, but the efficacy of physical therapy is limited. The spontaneous recovery of patients with BVF is relatively rare and incomplete. A permanent loss of vestibular function is the more frequent result; however, the thus-afflicted patient remains largely asymptomatic until confronted with high-frequency motion conditions or situations where proprioceptors or vision cannot replace the deficient vestibular system.

Vestibular neuritis

Acute unilateral (idiopathic) vestibular paralysis, also known as vestibular neuritis (VN), is a common cause of peripheral vestibular vertigo. It accounts for about 8% of the patients referred to a neurological dizziness unit (Table 46.7).

The chief symptom is the acute onset of prolonged severe rotatory vertigo, associated with spontaneous horizontal–rotatory nystagmus, postural imbalance, and nausea without concomitant auditory dysfunction. Caloric testing invariably shows ipsilateral hypo- or non-responsiveness (as a sign of horizontal semicircular canal paresis). Epidemic occurrence of the condition, the frequency of preceding upper respiratory tract infections, a small number of postmortem studies that found cell degeneration of one or more vestibular nerve trunks, and the demonstration of latent herpes simplex virus type I in human vestibular ganglia, all suggest that the cause may be a viral infection (or reactivation) of the vestibular nerve (Schuknecht & Kitamura, 1981; Arbusow et al., 1999), similar to those producing Bell's palsy and sudden sensorineural hearing loss.

VN is most likely a partial rather than a complete vestibular paresis, with predominant involvement of the horizontal and anterior semicircular canals (sparing the posterior semicircular canal). The condition mainly affects adults, ages 30 to 60, and has a natural history of gradual recovery within 1 to 6 weeks. Recovery is a product of combined (i) peripheral restoration of labyrinthine function (frequently incomplete); (ii) substitution for the unilateral vestibular deficit by contralateral vestibular input and the somatosensory and the visual systems; and (iii) central compensation of the vestibular tone imbalance (aided by physical exercise).

Diagnosis of VN is based on the simple assessment of an acute vestibular tone imbalance associated with a unilateral peripheral vestibular loss (bedside testing of high-frequency VOR; caloric testing) after clinical exclusion of a central neurological disorder. As this diagnostic procedure lacks selectivity, pathological processes other than VN which also cause an acute unilateral loss of peripheral labyrinthine function may be wrongly labelled. Thus, the term VN does not describe a well-defined clinical entity, but rather a syndrome in which peripheral vestibular paralysis can have a number of possible causes (usually viral or vascular). Some authors have proposed other sites for the lesion: peripheral labyrinth, vestibular nerve, or the insertion site of the root of the eighth nerve into the ponto-medullary brainstem (here an MS plaque can mimic VN). Differential diagnosis includes all other causes of acute loss of peripheral labyrinthine function.

Benign paroxysmal positional vertigo

Benign paroxysmal positioning vertigo (BPPV; also known as positioning vertigo) was initially defined by Bárány in 1921. BPPV is the most common cause of vertigo, particularly in the elderly. By age 70, about 30% of all elderly subjects have experienced BPPV at least once. This condition is characterized by brief attacks of rotatory vertigo and concomitant positioning rotatory–linear nystagmus which are elicited by rapid changes in head position relative to gravity. BPPV is a mechanical disorder of the inner ear in which the precipitating positioning of the head causes an abnormal stimulation, usually of the posterior semicircular canal (p-BPPV) of the undermost ear, less frequently of the horizontal (h-BPPV) or anterior (a-BPPV) semicircular canal.

Schuknecht (1969) hypothesized that heavy debris settle on the cupula (cupulolithiasis) of the canal, transforming it from a transducer of angular acceleration into a transducer of linear acceleration. It is now generally accepted that in the typical case the debris float freely within the endolymph of the canal ('canalolithiasis') (Parnes & McClure, 1991; Epley, 1992; Brandt & Steddin, 1993). The debris, possibly particles detached from the otoliths, congeal to form a free-floating clot (plug). Since the clot is heavier than the endolymph, it will always gravitate to the most dependent part of the canal during changes in head position which alter the angle of the cupular plane relative to gravity. Analogous to a plunger, the clot induces bidirectional (push or pull) forces on the cupula, thereby triggering the BPPV attack. Canalolithiasis explains all the features of BPPV: latency, short duration, fatigability (diminution with repeated positioning), changes in direction of nystagmus with changes in head position, and the efficacy of physical therapy (Brandt & Steddin, 1993).

In 1980 Brandt and Daroff proposed the first effective physical therapy (positioning exercises) for BPPV. Based on the assumption that cupulolithiasis was the underlying mechanism, the exercises were a sequence of rapid lateral head/trunk tilts, repeated serially to promote loosening and, ultimately, dispersion of the debris toward the utricular cavity. In 1988 Semont and coworkers introduced a single liberatory manoeuvre, and Epley promoted a variation in

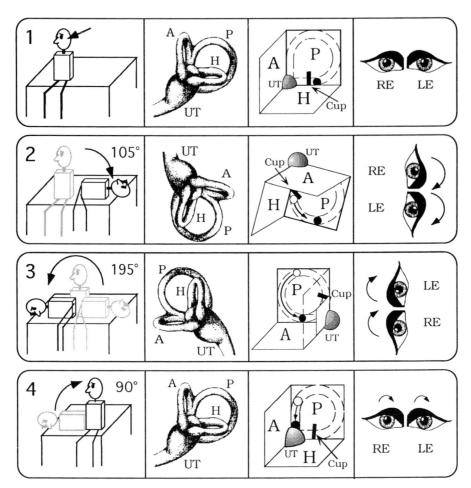

Fig. 46.3. Schematic drawing of the liberatory manoeuvre in a patient with typical BPPV of the left ear. Boxes from left to right: position of body and head, position of labyrinth in space, position and movement of the clot in the posterior canal and resulting cupula deflection, and direction of the rotatory nystagmus. The clot is depicted as an open circle within the canal; a black circle represents the final resting position of the clot. (i) In the sitting position, the head is turned horizontally 45° to the unaffected ear. The clot, which is heavier than endolymph, settles at the base of the left posterior semicircular canal. (ii) The patient is tilted approximately 105° toward the left (affected) ear. The change in head position, relative to gravity, causes the clot to gravitate to the lowermost part of the canal and the cupula to deflect downward, inducing BPPV with rotatory nystagmus beating toward the undermost ear. The patient maintains this position for 3 minutes. (iii) The patient is turned approximately 195° with the nose down, causing the clot to move toward the exit of the canal. The endolymphatic flow again deflects the cupula such that the nystagmus beats toward the left ear, now uppermost. The patient remains in this position for 3 minutes. (iv) The patient is slowly moved to the sitting position; this causes the clot to enter the utricular cavity. Abbreviations: A, P, and H = anterior, posterior, horizontal semicircular canals. Cup = cupula, UT = utricular cavity, RE = right eye, and LE = left eye. (From Brandt et al., 1994.)

1992. If performed properly, all three forms of therapy (Brandt–Daroff exercises and Semont and Epley's liberatory manoeuvre) are effective in BPPV patients (Herdman et al., 1993). The efficacy of physical therapy (Fig. 46.3) makes selective surgical destructions such as transsection of the posterior nerve (Gacek, 1984) or non-ampullary plugging of the posterior semicircular canal (Pace-Balzan & Rutka, 1991) largely unnecessary.

About 5–10% of BPPV patients suffer from horizontal canalolithiasis (h-BPPV; McClure, 1985). h-BPPV is elicited when the head of the supine patient is turned from side to side, around the longitudinal z-axis. Combinations are possible, and transitions from p-BPPV to h-BPPV occur, if the clot moves from one to the other semicircular canal. Transitions from canalolithiasis to cupulolithiasis in h-BPPV patients have been described (Steddin & Brandt,

1996). Most of the cases appear to be idiopathic (degenerative?), their incidence increasing with advancing age. Prolonged bedrest also facilitates their occurrence. Other cases arise due to trauma, vestibular neuritis, or inner ear infections.

The diagnosis of typical BPPV is simple and safe: the patient must have the usual history and exhibit positioning nystagmus toward the causative, undermost ear. Diagnosis is less easy in rare cases, for example, in patients with horizontal semicircular canal cupulolithiasis who exhibit positional nystagmus beating toward the uppermost ear for several minutes. Differential diagnosis includes different forms of central vestibular vertigo or nystagmus, vestibular paroxysmia, perilymph fistula, drug or alcohol intoxication, vertebrobasilar ischemia, Menière's disease and psychogenic vertigo.

Vestibular paroxysmia

Episodic vertigo and other vestibular syndromes can result from pathological excitation of various vestibular structures: the labyrinthine receptors, the vestibular nerve, the vestibular nuclei, and their ascending pathways to the thalamus and the cortex. There is evidence that neurovascular cross-compression of the eighth nerve is the probable cause of vestibular paroxysmia (also termed disabling positional vertigo), including both paroxysmal hyperactivity and progressive functional loss. Analogously to trigeminal neuralgia, vestibular paroxysmia is diagnosed by the occurrence of short attacks and series of rotational or to-and-fro vertigo, which are precipitated or modulated by changing head position and frequently associated with hypacusis and tinnitus (Brandt & Dieterich, 1994b).

This variable syndrome was first described by Jannetta (1975) and later labeled 'disabling positional vertigo' by the same authors (Jannetta et al., 1984; Møller et al., 1986).

Lacking a well-defined syndrome and a diagnostic test, the non-surgical clinician finds it difficult to believe in this disease. The increasing number of reports on vestibular paroxysmia prompt us to share our own preliminary experience with episodic vertigo, a treatable condition that has long escaped notice. The conservative therapeutic approach to the typical clinical syndrome of neurovascular compression of the eighth nerve is mainly based on the efficacy of treatment with carbamazepine, the recurrence of attacks following drug washout phases, and the exclusion of a central (particularly a demyelinating) disease. There is still no pathognomonic sign of the condition, and to date the current imaging techniques for identifying causative nerve-vessel contacts leave much to be desired,

since vessel contacts can also be imaged (even at root entry zones) in asymptomatic patients.

According to our findings, the diagnosis can be established on the basis of six characteristic features (Brandt & Dieterich, 1994b):
(i) short attacks of rotational or to-and-fro vertigo lasting for seconds to minutes,
(ii) attacks frequently provoked by particular head positions and whose duration is modified by changing head position,
(iii) hypacusis or tinnitus permanently or during the attack,
(iv) auditory or vestibular deficits measurable by neurophysiological methods,
(v) efficacy of carbamazepine, and
(vi) a central cause excluded by clinical, neurophysiological, and imaging investigations.

As distinct from typical trigeminal neuralgia – in which there is no significant sensory loss, vestibular paroxysmia is characterized by paroxysmal hyperactivity combined with some functional deficit in the attack-free interval.

Central vestibular disorders

Topographic diagnosis in neurology is frequently based on lesions along the course of long motor or sensory pathways. This is well established for the pyramidal tract and the visual pathways. Likewise, clinical studies of the differential effects of central vestibular pathway lesions have increasingly shown vestibular syndromes to be accurate indicators for a topographic diagnosis. Vestibular pathways run from the eighth nerve and the vestibular nuclei through ascending fibres, such as the ipsilateral or contralateral medial longitudinal fasciculus, the brachium conjunctivum, or the ventral tegmental tract to the oculomotor nuclei, the supranuclear integration centres in the rostral midbrain, and the vestibular thalamic subnuclei. From there they reach several cortex areas through the thalamic projection. Another relevant ascending projection reaches the cortex from vestibular nuclei via vestibular cerebellum structures, in particular the fastigial nucleus.

In the majority of cases, central vestibular vertigo syndromes are caused by dysfunction or a deficit of sensory input induced by a lesion. In a small proportion of cases they are due to pathological excitation of various structures, extending from the peripheral vestibular organ to the vestibular cortex. Since peripheral vestibular disorders are always characterized by a combination of perceptual, ocular motor, and postural signs and symptoms, central

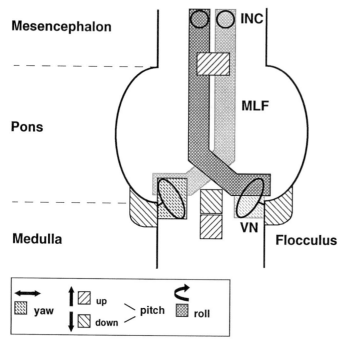

Fig. 46.4. Vestibular syndromes in roll, pitch, and yaw planes: critical areas are schematically represented based on our current knowledge of vestibular and ocular motor structures and pathways, a lesion of which causes a vestibular tone imbalance in one of the three major planes of action. The mere clinical sign of a vertical, torsional, or horizontal nystagmus, if central vestibular, allows a topographic diagnosis of the lesion, although the particular vestibular structures involved are still under discussion. Whereas a vestibular tone imbalance in the roll plane indicates unilateral brainstem lesions (a crossing in the pons), vertical nystagmus indicates bilateral lesions. Two separate causative loci are known for upbeat nystagmus: medullary or pontomesencephalic. Downbeat nystagmus indicates a bilateral paramedian lesion of the commissural fibres between the vestibular nuclei or a bilateral flocculus lesion. Horizontal nystagmus indicates unilateral pontomedullary lesions involving the vestibular nuclei. The differentiation of vestibular ocular motor signs according to the three major planes of action of the VOR and their mapping to distinct and separate areas in the brainstem are helpful for topographic diagnosis and for avoiding incorrect assignment of clinical signs to brainstem lesions identified with imaging techniques (INC = interstitial nucleus of Cajal, MLF = medial longitudinal fasciculus, VN = vestibular nucleus). (From Brandt & Dieterich, 1994.)

vestibular disorders may manifest as 'a complete syndrome' or with only single components. The ocular motor aspect, for example, predominates in the syndromes of upbeat or downbeat nystagmus. Lateral falls may occur without vertigo in vestibular thalamic lesions (thalamic astasia) or as lateropulsion in Wallenberg's syndrome.

Clinical classification (Fig. 46.4)

The 'elementary' neuronal network of the vestibular system is the di- or trisynaptic VOR. VOR properties are routinely tested in all patients who complain of dizziness (Leigh & Brandt, 1993) and are a part of the examination of the unconscious patient. There is evidence for a useful clinical classification of central vestibular syndromes according to the three major planes of action of the VOR: yaw, roll, and pitch (Brandt, 1991, Brandt & Dieterich 1994a).

Vestibular disorders in (horizontal) yaw plane
Yaw plane signs are horizontal nystagmus, past pointing, rotational and lateral body falls, deviation of perceived straight ahead.

Vestibular disorders in (frontal) roll plane
Roll plane signs are torsional nystagmus, skew deviation, ocular torsion, tilts of head, body, and perceived vertical.

Vestibular disorders in (sagittal) pitch plane
Pitch plane signs are upbeat/downbeat nystagmus, forward/backward tilts and falls, deviations of perceived horizontal.

The thus defined VOR syndromes allow for a precise topographic diagnosis of brainstem lesions as to their level and side (Brandt & Dieterich, 1994a).

- *A tone imbalance in yaw* indicates lesions of the lateral medulla including the root entry zone of the eighth nerve and/or the vestibular nuclei.
- *A tone imbalance in roll* indicates unilateral lesions (ipsiversive at pontomedullary level, contraversive at pontomesencephalic level).
- *A tone imbalance in pitch* indicates bilateral (paramedian) lesions or bilateral dysfunction of the flocculus.

It is hypothesized that signal processing of the VOR in roll and pitch is conveyed by the same rather than separate ascending pathways in the medial longitudinal fasciculus and the brachium conjunctivum. A unilateral lesion (or stimulation) of these 'graviceptive' pathways (which transduce input from vertical semicircular canals and otoliths) affects function in roll, whereas bilateral lesions (or stimulation) affects function in pitch. Thus, the vestibular system is able to change its functional plane of action from roll to pitch by switching from a unilateral to a bilateral mode of operation.

Pure syndromes in yaw are rare, since the small causative area covering the medial and superior vestibular nucleus is not only adjacent to but overlapped by the structures also subserving roll and pitch function. A lesion frequently

Table 46.8. Central vestibular syndromes

Site	Syndrome	Mechanism/Etiology
Vestibular cortex (multisensory)	Vestibular epilepsy	Vestibular seizures are auras (simple or complex partial multisensory seizures)
	Volvular epilepsy	Sensorimotor 'vestibular' rotatory seizures with walking in small circles
	Non-epileptic cortical vertigo	Rare rotatory vertigo in acute lesions of the parieto-insular vestibular cortex
	Spatial hemineglect (contraversive)	Multisensory horizontal deviation of spatial attention with (right) parietal or frontal cortex lesions
	Transient room-tilt illusions	Paroxysmal or transient mismatch of visual- and vestibular 3D spatial coordinate maps in vestibular brainstem, parietal, or frontal cortex lesions
	Tilt of perceived vertical with body lateropulsion (mostly contraversive)	Vestibular tone imbalance in roll with acute lesions of the parieto-insular vestibular cortex
Thalamus	Thalamic astasia	Dorsolateral vestibular thalamic lesions
	Tilt of perceived vertical (ipsiversive or contraversive) with body lateropulsion	Vestibular tone imbalance in roll
Mesodiencephalic brainstem	Ocular tilt reaction (contraversive; ipsiversive if paroxysmal)	Vestibular tone imbalance in roll (integrator-ocular tilt reaction with lesions of the interstitial nucleus of Cajal)
	Torsional nystagmus (ipsiversive or contraversive)	Ipsiversive in lesions of the interstitial nucleus of Cajal Contraversive in rostral lesions of the medial longitudinal fascicle
Mesencephalic brainstem	Skew torsion (contraversive)	Vestibular tone imbalance in roll with lesions of medial longitudinal fascicle
	Upbeat nystagmus	Vestibular tone imbalance in pitch in bilateral brachium conjunctivum lesions
Ponto-medullary brainstem	Tilt of perceived vertical, lateropulsion, ocular tilt reaction	Vestibular tone imbalance in roll with medial and/or superior vestibular nuclei lesions
	Pseudo 'vestibular neuritis'	Lacunar infarction or MS plaque at the root entry zone of the eighth nerve
	Downbeat nystagmus	Vestibular tone imbalance in pitch
	Transient room-tilt illusion	Acute severe vestibular tone imbalance in roll or pitch
	Paroxysmal room-tilt illusion in MS	Transversally spreading ephaptic axonal activity
	Paroxysmal dysarthria/ataxia in MS	Transversally spreading ephaptic axonal activation
	Paroxysmal vertigo evoked by lateral gaze	Vestibular nuclei lesion?
Medulla	Upbeat nystagmus	Vestibular tone imbalance in pitch? (nucleus prepositus hypoglossi)
Vestibular cerebellum	Downbeat nystagmus	Vestibular tone imbalance in pitch caused by bilateral flocculus lesions (disinhibition)
	Positional downbeat nystagmus	Disinhibited otolith–canal interaction in nodulus lesions?
	Familial episodic ataxia (EA1 with myokymia and EA2 with vertigo)	EA1 = autosomally dominant inherited potassium channelopathy EA2 = autosomally dominant inherited calcium channelopathy
	Encephalitis with predominant vertigo	Viral infection of cerebellum
	Epidemic vertigo	Viral infection of cerebellum

results in mixed (e.g. torsional and horizontal) nystagmus. The lesional sites of yaw syndromes are restricted to the pontomedullary level because of the short distance between the vestibular nuclei and the integration centre for horizontal eye movements in the paramedian pontine reticular formation. Syndromes in roll and pitch, however, may arise from brainstem lesions located in an area extending from the medulla to the mesencephalon, an area corresponding to the large distance between the vestibular nuclei and the integration centres for vertical and torsional eye movements in the rostral midbrain. Whereas vestibular tone imbalances in pitch, which involve bilateral pathways, may occur with various intoxications or metabolic disorders, this is an unusual etiology for tone imbalances in yaw or roll, which involve vestibular pathways unilaterally.

Some vestibular disorders are characterized by a simultaneously peripheral and central vestibular involvement. Examples are large acoustic neurinomas, infarctions of the anterior inferior cerebellar artery, head trauma, and syndromes induced by alcohol intoxication. Others may affect the vestibular nerve root in the brainstem (lacunar infarction, focal demyelination in MS).

Cortical vestibular syndromes include vestibular seizures (vestibular epilepsy) and lesional dysfunction with tilt of the perceived vertical, lateropulsion, rarely rotational vertigo. There is no primary vestibular cortex, but cortical vestibular function is embedded in a network of multisensory visual–vestibular–somatosensory functions and distributed over several separate and distinct areas in the temporo-parietal region.

The parieto-insular vestibular cortex (Guldin & Grüsser, 1996) seems to act as a kind of main integration centre. Dysfunction of this multisensory and sensorimotor cortex for spatial orientation and self-motion perception may be involved in spatial hemineglect and rare paroxysmal room-tilt illusions. Visual–vestibular interaction in self-motion perception is obviously based on reciprocal inhibitory interaction, a mechanism that makes perception of self-motion more robust and largely insensitive to visual–vestibular mismatches.

Most central vertigo syndromes have a specific locus (Table 46.8) but not a specific etiology.

Acknowledgment

I thank Judy Benson for copy-editing the manuscript.

References   * denotes key references

Arbusow, V., Strupp, M. & Brandt, T. (1998). Amiodarone-induced severe prolonged head-positional vertigo and vomiting. *Neurology*, **51**, 917.

Arbusow, V., Schulz, P., Strupp, M. et al. (1999). Distribution of herpes simplex virus type 1 in human geniculate and vestibular ganglia: implications for vestibular neuritis. *Am. Neurol.*, **46**, 416–19.

*Baloh, R.M. & Halmagyi, G.M. (eds.) (1996). *Disorders of the Vestibular System*. New York: Oxford University Press.

Baloh, R.W., Jacobson, K. & Honrubia, V. (1989). Idiopathic bilateral vestibulopathy. *Neurology*, **39**, 272–5.

Bárány, R. (1921). Diagnose von Krankheitserscheinungen im Bereiche des Otolithenapparates. *Acta Otolaryngol.* (Stockh.), **2**, 334–437.

Brandt, Th. (1991). Man in motion. Historical and clinical aspects of vestibular function. *Brain*, **114**, 2159–74.

*Brandt, T. (1999). *Vertigo: Its Multisensory Syndromes*, 2nd edn. London: Springer-Verlag.

Brandt, T. & Dieterich, M. (1994a). Vestibular syndromes in the roll plane: topographic diagnosis from brainstem to cortex. *Ann. Neurol.*, **36**, 337–47.

Brandt, Th. & Dieterich, M. (1994b). Vestibular paroxysmia: vascular compression of the eighth nerve? *Lancet*, **i**, 798–9.

Brandt, Th. & Steddin, S. (1993). Current view of the mechanism of benign paroxysmal positioning vertigo: cupulolithiasis or canalolithiasis? *J. Vestib. Res.*, **3**, 373–82.

Brandt, Th. & Daroff, R.B. (1980a). Physical therapy for benign paroxysmal positional vertigo. *Arch. Otolaryngol.*, **106**, 484–5.

Brandt, Th. & Daroff, R.B (1980b). The multisensory physiological and pathological vertigo syndromes. *Ann. Neurol.*, **7**, 195–203.

Brandt, Th., Steddin, S. & Daroff, R.B. (1994). Therapy for benign paroxysmal positioning vertigo, revisited. *Neurology*, **44**, 796–800.

*Bronstein, A.M., Brandt, T. & Woollacott, M. (1996). *Clinical Disorders of Balance, Posture and Gait*. London: Arnold.

*Curthoys, I.S. & Halmagyi, G.M. (1994). Vestibular compensation: a review of the oculomotor, neural, and clinical consequences of unilateral vestibular loss. *J. Vestib. Res.*, **5**, 67–107.

Dandy, W.E. (1941). The surgical treatment of Menière disease. *Surg. Gynecol. Obstet.*, **72**, 421–5.

*Dieringer, N. (1995). 'Vestibular compensation': neural plasticity and its relations to functional recovery after labyrinthine lesions in frogs and other vertebrates. *Prog. Neurobiol.*, **46**, 97–129.

Epley, J.M. (1992). The canalith repositioning procedure: for treatment of benign paroxysmal positional vertigo. *Otolaryngol. Head Neck Surg.*, **107**, 399–404.

Flohr, H., Bienhold, H., Abeln, W. & Macskovics, I. (1981). Concepts of vestibular compensation. In *Lesion-Induced Neuronal Plasticity in Sensorimotor Systems*, ed. H. Flohr & W. Precht, pp 153–72. New York: Springer.

Foster, C. & Baloh, R.W. (1996). Drug therapy for vertigo. In *Disorders of the Vestibular System*, ed. R.W. Baloh & G.M.

Halmagyi, pp. 541–50. Oxford University Press, Oxford : New York.

Gacek, R.R. (1984). Cupulolithiasis and posterior ampullary nerve transection. *Ann. Otol. Rhinol. Laryngol.* (Suppl. 112). **93**, 25–9.

*Guldin, W. & Grüsser, O-I. (1996). The anatomy of the vestibular cortices of primates. In *Le Cortex Vestibulaire*, ed. M. Collard, M. Jeannerod & Y. Christen, pp 17–26. Boulogne: Ipsen.

Hain, T.C., Fetter, M. & Zee, D.S. (1987). Head-shaking nystagmus in patients with unilateral peripheral vestibular lesions. *Am. J. Otolaryngol.*, **8**, 36–47.

Halmagyi, G.M. & Curthoys, I.S. (1988). A clinical sign of canal paresis. *Arch. Neurol.*, **45**, 737–9.

Herdman, S.J., Tusa, R.J., Zee, D.S., Proctor, L.R. & Mattox, D.E. (1993). Single treatment approaches to benign paroxysmal positional vertigo. *Arch. Otolaryngol. Head Neck Surg.*, **119**, 450–4.

Jannetta, P.J. (1975). Neurovascular cross-compression in patients with hyperactive dysfunction symptoms of the eighth cranial nerve. *Surg. Forum*, **26**, 467–8.

Jannetta, P.J., Møller, M.B. & Møller, A.R. (1984). Disabling positional vertigo. *N. Engl. J. Med.*, **310**, 1700–5.

Leigh, J. & Brandt, T. (1993). A reevaluation of the vestibulo-ocular reflex: new ideas of its purpose, properties, neural substrate, and disorders. *Neurology*, **43**, 1288–95.

McClure, J.A. (1985). Horizontal canal BPPV. *J. Otolaryngol.*, **14**, 30–5.

Manning, C., Scandale, L., Manning, E.J. & Gengo, F.M. (1992). Central nervous system effects of meclicine and dimenhydrinate: evidence of acute tolerance to antihistamines. *J. Clin. Pharmacol.*, **32**, 996–1002.

Møller, M.B., Møller, A.R., Jannetta, P.J. & Sekhar, L.N. (1986). Diagnosis and surgical treatment of disabling positional vertigo. *J. Neurosurg.*, **64**, 21–8.

Pace-Balzan, A. & Rutka, J.A. (1991). Non-ampullary plugging of the posterior semicircular canal for benign paroxysmal positional vertigo. *J. Laryngol. Otol.*, **105**, 901–6.

Parnes, L.S. & McClure, J.A. (1991). Posterior semicircular canal occlusion in the normal hearing ear. *Otolaryngol. Head Neck Surg.*, **104**, 52–7.

Rinne, T., Bronstein, A.M., Rudge, P., Gresty, M.A. & Luxon, L.M. (1995). Bilateral loss of vestibular function. *Acta Otolaryngol., (Stockh).* Suppl **520**, 247–50.

Schuknecht, H.F. (1969). Cupulolithiasis. *Arch. Otolaryngol.*, **90**, 765–78.

*Schuknecht, H.F. & Kitamura, K. (1981). Vestibular neuritis. *Ann. Otol. Rhinol. Laryngol.*, Suppl **90**, 1–19.

Semont, A., Freyss, G. & Vitte, E. (1988). Curing the BPPV with a liberatory maneuver. *Adv. Otorhinolaryngol.*, **42**, 290–3.

Steddin, S. & Brandt, T. (1996). Horizontal canal benign paroxysmal positioning vertigo (h-BPPV): transition of canalolithiasis to cupulolithiasis. *Ann. Neurol.*, **40**, 918–22.

Strupp, M., Arbusow, V., Maag, K.P., Gall, C. & Brandt, T. (1998). Vestibular exercises improve central vestbulo-spinal compensation after an acute unilateral peripheral vestibular lesion: a prospective clinical study. *Neurology*, **51**, 838–44.

Vibert, D., Liard, P. & Häusler, R. (1995). Bilateral idiopathic loss of peripheral vestibular function with normal hearing. *Acta Otolaryngol., (Stockh.)* **115**, 611–15.

Part V

Disorders of spine and spinal cord

47

Spinal cord injury and repair

John W. McDonald

Department of Neurology and Neurological Surgery, Center for the Study of Nervous System Injury,
Washington University School of Medicine, St. Louis MO, USA

Many victims of spinal cord injury are young and will live a near-normal lifespan (Fig. 47.1). Therefore, the toll to individuals and society is high. The average lifetime cost of treating a person with traumatic spinal cord injury in the United States runs between $500 000 and $2 million, depending on factors such as the extent of injury and where the cord is injured (higher levels correspond to greater disability and greater costs). Total direct costs of caring for Americans with spinal cord injury exceed $8 billion per year (DeVivo, 1997).

Current state of acute pharmacological treatment

This enormous human and economic toll calls for effective therapies. It was not until the 1990s, however, that the first proven therapy for spinal cord injury was introduced. A multicentre clinical study (National Acute Spinal Cord Injury Study, NASCIS 2) revealed that a high dose of the steroid methylprednisolone reduced disability when administered within 8 hours of the trauma (Bracken et al., 1990). Although the effectiveness of this drug was modest, the availability of any treatment for spinal cord injury was heartening. Subsequently, the multicentre NASCIS 3 trial compared treatment with methylprednisolone for 24 h (same treatment as in NASCIS 2) vs. treatment for 48 h. All patients treated with methylprednisolone within 3 hours of injury showed essentially identical rates of motor recovery. When treatment was initiated between 3 h and 8 h of injury, patients receiving the 48-hour protocol showed significantly more improvement in motor function. Therefore, the US standard of care is administration of methylprednisolone (bolus 30 mg/kg) within the first 8 h after injury. Treatment initiated within the first 3 h is continued (5.4 mg/kg/h) for 24 h, whereas treatment initiated between 3 h and 8 h is continued for 48 h.

Despite these studies, methylprednisolone remains controversial in other countries (Short et al., 2000). Additional experimental drugs, including SYGEN (GM-1 ganglioside), naloxone, and trilizad, have been tested in multicentre clinical trials, but primary endpoints were never achieved.

More recently, cellular and molecular advances in neurobiology have provided powerful insights into the nature of spinal cord injury and opened up new horizons for neural repair and restoration of function. In this chapter we describe how this rapidly burgeoning knowledge might be harnessed to help individuals with spinal cord unjury regain lost functions.

The working cord

The spinal cord is the primary pathway of communication between the brain and the body (Fig. 47.2, see colour plate section), and excellent reviews of its anatomy and physiology are available elsewhere (Byrne et al., 2000).

Millions of axons carry impulses up and down the spinal cord. Axons from neurons in the brain's motor cortex travel up to 1 metre to reach target neurons at each segmental level of the cord; the target neurons connect to relevant muscle cells in the body. Sensations from the skin and other organs travel as electrical signals in the reverse direction, relayed to the appropriate segment of the spinal cord and then up through axons within the cord to locations in the brain and cerebellum. These ascending sensory pathways allow you to feel the soft fur of a kitten, to sense pain when stung by a bee, to locate the position of your arm in the dark, and to know when to empty your bladder. The motor and sensory pathways are organized in a well-understood somatotopic manner, with sacral fibres tending to be more peripheral and cervical fibres more central. This discrete

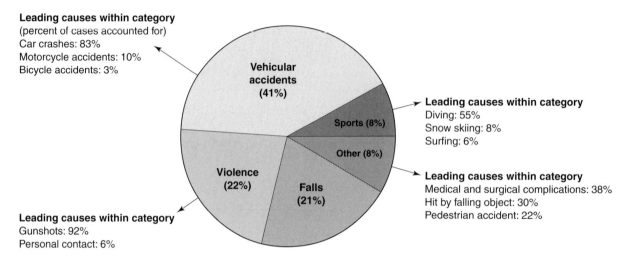

Leading causes within category
(percent of cases accounted for)
Car crashes: 83%
Motorcycle accidents: 10%
Bicycle accidents: 3%

Leading causes within category
Diving: 55%
Snow skiing: 8%
Surfing: 6%

Leading causes within category
Medical and surgical complications: 38%
Hit by falling object: 30%
Pedestrian accident: 22%

Leading causes within category
Gunshots: 92%
Personal contact: 6%

Fig. 47.1. Spinal cord injuries result from traumatic and non-traumatic causes (1994–1998), in roughly equal numbers. The following numbers and pie chart refer to traumatic cases in the United States. Incidence: 10 000 new cases per year. Prevalence: about 230 000. Men account for about 80% of cases. Most (43%) patients are injured between ages 16 and 30, whereas 28% are injured between ages 31 and 45. (Data were obtained from the National Spinal Cord Injury Statistical Center, University of Alabama, Birmingham.)

anatomical and physiological organization provides an ideal venue for research.

When injury strikes

Traumatic injury directly damages the delicate spinal cord with mechanical force, which typically is generated when broken fragments of vertebrae or soft tissue (ligament, herniated disc) impinge on the cord. Within minutes, small-blood vessels hemorrhage, and the spinal cord swells. These events obstruct the normal delivery of nutrients and oxygen to the injured part of the cord, causing many local neurons and glia to starve to death. This immediate damage is not the end of the destruction. A cascade of events triggered by the initial injury leads to secondary injury that progressively enlarges the damaged region during subsequent minutes, hours, and days (Fig. 47.3, see colour plate section). As a result of both initial and secondary injury, the cord can be left in disarray, with neuronal synaptic connections disrupted and many untraumatized axons rendered inactive by demyelination. With the exception of high velocity gunshot injuries and knife wounds, however, it is not common for trauma to completely sever the spinal cord. In postmortem studies, more than 60% of cases show some continuity of CNS tissue across the lesion (Bunge et al., 1993). Typically, a doughnut-shaped rim of white matter remains at the injury level (Bunge et al., 1993; Kakulas et al., 1998; Kakulas, 1999a,b) (Fig. 47.4). However,

scarring and the formation of a fluid-filled cavity (a syrinx) can occur, providing physical barriers to axon regeneration. Unlike many of the rodent contusion spinal cord injury models that reproducibly produce a central syrinx at the lesion site, only 20% to 30% of persons surviving traumatic spinal cord injury have a syrinx (Bunge et al., 1993).

What can be done about these barriers to functional recovery? Most laboratories are trying to accomplish two main therapeutic goals: limiting tissue damage, primarily by blocking important steps in the secondary injury cascade, and enhancing recovery, primarily by promoting the regeneration and reconnection of nerve cells. Accomplishing these goals in an optimal manner will require multiple interventions, administered in an orderly sequence, and involving a delicate balance between enhancing favourable (e.g. growth-promoting) factors and neutralizing unfavourable (e.g. growth-inhibiting) ones (Fig. 47.5, see colour plate section).

Terminology, classification and evolution of clinical approaches

To establish a foundation for understanding human spinal cord injury, we will provide clinical terminology and discuss outcomes. To convey severity, medical caregivers use the simple but accurate American Spinal Injury Association (ASIA) Impairment Scale (Table 47.1), a 5-category (A to E) system (ASIA, 1996). Although this classification scale has

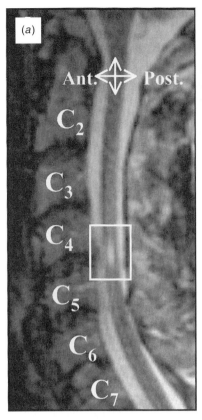

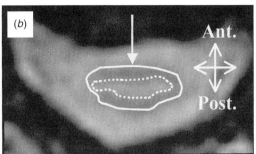

Fig. 47.4. When the spinal cord is damaged, conduction along axons is blocked, and the normal transfer of information to and from the brain is disrupted. (*a*) and (*b*) show a magnetic resonance image (MRI) of the cervical spinal cord of a patient who experienced a traumatic injury more than 20 years ago. It illustrates the presence of a fluid-filled cavity, called a syrinx, at the original injury site. (*a*) and (*b*) are T_2-weighted MRIs in sagittal (*a*) and axial (*b*) planes. The inset box in (*a*) highlights the injury level at C4/5 and demonstrates a fluid-filled syrinx (white) in the middle of the cord. (*b*) shows the syrinx more closely. The solid white line outlines the outer diameter of the spinal cord at the C4/5 level. The inner dotted white line outlines the fluid-filled syrinx. Therefore, the doughnut-shaped area between the two circles outlines the preserved cord tissue.

traditionally used the terms 'complete' and 'incomplete', there is no benefit to retaining such confusing, redundant, and outdated terminology. The terms mean little to individuals with spinal cord injury and, in most cases, are mistakenly believed to indicate the degree of anatomical connection (e.g. incomplete) or disconnection (severed cord; e.g. complete) of the spinal cord. Dimitrijevic and colleagues (Dimitrijevic, 1988; Dimitrijevic et al., 1983) introduced the term 'discomplete' to explain their finding of electrophysiological transmission of signals across a lesion in individuals with ASIA class A injuries (e.g. clinically complete, having lost all sensation and voluntary motor functions below the level of the lesion). Such a term is also not very useful because most injuries that do not physically separate the cord leave residual axonal connections across the lesion (Bunge et al., 1993; Kakulas, 1999a,b).

Our ability to accurately predict clinical outcomes based on early examination is very limited. The most important predictor of better outcomes is retention of sacral sensation (S4–5), particularly pinprick, 72 h to 1 week after injury (Waters et al., 1995; Marino et al., 1999). The most relevant generalities that can be drawn from the many years of outcome studies in the field are summarized in Table 47.2.

About 10% to 15% of individuals with ASIA A-grade lesions convert to ASIA B–D; however, only about 3% regain functional strength below the lesion level (ASIA D). Approximately 54% of individuals with initial sacral sensory sparing (ASIA B grade) gain substantial functional strength below the lesion (e.g. will convert to ASIA C–D).

Eighty-six per cent of those classified as ASIA C–D at 72 h regain useful motor function. Age is also a prognostic factor: in central cord syndromes, 91% of patients under age 50 recover ambulation, whereas only 41% over age 50 recover similar capabilities. Recovery of function is the most relevant endpoint for individuals with spinal cord injury and their caregivers. Table 47.3 outlines predicted functional recovery based on injury level for the more severe (A–C) ASIA grades.

When spinal cord damage results from trauma, most initial ER examinations reveal no function below the level of injury, primarily because of spinal shock. Spinal shock is an interesting but poorly understood phenomenon (Bachy-Rita & Illis, 1993) and this initial lack of function does not necessarily predict a poor outcome, and it should not influence medical and surgical decisions. The usefulness of tests such as motor and sensory evoked potentials,

Table 47.1. ASIA impairment scale

Scale grade	ASIA impairment scale
A	Complete: no motor or sensory function is preserved in the sacral segments S4–S5
B	Incomplete: sensory but not motor function is preserved below the neurologic level and includes the sacral segments S4–S5
C	Incomplete: motor function is preserved below the neurologic level, and more than half of key muscles below the neurologic level have a muscle strength grade <3
D	Incomplete: motor function is preserved below the neurologic level, and at least half of key muscles below the neurologic level have a grade of 3 or above
E	Normal: motor and sensory functions are normal.

cranial magnetic stimulation, and functional imaging is being examined, but these are still early days.

The recent rush of scientific advances in aspects of regeneration has changed the way we interact with individuals with spinal cord injury. We used to tell newly injured individuals that recovery was unlikely and that they should adapt to life in a wheelchair. This approach is no longer considered productive. Although the clinician's armamentarium for treating spinal cord injury remains limited by the lag between laboratory observations and clinical trials, we can now offer hope, because regeneration and some restoration of function are becoming achievable targets. The old view of limiting rehabilitation to ergonomics, adaptation, and strengthening is giving way to the idea that therapies that promote regeneration can restore additional function. Thus, studies of how environmental factors affect recovery from CNS injury are attracting attention (Ivanco & Greenough, 2000). The constraint-induced, forced-use studies in stroke rehabilitation (for review see Taub et al., 1999) and all the developmental data indicating the importance of patterned neural activity in preserving and (re-)generating the CNS, support the theory that modifying the environment to optimize neural activity is an important therapeutic goal.

Limiting secondary injury

As in conditions such as stroke (see 'Cellular mechanisms of neurological damage', 'Principles of neuroprotection',

Table 47.2. Summary of recovery in ASIA A–D patients

ASIA A

1. Most (60% to 90%) regain one motor level (Stauffer, 1984).
2. 0% to 11% will improve one or more ASIA grades (Frankel et al., 1969; Maynard et al., 1979; Wu et al., 1992; Bedbrook & Sakae, 1982; Stover & Fine, 1986; Ditunno et al., 1995).
3. 4% to 10% may undergo late conversion (after 30 days) to ASIA B or better (Waters et al., 1991, 1993). This can occur up to 2.5 yrs after injury.
4. Most motor recovery occurs during the first 6 months after injury, with the greatest rate of change during the initial 3 months. Motor strength can continue to improve during second year.
5. Muscles graded 1–3 in the zone of partial preservation (ZPP) will recover useful motor function.

ASIA B–D

6. Of ASIA B patients, sacral preservation of pinprick denotes better prognosis for recovery of functional ambulation than ability to sense light touch: 66% to 89% pinprick vs. 11% to 14% light touch (Foo et al., 1981; Folman & el Masri, 1989; Crozier et al., 1991; Waters et al., 1994; Katoh & el Masry, 1995).
7. Of ASIA C patients, 52% to 76% recover to ASIA D or E, compared with 20% to 28.3% of all ASIA B patients (Frankel et al., 1969; Ditunno et al., 1995; Bedbrook & Sakae, 1982; Stauffer, 1983).
8. Central cord syndromes (CCS): generally favourable prognosis (Merriam et al., 1986; Foo, 1986; Penrod et al., 1990; Roth et al., 1990), but age is a key determinant, with patients <50 yr having a better prognosis for ambulation than patients over 50 yr (97% vs. 41%). (Foo, 1986; Merriam et al., 1986; Penrod et al., 1990).
9. In general, Brown–Sequard syndrome (BSS) lesions recover more than central cord syndromes, which recover more than anterior cord syndromes (Stauffer, 1984).

and 'Principles of ischemic stroke management', Chapters 5, 14, 81, this volume and Volume 2), trauma to the spinal cord appears to induce additional neural cell death through a process called excitotoxicity (for review see Schwab & Bartholdi, 1996; Lee et al., 1999; McDonald et al., 1999). Glutamate, an amino acid neurotransmitter normally released in minute amounts from nerve terminals for signalling, is discharged excessively after neuronal injury (McAdoo et al., 1997). Building up in the extracellular space, it overactivates receptors on the membranes of neighbouring neurons and glial cells. These glutamate receptors open ion channels, admitting large amounts of

Table 47.3. Expected functional outcome based on injury level

Level (ASIA)	Breathing	Mobility	Driving	Transfers	Bowel	Bladder	Eating & grooming	Dressing upper extremities	Dressing lower extremities
C1–3	D	Power chair	N/A	D	D	D	D	D	D
C4	I	Power chair	N/A	D	D	D	D	D	D
C5	I	Power chair	Modified van	D	D	D	Partially D	Partially D	D
C6	I	Power and manual chair	Modified van	Perhaps I	I	I–O D–O	Partially D	Partially D	D
C7–8	I	Manual chair	Hand controls	I	I	I	I	I	Perhaps I
T1–12	I	Manual chair; bipedal ambulation with extensive bracing	Hand controls	I	I	I	I	I	I
L–S	I	Manual chair; bipedal ambulation with/without bracing	With/without hand controls	I	I	I	I	I	I

Notes:

D = dependent.

I = independent.

O = orthosis.

calcium and sodium into the cells. The resulting sustained elevation in intracellular calcium triggers a series of destructive events: protein-destroying enzymes are switched on, and bursts of oxygen free radicals damage cell membranes and intracellular organelles. Unable to withstand these insults, nerve cells die, compounding the direct damage from the initial mechanical injury.

As well as protecting neurons from excitotoxic injury, it is vital to protect spinal cord white matter, the outer ring of tissue that carries ascending and descending axons. It is not uncommon for a lesion to be confined to the central tissue, which contains nerve cell bodies (grey matter), while the surrounding white matter is spared. Such a central cord lesion confines motor and sensory disturbances to areas innervated at that level (for example, a C6 lesion affects the upper limbs) without much affecting function below that level, such as gait, bowel or bladder function. In contrast, destruction of white matter at the same segment, even if the injury spares grey matter, renders a person tetraplegic and incontinent.

Several studies of animal models of spinal cord injury suggest that anti-excitotoxic treatments can be beneficial (Faden & Simon, 1988; Wrathall et el., 1994). However, initial work that focused on the role of NMDA-type glutamate receptors documented preferential protection of grey matter, which did not bode well for functional improvements that depend on white matter preservation (most animal models involve thoracic spinal cord injury). More recent work has focused attention on the benefits of blocking a subclass of glutamate receptors called AMPA receptors (Wrathall et al., 1994, 1996). Such treatment protects white matter and improves locomotor function, but understanding of the cellular mechanism awaits later studies.

Although excitotoxicity has traditionally been thought to kill only neurons, recent studies suggest that it may also kill oligodendrocytes, which myelinate CNS axons. Thus, excitotoxic damage to oligodendrocytes contributes to white matter injury (Matute et al., 1997; McDonald et al., 1998a, 1998b, 1999; Li et al., 1999b; Li & Stys, 2000) and to demyelination and axonal conduction block often found in the injured spinal cord (Gledhill et al., 1973; Bresnahan, 1978; Bunge et al., 1993; Waxman, 1989, 1992).

In the past 5 years, recognition that a second form of cell death, programmed cell death or apoptosis, also occurs in the injured spinal cord, has opened new doors to protective strategies (Kerr et al., 1972; Wyllie et al., 1980). Apoptosis is essential to normal CNS development, when it removes unneeded cells, and it may be triggered inappropriately later in life when certain key structures, such as DNA, sustain damage (Johnson et al., 1996; Lee et al., 1999), leading to the unfortunate loss of nerve cells. Many of the neuroprotective effects of neurotrophins observed in animal and in vitro models of CNS injury prevent such apoptotic death of neurons and glia. Thus, NT-3 and BDNF have well-described injury-limiting effects in addition to prominent regenerative actions (see below).

Recent animal (Crowe et al., 1997; Liu et al., 1997; Shuman et al., 1997; Li et al., 1999a; Springer et al., 1999) and human (Emery et al., 1998) studies have revealed that a prominent wave of oligodendrocyte apoptosis may occur days to weeks after spinal cord injury, at quite remote sites. This delayed reaction may be triggered by a combination of early excitotoxic injury and a later loss of vital surface or trophic factor interactions as truncated axons slowly degenerate (for review see Beattie et al., 2000; Zipfel et al., 2000). Furthermore, administration of drugs or creation of dominant negative mutations that inhibit apoptosis permits rats and mice subjected to traumatic spinal cord injury to regain a better level of ambulation (Liu et al., 1997; Li et al., 2000).

Ultimately, treatments aimed at reducing secondary damage in the injured spinal cord will likely encompass multiple drugs delivered at different intervals and targeted at specific mechanisms of cell death in distinct cell populations. Almost certainly, the strategy of blocking excitotoxic and apoptotic death pathways will be augmented by delivery of trophic factors capable of promoting neuronal and glial cell survival. A great deal has been learned recently about the identities of these factors, their effects, and their mechanisms of action. Factors that regulate the production of neurotrophins and their receptors in oligodendrocytes, astrocytes, and microglia also have been discovered, and these may be useful for enhancing production of selected neurotrophins in the injured spinal cord.

Once interventions can limit secondary tissue injury as much as possible, the therapeutic focus will shift to promoting nerve cell regeneration and reconnection. The reminder of this article will summarize emerging concepts and potential strategies in this area. To obtain meaningful recovery of function, we will not need to completely shield the damaged spinal cord from secondary injury or entirely rebuild it. Preserving or re-establishing a fraction of the lost connections may enhance important functions, such as control of the bladder, bowel, and respiration. Studies from as early as the 1950s have indicated that preservation of less than 10% of the normal axon complement in the cat spinal cord can support walking (Blight, 1983), though this should not be viewed as the optimal requirement for restoring function. Moreover, detailed anatomical post-mortem studies of chronic human spinal cord injury reveal that small residual connections across the lesion can preserve some function (Kakulas, 1999a,b). In one individual with ASIA C spinal cord injury, only 1.17 mm^2 of white matter remained at the level of the lesion. One individual with some preserved motor function below the level of cervical injury had only 3175 corticospinal axons, less than 8% of the number (41 472) of similar axons in normal controls.

Injuries that are lower by just a single segment, at cervical level C6 instead of C5, for example (a difference of about 1.7 cm) also have fewer effects. Whereas a person with a C5 injury level has no upper extremity function other than limited motion at the shoulders, a person with a C6 injury can move shoulder and elbow joints, and surgical transfer of muscle tendons may restore partial hand function. Therefore, small anatomical gains can result in disproportionately higher functional gains Therapeutic implications of this observation are that small additive and stepwise treatments can be expected to produce large gains in function.

The critical balance

A complex constellation of signals is required for successful regeneration of spinal cord cells and for axons to reach their correct targets during development and regeneration. The fate of disconnected axons is determined by the balance between growth-promoting (chemoattractant) and growth-inhibiting (chemorepulsant) molecules in the local environment. The growth cone on the tip of a regenerating axon makes directional choices based on the multitude of guidance molecules it encounters.

Large families of guidance molecules have been discovered. They can be: (i) presented on the surface of a cell, (ii) fixed to the extracellular matrix, or (iii) secreted into extracellular fluid. Moreover, interactions can be simple or intricate. Some molecules act by altering the electrical charge of the local environment. Others work in a lock-and-key fashion, docking at specific receptors on target axons. These interactions can trigger a complex chemical cascade within the growth cone that makes the cone retreat, advance, or both, depending on the nature of the effectors. Soluble growth factors are being evaluated for their ability to stimulate regeneration after spinal cord injury, but the manipulation of substrate-bound guidance molecules lies largely in the future. Tipping the balance in favour of growth enhancement vs. growth inhibition will be the cornerstone of success.

Regrowth of nerve fibres: overcoming inhibition

Unlike developing neurons, mature peripheral nerves or certain networks in the CNS of invertebrates, fish, amphibians, and reptiles, mammals regenerate poorly after their axons are severed. This does not appear to be an intrinsic limitation of the adult neuron itself, however. In the 1980s,

Albert J. Aguayo and colleagues showed that adult rat neurons can regenerate when provided with a permissive environment. Using a piece of peripheral nerve from the leg as a graft, they constructed a bridge across the injured region of the spinal cord and redirected the cut axons across the graft. After many weeks, they observed robust axonal regeneration from the spinal cord into the graft, in some cases up to 30 to 40 mm (Richardson et al., 1980; David & Aguayo, 1981). But the credit for the first demonstration of the capacity of CNS neurons to regenerate predates these studies by 70 years (Tello, 1911); pieces of peripheral nerve were transplanted into the cortex of young rabbits, and several weeks later bundles of fibres entered the graft. These observations suggest that mammalian central neurons are reluctant to regrow after injury because of shortcomings in their immediate environment.

One promising approach to this problem is to study systems that can regenerate so factors that promote or inhibit regeneration can be identified. A particularly attractive system is the immature mammalian CNS. For example, spinal cord axons from the South American opossum, *Monodelphis domestica*, can regenerate after injury before, but not after, postnatal day 11 (for review see Nicholls & Saunders, 1996). The abrupt loss of regenerative capability appears in several cases to correlate with onset of myelination. Thus, motor axons in the hatchling chick regenerate if the spinal cord is cut before oligodendrocytes myelinate them (Steeves et al., 1994). Also, experimentally delaying myelination extends the period during which injured axons can regenerate (Keirstead et al., 1992). These studies suggest that myelin formation may be a key barrier to axon regeneration in the mature mammalian spinal cord.

More than a decade of work has focused on identifying specific nerve growth-preventing proteins in myelin (for review see Schwab et al., 1993; Schwab & Bartholdi, 1996), and the gene for one of these was recently cloned (Nogo A & B; Chen et al., 2000). Called myelin-associated neurite growth inhibitors, these proteins can prevent axonal outgrowth from cultured neurons (for review see Huber & Schwab, 2000). Applying a neutralizing antibody (termed IN–1, for inhibitor neutralizing antibody) induced axon growth from neurons cultured on the inhibitory molecules. Furthermore, infusing IN-1 into the injured rat spinal cord promoted long-distance regeneration in a small percentage of interrupted axons and improved the rats' ability to use their forepaws (Schnell & Schwab, 1990; von Meyenburg et al., 1998). In preparation for clinical trials, the active part of IN-1 has been cloned and re-engineered to be more acceptable to the human immune system. These recombinant humanized antibody fragments have recently been tested for their safety and regenerative properties in animal models of spinal cord injury (Brosamle et al., 2000).

Research has expanded the list of isolated inhibitory molecules to many families (Fitch & Silver, 1997; Kapfhammer, 1997), including the proteoglycans (for review, see Davies & Silver, 1998). In recent studies, regenerating axons from adult neurons stopped growing when confronted with a chondroitin sulfate proteoglycan-rich boundary, though they were able to cross the lesion and extend for long distances in the boundary's absence (Davies et al., 1997). Given the apparent multiplicity of molecules capable of inhibiting nerve fibre regeneration, a cocktail of drugs may be necessary to fully unmask the natural capacity of adult spinal cord neurons to regenerate after injury. As well as blocking inhibitory proteins (e.g. with antibody), it also might be possible to reduce inhibition by down-regulating production of these proteins. As the genes for key inhibitor molecules are cloned, researchers will be able to study their regulatory sites. This knowledge could be used to determine how expression of an inhibitory protein changes after injury and to devise methods for turning off the relevant gene.

Promoting outgrowth

As well as removing the inhibition of axonal regeneration, it might be possible to increase the availability of growth-promoting molecules. Major insights have come from studying axonal outgrowth during normal embryonic development. More than four decades ago, Rita Levi-Montalcini and Viktor Hamburger identified and isolated nerve growth factor (NGF), a small, soluble protein that supports the survival and development of sensory and sympathetic neurons. This pioneering work precipitated a successful search for additional neurotrophic factors, and NGF is now known to be one of a family of related neurotrophins that promote neuronal cell survival and axonal outgrowth during embryogenesis; several other families of trophic factors also have been identified (for review see Lindsay et al., 1994). However, synthesis of the messenger RNA needed to produce neurotrophic factors and their receptors can be depressed for weeks following spinal cord injury. Also, responses to neurotrophic factors can be selective for specific cell types and individual cell functions, depending on the location and expression of the receptors that are activated. For example, NT-3 selectively stimulates regrowth of injured corticospinal tract axons (Schnell et al., 1994; Grill et al., 1997; Houweling et al., 1998; von Meyenburg et al., 1998). It also can enhance cell survival and promote remyelination

(McTigue et al., 1998). In contrast, the fibroblast growth factor (FGF) family has more widespread effects, both in promoting growth and stimulating the formation of new cells from progenitors (see below). They also affect non-neural cell function. Growth-related factors such as platelet-derived growth factor (PDGF) can stimulate the replication of oligodendrocyte progenitors (for review, see Grinspan et al., 1994).

Considerable evidence suggests that endogenous production of growth factors in the injured cord falls short and that boosting the supply might improve cell survival and regeneration. This might be achieved by exogenous administration, endogenous delivery via gene transfer (see below), or modulating cellular production. Manipulating factors that regulate neurotrophin production might selectively enhance production of certain neurotrophins in the injured spinal cord and therefore promote regeneration. Promising results with many of the neurotrophic factors have been achieved in models of spinal cord injury (Schnell et al., 1994; Grill et al.;, 1997; Blesch et al., 1998; Houweling et al., 1998; von Meyenburg et al., 1998; McTigue et al., 1998; Zhang et al., 1998; Liu et al., 1999; Blits et al., 2000).

These efforts will need to be wary of unintended consequences, such as enhancing pain, already a common long-term complication of spinal cord injury (excellent reviews of this area are available: Beric, 1997; Christensen & Hulsebosch, 1997). Pain might increase because of aberrant axon sprouting within the CNS or by peripheral mechanisms such as growth factor-mediated sensitization of skin nociceptors (Mendell, 1999; Shu & Mendell, 1999). A paradoxical injury-enhancing effect of neurotrophins has also been recognized, in both culture and in vivo models of spinal cord injury (Koh et al., 1995; Gwag et al., 1995; McDonald et al., 2002).

Establishing correct functional connections

Promoting nerve outgrowth will be useful only if strategies to link regenerated axons with their suitable synaptic targets also can be developed. Powerful insights into axon guidance have come from studies of the developing nervous system, where a complex set of temporally and spatially regulated events coordinates the precise formation of intricate neural circuits. In the embryo, molecular signals that act directly on the leading tip (growth cone) of the lengthening axon choreograph outgrowth. Fortunately, the last several years have produced unprecedented advances in identifying many new families of targeting, guidance, and adhesion molecules that are expressed during development (for review see Leutwyler, 1995;

Tessier-Lavigne & Goodman, 1996; Guthrie & Varela-Echavarria, 1997; Walsh & Doherty, 1997; Terman & Kolodkin, 1999; Joosten & Bar, 1999; Quinn et al., 1999; Raper, 2000 (see also Chapter 97 by Compston in Volume 2)). Some are diffusible molecules released from cells. Their concentration gradients attract the growth cone, guiding it to another neuron or developing muscle fibre. Other signals are contained in the extracellular matrix (the material outside cells). For instance, a family of factors called netrins helps guide axons in the mammalian spinal cord by calling axons in one direction and repelling them from others (Serafini et al., 1994). By displaying netrins and other guidance molecules as if they were highway signs, the extracellular matrix acts as scaffolding that tells axons precisely where to go. Like highway signs, these signals must appear in the correct sequence; otherwise, an axon would lose its way. Unfortunately, we do not yet know how to reconstitute this sequence after injury. However, our present level of understanding may permit the design of interventions aimed at modulating the presentation of some of these guidance molecules, perhaps well enough to aid regeneration. Moreover, recent experiences with grafted fetal neurons have suggested that some axons can find appropriate targets even without additional chemical signals.

Building bridges

Since the demonstration that peripheral nerves can support the regrowth of CNS axons (Richardson et al., 1980; David & Aguayo, 1981) and, in one case, lead to the formation of functional synaptic connections, many research groups have explored the value of bridging the gap created by cord damage (Fig 47.5, see colour plate section). In one study, Schwann cells (the myelinating glia of the peripheral nervous system) transplanted into the spinal cord promoted axonal regeneration after a section of the spinal cord was completely removed (Xu et al., 1995). The Schwann cell produces a variety of growth factors and extracellular matrix molecules known to promote axon regeneration. Grown in culture and packed into a plastic-like tube, they have been used to connect the two ends of transected spinal cord. In combination with growth factor or methylprednisolone treatments, these grafts have allowed neurons to grow axons (Menei et al., 1998).

Knowledge of bridges and inhibitory factors has been combined to enhance behavioural recovery in spinal cord-injured rats. Peripheral nerves were grafted between the two ends of a severed spinal cord, and glue made of fibrin kept the nerves in place and released acidic fibroblast growth factor (aFGF) into the injured area (Cheng et al., 1996, 1997). The peripheral nerves were directed from white matter to the less inhibitory grey matter so regenerating axons would grow in that direction. Six months after this procedure, the corticospinal tract had partly regenerated. The rats also had regained some ability to walk. These studies have been difficult to replicate in other laboratories perhaps because of the complexity of the surgery.

Lessons learned from the Schwann cell have provided insights into what makes a good cellular candidate for supporting axonal regrowth (Bunge, 1993). An exciting example is the recent transplantation of olfactory ensheathing glial cells. These cells are found only in the olfactory nerve and bulb, and they reside in a unique area that permits axons to grow continually throughout adult life (for review, see Ramon-Cueto & Avila, 1998). In an early study, olfactory ensheathing glial cells were transplanted into the rat spinal cord where the corticospinal tract had been cut. After several months, there was partial regrowth of corticospinal axons and some improvement in the limb functions these nerves normally control (Li et al., 1997). In another study, transplanting ensheathing glia into cut cord stumps next to Schwann cell grafts led to long-distance axonal regeneration. It also improved growth of regenerated axons from graft into contiguous cord (Ramon-Cueto et al., 1998). Additional studies add to the intriguing concept that transplanted olfactory ensheathing glial cells might be competent escorts for regenerating axons in the damaged spinal cord (Ramon-Cueto & Nieto-Samparedo, 1994; Ramon-Cueto et al., 1994, 1998, 2000; Li et al., 1997, 1998; Perez et al., 1998; Navarro et al., 1999). Some work even suggests that these cells might be capable of myelinating single axons akin to Schwann cells (Li et al., 1997; Imaizumi et al., 1998, 2000; Barnett et al., 2000), but this finding remains controversial because these cells normally wrap groups of axons and their isolation is susceptible to contamination by Schwann cells. Understanding their regeneration-aiding properties is a next step for scientists. Armed with the why and how, researchers may be able to create or engineer cells that exhibit combinations of growth-promoting properties.

Replacing lost cells: cell transplants and genetic vectors

Cell transplants can serve three important functions (for review see Bjorklund & Lindvall, 2000). First, they can generate a local supply of key molecules, such as growth factors or guidance molecules, to promote cellular survival or regeneration. Secondly, they can provide mechanical stability and serve as a bridge (see above), supporting the regrowth of injured CNS axons. Third, they can replace lost neuronal or glial cells, restoring cellular functions such as signalling and axon myelination.

Adult neurons are unsuitable for transplantation because they neither divide nor survive isolation and relocation. Several different types of cells have been successfully transplanted into the injured spinal cord, however. They include fetal spinal cord tissue, immortalized neural cell lines, genetically engineered fibroblasts, CNS stem cells, and embryonic stem (ES) cells.

For several decades, pioneering groups have explored the transplantation of fetal CNS tissue into animal models of spinal cord injury. This tissue survives and partially integrates into the injured host cord, leading to limited segmental forms of functional recovery (Nygren et al., 1977; Buchanan & Nornes, 1986; Reier et al., 1986; Bernstein & Goldberg, 1987; Yakovleff et al., 1989; Jakeman & Reier, 1991; Bregman et al., 1993). Host fibres grow into the transplants, and transplanted neurons extend axons into host tissue. This valuable experience has emphasized the therapeutic potential of immature neuronal cells, but ethical dilemmas and the availability of suitable tissue limit the usefulness of this approach in humans. Another source of transplantable material is cell lines derived from central neurons that have been transformed by retroviral vectors. The cells are immature and capable of indefinite replication. They survive and respond to local environmental cues after transplantation; moreover, the adult CNS retains the capacity to direct their differentiation into more mature neurons (Park et al., 1999; Vescovi & Snyder, 1999; Whittemore, 1999). There is concern that such immortalized cells might undergo malignant transformation and become cancerous, however.

Other laboratories have used genetically engineered non-neuronal cells to obtain neurotrophic molecules and extracellular matrix molecules known to promote regeneration. This approach was recently applied to the injured spinal cord (Grill et al., 1997; McTigue et al., 1998). Fibroblasts were engineered to produce the neurotrophic molecule NT-3. After the cells were transplanted into the cut spinal cord, there was substantial regrowth of the corticospinal tract and improved stepping across the graft (Grill et al., 1997). Later work demonstrated enhanced myelination of regenerated axons in the graft (McTigue et el., 1998). The ability of this approach to provide effective bridges that support the regrowth of host axons is a particular strength that may well drive its incorporation into future therapies.

Another approach to cellular replacement is to take advantage of stem cells still present in the adult CNS. These retain the fetal capacity to survive isolation, replicate, and differentiate into mature cells. For many years, it was believed that the number of neurons in the mammalian brain and spinal cord is fixed at birth and that neurons cannot be replaced, unlike cells in organs such as skin or liver. As early as the 1960s, however, pioneering studies demonstrated that some cells in the adult hippocampal dentate gyrus divide, differentiating into neurons (Altman & Das, 1965). Such progenitor cells can be isolated from the mature brain, cultured, and transplanted back into adult brain, where they can turn into neurons. Recently, this approach has been expanded to cells isolated from the mature spinal cord (Shihabuddin et al., 1997; Horner et al., 2000).

Exciting recent work has demonstrated that formation of new neurons is a more universal and dynamic process that occurs even in adult humans (Eriksson et al., 1998; Del Bigio, 1999). The process appears to be influenced by the local physical and chemical environment (Kempermann et al., 1998; Kempermann and Gage, 1999; Gould et al., 1999a,b; Nilsson et al., 1999). However, we are just beginning to understand how to regulate progenitor cell birth and survival of subsequent differentiated neural cells, and endogenous production of sufficient numbers of cells to replace those lost from spinal cord injury is not feasible at present. The potential consequences of disturbing these neurotransmitter systems with the polypharmacy typically used to treat spinal cord injury should be carefully weighed against putative benefits.

How might stem cells be used for spinal cord repair? As we begin to understand the signals that determine when stem cells divide and how they commit to a particular cell fate (oligodendrocyte, astrocyte, or neuron), we may be able to isolate adult stem cells from a biopsy of the injured spinal cord, propagate them to gain adequate numbers, induce them to form the required cell types, and transplant them back into the same person's injured cord. Moreover, stem cells can be genetically engineered as easily as fibroblasts, so they could be made to function as biological timed-release capsules, delivering growth factors or guidance molecules at key stages of regeneration. Unlike fibroblasts, stem cells are capable of migrating and integrating into host tissue. Thus stem cells delivered to a single site might repopulate remote locations.

Other researchers are beginning to examine even more primordial stem cells, called embryonic stem cells, which are pluripotent (capable of forming any cell in the body) and immortal (living and dividing forever). Such cells have been isolated from rats, fish, chickens, Rhesus monkeys, and most recently from humans (Shamblott et al., 1998; Thomson et al., 1998; Itskovitz-Eldor et al., 2000; for review, see McDonald, 2002). When embryonic stem cells that were induced by retinoic acid to become neural precursors were transplanted into the contusion injury site of rat spinal cord 9 days after injury, they migrated long distances, differentiated into neurons, astrocytes, and oligodendrocytes, and promoted some recovery of locomotion (McDonald et al., 1999). That was an important result because no previous studies had demonstrated improved walking when transplantation was delayed for more than 24 hours. Subsequently, embryonic stem cells have been successfully coaxed to produce oligodendrocyte precursors that can myelinate axons in culture and when transplanted into the immature CNS (Brustle et al., 1999) and the injured adult spinal cord (Liu et al., 2000).

Neural xenotransplantation is another approach. It has been attempted in individuals with Huntington's disease (Philpott et al., 1997; Bachoud-Levi et al., 2000), Parkinson's disease (Kordower et al., 1995, 1998; Freeman et al., 1999), stroke (http://www.laytonbio.com; http://www.diacrin.com), epilepsy (http://www.diacrin.com), and spinal cord injury (Reier et al., 1994; Thompson et al., 1998; Wirth et al., 1999; http://www.diacrin.com). Xenotransplantation is favoured for use in human studies now since the greatest safety data is available. The major disadvantage of this approach is the possibility of rejection of the foreign tissue.

As an alternative to cell transplantation, replication-deficient viral vectors could transfer genes coding for desirable growth factors, blocking antibodies, or guidance molecules directly into surviving spinal cord cells. Virus-mediated gene transfer is most easily achieved into dividing cell types, but adenoviruses and lentiviruses have been used experimentally to transfer genes into non-dividing adult neurons (Suhr & Gage, 1999; Kafri et al., 2000). Maintaining high levels of foreign gene expression over time and limiting destruction by the host's immune system remain significant technical hurdles to clinical use. The recent development of 'gutless' adenoviruses, which lack the genes for immunoreactive coat molecules, and the design of strategies to protect infected cells by selectively repelling or killing invading immune cells are producing headway.

Finally, not all CNS diseases are equally amenable to cell replacement therapy. The best chance for success may lie in applications whose clinical efficacy is determined by a single defined biological mechanism, such as myelination to restore long-tract neurotransmission in spinal cord injury. We will do well, however, not to promise too much too early and to focus on therapies that would seem likely to work, such as those that have shown benefits in animal models. At present, achievable neuronal transplantation is limited to re-establishing local, short-distance connections (such as interneurons). Long-tract connections across a spinal cord lesion have not been seen in any animal model.

Perhaps the most success in animal models has been achieved by transplanting oligodendrocytes and their progenitors. Both the biology of the oligodendrocyte lineage and myelination are well understood, and this glial system is relatively simple compared with the neuronal system, which involves dozens of types of neurons and tens of thousands of interconnections. Therefore, the inherent risks associated with glial cells are limited compared with those associated with neurons.

Restoration of function: limited rebuilding, not cure

Fortunately, all available evidence indicates that the damaged spinal cord will not have to be completely rebuilt to obtain meaningful recovery. Animal studies suggest that less than 10% of functional long-tract connections are required to support locomotion (Blight, 1983). As previously mentioned, the preserved rim of white matter that carries long tracts between the brain and periphery of the body might be sufficient to restore meaningful function. Animal studies indicate that axons in this rim commonly remain anatomically intact but are non-functional because of focal demyelination or faulty myelination. Therefore, remyelinating intact connections seems like a reasonable approach to restoring function (Gledhill et al., 1973; Waxman, 1992; Bunge et al., 1993). Although such limited restoration may not enable people with spinal cord injury to walk, it might restore control over the bowel and bladder or improve limb mobility. Such gains facilitate independence.

Several research groups have suggested that some functional recovery may be possible without remyelination if conduction along existing dysfunctional axons can be improved. They used a potassium-channel blocker called 4-aminopyridine to enhance the flow of nerve impulses, allowing axons to transmit electrical information past demyelinated zones (Blight, 1989; Waxman, 1993). Some patients treated with 4-aminopyridine had encouraging improvement in aspects of sensory or motor function (Hansebout et al., 1993; Hayes et al., 1993, 1994).

Also, rats that sustained a lesion of the left corticospinal tract at the level of the brainstem were treated with IN-1. This antibody treatment improved movements of the forepaw (movements requiring corticospinal function) even though only a small fraction of the transected fibres regenerated. Recovery was probably attained by compensatory sprouting and reinnervation of denervated targets by unharmed fibre systems, a phenomenon not observed in untreated rats (Z'Graggen et al., 1998; Raineteau et al., 1999). Many other functions, such as gait or breathing, are partially controlled at the level of the spinal cord via central pattern generators. Recovery of limited supraspinal input is required to improve complex functions such as gait.

Rehabilitative strategies for rebuilding function

In addition to the new directions in pharmacologic, genetic, and transplantation research, there is important progress in clinical rehabilitation (for review see Sadowsky et al., 2002). For example, surgical reconstruction can provide important gains in function. Procedures include functional tendon transfers, peripheral nerve transplantation, and nerve splitting to reactive previously paralysed muscles. Functional electrical stimulation (FES) also has achieved considerable success and received FDA approval. It uses sophisticated electronics to activate intact but distant nerves, which then can regain control of muscles rendered useless by spinal cord injury. For example, FES can harness shoulder movements to move a paralysed hand (Fig. 47.6) (Freehand System; http://www.neurocontrol.com) or regain bowel and bladder control (Vocare System; http://www.neurocontrol.com; for review see Sadowsky et al., 2002). An FES system similar to the Freehand system can restore some simple functions to the legs, such as initiating standing to assist in transfers. Simpler FES systems restore diaphragmatic breathing by pacing the phrenic nerve, and they can aid coughing in patients whose respiration is impaired.

Additional research is altering the scope of rehabilitation by modifying neuronal circuitry. Several groups have shown that a distal region of the spinal cord that has been disconnected from the brain by injury is capable of learning and that early gait training may help promote walking abilities in a subset of individuals with spinal cord injury (Lovely et al., 1986; Barbeau & Rossignol, 1987; Wernig & Muller, 1992; for review see Barbeau et al., 1999). The central pattern generators can produce rhythmic, oscillating activity of limb flexor and extensor muscle groups without supraspinal or afferent input, and the molecular mechanisms that contribute to this phenomenon are being unravelled (Grillner et al., 1998; Barbeau et al., 1999). Gait patterns can be elicited by tapping into the central pattern generators via descending input and by sensory feedback. Such rehabilitative treatments may accomplish more than simple training; they may enhance regeneration. Taken together, studies of CNS development and regeneration suggest that optimal levels of patterned

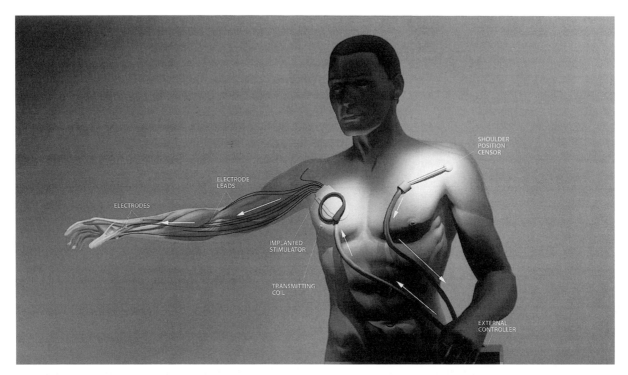

Fig. 47.6. The Freehand System is approved by the FDA for restoration of hand function in spinal cord injury. Particular movements by the opposite shoulder activate a detector that sends signals to an external control unit. That unit, in turn, relays the signals to an implanted transmitting coil connected to wires that terminate on selected arm and hand muscles. Shoulder movements then provide two types of hand function important for grasping a fork or a cup. (Reproduced with permission from *Scientific American* (McDonald et al., 1999).)

neural activity are important for many aspects of regeneration, including remyelination, new synapse formation, and the birth and survival of new progenitor cells. The enhanced functional recovery observed in the recent constraint-induced, forced-use stroke studies may represent such activity-dependent regeneration (Wolf et al., 1989; Miltner et al., 1999; van der Lee et al., 1999).

Development of systems that reduce environmental barriers to mobility and environmental control also is making major headway. For example, Johnson and Johnson recently developed a multicomputer-controlled wheelchair capable of ascending and descending stairs; it may be introduced as early as 2001. Continued progress in clinical rehabilitation will help maximize the benefits attained through advances in protective and regenerative drug therapies.

Acknowledgements

The author would like to thank Dennis Choi, MD, PhD and the members of the Christopher Reeves Paralysis Foundation Research Consortium for enlightening me to the field of spinal cord injury and for help in formulating many of the concepts that I have presented in this manuscript. I also thank Dr Cristina Sadowsky and Oksana Volshteyn for important comments on the manuscript. This work was supported by National Institute of Health grants NS01931, NS37927, NS40520, National Football Leagues, and the Keck Foundation.

References

Altman, J. & Das, G.D. (1965). Post-natal origin of microneurones in the rat brain. *Nature*, **207**, 953–6.

American Spinal Injury Association, International standards for neurological and functional classification of spinal cord injury, revised 1996. Chicago: American Spinal Injury Association, 1996.

Bachoud-Levi, A., Bourdet, C., Brugieres, P. et al. (2000). Safety and tolerability assessment of intrastriatal neural allografts in five patients with Huntington's disease. *Exp. Neurol.*, **161**, 194–202.

Bach-y-Rita, P. & Illis, L.S. (1993). Spinal shock: possible role of receptor plasticity and non synaptic transmission. *Paraplegia*, **31**, 82–7.

Barbeau, H. & Rossignol, S. (1987). Recovery of locomotion after chronic spinalization in the adult cat. *Brain Research*, **412**, 84–95.

Barbeau, H., McCrea, D.A., O'Donovan, M.J., Rossignol, S., Grill, W.M. & Lemay, M.A. (1999). Tapping into spinal circuits to restore motor function. *Brain Res. Rev.*, **30**, 27–51.

Barnett, S.C., Alexander, C.L., Iwashita, Y. et al. (2000). Identification of a human olfactory ensheathing cell that can effect transplant-mediated remyelination of demyelinated CNS axons. *Brain*, **123**, 1581–8.

Beattie, M.S., Farooqui, A.A. & Bresnahan, J.C. (2000). Review of current evidence for apoptosis after spinal cord injury. *J. Neurotrauma*, **17**, 915–26.

Bedbrook, G.M. & Sakae, T. (1982). A review of cervical spine injuries with neurological dysfunction. *Paraplegia*, **20**, 321–33.

Beric, A. (1997). Post-spinal cord injury pain states. *Pain*, **72**, 295–8.

Bernstein, J.J. & Goldberg, W.J. (1987). Fetal spinal cord homografts ameliorate the severity of lesion-induced hindlimb behavioural deficits. *Exp. Neurol.*, **98**, 633–44.

Bjorklund, A. & Lindvall, O. (2000). Cell replacement therapies for central nervous system disorders. *Nat. Neurosci.*, **3**, 537–44.

Blesch, A., Grill, R.J. & Tuszynski, M.H. (1998). Neurotrophin gene therapy in CNS models of trauma and degeneration. *Prog. Brain Res.*, **117**, 473–84.

Blight, A.R. (1983). Cellular morphology of chronic spinal cord injury in the cat: analysis of myelinated axons by line-sampling. *Neuroscience*, **10**, 521–43.

Blight, A.R. (1989). Effect of 4-aminopyridine on axonal conduction-block in chronic spinal cord injury. *Brain Res. Bull.*, **22**, 47–52.

Blits, B., Dijkhuizen, P.A., Boer, G.J. & Verhaagen, J. (2000). Intercostal nerve implants transduced with an adenoviral vector encoding neurotrophin-3 promote regrowth of injured rat corticospinal tract fibres and improve hindlimb function. *Exp. Neurol.*, **164**, 25–37.

Bracken, M.B., Shepard, M.J., Holdford, T.R. et al. (1990). A randomized, controlled trial of methylprednisolone or naloxone in the treatment of acute spinal-cord injury. Results of the Second National Acute Spinal Cord Injury Study. *N. Engl. J. Med.*, **322**, 1405–11.

Bregman, B.S., Kunkel-Bagden, E., Reier, P.J., Dai, H.N., McAtee, M. & Gao, D. (1993). Recovery of function after spinal cord injury: mechanisms underlying transplant-mediated recovery of function differ after spinal cord injury in newborn and adult rats. *Exp. Neurol.*, **123**, 3–16.

Bresnahan, J.C. (1978). An electron-microscopic analysis of axonal alterations following blunt contusion of the spinal cord of the rhesus monkey (*Macaca mulatta*). *J. Neurol. Sci.*, **37**, 59–82.

Brosamle, C., Huber, A.B., Fiedler, M., Skerra, A. & Schwab, M.E. (2000). Regeneration of lesioned corticospinal tract fibres in the adult rat induced by a recombinant, humanized IN-1 antibody fragment. *J. Neurosci.* **20**, 8061–8.

Brustle, O., Jones, K.N., Learish, R.D. et al. (1999). Embryonic stem cell-derived glial precursors: a source of myelinating transplants. *Science*, **285**, 754–6.

Buchanan, J. & Nornes, H.O. (1986). Transplants of embryonic brain-stem containing the locus coeruleus into spinal cord enhance the hindlimb flexion reflex in adult rats. *Brain Res.* **381**, 225–36.

Bunge, R.P. (1993). Expanding roles for the Schwann cell: ensheathment, myelination, trophism, and regeneration. *Curr. Opin. Neurobiol.*, **3**, 805–9.

Bunge, R.P., Puckett, W.R., Becerra, J.L., Marcillo, A. & Quencer, R.M. (1993). Observations on the pathology of human spinal cord injury. A review and classification of 22 new cases with details from a case of chronic cord compression with extensive focal demyelination. *Adv. Neurol.*, **59**, 75–89.

Byrne, T.N., Benzel, E.C. & Waxman, S.G. (2000). *Diseases of the Spine and Spinal Cord: Contemporary Neurology Series*, 58. New York, NY: Oxford University Press.

Chen, M.S., Huber, A.B., van der Haar, M.E. et al. (2000). Nogo-A is a myelin-associated neurite outgrowth inhibitor and an antigen for monoclonal antibody IN-1. *Nature*, **403**, 434–9.

Cheng, H., Cao, Y. & Olson, L. (1996). Spinal cord repair in adult paraplegic rats: partial restoration of hind limb function. *Science*, **273**, 510–13.

Cheng, H., Almstrom, S., Gimenez-Llort, L. et al. (1997). Gait analysis of adult paraplegic rats after spinal cord repair. *Exp. Neurol.*, **148**, 544–57.

Christensen, M.D. & Hulsebosch, C.E. (1997). Chronic central pain after spinal cord injury. *J. Neurotrauma*, **14**, 517–37.

Crowe, M.J., Bresnahan, J.C., Shuman, S.L., Masters, J.N. & Beattie, M.S. (1997). Apoptosis and delayed degeneration after spinal cord injury in rats and monkeys. *Nat. Med.*, **3**, 73–6.

Crozier, K.S., Graziani, V., Ditunno, J.F. Jr, & Herbison, G.J. (1991). Spinal cord injury: prognosis for ambulation based on sensory examination in patients who are initially motor complete. *Arch. Phys. Med. Rehabil.*, **72**, 119–21.

David, S. & Aguayo, A.J. (1981). Axonal elongation into peripheral nervous system 'bridges' after central nervous system injury in adult rats. *Science*, **214**, 931–3.

Davies, S.J. & Silver, J. (1998). Adult axon regeneration in adult CNS white matter. *Trends in Neurosci.*, **21**, 515.

Davies, S.J., Fitch, M.T., Memberg, S.P., Hall, A.K., Raisman, G. & Silver, J. (1997). Regeneration of adult axons in white matter tracts of the central nervous system. *Nature*, **390**, 680–3.

Del Bigio, M.R. (1999). Proliferative status of cells in adult human dentate gyrus. *Microscopic Res. Techniques*, **45**, 353–8.

DeVivo, M.J. (1997). Causes and cost of spinal cord injury in the United States. *Spinal Cord*, **35**, 809–13.

Dimitrijevic, M.R. (1988). Residual motor functions in spinal cord injury. In *Functional Recovery in Neurological Disease*, ed. S.G. Waxman, pp. 139–55. Raven Press: New York.

Dimitrijevic, M.R., Faganel, J. Lehmkuhl, D. & Sherwood, A. (1983). Motor control in man after partial or complete spinal cord injury. *Adv. Neurol.*, **39**, 915–26.

Ditunno, J.F., Cohen, M.S., Formal, C. & Whiteneck, G.G. (1995). Functional outcomes. In Stover S.I., DeLisa, J.A., Whiteneck, G.G., eds. *Spinal Cord Injury: Clinical Outcomes from the Model Systems*, pp. 170–84. Gaithersburg, MD: Aspen Publishers.

Emery, E., Aldana, P., Bunge, M.B. et al. (1998). Apoptosis after traumatic human spinal cord injury. *J. Neurosurg.*, **89**, 911–20.

Eriksson, P.S., Perfilieva, E., Bjork-Eriksson, T. et al. (1998). Neurogenesis in the adult human hippocampus. *Nat. Med.*, **4**, 1313–17.

Faden, A.I. & Simon, R.P. (1988). A potential role for excitotoxins in the pathophysiology of spinal cord injury. *Ann. Neurol.*, **23**, 623–6.

Fitch, M.T. & Silver, J. (1997). Glial cell extracellular matrix: boundaries for axon growth in development and regeneration. *Cell Tissue Res.*, **290**, 379–84.

Folman, Y. & Masri, W. (1989). Spinal cord injury: prognostic indicators. *Injury*, **20**, 92–3.

Foo, D. (1986). Spinal cord injury in forty-four patients with cervical spondylosis. *Paraplegia*, **24**, 301–6.

Foo, D., Subrahmanyan, T.S. & Rossier, A.B. (1981). Post-traumatic acute anterior spinal cord syndrome. *Paraplegia*, **19**, 201–5.

Frankel, H.L., Hancock, D.O., Hyslop, G. et al. (1969). The value of postural reduction in the initial management of closed injuries of the spine with paraplegia and tetraplegia. I. *Paraplegia*, **7**, 179–92.

Freeman, T.B., Vawter, D.E., Leaverton, P.E. et al. (1999). Use of placebo surgery in controlled trials of cellular-based therapy for Parkinson's disease. *N. Engl. J. Med.*, **341**, 988–92.

Gage, F.H. (1998). Cell Therapy. *Nature*, **392**, 18–24.

Geisler, F.H., Dorsey, F.C. & Coleman, W.P. (1991). Recovery of motor function after spinal-cord injury – a randomized, placebo-controlled trial with GM-1 ganglioside. *N. Engl. J. Med.*, **324**, 1829–38.

Gledhill, R.F., Harrison, B.M. & McDonald, W.I. (1973). Demyelination and remyelination after acute spinal cord compression. *Exp. Neurol.*, **38**, 472–87.

Gould, E., Beylin, A., Tanapat, P., Reeves, A. & Shors, T.J. (1999a). Learning enhances adult neurogenesis in the hippocampal formation. *Nat. Neurosci.*, **2**, 260–5.

Gould, E., Tanapat, P., Hastings, N.B. & Shors, T.J. (1999b). Neurogenesis in adulthood: a possible role in learning. *Trends in Cogn. Sci.*, **3**, 186–92.

Grill, R., Murai, K., Blesch, A., Gage, F.H. & Tuszynski, M.H. (1997). Cellular delivery of neurotrophin-3 promotes corticospinal axonal growth and partial functional recovery after spinal cord injury. *J. Neurosci.*, **17**, 5560–72.

Grillner, S., Ekeberg, E.E. Manira, A. et al. (1998). Intrinsic function of a neuronal network – a vertebrate central pattern generator. *Brain Res. Rev.*, **26**, 184–97.

Grinspan, J.B., Stern, J., Franceschini, B., Yasuda, T. & Pleasure, D. (1994). Protein growth factors as potential therapies for central nervous system demyelinative disorders. *Ann. Neurol.*, **36**, S140–2.

Guthrie, S. & Varela-Echavarria, A. (1997). Molecules making waves in axon guidance. *Genes Dev.*, **11**, 545–57.

Gwag, B.J., Koh, J.Y., Chen, M.M. et al. (1995). BDNF and IGF-1 potentiates free radical-mediated injury in cortical cell cultures. *NeuroReport*, **7**, 93–6.

Hansebout, R.R., Blight, A.R., Fawcett, S. & Reddy, K. (1993). 4-Aminopyridine in chronic spinal cord injury: a controlled, double-blind, crossover study in eight patients. *J. Neurotrauma*, **10**, 1–18.

Hayes, K.C., Blight, A.R., Potter, P.J. et al. (1993). Preclinical trial of 4-aminopyridine in patients with chronic spinal cord injury. *Paraplegia*, **31**, 216–24.

Hayes, K.C., Potter, P.J., Wolfe, D.L., Hsieh, J.T., Delaney, G.A. & Blight, A.R. (1994). 4-Aminopyridine-sensitive neurologic deficits in patients with spinal cord injury. *J. Neurotrauma*, **11**, 433–46.

Horner, P.J., Power, A.E., Kempermann, G. et al. (2000). Proliferation and differentiation of progenitor cells throughout the intact adult rat spinal cord. *J. Neurosci.*, **20**, 2218–28.

Houweling, D.A., Lankhorst, A.J., Gispen, W.H., Bar, P.R. & Joosten, E.A. (1998). Collagen containing neurotrophin-3 (NT-3) attracts regrowing injured corticospinal axons in the adult rat spinal cord and promotes partial functional recovery. *Exp. Neurol.*, **153**, 49–59.

Huber, A.B. & Schwab, M.E. (2000). Nogo-A, a potent inhibitor of neurite outgrowth and regeneration. *Biol. Chem.*, **381**, 407–19.

Imaizumi, T., Lankford, K.L., Waxman, S.G., Greer, C.A. & Kocsis, J.D. (1998). Transplanted olfactory ensheathing cells remyelinate and enhance axonal conduction in the demyelinated dorsal columns of the rat spinal cord. *J. Neurosci.*, **18**, 6176–85.

Imaizumi, T., Lankford, K.L. & Kocsis, J.D. (2000). Transplantation of olfactory ensheathing cells or Schwann cells restores rapid and secure conduction across the transected spinal cord. *Brain Res.*, **854**, 70–8.

Itskovitz-Eldor, J., Schuldiner, M., Karsenti, D. et al. (2000). Differentiation of human embryonic stem cells into embryoid bodies comprising the three embryonic germ layers. *Mol. Med.*, **6**, 88–95.

Ivanco, T.L. & Greenough, W.T. (2000). Physiological consequences of morphologically detectable synaptic plasticity: potential uses for examining recovery following damage. *Neuropharmacology*, **39**, 765–76.

Jakeman, L.B. & Reier, P.J. (1991). Axonal projections between fetal spinal cord transplants and the adult spinal cord: a neuroanatomical tracing study of local interactions. *J. Comp. Neurol.*, **307**, 311–34.

Jenkins, W.M. & Merzenich, M.M. (1987). Reorganization of neocortical representations after brain injury: a neurophysiological model of the basis of recovery from stroke. *Prog. Brain Res.*, **71**, 249–66.

Johnson, E.M., Deckwerth, T.L. & Deshmukh, M. (1996). Neuronal death in developing models: possible implications in neuropathology. *Brain Pathol.*, **6**, 397–409.

Joosten, E.A. & Bar, D.P. (1999). Axon guidance of outgrowing corticospinal fibres in the rat. *J. Anat.*, **194**, 15–32.

Kafri, T., van Praag, H., Gage, F.H. & Verma, I.M. (2000). Lentiviral vectors: regulated gene expression. *Mol. Therap.*, **1**, 516–21.

Kakulas, B.A., Lorimer, R.L. & Gubbay, A.D. (1998). White matter changes in human spinal cord injury. In ed. E. Stalberg, H.S. Sharma, Y. Olson, *Spinal Cord Monitoring*, Wien, New York: Springer-Verlag Publishers.

Kakulas, B.A. (1999a). The applied neuropathology of human spinal cord injury. *Spinal Cord*, **37**, 79–88.

Kakulas, B.A. (1999b). A review of the neuropathology of human spinal cord injury with emphasis on special features. *J. Spinal Cord Med.*, **22**, 119–24.

Kapfhammer, J.P. (1997). Restriction of plastic fibre growth after lesions by central nervous system myelin-associated neurite growth inhibitors. *Adv. Neurol.*, **73**, 7–27.

Katoh, S. & el Masry, W.S. (1995). Motor recovery of patients presenting with motor paralysis and sensory sparing following cervical spinal cord injuries. *Paraplegia*, **33**, 506–9.

Keirstead, H.S., Hasan, S.J., Muir, G.D. & Steeves, J.D. (1992). Suppression of the onset of myelination extends the permissive period for the functional repair of embryonic spinal cord. *Proc. Natl. Acad. Sci., USA*, **89**, 11664–8.

Kempermann, G., Brandon, E.P. & Gage, F.H. (1998). Environmental stimulation of 129/SvJ mice causes increased cell proliferation and neurogenesis in the adult dentate gyrus. *Curr. Biol.*, **8**, 939–42.

Kempermann, G. & Gage, F.H. (1999). New nerve cells for the adult brain. *Sci. Amer.*, **280**, 48–53.

Kerr, J.F.R., Wyllie, A.H. & Currie, A.R. (1972). Apoptosis: a basic biological phenomenon with wide-ranging implications in tissue kinetics. *Br. J. Cancer*, **26**, 239–57.

Koh, J-Y, Gwag, B.J., Lobner, D. & Choi, D. (1995). Potentiated necrosis of cultured cortical neurons by neurotrophins. *Science*, **268**, 573–5.

Kordower, J.H., Freeman, T.B., Snow, B.J. et al. (1995). Neuropathological evidence of graft survival and striatal reinnervation after the transplantation of fetal mesencephalic tissue in a patient with Parkinson's disease. *N. Engl. J. Med.*, **332**, 1118–24.

Kordower, J.H., Freeman, T.B., Chen, E.Y. et al. (1998). Fetal nigral grafts survive and mediate clinical benefit in a patient with Parkinson's disease. *Movem. Dis.*, **13**, 383–93.

Lee, J.M., Zipfel, G.J. & Choi, D.W. (1999). The changing landscape of ischaemic brain injury mechanisms. *Nature*, **399**, A7–14.

Leutwyler, K. (1995). The great attractors. Chemical guides direct young neurons to their final destinations. *Sci. Amer.*, **272**, 17–20.

Li, S. & Stys, P.K. (2000). Mechanisms of ionotrophic glutamate receptor-mediated excitotoxicity in isolated spinal cord white matter. *J. Neurosci.*, **20**, 1190–8.

Li, Y., Field, P.M. & Raisman, G. (1997). Repair of adult rat corticospinal tract by transplants of olfactory ensheathing cells. *Science*, **227**, 2000–2.

Li, Y., Field, P.M. & Raisman, G. (1998). Regeneration of adult rat corticospinal axons induced by transplanted olfactory ensheathing cells. *J. Neurosci.*, **18**, 10514–24.

Li, G.L., Farooque, M., Holtz, A. & Olsson, Y. (1999a). Apoptosis of oligodendrocytes occurs for long distances away from the primary injury after compression trauma to rat spinal cord. *Acta Neuropathol.*, **98**, 473–80.

Li, S., Mealing, G.A., Morley, P. & Stys, P.K. (1999b). Novel injury mechanism in anoxia and trauma of spinal cord white matter: glutamate release via reverse Na$^+$-dependent glutamate transport. *J. Neurosci.*, **19**, RC16.

Li, M., Ona, V.O., Chen, M. et al. (2000). Functional role and therapeutic implications of neuronal caspase-1 and -3 in a mouse model of traumatic spinal cord injury. *Neuroscience*, **99**, 333–42.

Lindsay, R.M., Wiegand, S.J., Altar, C.A. et al. (1994). Neurotrophic factors, from molecule to man. *Trends Neurosci.*, **17**, 182–90.

Liu, X.Z., Xu, X.M., Hu, R. et al. (1997). Neuronal and glial apoptosis after traumatic spinal cord injury. *J. Neurosci.*, **17**, 5395–406.

Liu, Y., Kim, D., Himes, B.T. et al. (1999). Transplants of fibroblasts genetically modified to express BDNF promote regeneration of adult rat rubrospinal axons and recovery of forelimb function. *J. Neurosci.*, **19**, 4370–87.

Liu, S., Qu, Y., Steward, T. et al. (2000). Embryonic stem cells differentiate into oligodendrocytes and myelinate in culture and after spinal cord transplantation. *Proc. Natl. Acad. Sci., USA*, **97**, 6126–31.

Lovely, R.G., Gregor, R.J., Roy, R.R. & Edgerton, V.R. (1986). Effects of training on the recovery of full weight-bearing stepping in the adult spinal cat. *Exp. Neurol.*, **92**, 421–35.

McAdoo, D.J., Hughes, M.G., Xu, G.Y., Robak, G. & de Castro, R. Jr. (1997). Microdialysis studies of the role of chemical agents in secondary damage upon spinal cord injury. *J. Neurotrauma*, **14**, 507–15.

McDonald, J.W. (2001). ES cells and neurogenesis. In *Stem Cells and CNS Development*, ed. M.S. Rao, pp. 207–61. Totowa NJ: Humana Press.

McDonald, J.W., Althomsons, S.P., Hyrc, K.L., Choi, D.W. & Goldberg, M.P. (1998a). Oligodendrocytes are highly vulnerable to AMPA/kainate receptor-mediated excitotoxicity. *Nat. Med.*, **4**, 291–7.

McDonald, J.W., Levine, J.M. & Qu, Y. (1998b). Multiple classes of the oligodendrocyte lineage are highly vulnerable to excitotoxicity. *NeuroReport*, **9**, 2757–62.

McDonald, J.W. and the Research Consortium of the Christopher Reeve Paralysis Foundation (1999). Repairing the damaged spinal cord. *Sci. Amer.*, **281**, 64–73.

McDonald, J.W., Liu, Z-X., Shin, H., Liu, S. & Choi, D.W. (2001). Neurotrophin-induced potentiation of spinal cord injury. *J. Neurosci.*, in press.

McKay, R. (1997). Stem cells in the central nervous system. *Science*, **276**, 66–71.

McTigue, D.M., Horner, P.J., Stokes, B.T. & Gage, F.H. (1998). Neurotrophin-3 and brain-derived neurotrophic factor induce oligodendrocyte proliferation and myelination of regenerating axons in the contused adult rat spinal cord. *J. Neurosci.*, **18**, 5354–65.

Marino, R.J., Ditunno, J.F., Donovan, W.H. & Maynard, F. (1999). Neurologic recovery after traumatic spinal cord injury: data from the model spinal cord injury systems. *Arch. Phys. Med. Rehabil.*, **80**, 1391–6.

Matute, C., Sanchez-Gomez, M.V., Martinez-Millan, L. & Miledi, R. (1997). Glutamate receptor-mediated toxicity in optic nerve oligodendrocytes. *Proc. Natl. Acad. Sci., USA*, **94**, 8830–5.

Maynard, F.M., Reynolds, G.G., Fountain, S., Wilmot, C. & Hamilton, R. (1979). Neurological prognosis after traumatic quadriplegia. Three-year experience of California Regional Spinal Cord Injury Care System. *J. Neurosurg.*, **50**, 611–16.

Maynard, F.M. Jr, Bracken, M.B., Creasey, G. et al. (1997).

International standards for neurological and functional classification of spinal cord injury. American Spinal Injury Association. *Spinal Cord*, **35**, 266–74.

Mendell, L.M. (1999). Neurotrophin action on sensory neurons in adults: an extension of the neurotrophic hypothesis. *Pain*, **6**, S127–32.

Menei, P., Montero-Menei, C., Whitemore, S.R., Bunge, R.P. & Bunge, M.B. (1998). Schwann cells genetically modified to secrete human BDNF promote enhanced axonal regrowth across transected adult rat spinal cord. *Eur. J. Neurosci.*, **10**, 607–21.

Merriam, W.F., Taylor, T.K., Ruff, S.J. & McPhail, M.J. (1986). A reappraisal of acute traumatic central cord syndrome. *J. Bone Joint Surg. (British Volume)*, **68**, 708–13.

Miltner, W.H., Bauder, H., Sommer, M., Dettmers, C. & Taub, E. (1999). Effects of constraint-induced movement therapy on patients with chronic motor deficits after stroke: a replication. *Stroke*, **30**, 586–92.

Navarro, X., Valero, A., Gudino, G. et al. (1999). Ensheathing glia transplants promote dorsal root regeneration and spinal reflex restitution after multiple lumbar rhizotomy. *Ann. Neurol.*, **45**, 207–15.

Nicholls, J. & Saunders, N. (1996). Regeneration of immature mammalian spinal cord after injury. *Trends Neurosci.*, **19**, 229–34.

Nilsson, M., Perfilieva, E., Johansson, U., Orwar, O. & Eriksson, P.S. (1999). Enriched environment increases neurogenesis in the adult rat dentate gyrus and improves spatial memory. *J. Neurobiol.*, **39**, 569–78.

Nygren, L-G., Olson, L. & Seiger, A. (1977). Monoaminergic reinnervation of the transected spinal cord by homologous fetal brain grafts. *Brain Res.*, **129**, 227–35.

Park, K.I., Liu, S., Flax, J.D., Nissim, S., Stieg, P.E. & Snyder, E.Y. (1999). Transplantation of neural progenitor and stem cells: developmental insights may suggest new therapies for spinal cord and other CNS dysfunction. *J. Neurotrauma*, **16**, 675–87.

Penrod, L.E., Hegde, S.K. & Ditunno, J.F. Jr (1990). Age effect on prognosis for functional recovery in acute, traumatic central cord syndrome. *Arch. Phys. Med. Rehabil.*, **71**, 963–8.

Perez, A., Wigley, C.G., Nacimiento, W., Noth, J. & Brook, G.A. (1998). Spontaneous orientation of transplanted olfactory glia influences axonal regeneration. *NeuroReport*, **9**, 2971–5.

Philpott, L.M., Kopyov, O.V., Lee, A.J. et al. (1997). Neuropsychological functioning following fetal striatal transplantation in Huntington's chorea: three case presentations. *Cell Transpl.*, **6**, 203–12.

Quinn, C.C., Gray, G.E. & Hockfield, S. (1999). A family of proteins implicated in axon guidance and outgrowth. *J. Neurobiol.*, **41**, 158–64.

Raineteau, O., Z'Graggen, W.J., Thallmair, M. & Schwab, M.E. (1999). Sprouting and regeneration after pyramidotomy and blockade of the myelin-associated neurite growth inhibitors NI 35/250 in adult rats. *Eur. J. Neurosci.*, **11**, 1486–90.

Ramon-Cueto, A. & Avila, J. (1998). Olfactory ensheathing glia: properties and function. *Brain Res. Bull.*, **45**, 175–89.

Ramon-Cueto, A. & Nieto-Sampedro, M. (1994). Regeneration into

the spinal cord of transected dorsal root axons is promoted by ensheathing glia transplants. *Exp. Neurol.*, **127**, 232–44.

Ramon-Cueto, A., Plant, G.W., Avila, J. & Bunge, M.B. (1998). Long-distance axonal regeneration in the transected adult rat spinal cord is promoted by olfactory ensheathing glia transplants. *J. Neurosci.*, **18**, 3808–15.

Ramon-Cueto, A., Cordero, M.I., Santos-Benito, F.F. & Avila, J. (2000). Functional recovery of paraplegic rats and motor axon regeneration in their spinal cord by olfactory ensheathing glia. *Neuron*, **25**, 425–35.

Raper, J.A. (2000). Semaphorins and their receptors in vertebrates and invertebrates. *Curr. Opin. Neurobiol.*, **10**, 88–94.

Reier, P.J., Bregman, B.S. & Wujek, J.R. (1986). Intraspinal transplantation of embryonic spinal cord tissue in neonatal and adult rats. *J. Comp. Neurol.*, **247**, 275–96.

Reier, P.J., Anderson, D.K., Young, W., Michel, M.E. & Fessler, R. (1994). Workshop on intraspinal transplantation and clinical application. *J. Neurotrauma*, **11**, 369–77.

Richardson, P.M., McGuinness, U.M. & Aguayo, A.J. (1980). Axons from CNS neurons regenerate into PNS grafts. *Nature*, **284**, 264–5.

Rosenberg, L.J., Teng, Y.D. & Wrathall, J.R. (1999). 2,3-Dihydroxy-6-nitro-7-sulfamoyl-benzo(*f*)quinoxaline reduces glial loss and acute white matter pathology after experimental spinal cord contusion. *J. Neurosci.*, **19**, 464–75.

Roth, E.J., Lawler, M.H. & Yarkony, G.M. (1990). Traumatic central cord syndrome: clinical features and functional outcomes. *Arch. Phys. Med. Rehabil.*, **71**, 18–23.

Sadowsky, C., Volshteyn, O. & McDonald, J.W. (2002). Spinal cord injury. *Disabil. Rehabil.*, in press.

Schnell, L. & Schwab, M.E. (1990). Axonal regeneration in the rat spinal cord produced by an antibody against myelin-associated neurite growth inhibitors. *Nature*, **343**, 269–72.

Schnell, L., Schneider, R., Kolbeck, R., Barde, Y.A. & Schwab, M.E. (1994). Neurotrophin-3 enhances sprouting of corticospinal tract during development and after adult spinal cord lesion. *Nature*, **367**, 170–3.

Schwab, M.E. & Bartholdi, D. (1996). Degeneration and regeneration of axons in the lesioned spinal cord. *Physiol. Rev.*, **76**, 319–70.

Schwab, M.E., Kapfhammer, J.P. & Bandtlow, C.E. (1993). Inhibitors of neurite growth. *Ann. Rev. Neurosci.*, **16**, 565–95.

Serafini, T., Kennedy, T.E., Galko, M.J., Mirzayan, C., Jessell, T.M. & Tessier-Lavigne, M. (1994). The netrins define a family of axon outgrowth-promoting proteins homologous to *C. elegans* UNC-6. *Cell*, **78**, 409–24.

Shamblott, M.J., Axelman, J., Wang, S. et al. (1998). Derivation of pluripotent stem cells from cultured human primordial germ cells. *Proc. Natl. Acad. Sci., USA*, **95**, 13726–31.

Shihabuddin, L.S., Ray, J. & Gage, F.H. (1997). FGF-2 is sufficient to isolate progenitors found in the adult mammalian spinal cord. *Exp. Neurol.*, **148**, 577–86.

Short, D.J., El Masry, W.S. & Jones, P.W. (2000). High dose methylprednisolone in the management of acute spinal cord injury – a systematic review from a clinical perspective. *Spinal Cord*, **38**, 273–86.

Shu, X.O. & Mendell, L.M. (1999). Neurotrophins and hyperalgesia. *Proc. Natl. Acad. Sci., USA*, **96**, 7693–6.

Shuman, S.L., Bresnahan, J.C. & Beattie, M.S. (1997). Apoptosis of microglia and oligodendrocytes after spinal cord contusion in rats. *J. Neurosci. Res.*, **50**, 798–808.

Springer, J.E., Azbill, R.D. & Knapp, P.E. (1999). Activation of the caspase-3 apoptotic cascade in traumatic spinal cord injury. *Nat. Med.*, **5**, 943–6.

Stauffer, E.S. (1983). Rehabilitation of posttraumatic cervical spinal cord quadriplegia and pentaplegia. In *Cervical Spine*, ed. Cervical Spine Research Society, Philadelphia, PA: pp. 317–22. JB Lippincott Co.

Stauffer, E.S. (1984). Neurologic recovery following injuries to the cervical spinal cord and nerve roots. *Spine*, **9**, 532–4.

Steeves, J.D., Keirstead, H.S., Ethell, D.W. et al. (1994). Permissive and restrictive periods for brainstem-spinal regeneration in the chick. *Prog. Brain Res.*, **103**, 243–62.

Stover, S.L. & Fine, F.R., eds. (1986). *Spinal Cord Injury: The Facts and Figures*. Birmingham, AL: University of Alabama at Birmingham.

Suhr, S.T. & Gage, F.H. (1999). Gene therapy in the central nervous system: the use of recombinant retroviruses. *Arch. Neurol.*, **56**, 287–92.

Taub, E., Uswatte, G. & Pidikiti, R. (1999). Constraint-induced movement therapy: a new family of techniques with broad application to physical rehabilitation – a clinical review. *J. Rehabil. Res. Dev.*, **36**, 237–51.

Tello, F. (1911). La influencia del neurotropismo en la regeneracion de los centros nerviosos. *Trab. Lab. Invest. Biol.*, **9**, 123–59.

Terman, J.R. & Kolodkin, A.L. (1999). Attracted or repelled? Look within. *Neuron*, **23**, 193–5.

Tessier-Lavigne, M. & Goodman, C.S. (1996). The molecular biology of axon guidance. *Science*, **274**, 1123–33.

Thompson, F.J., Uthman, B., Mott, S. et al. (1998). Neural tissue transplantation in syringomyelia patients: Neurophysiological assessments. Paper presented at the fifth annual conference of the American Society for Neuronal Transplantation, **4**, 33.

Thomson, J.A., Itskovitz-Eldor, J., Shapiro, S.S. et al. (1998). Embryonic stem cell lines derived from human blastocysts. *Science*, **282**, 1145–7.

van der Lee, J.H., Wagenaar, R.C., Lankhorst, G.J., Vogelaar, T.W., Deville, W.L., Bouter, L.M. (1999). Forced use of the upper extremity in chronic stroke patients: results from a single-blind randomized clinical trial. *Stroke*, **30**, 2369–75.

Vescovi, A.L. & Snyder, E.Y. (1999). Establishment and properties of neural stem cell clones: plasticity in vitro and in vivo. *Brain Pathol.*, **9**, 569–98.

von Meyenburg, J., Brösamle, C., Metz, G.A.S. & Schwab, M.E. (1998). Regeneration and sprouting of chronically injured corticospinal tract fibers in adult rats promoted by NT-3 and the mAb IN-1, which neutralizes myelin-associated neurite growth inhibitors. *Exp. Neurol.*, **154**, 583–94.

Walsh, F.S. & Doherty, P. (1997). Neural cell adhesion molecules of the immunoglobulin superfamily: role in axon growth and guidance. *Ann. Rev. Cell Dev. Biol.*, **13**, 425–56.

Waters, R.L., Adkins, R.H. & Yakura, J.S. (1991). Definition of complete spinal cord injury. *Paraplegia*, **29**, 573–81.

Waters, R.L., Adkins, R.H., Yakura, J.S. & Sie, I. (1993). Motor and sensory recovery following complete tetraplegia. *Arch. Phys. Med. Rehabil.*, **74**, 242–7.

Waters, R.L., Adkins, R.H., Yakura, J.S. & Sie, I. (1994). Motor and sensory recovery following incomplete tetraplegia. *Arch. Phys. Med. Rehabil.*, **75**, 306–11.

Waters, R.L., Sie, I., Adkins, R.H. & Yakura, J.S. (1995). Injury pattern effect on motor recovery after traumatic spinal cord injury. *Arch. Phys. Med. Rehabil.*, **76**, 440–3.

Waxman, S.G. (1989). Demyelination in spinal cord injury. *J. Neurol. Sci.*, **91**, 1–14.

Waxman, S.G. (1992). Demyelination in spinal cord injury and multiple sclerosis: what can we do to enhance functional recovery? *J. Neurotrauma*, **9**, S105–17.

Waxman, S.G. (1993). Aminopyridines and the treatment of spinal cord injury. *J. Neurotrauma*, **10**, 19–24.

Wernig, A. & Muller, S. (1992). Laufband locomotion with body weight support improved walking in persons with severe spinal cord injuries. *Paraplegia*, **30**, 229–38.

Wirth, E.D. III, Fessler, R.G., Reier, P.J. et al. (1999). Neural tissue transplantation in patients with syringomyelia: update on feasibility and safety. *Prog. Abst. Am. Soc. Neural Transpl. Repair*, **5/6**, 22.

Whittemore, S.R. (1999). Neuronal replacement strategies for spinal cord injury. *J. Neurotrauma*, **16**, 667–73.

Whittemore, S.R. & Snyder, E.Y. (1996). Physiological relevance and functional potential of central nervous system-derived cell lines. *Mol. Neurobiol.*, **12**, 13–38.

Wolf, S.L., Lecraw, D.E., Barton, L.A. & Jann, B.B. (1989). Forced use of hemiplegic upper extremities to reverse the effect of learned nonuse among chronic stroke and head-injured patients. *Exp. Neurol.*, **104**, 125–32.

Wrathall, J.R., Choiniere, D. & Teng, Y.D. (1994). Dose dependent reduction of tissue loss and functional impairment after spinal cord trauma with the AMPA/kainate antagonist NBQX. *J. Neurosci.*, **14**, 6598–607.

Wrathall, J.R., Teng, Y.D. & Choiniere, D. (1996). Amelioration of functional deficits from spinal cord trauma with systemically administered NBQX, an antagonist of non-N-methyl-D-aspartate receptors. *Exp. Neurol.*, **137**, 119–26.

Wu, L., Marino, R.J., Herbison, G.J. & Ditunno, J.F. Jr (1992). Recovery of zero-grade muscles in the zone of partial preservation in motor complete quadriplegia. *Arch. Phys. Med. Rehabil.*, **73**, 40–3.

Wyllie, A.H., Kerr, J.F. & Currie, A.R. (1980). Cell death: the significance of apoptosis. *Int. Rev. Cytol.*, **68**, 251–306.

Xu, X.M., Guenard, V., Kleitman, N. & Bunge, M.B. (1995). Axonal regeneration into Schwann cell-seeded guidance channels grafted into transected adult rat spinal cord. *J. Comp. Neurol.*, **351**, 145–60.

Yakovleff, A., Roby-Brami, A., Guezard, B. et al. (1989). Locomotion in rats transplanted with noradrenergic neurons. *Brain Res. Bull.*, **22**, 115–21.

Z'Graggen, W.J., Metz, G.A., Kartje, G.L., Thallmair, M. & Schwab, M.E. (1998). Functional recovery and enhanced corticofugal plasticity after unilateral pyramidal tract lesion and blockade of myelin-associated neurite growth inhibitors in adult rats. *J. Neurosci.*, **18**, 4744–57.

Zhang, Y., Dijkhuizen, P.A., Anderson, P.N., Lieberman, A.R. & Verhaagen, J. (1998). NT-3 delivered by an adenoviral vector induces injured dorsal root axons to regenerate into the spinal cord of adult rats. *J. Neurosci. Res.*, **54**, 554–62

Zipfel, G.J., Babcock, D.J., Lee, J.M. & Choi, D.W. (2000). Neuronal apoptosis after CNS injury: the roles of glutamate and calcium. *J. Neurotrauma*, **17**, 857–70.

48

Myelopathies

Philip D. Thompson[1] and Peter C. Blumbergs[2]

[1] University Department of Medicine, University of Adelaide and Department of Neurology, Royal Adelaide Hospital and
[2] Department of Neuropathology, Institute of Medical and Veterinary Science and University Department of Medicine, University of Adelaide, South Australia

An etiological classification of myelopathies yields an extensive list of diverse conditions (Table 48.1). In clinical practice, myelopathies are classified into spinal cord syndromes, based on patterns of neurological symptoms and signs, which identify the anatomical location and distribution of spinal cord pathology. The time course of symptoms is useful in distinguishing between different etiologies. Vascular lesions generally present with acute onset or rapid progression of symptoms. Inflammatory disease evolves in a subacute manner and may fluctuate over days or weeks. Compressive lesions also may present with a subacute onset and generally have a progressive course. Degenerative myelopathies are usually slowly progressive over months or years. The evolution and type of spinal cord syndrome suggest certain diagnostic possibilities and guide appropriate investigation.

Symptoms and signs of spinal cord disease

Motor symptoms and signs

The clinical presentation of an evolving myelopathy often is precipitated by limb weakness and spasticity due to corticospinal tract involvement. Arm and leg weakness suggests a cervical cord lesion. A paraparesis, with leg weakness or walking difficulty alone, suggests a lesion of the thoracic spinal cord or below. Progressive cervical cord lesions may evolve in a sequence, beginning with weakness of the arm ipsilateral to the lesion, followed by weakness of the ipsilateral then contralateral leg, and finally the contralateral arm.

Exacerbation of symptoms by exercise, or during increases in body temperature (hot weather or a hot bath) suggests demyelination, but may also occur in dural arteriovenous malformations of the spinal cord.

Motor signs of spinal cord disease reflect involvement of the long tracts of the spinal cord with increased muscle tone, brisk tendon reflexes, extensor plantar responses and weakness of hip and knee flexion and ankle dorsiflexion. Involvement of the anterior horn cells or anterior (motor) spinal nerve roots produces additional lower motor neuron signs of segmental wasting and weakness (Table 48.2).

Sensory symptoms and signs

Back pain

Back pain is often an early complaint of a myelopathy, preceding any motor symptoms. The site of pain may localize the level of a focal structural lesion such as a spinal epidural abscess, vertebral body collapse or intervertebral disc prolapse. Dull, poorly localized backache is common in intrinsic spinal lesions but is of little localizing or diagnostic value. An increase in pain when coughing and straining or exacerbation of pain with movement suggests an extramedullary (extradural) compressive lesion. Nocturnal back pain when recumbent occurs in extradural spinal lesions such as a thoracic meningioma or a benign spinal nerve root sheath tumour (schwannoma/neurofibroma). Severe thoracic or interscapular pain may be the presenting feature of inflammatory transverse myelitis.

Radicular symptoms and signs

Compression of posterior spinal roots by extrinsic spinal cord lesions or infiltration of the posterior root entry zone by intrinsic cord lesions, causes radicular pains which radiate along the affected dermatome, localizing the level of spinal pathology (Fig. 48.1). Radicular pains are typically sharp or knife-like and accompanied by cutaneous burning dysesthesia or hyperesthesia over the affected skin. Thoracic sensory root involvement can produce constricting chest or

Table 48.1. Etiological classification of myelopathies

Trauma

Vascular
   Anterior spinal artery thrombosis
   Spinal arteriovenous malformation
   Dural arteriovenous malformation
   Epidural hematoma
   Hematomyelia
   Arteritis (polyarteritis nodosa, systemic lupus erythematosus)

Inflammatory
   Idiopathic transverse myelitis
   Multiple sclerosis, Devic's disease
   Postinfectious encephalomyelitis
   Idiopathic necrotic myelopathy

Infectious
   Neurotropic viruses
      Herpes zoster, Herpes simplex, Polio
   Coxsackie, echovirus, cytomegalovirus, Epstein–Barr
   Retrovirus myelopathies
      Human immunodeficiency virus (HIV) vacuolar myelopathy
      Human T-lymphotrophic virus type I (HTLV I) tropical
         myelopathies
   Mycoplasma myelopathy
   Spinal epidural abscess
   Syphilitic meningomyelitis
   Tuberculosis
      Osteitis (Pott's disease)
      Radiculomyelitis
   Schistosoma myelopathy

Granulomatous
   Sarcoidosis

Neoplastic
   Primary
      Intramedullary – astrocytoma, ependymoma
      Extramedullary – neurofibroma, meningioma
   Secondary
      Intramedullary metastasis (rare)
      Extradural metastasis
      Contiguous spread – paravertebral neuroblastoma,
         lymphoma
Paraneoplastic
   Necrotic myelopathy
   Myeloradiculoneuropathy

Degenerative
   Motor neuron disease

Vertebral disease with myelopathy
   Cervical spondylotic myelopathy
   Intervertebral disc prolapse
   Rheumatoid arthritis (atlantoaxial subluxation)
   Psoriatic arthropathy
   Achondroplasia
   Mucopolysaccharidoses
   Paget's disease

Table 48.1 (*cont.*)

Congenital
   Spinal dysraphism:
      Spina bifida
      Diastematomyelia
   Syringomyelia

Hereditary
   Hereditary spastic paraplegia
   Friedreich's ataxia
   Spinal muscular atrophy

Nutritional
   Malabsorption syndromes with myelopathy
      Vitamin B12 deficiency (subacute combined degeneration)
      Vitamin E deficiency (Bassen–Kornzweig disease)

Toxins
   Tropical spastic paraparesis (such as cassava)
   Lathyrism (chick pea – *Lathyrus sativa*)

Miscellaneous
   Caisson disease (decompression myelopathy in divers)
   Myelopathy of systemic disease (liver failure)
   Radiation myelopathy

Table 48.3. Segmental innervation of muscles

C3, 4	Trapezius
C4, 5	Rhomboids
C5	Deltoid
C5, 6	Supraspinatus, Infraspinatus, Biceps
C6	Brachioradialis
C7	Triceps, Extensor digitorum
C8	Flexor digitorum superficialis and profundus
T1	Intrinsic hand muscles
T7–10	Upper rectus abdominis
T10–12	Lower rectus abdominis
L1	Iliopsoas
L2	Adductor magnus
L3, L4	Quadriceps femoris
L4	Tibialis anterior
L5	Extensor hallucis longus
L5, S1	Hamstrings
S1	Extensor digitorum brevis
S1, S2	Soleus, gastrocnemius

abdominal pain, severe enough to suggest myocardial infarction, aortic dissection or an acute abdomen. Extradural spinal lesions (metastatic carcinoma, abscess) produce radicular pain, local tenderness and restriction of movement at the affected level before spinal cord compression develops and long tract signs appear. Intramedullary spinal lesions such as primary spinal tumours produce long

Table 48.3. Segmental sensory and motor innervation of tendon and cutaneous reflexes

Biceps reflex	C5, 6
Brachioradialis reflex	C6
Triceps reflex	C7
Finger reflexes	C8
Abdominal reflexes	
upper	T8–12
lower	T10–12
Knee (patellar) reflex	L3, 4
Adductor reflex	L2
Cremasteric reflex	L1, 2
Plantar reflex	L5
Ankle reflex	S1
Anal reflex	S4, 5

tract symptoms and signs early in the illness while root involvement is unusual and occurs late. In contrast to the severity of radicular pain, examination may reveal only subtle sensory loss in radicular lesions. Depression or absence of a tendon or cutaneous reflex may also be a valuable sign of a radicular sensory lesion (Table 48.3).

Sensory tract symptoms and signs

Paresthesiae (tingling, 'pins and needles') and loss of sensation are common in diseases of the long spinal sensory tracts. The distribution and extent of sensory tract symptoms depend on the site and size of the lesion. The trunk is frequently involved and is an important clinical clue to a sensory tract lesion. In progressive myelopathies, a sensory tract disturbance may evolve, ascending from the legs onto the trunk, or decending down the trunk to the legs. The pattern of spread occurs as the lesion enlarges and encroaches on adjacent laminated sensory fibres in the sensory tracts (Fig. 48.2). The combination of trunkal, upper and lower limb sensory symptoms indicates cervical cord involvement. Leg and trunk symptoms alone point towards thoracic or lumbar cord involvement.

Spinothalamic tract symptoms and signs

Cutaneous dysesthesia (burning, prickling, itching), abnormal warm or cold sensations, hyperesthesia (enhanced sensitivity to minor or trivial sensory stimuli) and hyperpathia are characteristic of a spinothalamic tract sensory disturbance. Spontaneous deep, poorly localized pain may be felt in areas of sensory loss (anaesthesia dolorosa). The patient may be unaware of the sensory deficit and sustain burns, accidental soft tissue injury or bony damage (Charcot's

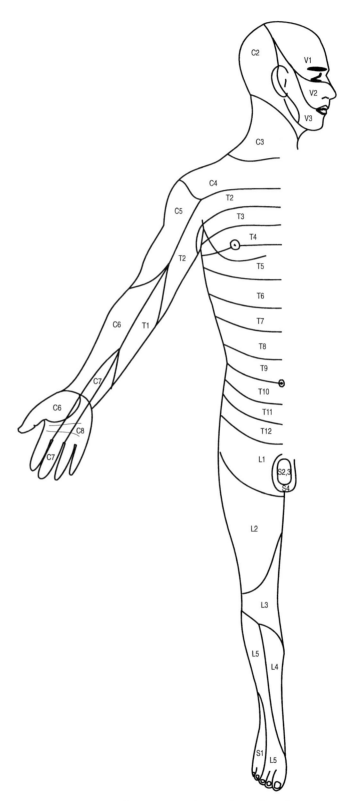

Fig. 48.1. Distribution of dermatomes on the anterior surface of the body.

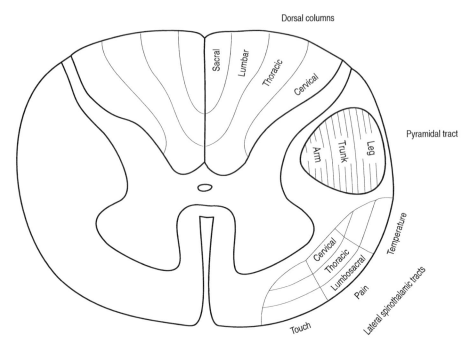

Fig. 48.2. Cross section of the cervical spinal cord demonstrating the lamination of the long sensory and motor tracts.

joints) in areas of impaired pain and temperature perception.

A lateral spinothalamic tract lesion results in contralateral pain and temperature loss (dissociated), sensory loss beginning two or three segments below the lesion. The upper limit of a spinothalamic sensory loss is often marked by a rim of hyperesthesia (Fig. 48.3). Pain and temperature fibres decussate shortly after entry into the spinal cord and ascend in the spinothalamic tract. A discrete central cord lesion may therefore only interrupt sensation from a few adjacent segments, producing a suspended, dissociated cape or breastplate sensory loss (Fig. 48.3). Lamination of the spinothalamic tract fibres leads to sparing of sacral sensation in intramedullary lesions (sacral sparing) and sensory levels that can be well below the actual lesion (Fig. 48.2). Accordingly, a spinothalamic sensory level can be misleading in assessing the site of a spinal lesion. The pattern of sensory loss also does not distinguish between intramedullary and extramedullary lesions. The precise lesion level is best obtained from magnetic resonance imaging of the whole spinal cord.

Posterior column symptoms and signs

Posterior column lesions give rise to paresthesiae and numbness often accompanied by sensations of limb swelling, constricting bands around the limbs and trunk or a sensation that a limb is 'encased in plaster'. Discrete lesions of the laminated dorsal column fibres may affect sensation in isolated body segments at the level of the lesion or several segments distal to the level of the lesion (Fig. 48.2). For example, dorsal column lesions in the cervical cord can lead to bilateral symmetrical loss of discriminatory sensation in the hands or tight bands around a leg or the trunk. Loss of proprioception (deafferentation) results in clumsiness of hand or foot movement (sensory ataxia), that may be misinterpreted as weakness. A characteristic symptom of dorsal column lesions is 'electric' paresthesiae radiating down the back, induced by neck flexion (L'hermitte's phenomenon).

Sphincters

Urinary retention and constipation may precede the onset of overt paralysis in a spinal cord syndrome, particularly when the conus medullaris or cauda equina are involved. Sphincter involvement is an early feature in intrinsic or intramedullary spinal lesions and a late feature in extrinsic compression of the spinal cord, after the appearance of motor symptoms.

Patterns of spinal cord syndromes

In lesions of the thoracic and cervical spinal cord, certain patterns of abnormality are well recognized (Fig. 48.3).

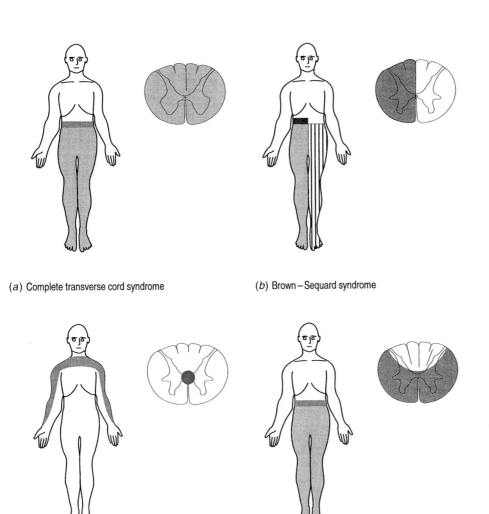

(a) Complete transverse cord syndrome

(b) Brown–Sequard syndrome

(c) Central cord syndrome

(d) Anterior cord syndrome

Fig. 48.3. Patterns of spinal cord disease. (a) Complete transection of the spinal cord produces paralysis and anesthesia below the level of the lesion. There is often a rim of hyperesthesia at the upper level of the sensory loss. (b) In a Brown–Sequard or hemicord syndrome, upper motor neurone signs including weakness and dorsal column signs are found below the lesion on the same side, and there is a contralateral loss of spinothalamic sensory modalities (vertical stripes). Again, there may be a rim of hyperesthesia on the side of the spinal lesion. (c) A central cord syndrome interrupts decussating spinothalamic fibres over a few spinal segments and produces a suspended dissociated sensory loss. In this example, C4, 5, 6 dermatomes are affected. (d) An anterior cord syndrome produces upper motor neurone signs below the level of the lesion with impaired spinothalamic sensation. A rim of hyperesthesia at the upper level of the spinothalamic sensory level is also shown. Dorsal column function is spared. Lower motor neuron signs may also be present if the cervical or lumbar cord is affected.

Hemicord (Brown–Séquard) syndrome

A unilateral lesion of the spinal cord results in a contralateral loss of spinothalamic sensation (pain and temperature), ipsilateral weakness with upper motor neuron signs, and ipsilateral dorsal column (proprioception) sensory loss (Brown–Séquard syndrome). Light touch is preserved. The syndrome may be partial or complete. Demyelination, knife or bullet injuries, and cord compression are common causes.

Anterior cord syndromes

The anterior cord syndrome consists of paralysis with upper and lower motor neuron signs, a bilateral spinothalamic (pain and temperature) sensory loss and sphincter paralysis. Posterior column sensory modalities are spared. Ischemia in the territory of the anterior spinal artery is the commonest cause.

Central (cervical) cord syndromes

A central cervical cord syndrome produces a combination of lower motor neuron signs of muscle wasting and weakness and depressed or absent tendon reflexes in the arms, a paraparesis and a suspended dissociated sensory loss over the arms and trunk. Acute central cervical cord lesions produce bilateral arm weakness, pain and hyperpathia. Rarely, central cord lesions may result in segmental muscle rigidity and spasms. Central cord lesions are caused by flexion–extension spinal trauma, neoplasms, watershed (hypotensive) cord ischemia and syringomyelia.

Radiculomyelopathy syndromes

Radiculomyelopathies present two broad clinical scenarios. The first comprises a sensory or motor radicular lesion at the upper level of an extrinsic compressive or intrinsic infiltrative myelopathy. Segmental amyotrophy or sensory radiculopathy are evident at the level of the lesion and upper motor neuron and sensory tract signs are found below. In the second, multiple spinal levels are involved and a combination of upper and lower motor neuron signs and sensory root and tract signs are evident. The common causes of radiculomyelopathies are listed in Table 48.4.

Spinal shock

Segmental reflex activity is abolished below the level of an acute spinal lesion (spinal shock) for 1 to 6 weeks after the injury. Areflexic quadriplegia in cervical cord lesions or

Table 48.4. Causes of radiculomyelopathy classified according to whether one or multiple spinal levels are involved

Single level	
Acute transverse myelitis	
Vascular	Spinal cord infarction (anterior spinal artery thrombosis)
	Spinal arteriovenous malformation
Neoplastic	Primary spinal tumour
	Extradural metastatic carcinoma
	Carcinomatous meningitis
Infective	Spinal epidural abscess
Multiple levels	
Cervical and lumbar spondylosis	
Necrotic myelopathy	
Chronic meningitis (infectious or granulomatous)	
Spinal arachnoiditis	
Neoplastic	Carcinomatous or lymphomatous meningitis
Paraneoplastic	Carcinomatous neuromyopathy

paraplegia in thoracic cord lesions is accompanied by abnormal autonomic control below the lesion, with loss of vasomotor tone, profuse sweating and piloerection. Return of spinal reflex activity is marked by the appearance of upper motor neuron signs, exaggerated tendon reflexes and enhanced cutaneous flexor reflexes, which become the dominant physical signs of a chronic spinal cord lesion. Minor cutaneous stimuli may elicit flexor spasms, reflex defecation or micturition and profuse sweating.

Specific spinal cord syndromes

Foramen magnum lesions

A slowly evolving asymmetric quadriparesis, lower cranial nerve (accesssory and hypoglossal) palsies, neck stiffness, abnormal posturing of the neck, a Horner's syndrome and subtle sensory changes occur in foramen magnum lesions and may escape detection in the early stages. Compression of the upper cervical sensory roots and distortion of the spinal cord produce neck and occipital pain in the C2–4 dermatomes, sensory impairment in the first division of the trigeminal nerve and contralateral spinothalamic sensory loss. Downbeat nystagmus is characteristic of lesions at this site. In addition to an asymmetric quadriparesis, high cervical lesions may produce lower motor neuron signs of wasting and weakness in intrinsic hand muscles, due to venous stasis with ischemia in the distal

C8–T1 spinal segments (Stark et al., 1981). Phrenic nerve involvement may interfere with diaphragm function and ventilation. Causes include a benign nerve root sheath tumour (schwannoma/neurofibroma), anterior atlanto-axial subluxation in rheumatoid arthritis and psoriatic arthropathy, achondroplasia and the mucopolysaccharidoses.

Cervical spinal cord lesions

Lesions of the cervical spinal cord produce a myeloradiculopathy with a combination of upper and lower motor neuron signs in the arms, a spastic paraparesis, sensory loss in the arms and sensory tract signs over the trunk and lower limbs. Clinical guides to the level of the lesion include the highest motor and sensory segments affected and lower motor neuron signs (muscle wasting, weakness, and fasciculation) (Table 48.2). The pattern of muscle tone and tendon reflex change in the arms (Table 48.3) is determined by the level of the lesion. Lower motor neuron signs (muscle wasting, weakness), depression or absence of tendon reflexes and sensory loss will be evident at the level of the lesion while upper motor neurone signs (increased muscle tone, brisk tendon reflexes) will be evident below the lesion.

Sensory loss in cervical lesions may be radicular and limited to a dermatome with loss of light touch, or extend over several segments in a spinothalamic or posterior column tract distribution, with preservation of light touch.

Thoracic spinal cord lesions

The upper border of a thoracic spinothalamic sensory level lies two or three segments below the approximate level of the thoracic lesion. Radicular pain provides a more accurate thoracic level, but radicular sensory loss may be difficult to elicit. In addition to paraplegia, thoracic cord lesions may produce trunkal weakness due to either upper or lower motor neuron involvement. Signs of abdominal weakness include loss of abdominal muscle tone with paradoxical protrusion of the abdominal wall during coughing, exhalation and attempted trunkal flexion (when sitting up). Thoracic cord lesions below T10 produce differential weakness of lower abdominal muscles so that on sitting up or lifting the head when supine, contraction of the upper recti (innervated by T7–T10) will be unopposed by the paralysed lower recti (T10–T12) resulting in an upward movement of the umbilicus (Beevor's sign). Superficial abdominal reflexes are abolished below the level of the spinal lesion.

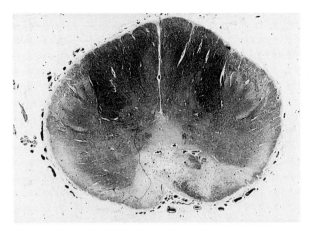

Fig. 48.4. Old cystic ischemic necrosis C4 cord in the territory of the anterior spinal artery (Weil stain for myelin ×7 magnification).

Conus medullaris and cauda equina lesions

Conus lesions result in early and prominent sphincter impairment (urinary retention and constipation), sacral sensory loss affecting lower perineal segments (S3–S5) more than leg segments (L5–S2) and impotence. Leg muscle weakness is variable in conus lesions and may be mild unless the lesion extends higher in the lumbar cord. An extensor plantar response implies the lesion affects the spinal cord above the L5 segment (innervating the extensor digitorum longus muscle). Reflex change will be determined by the level of the lesion.

An asymmetric, flaccid, areflexic paralysis with radicular sensory loss, urinary or fecal incontinence and loss of anal tone points towards predominant involvement of the cauda equina. Muscle wasting with fasciculation indicates a chronic lesion.

Causes of myelopathy

Vascular myelopathies

Spinal cord infarction

Anterior spinal artery occlusion
Infarction of the spinal cord typically involves the territory of the anterior spinal artery, which supplies the anterior two-thirds of the spinal cord and results in an anterior cord syndrome with paraplegia, a mid-thoracic spinothalamic sensory level and sphincter paralysis (Fig. 48.4). A mid-thoracic level (T4–T6) is most common, as it lies in

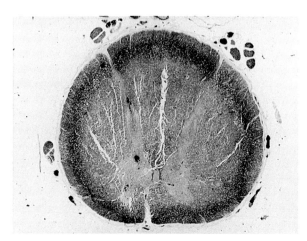

Fig. 48.5. Recent ischemic necrosis of central cord affecting central grey matter and surrounding white matter of T5 spinal cord secondary to prolonged hypotension. Only a peripheral rim of myelin is preserved (Weil stain for myelin ×8 magnification).

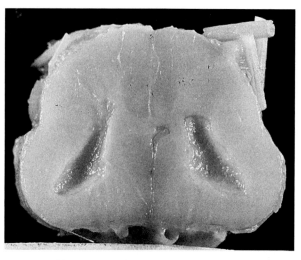

Fig. 48.6. Old central spinal cord infarction with cystic necrosis of anterior grey matter (×8 magnification).

the critical rostrocaudal watershed zone of the spinal circulation which is derived from segmental arteries between T10 and L3 (the artery of Adamkiewicz) and descending branches from the vertebral and ascending cervical arteries. The vascular pathology is usually thromboembolic occlusion of spinal segmental arteries, such as the artery of Adamkiewicz, or aortic disease (dissection, clamping in surgery, severe atheroma). Primary atheromatous occlusion of the anterior spinal artery itself is uncommon, but the vessel may be occluded by vasculitis or systemic embolism.

Segmental artery occlusion

Occlusion of cervical segmental arteries causing infarction of the cervical cord and quadriplegia is rare. Lumbosacral radicular artery thromboembolism (Anderson & Willoughby, 1987) and compression of lumbosacral radicular arteries by a prolapsed intervertebral disc (Lazorthes, 1972) may cause infarction of the conus medullaris.

Central cord infarction

Profound hypotension, aortic dissection or surgical clamping of the aorta may lead to painless watershed infarction of the central grey matter of the low thoracic and lumbosacral spinal cord (Blumbergs & Byrne, 1980) (Fig. 48.5). This selective damage produces paraparesis, patchy upper and lower motor neuron signs in the legs, dissociated sensory loss, and sphincter paralysis. Central cord ischemia may involve the interneurons in spinal grey matter (Fig. 48.6) leading to rigidity and myoclonus of

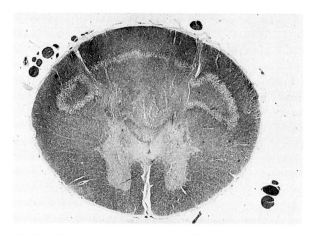

Fig. 48.7. Watershed ischemic necrosis of T3 spinal cord secondary to prolonged hypotension from a dissecting aortic aneurysm (Weil stain for myelin ×8 magnification).

spinal origin. Rarely, watershed infarction occurs at the boundary of the intrinsic anterior and posterior vascular territories of the mid thoracic spinal cord (Fig. 48.7).

Spinal vascular malformations

Intradural (especially intramedullary) spinal arteriovenous malformations present with the sudden onset of neck pain, limb weakness, radicular or tract sensory loss and sphincter disturbance due to spinal subarachnoid hemorrhage or hematomyelia. These malformations involve the cervical and thoracic spinal cord. Symptoms appear in the first and second decades (Rosenblum et al., 1987). In contrast, dural

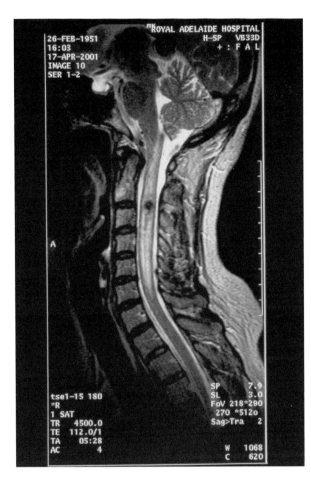

Fig. 48.8. Magnetic resonance image of the cervical spinal cord in a 50-year-old woman who presented with an acute hematomyelia resulting in transient quadriplegia with a sensory level at C4 showing a cavernous angioma (cavernoma).

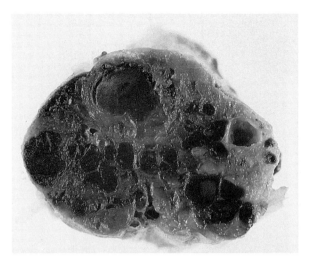

Fig. 48.9. Cavernous angioma of T5 spinal cord.

arteriovenous fistulae occur in the low thoracic and lumbar cord, most commonly in elderly men. A slowly progressive paraparesis with upper and lower motor neuron signs, sensory symptoms including pain and sphincter disturbances evolve slowly over months to years (Logue, 1979). These deficits are caused by prolonged venous hypertension (Kendall & Logue, 1977). Symptoms may be exacerbated by exercise. A spinal cavernous angioma may present with an acute cord syndrome due to hemorrhage and hematomyelia (Fig. 48.8) or a slowly progressive myelopathy secondary to the intraspinal mass lesion (Fig. 48.9) (Deutsch et al., 2000). Neurocutaneous manifestations, such as vertebral anomalies, scoliosis, cutaneous angiomata and spinal dysraphism may accompany spinal vascular malformations (Aminoff & Logue, 1974).

Inflammatory myelopathies – acute transverse myelitis

Acute or subacute transverse myelitis due to inflammatory demyelination may occur in multiple sclerosis or in a monophasic postinfectious encephalomyelitis. Symptoms include paresthesiae ascending from the legs onto the trunk and a thoracic sensory level (both cervical and thoracic cord can be affected), paraparesis or quadriparesis and sphincter disturbance. Ropper and Poskanzer (1978) identified three groups of acute transverse myelitis. In the first, ascending sensory symptoms evolve over 1–14 days, followed by good recovery. The second, characterized by an acute onset and rapid progression with back pain and paraplegia, had a poor outcome. A third group present with the gradual onset and stuttering progression of symptoms over weeks and have a similar outcome to the first group. This syndrome appears to represent a distinct entity. Cerebrospinal fluid may show a lymphocytic pleocytosis with raised protein but not oligoclonal bands. Magnetic resonance imaging of the spinal cord reveals extensive or confluent high signal lesions extending over several segments (Fig. 48.10). Less than 10% of cases progress to develop multiple sclerosis. This number may be even lower if cases with cerebrospinal fluid oligoclonal bands and cerebral white matter lesions on imaging, both of which favour a diagnosis of multiple sclerosis, are excluded. Acute myelopathies in multiple sclerosis tend to be of gradual evolution with partial, asymmetric spinal cord syndromes (Miller et al., 1987).

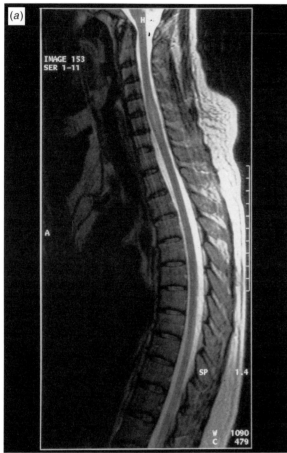

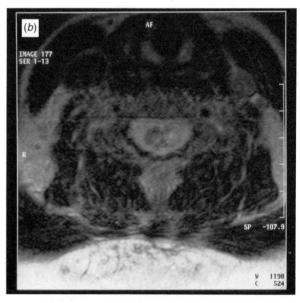

Fig. 48.10. Magnetic resonance image of the cervical spinal cord in a 53-year-old woman presenting with a left Brown–Sequard syndrome and an elongated area of high signal in the central and right side of the cervical spinal cord. The transverse view was taken at the level of C5.

Infectious myelopathies

A wide range of infections are associated with acute myelopathy, either by direct invasion, postinfectious demyelination or abscess formation. Systemic bacterial infections may be complicated by an epidural or extradural abscess. These present with back and root pain, fever and local tenderness which precedes the development of spinal cord compression by a few days. Tuberculous osteitis destroys thoracic vertebral bodies and intervertebral discs over a period of months leading to a progressive kyphosis, spinal cord compression and paraplegia (Pott's paraplegia). Schistosoma myelopathy involving the conus medullaris progresses to paraplegia over days to weeks (Scrimgeour & Gajdusek, 1985). Mycoplasma infections may be complicated by meningoencephalitis and transverse myelopathy.

Several viruses (coxsackie, echovirus, cytomegalovirus, Epstein–Barr) have also been reported to produce transverse myelitis. Neurotropic viruses (herpes zoster, poliomyelitis, herpes simplex) affect predominantly the grey matter of the spinal cord with anterior horn cell loss, resulting in segmental lower motor neuron signs of muscle fasciculation, wasting and weakness. A vacuolar myelopathy, affecting white matter tracts of the thoracic cord, particularly the posterior columns and corticospinal tract, occurs in up to 20% of patients with the acquired immune deficiency syndrome (AIDS) and HIV (human immunodeficiency virus) infection (Petito et al., 1985). Pathological changes of myelin vacuolation sparing axons is found in 50% of cases of AIDS (Shepherd et al., 1999). Asymmetric limb weakness develops over several weeks followed by sensory signs and sphincter involvement. Tropical spastic paraparesis, or myelopathy associated with human T-lymphotropic virus type I (HTLV I) infection (Johnson, 1987) (HAM), is a common cause of paraparesis in tropical regions such as the Caribbean, and also Japan. Paraparesis evolves in a slow but progressive manner with upper motor neuron signs and prominent sphincter involvement. Upper limb reflexes are brisk but arm weakness is uncommon. Loss of vibration sense, peripheral sensory impairment and depressed or absent ankle jerks suggesting a neuropathy are common. A thoracic sensory level may be observed in some cases and sensory symptoms may herald the onset of HAM. Pathologically, the spinal lesions are characterized by degeneration of myelin and axons in the anterolateral and posterior columns and an inflammatory process presumably directed against HTLV-1 infected T-lymphocytes (Izumo et al., 2000).

Myelopathy in neoplasia

Secondary extradural metastases from lung, breast or prostate carcinoma in vertebral bodies extend into the extradural space causing focal back pain, radicular pain and subsequently spinal cord compression, evolving over weeks to months. The thoracic cord is most commonly involved. Once spinal compression begins, paraplegia evolves over days with sphincter disturbances. Neoplastic destruction of vertebral bodies may lead to vertebral collapse, dislocation and increasing angular deformity further compromising cord function. A similar progressive myelopathy may accompany intramedullary spinal metastases, which are rarer than extradural metastases and not accompanied by vertebral body destruction.

Carcinomatous meningitis due to neoplastic infiltration of the leptomeninges presents with a subacute onset of lower motor neuron signs, absent tendon reflexes, extensor plantar responses, and a peripheral sensory loss (Olson et al., 1974). Pain and multifocal involvement of the central nervous system are additional clues to the diagnosis.

Primary spinal tumours, intramedullary ependymoma and astrocytoma, or extramedullary neurofibroma and meningioma evolve slowly over months and years. Symptoms are produced by internal disruption of the long tracts of the spinal cord or the development of syringomyelia in intramedullary tumours and spinal nerve root or spinal cord compression in extramedullary tumours.

Necrotizing myelopathies

A subacute necrotic myelopathy developing over weeks occurs as a rare paraneoplastic event (Mancall & Rosales, 1964), but also may appear as an isolated myelopathy in the absence of other systemic disease (Katz & Ropper, 2000). Sensory symptoms, including pain, are prominent early and may ascend from the lower limbs or descend down the trunk. Progression may occur in a stepwise manner. Upper and lower motor neuron signs are common. Imaging studies reveal cord swelling and cavitation. Spinal cord necrosis is evident on pathological examination (Fig. 48.11).

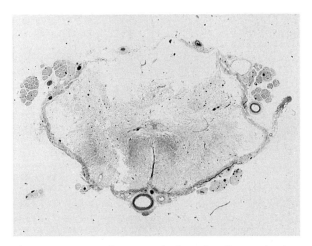

Fig. 48.11. T10 necrotic paraneoplastic myelopathy associated with renal cell carcinoma (Trichrome ×8 magnification).

Cervical spondyslosis and myelopathy

Degenerative cervical spondylosis with myelopathy is a common cause of cervical cord disease. The most frequently affected levels, in descending order of frequency are C5–C6, C6–C7, and C4–C5. The clinical picture is of a myeloradiculopathy. Wasting of intrinsic hand muscles rarely occurs in cervical spondylosis, since the levels commonly involved (C5–6, C6–7) are above the T1 spinal segment. Prominent hand wasting in association with a cervical cord syndrome suggests intrinsic spinal disease such as motor neuron disease or syringomyelia rather than cervical spondylosis. Sensory symptoms are often not prominent in cervical spondylosis and myelopathy. Pain and radicular sensory loss in the distribution of (C5, 6 or 7) dermatomes suggests a lateral cervical disc protrusion, though objective sensory loss may be subtle and less dramatic than symptoms. Reduced vibration and joint position sense in the feet reflect dorsal column involvement. Dorsal column involvement occasionally leads to loss of joint position sense and clumsy deafferented hands (Fig. 48.12). Spinothalamic involvement may manifest as a painful central cord syndrome or occasionally a distal symmetrical loss of pain and temperature mimicking a small fibre peripheral neuropathy.

Syringomyelia

The classical clinical presentation of syringomyelia is a progressive dissociated sensory loss involving pain and temperature, accompanied by loss of tendon reflexes, muscle wasting and weakness in one or both upper limbs,

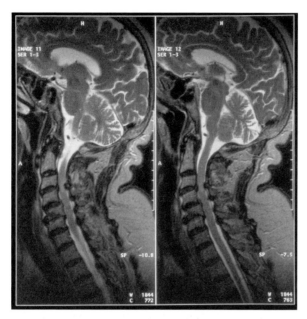

Fig. 48.12. Magnetic resonance image of the cervical spinal cord in an 83-year-old woman with progressive sensory ataxia of the hands and a paraparesis showing multiple levels of spondylosis and marked canal stenosis at C3, 4, C4, 5 and C5, 6 with cord compression and distortion at these levels.

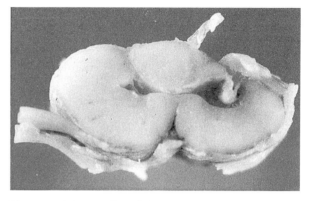

Fig. 48.13. Syringomyelia with the syrinx at C4 level involving the right lateral and dorsal white matter columns, right posterior horn of the central grey matter, base of the left dorsal white matter and adjacent left dorsal horn.

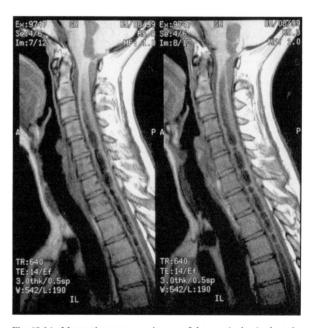

Fig. 48.14. Magnetic resonance image of the cervical spinal cord and craniocervical junction in a 32-year-old woman with loss of pain and temperature sensation and a deep burning discomfort in the C4–8 dermatomes of both arms and a mild spastic paraparesis, showing an extensive syrinx throughout the cervical spinal cord, extending into the brainstem above and the thoracic cord below.

particularly the hands. Sensory loss over the limbs and trunk is 'suspended' in a cape, hemicape or breastplate distribution reflecting interruption of decussating spinothalamic fibres over a series of adjacent segments (Fig. 48.3). Deep aching neck and radicular pain are common. There may be a spastic paraparesis. Considerable variation occurs in the extent of these signs, depending on the diameter and length of the syrinx (Fig. 48.13). The advent of MRI has greatly improved the diagnosis of syringomyelia and increased recognition of variants (Fig. 48.14). Other features include soft tissue and bony damage secondary to loss of pain and temperature sensation with painless burns, thickening and discoloration of the skin, hyperhidrosis, arthropathy (Charcot's joints) and scoliosis. Occasionally, proprioceptive loss is evident if the cavity encroaches on the posterior columns.

The cervical spinal cord is the commonest site for development of a syrinx. In many cases a craniocervical junction developmental defect, such as an Arnold Chiari malformation is present. A syrinx may develop in association with intraspinal tumours or follow significant spinal trauma. Post-traumatic syringomyelia may develop many years after spinal trauma, presenting with a painless deterioration in motor function and an ascending sensory level (Rossier et al., 1985).

Connective tissue disease

Myelopathy is a rare complication of connective tissue disease. Systemic lupus erythematosus may present with myelopathy. Sjogren's syndrome and mixed connective tissue disease also may be complicated by myelopathy. The presentation of myelopathy may take the form of acute transverse myelitis or evolve in a chronic progressive manner affecting predominantly the corticospinal tracts. MRI of the spinal cord may show patchy areas of increased signal or no abnormality. Pathological examination reveals microscopic perivascular inflammation, fibrinoid necrosis of arterioles and degeneration of white matter tracts. Necrotizing vasculitis affecting the anterior spinal artery and spinal subarachnoid hemorrhage have also been described.

Toxic myelopathies

Lathyrism, caused by a toxin derived from *Lathyrus sativa*, the chickling pea produces a spastic paraparesis in southern India and other tropical countries (Ludolph et al., 1987).

Nutritional deficiencies and myelopathy

Vitamin B12 deficiency and subacute combined degeneration of the cord

The myelopathy of subacute combined degeneration affects the posterior and lateral columns of the spinal cord. Neuropathy may also develop leading to a combination of upper motor neuron signs, depressed or absent ankle jerks and distal sensory impairment with prominent dorsal column sensory loss. Symptoms may begin in the upper limbs and include L'Hermitte's sign, indicating a predilection for cervical spinal cord involvement.

Increasingly recognized is the myeloneuropathy similar to subacute combined degeneration that results from prolonged exposure to nitrous oxide. Posterior and lateral columns are affected and accompanied by an axonal neuropathy and megaloblastic anemia. Nitrous oxide inhibits methionine synthetase mimicking the effect of vitamin B12 deficiency.

Radiation myelopathy

Inclusion of the spinal cord in the radiotherapy field when treatment involves radiation doses greater than 3, 500 rads predisposes to the development of radiation myelopathy. Myelopathy develops after an interval of 6 months or even years and progresses slowly over weeks to months. Initial

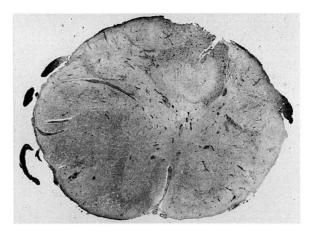

Fig. 48.15. Radiation necrosis of the C1 cord with swelling of the cord and loss of myelin (Weil stain for myelin ×5 magnification).

symptoms may be sensory or a progressive quadriparesis culminating in a complete transverse cord syndrome (Fig. 48.15).

Decompression myelopathy

Myelopathy, presenting with predominantly sensory symptoms beginning within 6 hours of the last dive, is common in decompression sickness (Caisson disease).

References

Aminoff, M.J. & Logue, V. (1974). Clinical features of spinal vascular malformations. *Brain*, **97**, 197–210.

Anderson, N.E. & Willoughby, E.W. (1987). Infarction of the conus medullaris. *Ann. Neurol.*, **21**, 470–4.

Blumbergs, P.C. & Byrne, E. (1980). Hypotensive central infarction of the spinal cord. *J. Neurol., Neurosurg., Psychiatry*, **43**, 751–3.

Deutsch, H., Jallo, G.I., Faktorovich, A. & Epstein, F. (2000). Spinal intramedullary cavernoma: clinical presentation and surgical outcome. *J. Neurosurg.*, **93**, 65–70.

Izumo, S., Umehara, F. & Osame, M. (2000). HTLV-1 associated myelopathy. *Neuropathology*, **20**, Suppl., S65–68.

Johnson, R. (1987). Myelopathies and retroviral infections. *Ann. Neurol.*, **21**, 113–16.

Katz, J. & Ropper, A.H. (2000). Progressive necrotic myelopathy. *Arch. Neurol.*, **57**, 355–61.

Kendall, B.E. & Logue, V. (1977). Spinal epidural angiomatous malformations draining into intrathecal veins. *Neuroradiology*, **13**, 181–9.

Lazorthes, G. (1972). Pathology, classification and clinical aspects of vascular diseases of the spinal cord. In *Handbook of Clinical*

Neurology, Vol. 12. ed. P.J. Vinken & G.W. Bruyn, pp. 492–506. Amsterdam: North Holland.

Logue, V. (1979). Angiomas of the spinal cord: review of the pathogenesis, clinical features and results of surgery. *J. Neurol., Neurosurg., Psychiatry*, **13**, 181–9.

Ludolph, A.C., Hugon, J., Duivedi, M.P., Schoenberg, H.H. & Spencer, P.S. (1987). Studies on the aetiology and pathogenesis of motor neuron diseases: 1. lathyrism: clinical findings in established cases. *Brain*, **110**, 149–65.

Mancall, E.J. & Rosales, E.K. (1964). Necrotizing myelopathy associated with visceral carcinoma. *Brain*, **87**, 639–56.

Miller, D.H., McDonald, W.I., Blumhardt, L.D. et al. (1987). Magnetic resonance imaging in isolated non-compressive spinal cord syndromes. *Ann. Neurol.*, **22**, 714–23.

Olson, M.E., Chernik, N.L. & Posner, J.B. (1974). Infiltration of the leptomeninges by systemic cancer: a clinical and pathological study. *Arch. Neurol.*, **30**, 122–37.

Petito, C.K., Navia, B.A., Cho E-S. et al. (1985). Vacuolar myelopathy pathologically resembling subacute combined degeneration in patients with the acquired immunodeficiency syndrome. *N. Engl. J. Med.*, **312**, 874–9.

Ropper, A.H. & Poskanzer, D.C. (1978). The prognosis of acute and subacute transverse myelopathy based on early signs and symptoms. *Ann. Neurol.*, **4**, 51–9.

Rosenblum, B., Oldfield, E.H., Doppman, J.L. & DiChiro, G. (1987). Spinal arteriovenous malformations: a comparison of dural arteriovenous fistulas and intradural AVMs in 81 patients. *J. Neurosurg.*, **67**, 795–802.

Rossier, A.B., Foo, D., Shillito, J. & Dyro, F.M. (1985). Post traumatic syringomyelia. *Brain*, **108**, 39–62.

Scrimgeour, E.M. & Gajdusek, D.C. (1985). Involvement of the central nervous sytem in *Schistosoma mansoni* and *S. haematobium* infection. *Brain*, **108**, 1023–38.

Shepherd, E., Brettle, R., Liberski, P.P. et al. (1999). Spinal cord pathology and viral burden in homosexuals and drug users with AIDS. *Neuropathol. Appl. Neurobiol.*, **25**, 2–10.

Stark, R.J., Kennard, C. & Swash, M. (1981). Hand wasting in spondylotic high cord compression: an electromyographic study. *Ann. Neurol.*, **9**, 58–62.

49

Diseases of the vertebral column

Simon F. Farmer and Lucinda J. Carr

Department of Neurology, St Mary's Hospital, London, National Hospital for Neurology and Neurosurgery,
London and Department of Neurology, Great Ormond Street Hospital for Children, London, UK

Abnormalities of the vertebral column

Embryology of the spine

Interpretation of congenital and acquired anomalies of the vertebral column is aided by an understanding of normal development. In early fetal life the ectodermal germ layer gives rise to the primitive neural tube. This normally closes by the end of the fourth intrauterine week; failure of this primary neurulation results in fusion defects such as anencephaly or spina bifida. By this time the primary brain vesicles are present, representing forebrain, midbrain and hindbrain. Mesoderm lies around the neural tube and by the end of the fifth intrauterine week will have completed segmentation into 42–44 recognizable somite pairs (occipital to coccygeal). Once established, the epithelioid cells of these somites rapidly transform and migrate towards the notochord where they differentiate into three distinct cell lines: sclerotomes (from which connective tissue, cartilage and bone are derived), myotomes (providing segmental muscle) and dermatomes (providing segmental skin). Chondrification of the sclerotomes leads to the development of ossification centres, with an anterior and posterior centre for each vertebral body and a pair for each arch. The process is largely complete by the end of the third month of fetal development. Disruption during these early stages accounts for many of the vertebral and craniocervical anomalies. There is increasing interest in the possible role of abnormal notochord signalling and Pax-1 gene expression in these segmentation defects (see for example, David et al., 1997). After the third month of gestation the vertebral column and dura lengthen more rapidly than the spinal cord resulting in regression of the cord tip, leaving the filum terminale below. By term the cord tip typically lies at the L2–3 interspace. Failure of normal cord ascent may lead to tethering of the spinal cord.

Idiopathic scoliosis

Scoliosis refers to a lateral deviation of the spine and is always abnormal. It may be classified on the basis of clinical examination into structural and non-structural forms. In a structural scoliosis there is a rotational component to the curve which is best seen on forward flexion when prominence of rib or loin musculature becomes apparent. This is not the case in non-structural scoliosis, where there is no rotational element. Non-structural scoliosis may be a marker of other pathology such as leg length discrepancy or muscle spasm but is rarely of clinical significance in itself. If associated with underlying neurological disease it may progress to a structural deformity.

Once a structural scoliosis is diagnosed, the severity and potential for progression must be assessed. Erect postero-anterior and lateral X-rays should be taken in a standardized manner so that serial films can be compared. The severity of the curve is given by the Cobb angle, which describes the angle created by the intersection of lines drawn across the end plates of the upper and lowermost vertebrae delineating the curve i.e those with the greatest opposing tilt as illustrated in Fig. 49.1. Angles >20° in skeletally immature children demand particular vigilance; it is during periods of rapid growth that scoliosis may progress significantly, thus scoliosis presenting in younger children has a greater risk of progression. Progression in adults is less common, although underlying neuromuscular disease, pregnancy and osteoporosis pose increased risks.

The major causes of structural scoliosis are given in Table 49.1. The commonest type is idiopathic scoliosis which accounts for around 70% of all cases. The child is otherwise healthy and no underlying pathology is found. The prevalence of adolescent scoliosis, the commonest form, is approximately 4% of the population if mild cases are included (Dickens, 1997). The majority are right sided,

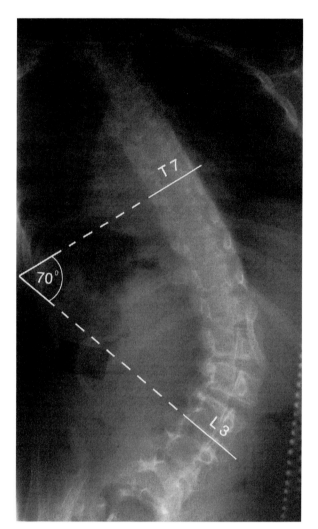

Fig. 49.1. Plain antero-posterior spine X-ray showing thoroco-lumbar scoliosis in an adolescent with a spino-cerebellar syndrome. The Cobb angle drawn between the apices of the curve measures 70 degrees.

Table 49.1. Causes of structural scoliosis

Idiopathic scoliosis
Infantile <3 years
Juvenile 3–10 years
Adolescent >10 years

Congenital scoliosis
Failure of vertebral segmentation and/or formation

Neuromuscular scoliosis
Neuropathic
    Upper motoneuron, e.g. Cerebral palsy
    Lower motoneuron, e.g. Spinomuscular atrophy, Poliomyelitis
    Mixed, e.g. Myelomeningocoele and spinal dysraphism
Myopathic
    Hereditary neuropathies and dysautonomias
    Congential myopathies
    Muscular dystrophies, e.g. Duchenne

Miscellaneous causes
Skeletal dysplasias
Marfan syndrome
Neurofibromatosis
Spinocerebellar degenerations including Freidrich's ataxia
Arthrogryposis
Rett's syndrome
Metabolic bone disease
Dystonia
Parkinson's disease and parkinsonian syndromes
Craniocervical junction anomalies especially if associated with syringomyelia
Spinal tumours/trauma/irradiation

thoracic and painless. An MRI scan is advised if features are atypical or neurological signs are present, for example a left-sided lumbar curve or absent abdominal reflexes, as these features may indicate underlying pathology such as spinal cord tumours or Chiari malformation. The infantile and juvenile forms of idiopathic scoliosis are uncommon.

The cause of idiopathic scoliosis is multifactorial and the development and progression of the scoliosis may have different mechanisms. There is often a positive family history of scoliosis, with girls eight times more likely than boys to require treatment (Dickens, 1997). The inheritance can be described by a dominant major gene diallele model (the gene is as yet unidentified) with incomplete pene-trance (Axenovich et al., 1999). Progression of the curve is more common in thoracic or large curves (>35°) with skel-etal maturity another important consideration. The conse-quences of severe idiopathic scoliosis are cosmetic deformity, cardiopulmonary compromise and back pain.

Congenital scoliosis

In congenital scoliosis the vertebrae are anomalous due either to a failure of natural segmentation, leading to asymmetric fusion, or to failure of formation, in which only part of the vertebra is formed. Often there is a combination of both pathologies. In congenital scoliosis there is a high incidence of associated anomalies. These include neuraxis anomalies in up to 40% of patients, renal and gastrointes-tinal tract abnormalities in around 20% and congenital heart defects in approximately 10% (McMaster & Ohtsukak, 1982). Sometimes the scoliosis is part of a syndromic diagnosis such as in the Klippel–Feil and Noonan syndromes. Clinically the scoliosis may vary from a mild non-progressive deformity to a severe and rapidly progressive curve that compromises the spinal cord. There is often an associated kyphosis.

Neuromuscular scoliosis

Spinal deformity is common in many of the neuromuscular disorders. In the developed world cerebral palsy, spina bifida and Duchenne muscular dystrophy are the most common causes of neuromuscular scoliosis, although poliomyelitis is still an important cause in developing countries. Because of the underlying condition, the spinal curvature, in contrast to idiopathic scoliosis, generally presents earlier, is more extensive and is more likely to deteriorate through childhood and into adult life. Other systems are often already compromised; for example, there may be muscle imbalance, cardiopulmonary insufficiency, poor nutrition, insensate skin and osteoporosis. These problems may be further exacerbated by the physical and functional effects of the scoliosis itself. In addition, the scoliosis may adversely affect walking and seating and cause pain as the ribs abut the iliac crest. This is often compounded by coexisting pelvic obliquity, particularly in the non-ambulant patient.

Kyphosis and lordosis

The spine naturally shows some curvature in the antero-posterior plane, seen as a kyphosis in the thoracic region and lordosis at the lumbar spine. A normal lumbar lordosis shows full correction on forward flexion. Excessive lordosis may occur postlaminectomy, in the neuromuscular conditions, or when there is fixed flexion deformity at the hip.

A kyphosis >40° is abnormal. It may be congenital, due to a lack of fusion of the vertebral bodies anteriorly or a lack of formation of one or more anterior bodies. Although less common than congenital scoliosis, it carries a more severe prognosis as a higher proportion of patients will develop progressive deformity and myelopathy particularly during the adolescent growth spurt (McMaster & Singh, 1999). Patients with anterior failure of vertebral body formation, who present with a sharp angle kyphosis, are at particular risk of rapid progression and spinal cord compression. Early arthrodesis is indicated in these cases. Schuermann's kyphosis is the most common form of acquired kyphosis, presenting in adolescents it is generally benign. Kyphosis only occasionally progresses once skeletal maturity is reached.

Miscellaneous causes of spinal deformity

A number of primary diseases of bone and connective tissue produce pathology of the spine and craniocervical junction. Those that present neurological problems are classified into four broad categories:

Osteopenic disorders

In these bone mineralization is reduced. These include endocrine diseases such as hyperparathyroidism, Cushing's disease, osteomalacia, primary osteoporosis and osteogenesis imperfecta.

Osteogenesis imperfecta (OI) is a heritable disorder of collagen that results in osteopenia and increased bone fragility. In the majority of patients mutations are found in the genes encoding the $\alpha 1$ and $\alpha 2$ collagen chains. These result in reduced amounts of collagen which is often structurally abnormal. To date, over 200 mutations have been described (Dalgleish, 1997); however, there is no close correlation between the molecular abnormalities and the clinical manifestations which are highly variable. Prenatal diagnosis is available for some forms of the disease. The Sillence classification delineates four major phenotypes on the basis of bone fragility, growth and the presence or absence of additional features such as blue sclerae, dentinogenesis imperfecta and presenile hearing loss (Sillence, 1981). Progressive skeletal deformity is a particular feature of OI type III and often requires orthopedic intervention. Basilar invagination is a rare but important complication of OI. This may be associated with ventral brainstem compression, hydromyelia and hydrocephalus. It generally presents in early adult life with progressive neurological symptoms and signs, the commonest being headache and lower cranial nerve dysfunction, particularly atypical trigeminal neuralgia. Other features include quadriparesis, ataxia and nystagmus (Sawin & Menezes, 1997). Trigeminal pain, if intractable, may require stereotactic surgery. The treatment of myelopathy involves ventral decompression and occipito-cervical fusion, with or without decompression of the foramen magnum (Lynch & Crockard, 1999).

Currently, there is much interest in the role of bisphosphonates in the management of OI. There is evidence that these drugs reduce bone pain, improve both bone density and vertebral height (Glorieux et al., 1998). However, long-term benefits on disease progression, function and quality of life have yet to be demonstrated.

Skeletal dysplasias

Menezes has classified these into 5 categories, the largest being the osteochondrodysplasias and the dysostoses (Menezes & Ryken, 1992). Osteochondrodysplasias are defined as abnormalities of cartilage or bone growth and development. They generally present as short-limbed dwarfism, with achondroplasia the commonest form. Around 50% of children with achondroplasia have a thoracolumbar kyphosis in infancy and there is a risk of spinal cord stenosis. Patients characteristically have macrocephaly but a small mid face and small foramen magnum. These abnormalities place them at risk of symptomatic stenosis and hydrocephalus. Sleep apnea is seen in the majority of patients, which may have a central or respiratory cause. Cervicomedullary decompression with resection of the foramen magnum may be necessary. Atlantoaxial instability has been increasingly recognized in the skeletal dysplasias.

The dysostoses are defined as malformations of individual bones singly or in combination. These include the craniosynostoses (Crouzon and Apert syndromes) in which vertebral anomalies are commonly recognized and Klippel–Feil syndrome which is discussed later.

The metabolic storage disorders

These include the mucopolysaccharidoses, the glycoprotein storage disorders, the gangliosidoses and the mucolipidoses. These neurodegenerative diseases vary in their severity but show characteristic skeletal dysplasias, such as 'hooked' vertebrae, broad ribs and flared pelvis. Thoracolumbar kyphosis is common, with a risk of spinal cord compression. Other neurological complications include cognitive deterioration, carpal tunnel syndrome and deafness. In Morquio's syndrome (mucopolysaccharidosis IV) the os odontium is dysplastic or absent. These patients also have striking ligamentous laxity which gives a particularly high risk of atlantoaxial instablity and spinal cord compression.

Mesenchymal and connective tissue disorders

Neurofibromatosis is considered in detail in Chapter 128. Around 30% of patients will develop scoliosis, of which 40% will have associated cervical spine abnormalities. The scoliosis often manifests as an acute-angled short segment kyphoscoliosis which will inevitably progress unless fusion is performed (Winter et al., 1979). Approximately 50% of patients with Marfan's syndrome will develop significant scoliosis.

Management of spinal deformity

Patient management varies from case to case and will be influenced by the underlying diagnosis, current levels of function especially ambulatory abilities, life expectancy and concomitant medical problems.

In kyphosis bracing is advocated for skeletally immature patients with progressive curves <60°. Surgery is often required if the curve exceeds 60°.

In patients with idiopathic scoliosis bracing may delay or arrest scoliosis progression in the skeletally immature child. Indications for bracing are curves >30° or earlier if there is radiological progression. Bracing is rarely effective once the curve exceeds 45°. It may improve pain in adults with scoliosis. A thoracolumbar spinal orthosis is generally used, with an added cervical extension (as in the Milwaukee brace) if the apex of the curve is above T8. If bracing is not appropriate, or fails to control the scoliosis, surgical stabilization is necessary, although this may be at the cost of spinal growth.

In congenital or neuromuscular scoliosis there may be a role for bracing but given the relentless progression of the scoliosis in many of these conditions, early surgery is often indicated. In non-ambulant patients the spinal fusion should involve the pelvis. Surgical risk, particularly of hemostasis and postoperative chest infection, is high in this patient group.

A solid arthrodesis is the primary goal of surgery, often requiring joint excision, decortication and bone grafts. Instrumentation is added to achieve and maintain correction as well as providing stability to the fusion mass. Surgical procedures will vary but are largely determined by the underlying pathology. The reader is referred to standard orthopedic texts (see Moe's textbook of scoliosis, 1994). Good results are dependent on meticulous patient selection at all stages, with multidisciplinary preoperative assessment, intraoperative neurophysiological spinal cord monitoring and intensive care support postoperatively. Complications include immediate perioperative problems such as hemorrhage and pneumothorax. Infection occurs in up to 2% of patients. Paraplegia occurs in <1% of patients and postoperative paraparesis warrants urgent removal of any instrumentation. Up to 5% of patients experience failure of graft implantation usually due to pseudarthrosis.

Craniovertebral junction anomalies

The pathophysiology of the craniocervical junction anomalies is complex. A useful classification is proposed by Menezes (1999), reproduced in Table 49.2, subdivides the anomalies into congenital, developmental and acquired causes.

Clinical features of craniocervical junction anomaly

Symptoms and signs may be insidious or of rapid onset. Clinical presentation is diverse as dysfunction may occur

Table 49.2. Causes of craniovertebral anomalies

1. Congenital anomalies and malformations
   A. Occipital sclerotome malformations – atlas assimilation, proatlas remnants
   B. Atlas malformations – bifid atlas, assimilation, fusion, absent arches
   C. Axis malformations – segmentation defects, odontoid dysplasias
2. Developmental and acquired anomalies
   A. Foramen magnum abnormalities
      (i) foramen stenosis, e.g. Achondroplasia
      (ii) secondary invagination, e.g. Ostoeogenesis Impefecta, Paget's
   B. Atlantoaxial instability
      (i) Down's syndrome
      (ii) metabolic disorders, e.g. Morquio, Hurler syndromes
      (iii) Infections, e.g. Grisel's syndrome, Tuberculosis
      (iv) Trauma
      (v) Inflammation, e.g. rheumatoid arthritis, Reiter's syndrome
      (vi) Tumour, e.g. osteoblastoma, neurofibromatosis
      (vii) Miscellaneous, e.g. syringomyelia

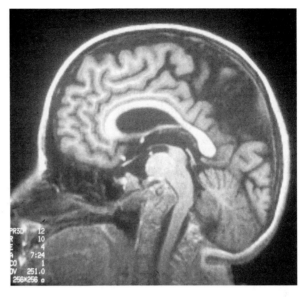

Fig. 49.2. Sagittal MRI brain demonstrating basilar impression in an adolescent with severe (type III) osteogenesis imperfecta (OI).

at many levels: the lower brainstem, cranial nerves, cervical roots and upper cervical cord may be compromised by pressure from bone or soft tissue, there also may be indirect compromise of the blood supply. Congenital anomalies of the craniocervical junction are often associated with dysmorphic features and obvious skeletal anomalies. Patients most commonly complain of headache and neck pain worsened by movement and coughing. Pain characteristically originates in the suboccipital region and radiates to the vertex, in a C2 distribution. Head tilt and 'torticollis' are common. In children with craniocervical junction anomalies hearing loss is the most common cranial nerve symptom. In adults, trigeminal distribution pain and neuralgia may result from direct compression of the V nerve or compression of the V nerve nuclei in the upper cervical cord. Lesions of other cranial nerves particularly IX, X, XI and XII are also seen. Spinal cord compression produces a myelopathic picture with upper motor neuron features, often progressing to loss of bladder and bowel control. Occasionally, the myelopathy is confined to the upper limbs. Sometimes there is a predilection for the dorsal columns, producing marked joint position sense loss. Brainstem involvement may produce dysphagia, dysarthria, internuclear ophthalmoplegia and nystagmus (most commonly horizontal but more classically down beating). Central apnea, drop attacks and syncope are important additional features. The intimate relationship of

the vertebral arteries to the upper cervical spine and foramen magnum may increase the risk of basilar migraine and vertebro-basilar ischemia.

There are three principal mechanisms by which the craniocervical junction anomalies lead to neurological signs. Frequently, more than one mechanism coexists.

Direct compression

This may result from developmental abnormalities of the odontoid process. Of particular importance is the condition os odontoidium where the odontoid and the body of the axis are not fused. Atlas assimilation, where there is failure of segmentation between the fourth occipital and first spinal sclerotomes, is relatively common and is particularly associated with the Chiari malformations. Direct compression may also result from abnormal articulation around cervical vertebral blocks as is seen in the Klippel–Feil syndrome.

Structural

Basilar invagination describes deformity of the osseous structures of the skull base which leads to upward displacement of the edge of the foramen magnum (see Fig. 49.2). In its primary congenital form it is often associated with platybasia where the clivus and anterior skull base are abnormally flattened. It may be associated with more subtle developmental bony anomalies and associated neurodysgeneses such as hindbrain herniation (particularly Chiari malformations) and syringohydromyelia. The foramen magnum itself may be narrow, usually as a feature of underlying skeletal dysplasia, as in achondroplasia. Acquired forms of basilar invagination are more common and result from any bone softening condition. The most important causes are osteogenesis imperfecta (see Fig. 49.2) and Paget's disease. Diagnosis of basilar invagination on cervical spine X-ray involves measuring the position of the odontoid tip with respect to either the foramen magnum itself (McRae's line) or from lines drawn between the roof of the hard palate and either the posterior lip of the foramen magnum (Chamberlain's line) or the caudal part of the occipital bone (McGregor's line).

Atlantoaxial instability

Atlantoaxial dislocation results from incompetence of the transverse ligaments or abnormalities of the dens itself (Stevens et al., 1994). Instability is defined by an atlanto-dens interval >5 mm, and is demonstrated by flexion/extension X-rays of cervical spine or 3D CT reconstruction, the latter also allows assessment of any rotational component. Instability may occur spontaneously or develop secondarily due to inflammation or trauma. It is a recognized feature of the complex developmental craniofacial and cranio-vertebral anomalies, particularly if there is atlas assimilation and segmentation failure as in the Klippel–Feil syndrome. Syndromes which are also associated with ligamentous laxity carry a particular risk of dislocation; such as the mucopolysaccharidoses and Down's syndrome (Fig. 49.3).

The surgical treatment of craniocervical junction anomaly is complex and beyond the scope of this chapter (see Robertson & Coakham, 1999). If neurological symptoms and signs of brain stem compression occur surgery is usually indicated. Treatment of basilar invagination, for example, due to osteogenesis imperfecta involves ventral decompression and dorsal occipitocervical fusion.

Down's syndrome

Trisomy 21 occurs in around one in 650 live births and is the single most common cause of severe learning difficulties. It initially presents with characteristic dysmorphic features and hypotonia, often with associated cardiac and gastrointestinal anomalies. It is estimated that up to 25% of patients with Down's syndrome have asymptomatic atlantoaxial instability. Only around 1% are symptomatic (Pueschal & Scola, 1987). Recognized presentations include mild pyramidal tract signs with gait disturbance or the precipitous onset of cord compression. In the absence of signs or symptoms, screening of the atlanto-dens inter-

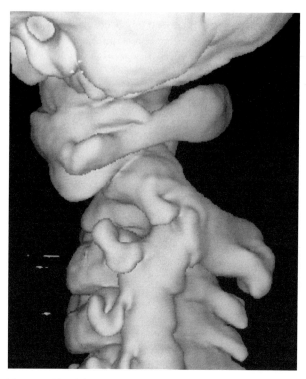

Fig. 49.3. Three dimensional CT reconstruction showing atlanto-axial subluxation in an 8-year-old child with Down's syndrome.

val is no longer routine, however sports such as trampolining and somersaults should be avoided. Once symptoms are present, surgical stabilization is recommended.

Chiari malformations

Chiari described four types of hindbrain malformation. The Chiari I malformation is demonstrated on neuroimaging by the dorsal extension of the cerebellar tonsils below the level of the foramen magnum (Fig. 49.4). Some studies report the prevalence of tonsillar descent (3–5 mm below the foramen magnum) on sagittal MRI in asymptomatic individuals to be as high as 20%. However, more definitive volumetric reconstruction of coronal MRI demonstrates that the complex shape of the rostral cerebellum may lead to sagittal MRI overestimating tonsillar descent (Savy et al., 1994). The true prevalence of Chiari I in asymptomatic individuals is probably less than 1%, although it rises if tonsillar descent on sagittal MRI is associated with appropriate symptoms or other hind brain anomalies and in around 50% of cases of true cerebellar ectopia there is elongation of the medulla. Approximately 50% of Chiari I malformations are associated with craniocervical anomalies and

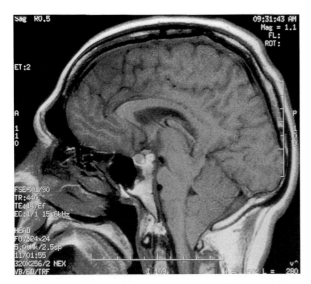

Fig. 49.4. Sagittal MRI brain showing Chiari I malformation.

lus in >90% of cases and generally manifests in the neonatal period. It consists of caudal displacement of the medulla and cerebellum (particularly vermis) into the cervical canal overriding the spinal cord often accompanied by partial herniation of the fourth ventricle and distortion of midbrain tectum. Associated abnormalities of supratentorial and midbrain structures are common. Chiari III is analogous to type II but describes downward displacement of the cerebellum into a posterior encephalocele, again with elongation and herniation of the fourth ventricle. Clinical features are severe and often life threatening, particularly where there is cranial nerve dysfunction.

The Chiari IV malformation describes cerebellar hypoplasia and on current understanding is not part of the Chiari spectrum.

syringomyelia (Milhorat et al., 1999). The development of Chiari I is likely to be multifactorial. It has been postulated on the basis of familial aggregation that Chiari I is a disorder of para-axial mesoderm (Milhorat et al., 1999). However, unlike Chiari II–IV there are clear examples of acquired Chiari I in which serial MRI has demonstrated postnatal development of the anomaly (Huang & Constantine, 1994). Furthermore, lowering of CSF pressure following lumbar puncture or lumbar peritoneal shunting may be a risk factor for cerebellar tonsil descent (Chumas et al., 1993; Payner et al., 1994). There are well-documented examples of 'Chiari' or 'pseudo-Chiari' malformations improving following treatment of abnormally low CSF pressure due to CSF leakage (Samii et al., 1999).

The symptoms and signs resulting from Chiari I overlap with those associated with other craniocervical anomalies (see above). These include headache especially cough headache, nystagmus and quadriplegia. Additional symptoms and signs may result from associated hydrocephalus or syringomyelia. The condition is rarely symptomatic in childhood. Unusual presentations of Chiari I have been described. These include sudden death, syncope, ventricular fibrillation due to head movement, lingual myoclonus, pulsatile tinnitus, Menière's-type symptoms, acquired esotropia, central apnea and paroxysmal rage. Surgical treatment involves decompression of the foramen magnum and should be offered on the basis of significant and relevant symptoms, e.g. severe cough headache, or the presence of physical signs indicating neurological compromise.

Chiari II malformation is a congenital anomaly which is associated with myelomeningocele and hydrocepha-

Spinal dysraphism

Spinal dysraphic states are caused by localized failure of neural tube closure during fetal development. Myelomeningocele is the most common form, with an incidence of 0.8/1000 live births. There are marked regional variations in its incidence and the condition is heterogeneous. There are strong genetic components and recurrence risks rise from 1–2% after one affected child to 10% with two affected children (Todorov, 1982). The process of neuralation may be disrupted by teratogenic agents and in particular by maternal and/or fetal folate deficiency. Early folic acid supplementation reduces the incidence of neural tube defects, so that all women are recommended to take supplemental folate prior to conception and during the first trimester. This advice is especially important for women with a previously affected pregnancy or those taking anticonvulsants in whom the incidence of neural tube defects is around 1% of pregnancies, larger amounts of folic acid are recommended for these women. Routine antenatal screening provides a prenatal diagnosis in many cases; raised maternal serum α fetoprotein is associated with open neural tube defects and fetal ultrasonography allows cranial and vertebral structures to be visualized directly. Prenatal counselling and termination can then be offered.

Myelomeningocele and myeloscisis comprise 95% of cases of spinal dysraphism, with exposed neural tissue a common feature (Fig. 49.5). In a meningocele and in spina bifida occulta neural elements are covered by skin. The clinical features are determined by the extent of the myelocele and the presence of associated abnormalities, which may include both neural and extraneural anomalies.

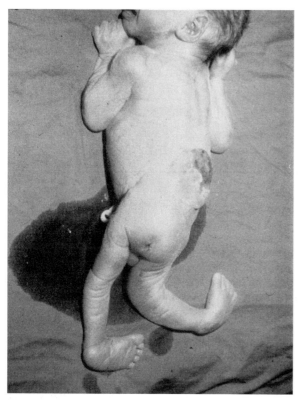

Fig. 49.5. A new born infant with thoroco-lumbar myelomeningocele. He has a neuropathic bladder, patulous anus and flaccid lower limbs with bilateral talipes.

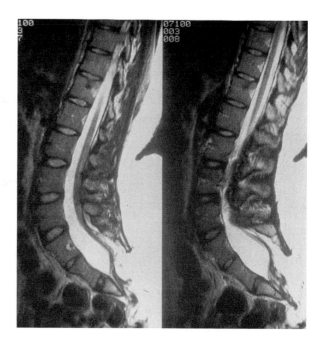

Fig. 49.6. Sagittal MRI of lumbar–sacral spine showing a lipomyelomeningocele.

Progressive hydrocephalus requiring surgical treatment is present in 90% of cases and around 70% have a Chiari II malformation. Learning difficulties are common, one-third have an IQ < 80. Syringomyelia is present in up to 75% of cases and is often associated with severe scoliosis. Approximately a third of patients have diastematomyelia.

Approximately 80% of open spina bifida defects are located in the lumbosacral area. The sensory level indicates the upper level of the lesion. Lesions above L3 result in complete paraplegia, but motor deficits may otherwise be patchy with a mixed pattern of upper and lower motoneuron signs. Sphincter and detrusor function is always compromised and careful urological assessment is required. Surgical closure is undertaken within 48–72 hours of delivery to reduce the risk of ascending infection and protect viable neural tissue within the placode. Following closure delayed hydrocephalus is likely. Patients generally require ongoing medical care by a multidisciplinary team.

Spina bifida occulta describes occult dysraphism, where neural structures have not herniated through the mesenchymal defect. It includes diastematomyelia, terminal myelo-

cystocele and tight filum terminale. Lipomyelomeningocele and dermal sinuses are often included in this classification as they also result from abnormal neurulation. Spina bifida occulta is often neurologically asymptomatic. The majority of patients have associated cutaneous abnormalities such as a tuft of hair or a dimple over the region, and plain X-rays show underlying vertebral anomalies. MRI scan then confirms the diagnosis (Fig. 49.6). Two neurological presentations are recognized. First, a congenital asymmetric weakness and atrophy of the lower limbs and second the 'tethered cord syndrome' with progressive and sometimes precipitous onset of weakness and spasticity. The latter often presents in childhood or during the adolescent growth spurt and is an important cause of toe walking in childhood. Both presentations may be associated with sphincter disturbance. Treatment is primarily neurosurgical, with release of the spinal cord from the tethering lesion, with full preoperative neurological and urological assessment. Orthopedic, orthotic and physiotherapy management of lower limb deformity is also important.

Klippel–Feil syndrome

Described in 1912, the disorder is characterized by a short neck, impaired neck mobility and a low hairline (Klippel & Feil, 1912). The incidence is approximately 1 : 40 000 births. The skeletal abnormalities include fusion of two or more

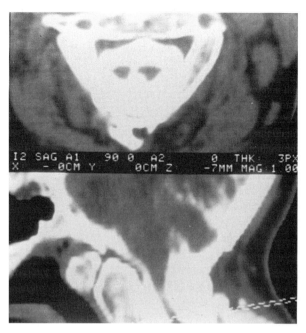

Fig. 49.7. Axial CT myelogram with sagittal reconstruction showing split cervical spinal cord in a patient with Klippel–Feil syndrome.

cervical or cervicothoracic vertebrae. The syndrome is heterogeneous; differing numbers and positions of fused vertebrae are described and the associated anomalies are highly variable (Clarke et al., 1998). The condition may be familial: dominant, recessive and X-linked inheritance patterns have been proposed. A dominant form in which there is chromosome 8 inversion is described (Clarke et al., 1995). Despite the sometimes dramatic spinal abnormalities, a follow-up study over a 10-year period has indicated that only 20% of patients experienced significant cervical spine symptoms and only 6% required surgical intervention (Theiss et al., 1997).

Extravertebral anomalies associated with Klippel–Feil syndrome affect multiple systems. Skeletal and systemic abnormalities include: scoliosis, scapula elevation, rib anomalies, cranio-facial dysmorphology, pulmonary, cardiac, gastrointestinal and urogenital anomalies. Neurological problems include syringomyelia, cranial nerve abnormalities, Duane's retraction syndrome, deafness, acquired myelopathy due to the spinal abnormality, thin corpus callosum, split cervical spinal cord (see Fig. 49.7) and failure of pyramidal tract decussation (Gunderson & Solitaire, 1968; Schott & Wyke, 1981; David et al., 1996). The latter anomaly is particularly interesting as it may underlie the intense congenital mirror movements which affect a number of these patients.

Congenital mirror movements

These are intense involuntary movements, primarily of distal upper limb muscles, which mirror the voluntary unilateral movement. They cannot be suppressed and typically do not occur during passive movement. Mirror movements occur normally during a child's motor development, however, they are rarely intense and disappear by the age of 6 years. Pathological mirror movements are rarely disabling and patients learn adaptive proximal movements so as to avoid inappropriate finger movements, for example wrong key strikes whilst typing. Neurophysiological study of mirror movements has provided new insights into central motor control and plasticity.

A single subject with Klippel–Feil syndrome and mirror movements has been studied in detail (Farmer et al., 1990). Similar neurophysiological findings have been reported in patients with congenital mirror movements and mirror movements in association with X-linked Kallman syndrome (Cohen et al., 1991; Mayston et al., 1997). Unilateral focal electrical or magnetic brain stimulation of either left or right primary motor cortex at threshold in non-mirroring subjects evokes contralateral short latency EMG responses due to rapid conduction through pyramidal tract pathways (see Fig. 49.8). In contrast, mirroring individuals show simultaneous bilateral short latency EMG responses following unilateral motor cortex stimulation. Abnormal bilateral EMG responses indicate that in subjects with mirror movements the corticospinal tract is aberrant and bilaterally represented. In mirroring subjects the short latency (N20) component of the somatosensory evoked potential is confined to the contralateral sensory cortex. Spinal (short) latency cutaneomuscular (CMR) and stretch reflexes are confined, as in normal subjects, to the stimulated side. However, in mirroring subjects the long-latency components of the CMR and stretch reflexes are simultaneously present in both the stimulated and non-stimulated limbs (Farmer et al., 1990; Matthews et al., 1990; Capaday et al., 1991). This abnormal crossing of the long-latency CMR and stretch reflexes in mirroring subjects has provided strong evidence in support of the view that in human hand muscles long-latency reflexes are transmitted via a transcortical loop (see Fig. 49.8). Cross-correlation analysis of EMG activity recorded simultaneously from homologous muscles of left and right hands, reveals, in contrast to healthy subjects, the presence of a short duration peak at time zero, indicating that during normal muscle contraction both hands receive abnormal common presynaptic drive (see Fig. 49.8). This abnormal drive can be shown to be highly muscle specific, indicating that abnormal bilateral corticospinal axons innervate the

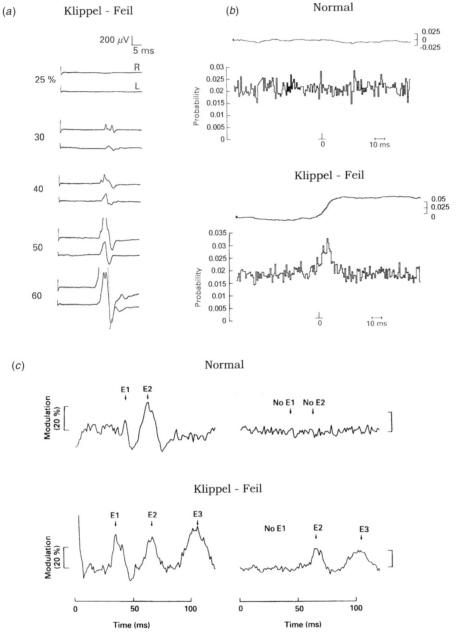

Fig. 49.8. Neurophysiological data from a normal subject and a subject with Klippel–Feil syndrome and mirror movements. (*a*) Abnormal bilateral short-latency muscle responses to focal transcutaneous electrical stimulation of the left motor cortex in the Klippel–Feil subject. (*b*) Cross-correlation histograms and CUSUM constructed between simultaneous left and right hand muscle EMGs in the normal subject and the Klippel–Feil subject. The abnormal peak in the Klippel–Feil subject data reflects abnormal common presynaptic drive to left and right spinal motoneurons. (*c*) Cutaneomuscular reflexes in the normal subject and Klippel–Feil subject. In contrast to normal subjects, those with mirror movements show crossing of long-latency reflex activity (E2 and E3 components), similar results are found for the long-latency stretch reflex, indicating that late reflex components are generated by a transcortical loop.

equivalent motoneuron pools, e.g. those of first dorsal interosseous muscle on left and right sides of the spinal cord. These findings indicate that voluntary and long-loop reflex activity in abnormal central motor pathways produces the mirror movements of Klippel–Feil syndrome.

Mirror movements in childhood hemiplegia

Neurophysiological studies of mirror movements have been extended to include childhood hemiplegia. Intense mirror movements are a recognized feature of childhood hemiplegia and have been proposed to represent a physical sign of corticospinal tract re-wiring following early brain damage (Woods & Teuber, 1978). Children with hemiplegia and mirror movements have been studied using the approach outlined above for Klippel–Feil syndrome. The findings are similar except that the corticospinal axons reach both sides of the spinal cord from the undamaged motor cortex (Farmer et al., 1991; Carr et al., 1993). The presence of mirror movements with characteristic neurophysiological findings is associated with MRI scans in which there is no gliosis in response to the cerebral injury, suggesting that antenatal insults before gestational age 28 weeks causing hemiplegia are associated with pyramidal tract plasticity and mirror movements. This remarkable central nervous reorganization may help to sustain function of the child's hemiplegic hand albeit at the expense of mirror movements (Carr et al., 1993).

Paget's disease

The disorder is rare before the age of 40 but becomes increasingly common with time, affecting 10% of 90-year-olds. The clinical features are those of bone pain, local deformity, bone enlargement, pathological fracture and a predisposition to sarcomatous change. The disorder often affects the skull and spine and as a result neurological involvement is common. Diagnosis is made by typical radiological appearances and the finding of an elevated serum alkaline phosphatase. The disease is one of excessive bone resorption with excessive osteoblastic and osteolytic activity. A genetic predisposition is described and some familial cases have been linked to chromosome 18q (Cody et al., 1997). Pagetic osteoclasts contain nuclear inclusions and osteoclastic infection with paramyxoviruses is one postulated cause of the disease (Singer, 1999).

There are a numerous potential neurological sequelae of Paget's disease. Direct compression by Pagetic bone may lead to the following: headache, dementia, brainstem and cerebellar dysfunction, cranial neuropathies, myelopathy, cauda equina syndrome, and radiculopathies. The most

common cranial neuropathy is sensorineural deafness; optic atrophy, trigeminal neuralgia and hemifacial spasm are also described. Pagetic softening of the skull may lead to basilar invagination resulting in brain stem and high cervical compression syndromes and occasionally hydrocephalus. The brain and spinal cord can become acutely compressed due to epidural hematoma. The vascularity of Pagetic bone may lead to cerebral ischemia as part of a steal syndrome (compared to normal bone, blood flow in Pagetic bone is increased threefold). Neurological syndromes may also develop due to compression of blood vessels.

Paget's disease generally responds to treatment with bisphosphonates although a relative resistance to these drugs is described (Gutteridge et al., 1999). First-line treatment is with potent oral bisphosphonates. Second-line treatment regimes include calcitonin, etidronate and intravenous bisphonsphonates (Poncelet, 1999). Bone pain in particular can resolve within 1–2 weeks of commencement of treatment, treatment efficacy may be monitored by serum alkaline phosphatase levels and a therapeutic response may be expected in approximately 80% of patients treated. Neurological syndromes often improve with medical treatment. Rapidly progressive neurological syndromes require high dose intravenous bisphosphonate therapy and/or treatment with calcitonin. However, hydrocephalus generally requires shunting. Surgical decompression for basilar invagination, cranial nerve lesions, spinal cord and root compression is indicated if neurological symptoms and signs progress rapidly or despite best medical treatment (Poncelet, 1999). Medical treatment prior to surgical intervention may reduce bone vascularity and thus the risk of perioperative hemorrhage.

Rheumatoid arthritis

Rheumatoid arthritis is a chronic, inflammatory, immune-mediated symmetrical polyarthritis with a predilection for the distal joints. Females are affected twice a commonly as males and the prevalance ranges from 0.2–2 % of the population. The inflamed synovium is termed the pannus; it is characterized by T and B cell activation, cytokine release, immune complex deposition, angiogenesis, and cellular proliferation. This inflammatory process leads to damage and destruction of bone, cartilage and ligaments. Aggressive immunosuppressive therapy with disease modifying drugs (in particular sulfasalazine and methotrexate) improves the prognosis of rheumatoid arthritis (Madhok et al., 2000), it is not yet known whether this approach reduces the incidence of neurological complications of the disease.

Neurological manifestations of rheumatoid arthritis include entrapment neuropathy, vasculitic neuropathy, myopathy and ischemic syndromes due to vasculitis, these are discussed further in Chapter 94 on the vasculitides. The spinal cord manifestations result from ligamentous disruption, bone destruction and secondary osteoporosis. A rare syndrome of diffuse dural infiltration with inflammatory cells producing a pachymeningitis has been described.

Patients with rheumatoid arthritis of the cervical spine frequently experience headache and neck pain. The most feared neurological complication of rheumatoid arthritis is upper cervical cord and brainstem compression. Involvement of the atlanto-axial ligament often combined with local pannus formation and bone destruction produces subluxation. Atlanto-axial subluxation affects 25% of rheumatoid patients of whom 25% have neurological signs. Atlanto-axial subluxation may occur in lateral, rotational, anterior, posterior and vertical directions; the latter three directions being the most neurologically significant. Rheumatoid arthritis may affect the spinal cord caudal to the C1/C2 level independently or in association with a high cord lesion. Postmortem studies of myelopathy show necrosis, gliosis and Wallerian degeneration within ascending and descending white matter (Fujiwara et al., 1999). The degree of atlanto-axial subluxation is well characterized by plain flexion–extension radiography; however, because a large part of the compression is due to inflammatory soft tissue proper assessment requires magnetic resonance imaging (Rogers et al., 1994).

In a series of 235 rheumatoid patients referred for neurosurgical assessment of craniocervical junction instability 60% had myelopathy, the majority of these either had motor or mixed motor and sensory long-tract signs; in approximately 10% the predominant deficits were loss of joint position and Rombergism, indicating a mainly posterior compression. Cranial nerve signs and nystagmus were rare and in this series were associated with other pathologies especially Chiari malformation (Rogers et al., 1994). The combination of mild neurological impairment and rheumatological/orthopedic problems puts rheumatoid patients at increased risk of falls and even minor cervical injury can produce catastrophic neurological deterioration. Atlanto-axial subluxation increases the anesthetic risk due to neck extension during artificial ventilation. Surgical treatment of these patients requires posterior stablization. However, in patients with irreducible subluxation and anterior neuroaxis compression, transoral decompression is undertaken first.

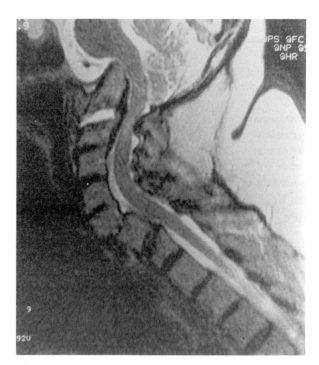

Fig. 49.9. Sagittal MRI of a patient with rheumatoid arthritis showing hind-brain compression from atlanto-axial involvement and multilevel degenerative disease of the cervical spine.

Selection of appropriate patients for surgical intervention presents a major clinical problem. The policy of waiting until rheumatoid patients with atlanto-axial subluxation develop signs of serious myelopathy has been strongly challenged on the basis that once spinal cord damage has been sustained it is rarely reversible (Fig. 49.9). In a prospective trial it has been shown that, following surgical stabilization with or without transoral anterior decompression, approximately 60% of ambulant patients will show stabilization or improvement of their functional status, in contrast only 20% of non-ambulant patients will show any recovery (Casey et al., 1996). Furthermore, surgical morbidity and mortality were found to be significantly higher in the non-ambulant (12.7%) compared to the ambulant group (8.9%).

Spondyloarthropathies

The inflammatory spondyloarthropathies include ankylosing spondylitis, psoriatic arthritis, arthritis associated with inflammatory bowel disease and reactive arthritis, e.g. Reiter's disease. Low back pain is common to all conditions. The primary neurological manifestations are best represented through consideration of ankylosing spondylitis, although they may also occur in association with the other spondyloarthritides.

Ankylosing spondylitis usually presents with gradual onset low back pain and stiffness of the large joints. The condition can affect other organ systems. Men are affected more than women. Disease onset is typically before age 40. HLA B27 is strongly associated with in excess of 90% of patients expressing the antigen. The pathological hallmark is the development of enthesopathy, that is inflammation around sites of tendonous insertion. In the spine syndesmophytes form at the point where spinal ligaments attach to the vertebral bodies.

The neurological manifestations of ankylosing spondylitis are usually a late stage complication. Loss of spinal movement is associated with vertebral body squaring and extensive loss of ligamentous laxity due to syndesmophyte formation. This process produces a rigid spine with kyphosis. Spinal involvement may produce atlanto-axial subluxation, pathological vertebral fracture, discovertebral destruction, spinal canal especially lumbar canal stenosis and a cauda equina syndrome. Atlanto-axial subluxation is rarer than in rheumatoid arthritis; the management issues, however, are similar. Spinal rigidity and disco-vertebral problems predispose to cord compression. Acute spinal cord compression due to epidural hematoma is a recognized problem.

Cauda equina syndrome is a rare late stage complication of ankylosing spondylitis. It presents gradually with leg pain, leg weakness, sensory disturbance and sphinteric dysfunction. On imaging studies posterior lumbar–sacral diverticulae are present. An arachnoiditis may also contribute to the development of the cauda equina syndrome, the presence of the diverticulae, however, indicates that ankylosing spondylitis is the likely cause rather than some other form of arachnoiditis. It is important to remember that spinal irradiation was used to treat ankylosing spondylitis and late radiation neurological damage and bone sarcoma may result.

Superficial siderosis

This is a condition in which there is abnormal subarachnoid hemosiderin deposition. The condition affects many neurological systems and when taken together the symptoms and signs form a coherent and recognizable clinical picture. A recent literature review of 87 cases (Fearnley et al., 1995) revealed the following clinical features: sensorineural deafness (95%), cerebellar ataxia (88%), pyramidal signs (76%), dementia (24%), bladder disturbance (24%),

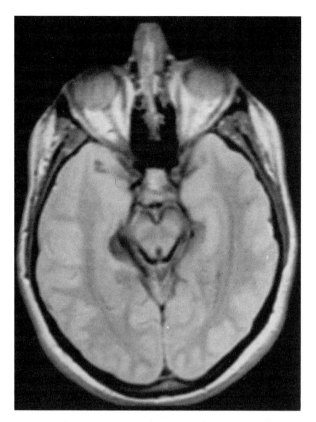

Fig. 49.10. Axial MRI of the brain in a patient with superficial siderosis showing a dark rim around dorsal and ventral mid-brain structures due to iron deposition.

anosmia (at least 17%), aniscoria (at least 10%) and sensory signs (13%). Less frequent features included extraocular motor palsies, and lower motor neuron signs (5–10% each). Neck pain, low back pains and sciatic type pain were well-recognized clinical features. T2-weighted MRI studies of these patients reveal a dark rim, representing the paramagnetic affects of iron deposition, particularly around posterior fossa structures, the spinal cord and occasionally the cerebral hemispheres (Fig. 49.10).

Previous spinal surgery is a recognized cause of superficial siderosis with chronic subarachnoid bleeding due to small blood vessel anomaly. Local spinal pathology affecting the dura such as a root lesion or vascular anomaly is a recognized cause of the condition. The remainder of cases in which a cause may be identified result from subarachnoid hemorrhage or the consequences of hemispherectomy. The serious long-term prognosis of the disorder means an exhaustive search for a bleeding source should be undertaken. This may involve exploratory surgery of a region from which chronic bleeding may occur, for example the site of previous surgery. Successful surgical ablation of a bleeding source has, in anecdotal accounts, produced arrest of the condition. The role of medical treatment with chelation therapy (trientene) is not established although again anecdotal accounts suggest such treatment may have a role in slowing disease progression.

In conclusion, diseases of the vertebral column are relatively common. However, the neurologist or neurosurgeon will tend to see only those cases at the severe end of the spectrum. A good understanding of these conditions is necessary for diagnosis both of the condition, its neurological sequelae and optimal medical and surgical management.

Acknowledgments

We thank Dr J. Stevens and Mr D. Thompson who provided many of the figures and valuable advice during preparation of this chapter.

References   * denotes key references

*Axenovich, T.I., Zaidman, A.M., Zorkoltseva, I.V. & Borodin, P.M. (1999). Segregation analysis of idiopathic scoliosis: demonstration of a major gene effect. *Am. J. Hum. Genet.*, **86**, 389–94.

Capaday, C., Forget, R., Fraser, R. & and Lamarre, Y. (1991). Evidence for a contribution of the motor cortex to the long-latency stretch reflex of the human thumb. *J. Physiol.*, **440**, 243–55.

Carr, L.J., Harrison, L.M., Evans, A.I. & Stephens, J.A. (1993). Patterns of central nervous reorganization in hemiplegic cerebral palsy. *Brain*, **116**, 1223–47.

*Casey, A.T., Crockard, H.A., Bland, J.M., Stevens, J., Moskovich, R. and Ransford, A.O. (1996). Surgery on the rheumatoid cervical spine for the non-ambulant myelopathic patient-too much, too late? *Lancet*, **347** (9007), 1004–7.

Chumas, P.D., Armstrong, D.C., Drake, J.M. et al. (1993). Tonsillar herniation: the rule rather than the exception after lumboperitoneal shunting in the pediatric population. *J. Neurosurg.*, **78**, 568–73.

Clarke, R.A., Kearsley, J.H., Singh, L.S. & Yip, M. (1995). Familial Klippel–Feil syndrome and paracentric inversion inv(8) (q 22.2 q23.3). *Am. J. Hum. Genet.*, **57**, 1364–70.

Clarke, R.A., Catalan, G., Diwan, A.D. & Kearsly, J.H. (1998). Heterogenicity in Klippel Feil syndrome: a new classification. *Paediatr. Radiol.*, **28**, 967–74.

Cody, J.D., Singer, F.R., Roodman, G.D. et al. (1997). Genetic linkage of Paget's disease of bone to chromosome 18q. *Am. J. Hum. Genet.*, **61**, 1117–22.

Cohen, L.J., Meer, J., Tarkka, I. et al. (1991). Congenital mirror movements. Abnormal organization of motor pathways in two patients. *Brain*, **114**, 381–401.

Dalgleish, R. (1997). The human type I collagen mutation database. *Nucl. Acid Res.*, 25, 181–7.

David, K.M., Copp, A.J., Stevens, J.M., Hayward, R.D. & Crockard, H.A. (1996). Split cervical spinal cord with Klippel–Feil syndrome: seven cases. *Brain*, **119**, 1859–72.

David, K.M., Thorogood, P., Stevens, J.M., Einstein, S., Ransford, A.O. & Crockard, H.A. (1997). The one bone spine: a failure of notochord/sclerotome signalling. *Clini. Dysmorphol.*, **64**, 303–14.

Dickens, D.R.V. (1997). The spine. In *A Textbook of Paediatric Orthopedics*, ed. N.S. Broughton. pp. 267–81. London: WB Saunders & Co.

*Farmer, S.F., Ingram, D.A. & Stephens, J.A. (1990). Mirror movements studied in a patient with Klippel–Feil syndrome. *J. Physiol.*, **428**, 467–84.

Farmer, S.F., Harrison, L.M., Ingram, D.A. & Stephens, J.A. (1991). Plasticity of central motor pathways in children with hemiplegic cerebral palsy. *Neurology*, **41**, 1505–10.

*Fearnley, J.M., Stevens, J.M. & Rudge, P. (1995). Superficial siderosis of the central nervous system. *Brain*, **118**, 1051–66.

Fujiwara, K., Fujimoto, M., Yonenobu, K. & Ochi, A. (1999). A clinicopathological study of cervical myelopathy in rheumatoid arthritis: post-mortem analysis of two cases. *Eur. Spine J.*, **8**, 46–53.

*Glorieux, F.H., Bishop, N.J., Plotkin, H., Chabot, G., Lanque, G. & Travers, R. (1998). Cyclic administration of Pamidronate in children with severe *Osteogenesis imperfecta*. *N. Engl. J. Med.*, **339**, 947–52.

Gunderson, C.H. & Solitare, G.B. (1968). Mirror movements in patients with Klippel-Feil syndrome. *Arch. Neurol.*, **18**, 675–9.

Gutteridge, D.H., Ward, L.C., Stewart, G.O. et al. (1999). Paget's disease: Acquired resistance to one aminobisphosphonate with retained response to another. *J. Bone Min. Res.*, **14** (Suppl. 2), 79–84.

Huang, P.P. & Constantine, S. (1994). 'Acquired' Chiari I malformations. *J. Neurosurg.*, **80**, 1099–102.

Klippel, M. & Feil, A. (1912). Anomole de la colonne vertebrale par l'absence des vertebres cervicales: cage thoracic remontant jusqua a la base du crane. *Bull. Hem. Soc. Anat., Paris*, **87**, 185–8.

Lynch, J.J. & Crockard, H.H. (1999). Primary bone disease of the skull base. In *Cranial Base Surgery – Management, Complications and Outcome*. ed. J. Robertson & H. Coakham. pp. 659–73. New York: Churchill Livingstone.

*McMaster, M.J. & Ohtsukak, K. (1982). The natural history of congenital scoliosis. *J. Bone Joint Surg.*, **64A**, 1128–47.

McMaster, M.J. & Singh, H. (1999). Natural history of congenital kyphosis and kyphoscoliosis. *J. Bone Joint Surg.*, **81A**, 1367–83.

Madhok, R., Kerr, H. & Capell, H.A. (2000). Recent advances-Rheumatology. *Br. Med. J.*, **321**, 892–85.

Matthews, P.B.C., Farmer, S.F. & Ingram, D.A. (1990). On the localization of the stretch reflex in a patient with mirror movements. *J. Physiol.*, **428**, 561–77.

Mayston, M.J., Harrison, L.M., Quinton, R., Stephens, J.A., Krams, M. & Bouloux, P-M.G. (1997). Mirror movements in X-linked Kallmann's syndrome: 1. A neurophysiological study. *Brain*, **120**, 1199–216.

Menezes, A.H. (1999). Craniocervical anomalies and syringomyelia. In *Pediatric Neurosurgery*. ed. M. Choux, C. DiRocco, A. Hockley & M. Walker. pp. 151–84. New York: Churchill Livingstone.

Menezes, A. H. & Ryken, T.C. (1992). Craniovertebral abnormalities in Down's syndrome. *Paediat. Neurosurg.*, **18**, 24–33.

*Milhorat, T.H., Chou, M.W., Trinidad, E.M. et al. (1999). Chiari I malformation redefined: clinical and radiographic findings for 364 symptomatic patients. *Neurosurgery*, **44**, 1005–17.

Moe's Textbook of Scoliosis and Other spinal Deformities. (1994). 3rd edn., eds. Lonstien, Winter, Bradford, Ogilvie. WD Saunders & Co.

Payner, T.D., Prenger, E., Beger, T.S. & Crone, K.R. (1994). Acquired Chiari malformations: incidence, diagnosis and management. *Neurosurgery*, **34**, 429–34.

Poncelet, A. (1999). The neurological complications of Paget's disease. *J. Bone Mineral Res.*, **14** (Suppl. 2), 88–91.

Pueschal, S.M. & Scola F. (1987). Atlantoaxial instability in individuals with Down's syndrome: epidemiologic, radiographic and clinical studies. *Pediatrics*, **80**, 555.

Robertson, J. & Coakham, H., ed. (1999). *Cranial Base Surgery – Management, Complications and Outcome*. New York: Churchill Livingstone.

Rogers, M.A., Crockard, H.A., Moskovich, R. et al. (1994). Nystagmus and joint position sensation: Their importance in posterior occipitocervical fusion in rheumatoid arthritis. *Spine*, **19**, 16–20.

Samii, C., Mobius, E., Weber, E., Heinbrok, H.W. & Berlit, P. (1999). Pseudo Chiari type I malformation secondary to cerebrospinal fluid leakage. *J. Neurol.*, **246**, 162–4.

Savy, L.E., Stevens, J.M., Taylor, D.J. & Kendall, B.E. (1994). Apparent cerebellar ectopia: a reappraisal using volumetric MRI. *Neuroradiology*, **36**, 360–3.

Sawin, P.D. & Menezes, A.H. (1997). Basilar invagination in osteogenesis imperfecta and related osteochondrodysplastias: medical and surgical management. *J. Neurosurg.*, **86**, 950–60

Schott, G.D. & Wyke, M.A. (1981). Congenital mirror movements. *J. Neurol. Neurosurg. Psychiatry*, **44**, 586–99.

*Sillence, D. (1981). Osteogenesis imperfecta: an expanding panorama of variants. *Clin. Orthop.*, **159**, 11–25.

Singer, F.R. (1999). Update on the viral etiology of Paget's disease of bone. *J. Bone Mineral Res.*, **14** (Suppl. 2), 29–33.

Stevens, J.M., Chong, W.K., Barber, C., Kendell, B.E. & Crockard, H.A. (1994). A new appraisal of abnormalities of the odontoid process associated with atlanto-axial subluxation and neurological disability. *Brain*, **117**, 133–48.

*Theiss, S.M., Smith, M.D. & Winter, R.B. (1997). The long-term follow up of patients with Klippel–Feil syndrome and congenital scoliosis. *Spine*, **22**, 1219–22.

Todorov, A.B. (1982). Genetic aspects of neurosurgical problems. In *Neurological Surgery*. Vol 3. 2nd edn. ed. J.R. Youmans, pp. 1207–1235. Philadelphia: WB Saunders.

Winter, R., Moe, J., Bradford, D., Lonstein, J., Pedras, C. & Weber, A. (1979). Spine deformity in neurofibromatosis. A review of one hundred and two patients. *J. Bone Joint Surg.*, **61A**, 677–94.

Woods, B.T. & Teuber, H-L. (1978). Mirror movements after childhood hemiparesis. *Neurology*, **28**, 1152–8.

50

Cervical pain

Nikolai Bogduk

Newcastle Bone and Joint Institute, University of Newcastle, Royal Newcastle Hospital, New South Wales, Australia

Several terms apply to pain of cervical origin. These include radiculopathy, radicular pain or brachialgia, neck pain, and somatic referred pain. In the past and to some extent still, these terms have been confused, and sometimes used wrongly as equivalent and referring to the same phenomenon. The conditions or symptoms to which these terms refer differ in mechanism and cause; they differ with respect to the investigations required and the treatment that is appropriate. It is important, therefore, not just for taxonomic purposes (Merskey & Bogduk, 1994) but also for clinical purposes, to define how the terms should correctly be used.

Radiculopathy is a condition in which conduction along peripheral nerves is blocked at the level of the spinal nerve or its roots (Merskey & Bogduk, 1994). It is manifest clinically as numbness and/or weakness in a segmental distribution. Reflexes may be impaired according to whether conduction is blocked in Ia afferents or motor efferents or both. Paresthesiae may be another feature, and are indicative of the spinal nerve or its roots becoming ischemic. In essence, radiculopathy is a classical neurological disorder, manifest by objective neurological signs in a segmental distribution. Although pain may be an accompanying feature, it is not a necessary criterion. The diagnosis of radiculopathy is based on the objective neurological signs.

Radicular pain is pain arising from a disorder of a spinal nerve or nerve root (Merskey & Bogduk, 1994). It is perceived in the distribution of that nerve. Accordingly, cervical radicular pain is perceived in the upper limb. For that reason cervical radicular pain is not neck pain. Although neck pain may be a small component of radicular pain, radicular pain is never perceived exclusively in the neck. Its cardinal distribution is in the arm and forearm. Radicular pain may occur in association with radiculopathy, and for that reason it has been customary to group the two into one entity. Doing so, however, creates misconceptions, for not all pain that is associated with radiculopathy is necessarily radicular pain; radicular pain can occur without features of radiculopathy; and radiculopathy can occur without pain.

Neck pain is pain perceived in the cervical region of the spine, i.e. anywhere in the region bounded superiorly by the superior nuchal line, inferiorly by an imaginary transverse line through the T1 spinous process, and laterally by the margins of the posterior cervical muscles (Merskey & Bogduk, 1994). In this regard, it is clearly distinguished from radicular pain for, by definition, it is not perceived in the upper limb. Moreover, neck pain and radicular pain differ in mechanism. Neck pain is nociceptive, i.e. it arises as a result of stimulation of nerve endings in the structure that is the source of pain. In contrast, radicular pain is produced by the generation of ectopic impulses in the affected nerve.

Somatic referred pain is pain perceived in a region innervated by nerves, or branches of nerves, other than those that innervate the actual source of pain (Merskey & Bogduk, 1994). It does not involve the stimulation of nerve roots. Its mechanism involves convergence within the central nervous system between afferents from the two disparate sites. In that regard it is an extension of nociceptive pain. Its causes are the same as those of neck pain.

From the cervical spine, somatic pain can be referred to the head, to the anterior chest wall, to the upper limb girdle, and into the upper limb itself. In this latter distribution it can be confused with, and may be difficult to distinguish from, cervical radicular pain. It is that confusion, in the past, that has perhaps caused disappointment to physicians and their patients. Failure to recognize the difference between somatic referred pain and cervical radicular pain can result in investigations being pursued and treatments being applied for radicular pain when the patient has somatic referred pain; the result being either negative results, or false positive results and failed treatment.

Table 50.1. Less common causes of cervical radiculopathy, listed by structure and pathology

Structure	Pathology
Zygapophysial joint	Ganglion
	Tumour
	Inflammation
	Rheumatoid arthritis
	Gout
	Ankylosing spondylitis
	Fracture
Vertebral body	Primary tumour
	Secondary tumour
	Paget's disease
	Fracture
	Osteomyelitis
	Hydatid
	Hyperparathyroidism
Meninges	Cysts
	Meningioma
	Dermoid cyst
	Epidermoid cyst
Blood vessels	Angioma
	Arteritis
Nerve sheath	Neurofibroma
	Schwannoma
Nerve	Neuroblastoma
	Ganglioneuroma

Source: From Bogduk, 1999.

Radiculopathy

Pathology

There is a large number of possible causes of cervical radiculopathy. In essence, any space-occupying lesion that compromises a cervical spinal nerve or its roots can cause radiculopathy (Bogduk, 1999), (Table 50.1). Rare causes of cervical radiculopathy include conditions that affect the nerve intrinsically or do not involve the anatomic relations of the nerve. These include: giant-cell arteritis (Sanchez et al., 1983), sarcoidosis (Atkinson et al., 1982), Pancoast tumour (Vargo & Flood, 1990), and even intracranial tumour (Clar & Cianca, 1998). However, by far the most common causes of cervical radiculopathy are disc protrusions and cervical spondylosis.

Disc protrusions are described as 'soft' or 'hard'. Soft protrusions consist of nuclear material that is extruded into the vertebral canal in a fairly focal manner. Hard protru-

sions are masses of disc material, usually in the form of a transverse bar or ridge, and which consist of fibrocartilage or are otherwise rendered hard by being ossified or encased by osteophytes from the vertebral margins.

Disc protrusions are also classified as medial or lateral, according to their principal location and the structures that they affect. Medial protrusions narrow the vertebral canal and affect the spinal cord. They typically cause myelopathy and so, are manifest by long tract signs. Lateral protrusions narrow the intervertebral foramen, and cause radiculopathy. They occur most commonly at the C5–6 and C6–7 levels, less commonly at C4–5, and all but rarely at C3–4 and C7–T1 (Odom et al., 1958; Yamano, 1985; Yoss et al, 1957; Henderson et al., 1983).

Cervical spondylosis is characterized by hard disc protrusions and osteophytes from the uncovertebral region or the zygapophysial joints. These can cause radiculopathy if and when they compromise the spinal nerve in the intervertebral foramen.

Mechanism

There are no experimental data that explicitly reveal the mechanism of radiculopathy. The prevailing view is that conduction block in the affected nerve is produced by compression of the nerve. Either the axons are compressed directly or their blood supply is compromised by the compression. Post-inflammatory scarring is another possibility, but its incidence has not been explicitly determined.

It is probably important not to extrapolate to the cervical spine data from experimental and clinical studies in the lumbar spine. In the lumbar spine, the evidence points to inflammatory processes being cardinal amongst the mechanisms of lumbar radiculopathy (Bogduk & Govind, 1999), but this may not pertain to the cervical spine. Lumbar disc prolapse is an acute event that involves an inflammatory response to the prolapsed material. Whereas this may be analogous to soft protrusions in the neck, it is not analogous to hard protrusions or spinal nerve compression by osteophytes, for which there is no evidence of an inflammatory process.

Clinical features

The characteristic features of cervical radiculopathy are numbness, weakness, paresthesiae, and hyporeflexia, in some combination. Different studies attest to a different relative incidence of these features in patients with surgically proven radiculopathy (Table 50.2), but this may reflect differences in the criteria used by surgeons to justify operation, rather than real differences in incidence.

Table 50.2. Proportion of patients with radiculopathy presenting with the neurological features listed

Ref	N	Numbness	Weakness	Paresthesiae	Hyporeflexia
Gregorius et al., 1976	41	0.60	0.70	–	–
Lunsford et al., 1980	295	0.50	0.35	0.26	0.55
Yoss et al., 1957	100	0.24	0.10	0.65	0.65
Honet and Puri, 1976	82	0.59	0.51	–	0.52
Henderson et al., 1983	841	0.85	0.68	0.99	0.71

Clinical diagnosis

The presence of numbness, weakness, or paresthesiae allows the diagnosis of radiculopathy to be made clinically. Testing for numbness is a reasonably reliable procedure, carrying a kappa score of between 0.45 and 0.64 (Viikari-Juntura, 1987). The validity of clinical examination is also reasonable, but differs according to the criterion standard used (Bogduk, 1999). If the criterion standard is evidence of nerve root compression on CT myelography, neurological signs have high sensitivity, but only moderate to good specificity (Viikari-Juntura et al., 1989), resulting in positive likelihood ratios of only between 2 and 4 (Bogduk, 1999). Better figures arise when surgical findings are used as the criterion standard, and in the context of determining the segmental level.

For correctly detecting a C6 radiculopathy, the likelihood ratio of numbness in the C6 dermatome is 2.7, and that of biceps weakness is 3.4. For a decreased biceps jerk the likelihood ratio is 4.8, and that of paresthesiae in the C6 dermatome is 3.2 (Bogduk, 1999). For correctly detecting C7 radiculopathy, the likelihood ratio of C7 numbness is 4.4; that of triceps weakness is only 2.0; but that of a decreased triceps reflex is 3.8 (Bogduk, 1999). Paresthesiae in the C7 dermatome has a likelihood ratio of 7.7, and is therefore the strongest indicator of C7 radiculopathy (Bogduk, 1999).

The axial compression test (An, 1996; Spurling & Scoville, 1944) has good reliability (Viikari-Juntura, 1987). Adding the compression test to the neurological examination increases diagnostic confidence considerably, by increasing specificity (Viikari-Juntura et al., 1989), and raising the likelihood ratio to more than 8.0 (Bogduk, 1999). Other tests, such as the arm abduction test (Beatty et al., 1987; Davidson et al., 1981; Fast et al., 1989), and manual traction on the neck (Viikari-Juntura et al., 1989) are highly specific but poorly sensitive (Viikari-Juntura et al., 1989); and when added to the examination do not improve diagnostic confidence (Bogduk, 1999).

In essence, radiculopathy can be strongly suspected when the patient presents with some combination of numbness, weakness, paresthesiae, and hyporeflexia, in a segmental distribution. Diagnostic confidence is increased if a compression test is added, but other clinical tests are not contributory and are superfluous. The affected segment can be determined quite well from a good clinical examination alone.

Investigations

Nerve conduction tests do not aid in establishing the diagnosis of cervical radiculopathy (Bogduk, 1999). Clinical examination provides sufficient diagnostic confidence to make 'confirmation' by nerve conduction tests superfluous. Nor does electromyography help in pinpointing the affected segment (Bogduk, 1999). Nerve conduction tests are required only when the clinical picture is not distinctly one of radiculopathy, and the possibility arises of a peripheral neuropathy being the cause of the symptoms and signs.

Nor is medical imaging required to make the diagnosis of radiculopathy, in the first instance. Its role, rather, is to identify the actual cause of the radiculopathy. For this purpose, MRI has a greater sensitivity and specificity than CT or CT myelography, for it can better resolve soft-tissue lesions, and detect them sooner (Bogduk, 1999). Any deficiency of MRI in resolving small bony lesions can be overcome by supplementing MRI with a plain film (Kaiser & Holland, 1998).

Treatment

In considering treatment, it is important to distinguish radiculopathy from radicular pain. If radiculopathy is due to compression of nerve roots, there is no reason, *a priori*, to believe or to expect that physical therapy, drug therapy, or exercise will somehow relieve that compression. Indeed, there are no data from descriptive studies, let alone from controlled trials, to indicate that any form of conservative therapy is of benefit expressly for cervical radiculopathy. Surgical decompression is the only definitive form of management.

Radicular pain

Causes

No literature explicitly lists the causes of cervical radicular pain. Instead, because radicular pain has usually been considered in conjunction with radiculopathy, radicular pain has conventionally been attributed to the same conditions as cause radiculopathy. Accordingly, the most common causes of cervical radicular pain are cervical disc protrusions and cervical spondylosis.

Mechanisms

There are also no data on the mechanisms explicitly of cervical radicular pain. Such experiments as have been conducted, both in animals (Howe, 1979; Howe et al., 1977) and in human subjects (MacNab, 1972; Smyth & Wright, 1959), pertain to lumbar radicular pain. Those experiments show that compression or traction of normal nerve roots evokes paresthesiae or numbness, but does not cause pain. For a nerve root to produce pain it has to be inflamed. However, compression of a dorsal root ganglion does evoke activity in nociceptive afferents. Therefore, it would seem that for compression to be a mechanism of cervical radicular pain, the dorsal root ganglion of the affected nerve has to be compressed. The specific pathophysiological mechanism would appear to be the generation of ectopic impulses from the ganglion, although this has yet to be explicitly demonstrated experimentally.

Clinical features

Rules that maintain that radicular pain follows a dermatomal pattern (Ahlgren & Garfin, 1996) are wrong. Experimental studies, in which cervical nerves have been stimulated mechanically with a needle, show that radicular pain is perceived widely over areas not encompassed by any single dermatome (Slipman et al., 1998). Moreover, regardless of the segment involved, cervical radicular pain is perceived proximally over the scapular region and shoulder girdle, where the corresponding dermatome is not represented. Furthermore, it is perceived deeply and, indeed, more so than in areas of skin.

This should not be surprising, even though it may seem contrary to popular wisdom. If a dorsal root ganglion is compressed and causes pain, all afferents subtended by that ganglion are likely to be affected, not just those from the corresponding dermatome. That includes afferents from deep tissues such as muscles, ligaments and joints. This would seem to be the basis of the deep, gnawing

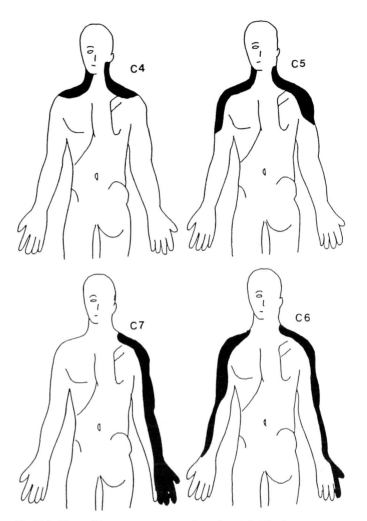

Fig. 50.1. Maps of the most common and consistent distributions of pain evoked by mechanical stimulation of the C4, C5, C6, and C7 spinal nerves. (Based on Slipman et al., 1998. Reproduced, with permission, from Bogduk, 1999.)

pain that accompanies stimulation of a cervical spinal nerve.

Although cervical radicular pain is not dermatomal, it can be portrayed as following a nevertheless segmental pattern, referred to as dynatomal (Slipman et al., 1998). Although the pain may extend to other areas, and although particular dynatomes differ from individual to individual, the areas in which radicular pain is most often and most consistently perceived are illustrated in Fig. 50.1. Quite clearly, the areas are not dermatomes, even though some do overlap the corresponding dermatome, although only in part. Conspicuously, the dynatomes for C6 and for C7 radiate from over the shoulder into the distal upper limb. They are not restricted to the forearm and hand. The dynatomes for C4 and C5 are not distinguishable from one another clinically; but those of C6 and C7 are distinguished from C5 by their distal extent. However, although the C7 dynatome extends somewhat more posteriorly over the forearm than does the C6 dynatome, C7 radicular pain cannot be reliably distinguished from C6 pain.

Diagnosis

An important realization is that not all pain in the upper limb is necessarily radicular pain. Radicular pain needs to be distinguished from somatic referred pain (q.v.). This becomes particularly pertinent when pain is the only clinical feature, i.e. neurological signs are absent.

If features of radiculopathy are present, any accompanying pain in the upper limb is likely to be radicular in origin, particularly if it extends distally into the forearm. In that event, however, the pain and its distribution do not bear on the diagnosis. The diagnosis rests on the features of the radiculopathy. It is the segmental distribution of numbness, weakness, paresthesiae, and hyporeflexia that implicate a radiculopathy and its segmental level. It is only the association with radiculopathy that permits the assumption that the pain is radicular.

Investigations

No investigations confirm or help in the diagnosis of cervical radicular pain. Nerve conduction tests and medical imaging may be applied in the pursuit of radiculopathy, but they demonstrate nothing about pain. If medical imaging demonstrates nerve root compression, it explains the radiculopathy. Any relationship with pain is only inferential. Medical imaging does not show pain. Indeed, cervical radicular pain bears only a weak relationship with radiological signs of nerve root compression (Viikari-Juntura et al., 1989). Neither is dependably predictive of the other. Therefore, whereas it may be appropriate to undertake medical imaging for radiculopathy, it is not appropriate for the investigation of pain.

Natural history

There are few data on the natural history of cervical radicular pain. On the basis of anecdotal reports, cervical radicular pain seems to have a favourable natural history (Dillin et al., 1986; Persson et al., 1997). In studies of conservative therapy, some 70% of patients treated with placebo improve, and 20% lose all symptoms (British Association of Physical Medicine, 1966). In one survey of 561 patients,

90% were considered normal or only mildly incapacitated at 5 years (Radhakrishan et al., 1994).

Treatment

It has been traditional to treat cervical radicular pain conservatively. However, the literature is quite vague about what constitutes conservative therapy. By default, it is any therapy that occurs before surgery. The literature that provides information embraces various combinations of drug therapy, physical therapy, traction, collars, bed rest, exercise and transcutaneous electrical nerve stimulation (Bogduk, 1999).

The few controlled trials available paint a sobering picture of the efficacy of conservative therapy for cervical radicular pain. One study found no difference in outcome for patients treated with traction, sham traction, collar, heat, or placebo (British Association of Physical Medicine, 1966). Another study compared neck exercises, traction, and no treatment (Goldie & Landquist, 1970). According to the patients, a greater proportion of those receiving no treatment failed to improve. According to the physician's assessment, there was no difference between the three groups. In a rigorous study of patients with chronic radicular pain due to cervical spondylosis, weighted traction proved no better than placebo traction, in terms of pain scores, sleep disturbance, social dysfunction, and activities of daily living (Klaber-Moffett et al., 1990).

Some studies in the pain literature promote the use of epidural injections of steroids for cervical radicular pain. No controlled studies validate this therapy, and the descriptive studies are far from compelling. Collectively, they attest to between 0% and 30% of patients obtaining complete relief, and a similar proportion of patients obtaining 75% relief (Bogduk, 1999). One descriptive study has promoted fluroscopically-guided, transforaminal injection of steroids, but provides incomplete data on efficacy (Bush & Hillier, 1996).

Surgery is ultimately the mainstay of treatment for cervical radicular pain. According to descriptive studies it offers a high yield of successful results, irrespective of the technique used (Bogduk, 1999). There has been only one controlled study of surgery for cervical radicular pain (Persson et al., 1997). Patients were randomly allocated to treatment by physiotherapy, a collar, or surgery. At 4 months follow-up, all groups had improved, and the surgery group had less pain; but this difference was extinguished by 12 months. However, fewer than 10% of patients in each group were free of pain at 12 months. This low success rate is inconsistent with the reputed efficacy of surgery for cervical radicular pain.

Somatic referred pain

The early clinical experiments on somatic referred pain determined the distribution of pain when noxious stimuli were administered to interspinous muscles in normal volunteers (Kellgren, 1939; Feinstein et al., 1954). The patterns of distribution observed were segmental, but did not correspond to dermatomes (Fig. 50.2). The significance of these studies was that they showed that pain referred into the upper limb could be produced by means other than the stimulation of spinal nerves or nerve roots. For clinical purposes, these studies established that not all pain referred to the upper limb was necessarily radicular.

More recent studies have examined the patterns of distribution of pain in normal volunteers from particular structures in the cervical spine other than the interspinous muscles. These include the atlanto-axial and atlanto-occipital joints (Dreyfuss et al., 1994), and the cervical zygohypophyseal joints (Dwyer et al., 1990). The patterns observed are quasi-segmental but unrelated to dermatomes (Fig. 50.3). Similar patterns of pain have been noted in patients with neck pain undergoing cervical disc stimulation (Grubb & Kelly, 2000). This similarity indicates that patterns of referred pain do not reflect the structure that is the source of pain, but they do relate to its innervation. Structures with the same segmental innervation will produce referred pain in similar areas.

Somatic referred pain is not a separate diagnostic entity. It is just a physiological phenomenon. Since it can arise from virtually any structure in the neck its sources and causes are the same as those of neck pain.

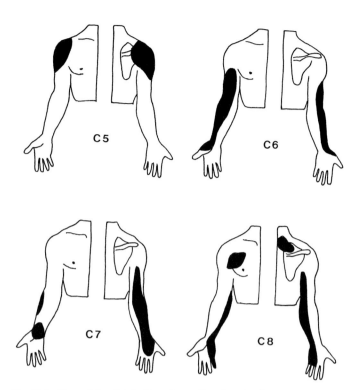

Fig. 50.2. Maps of the distribution of somatic referred pain elicited in normal volunteers by noxious stimulation of the interspinous ligaments. (Based on Kellgren, 1939.)

Neck pain

Epidemiology

Neck pain is common. Acute neck pain affects some 10% of the community, and the prevalence of chronic neck pain is about 14% (Bovim et al., 1994; Makela et al., 1991; van der Donk et al., 1991; Lawrence, 1969). It is more common among manual workers, office workers, secretaries and sewing machine operators (Vasseljen & Westgaard, 1995; Kamwendo et al., 1991; Westgaard & Jansen, 1992).

Etiology

The possible causes of neck pain can be classified as serious or non-threatening conditions, and as common or uncommon conditions (Table 50.3). Known causes involving demonstrable pathology are uncommon.

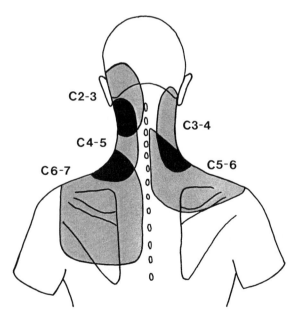

Fig. 50.3. Maps of the distribution of referred pain elicited in normal volunteers by noxious distension of the cervical zygapophysical joints. (Based on Dwyer et al., 1990.)

Table 50.3. The causes of neck pain grouped according to whether they are common and serious

	Non-threatening	Serious
Uncommon	Rheumatoid arthritis	Fractures
	Ankylosing spondylitis	Tumours
	Reiter's syndrome	Spinal infections
	Psoriatic arthritis	Dissecting aneurysms
	Crystal arthropathies	Spinal hematomas
		Metabolic disorders
Common	Cervical spinal pain of unknown origin	
	Acceleration-deceleration Injuries of the neck	
	Zygapophysial joint pain	
	Discogenic pain	

Neck pain can occur in patients with rheumatoid arthritis, but it is unlikely to be the sole presenting feature. Fewer than 2% of patients with rheumatoid arthritis have neck pain as their only feature (Sharp et al., 1958). Rheumatoid arthritis becomes potentially serious if it affects the C1–2 joints, but even then the prognosis is favourable (Isdale & Conlon, 1971). Some 10% of patients with ankylosing spondylitis may present with neck pain (Hochberg et al., 1978), but the rarity of ankylosing spondylitis renders it an uncommon cause of neck pain.

Tumours, infections and metabolic disorders are very uncommon causes of neck pain. Although their prevalence has not been explicitly established, the failure of large radiological surveys to detect such conditions (Heller et al., 1983; Johnson & Lucas, 1997) implies that their prevalence is less than 0.4% in primary care.

Headache is the most common presenting feature of internal carotid artery dissection, but neck pain has been the sole presenting feature in some 6% of cases (Silbert et al., 1995; Biousse et al., 1994). In 17% of patients headache may occur in combination with neck pain (Biousse et al., 1994). Neck pain has been the initial presenting feature in 50% to 90% of patients with vertebral artery dissection, but is usually also accompanied by headache, typically in the occipital region although not exclusively so (Silbert et al., 1995; Sturzenegger, 1994). Although the typical features of dissecting aneurysms of the aorta are chest pain and cardiovascular distress, neck pain has been reported as the presenting feature in some 6% of cases (Garrard & Barnes, 1996; Hirst et al., 1958).

Although considered common, and feared as a cause of neck pain (for medicolegal reasons), fractures of the neck are actually not common. In accident and emergency set-tings, only about 3% of patients suspected of having a fracture prove to have fractures upon cervical radiography (MacNamara, 1988; Bachuklis et al., 1987; Roberge et al., 1988; Kreipke et al., 1989; Hoffman et al., 1992; Gerrelts et al., 1991).

Missing from Table 50.3 are cervical spondylosis and cervical osteoarthrosis. Although hallowed by tradition, these entities defy legitimate diagnosis. Clinically, they are indistinguishable from any other cause of neck pain. The only available diagnostic criterion are the radiological features of these conditions, but these features are only age-changes. They correlate poorly with neck pain (Heller et al., 1983). Indeed, cervical osteoarthrosis is more common in patients with no neck pain (Fridenberg & Miller, 1963).

For patients with neck pain whose cause is not apparent, the International Association for the Study of Pain recommends the rubric: cervical spinal pain of unknown origin, as an honest diagnosis (Merskey & Bogduk, 1994). Acceleration– deceleration injury, or whiplash, is perhaps the most common traumatic basis for neck pain. However, it does not constitute a diagnosis in a patho-anatomic sense. It is a label that simply recognizes the reported circumstances of onset of neck pain. Zygapophysial joint pain and discogenic pain are specific subsets of what otherwise might be known as 'mechanical' neck pain but their diagnosis requires invasive procedures such as zygapophysial joint blocks and disc stimulation (q.v.).

Although favoured by many, there is no evidence that trigger points are a cause of neck pain. Even in the hands of experts, the diagnosis is unreliable (Wolfe et al., 1992); and the absence of a criterion standard means that its validity cannot be tested. Furthermore, trigger points in the neck do not satisfy the prescribed criteria for a trigger point. They are characterized solely by tenderness and reproduction of pain, in which regard they cannot be distinguished from tenderness of underlying zygapophysial joints (Bogduk & Simons, 1993).

Whiplash

Neck pain due to whiplash is distinguished by an onset attributed to a motor vehicle accident. In western societies the incidence of reported whiplash accidents is about 1 per 1000 population per year (Barnsley et al., 1994a, 1998). However, that is not to say that all cases develop neck pain. The natural history of neck pain attributed to whiplash is quite benign. Within 12 months some 75% of victims are asymptomatic, with the figure rising to 82% by 2 years. This leaves some 20% of patients still with symptoms, but only 4% are severely disabled (Radanov et al., 1995). The prevalence, in the general community, of chronic neck pain due to whiplash has been calculated as about 1% or less, making it only a fraction of the causes of chronic neck pain (Barnsley et al., 1994a, 1998).

Given the natural history of neck pain after whiplash, the majority of patients must sustain no substantive injury to their neck. Perhaps they suffer a minor muscle sprain, or simply jarring of their neck. However, a minority of patients suffer definite injuries.

Rare injuries include disruption of the alar ligaments, prevertebral hematoma, perforation of the oesophagus, tears of the sympathetic trunk, damage to the recurrent laryngeal nerve, spinal cord injury, periplymph fistula, thrombosis or traumatic aneurysms of the vertebral or internal carotid arteries, retinal angiopathy, and anterior spinal artery syndrome (Barnsley et al., 1994a, 1998). Fractures after whiplash are so uncommon as to be rare. Such fractures as have been attributed to whiplash have been reported only in case studies or small, descriptive series. These fractures may be difficult to detect on conventional investigations, and special attention needs to be paid to their possibility if they are to be detected. The majority involve the upper cervical spine, and include fractures of the odontoid process (Seletz, 1958; Signoret et al., 1986), the laminae and articular processes of C2 (Seletz, 1958; Signoret et al., 1986; Craig & Hodgson, 1991), and the occipital condyles (Stroobants et al., 1994). In one study of 283 patients with acute neck pain after whiplash, however, no fractures were found on plain radiography (Hoffman et al., 1992). This result implies a prevalence of less than 1.3%.

The most likely lesions that underlie chronic neck pain after whiplash are injuries to the intervertebral discs and zygapophysial joints. Cineradiography studies in normal volunteers undergoing simulated whiplash collisions reveal that at some 100 msec after impact, the cervical spine undergoes a sigmoid deformation, during which the lower cervical vertebrae undergo extension about an abnormal axis of rotation (Kaneoka et al., 1999). The movement is such that the anterior edges of the vertebral bodies separate and the zygapophysial joints impact. These movements indicate that the anterior anulus fibrosus can be sprained while the zygapophysial joints can suffer impaction fractures or contusions to their meniscoids (Kaneoka et al., 1999). These are the very lesions that have been demonstrated in postmortem studies of victims of motor vehicle accidents (Jonsson et al., 1994; Taylor & Twomey, 1993; Taylor & Taylor, 1996).

Clinical diagnosis

Critical to the clinical assessment of neck pain is a thorough and careful history. A history of substantial trauma warns of the possibility of fracture, or of vascular injury. Past medical history, current general health, and associated features provide clues to possible serious causes of neck pain. A past history of cancer, weight loss, and ill health, warn of tumour. Transient ischemic episodes warn of vertebral or carotid aneurysms. Arthropathy elsewhere in the body warns of inflammatory joint disease. Neck pain in the elderly warrants consideration of myeloma and Paget's disease. Hyperparathyroidism is a possible cause of spinal pain that is easily overlooked because of its rarity. Neurological symptoms, however, convert the presentation from one of neck pain to one of a neurological disorder. In most cases, however, history reveals no medical disorder; the presentation is simply one of neck pain.

Physical examination offers little towards the diagnosis of neck pain. Typically, the patient will be tender in the cervical spine, and will exhibit restriction of neck movements because of pain. Neither of these features, however, is a valid indicator of any particular source or cause of pain.

In this context, neurological examination is immaterial in the assessment of neck pain, for it is not a neurological disorder. Neurological examination is pertinent if the patient has neurological symptoms, but not if pain is the only presenting feature. In that event, a screening neurological examination, looking for weakness or numbness, is all that is warranted.

Special techniques of examination, such the detection of cervical intersegmental motion, have either not been shown to be valid, or have been found to lack reliability, validity or both. For the detection of tenderness over the zygapophysial joints, inter-observer agreement is good, with a kappa score of 0.68 (Hubka & Phelan, 1994). For other signs, particularly those espoused by chiropractors, observer agreement is poor (Gross et al., 1996; Levoska et al., 1991; Sandmark & Nisell, 1995; De Boer et al., 1985; Nansel et al., 1989; Mior et al., 1985; Smedmark et al., 2000).

Plain radiography

Plain radiography for neck pain is indicated only if the physician has grounds to suspect a fracture or some other serious condition. In the absence of such clinical indicators, different guidelines apply. In two large studies, each involving over 1000 patients with neck pain, no instances of unexpected malignancy or infection were found (Heller et al., 1983; Johnson & Lucas, 1997). The British study concluded that 'the request for X-ray films of the cervical spine "just in case" such a finding is present is probably unjustified.' (Heller et al., 1983). The US study found that upon 5-year follow-up 'no medically dangerous diagnoses would have been missed if the cervical spine series had not been done'. (Johnson & Lucas, 1997).

What plain radiography is likely to reveal in a patient with neck pain is either a normal cervical spine or cervical spondylosis. The features of cervical spondylosis, however, are simply age-related changes. In some studies cervical spondylosis occurs somewhat more commonly in symptomatic individuals than in asymptomatic individuals (van der Donk et al., 1991; Heller et al., 1983), but the odds ratios for disc degeneration or osteoarthritis as predictors of neck pain are only 1.1 and 0.97, respectively, for women, and 1.7 and 1.8 for men (van der Donk et al., 1991). In other studies, the prevalence of disc degeneration, at individual segments of the neck, is not significantly different between symptomatic patients and asymptomatic controls (Fridenberg & Miller, 1963). Non-covertebral osteophytes and osteoarthrosis are less prevalent in symptomatic individuals (Fridenburg & Miller, 1963).

Loss of lordosis is a feature sometimes reported in cervical spine films, but this phenomenon is a normal variant, and carries no diagnostic implication. It is equally prevalent amongst patients with acute neck pain, chronic neck pain and no neck pain (Helliwell et al., 1994). It is independent of age and symptoms but is more common in females (Helliwell et al., 1994).

CT scanning

No data, and no studies, justify the use of CT as a screening test for undiagnosed neck pain. CT may be of use in better defining known or suspected pathology, such as fractures or tumours; it may be of value in defining the cause of radicular pain; but it offers no value in the pursuit of uncomplicated neck pain. Nothing that might be evident on CT has been shown to correlate with any known cause of neck pain.

MRI

In the context of neck pain, magnetic resonance imaging offers little prospect of a positive diagnosis. Nevertheless, because of its high sensitivity for unusual disorders it is the premier screening tool for chronic, undiagnosed neck pain. In that context, however, its utility lies in ruling out undetected disorders rather than in pinpointing the cause of pain. For finding the cause of pain, MRI is as useless as CT. Moreover, it is confounded by the high incidence of so-called abnormalities in totally asymptomatic individuals.

Disc degeneration, disc bulges, spinal stenosis, and even spinal cord impingement occur in asymptomatic individ-

uals, and with increasing frequency with age (Boden et al., 1990; Teresi et al., 1987). Finding such abnormalities does not provide a diagnosis. In the context of whiplash, multiple studies have failed to detect any diagnostic abnormality in patients with uncomplicated neck pain (Ellertsson et al., 1978; Pettersson et al., 1994; Fagerlund et al., 1995; Borchgrevink et al., 1995; Ronnen et al., 1996; Voyvodic et al., 1997).

SPECT scanning

A small study has provided encouraging news concerning the possible utility of single-positron emission tomography (Seitz et al., 1995). It found that, in patients with acute neck pain after whiplash, SPECT could reveal small fractures undetected by plain radiography or obscured by osteoarthrosis of the joint affected. The fractures consisted of small articular fractures and avulsions of the vertebral rims. The optimum time for using SPECT would seem to be at about four to six weeks after injury. However, the utility of SPECT needs to be determined by larger studies before its wholesale application can be justified.

In the context of chronic neck pain, the one study published on SPECT scanning reported no correlation between whether a zygapophysial joint appeared active or not and whether or not it was painful (Barnsley et al., 1992). Thus, there is no proven utility of SPECT in chronic neck pain.

Invasive techniques

It is not surprising that medical imaging lacks utility for the vast majority of patients with neck pain. Pain is a symptom. It cannot be seen on morphological tests. It requires physiological tests. In this regard, two such tests have been advocated.

Disc stimulation

Disc stimulation is a test designed to determine if an intervertebral disc is painful or not. It involves introducing a needle into the centre of the suspected disc, through which contrast medium is injected in order to stress the disc by distending it from within (Bogduk et al., 1995). The recommended criteria for a diagnosis of discogenic pain are that stressing a particular disc reproduces the patient's pain but provided that stressing adjacent discs does not (Merskey & Bogduk, 1994; Bogduk et al., 1995).

Although championed in some quarters, cervical disc stimulation is fraught with persisting problems. Cervical discs are painful even in asymptomatic individuals.

However, they are not particularly painful. Therefore, it is recommended that the criteria for discogenic pain include reproduction of pain to a level of at least 7 on a 10-point visual analogue scale (Schellhas et al., 1996).

Even so, cervical disc stimulation is compromised by false-positive responses. Disc stimulation can be positive in patients in whom the zygapophysial joints of the same segment are actually the source of pain (Bogduk & Aprill, 1993). Consequently, discogenic pain cannot be diagnosed unless it is shown that other joints in the same segment are not painful.

Furthermore, a recent study has shown that cervical discs are infrequently symptomatic at single levels (Grubb & Kelly, 2000). Positive responses are commonly encountered at two, three, and even four levels or more. The assessment of the patient is, therefore, not complete unless and until all levels are studied; which makes cervical disc stimulation a demanding procedure. If disc stimulation is undertaken at only one, two, or three, preferred or habitual levels, the likelihood of a false-positive result is high.

The one virtue of cervical disc stimulation is that, if multiple discs are found to be symptomatic, surgery is not indicated. Disc stimulation, therefore, plays an important role in reducing unnecessary and futile cervical surgery (Grubb & Kelly, 2000).

Zygohypophyseal joint blocks

Zygohypophyseal (Z joint) blocks can be used to test if a zygohypophyseal joint is the source of a patient's neck pain. They involve anesthetizing, under fluoroscopic control, the small nerves that innervate the target joint, each with not more than 0.3 ml of local anesthetic (Bogduk & Lord, 1998). Z joint blocks have face-validity, in that they selectively anesthetize the target nerves, and do not anesthetize any nearby structures that realistically might be the source of pain (Barnsley & Bogduk, 1993). Single diagnostic blocks, however, are not valid. They carry a false-positive rate of some 27% (Barnsley et al., 1993a). Controls are, therefore, required in each and every patient. When performed under controlled conditions, Z joint blocks have proven construct validity (Barnsley et al., 1993b).

Depending on the circumstances, either placebo controls or comparative diagnostic blocks can be used (Bogduk & Lord, 1998). Comparative blocks involve the administration, on separate occasions, of local anesthetic agents with differing durations of action (Barnsley et al., 1993a). A valid response is one in which the patient obtains a duration of relief concordant with the expected duration of action of the agent administered, i.e. long-lasting relief when a long-acting agent is used, and short-lasting relief when a short-acting agent is used. Controlled studies have shown that diagnostic decisions based on this paradigm are robust (Lord et al., 1995).

Epidemiological studies, using double-blind, controlled, diagnostic blocks, have shown that zygapophysial joint pain is the single most common basis of chronic neck pain after whiplash. On worst-case figures, it accounts for at least 49% of patients (Barnsley et al., 1995; Lord et al., 1996a). In patients with neck pain after severe motor vehicle accidents, the prevalence of Z joint pain is as high as 80% (Gibson et al., 2000). The joints most commonly involved are C5–6 and C6–7 in patients with neck pain and somatic referred pain to the shoulder girdle, and C2–3 in patients with neck pains and headache (Lord & Bogduk, 1996). In patients in whom headache is the dominant symptom, the source of pain can be traced to the C2–3 joint in some 53% of cases (Lord et al., 1994).

Of all the possible diagnostic tests that might be applied to a patient with neck pain, Z joint blocks are the only validated test. Of all the possible causes of chronic neck pain, Z joint pain is the only proven entity, and is the most common cause after whiplash.

Conservative therapy

Many treatments have been used and recommended for neck pain (Bisbee & Hartsell, 1993; Greenman, 1993; Tessell et al., 1993). These include, rest, collars, exercises, posture control, physical therapy, traction, manual therapy, analgesics, trigger point injection, epidural steroids, craniosacral manipulation, and manipulation under general anesthesia. Compelling evidence of efficacy is lacking for most of these interventions. For others the evidence indicates lack of efficacy.

A systematic review of physical and manual therapies (Aker et al., 1996) detailed the positive and negative studies and, where possible, calculated effect sizes of various therapies. Some therapies were reported as having no effect above comparison therapies; others were found to have a positive effect. However, the review did not address the duration of positive effects or their clinical significance; nor did it address outcome measures such as the proportion of patients obtaining complete relief. The only outcome measure used to identify positive effects was improvement of pain, in terms of the mean or median scores on a visual analogue scale. The review was satisfied with statistically significant improvement beyond control as the cardinal, if not only, measure of successful therapy.

Despite its graciousness in this regard, the review nonetheless concluded that:

> there is early evidence to support the use of manual treatments in combination with other treatments for short term pain relief, but in general, conservative interventions have not been studied in enough detail to assess efficacy or effectiveness adequately (Aker et al., 1996).

A less gracious appraisal of the literature (Bogduk, 1998) provides a more alarming view. For acute neck pain not due to whiplash, spray and stretch therapy (Snow et al., 1992) and laser acupuncture (Thorsen et al., 1992) are no more effective than placebo. Traction is not discernibly more effective than isometric exercises (Goldie & Landquist, 1970), and when combined with other interventions, traction offers no advantage over traction alone (Caldwell & Krusen, 1962). Neck school is no better than no treatment (Kamwendo & Linton, 1991). One study reported that, immediately after treatment, manipulation combined with azopropazone afforded greater relief of pain than treatment with azopropazone alone, but the difference was extinguished one and three weeks later (Howe et al., 1983). In another study, there was no significant difference at 3 weeks between patients receiving one to three manipulations and those treated with a muscle relaxant (Sloop et al., 1982).

For chronic neck pain not due to whiplash, there are no studies of the efficacy of exercise, collars, TENS, neck school, spray and stretch, or traction. Wearing magnetic necklaces is no more efficacious than placebo (Hong et al., 1982). Laser acupuncture is no more effective than sham transcutaneous electrical nerve stimulation (TENS) (Lewith & Machin, 1981); and needle acupuncture is no more effective than sham acupuncture or an injection of diazepam (Thomas et al., 1991), or sham TENS (Petrie & Langley, 1983; Petrie & Hazelman, 1986). Compared to no treatment, a programme of gymnastics was found to offer no therapeutic benefit (Takala et al., 1994).

In a study that focused on manipulation for back pain, 64 patients with neck pain were treated (Koes et al., 1992). Separate data on these patients were not reported in the original publication, but subsequent analysis found no statistically significant differences in response between those patients receiving manual therapy and those receiving physiotherapy and general practice care (Hurwitz et al., 1996). Another study compared manipulation, physiotherapy, and being treated with salicylate (Brodin, 1984, 1985). It reported a statistically significant benefit from manipulation. Analysis of the data, however, reveals that the difference arose because of poorer outcomes in the patients treated with physiotherapy. Between the outcomes of patients treated with manipulation and those treated with salicylate, there was no statistically significant difference.

In a methodologically strong study (Foley-Nolan et al., 1990) pulsed electromagnetic therapy delivered through a collar was found to have a significantly greater effect on pain than a collar alone. The difference arose, however, because of a greater proportion of patients in the active treatment group reporting 'moderately better' as opposed to 'no change' in the control group. The number of patients 'completely well' or 'much better' was not significantly different in the two groups. The study did not report the duration of effect for any period after cessation of treatment.

For acute neck pain after whiplash, the Quebec Task Force on Whiplash Associated Disorders attempted a major synthesis of the literature available up to September 1993, but was unable to compose a systematic review or meta-analysis (Spitzer et al., 1995). Out of 10382 potentially relevant articles, only 62 were accepted as both relevant and scientifically meritorious. The Task Force concluded that: 'the evidence was found to be sparse and generally of unacceptable quality' (Spitzer et al., 1995).

Rest and analgesia (McKinney et al., 1989), combinations of TENS, ultrasound and pulsed electromagnetic therapy (Provinciali et al., 1996), and soft collars (McKinney et al., 1989; Foley-Nolan et al., 1992; Mealy et al., 1986), have each been used in controlled studies as reference treatments, and each has been found to be inferior to other interventions. Traction offers no additional benefit when added to instruction, moist heat and exercise (Zylbergold & Piper, 1985), and is no better than rest in a collar (Pennie & Agambar, 1990). Receiving pulsed electromagnetic therapy delivered from a device implanted in a collar affords greater improvement in pain than wearing the same collar with a dummy device (Foley-Nolan et al., 1992); but the difference is apparent only for the first four weeks of treatment; by 12 weeks electromagnetic therapy affords no advantage.

The application of ice for the first 24 hours after injury, followed by mobilization, local heat, exercises and analgesia is superior to rest, analgesia and a soft collar (Mealy et al., 1986), at 4 weeks and 8 weeks after treatment, but no long-term data are available. Active out-patient physiotherapy (consisting of a tailored programme of hot and cold applications, short-wave diathermy, hydrotherapy, traction, and mobilization), and a home-exercise programme both achieve greater improvements than rest and analgesia, at one month and two months after treatment, but active physiotherapy is not superior to home exercises alone (Provinciali et al., 1996). In a long-term follow-up, however, home exercises achieved a greater proportion of patients free of pain (McKinney, 1989).

So-called 'multimodal therapy', consisting of relaxation training, reduction of cervical lordosis, psychological support, eye fixation exercises, and massage and mobilization, is superior to applications of TENS, pulsed electromagnetic therapy, ultrasound, and calcic iontophoresis, at 2 weeks and 4 weeks after therapy (Provinciali et al., 1996); but in the long term, results are no better than those achieved by other and simpler means, including rest and analgesia and wearing a collar.

In essence, the combined data on physical and manual therapy, do show that intervention is superior to rest and analgesia, but the impact pertains to a decrease in average pain score, and is evident only at 4 to 8 weeks after onset of pain. Thereafter, either there are no data or the suggestion that patients not treated actively eventually achieve the same degree of recovery. The impact of physical and manual therapy is to achieve not resolution in a greater proportion of patients but a more rapid resolution in the early weeks after onset of pain. The only long-term data indicate that a greater proportion of patients achieve complete recovery when treated with home exercise.

A challenging observation has been a study in which an index treatment was compared with rest, analgesia and a collar. At 6 months and at 1 year after treatment, there were few differences, but the results favoured the index treatment. That treatment was reassurance, a direction to resume normal activities, and denial of sick-leave (Borchgrevink et al., 1998).

For chronic neck pain after whiplash, there is no evidence of the efficacy of any conservative therapy. Even the Quebec Task Force (Spitzer et al., 1995), in its consensus approach, recommended no specific therapy. For patients still unresolved by 12 weeks, it recommended only evaluation by a multidisciplinary team, without venturing what sort of management this might result in, and without offering any evidence of the efficacy of multidisciplinary pain management.

Medical therapy

There are no data explicitly demonstrating the efficacy of analgesics, non-steroidal anti-inflammatory agents, or other drugs, for neck pain of any nature (Spitzer et al., 1995). If such agents are used, it is on the basis of presumed efficacy, but should be in the full knowledge that, for neck pain, they may be no more effective than placebo.

No studies have demonstrated the efficacy for neck pain of any form of injection into the neck, be that using local anesthetic, sclerosing agents, or corticosteroids. For chronic neck pain stemming from the zygapophysial joints, intra-articular injections of corticosteroids are no more effective than injections of local anesthetic, and both treatments fail to achieve sustained relief in more than a minority of patients (Barnsley et al., 1994b).

Surgical therapy

There is no compelling evidence of the efficacy of cervical fusion for neck pain. Such studies as have reported on this therapy claim success (Kikuchi et al., 1981; Whitecloud & Seago, 1987) but outcome measures are few and lacking in rigour. Some studies report disheartening results (De Palma et al., 1972), particularly for surgical therapy of neck pain after whiplash (Algers et al., 1993).

The one surgical procedure that has withstood scientific scrutiny is percutaneous, radiofrequency, medial branch neurotomy. In this procedure, the nerves that innervate the cervical zygapophysial joints are coagulated in an effort to relieve pain stemming from these joints (Lord et al., 1998). Under double-blind, controlled conditions, the procedure has proven not to be a placebo (Lord et al., 1996b). Moreover, it is the only treatment for neck pain that has been shown to achieve complete relief of pain, and restoration of activities of daily living (Lord et al., 1996b; 1998). Furthermore, relief of pain is attended by complete resolution of psychological distress (Wallis et al., 1997). A limitation of the procedure, however, is that pain recurs as the nerves regenerate. However, in that event, the procedure can be repeated and the pain once again completely relieved. Long-term studies have shown that continued, repeated relief can be sustained for up to 2000 days (McDonald et al., 1999).

Recommendations

In the light of the available evidence, the best recommendations that might be offered are:
For acute neck pain,
- Simple analgesics or non-steroidal anti-inflammatory agents might be used to provide analgesia while patients undergo natural recovery, but in the knowledge that the efficacy of these agents may be no greater than placebo.
- There is no evidence to justify the use of major tranquillizers or tricyclic antidepressants.

For neck pain after whiplash, during the first 8 weeks after injury,
- Patients could be treated with rest and analgesia, but
- A more rapid resolution of pain might be achieved by the use of ice, and passive mobilization, although
- A home-exercise programme offers just as much chance

of rapid resolution and a greater chance of being pain-free at 2 years; however,

- Firm reassurance, and insistence to resume normal activities, may be as effective as any other measure.

In the face of refuting data, and given the availability of a proven alternative,

- Traction, electromagnetic therapy, collars, TENS, ultrasound, neck school, spray and stretch, laser therapy, or traction, should not be used in the treatment of acute neck pain.

For chronic neck pain,

- No physical therapy is justified on the basis of available evidence.
- The use of analgesics might be justified on humanitarian grounds but not on the basis of evidence of efficacy.
- If NSAIDs are used their efficacy should be determined, and patients carefully monitored for side effects.
- Intra-articular injections of corticosteroids into the cervical zygapophysial joints should not be used unless it can be shown that the patient can achieve lasting and worthwhile relief that is cost-effective.
- Disc excision and fusion for neck pain without neurological signs might be entertained on the basis of uncontrolled clinical trials of this procedure, but this form of therapy would best be reserved for the context of clinical trials approved by an ethics committee or an institutional review board, and designed to determine its efficacy and safety.
- Radiofrequency neurotomy can be used to provide complete relief of pain in patients diagnosed rigorously as suffering from cervical zygapophysial joint pain, but the use of this procedure should be restricted to trained and accredited providers.

Resolving a dilemma

Quite clearly, neck pain is not radicular pain. Neck pain is perceived in the cervical region, not in the upper limb. Neck pain, however, can be associated with referred pain; and it is this somatic referred pain that can be difficult to distinguish from radicular pain.

The patterns observed for referred pain from cervical joints in normal volunteers (Fig. 50.3) were more restricted than those reported for interspinous ligaments (Fig. 50.2). The pain was restricted to the immediate vicinity of the neck and shoulder girdle, and did not extend distally into the upper limb. One reason for this difference is perhaps that the stimuli used were more restrained and less intense. Whereas the interspinous ligaments were stimulated with injections of hypertonic saline, the cervical

joints were stimulated with injections of contrast medium to distend the joint. In order not to disrupt the joint, injections were terminated immediately once pain was elicited. In essence, the stimulus was minimal. It may be, therefore, wider areas of referral could occur from cervical joints or discs if stronger noxious stimuli were applied to these structures. However, this has not been tested experimentally; nor has it been borne out clinically.

No clinical studies have reported relief of somatic referred pain in the distal upper limb. Patients in whom somatic referred pain has been relieved by injections of local anesthetic into the neck have had referred pain no further than the shoulder girdle (Barnsley et al., 1995; Lord et al., 1996a). It seems, therefore, in practice, that somatic referred pain from the neck does not commonly extend beyond the region of the shoulder girdle. This empirical fact bears on the distinction between somatic referred pain and cervical radicular pain.

Since somatic referred pain from C6 or C7 does not commonly extend into the forearm, yet C6 and C7 radicular pain does, it is reasonable to deduce that referred pain that extends into the forearm is more likely to be radicular in origin than to be somatic referred pain. In contrast, C5 radicular pain typically extends only over the shoulder girdle (Fig. 50.1), and in that regard cannot be distinguished from somatic referred pain stemming from C5,6 structures (Fig. 50.3). However, epidemiologically, C5 radicular pain is not common (Merskey & Bogduk, 1994) but C5,6 somatic referred pain is (Barnsley et al., 1995; Lord et al., 1996a; Lord & Bogduk, 1996). Therefore, the pre-test probability of pain over the shoulder girdle favours somatic referred pain. Consequently, physicians should be guarded in diagnosing pain over the shoulder girdle as radicular pain.

The cardinal distinction between cervical radicular pain and somatic referred pain is that somatic referred pain is not associated with neurological signs; yet radicular pain usually is. Therefore, the presence of neurological signs favours a diagnosis of radicular pain, and in the case of pain extending into the forearm, neurological signs all but confirm the diagnosis of radicular pain.

These guidelines, however, are not absolute. Physicians need to heed that a patient's pain may not necessarily be entirely radicular; they may have components both of radicular pain and of somatic referred pain. It may be that a patient suffers a condition that by different, and parallel, mechanisms produces different clinical features. The condition may produce nociceptive pain, which if severe may radiate as somatic referred pain. Meanwhile, the same condition may also mechanically compromise a spinal nerve and produce both radicular pain and radiculopathy. For example, an arthritic C6–7 zygapophysial joint may be locally painful and produce neck pain; it may produce somatic referred pain to the shoulder region; but its osteophytes may also compress the C6 spinal nerve to produce C6 radicular pain and C6 radiculopathy. In that event, the neurological signs and the forearm pain can be attributed to the radicular component of the diathesis; the neck pain stems from the joint itself, and not from nerve root irritation; but the pain across the shoulder is a mixture of somatic referred pain and the proximal component of the radicular pain.

Such combinations may underlie treatment failures. If all of the patient's symptoms are summarily attributed to radiculopathy and are treated as such, the radicular components may well be relieved; but the somatic components may not; and the patient will be left with neck pain and somatic referred pain. It is for such reasons that each of the patient's symptoms and signs should be analysed separately, and if necessary investigated and treated separately.

References

Ahlgren, B.D. & Garfin, S.R. (1996). Cervical radiculopathy. *Orthop. Clin. North Am.*, **27**, 253–63.

Aker, P.D., Gross, A.R., Goldsmith, C.H. & Peloso, P. (1996). Conservative management of mechanical neck pain: systematic overview and meta-analysis. *Br. Med. J.*, **313**, 1291–6.

Algers, G., Pettersson, K., Hildingsson, C. & Toolanen, G. (1993). Surgery for chronic symptoms after whiplash injury. Follow-up of 20 cases. *Acta Orthop. Scand.*, **64**, 654–6.

An, H.S. (1996). Cervical root entrapment. *Hand Clinics*, **12**, 719–30.

Atkinson, R., Ghelman, B., Tsairis, P., Warren, R.F., Jacobs, B. & Lavyne, M. (1982). Sarcoidosis presenting as cervical radiculopathy: a case report and literature review. *Spine*, **7**, 412–16.

Bachulis, B.L., Long, W.B., Hynes, G.D. & Johnson, M.C. (1987). Clinical indications for cervical spine radiographs in the traumatized patient. *Am. J. Surg.*, **153**, 473–7.

Barnsley, L. & Bogduk, N. (1993). Medial branch blocks are specific for the diagnosis of cervical zygapophysial joint pain. *Regional Anesth.*, **18**, 343–50.

Barnsley, L., Bogduk, N., Thomas, P., Chahl, J. & Southee, A. (1992). SPECT bone scans for the diagnosis of symptomatic cervical zygapophysial joints. *Aust. NZ J. Med.*, **22**, 735 (Abstract).

Barnsley, L., Lord, S., Wallis, B. & Bogduk, N. (1993a). False-positive rates of cervical zygapophysial joint blocks. *Clin. J. Pain*, **9**, 124–30.

Barnsley, L., Lord, S. & Bogduk, N. (1993b). Comparative local anaesthetic blocks in the diagnosis of cervical zygapophysial joints pain. *Pain*, **55**, 99–106.

Barnsley, L., Lord, S. & Bogduk, N. (1994a). Clinical review: whiplash injuries. *Pain*, **58**, 283–307.

Barnsley, L., Lord, S.M., Wallis, B.J. & Bogduk, N. (1994b). Lack of

effect of intraarticular corticosteroids for chronic pain in the cervical zygapophysial joints. *N. Engl. J. Med.*, **330**, 1047–50.

Barnsley, L., Lord, S.M., Wallis, B.J. & Bogduk, N. (1995). The prevalence of chronic cervical zygapophysial joint pain after whiplash. *Spine*, **20**, 20–6.

Barnsley, L., Lord, S. & Bogduk, N. (1998). The pathophysiology of whiplash. In *Cervical Flexion–Extension/Whiplash Injuries. Spine: State of the Art Reviews*, ed. G.A. Malanga, vol. 12, pp. 209–42. Philadelphia: Hanley & Belfus.

Beatty, R.M., Fowler, F.D. & Hanson, E.J. (1987). The abducted arm as a sign of ruptured cervical disc. *Neurosurgery*, **21**, 731–2.

Biousse, V., D'Anglejan-Chatillon, J., Massiou, H. & Bousser, M.G. (1994). Head pain in non-traumatic carotid artery dissection: a series of 65 patients. *Cephalalgia*, **14**, 33–6.

Bisbee, L.A. & Hartsell, H.D. (1993). Physiotherapy management of whiplash injuries. *Spine: State of the Art Rev.*, **7**, 501–16.

Boden, S.D., McCowin, P.R., Davis, D.G., Dina, T.S., Mark, A.S. & Wiesel, S. (1990). Abnormal magnetic-resonance scans of the cervical spine in asymptomatic subjects: a prospective investigation. *J. Bone Joint Surg.*, **72A**, 1178–84.

Bogduk, N. (1998). Treatment of whiplash injuries. In *Cervical Flexion–Extension/Whiplash Injuries. Spine: State of the Art Reviews*, ed. G.A. Malanga, vol. 12, pp. 469–83. Philadelphia: Hanley & Belfus.

Bogduk, N. (1999). *Medical Management of Cervical Radicular Pain. An Evidence-Based Approach*. Newcastle: Newcastle Bone and Joint Institute.

Bogduk, N. & Aprill, C. (1993). On the nature of neck pain, discography and cervical zygapophysial joint pain. *Pain*, **54**, 213–17.

Bogduk, N. & Govind, J. (1999). *Medical Management of Acute Lumbar Radicular Pain. An Evidence-Based Approach*. Newcastle: Newcastle Bone and Joint Institute.

Bogduk, N. & Lord, S.M. (1998). Cervical zygapophysial joint pain. *Neurosurg. Quarterly*, **8**, 107–17.

Bogduk, N. & Simons, D.G. (1993). Neck pain: joint pain or trigger points. In *Progress in Fibromyalgia and Myofascial Pain*, ed. H. Vaeroy & H. Merskey, pp. 267–73. Amsterdam: Elsevier.

Bogduk, N., Aprill, C. & Derby, R. (1995). Discography. In *Spine Care, Volume One: Diagnosis and Conservative Treatment*, ed. A.H. White, pp. 219–38. St Louis: Mosby.

Borchgrevink, G.E., Smevik, O., Nordby, A., Rinck, P.A., Stiules, T.C. & Lereim, I. (1995). MR imaging and radiography of patients with cervical hyperextension–flexion injuries after car accidents. *Acta Radiol.*, **36**, 425–8.

Borchgrevink, G.E., Kaasa, A., McDonagh, D., Stiles, T.C., Haraldseth, O. & Lereim, I. (1998). Acute treatment of whiplash neck sprain injuries: a randomized trial of treatment during the first 14 days after a car accident. *Spine*, **23**, 25–31.

Bovim, G., Schrader, H. & Sand, T. (1994). Neck pain in the general population. *Spine*, **19**, 1307–9.

British Association of Physical Medicine (1966). Pain in the neck and arm: a multicentre trial of the effects of physiotherapy. *Br. Med. J.*, **1**, 253–8.

Brodin, H. (1984). Cervical pain and mobilization. *Int. J. Rehab. Res.*, **7**, 190–1.

Brodin, H. (1985). Cervical pain and mobilization. *Man. Med.*, **2**, 18–22.

Bush, K. & Hillier, S. (1996). Outcome of cervical radiculopathy treated with periradicular/epidural corticosteroid injections: a prospective study with independent clinical review. *Eur. Spine J.*, **5**, 319–25.

Caldwell, J.W. & Krusen, E.M. (1962). Effectiveness of cervical traction in treatment of neck problems: evaluation of various methods. *Arch. Phys. Med. Rehab.*, **43**, 214–21.

Clar, S.A. & Cianca, J.C. (1998). Intracranial tumor masquerading as cervical radiculopathy: a case study. *Arch. Phys. Med. Rehabil.*, **79**, 1301–2.

Craig, J.B. & Hodgson, B.F. (1991). Superior facet fractures of the axis vertebra. *Spine*, **16**, 875–77.

Davidson, R.I., Dunn, E.J. & Metzmaker, J.N. (1981). The shoulder abduction test in the diagnosis of radicular pain in cervical extradural compressive monoradiculopathies. *Spine*, **6**, 441–6.

De Boer, K.F., Harman, R., Tuttle, C.D. & Wallace, H. (1985). Reliability study of detection of somatic dysfunctions in the cervical spine. *J. Manip. Physiol. Ther.*, **8**, 9–16.

De Palma, A.F., Rothman, R.H., Levitt, R.L. & Hamond, N.L. (1972). The natural history of severe cervical disc degeneration. *Acta Orthop. Scand.*, **43**, 392–6.

Dillin, W., Booth, R., Cuckler, J., Balderston, Simeone, F. & Rothman, R. (1986). Cervical radiculopathy: a review. *Spine*, **11**, 988–91.

Dreyfuss, P., Michaelsen, M. & Fletcher, D. (1994). Atlanto-occipital and lateral atlanto-axial joint pain patterns. *Spine*, **19**, 1125–31.

Dwyer, A., Aprill, C. & Bogduk, N. (1990). Cervical zygapophysial joint pain patterns I: a study in normal volunteers. *Spine*, **15**, 453–7.

Ellertsson, A.G., Sigurjonsson, K. & Thorsteinsson, T. (1978). Clinical and radiographic study of 100 cases of whiplash injury. *Acta Neurol. Scand. Supp.*, **67**, 269.

Fagerlund, M., Bjornebrink, J., Pettersson, K. & Hildingsson, C. (1995). MRI in acute phase of whiplash injury. *Eur. Radiol.*, **5**, 297–301.

Fast, A., Parikh, S. & Marin, E.L. (1989). The shoulder abduction relief sign in cervical radiculopathy. *Arch. Phys. Med. Rehabil.*, **70**, 402–3.

Feinstein, B., Langton, J.B.K., Jameson, R.M. & Schiller, F. (1954). Experiments on referred pain from deep somatic tissues. *J. Bone Joint Surg.*, **36A**, 981–97.

Foley-Nolan, D., Barry, C., Coughlan, R.J., O'Connor, P. & Roden, D. (1990). Pulsed high frequency (27mHz) electromagnetic therapy for persistent pain: a double blind, placebo-controlled study of 20 patients. *Orthopaedics*, **13**, 445–51.

Foley-Nolan, D., Moore, K., Codd, M., Barry, C., O'Connor, P. & Coughlan, R.J. (1992). Low energy high frequency pulsed electromagnetic therapy for acute whiplash injuries. *Scand. J. Rehab. Med.*, **24**, 51–9.

Fridenberg, Z.B. & Miller, W.T. (1963). Degenerative disc disease of the cervical spine. A comparative study of asymptomatic and symptomatic patients. *J. Bone Joint Surg.*, **45A**, 1171–8.

Garrard, P. & Barnes, D. (1996). Aortic dissection presenting as a neurological emergency. *J. R. Soc. Med.*, **89**, 271–2.

Gerrelts, B.D., Petersen, E.U., Mabry, J. & Petersen, S.R. (1991). Delayed diagnosis of cervical spine injuries. *J. Trauma*, **31**, 1622–6.

Gibson, T., Bogduk, N., Macpherson, J. & McIntosh, A. (2000). Crash characteristics of whiplash associated chronic neck pain. *J. Musculoskeletal Pain*, **8**, 87–95.

Goldie, I. & Landquist, A. (1970). Evaluation of the effects of different forms of physiotherapy in cervical pain. *Scand. J. Rehab. Med.*, **2–3**, 117–21.

Greenman, P.E. (1993). Manual and manipulative therapy in whiplash injuries. *Spine: State of the Art Rev.*, **7**, 517–30.

Gregorius, F.K., Estrin, T. & Crandall, P.H. (1976). Cervical spondylotic radiculopathy and myelopathy: a long-term follow-up study. *Arch. Neurol.*, **33**, 618–25.

Gross, A.R., Aker, P.D. & Quartly, C. (1996). Manual therapy in the treatment of neck pain. *Rheum. Dis. Clin. North Am.*, **22**, 579–98.

Grubb, S.A. & Kelly, C.K. (2000). Cervical discography: clinical implications from 12 years of experience. *Spine*, **25**, 1382–9.

Heller, C.A., Stanley, P., Lewis-Jones, B. & Heller, R.F. (1983). Value of x ray examinations of the cervical spine. *Br. Med. J.*, **287**, 1276–8.

Helliwell, P.S., Evans, P.F. & Wright, V. (1994). The straight cervical spine: does it indicate muscle spasm? *J. Bone Joint Surg.*, **76B**, 103–6.

Henderson, C.M., Hennessy, R.G., Shuey, H.M. & Shackelford, E.G. (1983). Posterior-lateral foraminotomy as an exclusive operative technique for cervical radiculopathy: a review of 846 consecutively operated cases. *Neurosurgery*, **13**, 504–12.

Hirst, A.E., Johns, V.J. & Kime, F.W. (1958). Dissecting aneurysm of the aorta: a review of 505 cases. *Medicine*, **37**, 217–75.

Hochberg, M., Borenstein, D. & Arnett, F. (1978). The absence of back pain in classic ankylosing spondylitis. *Johns Hopkins Med. J.*, **143**, 181–3.

Hoffman, J.R., Schriger, D.L., Mower, W., Luo, J.S. & Zucker, M. (1992). Low-risk criteria for cervical-spine radiography in blunt trauma: a prospective study. *Ann. Emerg. Med.*, **21**, 1454–60.

Honet, J.C. & Puri, K. (1976). Cervical radiculitis: treatment and results in 82 patients. *Arch. Phys. Med. Rehabil.*, **57**, 12–16.

Hong, C.Z., Lin, J.C., Bender, L.F., Schaeffer, J.N., Meltzer, R.J. & Causin, P. (1982). Magnetic necklace: its therapeutic effectiveness on neck and shoulder pain. *Arch. Phys. Med. Rehabil.*, **63**, 426–66.

Howe, D.H., Newcombe, R.G. & Wade, M.T. (1983). Manipulation of the cervical spine – pilot study. *J. Roy. Coll. Gen. Pract.*, **33**, 574–9.

Howe, J.F. (1979). A neurophysiological basis for the radicular pain of nerve root compression. In *Advances in Pain Research and Therapy*, J.J. Bonica, J.C. Liebeskind & D.G. Albe-Fessard, Vol 3, pp. 647–57. New York: Raven Press.

Howe, J.F., Loeser, J.D. & Calvin, W.H. (1977). Mechanosensitivity of dorsal root ganglia and chronically injured axons: a physiological basis for the radicular pain of nerve root compression. *Pain*, **3**, 25–41.

Hubka, M.J. & Phelan, S.P. (1994). Interexaminer reliability of palpation for cervical spine tenderness. *J. Manip. Physiol. Ther.*, **17**, 591–5.

Hurwitz, E.L., Aker, P.R., Adams, A.H., Meeker, W.C. & Shekelle, P.G.

(1996). Manipulation and mobilization of the cervical spine: a systematic review of the literature. *Spine*, **21**, 1746–60.

Isdale, I.C. & Conlon, P.W. (1971). Atlanto-axial subluxation. A six-year follow-up report. *Ann. Rheum. Dis.*, **30**, 387–9.

Johnson, M.J. & Lucas, G.L. (1997). Value of cervical spine radiographs as a screening tool. *Clin. Orthop.*, **340**, 102–8.

Jonsson, H., Cesarini, K., Sahlstedt, B. & Rauschning, W. (1994). Findings and outcomes in whiplash-type neck distortions. *Spine*, **19**, 2733–43.

Kaiser, J.A. & Holland, B.A. (1998). Imaging of the cervical spine. *Spine*, **23**, 2701–12.

Kamwendo, K. & Linton, S.J. (1991). A controlled study of the effect of neck school in medical secretaries. *Scand. J. Rehab. Med.*, **23**, 143–52.

Kamwendo, K., Linton, S.J. & Moritz, U. (1991). Neck and shoulder disorders in medical secretaries. Part I. Pain prevalence and risk factors. *Scand. J. Rehab. Med.*, **23**, 127–33.

Kaneoka, K., Ono, K., Inami, S. & Hayashi, K. (1999). Motion analysis of cervical vertebrae during whiplash loading. *Spine*, **24**, 763–70.

Kellgren, J.H. (1939). On the distribution of pain arising from deep somatic structures with charts of segmental pain areas. *Clin. Sci.*, **4**, 35–46.

Kikuchi, S., Macnab, I. & Moreau, P. (1981). Localisation of the level of symptomatic cervical disc degeneration, *J. Bone Joint Surg.*, **63B**, 272–7.

Klaber Moffett, J.A., Hughes, G.I. & Griffiths, P. (1990). An investigation of the effects of cervical traction. Part 1: clinical effectiveness. *Clin. Rehab.*, **4**, 205–11.

Koes, B.W., Bouter, L.M., van Mameren, H. et al. (1992). The effectiveness of manual therapy, physiotherapy, and treatment by the general practitioner for nonspecific back and neck complaints: a randomized clinical trial. *Spine*, **17**, 28–35.

Kreipke, D.L., Gillespie, K.R., McCarthy, M.C., Mail, J.T., Lappas, J.C. & Broadie, T.A. (1989). Reliability of indications for cervical spine films in trauma patients. *J. Trauma*, **29**, 1438–9.

Lawrence, J.S. (1969). Disc degeneration: its frequency and relationship to symptoms. *Ann. Rheum. Dis.*, **28**, 121–38.

Levoska, S., Keinanen-Kiukaanniemi, S. & Bloigu, R. (1991). Repeatability of measurement of tenderness in the neck-shoulder region by a dolorimeter and manual palpation. *Clin. J. Pain*, **9**, 229–35.

Lewith, G.T. & Machin, D. (1981). A randomised trial to evaluate the effect of infra-red stimulation of local trigger points, versus placebo on the pain caused by cervical osteoarthrosis. *Acupuncture Electro-Therapeut. Res. Int. J.*, **6**, 277–84.

Lord, S.M. & Bogduk, N. (1996). The cervical synovial joints as sources of post-traumatic headache. *J. Musculoskeletal Pain*, **4**, 81–94.

Lord, S., Barnsley, L., Wallis, B. & Bogduk, N. (1994). Third occipital nerve headache: a prevalence study. *J. Neurol. Neurosurg., Psychiatry*, **57**, 1187–90.

Lord, S.M., Barnsley, L., Bogduk, N. (1995). The utility of comparative local anaesthetic blocks versus placebo-controlled blocks for the diagnosis of cervical zygapophysial joint pain. *Clin. J. Pain*, **11**, 208–13.

Lord, S.M., Barnsley, L. & Wallis, B.J. & Bogduk, N. (1996a). Chronic cervical zygapophysial joint pain after whiplash: a placebo-controlled prevalence study. *Spine*, **21**, 1737–45.

Lord, S.M., Barnsley, L., Wallis, B.J., McDonald, G.J. & Bogduk, N. (1996b). Percutaneous radio-frequency neurotomy for chronic cervical zygapophysial-joint pain. *N. Engl. J. Med.*, **335**, 1721–6.

Lord, S.M., McDonald, G.J. & Bogduk, N. (1998). Percutaneous radiofrequency neurotomy of the cervical medial branches: a validated treatment for cervical zygapophysial joint pain. *Neurosurg. Quart.*, **8**, 288–308.

Lunsford, L.D., Bissonette, D.J., Jannetta, P.J., Sheptak, P.E. & Zorub, D.S. (1980). Anterior surgery for cervical disc disease. Part 1: treatment of lateral cervical disc herniation in 253 cases. *J. Neurosurg.*, **53**, 1–11.

MacNab, I. (1972). The mechanism of spondylogenic pain. In *Cervical Pain*, ed. C. Hirsch & Y. Zotterman, pp. 89–95. Pergamon, Oxford.

Makela, M., Heliovaara, M., Sievers, K., Impivaara, O., Knekt, P. & Aromaa, A. (1991). Prevalence, determinants and consequences of chronic neck pain in Finland. *Am. J. Epidemiol.*, **124**, 1356–67.

McDonald, G., Lord, S.M. & Bogduk, N. (1999). Long-term follow-up of cervical radiofrequency neurotomy for chronic neck pain. *Neurosurgery*, **45**, 61–8.

McKinney, L.A. (1989). Early mobilisation and outcomes in acute sprains of the neck. *Br. Med. J.*, **299**, 1006–8.

McKinney, L.A., Dornan, J.O. & Ryan, M. (1989). The role of physiotherapy in the management of acute neck sprains following road-traffic accidents. *Arch. Emerg. Med.*, **6**, 27–33.

McNamara, R.M. (1988). Post-traumatic neck pain: a prospective and follow-up study. *Ann. Emerg. Med.*, **17**, 906–11.

Mealy, K., Brennan, H. & Fenelon, G.C.C. (1986). Early mobilisation of acute whiplash injuries. *Br. Med. J.*, **292**, 656–7.

Merskey, H. & Bogduk, N. (ed.) (1994). *Classification of Chronic Pain. Descriptions of Chronic Pain Syndromes and Definition of Pain Terms*, 2nd edn. Seattle: IASP Press.

Mior, S.A., King, R.S., McGregor, M. & Bernard, M. (1985). Intra and interexaminer reliability of motion palpation in the cervical spine. *J. Can. Chiro. Assoc.*, **29**, 195–8.

Nansel, D.D., Peneff, A.L., Jansen, R.D. & Cooperstein, R. (1989). Interexaminer concordance in detecting joint-play asymmetries in the cervical spines of otherwise asymptomatic subjects. *J. Manip. Physiol. Ther.*, **12**, 428–33.

Odom, G.L., Finney, W. & Woodhall, B. (1958). Cervical disk lesions. *J. Am. Med. Assoc.*, **166**, 23–8.

Pennie, B.H. & Agambar, L.J. (1990). Whiplash injuries: a trial of early management. *J. Bone Joint Surg.*, **72B**, 277–9.

Persson, L.C.G., Carlsson, C.A. & Carlsson, J.Y. (1997). Long-lasting cervical radicular pain managed with surgery, physiotherapy or a cervical collar: a prospective, randomized study. *Spine*, **22**, 751–8.

Pettersson, K., Hildingsson, C., Toolanen, G., Fagerlund, M. & Bjornebrink, J. (1994). MRI and neurology in acute whiplash trauma. *Acta Orthop. Scand.*, **65**, 525–8.

Petrie, J.P. & Hazleman, B.L. (1986). A controlled study of acupuncture in neck pain. *Br. J. Rheumatol.*, **25**, 271–5.

Petrie, J.P. & Langley, G.B. (1983). Acupuncture in the treatment of chronic cervical pain: a pilot study. *Clin. Exp. Rheumatol.*, 1, 333–5.

Provinciali, L., Baroni, M., Illuminati, L. & Ceravolo, G. (1996). Multimodal treatment to prevent the late whiplash syndrome. *Scand. J. Rehab. Med.*, 28, 105–11.

Radanov, B.P., Sturzenegger, M. & Di Stefano, G. (1995). Long-term outcome after whiplash injury: a 2-year follow-up considering features of injury mechanism and somatic, radiologic, and psychosocial findings. *Medicine*, 74, 281–97.

Radhakrishan, K., Litchy, W.J., O'Fallon, M. & Kurland, L.T. (1994). Epidemiology of cervical radiculopathy. A population-based study from Rochester, Minnesota, 1976 through 1990. *Brain*, 117, 325–35.

Roberge, R.J., Wears, R.C., Kelly, M. et al. (1988). Selective application of cervical spine radiography in alert victims of blunt trauma: a prospective study. *J. Trauma*, 28, 784–8.

Ronnen, H.R., de Korte, P.J., Brink, P.R.G., van der Bijl, H.J., Tonino, A.J. & Franke, C.L. (1996). Acute whiplash injury: is there a role for MR imaging? A prospective study of 100 patients. *Radiology*, 201, 93–6.

Sanchez, M.C., Arenillas, J.I.C., Gutierrez, D.A., Alonso, J.L. & Alvarez, J. de P. (1983). Cervical radiculopathy: a rare symptom of giant cell arteritis. *Arth. Rheum.*, 26, 207–9.

Sandmark, H. & Nisell, R. (1995). Validity of five common manual neck pain provoking tests. *Scand. J. Rehab. Med.*, 27, 131–6.

Schellhas, K.P., Smith, M.D., Gundry, C.R. & Pollei, S.R. (1996). Cervical discogenic pain: prospective correlation of magnetic resonance imaging and discography in asymptomatic subjects and pain sufferers. *Spine*, 21, 300–12.

Seitz, J.P., Unguez, C.E., Corbus, H.F. & Wooten, W.W. (1995). SPECT of the cervical spine in the evaluation of neck pain after trauma. *Clin. Nucl. Med.*, 20, 667–73.

Seletz, E. (1958). Whiplash injuries: neurophysiological basis for pain and methods used for rehabilitation. *J. Am. Med. Assoc.*, 168, 1750–5.

Sharp, J., Purser, D.W. & Lawrence, J.S. (1958). Rheumatoid arthritis of the cervical spine in the adult. *Ann. Rheum. Dis.*, 17, 303–13.

Signoret, F., Feron, J.M., Bonfait, H. et al. (1986). Fractured odontoid with fractured superior articular process of the axis. *J. Bone Joint Surg.*, 68B, 182–4.

Silbert, P.L., Makri, B. & Schievink, W.I. (1995). Headache and neck pain in spontaneous internal carotid and vertebral artery dissections. *Neurology*, 45, 1517–22.

Slipman, C.W., Plastaras, C.T. Palmitier, R.A., Huston, C.W. & Sterenfeld, E.B (1998). Symptom provocation of fluoroscopically guided cervical nerve root stimulation: are dynatomal maps identical to dermatomal maps? *Spine*, 23, 2235–42.

Sloop, P.R., Smith, D.S., Goldberg, E. & Dore, C. (1982). Manipulation of chronic neck pain: a double-blind controlled study. *Spine*, 7, 532–5.

Smedmark, V., Wallin, M. & Arvidsson, I. (2000). Inter-examiner reliability in assessing passive intervertebral motion of the cervical spine. *Man. Ther.*, 5, 97–101.

Smyth, M.J. & Wright, V. (1959). Sciatica and the intervertebral disc. An experimental study. *J. Bone Joint Surg.*, 40A, 1401–18.

Snow, C.J., Aves Wood, R., Dowhopouuk, H. et al., (1992). Randomized controlled clinical trial of spray and stretch for relief of back and neck myofascial pain. (Abstract). *Physiother. Canada*, 44, (2)S8.

Spitzer, W.O., Skovron, M.L., Salmi, L.R. et al. (1995). Scientific monograph of the Quebec task force on whiplash-associated disorders: redefining 'whiplash' and its management. *Spine*, 20, 1S–73S.

Spurling, R.G. & Scoville, W.B. (1944). Lateral rupture of the cervical intervertebral discs. *Surg. Gynec. Obstet.*, 78, 350–8.

Stroobants, J., Fidler, L., Storms, J.L., Klaes, R., Dua, G. & van Hoye, M. (1994). High cervical pain and impairment of skull mobility as the only symptoms of an occipital condyle fracture. *J. Neurosurg.*, 81, 137–8.

Sturzenegger, M. (1994). Headache and neck pain: the warning symptoms of vertebral artery dissection. *Headache*, 34, 187–93.

Takala, E.P., Viikari-Juntura, E. & Tynkkynen, E.M. (1994). Does group gymnastics at the workplace help in neck pain? *Scand. J. Rehab. Med.*, 26, 17–20.

Taylor, J.R. & Taylor, M.M. (1996). Cervical spinal injuries: an autopsy study of 109 blunt injuries. *J. Musculoskeletal Pain*, 4, 61–79.

Taylor, J.R. & Twomey, L.T. (1993). Acute injuries to cervical joints: an autopsy study of neck sprain. *Spine*, 9, 1115–22.

Tessell, R.W., Shapiro, A.P. & Mailis, A. (1993). Medical management of whiplash injuries. *Spine: State of the Art Rev.*, 7, 481–99.

Teresi, L.M., Lufkin, R.B., Reicher, M.A. et al. (1987). Asymptomatic degenerative disk disease and spondylosis of the cervical spine: MR imaging. *Radiology*, 164, 83–8.

Thomas, M., Eriksson, S.V. & Lundberg, T. (1991). A comparative study of diazepam and acupuncture in patients with osteoarthritis pain: a placebo controlled study. *Am. J. Chin. Med.*, 19, 95–100.

Thorsen, H., Gam, A.N., Svensson, B.H. et al. (1992). Low level laser therapy for myofascial pain in the neck and shoulder girdle. A double-blind, cross-over study. *Scand. J. Rheumatol.*, 21, 139–42.

Van der Donk, J., Schouten, J.S.A.G., Passchier, J., van Romunde, L.K.J. & Valkenburg, H.A. (1991). The associations of neck pain with radiological abnormalities of the cervical spine and personality traits in a general population. *J. Rheumatol.*, 18, 1884–9.

Vargo, M.M. & Flood, K.M. (1990). Pancoast tumour presenting as cervical radiculopathy. *Arch. Phys. Med. Rehabil.*, 71, 606–9.

Vasseljen, O. & Westgaard, R.H. (1995). A case-control study of trapezius muscle activity in office and manual workers with shoulder and neck pain and symptom-free controls. *Int. Arch. Occup. Environ. Health*, 67, 11–18.

Viikari-Juntura, E. (1987). Interexaminer reliability of observations in physical examinations of the neck. *Phys. Ther.*, 67, 1526–32.

Viikari-Juntura, E., Porras, M. & Laasonen, E.M. (1989). Validity of clinical tests in the diagnosis of root compression in cervical disc disease. *Spine*, 14, 253–7.

Voyvodic, F., Dolinis, J., Moore, V.M. et al. (1997). MRI of car occupants with whiplash injury. *Neuroradiology*, 39, 25–40.

Wallis, B.J., Lord, S.M. & Bogduk, N. (1997). Resolution of psychological distress of whiplash patients following treatment by radiofrequency neurotomy: a randomised, double-blind, placebo-controlled trial. *Pain*, **73**, 15–22.

Westgaard, R.H. & Jansen, T. (1992). Individual and work related factors associated with symptoms of musculoskeletal complaints. II Different risk factors among sewing machine operators. *Br. J. Ind. Med.*, **49**, 154–62.

Whitecloud, T.S. & Seago, R.A. (1987). Cervical discogenic syndrome. Results of operative intervention in patients with positive discography. *Spine*, **12**, 313–16.

Wolfe, F., Simons, D.G., Fricton, J. et al. (1992). The fibromyalgia and myofascial pain syndromes: a preliminary study of tender points and trigger points in persons with fibromyalgia, myofascial pain and no disease. *J. Rheumatol.*, **19**, 944–51.

Yamano, Y. (1985). Soft disc herniation of the cervical spine. *Int. Orthop.*, **9**, 19–27.

Yoss, R.E., Corbin, K.B., MacCarthy, C.S. & Love, J.G. (1957). Significance of symptoms and signs in localization of involved root in cervical disk protrusion. *Neurology*, **7**, 673–83.

Zylbergold, R.S. & Piper, M.C. (1985). Cervical spine disorders: a comparison of three types of traction. *Spine*, **10**, 867–71.

51

Diagnosis and management of low back pain

Donlin M. Long and Mohammed BenDebba

Department of Neurosurgery, Johns Hopkins School of Medicine, Baltimore, Maryland, USA

Low back pain (with or without sciatica) is one of the most common complaints of patients in all developed countries (Ackerman et al., 1997a; BenDebba et al., 1997; Deyo & Tsui-Wu, 1987; Fredrickson et al., 1984; Long, 1989; Long et al., 1979). In the USA, it is the second most common reason to see a physician (Carey et al., 1995), and the most common reason for Workmen's Compensation claims (Long et al., 1996). Surgery on the spine now ranks third among procedures in the Medicare population (Zeidman & Long, 1996).

Thus, it is surprising to discover that there is no complete classification system for low back pain with or without sciatica, and standards for diagnosis, treatment, and assessment of outcomes of therapy have not been established (BenDebba et al., 1997; Merskey & Bogduk, 1994).

One of the principal reasons why this situation exists is that for most patients, the causes of low back pain remain unknown, and the value of therapy is uncertain (Bigos et al., 1994; Waddell et al., 1984). The magnitude of the problem and the huge expenditures required for low back pain make it particularly important to understand what is currently known and not known about back pain, so that treatment is rational and based upon the most up-to-date information and guidelines.

Classification of low back pain

Classifications may be etiologic, based upon anatomical descriptions, or may use surrogate descriptors when anatomical and pathological details are not well understood. The most common classification system for low back pain is temporal and relates to descriptions of patients, rather than to pathological processes (BenDebba, 1997; Bigos et al., 1994; Long et al., 1996). This practical system is of real value in managing patients, although it does not provide

the desired etiologic accuracy that is available with anatomical and pathological classifications (Bogduk, 1997; Main et al., 1992).

Transient low back pain

Transient low back pain is that which occurs so briefly that the patient does not seek medical attention. The etiologies of these brief periods of low back pain remain unknown, but will be discussed in greater detail later in the chapter.

Acute low back pain

Acute low back pain lasts for a longer period of time, usually a few days, and often brings the patient to medical attention. These patients have been addressed in guidelines promulgated by the consensus method from the National Institute for Health Policy Research (Bigos et al., 1994). Such patients require a careful history with the intent to determine if there are danger signals suggesting that this episode of back pain is a symptom of a serious underlying disease or the result of major trauma. It is unlikely that the history will be important otherwise, but in the acute phase, the primary concern is that an important intercurrent disease such as trauma with resultant fracture or instability, infection, or neoplasm may be missed. The physician needs to ensure that the back pain is not referred from gastrointestinal or renal disease and is not a symptom of vascular disease such as aortic aneurysm. Back pain as a part of an arthritic syndrome, such as ankylosing spondylitis or rheumatoid arthritis is possible, but generally such a diagnosis is less critical in the acute phase.

The physical examination requires inspection of the back, palpation for assessment of muscle spasm and local tenderness, assessment of range of motion, and/or a neurological evaluation that examines reflexes, strength, and sensation in the lower extremities. Any acute neurological loss is important, but only severe deficits are likely to precipitate immediate therapy. Patients usually know about bowel or bladder dysfunction, but it is important to ask even though definitive testing is not required in the absence of complaints. A key issue in the neurological examination is the differential diagnosis, which should separate lumbar radicular abnormalities from other neurological deficits (Deyo et al., 1992; Dreyfuss et al., 1996; Mooney, 1987).

Management of acute low back pain

If there are no indications of intercurrent disease and no evidence of significant neurological loss, consensus guidelines indicate that no further evaluation is required (Bigos et al., 1994). Specifically, imaging studies need not be done. Indications for imaging of any kind are: a history of significant trauma, the presence of known or suspected intercurrent disease, and the presence of a significant neurological deficit. Without them, treatment is expectant. Patients should be prescribed rest or limited activity for a few days until improvement begins. Adequate analgesia is important (Long et al., 1979; Solomon et al., 1980). No other treatment is required because spontaneous recovery will occur in most patients within a few days. In fact, patients should be returned to full function as soon as possible (Turner, 1996). There is good evidence that recovery is hastened by increased activity as tolerated (van den Hoogen et al., 1998). Most patients will recover substantially within the first month. If they do not, or if any new important neurological or other symptomatic changes occur, imaging is then reasonable (Bigos et al., 1994; Liang & Komaroff, 1982). Plain films with flexion/extension and MRI give the most information. CT is a reasonable substitute, but will provide less information about soft tissue changes than MRI. The purpose of imaging is not necessarily to make a diagnosis, but rather to determine if a surgically remediable abnormality or otherwise treatable disease is present (Ackerman et al., 1997b,c; Lindstrom et al., 1992). There is little evidence to support the use of physical therapy, manipulation therapy, or any alternative medicine treatments at any time in the management of acute low back pain. The cost is substantial and the benefit marginal even in the most favourable studies (American Academy of Orthopedic Surgeons and North American Spine Society, 1996; Anderson et al., 1999; Bigos et al., 1994; Cherkin et al., 1996b, 1998; Koes et al., 1991a,b, 1994; Koes & van den Hoogen, 1994; Linton & Kamwendo, 1987).

Many experienced practitioners use a short course of oral steroids when an acute radicular syndrome is present without neurological deficit (Sonne et al., 1985). There is no definitive study supporting this practice, but many practitioners find that a short course of oral steroids will rapidly relieve radicular pain. Some clinicians use epidural steroids for the same purpose. It has always been our contention that the evidence for substantial improvement is meagre and that the procedure is not without risk. We use oral steroids for acute radicular syndromes, but have discouraged the use of epidural steroids because we believe that their limited benefits do not clearly justify the cost and risks associated with them. Since most patients recover spontaneously, the least intervention possible in acute syndromes is best (American Academy of Orthopedic Surgeons and North American Spine Society, 1996; Bigos et al., 1994; Carey et al., 1995; Indahl, 1995; Long & Watts, 1996; Long & Zeidman, 1994; van Tulder et al., 1997).

The persistent low back pain syndrome

Not all patients recover spontaneously (Lindstrom et al., 1995). Recently, we identified a subgroup in which symptoms persist after 3 months and apparently become permanent (Ackerman et al., 1997c; Long et al., 1996; Long & Watts, 1996; Long & Zeidman, 1994). For these patients who still complain of substantial pain and disability after 3 months, it is appropriate to carry out an immediate investigation to identify the cause of the pain. Although there are specific constellations of signs that denote specific root involvement, they occur rarely and the neurological examination is seldom diagnostic. The most important sign is the positive straight leg-raising test. When present, this strongly suggests root compression, but does not suggest the cause (Long et al., 1996).

The imaging evaluation begins with flexion and extension plain films and MRI (Ackerman et al., 1997c; American Academy of Orthopedic Surgeons, 1995). CT of the lumbar spine is indicated when the disease is thought to have a significant bony involvement. CT myelogram, which was the major diagnostic test until fairly recently, is now rarely indicated. It is used principally when intradural pathology is suspected or when a patient cannot tolerate MRI and plain CT does not provide adequate information (Fullenlove & Williams, 1957; Loisel et al., 1997; Scavone et al., 1981).

Of interest is that in an extensive prospective review of nearly 4,000 patients, we found no clinically significant psychological dysfunction in patients with persistent low back pain complaints (BenDebba et al., 1997; Long et al., 1996).

The chronic pain syndrome

The group described above is quite different from a group of patients identified well over 30 years ago in whom pain complaints with clinically significant psychological dysfunction produce a completely disabling syndrome (Morley et al., 1999; Waddell et al., 1984). These patients, who have high levels of psychological distress and are disabled by pain without evidence of physical impairment, differ from patients with the persistent pain syndrome (Bigos et al., 1991; Main et al., 1992). Their evaluation and treatment has been studied intensively in multidisciplinary pain treatment centres (Long et al., 1981, 1988; Long, 1992). At Johns Hopkins, we evaluate this group by using a medical model that comprises an exhaustive investigation of possible causes of the pain, assessment of physical impairment, and careful assessment of psychological dysfunction. Treatment consists of a multidisciplinary approach that involves eliminating the cause of the pain, improving physical functioning, and attending to psychological needs (Loisel et al., 1997; Long 1991a,b; Phillips & Grant, 1991a; Zeidman & Long, 1996).

Etiologies of low back pain

The major problem in classifying low back pain is that it is a symptom of many diseases for which correlations are excellent, but the underlying causative factors are not understood (Bogduk & Long, 1979). Obviously, the pain is generated through the activation of nociceptors serving the abnormal areas (Ackerman et al., 1997c; Long, 1989; Merskey & Bogduk, 1994). What activates these nociceptors, however, is unclear (Mooney, 1987). Most experts agree that compression of individual lumbar nerve roots will produce pain, both localized in the spine and with a radicular character (Smyth & Wright, 1959). Relief of the compression usually improves the pain. Severe degrees of dislocation with movement also produce pain (Fredrickson et al., 1984). Nevertheless, there is no consensus about what minimal degree of subluxation is required to be either pathological or painful. Some believe that small movements that are not discernible on imaging studies may be sufficient to cause chronic pain (Mooney & Robertson, 1976; Morley et al., 1999); others suggest that the mediators are the chemical components of the inflammatory cascade that may occur acutely or may be a part of the spondylotic process (Mooney, 1987). Definitive data do not exist to prove or disprove these hypotheses. Although, there is a strong association of back pain with spondylotic disease in the majority of sufferers, this correlation is clearly not absolute. Moreover, several authors have demonstrated that patients with significant spondylotic disease may be asymptomatic (Ackerman et al., 1997b; Fullenlove & Williams, 1957; Splinthoff, 1953).

In the absence of definitive data, it is necessary to define clinical hypotheses for the origins of back pain and direct treatments empirically. The fundamental hypothesis that leads to surgery is that some patients have back and leg pain associated with nerve root compression, instability of the spine, or both, and that these are the only conditions currently known that surgery can ameliorate (Long, 1978, 1985, 1987; Long et al., 1988). Only a small minority of patients with back pain have either of these conditions demonstrated. So, for the majority of patients, the cause of their complaint remains unknown and assumptions about primary or secondary painful phenomena remain descriptive (Bogduk & Long, 1979; Dreyfuss et al., 1996; Hirschberg et al., 1979; Ingpen & Burry, 1970; Johnson, 1989).

Specific conditions associated with back pain

Back pain as a consequence of systemic disease

Back pain may occur as a consequence of a number of organ-specific diseases that manifest themselves in or near the lumbar spine, particularly in the retroperitoneal space. These include aortic aneurysm, metastatic or locally invasive neoplasm, inflammatory disease of the bowel, kidney diseases of many kinds, pelvic neoplasia and inflammatory disease, and endometriosis. Hip disease, lower extremity occlusive vascular disease, and sensory motor neuropathies can mimic lumbar radiculopathy. In a study of nearly 4000 patients, however, only 3% had back pain as a symptom of intercurrent disease and almost all of these were previously undetected metastatic cancer (Long et al., 1996; Magora & Schwartz, 1976). Intradural spinal cord tumours are occasionally present with back pain. In all these instances, the history usually reveals that this pain differs from the usual back pain of unknown etiology (Ackerman et al., 1997c; Deyo et al., 1992; Deyo & Tsui-Wu, 1987; Phillips & Grant, 1991b; van den Hoogen et al., 1998; von Korff, 1994).

Infections

Lumbar diskitis, with or without paravertebral abscess, is an unusual and extremely serious cause of back pain (Waldvogel & Vasey, 1980; Zeidman & Long, 1996). The most common infective agents are tuberculosis and infections spread from other sources, such as dental or kidney infections. Most patients have a history suggestive of infection, including malaise, chills, and fever, but sometimes pain is the only or predominant symptom and fever does not occur. Imaging studies based upon symptoms indicative of infection will invariably make the diagnosis, except in the most acute cases.

Arthritis and spondylitis

Severe back pain is the defining symptom in a number of spondylitic and arthritic diseases, the most common of which is rheumatoid arthritis. Ankylosing spondylitis in males is another well-known disease. Arthropathy of zygapophyseal joints occurs in psoriasis, and in both gout and pseudo-gout. Inadequately treated acromegaly is often complicated by intractable back pain. Most of the less frequently encountered arthritides can also present with back pain. Back pain and spinal stenosis are common early mid-life complications in achondroplasia. Imaging studies and an appropriate diagnosis of the underlying arthritic condition usually establish the cause of the pain (Long, 1978, 1991a).

Back strain and fibromyalgia

The most common cause of acute back pain is generally assumed to be muscular strain and/or muscular-ligamentous inflammation (Ingpen & Burry, 1970; Johnson, 1989). The assumption is made because of the presence of focal tender points and spasm in muscles. Since no clearly defined structural abnormalities are found, back strain, myositis, fibromyalgia, or any of several other descriptive diagnoses are commonly made (Johnson, 1989). There is no definitive evidence that these are real entities; they are inferred because of local nonspecific findings. Clearly, all of these local changes exist in patients, but whether they are primary causes of the problem or simply secondary to the, as yet, undefined abnormalities of the lumbar spine is not known. Still, patients improve with treatment of these local abnormalities, whether they are primary or epiphenomena (Anderson et al., 1999; Cherkin et al., 1998; Fordyce et al., 1986; Indahl et al., 1995). Treatment consists of analgesic and anti-inflammatory agents, and passive measures such as heat, massage, ultrasound, electrical stimulation, and local analgesic and/or steroid injection. Bed rest is often helpful for a few days, as well as some restriction of activities that aggravate the pain (Bigos et al., 1994; Deyo, 1996; Long, 1989).

The argument over the reality of a primary diagnosis of fibromyalgia persists. Those who believe in a unifying diagnosis have not yet demonstrated diagnostic features that reliably define a disease process. In practical terms, it makes little difference, because the treatments are all symptomatic (Wheeler & Hanley, 1995).

Surgery is indicated for very specific diagnoses and all other treatments for spinal problems are either expectant, awaiting spontaneous resolution, or symptomatic (American Academy of Orthopedic Surgeons, 1995). For this reason, the most important issues for patients with persistent or chronic low back pain are to be certain that there is no treatable underlying pathology, that there is no evidence of serious intercurrent disease, and to determine if surgical therapy can change the structural abnormalities found in the spine. When all three issues are addressed and nothing treatable is found, use of symptomatic therapies is routine. The evidence that these symptomatic therapies are valuable is marginal. The best published data suggest that weight loss, general conditioning, and a specific exercise program aimed at strengthening lumbar and abdominal muscles will be beneficial (Forssell, 1981; Indahl et al., 1998; Jackson & Brown, 1983; Lindstrom et al., 1992; Moffett et al., 1999). Our data strongly suggest that most of the currently used symptomatic therapies will not result in significant improvement (Cherkin et al., 1996a; Frymoyer & Cats-Baril, 1987; Koes et al., 1991a,b, 1994).

Degenerative disc disease and spondylosis

The majority of patients with persistent low back pain have general spondylotic changes that are characterized by loss of disc hydration, inflammatory and hypertrophic changes in bones and ligaments, fissures and tears in the annulus, fibrosis, loss of disc height, facet arthropathy including synovial cyst formation, and changes in spinal alignment including spondylolisthesis, retrolisthesis, and many variations of scoliosis. The simplest expression is lumbar disc herniation.

The herniated lumbar disc

Disc herniations are usually heralded by back pain and radicular pain in the distribution of the nerves affected, with or without neurological changes related to those same nerves. Herniation may be traumatic or spontaneous. It may be preceded by a long history of lesser back problems or may occur as a first-time event. Herniation occurs most commonly at L4–L5 and L5–S1 with higher levels being involved only about 15% of the time. Typical herniations are midline, lateral within the spinal canal, or far lateral in the foramen or beyond. The most important feature is the history of radicular pain. Massive disc herniations may also compromise bowel, bladder, and sexual functions, but the typical disc affects one or two nerve roots only.

Herniations at L5–S1 may affect either nerve root or both. Involvement of the S1 nerve root produces sciatica with pain reaching the lateral side of the foot and sole. The ankle reflex is diminished or absent. Sensory loss occurs in the lateral two toes, lateral foot, and sole. Motor loss produces weakness of extension of the foot. Involvement of the L5 nerve root produces sciatica that reaches the top of the foot, the medial foot, and first three toes, in particular the great toe. There is no associated reflex change. Sensory loss occurs in the top of the foot and specifically in the web space between the first and second toes. Weakness is manifested by impaired ability to flex foot and toes. Straight leg-raising is a strong confirmatory sign. With a patient lying flat, the painful leg is raised slowly while extended. Sciatic pain must be reproduced for the test to be positive. When the non-painful leg is raised and contralateral pain occurs, this is called positive crossed straight leg-raising and is a very reliable sign of nerve root compression. In all patients with disc herniation, there may be associated non-specific findings of muscle spasm, paravertebral muscle tenderness, sciatic notch and sciatic nerve tenderness, but these do not aid in the diagnosis.

Involvement of the L4 nerve root causes absence or diminution of the knee reflex, sensory loss in the anterior thigh and lateral leg, and weakness of leg extension. Sciatic stretch by straight leg-raising may be positive. The femoral stretch, which is assessed by passively moving the leg posteriorly, may also be positive.

Higher disc herniations affecting the upper lumbar roots have no associated reflex changes. Sensory and motor changes are those appropriate for the roots involved. Femoral stretch will be positive, but straight leg-raising will be negative.

Far lateral disc herniations may have a special characteristic. Because the dorsal root ganglion is affected, the pain is perceived as burning and particularly unpleasant. Such a sign is suggestive only.

Most acute disc herniations relent with time and do not require surgery. Indications for urgent operation are intractable pain that cannot be relieved with reasonable analgesics; a lower extremity neurological loss that would be undesirable if permanent; and significant change in bowel, bladder or sexual function. Otherwise, most patients can be treated expectantly with adequate analgesia, bed rest, and then restriction of activities until recovery occurs. Most patients begin to improve within a few days and many show signs of recovery within the first week. Substantial improvement is probable within the first month. Most patients recover completely within 3 months. In the acute situation, imaging studies are not required immediately unless pain or neurological deficits are severe. If a patient fails to follow the expected course of spontaneous improvement, MRI is the imaging study of choice. Surgical therapy should proceed when it is clear the patient's symptoms warrant intervention and spontaneous recovery is not likely to occur. There is no evidence that interposing physical therapy, manipulation, or any form of alternative medicine will alter the natural history of the disc herniation. For many years, the standard practice has been to interpose physical therapy as a requirement for surgery. The evidence that this is beneficial is marginal (Long, 1987; Long et al., 1996).

New treatments for the herniated lumbar disc are introduced continually (Solomon et al., 1980; van Tulder et al., 1997). Intradiscal therapies have included the injection of steroids, agents that dissolve the nucleus pulposus, and sclerosing agents to strengthen ligaments. Percutaneous removal of disc material has been attempted with lasers, nucleotones, and more typical surgical instruments controlled by endoscopes. A recent addition to this percutaneous armamentarium has been the concept of intradiscal heat coagulation, which is thought to strengthen the internal structure of the disc and which some postulate may destroy sensory nociceptors. Most of these techniques come and go without being subjected to rigorous clinical trials. Because the natural history of acute back pain and sciatica is one of spontaneous improvement, it is easy for practitioners and patients to believe that the prescribed treatments have produced the observed improvement (Wheeler & Hanley, 1995).

Spinal stenosis

Another common spondylitic syndrome is spinal stenosis. The disease usually appears in patients who begin with congenitally short pedicles and then have further compromise of the central spinal canal and neural foramina by age-related spondylotic changes. The typical syndrome combines back pain with a leg pain complex known as claudication. With activity, leg pain generally worsens and a transient neurological deficit may occur. The syndrome is very similar to vascular claudication, but examination of the vascular system usually reveals no significant abnormality. Neurological findings are variable and the history is more important because the neurological abnormalities are often transient and related to exercise or position. In severe cases simply standing is enough to precipitate symptoms. Diagnosis is obvious on MRI. In severely incapacitated patients, surgical decompression with restoration of an adequate canal and/or foraminal capacity is, typically, highly efficacious (Long & Watts, 1996).

Spinal instability

There is much debate about what constitutes spinal instability. Pain associated with obvious subluxation of spinal elements with movement is well-documented (Schneiderman et al., 1995), but how to define the degree of movement required to diagnose instability is uncertain (Bogduk, 1997; Bogduk & Long, 1979, 1980). So-called glacial instability that changes perceptibly over months or years is also generally thought to be painful, but definitive supportive clinical data are lacking (Phillips & Grant, 1991b). All spinal fusions are based upon the elimination of instability or correction of biomechanical deformity (Indahl et al., 1998). Correction of significant and/or progressive scoliosis in all its forms and stabilization of obvious subluxation are well accepted. The value of fusion procedures in less obvious instability situations is less well demonstrated (Moreton, 1966).

Degenerative disc and spondylotic abnormalities without instability or root compression

Degenerative changes have been observed on imaging studies in many people. Loss of disc hydration begins in late youth to early middle age in a large percentage of the population. This so-called degenerative disc disease continues to progress to late middle age and then usually stabilizes. In some people progressive changes continue to occur. Nevertheless, many people with substantial degenerative changes have no symptoms, and many people with significant symptoms have few, if any, degenerative changes. It is generally accepted that these degenerative disc changes are causally related to pain, but the cause of the pain is unknown. Because of the poor correlation between clinical syndrome and imaging findings, a large variety of treatment modalities have been used without strong evidence of their efficacy. Therapy is usually symptomatic, of limited value, so it is not surprising that there are many treatment schemes touted to be the answer for low back pain (Moffett et al., 1999). The appearance of new explanations and new treatments has been a cyclical event.

The national low back pain study (NLBPS)

Our concepts of treatment are based on the results of an eight-centre nationwide study of patients with significant persisting back and/or leg pain, known as the NLBPS. The study began more than 10 years ago and is still ongoing. Our goal was to study those patients who were seriously incapacitated by low back pain uncomplicated by multiple interventional treatments or previous surgery. As already stated, most acute back and leg pain is self-limited and does not require significant treatment. Therefore, we identified a group of patients with pain persisting for 3 months or longer, who were referred to orthopedic or neurological surgeons for evaluation and possible surgical treatment. Complete history and a thorough physical examination, as well as imaging studies, were used to establish the diagnosis thought most likely to account for each patient's pain and functional impairment. The outcome of therapy was monitored over a 2-year period with a battery of tests that assess all the characteristics of the complaint: pain severity, function disability, psychological status, symptoms other than pain, and healthcare utilization. This was an effectiveness study that examined the value of all therapies employed, but did not allow comparisons between therapies.

The demographic make-up of the patient population proved to mimic that of the general population. Of the more than 2300 patients enrolled in the study, 1441 were prescribed conservative care, 332 were prescribed no treatment, and 331 were prescribed immediate surgical care. Another 254 patients went to surgery after failure of conservative care.

All the patients in the study were significantly disabled by their problem, such that they had been referred to an orthopedic or neurological surgeon for possible surgery. Over 80% had a final diagnosis implicating spondylotic disease as the cause of their symptoms, and 60% had a diagnosis of nerve root compression syndrome. Nevertheless, only 25% of the entire study population were selected for surgery.

Instability was infrequently diagnosed, occurring in only 10% of the patients. It was surprising to discover that the physical examination was irrelevant to the diagnosis. The history was the most important diagnostic determinant, and as expected, sciatica was the predominant symptom leading to surgery. The only physical finding consistently predictive of nerve root compression was a positive straight leg-raising test. Most patients had no neurological abnormalities. Reflex, motor, or sensory changes occurred in about one third of the patients, and the classic triad taught to be diagnostic of lumbar disc disease was observed in less than 1% of patients. Whereas significant neurological deficits are certainly indications for surgery, we found such cases to be rare even in patients with significant disc protrusion (Long et al., 1996).

The patients' psychological profile was consistent with that of a typical ill patient population. There was no evidence for psychopathology in the genesis of the complaint of low back pain (BenDebba et al., 1997; Phillips Grant, 1991a).

The first important finding from the follow-up studies was that there was no significant spontaneous improvement with time. The entire cohort was followed for 2 years and a subset was followed for 5 years. Spontaneous improvement was observed in neither. Thus, we believe we have identified a group of patients who comprise a consistent syndrome. These are patients who do not improve spontaneously; but usually have episodic pain for years. We have referred to them as persistent back pain patients to differentiate them from acute and chronic low back pain patients. No conservative care modality, whether recommended by the study physicians, other physicians, or chosen independently by patients, had any significant effect on the complaint of back pain and sciatica. Since none were of significant value, there is little evidence to suggest that using any of the so-called conservative care measures could prevent surgery (Long et al., 1996).

It is important not to misunderstand these statements. They apply only to persistent back pain patients. Most patients with acute low back pain and sciatica, even with demonstrated disc herniation, will improve spontaneously with no more than symptomatic treatment (Bigos et al., 1994). Surgery is rarely required, unless pain is intolerable or a significant neurological deficit is present. Our data indicate that when spontaneous recovery does not occur, it is unlikely that any of the conservative care measures will change the natural history of the disease, or give the patient symptomatic relief. This is a radical departure from the usual treatment approach and will require long-term validation.

The outcome of surgery was quite different and very satisfactory. However, the experts in spinal surgery involved in our study chose only a small number of the referred patients for surgical treatment. The most common indication for surgery was unrelieved radicular pain (BenDebba et al., 2000). For most patients, the severity of pain led to the surgical decision, and most of the surgeries were complex procedures. The goal was to relieve nerve root compression, and/or eliminate instability. Twenty per cent of the surgically treated patients has a fusion.

Outcomes for the surgically treated patients were excellent, with over 90% of patients being satisfactorily relieved of pain without mortality and without significant morbidity. Only 2% of patients were unchanged or worse, and only 5% required reoperation. These outcomes persisted throughout the follow-up period. Thus, it appears that patients with sciatica secondary to disc herniation, spinal stenosis, or spondylolisthesis, whose pain is severe enough to warrant surgery, can be predictably relieved with little or no risk. Nevertheless, these patients constitute a small minority, even among those who are referred to orthopedic and neurological surgeons who are knowledgeable about spinal problems (Long et al., 1996).

Diagnostic blocks in decision-making in low back pain

Diagnostic blockade is widely used in patients with low back and leg pain as an adjunct in the decision-making process (Bogduk & Long, 1979, 1980). The rationale is sound, but clinical correlations are as tenuous as those between radiological findings and clinical syndromes. The concept is that if a specific structure in the spine is anesthetized with a local anesthetic, the pain originating in or mediated by that structure should be relieved. In an effort to make the blocks more helpful, a second parameter, the provocation of the patient's own pain syndrome, has been added to the interpretation. Thus, with provocative diagnostic blockade, the patient is queried about the reproduction of their usual pain syndrome during needle placement and during injection. Relief of pain is assessed after injection. The most significant block is the one that both provokes and relieves pain. Blocks in common usage include lumbar zygapophyseal joints, individual nerve roots, and intradiscal blocks. Although these applications are rational and intuitively correct, there are two problems with their utilization: first, selectivity and specificity are weak; second, clinical correlations between the results of blocks and treatment outcomes are lacking. Bogduk has studied specificity and selectivity of cervical blocks in great detail. The most reliable blocks include placebo controls. Uncontrolled blocks, and blocks of adjacent nerves or major nerve trunks made up of overlapping root origins are less specific. Currently, in our clinic, provocative blocks are used as adjuncts to strengthen clinical decisions already made on other grounds. They are never used alone to guide surgery. Much more data will be required before these provocative blocks can be considered more than adjunctive in the diagnostic and decision-making process.

Impairment, disability, litigation, and the compensation process

The problem of low back pain in the United States and in most developed nations is complicated by its intimate relationship with disability and litigation (Bigos et al., 1991; Frank et al., 1998; Mayer et al., 1987; Scheer et al., 1995). The impairment guides of The American Medical Association are used 94% of the time for the spine. It is clear to most experts that patients involved in litigation and disability claims do not recover as well as those without such claims. In our own national low back pain study, all patients employed at the time of surgery returned to work at the same job without restrictions; virtually none of the patients involved in disability returned to work. Those involved in litigation complained much more, used more medical resources, and were much less likely to return to work when compared with similar patients without litigation, although no significant differences between the two

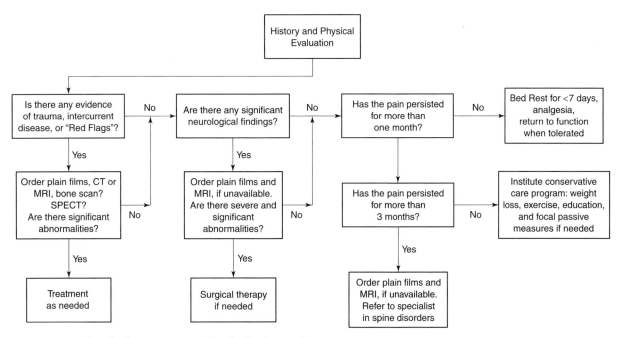

Fig. 51.1. A paradigm for the management of low back pain complaints.

groups in terms of diagnoses or therapies could be discerned. Nevertheless, physicians complicate the social issues through diagnoses and choice of treatments. The social and political issues surrounding the disability question are complex and well beyond the scope of this chapter. There is no doubt, however, that the presence of claimed disability increases complaints, leads to greater medical utilization, and greatly reduces the vocational capabilities of patients after apparently successful surgery. Patients with disability claims should not be deprived of surgical treatments for diseases known to respond well to surgery, nor should the indications for surgery be expanded for them.

A management paradigm for low back pain

Our current paradigm, illustrated in Fig. 51.1, follows the rules for management of acute low back pain with or without leg pain promulgated by the Agency for Health Policy and Research. This means no evaluation for the majority of patients acutely, but adequate symptomatic relief. Rapid return to function is important. Patients are restricted from aggressive practitioners who use any form of surgical or conservative care, and spontaneous healing is allowed to occur. When patients do not improve spontaneously within 1 month, or if symptoms remain incapacitating for more than a short period of time, evaluation

proceeds. Surgery is performed immediately for those with sufficient symptoms and clear-cut root compression or instability. There is no reason to implement any conservative care program since none will be of value. When surgery is contemplated it should proceed only after 3 months of waiting, unless symptoms preclude such a wait. The majority of patients will not be candidates for surgery. The best evidence suggests that most patients do not respond to conventional conservative programs, but can benefit by an intensive program that includes weight control, local measures for relief of muscular and ligamentous pain, and a vigorous functional exercise program that restores them to their maximum capabilities.

References

Ackerman, S.J., Steinberg, E.P., Bryan, R.N., BenDebba, M. & Long, D.M. (1997a). Patient characteristics associated with diagnostic imaging evaluation of persistent low back problems. *Spine*, **22**, 1634–40.

Ackerman, S.J., Steinberg, E.P., Bryan, R.N., BenDebba, M. & Long, D.M. (1997b). Persistent low back pain in patients suspected of having herniated nucleus pulposus: radiologic predictors of functional outcome – implications for treatment selection. *Radiology*, **203**, 815–22.

Ackerman, S.J., Steinberg, E.P., Bryan, R.N., BenDebba, M. & Long, D.M. (1997c). Trends in diagnostic imaging for low back pain: has MR imaging been a substitute or add-on? *Radiology*, **203**, 533–8.

American Academy of Orthopaedic Surgeons (1995). Evidence-based recommendations for patients with acute activity intolerance due to low back symptoms. *Orthop. Update*, **5**, 625–32.

American Academy of Orthopaedic Surgeons and North American Spine Society (1996). *Draft Clinical Algorithm on Low Back Pain.*

Anderson, G.B.J., Lucente, T., Davis, A.M., Kappler, R.E., Lipton, J.A. & Leurgans, S. (1999). A comparison of osteopathic spinal manipulation with standard care for patients with low back pain. *N. Engl. J. Med.*, **341**, 1426–31.

BenDebba, M., Torgerson, W.S. & Long, D.M. (1997). Personality traits, pain duration and severity, functional impairment, and psychological distress in patients with persistent low back pain. *Pain*, **72**, 115–25.

BenDebba, M., Torgerson, W.S. & Long, D.M. (2000). A validated, practical classification procedure for many persistent low back pain patients. *Pain*, **87**, 89–97.

Bigos, S.J., Battie, M.C., Spengler, D.M. et al. (1991). A prospective study of work perceptions and psychosocial factors affecting the report of back injury. *Spine*, **16**, 1–6.

Bigos, S.J. et al. (1994). *Acute Low Back Pain Problems in Adults. Clinical Practice Guidelines*, **Quick Reference Guide Number 14**. Rockville, MD: US Department of Health and Human Services, Public Health Service, Agency for Health Care Policy and Research.

Bogduk, N. (1997). *Clinical Anatomy of the Lumbar Spine and Sacrum.*, 3rd edn. Edinburgh: Churchill Livingstone.

Bogduk, N. & Long, D.M. (1979). Anatomy of the so-called articular nerves and their relationship to facet denervation in the treatment of low back pain. *J. Neurosurg.*, **51**, 172–7.

Bogduk, N. & Long, D.M. (1980). Percutaneous lumbar medial branch neurotomy. A modification of facet denervation. *Spine*, **5**, 193–200.

Carey, T.S., Garrett, J., Jackman, A., McLaughlin, C., Fryer, J. & Smucker, D.R. (1995). The outcomes and costs of care for acute low back pain among patients seen by primary care practitioners, chiropractors, and orthopaedic surgeons. *N. Engl. J. Med.*, **333**, 913–17.

Cherkin, D.C., Deyo, R.A., Street, J. & Barlow, W. (1996a). Predicting poor outcomes for back pain seen in primary care using patients' own criteria. *Spine*, **21**, 1900–7.

Cherkin, D.C., Deyo, R.A., Street, J.H., Hunt, M. & Barlow, W. (1996b). Pitfalls of patient education. Limited success of a program for back pain in primary care. *Spine*, **21**, 345–55.

Cherkin, D.C., Deyo, R.A., Battie, M., Street, J. & Barlow, W. (1998). A comparison of physical therapy, chiropractic manipulation, and provision of an educational booklet for the treatment of patients with low back pain. *N. Engl. J. Med.*, **339**, 1021–9.

Deyo, R.A. (1996). Drug therapy for back pain. Which drugs help which patients? *Spine*, **21**, 2840–50.

Deyo, R.A. & Tsui-Wu, Y.J. (1987). Descriptive epidemiology of low-back pain and its related medical care in the United States. *Spine*, **12**, 264–8.

Deyo, R.A., Rainville, J., & Kend, D.L. (1992). What can the history and physical examination tell us about low back pain? *J. Am. Med. Assoc.*, **268**, 760–5.

Dreyfuss, P., Michaelsen, M., Pauza, K., McLarty, J. & Bogduk, N. (1996). The value of history and physical examination in diagnosing sacroiliac joint pain. *Spine*, **21**, 2594–602.

Fordyce, W.E., Brockway, J.A., Bergman, J.A. & Spengler, D. (1986). Acute back pain: a control-group comparison of behavioural vs. traditional management methods. *J. Behav. Medi.*, **9**, 127–40.

Forssell, M.Z. (1981). The back school. *Spine*, **6**, 104–6.

Frank, J., Sinclair, S., Hogg-Johnson, S. et al. (1998). Preventing disability from work-related low-back pain – new evidence gives new hope – if we can just get all the players onside. *Can. Med. Assoc. J.*, **158**, 1625–31.

Fredrickson, B.E., Baker, D., McHolick, W.J., Yuan, H.A & Lubicky, J.P. (1984). The natural history of spondylolysis and spondylolisthesis. *J. Bone Joint Surg.-Amer. Vol.*, **66A**, 699–707.

Frymoyer, J.W. & Cats-Baril, W. (1987). Predictors of low back pain disability. *Clin. Orthop. Rel. Res.*, 89–98.

Fullenlove, T.M. & Williams, A.J. (1957). Comparative roentgen findings in symptomatic and asymptomatic backs. *Radiology*, **68**, 572–4.

Hirschberg, G.G., Froetscher, L. & Naeim, F. (1979). Iliolumbar syndrome as a common cause of low back pain: diagnosis and prognosis. *Arch. Phys. Med. Rehabil.*, **60**, 415–19.

Indahl, A., Velund, L. & Reikeraas, O. (1995). Good prognosis for low back pain when left untampered: a randomized clinical trial. *Spine*, **20**, 473–7.

Indahl, A., Haldorsen, E.H., Holm, S., Reikeras, O. & Ursin, H. (1998). Five-year follow-up study of a controlled clinical trial using light mobilization and an informative approach to low back pain. *Spine*, **23**, 2625–30.

Ingpen, M.L. & Burry, H.C. (1970). A lumbo-sacral strain syndrome. *Ann. Phys. Med.*, **10**, 270–4.

Jackson, C.P. & Brown, M.D. (1983). Is there a role for exercise in the treatment of patients with low back pain? *Clin. Orthop. Rel. Res.*, 39–45.

Johnson, E.W. (1989). The myth of skeletal muscle spasm. *Am. J. Phys. Med. Rehabil.*, **68**, 1–1.

Koes, B.W. & van den Hoogen, H.J.M. (1994). Efficacy of bed rest and orthoses of low-back pain. A review of randomized clinical trials. *Eur. J. Phys. Med. Rehabil.*, **4**, 86–93.

Koes, B.W., Assendelft, W.J.J., van der Heijden, G.J.M.G., Bouter, L.M. & Knipschild, P.G. (1991a). Spinal manipulation and mobilization for back and neck pain: a blinded review. *Br. Med. J.*, **303**, 1298–303.

Koes, B.W., Bouter, L.M., Beckerman, H., van der Heijden, G.J.M.G. & Knipschild, P.G. (1991b). Physiotherapy exercise and back pain: a blinded review. *Br. Med. J.*, **302**, 1572–6.

Koes, B.W., Van Tulder, M.W., van der Windt, D.A.W.M. & Bouter, L.M. (1994). The efficacy of back schools – a review of randomized clinical trials. *J. Clin. Epidemiol.*, **47**, 851–62.

Liang, M. & Komaroff, A.L. (1982). Roentgenograms in primary care patients with acute low-back-pain – a cost-effectiveness analysis. *Arch. Intern. Med.*, **142**, 1108–12.

Lindstrom, I., Ohlund, C., Eek, C., Wallin, L., Peterson, L.E. &

Nachemson, A. (1992). Mobility, strength, and fitness after a graded activity program for patients with subacute low-back-pain – a randomized prospective clinical-study with a behavioral-therapy approach. *Spine*, **17**, 641–52.

Lindstrom, I., Ohlund, C. & Nachemson, A. (1995). Physical performance, pain, pain behavior and subjective disability in patients with subacute low-back-pain. *Scand. J. Rehabil. Med.*, **27**, 153–60.

Linton, S.J. & Kamwendo, K. (1987). Low-back-pain schools – a critical review. *Phys. Ther.*, **67**, 1375–83.

Loisel, P., Abenhaim, L., Durand, P.E.J.M. et al. (1997). A population-based, randomized clinical trial on back pain management. *Spine*, 2911–18.

Long, D.M. (1978). Functional neurosurgery. In *Metabolic Surgery, Modern Surgical Monographs*, ed. H. Buchwald & R.L.Varco, pp. 229–54, New York, NY: Grune & Stratton Publishers.

Long, D.M. (1985). Low back pain and sciatica. In *Current Therapy in Neurologic Disease 1985–1986*, ed. R.T. Johnson, pp. 69–72, Philadelphia, PA: B.C. Decker.

Long, D.M. (1987). Laminotomy for lumbar disc disease. In *Lumbar Discectomy and Laminectomy Principles and Techniques in Spine Surgery*, ed. R.G.Watkins & J.S.Collis, Jr., pp. 173–7, Rockville: Aspen Publisher.

Long, D.M. (1989). Nonsurgical therapy for low back pain and sciatica. *Clin. Neurosurg.*, **35**, 351–9.

Long, D.M. (1991a). Failed back surgery syndrome. In *Neurosurgery Clinics of North America*, Vol. 2, ed. H.R. Winn, M.R. Mayberg & J.D. Loeser, pp. 899–919, Philadelphia, PA: Saunders.

Long, D.M. (1991b). Fifteen years of transcutaneous electrical stimulation for pain control. *Stereotactic Funct. Neurosurg.*, **56**, 2–19.

Long, D.M. (1992). Chronic adhesive spinal arachnoiditis: pathogenesis prognosis and treatment. *Neurosurg. Quart.*, **2**, 296–319.

Long, D.M. & Watts, C. (1996). Lessons from recent national back pain projects. In *Current Techniques in Neurosurgery*, ed. M. Saloman, 2nd edn, pp. 171–82, Philadelphia, PA: Current Medicine.

Long, D.M. & Zeidman, S.M. (1994). Outcome of low back pain therapy. In *Perspectives in Neurological Surgery*, Vol. 5, ed. M.N. Handley, pp. 41–51, Lt. Louis, MI: Quality Medical Publishing.

Long, D.M., Campbell, J.N. & Gucer, G. (1979). Transcutaneous electrical stimulation for relief of chronic pain. In *Advances in Pain Research and Therapy*, Vol. 3, ed. J.J. Bonica, pp. 593–9, New York: Raven Press.

Long, D.M., Erickson, D., Campbell, J. & North, R. (1981). Electrical stimulation of the spinal cord and peripheral nerves for pain control. A 10-year experience. *Appl. Neurophysiol.*, **44**, 207–17.

Long, D.M., Filtzer, D.L., BenDebba, M. & Hendler, N.H. (1988). Clinical features of the failed-back syndrome. *J. Neurosurg.*, **69**, 61–71.

Long, D.M., BenDebba, M., Torgerson, W.S. et al. (1996). Persistent back pain and sciatica in the United States: patient characteristics. *J. Spinal Disord.*, **9**, 40–58.

Magora, A. & Schwartz, A. (1976). Relation between the low back pain syndrome and X-ray findings. *Scandinavian Journal of Rehabilitation Medicine*, **8**, 115–26.

Main, C.J., Wood, P.L., Hollis, S., Spanswick, C.C. & Waddell, G. (1992). The distress and risk assessment method: a simple patient classification to identify distress and evaluate the risk of poor outcome. *Spine*, **17**, 42–52.

Mayer, T.G., Gatchel, R.J., Mayer, H., Kishino, N., Keeley, J. & Mooney, V. (1987). A prospective two-year study of functional restoration in industrial low back injury. *J. Am. Med. Assoc.*, **258**, 1763–7.

Merskey, H. & Bogduk, N. (1994). *Classification of Chronic Pain: Descriptions of Chronic Pain Syndromes and Definitions of Pain Terms*, 2nd edn. Seattle: IASP Press.

Moffett, J.K., Torgerson, D., Bell-Syer, S. et al. (1999). Randomized controlled trial of exercise for low back pain: clinical outcomes, costs, and preferences. *Bri. Med. J.*, **319**, 279–83.

Mooney, V. (1987). When is the pain coming from? *Spine*, **12**, 754–9.

Mooney, V. & Robertson, J.T. (1976). The facet syndrome. *Clin. Orthop.*, **115**, 149–56.

Moreton, R.D. (1966). Spondylolysis. *J. Am. Med. Assoc.*, **195**, 671–4.

Morley, S., Eccleston, C. & Williams, A. (1999). Systematic review and meta-analysis of randomized controlled trials of cognitive behaviour therapy and behaviour therapy for chronic pain in adults, excluding headache. *Pain*, **80**, 1–13.

Phillips, H.C. & Grant, L. (1991a). Acute back pain: a psychological analysis. *Behav. Res. Ther.*, **29**, 429–34.

Phillips, H.C. & Grant, L. (1991b). The evolution of chronic back pain problems: a longitudinal study. *Behav. Res. Ther.*, 435–41.

Scavone, J.G., Latshaw, R.F. & Weidner, W.A. (1981). Anteroposterior and lateral radiographs: an adequate lumbar spine examination. *Am. J. Roentgenol.*, **136**, 715–17.

Scheer, S.J., Radack, K.L. & O'Brien, D.R., Jr. (1995). Randomized controlled trials in industrial low back pain relating to return to work. Part 1. Acute interventions. *Arch. Phys. Med. Rehabil.*, **76**, 966–73.

Schneiderman, G.A., McLain, R.F., Hambly, M.F. & Nielsen, S.L. (1995). The pars defect as a pain source. A histologic study. *Spine*, **20**, 1761–4.

Smyth, M.J. & Wright, V. (1959). Sciatica and the intervertebral disc. An experimental study. *J. Bone Joint Surg.*, 1401–18.

Solomon, R.A., Viernstein, M.C. & Long, D.M. (1980). Reduction of postoperative pain and narcotic use by transcutaneous electrical nerve stimulation. *Surgery*, **87**, 142–6.

Sonne, M., Christensen, K., Hansen, S.E. & Jensen, E.M. (1985). Injection of steroids and local anesthetics as therapy for low-back pain. *Scand. J. Rheumatol.*, **14**, 343–5.

Splinthoff, C.A. (1953). Lumbosacral junction: roentgenographic comparison of patients with and without backaches. *J. Am. Med. Assoc.*, 1610–13.

Turner, J.A. (1996). Educational and behavioral interventions for back pain in primary care. *Spine*, **21**, 2851–7.

van den Hoogen, H.J.M., Koes, B.W., van Eijk, J.T.M., Bouter, L.M. & Deville, W. (1998). On the course of low back pain in general practice: a one year follow up study. *Ann. Rheum. Dis.*, **57**, 13–19.

van Tulder, M.W., Koes, B.W. & Bouter, L.M. (1997). Conservative treatment of acute and chronic nonspecific low back pain. A systematic review of randomized controlled trials of the most common interventions. *Spine*, **22**, 2128–56.

von Korff, M. (1994). Studying the natural history of back pain. *Spine*, **19**, 2041S–6S.

Waddell, G., Main, C.J., Morris, E.W., Dipaola, M. & Gray, I.C.M. (1984). Chronic low back pain, psychological distress, and illness behavior. *Spine*, **9**, 209–13.

Waldvogel, F.A. & Vasey, H. (1980). Osteomyelitis – the past decade. *N. Engl. J. Med.*, **303**, 360–70.

Wheeler, A.H. & Hanley, E.N. (1995). Spine update nonoperative treatment for low-back-pain – rest to restoration. *Spine*, **20**, 375–8.

Zeidman, S.M. & Long, D.M. (1996). Failed back surgery syndrome. In *Principles of Spinal Surgery*, ed. A.H. Menezes & V.K.H. Sonntag, pp. 657–79, New York, NY: McGraw-Hill Publishers.

Part VI

Disorders of body functions

52

Autonomic function and dysfunction

Christopher J. Mathias

Neurovascular Medicine Unit, Division of Neuroscience and Psychological Medicine
Imperial College of Science, Technology & Medicine at St Mary's, and Autonomic Unit, National Hospital for Neurology and Neurosurgery, Queen Square/
University Department of Clinical Neurology, Institute of Neurology, University College London, London, UK

The autonomic nervous system is a dynamic system intimately involved with the function of every organ in the body. In addition, it plays a key role in integrative function, such as control of the circulation and regulation of body temperature. Its motor (efferent) components, consist of the parasympathetic nervous system with a cranial and sacral spinal outflow, and the sympathetic nervous system with a thoraco-lumbar spinal outflow (Fig. 52.1). However, there is interaction at various levels of the neural axis. Thus, virtually every afferent in the body, through relays at a cerebral or spinal level, influences function of the autonomic nervous system. Centres in the brain can activate autonomic pathways directly or by stimulating spinal autonomic centres. There are multiple neurotransmitters at different synapses and ganglia that are better defined in the periphery than centrally (Fig. 52.2). Complex processes at parasympathetic and sympathetic nerve terminals influence the synthesis, release and re-uptake of various transmitters (Figs 52.3 and 52.4). The autonomic supply to the gut and pelvic viscera (enteric nervous system) additionally is richly endowed with peptides, amines and purines involved in neurotransmission and neuromodulation; they also have direct effects, especially upon the gastrointestinal tract and splanchnic circulation.

Classification of autonomic disorders

An outline classification is provided (Table 52.1). There are primary disorders where the etiology is not known; examples are pure autonomic failure (PAF) and multiple system atrophy (MSA). A large number of secondary autonomic disorders may be hereditary, associated with disease (such as diabetes mellitus), due to a specific deficit (dopamine beta-hydroxylase deficiency) or the result of trauma. A variety of drugs, poisons and toxins cause autonomic dys-

function by directly influencing sympathetic or parasympathetic activity, or by causing an autonomic neuropathy. In neurally mediated syncope, autonomic function is intermittently abnormal with either overactivity (such as increased vagal tone causing bradycardia) or underactivity (sympathetic withdrawal causing hypotension); the most common is vasovagal syncope. A recently described disorder is postural tachycardia syndrome (PoTS).

In many of these autonomic disorders there is involvement of different organs or systems. Some are localized, predominantly affecting one organ, area or system, such as the pupil in the Holmes–Adie syndrome, the face in Horner's syndrome and sweat glands in essential hyperhidrosis.

Clinical manifestations

Characteristic features follow dysfunction affecting the sympathetic and parasympathetic nervous systems. Sympathetic adrenergic failure results in orthostatic (postural) hypotension and ejaculatory failure, while sympathetic cholinergic failure causes anhidrosis. The reverse, sympathetic overactivity, may result in hypertension, tachycardia and hyperhidrosis. Parasympathetic failure causes a fixed heart rate, an atonic urinary bladder, a sluggish large bowel and erectile failure; overactivity can result in bradycardia and even cardiac arrest. Thus, a wide spectrum of manifestations can occur in autonomic dysfunction (Table 52.2), with various combinations depending upon the extent of the lesion, the associated disorder and the ensuing functional deficit. In disorders such as multiple system atrophy, there may be difficulties in diagnosis, as non-automic disorders may result in similar symptoms.

In the Riley–Day syndrome (familial dysautonomia), there usually is a history of consanguinity and an Ashkenazi

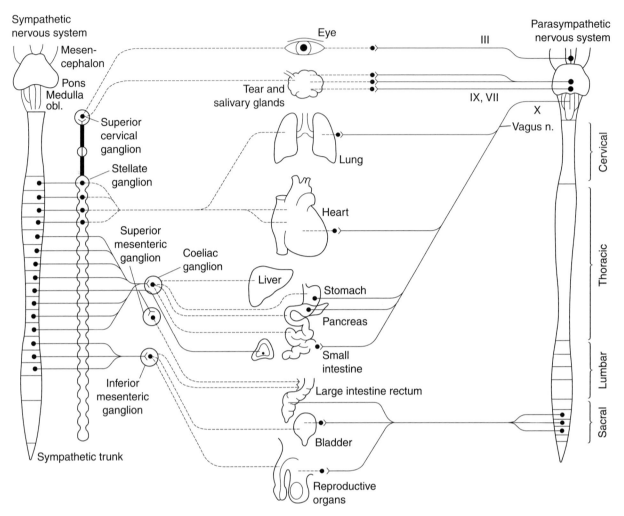

Fig. 52.1. Parasympathetic and sympathetic innervation of major organs. (From Janig, 1987.)

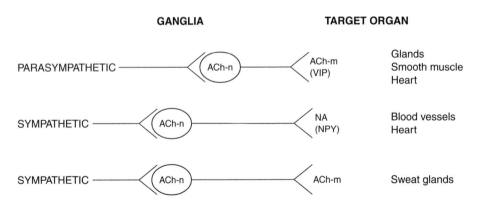

Fig. 52.2. Outline of the major transmitters at autonomic ganglia and postganglionic sites on target organs supplied by the sympathetic and parasympathetic efferent pathways. The acetylcholine receptor at all ganglia is of the nicotinic subtype (ACh-n). Ganglionic blockers such as hexamethonium thus prevent both parasympathetic and sympathetic activation. Atropine, however, acts only on the muscarinic (ACH-m) receptor at postganglionic parasympathetic and sympathetic cholinergic sites. The cotransmitters along with the primary transmitters are also indicated (NA = noradrenaline; VIP = vasoactive intestinal polypeptide; NPY = neuropeptide Y). (From Mathias, 2000a.)

Table 52.1. Outline classification of autonomic disorders

Primary
  Acute/subacute autonomic neuropathy
  Chronic autonomic failure
    – pure autonomic failure
    – multiple system atrophy

Secondary
  Hereditary
    – Riley–Day syndrome
    – familial amyloid polyneuropathy
  Metabolic
    – diabetes mellitus
  Enzyme deficiency
    – dopamine beta-hydroxylase deficiency
  Inflammatory
    – Guillain–Barré syndrome
  Infectious
    – Chagas disease
  Trauma
    – spinal cord transection

Drugs, poisons and toxins
  Direct effects
  Autonomic neuropathy
    – alcohol

Neurally-mediated syncope
  Vasovagal syncope
  Carotid sinus hypersensitivity
  Miscellaneous causes
    – micturition syncope

Postural tachycardia syndrome

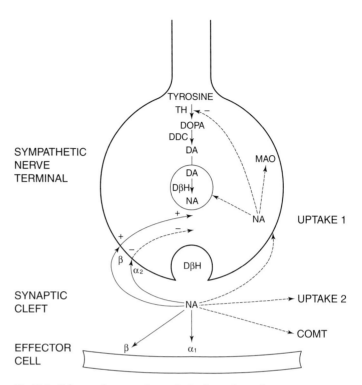

Fig. 52.3. Schema of some pathways in the formation, release and metabolism of noradrenaline from sympathetic nerve terminals. Tyrosine is converted into dihydroxyphenylalanine (DOPA) by tyrosine hydroxylase (TH). DOPA is converted into dopamine (DA) by dopadecarboxylase. In the vesicles DA is converted into noradrenaline (NA) by dopamine beta-hydroxylase (DβH). Nerve impulses release both DβH and NA into the synaptic cleft by exocytosis. NA acts predominantly on alpha$_1$-adrenoceptors but has actions on beta-adrenoceptors on the effector cell of target organs. It also has presynaptic adrenoceptor effects. Those acting on alpha$_2$ adrenoceptors inhibit NA release; those on beta-adrenoceptors stimulate NA release. NA may be taken up by a neuronal (uptake 1) process into the cytosol, where it may inhibit further formation of DOPA through the rate-limiting enzyme TH. NA may be taken into vesicles or metabolized by monoamine oxidase (MAO) in the mitochondria. NA may be taken up by a higher capacity but lower affinity extraneuronal process (uptake 2) in peripheral tissues, such as vascular and cardiac muscle and certain glands. NA is also metabolized by catechol-o-methyl transferase (COMT). NA measured in plasma is the overspill not affected by these numerous processes. (From Mathias, 2000a.)

Jewish origin; the disorder often is recognized at birth. Vasovagal syncope presents commonly in the teenage years, while familial amyloid polyneuropathy begins in early adulthood and middle age. Neurodegenerative disorders such as multiple system atrophy present in the mid- to late 50s. There may be a gender preponderance; vasovagal syncope is more common in females. A detailed history is essential and must include drug medication intake and previous exposure to chemical substances.

In secondary autonomic disorders and those caused by drugs, the features of the underlying or associated disorder need consideration as these may exacerbate autonomic manifestations. Individual assessments are necessary, especially of psyche, in conditions such as vasovagal syncope, also know as emotional syncope.

The clinical findings may be confined to an area, organ or involve a system. In essential hyperhidrosis only the palms and soles may be affected, while in the Holmer – Adie pupil there is impairment of parasympathetic function of the iris musculature. In generalized disorders a cardinal feature is orthostatic (postural) hypotension (Fig. 52.5). This is defined as a decrease in systolic blood pressure of more than 20 mm Hg, or a fall in diastolic blood pressure of more than 10 mm Hg, while either standing or during head-up tilt to 60° for at least 3 minutes (Schatz et al., 1996). A variety of

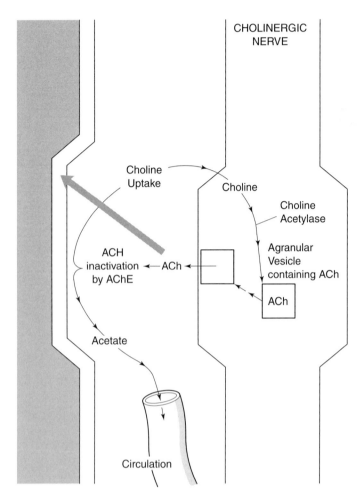

CHOLINERGIC
NERVE

Choline
Uptake

Choline

Choline
Acetylase

ACH
inactivation ← ACh
by AChE

Agranular
Vesicle
containing ACh

ACh

Acetate

Circulation

Fig. 52.4. Schema of pathway in the formation of acetylcholine (AChL) from choline and its inactivation by acetylcholine esterases (from Appenzeller & Oribe, 1997).

Table 52.2. Some clinical manifestations of autonomic dysfunction

Cardiovascular	
Postural hypotension	Supine hypertension
Lability of blood pressure	Paroxysmal hypertension
Tachycardia	Bradycardia
Sudomotor	
Hypohidrosis or anhidrosis	Hyperhidrosis
Gustatory sweating	
Hyperpyrexia	Heat intolerance
Alimentary	
Xerostomia	Dysphagia
Gastroparesis	Dumping syndrome
Constipation	Diarrhea
Urinary	
Nocturia	Frequency
Urgency	
Retention	Incontinence
Sexual	
Erectile failure	Ejaculatory failure
Retrograde ejaculation	
Eye	
Pupillary abnormalities	Partial ptosis
Alacrima	Lachrymation with food ingestion

symptoms accompany the fall in blood pressure (Mathias et al., 1999) (Table 52.3). These depend upon the rapidity and degree of fall in blood pressure, the extent to which compensatory factors come into play and the underlying disorder; additionally many factors influence orthostatic hypotension (Table 52.4). These range from stimuli in daily life such as food ingestion and mild exercise (Figs. 52.6 and 52.7) that can accentuate or exaggerate orthostatic hypotension. Determination of the mechanisms contributing to orthostatic hypotension is of importance in management.

Investigation of autonomic function and dysfunction

Activity may be measured directly or indirectly; sympathetic neural activity is measured electrophysiologically

(using microneurography) or biochemically (by measuring plasma levels of noradrenaline and adrenaline or using spillover techniques) (Wallin et al., 1996). Each has its limitations, especially as measurements in a particular territory may not reflect activity either in the whole body or in other regions. In clinical practice, functional effects are measured with investigation directed to systems and organs (Mathias & Bannister, 1999a, b) (Table 52.5). Screening tests have been developed for evaluating cardiovascular autonomic function. They utilize safe and mainly non-invasive techniques and in combination with the clinical history and examination determine if further or detailed investigation is needed. The main objectives of investigation are:
(i)   to assess if autonomic function is normal or abnormal;
(ii) if the latter, to ascertain the degree of autonomic dysfunction with an emphasis on the site of lesion and functional deficit;
(iii) to determine the underlying or associated disease as this will need concurrent treatment with management of autonomic dysfunction.
Non-autonomic tests may be needed to diagnose or delineate the underlying disorder. These include MRI scans of

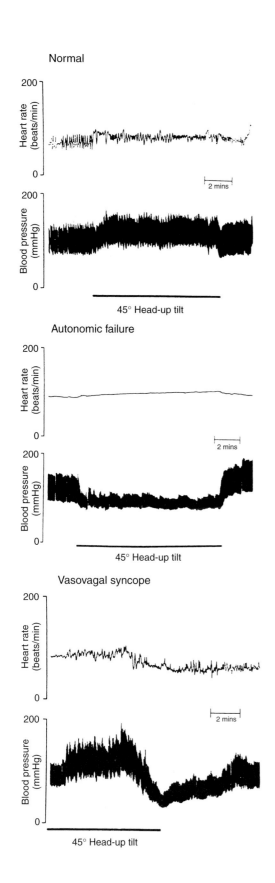

Table 52.3. Some of the various symptoms resulting from orthostatic hypotension and impaired perfusion of various organs

---

Cerebral hypoperfusion
- Dizziness
- Visual disturbances
  - Blurred
  - Tunnel
  - Scotoma
  - Greying out
  - Blacking out
  - Colour defects
- Loss of consciousness
- Impaired cognition

Muscle hypoperfusion
- Paracervical and suboccipital ('coathanger') ache
- Lower back/buttock ache
- Calf claudication

Cardiac hypoperfusion
- Angina pectoris

Spinal cord hypoperfusion

Renal hypoperfusion
- Oliguria

Non-specific
- Weakness, lethargy, fatigue
- Falls

Source: Adapted from Mathias (2000a).

Fig. 52.5. Blood pressure and heart rate before, during and after head-up tilt in a normal subject (uppermost panel), a patient with pure autonomic failure (middle panel), and a patient with vasovagal syncope (lowermost panel). In the normal subject there is no fall in blood pressure during head-up tilt, unlike the patient with autonomic failure in whom blood pressure falls promptly and remains low with a blood pressure overshoot on return to the horizontal. In the patient with autonomic failure there is only a minimal change in heart rate despite the marked blood pressure fall. In the patient with vazovagal syncope there was initially no fall in blood pressure during head-up tilt; in the latter part of tilt, as indicated inthe record, blood pressure initially rose and then markedly fell, to extremely low levels, so that the patient had to be returned to the horizontal. Heart rate also fell. In each case continuous blood pressure and heart rate were recorded with the Portapress II. (From Mathias & Bannister, 1999a).

Table 52.4. *Factors influencing postural (orthostatic) hypotension*

Speed of positional change

Time of day (worse in the morning)

Prolonged recumbency

Warm environment (hot weather, central heating, hot bath)

Raising intrathoracic pressure – micturition, defecation or coughing

Food and alcohol ingestion

Water ingestion[a]

Physical exertion

Manoeuvres and positions[b] (bending forward, abdominal compression, leg crossing, squatting, activating calf muscle pump)

Drugs with vasoactive properties (including dopaminergic agents)

Notes:

[a] May raise blood pressure, unlike food and alcohol.

[b] Usually reduce the postural fall in blood pressure.

Source: Adapted from Mathias and Bannister (1999).

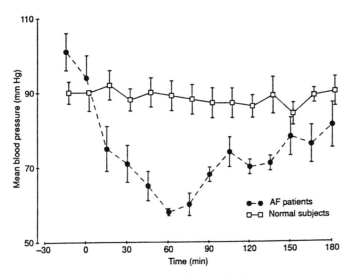

Fig. 52.6. Percentage change in mean blood pressure in a group of patients with chronic autonomic failure (dashed line, filled circles) and normal subjects (continuous line, open square) before and after food ingestion at time 0. The indicate mean ± SEM. (From Mathias et al., 1989.)

Table 52.5. *Outline of investigations in autonomic failure*

Cardiovascular	
Physiological	Head-up tilt (45°)[a]; standing[a]; Valsalva[a] manoeuvre[a]
	Pressor stimuli – isometric exercise[a], cold pressor[a], mental arithmetic[a]
	Heart rate responses – deep breathing[a], hyperventilation[a], standing[a], head-up tilt[a], 30: 15 ratio
	Liquid meal challenge
	Exercise testing
	Carotid sinus massage
Biochemical	Plasma noradrenaline – supine and head-up tilt or standing; urinary catecholamines; plasma renin activity and aldosterone
Pharmacological	Noradrenaline – α-adrenoceptors – vascular
	Isoprenaline – β-adrenoceptors – vascular and cardiac
	Tyramine – pressor and noradrenaline response
	Edrophonium – noradrenaline response
	Atropine – parasympathetic cardiac blockade
Sudomotor	Central regulation – thermoregulatory sweat test
	Sweat gland response – intradermal acetylcholine, quantitative sudomotor axon reflex test (Q-SART), localized sweat test
	Sympathetic skin response
Gastrointestinal	Barium studies, video-cine-fluoroscopy, endoscopy, gastric emptying studies
Renal function and urinary tract	Day and night urine volumes and sodium/potassium excretion
	Urodynamic studies, intravenous urography, ultrasound examination, sphincter electromyography
Sexual function	Penile plethysmography
	Intracavernosal papaverine
Respiratory	Laryngoscopy
	Sleep studies to assess apnea/oxygen desaturation
Eye	Lachrymal function – Schirmer's test
	Pupil function – pharmacological and physiological

Notes:

[a] Indicates screening tests used in our Units.

Source: From Mathias and Bannister (1999a).

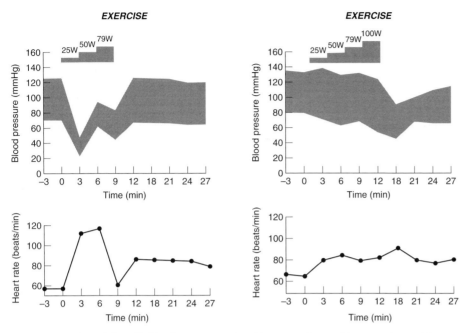

Fig. 52.7. Systolic and diastolic blood pressure (top) and heart rate (bottom) in two patients with autonomic failure before, during and after bicycle exercise performed with the patients in the supine position at different workloads, ranging from 25 to 100 watts. In the patient on the left there is a marked fall in blood pressure on initiating exercise; she had to crawl upstairs because of severe exercise induced hypotension. In the patient on the right, there are minor changes in blood pressure during exercise, but a marked decrease soon after stopping exercise. This patient was usually asymptomatic while walking, but developed postural symptoms when he stopped walking and stood still. It is likely that the decrease in blood pressure postexercise was due to vasodilatation in exercising skeletal muscle, not opposed by the calf muscle pump. (From Mathias & Williams, 1994.)

the brain in neurodegenerative disorders, sural nerve or cutaneous nerve biopsy in peripheral nerve disorders, genetic testing in familial amyloid polyneuropathies, and a range of non-neurological investigations, from HIV testing to defining the site of the primary in paraneoplastic autonomic neuropathy.

Management of autonomic disorders

A comprehensive approach is needed, especially in autonomic disorders that involve multiple systems and organs. The principles outlined for the management of orthostatic hypotension involve a combination of non-pharmacological and pharmacological measures (Table 52.6), that are based on pathophysiological mechanisms (Mathias & Kimber, 1999). In neurogenic orthostatic hypotension cure usually is not possible, and management in the individual patient should be directed to reducing disability, enabling independence and ensuring a reasonable quality of life whilst providing advice that is practical, and drugs that are safe. A similar approach

should be used for impairment of sudomotor, gastrointestinal, urinary bladder and sexual function (Table 52.7) and modified accordingly.

Surgical intervention may be needed, such as tracheostomy in MSA with laryngeal abductor paresis or insertion of a percutaneous enterogastrotomy tube for severe dysphagia. Complex procedures, such as hepatic transplantation reduce levels of variant transthyretin in familial amyloid polyneuropathy and halt deposition of amyloid in nerves, while pancreatic (usually in combination with renal) transplantation improves certain features in diabetic autonomic neuropathy. In essential hyperhidrosis there is a role for percutaneous endoscopic sympathectomy; botulism toxin has been proved useful (Naumann et al., 1997).

In addition to autonomic deficits, attention should be paid to associated features, such as depression in the parkinsonian syndromes, or anxiety and phobia in vasovagal syncope. Education of the patient is of importance as increased knowledge of the disorder and its mechanisms improves patient compliance and management. In disorders such as MSA, education of the spouse, carers and medical therapists is important.

Table 52.6. Management of orthostatic hypotension

Non-pharmacological measures
To be avoided
– Sudden head-up postural change (especially on waking)
– Prolonged recumbency
– Straining during micturition and defecation
– High environmental temperature (including hot baths)
– 'Severe' exertion
– Large meals (especially with refined carbohydrate)
– Alcohol
– Drugs with vasodepressor properties

To be introduced
– Head-up tilt during sleep
– Small, frequent meals
– High salt intake
– Judicious exercise (including swimming)
– Body positions and manoeuvres

To be considered
– Elastic stockings
– Abdominal binders
– Water ingestion

Pharmacological measures
Starter drug:
– fludrocortisone

Sympathomimetics
– ephedrine, midodrine, l-dihydroxyphenylserine

Specific Targeting
– desmopressin for nocturnal polyuria
– octreotide for postprandial hypotension
– erythopoietin for anemia

Sources: Adapted from Mathias and Kimber (1999).

Primary autonomic failure syndromes

These include the acute/sub-acute dysautonomias and chronic autonomic failure syndromes (Table 52.8).

Acute/subacute dysautonomia

These are relatively rare disorders. In pure pandysautonomia, there are features of both sympathetic and parasympathetic failure. Orthostatic hypotension often is a major problem. The peripheral nerves may be affected in pure dysautonomia with other neurological features. The prognosis in pandysautonomia is variable, with complete recovery in some. The response to immunoglobulin therapy (Heafield et al., 1996; Smit et al., 1997) suggests an immunological etiology.

Table 52.7. Outline of management strategies in autonomic failure when different systems are involved, as in MSA

Specific	for orthostatic hypotension and bladder, bowel and sexual dysfunction: non-pharmacological and pharmacological therapy for respiratory abnormalities: to consider tracheotomy for oropharyngeal dysphagia: to consider percutaneous endoscopic gastrotomy
General	for depression etc.
Education	of patient, partners, relatives, carers, practitioners (medical and supportive therapists, to include physiotherapists, occupational therapists, speech therapists, dietitians)
Patient support groups	to disseminate information and increase awareness. They include: Shy–Drager Association in USA Autonomic disorders Association Sarah Matheson Trust in UK
Integrative approaches	Autonomic nurse specialist or autonomic liaison nurse to co-ordinate and promote seamless management

Pure cholinergic dysautonomia is an even rarer condition mainly affecting children and young adults. There are symptoms of parasympathetic failure (blurred vision, dry eyes, xerostomia, dysphagia involving mainly the lower esophagus, constipation and urinary retention), and sympathetic cholinergic failure (anhidrosis and a tendency to hyperthermia). The signs include dilated pupils, raised heart rate, dry and hot skin, a distended abdomen and a palpable urinary bladder. Orthostatic hypotension is absent as sympathetic vasoconstrictor function is not impaired. Recovery from the defect is unlikely. Therapy should include maintenance of fluid balance and body temperature. A barium meal examination must be avoided as it will be retained in the colon. The differential diagnosis includes anticholinergic drugs that may cause similar features, but with recovery in a few days. A variant of botulinum (botulism B) affects cholinergic pathways alone with sparing of the motor pathways; substantial recovery often occurs within a few months.

Chronic autonomic failure syndromes

The main disorders, along with diseases with overlapping features, are schematically outlined in Fig. 52.8.

Table 52.8. Primary autonomic failure syndromes

Acute/subacute autonomic neuropathy
- Pure pandysautonomia
- Pandysautonomia with additional neurological features
- Pure cholinergic dysautonomia

Chronic autonomic failure
- Pure autonomic failure
- Multiple system atrophy
- Parkinson's disease with autonomic failure
- Diffuse Lewy Body Disease

Table 52.9. Clinical manifestations and possible presenting features of syndromes of primary chronic autonomic failure

System affected	Clinical features
Cardiovascular	Orthostatic hypotension
Sudomotor	Anhidrosis, heat intolerance
Gastrointestinal[a]	Constipation, occasionally diarrhea, dysphagia
Renal and urinary bladder	Nocturia, frequency, urgency, incontinence, retention of urine
Reproductive	Erectile and ejaculatory failure
Ocular	Anisocoria, Horner's syndrome
Respiratory[a]	Stridor, inspiratory gasps, apneic episodes
Neurologic	Parkinsonian, cerebellar and pyramidal

Notes:
[a] Certain features, such as oropharyngeal dysphagia and respiratory abnormalities (including those resulting from laryngeal-abductor paresis), occur in multiple system atrophy rather than in pure autonomic failure.
Source: From Mathias (1997).

Pure autonomic failure

These patients often are over the age of 50 at presentation. In the majority the diagnosis usually is considered when orthostatic hypotension is detected. The onset may be insidious as a number of compensatory mechanisms, often unwittingly used, help reduce the symptoms of orthostatic hypotension. Alternative diagnoses, ranging from epilepsy to a psychiatric disorder, may be considered erroneously. In males, impotence is common. Nocturia (rather than the urinary symptoms listed in Table 52.6) is frequent, along with constipation. Impairment of sweating may not be recognized in temperate climates. Heat intolerance and collapse may occur in tropical areas. The clinical and laboratory features include widespread sympathetic failure, usually with parasympathetic deficits. The physiological and biochemical tests indicate a peripheral autonomic lesion which is consistent with the neuropathological data available (Matthews, 1999). Lewy bodies have been reported in autonomic ganglia.

In PAF, management of orthostatic hypotension is of importance as it contributes to morbidity and may result in injury. Control of bowel and bladder function, and in males sexual function, may need to be addressed. The overall prognosis in PAF is good, with a life expectancy not dissimilar to healthy individuals of an equivalent age.

Multiple system atrophy

This probably is the most common neurodegenerative condition affecting the autonomic nervous system in humans. It is synonymous with the Shy–Drager syndrome and is a sporadic non-familial disorder with autonomic, parkinsonian, cerebellar and pyramidal features that occur in any combination over a varying time scale (Mathias & Williams, 1994; Wenning et al., 1994; Gilman et al., 1998) (Table 52.9). It is a progressive disorder but with an unpredictable rate of progression; this adds to difficulties in diagnosis. The majority with MSA have parkinsonian features at

some stage of the disease. When parkinsonism is a presenting feature there are difficulties in distinguishing MSA from Parkinson's disease (PD). This accounts for why up to 25% of patients diagnosed in vivo as IPD were found at postmortem to have the characteristic neuropathological features of MSA. In the early stages, depending on the presentation, patients may consult a range of specialists, from neurologists and cardiologists to urologists and psychiatrists.

There are three major subgroups in MSA based on their neurological features; the parkinsonian form (MSA-P; where the neuropathological findings include striatonigral degeneration), the cerebellar form (MSA-C; with olivopontocerebellar degeneration) and the mixed form, with a combination of neurological features (MSA-M); with striatonigral and olivopontocerebellar degeneration (Daniel, 1999). A key neuropathological feature is the presence of intracytoplasmic argyrophyllic inclusions in oligodendrocytes, within defined areas of the brain and spinal cord. Programmed cell death (apoptosis) appears to be specific for oligodendrocytes in MSA (Probst-Cousin et al., 1998). Cell loss in various brainstem nuclei (including the vagus), the intermediolateral cell mass in the thoracic and lumbar spinal cord, and Onuf's nucleus in the sacral spinal cord account for various abnormalities. The paravertebral ganglia and visceral (enteric) plexuses are not affected.

In MSA, the additional neurological features do not necessarily help distinction from overlapping syndromes. In

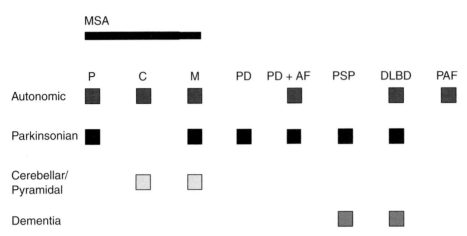

Fig. 52.8. The major clinical features in parkinsonian syndromes and allied disorders with autonomic failure. These include the three major neurologic forms of multiple system atrophy – the parkinsonian form (MSA-P, also called striatonigral degeneration), the cerebellar form (MSA-C, also olivoponocerebellar atrophy) and the multiple or mixed form (MSA-M, which has features of both other forms); idiopathic Parkinson's disease (PD), Parkinson's disease + autonomic failure (PD + AF); progressive supranuclear palsy (PSP), diffuse Lewy body disease (DLBD) and pure autonomic failure (PAF). (Adapted from Mathias, 1997.)

the parkinsonian forms, the onset of bradykinesia and rigidity is often bilateral, with minimal or no tremor, unlike PD. Lack of a motor response to dopaminergic drugs alone is not helpful, as two-thirds of MSA patients respond favourably initially, although side effects and refractoriness to the motor benefits with time lowers this to a third or less. The presence of autonomic failure (especially cardiovascular and genitourinary) in a patient with parkinsonism should alert one to the possibility of MSA. Respiratory abnormalities and oropharyngeal dysphagia favour MSA, and often occur as the disease advances.

Investigation aids diagnosis and management (Table 52.10). Neuroimaging (especially positron emission tomography, MR scanning of the brain and proton magnetic resonance spectroscopy of the basal ganglia), may help distinguish MSA from other parkinsonian syndromes. The presence of orthostatic hypotension does not necessarily indicate autonomic failure (Table 52.11), although its recording is of importance for management. Cardiac sympathetic denervation is not observed in MSA, and this is consistent with a central, preganglionic lesion. The sympathetic skin response often is abnormal in the mixed form, but up to a third of either MSA-P or MSA-C have a preserved SSR, excluding it as a diagnostic test in the early stages. The combined neuropharmacological–neuroendocrine approach using clonidine-growth hormone (GH) testing separates central from peripheral autonomic failure (Thomaides et al., 1992). The centrally acting alpha-2 adrenoceptor agonist clonidine stimulates hypothalamic GH releasing hormone that acts on the anterior pituitary to

release GH (Fig. 52.9(a),(b)). After clonidine, levels of GH rise in PAF, where there is no central autonomic abnormality. In the different forms of MSA there is no GH response to clonidine. However, another GH secretagogue, L-dopa, raises GHRH and GH levels in MSA (Kimber et al., 1999) while apomorphine raises GH in MSA with a greater response in PD (Friess et al., 2001), indicating that the abnormal response is not the result of widespread and hypothalamic neuronal fall-out, and probably indicates a specific alpha-2 adrenoceptor-hypothalamic deficit. Early reports indicate preservation of the clonidine-GH response in non-drug treated PD (Kimber et al., 1997a); this may not apply to drug-treated PD. Whether the clonidine-GH test will distinguish MSA from other parkinsonian and peripheral autonomic syndromes at an early stage remains to be determined. In MSA, the urethral or anal sphincter electromyograph is usually abnormal, characteristically indicating denervation and reinnervation (Palace et al., 1997). False positives include prostatic surgery in the male and multiparous females; it also may be abnormal in progressive supranuclear palsy (PSP). The combination of orthostatic hypotension and an abnormal urethral/anal sphincter electromyograph, in conjunction with the characteristic clinical features, are virtually confirmatory of MSA.

The prognosis in MSA is poor compared with PD and PAF, as the motor and autonomic deficits progressively worsen. There is a refractoriness to anti-parkinsonian agents; orthostatic hypotension may further impair mobility. Communication becomes increasingly difficult. In the cerebellar form, worsening truncal ataxia may cause falls

Table 52.10. *Some of the investigations used in parkinsonism to evaluate autonomic function and separate MSA from IPD*

Neuroimaging studies
– Magnetic resonance imaging
– Magnetic resonance spectroscopy
– Positron emission tomography – with various ligands

Autonomic screening tests
– to determine if orthostatic hypotension is present
– to assess sympathetic vasoconstrictor responses
– to evaluate parasympathetic cardiac responses

Additional autonomic tests
– food and exercise challenge
– 24-hour ambulatory blood pressure and heart rate profile

Cardiac sympathetic evaluation
– meta-iodo-benzyl-guanidine and gamma scintiscanning
– 6-Fluorodopamine and positron emission tomography scanning

Sympathetic skin response

Clonidine-growth hormone stimulation test

Urethral or anal sphincter electromyography

Table 52.11. *Some of the possible causes of orthostatic hypotension in a patient with parkinsonian features*

Side effects of anti-parkinsonian therapy
   L-DOPA, bromocriptine, pergolide
   the combination of L-DOPA and COMT inhibitors (tolcapone)
   the MAO 'b' inhibitor, selegiline

Coincidental disease causing autonomic dysfunction
   e.g. diabetes mellitus

Coincidental administration of drugs for an allied condition
   Antihypertensives
      α-adrenoceptor blockers (for benign prostatic hypertrophy)
   Vasodilators (for ischemic heart disease)
   Diuretics (for cardiac failure)

Multiple system atrophy (Shy–Drager syndrome)

Parkinson's disease with autonomic failure

Diffuse Lewy body disease

Source: Adapted from Mathias and Kimber (1999).

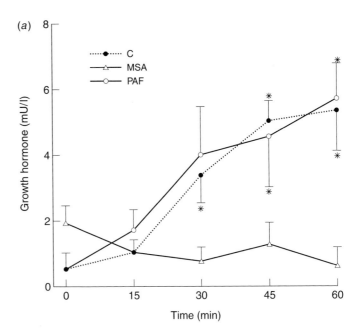

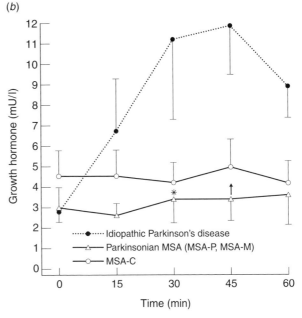

Fig. 52.9. (*a*) Serum growth hormone (GH) concentrations before (0) and at 15 min intervals for 60 min after clonidine (2 μg/kg/min) in normal subjects (C, controls) and in patients who have multiple system atrophy (MSA) and pure autonomic failure (PAF). GH concentrations rise in controls and in patients who have PAF with a peripheral lesion; there is no rise in patients with MSA with a central lesion. (From Thomaides et al., 1992.)

(*b*) Lack of serum GH response to clonidine in the two forms of MSA (the cerebellar form, MSA-C and the parkinsonian forms, MSA-P and MSA-M) in contrast to patients with idiopathic Parkinson's disease with no autonomic deficit, in whom there is a significant rise in GH levels. (From Kimber et al., 1997a.)

and an inability to stand upright; incoordination in the upper limbs, speech deficits and nystagmus add to the disability. Oropharyngeal dysphagia enhances the risk of aspiration, especially as many have vocal cord abnormalities; a percutaneous feeding gastrostomy may be needed. Respiratory abnormalities that include obstructive (due to laryngeal abductor cord paresis) and central apnea, may necessitate a tracheostomy.

In MSA there currently is no means of reversing the neurological decline. Supportive therapy is an essential component in management and should incorporate the family, therapists and community. Many autonomic features can be helped, and this includes orthostatic hypotension, bowel, bladder and sexual dysfunction.

Idiopathic Parkinson's disease and other parkinsonian disorders

In PD, autonomic features usually are not prominent, especially in the early stages. Orthostatic hypotension if present, may be related to increased duration of disease, age and multiple drug therapy. A varying prevalence has been described, from rare to high (58% with 38.5% symptomatic) (Mathias, 1998a,b). Meta-iodo-benzylguanidine with gamma scintiscanning, and fluorodopamine with positron emission tomographic scanning, of the heart indicate that cardiac sympathetic denervation may occur early in the disorder, often without other detectable autonomic features (Goldstein et al., 1997, Orima et al., 1999). The implications of this observation are unclear and have relevance to cardiac arrhythmias and drug therapy in PD. Whether the urinary and gastrointestinal features are due to autonomic or other mechanisms is unclear. In PD Lewy bodies are present in the esophageal and colonic myenteric plexuses with reduction of dopaminergic neurons in the latter.

There is a smaller group, often of older patients with apparently classic PD, who have been successfully treated with l-dopa for many years and then develop features of autonomic failure, usually with severe postural hypotension. They thus differ from the majority of patients with PD in whom autonomic deficits, if present, are relatively mild. Cardiac scanning techniques indicate sympathetic denervation, favouring a peripheral lesion similar to PAF (Goldstein et al., 1997). These patients also have low basal plasma noradrenaline levels and their orthostatic hypotension does not respond to yohimbine (whose actions are dependent on intact sympathetic nerves). The etiology of PD with AF is unknown. It may be a coincidental association of a common condition with an uncommon disorder (PAF), or an indication of vulnerability to autonomic degeneration in a sub-group of PD, that may be linked to increasing age, chronic anti-parkinsonian drug therapy, an inherent metabolic susceptibility, or to a combination of these factors. These patients do not appear to suffer from the many complications of MSA and clinically appear to differ from them.

Dizziness and orthostatic hypotension is more common in diffuse Lewy body disease(DLBD), than previously recognized. Some patients may be mistakenly diagnosed as PAF or MSA. In PAF, Lewy bodies are also present in the peripheral autonomic nervous system, raising the possibility that it may be a forme fruste, or an early stage, of DLBD. In PSP, unlike previous reports, more recent studies indicate lack of orthostatic hypotension and cardiovascular autonomic features, which has now been proposed as an exclusionary feature in the diagnosis of this disorder (Kimber et al., 2000). Urinary abnormalities and an abnormal sphincter electromyograph may be present; there is evidence of degeneration of Onuf's nucleus in the sacral cord. In Huntingdon's disease, defects in vasoregulation have been described and attributed to involvement of suprabulbar structures including caudate nuclei, but there is no significant cardiovascular abnormality; however, hyperhidrosis, diarrhea and sphincter disturbances may occur. In Guamanian parkinsonism and parkinsonian–dementia complex, there are autonomic abnormalities affecting the cardiovascular system that are greater than usually observed in PD and less than MSA but may be confounded by diabetes and antihypertensive drug therapy. Whether there are autonomic abnormalities of significance in other parkinsonian syndromes remains to be determined.

Secondary autonomic failure

There is a wide range of secondary disorders (Table 52.12). Some are described briefly below.

Hereditary

Riley–Day syndrome; familial dysautonomia

This occurs in children of Ashkenazi–Jewish extraction (Axelrod, 1999). They have absent fungiform papillae, lack of corneal reflexes, decreased deep tendon reflexes and a diminished response to pain. This is often observed at birth. An abnormal intradermal histamine skin test (with an absent flare response) and pupillary hypersensitivity to cholinomimetics, confirms the diagnosis. The defective gene has been mapped to the long arm of chromosome 9 (q31).

Table 52.12. Secondary autonomic failure

Congenital
– Nerve growth factor deficiency

Hereditary
Autosomal dominant
– Familial amyloid neuropathy
– Porphyria

Autosomal recessive
– Familial dysautonomia (Riley–Day syndrome)
– Dopamine beta-hydroxylase deficiency
– Aromatic L-amino acid decarboxylase deficiency

X-linked recessive
– Fabry's disease

Metabolic diseases
– Diabetes mellitus
– Chronic renal failure
– Chronic liver disease
– Vitamin B_{12} deficiency
– Alcohol-induced

Inflammatory
– Guillain–Barré syndrome
– Transverse myelitis

Infections
– Bacterial   – tetanus, leprosy
– Viral   – human immuno-deficiency virus infection
– Parasitic   – Chagas' disease
– Prion   – fatal familial insomnia

Neoplasia
– Brain tumours – especially of third ventricle or posterior fossa
– Paraneoplastic, to include adenocarcinomas – lung, pancreas and Lambert–Eaton syndrome

Connective tissue disorders
– Rheumatoid arthritis
– Systemic lupus erythematosus
– Mixed connective tissue disease

Surgery
– Regional sympathectomy – upper limb, splanchnic
– Vagotomy and drainage procedures – 'dumping syndrome'
– Organ transplantation – heart, kidney

Trauma
– Spinal cord transection

A variety of symptoms, resulting from both autonomic underactivity and overactivity may occur. These include a labile blood pressure (with hypertension and postural hypotension), parasympathetic abnormalities (with periodic vomiting, dysphagia, constipation and diarrhea) and urinary bladder disturbances. Neurological abnormalities, associated skeletal problems (scoliosis) and renal failure previously contributed to a poor prognosis. The ability to anticipate complications and provide adequate support and therapy has resulted in a number of children now reaching adulthood.

Amyloid polyneuropathy

Both light chain (AL) and familial amyloid polyneuropathy (FAP) result in autonomic dysfunction (Reilly & Thomas, 1999). In the AL form, amyloid is derived from monoclonal light chains, secondary to multiple myeloma, malignant lymphoma or Waldenstrom's macroglobulinemia. The features vary with an overall poor prognosis. In FAP, symptoms usually occur in adulthood. Sensory, motor and autonomic abnormalities result from deposition in peripheral nerves of mutated amyloid protein, mainly produced in the liver. Motor and sensory neuropathy often begins in the lower limbs. Classification of FAP is now based on the chemical and molecular nature of the constituent proteins and not on clinical presentation. There are various forms; transthyretin (TTR) FAP; FAP Ala 60 (Irish/ Appalachian) and FAP Ser 84 and His 58. The cardiovascular system, gut and urinary bladder can be affected at any stage. The disease relentlessly progresses but at a variable rate. There may be dissociation of autonomic symptoms from functional deficits; this is of importance, as evaluation and treatment of cardiovascular autonomic abnormalities is essential in reducing morbidity and mortality especially during hepatic transplantation. Currently, this is the only way to reduce levels of variant transthyretin and its deposition in nerves; it prevents progression of, and may reverse some, neuropathic features. It may be of greater value if performed before nerve damage occurs.

Dopamine beta-hydroxylase deficiency

This rare disorder, recognized in the mid-1980s, has been described in seven patients, two of whom are siblings (Mathias & Bannister, 1999c). Symptoms began in childhood, although an autonomic disorder was not considered until they became teenagers, when orthostatic hypotension was first recognised. Whether the symptoms become more prominent, or are easier to detect at this time, is unclear. The clinical features indicate sympathetic adrenergic failure with sparing of sympathetic cholinergic and parasympathetic function. Sweating is preserved and

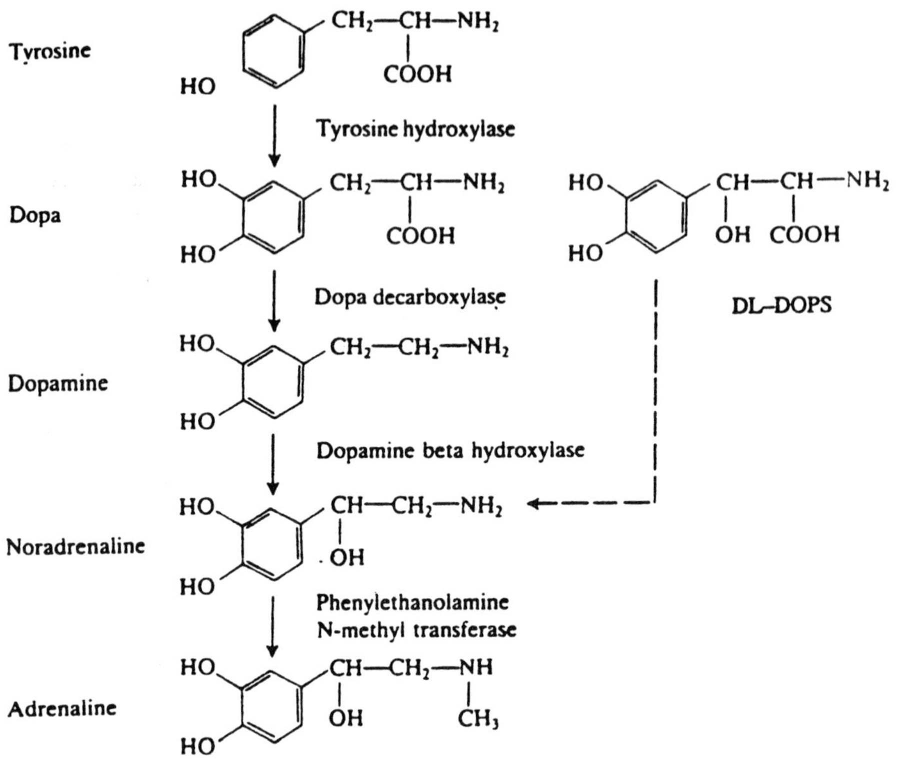

Fig. 52.10. Biosynthetic pathway in the formation of noradrenaline and adrenaline. The structure of DL-DOPS is indicated on the right. It is converted directly to noradrenaline by dopa decarboxylase, thus bypassing dopamine β-hydroxylase.

urinary bladder and bowel function is normal; in one of the males erection was possible but ejaculation was difficult to achieve. The diagnosis may be made from basal levels of plasma catecholamines, as noradrenaline and adrenaline levels are undetectable while dopamine levels are elevated. The enzymatic defect is highly specific, with the sympathetic nerve pathways and terminals otherwise intact, as has been demonstrated by both electron microscopy and preservation of muscle sympathetic nerve activity using microneurography. These subjects, therefore, are a unique model of superselective sympathetic adrenergic failure. Treatment is with the pro-drug L-dihydroxyphenylserine (Fig. 52.10), which has a structure similar to noradrenaline except for a carboxyl group that is acted upon by the enzyme dopadecarboxylase (abundantly present in extraneuronal tissues such as the liver and kidneys), thus transforming it into noradrenaline. This reduces orthostatic hypotension and has resulted in remarkable improvements in their ability to lead active lives.

Diabetes mellitus

There is a high incidence of both peripheral and autonomic neuropathy, especially in older, long-standing diabetics on insulin therapy (Watkins, 1998). Their morbidity and mortality is considerably higher than in those without a neuropathy. It initially often involves the vagus, with characteristic features of cardiac vagal denervation. This may occur in conjunction with partial preservation of the cardiac sympathetic and may predispose diabetics, many of whom have ischemic heart disease, to sudden death from cardiac dysrhythmias. In some, sympathetic failure may cause orthostatic hypotension, that may be enhanced by insulin (Fig. 52.11). Awareness of hypoglycemia, that depends on autonomic activation, is diminished. There may be involvement of the gastro-intestinal tract (gastroparesis diabeticorum and diabetic diarrhea), the urinary bladder (diabetic cystopathy) and in the male, impotence. Sudomotor abnormalities include gustatory sweating. Damage to other organs may occur through non-neuropathic factors and compounds the problems caused by the neuropathy. Diabetic foot problems may result from a combination of neuropathy and ischemia. Other than maintaining normoglycemia, there is no known means to prevent and reverse the neuropathy except possibly by pancreatic transplantation.

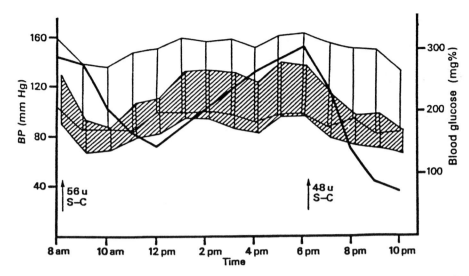

Fig. 52.11. Diurnal variation of lying and standing blood pressure in a 48-year-old man with severe diabetic autonomic neuropathy. Insulin was given subcutaneously (S-C) at times shown by the vertical arrows. The unhatched area shows supine blood pressure, the hatched area the standing blood pressure, and the continuous line the blood glucose. (From Watkins & Edmonds, 1999.)

Spinal cord diseases

Autonomic dysfunction affecting various systems occurs in spinal cord disease, as the entire sympathetic and the sacral sympathetic outflow is from the spinal cord (Mathias & Frankel, 1999). The level of completeness of lesion determines the degree of dysfunction.

Cardiovascular autonomic dysfunction can contribute to morbidity and mortality, especially in cervical and high thoracic spinal cord lesions. Orthostatic hypotension results from the inability of the brain to activate efferent sympathetic pathways, despite preservation of baroreceptor afferent and central connections. In these subjects the reverse, paroxysmal hypertension, may occur following large bowel and urinary bladder contraction as part of the mass reflex, in the syndrome of autonomic dysreflexia (Fig. 52.12). This is due to isolated spinal cord reflex activity (without the restraint of cerebral control) and can be induced by a variety of stimuli, from cutaneous, skeletal muscle or visceral sources, below the level of the lesion. In the acute phase after injury, such patients may have a different set of clinical problems, because of 'spinal shock' and the absence of even isolated spinal sympathetic activity; some of these result also from excessive cardiac vagal activity causing bradycardia or even cardiac arrest.

A combination of autonomic underactivity and overactivity may occur in non-spinal disorders. In the Guillain–Barré syndrome both autonomic hyperactivity and underactivity may occur (Asahina et at., 2001); tachycardia and hypotension may alternate with bradycardia and hypertension. The precise mechanisms are unclear and the possibilities should be anticipated as appropriate

drugs may be needed. Cardiovascular disturbances of a similar nature may occur in tetanus, especially in those who suffer muscle paralysis and are on assisted respiration.

Drugs, chemicals, toxins

Drugs may cause autonomic dysfunction through their recognized pharmacological effects, such as sympatholytic agents (Table 52.13). A side effect of a drug may cause clinical problems when used in high dosage or over a prolonged period (such as the anticholinergic effects of antidepressants), or when autonomic deficits are unmasked or induced in susceptible individuals. Examples of the latter include L-dopa worsening orthostatic hypotension in MSA (Fig. 52.13), the ability of pressor agents to cause severe hypertension in autonomic failure because of denervation supersensitivity (Fig. 52.6), and the antiarrhythmic disopyramide inducing urinary retention in subjects with benign prostatic hypertrophy. Drugs such as perhexeline maleate, vincristine and alcohol may induce autonomic dysfunction independently of their pharmacological properties, by causing an autonomic neuropathy.

Neurally mediated syncope

These disorders are characterized by an intermittent cardiovascular autonomic abnormality resulting in syncope (loss of consciousness synonymous with fainting, blackouts) (Kapoor, 2000; Mathias et al., 2001) (Table 52.14). An

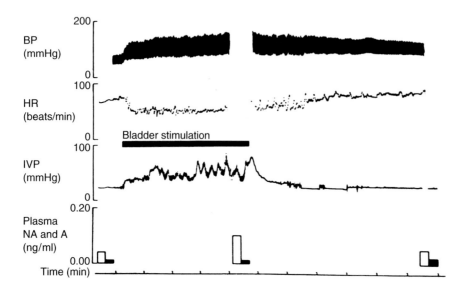

Fig. 52.12. Blood pressure (BP), heart rate (HR), intravesical pressure (IVP), and plasma noradrenaline (NA; open histogram) and adrenaline (A; filled histogram) levels in a tetraplegic patient before, during and after bladder stimulation induced by suprapubic percussion of the anterior abdominal wall. The rist in BP is accompanied by a fall in heart rate as a result of increased vagal activity in response to the rise in blood pressure. Levels of plasma NA, but not A rise, suggesting an increase in sympathetic neural activity independently of adrenomedullary activation. (From Mathias & Frankel, 1999.)

increase in cardiac parasympathetic activity causes severe bradycardia or cardiac arrest (cardio-inhibitory form) and withdrawal of sympathetic nerve activity results in hypotension (vasodepressor form). The two may occur separately, or together as the mixed form (Fig. 52.14). Between episodes there may be no abnormalities detected on routine autonomic testing.

In the young, the more common condition is vasovagal syncope. There is often a family history of a similar disorder (Mathias et al., 1998). It is more common in women. It may be induced by various stimuli, from fear and the sight of blood, to venepuncture and at times even discussion of venepuncture. Standing still, a warm environmental temperature and other factors that promote vasodilation, including gravitational pooling, can induce syncope. Modified testing, which includes prolonged tilt-table testing and, in some, application of a provocative stimulus (including venepuncture or pseudo-venepuncture), may induce an episode. Cardiac conduction disorders and other causes of syncope need to be excluded. Some advocate supraphysiological (head-up tilt and lower body negative pressure) and pharmacological (head-up tilt and isoprenaline infusion) testing; these stimuli however, may provoke an attack in subjects who have never fainted (El-Bedawi & Hainsworth, 1994; Morillo et al., 1995). Management includes reducing or preventing exposure to precipitating

causes although these may be unclear; in some behavioural therapy (especially in those with phobias), is needed. A high salt diet, exercise and various drugs such as fludrocortisone, vasopressor agents, and antidepressants (including the serotonin-uptake release inhibitors), have been used with varying success. In some with the cardio-inhibitory form, a cardiac demand pacemaker is of value. The long-term prognosis is favourable and in many, attacks do not occur after the third decade.

In the elderly, carotid sinus hypersensitivity may be more common than previously thought; it may be a major cause of unexplained falls (McIntosh et al., 1993). There may be a classical history of syncope induced by head movements or collar tightening; in many the precipitating factors are unclear. Investigation should include carotid sinus massage performed with requisite precautions in the laboratory with adequate resuscitation facilities, ideally using beat-by-beat blood pressure and heart rate recording. Carotid massage also should be performed with the subject tilted head-up, as hypotension is more likely to occur in situations when sympathetic nerve activity is needed. In the cardio-inhibitory form a cardiac demand pacemaker is used. The vasodepressor forms are more difficult to manage and pressor agents have been used. Denervation of the carotid sinus may be used especially in unilateral hypersensitivity.

Table 52.13. Drugs/chemicals/poisons/toxins

DECREASING SYMPATHETIC ACTIVITY

Centrally acting
- Clonidine
- Methyldopa
- Reserpine
- Barbiturates
- Anesthetics

Peripherally acting
- Sympathetic nerve ending (guanethidine, bethanadine)
- Alpha-adrenoceptor blockade (phenoxybenzamine)
- Beta-adrenoceptor blockade (propranolol)

INCREASING SYMPATHETIC ACTIVITY
- Amphetamines
- Releasing noradrenaline (tyramine)
- Uptake blockers (imipramine)
- Monoamine oxidase inhibitors (tranylcypromine)
- Beta-adrenoceptor stimulants (isoprenaline)
- Following drug withdrawal (clonidine, alcohol, opiates)

DECREASING PARASYMPATHETIC ACTIVITY
- Antidepressants (imipramine)
- Tranquillizers (phenothiazines)
- Antidysrhythmics (disopyramide)
- Anticholinergics (atropine, probanthine, benztropine)
- Toxins (botulinum)

INCREASING PARASYMPATHETIC ACTIVITY
- Cholinomimetics (carbachol, bethanechol, pilocarpine, mushroom poisoning)
- Anticholinesterases
- Reversible carbamate inhibitors (pyridostigmine, neostigmine)
- Organophosphorus inhibitors (parathion)

Miscellaneous
- Alcohol, thiamine (vitamin B$_1$ deficiency)
- Vincristine, perhexiline maleate
- Thallium and arsenic
- Mercury poisoning (Pink disease)
- Cyclosporin
- CNS serotonergic syndrome
- Ciguatera (reef fish) toxicity
- Jelly fish and marine animal venoms

Table 52.14. Neurally mediated syncope

Vasovagal syncope

Carotid sinus hypersensitivity

Variants of reflexly induced syncope
Tracheal stimulation in spinal shock
Swallow syncope
Glossopharyngeal vagal irritation
Pelvic examination/instrumentation
Defecation syncope
Micturition syncope
Cough syncope
Laughter-induced syncope
Fainting lark (Mess trick)

Associations with
Children (vagotonia)
Athletes (postexercise)
Weight lifters
Oarsmen

Drug-induced (Bezold–Jarisch reflex)
First dose effect of angiotensin-1 converting enzyme inhibitors and prazosin

A variety of stimuli and circumstances may induce neurally mediated syncope. In some, reflexly induced exaggeration of vagal activity is responsible, as in cardiac arrest caused by tracheal stimulation in tetraplegics on artificial respiration, where increased vagal tone is not opposed by sympathetic activity or the pulmonary inflation reflex (Fig. 52.15). Syncope induced by swallowing (in some in association glossopharyngeal neuralgia) (Deguchi & Mathias, 1999) and, caused by pelvic and rectal examinations or instrumentation, are other examples. Malignancies in the pharynx and thorax may increase the tendency to reflexly induced syncope. In micturition and defecation syncope changes in intrathoracic pressure may contribute as in cough and laughter-induced, trumpet blowing and voluntary syncope ('fainting lark'). In extremely fit subjects, such as sportsmen, increased vagal tone, as occurs in children, also may contribute to syncope. The first-dose hypotensive effect of certain drugs may be neurally mediated, via the Bezold–Jarisch reflex.

Postural tachycardia syndrome (PoTS)

The postural tachycardia syndrome (PoTS) is a disorder mainly affecting women between the ages of 20 and 50, with symptoms of orthostatic intolerance (light headedness and other manifestations of cerebral hypoperfusion), often with palpitations (Low et al., 1995). The symptoms disappear on sitting or lying down. Investigations exclude orthostatic hypotension and autonomic failure. During postural challenge heart rate increases by 30 beats per minute or over. There are similarities with the syndromes initially described by Da Costa & Lewis (also known as

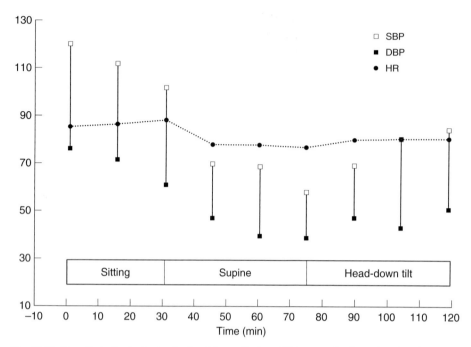

Fig. 52.13. The effect of a single standard oral dose of L-dopa (250 mg) and a dopa-decarboxylase inhibitor carbidopa (25 mg) given at time zero, on the blood pressure of a patient with parkinsonian features. There was a marked fall in blood pressure after 30 mins, resulting in the patient first being placed supine and then head-down. On investigation the patient had autonomic failure, with orthostatic hypotension unmasked by L-dopa; the final diagnosis was the parkinsonian form of multiple system atrophy. SBP, systolic blood pressure; DBP, diastolic blood pressure; HR, heart rate. (From Mathias, 2000b.)

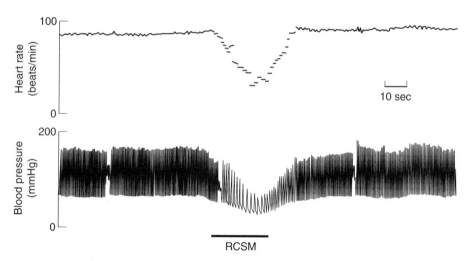

Fig. 52.14. Heart rate and blood pressure before, during and after right carotid sinus massage (RCSM) in a patient with syncopal episodes. There is a fall in both heart rate and blood pressure during carotid sinus massage, typical of the mixed (cardioinhibitory and vasodepressor) form of this disorder. The breaks in the record indicate calibration at intervals by the Finapres machine. (From Mathias, 2000a.)

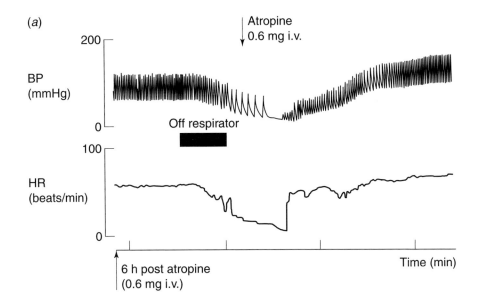

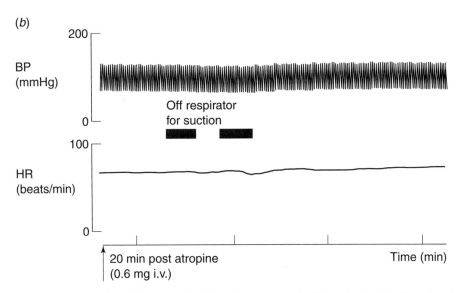

Fig. 52.15. (*a*) The effect of disconnecting the respirator (as required for aspirating the airways) on the blood pressure (BP) and heart rate (HR) of a recently injured tetraplegic patient (C4/5 lesion) in spinal shock, 6 hours after the last dose of intravenous atropine. Sinus bradycardia and cardiac arrest (also observed on the electrocardiograph) were reversed by reconnection, intravenous atropine and external cardiac massage. (From Frankel et al., 1975.)

(*b*) The effect of tracheal suction, 20 minutes after atropine. Disconnection from the respirator and tracheal suction did not lower either heart rate or blood pressure. (From Mathias, 1976.)

soldier's heart syndrome or neurocirculatory esthenia), mitral valve prolapse syndrome, chronic fatigue syndrome (Schondorf & Freeman, 1999) and deconditioning following prolonged bed rest and microgravity during spaceflight. The condition appears heterogenous (Khurana, 1995). In some the disorder appears to follow a viral infection. There may be features of a partial autonomic neuropathy, with lower limb denervation (Schondorf & Low, 1993; Jacob et al., 2000). In a family with affected twins, a genetic basis, with a defect in the noradrenaline transporter system, has been described which accounted for the raised basal noradrenaline levels. A mutation of the gene encoding the noradrenaline transporter was thought responsible for the hyperadrenergic state (Shannon et al., 2000). Hypovolemia may contribute.

The prognosis is variable, and some patients may recover with time. A variety of drugs, including beta blockers and drugs used in the treatment of orthostatic hypotension need to be considered; methods to increase volume expansion appear beneficial.

Localized autonomic disorders

Examples of these are listed in Table 52.15 with a brief description of a few.

The Holmes–Adie pupil is characteristically dilated and sluggishly responsive to light but responds to near vision, hence the descriptive term 'near-light dissociation'. It results from parasympathetic denervation, probably of the ciliary ganglia, with supersensitivity of the iris musculature to locally applied cholinomimetics. The term Holmes–Adie syndrome is used when associated with absent tendon reflexes; this probably is due to involvement of dorsal root ganglia, accounting for the absent H reflex on electrophysiological testing. Some patients have areas of anhidrosis, although they often complain of hyperhidrosis that is likely to be compensatory in nature (Ross syndrome). Others may have cardiovascular autonomic deficits, a chronic dry cough and diarrhea (Kimber et al., 1998). Although considered benign, in some the disorder may be progressive, with baroreceptor reflex dysfunction causing labile hypertension and also orthostatic hypotension.

In Horner's syndrome, there is partial ptosis and a small pupil as the sympathetic fibres to the face are affected. It may result from a lesion along the course of the facial sympathetic supply, in the brain, spinal cord, the upper thoracic ganglia or post-ganglionic efferents that follow the vasculature. Although it causes few, if any, symptoms it may be a harbinger of a serious underlying disorder.

Table 52.15. Examples of localized autonomic disorders

Holmes – Adie pupil
Horner's syndrome
Crocodile tears (Bogorad's syndrome)
Gustatory sweating (Frey's syndrome)
Essential (primary) hyperhidrosis
Reflex sympathetic dystrophy
Hirchsprung's disease (congenital megacolon)
Chagas' disease (*Trypanosomiasis cruzii*)
Surgical procedures[a]
– Sympathectomy – regional
– Vagotomy and gastric drainage procedures in 'dumping syndrome'
– Organ transplantation – heart, lungs

Notes:
[a] Surgery may cause some of the disorders listed above (such as Frey's syndrome following parotid surgery).

The lachrymal glands have a rich autonomic innervation. Alachryma may occur as part of a generalized autonomic disorder. 'Crocodile' tears may result from aberrant reinnervation of the lachrymal gland with fibres from the salivary glands. The mechanisms are similar to gustatory sweating, due to aberrant reinnervation between salivary and facial sweat glands; in both acetylcholine is the neurotransmitter. In essential (primary) hyperhidrosis there is no peripheral neural abnormality; whether hypothalamic dysfunction or altered behavioural responses are the trigger to hyperhidrosis is unclear. The treatment of hyperhidrosis, especially of the palms and face includes percutaneous endoscopic transthoracic sympathectomy, with bilateral ablation of ganglia between T2 and T4; compensatory hyperhidrosis affecting the trunk and lower limbs may occur postsurgery and in some may be worse than the original complaint. Injection of botulinum toxin especially into small areas such as the palm, face and axillae has been successfully used, but needs to be repeated and long-term benefits are unknown (Naumann et al., 1997). In reflex sympathetic dystrophy (chronic regional pain syndrome; CRPS type 2), there is debate about whether features such as sweating and vascular changes have an autonomic basis (Kimber et al., 1997b; in some these abnormalities are relieved by sympatholytic (guanethidine) blockade.

Localized disorders of the gut include Hirschsprung's disease. In Chagas' disease (after infection with *Trypanosoma cruzii*) the intrinsic autonomic ganglia in the esophagus, colon and heart are specifically targeted, probably by an immunological process. Various surgical procedures may be complicated by autonomic dysfunction, an example being the dumping syndrome complicating vagot-omy and gastric drainage procedures. Denervation of trans-planted organs such as heart or kidneys also may result in dysfunction; reinnervation may occur in due course.

References

Appenzeller, O. & Oribe, E. (1997). *The Autonomic Nervous System*, 5th edn, Amsterdam: Elsevier.

Asahina, M., Kuwabara, S., Suzuki, A. & Hattori, T. (2001). Autonomic function in demyelinating and axonal subtypes of Guillain–Barre syndrome. *Acta Neurol. Scand.*, **105**, 1–7.

Axelrod, F.B. (1999). Familial dysautonomia. In *Autonomic Failure: A Textbook of Clinical Disorders of the Autonomic Nervous System*, ed. C.J. Mathias & R. Bannister, 4th edn, pp. 402–9. Oxford: Oxford University Press.

Daniel S. (1999). The neuropathology and neurochemistry of multiple system atrophy. In *Autonomic Failure: A Textbook of Clinical Disorders of the Autonomic Nervous System*, ed. C.J. Mathias & R. Bannister, 4th edn, pp. 321–8. Oxford: Oxford University Press.

Deguchi, K. & Mathias, C.J. (1999). Continuous haemodynamic monitoring in an unusual case of swallow-induced syncope. *J. Neurol. Neurosurg. Psychiatry*, **67**, 220–3.

El-Bedawi, K.M. & Hainsworth, R. (1994). Combined head-up tilt and lower body suction: a test of orthostatic intolerance. *Clinical Autonomic Research*, **4**, pp. 41–7.

Frankel, H.L., Mathias, C.J. & Spalding, J.M.K. (1975). Mechanisms of reflex cardiac arrest in tetraplegic patients. *Lancet*, **ii**, 1183–5.

Friess, E., Kuempfel, T., Winkelmann, J. et al. (2001). Increased growth hormone response to apomorphine in Parkinson Disease compared with multiple system atrophy. *Arch. Neurol.*, **58**, 241–6.

Gilman, S., Low, P., Quinn, N. et al. (1998). Consensus statement on the diagnosis of multiple system atrophy. *Clin. Autonom. Res.* **8**, 359–62.

Goldstein, D.S., Holmes, C., Cannon, R.O. III, Eisenhofer, G & Kopin, I.J. (1997). Sympathetic cardioneuropathy in dysautono-mias. *N. Engl. J. Med.*, **336**, 696–702.

Heafield, M.T., Gammage, M.D., Nightingale, S. & Williams, A.C. (1996). Idiopathic dysautonomia treated with intravenous gam-maglobulin. *Lancet*, **347**, 28–9.

Jacob, G., Costa, F., Shannon, J.R. et al. (2000). The neuropathic postural tachycardia syndrome. *N. Engl. J. Med.*, **343**, 1008–14.

Janig, W. (1987). Autonomic nervous system. In *Human Physiology*, 2nd edn., ed. R.F. Schmidt & G. Thews, pp. 333–70. Berlin: Springer-Verlag.

Kappoor, W.N. (2000) Syncope. *N. Engl. J. Med.*, **343**, 1856–62.

Khurana, R.K. (1995). Orthostatic intolerance and orthostatic tach-ycardia: a heterogeneous disorder. *Clin. Autonom. Res.*, **5**, 12–18.

Kimber, J.R., Mathias, C.J. (1999). Neuroendocrine responses to Levodopa in multiple system atrophy (MSA). *Movement Dis.*, **14**, 981–87.

Kimber, J., Smith, G.D.P. & Mathias, C.J. (1997a). Reflex sympa-thetic dystrophy in a pateint with peripheral sympathetic dener-vation. *Europ. J. Neurol.*, **4**, 315–17.

Kimber, J.R., Watson, L. Mathias, C.J. (1997). Distinction of idio-pathic Parkinson's disease from multiple system atrophy by stimulation of growth hormone release with clonidine. *Lancet*, **349**, 1877–81.

Kimber, J., Mitchell, D. & Mathias, C.J. (1998). Chronic cough in the Holmes–Adie syndrome: association in five cases with auto-nomic dysfunction. *J. Neurol., Neurosurg. Psychiatry*, **65**, 583–6.

Kimber, J., Watson, L. & Mathias, C.J. (1999). Neuroendocrine responses to levodopa in multiple system atrophy. *Movem. Disorders*, **14**, 981–7.

Kimber, J., Mathias, C.J., Lees A.J. et al. (2000). Physiological, phar-macological and neurohormonal assessment of autonomic function in progressive supranuclear palsy. *Brain*, **123**, 1422–30.

Low, P.A., Opfer-Gehrking, T.L., Textor, S.C. et al. (1995). Postural tachycardia syndrome (POTS). *Neurology*, **45**, S19–25.

McIntosh, S.J., Lawson, J. Kenny, R.A. (1993). Clinical characteris-tics of vasodepressor, cardioinhibitory and mixed carotid sinus syndrome in the elderly. *Am. J. Med.*, **95**, 203–8.

Mathias, C.J. (1998a). Autonomic disorders. In *Textbook of Neurology*, ed. J. Bogousslavsky & M. Fisher, pp. 519–45. Massachusetts: Butterworth Heinemann.

Mathias, C.J. (1976). Bradycardia and cardiac arrest during tracheal suction – mechanisms in tetraplegic patients. *Eur. J. Intens. Care Med.*, **2**, 147–56.

Mathias, C.J. (1997). Autonomic disorders and their recognition. *N. Engl. J. Med.*, **10**, 721–4.

Mathias, C.J. (1998b). Cardiovascular autonomic dysfunction in parkinsonian patients. *Clin. Neurosci.*, **5**, 153–66.

Mathias, C.J. (2000a). Disorders of the autonomic nervous system. In *Neurology in Clinical Practice*, 3rd edn, ed. W.G. Bradley, R.B. Daroff, G.M. Fenichel, C.D. Marsden, pp. 2131–65. Boston, USA: Butterworth-Heinemann.

Mathias, C.J. (2000b). Autonomic dysfunction. In *Oxford Textbook of Geriatric Medicine*, 2nd edn, ed. J. Grimley-Evans, T. Franklin Williams, B. Lynn Beattie, J.-P. Michel & G.K. Wilcock, pp. 833–52. Oxford: Oxford University Press.

Mathias, C.J. & Frankel, H. (1999). Autonomic disturbances in spinal cord lesions. In *Autonomic Failure: A Textbook of Clinical Disorders of the Autonomic Nervous System*, ed. C.J. Mathias & R. Bannister, 4th edn, pp. 494–513. Oxford: Oxford University Press.

Mathias, C.J. & Bannister, R. (1999a). Investigation of autonomic disorders. In *Autonomic Failure: A Textbook of Clinical Disorders of the Autonomic Nervous System*, ed. C.J. Mathias & R. Bannister, 4th edn, pp. 169–95. Oxford: Oxford University Press.

Mathias, C.J. & Bannister, R. (1999b). Dopamine β-hydroxylase deficiency – with a note on other genetically determined causes of autonomic failure. In *Autonomic Failure: A Textbook of Clinical Disorders of the Autonomic Nervous System*, ed. C.J. Mathias & R. Bannister, 4th edn, pp. 387–401. Oxford: Oxford University Press.

Mathias, C.J. & Kimber, J.R. (1999). Postural hypotension – causes, clinical features, investigation and management. *Ann. Rev. Med.*, **50**, 317–36.

Mathias, C.J. & Williams, A.C. (1994). The Shy Drager syndrome (and multiple system atrophy). In *Neurodegenerative Diseases*, ed. D.B. Calne, 1st edn, vol. 43, pp. 743–68. Philadelphia, Pennsylvania, USA: W. B. Saunders Co.

Mathias, C.J., da Costa, D.F., Fosbraey, P. et al. (1989). Cardiovascular, biochemical and hormonal changes during food induced hypotension in chronic autonomic failure. *J. Neurol. Sci.*, **94**, 255–69.

Mathias, C.J., Deguchi, K., Bleasdale-Barr, K. & Kimber, J.R. (1998). Frequency of family history in vasovagal syncope. *Lancet*, **352**, 33–4.

Mathias, C.J., Mallipeddi, R. & Bleasdale-Barr, K. (1999). Symptoms associated with orthostatic hypotension in pure autonomic failure and multiple system atrophy. *J. Neurol.*, **246**, 893–8.

Mathias, C.J., Deguchi, K. & Schatz, I.J. (2001). Observations on recurrent syncope and presyncope in 641 patients. *Lancet*, **357**, 348–53.

Matthews, M. (1999). Autonomic ganglia and preganglionic neurones in autonomic failure. In *Autonomic Failure: a Textbook of Clinical Disorders of the Autonomic Nervous System*, ed. C.J. Mathias & R. Bannister, 4th edn, pp. 329–39. Oxford: Oxford University Press.

Morrillo, C.A., Klein, G., Zandri, S. & Yee, R. (1995). Diagnostic accuracy of a low dose isoprotenerol head up tilt protocol *Am. Heart J.*, **129**, 901–6.

Naumann, M., Flachenecker, P., Brocker, E-B. et al. (1997). Botulinum toxin for palmar hyperhidrosis. *Lancet*, **349**, 252.

Orima, S., Ozawa, E., Nakade, S., Sugimoto, T. & Mizusawa, H. (1999). ^{123}I-meta-iodobenzylguanidine myocardial scintigraphy in Parkinson's disease. *J. Neurol. Neurosurg. Psychiatry*, **67**, 189–94.

Palace, J., Chandiramani, V.A. & Fowler, C.J. (1997). Value of sphincter EMG in the diagnosis of multiple system atrophy. *Muscle and Nerve*, **20**, 1396–403.

Probst-Cousin, S., Rickert, C.H., Schmid, K.W. & Gullotta, F. (1998). Cell death mechanisms in multiple system atrophy. *J. Neuropath. Experiment. Neurol.*, **57**, 814–21.

Reilly, M.M. & Thomas, P.K. (1999). Amyloid polyneuropathy. In *Autonomic Failure: A Textbook of Clinical Disorders of the Autonomic Nervous System*, ed. C.J. Mathias & R. Bannister, 4th edn., pp. 410–20. Oxford: Oxford University Press.

Schatz, I.J., Bannister, R., Freeman, R.L. et al. (1996). Consensus statement on the definition of orthostatic hypotension, pure autonomic failure and multiple system atrophy. *Clin. Autonom. Res.*, **6**, 125–6.

Schondorf, R. & Low, P.A. (1993). Idiopathic postural tachycardia syndrome: an attenuated form of acute pandysautonomia? *Neurology*, **43**, 132–37.

Schondorf, R. & Freeman, R. (1999). The importance of orthostatic intolerance in the chronic fatigue syndrome. *Am. J. Med. Sci.*, **317**, 117–23.

Shannon, J.R., Flatten, N.L., Jordan, J. et al. (2000). Orthostatic intolerance and tachycardia associated with norepinephrine-transporter deficiency. *N. Eng. J. Med.*, **342**, 541–9.

Smit, A.A., Vermeulen, M., Koelman, J.H. & Wieling, W. (1997). Unusual recovery from acute panautonomic neuropathy after immunoglobulin therapy. *Mayo Clin. Proc.* **72**, 333–5.

Thomaides, T., Chaudhuri, K.R., Maule, S., Watson, L., Marsden, C.D. & Mathias, C.J. (1992). The growth hormone response to clonidine in central and peripheral primary autonomic failure. *Lancet*, **340**, 263–66.

Wallin, B.G., Thompson, J.M., Jennings, G.I. & Esler, M.D. (1996). Renal noradrenaline spillover correlates with muscle sympathetic activity in humans. *J. Physiol. (Lond.)* **491**, 881–7.

Watkins, P.J.K. (1998). The enigma of autonomic failure in diabetes. *J. Roy. Coll. Phys.*, **32**, 360–5.

Watkins, P.J. & Edmunds, M.E. (1999). Diabetic autonomic failure. In *Autonomic Failure. A Textbook of Clinical Disorders of the Autonomic Nervous System*, ed C.J. Mathias & R. Bannister, 4th edn, pp. 378–86. Oxford, UK: Oxford University Press.

Wenning, G.K., Ben-Schlomo, U., Magalhaes, M. Daniel, S.E. & Quinn, N.P. (1994). Clinical features and natural history of multiple system atrophy. An analysis of 100 cases. *Brain*, **117**, 835–45

53

Human brain–gut interactions: mechanisms of swallowing, visceral perception, and anal continence in health and disease

Shaheen Hamdy

Department of GI Science, Hope Hospital, Salford, Manchester, UK

It is now increasingly recognized that the brain plays an important role in modulating gut function. For example, alterations in emotional state can lead to disturbed gastrointestinal symptoms such as diarrhea, dyspepsia and even abdominal pain. Furthermore, alterations in gastrointestinal motility have been described after lesions to the central nervous system, for instance symptoms such as dysphagia after stroke, anal incontinence in cerebrovascular disease and multiple sclerosis and even alterations in small bowel motility following brainstem damage.

In this chapter I will describe current knowledge of human brain–gut interactions both in health and disease in relation to three specific areas: mechanisms of swallowing, mechanisms of anal continence and mechanisms of visceral perception. Particularly, I aim to bring the reader up to date with some newer concepts in relation to the neurophysiology of human cortical swallowing and anal motor function as well as touching on the newer areas of visceral sensitivity and functional bowel disorders. Finally, I will look at future directions specifically looking at potential therapies which may help in disease states that disrupt the human brain–gut axis.

Basic anatomy and physiology of the brain–gut axis

The enteric nervous system

The human brain–gut axis is a complex sensory motor system which has both extrinsic and intrinsic neural elements. At the intrinsic level the enteric nervous system represents an integrative system of neurons and interneurons with structural complexity and functional heterogenicity similar to that of the brain and spinal cord (Gershon, 1981). The principal role of the enteric nervous system

(ENS) is to control and coordinate gut functions, including motility, secretion, mucosal transport and blood flow as necessary for normal digestive processes. These functions are mediated by the ENS via motor neurons located within enteric ganglia which form the final common pathway to the effector cells of the GI tract. The ENS houses a matrix of differing cell populations, which each play a role in maintaining intrinsic gastrointestinal sensory motor activity and include mast cells, smooth muscle cells, interstitial cells of Cajal, enteric enteroenteric cells and motor neurons. These also are subject to the release of various neurotransmitters, growth factors and cytokines which result in an enteric micro-environment that controls GI motility in an autonomous manner.

Vagal and spinal innervation

Whilst the enteric nervous system is almost autonomous it does receive input from extrinsic pathways via the central nervous system (CNS) via both vagal and spinal pathways linking it with the brain and spinal cord (Fig. 53.1). As a result this has led to the concept of the brain–gut axis revolving around both the 'big brain' and the 'little brain' representing the CNS and the ENS, respectively (Aziz & Thompson, 1998). The connecting pathways intervening can be conveniently divided into vagal (para-sympathetic) pathways and spinal (sympathetic) pathways.

Vagal pathways

The vagus nerve conveys a large amount of information between viscera and the brainstem, and contains both afferent and efferent fibres which in man innervate the entire gut as far as the distal third of the colon (Roman & Gonella, 1987). Approximately 90% of fibres within the vagal trunks are unmyelinated afferent neurons with cell bodies located in the nodose ganglion which lies just below

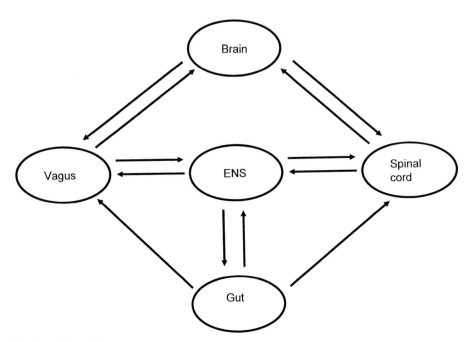

Fig. 53.1. Schematic representation of the intrinsic and extrinsic innervation of the gut.

the jugular foramen. There resides within the nodose ganglia a crude viscerotopic organization corresponding to sensory neurons projecting to soft palate and pharynx located superiorly and those projecting to the stomach, small bowel and lower GI tract which are located more caudally (Altschuler et al., 1989). Afferent fibres from the nodose ganglia then terminate in the brainstem within the medial division of the nucleus tractus solitarius (NTS), where a further viscerotopic organization within distinct subnuclei is displayed. Vagal afferents are believed to mediate non-noxious physiological sensation, such as anxiety and nausea and have a relatively low threshold of response to mechanical and electrical stimulation. There is also increasing evidence that vagal afferents may play a role in the modulation, at least, of nociceptive input from the bowel (Randich & Gebhart, 1992).

The other 10% of the vagal fibres are efferents that project from both the nucleus ambiguous and the dorsal motor nucleus representing the vagal motor nuclei complex. The nucleus ambiguous (NA) is located in the ventrolateral medulla and tends to innervate the striated musculature of the upper GI tract including the pharynx, larynx and upper esophagus and thus plays an important role in the complex motor act of swallowing. By comparison, the dorsal motor nucleus (DMN) of the vagus provides efferents to smooth muscle regions of the gut in association with myenteric plexus neurons. DMN motor neurons display extensive dendritic arborizations allowing some degree of coordination of efferent activity. These dendrites not only innervate specific viscera but also have linkages with NTS resulting in organ specific monosynaptic interactions between the NTS and the DMN and functionally provide the circuitry for 'the vasovagal' reflexes, such as the gastro-gastric reflex, the enterogastric reflex, the hepato-pancreatic reflex and the gastrocolic reflex (Gillis et al., 1989). In both the DMN and NA there is some topographic subnuclei organization both in terms of the striated muscle of the gut in the nucleus ambiguous and in abdominal viscera in the dorsal motor nucleus.

In addition to the vagus there is a second 'parasympathetic' innervation of the GI tract which will be further described in this chapter as sacral pathways. These are projections from pre-ganglionic neurons located in the intermediate grey matter of the sacral cord segments (S1 to S5) and innervate the distal colon, rectum and internal anal sphincter via pelvic ganglia from where postganglionic pelvic nerve fibres innervate the enteric ganglia. As with the vagus, there are both afferent and efferent pathways with the afferent fibres from the colon going via the pelvic nerve afferents to the dorsal root ganglia of the sacral segments. Some of these fibres then send projections to preganglionic neurons to the ENS of the lower colon and result in spinal reflexes that regulate colonic motility and defecation. A somatic component of this innervation is the pudendal nerve which has motor neurons located in the ventral horn of S1 and S2 segments and innervates the external anal sphincter while pudendal afferents relay sensory information from the anal sphincter margin and canal back to the spinal cord.

Spinal pathways

In addition to the vagal pathways innervating the gastrointestinal tract, there are also spinal visceral afferents which have been wrongly termed 'sympathetic' pathways as they pass via prevertebral and paravertebral ganglia of the sympathetic system to the spinal cord but importantly have their cell bodies in the dorsal root ganglia of the cervical, thoracic, and upper lumbar spinal segments. These spinal afferents are predominately unmyelinated C and A-delta fibres and relay predominantly mechanoreceptive and chemical stimuli to a noxious level (Sengupta & Gebhart, 1994). It is important to recognize that considerable segmental overlap exists in the spinal cord in relation to the spinal afferents which partially explains the poor viscerotopic localization of sensation from the GI tract. Furthermore, because there is convergence of such spinal afferents with somatic afferents, the result is some degree of referred pain from a particular organ to a corresponding cutaneous area on the body surface. As with other spinal afferents, visceral spinal afferents are then transmitted proximally within the spinal cord via a number of tracts of which the spinothalamic and the dorsal column pathways are most important. Thus the role of visceral spinal afferents is one predominantly of transmission of nociceptive information; however, it is likely that these afferents have stimulus response functions that cover both physiological and nociceptive ranges of stimulation so that they play the major role in visceral perception and sensitivity.

In addition to spinal afferents there are also associated sympathetic efferent pathways from the cervical, thoracic and lumbar segments of the spinal cord. These have preganglionic and postganglionic synaptic connections the latter of which most prominently represent the celiac and superior mesenteric ganglia and the inferior mesenteric ganglion which innervate the proximal bowel and the distal bowel respectively. It is likely that these sympathetic efferent connections result in an inhibition of GI function and consequently a reduction in motility via the release of acetylcholine.

Supra spinal and higher centre influences on intrinsic and extrinsic neural pathways to the gut

Both the vagal and spinal pathways and consequently the enteric nervous system are under the influence of higher centre regulatory processing. The vagus nerve carries afferent projections via the NTS to higher brain regions via a relay in the pons and medulla, from where there appear to be at least four levels of input. The first are direct projections to autonomic motor nuclei involving both parasympathetic and sympathetic preganglionic neurons in the dorsal motor nucleus and the nucleus ambiguous of the vagus as well as the intermediolateral cell column of the spinal cord. These projections provide the anatomical substrate for short autonomic reflex loops. Secondly, the NTS sends relays to the motor components for ingestion found in the trigeminal, facial, and hypoglossal nuclei and also in the nucleus ambiguous. Thirdly, visceral information is relayed to more rostral regions of the brainstem such as the parabrachial nuclei, which are in turn connected to higher centres. Fourthly, long projections terminate in the thalamus, hypothalamus and limbic and insular cortical regions that mediate autonomic neuroendocrine and behavioural functions. These regions all have reciprocal connections with other brain regions such as the area prostrema, the parabrachial nucleus, hypothalamus, amygdala and the orbitofrontal, insular and inferior limbic and cingulate cortex (Sawchenko, 1983). These connections integrate sensory input arriving from the nucleus of the tractus solitarius with descending influences from higher brain centres and provide the circuitry for visceral reflex loops. This integration presumably results in the orchestration of autonomic reflexes involving GI, cardiovascular and respiratory activities such as that which occur in vomiting. Visceral spinal afferents also project to higher centres via relays in the brainstem and thalamus. From the thalamus, sensory information passes to the insular cortex, the primary somatosensory cortex and the prelimbic, limbic and infra-limbic areas of the medial pre-frontal cortex. It is likely that these pathways are responsible for the integration of somatic and visceral input from wide areas of the body.

Vagal motor pathways also receive direct connections from anterolateral motor strip, premotor cortex, insula and probably a number of other areas including the supplementary motor cortex, all of which have been associated with the motor control of swallowing and other GI functions. In a similar manner, sacral motor pathways appear to have direct connections via cortical spinal tracts from more medial aspects of the motor strip as well as areas similar to that which have already been mentioned to the vagus nerve. Finally, sympathetic efferents are recognized to have connections via projections from the hypothalamus, medial forebrain, anterior sigmoid and orbital and cingulate gyri of the cerebral cortex, which when stimulated can result in inhibition of colonic motility (Rostad, 1973).

Mechanisms of swallowing

The process of swallowing is a complex neuromuscular activity which allows the safe transport of material from the mouth to the stomach for digestion without compromising the airway. This is a fairly simplistic description as the act of swallowing requires a sophisticated integration of both central control and anatomical structures to produce the sensory motor output that we call the swallow. In addition to transporting food, swallowing is also concerned with the protection of the airway, ejection of noxious ingested substances and the preparation of food material. Therefore, when considering swallowing it is important to consider both the anatomy, physiology and the neurophysiology behind this exquisitely complex function.

Anatomy of the swallowing tract

The anatomy of the swallowing tract encompasses the oral cavity, the pharynx which is functionally linked with the larynx and the esophagus. In total, there are at least 32 pairs of muscles which act synergistically to produce the swallow, thereby making it one of the most superior 'reflexes' in the human body. The oral cavity is surrounded by supportive structures including the mandible, maxilla, hard palate and alveolar ridges which house dentition. The mouth itself is enclosed by various muscles including those of mastication and facial expression as well as the intrinsic and extrinsic muscles of the tongue and soft palate. The pharynx supported by pharyngo-basilar fascia comprises three sequentially placed constrictor muscles with the cricopharyngeus distally and stylopharyngeus proximally. Anterior to this, on the anterior wall of the hypopharynx is a cartilaginous box known as the larynx which is surrounded and connected to the hyoid bone and thyroid fascia by the strap muscles of the neck. Intrinsically, the larynx contains eight pairs of muscles of which only two pairs (the aryepiglottic muscles or 'false vocal cords' and the lateral cricoarytenoid muscles or 'true vocal cords') are responsible predominantly for airway protection during swallowing. Extending posteriorly and rostrally is the epiglottis, which forms the base of the tongue and is at its apex connected with the larynx. Beyond the pharynx and the high pressure zone of the upper esophageal sphincter is a 20 cm long muscular tube known as the esophagus. The esophagus consists of predominately striated muscle fibres in its proximal one-third, mixed smooth muscle and striated muscle fibres in its middle third, and predominantly smooth muscle fibres in its distal third which merge with the cardia of the stomach at the level of the lower esophageal sphincter.

The physiological events of swallowing

Swallowing is commonly described as having three distinct phases or stages which comprise the oral phase, the pharyngeal phase and the esophageal phase (Kennedy & Kent, 1988). It was generally thought that the oral phase is voluntary, whereas the pharyngeal and esophageal phases are involuntary; however, it is now accepted that higher inputs can influence both these latter two phases, probably more in a modulatory capacity. Humans swallow on average once every minute which is supplemented by the production of saliva which when absent or reduced inhibits the ability to swallow. Swallowing almost completely tails off during deep (stage 4) sleep but does occur during REM sleep, indicating that a level of arousal is necessary for swallowing to take place (Lichter & Muir, 1975). The oral phase is sometimes described as being preceded by the preparatory phase, particularly when solid or semisolid foods are ingested. Mastication and mixing with saliva occurs at this point and the bolus is then cupped in the anterior portion of the tongue before being propelled by an upward and compressing force initiated by the tongue against the hard palate to 'squeeze' the bolus into the pharynx. During this phase, the soft palate rises to seal off the naso-pharynx and thus completes the oral phase which lasts 0.6 to 1.2 seconds.

The pharyngeal phase typically begins as the bolus reaches the faucial pillars of the hypopharynx. Simultaneously, the larynx and hyoid bone are lifted upwards and forwards by contraction of the strap muscles of the neck and in so doing enlarges the space available for the pharynx to receive the incoming bolus. The bolus is then propelled aborally by sequential contractions of the constrictor muscles of the pharynx and this is associated with a reflex relaxation of the normally high toned upper esophageal sphincter to allow passage of the bolus into the esophagus. During transport through the pharynx, respiration is momentarily halted, the swallow usually occurring whilst in expiration. Concurrently, a protective mechanism of aryepiglottic fold closure and approximation of the arytenoid and epiglottic cartilage by contraction of the intrinsic muscles of the larynx then occurs. The whole pharyngeal phase usually takes less than 0.6 seconds.

Thus commences the esophageal phase of swallowing which comprises a propagated peristaltic wave which propels the bolus at approximately 2 to 4 cm per second. As the bolus passes through the esophageal body, the lower esophageal sphincter relaxes and the bolus enters the stomach, the esophageal phase lasts between 6 and 10 seconds, and the whole process of swallowing usually 12 seconds in total.

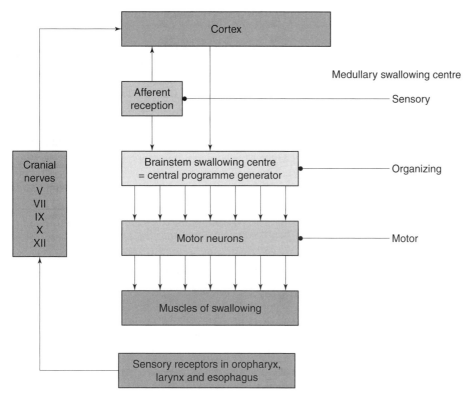

Fig. 53.2. The hierarchical organization of the central regulation of swallowing. Input from the periphery and higher centres converge onto interneurons in the brainstem swallowing centre, which generates the sequenced pattern of swallowing via the bulbar motor nuclei.

The neurophysiology of swallowing

The central neural control of swallowing can be divided into essentially three basic components: an afferent system, a central processor and regulating system and an efferent system (Fig. 53.2). At this point it is important to emphasize that the central processing system has at least three levels including the brainstem swallowing centre, subcortical structures and the cortex itself.

The afferent system

Afferent input comes from three cranial nerves innervating the muscles of the swallowing tract and includes the trigeminal nerve, the glossopharyngeal nerve and the vagus nerve, of which its superior laryngeal branch appears to have most importance. Stimulation of any of these nerves can initiate or modulate a swallow (Miller, 1982). These afferent fibres terminate centrally at the level of the brainstem in the tractus solitarius and in the nucleus of the spinal trigeminal system before converging in the NTS. There is however, a second projection which ascends via a pontine relay to the level of the cortex without transgress-

ing the NTS (Car et al., 1975). The most potent trigger for swallowing is the superior laryngeal nerve which is only matched by direct stimulation of the nucleus of the tractus solitarius, suggesting that the solitary system is a major contributor of swallowing afferent input (Jean, 1984). Importantly, anesthesia of areas innervated by these cranial nerve afferents will disrupt but will not necessarily completely abolish the ability to swallow (Mansson & Sandberg, 1974). Sensation from the oral, pharyngeal and laryngeal regions includes a broad range of modalities including two point discrimination, vibrotactile detection, somesthetic sensitivity, proprioception, nociception, chemical sensitivity and thermal sensitivity (Miller, 1999). The oral, pharyngeal and laryngeal mucosae possess an epithelium innervated by both free nerve endings and within deeper layers more organised sensory receptors. Of interest there appear to be chemosensitive receptors that are specifically water responsive which will not trigger at isotonic levels. There also appear to be different groups of cold responsive sensory fibres which discharge at around 25 to 30 °C. Mechanical stimuli appear to be the most effective stimuli for exciting NTS neurons within receptive fields of the oral cavity and epiglottis, a moving mechanical stimulus excites more neurons than a static stimulus. When comparing the receptive field responsiveness within the oral cavity, it appears that mechanical stimulation is more potent than chemical stimulation which in turn is greater than thermal stimulation (Miller, 1999).

The efferent system

The efferent system comprises motor neuron pools, consisting of the facial motor nucleus, the hypoglossal motor nucleus, the trigeminal motor nucleus, and the vagal motor nuclei. Inputs from the brainstem central pattern generator and from supra-bulbar regions impinge on these motor nuclei in a manner which synergistically produces the swallow. The cranial motor nuclei mentioned above have subdivisions based on the motor neurons innervating specific muscles. The facial motor nucleus is involved with the labial muscles for which there are several functions both in swallowing and speech as well as chewing. The hypoglossal nucleus contains the motor neurons innervating the intrinsic and extrinsic muscles of the tongue, which are involved in numerous motor functions including speech, respiration, licking, mastication as well as swallowing. The trigeminal motor nucleus contains the motor neuron pools that innervate the mandibular muscles and can be divided into four nuclei which appear to develop at different times during development in the fetus (Miller, 1999). The nucleus ambiguous is also subdivided into at least four layers including the compact layer, semicompact layer, the loose layer and the external formation. These motor neurons innervate the palatal, pharyngeal, laryngeal and esophageal muscles. Finally the dorsal motor nucleus of the vagus contains neurons that innervate the esophagus and portions of the proximal gastrointestinal tract. It appears that the earliest motor neuron to develop during swallowing in the fetus is probably the hypoglossal nerve (Miller, 1999) as tongue activities are present in the fetus at about the same time as the jaw opening reflex. Indeed by the eleventh week of development of the human fetus, the first pharyngeal motor responses can also be detected.

Whilst lesions to the facial motor nucleus do not implicitly result in dysphagia, lesions to the nucleus ambiguous and to a lesser extent the hypoglossal and trigeminal motor nuclei result in more significant dysphagic symptoms (Miller, 1999). Thus, as a result of input from the NTS and higher centres to the dorsal region of the medulla and the brainstem swallowing centre, motoneurons in this region will provide the patterned sequential discharge activating the oral pharyngeal and esophageal phases of swallowing.

Central and supra-bulbar regulatory systems

Brainstem swallowing centre

Much of the research pertaining to the central regulation of human swallowing has focused on the issue of the brainstem swallowing centre. This important swallowing region is central to the regulation of human swallowing and is distributed within the reticular formation just dorsal to the inferior olive either side of the midline in the medulla (Jean, 1990). It is believed that this network of neurons and interneurons integrates incoming information from other levels, both central and peripheral, before activating a pre-programmed sequence of responses which then dictate the pattern of swallowing. The concept of a central pattern generator within the brainstem is supported by the fact that even after disruption of both afferent and efferent fibres to this region, the pattern of swallowing remains essentially unchanged when studied in animals (Jean, 1990).

It appears that the circuitry of the central pattern generator has different populations of interneurons responsible for the different temporal stages of swallowing and termed 'early' 'late' and 'very late' neurons which closely correspond to their muscular counterparts within the oropharynx, lower pharynx and striated muscle portion of the esophagus, and the smooth muscle esophagus respectively (Jean, 1984). Functionally, it appears that the brainstem swallowing centre can be divided into two, the dorsal medullary region and the ventral medullary region. The dorsal medullary region provides the neurons that initiate the sequential activity of swallowing and can be defined as generating neurons. The ventral medullary region which includes an area around the nucleus ambiguous appears to play a switching role in modifying and activating the motor neuron pools controlling swallowing output. In between these two regions there is a short interneuronal network that has both excitatory and inhibitory components and which relays information from the dorsal region to the ventral region.

Within both regions of the medulla there are a number of neurotransmitter substances which appear to have relevant roles (Bieger, 1993); for example, the injection of glutamate into the dorsal region of the brainstem evokes pharyngeal swallowing suggesting that it is excitatory. By comparison, injection of dopamine or noradrenalin appears to inhibit the elicitation of pharyngeal swallowing. It also appears likely that gamma-aminobutyric acid, acetylcholine, n-methyl D-aspartate and nitric oxide probably play an important role in the inhibitory and excitatory regulation of swallowing.

In addition to the medullary brainstem swallowing centre, there appears to be a separate area within the pontine reticular formation which will also when stimulated evoke swallowing. This region, when stimulated at low intensity will evoke both swallowing and rhythmic jaw movements but at high intensity results in more inhibitory effects. It is likely that pathways from the afferent innervation of swallowing project to this region as well as the medullary area on their way to the antero-lateral cortex. Activation of the pontine region may in fact result in a transcortical reflex to evoke the swallow rather than the pontine area being directly involved in the initiation of swallowing.

Supra-bulbar regions influencing swallowing

There is extensive experimental evidence to support the role of subcortical structures in the control and modulation of swallowing (Bieger & Hochman, 1976). These regions can be anatomically divided into the hindbrain, comprising the cerebellum, the midbrain, comprising the substantia nigra and the ventral tegmentum and basal forebrain, comprising the hypothalamus, amygdala and basal ganglia. In animals, activation of all these sites has been shown to facilitate the swallow response when combined with either superior laryngeal nerve stimulation or cortical stimulation. Evidence from human studies also suggests an important contribution from subcortical areas, such as the basal ganglia, where dysphagia is a common consequence of Parkinson's disease (Bernheimer et al., 1973). In a recent functional imaging study of human swallowing it was demonstrated that areas including the left amygdala and the left cerebellum as well as the dorsal brainstem show increased regional cerebral blood flow during volitional swallowing (Hamdy et al., 1999). The lateralized nature of these activations was of interest and supported the possibility that swallowing displays significant interhemispheric asymmetry in its motor control.

The cerebral cortex has been strongly implicated in the control of swallowing where numerous investigators have observed a stimulation of the cerebral cortex both in animals and humans can elicit the full swallow sequence (Martin & Sessle, 1993; Penfield & Boldery, 1937). The areas implicated in these studies seem to be the dorsolateral and antero-lateral frontal cortex as well as the premotor cortex, the frontal operculum and also the insula. Much of the information regarding the cerebral localization of human swallowing has relied on inference from studies of swallowing abnormalities following cerebral injury (Veis & Logemann, 1985; Gordon et al., 1987; Horner & Massey, 1988). From these reports a rather diffuse picture has emerged of those areas of the brain considered important, for example, lesions located in the thalamus, pyramidal tracts, frontal operculum and the insula have all been associated with dysphagia. More recently, functional imaging has also established a clear role for the lateral sensorimotor cortex and, in particular, the right insula during the process of swallowing (Hamdy et al., 1999). More information has come from the studies of transcranial magnetic stimulation of the human precentral gyrus in understanding the cortical control of swallowing (Hamdy et al., 1996, 1997b, 1998a). Transcranial magnetic stimulation uses a very short rapidly changing magnetic field to induce electric current in the brain beneath the stimulator. These studies usually employ single shocks given several seconds apart and, following stimulation, the cortical evoked motor response can be recorded as electromyographic activity from electrodes housed within an intraluminal catheter inserted into pharynx and esophagus. Following cortical stimulation, the type of response observed is usually a simple EMG potential which has a latency of about 8 to 10 milliseconds, compatible with a fairly direct and rapidly conducting pathway from cortex to the muscle (Fig. 53.3). During these magnetic stimulation mapping studies the projections to the various swallowing muscles were demonstrated to be somatotopically arranged in the motor strip with the oral muscles most lateral and the pharynx and esophagus more medial. A more interesting finding from a large group of healthy subjects studied was that in the majority of individuals, the projection from one hemisphere tended to be larger than the other suggesting an asymmetric representation for swallowing between the two hemispheres, independent of handedness. These findings have also been validated with functional imaging techniques such as positron emission tomography (PET) and functional magnetic resonance imaging (fMRI) where cerebral lateralization has been also observed (Hamdy et al., 1996, 1999). These functional imaging studies have, however, identified a number of other cortical areas associated with swallowing including anterior cingulate cortex, premotor cortex (including the supplementary motor cortex), the insular cortex, frontal opercular cortex and the temporal cortex. Taken together these observations suggest that swallow-related cortical activity is multidimensional, recruiting brain areas implicated in the processing of motor, sensory and presumably attention/affective aspects of the task.

Swallowing dysfunction after injury to the central nervous system

Difficulty in swallowing can occur as a consequence of disease to either the anatomical structures involved in swallowing or more commonly to the central nervous system controlling swallowing (neurogenic dysphagia).

Right hemisphere   **Left hemisphere**

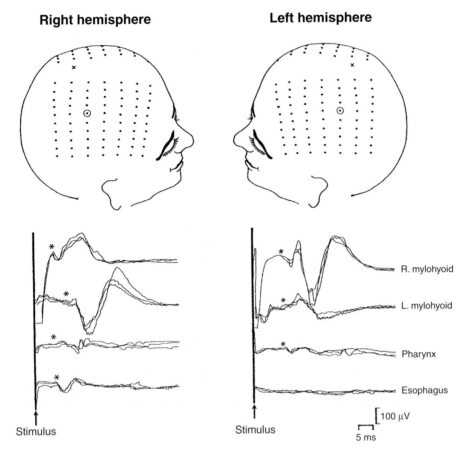

Fig. 53.3. Schematic representations of the sites of stimulation on a scalp grid in relation to the head surface are shown above. The cranial vertex is marked by X. The cortically evoked EMG responses recorded in one normal subject from: right mylohyoid muscle, left mylohyoid muscle, pharynx, and esophagus, following transcranial magnetic stimulation of the right and left hemispheres are shown below. The sites of stimulation on the grid from which these responses were obtained are indicated by the open circle. Responses to three stimuli have been superimposed to show reproducibility. It is evident, however, that the pharyngeal and esophageal responses obtained from the right hemisphere are larger than those from the left hemisphere. (* indicates onset of EMG response.)

The anatomical problems which disrupt swallowing are myriad and include almost any gastrointestinal disease process which affects the oral cavity through to the duodenum. It is therefore important to exclude any intrinsic disease to the gut before making a diagnosis of neurogenic dysphagia in someone presenting with symptoms of swallowing difficulty.

There are many neurological conditions that can disrupt swallowing including diseases of the muscle or neuro muscular junction, e.g. polymyositis, myasthenia gravis and the muscular dystrophies; diseases of the peripheral nerves, e.g. Guillain–Barré syndrome, polio and diptheria; and disease affecting the central swallowing centres, e.g. stroke, head injuries, motor neuron disease, Parkinson's disease, multiple sclerosis and other neurologic diseases. In addition, it is important to recognise that any pharmac-

ological agent which alters neuromuscular function can produce dysphagia. It is beyond the scope of this chapter to go into detail of the many neurological conditions which can affect swallowing and for the rest of this section I will discuss the clinical consequences and underlining mechanisms related to dysphagia following cerebrovascular disease, specifically stroke.

Injury to swallowing areas of motor cortex and/or their connections to the brainstem will usually result in problems with swallowing (dysphagia). The commonest reason for dysphagia is now stroke. Traditionally, it had been assumed that only strokes producing brainstem or bilateral cortical damage are associated with dysphagia; however, since the 1970s it has been increasingly recognized that unilateral cerebral lesions can also cause dysphagia (Barer, 1989; Meadows, 1973; Daniels & Foundas,

1997). Up to half of all stroke patients experience dysphagia, which is associated with the life-threatening complications of pulmonary aspiration and malnutrition. Dysphagia leads to increased lengths of stay in hospital and greater demands on health service resources.

Diagnosing dysphagia following cerebral injury can be difficult and therefore requires a high level of clinical suspicion. The pattern of disordered swallowing after stroke is usually a combination of oral and pharyngeal abnormalities, typically delayed swallow reflex with pooling or stasis of residue in the hypopharynx associated with reduced pharyngeal peristalsis and weak tongue control but occasionally esophageal abnormalities may be apparent. Clinical suspicion of swallowing difficulty should be followed up by thorough bedside swallowing assessment and where appropriate imaging of the swallowing process such as videofluoroscopy. The bedside examination incorporates a number of clinical measures including assessment of the patient's feeding status, posture, breathing and cooperation levels before examining the patients oral musculature, oral reflexes, pharyngeal swallow and usually a trial feed with 5 to 10 ml of water given either by spoon or in a beaker. The bedside assessment is cheap and relatively easy to perform and has the advantage of involving no radiation exposure. However, it lacks sensitivity and does not give detailed information of the pharyngeal stage of swallowing making it prone to missing significant aspiration, especially silent aspiration. When the diagnosis is in doubt, videofluoroscopy can give a detailed anatomical assessment of the pharyngeal swallow and has the advantage of detecting silent aspiration and other abnormalities of the swallow anatomy. However it is expensive, involves radiation and uses a non-physiological medium i.e. barium, which may not give a true picture of the patients swallowing performance. A recent advance is the introduction of flexible endoscopic evaluation of swallowing (FEES). FEES involves the passing of a nasoendoscope into the oropharynx while a small volume of a coloured physiological meal or liquid is ingested. This allows the anatomy of the pharyngeal swallow to be directly visualized and the swallowing mechanism assessed.

The management of dysphagia after stroke is therefore critical. With severe dysphagia the risk of aspiration is high and the patient is therefore kept nil by mouth with early commencement of parenteral fluids. With less severe dysphagia, based upon videofluoroscopic and bedside swallowing assessment outcomes, there are a number of therapeutic interventions which can be tried. These interventions include changing diet, posture and food placement adjustment as well as methods for sensitizing or de-sensitizing the oropharynx to alter the swallow reflex.

Unfortunately, the efficacy of these therapeutic manoeuvres is a matter of some controversy: at present there are no randomized controlled trials of these interventions to show proven efficacy in improving the swallow after stroke. Consequently, patients often require nasogastric tube or gastrostomy feeding until swallowing improves spontaneously.

Mechanism for dysphagia following stroke

Whilst it is relatively easy to appreciate the mechanisms behind dysphagia following bilateral cortical stroke or brainstem disease the mechanism underlying dysphagia after unilateral cerebral injury particularly after hemispheric injury has remained unclear. Speculated suggestions include occult disease in the unaffected hemisphere, cerebral edema leading to pressure on the adjacent hemisphere or brainstem, and the possibility that swallowing, like speech, may show significant cerebral lateralization. Indeed, in a transcranial magnetic stimulation study of the projections from both hemispheres to the swallowing musculature in a large series of pure unilateral hemispheric stroke patients, of which half had dysphagia, it was observed that whilst stimulation of the damaged hemisphere produced little or no response in either dysphagic or non-dysphagic patients, stimulation of the undamaged hemisphere evoked much larger responses in the non-dysphagic than in the dysphagic subjects (Hamdy et al., 1997a). The conclusion from this study was that the size of the hemispheric projection of the undamaged side to swallowing muscles determined the presence or absence of dysphagia with the implication that dysphagia would occur if damage had affected the side of the brain with the largest or dominant projection. This observation supported the concept that swallowing is lateralized within the cerebral cortex.

Mechanisms of recovery of swallowing after cerebral injury

Given sufficient time, a large proportion of dysphagic stroke patients eventually recover the ability to swallow again (Barer, 1989). The mechanism for this recovery, seen in as many as 90% of the initially dysphagic stroke patients has, however, remained controversial. In a recent study of stroke using transcranial magnetic stimulation both dysphagic and non-dysphagic patients were serially mapped over several months while swallowing recovered (Hamdy et al., 1998a). The findings of this study showed that the area of pharyngeal representation in the undamaged hemisphere increased markedly in patients who recovered whilst there was no change in patients who had persistent dysphagia or in patients who were non-dysphagic. Furthermore no changes were seen in the damaged hemisphere in any of the groups of patients. These observations imply that over a period of weeks, the recovery of swallowing after stroke depends on compensatory reorganization in the undamaged hemisphere. The situation appears to differ from that in the limb muscles where some magnetic stimulation studies have indicated that limb recovery after hemiparesis is more likely to result from an increase in the activity of the remaining viable cortex in the damaged hemisphere (Turton et al., 1996). In such cases, scope for expansion of a normal connection from the undamaged part of the brain may be a limiting factor in recovery.

Mechanisms of anal continence

The anal sphincter is a midline muscular structure at the terminus of the gastrointestinal tract that functions to maintain fecal continence. It has two components, the internal sphincter and the external sphincter. Whereas the internal anal sphincter consists of circular smooth muscle and is innervated predominately by autonomic fibres from the pelvic plexus and sacral spinal cord, the external sphincter is of striated muscle and is innervated by the somatic fibres of the second, third and fourth sacral segments via the pudendal nerve. The neural control of anal continence therefore has sensorimotor contributions from both intrinsic and extrinsic reflexes, the former predominately via myenteric interaction within the internal anal sphincter, and the latter via strong descending volitional interactions with the motor neurons innervating the external anal sphincter (Christensen, 1983).

The neurophysiology of anal continence

Anal continence represents an important physiological and socially essential gastrointestinal function which is regulated by sensorimotor interactions within the anal sphincter and pelvic floor. In particular, contraction of the external anal sphincter serves to increase anal canal pressure both voluntarily, when the urge to defecate becomes strong and via more involuntary reflexes, for instance during coughing when intra abdominal pressure suddenly rises. In either case, the cerebral cortex is able to modulate this activity via powerful descending inputs to the pelvic plexus and sacral nerves so defecation can be resisted until a socially convenient opportunity arises. The importance of cortical influences in the control of the external anal sphincter is well recognized, direct stimulation of the most medial motor cortex adjacent to the interhemispheric fissure will induce anal sphincter contractions (Leyton & Sherrington, 1917). More recent experiments in humans have shown that the corticofugal pathways to the external anal sphincter can be studied non-invasively by recording the electro-myographic and manometric responses evoked by transcranial electric and magnetic stimulation of the motor cortex (Merton et al., 1982; Turnbull et al., 1999). These studies have suggested that the motor cortical representation of anal sphincter function is bilateral and may display, as with swallowing, an interhemispheric asymmetry.

The peripheral innervation of the external anal sphincter comes from the pudendal nerve. Anatomical and electrical physiological studies of the innervation of the external anal sphincter in animals has shown that most of the pudendal projections to and from the external anal sphincter are centrally organized to spinal segments L6 to S3 with the majority with the S1, S2 segments (Thor et al., 1989). Furthermore the motor neurons innervating the external anal sphincter, are particularly located in the dorsomedial and ventromedial divisions of Onuf's nucleus in the ventral horn of the spinal cord while the afferent axonal projections appear to cluster within the marginal zone, intermediate grey and dorsal grey surrounding the nucleus gracile of the dorsal column and laminal 1, around the dorsal horn of the spinal cord. Of interest is the observation that, while there is clear unilateral spinal predominance of these projections during retrograde tracing studies of a single nerve, in both the efferent and afferent pathways, there is contralateral axonal connectivity across the midline, suggesting degrees of bilateral convergence. In a recent study of pudendal nerve function it was found in a number of healthy volunteers that the evoked muscle potential to pudendal nerve stimulation can be quite asymmetric between the two sides (Hamdy et al., 1999). Furthermore, when pudendal or even lumbar sacral stimulation was used to condition the peripheral pathway, cortical stimulation of the anal region of the motor strip induced much greater responses in the anal sphincter compared to no conditioning (Hamdy et al., 1998b). Importantly, stimulation of the pudendal nerve with the larger response induced significantly more facilitation of the cortico-anal pathway than stimulation of the pudendal with the smaller response. This suggested that there may indeed be some functional asymmetry in the pudendal pathways to the anal sphincter possibly in conjunction with asymmetry at higher levels.

Anal incontinence

Anal incontinence represents a distressing complication of disease to the central nervous system, for example injury to the pelvic nerves, as in instrumental deliveries at child birth, will result in significant anal sphincter dysfunction, as well as disruption of the brain–gut axis from cortex to sphincter seen in conditions such as stroke, multiple sclerosis and spinal injury. In the case of the former, anal incontinence has been attributed to pudendal nerve damage where a number of studies have shown clear abnormalities in pudendal nerve function (as determined by prolonged nerve conduction terminal latency) in incontinent female patients following vaginal delivery both with and without instrumental intervention (Snooks et al., 1984). It is important to mention at this stage that more detailed evaluation of these patients, however, often reveals underlying anatomical defects of the anal sphincter as a consequence of the delivery and which also explains the incontinence in many cases (Sultan et al., 1993). Nonetheless electrophysiologic assessment of pudendal nerve function remains of some importance as this parameter may be clinically relevant in differentiating patients with fecal leakage from solid stool incontinence and there exist patients without external anal sphincter defects who have significant continence problems and whose only demonstrable abnormality is that of pudendal neuropathy.

Fecal incontinence can present in the setting of central nervous system damage such as in patients with stroke or frontal lobe damage, for example it has been demonstrated that the fecal incontinence is strongly associated with larger strokes and particularly when the cerebral cortex is involved (Nakayama et al., 1997). Fecal incontinence is also frequently encountered in patients with multiple sclerosis and one survey of anorectal function in subjects with multiple sclerosis has suggested that there may be central motor mechanisms involved (Jameson et al., 1994).

Functional bowel disorders

An increasingly common condition seen by both general practitioners and hospital doctors is that of functional bowel disorder, of which the most important is irritable bowel syndrome. This and its associated conditions including non-ulcer dyspepsia, non-cardiac chest pain and proctalgia are likely to have some degree of commonality in both their physiological mechanisms and treatment approaches. Irritable bowel syndrome (IBS) has often been characterized into a syndrome consisting of abdominal pain or discomfort for at least 12 weeks in the preceding 12 months and two of the following: pain relief with defecation; onset associated with change in frequency of stool; onset associated with change in form (appearance of) stool. As many as 15% of all people expe-

rience a mild version of irritable bowel syndrome although only a small minority seek medical care. The speculated underlying mechanisms behind irritable bowel include a disturbance of colonic motility, visceral hyper-algesia and an abnormality of processing sensory information from the gut within the cerebral cortex (Mayer & Raybould, 1990). Whilst the pathophysiology of IBS remains a matter of controversy it is likely that the condition is multifactorial involving all three potential mechanisms as well as other factors including genetics, environment, psychological factors including life stress, psychological state, coping mechanisms and social support. Therefore, the treatment of functional bowel disorders such as IBS revolves around both psychologic and pharmacological treatments. These include education and reassurance, potential lifestyle and dietary modifications and then pharmacological agents, which may act on gut motility and sensation, such as either laxatives or antidiarrheal agents and for more severe cases, psychological treatment including antidepressants.

Future directions in human brain–gut interactions

With the advent of functional non-invasive brain imaging techniques it is likely that future understanding of the mechanisms underlying visceral sensitivity, functional bowel disorders and indeed understanding mechanisms behind dysphagia after cerebral injury and incontinence after central nervous system injury will be further elucidated. For example, it has been recently demonstrated that sensory stimulation of the pharynx can induce reorganizational changes in swallowing areas of the motor cortex which outlast the period of stimulation by several minutes (Hamdy et al., 1998a,b,c). The changes recorded to pharyngeal stimulation appear reminiscent of the spontaneous changes associated with swallowing recovery after stroke. It is possible therefore that sensory stimulation techniques may hold an attractive therapeutic approach for treating dysphagia after stroke. Furthermore, lumbo-sacral stimulation which normally induces sphincter contraction in the external anal sphincter, may in future play a role in conditioning anal sphincter muscles in a way which aids anal function in patients with fecal incontinence. Finally functional imaging techniques such as fMRI and PET as well as magnetoencephalography may also allow the dissection of mechanisms underlying functional bowel disorders including influences such as emotion, attention and other psychological constructs. The ability of PET studies to provide ligand information on the neuropharmacology of the brain processing of visceral sensation as well as the motor control of swallowing and anal continence may well allow future drug treatment to be developed which may be able to target abnormal processing of visceral areas with a view to either enhancing function or blocking aberrant function within the human brain–gut axis.

References   * denotes key references

*Altschuler, S.M., Bao, X., Bieger, D., Hopkins, D.A. & Miselis, R.R. (1989). Viscerotopic representation of the upper alimentary tract in the rat: sensory ganglia and nuclei of the solitary and spinal trigeminal tracts. *J. Comp. Neurol.*, **283**, 248–68.

*Aziz, Q. & Thompson, D.G. (1998). The brain–gut axis in health and disease. *Gastroenterology*, **114**, 559–78.

Barer, D.G. (1989). The natural history and functional consequences of dysphagia after hemispheric stroke. *J. Neurol. Neurosurg., Psychiatry*, **52**, 236–41.

Bernheimer, H., Birkmayer, H. & Hornkiewicz, R. (1973). Brain dopamine and the syndromes of Parkinson and Huntington; clinical, morphological and neurochemical correlations. *J. Neurol. Sci.*, **20**, 415–55.

Bieger, D. & Hockman, C.H. (1976). Suprabulbar modulation of reflex swallowing. *Exp. Neurol.*, **52**, 311–24.

Bieger, D. (1993). Central nervous system control mechanisms of swallowing: a neuropharmacological perspective. *Dysphagia*, **8**(4), 308–10.

Car, A., Jean, A. & Roman, C. (1975). A pontine primary relay for ascending projections of the superior laryngeal nerve. *Exp. Brain Res.*, **22**, 197–210.

Christensen, J. (1983). Motility of the colon. In *Physiology of the Gastrointestinal Tract*, ed. L.R. Johnson, pp. 445–72. New York: Raven.

Daniels, S.K. & Foundas, A.L. (1997). The role of the insular cortex in dysphagia. *Dysphagia*, **12**, 146–56.

Gershon, M.D. (1981). The enteric nervous system. *Ann. Rev. Neurosci.*, **4**, 227–72.

Gillis, R.A., Quest, J.A., Pagini, F.D. & Norman, W.P. (1989). Control of centres in the central nervous system for regulating gastrointestinal motility. In *Handbook of Physiology*. Section 6. *The Gastrointestinal System*, ed. S.G. Schultz, J.D. Wood & B.B. Rauner, pp. 621–83. New York: Oxford University.

Gordon, C., Langton-Hewer, R. & Wade, D.T. (1987). Dysphagia in acute stroke. *Br. Med. J.*, **295**, 411–14.

*Hamdy, S., Aziz, Q., Rothwell, J.C. et al. (1996). The cortical topography of human swallowing musculature in health and disease. *Nat. Med.*, **2**, 1217–24.

Hamdy, S., Aziz, Q., Rothwell, J.C. et al. (1997a). Explaining oropharyngeal dysphagia after unilateral hemispheric stroke. *Lancet*, **250**, 686–92.

Hamdy, S., Aziz, Q., Rothwell, J.C., Hobson, A., Barlow, J. & Thompson, D.G. (1997b). Cranial nerve modulation of human cortical swallowing motor pathways. *Am. J. Physiol.*, **272**, G802–8.

*Hamdy, S., Aziz, Q., Rothwell, J.C. et al. (1998a). Recovery of swallowing after dysphagic stroke relates to functional reorganisation in intact motor cortex. *Gastroenterology*, **5**, 1104–12.

Hamdy, S., Enck, P., Aziz, Q. et al. (1998b). Spinal and pudendal nerve modulation of human cortico-anal motor pathways. *Am. J. Physiol.*, **274**, G419–23.

*Hamdy, S., Rothwell, J.C., Aziz, Q., Singh, K.D. & Thompson, D.G. (1998c). Long-term reorganisation of human motor cortex driven by short-term sensory stimulation. *Nat. Neurosci.*, **1**(1), 64–8.

Hamdy, S., Enck, P., Aziz, Q., Uengorgil, S., Hobson, A. & Thompson, D.G. (1999). Laterality effects of human pudendal nerve stimulation on cortico-anal pathways: Evidence for functional asymmetry. *Gut*, **45**, 58–63.

Hamdy, S., Mikulis, D.J., Crawley, A. et al. (1999). Cortical activation during human volitional swallowing: an event related fMRI study. *Am. J. Physiol.*, **277**, G219–25.

Hamdy, S., Rothwell, J.C., Brooks, D.J. et al. (1999). Identification of the cerebral loci processing human swallowing using H_2O^{15} PET activation. *J. Neurophysiol.*, **81**, 1917–26.

Horner, J. & Massey, E.W. (1988). Silent aspiration following stroke. *Neurology*, **38**, 317–19.

Jameson, J.S., Rogers, J., Chia, Y.W., Misiewicz, J.J., Henry, M.M. & Swash, M. (1994). Pelvic floor function in multiple sclerosis. *Gut*, **35**, 388–90.

Jean, A. (1984). Brainstem organisation of the swallowing network. *Brain Behav. Evol.*, **25**, 109–16.

*Jean, A. (1990). Brainstem control of swallowing: localisation and organisation of central pattern generator of swallowing. In Neurophysiol. Jaws Teeth, ed. A. Taylor, pp. 294–321. London: MacMillan Press.

Kennedy, J.G. & Kent, R.D. (1988). Physiological substrates of normal deglutition. *Dysphagia*, **3**, 24–37.

Leyton, A.S.F. & Sherrington, C.S. (1917). Observations on the excitable cortex of the chimpanzee, orangutan and gorilla. *Q. J. Exp. Physiol.*, **11**, 135–222.

Lichter, J. & Muir, R.C. (1975). The pattern of swallowing during sleep. *Electroencephalog. Clin. Neurophysiol.*, **38**, 427–32.

Mansson, I. & Sandberg, N. (1974). Effects of surface anaesthesia on deglutition in man. *Laryngoscope*, **84**, 427–37.

*Martin, R.E. & Sessle, B.J. (1993). The role of the cerebral cortex in swallowing. *Dysphagia*, **8**, 195–202.

*Mayer, E.A. & Raybould, H.E. (1990). Role of visceral afferent mechanisms in functional bowel disorders. *Gastroenterology*, **99**, 1688–704.

Meadows, J. (1973). Dysphagia in unilateral cerebral lesions. *J. Neurol., Neurosurg., Psychiatry*, **36**, 853–60.

Merton, P.A., Morton, H.B., Hill, D.K. & Marsden, C.D. (1982). Scope of a technique for electrical stimulation of the human brain, spinal cord and muscle. *Lancet*, **2**, 597–600.

*Miller, A.J. (1982). Deglutition. *Physiol. Rev.*, **52**, 129–84.

Miller, A.J. (1999). *The Neuroscientific Principles of Swallowing and Dysphagia*. San Diego: Singular Publishing Group, Inc.

Nakayama, H., Jorgensen, H.S., Pedersen, P.M., Raaschou, H.O. & Olsen, T.S. (1997). Prevalence and risk factors of incontinence after stroke. *Stroke*, **28**, 58–62.

Penfield, W. & Boldery, E. (1937). Somatic motor and sensory representation in the cerebral cortex of man as studied by electrical stimulation. *Brain*, **60**, 389–443.

Randich, A. & Gebhart, G.F. (1992). Vagal afferent modulation of nociception. *Brain Res. Rev.*, **17**, 77–99.

Roman, C. & Gonella, J. (1987). Extrinsic control of digestive tract motility. In *Physiology of the Gastrointestinal Tract*, 2nd edn, ed. L.R. Johnson, pp. 507–53. New York: Raven.

Rostad, H. (1973). Colon motility in the cat. IV. Peripheral pathways mediating the effects induced by hypothalamic and mesencephalic stimulation. *Acta Physiol. Scand.*, **89**, 154–68.

Sawchenko, P.E. (1983). Central connections of the sensory and motor nuclei of the vagus nerve. *J. Auton. Nerv. Syst.*, **9**, 13–26.

Sengupta, J.N. & Gebhart, G.F. (1994). Gastrointestinal afferent fibres and sensation. In *Physiology of the Gastrointestinal Tract*, 3rd edn, ed. L.R. Johnson, pp. 483–519. New York: Raven.

*Snooks, S.J., Setchell, M., Swash, M. & Henry, M.M. (1984). Injury to innervation of pelvic floor musculature in childbirth. *Lancet*, **ii**, 546–50.

*Sultan, A.H., Kamm, M.A., Hudson, C.N., Thomas, J.M. & Bartram, C.I. (1993). Anal sphincter disruption during vaginal delivery. *N. Engl. J. Med.*, **329**(26), 1905–11.

Thor, K.B., Morgan, C., Nadelhaft, I., Houston, M. & De Groat, W.C. (1989). Organization of afferent and efferent pathways in the pudendal nerve of the female cat. *J. Comp. Neurol.*, **288**, 263–79.

*Turnbull, G.K., Hamdy, S., Aziz, Q., Singh, K.D. & Thompson, D.G. (1999). The cortical topography of human ano-rectal musculature. *Gastroenterology*, **117**, 32–9.

Turton, A., Wroe, S., Trepte, N., Fraser, C. & Lemon, R.N. (1996). Contralateral and ipsilateral EMG responses to transcranial magnetic stimulation during recovery of arm and hand function after stroke. *Electroencephalog. Clin. Neurophysiol.*, **101**(4), 316–28.

Veis, S.L. & Logemann, J.S. (1985). Swallowing disorders in persons with cerebrovascular accident. *Arch. Phys. Med. Rehabil.*, **66**, 372–5.

54

Eating disorders: neurobiology and symptomatology

David C. Jimerson and Barbara E. Wolfe

Department of Psychiatry, Beth Israel Deaconess Medical Center and Harvard Medical School, Boston, MA, USA

The 1990s have witnessed a remarkable upsurge in research on neurochemical pathways in the central nervous system (CNS) that contribute to the regulation of food intake and body weight homeostasis. These investigations have been driven in part by increasing recognition that obesity, anorexia nervosa and bulimia nervosa represent major public health concerns. Moreover, advances in molecular neurobiology have accelerated the identification of new peptides, proteins and their receptors in the hypothalamus and other brain regions critical to the regulation of ingestive behaviour. This chapter begins with a clinical overview of anorexia nervosa and bulimia nervosa, including brief summaries of diagnostic criteria and therapeutic considerations. Subsequent sections highlight promising areas of research on the clinical neurobiology of these disorders. Findings to date suggest that alterations in regulatory systems involving serotonin, cholecystokinin (CCK) and leptin may contribute to the initial onset or perpetuation of eating disorder symptoms.

Anorexia nervosa

Symptom patterns and diagnostic criteria

Descriptions of anorexia nervosa as a disorder of unexplained weight loss first appeared in the medical literature more than a century ago. The central psychological symptom of the disorder is 'refusal to maintain body weight at or above a minimally normal weight for age and height' (Table 54.1) (American Psychiatric Association, 2000). Patients demonstrate a persistent preoccupation with body shape and weight, with an underlying pervasive fear of becoming fat. Clinical observations and laboratory studies have shown that patients with anorexia nervosa do not suffer from loss of appetite, however (Sunday & Halmi,

1996). The characteristic amenorrhea appearing in postmenarcheal women is generally thought to be a consequence of malnutrition, although in some cases the loss of menstrual cycles can precede the onset of significant weight loss.

In most survey data, the prevalence of anorexia nervosa is approximately 0.5% among adolescent girls and young women. The typical age of onset is 18 years, and the prevalence in boys and young men is estimated to be 10% of that in females (Lucas et al., 1991; Whitaker et al., 1990). Episodes of recurrent dieting typically precede the onset of an eating disorder, and psychological and cultural factors contributing to increased preoccupation with body weight and appearance are thought to play a role in the etiology of anorexia nervosa. Behavioural risk factors include perfectionism and negative self-esteem (Fairburn et al., 1999). Based on family and twin studies, heritability estimates for the disorder are approximately 60% (Wade et al., 2000).

Anorexia nervosa is often a chronic illness, with multiple episodes of weight recovery and relapse. Studies of the natural course of the disorder have shown that 50% or more of patients recover after 10 years. Up to 20% or more of patients are likely to have a poor outcome (Eckert et al., 1995; Hsu, 1996; Strober et al., 1997b), with an aggregate mortality rate of approximately 6% per decade (Sullivan, 1995). There are few predictors of clinical outcome, although very early onset and very low weight at initial assessment may be associated with less favourable outcomes.

Clinical assessment and therapeutic approaches

In the clinical evaluation of patients with an eating disorder, it is useful to obtain detailed information about the individual's daily eating patterns, quantity of foods consumed, eating-related rituals and perceptions, and associated feelings of anxiety. Although the prototypical

Table 54.1. Diagnostic criteria for anorexia nervosa[a]

A. Refusal to maintain body weight at or above a minimally normal weight for age and height (e.g. weight loss leading to maintenance of body weight less than 85% of that expected; or failure to make expected weight gain during period of growth, leading to body weight less than 85% of that expected).

B. Intense fear of gaining weight or becoming fat, even though underweight.

C. Disturbance in the way in which one's body weight or shape is experienced, undue influence of body shape and weight on self-evaluation, or denial of the seriousness of current low body weight.

D. In postmenarcheal females, amenorrhea, i.e. the absence of at least three consecutive menstrual cycles. (A woman is considered to have amenorrhea if her periods occur only following hormone, e.g. estrogen, administration.)

Specify type:

Restricting type: during the episode of anorexia nervosa, the person has not regularly engaged in binge-eating or purging behaviour (i.e. self-induced vomiting or the misuse of laxatives, diuretics or enemas)

Binge-eating/Purging type: during the current episode of anorexia nervosa, the person has regularly engaged in binge-eating or purging behaviour (i.e. self-induced vomiting or the misuse of laxatives, diuretics or enemas)

Notes:

[a] Diagnostic criteria in Tables 54.1 and 54.2 are reprinted with permission from the Diagnostic and Statistical Manual of Mental Disorders, 4th edn, Text Revision. © 2000 American Psychiatric Association.

Table 54.2. Diagnostic criteria for bulimia nervosa[a]

A. Recurrent episodes of binge eating. An episode of binge eating is characterized by both of the following:
(1) eating, in a discrete period of time (e.g. within any 2-hour period), an amount of food that is definitely larger than most people would eat during a similar period of time and under similar circumstances
(2) a sense of lack of control over eating during the episode (e.g. a feeling that one cannot stop eating or control what or how much one is eating)

B. Recurrent inappropriate compensatory behaviour in order to prevent weight gain, such as self-induced vomiting; misuse of laxatives, diuretics, enemas or other medications; fasting; or excessive exercise.

C. The binge eating and inappropriate compensatory behaviours both occur, on average, at least twice a week for 3 months.

D. Self-evaluation is unduly influenced by body shape and weight.

E. The disturbance does not occur exclusively during episodes of anorexia nervosa.

Specify type:

Purging type: during the current episode of bulimia nervosa, the person has regularly engaged in self-induced vomiting or the misuse of laxatives, diuretics or enemas.

Non-purging type: during the current episode of bulimia nervosa, the person has used other inappropriate compensatory behaviours, such as fasting or excessive exercise, but has not regularly engaged in self-induced vomiting or the misuse of laxatives, diuretics or enemas

patient is often described as food avoidant, approximately half of women with anorexia nervosa develop recurrent binge eating episodes, often after about a year of the disorder. To facilitate increased understanding of clinical and biological correlates of these patterns, diagnostic criteria include designations for patients with 'restricting' and 'binge-eating/purging' types (Table 54.1).

A detailed psychiatric history is important for evaluation of comorbid major psychiatric disorders. Major depression occurs in more than half of patients with anorexia nervosa, although depressed mood can also be a consequence of weight loss *per se* and may resolve spontaneously with weight gain. Attention should be given to the evaluation of suicidality, anxiety disorders (including obsessive–compulsive disorder) and substance use disorders. The clinician also needs to be alert to the possibility of other neuropsychiatric syndromes (e.g. psychotic disorders) which can in rare instances present with unexplained weight loss. Assessment of psychosocial stressors, family history and, for younger patients, family relationships can be important in planning therapeutic interventions.

The initial assessment of a patient with anorexia nervosa includes a careful medical history and physical examination, with particular attention to possible medical or neurological causes for altered eating patterns and malnutrition. Physical examination commonly reveals signs of cachexia, e.g. bradycardia and hypotension. Basic laboratory tests include complete blood count, urinalysis, evaluation of serum electrolyte, blood urea nitrogen, and creatinine levels, and thyroid function tests (American Psychiatric Association Workgroup on Eating Disorders, 2000). An electrocardiogram is often part of the initial evaluation. Inclusion of additional laboratory tests, as well as evaluation for osteopenia and osteoporosis, is related to the extent and duration of malnutrition. Endocrine abnormalities are commonly present, including elevated serum cortisol, decreased thyroid hormone levels, and decreases in gonadal hormone levels (Stoving et al., 1999). Neurological complications include myopathy (McLoughlin et al., 1998), or central pontine myelinolysis (Copeland, 1989).

Neuroimaging studies may be included in the clinical assessment for the evaluation of neurological or atypical behavioural symptoms (American Psychiatric Association Workgroup on Eating Disorders, 2000). Brain imaging studies have shown that low weight anorexic patients have decreased cortical size reflected in enlargement of cerebral ventricles and cortical sulci (Jimerson et al., 1998). These patterns usually normalize with weight restoration, although there is some evidence for persistent changes (Lambe et al., 1997). Studies of cerebral blood flow with single-photon emission computed tomography (SPECT) and cerebral metabolic rate with positron emission tomography (PET) have reported unilateral decreases in temporal lobe blood flow (Gordon et al., 1997), and trends toward alterations in frontal and parietal cortical metabolic rates that persist following weight restoration (Delvenne et al., 1996).

Treatment planning for anorexia nervosa generally includes the collaborative efforts of a primary care physician and a mental health professional. Interventions commonly involve individual psychotherapy, family therapy (particularly for the younger patient) and nutritional consultation. Hospitalization may be necessitated for medical stabilization or for monitoring of severe psychiatric symptomatology such as suicidal ideation. Although the recent trend has been toward relatively brief inpatient stays, specialized inpatient programmes based on behavioural and cognitive–behavioural interventions can be of significant benefit to the severely underweight patient. Participation in a day treatment programme can facilitate the transition from hospitalization to outpatient treatment.

In controlled trials, pharmacological treatments including antidepressants and neuroleptic medications have generally demonstrated very limited benefit as an adjunct to inpatient-based weight restoration programmes (Jimerson et al., 1996). Similarly, recent studies have failed to demonstrate a significant benefit for selective serotonin reuptake inhibitor (SSRI) antidepressant medications in weight restoration programmes (Attia et al., 1998; Ferguson et al., 1999; Strober et al., 1999). Preliminary studies have provided mixed evidence regarding the possible efficacy of an SSRI in the prevention of relapse following weight restoration (Kaye et al., 1998a; Strober et al., 1997a).

Bulimia nervosa

Symptom patterns and diagnostic criteria

In the 1970s, clinicians recognized a syndrome in normal weight individuals characterized by recurrent episodes of binge eating accompanied by compensatory weight-control measures. Initially conceptualized as a variant of anorexia nervosa, bulimia was included in the psychiatric diagnostic criteria in 1980. Current diagnostic criteria specify that binge eating episodes occur on average twice per week, and that abnormal eating patterns are accompanied by psychological symptoms involving preoccupation with body shape and weight (Table 54.2) (American Psychiatric Association, 2000). Survey studies have suggested that important clinical characteristics of bulimia nervosa may be manifested by individuals with subclinical forms of the disorder (e.g. individuals who meet all criteria except that their average frequency of binge eating is only once per week).

Bulimia nervosa has a prevalence of approximately 2–3% among adolescent girls and young women (Kendler et al., 1991), and resembles anorexia nervosa in the average age of onset (approximately 18 years) and in the ten-fold increased prevalence in girls and young women in comparison to boys and young men. Psychological and cultural factors resulting in increased preoccupation with slimness, as well as a history of obesity, are thought to play a role in the onset of bulimia nervosa (Fairburn et al., 1997). There is an increased risk of eating disorders in family members of bulimic patients (Kassett et al., 1989), and twin studies have shown heritability of approximately 55% (Kendler et al., 1991). Naturalistic follow-up studies indicate that approximately three-quarters of patients have recovered by seven years following initial assessment (Herzog et al., 1999).

Provisional criteria for 'binge eating disorder' have been included in an appendix listing in DSM-IV-TR (American Psychiatric Association, 2000). As recently reviewed, this disorder is characterized by recurrent binge eating in the absence of compensatory weight control behaviours, resulting in patients who tend to be overweight (Devlin, 1996).

Clinical assessment and therapeutic approaches

During the initial clinical assessment, it is valuable for the clinician to inquire specifically regarding eating patterns, frequency and type of purging behaviours, and body weight fluctuations. Clinical observations and laboratory studies have demonstrated that patients with bulimia nervosa have impaired postingestive satiety, possibly contributing to the large size of binge meals (Kissileff et al., 1996). Although 'objectively' large binge eating episodes are required by the diagnostic criteria (Table 54.2), some patients may describe 'subjective' binge episodes which have similar psychological characteristics but are smaller in size. A detailed psychiatric history is important to identify comorbid major psychiatric disorders, including major depression, which occurs in more than half of patients with bulimia nervosa, suicidal ideation, substance use disorders and anxiety disorders. As with anorexia nervosa, review of family history and psychosocial stressors is important in planning therapeutic interventions.

The scope of the medical assessment is based on the patient's symptoms and the clinical setting. In reviewing the clinical history, the clinician should be alert to atypical symptoms suggestive of an underlying medical or neurological disorder (e.g. Kleine–Levin syndrome). The physical examination may reveal findings such as bradycardia and hypotension associated with nutritional abnormalities, or erosion of the dental enamel or parotid gland swelling associated with binge eating and purging behaviours. Based on symptom patterns, initial laboratory tests may include serum electrolytes, blood urea nitrogen levels, creatinine levels, thyroid function tests, complete blood count, urinalysis, and electrocardiogram (American Psychiatric Association Workgroup on Eating Disorders, 2000). Although abnormal results are less common than for anorexia nervosa, bulimia nervosa is associated with hypokalemia (Wolfe et al., 2001), which could contribute to life-threatening cardiac arrhythmias. Atypical behavioural symptoms or abnormal findings on neurological examination may necessitate neuroimaging studies.

Since 1990 there have been extensive studies of psychotherapeutic and psychopharmacological interventions for bulimia nervosa (Jimerson et al., 1996; Mitchell et al., 1997). For many patients, the initial intervention is a trial of short-term psychotherapy, with recent studies of cognitive–behavioural therapy or interpersonal therapy showing an approximately two-thirds decrease in frequency of binge eating. Efficacy of antidepressant medications has also been demonstrated in double-blind, controlled trials, the largest of which showed significant therapeutic response to an SSRI medication (fluoxetine). Relatively early intervention with antidepressant medications is often considered for patients who do not respond during the initial phases of psychotherapy (Agras et al., 2000), and for patients who have comorbid psychiatric disorders such as major depression. In spite of the effectiveness of current treatment approaches, only a minority of patients achieve full abstinence from binge eating and purging during short-term treatments. In planning medication treatment for an individual patient, consultation with a specialist may assist in considering choice and dose of medication, and special side effects issues in this patient group.

Neurobiology of the eating disorders

Serotonin

Hypotheses linking abnormal regulation of CNS serotonin with the eating disorders resulted from preclinical obser-vations showing that this neurotransmitter, as well as the catecholamines, play an important role in the regulation of ingestive behaviour (Blundell, 1986; Samanin & Garattini, 1996). Activation of serotonergic pathways in the medial basal hypothalamus was shown to limit meal size by enhancing postingestive satiety (Leibowitz & Alexander, 1998). Conversely, activation of inhibitory serotonin-1A somato-dendritic autoreceptors on cell bodies in the raphe nuclei decreases hypothalamic serotonin release and enhances food intake. Serotonin-2C receptors are thought to play an important role in the satiety response, given that mutant mice deficient in serotonin-2C receptors have significantly increased food intake, with resulting obesity (Tecott et al., 1995). Studies in healthy volunteers have shown that serotonin receptor agonist drugs such as m-chlorophenylpiperazine (mCPP) decrease food intake (Brewerton et al., 1994). The indirect serotonin agonist dexfenfluramine, which was used in the treatment of obesity prior to its withdrawal from the market because of cardiac side effects, was thought to decrease food intake through facilitation of CNS serotonergic transmission.

Based on these observations, clinical investigators hypothesized that increased serotonin function could contribute to small meal size and weight loss in anorexia nervosa (Jimerson et al., 1990). Cerebrospinal fluid (CSF) concentrations of the major serotonin metabolite 5-hydroxyindole acetic acid (5-HIAA) were abnormally low in anorexia nervosa, however (Kaye et al., 1984). Responsiveness of CNS serotonin pathways, assessed by measuring the release of prolactin and cortisol following the administration of serotonin agonist drugs, was also diminished in low weight anorexic patients. As patients gained weight, CSF metabolite and neuroendocrine response measures returned towards normal, suggesting that abnormalities in the low weight patients could be a result of malnutrition (Brewerton & Jimerson, 1996; Hadigan et al., 1995; Monteleone et al., 1998; O'Dwyer et al., 1996). Studies showing elevated CSF 5-HIAA levels and abnormal test meal responses in patients who have achieved stable weight restoration suggest that anorexia nervosa may be associated with abnormalities of serotonin regulation independent of nutritional status (Kaye et al., 1991; Ward et al., 1998). There has also been considerable interest in genetic linkage studies in anorexia nervosa (Gorwood et al., 1998), with preliminary findings suggesting a possible association with an altered serotonin-2A receptor gene promoter polymorphism (Collier et al., 1997).

Diminished serotonergic responsiveness in bulimia nervosa is thought to contribute to impaired satiety and binge eating, and to the efficacy of antidepressant medications. Thus, patients with severe symptoms of bulimia nervosa have low CSF 5-HIAA concentrations (Jimerson et al., 1992), and diminished neuroendocrine responses following single dose administration of serotonin agonist drugs (Brewerton et al., 1992; Jimerson et al., 1997; Levitan et al., 1997; Monteleone et al., 1998). Differences were observed following careful matching of controls for such clinical parameters as height-adjusted body weight, age, and menstrual cycle phase. Patients who have recovered from bulimia nervosa also demonstrate abnormal serotonin-related behavioural responses, although neuroendocrine hormone release appears to be normal (Kaye et al., 1998b; Smith et al., 1999; Wolfe et al., 2000). Recent studies have begun to explore whether recurrent dieting episodes may promote the onset of bulimia nervosa by decreasing CNS serotonin synthesis (Cowen et al., 1996).

Cholecystokinin

Normal regulation of body weight is dependent on a homeostatic balance between energy expenditure and food intake. While initial investigations of the CNS control of eating behaviour focused on the role of the monoamine neurotransmitters, studies of peripheral influences on eating behaviour revealed that the gut-related peptide CCK is involved in limiting meal size (Gibbs et al., 1973). In humans, exogenous CCK administration decreased meal size through augmentation of postingestive satiety (Kissileff et al., 1981). These effects are thought to be mediated in part through inhibition of gastric emptying, with resultant satiety-related signalling relayed to the CNS via vagal afferent pathways. Additionally, CCK released into the circulation may act at selective receptors in brain regions where the blood–brain barrier is relatively permeable to peptides (Moran et al., 1986).

It has been postulated than an increase in postingestive CCK release might contribute to small meal size in anorexia nervosa. However, CCK response to a test meal does not appear to be abnormal in patients with anorexia nervosa (Geracioti, Jr. et al., 1992; Pirke et al., 1994). Variability in responses across studies has been noted, possibly a result of differences in patient characteristics and peptide assay methodology. Other related studies in anorexia nervosa have shown normal CCK-like immunoreactivity in CSF (Gerner & Yamada, 1982), and low T-lymphocyte concentrations of cholecystokinin octapeptide (Brambilla et al., 1996).

Studies in bulimia nervosa indicate that diminished CCK responsiveness may contribute to attenuated postingestive satiety. Thus, in comparison to healthy controls, patients with bulimia nervosa have shown significantly attenuated responses in plasma CCK concentrations and in satiety ratings (Geracioti, Jr. & Liddle, 1988; Pirke et al.,

1994; Devlin et al., 1997). Further studies are needed to evaluate the extent to which these changes may be a consequence of abnormal eating patterns and related changes in gastric physiology (Geliebter et al., 1992). Other findings in bulimia nervosa include decreased concentrations of CCK octapeptide in CSF (Lydiard et al., 1993) and in T-lymphocytes (Brambilla et al., 1996). Thus, current studies indicate that changes in CCK function may help to perpetuate recurrent binge eating in bulimia nervosa.

Leptin

An important new chapter in research on the regulation of food intake and body weight opened with the discovery of the adipose tissue hormone leptin (Zhang et al., 1994). Leptin acts in the CNS to decrease food intake, and in the periphery to increase energy metabolism (Friedman & Halaas, 1998; Schwartz et al., 1999; Tang-Christensen et al., 1999). Leptin administration decreases meal size in rodents (Kahler et al., 1998; Flynn et al., 1998), suggesting a role in mechanisms related to satiety. Leptin may be particularly involved in the longer-term regulation of body weight, acting as a feedback signal to the CNS conveying information related to adipose stores (Woods et al., 2000).

The effects of leptin on eating behaviour are likely to be mediated in the medial hypothalamus, where there are relatively high concentrations of the signalling, long-form of the leptin receptor. Activation of leptin receptors in the arcuate nucleus is thought to inhibit the release of the orexigenic peptide NPY in the paraventricular nucleus of the hypothalamus (Schwartz et al., 1996). On-going studies have delineated complex interactions between a number of other CNS neuropeptides, such as the melanocortins and their antagonists, in the regulation of feeding (Elmquist et al., 1999). There is also recent evidence that hypothalamic regulation of food intake may be influenced by alterations in fatty acid synthesis. Thus, inhibition of fatty acid synthase in mice through peripheral administration of C75, a synthetic derivative of cerulenin, resulted in marked weight loss which was not dependent on leptin (Loftus et al., 2000). This observation may reflect a novel mechanism for body weight homeostatis, and a possible future direction for therapeutic intervention research in obesity.

While a role for leptin deficiency has been demonstrated in animal models of obesity, the role of abnormal leptin regulation in human obesity is uncertain. In healthy volunteers and overweight individuals, there is a high correlation of leptin with body mass index or percentage body fat (Considine et al., 1996). In general, obese patients do not have decreased leptin levels, so it has been proposed that obesity may involve postreceptor forms of leptin resistance. Preliminary clinical trials in obese patients have shown a modest effect of leptin in decreasing body weight (Heymsfield et al., 1999).

In anorexia nervosa, leptin levels are markedly reduced and increase to normal levels following weight restoration (Hebebrand et al., 1995; Grinspoon et al., 1996; Mantzoros et al., 1997; Eckert et al., 1998). A disproportionate rise in leptin levels during treatment could contribute to the commonly observed resistance to weight restoration (Mantzoros et al., 1997). Leptin may play a role in some of the neuroendocrine alterations (e.g. decreased gonadal hormones and decreased thyroid hormone levels) observed in low weight anorexic patients (Flier, 1998).

In comparison to controls matched for age, gender and body weight, patients with bulimia nervosa have significantly decreased leptin levels (Brewerton et al., 2000; Jimerson et al., 2000; Monteleone et al., 2000). Moreover, there appears to be a persistent decrease in leptin levels in patients who have achieved stable remission from bulimia nervosa, suggesting a trait-related characteristic (Jimerson et al., 2000). Follow-up studies are needed to assess whether diminished leptin function contributes to impaired satiety, decreased thyroid hormone levels, and decreased resting metabolic rate in this disorder (Obarzanek et al., 1991), possibly reflecting a biological risk factor for the onset of bulimia nervosa.

References

Agras, W.S., Crow, S.J., Halmi, K.A., Mitchell, J.E., Wilson, G.T. & Kraemer, H.C. (2000). Outcome predictors for the cognitive behavior treatment of bulimia nervosa: data from a multisite study. *Am. J. Psychiatry*, **157**, 1302–8.

American Psychiatric Association (2000). *Diagnostic and Statistical Manual of Mental Disorders, Fourth Edition, Text Revision*. Washington, DC: American Psychiatric Association.

American Psychiatric Association Workgroup on Eating Disorders (2000). Practice guideline for the treatment of patients with eating disorders (revision). *Am. J. Psychiatry*, **157**, 1–39.

Attia, E., Haiman, C., Walsh, B.T. & Flater, S.R. (1998). Does fluoxetine augment the inpatient treatment of anorexia nervosa? *Am. J. Psychiatry*, **155**, 548–51.

Blundell, J.E. (1986). Serotonin manipulations and the structure of feeding behaviour. *Appetite*, **7 Suppl.**, 39–56.

Brambilla, F., Ferrari, E., Brunetta, M. et al. (1996). Immunoendocrine aspects of anorexia nervosa. *Psychiatry Res.* **62**, 97–104.

Brewerton, T.D. & Jimerson, D.C. (1996). Studies of serotonin function in anorexia nervosa. *Psychiatry Res.*, **62**, 31–42.

Brewerton, T.D., Mueller, E.A., Lesem, M.D. et al. (1992).

Neuroendocrine responses to *m*-chlorophenylpiperazine and L-tryptophan in bulimia. *Arch. Gen. Psychiatry*, **49**, 852–61.

Brewerton, T.D., Murphy, D.L. & Jimerson, D.C. (1994). Testmeal responses following *m*-chlorophenylpiperazine and L-tryptophan in bulimics and controls. *Neuropsychopharmacology*, **11**, 63–71.

Brewerton, T.D., Lesem, M.D., Kennedy, A. & Garvey, W.T. (2000). Reduced plasma leptin concentrations in bulimia nervosa. *Psychoneuroendocrinology*, **25**, 649–58.

Collier, D.A., Arranz, M. J., Li, T., Mupita, D., Brown, N. & Treasure, J. (1997). Association between 5-HT2A gene promoter polymorphism and anorexia nervosa [letter]. *Lancet*, **350**, 412.

Considine, R.V., Sinha, M.K., Heiman, M.L. et al. (1996). Serum immunoreactive-leptin concentrations in normal-weight and obese humans. *N. Engl. J. Med.*, **334**, 292–5.

Copeland, P.M. (1989). Diuretic abuse and central pontine myelinolysis. *Psychother. Psychosom.*, **52**, 101–5.

Cowen, P.J., Clifford, E.M., Walsh, A.E., Williams, C. & Fairburn, C.G. (1996). Moderate dieting causes 5-HT2C receptor supersensitivity. *Psychol. Med.*, **26**, 1155–9.

Delvenne, V., Goldman, S., De Maertelaer, V., Simon, Y., Luxen, A. & Lotstra, F. (1996). Brain hypometabolism of glucose in anorexia nervosa: normalization after weight gain. *Biol. Psychiatry*, **40**, 761–8.

Devlin, M.J. (1996). Assessment and treatment of binge-eating disorder. *Psychiatr. Clin. North Am.*, **19**, 761–72.

Devlin, M.J., Walsh, B.T., Guss, J.L., Kissileff, H.R., Liddle, R.A. & Petkova, E. (1997). Postprandial cholecystokinin release and gastric emptying in patients with bulimia nervosa. *Am. J. Clin. Nutr.*, **65**, 114–20.

Eckert, E.D., Halmi, K.A., Marchi, P., Grove, W. & Crosby, R. (1995). Ten-year follow-up of anorexia nervosa: clinical course and outcome. *Psychol. Med.*, **25**, 143–56.

Eckert, E.D., Pomeroy, C., Raymond, N., Kohler, P.F., Thuras, P. & Bowers, C.Y. (1998). Leptin in anorexia nervosa. *J. Clin. Endocrinol. Metab.*, **83**, 791–5.

Elmquist, J.K., Elias, C.F. & Saper, C.B. (1999). From lesions to leptin: hypothalamic control of food intake and body weight. *Neuron*, **22**, 221–32.

Fairburn, C.G., Welch, S.L., Doll, H.A., Davies, B.A. & O'Connor, M.E. (1997). Risk factors for bulimia nervosa. A community-based case-control study. *Arch. Gen. Psychiatry*, **54**, 509–17.

Fairburn, C.G., Cooper, Z., Doll, H.A. & Welch, S.L. (1999). Risk factors for anorexia nervosa: three integrated case-control comparisons. *Arch. Gen. Psychiatry*, **56**, 468–76.

Ferguson, C.P., La Via, M.C., Crossan, P.J. & Kaye, W.H. (1999). Are serotonin selective reuptake inhibitors effective in underweight anorexia nervosa? *Int. J. Eat. Disord.*, **25**, 11–17.

Flier, J.S. (1998). Clinical review 94: What's in a name? In search of leptin's physiologic role. *J. Clin. Endocrinol. Metab.*, **83**, 1407–13.

Flynn, M.C., Scott, T.R., Pritchard, T.C. & Plata-Salaman, C.R. (1998). Mode of action of OB protein (leptin) on feeding. *Am. J. Physiol.*, **275**, R174–9.

Friedman, J.M. & Halaas, J.L. (1998). Leptin and the regulation of body weight in mammals. *Nature*, **395**, 763–70.

Geliebter, A., Melton, P.M., McCray, R.S., Gallagher, D.R., Gage, D. & Hashim, S.A. (1992). Gastric capacity, gastric emptying, and test-meal intake in normal and bulimic women. *Am. J. Clin. Nutr.*, **56**, 656–61.

Geracioti, T.D., Jr. & Liddle, R.A. (1988). Impaired cholecystokinin secretion in bulimia nervosa. *N. Engl. J. Med.*, **319**, 683–8.

Geracioti, T.D., Jr., Liddle, R.A., Altemus, M., Demitrack, M.A. & Gold, P.W. (1992). Regulation of appetite and cholecystokinin secretion in anorexia nervosa. *Am. J. Psychiatry*, **149**, 958–61.

Gerner, R.H. & Yamada, T. (1982). Altered neuropeptide concentrations in cerebrospinal fluid of psychiatric patients. *Brain Res.*, **238**, 298–302.

Gibbs, J., Young, R.C. & Smith, G.P. (1973). Cholecystokinin decreases food intake in rats. *J. Comp. Physiol. Psychol.*, **84**, 488–95.

Gordon, I., Lask, B., Bryant-Waugh, R., Christie, D. & Timimi, S. (1997). Childhood-onset anorexia nervosa: towards identifying a biological substrate. *Int. J. Eat. Disord.*, **22**, 159–65.

Gorwood, P., Bouvard, M., Mouren-Simeoni, M.C., Kipman, A. & Ades, J. (1998). Genetics and anorexia nervosa: a review of candidate genes. *Psychiatr. Genet.*, **8**, 1–12.

Grinspoon, S., Gulick, T., Askari, H. et al. (1996). Serum leptin levels in women with anorexia nervosa. *J. Clin. Endocrinol. Metab.*, **81**, 3861–3.

Hadigan, C.M., Walsh, B.T., Buttinger, C. & Hollander, E. (1995). Behavioral and neuroendocrine responses to *meta*CPP in anorexia nervosa. *Biol. Psychiatry*, **37**, 504–11.

Hebebrand, J., van der Heyden, J., Devos, R. et al. (1995). Plasma concentrations of obese protein in anorexia nervosa [letter]. *Lancet*, **346**, 1624–5.

Herzog, D.B., Dorer, D.J., Keel, P.K. et al. (1999). Recovery and relapse in anorexia and bulimia nervosa: a 7.5-year follow-up study. *J. Am. Acad. Child Adolesc. Psychiatry*, **38**, 829–37.

Heymsfield, S.B., Greenberg, A.S., Fujioka, K. et al. (1999). Recombinant leptin for weight loss in obese and lean adults: a randomized, controlled, dose-escalation trial. *J. Am. Med. Assoc.*, **282**, 1568–75.

Hsu, L.K. (1996). Epidemiology of the eating disorders. *Psychiatr. Clin. North Am.*, **19**, 681–700.

Jimerson, D.C., Lesem, M.D., Hegg, A.P. & Brewerton, T.D. (1990). Serotonin in human eating disorders. *Ann. N.Y. Acad. Sci.*, **600**, 532–44.

Jimerson, D.C., Lesem, M.D., Kaye, W.H. & Brewerton, T.D. (1992). Low serotonin and dopamine metabolite concentrations in cerebrospinal fluid from bulimic patients with frequent binge episodes. *Arch. Gen. Psychiatry*, **49**, 132–8.

Jimerson, D.C., Wolfe, B.E., Brotman, A.W. & Metzger, E.D. (1996). Medications in the treatment of eating disorders. *Psychiatr. Clin. North Am.*, **19**, 739–54.

Jimerson, D.C., Wolfe, B.E., Metzger, E.D., Finkelstein, D.M., Cooper, T.B. & Levine, J.M. (1997). Decreased serotonin function in bulimia nervosa. *Arch. Gen. Psychiatry*, **54**, 529–34.

Jimerson, D.C., Wolfe, B.E. & Naab, S. (1998). Anorexia nervosa and bulimia nervosa. In *Textbook of Pediatric Neuropsychiatry*, ed. C.E. Coffee & R.A. Brumback, pp. 563–78. Washington, DC: American Psychiatric Press.

Jimerson, D.C., Mantzoros, C., Wolfe, B.E. & Metzger, E.D. (2000). Decreased serum leptin in bulimia nervosa. *J. Clin. Endocrinol. Metab.*, **85**, 4511–14.

Kahler, A., Geary, N., Eckel, L.A., Campfield, L.A., Smith, F.J. & Langhans, W. (1998). Chronic administration of OB protein decreases food intake by selectively reducing meal size in male rats. *Am. J. Physiol.*, **275**, R180–5.

Kassett, J.A., Gershon, E.S., Maxwell, M.E. et al. (1989). Psychiatric disorders in the first-degree relatives of probands with bulimia nervosa. *Am. J. Psychiatry*, **146**, 1468–71.

Kaye, W.H., Gwirtsman, H.E., George, D.T. & Ebert, M.H. (1991). Altered serotonin activity in anorexia nervosa after long-term weight restoration. Does elevated cerebrospinal fluid 5-hydroxyindoleacetic acid level correlate with rigid and obsessive behavior? *Arch. Gen. Psychiatry*, **48**, 556–62.

Kaye, W.H., Ebert, M.H., Raleigh, M. & Lake, R. (1984). Abnormalities in CNS monoamine metabolism in anorexia nervosa. *Arch. Gen. Psychiatry*, **41**, 350–5.

Kaye, W., Gendall, K. & Strober, M. (1998a). Serotonin neuronal function and selective serotonin reuptake inhibitor treatment in anorexia and bulimia nervosa. *Biol. Psychiatry*, **44**, 825–38.

Kaye, W.H., Greeno, C.G., Moss, H. et al. (1998b). Alterations in serotonin activity and psychiatric symptoms after recovery from bulimia nervosa. *Arch. Gen. Psychiatry*, **55**, 927–35.

Kendler, K.S., MacLean, C., Neale, M., Kessler, R., Heath, A. & Eaves, L. (1991). The genetic epidemiology of bulimia nervosa. *Am. J. Psychiatry*, **148**, 1627–37.

Kissileff, H.R., Pi-Sunyer, F.X., Thornton, J. & Smith, G.P. (1981). C-terminal octapeptide of cholecystokinin decreases food intake in man. *Am. J. Clin. Nutr.*, **34**, 154–60.

Kissileff, H.R., Wentzlaff, T.H., Guss, J.L., Walsh, B.T., Devlin, M.J. & Thornton, J.C. (1996). A direct measure of satiety disturbance in patients with bulimia nervosa. *Physiol. Behav.*, **60**, 1077–85.

Lambe, E.K., Katzman, D.K., Mikulis, D.J., Kennedy, S.H. & Zipursky, R.B. (1997). Cerebral gray matter volume deficits after weight recovery from anorexia nervosa. *Arch. Gen. Psychiatry*, **54**, 537–42.

Leibowitz, S.F. & Alexander, J.T. (1998). Hypothalamic serotonin in control of eating behavior, meal size, and body weight. *Biol. Psychiatry*, **44**, 851–64.

Levitan, R.D., Kaplan, A.S., Joffe, R.T., Levitt, A.J. & Brown, G.M. (1997). Hormonal and subjective responses to intravenous meta-chlorophenylpiperazine in bulimia nervosa. *Arch. Gen. Psychiatry*, **54**, 521–7.

Loftus, T.M., Jaworsky, D.E., Frehywot, G.L. et al. (2000). Reduced food intake and body weight in mice treated with fatty acid synthase inhibitors. *Science*, **288**, 2379–81.

Lucas, A.R., Beard, C.M., O'Fallon, W.M. & Kurland, L.T. (1991). 50-year trends in the incidence of anorexia nervosa in Rochester, Minn.: a population-based study. *Am. J. Psychiatry*, **148**, 917–22.

Lydiard, R.B., Brewerton, T.D., Fossey, M.D. et al. (1993). CSF cholecystokinin octapeptide in patients with bulimia nervosa and in normal comparison subjects. *Am. J. Psychiatry*, **150**, 1099–101.

McLoughlin, D.M., Spargo, E., Wassif, W.S. et al. (1998). Structural and functional changes in skeletal muscle in anorexia nervosa. *Acta Neuropathol.(Berl.)*, **95**, 632–40.

Mantzoros, C., Flier, J.S., Lesem, M.D., Brewerton, T.D. & Jimerson, D.C. (1997). Cerebrospinal fluid leptin in anorexia nervosa: correlation with nutritional status and potential role in resistance to weight gain. *J. Clin. Endocrinol. Metab.*, **82**, 1845–51.

Mitchell, J.E., de Zwaan, M. & Crow, S. (1997). Psychopharmacology of eating disorders. *Ballière's Clinical Psychiatry*, **3**, 217–34.

Monteleone, P., Brambilla, F., Bortolotti, F., Ferraro, C. & Maj, M. (1998). Plasma prolactin response to D-fenfluramine is blunted in bulimic patients with frequent binge episodes. *Psychol. Med.*, **28**, 975–83.

Monteleone, P., Di Lieto, A., Tortorella, A., Longobardi, N. & Maj, M. (2000). Circulating leptin in patients with anorexia nervosa, bulimia nervosa or binge-eating disorder: relationship to body weight, eating patterns, psychopathology and endocrine changes. *Psychiatry Res.*, **94**, 121–9.

Moran, T.H., Robinson, P.H., Goldrich, M.S. & McHugh, P.R. (1986). Two brain cholecystokinin receptors: implications for behavioral actions. *Brain Res.*, **362**, 175–9.

Obarzanek, E., Lesem, M.D., Goldstein, D.S. & Jimerson, D.C. (1991). Reduced resting metabolic rate in patients with bulimia nervosa. *Arch. Gen. Psychiatry*, **48**, 456–62.

O'Dwyer, A.M., Lucey, J.V. & Russell, G.F. (1996). Serotonin activity in anorexia nervosa after long-term weight restoration: response to D-fenfluramine challenge. *Psychol. Med.*, **26**, 353–9.

Pirke, K.M., Kellner, M.B., Friess, E., Krieg, J.C. & Fichter, M.M. (1994). Satiety and cholecystokinin. *Int. J. Eat. Disord.*, **15**, 63–9.

Samanin, R. & Garattini, S. (1996). Pharmacology of ingestive behaviour. *Therapie*, **51**, 107–15.

Schwartz, M.W., Seeley, R.J., Campfield, L.A., Burn, P. & Baskin, D.G. (1996). Identification of targets of leptin action in rat hypothalamus. *J. Clin. Invest.*, **98**, 1101–6.

Schwartz, M.W., Baskin, D.G., Kaiyala, K.J. & Woods, S.C. (1999). Model for the regulation of energy balance and adiposity by the central nervous system. *Am. J. Clin. Nutr.*, **69**, 584–96.

Smith, K.A., Fairburn, C.G. & Cowen, P.J. (1999). Symptomatic relapse in bulimia nervosa following acute tryptophan depletion. *Arch. Gen. Psychiatry*, **56**, 171–6.

Stoving, R.K., Hangaard, J., Hansen-Nord, M. & Hagen, C. (1999). A review of endocrine changes in anorexia nervosa. *J. Psychiatr. Res.*, **33**, 139–52.

Strober, M., Freeman, R., DeAntonio, M., Lampert, C. & Diamond, J. (1997a). Does adjunctive fluoxetine influence the post-hospital course of restrictor-type anorexia nervosa? A 24-month prospective, longitudinal followup and comparison with historical controls. *Psychopharmacol. Bull.*, **33**, 425–31.

Strober, M., Freeman, R. & Morrell, W. (1997b). The long-term course of severe anorexia nervosa in adolescents: survival analysis of recovery, relapse, and outcome predictors over 10–15 years in a prospective study. *Int. J. Eat. Disord.*, **22**, 339–60.

Strober, M., Pataki, C., Freeman, R. & DeAntonio, M. (1999). No effect of adjunctive fluoxetine on eating behavior or weight phobia during the inpatient treatment of anorexia nervosa: an historical case-control study. *J. Child Adolesc. Psychopharmacol.*, **9**, 195–201.

Sullivan, P.F. (1995). Mortality in anorexia nervosa. *Am. J. Psychiatry*, **152**, 1073–4.

Sunday, S.R. & Halmi, K.A. (1996). Micro- and macroanalyses of patterns within a meal in anorexia and bulimia nervosa. *Appetite*, **26**, 21–36.

Tang-Christensen, M., Havel, P.J., Jacobs, R.R., Larsen, P.J. & Cameron, J.L. (1999). Central administration of leptin inhibits food intake and activates the sympathetic nervous system in rhesus macaques. *J. Clin. Endocrinol. Metab.*, **84**, 711–17.

Tecott, L.H., Sun, L.M., Akana, S.F. et al. (1995). Eating disorder and epilepsy in mice lacking 5-HT2c serotonin receptors. *Nature*, **374**, 542–6.

Wade, T.D., Bulik, C.M., Neale, M. & Kendler, K.S. (2000). Anorexia nervosa and major depression: shared genetic and environmental risk factors. *Am. J. Psychiatry*, **157**, 469–71.

Ward, A., Brown, N., Lightman, S., Campbell, I.C. & Treasure, J. (1998). Neuroendocrine, appetitive and behavioural responses to d-fenfluramine in women recovered from anorexia nervosa. *Br. J. Psychiatry*, **172**, 351–8.

Whitaker, A., Johnson, J., Shaffer, D. et al. (1990). Uncommon troubles in young people: prevalence estimates of selected psychiatric disorders in a nonreferred adolescent population. *Arch. Gen. Psychiatry*, **47**, 487–96.

Wolfe, B.E., Metzger, E.D., Levine, J.M., Finkelstein, D.M., Cooper, T.B. & Jimerson, D.C. (2000). Serotonin function following remission from bulimia nervosa. *Neuropsychopharmacology*, **22**, 257–63.

Wolfe, B.E., Metzger, E.D., Levine, J.M. & Jimerson, D.C. (2001). Laboratory screening for electrolyte abnormalities and anemia in bulimia nervosa: a controlled study. *Int. J. Eat. Disord.*, **30**, 288–93.

Woods, S.C., Schwartz, M.W., Baskin, D.G. & Seeley, R.J. (2000). Food intake and the regulation of body weight. *Annu. Rev. Psychol.*, **51**, 255–77.

Zhang, Y., Proenca, R., Maffei, M., Barone, M., Leopold, L. & Friedman, J.M. (1994). Positional cloning of the mouse obese gene and its human homologue. *Nature*, **372**, 425–32.

55

Sleep and its disorders

Robert Y. Moore, and Eric A. Nofzinger

Departments of Neurology, Psychiatry and Neuroscience, University of Pittsburgh, PA 15213, USA

Sleep is a necessary behaviour

Our lives are dominated by daily cycles of sleep and wake. The origin of these cycles begins with the earliest life on this planet. Life requires energy and the only available source of energy for the earliest life was the sun. Because of the cyclic availability of solar energy, prokaryotes evolved adaptations to use energy during the solar day, and to carry out other functions at night. With the evolution of nervous systems in primitive animals, this pattern of adaptation was maintained as rest–activity cycles. Recent studies indicate that, even in an invertebrate such as the fruit fly, *Drosophila*, the rest–activity cycles bear a striking resemblance to sleep–wake cycles in mammals. Sleep has long been recognized to have a restorative function and sleep is required to maintain life. Total deprivation of sleep results in death and even relatively brief periods of sleep deprivation, when repeated over several days, produce profound decrements in vigilance, psychomotor performance and mood. One of the commonest, transient forms of sleep disruption, that occurring with jet lag, can produce cognitive impairment and structural brain changes when it is chronic. Thus, sleep is necessary for life and successful adaptive, waking behaviour.

Sleep disorders are common and important

Loss of sleep is a major problem in our industrialized society, with an immense impact on health and productivity. This occurs as a conseqeunce of economic pressures and the pace of modern life but also results from environmental constraints that alter the normal pattern of the rest–activity cycle; shift work is an important example. Further, common medical and psychiatric illnesses impair sleep resulting in insomnia and chronic sleep deprivation. Finally, we now recognize that there are many primary sleep disorders that have a significant impact on health and normal function. In this chapter, we will review the neurobiology of sleep and important sleep disorders.

Neurobiology of sleep

Behaviour is divided into three states, waking, REM sleep and non-REM (NREM) sleep

With the development of electroencephalography (EEG) in the first half of the twentieth centry, it became possible to record brain activity continuously and to correlate the activity obtained from surface scalp electrodes with behavioural state. With this it was quickly recognized that the waking state is associated with desynchronized, low voltage EEG dominated by high frequency activity, predominantly in the 8–12 Hz range. As sleep supervenes, the EEG activity increases in voltage but decreases in frequency progressively over time with increasing synchrony until, with deep sleep, the very high voltage, slow activity of non-REM (NREM), or slow wave, sleep is evident. In a normal, young individual, sleep is initiated with a gradual slowing of EEG activity accompanied by a loss of responsiveness. Sleep is initiated with NREM sleep which is typically described to have four stages, designated stages 1–4, which are characterized by increasing unresponsiveness and slowing of the EEG. After 60–75 minutes of NREM sleep, REM sleep, a state characterized by an activated EEG, irregular, rapid eye movements (REM), muscular atonia, and unresponsiveness to sensory stimuli replaces it (Fig. 55.1). Work by several investigators, particularly Nathaniel Kleitman and his associates, demonstrated that the activated EEG of REM sleep is essentially equivalent to that of waking and that dreaming is the behavioural concomitant of the activated cortex of REM sleep.

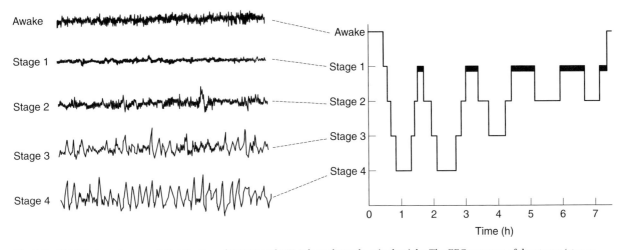

Fig. 55.1. NREM sleep stages and distribution of NREM and REM sleep through a single night. The EEG patterns of the stages (stages 1–4) of NREM sleep are shown on the left. On the right is the transition from NREM to REM sleep over the course of the sleep period. REM sleep epochs are designated by the dark bars above NREM stage 1 (▬▬).

Waking is an active state with behavioural adaptation

The waking state is associated with a conscious perception of environmental events and ongoing integrative activities of learning, problem solving, cognition and emotion and a motor output which includes speech, writing and a panoply of simple and complex motor acts. The essential feature of human adaptive waking behaviour is its complexity. It was assumed early in the twentieth century that waking was maintained by sensory information transmitted through the well-known lemniscal sensory pathways. This view was revised in the late 1940s when Giuseppi Moruzzi and Horace Magoun showed that the rostral brainstem reticular formation is critical to maintaining the waking state. Animals with lesions destroying the midbrain reticular formation, but preserving lemniscal sensory pathways, particularly visual and olfactory input, remained in a constant, unresponsive state with a high voltage, low frequency EEG. The same state is observed in humans with similar lesions. These observations led to the concept of an 'ascending reticular activating system', which has been extended and amplified over the last 50 years. The components of this system and the pathways through which it activates the cerebral cortex are shown in Fig. 55.2. Activity in the reticular activating system is driven, at least in part, by sensory input from all primary modalities. The reticular activating system provides input to activating-arousal systems in brainstem (locus ceruleus, midbrain raphe nuclei, pontine cholinergic nuclei), hypothalamus (posterior and lateral hypothalamus), thalamus and basal forebrain. These systems provide input to the cerebral cortex to maintain it in an activated state which permits the elaboration of the varieties of adaptive, and sometimes maladaptive, behaviours that characterize the waking state. The contribution of each of these systems to arousal and the waking state is different, and not yet thoroughly understood. Recent work, which will be described in greater detail in a discussion of narcolepsy, has emphasized the role of the hypothalamus. This was first appreciated by Constantine von Economo in the pathology of encephalitis lethargica and demonstrated experimentally by Walle Nauta who showed prolonged and profound deficits in arousal in animals with posterior hypothalamic lesions. The important role of the hypothalamus in sleep–wake regulation was neglected for many years but is now more fully appreciated. The hypothalamus contains both arousal/wake-promoting areas and sleep-promoting areas (for review, see Jones, 2000). Lesions involving the anterior hypothalamus result in diminished arousal. Recent work has shown a small group of ventrolateral preoptic neurons that are activated during NREM sleep and, as we will see in sections to follow, the posterior hypothalamus contains several areas which appear to function in waking and arousal.

In the 1960s, the noradrenaline neurons of the locus ceruleus and the serotonin neurons of the midbrain raphe were shown to project widely over the forebrain, including to the entire cerebral cortex, a pattern of projection that indicates a role in behavioural state regulation. Neurons of the locus ceruleus fire continuously during waking. They respond particulary to stimuli that produce behavioural vigilance and may have a special function in producing the heightened capacity for adaptive behaviour that accompanies

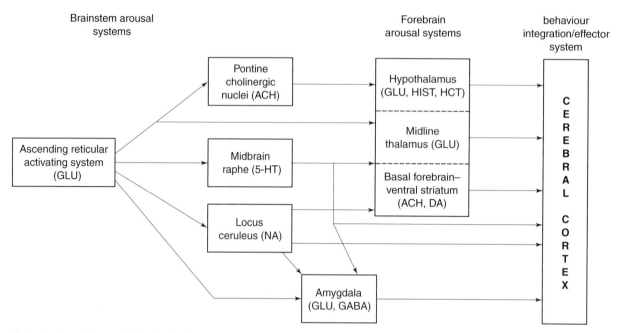

Fig. 55.2. Arousal systems in the human brain (see text for description). The transmitters associated with each system are abbreviated: ACH, acetylcholine; DA, dopamine; GABA, gamma aminobutyric acid; GLU, glutamate; HIST, histamine; HYP, hypocretin; NA, noradrenaline; 5HT, serotonin.

vigilance. During NREM sleep, the firing of locus ceruleus neurons diminishes compared to waking and they cease firing in REM sleep. The firing of midbrain raphe neurons projecting to forebrain has a similar pattern except that they typically do not respond to sensory input. Both of these systems, the noradrenaline neurons of the locus ceruleus and the serotonin neurons of the midbrain raphe nuclei, have widespread projections to diencephalon, basal forebrain and cerebral cortex. The action of norepinephrine and serotonin at synapses is predominantly modulatory and its seems likely that the action of these systems is to alter the responsiveness of forebrain neurons to other inputs and to contribute to induction of arousal and the maintenance of the waking state in this manner. In contrast, the cholinergic input from basal forebrain and the glutamatergic inputs from thalamus and hypothalamus play a more direct role in arousal and maintaining the waking state.

Sleep–wake regulation requires circadian and homeostatic factors

Circadian timing is crucial to sleep–wake regulation

The solar cycle of light and dark is the most pervasive, cyclic stimulus in the environment. Animals have evolved

rest–activity cycles, sleep–wake cycles in higher vertebrates, to maximize adaptation to their environment. These cycles have two predominant features: (i) in a normal solar cycle, they are exactly 24 hours in length and exhibit a precise phase relationship to the solar cycle, a phenomenon termed 'entrainment'; (ii) in the absence of a light–dark cycle, they are maintained by endogenous timing mechanisms, or clocks. These features predict the fundamental organization of a circadian timing system, a set of related neural structures which functions to provide a precise temporal organization of physiological processes and behaviour. The circadian timing system has three components: (i) photoreceptors that transduce photic information into neural information that is conveyed to circadian pacemakers by entrainment pathways; (ii) pacemakers which receive entrainment information and contain genetically determined molecular timing mechanisms that generate a cellular circadian output; (iii) efferent pathways from the pacemakers to effector systems that are under circadian control. The components of the circadian timing system are shown in Fig. 55.3. Photic information appears to be transduced by a unique set of photoreceptors which appear to be neither rods nor cones. These photoreceptors are connected by as yet unknown retinal elements to a subset of retinal ganglion cells distributed over the entire retina that project only to the circadian timing system through the retinohypotha-

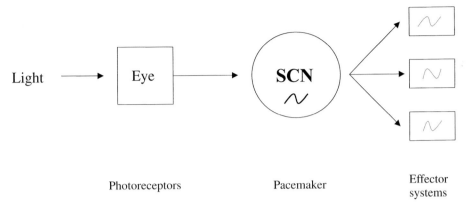

Fig. 55.3. Components of the circadian timing system. See text for description.

lamic tract. Destruction of the retinohypothalamic tract eliminates circadian rhythm entrainment without affecting other aspects of visual function, providing the basis for a disorder of entrainment as a specific sleep disorder (see below).

The circadian pacemaker in mammals that controls most circadian rhythms, particularly the sleep–wake rhythm, is the suprachiasmatic nucleus (SCN) of the hypothalamus. Lesions of the SCN eliminate most circadian rhythms, including the rhythm in sleep–wake behaviour. Neurons of the SCN exhibit a circadian rhythm in firing rate, both in vivo and in vitro and transplantation of fetal SCN into the brains of animals rendered arrhythmic by SCN lesions restores circadian control of sleep–wake behaviour. The output of the SCN is predominantly to hypothalamus and different pathways provide circadian control of separate functions. For example, SCN projections to paraventricular hypothalamic nucleus neurons which, in turn, project to the upper thoracic intermediolateral cell column provide circadian control of melatonin secretion through superior cervical ganglion sympathetic innervation of the pineal gland. Similarly, a separate set of SCN projections to parvocellular corticotropin releasing hormone (CRH) neurons of the paraventricular hypothalamic nucleus controls the production and secretion of CRH at the median eminence with downstream control of pituitary corticotropins and cortisol producing cells of the adrenal cortex. Until recently, the pathways involved in sleep–wake regulation were not well understood. It now seems clear that SCN projections to neuron groups in the posterior and lateral hypothalamus promoting arousal and wakefulness (Fig. 55.2) mediate this function. The function of the SCN in controlling the sleep–wake cycle is one of maintaining arousal against homeostatic drive for sleep. Thus, the circadian system, particularly the SCN, could be viewed as the component of the hypothalamic arousal/waking system depicted in Fig. 55.2.

Homeostatic drive for sleep interacts with circadian control of waking

It is apparent to all humans that a need for sleep, termed homeostatic drive, increases as a function of the waking time since the last period of sleep. Early in the study of sleep control, it was assumed that this was the principal mechanism controlling sleep onset and duration. The role of the circadian system was first recognized to interact with homeostatic mechanisms in a systematic way by Alexander Borbély and Sergei Daan and their associates (Borbély et al., 1989). The homeostatic mechanisms can be conceptualized as a simple, time-dependent accumulation of a sleep-promoting substance, S, which continues to accumulate until it is dissipated by sleep. The extent to which S is lost is a function of the duration of the sleep period.

The nature of S, of whether it is a simple mechanism or multiple factors, is not known. For many years, there have been proposals that the homeostatic propensity for sleep reflects the build-up of sleep-promoting substances in brain. A number of studies have implicated a variety of neuroactive peptides and cytokines as sleep promoting. Perhaps the most intriguing molecule is adenosine. The effects of caffeine and related adenosine-receptor blockers are well known. Adenosine has been shown to accumulate in brain with sleep deprivation, including in areas important for the maintenance of arousal, further supporting this compound as a sleep-promoting substance.

NREM sleep facilitates adaptive, waking behaviour

NREM, or slow wave, sleep is a behavioural state characterized by a lack of response to environmental stimuli, minimal movements and a reduction of brain activity. The majority of total sleep time, which averages 7.5–8.5 hours a day in normal young adults, is spent in NREM sleep. Sleep is typically consolidated with approximately 95% of the night spent asleep in normal young individuals. NREM sleep occupies 75 to 80% and REM 20 to 25% of the total sleep period. NREM and REM sleep alternate in approximately 90-minute epochs with NREM periods becoming shorter and REM periods longer over the night. The proportion of total sleep time in NREM sleep gradually increases over the lifespan as REM sleep diminishes and aging is typically associated with less stage 3 and 4 NREM sleep and more sleep interruptions. Although dreaming is associated primarily with REM sleep, it is well established that dreams can occur in NREM sleep. In general, dreams in NREM sleep are much less frequent, briefer and less complex than those occurring with REM sleep. Although there continues to be speculation about the function of REM sleep (see below), it is generally accepted that NREM sleep has a restorative function that promotes successful adaptive waking behaviour. This includes both a permissive role in restoring a variety of somatic functions and one in restoring brain function. There is substantial support for a hypothesis that NREM sleep works to restore effective brain energy metabolism. Recent data indicate that memory consolidation is an important concomitant of NREM sleep.

Brain activity is reduced in NREM sleep

Consonant with the view that NREM sleep is restorative, the onset of NREM sleep is heralded by increased voltage, slow activity that reflects a synchronous discharge of populations of thalamocortical neurons. And, with positron emission tomography (PET), global cerebral blood flow (CBF) and glucose utilization are shown to be reduced indicating a decrease in information processing as that is reflected in the energy requirements of synaptic activity. CBF decreases by approximately 25% in stages 3–4 NREM sleep in comparison to waking. With analysis of regional blood flow (rCBF), decreases are found in cerebellum, brainstem, thalamus, basal ganglia, basal forebrain and over much of the cortex with only primary sensory areas maintaining waking levels of rCBF (Braun et al., 1997). Extensive electrophysiological analysis since 1985, particularly by Mircea Steriade and David McCormick and their collaborators (for review, see McCormick & Bal, 1997), has shown that NREM sleep represents an interaction between the neurons of thalamic relay nuclei which each project to cerebral cortex with collaterals to thalamic reticular nucleus, cortical neurons projecting to thalamic reticular nucleus and thalamic relay nuclei and the inhibitory pro-

jections of thalamic reticular nucleus to relay nuclei. With the sleep-promoting effects of the sleep homeostatic control mechanisms, there is a gradual hyperpolarization of the components of the thalamocortical system that results in synchronous firing with consequent EEG changes of sleep spindle formation and slow waves which result in the NREM state.

REM sleep reflects an activated forebrain

The typical pattern of sleep is onset with NREM sleep followed by REM sleep in epochs of 90–100 minutes. Through the night the NREM component decreases while the REM component increases and awakening typically occurs from REM sleep. In REM sleep, individuals are unresponsive but the EEG is essentially indistinguishable from waking with low voltage, desynchronized activity. REM sleep is also associated with muscular hypotonia and with saccadic eye movements, the 'REM' of REM sleep. The behaviour of REM sleep is dreaming. When individuals are awakened from REM sleep, approximately 80% report having a dream. There is an extensive literature, beginning particularly with the Freudian psychoanalytic era in psychiatry, reporting analysis of the content of dreams. More recently, attempts have been made to provide a formal, scientific analysis of dream content (for review see Hobson et al., 1998). The content of dreams typically includes visual and motor material which, since sensory input and motor output are inhibited in REM, represent hallucinations. Dream imagery is often bizarre and it is typical to have abrupt transitions in content. There is increased and intensified emotion associated with dream content, particularly fear–anxiety. Dream content proceeds without volitional control. This changing, vivid material of dreams is consonant with an activated cerebral cortex, as is indicated by the nature of REM sleep EEG activity and the fact that glucose utilization in the cortex in REM sleep is equivalent to that in waking. It seems likely that dream content reflects an activated state, and the fact that the cortex is isolated from sensory input and motor output. The other constant feature of dreams is that they are forgotten, lost to conscious recall, unless the individual awakens from a dream and immediately recounts the dream content in the waking state. Since dreams appear to represent a process of cortical activation superimposed on the relatively quiescent state of NREM sleep, the content of the dream can only reflect an ensemble activity of cortical neuronal populations. The mental content of that activity, in turn, must be founded in the experience of that individual and the specific patterns of brain activation occurring in the REM state.

Recent PET studies have provided new insight into the neurobiology of REM sleep. Although there are some small differences among the studies, all show that REM sleep, in comparison to waking, is associated with increased activity in the pons and midbrain, the basal ganglia, hypothalamus and a set of limbic–paralimbic structures including the anterior cingulate and subgenual cortex, orbitofrontal cortex, parahippocampal cortex, and amygdala either as increased cerebral blood flow or as increased glucose utilization. This pattern of increased regional activity in REM is strikingly different from the regional pattern in waking, and that in NREM sleep.

The mechanisms that initiate the onset of REM sleep are unknown, but also probably reflect a combination of homeostatic and circadian factors. The onset of REM sleep occurs with the coincidence of two sets of events, firing from a group of cholinergic REM-on neurons in the pontine reticular formation and diminished firing of the aminergic neurons of the locus ceruleus and raphe nuclei. The firing of the pontine cholinergic neurons generates the forebrain activation of REM sleep and this appears to occur as a consequence of the removal of a tonic inhibition of these neurons by the locus and raphe.

Sleep disorders

Disturbances of sleep are among the most frequent complaints brought to physicians. Sleep disorders are both common and have an extensive morbidity, interfering with performance on the job and in social and family interactions and leading to accidents at work and while driving. And sleep disorders exacerbate medical and psychiatric illnesses. Patients with sleep disorders typically complain of one or more of three types of problems, insomnia, excessive daytime sleepiness or abnormal movements, sensations and behaviours during sleep or at nocturnal awakenings. The approach to these complaints requires a detailed history, physical and neurological examination including an assessment of mental status and the appropriate laboratory tests. Sleep disorders medicine has evolved into a subspeciality with a board examination. There is an International Classification of Sleep Disorders: Diagnostic and Coding Manual (1997) which has four categories of disorders: (i) dyssomnias, disorders of initiating and maintaining sleep and disorders of excessive daytime sleepiness; (ii) parasomnias, disorders which do not present with insomnia or excessive daytime sleepiness; (iii) disorders associated with medical or psychiatric illnesses; (iv) proposed sleep disorders, ones for which there is insufficient current evidence to definitively establish them as sleep disorders. Major examples of the first three categories will be presented below.

Dyssomnias

Sleep apnea syndrome

Sleep apnea syndrome refers to episodes of transient cessation of breathing during sleep (≥ 10 seconds) that disrupt sleep and thereby lead to excessive daytime sleepiness. In most cases, this is related to occlusion of the pharyngeal airway and is referred to as an obstructive sleep apnea syndrome. In other cases, there is reduced ventilatory effort during sleep in the absence of any discrete airway obstruction, and this is referred to as a central sleep apnea syndrome. A third condition, the upper airway resistance syndrome (UARS), consists of increased respiratory effort in the absence of discrete apneic events. This increased effort leads to non-restorative sleep which, in turn, produces daytime sleepiness.

These syndromes occur most commonly in obese, aging men but are not restricted to these Pickwickian types. Epidemiological studies suggest that roughly 4% of men and 2% of women ages 30 to 60 will meet minimal diagnostic criteria for obstructive sleep apnea syndrome. The most common clinical symptoms reported are daytime sleepiness in the presence of sleep-related snoring with occasional pauses in breathing or 'gasping' for breath during sleep. Other daytime symptoms include fatigue, morning headaches, and cognitive changes such as reduced concentration and attention. The sleepiness of sleep apnea is differentiated from the sleepiness of narcolepsy by the constant, unrelenting nature of the sleepiness, whereas, in narcolepsy, the sleepiness is qualitatively more sudden in onset and offset. The constant sleepiness and fatigue need to be differentiated from similar sleep symptoms in psychiatric patients by the concurrent changes in mood or personality found in psychiatric disorders that are not found in the isolated apneic patient.

The pathophysiology of obstructive sleep apnea syndrome is related to the anatomic factors that maintain airway patency during sleep. The site of airway obstruction in obstructive sleep apnea syndrome is in the pharynx. Whether this airway will close during sleep reflects the balance between forces that narrow the airway, such as intrapharyngeal suction during inspiration, and forces that dilate the airway, such as the tone of pharyngeal airway muscles. Anatomical abnormalities found in apneic patients in this area include the manifestations of obesity, enlarged tonsils, and facial bony abnormalities. Additionally, sleep itself is associated with a loss of tone in pharyngeal muscles that maintain the outward pressure necessary for airway patency. Alcohol may contribute to symptoms by acting as an extrinsic suppressant of pharyngeal muscle tone that exacerbates apnea by reducing the outward pressure on the pharyngeal airway.

Central sleep apnea syndrome refers to the periodic loss of ventilatory effort with associated cessation of breathing during sleep. This is differentiated from obstructive type apneas in which there is a loss of breathing despite persistent attempts at ventilation. These patients constitute less than 10% of apneic patients. The pathogenesis of central sleep apnea is likely to be diverse, given the broad conditions that produce this type of breathing during sleep such as central alveolar hypoventilation, congestive heart failure, nasal obstruction and dysautonomias. In general, a final common pathway appears to be some disturbance in the respiratory control system that includes sensors for hypoxia and hypercapnia and brainstem and forebrain centres that influence respiratory function in response to metabolic and behavioural demands. Clinically, patients with alveolar hypoventilation present with signs of respiratory failure, whereas non-hypercapnic patients may present with insomnia, normal body habitus and awakenings with gasping for breath. Diagnosis is definitively made in the research setting by the use of an esophageal balloon. Treatment for the hypercapnic patient with hypoventilation during waking requires ventilation at night using a nasal mask and a pressure-cycled ventilator. For the non-hypercapnic patient, treatment consists of correcting the underlying problem (e.g. nasal obstruction, congestive heart failure) or watchful waiting as approximately 20% may resolve spontaneously. Nasal CPAP can be tried if the patient is obese, snores and has heart failure. Oxygen administration may be helpful if the apneic events are associated with hypoxemia. If symptoms are persistent, a carbonic anhydrase inhibitor can be useful.

Primary insomnia

Insomnia is the experience of inadequate or poor quality of sleep and is characterized by one or more of the following: difficulty falling asleep, difficulty maintaining sleep and/or awakening earlier than one would prefer. Additionally, patients have daytime dysfunction that may include fatigue, altered mood and difficulty with cognitive functions that require attention and concentration. Roughly 10% of the adult population suffers from chronic insomnia and 30 to 50% will experience transient insomnia at some point in their life. Females appear to be more affected across the lifespan and the elderly are particularly vulnerable. Consequences of insomnia may include poor daytime performance, an increased likelihood of subse-

quent development of a mental disorder such as depression or anxiety, and increased medical morbidity and mortality. Insomnias may be classified as either short term (transient) or long term (chronic) and as either primary or secondary to another general medical or mental disorder.

Transient insomnias occur in otherwise healthy individuals and are usually related to sleeping in an unfamiliar environment, an environment that is temporarily disrupted by noises, sounds or temperature changes, a recent life stressor, a change in the timing of bedtime related to travel across time zones or shift work, or to acute administration or withdrawal of a medication that affects the sleep/wake cycle. In each case, identification of the etiology is important. Short-term (1 to 4 weeks) sedative hypnotic use may be indicated. Care should be taken to taper and discontinue this medication following resolution of the acute event to avoid the development of psychological or physiological dependence on the hypnotic.

Chronic primary insomnias are by definition primary and not secondary to other medical or mental disorders. Other terms that have been used to define this population include pyschophysiological insomnia, sleep state misperception and idiopathic insomnia. The term psychophysiological insomnia stems from a literature which suggests that insomnia patients suffer from psychophysiological 'hyperarousal'. A vicious cycle of precipitating event, increased arousal, difficulty sleeping, preoccupation with inability to sleep leading to even more arousal and inability to sleep defines the pathophysiology of these patients. The neurobiology of the concept of 'hyperarousal' however, remains poorly defined. In part, the presence of an excessive amount of high frequency EEG activity within the sleep period is used in support of the concept of hyperarousal. Sleep state misperception refers to the subjective perception of being awake throughout the night, despite the presence of polysomnographically determined sleep. In general, primary insomnia patients tend to underestimate the actual amount of sleep they are getting in a night. These observations raise the likelihood that the sleep that insomniac patients experience may not represent the restorative sleep that non-insomniac patients receive each night. The presence of high frequency EEG activity within polysomnographically determined sleep may represent a less differentiated behavioural state that includes components of both sleep and wakefulness in the same individual. Treatment of insomnia is multifaceted and includes behavioural and pharmacological approaches. Historically, there should be no evidence that the insomnia is secondary, and if so, the underlying disorder should be evaluated and treated. Several behavioural strategies are available. Relaxation techniques include progressive muscle relaxation, EMG biofeedback, meditation, and guided imagery. Stimulus control therapy follows from a learning model of insomnia. In this model, insomniacs develop negative associations to the bedroom, and the sleeping environment that when exposed to, produce increased arousal and subsequent insomnia. Stimulus control instructions include: 'lie down only when you feel sleepy', 'use the bed and bedroom for sleep and sex only', and 'get out of bed and go to another room if you are not sleeping'. Along with these instructions include prescriptions to maintain the same clock times for going to bed and getting out of bed the next day as well as to avoid daytime napping, irrespective of how much sleep had been obtained on the preceding night. Sleep restriction therapy refers to restricting the amount of time in bed to the time that a person believes he/she is actually sleeping. For example, a schedule for someone who believes he/she is sleeping for 6 hours might be set for midnight to 6 am; for 4 hours from 1 am to 5 am; or for 8 hours from 10 pm to 6 am. These individuals should also be instructed to avoid daytime napping. This counters the natural tendency of insomniac patients to nap or prolong their times in bed in an effort to obtain more sleep. This is often counterproductive as it lightens the sleep that they do get, increasing the likelihood of middle of the night and early morning awakenings. Cognitive therapy for insomnia includes questioning erroneous beliefs that an insomniac patient may have regarding the catastrophic consequences of insomnia and beliefs regarding the inadequacy of sleep that they are having.

Narcolepsy

Narcolepsy is a sleep disorder, recognized as a distinct entity for more than a century, characterized by excessive daytime sleepiness and the intrusion of REM sleep phenomena, particularly cataplexy (muscle atonia induced by emotion-provoking stimuli), into waking. Individuals with narcolepsy may fall asleep at any time during the day, often very abruptly. These uncontrollable episodes of daytime sleeping are the necessary and predominant manifestation of narcolepsy in most affected individuals and this symptom, particularly when associated with cataplexy, produces severe impairment of function in social interactions and work performance and a very diminished quality of life. Despite the occurrence of daytime sleep episodes, total daily sleep time is unaltered because night sleep is reduced proportionately to that occurring during the day. The diagnosis of narcolepsy is often difficult because there are many causes of excessive daytime sleepiness, and this problem is accentuated because a lack of understanding of

the pathophysiology of the disease has prevented development of a simple and reliable diagnostic test. It appears, however, that this situation will change in the near future. A series of recent studies indicates that narcolepsy will be a model for the application of molecular genetics and molecular biology to the understanding of disease.

Unfolding the basis for narcolepsy began in 1998 with the discovery of a new gene, expressed in the hypothalamus, that codes for new peptides termed hypocretins, or orexins. The term 'orexin' appears inappropriate as it was applied with the view that the peptides function primarily in the control of feeding and this clearly is not the case. 'Hypocretin' was applied to signify that the gene is expressed in the hypothalamus and that the peptide product belongs to the secretin family of peptides. Following discovery of the hypocretin gene, and characterization of the peptide, immunohistochemical studies showed that hypocretin neurons are located exclusively in the posterior and lateral hypothalamus with axonal projections distributed widely over the neuraxis, particularly to areas involved in arousal and to the entire neocortex in rodents and the human. Transgenic mice with deletion of the hypocretin gene exhibit a behavioural phenotype consistent with narcolepsy, and a well-characterized canine model of narcolepsy was found to carry a mutation in the gene for a hypocretin receptor. Analysis of CSF from narcoleptic patients demonstrated a marked reduction in hypocretin content in comparison to controls. Finally, immunohistochemical analysis of narcoleptic brains shows a striking loss of hypocretin neurons and their axonal plexuses in the hypothalamus. Thus, in less than 2 years we progressed from almost no understanding of the pathophysiology of narcolepsy to a detailed account of a very selective neuropathology. The principal issues remaining are to determine the basis for the hypocretin neuron pathology and how this results in the manifestations of the disease. Although there are instances of familial cases, narcolepsy is predominantly a sporadic disease. Until the recent work on the hypocretin neuron pathology, the only known biological association was the finding that over 90% of narcoleptics have the histocompatibility marker HLA-DQB1 0602. This suggests that the hypocretin neuron pathology may occur on an autoimmune basis; that is, the fundamental basis of the pathophysiology is a genetically determined immune system status that results in a predilection to autoimmune responses in which individuals produce antibodies against hypocretin. This is an attractive hypothesis but it remains to be established.

There are two independent clusters of symptoms that may require treatment in narcoleptic patients. The first is daytime sleepiness. Given the severity of the sleepiness, it would be unusual for behavioural interventions to be completely effective. Some patients find that adding periodic, brief daytime naps reduces some of the sleep attacks. Allowing for adequate sleep at night is advised, and occasionally, these patients will demonstrate insomnia, or nightmares, that require the use of a sedative hypnotic medication. The primary treatment for sleepiness, however, consists of the use of either a stimulant medication or a medication that promotes wakefulness. The commonly used stimulants include methylphenidate, dextroamphetamine, and pemoline, in descending order of stimulant potency. Short-acting preparations last around 4 hours and longer-acting preparations extend this effect a few hours. Consequently, these medications are often prescribed at least at morning and around lunchtime. Occasionally, a patient may need a late afternoon dose if he/she anticipates being involved in activities during the evening that require full attention. Often, the development of tolerance to low doses forces escalation to effective levels. Side effects such as nervousness, affective symptoms and nocturnal insomnia require monitoring. An alternate medication is modafinil. This medication often reduces daytime sleep and benefits most patients. Some patients, however, do not obtain full relief of their sleepiness with modafinil and require addition of a stimulant. Modafinil is an interesting addition to the treatment of narcolepsy in that it does not appear to act via the dopamine systems, has very limited potential for abuse and does not appear to induce tolerance.

The second cluster of symptoms that require treatment includes cataplexy, hypnagogic hallucinations and sleep onset paralysis. Of these, the cataplexy is the most significant symptom clinically, as it is associated with considerable limitation in psychosocial function and potential danger to the individual as a result of personal injury from falls. These symptoms are generally effectively managed with the use of antidepressant agents such as clomipramine, the selective serotonin reuptake inhibitors, or venlafaxine. Dosages that relieve cataplexy are generally lower than those used to treat depression. Tolerance to these agents can develop which may require switching to an alternative agent.

Disorders of circadian function

The function of the CTS is to provide a temporal organization of physiological processes and behaviour to promote effective adaptation to the environment. At the behavioural level, this is expressed in regular cycles of sleep and waking and disorders of circadian function are typically characterized by disturbances of sleep and waking and by other behavioural symptoms that reflect both the sleep disturbances and alterations of circadian regulation of waking adaptive behaviour. From the organization of the CTS, we would expect three types of circadian disorder: abnormalities of entrainment, pacemaker function and pacemaker coupling to effector systems (for recent review, see Moore, 1998).

Disorders of entrainment

Blindness (non-24 hour sleep–wake syndrome)

Congenital and acquired blindness provide instances of pure disorders of entrainment. Individuals who are blind typically attempt to adapt their behaviour to that of their community. For a number of years it was believed that the blind accomplished this by entraining their circadian system to the social cues of the environment, but it now appears that many are not able to do so. Blind subjects fall into two categories. The first is composed of individuals with a free-running melatonin rhythm indicating that they were not entrained to the environmental light–dark cycle. These individuals typically maintain 24-hour sleep–wake cycles, however, and when their melatonin rhythm peaks during sleep, they report sleeping well and feeling well. When their melatonin and sleep periods are out of phase, they experience sleep disturbances and other symptoms indicative of disturbed circadian regulation. The second blind group has entrained melatonin rhythms and sleep–wake cycles and reports no symptoms of sleep disturbance or those related to circadian disruption. Some of these individuals show a normal suppression of peak melatonin levels by light even though they are totally blind. The nocturnal suppression of peak melatonin levels is a function of the retinohypothalamic projections so that we must conclude that, in these individuals, the retinal phototransduction mechanisms are intact through those pathways even though all other retinal mechanisms are non-functional. The mirror image of this is individuals who are not blind but exhibit the free-running rhythms and symptoms of the non-24-hour sleep–wake syndrome. Although this remains to be established, we would presume that these individuals lack the specific circadian phototransduction process. There are also blind individuals who are normally entrained but lack light suppression of melatonin. It is assumed that these individuals employ a non-photic entrainment process.

Rapid time zone change syndrome (jet lag)

The jet lag syndrome is a disorder of modern life. Symptoms of rapid time zone change occur in some individuals with changes of as little as 3 hours but at least a 5-hour change is required for most. The typical symptoms of jet lag include sleep disruption, fatigue, difficulty concentrating, gastrointestinal distress, impaired psychomotor coordination, reduced cognitive skills and alterations of mood. The symptoms remit spontaneously over days with their duration determined by the direction of travel, west to east produces more impairment than east to west, and the number of time zones crossed. Numerous measures have been reported to ameliorate jet lag but the evidence is usually anecdotal. Recent studies done with a placebo control indicate that melatonin is an effective treatment, presumably by acting on the SCN pacemaker. An interesting recent study has reported both cognitive changes and temporal lobe atrophy in individuals with chronic jet lag (Cho, 2001).

Work shift syndrome

Many workers in industrialized countries perform their occupation at unusual hours. This is particularly true of health care workers, police and security guards, truck drivers and some workers in heavy industry. The factors involved in adjusting to shift work are complex and disruption of circadian mechanisms is only one of those involved. The major symptom of work shift disorder is impaired sleep and attendant impairment of function. There have been recent descriptions of the use of bright light and melatonin to treat the circadian abnormalities associated with shift work.

Delayed sleep phase syndrome

This is a syndrome characterized by a persistent inability to fall asleep and arise at conventional clock times. This reflects a delay in the phase of the sleep–wake cycle. Sleep onset is usually delayed to early morning hours with a consequent delay in arising. If individuals attempt to go to bed earlier, they are unable to go to sleep until their usual time and, if they attempt to maintain a normal schedule, they suffer insomnia and daytime fatigue. This syndrome has customarily been viewed as a consequence of choice, or lifestyle, so-called 'night' people. It often begins in the teenage years which, with the other behavioural manifestations of this difficult period, has tended to reinforce this view. While the symptoms clearly represent lifestyle in some individuals, it is also clearly a disorder of entrainment in others in which there appears to be an alteration of normal pacemaker sensitivity to entraining stimuli.

Advanced sleep phase syndrome

This is the mirror image of the delayed sleep phase syndrome. Individuals with the advanced sleep phase syndrome have persistent early onset of sleep, usually around 7–9 pm with a consequent awakening at 3–5 am. Attempts to delay sleep onset are usually met with failure and complaints of an inability to stay awake for social events in the evening, and being alone without companionship in the early morning, are typical. If they try to maintain a normal bedtime, they have difficulty with severe evening fatigue. This syndrome is most often reported in the elderly.

Disorders of pacemaker function and pacemaker–effector coupling

There are two types of disorders associated with pacemaker dysfunction. The first is a loss of circadian function; arrhythmicity similar to that seen in animals with destruction of the pacemaker. The second is an alteration of normal pacemaker output. A diminution of the amplitude of circadian rhythms is characteristic of aging. In this circumstance, however, it is unclear whether the problem is at the level of the pacemaker or reflects a partial inability of effector systems to respond to a normal pacemaker input.

Irregular sleep–wake pattern syndrome

This is a relatively uncommon syndrome in which affected individuals have an irregular distribution of sleep and wake with numerous interruptions. These individuals complain both of their difficult schedule and insomnia and of daytime fatigue, and appear to be arrhythmic. In some instances in which 24-hour recordings have been made, there is no discernible rhythm in core body temperature. This may occur in two situations, with evident hypothalamic pathology such as a tumour compressing the anterior hypothalamus, and spontaneously without evident neuropathology.

Syndrome associated with decreased amplitude

In many elderly individuals, there is increased fragmentation of sleep and less sleep in the deeper stages of slow wave sleep, decreased amplitude of the body temperature rhythm and decreased amplitude of the cortisol and melatonin rhythms as well as the advance in phase described above. These observations suggest that there is a decrease in pacemaker output in aging and that the symptomatic expression of this abnormality is insomnia. It has been reported recently that melatonin therapy, which should improve pacemaker coupling, is significantly better than placebo in treating sleep disturbances in the elderly. It is not possible to state, however, that the sleep disturbances of the elderly do not include problems of pacemaker coupling to output systems. It seems likely that a complex interaction of decreased pacemaker output and decreased responsiveness of effector systems to pacemaker output are operative in many of the circadian disturbances of the elderly.

Parasomnias

Restless legs syndrome/periodic limb movement disorder

The restless legs syndrome (RLS) and periodic limb movement disorder are related sleep disorders. Restless legs refers to a waking complaint that interferes with sleep onset, whereas periodic limb movements are found during sleep and may interfere with restorative sleep. The restless legs complaint is a dysesthesia described as an uncomfortable restless, or creeping and crawling sensation in the lower legs. This sensation is only relieved with vigorous movement of the legs, often requiring the patient to get out of bed. The disorder affects between 5 and 10% of the population, beginning generally in mid-life. Periodic limb movements during sleep often occur with restless legs syndrome, but may be found in isolation. In this disorder, stereotypic periodic (every 20–40 seconds) limb movements (0.5 to 5 second extensions of the big toe and dorsiflexion of the foot at the ankle are often associated with signs of arousal from sleep, such as K complexes followed by alpha EEG waves. The degree to which PLMS is a disorder that either impairs sleep or that requires any intervention remains unclear, however, since roughly 11% of the normal population without sleep complaints, especially the aged, will demonstrate PLMS on polysomnographic assessment.

The pathophysiology of RLS and PLMS has not been well defined. The effectiveness of dopamine agonists and levodopa in the treatment of RLS-PLMS suggests that abnormal dopaminergic function in the CNS may play a role. The efficacy of opiates in the treatment of the disorder suggests a role for the endogenous opiate system. Associated medical conditions for RLS include uremia, iron deficiency anemia, peripheral neuropathy, fibromyalgia, magnesium deficiency, rheumatoid arthritis and post-traumatic stress disorder. Medications that exacerbate RLS or PLMS include lithium, tricyclic and SSRI medications as well as withdrawal from anticonvulsants, benzodiazepines and barbiturates. Bupropion is one antidepressant that has been associated with a reduction in periodic limb movements, perhaps related to its dopaminergic activity.

The treatment of RLS and PLMS is primarily dopaminergic agonists, or levodopa/carbidopa, administered at bedtime. The relatively short duration of action of these drugs often requires a second dose during the night unless the sustained release preparation is used. Benzodiazepines and traditional sedative/hypnotics consolidate sleep and may reduce arousal secondary to the PLMS. Opiate medications are useful in the treatment of these disorders but, given their abuse potential, they should be employed as a last measure. Less information is available to support the use of other agents such as carbamazepine, clonidine and gabapentin.

NREM parasomnias

Three related sleep disorders, or sleep syndromes, fall into a category of NREM parasomnias: confusional arousals, sleep terrors and sleepwalking. Each is thought to represent a 'disorder or arousal'. As a group, these disorders tend to occur normally in children below the age of 5 when behavioural state regulation is not yet well differentiated. There appears to be a genetic tendency for these disorders as a group. Persistence into adulthood is not the norm, but when they do, they can interfere with psychosocial functioning. They each tend to occur out of a deeper NREM sleep stage (slow wave sleep) early in the night and each is associated with amnesia for the event.

Confusional arousals refer to periods of partial sleep and partial waking behaviour with amnesia for the events on full awakening. The individual will have the appearance of being confused, disoriented with incomplete responsiveness to their surroundings. These episodes may last from a few seconds to a few minutes with return to sleep.

Sleep terrors refer to periods in which the individual seems to be in the midst of a panic-like state with crying out, sitting erect in bed with acute autonomic arousal such as increases in heart rate, respiration and sweating. No recall of the event is noted.

Sleep walking refers to the appearance of motor behaviour during sleep that can lead to an individual getting out of bed and walking around his/her environment. Occasionally the motor behaviour is isolated to the bed, with uncomplicated, brief, automatic behaviours. At other times, the behaviour can be very complex, including walking around the bedroom performing some stereotypic act, or leaving the bedroom and walking around the house. Sleep-related eating episodes are not uncommon. On rare occasions, a sleepwalker may leave his/her immediate home, walk around the neighbourhood or even drive a car. In general, the individual returns to bed voluntarily, either on completion of the episode, or after full awakening from the episode. The individual is often somewhat difficult to arouse and only partially responsive to environmental stimuli. Complete amnesia for the events is most common.

The pathophysiology for all of the confusional arousals is unclear. A strong genetic component is recognized for both sleep terrors and sleepwalking. Aside from this, factors which are associated with increasing the depth of sleep, such as sleep deprivation, or dissociating sleep, such as acute toxic/metabolic changes, or stressing an individual may increase the likelihood that these episodes will occur in genetically predisposed individuals. Presumably, these episodes occur when there is dissociation between the brain mechanisms that regulate cortical activation or behavioural arousal and those that regulate motor behaviour. It remains unclear whether there is an association between these events and psychopathology. Any association may simply be related to the observations that mental disorders are themselves associated with disruptions in sleep continuity, factors that would be expected to increase the frequency of such events in susceptible individuals.

The diagnosis of each of these disorders is generally a clinical one. Reports of parasomnias in the first third of the night with specific features as described above support the diagnoses. Polysomnography can be performed, although it is infrequently helpful given the difficulty of 'capturing' one of the episodes in the sleep laboratory. Attempts to precipitate an episode in the lab by forced arousals from delta sleep may aid in diagnosis. In cases where a seizure disorder may be suspected, one or several daytime diagnostic EEGs and an EEG during sleep may be performed to detect epileptiform activity.

Treatment of these disorders is largely conservative and educational in nature, informing the patient and his/her family about sleep and the generally benign longitudinal course of parasomnic behaviours. At the time of occurrence, the individuals should not be disturbed, but rather the parasomnic events should be allowed to self-terminate. Occasionally, forced arousals during an event can precipitate an unconscious aggressive attack. Minimizing sleep deprivation, stressors and medications or dietary factors that may interfere with sleep integrity (e.g. alcohol, caffeine, antidepressant medications) are recommended. If there is reason to suspect that the behaviours may be interfering with either sleep integrity or with daytime functioning, occasional use of sleep consolidating medications such as the benzodiazepines may be effective in preventing the escalation of these partial arousals into more complex behaviours during sleep. If an underlying mental disorder is present that appears to be interfering with sleep continuity, this can be referred for appropriate intervention, either psychotherapy or pharmacotherapy with non-alerting antidepressant medications. If there is a history of either self- or other- injury during the events, steps should be taken to 'sleepwalker-proof' the bedroom and surrounding environment. This may include the removal of potentially dangerous objects, locking doors and separating bed-partners from the sleepwalker.

Nightmares

The term 'nightmare' implies a vivid dream in which something catastrophic or frightening is happening either to the dreamer or to someone else. Often, this term also implies an awakening from the frightening dream in a fearful state. There is no clear distinction, however, between a nightmare and a dream. Nearly everyone has experienced a nightmare suggesting that this is a normal phenomenon of sleep. In general, the causal occurrence of nightmares does not come to the attention of the medical community and no interventions are required. Nightmares are more common in childhood than in adulthood and more common in girls than in boys. The prevalence of a nightmare disorder is difficult to define, however, given the difficulty in defining a separate disorder from the more common occurrence of having bad dreams.

The pathophysiology of nightmares is unknown. Human brain imaging studies performed during REM sleep consistently reveal selective activation of anterior limbic and paralimbic structures, regions thought to play a significant role in emotional behaviour, although no comparative studies have been performed to differentiate regional cerebral function during REM sleep in healthy subjects vs. nightmare disorder subjects. Elevations in autonomic arousal prior to awakening with a nightmare have been observed. Behavioural studies suggest that individuals with 'thin' interpersonal boundaries, defined as more open, sensitive and vulnerable to intrusions, are more susceptible to suffering from nightmares. Numerous drugs that affect sleep, and REM sleep specifically, such as many antidepressant medications, are known to precipitate nightmares. Alcohol withdrawal is particularly associated with bizarre vivid dreaming. Subjects with post-traumatic stress disorder have recurrent intrusive nightmares related to their traumatic life experience as part of their diagnostic criteria.

Given the diverse etiologies of nightmares, there is no uniform therapy. Identification and removal of precipitating factors including toxic/metabolic or drug induced is often the simplest treatment. There have been no empirical medication trials to determine the efficacy of any medication treatment for nightmare sufferers and clinical experience would suggest that response is highly individual. Psychotherapy may be of some benefit in cases where the nightmare appears to reflect an unsuccessful attempt at some type of emotionally adaptive behaviour to a stressful life situation.

REM sleep behaviour disorder

Clinically, REM sleep behaviour disorder (RBD) refers to a parasomnia in which there are sleep-related behaviours associated with elaborate dream mentation. Depending on the elaborateness of the behaviour and the aggressiveness of the dream, these behaviours can result in accidental self- or other injury. In general, the nature of the dream enactments is out of character for the person's waking behaviour. Often, the presenting complaint comes from the bed-partner who is concerned about the behaviours rather than the actual patient who often is unaware that anything unusual has happened during sleep. The disorder most often occurs in men and is more common in aging.

The pathophysiology of the disorder can best be understood, based on an understanding of the normal physiology of REM sleep. REM sleep occurs periodically throughout the night, alternating with NREM sleep in roughly 90-minute cycles. During REM sleep the brain is in an active behavioural state in which cerebral metabolism and other signs of cortical activation are comparable to those of waking. Two exceptions include the absence of conscious awareness and the near complete immobilization of skeletal musculature via an active inhibition of motor activity by pontine centres in the locus ceruleus region. These exert an excitatory influence on the magnocellular reticular nucleus of the medulla. This nucleus in turn, hyperpolarizes spinal motor neurons. It is inferred that a defect in some aspect of this REM sleep atonia system is disturbed in patients suffering from REM sleep behaviour disorder.

Acute toxic/metabolic RBD has been associated with alcohol and benzodiazepine Withdrawal, or an adverse effect associated with administration of tricyclic antidepressants, monoamine oxidase inhibitors, selective serotonin reuptake inhibitors and clomipramine. Chronic RBD is either idiopathic (estimated to be around 40%) or associated with some form of neurologic insult. These can be from a variety of etiologies including vascular, malignant, infectious and degenerative. The specific pathology in each case, although presumed to have a final common pathway on the REM sleep atonia system is not known.

Diagnosis is suspected based on a clinical report of potentially harmful sleep-related behaviours in which there appears to be an acting out of some dream sequence. Diagnosis is confirmed in a polysomnographic study that shows increased tone, or increased twitching in the chin EMG channel. Videotaping sleep-related behaviours is helpful diagnostically when increased movements are seen during a polysomnographically identified REM sleep period.

The most widely supported treatment for RBD is administration of clonazepam at bedtime beginning with small doses and titrating upwards to achieve clinical benefit. In general, tolerance is not seen and this medication is reported to be helpful in over 90% of cases.

Medical–psychiatric sleep disorders

Sleep disorders associated with psychiatric illness

We turn now to characterizing the sleep disturbances in the major mental disorders, where the vast majority of research has been in the areas of depression and schizophrenia.

Depression

The majority of patients with mood disorders describe difficulty falling asleep, difficulty staying asleep, and difficulty returning to sleep after early morning awakenings. Clinically, they report a paradoxical state of physical daytime fatigue, yet with persistent mental activity that makes it difficult for them to fall asleep at night. Whereas insomnia characterizes the melancholia of middle age and elderly unipolar depression, younger patients and bipolar depressed patients will often describe difficulty getting up in the morning and hypersomnia during the daytime.

An extensive literature describes the changes in electroencephalographic (EEG) sleep in patients with depression. Measures derived from the EEG sleep recordings that have been found to differ between healthy and depressed subjects include measures of sleep continuity, measures of visually scored EEG sleep stages, and automated measures of characteristics of the EEG waveform across the sleep period such as period amplitude or EEG spectral power measures.

The changes in subjective sleep complaints are paralleled by EEG measures of sleep. These include increases in sleep latency and decreases in sleep continuity. In terms of EEG sleep stages or 'sleep architecture', depressed patients often show reduced state 3 and 4 NREM sleep. Several changes in REM sleep have also been noted. These include an increase in the amount of REM sleep, a shortening of the time to onset of the first REM period of the night, a shortened REM latency, and an increase in the frequency of eye movements within a rapid eye movement period. Depressed women appear to have relative preservation of stages 3 and 4 slow wave sleep in relation to depressed men.

Other studies have correlated the severity of psychopathology with sleep abnormalities in depression. Patients with psychotic depression have particularly severe EEG sleep disturbances and very short REM sleep latencies. Patients with recurrent depression have more severe REM sleep disturbances than patients in their first episode and sleep continuity and REM sleep disturbances are more prominent early in a recurrent depressive episode. EEG sleep findings help to inform our understanding of the neurobiology of longitudinal course and treatment outcome in depression. Although severely reduced REM latencies, phasic REM measures and sleep continuity disturbances generally move toward control values after remission of depression, most sleep measures show high correlations with clinical manifestations across the course of an episode. Reduced REM latency is associated with increased response rates to pharmacotherapy, but not to psychotherapy. Depressed patients with abnormal sleep profiles (reduced REM latency, increased REM density and poor sleep continuity) are significantly less likely to respond to cognitive behaviour therapy and interpersonal therapy than patients with a 'normal' profile. Reduced REM latency and decreased delta EEG activity in the first episode appear to be associated with increased likelihood, or decreased time until recurrence, of depression in patients treated with medications or psychotherapy.

Each of the major neurotransmitter systems which has been shown to modulate the ascending activation of the cortex, i.e. the cholinergic, noradrenergic and serotonergic systems, have been implicated in the pathophysiology of mood disorders. Nearly all effective antidepressant medications show a pronounced inhibition of REM sleep including a prolongation of the first REM cycle and a reduction in the overall percentage of REM sleep except for nefazadone and bupropion which do not suppress REM sleep. Enhanced cholinergic function concurrent with reduced monoaminergic tone in the central nervous system has been proposed as a pharmacologic model for depression. In an exaggerated sense, the state of REM sleep mimics the formulation. REM can be viewed as a cholinergically driven state with reduced firing of noradrenergic and serotonergic neurons. Cholinergic agents such as the muscarinic agonist, arecoline, physostigmine and scopolamine produce exaggerated REM sleep effects in depressed patients in comparison to patients with eating disorders, personality disorders, anxiety disorders, and healthy controls. These studies suggest that there may be a supersensitivity of the cholinergic system driving REM sleep in depressed patients, although an alternative plausible hypothesis is that there may be reduced monoaminergic (5-HT and/or NA) inhibition of the brainstem cholinergic nuclei. Selective serotonin reuptake inhibitors (SSRIs) are known to have prominent REM suppressing activity, most notably early in the night when alterations in REM sleep are most common in depression. A tryptophan-free diet, which depletes central serotonin activity, is noted to decrease REM latency in healthy controls and in depressed patients and ipsaparone, a 5-HT1a agonist, is noted to prolong REM latency in both normal controls and in depressed patients. Anatomically, 5-HT1a receptors have been conceptualized as the limbic receptors given their high densities in the hippocampus, the septum, the amygdala, and cortical paralimbic structures. The action of serotonin in these structures is largely inhibitory. Given the importance of limbic and paralimbic structures in REM sleep modulation, the influence of SSRIs may be mediated by these limbic receptors. Importantly, in the brainstem laterodorsal tegmental nucleus, a cholinergic cell group involved in the generation of REM sleep, bursting cholinergic neurons are inhibited by the action of serotonin on 5-HT1a receptors. The 5-HT1a antagonist pindolol reduces REM sleep in healthy subjects. This has been interpreted to be a consequence of a reduction in midbrain raphe serotonin neuron autoregulation resulting in increased serotonergic input to pontine cholinergic centres which inhibits REM sleep.

Given the selective activation of limbic and paralimbic structures during REM sleep in healthy subjects, the study of the functional neuroanatomy during REM sleep in depressed patients may provide insight into the pathophysiology of depression. In contrast to healthy controls, depressed patients fail to activate anterior paralimbic structures (anterior cingulate and medial prefrontal cortices) from waking to REM sleep and show large activations in the dorsal tectum and activations in the sensorimotor cortex, inferior temporal cortex, uncus, amygdala, and subicular complex during REM sleep. These findings indicate that depressed patients have patterns of brain activation from waking to REM sleep that differ markedly from healthy controls. In the context of models relating forebrain function during REM sleep to attention, motivation, emotion and memory, these results suggest that REM sleep abnormalities in depressed patients are associated with alterations in limbic and paralimbic forebrain function which reflect the basic pathophysiology of depression (Fig. 55.4, see colour plate section).

Functional neuroimaging of sleep in depressed subjects would be expected to provide insight into homeostatic regulation of sleep in mood disorders patients since this is a time in which the build-up of a sleep-dependent process, process S, is discharged and during which growth hormone secretion occurs. Whole brain and regional cerebral glucose metabolism are elevated during the first NREM period of the night for depressed men in relation to healthy men suggesting a reduction of homeostatic mechanisms secondary to cortical hyperarousal. Other studies have shown that reductions in delta sleep in depressed patients are associated with reductions in afternoon waking relative and global blood flow. This suggests that the elevations in glucose metabolism during NREM sleep in depressed patients are not related to a waking hypermetabolic state. Studies across waking and NREM sleep are needed in order to clarify this notion. Depression symptoms respond to acute sleep deprivation and imaging studies have shown that depressed patients who have high pre-treatment relative glucose metabolic rates in the medial prefrontal cortex are more likely to respond to sleep deprivation. Further, a reduction in relative metabolism in this region was found following sleep deprivation.

Schizophrenia

The predominant current view in biological psychiatry is that schizophrenia is a developmental brain disorder with many of its manifestations the consequence of selective, early onset neuronal degeneration. Early sleep studies sought to test the intriguing hypothesis that aspects of the thought disorder in schizophrenia are a spillover of the dream state into wakefulness. No evidence has accrued to support this view, but subtle alterations in architecture of REM sleep have been reported. These are difficult to interpret, however, as studies examining treatment of naïve schizophrenia patients show no increases in REM sleep and the increases in REM sleep observed in previously treated subjects probably reflect effects of medication withdrawal, and/or changes related to the acute psychotic state.

Slow wave sleep is of particular interest to schizophrenia because of the implication of the prefrontal cortex in this disorder and in the generation of NREM sleep. Several studies have shown a reduction of NREM sleep in schizophrenic patients. NREM sleep deficits have been seen in acute, chronic, and remitted states and in never-medicated, neuroleptic-treated and unmedicated patients. Research since 1990 has focused increasingly on both the positive and negative syndromes of schizophrenia, a conceptual distinction of particular importance to understanding its pathophysiology. In a longitudinal study, alterations of NREM sleep appeared to be stable when polysomnographic studies were repeated at 1 year, but the REM sleep parameters appeared to change. These observations suggest that NREM sleep deficits in schizophrenia might be trait related. Consistent with this view, delta sleep abnormalities have been found to correlate with negative symptoms and with impaired outcome at one and at two years.

In general, it has been difficult to determine a clear abnormality in sleep–wake regulation in schizophrenia.

Alzheimer's disease

Disturbances in sleep commonly accompany Alzheimer's disease. These disturbances are a significant cause of distress for caregivers often leading to institutionalization of these patients. The changes in sleep often parallel the changes in cognitive function in demented patients. Also, daytime agitation has been associated with sleep quality at night. A large-scale community-based study of Alzheimer's disease patients reported that sleeping more than usual and early morning awakenings were the most common sleep disturbances in non-institutionalized patients. Night-time awakenings, however, were more disturbing to caregivers. Night-time awakenings were associated with male gender, and greater memory and functional declines. Three groups of subjects were identified in association with nocturnal awakenings: (i) patients with only daytime inactivity; (ii) patients with fearfulness, fidgeting and occasional sadness; and (iii) patients with multiple behavioural problems including frequent episodes of sadness, fearfulness, inactivity, fidgeting and hallucinations.

In terms of sleep laboratory-based evaluations, sleep continuity disturbances in these patients include decreased sleep efficiencies, increased lighter stage 1 NREM sleep, and an increased frequency of arousals and awakenings. Sleep architecture abnormalities include decreases in stages 3 and 4 NREM sleep and some reports of decreases in REM sleep. Loss of sleep spindling and K complexes have also been noted in dementia. Sleep apnea has been observed in 33 to 53% of patients with probable Alzheimer's disease. It is unclear if there is an increased prevalence of sleep apnea, however, in Alzheimer's patients in relation to age- and gender-matched controls. Nocturnal behavioural disruptions, or 'sun-downing' are reported commonly in the clinical management of Alzheimer's patients, although specific diagnostic criteria for a 'sun-downing' episode have been difficult to define. Despite extensive clinical research in this area, the pathophysiology of sun-downing, including its relationship with brain mechanisms that control sleep/wake and circadian regulation remain unclear. Overall, the literature on sleep in Alzheimer's disease suggests that the primary defect in this disease is the more general neurodegenerative changes that lead to the profound cognitive and functional declines of this disease and that the sleep changes are secondary manifestations of the disorder. If sleep is viewed as generated by core sleep systems that then require a relatively intact neural cortex and subcortical areas for expression of behavioural states, then the sleep changes in Alzheimer's disease are most likely related to end-organ failure, in the cortex, as opposed to pathology in key sleep or circadian systems themselves.

Parkinson's disease

Light, fragmented sleep occurs frequently in Parkinson's disease patients. Sleep problems have been reported in as high as 74–96% of patients. Complaints included frequent awakenings, early awakening, nocturnal cramps, pains, nightmares, vivid dreams, visual hallucinations, vocalizations, somnambulisms, impaired motor function during sleep, myoclonic jerks, excessive daytime sleepiness, REM sleep behaviour disorder, sleep-related violence leading to injury. These changes may result from the disease itself, or to complications from treatment with dopaminergic agents. Additionally, depression is common in Parkinson's disease and the sleep disruption may in part be related to this comorbid disorder.

Sleep architecture abnormalities include increased awakenings, reductions in stages 3 and 4 sleep, REM sleep and sleep spindles. Reductions in REM latency have been observed. Increased muscular activity, contractions and periodic limb movements may prevent slow-wave sleep and foster light fragmented sleep. Disorganized respiration is also found. Recent studies have raised concern about abrupt onset daytime sleep episodes in Parkinson's disease in association with treatment with newer dopamine agonists. Although this requires further analysis, it is unclear whether the sleep episodes are more frequent with dopamine agonist therapy than in the Parkinson's disease population.

In conclusion, sleep disorders are common and carry a substantial morbidity and cost to society. They occur as primary disorders, responses to the environmental demands of modern society, major manifestations of psychiatric diseases and important complications of medical illnesses, including neurological diseases. Understanding the neurobiology of sleep and sleep disorders is critical to the practice of neurology.

General Reference

Kryger, M.H., Roth, T., Dement, W.C. *Principles and Practice of Sleep Medicine*. 3rd Edn, Saunders, Philadelphia, 2000.

References

Bazhenov, M., Timofeev, I., Steriade, M. & Sejnowski, T. (2000). Spiking-bursting activity in the thalamic reticular nucleus initiates sequences of spindle oscillations in thalamic networks. *J. Neurophysiol.*, **84**, 1076–87.

Bennington, J.H. & Heller, H.C. (1994). REM-sleep timing is controlled homeostatically by accumulation of REM-sleep propensity in non-REM sleep. *Am. J. Physiol.*, **266**, R1992–2000.

Bennington, J.H. & Heller, H.C. (1995). Restoration of brain energy metabolism as the function of sleep. *Prog. Neurobiol.*, **45**, 347–60.

Bliwise, D.L., Hughes, M., McMahon, P.M. et al. (1995). Observed sleep/wakefulness and severity of dementia in an Alzheimer's disease special care unit. *J. Gerontol.*, **50**, M303–6.

Borbély, A.A., Tobler, I., Loepfe, M. et al. (1984). All-night spectral analysis of the sleep EEG in untreated depressives and normal controls. *Psychiatry Res.*, **12**, 27.

Borbély, A.A., Ackerman, P., Trachsel, L. & Tobler, I. (1989). Sleep initiation and initial sleep intensity: interactions of homeostatic and circadian mechanisms. *J. Biol. Rhythms*, **4**, 149–60.

Braun, A.R., Balkin, T.J., Wesensten, N.J. et al. (1997). Regional cerebral blood flow throughout the sleep–wake cycle: an H$_2$, ^{15}O PET study. *Brain*, **120**, 1173–97.

Cho, K. (2001). Chronic 'jet lag' produces temporal lobe atrophy and spatial cognitive deficits. *Nat. Neurosci.* **4**, 567–8.

Dijk, D.J. & Czeisler, C.A. (1994). Paradoxical timing of the circadian rhythm of sleep propensity serves to consolidate sleep and wakefulness in humans. *Neurosci. Lett.*, **166**, 63–8.

Ganguli, R., Reynolds, C.F. & Kupfer, D.J. (1987). Electroencephalographic sleep in young, never medicated schizophrenics. *Arch. Gen. Psychiatry*, **44**, 36.

Ho, A.P., Gillin, J.C., Buchsbaum, M.S. et al. (1996). Brain glucose metabolism during non-rapid eye movement sleep in major depression: a positron emission tomography study. *Arch. Gen. Psychiatry*, **53**, 645.

Hobson, J.A., Stickgold, R. & Pace-Schott, E.F. (1998). The neuropychology of REM sleep dreaming. *NeuroReport*, **9**, R1–R14.

Jones, B.E. (2000). Basic mechanisms of sleep–wake states. In *The Principles and Practice of Sleep Medicine*, 3rd edn, ed. M. Kryger et al., pp. 134–54.

Keshavan, M.S., Reynolds, C.F., Ganguli, R. et al. (1991). Electroencephalographic sleep and cerebral morphology in functional psychoses: a preliminary study with computed tomography. *Psychiatry Res.*, **39**(293).

Kripke, D.F., Simons, P.N., Garfinkel, L. & Hammond, E. (1979). Short and long term sleep and sleeping pills: is increased mortality associated? *Arch. Gen. Psychiatry*, **36**, 103–16.

Lebowitz, M.D. & Pickering, T.G. (2000). Association of sleep-disordered breathing, sleep apnea and hypertension in a large community-based study. *J. Am. Med. Assoc.*, **283**, 1829–36.

Leger, D. (2000). Public health and insomnia: economic impact. *Sleep*, **23**, 569–76.

Loube, D.I., Gay, P.C., Strohl, K.P., Pack, A.I., White, D.P. & Collop, N.A. (1999). Indications for positive airway pressure treatment of adult obstructive sleep apnea patients. *Chest*, **115**, 863–6.

Maquet, P., Peters, J-M., Aerts, J. et al. (1996). Functional neuroanatomy of rapid-eye movement sleep. *Nature*, **383**, 163–6.

McCormick, D.A. & Bal, T. (1997). Sleep and arousal: thalamocortical mechanisms. *Ann. Rev. Neurosci.*, **20**, 185–212.

Moore, R.Y. (1998). Circadian rhythms: basic neurobiology and clinical applications. *Am. Rev. Med.*, **48**, 253–66.

Nieto, F.J., Young, T.B., Lind, B.K. et al. (1997). The morbidity of insomnia uncomplicated by psychiatric disorders. *Gen. Hosp. Psychiatry*, **19**, 245–50.

Nofzinger, E.A., Mintun, M.A., Wiseman, M.B., Kupfer, D.J. & Moore, R.Y. (1997). Forebrain activation in REM sleep: an FDG PET study. *Brain Res.*, **770**, 192–201.

Nofzinger, E.A., Nichols, T.E., Meltzer, C.C. et al. (1999). Changes in forebrain function from waking to REM sleep in depression: Preliminary analyses of [18F] FDG PET studies. *Psychiatry Res. Neuoimaging*, **91**, 59.

Nofzinger, E.A., Price, J.C., Meltzer, C.C. et al. (2000). Towards a neurobiology of dysfunctional arousal in depression: the relationship between beta EEG power and regional cerebral glucose metabolism during NREM sleep. *Psychiatry Res. Neuroimaging*, **98**, 71.

Prinz, P.N., Peskind, E.R., Vitaliano, P.P. et al. (1982). Changes in the sleep and waking EEGs of nondemented and demented elderly subjects. *J. Am. Geriatr. Soc.*, **30**, 86.

Reynolds, C.F., Monk, T.H., Hoch, C.C. et al. (1991). Electroencephalographic sleep in the healthy 'old old': A comparison with the 'young old' in visually scored and automated measures. *J. Gerontol.*, **46**, M39–46.

Sejnowski, T.J. & Destexhe, A. (2000). Why do we sleep? *Brain Res.*, **886**, 208–23.

Shermin, J.E. Shiromani, P.J., McCarley, R.W. & Saper, C.B. (1999). Activation of ventrolateral preoptic neurons during sleep. *Science*, **271**, 216–19.

Tandberg, E., Larsen, J.P. & Karlsen, K.A. (1998). A community-based study of sleep disorders in patients with Parkinson's disease. *Mov. Disord.*, **13**, 895.

Wehr, T.A. (1990). Effects of wakefulness and sleep on depression and mania. In *Sleep and Biological Rhythms: Basic Mechanisms and Applications to Psychiatry*, ed. J. Montplaisir & R. Godbout, p. 42. New York: Oxford University Press.

Wu, J., Buchsbaum, M.S., Gillin, J.C. et al. (1999). Prediction of antidepressant effects of sleep deprivation by metabolic rates in the ventral anterior cingulate and medial prefrontal cortex. *Am. J. Psychiatry*, **156**, 1149.

56

Bladder and sexual dysfunction

Oliver J. Wiseman and Clare J. Fowler

Institute of Neurology, Queen Square, London WC1N 3BG, UK

Control of bladder function

The bladder performs only two functions, storage and voiding of urine. Control of these two mutually exclusive activities requires intact central and peripheral neural pathways. Neural programmes for each exist in the dorsal tegmentum of the pons, and suprapontine influences act to switch from one state to the other. The decision as to when to initiate voiding is determined by the perceived state of bladder filling and an assessment of the social circumstances.

As an individual may micturate once every 4 or so hours, and take only one or two minutes to void, the bladder is in storage mode for most of the time. During the storage phase, contraction of the detrusor smooth muscle in the bladder is prevented by inhibiting parasympathetic outflow. Closure of the bladder outlet is maintained by sympathetic influences on the detrusor smooth muscle in the bladder neck region and by contraction of the striated muscle of the urethral sphincter and pelvic floor innervated by the pudendal nerve. Voiding is initiated by a complete relaxation of the urethral sphincter and the reciprocal action of a sustained detrusor contraction, so that urine is effectively expelled.

To effect both storage and voiding, connections between the pons and the sacral spinal cord must be intact as well as the peripheral innervation which arises from the most caudal segments of the sacral cord (reviewed in Chapter 53). From there the peripheral innervation passes through the cauda equina to the sacral plexus and via the pelvic and pudendal nerves to innervate the bladder and sphincter. Thus the innervation needed for control of the bladder is extensive, requiring suprapontine inputs, intact spinal connections between the pons and the sacral cord, as well as intact peripheral nerves. Urinary continence is thus a severe test of neurological integrity.

An excellent review on the control of bladder function is available (de Groat, 1999).

Bladder dysfunction in neurological disease

Cortical lesions

Anterior regions of the frontal cortex are crucial for bladder control. This was shown by a series of patients with disturbed bladder control who had had various frontal lobe disturbances, including intracranial tumours, intracranial aneurysm rupture, penetrating brain injuries or prefrontal lobotomy (Andrew & Nathan, 1964). The typical clinical picture of frontal lobe incontinence is of a patient with normally coordinated micturition who has severe urgency, urge incontinence and frequency, or loss of sensation of impending micturition but who is not demented such that they are aware of and embarrassed by the incontinence. Micturition is normally coordinated, indicating that the disturbance is in the higher control of these processes.

Six cases were described with disturbances of micturition due to aneurysms of anterior communicating or anterior cerebral arteries (Andrew et al., 1966). The authors hypothesize that the disconnection of the frontal or anterior cingulate regions from the septal and hypothalamic areas allows micturition to proceed automatically and involuntarily following brain damage. In an earlier paper Ueki analysed the urinary symptoms of 462 patients being operated upon for brain tumours, 34 cases of frontal lobectomy and 16 cases of bilateral anterior cingulectomy. He concluded that there was a strong positive influence on micturition by an area in the pons and an inhibitory input from the frontal lobe and bilateral paracentral lobules (Ueki, 1960).

Positron emission tomography (PET) studies of male and females voiding have shown that there is significant activity in the right inferior frontal gyrus during voiding that is not present during the withholding phase (Blok et. al., 1997).

It should be noted that, as well as urinary incontinence, urinary retention has also been described in patients with right frontal lobe pathology, with restoration of normal voiding after successful treatment of the lesions.

Head injuries

There are a few reports of bladder dysfunction occurring after minor head injuries. However, serious traumatic head injury is typically followed by a period of detrusor areflexia, followed by detrusor hyperreflexia (McGuire, 1984). In 17 patients in a vegetative state 1–6 months after injury, urodynamics revealed that all patients had detrusor hyperreflexia (Krimchansky et al., 1999).

Cerebrovascular disease

The effects of a stroke on bladder function depend upon the size and site of the disruption caused to cerebral tissue and pathways. During the early stages of injury, a period of detrusor areflexia may occur, resulting in acute urinary retention, but after this initial period most commonly detrusor hyperreflexia develops (Khan et al., 1990; Wein & Barrett, 1988). Urodynamic studies show that voiding is mostly normally coordinated, with the most common cystometric finding being detrusor hyperreflexia. The patient complains of frequency and urgency, and may also have urge incontinence. The presence of urinary incontinence within seven days of a stroke is actually a stronger prognostic indicator of poor survival than a depressed level of consciousness (Wade & Langton-Hewer, 1985).

Epilepsy

Urinary incontinence is a common feature of generalized tonic clonic seizures, and occurs due to relaxation of the external sphincter (Gastaut et al., 1974). However, urinary incontinence and ictal urination are rare during focal seizures (Freeman & Schachter, 1995; Liporace & Sperling, 1997). Symptoms of detrusor overactivity may occur with seizures, manifested by urgency and urge incontinence. Urinary urgency may be seen during typical absence seizures, and urodynamics have revealed detrusor hyperreflexia during such seizures (Gastaut et al., 1964). 'Ictal urinary urge' is a rare symptom during temporal lobe seizures (Baumgartner et al., 2000).

Basal ganglia

Bladder dysfunction may occur for a number of different reasons in patients with parkinsonism.

In idiopathic Parkinson's disease (IPD), bladder symptoms usually occur later, and thus in elderly men bladder overflow obstruction caused by benign prostatic hyperplasia is usually the cause of urinary symptoms. Patients with IPD typically complain of frequency and urgency. They may also suffer from urge incontinence because with poor mobility they may not have time to reach a toilet. The most common urodynamic finding is detrusor hyperreflexia (DH), because in health the basal ganglia have an inhibitory effect on the micturition reflex. Animal studies have supported this, concluding that the D1 receptor is the main inhibitory influence (Yoshimura et al., 1992).

In patients with mild parkinsonism but disproportionately severe urinary symptoms, or where urinary symptoms precede the development of neurological involvement, a diagnosis of multiple system atrophy (MSA) must be considered. A retrospective study of 62 patients diagnosed with MSA showed that bladder symptoms and erectile dysfunction preceded the diagnosis of MSA by 4–5 years, and the onset of neurological symptoms by 2 years. Almost half the male patients had had a transurethral prostatectomy (TURP), from which few benefited (Beck et al., 1994).

That urinary complaints are so severe early on in patients with MSA may be explained by the fact that the disease affects several locations in the central nervous system which are important for bladder control. Both DH and incomplete bladder emptying may be seen in these patients, the former tending to present first, followed by increasing post micturition residuals over time. DH may be explained by neuronal loss in the pontine region, and incomplete bladder emptying by degeneration of the parasympathetic input to the detrusor following neuronal loss in the intermediate grey matter of the sacral cord segments (S_1–S_5). In addition to the hyperreflexia and increasing residuals, these patients also develop sphincteric weakness due to anterior horn cell loss in Onuf's nucleus, exacerbating their incontinence (Kirby et al., 1986).

The reports of poor outcome of patients with Parkinson's disease from prostatic surgery may well have been due to the inclusion of some patients with MSA, and a TURP should be considered only if there is convincing evidence of bladder outflow obstruction in a man with a definite diagnosis of IPD.

Spinal cord

Interruption of the spinal pathways which connect the pontine micturition centre (PMC) with the sacral cord has severe consequences for micturition, and spinal cord pathology is the most common cause of neurogenic bladder dysfunction. As the innervation of the bladder arises more caudally than that of the lower limbs, unless the lesion is entirely confined to the conus, patients with bladder dysfunction due to spinal cord disease will almost always have neurological signs in their lower limbs.

Patients develop detrusor hyperreflexia due to the emergence of new spinal segmental reflexes, and experimental work in cats suggests C fibres become the major afferents (de Groat, 1998). Patients complain of frequency and urgency due to their small bladder capacity and may also suffer from urge incontinence if DH is severe and/or they have poor mobility. Decreased sacral neural input to the detrusor in these patients can lead to decreased bladder emptying. Residual urine can exacerbate the symptoms due to detrusor hyperreflexia.

Reciprocal activity of the detrusor and external urethral sphincter, which is required for normal voiding, needs intact connections between the sacral spinal cord and the PMC. When these are lost, uncoordinated activity results, with the sphincter contracting during detrusor contraction, a condition known as detrusor sphincter dyssynergia (DSD) (Betts, 1999). Although the voiding process may have been as severely disrupted as the storage process, it is usually symptoms related to the latter that the patient complains of. Symptoms of hesitancy and an interrupted stream may only be elicited on direct questioning. Approximately 75% of patients with MS have bladder dysfunction, a similar percentage to those who have been shown to have spinal cord involvement. Patients most commonly complain of urgency, and several series of urodynamic studies have shown that this is due to DH.

Patients with MS rarely develop upper tract problems, in contrast to patients with spinal cord injury (SCI). The reason for this is unknown, but treatment of these patients must therefore be directed towards symptomatic relief. This can be hard to achieve, as with disease progression DH worsens as does the inability to effect bladder emptying. The deterioration in bladder function occurs against a background of decreasing mobility and possibly cognitive decline, making symptomatic relief and the avoidance of urge incontinence a difficult goal (Fowler, 1997).

Bladder dysfunction also occurs in other non-traumatic forms of spinal cord disease. In transverse myelitis bladder dysfunction may typically be the only remaining neurological remnant of a condition that, during the acute illness, may have required artificial ventilation and caused a quadraparesis (Sakakibara et al., 1996). The reason for this is unknown. Patients with tropical spastic paraparesis, a progressive myelopathy caused by infection with HTLV-1, may have DH as a presenting symptom.

Management of patients with traumatic spinal cord injury (SCI) necessarily has a different focus as, in this group, upper tract damage can occur (Arnold, 1999). Renal failure arises secondary to DH and loss of compliance which causes ureteric reflux, hydonephrosis and subsequent upper tract damage. Thus these patients, who are often young and otherwise fit, need to have their bladder problems managed aggressively. They often have surgical rather than solely medical management.

Spina bifida

Open and closed spina bifida are the commonest causes of neurogenic bladder dysfunction in childhood, and can also cause significant problems in adults (Borzyskowski, 1999).

Patients may develop similar complications from bladder dysfunction to those patients with spinal cord injury, namely DH, ureteric reflux, and subsequent renal failure. However the advent of CISC, anticholinergic medication and newer surgical techniques has decreased the morbidity from urological problems. Even so, the most common reason for hospital admission in these patients remains urological problems. Three types of bladder dysfunction, detailed below, have been identified, and these are classified according to detrusor behaviour (Rickwood et al., 1982). Urethral dysfunction is almost universal across the three groups, being dyssynergic in the first group and static in the other two groups.

The first type is 'contractile', where patients exhibit DH with a normal bladder. DSD is commonly seen. The majority of patients have decreased capacity and incomplete bladder emptying and incontinence. The risk of upper tract damage is significant if vesicoureteric reflux is present.

'Intermediate' is the commonest type of dysfunction, and also has the highest risk of upper tract damage. Intravesical pressure is continuously raised as bladder wall compliance is reduced. The distal sphincter mechanism is defective, both incompetent and obstructive, and this, combined with poor detrusor function leads to incomplete bladder emptying and incontinence. Surgery is frequently required to protect the upper tracts.

The final type of dysfunction is 'acontractile', where the detrusor is atonic. This, together with the incompetent bladder neck and dysfunctional sphincter mechanism leads to overflow and stress incontinence. The upper tracts are relatively safe in this group of patients.

Cauda equina

Sacral sympathetic outflow and somatic efferent and afferent fibres travel in the cauda equina, with damage to it therefore resulting in loss of sensation in the perineal saddle area as well as parasympathetic loss to the bladder, bowel and sexual organs.

Bladder dysfunction is unpredictable. Many patients report a reduced flow, incomplete bladder emptying, and in severe cases retention with overflow incontinence due to urodynamically confirmed detrusor areflexia. However, some have symptoms related to DH which has also been reported on urodynamics. Bladder neck incompetence may make stress incontinence an added problem for these patients.

Urodynamics in patients with tethered spinal cord reveals DH together with incomplete bladder emptying. Surgery to release the cord has been claimed to improve bladder dysfunction, but the operation is usually performed to treat pain or prevent neurological progression.

Peripheral innervation

Diabetic neuropathy

Bladder involvement is common as evidenced by cystometry, but is often asymptomatic. Both bladder afferents and detrusor efferents may be involved, and patients symptoms result from a decreased sensation of bladder filling and increasingly ineffective emptying, resulting in overflow incontinence and chronic low-pressure urinary retention. These patients mostly have signs and symptoms of generalized neuropathy, especially affecting the feet. This is because the peripheral small fibres are affected in a length-dependent manner, such that when the bladder is affected, the longer fibres subserving sensation to the lower limbs have also been affected. Urodynamics confirms decreased sensation of bladder filling, impaired detrusor contractility and incomplete emptying.

Amyloid neuropathy

Urogenital dysfunction may result in patients with both inherited familial polyneuropathy and amyloidosis secondary to benign plasma cell dyscrasia or myeloma. Amyloid deposition in the pelvic autonomic nerves can lead to similar symptoms as seen in patients with urogenital dysfunction secondary to diabetes. By the time pelvic autonomic dysfunction results however, there will typically be symptoms or signs related to somatic sensory involvement.

Immune mediated neuropathies

In severe cases of Guillain–Barré syndrome bladder dysfunction may result, and cystometry has shown delay in the initial sensations of bladder filling and detrusor areflexia, indicating damage to both bladder afferent and detrusor efferent nerves. Not all patients will recover bladder function, and recovery may take some months in those who do.

Pelvic nerve injury

Peripheral innervation of the pelvic organs may become damaged during pelvic surgery, such as anterior resection, radical prostatectomy or radical hysterectomy. Lower urinary tract dysfunction after the latter two is reported at rates between 10 and 60%, and in approximately one-fifth of these, the dysfunction may be permanent (McGuire, 1984). This injury may be the result of simple denervation, or nerve tethering or encasement in scar tissue, direct bladder or urethral trauma, or bladder devasularization.

The basis of the voiding dysfunction in patients with permanent dysfunction following radical pelvic surgery is a failure of detrusor contraction, with obstruction by the residual fixed striated urethral sphincter.

Urinary incontinence that follows a radical prostatectomy is due to damage to the innervation of the striated urethral sphincter.

Retention in women

Urinary retention and dysfunctional voiding in young women without any evidence of neurological disease has posed diagnostic difficulties for urologists and neurologists for some time, and such retention was often referred to as 'psychogenic', physicians believing that there was no organic underlying cause. The combination of urinary retention, abnormal sphincter EMG and polycystic ovaries was first described in 1988 (Fowler et al., 1988), and the hypothesis is that in these patients the primary abnormality exists in the striated urethral sphincter, which is overactive and which has impaired ability to relax.

Patients are typically premenopausal (mean age 26 years) and often present, following an operative procedure, in painless urinary retention, with a bladder capacity in excess of 1 litre. On direct questioning of these patients in one study, 78% claimed to have abnormal voiding prior to the onset of complete retention, and of those who had undergone pelvic ultrasonography, 50% were found to have polycystic ovaries (Swinn et al., 2002).

Urethral sphincter EMG of these patients typically reveals abnormal excitatory activity, with decelerating bursts and complex repetitive discharges. Many of these patients have to manage their voiding dysfunction by performing CISC, but this group of patients appears to respond particularly well to sacral neuromodulation (Swinn et al., 2000).

Investigation of bladder dysfunction in neurologic disease

When faced with a patient with bladder dysfunction and known neurological disease, it is important to ensure that the symptoms the patient is experiencing are not due to 'other' pathology, such as a bladder tumour, or bladder outflow obstruction caused, for example, by an enlarged prostate gland. A thorough history together with the investigations detailed below are sufficient in the initial evaluation of these patients.

History

Table 56.1 shows what bladder symptoms might be expected from neurological disease at different levels. Also shown are the other symptoms of pelvic organ dysfunction with a lesion at each level since clustering of symptoms is important in trying to decide if pelvic organ complaints are due to 'ordinary', local pathology or are neurogenic. For example, in a patient with spinal cord disease, bladder and sexual dysfunction are usually present together whereas, if bladder symptoms are due to prostatic outflow obstruction, sexual function is usually preserved. Therefore, when taking the history, attention should focus on identifying whether bladder complaints are isolated or are part of a pelvic organ symptom complex.

Investigations

Urine examination is important. A simple bedside dipstick test will help determine if the patient has a urinary tract infection accounting for, or resulting in, an exacerbation of their bladder symptoms. If positive, the urine should then be sent off for formal microscopy and culture. Dipstick examination may also reveal the presence of hematuria, a finding which, in the absence of an infection, requires full urological assessment. This is to investigate the possibility that local bladder pathology such as a ureteric or bladder stone or transitional cell cancer may be the cause of the patient's symptoms.

'Urodynamic investigations' is a term which includes all investigations of the lower urinary tract function, but it is often incorrectly used as a synonym of cystometry.

Uroflowmetry is the simplest urodynamic investigation. It is non-invasive and involves recording the rate of urine flow during voiding per unit time. A uroflow trace is generated during the test, and parameters of the flow rate calculated, including the maximum flow rate, mean flow rate, flow time and the volume voided. For a flow trace to be meaningful, the volume voided should be over 150 ml. Useful, but limited information may be ascertained from uroflowmetry. A normal flow curve is bell shaped, but may be flattened, with a low maximum flow rate (Q_{max}), in patients with either an element of bladder outflow obstruction, due to an enlarged prostate gland or a urethral stricture, or a hypocontractile detrusor muscle. A normal uroflow trace is shown in Fig. 56.1, with a trace below it showing the curve seen in a patient who has bladder outflow obstruction due to an enlarged prostate.

Ultrasonography is one of the most important investigations in a patient with neurogenic bladder dysfunction, and often this is combined with uroflowmetry. It is used to assess residual urine, with a postmicturition volume of greater than 100 ml being significant. Ultrasonography may also be used to assess upper tract dilatation, which may occur in some patients who have neurogenic bladder dysfunction. While residual urine volume may be measured with relative ease by clinic staff, an upper tract ultrasound needs to be performed by a radiologist.

Often uroflowmetry combined with an ultrasound scan of the bladder to assess residual urine volume is all that is required in patients who have established neurological disease and bladder dysfunction but in others, full cystometry is indicated. Such cases may be in patients with an unusual collection of urological symptoms, or in whom the neurological basis of their disease is unclear. Cystometry requires urethral catheterization with a filling catheter and an intravesical pressure catheter, although single dual lumen catheters are now available, which will provide both functions. A rectal pressure line is also inserted. Subtraction of the measured rectal pressure from the intravesical pressure gives the pressure generated by the smooth muscle of the bladder, the detrusor (Fig. 56.2). During the investigation, the bladder is filled at a controlled rate by an infusion pump, and while the rate of filling is variable, it should be remembered that rapid filling may provoke a rise in detrusor pressure. During the study, recordings are made of the intravesical and intra-abdominal pressures, and the detrusor pressure calculated from this. Once filling is complete, the patient voids with the pressure lines *in situ*, and the pressures are once again recorded, as is the flow rate.

The commonest abnormality shown by cystometry in neurogenic incontinence is detrusor hyperreflexia, which is an involuntary phasic rise in detrusor pressure associated with urgency. If this pressure exceeds urethral pressure, involuntary loss of urine will result (Fig. 56.2). However, bladder outflow obstruction which is indicative of an obstructing prostate or a urethral stricture may also be identified. This may mimic some of the bladder symptoms seen in patients with neurogenic bladder dysfunction which is important, as correct identification may allow treatment of the condition, thus alleviating the patient's symptoms.

Table 56.1. Pelvic organ dysfunction resulting from neurological pathology at different sites

Level of lesion	Neurological causes	Pelvic organ dysfunction
Suprapontine: Cortical	Dementia CVA Tumour	DH Fecal incontinence (very rare) Altered sexuality/sexual apathy
Extrapyramidal	IPD MSA Note: DH occurs without DSD	DH (early in MSA) Incomplete emptying Constipation MED (early in MSA) Note: Signs of Parkinsonism advanced in IPD, minor in MSA
Suprasacral: Spinal	Multiple sclerosis Spinal cord injury (trauma) Compression (e.g. tumour) Transverse myelitis AV malformation Spina bifida[a] Note: DH may occur with DSD	DH Incomplete bladder emptying Difficulty with bowel evacuation (in advanced disease), with poor sphincter control MED, FSD
Infrasacral: Conus	Spina bifida[a] Tethered cord	Various forms of lower urinary tract dysfunction exist (see text) Constipation, soiling MED
Cauda equina	Trauma Central disc prolapse AV malformation Congenital	Detrusor areflexia or DH Stress urinary incontinence Constipation Fecal incontinence/difficulty with evacuation MED, FSD Note also: Saddle sensory impairment and sexual sensory loss
Peripheral innervation	Diabetes mellitus Amyloid polyneuropathy Immune-mediated neuropathy	Detrusor areflexia Diarrhea MED (early)
Innervation within pelvis	Pelvic surgery Childbirth injury	Detrusor areflexia, with external sphincter damage and thus stress incontinence MED, sometimes FSD

Note:

[a] Patients with spina bifida may have a combination of suprasacral and infrasacral pathologies.

DH = detrusor hyperreflexia, MED = male erectile dysfunction, FSD = female sexual dysfunction, IPD = idiopathic Parkinson's disease, MSA = multiple system atrophy, DSD = detrusor sphincter dyssynergia.

Neurophysiological investigations

Various neurophysiological investigations of the pelvic floor and the sphincters have been developed and used over the years. Currently, those thought to be useful include anal sphincter EMG to recognize changes of chronic reinnervation in MSA, and the use of urethral sphincter EMG to recognize a primary disorder of sphincter relaxation in young women with isolated urinary retention (Vodusek & Fowler, 1999).

Needle electrode EMG of either the anal or urethral sphincter can be performed to show evidence of sacral segment or root damage in much the same way as EMG is used at somatic sites. However, because motor units in the sphincter fire tonically it is difficult to recognize changes of denervation and most often changes of reinnervation are sought, based on the analysis of individual motor units captured using a trigger and delay line. In general, EMG is held to be the most valuable of the pelvic floor investigations to detect lower motor neuron damage. EMG of the

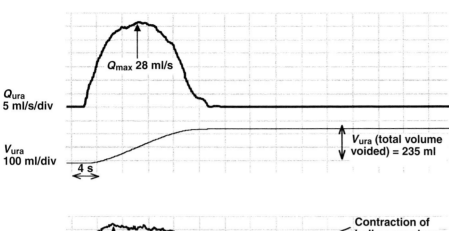

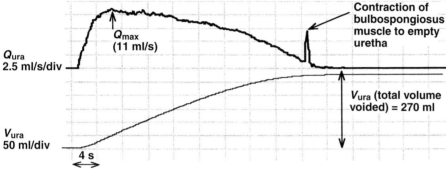

Fig. 56.1. Uroflow traces. The upper trace shows a normal uroflow trace. Note the smooth shape to the uroflow curve. The lower trace shows a flattened curve, as may be seen in a patient with a bladder outflow obstruction. Q_{ura} = urine flow rate (ml/s); Q_{max} = maximum urinary flow rate (ml/s); V_{ura} = volume voided.

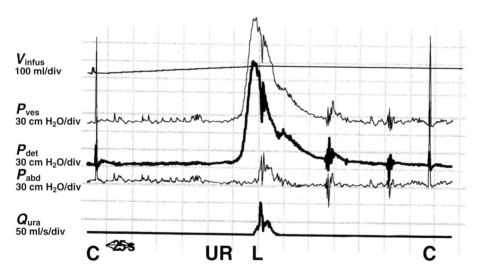

Fig. 56.2. Cystometrogram trace from a patient with MS, demonstrating detrusor hyperreflexia and urge incontinence. After 80 ml had been instilled (V_{infus}), the patient experienced urgency (UR) that was associated with an uninhibitable detrusor contraction (P_{det}) and involuntary leakage of urine occurred (L). The transient rises seen in P_{det} and P_{abd} are due to the patient coughing at intervals to ensure the lines are still in place and recording accurately (C). P_{ves} = intravesical pressure; P_{abd} = intra-abdominal pressure; P_{det} = detrusor pressure; Q_{ura} = urine flow rate.

striated musculature of the pelvic floor can demonstrate changes of denervation and chronic reinnervation in patients with cauda equina lesions as well as those with suspected MSA. Changes of reinnervation in MSA are non-specific and some caution must be exercised in interpreting EMG findings in multiparous women or in patients who have had extensive pelvic surgery. There is some controversy as to the value of the test in distinguishing between MSA and IPD, but extreme prolongation of the mean of ten motor units in a patient with early minor parkinsonism and severe urinary incontinence and erectile dysfunction is strongly indicative of MSA (Palace et al., 1997).

Urethral sphincter EMG may be used to further investigate young women with urinary retention. When a concentric needle electrode is used to record from the striated urethral sphincter in some of these women, abnormal EMG activity may be recorded. This consists of complex repetitive discharges and decelerating bursts (Fowler et al., 1985). A syndrome consisting of this abnormal activity, urinary retention, and polycystic ovaries has been described (Fowler et al., 1988), and the hypothesis is that the primary abnormality lies in the striated sphincter muscle, which is overactive and causes a feedback inhibition of the detrusor muscle, such that these patients are unable to void.

Treatment of bladder dysfunction in neurologic disease

The mainstay of management of neurological bladder dysfunction is a conservative approach consisting of first the treatment of detrusor hyperreflexia, and secondly the management of incomplete emptying.

Treatment of detrusor hyperreflexia (DH)

Oral agents

Most patients with detrusor hyperreflexia respond well to oral anticholinergics (Chapple, 2000), of which the most widely prescribed is oxybutynin (Yarker et al., 1995). It should be commenced at a dose of 2.5 mg twice daily, with the dosage being increased as necessary up to a maximum of 20 mg per day in divided doses. Oxybutinin, however, has the disadvantage of troublesome antimuscarinic side effects, which include a dry mouth, constipation and blurred vision. A dry mouth is the most problematic and common of these reported, even on low doses, and a patient not experiencing this is probably not achieving therapeutic concentrations. A single dose, taken when required, provides adequate treatment for patients who require treatment only occasionally, when for example they know that they will not have toilet access for a while, such as prior to a long car or train journey.

Controlled release oxybutinin is now available as a single daily dose of between 5 and 30 mg. The drug is released over a 24-hour time period, leading to a smoother plasma concentration–time profile, with a significantly reduced incidence of a dry mouth, and comparable efficacy to the immediate release formulation. A multicentre, prospective trial has shown that patients are able to tolerate a higher dose of controlled release oxybutinin than of the conventional preparation, which may lead to a more effective control of symptoms (Anderson et al., 1999).

More recently, tolterodine, a more 'bladder selective' anticholinergic has been introduced, which in clinical studies led to fewer treatment withdrawals compared to oxybutinin. In this study a troublesome dry mouth was reported in 60% of oxybutinin-treated patients, compared to 17% of those taking tolterodine (Appell, 1997). It may be given at a dose of up to 2 mg, twice daily.

Propiverine hydrochloride, at doses of up to 15 mg four times a day, is another effective treatment for DH (Madersbacher et al., 1999). It has both anticholinergic and calcium antagonistic properties, and has been shown to be as effective as oxybutinin in controlling urgency and urge incontinence. The drug is associated with a lower incidence of dry mouth compared to oxybutinin.

Propantheline may be used in some cases when other treatments are unavailable. The addition of a tricyclic antidepressant with antimuscarinic properties such as imipramine, amitriptyline or nortriptyline is sometimes helpful in patients who fail to respond to oxybutynin alone.

Desmopressin, an analogue of ADH, may be used as a nasal spray (Desmospray) or tablets (Desmotabs) to reduce troublesome nocturia in patients not responding to anticholinergics alone (Valiquette et al., 1996). It acts on the kidney, increasing water resorption at the collecting tubule, and thus reducing urine formation. Because of the risk of dilutional hyponatremia, which if it occurs usually does so within the first week or so of starting treatment, it is advisable to check serum sodium levels if the patient experiences any adverse effects. Even though recovery of sodium levels occurs promptly once the medication is stopped, it should be used with caution in patients with compromised renal or cardiovascular function, and avoided in the elderly.

Intravesical agents

There are a number of intravesical agents which have been used to treat detrusor hyperreflexia in patients who do not respond to oral anticholinergic medication, or who find the side effects of such medication limiting (Fowler, 2000). Two different types of treatment have been used. The first of these blocks cholinergic transmission between the pelvic nerve and detrusor muscle and includes oxybutinin and atropine, while the second group includes agents which act on afferent innervation of the bladder, such as the vanilloids capsaicin and resiniferatoxin.

Oxybutinin acts intravesically by interfering with cholinergic transmission, as well as having a local anesthetic effect. It has been shown to be effective in children and adults with resistant detrusor hyperreflexia, and patients did not report the level of side effects that they experienced with the oral formulation of the drug. Thus for those patients unable to tolerate the oral preparation of the drug, intravesical oxybutinin may be advantageous, but with the normal dose being 5 mg (30 ml of solution) intravesically three times a day, it requires frequent catheterization and is only a realistic option for those patients who are performing clean intermittent self-catheterization already.

Intravesical capsaicin, a member of a group of compounds with a common chemical structure of a vanillyl ring called vanilloids, is a pungent ingredient of the red hot chilli pepper and has been used to treat intractable detrusor hyperreflexia due to spinal cord disease (Fowler et al., 1994). It is a C fibre neurotoxin, affecting those afferent neurons that are responsible for the signals that trigger detrusor activity in patients with DH. It has been shown to increase bladder capacity and reduce the amplitude of hyperreflexic contractions in some patients, with a benefit that lasts for an average of 3–4 months.

Resiniferatoxin is another member of the vanilloid group, and has been demonstrated to be 1000 times more neurotoxic than capsaicin. Initial reports of the use of RTX to deafferent the bladder of patients with detrusor hyperreflexia have been promising (Lazzeri et al., 1998; Silva et al., 2000).

Incomplete bladder emptying or urinary retention

In patients with detrusor hyperreflexia and a significant postmicturition residual, the treatment of incomplete bladder emptying is central, as any treatment to reduce detrusor overactivity is unlikely to be effective in the presence of large residual volumes. In patients with hypo- or acontractile bladders, ensuring bladder emptying is crucial.

Many neurological patients with voiding problems develop their own method of assisting bladder emptying but the best option to deal with significant residual volumes in these patients is clean intermittent self-catheterization (CISC). Patients are often unaware of the extent to which they fail to empty their bladder, and for this reason the measurement of residual volume is the single most important measurement to be made when planning bladder management (Fig. 56.3). A generally accepted figure for significant residual volume is 100 ml, with volumes greater than this requiring drainage.

The patient should be taught CISC by someone experienced in the method and nurse specialist continence advisors are particularly expert. A main requirement for success with this technique is patient motivation; a degree of physical disability may be overcome provided the patient is sufficiently determined. Sometimes impaired visual acuity or other symptoms related to their neurological disease such as spasticity, tremor or rigidity might make it impossible for the patient to perform self-catheterization and in such circumstances it may be performed by a partner if they and the patient are willing, or a care assistant. Most patients are advised initially to perform it at least twice a day.

In spinal cord disease, a combination of intermittent self-catheterization together with an oral anticholinergic manages both aspects of bladder malfunction, namely incomplete emptying and detrusor hyperreflexia. In a patient with a borderline significant residual volume, starting an anticholinergic may have the effect of further impairing bladder emptying. This should be suspected if the anticholinergic has some initial efficacy which then disappears. In any case, however, the residual volume should be checked after initiation of anticholinergic therapy. The management algorithm for the initial treatment of patients with neurogenic incontinence is summarized in Fig. 56.3.

Permanent indwelling catheters/collection devices

Although a combination of anticholinergic medication together with intermittent catheterization is the optimal management for patients with DH and incomplete bladder emptying, there comes a point with worsening neurological disease when the patient is no longer able to perform self-catheterization, or when urge incontinence and frequency are unmanageable. At this stage an indwelling catheter may help greatly with management of bladder symptoms.

Problems with permanent catheterization such as infection, catheter blockage, urinary leakage or expulsion are common. Another major problem may be leakage of urine around the catheter. Bladder stones and recurrent, resistant infections are also more common in patients with a

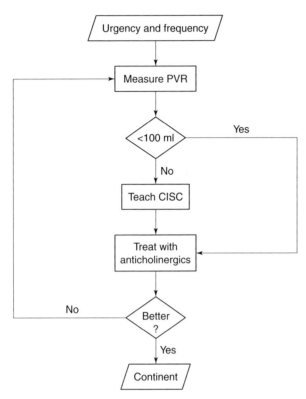

Fig. 56.3. Algorithm for management of detrusor hyperreflexia.

permanent indwelling catheter compared to those who perform CISC.

A preferred alternative to an indwelling urethral catheter is a suprapubic catheter, which can be inserted under local anesthetic. Although by no means a perfect system, a suprapubic catheter is a better alternative to an indwelling urethral catheter and is often the method of choice in managing incontinence in patients for whom other means are no longer effective.

There are some patients in whom medical management is not successful and who then require practical help with their continuing continence problems. The priority in most cases is usually containment of any urine leakage, and the continence advisor is best placed to recommend whether absorbent pads or, in men, an external collecting device may be the best option. A review of these can be found elsewhere (Dasgupta & Haslam, 1999).

Neural stimulation

At present, two different forms of treatment modalities are available. In patients with urge incontinence or voiding dysfunction, neuromodulation of the S3 nerve with an extradural implantable pulse generator (IPG) has been

shown to be effective (Shaker & Hassouna, 1998; Swinn et al., 2000). In patients with spinal cord injury, posterior sacral root rhizotomies with implantation of Brindley stimulators on the anterior sacral roots may improve voiding (Brindley et al., 1986; van Kerrebroeck & Debruyne, 1993).

Urological surgery

Various urological procedures can be carried out to treat incontinence (Walsh et al., 1998). Although surgical procedures to deal with urine leakage in an otherwise fit patient are often successful, caution must be exercised before using such measures on those patients with progressive neurological disease. When the bladder symptoms of these patients are becoming unmanageable by using a combination of intermittent catheterization and anticholinergics or even intravesical agents, their neurological disease may be so advanced that urological surgery is not appropriate. However, in some cases, such as those patients with traumatic spinal cord injury, surgery may be the best option for long-term bladder management.

Control of sexual function

Similarities do exist in the neurological control of sexual function in men and women, though that of women is less well understood.

There are two major neurologic pathways of erection, reflexogenic and psychogenic. Reflexogenic erections are the result of direct genital stimulation, with afferent impulses carried in the pudendal nerve to S2–S4, and the efferent arm using the same pathway. Preservation of reflex erections is seen in men with lesions above T11.

Psychogenic erections occur in response to input from higher centres, and require intact long tracts between cortex, spinal cord and autonomic outflow. Somatic sensory afferents deliver information on tactile sexual stimuli which, after synapsing in the sacral spinal cord, pass information centrally leading to awareness of sexual stimulation, and locally to induce the sexual responses dependent upon increased blood flow. Parasympathetic efferents from S2–S4 spinal segments travelling through the pelvic plexus and cavernosal nerves, initiate erection. Blood flow in the penile artery, and the corresponding artery in the clitoris, increases. The smooth muscle of the cavernous sinuses in the penile corpora relax and the sinuses fill with blood. The increased pressure in the corporal bodies reduces venous outflow by compression of the subtunical veins, with the combined reaction resulting in erection. Continued sacral parasympathetic activity maintains this erection.

Seminal emission begins during arousal (Mitsuya et al., 1960) and with continued sensory stimulation, orgasm is triggered with ejaculation resulting from the rhythmic phasic contractions of perineal and pelvic floor muscles. Ejaculation is effected by integrated sympathetic outflow from T11–L2 segments travelling through the sympathetic chain and hypogastric plexus, and along the pelvic and pudendal nerves and somatic efferents travelling through the pudendal nerves. Sympathetic outflow causes smooth muscle contraction in the seminal vesicles, vas deferens and prostate to deliver seminal fluid to the posterior urethra, and bladder neck contraction to prevent retrograde ejaculation. In women parasympathetic activity causes clitoral erection, engorgement of labia, and vaginal lubrication. In the periphery, the main proerectile transmitter is nitric oxide which is colocalized with vasoactive intestinal peptide and acetylcholine (Rajfer et al., 1992). The same mechanisms are thought to be responsible for clitoral erection and nitric oxide synthetase activity has been demonstrated in nerve fibres within the human glans and corpora cavernosa of the clitoris (Burnett et al., 1997).

Orgasmic sympathetic activity results in rhythmic contractions of uterus, fallopian tubes, and paraurethral glands, and the somatic motor activation in rhythmic contractions of pelvic floor muscles (Berard, 1989; Bohlen et al., 1982). Motor innervation of the pelvic floor muscles as well as the ischiocavernosus and bulbocavernosus muscles is conveyed through pudendal nerve branches from below. However, there is also a motor innervation of the pelvic floor muscles directly from the sacral plexus.

Sensory information from the glans and the skin of the penis and clitoris is conveyed through bilateral branches of the pudendal nerve. The afferents from the root of the penis (and from the anterior part of scrotum) join the ilioinguinal nerve.

The role of the cerebral hemispheres, the brainstem, and even of the spinal cord in controlling human sexual behaviour has not been fully elucidated. The forebrain areas regulate initiation and execution of sexual behaviour; the medial preoptic area integrates sensory and hormonal signals, and the amygdala and other nuclei play a role in the execution and reward aspects of sexual function.

Sexual dysfunction in neurological disease

Cortical lesions

Much remains to be discovered about the cortical control of sexual function, and it is thought that cerebral processing determines libido and desire.

Animal experiments have shown that the limbic system is important for sexual responses, and the medial preoptic hypothalamic area has an integrating function. Observations of patients with brain lesions indicate that temporal or frontal disease may cause disturbances in sexuality.

Head injuries

Disability, cognitive impairment and personality change may occur often after a traumatic brain injury, and be accompanied by sexual dysfunction either as a consequence of the cerebral lesion or as a consequence of psychological factors (Elliott & Biever, 1996). In a group of patients with closed head injury admitted for 24 hours or more, an incidence of significant sexual dysfunction in 50% over a 15 years time span was found (O'Carroll et al., 1991). Decreased and increased sexual desire, erectile failure, and retarded ejaculation have been reported (Kreutzer & Zasler, 1989; Meyer, 1955). Lesions of the frontal and temporal lobe seem to result more often in sexual problems than do lesions of the parieto-occipital part of the brain. Hypersexuality, disinhibited and inappropriate sexual behaviour, and changes in sexual preference have been reported with basal frontal and limbic brain injury (Miller et al., 1986).

Cerebrovascular disease

One measure of sexual impairment following stroke is decline in frequency of intercourse. In some studies about 75% of patients who were sexually active before the stroke reported an abrupt and permanent decrease in coital frequency (Boldrini et al., 1991). Furthermore, the majority of men (50–65%) have erectile dysfunction after a stroke (Monga et al., 1986a; Boldrini et al., 1991) and orgasmic dysfunction after stroke is common in men. Whereas 88% of men were able to ejaculate before stroke, only 29% could achieve this afterwards in one study (Bray et al., 1981). However, in another study both erections and ejaculation returned to approximately 60% of men 8 months after the stroke (Boldrini et al., 1991).

Hypersexuality has also been reported after stroke, associated with temporal lobe damage and seizures (Monga et al., 1986b). An overall change in sexual life is reported more frequently by men but changes also occur in women after stroke. In one study 63% of women reported normal vaginal lubrication before, but only 29% did so after the stroke. Similarly only 34% failed to achieve orgasm before stroke, but 77% did so afterwards (Monga et al., 1986a). However, in another study, only one-third of women who remained sexually active after a stroke suffered a decline in ability to achieve orgasm (Boldrini et al., 1991).

Epilepsy

Sexual dysfunction

It has long been known that epilepsy is associated with sexual problems, more so in men than women. Various types of abnormal behaviour, more commonly hyposexuality, but also hypersexuality, are reported, particularly in temporal lobe epilepsy (Shukla et al., 1979) and basal–medial frontal lobe lesions. Both men and women with epilepsy often suffer from loss of sexual desire, reduced sexual activity, or inhibited sexual arousal; percentages vary in different studies (Morrell et al., 1994; Guldner & Morrell, 1996). It has been suggested that subclinical hypogonadotrophic hypogonadism is the underlying condition, induced by temporal lobe dysfunction (Murialdo et al., 1995).

However, in some men with temporal lobe damage and epilepsy, desire may be preserved with loss of erectile function (Hierons & Saunders, 1966). Apart from inability to maintain an erection, ejaculatory dysfunction, decreased satisfaction with sexual life, and reduced sexual fantasies, dreams and initiatives have all been reported in patients with complex partial epilepsy and a mesiobasal temporal spike focus (Shukla et al., 1979). Loss of nocturnal tumescence has been reported in such patients (Guldner & Morrell, 1996). Surgery for epilepsy rarely restores function (Blumer & Walker, 1967), and antiepileptic drugs including carbamazepine, phenytoin, and phenobarbitone may influence both sexual desire and performance (Isojärvi et al., 1995).

Basal ganglia

Dopaminergic mechanisms are involved in both inducing penile erection and determining libido. The medial preoptic area of the hypothalamus has been shown to regulate sexual drive in animal studies, with D2 receptors being involved. Patients with Parkinson's disease commonly display decreased sexual desire, and sexual dysfunction is also frequent in their partners (Brown et al., 1990).

Erectile dysfunction (ED) is a considerable problem for patients with Parkinson's disease. In one study, 60% of a group of men with IPD were affected compared with 37.5% of an age-matched healthy group (Singer et al., 1992). ED usually affects men with IPD some years after the onset of neurological disease, whereas in men with MSA, ED may be the first symptom. Further adding to their sexual dys-

function, many men with IPD are also unable to ejaculate or to reach orgasm.

Treatment of Parkinson's disease with dopaminergic compounds may result in an apparent increase, or rather a normalization, of sexual desire (Uitii et al., 1989) without corresponding improvement of the movement disorder. Dopaminergic agonists have been shown to induce erection in animal species, and spontaneous erections have been seen in patients treated with L-dopa. Apomorphine, in both subcutaneous and sublingual preparations, has been reported to increase erectile function in some patients (O'Sullivan & Hughes, 1998). There are also reports of hypersexuality in a proportion of patients treated with anti-Parkinsonian medication (Uitti et al., 1989) and this can be of considerable concern to families looking after these patients.

Erectile failure is almost universal among patients with MSA and in a retrospective study of the duration of symptoms in 46 men clinically diagnosed as suffering from MSA, 96% had erectile dysfunction at the time of diagnosis. Erectile dysfunction alone was the first symptom in 37% but was part of the presenting symptom complex in 59% (Beck et al., 1994). The onset of ED usually predated the onset of other neurological symptoms by several years, many of the men having developed ED in their early 50s or late 40s. The reason for the early selective involvement of erectile function in patients with MSA is not known, but preserved erectile function is a clinical feature which suggests a diagnosis of MSA should be reconsidered. There are insufficient clinical grounds for attributing it to part of a general autonomic failure because symptomatic or laboratory-proven autonomic failure occurred much later in most instances (Kirchhof et al., 2000).

Spinal cord

In men, the level and completeness of spinal cord injury determines sexual function. In high spinal cord lesions, while the ability to have psychogenic erections may be lost, reflexogenic erections should be intact. In theory, a lesion below L2 should leave psychogenic erections intact, but in practice the quality of the erection is often insufficient for intercourse. Psychogenic erections are more likely to be preserved if spinal cord damage at any level is incomplete. With lower spinal cord damage, especially if the cauda equina is involved, there may be little or no erectile capacity.

Estimates of the prevalence of ED in MS vary between 35 and 80% (Mattson et al., 1995; Ghezzi et al., 1996), usually in combination with bladder dysfunction as well. Early in the disease process the initial complaint is of trouble sustaining erections, and with advancing disease, erectile function may totally cease. Problems with ejaculation are also common in men with MS, affecting approximately 40% of patients (Valleroy & Kraft, 1984) (Minderhoud et al., 1984). One paper (Vas, 1969) reported that all men with complete ED had lost ejaculation, and one-third of those with partial ED also had ejaculatory problems.

In women with MS, sexual dysfunction is a common problem affecting up to 60% of patients. A decrease in lubrication, altered pelvic sensation and inability to reach orgasm are three of the commoner complaints (Shaughnessy et al., 1997), and fatigue, lower limb spasticity and fear of urinary and bowel incontinence may contribute adversely to the situation. A reduction in sexual desire is also commonly reported.

Over 50% of all SCI men have ED (Bors & Comarr, 1960). Reflexogenic, psychogenic, and mixed erections are well described in SCI men, and the percentage of patients achieving such erections varies in different reports (Beretta et al., 1986; Tsuji et al., 1961; Yarkony, 1990). The level of SCI and the completeness of the lesions may have a bearing on the likelihood of ED, although there is much individual variation and an accurate prognosis for future sexual function in the individual may not be possible.

As well as ED, the ability to ejaculate by masturbation or sexual intercourse is impaired in most men with SCI and, consequently, men with SCI rarely father children without medical intervention (Martinez-Arizala & Brackett, 1994). Reduced fertility cannot be attributed completely to ejaculatory dysfunction because semen obtained from SCI men by methods of assisted ejaculation is of poor quality (Brackett et al., 1998; Sønksen et al., 1999). Ejaculation is generally more likely to be preserved among SCI men with incomplete rather than complete lesions.

Although orgasm has been noted to occur in men with SCI, it may differ in quality compared to before the injury (Alexander et al., 1993). Surprisingly, some women with complete SCI may retain their ability to achieve orgasm possibly because of afferents from cervix travelling with the vagus nerve (Whipple & Komisaruk, 1997).

Sympathetic thoracolumbar outflow

Retroperitoneal lymph node dissection may damage the sympathetic thoracolumbar outflow, which leaves the spinal cord at T10–L2 to pass retroperitoneally and enter the pelvic plexus. Loss of this innervation causes disorders of ejaculation, with the result that there is either no emission, or retrograde ejaculation occurs due to the inability of the normally sympathetically innervated bladder neck to contract. However, nerve sparing approaches in retroperi-

toneal dissection have been developed with considerable success (Donohue et al., 1990).

Spina bifida

As patients with spina bifida now have increased life expectancy and erectile dysfunction is a common problem, it is now recognized as an important quality of life issue (Joyner et al., 1998).

Cauda equina

Erectile dysfunction is commonly seen in men with cauda equina damage (Bors & Comarr, 1960), and sexual dysfunction in women is also a problem with both genders having a severe problem with loss of genital sensation.

Traumatic cauda equina lesions are generally considered with SCI. A complete lesion of the cauda equina will damage the parasympathetic erectile pathways to the penis. However, approximately one-quarter of men may still be able to achieve an erection psychogenically (Bors & Comarr, 1960). This is thought to be mediated by a sympathetic erectile pathway via the hypogastric plexus. Ejaculatory disturbances, penile sensory loss, and pain syndromes have also been described.

Women report loss of lubrication, dyspareunia, diminished sensation, difficulties in achieving orgasm, as well as changes in the qualities of orgasm. The effects on vaginal lubrication and orgasm are related to the level and completeness of the lesion (Berard, 1989). Patients with incomplete SCI retain the ability for psychogenic genital vasocongestion if pinprick sensation is preserved in the T11–12 segments; only reflexogenic responses are obtained in those with complete SCI (Sipski et al., 1995, 1997).

Peripheral innervation

Diabetic neuropathy

Diabetes is the commonest cause of erectile dysfunction, with this as the underlying diagnosis in approximately 25% of patients attending ED clinics. The prevalence of ED in diabetic men is between 30 and 60% (Kolodny et al., 1979; McCulloch et al., 1980) and is higher in patients with longstanding diabetes and in those who have developed some of the other complications of the disease. Neuropathy may not be the only cause, and both microvascular disease and the effect of formation of advanced glycation end products of neurotransmitters involved may play a role. Retrograde ejaculation may occur in patients who have diabetic cystopathy, due to neuropathy of the sympathetic nerves supplying the bladder neck (Ellenberg, 1966).

Female sexual dysfunction has been studied to a lesser degree, but studies suggest that diabetic women may also be affected by specific disorders of sexual function, which may include decreased lubrication (Tyrer et al., 1983) and inability to reach orgasm, as well as dyspareunia and vaginal fungal infections.

Immune mediated neuropathies

Autonomic involvement may lead to ED in Guillain–Barré syndrome, and Guillain reported this in his original description.

Pelvic nerve injury

The peripheral autonomic nerves to the genital organs may be injured, for example by surgical procedures, leading to ED or ejaculatory problems in men, and loss of lubrication in women. The sympathetic thoracolumbar fibres may be injured by retroperitoneal lymph node dissections. Pelvic plexus and cavernosal nerves may be injured in surgery, such as by abdominoperineal resection of carcinoma, hysterectomy, radical prostatectomy, or sphincterotomy. Surgeons are increasingly aware of these possibilities and have developed 'nerve sparing' operations. In the case of radical prostatectomy, prior to development of nerve sparing techniques almost all patients were impotent post-operation. In one series of patients followed up after nerve sparing radical prostatectomy, erectile dysfunction was reported in almost 60% at 18 months (Stanford et al., 2000). ED has also been reported after injection of sclerosing agents to treat hemorrhoids (Bullock, 1997), and subtrigonal injections to treat a hypersensitive bladder (Bennani, 1994).

Investigation of sexual dysfunction in neurologic disease

In many patients with neurological disease and bladder dysfunction, sexual dysfunction often coexists (See Table 56.1). In some patients investigations are contributory, but in the majority a thorough history and clinical examination are sufficient to attribute the dysfunction to the established neurological disease.

History

In patients with sexual dysfunction secondary to neurological disease there are usually other neurological symptoms.

The temporal association of sexual dysfunction with onset or progression of their neurological disease is often strong. Depression which may accompany neurological disease may result in sexual dysfunction as well, as may antidepressant medication or a range of other medications including some diuretics, antihypertensives, H2 antagonists, and a high intake of recreational drugs such as alcohol and marijuana. Normal sexual function with a different partner or during differing sexual activities strongly suggest a psychogenic explanation for erectile dysfunction. It is possible for patients with spinal cord disease to have reflexogenic erections from genital stimulation, but be unable to have psychogenic erections and thus preserved nocturnal and early morning erections need not mean that erectile dysfunction has a psychogenic basis.

Clinical examination

Sexual dysfunction has many different possible neurological causes. However there are also a number of non-neurological causes of which the clinician must be aware. In a neurological patient with sexual dysfunction in whom there are no clues from the history as to the underlying diagnosis, it is necessary to perform a full neurological examination, looking for evidence of neurological disease. Because normal sexual function is highly dependent on the integrity of the spinal cord, examination of the lower limbs should be especially thorough. This should include sensation and vibration perception which, if deficient, may indicate an underlying peripheral neuropathy. In cases of cauda equina injury sensation in the saddle area should be tested, as should anal tone. Erectile dysfunction may occur as the first symptom of multiple system atrophy, and early signs of extrapyramidal or cerebellar dysfunction should therefore be carefully sought.

Inspection of the distribution of body hair may indicate if there is an underlying hormonal basis for erectile dysfunction, as may the finding of gynaecomastia. The patient's leg pulses should always be checked to rule out the possibility of peripheral vascular disease as being the underlying cause of the dysfunction, and the patient's blood pressure checked. It should also be remembered that there are several urological causes of erectile dysfunction.

Investigations

Dipstick examination of the urine may reveal glycosuria, indicating that diabetes may be the underlying cause of sexual dysfunction. Routine laboratory tests should be performed, and these should include serum HbA_1C, also to

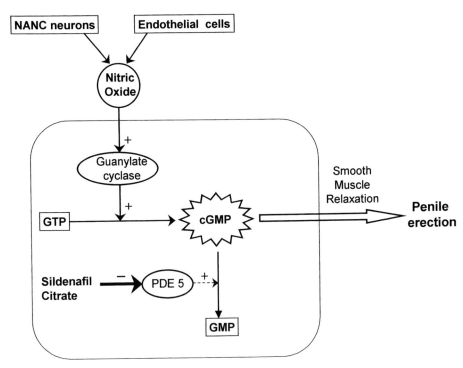

Fig. 56.4. Nitric oxide-cGMP mechanism of corpus cavernosal smooth muscle relaxation and penile erection. Sexual stimulation results in the release of nitric oxide from corporal vascular endothelium and non-adrenergic–non-cholinergic (NANC) neurons. PDE 5 = cGMP-specific phosphodiesterase type 5.

exclude underlying diabetes as a cause, as well as serum testosterone if the history or examination suggest possible hypogonadism. Prolactin should be measured if the serum testosterone is low, or if there is a loss in libido, and LH should be measured if testosterone is low. A hemoglobinopathy screen should be performed in Afro-Caribbean patients, to exclude sickle cell disease, as erectile dysfunction may follow an episode of priapism.

Other investigations, which are really the remit of a urologist with an interest in andrology may include nocturnal penile tumescence monitoring, a Rigiscan which is a home monitoring device capable of continuously monitoring penile circumference and rigidity, or a colour duplex Doppler ultrasound to investigate an underlying vascular cause.

Treatment of sexual dysfunction in neurologic disease

Recent advances in knowledge of the physiology and pharmacology of erection have led to the development of drug treatments by the oral, intracavernous and intraurethral routes. As a last resort, surgical treatment is also possible.

Such treatment is available also for neurologically impaired patients.

Oral agents

Since the introduction of sildenafil citrate (Viagra) in 1997, the management of erectile dysfunction has been revolutionized. It is an orally active potent inhibitor of PDE5, thus prolonging the effect of cyclic GMP, increasing the relaxation of smooth muscle in the corpora cavernosa (See Fig. 56.4). In response to sexual stimuli, cavernous nerves and endothelial cells release nitric oxide, which stimulates the formation of cyclic GMP. In turn, this leads to smooth muscle relaxation, and the cGMP is then metabolized by cyclic GMP specific phosphodiesterase type 5 (PDE5). Viagra has been shown to be effective in treating erectile dysfunction of various different etiologies (Goldstein et al., 1998), and has been particularly effective in patients with MS. In one study, 90% of patients reported improvements in erections compared to 24% of those on placebo (Fowler et al., 1999) and had a demonstrable improvement in quality of life (Miller et al., 1999). In addition to MS, it has also been shown to successfully treat ED in men with spinal cord lesions (Guiliano et al., 1999; Schmid et al., 2000). However, the efficacy depended on sparing of either sacral (S2–S4) or thoracolumbar (T10–L2) spinal segments which, in this study, was shown to be of relevance in mediating psychogenic erections in male SCI patients. Other studies have shown the beneficial effect of sildenafil in patients with spina bifida (Palmer et al., 2000), and Parkinson's Disease (Zesiewicz et al., 2000; Hussain et al., 2000). A note of caution should be sounded, however, in patients with MSA, as profound decreases in blood pressure have been shown following administration of sildenafil in these patients (Hussain et al., 2000).

The use of sildenafil in women with sexual dysfunction secondary to neurological disease is currently an area of research interest. It is believed that the nitric oxide–cGMP pathway which Viagra has been shown to affect so successfully by inhibition of phosphodiesterase type 5 (PDE5) in the male (Fig. 56.4) may be important in the female sexual response, producing clitoral engorgement and vaginal lubrication in the female during sexual stimulation. This may provide a treatment option for women with sexual dysfunction and multiple sclerosis, and trials are currently being undertaken.

Sildenafil is well tolerated with a low side effect profile, which includes headache, flushing and dyspepsia. It is however not suitable for those patients taking nitrates, or patients with severe hepatic disease or hereditary retinal disorders.

Intracavernous injection therapy

Now the most widely used agent for intracavernosal injection therapy is alprostadil, Prostaglandin E1. It is highly effective in treating erectile dysfunction, and produces erections satisfactory for intercourse in 66% of patients self-injecting at home (Godschalk et al., 1994) 94% of the time (Linet & Ogrinc, 1996). It has few contraindications or interactions, is rapidly effective and has high rates of partner satisfaction.

Potential problems with this treatment include the manual dexterity required to give such injections, which is particularly pertinent in a neurological patient population, together with penile pain on injection (Linet & Ogrinc, 1996), and the occurrence of fibrosis, which has reported incidences of up to 20%. There is also a reported incidence of priapism, a urological emergency, of up to 1% (Chew et al., 1997).

Intraurethral therapy

Transurethral therapy with alprostadil (MUSE) has been reported to be effective in the treatment of ED. In a study of over 1500 men with ED of various etiologies, use of MUSE resulted in 65.9% having erections satisfactory for intercourse (Padma-Nathan et al., 1997). However, other reports indicate that this treatment is not very effective, with 63% of men not achieving erections satisfactory for intercourse in one study (Werthman & Rajfer, 1997). Despite this, compared to intracavernosal treatment the risk of priapism is lower, and MUSE may be suitable for patients who have difficulty either in preparing or administering intracavernosal alprostadil. However, it is slower acting than injection therapy, with lower efficacy (Werthman & Rajfer, 1997; Porst, 1997). The reported side effects include mild penile pain and urethral discomfort.

Vacuum devices

A vacuum device consists of an external cylinder which fits over the penis, and then air is pumped out. This results in blood flow into the penis, following which a constriction ring is fitted around the base of the penis to maintain the erection. This type of treatment has a long history; achievement of adequate rigidity for penetration has been reported in 90% of patients with neurogenic ED (Seckin et al., 1996; Denil et al., 1996). The most common complaints are of premature loss of rigidity and difficulty in placing and removing the constriction bands and the most common complications are bruising, petechiae, and skin edema. Severe complications such as penile gangrene, severe erosions, and cellulitis can occur and are associated with prolonged constriction-band wearing (Rivas & Chancellor, 1994).

Penile prostheses

Penile prostheses are semirigid, inflatable or malleable implants that are surgically inserted into the penis to allow an erect state. They are suitable for patients who have an organic basis to their erectile dysfunction who have failed to respond to other treatments. Once placement of a prosthesis is undertaken, other treatments for erectile dysfunction are ruled out. Inflatable prostheses require manual dexterity by the patient or his partner. They allow a flaccid penis when not inflated, which is more practical for everyday life. Most reports in the literature deal with the semirigid type of prosthesis (Evans, 1998). Complications include prosthesis extrusion leading to explantation and prosthesis failure. However this incidence may be higher in neurogenic patients due to the increased risk of erosion because of sensory loss. The biggest disadvantage of this treatment is that it requires an operative procedure, which is invasive and has its own set of potential complications.

References

Alexander, C.J., Sipski, M.L. & Findley, T.W. (1993). Sexual activities, desire and satisfaction in males pre- and post-spinal cord injury. *Arch. Sex. Behav.* **22**, 217–28.

Anderson, R.U., Mobley, D., Blank, B., Saltzstein, D., Susset, J. & Brown, J.S. (1999). Once daily controlled versus immediate release oxybutynin chloride for urge urinary incontinence. OROS Oxybutynin Study Group. *J. Urol.,* **161**(6), 1809–12.

Andrew, J. & Nathan, P.W. (1964). Lesions of the anterior frontal lobes and disturbances of micturition and defecation. *Brain*, **87**, 233–62.

Andrew, J., Nathan, P. & Spanos, N. (1966). Disturbances of micturition and defaecation due to aneurysms of anterior communication or anterior cerebral arteries. *J. Neurosurg.*, **24**, 1–10.

Appell, R.A. (1997). Clinical efficacy and safety of tolterodine in the treatment of overactive bladder: a pooled analysis. *Urology*, **50**(6A Suppl), 90–6; discussion 97–9.

Arnold, E.P. (1999). Spinal cord injury. In *Neurology of Bladder, Bowel and Sexual Dysfunction*, ed. C. J. Fowler, pp. 275–88. Boston: Butterworth-Heinemann.

Baumgartner, C., Groppel, G., Leutmezer, F. et al. (2000). Ictal urinary urge indicates seizure onset in the nondominant temporal lobe. *Neurology*, **55**(3), 432–4.

Beck, R.O., Betts, C.D. & Fowler, C.J. (1994). Genito-urinary dysfunction in Multiple System Atrophy: clinical features and treatment in 62 cases. *J. Urol.*, **151**: 1336–41.

Bennani, S. (1994). [Evaluation of sub-trigonal injections in the treatment of the hyperactive bladder]. *Ann. Urol. (Paris)*, **28**(1), 13–19.

Berard, E.J. (1989). The sexuality of spinal cord injured women: physiology and pathophysiology. A review. *Paraplegia*, **27**(2), 99–112.

Beretta, G., Zanollo, A., Fanciullacci, F. & Catanzaro, F. (1986). Intracavernous injection of papaverine in paraplegic males. *Acta Eur. Fertil.,* **17**, 283–4.

Betts, C.D. (1999). Bladder and sexual dysfunction in multiple sclerosis. In *Neurology of Bladder, Bowel and Sexual Dysfunction*. ed. C.J. Fowler, pp. 289–308. Boston: Butterworth-Heinemann.

Blok, B., Willemsen, T. & Holstege, G. (1997). A PET study of brain control of micturition in humans. *Brain*, **120**, 111–21.

Blumer, D. & Walker, A. (1967). Sexual behavior in temporal lobe epilepsy. *Arch. Neurol.*, **16**, 37–43.

Bohlen, J.G., Held, J.P., Sanderson, M.O. & Ahlgren, A. (1982). The female orgasm: pelvic contractions. *Arch. Sex. Behav.*, **11**(5), 367–86.

Boldrini, P., Basaglia, N. & Calancq, M. (1991). Sexual changes in hemiparetic patients. *Arch. Phys. Med. Rehabil.*, **72**, 202–7.

Bors, E. & Comarr, A. (1960). Neurological disturbances of sexual function with special references to 529 patients with spinal cord injury. *Urol. Survey*, **10**, 191–222.

Borzyskowski, M. (1999). Spina bifida. In *Neurology of Bladder, Bowel and Sexual Dysfunction*, ed. C. J. Fowler, pp. 353–66. Boston, Butterworth-Heinemann.

Brackett, N.L., Bloch, W.E. & Lynne, C.M. (1998). Predictors of necrospermia in men with spinal cord injury. *J. Urol.*, **159**, 844–7.

Bray, G., DeFrank, R. & Wolfe, T. (1981). Sexual functioning in stroke survivors. *Arch. Phys. Med. Rehabil.,* **62**, 286–8.

Brindley, G.S., Polkey, C.E., Rushton, D.N. & Cardozo, L. (1986). Sacral anterior root stimulators for bladder control in paraplegia: the first 50 cases. *J. Neurol., Neurosurg. Psychiatry*, **49**, 1104–14.

Brown, R.G., Jahanshahi, M., Quinn, N. & Marsden, C.D. (1990). Sexual function in patients with Parkinson's disease and their partners. *J. Neurol., Neurosurg., Psychiatry*, **53**(6), 480–6.

Bullock, N. (1997). Impotence after sclerotherapy of haemorrhoids: case reports. *Br. Med. J.,* **314**(7078), 419.

Burnett, A.L., Calvin, D.C., Silver, R.I., Peppas, D.S. & Docimo, S.G. (1997). Immunohistochemical description of nitric oxide synthase isoforms in human clitoris. *J. Urol.,* **158**(1), 75–8.

Chapple, C.R. (2000). Muscarinic receptor antagonists in the treatment of overactive bladder [see comments]. *Urology*, **55**(5A Suppl), 33–46; discussion 50.

Chew, K.K., Stuckey, B.G., Earle, C.M., Dhaliwal, S.S. & Keogh, E.J. (1997). Penile fibrosis in intracavernosal prostaglandin E1 injection therapy for erectile dysfunction [see comments]. *Int. J. Impot. Res.*, **9**(4), 225–9; discussion 229–30.

Dasgupta, P. & Haslam, C. (1999). Treatment of neurogenic bladder dysfunction. In *Neurology of Bladder, Bowel and Sexual Dysfunction*, ed. C. J. Fowler, pp. 163–83. Boston: Butterworth-Heinemann.

de Groat, W.C. (1998). Developmental and injury induced plasticity in the micturition reflex pathway. *Behav. Brain Res.*, **92**, 127–40.

de Groat, W.C. (1999). Neural control of the urinary bladder and sexual organs. In *Autonomic Failure*, ed. C. Mathias & R. Bannister, pp. 151–68. Oxford: Oxford University Press.

Denil, J., Ohl, D.A. & Smythe, C. (1996). Vacuum erection device in spinal cord injured men: patient and partner satisfaction. *Arch. Phys. Med. Rehabil.*, **77**(8), 750–3.

Donohue, J.P., Foster, R.S., Rowland, R.G., Bihrle, R., Jones, J. & Geier, G. (1990). Nerve-sparing retroperitoneal lymphadenectomy with preservation of ejaculation. *J. Urol.,* **144**(2 Pt 1), 287–91; discussion 291–2.

Ellenberg, M.W.H. (1966). Retrograde ejaculation in diabetic neuropathy. *Ann. Intern. Med.*, **65**, 1237–46.

Elliott, M. & Biever, L. (1996). Head injury and sexual dysfunction. *Brain Injury*, **10**, 703–17.

Evans, C. (1998). The use of penile prostheses in the treatment of impotence. *Br. J. Urol.*, **81**(4), 591–8.

Fowler, C.J. (1997). The cause and management of bladder, bowel and sexual dysfunction in multiple sclerosis. In *Bailliere's Clinical Neurology*, ed. D. Miller, **vol 6**(3), pp. 447–65. London: Harcourt Brace & Company Ltd.

Fowler, C. (2000). Intravesical treatment of the overactive bladder. *Urology*, **55**(5A Suppl), 60–4.

Fowler, C.J., Kirby, R.S. & Harrison, M.J.G. (1985). Decelerating bursts and complex repetitive discharges in the striated muscle of the urethral sphincter associated with urinary retention in women. *J. Neurol., Neurosurg., Psychiatry*, **48**, 1004–9.

Fowler, C.J., Christmas, T.J., Chapple, C.R., Fitzmaurice, P.H., Kirby,

R.S. & Jacobs, H.S. (1988). Abnormal electromyographic activity of the urethral sphincter, voiding dysfunction, and polycystic ovaries: a new syndrome? *Br. Med. J.*, **297**, 1436–8.

Fowler, C., Beck, R., Gerrard, S., Betts, C. & Fowler, C. (1994). Intravesical capsaicin for treatment of detrusor hyperreflexia. *J. Neurol. Neurosurg., Psychiatry*, **57**, 169–73.

Fowler, C., Miller, J. & Sharief, M. (1999). Viagra (Sildenafil Citrate) for the treatment of erectile dysfunction in men with multiple sclerosis. *Ann. Neurol.*, **46 (3)**, 497.

Freeman, R. & Schacter, S. (1995). Autonomic Epilepsy. *Semin. Neurol.*, **15**, 158–66.

Gastaut, H., Batini, C., Broughton, R., Lob, H. & Roger, J. (1964). Polygraphic study of enuresis during petit mal absences. *Electroencephalogr. Clin. Neurophysiol.*, **16**, 626.

Gastaut, H., Broughton, R., Roger, J. & Tassinari, C. (1974). Generalised non-conclusive seizures without local onset. In *Handbook of Clinical Neurology*, ed. P. Vinken & G. Bruyn, pp. 130–44. New York.

Ghezzi, A., Zaffaroni, M., Baldini, S. & Zibetti, A. (1996). Sexual dysfunction in multiple sclerosis male patients in relation to clinical findings. *European Neurology*, **3**, 462–6.

Giuliano, F., Hultling, C., El Masry, W.S. et al. (1999). Randomized trial of sildenafil for the treatment of erectile dysfunction in spinal cord injury. Sildenafil Study Group. *Ann. Neurol.*, **46**(1), 15–21.

Godschalk, M.F., Chen, J., Katz, P.G. & Mulligan, T. (1994). Treatment of erectile failure with prostaglandin E1: a double-blind, placebo-controlled, dose–response study. *J. Urol.*, **151**(6), 1530–2.

Goldstein, I., Lue, T., Padma-Nathan, H. et al. (1998). Oral sildenafil in the treatment of erectile dysfunction. *N. Engl. J. Med.*, **338**, 1397–404.

Guldner, G. & Morrell, M. (1996). Nocturnal penile tumescence and rigidity evaluation in men with epilepsy. *Epilepsia*, **37**, 1211–14.

Hierons, R. & Saunders, M. (1966). Impotence in patients with temporal lobe lesions. *Lancet*, **ii**, 761.

Hussain, I., Brady, C. & Fowler, C.J. (2000). Sildenafil in the treatment of erectile dysfunction in parkinsonism. *Br. J. Urol. Int.*, **85** Suppl. 5, 14.

Isojärvi, J.T., Repo, M., Pakarinen, A.J., Lukkarinen, O. & Myllyla, V.V. (1995). Carbamazepine, phenytoin, sex hormones, and sexual function in men with epilepsy. *Epilepsia*, **36**, 366–70.

Joyner, B., McLorie, G. & Khoury, A. (1998). Sexuality and reproductive issues in children with Myelomeningocele. *Eur. J. Paediatr. Surg.*, **8**, 29.

Khan, Z., Starer, P., Yang, W. & Bhola, A. (1990). Analysis of voiding disorders in patients with cerebrovascular accidents. *Urology*, **35**, 263–70.

Kirby, R.S., Fowler, C.J., Gosling, J. & Bannister, R. (1986). Urethro-vesical dysfunction in progressive autonomic failure with multiple system atrophy. *J. Neurol., Neurosurg., Psychiatry*, **49**, 554–62.

Kirchhof, K., Matthias, C.J. & Fowler, C.J. (2000). The relationship of uro-genital dysfunction to other features of autonomic failure in MSA. *Clin. Auton. Res.*, **9**(1), 28.

Kolodny, R.C., Masters, W.H. & Johnson, V.E. (1979). Sex and the handicapped. In *Textbook of Sexual Medicine.*, ed. R. C. Kolodny, W. H. Masters & V. E. Johnson, pp. 353–80. Boston: Little Brown.

Kreutzer, J. & Zasler, N. (1989). Psychosexual consequences of traumatic brain injury. *Brain Injury*, **3**, 177–86.

Krimchansky, B.Z., Sazbon, L., Heller, L., Kosteff, H. & Luttwak, Z. (1999). Bladder tone in patients in post-traumatic vegetative state. *Brain Inj.*, **13**(11), 899–903.

Lazzeri, M., Spinelli, M., Beneforti, P., Zanollo, A. & Turini, D. (1998). Intravesical resiniferatoxin for the treatment of detrusor hyper-reflexia refractory to capsaicin in patients with chronic spinal cord diseases. *Scand. J. Urol. Nephrol.*, **32**(5), 331–4.

Linet, O.I. & Ogrinc, F.G. (1996). Efficacy and safety of intracaver-nosal alprostadil in men with erectile dysfunction. The Alprostadil Study Group [see comments]. *N. Engl. J. Med.*, **334**(14), 873–7.

Liporace, J. & Sperling, M. (1997). Simple Autonomic Seizures. In *Epilepsy: a Comprehensive Textbook*, ed. J.J. Engel & T. Pedley, pp. 549–55. Philadelphia: Lippincott-Raven.

McCulloch, D., Campbell, I., Wu, F., Prescott, R. & Clarke, B. (1980). The prevalence of diabetic impotence. *Diabetologia*, **18**, 279–83.

McGuire, E.J. (1984). Clinical evaluation and treatment of neurogenic vesical dysfunction. In *International Perspectives in Urology*, ed. L. J. Baltimore: Williams and Wilkins Co. **vol. 11**.

Madersbacher, H., Halaska, M., Voigt, R., Alloussi, S. & Hofner, K. (1999). A placebo-controlled, multicentre study comparing the tolerability and efficacy of propiverine and oxybutynin in patients with urgency and urge incontinence. *Br. J. Urinol. Int.*, **84**(6), 646–51.

Martinez-Arizala, A. & Brackett, N.L. (1994). Sexual dysfunction in spinal injury. In *Sexual Dysfunction: A Neuro-Medical Approach*, ed. C. Singer & W. Weiner, pp. 135–53. Armonk, NY: Futura Publishing Company Inc.

Mattson, D., Petrie, M., Srivastava, D. &. McDermott, M. (1995). Multiple sclerosis. Sexual dysfunction and its response to medications. *Arch. Neurol.*, **52**, 862–8.

Meyer, J. (1955). Die sexuellen Störungen der Hirnverletzten. *Arch. Psychiat. Zschr. Nervenheilk.*, **193**, 449–69.

Miller, B., Cummings, J. & McIntyre, H. (1986). Hypersexuality or altered sexual preference following brain injury. *J. Neurol. Neurosurg. Psychiatry*, **49**, 867–73.

Miller, J., Fowler, C. & Sharief, M. (1999). Effect of sildenafil citrate (Viagra) on quality of life in men with erectile dysfunction and multiple sclerosis. *Ann. Neurol.*, **46 (3)**, 496–7.

Minderhoud, J.M., Leemhuis, J.G., Kremer, J., Laban, E. & Smits, P.M.L. (1984). Sexual disturbances arising from multiple sclerosis. *Acta. Neurol. Scand.*, **70**, 299–306.

Mitsuya, H., Asai, J., Suyama, K., Ushida, T. & Hosoe, K. (1960). Application of X-ray cinematography in urology. 1. Mechanisms of ejaculation. *J. Urol.*, **83**, 86–92.

Monga, T., Lawson, J. & Inglis, J. (1986a). Sexual dysfunction in stroke patients. *Arch. Phys. Med. Rehabil.*, **67**, 19–22.

Monga, T.N., Monga, M., Raina, M.S. & Hardjasudarma, M. (1986b). Hypersexuality in stroke. *Arch. Phys. Med. Rehabil.*, **67**, 415.

Morrell, M.J., Sperling, M.R., Stecker, M. & Dichter, M.A. (1994).

Sexual dysfunction in partial epilepsy: a deficit in physiological arousal. *Neurology*, **44**, 243–7.

Murialdo, G., Galimberti, C. Fonzi, S. et al. (1995). Sex hormones and pituitary function in male epileptic patients with altered or normal sexuality. *Epilepsia*, **36**, 360–5.

O'Carroll, R., Woodrow, J. & Maroun, F. (1991). Psychosexual and psychosocial sequelae of closed head injury. *Brain Injury*, **5**, 303–13.

O'Sullivan, J. & Hughes, A.(1998). Apomorphine-induced penile erections in Parkinson's disease. *Movem. Dis.*, **13**, 536–9.

Padma-Nathan, H., Hellstrom, W.J., Kaiser, F.E. et al. (1997). Treatment of men with erectile dysfunction with transurethral alprostadil. Medicated Urethral System for Erection (MUSE) Study Group [see comments]. *N. Engl. J. Med.*, **336**(1), 1–7.

Palace, J., Chandiramani, V.A. & Fowler, C.J. (1997). Value of sphincter EMG in the diagnosis of multiple system atrophy. *Muscle Nerve*, **20**, 1396–403.

Palmer, J., Kaplan, W. & Firlit, C. (2000). Erectile dysfunction in patients with spina bifida is a treatable condition. *J. Urol.*, **164**, 958–61.

Porst, H. (1997). Transurethral alprostadil with MUSE (medicated urethral system for erection) vs intracavernous alprostadil – a comparative study in 103 patients with erectile dysfunction [see comments]. *Int. J. Impot. Res.*, **9**(4), 187–92.

Rajfer, J., Aronson, W.J., Bush, P.A., Dorey, F.J. & Ignarro, L.J. (1992). Nitric oxide as a mediator of relaxation of the corpus cavernosum in response to nonadrenergic, noncholinergic neurotransmission. *N. Engl. J. Med.*, **326**(2), 90–4.

Rickwood, A.M.K., Thomas, D.G., Philp, N.M. & Spicer, R.D. (1982). Assessment of congenital neuropathic bladder by combined urodynamic and radiologic studies. *Br. J. Urol.*, **54**, 512–18.

Rivas, D.A. & Chancellor, M.B. (1994). Complications associated with the use of vacuum constriction devices for erectile dysfunction in the spinal cord injured population. *J. Am. Paraplegia Soc.*,**17**(3), 136–9.

Sakakibara, R., Hattori, T., Yasuda, K. & Yamanishi, T. (1996). Micturition disturbance in acute transverse myelitis. *Spinal Cord*, **34**, 481–5.

Schmid, D.M., Schurch, B. & Hauri, D. (2000). Sildenafil in the treatment of sexual dysfunction in spinal cord-injured male patients. *Eur. Urol.*, **38**(2), 184–93.

Seckin, B., Atmaca, I., Ozgok, Y., Gokalp, A. & Harmankaya, C. (1996). External vacuum device therapy for spinal cord injured males with erectile dysfunction. *Int. Urol. Nephrol.*, **28**(2), 235–40.

Shaker, H. & Hassouna, M. (1998). Sacral nerve root neuromodulation, an effective treatment for refractory urge incontinence. *J. Urol.*, **159**, 1516–19.

Shaughnessy, L., Schuchman, M., Ghumra, M., Daily, P. & Burks, J.S. (1997). Sexual dysfunction in multiple sclerosis. In *Sexual and Reproductive Neurorehabilitation*, ed. M. Aisen, pp. 169–95. Totowa, New Jersey: Humana Press Inc.

Shukla, G., Srivastava, O. & Katiyar, B. (1979). Sexual disturbance in temporal lobe epilepsy, a controlled study. *Br. J. Psychiatry*, **134**, 288–92.

Silva, C., Rio, M-E. & Cruz, F. (2000). Desensitization of bladder sensory fibres by intravesical resiniferatoxin, a capsaicin analogue, long-term results for the treatment of detrusor hyperreflexia. *Eur. Urol.*, **38**(4), 444–52.

Singer, C., Weiner, W.J. & Sanchez-Ramos, J.R. (1992). Autonomic dysfunction in men with Parkinson's disease. *Eur. Neurol.*, **32**(3), 134–40.

Sipski, M.L., Alexander, C.J. & Rosen, R.C. (1995). Physiological parameters associated with psychogenic sexual arousal in women with complete spinal cord injuries. *Arch. Phys. Med. Rehabil.*, **76**(9), 811–18.

Sipski, M.L., Alexander, C.J. & Rosen, R.C. (1997). Physiologic parameters associated with sexual arousal in women with incomplete spinal cord injuries. *Arch. Phys. Med. Rehabil.*, **78**(3), 305–13.

Sønksen, J., Ohl, D.A., Giwercman, A., Biering-Sorensen, F., Skakkebaek, N.E. & Kristensen, J. K. (1999). Effect of repeated ejaculation on semen quality in spinal cord injured men. *J. Urol.*, **161**, 1163–5.

Stanford, J.L., Feng, Z., Hamilton, A.S. et al. (2000). Urinary and sexual function after radical prostatectomy for clinically localized prostate cancer, the Prostate Cancer Outcomes Study [see comments]. *J. Am. Med. Assoc.*, **283**(3), 354–60.

Swinn, M.J., Wiseman, O.J., Lowe, E. & Fowler, C.J. (2002). The cause and natural history of isolated retention in young women. *J. Urol.*, **167**(1), 165–8.

Swinn, M.J., Kitchen, N.D., Goodwin, R.J. & Fowler, C.J. (2000). Sacral neuromodulation for women with Fowler's syndrome [In Process Citation]. *Eur. Urol.*, **38**(4), 439–43.

Tsuji, I., Nakajima, F., Morimoto, J. & Nounaka, Y. (1961). The sexual function in patients with spinal cord injury. *Urol. Int.*, **12**, 270–80.

Tyrer, G., Steele, J.M., Ewing, D.J., Bancroft, J., Warner, P. & Clarke, B.F. (1983). Sexual responsiveness in diabetic women. *Diabetologia*, **24**, 166–71.

Ueki, K. (1960). Disturbances of micturition observed in some patients with brain tumour. *Neurol. Med. Chir.*, **2**, 25–33.

Uitti, R.J., Tanner, C.M., Rajput, A.H., Goetz, C.G., Klawans, H.L. & Thiessen, B. (1989). Hypersexuality with antiparkinsonian therapy. *Clin. Neuropharmacol.*, **12**(5), 375–83.

Valiquette, G., Herbert, J. & Meade-D'Alisera, P. (1996). Desmopressin in the management of nocturia in patients with multiple sclerosis. *Arch. Neurol.*, **53**, 1270–5.

Valleroy, M.L. Kraft, G.H. (1984). Sexual dysfunction in multiple sclerosis. *Arch. Phys. Med. Rehabil.*, **65**, 125–8.

van Kerrebroeck, P. & Debruyne, F. (1993). World wide experience with the Finetech–Brindley sacral anterior root stimulator. *Neurourol. Urodynamics*, **12**, 497–503.

Vas, C.J. (1969). Sexual impotence and some autonomic disturbances in men with multiple sclerosis. *Acta. Neurol. Scand.*, **45**, 166–82.

Vodusek, D.B. & Fowler, C.J. (1999). *Clinical Neurophysiology*. Boston: Butterworth Heinemann.

Wade, D. & Langton-Hewer, R. (1985). Outlook after an acute stroke: urinary incontinence and loss of consciousness compared in 532 patients. *Qu. J. Med.*, **56**, 601–8.

Walsh, P., Retik, A., Darracott Vaughan, E. & Wein, A. (1998). *Campbell's Urology.* Philadelphia, W.B. Saunders Co.

Wein, A. & Barrett, D. (1988). *Voiding Function and Dysfunction. A Logical and Practical Approach.* Chicago: Year Book Medical Publishers.

Werthman, P. & Rajfer, J. (1997). MUSE therapy, preliminary clinical observations. *Urology,* **50**(5), 809–11.

Whipple, B. & Komisaruk, B.R.(1997). Sexuality and women with complete spinal cord injury. *Spinal Cord,* **35**, 136–8.

Yarker, Y.E., Goa, K.L. & Fitton, A. (1995). Oxybutynin. A review of its pharmacodynamic and pharmacokinetic properties, and its therapeutic use in detrusor instability. *Drugs Aging,* **6**(3), 243–62.

Yarkony, G.M. (1990). Enhancement of sexual function and fertility in spinal cord-injured males. *Am. J. Phys. Med. Rehabil.,* **69**, 81–7.

Yoshimura, N., Sas, M., Yoshida, O. & Takaori, S. (1992). Dopamine D1 receptor-mediated inhibition of micturition reflex by central dopamine from the substantia nigra. *Neurourol. Urodynamics,* **11**, 535–45.

Zesiewicz, T.A., Helal, M. & Hauser, R.A. (2000). Sildenafil citrate (Viagra) for the treatment of erectile dysfunction in men with Parkinson's disease. *Mov. Disord.,* **15**(2), 305–8.

57

Hypothalamic/pituitary function and dysfunction

Roberto Salvatori and Gary S. Wand

Department of Medicine, The Johns Hopkins University School of Medicine, Baltimore, Maryland, USA

The hypothalamus and pituitary gland are a functional unit forming an interface between the nervous and endocrine systems. The hypothalamic–pituitary axes regulate several endocrine glands (e.g. thyroid, adrenal, and gonad) and many metabolic processes. Abnormalities of the pituitary gland present in three ways. First, a mass within the sella can compress the normal pituitary gland causing varying degrees of hypopituitarism. The spectrum of presentation includes non-specific complaints, slowly progressive constitutional symptoms and acute, life-threatening consequences of hormonal deficiencies. Secondly, an expanding sellar mass can injure contiguous structures resulting in visual field abnormalities, diminished acuity, diplopia, headache, and other neurologic symptoms. Thirdly, secretory pituitary adenomas can cause unusual clinical syndromes including acromegaly, Cushing disease, amenorrhea/galactorrhea syndrome or thyroid toxicosis. Sellar abnormalities are also incidentally discovered when radiographic tests are ordered for other reasons. In rare patients, pituitary adenoma is part of the familial multiple endocrine neoplasia syndrome, Type 1 (MEN 1), which also includes hyperparathyroidism and pancreatic islet cell adenomas.

Hypothalamic disorders (e.g. tumours, infiltrative disease or genetic abnormalities) often affect pituitary function, generally causing panhypopituitarism or monohormonal failure (e.g. Kallman's syndrome causing gonadal failure or growth hormone releasing hormone deficiency causing growth retardation). Less frequently hypothalamic disorders are associated with hyperfunction of the pituitary gland (e.g. precocious puberty).

Normal pituitary function

The pituitary gland receives its blood supply from the superior and inferior hypophysial arteries. The superior

Table 57.1. Hypothalamic factors and the pituitary hormones they regulate

Hypothalamic hormones	Anterior pituitary hormones
Growth hormone-releasing hormone (GHRH)	Stimulates growth hormone
Somatostatin	Inhibits growth hormone
Dopamine	Inhibits prolactin
Thyrotropin-releasing hormone (TRH)	Stimulates thyrotropin (TSH)
Corticotropin releasing hormone (CRH)	Stimulates ACTH and other POMC products
Gonadotropin-releasing hormone (GnRH)	Stimulates luteinizing hormone (LH) and follicle-stimulating hormone (FSH)

hypophysial artery, a branch of the internal carotid artery, forms a capillary plexus surrounding the hypothalamus and infundibulum and drains into the hypophysial–portal system. The hypothalamic releasing and inhibiting factors, which modulate anterior pituitary function, are secreted into this capillary plexus and are carried by the hypophysial–portal circulation to the anterior pituitary, their site of action. Once reaching the anterior pituitary, the hypothalamic releasing and inhibiting factors bind to specific membrane receptors and modulate synthesis, release and sometime posttranslational processing of anterior pituitary hormones. The pituitary gland synthesizes and secretes at least six hormones, and each is under some form of hypothalamic control (Table 57.1). In addition, it is possible for blood to flow retrograde up the infundibulum to the median eminence and thereby provide a route for pituitary hormones to control their own release by positive and negative feedback mechanisms. The posterior pituitary receives a direct arterial blood supply from the inferior hypophysial artery. This portion of the pituitary does not manufacture hormones but rather is a storage depot for vasopression and oxytocin synthesized in specific hypothalamic nuclei.

Hypothalamic–pituitary–adrenal (HPA) axis

The HPA axis is responsible for generating the glucocorticoid component of the stress response and for stimulating adrenal androgen production. Secretion of ACTH is primarily stimulated by corticotropin-releasing factor (CRH). In response to stress, the hypothalamus secretes CRH, which in turn stimulates the release of ACTH from the pituitary. ACTH is the primary regulator of adrenocortical function and increases cortisol, androgen and to a lesser extent, aldosterone secretion. Cortisol participates in its own regulation through a negative feedback loop inhibiting ACTH at the pituitary level and CRH at the hypothalamus. ACTH secretion has a diurnal cycle, with the highest levels occurring in the early morning before awakening and preceding the early-morning rise in cortisol.

ACTH is 49-amino acid peptide synthesized in the pituitary as part of a larger prohormone, proopiomelanocortin (POMC). POMC is a 265-amino-acid peptide that contains the sequence of ACTH, β-LPH, α-MSH, β-endorphin and other peptides. The endocrine role of ACTH is well understood, but the roles of β-LPH and the other mature peptide derived from POMC precursor are uncertain. The main hypothalamic regulator of ACTH is CRH. This peptide is expressed primarily in the paraventricular nucleus of the hypothalamus. The CRH neurons within the paraventricular nucleus are under regulation by several neurotransmitter systems. Hypothalamic β-endorphin and γ-aminobutyric acid (GABA) inhibit the release of CRH, whereas serotonin and α-adrenergic input stimulates CRH release. Vasopressin (AVP) is co-secreted from paraventricular neurons with CRH and potentiates the action of CRH on ACTH secretion. Angiotensin II, another neuropeptide released during stress, increases ACTH secretion.

Hypothalamic–pituitary–gonadal (HPG) axis

The HPG axis is responsible for maintaining normal gonadal function. Luteinizing hormone (LH) and follicle-stimulating hormone (FSH) are the main regulators of gonadal steroidogenesis (e.g. estrogen and testosterone). Both hormones are glycoproteins composed of α and β subunits. The β subunits of LH, FSH, TSH, and the placental peptide human chorionic gonadotropin are identical. Immunologic activity for detection of the intact hormone in radioimmunoassys depends on the integrity of the β subunit, whereas biologic activity depends on association of the α and β subunits and appropriate post-translational glycosylation of the subunits.

The decapeptide, gonadotrophin-releasing hormone (GnRH) is the main hypothalamic-stimulating factor for the secretion of LH and FSH. GnRH stimulates the release of both LH and FSH. In turn, LH and FSH stimulate the gonads to produce sex-steroid hormones. Through a sensitive negative feedback loop, estrogen and testosterone participate in their own regulation by inhibiting LH, FSH and GnRH release. The pituitary hormone prolactin (PRL) can also inhibit the release of GnRH accounting for the hypogonadism associated with hypoprolactinemia.

Hypothalamic–pituitary–thyroid (HPT) axis

The HPT axis is responsible for maintaining normal thyroid homeostatis. Thyroid-stimulating hormone (TSH) is a glycoprotein that regulates thyroid gland function. It has a molecular weight of 28 000 and like LH and FSH is composed of two non-covalently linked chains, the α and β subunits. Triiodothyronine (T_3) is the main hormone regulating TSH secretion. Through negative feedback, this thyroid hormone inhibits TSH and hypothalamic thyroid releasing hormone (TRH) synthesis and release. Although some T_3 comes directly from the thyroid, most is derived from the conversion of L-thyroxine (T_4) into T_3 by type II thyroxine 5-deiodinase within the pituitary gland.

The most important peptide regulating TSH is hypothalamic TRH. This simple tripeptide is found throughout the nervous system, but is enriched in TRH-secreting neurons within the median eminence. Like TSH, TRH secretion is inhibited by T3. TRH administration induces a dose-dependent increase in TSH secretion. Although rarely needed, failure of TSH to respond to synthetic TRH is one of the most sensitive clinical tests for hyperthyroidism. TRH can also be used to assess TSH reserve in patients with pituitary disease. In addition to T3 and TRH regulation of TSH, the hypothalamic inhibitory factor, somatostatin, also inhibits TSH secretion.

Somatotroph axis

Somatic growth is regulated by growth hormone (GH), a 21 500 Da protein. Most of the growth promoting effects of GH are mediated through GH-induced release of insulin-like growth factor (IGF-I), a protein made predominantly by the liver but also by other tissues. GH and IGF-I are required for normal growth and development during childhood. The presence of both factors is necessary for normal adult metabolic processes (e.g. muscle mass, lipid profile, and cognitive function).

Hypothalamic control of GH secretion is mediated by at least two peptides: somatostatin, which inhibits GH and growth hormone-releasing hormone (GHRH), which stimulates GH release. A recently identified third factor, Ghrelin, also stimulates GH secretion (Kojima et al., 1999). The GH inhibiting factor, somatostatin is a 14-amino-acid peptide present in the hypothalamus and distributed widely throughout the human central nervous system. Somatostatin blocks the release of GH induced by exercise, amino acids, and hypoglycemia. Somatostatin is also effective in reducing elevated GH and TSH levels in GH- and TSH secreting pituitary tumours, respectively. In normal humans, dopamine stimulates GH release. In patients with acromegaly (e.g. GH-secreting pituitary tumour), dopamine inhibits GH release. This inhibitory effect of dopaminergic agonists has been exploited in the treatment of acromegaly. Stress, exercise and slow wave sleep induce GH release. In normal individuals, glucose suppresses GH, whereas certain amino acids (e.g. arginine) stimulate GH secretion. In acromegalic patients glucose does not generally suppress GH and often, paradoxically stimulates GH. This difference in GH responses to a carbohydrate load between normals and patients with acromegaly forms the basis for the glucose-GH suppression test, a study employed to diagnosis acromegaly.

Prolactin

Prolactin, a 22 000 Da molecular weight protein, induces breast milk production in the presence of estrogens. In contrast to all other pituitary hormones, prolactin is primarily under inhibitory control by dopamine synthesized within tubero-infundibular neurons of the hypothalamus. In addition, the prohormone for GnRH contains a 56-amino-acid sequence that strongly inhibits the release of prolactin. This peptide is coreleased with GnRH and may serve to reduce prolactin levels.

The rise in prolactin induced by suckling, sleep, stress, and exercise is thought to be mediated through serotonergic input. Endogenous opioids (e.g. endorphin and enkephalins) stimulate prolactin secretion. Moreover, a variety of peptides (e.g. cholecystokinin, vasoactive intestinal polypeptide, neurotensin, and substance P) stimulate prolactin release. However, the physiologic significance of these effects remains uncertain. Estrogen modulates prolactin secretion. It acts on the hypothalamus to regulate dopamine turnover and at the level of the pituitary.

Disorders of the hypothalamic–pituitary unit

Precocious puberty

Precocious puberty results from the activation of the hypothalamic–pituitary–gonadal axis (Lee, 1999). While often observed after the development of a hypothalamic lesion, it can also be idiopathic. Precocious puberty has been described in the setting of various hypothalamic lesions but is most often observed in the presence of hamartomas, teratomas, germinomas and ependymomas. Other types of tumours associated with precocious puberty include optic nerve gliomas, astrocytomas, chorioepitheliomas, and neurofibroma (as part of von Recklinghausen's syndrome). These tumours both synthesize and secrete GnRH or stimulate the hypothalamus to prematurely release GnRH in a pulsatile manner.

Long-acting GnRH analogues are used to treat central precocious puberty because after a brief period of stimulation of LH and FSH, the analogues result in long-term inhibition of LH and FSH (Schally, 1999). GnRH analogues have the advantage of not causing other pituitary dysfunction, and prevent premature closure of the epiphyses (leading to short stature) that can be caused by the gonadal steroids.

McCune–Albright syndrome

The McCune–Albright syndrome is characterized by irregular pigmented areas (e.g. café-au-lait spots) on the trunk and polyostotic fibrous dysplasia of bone (De Sanctis et al., 1999). Precocious puberty and other endocrine hypersecretory syndromes (e.g. acromegaly, hyperthyroidism) can also be manifestations of the disorder. The hypersecretory states seen in McCune–Albright syndrome are the product of a somatic mutation in the Gs alpha gene leading to the constitutive activation of adenylyl cyclase signal transduction. This same mutation also accounts for approximately 30–40% of sporadically occurring GH-secreting pituitary tumours.

Pituitary adenomas

Pituitary adenomas are almost always benign accounting for 90% of sellar lesions and 10% of intracranial neoplasms. Pituitary adenomas are classified as microadenomas if their diameter is less than 1 cm, and macroadenomas if they are 1 cm or larger. This distinction is made because lesions greater than 1 cm often extend out of the sella and injure surrounding structures (e.g. optic chiasm). One can appreciate the potential symptoms (Table 57.2) created by

Table 57.2. Presentations of pituitary tumours

Increased hormone production
    Hyperprolactinemia
    Acromegaly (growth hormone)
    Cushing's disease (adrenocorticotropin (ACTH))
    Hyperthyroidism (thyroid-stimulating hormone (TSH))
Compression of adjacent structures
    Headache
    Visual field defects (classically, superior bitemporal)
    Cranial nerve deficits
Hypopituitarism
    Hypothyroidism
    Hypogonadism
    Adrenal dysfunction
    GH deficiency
Incidental radiographic detection
    Microadenoma
    Macroadenoma

an expanding sellar mass by remembering the structures adjacent to the pituitary (Fig. 57.1). As a sellar lesion expands it may induce (i) sign/symptoms of hypopituitarism resulting from compression of the normal pituitary gland; (ii) signs/symptoms secondary to extension of the mass into surrounding structures (e.g. optic chiasm); and (iii) clinical manifestations resulting from excess hormone secretion by the sellar mass. The pituitary gland 'sits' in a cavity, the sella turcica (Turkish saddle). This boney structure surrounds the anterior, ventral (floor) and posterior portions of the pituitary gland. The gland is also attached to hypothalamus by the stalk or infundibulum. However, the pituitary is on the peripheral side of the blood-brain barrier. In the superior direction, the gland is separated from CSF, optic chiasm and hypothalamus by a thin section of dura, the diaphragm sellae. Under normal circumstances, this boundary does not allow CSF to enter the sella turcica. Laterally, the pituitary is separated from both cavernous sinuses by thickened dura. The cavernous sinus contains cranial nerves III, IV, VI and the first two divisions of cranial nerve V. The carotid artery passes through the cavernous sinus and parasympathetic nerves inducing pupillary constriction ride on the surface of the carotids within the cavernous sinus. Below the floor of the sella is the sphenoid sinus.

Similar to any mass within a closed space, the expanding pituitary adenoma usually takes the path of least resistance, which is the superior direction. The lesion may compress the normal pituitary cells and induce various degrees

of hypopituitarism (e.g. hypothyroidism, hypogonadism, adrenal insufficiency and GH deficiency). The mass can also stretch the diaphragm sella and induce dull frontal headaches. If the lesion continues to expand in the superior direction, it will compress the optic chiasm causing visual abnormalities. Loss of vision can be the sole presenting symptom of pituitary adenoma. The subtlest visual abnormality is colour desaturation in the superior temporal fields, caused by compression of the medial inferior portion of the optic chiasm. However, some patients describe their vision as dim or foggy, or feel as though they have a veil over their eyes. Many patients have only vague complaints, like loss of depth perception. Some are unaware of their visual loss because peripheral vision is typically affected first. However, they may acknowledge problems with driving, which requires peripheral vision, or may complain that they are bumping into furniture or other people. If the tumour continues to grow, patients may suffer bitemporal hemianopia, optic atrophy, and loss of visual acuity. Papilledema is rare. In a few patients, an expanding tumour impinges on the hypothalamus, disturbing consciousness or temperature regulation, or causing hyperphagia. Tumour obstructing the third ventricle and cerebrospinal fluid flow can lead to hydrocephalus.

Less commonly the tumour will erode through the floor of the sella or into either cavernous sinus. Cavernous sinus invasion can result in injury to cranial nerves III, IV, V, and VI causing diplopia, ophthalmoplegias or facial numbness. Compression of the carotid artery may cause pupillary dilatation by injury to parasympathetic nerves on the surface of the vessel. Lastly, pituitary adenomas may cause a variety of syndromes secondary to excess hormone secretion.

Prolactin-searching and non-functional adenomas are the most common pituitary lesions. Less common are growth hormone-secreting adenomas, mixed prolactin- and growth hormone-secreting adenomas, ACTH secreting adenomas, and gonadotropin-secreting adenomas. Rare adenomas secrete TSH.

Prolactin-secreting adenomas and hyperprolactinemia

Patients with prolactin-secreting pituitary adenomas present with complaints resulting from the hormonal consequences of hyperprolactinemia and/or from tumour expansion (Molitch, 1995). The most common symptom is galactorrhea (non-puerperal lactation). However, this complaint is non-specific, affecting upwards of 20% of all previously pregnant premenopausal women. Most hyperprolactinemica women also have irregular menses. In fact,

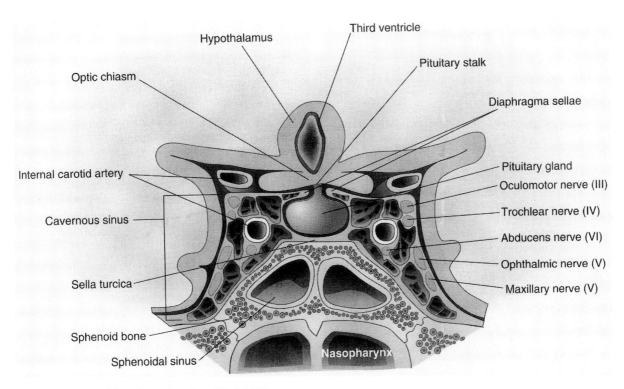

Fig. 57.1. Anatomy of the sellar region. (From Ward, 1996.)

15% of women presenting for evaluation of amenorrhea, 25% with galactorrhea, 35% with infertility and 75% with amenorrhea and galactorrhea have hyperprolactinemia. The prevalence of prolactinoma is approximately 5 cases per 10 000.

While menstrual dysfunction often leads women to seek medical help and permits early detection of prolactin-secreting adenomas, men less frequently complain to physicians about their core symptoms of hyperprolactinemia: impotence and decreased libido. At the time of diagnosis, men's tumours tend to be larger than women's. Hyperprolactinemia suppresses GnRH and therefore plasma LH and FSH levels, resulting in low circulating gonadal steroids causing diminished libido and vasomotor flushing in either sex. Relatively few men present with galactorrhea and gynecomastia.

It is important to consider physiologic and other pathologic causes of hyperprolactinemia and not assume that an elevated prolactin is always associated with prolactinoma (Table 57.3). The most common cause of hyperprolactinemia in women is pregnancy. Other important causes of hyperprolactinemia are (i) sellar or suprasellar lesions that block dopamine transport from hypothalamus to the pituitary (e.g. hypothalamic glioma, craniopharyngioma, and large non-functioning pituitary adenomas); (ii) medica-tions that deplete dopamine synthesis or block the D2-dopamine receptor (e.g. phenothiazines, Reglan[R]) (iii) kidney failure; and (iv) liver failure. In rare patients, severe primary hypothyroidism causes hyperprolactinemia. In this setting hypothyroidism may mimic a prolactin-secreting pituitary tumour by causing amenorrhea, galactorrhea, and even sellar enlargement due to thyrotropin-secreting cell hypertrophy. A TSH level should be checked in all patients with hyperprolactinemia to exclude primary hypothyroidism. In some patients, hyperprolactinemia is caused by chest wall injury or irritation (e.g. herpes zoster), which activate the neurologic circuitry responsible for elevations in prolactin induced by suckling.

Serum prolactin levels usually distinguish prolactin-secreting macroadenomas from other causes of hyperprolactinemia. Most prolactin-secreting macroadenomas produce serum prolactin levels above 250 ng/ml. Prolactin levels in microadenomas and other hyperprolactinemic disorders are generally lower.

Medical intervention with a dopamine agonist is first line treatment of prolactinoma regardless of size. Cabergoline (Dostinex[R]) and bromocriptine (Parlodel[R]) are the most frequently used dopamine agonists in this setting. Dopamine agonists normalize serum prolactin level in more than 90% of patients with microadenomas

Table 57.3. Causes of hyperprolactinemia

Physiologic
Pregnancy
Suckling
Exercise
Sleep
Postprandial

Pathologic
Prolactin-secreting tumours
Lesions interfering with hypothalamic dopaminergic tone
   Hypothalamic diseases, e.g. sarcoidosis, tumour
   Suprasellar lesions, e.g. craniopharyngioma
   Non-functioning pituitary adenoma
Acromegaly (cosecretion of prolactin in 25% of patients)
Kidney failure
Liver failure
Hypothyroidism
Chest wall stimulation, e.g. by herpes zoster, surgery, trauma
Chronic anovulatory syndrome

Pharmacologic
Dopamine-blocking agents, e.g. phenothiazines,
   metoclopramide
Catecholamine-depleting drugs, e.g. reserpine
Certain other intravenous drugs, e.g. cimetidine, verapamil

and 75% with macroadenomas. In both sexes, unless the tumour has destroyed the gonadotroph cells, both drugs reverse the hypogonadotropic hypogonadism that accompanies hyperprolactinemia. By reversing hypogonadism, medical therapy can halt or partially reverse decreased bone mineralization associated with hyperprolactinemia (Schlechte et al., 1992). In women, estrogen deficiency and galactorrhea production stops. This is accompanied by a return in ovulatory menstrual cycles. In men, normalization in prolactin is accompanied by a return of serum testosterone into the normal range. This is followed by restoration of libido, potency, spermatogenesis and fertility.

Importantly, dopamine agonists significantly shrink more than two-thirds of prolactin-secreting tumours. In most cases the drug needs to be taken indefinitely. The most common side effects are nausea, dizziness, nasal congestion and headache. In most cases, the side effects will abate after several weeks of therapy. In cases where tumours are resistant to dopamine agonists or the patient cannot tolerate medical intervention, transphenoidal surgery should be considered. However, the surgical cure rate is 50% for microadenomas and less than that for macroadenomas. Radiation therapy is efficacious in pre-

venting tumour growth but is not effective in normalizing the serum prolactin level.

Special consideration should be given to women with prolactinomas that become pregnant during medical therapy (Molitch, 1998). Under the influence of high estrogen levels, prolactinomas grow during pregnancy. Upward of 30% of macroadenomas and a small subset of microadenomas will grow to the extent that hypopituitarism or neurological defects occur. For this reason, most endocrinologists maintain macroadenoma patients on bromocriptine during pregnancy. Retrospective studies have strongly suggested that bromocriptine is not teratogenic nor does it induce spontaneous abortion. The safety of cabergoline during pregnancy has not been established at the time of this writing.

Growth hormone-secreting adenomas and acromegaly

Acromegaly is a syndrome caused by GH-secreting pituitary tumours (Klibanski & Zervas, 1991). The prevalence of acromegaly is approximately 7 cases per 100 000. Acromegaly is easy to diagnose when the manifestations are severe, but more often, there is a considerable delay between disease onset and diagnosis. This is because GH-induced changes in appearance occur insidiously and these subtle alterations evolve gradually over time. Indeed, family members and physicians often do not notice the gradual change in appearance. It has been estimated that, on average, 8 years separate the time of diagnosis from the onset of the syndrome. It is helpful for physicians to review old photographs of the patient. Unfortunately, by the time most GH secreting tumours are discovered, they are larger than 1 cm (e.g. macroadenoma) and have already caused local compressive effects. Moreover, the larger tumours are more difficult to cure.

Although 99% of acromegaly results from GH-secreting pituitary tumours, if a pituitary tumour is not identified by MRI, the physician must consider other causes. For example, eutopic overproduction of growth hormone-releasing hormone by the hypothalamus or ectopic production of this hormone by a peripheral tumour (e.g. islet cell tumour) can cause excess GH secretion and the syndrome of acromegaly.

Acromegalic patients first develop soft-tissue hypertrophy causing a generalized coarsening of the facial features, thickening of lips, tongue (macroglossia), ear lobes and skin (Table 57.4). Malodorous hyperhidrosis is an early symptom. With time, undiagnosed patients may complain of increasing ring, glove or shoe size resulting from enlargement of hands and feet. They may also develop a

Table 57.4. Common clinical features of acromegaly

Headaches
Impaired glucose tolerance or overt diabetes mellitus
Acral growth and prognathism
Coarsening of facial features
Hypertrophy of the frontal sinuses (frontal bossing)
Deepening of the voice
Hypertension
Arthritic complaints
Menstrual irregularities
Carpal tunnel syndrome
Thick skin
Visceromegaly
Hyperhidrosis
Hypertrichosis

deepening voice (hypertrophy of the vocal cords), snoring, sleep apnea, carpal tunnel syndrome and organomegaly. Approximately 40% of growth hormone-secreting tumours also secrete prolactin and therefore patients may complain of breast secretion (galactorrhea). Over time significant boney changes occur resulting in arthritis, enlargement of the mandible (prognathism), wide spacing of the teeth, and hypertrophy of the frontal sinuses (frontal bossing). Metabolic abnormalities can include glucose intolerance, hypertension, hyperphosphatemia and hypercalciuria. If acromegaly begins prior to closure of the epiphyseal growth plates, then excess growth hormone secretion will result in gigantism.

Because GH is secreted in pulses, a single serum growth hormone determination is not an accurate indicator of acromegaly unless markedly elevated. Glucose challenge testing is more reliable. In normal people, 50–100 grams of glucose suppresses GH to undetectable levels; acromegalics typically have either inadequate suppression or a paradoxical rise in GH following a carbohydrate load. Insulin-like growth factor I (IGF-I) synthesized in the liver, is a major mediator of growth hormone action. This protein has a long plasma half-life and is not secreted in a pulsatile manner. Therefore a single elevated plasma IGF-I determination can also be diagnostic, although elevations are found in some normal young adults.

Growth hormone-secreting tumours are usually first treated surgically, by transphenoidal resection through the nasal cavity and sphenoid sinus (Laws & Thapar, 1999). In the hands of an experienced neurosurgeon, approximately 80–90% of microadenomas and 20–50% of macroadenomas are cured. Similar to transphenoidal surgery for any pituitary tumour, fewer than 5% of acromegalics will

develop hemorrhage, infection, cerebrospinal fluid leak or injury to the anterior pituitary. However, transient diabetes insipidus occurs in about 25% of patients with permanent diabetes insipidus in fewer than 3%.

Recent studies have established new guidelines for defining cure of this syndrome. These guidelines were revised following reports showing that treated acromegalics still have two- to three-fold higher incidence of mortality compared to the general population unless serum GH levels are 1 μg or less and the IGF-I levels are in the normal range. Patients who still have elevated GH or IGF-I levels after surgery should be given a trial of a somatostatin analogue. Somatostatin analogs (e.g. Octreotide[R]) normalize growth hormone levels in about two-thirds of patients and occasionally induce tumour shrinkage. Dopamine agonists also have some efficacy. Pegvisomant, a newly developed GH receptor antagonist, is a promising therapy for patients who had unsuccessful surgery (Trainer et al., 2000).

When patients are not cured by medical and surgical therapy, the remaining option is radiation therapy. However, conventional radiation may take 2–5 years to work, it does not cure all patients, and in 30–50% of patients it induces hypopituitarism. Radiotherapy for Acromegaly is often combined with medical treatment. All patients need periodic follow-up of their pituitary function. Ongoing studies are evaluating the efficacy of gamma knife radiation in the treatment of Acromegaly (Jackson & Noren, 1999).

ACTH-secreting adenomas and Cushing disease

Cushing syndrome results from hypercortisolism from any source: ACTH-secreting pituitary adenomas, ectopic production of ACTH by peripheral tumours, autonomies, cortisol secreting adrenal adenomas and autominously administered corticosteroids (Table 57.5). Cushing disease specifically defines hypercortisolism caused by an ACTH-secreting pituitary adenoma. It has a prevalence of approximately 4 cases per 100000. Cushing disease accounts for approximately 80% of all causes of endogenous Cushing syndrome (Aron & Tyrrell, 1994). The ACTH-secreting pituitary tumour most often afflicts women in their childbearing years. Signs and symptoms include truncal obesity, cervicodorsal fat pad (buffalo hump), moon facies, plethora, purple striae, proximal muscle wasting and weakness, easy bruising, amenorrhea, psychiatric disturbances, and hirsutism (Table 57.6). Many ACTH-secreting pituitary adenomas are less than 0.5 cm in diameter and up to 70% cannot be visualized by MRI.

The diagnosis of Cushing syndrome requires the patient to undergo a low dose dexamethasone suppression test;

Table 57.5. Causes of Cushing's syndrome

ACTH dependent
Administration of exogenous ACTH
ACTH-producing pituitary adenoma
Corticotrophin cell hyperplasia
  Idiopathic
  Secondary to production of CRH
Ectopic ACTH production

ACTH independent
Administration of glucocorticoids
Associated with alcoholism
Adrenal
  Benign adenoma
  Adrenal carcinoma
  Hyperplasia–non-ACTH induced (rare)

Table 57.6. Common clinical features of hypercortisolism

Obesity–centripetal
Hypertension
Impaired glucose tolerance or diabetes mellitus
Menstrual irregularities or amenorrhea; sexual dysfunction
Hirsutism and acne
Striae
Proximal muscle weakness
Osteoporosis
Easy bruisability
Psychiatric disturbance

the details of which are beyond the scope of this text. Once Cushing syndrome is firmly established, the diagnosis of Cushing disease is made by performing the high dose dexamethasone. Inferior petrosal sinus sampling can be used to diagnosis of Cushing disease, when results from the high dose suppression tests are ambiguous and there is no evidence of a pituitary lesion on MRI.

First-line therapy of Cushing's disease is transphenoidal resection of the tumour, curing upwards of 80% of patients. The remainder can be given a combination of pituitary radiation and 'medical adrenalectomy' with one or more drugs that inhibit adrenal glucocorticoid biosynthesis, for example, Ketoconazole[R], metyrapone, aminoglutethimide, Trilostane[R], and o,p-DDD. However, none of these agents easily normalizes glucocorticoid secretion, and all have side effects. By 5 years, radiotherapy cures only 50% of adults, but more than 50% of children.

If pituitary surgery, radiotherapy, and medical therapy fail to control hypercortisolism, the last option is bilateral adrenalectomy. This commits patients to lifelong glucocorticoid and mineralocorticoid replacement. About 10% of patients who undergo bilateral adrenalectomy develop Nelson's syndrome, which is a progressive enlargement of the pituitary tumour, hyperpigmentation, and very high plasma ACTH levels unleashed by loss of cortisol-negative feedback. Such tumours can be aggressive and difficult to cure. Tumours causing Nelson's syndrome can be detected radiographically as well as by extremely high ACTH levels. All patients who have undergone bilateral adrenalectomy should be monitored closely.

Gonadotroph-secreting tumours

Many pituitary tumours secrete immunoreactive LH and/or FSH (Snyder, 1995). At the time of diagnosis, most are large and cause local compressive symptoms. Typical patients present with hypogonadism despite their high serum FSH or LH levels, because the hormones produced by the tumour have reduced biological activity. The gonadotroph tumour does not respond to medical therapy and is managed with surgery followed by radiotherapy if a significant tumour remnant remains.

TSH-secreting tumours

The least common pituitary adenomas secrete TSH and usually cause hyperthyroidism (Mindermann & Wilson, 1993). Unlike typical patients with primary hyperthyroidism, for example, from Graves' disease, in whom circulating TSH levels are undetectable, patients with hyperthyroidism from TSH-secreting adenomas have either elevated or inappropriately normal serum TSH levels (inappropriate secretion of thyroid hormone) at the same time that they have high serum T4 and T3 levels. Most TSH-secreting adenomas are managed with surgery; many patients also need antithyroid drugs and radioactive iodine. Somatostatin analogues have been shown to reduce TSH secretion from these tumours.

A cause of inappropriate TSH secretion that is not associated with a pituitary adenoma is the thyroid hormone resistance syndrome, a rare genetic disorder (Refetoff, 1996). When thyroid hormone resistance is more pronounced in the pituitary gland compared to peripheral tissues, patients have an appropriate elevation in TSH and are either euthyroid or hyperthyroid. However, when thyroid hormone resistance exists in the periphery and in the pituitary gland, patients present with unsuppressed TSH levels and features of hypothyroidism.

Non-functional pituitary tumours

Approximately 40% of pituitary adenomas are classified as non-functional because they produce no clinical syndrome resulting from hormone excess (Shimon & Melmed, 1998). However, the majority of non-functional adenomas do synthesize and secrete hormones, albeit at low levels. These tumours are managed with surgery followed by ratiotherapy if a significant tumour remnant remains. Medical therapy is not effective.

Pituitary incidentalomas

Pituitary adenomas that cause symptoms resulting from mass effect or hormone hypersecretion are uncommon. The prevalence of these lesions is approximately 20 cases per 100 000. However, clinicians are increasingly encountering incidental pituitary adenomas on CT and MRI scanning (Aron & Howell, 2000). The prevalence of pituitary incidentalomas found by CT ranges from 4% to 20%, and the prevalence found by MR imaging is approximately 10% (Katzman et al., 1999).

Given the high incidence of incidentalomas and the low incidence of potentially problematic lesions, an assessment algorithm would be helpful. Unfortunately, the optimal strategy for assessing patients with incidental adenomas has not been established. However, it has been suggested that any patient with an incidentaloma and clinical signs or symptoms suggestive of hormone hypersecretion should undergo appropriate testing as described above. Also, the asymptomatic patient with an incidentally discovered microadenoma should undergo limited hormonal testing. Most neuroendocrinologists would recommend that at least a serum prolactin be obtained. Evaluation of subclinical growth hormone or ACTH excess is not recommended in the absence of any signs or symptoms of these disorders. However, these patients require follow-up and if signs or symptoms of pituitary disease emerge, further evaluation is warranted.

In the presence of an incidentally discovered non-functional macroadenoma, some degree of hypopituitarism is not uncommon. Therefore, hormonal screening is suggested to detect potential deficiency of ACTH, TSH, GH, and gonadotropins. Patients with syndromes of hormonal excess should receive specific therapy as detailed below. These patients require formal visual field testing. Patient with evidence of visual field defects or cranial nerve injury should undergo surgery. For patients with non-functional

macroadenomas and no signs of visual abnormalities or hypopituitarism, optimal management is unclear. If the lesion is abutting the optic chiasm, surgery is strongly suggested. If the lesion does not extend into the suprasellar cistern a 'watch and wait' approach is reasonable. However, evidence of tumour growth or hypopituitarism should result in surgical intervention. If there is no evidence of growth of the lesion, the time period between scans can be lengthened.

Empty sella syndrome

The empty sella syndrome is a symmetric enlargement of the sella turcica caused by invagination of the diaphgram sella by CSF, putting pressure on adjacent bone, and compressing the pituitary gland towards the floor of the sella (Vance, 1997). In spite of this pressure, pituitary function is generally normal, although hyperprolactinemia or some degree of hypopituitarism is observed approximately 5% of the time. The empty sella syndrome most often affects obese hypertensive women. It is also seen following pituitary apoplexy and rarely in patients with neurosarcoidosis. MRI of the sella can distinguish it from a pituitary tumour. Empty sella must be distinguished from a Rathke's cleft cyst since the former is never treated surgically whereas enlarging pituitary cysts may require surgical intervention.

Other sellar lesions

In addition to pituitary adenomas, the sellar and suprasellar regions can harbour other types of neoplasm (Albrecht et al., 1995). Craniopharyngiomas are squamous epithelial tumours that arise from the upper part of the pituitary stalk, hypothalamus or third ventricle (Hayward, 1999). They are partly cystic and the cysts often contain a viscous fluid. These lesions have a peak incidence in childhood but can occur any time in life. The craniopharyngioma is treated by surgery, often requiring craniotomy. Other hypothalamic lesions that can alter pituitary function include hamartomas, teratomas, germinomas, ependymomas, gliomas, astrocytomas, chorioepitheliomas and neurofibroma. Metastases from breast and lung cancers, lymphoma, and melanoma are other uncommon hypothalamic and pituitary lesions affecting pituitary function.

Rarely, autoimmune, infiltrative, and infectious diseases involve the pituitary, sometimes mimicking a tumour. Lymphocytic hypophysitis predominantly affects young women in late pregnancy or postpartum, and is thought to have an autoimmune pathogenesis (Beressi et al., 1999).

Infiltrative and infectious processes that can damage the hypothalamus and pituitary include sarcoidosis, Langerhans' histiocytosis, and tuberculosis.

Hypopituitarism

There are numerous causes and various ways patients present with hypopituitarism. Pituitary dysfunction can occur gradually with insidious symptoms or suddenly with a catastrophic event. The most frequent causes of hypopituitarism are listed in Table 57.7. As the posterior pituitary only functions as a storehouse for ADH and oxytocin, the presence of diabetes insipidus usually indicates the involvement of the hypothalamus in the pathological process (Freda & Post, 1999).

Presenting signs and symptoms

Injury to LH- and FSH-secreting cells causes secondary ('central') hypogonadism. In children, this delays or prevents puberty. In adult men, it causes impotence, decreased libido, and infertility. In women, it leads to menstrual irregularities, amenorrhea, infertility, hot flushes, decreased libido, vaginal dryness, and dyspareunia. Deficient prolactin secretion makes women unable to lactate postpartum.

Injury to ACTH-secreting cells causes secondary adrenal insufficiency. Many patients complain of weight loss, anorexia, nausea, weakness, arthralgia, and myalgia. The degree of adrenal insufficiency is often milder than observed in patients with primary adrenal failure, and it is not unusual to observe symptoms only during times of physical stress, when the cortisol requirements are higher (Oelkers, 1996). Decreased adrenal androgen production diminishes women's axillary and pubic hair. Patients with secondary adrenal insufficiency do not have hyperpigmentation, which is a common feature of primary adrenal insufficiency. Further, since ACTH is not the primary regulator of the mineralocorticoid axis, patients with secondary insufficiency do not have extracellular fluid volume depletion and hyperkalemia, which are often seen in primary adrenal insufficiency. Many patients do have hyponatremia; this is caused by impaired renal free water clearance, which is dependent on glucocorticoid action, and by the frequent co-existence of central hypothyroidism. Patients are typically sensitive to infection and other stresses, which can quickly precipitate hypoglycemia, hypotension, circulatory collapse, and death.

The most frequent cause of secondary adrenal insufficiency is long-term exposure to exogenous glucocorticoids, which may last for several months after

Table 57.7. Causes of pituitary failure

Hypothalamic
1. Developmental
   Kallman syndrome, septo-optic dysplasia, anencephaly
2. Traumatic
3. Neoplastic
   chraniopharingiomas, hamartomas, gliomas, astrocytomas, teratomas, germinomas, ependymomas, chorioepitheliomas
   metastatic disease (lymphomas, leukemias)
4. Inflammatory/infiltrative
   sarcoidosis, tuberculosis, histiocytosis X
5. Radiation therapy

Pituitary
1. Neoplastic
   pituitary adenomas or metastatic disease (breast, lung, melanoma)
2. Hereditary
   multi-hormonal: mutations in Pit-1 or Prophet of Pit-1 transcription factors
3. Developmental
   aplasia, ectopia, Rathke's cleft cyst, arachnoid cysts
4. Traumatic
5. Postsurgical
6. Inflammatory or infiltrative
   Tubercolosis, fungal, syphilis, sarcoidosis, hemochromatosis, lymphocytic hypophysitis
7. Vascular
   Sheehan's syndrome (postpartum pituitary necrosis), pituitary infarction or apoplexy
8. Other
   Empty sella syndrome

Extrasellar diseases
1. Parasellar neoplasms
   meningioma, chordoma, optic nerve glioma
2. Aneurysms of the internal carotid artery
3. Nasopharyngeal carcinoma

glucocorticoids are discontinued. Every patient who has been treated with supraphysiological doses of glucocorticoids for 3 weeks or longer needs to be suspected to be adrenal insufficient (Krasner, 1999).

Injury to TSH-secreting cells causes secondary hypothyroidism. Symptoms include fatigue, cold intolerance, dry skin, constipation, weight gain, impaired mentation, and menstrual irregularities in women. These manifestations resemble those of primary hypothyroidism, but are usually less severe.

Growth hormone deficiency impairs skeletal growth if the epiphyses have not fused. Infants with GH deficiency are prone to hypoglycemia. Growth hormone-deficient adults can lose muscle mass and strength, have reduced bone mineral density, increased adipose mass, hypercholesterolemia and reduced sensation of well being, often associated with emotional lability and feelings of social isolation (Carrol & Christ, 1998). Treatment with recombinant GH at a dose sufficient to normalize IGF-1 has been proven to improve all the above changes (Gibney et al., 1999).

Diagnosis of hypopituitarism

When a patient develops pituitary failure from compression by a sellar mass, the first anterior pituitary hormone to fail is usually GH, followed by LH and FSH, TSH and ACTH. However, especially in the case of radiation-induced-hypopituitarism, this order can be inverted, and it is not unusual to observe isolated deficit of TSH or ACTH.

If a patient is diagnosed with partial or complete hypopituitarism secondary to a pituitary macroadenoma, hormonal function needs to be reassessed after neurosurgical treatment, as it may improve or worsen postoperatively (Webb et al., 1999).

In evaluation of a patient with suspected hypopituitarism, the physician must identify the patient's hormone deficiencies and determine whether they are caused by pituitary failure (secondary, 'central' hormone deficiencies) or target gland dysfunction (primary, 'peripheral' hormone deficiencies). Levels of target gland hormones – T4, cortisol, and estradiol or testosterone – can be low in both primary and secondary endocrine disorders. Distinguishing between peripheral and central failure depends, then, on the level of the pituitary trophic hormone. For example, T4 levels are low in both primary and secondary hypothyroidism, so one must look to the pituitary trophic hormone, TSH. In primary hypothyroidism, diminished negative feedback causes the TSH to be high, while in secondary hypothyroidism, pituitary injury makes the TSH either low or inappropriately normal. Analogous patterns allow the physician to distinguish between primary and secondary adrenal insufficiency and between primary and secondary hypogonadism.

In addition to a careful history and physical examination, evaluation of patients with a possible sellar lesion usually requires a focused hormone assessment, imaging studies, and visual field analysis.

Suspected GH deficiency in children
Growth failure is particularly suspicious when a deflection in growth velocity is observed in a child with previously normal growth curve. Several systemic diseases can also cause growth failure. Therefore, renal failure, malabsorption or hypothyroidism, need to be ruled out before GH secretion is evaluated.

GH deficiency can be isolated or part of multihormonal pituitary failure. Isolated GH deficiency in children manifests itself as growth failure and may be caused by any hypothalamic or pituitary disease. However, structural abnormalities are evident via MRI only in 12.5% of children affected by isolated GH deficiency (Cacciari et al., 1990). Genetic abnormalities (mutations in the GH gene or the GHRH-receptor gene) are present only in a minority of patients, leaving the vast majority classified as idiopathic. The clinical presentation includes growth failure, abdominal fat accumulation and delayed bone age. Several genetic syndromes (such as Turner syndrome, Silver Russel syndrome or Noonan syndrome) also present with short stature, and a careful physical examination in search of dysmorphic characters needs to be performed. Insulin-like growth factor-1 (IGF-1) is produced by the liver under the influence of GH and mediates most of the effects of GH. It circulates as a ternary complex bound to IGF-binding protein 3 (IGF-BP3) and to the acid labile subunit (ALS), whose synthesis is also under control of GH. Therefore, an indirect evidence of GH deficiency may be provided by measurement of serum IGF-1 or IGF-BP3 levels (ALS is not routinely used at the present time). However, confirmation of GH deficiency needs to be obtained via one of the many stimulation tests (insulin-induced hypoglycemia, GHRH, arginine, L-dopa, clonidine or combinations of the above) (Vance & Mauras, 1999). Although the cutoff of normal response is debated, usually a peak value below 7 ng/ml is considered diagnostic of GH deficiency. As each one of these tests has false positives, it is preferable to confirm GH deficiency with two tests before committing a child to a long and expensive injectable therapy.

Suspected GH deficiency in adults
The vast majority of adults with GH deficiency have overt pituitary disease. Among patients with pituitary tumours, those with deficiency in other hormones are very likely to be GH deficient. The likelihood of GH deficiency is close to 100% in a patient with deficit of gonadotropins, TSH and ACTH. Adults with a history of childhood onset isolated GH deficiency need to be retested, as more than 50% have normal GH secretion when retested as adults (Tauber et al., 1997). Serum IGF-1 and IGFBP3 levels are not reliable in diagnosing GH deficiency in adult, particularly in older patients, as a large overlap exists between subjects with normal and abnormal GH secretory reserve. Stimulation tests are often needed: insulin-induced hypoglycemia is the 'gold standard' in adults as well (except for patients

with known or suspected coronary artery disease and in patients with history of seizures). Alternatively, arginine, GHRH or GHRH plus arginine or clonidine can be used. At present, as the long term side effects of GH therapy in adults are not known, it is recommended that only patients with severe GH deficiency (peak GH after insulin <3 ng/ml) be treated (Bengtsson et al., 2000). The usual starting dose is 3–4 mcg/kg/day for males and 4–5 µg/kg/day for females. Side effects are usually dose dependent, limited to edema and arthralgia or myalgia. Absolute contraindications to GH treatment are active malignancy, proliferative or preproliferative diabetic retinopathy and benign intracranial hypertension (Growth Hormone Research Society, 1998).

Suspected secondary adrenal insufficiency

A basal morning cortisol is generally not a useful screening test for adrenal insufficiency, unless the level is above 20 µg/dl (indicating normal HPA axis) or below 3 µg/dl during the morning hours (indicating adrenal insufficiency). Therefore, most patients need to have a dynamic test. The available tests are the ITT, the overnight metyrapone test, the CRF tests and the ACTH tests.

The insulin tolerance test is the gold standard for diagnosing secondary adrenal insufficiency because it assesses the integrity of the entire hypothalamic–pituitary–adrenal (HPA) axis (Abdu et al., 1999). It has the additional advantage of simultaneously testing GH reserve when needed. It is, however, dangerous in patients above 60, or with history of seizures or known or suspected coronary artery disease.

The metyrapone test is an accurate way to diagnose acute secondary adrenal insufficiency as it evaluates both the pituitary and the adrenal cortex. It takes advantage of the ability of metyrapone to reduce serum cortisol by blocking the enzyme 11-beta-hydroxylase, which catalyses the last step in cortisol biosynthesis. Metyrapone (30 mg/kg; maximal dose 3 gm) is given at midnight and a single blood sample is drawn at 8 am the following morning. When cortisol synthesis is inhibited, a normal pituitary responds by secreting more ACTH, thereby raising plasma levels of 11-deoxycortisol, the immediate precursor to cortisol, above 7.5 µg/dl. Patients with secondary adrenal insufficiency have blunted ACTH and 11-deoxycortisol responses. This test needs to be performed with overnight hospitalization because of the theoretical risk of inducing an adrenal crisis (Fiad et al., 1994).

The rapid ACTH stimulation test detects pituitary–adrenal dysfunction only when secondary adrenal insufficiency has been chronic (>6 weeks). Traditionally patients are given 250 µg of synthetic ACTH and one hour later a serum cortisol value >20 µg/dl defines a normal response. Even more sensitive is the low dose of ACTH test where patients receive 1 µg of synthetic ACTH and 30 minutes later a serum cortisol >18.6 µg/dl defines a normal response (Abdu et al., 1999).

The CRF test utilizes the ability of ovine CRF of causing a raise in ACTH and cortisol. It is safe but expensive (CRF costs about $300/vial) and it is not yet well standardized.

Suspected secondary hypothyroidism

The physician should measure the free T4 (by T4 radioimmunoassay or free T4 index) and serum TSH concentrations. In secondary hypothyroidism, the free thyroxine is low, while the serum TSH is low or inappropriately normal. A normal TSH level in a patient with secondary hypothyroidism is explained by the fact that TSH produced in patients with pituitary and hypothalamic diseases is less biologically active than normal. In rare cases a TRH stimulation test (showing reduced TSH response to TRH) may help confirming the diagnosis of central hypothyroidism. As opposed to the treatment of primary hypothyrodism, TSH is not a reliable marker in patients with central hypothyroidism. Appropriateness of L-thyroxine replacement therapy must be assessed clinically and by measuring free T4 levels.

Suspected secondary hypogonadism

The gonadal axis can be evaluated by measuring the LH, FSH, and estradiol or testosterone. Secondary deficiency is marked by LH and FSH levels that are inappropriately low relative to low sex steroid levels. Normal LH and FSH levels in a postmenopausal woman who is not on estrogen replacement, rather than the expected elevations, also suggest hypopituitarism, especially in the initial postmenopausal years (Santoro et al., 1998).

Imaging and visual field testing

Imaging of the sella turcica, preferably by MRI, reveals sellar lesions, defines their size, and occasionally suggests the specific tumour type. For example, a craniopharyngioma can often be predicted by calcification (better detected by CT than MRI) and cystic degeneration as well as by its suprasellar position (Naidich & Russell, 1999). Because many people have clinically irrelevant nonsecretory pituitary adenomas ('pituitary incidentalomas', see above), pituitary imaging should be deferred until hormonal or neurologic findings confirm that there is reason to suspect a clinically significant sellar lesion.

If imaging studies show a macroadenoma, the patient should have visual field tests to detect possible optic nerve abnormalities. Although routine physical exam can reveal gross defects in peripheral vision, formal ophthalmologic evaluation is essential to find subtle abnormalities. Furthermore, visual field test is a sensitive indicator of rapid changes in size of a pituitary mass (such as the growth that may occur after hemorrhage of a macroadenoma or the shrinkage of a macroprolactinoma in response to dopaminergic therapy).

Pituitary apoplexy

About 5–20% of pituitary adenomas hemorrhage spontaneously. About one-third of these hemorrhages are recognizable as pituitary apoplexy, a syndrome of sudden, severe headache, neurologic symptoms and signs, and acute adrenal insufficiency (Randeva et al., 1999). Neurologic problems characteristically include vision loss, diplopia, ptosis, and pupil abnormalities. Within hours, lack of ACTH and cortisol production (present in two-thirds of the cases) may cause nausea, vomiting, and hypotension. If necrotic tissue and blood enter the cerebrospinal fluid, the patient may also develop meningismus, hyperpyrexia, and coma. CSF analysis may show pleiocytosis and increased protein concentration. The diagnosis of pituitary apoplexy is often delayed because 60% of the patients presenting with this syndrome have previously undiagnosed pituitary adenomas. Furthermore, symptomatology often can mimic the symptoms of subarachnoid hemorrhage and meningitis; and differentiating these disorders requires imaging of the sella. Although CT scan of the brain reveals a pituitary mass in about 90% of the cases, MRI is superior in diagnosing pituitary hemorrhage. Treatment requires urgent administration of intravenous glucocorticoids to treat acute adrenal insufficiency. Surgical decompression of the sella is required in the presence of reduced vision (symptom of acute chiasmal compression) and altered level of consciousness (symptom of increased intracranial pressure). Extraocular motor palsies do not constitute indication for surgery, as they revert spontaneously in most cases. Some authors believe that early (within a week) surgical decompression reduces the incidence of long-term hypopituitarism (Arafah et al., 1988) and visual deficit (Bills et al., 1993), but no prospective study is available to support these opinions. Acute pituitary failure is often transient, and patient's hormonal function needs to be re-evaluated weeks after the acute event.

The posterior pituitary

The posterior pituitary is a storehouse for the hormones antidiuretic hormone (ADH) (or vasopressin) and oxytocin produced by neurosecretory cells whose bodies are located in the supraoptic and paraventricular nuclei of the hypothalamus. The axonal processes of these neurons extend into the posterior pituitary where they carry the secretory material, containing the hormones and the associated protein neurophysins. A second secretory pathway releases vasopressin in the portal hypophysial system, where this hormone is believed to play a role in the secretion of ACTH from the anterior pituitary.

The secretion of ADH is mainly regulated by osmotic factors. Osmotic receptors are present in the CNS, and can detect very subtle changes in serum osmolarity. The amount of ADH released is proportional to the increase in plasma osmolarity. Increased osmolarity also stimulates ADH gene expression. ADH causes increase in urinary osmolarity. A 2% increase or decrease in serum osmolarity causes maximal concentration (>1000 mmol/kg) or maximal dilution (<100 mmol/kg) of the urine, respectively. As the onset of thirst occurs at values of plasma osmolarity similar to those of the threshold of ADH release, in a normal subject with access to water plasma osmolarity is tightly regulated.

ADH release is also regulated by baroreceptors located in the left atrium, aortic arch and carotid sinus. Stimulation of these receptors via ascending neural pathways suppresses ADH release, while reduced activity, as seen in hypovolemia or hypotension, causes increase in ADH release. The threshold for activation is much higher than for osmotically stimulated thirst and ADH secretion. Finally, ADH release is negatively regulated by glucocorticoids and stimulated by opioids, nausea and vomiting.

The effects of ADH on the renal collecting ducts (increase in water permeability) is mediated by a specific V2 receptor which activates water channels called aquaporins (Agre, 2000). ADH has a dual effect: a short-term one, triggering the translocation of aquaporin-containing intracellular vesicles to the plasma membrane, and a long-term one, increasing the number of aquaporin-containing vesicles (Knepper et al., 1997). However, it is the inner medullary-concentrating gradient that determines the degree of urine concentration in the presence of maximal ADH activity.

The effect of oxytocin is to cause contraction of the myoepithelial cells in the lactating mammary gland and to stimulate uterine contraction during parturition and expulsion of the placenta. The only two known stimuli for oxytocin secretion are nipple suckling and vaginal distention.

Diabetes insipidus

Disorders of the posterior pituitary lead to syndromes caused by inadequate (diabetes insipidus) or excessive

(SIADH) secretion of ADH. Diabetes insipidus is a polyuric syndrome of excessive excretion of dilute urine, with secondary polydipsia (Bichet, 1995). Diabetes insipidus can result from either inadequate ADH production ('central' or 'neurogenic' diabetes insipidus) or renal disease impairing responsiveness to ADH ('nephrogenic' diabetes insipidus). Central diabetes insipidus develops when the posterior lobe of the pituitary fails to secrete sufficient amount of ADH. In 10–30% of the cases the disorder is idiopathic; the major known causes are hypothalamic tumours, head trauma, central nervous system infiltrative disorders (e.g. sarcoidosis) or infection (e.g. tuberculosis), and transphenoidal surgery. Primary disease of the pituitary gland is rarely the culprit, because the posterior pituitary is merely a storage site for ADH after its synthesis in the hypothalamus. Thus, diabetes insipidus accompanying anterior pituitary dysfunction suggests underlying hypothalamic disease. Rarely, diabetes insipidus can be caused by very large pituitary tumours, pituitary apoplexy or lymphocytic hypophisitis. Rare familial autosomal dominant forms have been described, caused by mutations in the ADH signal peptide or in the neurophysins.

Patients with central diabetes insipidus require MR imaging of the sellar region to rule out secondary causes. The posterior pituitary usually appears as a bright spot, corresponding to the presence of stored ADH. In patients with idiopathic diabetes insipidus such a bright spot is usually absent. However, the presence of a normal bright spot does not rule out the diagnosis of diabetes insipidus.

In contrast, nephrogenic diabetes insipidus is caused by kidney disorders in which the renal tubules do not respond normally to ADH. The condition can be familial or acquired through electrolyte derangements (e.g. hypokalemia, hypercalcemia), diseases of the renal interstitium that disrupt medullary concentrating mechanisms, or drugs that impair renal tubular function (e.g. lithium carbonate or demeclocycline). Familial nephrogenic diabetes insipidus can be transmitted as an X-linked character (due to defects in the ADH receptor gene) or, less frequently, autosomal recessive (due to defects in the gene encoding for the vasopressin-sensitive water channel aquaporin-2) (Bichet, 1998).

Differential diagnosis

Polyuria is not pathognomonic for diabetes insipidus, and the physician must consider other conditions when a patient presents with excessive urination. Polyuria can reflect primary renal diseases, diuretic therapy, and diabetes mellitus. The cause can also be compulsive water drinking, also known as 'psychogenic' or 'primary' polydipsia. Such chronic excessive water drinking can lead to temporary loss of renal medullary hypertonicity, which then

impairs urine concentration even when the drinking is temporarily interrupted and plasma ADH levels rise, resembling nephrogenic diabetes insipidus. Primary polydipsia is usually diagnosed in young women with known psychiatric disease; in rare patients, the cause is a structural lesion in the hypothalamus. It needs to be suspected particularly in polyuric patients who have hyponatremia, never caused by diabetes insipidus.

The physician evaluating a patient with polyuria must first exclude an osmotic diuresis, such as the glycosuria of diabetes mellitus. The history and routine laboratory findings can generally exclude diabetes mellitus, primary renal diseases, drug effects, and electrolyte disturbances. The degree of polyuria can vary, up to 16–18 litres a day in case of total lack of ADH. Special tests are needed for certain systemic diseases that affect renal interstitial function, for example, sickle cell disease, amyloidosis, multiple myeloma, and Sjögren's syndrome. It is important to remember that lithium can cause a transient and a permanent form of nephrogenic diabetes insipidus. Therefore, lithium exposure needs to be considered as a possible etiology even if the medication has been discontinued.

Most patients need a water deprivation test to confirm diabetes insipidus and to distinguish central from nephrogenic diabetes insipidus. Fluids and food are withheld, starting in the morning to avoid dangerous nocturnal dehydration. Over the next 4–8 hours, hourly measurements of urine and plasma should show increasing osmolality and a two- to four-fold greater increase in urine osmolality than plasma osmolality. When plasma osmolality exceeds 295 mosm/l or urine osmolality stops rising, blood is drawn for ADH level and patients are given aqueous ADH or its analogue dDAVP. In normal people, endogenous ADH is already maximally stimulated, so exogenous ADH does not cause further urine concentration. Patients with complete central diabetes insipidus do not concentrate their urine despite a rising plasma osmolality, but do respond to exogenous ADH with a rise in urine concentration. Patients with nephrogenic diabetes insipidus also maintain dilute urines despite dehydration, and when they receive exogenous ADH, their urine osmolality does not rise above that of plasma. In selected cases with partial diabetes insipidus, a short administration of hypertonic saline may be needed to reach a serum osmolality of 295 mosm/l.

When central diabetes insipidus is diagnosed, patients should have a MRI scan to check the hypothalamic and pituitary regions for the presence of tumour or infiltrative diseases.

Patients with primary polydipsia may be difficult to identify with the water deprivation test because chronic dilution

Table 57.8. Distinguishing primary polydipsia from diabetes insipidus (DI)

Feature	Primary polydipsia	Diabetes insipidus
Onset of polyuria	Gradual	Sudden
Nocturia	Unusual	Common
Random plasma osmolality	Sometimes <285 mOsm/l	Normal or elevated
Morning plasma osmolality	Normal	Elevated
Morning urine osmolality	Normal	Inappropriately low
Plasma ADH concentration	Normal relative to plasma osmolality	Low relative to plasma osmolality (in neurogenic DI)

of their renal medullary osmolar gradient can prevent them from responding properly to either endogenous or exogenous ADH. However, other features may distinguish primary polydipsia from diabetes insipidus (Table 57.8). Polyuria usually begins gradually in primary polydipsia, but suddenly in diabetes insipidus. Patients with primary polydipsia may not have much nocturia, but most patients with diabetes insipidus have a constant urine output. Compulsive water drinkers do not share the high plasma osmolality and inappropriately low urine osmolality seen after overnight fasting in patients with central or nephrogenic diabetes insipidus. Most patients with primary polydipsia have at least one random plasma sample documenting an osmolality below 285 mosm/l (dilutional hyponatremia). Plasma ADH levels are normal relative to plasma osmolality in patients with primary polydipsia, but are low in patients with central diabetes insipidus.

Management

Patients with mild diabetes insipidus may not need drug treatment as long as they have an intact thirst mechanism and free access to water. However, patients with diabetes insipidus who are temporarily deprived of water can quickly develop circulatory collapse and hypertonic encephalopathy. Treatment is usually indicated when urine volumes exceed 5 l per day or when nocturia interferes with restful sleep.

DDAVP (Desmopressin^R), a long-acting synthetic analog of ADH, is the treatment of choice for central diabetes insipidus. The drug is usually given orally (0.1–0.2 mg once or twice a day) or by nasal insufflation (10 µg/spray, 1–2 spray a day). Subcutaneous injections (1 µg SQ 1–2 times a day) are available for situations in which oral or nasal administrations are not possible. The dose–effect equivalence between oral, intranasal and SQ administration is approximately 1/10/200. If patients with partial central diabetes insipidus require treatment, many can be successfully managed with chlorpropamide, which augments ADH release and potentiates its action on renal tubular cells. Most patients with normal glucose tolerance can take chlorpropamide in the low dose required, without developing symptomatic hypoglycemia. Clofibrate and carbamazepine can also augment ADH release. During pregnancy the dose requirement of DDAVP may increase, due to vasopressinase produced by the placenta.

There is no good treatment for nephrogenic DI. Some patients show a partial response to high doses of DDAVP, but most are treated with volume contraction (thiazide diuretics) to decrease glomerular filtration rate.

Syndrome of inappropriate secretion of ADH (SIADH)

Differential diagnosis

Excessive secretion of ADH, termed the 'syndrome of inappropriate secretion of antidiuretic hormone' (SIADH), leads to excessive water retention and hyponatremia. SIADH is the most common cause of non-iatrogenic hyponatremia. The major causes of SIADH are ectopic secretion of ADH (e.g. by a small cell carcinoma), neurologic disorders, pulmonary diseases, and certain drugs (Table 57.9). Cardinal features of the syndrome are hyponatremia and serum hypo-osmolality resulting from an inappropriately concentrated urine.

Patients with mild SIADH may have few symptoms and signs, especially if hyponatremia develops slowly. But when the serum sodium falls below 130 meq/l, patients can become anorexic, lethargic, and confused, with nausea and muscle cramping. When the serum sodium falls below 115 meq/l, patients can become obtunded and develop seizures. The severity of symptoms generally corresponds to the degree of hypo-osmolality and the rate at which hyponatremia develops. Premenopausal women seem to be more sensitive to rapid fluxes in serum sodium than are men and postmenopausal women and have a higher risk of permanent neurologic damage following hyponatremic encephalopathy.

Table 57.9. Common causes of the syndrome of inappropriate secretion of antidiuretic hormone

1. Central nervous system diseases
Meningitis
Encephalitis
Brain abscess
Subarachnoid hemorrage
Postoperative (5–7 days after pituitary surgery)

2. Pulmonary diseases
Lung abscess
Pneumonia
Positive pressure ventilation

3. Tumours
Lung carcinoma (especially small cell)
Gastrointestinal malignancies
Prostate cancer
Thymoma
Lymphoma

4. Drugs
Vincristine
Chlorpropramide
Narcotics
Clofibrate
Carbamazepine
Nicotine
Phenothiazine
Cyclophosphamide

Hyponatremia is the most common form of electrolyte abnormality in hospitalized patients. Other causes of hyponatremia must be considered in the differential diagnosis of SIADH. Sodium may be falsely low ('pseudohyponatremia') in case of severe hypertriglyceridemia or marked increase in serum protein concentration. Hyperglycemia can cause hyponatremia by attracting free water in the extracellular space. Plasma glucose will generally decrease plasma sodium concentration by 1.6 meq/l for every 100 mg/dl increase in glucose above 100 mg/dl. The physician should determine clinically whether hyponatremic patients are euvolemic (normal water volume), hypervolemic, or hypovolemic. Although patients with SIADH do have modest volume expansion, they are not edematous. In patients with edema, the physician should consider the major causes of hypervolemic hyponatremia such as liver cirrhosis, heart failure, and kidney failure. Patients with glucocorticoid or thyroid hormone deficiencies can develop hyponatremia because these hormones are essential for normal renal tubular function and free water excretion by the kidney. Thus, the diagnosis of

SIADH cannot be established until hypothyroidism has been excluded by measurement of the serum free T4 and TSH concentrations, adrenal insufficiency has been excluded, and kidney disease has been excluded by renal function tests. The physician should also seek a history of medications (chlorpropramide, carbamazepine, vincristin), neoplasia, pulmonary disease, and neurologic disorders known to be associated with SIADH.

In SIADH, urine sodium is generally above 20 meq/l, but it is usually below 20 meq/l in conditions with intravascular volume contraction or decreased effective plasma volume, for example, congestive heart failure, cirrhosis, and the nephrotic syndrome (Chung et al., 1987). The blood urea nitrogen and uric acid are low in SIADH but high in volume-contracted states. Lastly, in SIADH the urine is less than maximally dilute (50–100 mosm/kg) despite plasma hypo-osmolality. Occasionally the water load test helps the diagnosis of SIADH. After drinking 20 ml/kg of water, normal individuals reach maximally diluted urine (<100 mosm/kg) and eliminate 80–90% of the water load within 4 hours. This test should not be performed if serum sodium is <125 meq/l.

Management

The aims of treating SIADH are to correct hypo-osmolality and hyponatremia, and to diagnose and, when possible, treat the underlying disorder. It is important to understand that the brain can adapt to hyponatremia by releasing osmoles, provided that it develops slowly. Therefore, it is not unusual to find patients with marked hyponatremia who are absolutely asymptomatic. For the asymptomatic patient, water restriction to 500–1000 cc a day corrects hyponatremia at a rate of about 5 meq/l a day. Infusions of normal saline do not correct hyponatremia because the sodium is promptly excreted in the urine. Only symptomatic hyponatremia is treated with hypertonic saline (3% NaCl) until the serum sodium concentration reaches 125 meq/l (Verbalis & Martinez, 1991). An approximate way of calculating the rate (cc/hour) of hypertonic solution infusion is to multiply the ideal body weight by the desired hourly increase in serum sodium concentration. In a 70 kg patient, if an increase of 0.5 meq/l/hour is desired, the rate of infusion should be 70 × 0.5 = 35 cc/hour. Serum osmolarity should not be corrected faster than 12 meq/l in 24 hours, because of risk of potentially fatal central pontine myelolysis. Therefore, plasma sodium level should be monitored very closely during hypertonic solution infusion. Once a level of 125 is reached, hypertonic solution should be discontinued and plasma osmolality is restored gradually by water restriction alone. For many patients with chronic SIADH in whom hyponatremia cannot be controlled with fluid restriction only, demeclocycline normalizes serum sodium by inhibiting ADH action in the kidney. Lithium carbonate acts similarly but is rarely used because it can be more toxic.

Fluid abnormalities after pituitary surgery

Manipulation of the pituitary gland during transphenoidal or transcranial pituitary surgery may cause transient or permanent abnormalities in ADH production, leading to diabetes insipidus or hyponatremia. Although a classical triphasic pattern is often reported when the posterior pituitary is permanently damaged (with transient diabetes insipidus followed by a SIADH phase and ultimately by permanent diabetes insipidus) the possible patterns are way more variable. In a large analysis of 1571 transphenoidal pituitary surgery done by Hensen et al. (1999) the classical triphasic pattern was observed only in 1.1% of patients. However, 8.4% developed hyponatremia (symptomatic in 2.1%) at some point during the first 10 postoperative days. Patients with Cushing's disease seem to have a particular high prevalence of polyuria and hyponatremia, and should be monitored particularly closely.

References

Abdu, T.A.M., Neary, T.S. & Clayton, R.N. (1999). Comparison of the low dose short synachten test (1 μg), the conventional dose short synachten test (250 μg), and the insulin tolerance test for assessment of the hypothalamo-pituitary-adrenal axis in patients with pituitary disease. *J. Clin. Endocrinol. Metab.*, **84**, 838–43.

Agre, P. (2000). Aquaporin water channels in kidney. *J. Am. Soc. Nephrol.*, **11**, 764–77.

Albrecht, S., Bilboa, J. & Kovacs, K. (1995). Nonpituitary tumours of the sella region. In *The Pituitary*, ed. S. Melmed, pp. 576–95. Cambridge, MA: Blackwell Science.

Arafah, B.M., Harrington, F., Madhoun, Z.T. et al. (1988). Improvement of pituitary function after surgical decompression for pituitary tumour apoplexy. *J. Clin. Endocrinol. Metab.*, **71**, 323–7.

Aron, D.C. & Howell, T. (2000). Pituitary incidentalomas. *Endocrinol. Clin. North Am.*, **29**, 205–20.

Aron, D.C. & Tyrrell, J.B. (1994). Cushing's syndrome. *Endocrinol. Clin. North Am.*, **23**, 451–691.

Bengtsson, B-A., Johannsson, G., Shalet, S.M. et al. (2000). Treatment of growth hormone deficiency in adults. *J. Clin. Endocrinol. Metab.*, **85**, 933–46.

Beressi, N., Beressi, J.P., Cohen, R. et al. (1999). Lymphocytic hypophysitis. A review of 145 cases. *Ann. Med. Interne (Paris)*, **150**(4), 327–41.

Bichet, D.G. (1995). The posterior pituitary, In *The Pituitary*, ed. S. Melmed, pp. 277–306. Cambridge, MA: Blackwell Science.

Bichet, D.G. (1998). Nephrogenic diabetes insipidus. *Am. J. Med.*, **105**, 431–42.

Bills, D.C., Meyer, F.B., Laws, E.R. Jr. et al. (1993). A retrospective analysis of pituitary apoplexy. *Neurosurgery*, **33**, 602–9.

Cacciari, E., Zucchini, S., Carla, G. et al. (1990). Endocrine function and morphological findings in patients with disorders of the hypothalamo-pituitary area: a study with magnetic resonance. *Arch. Dis. Child*, **65**, 1199–202.

Carrol, P.V. & Christ, E.R. (1998). Growth hormone deficiency in adulthood and the effects of growth hormone replacement: a review. *J. Clin. Endocrinol. Metab.*, **83**, 382–95.

Chung, H.M., Kluge, R., Schrier, R.W. & Anderson, R.J. (1987). Clinical assessment of extracellular fluid volume in hyponatremia. *Am. J. Med.*, **83**, 905–8.

De Sanctis, C., Lala, R., Matarazzo, P. et al. (1999). McCune–Albright syndrome: a longitudinal clinical study of 32 patients. *J. Pediatr. Endocrinol. Metab.*, **12**(6), 817–26.

Fiad, T.M., Kirby, J.M., Cunningham, S.K. & Mckenna, T.J. (1994). The overnight single-dose metyrapone test is a simple and reliable index of the hypothalamic–pituitary–adrenal axis. *Clin. Endocrinol. (Oxf.)*, **40**, 603–9.

Freda, P.U. & Post, K.D. (1999). Differential diagnosis of sellar masses. *Endocrinol. Metab. Clin. N. Am.*, **28**, 81–117.

Gibney, J., Wallace, J.D., Spinks, T. et al. (1999). The effects of 10 years of recombinant human growth hormone (GH) in adult GH-deficient patients. *J. Clin. Endocrinol. Metab.*, **84**, 2596–602.

Growth Hormone Research Society. (1998). Consensus guidelines for the diagnosis and treatment of adults with growth hormone deficiency: summary statement of the adult growth hormone research society workshop on adult growth hormone deficiency. *J. Clin. Endocrinol. Metab.*, **83**, 379–81.

Hayward, R. (1999). The present and future management of childhood craniopharyngioma. *Childs Nerv. Syst.*, **15**(11–12), 764–9.

Hensen, J., Henig, A., Fahlbush, R. et al. (1999). Prevalence, predictors and patterns of postoperative polyuria and hyponatremia in the immediate course after transsphenoidal surgery for pituitary adenomas. *Clin. Endocrinol. (Oxf.)*, **50**, 431–9.

Jackson, I.M.D. & Noren, G. (1999). Role of gamma knife radiosurgery in acromegaly. *Pituitary*, **2**, 71–7.

Kattzman, G.L., Dagher, A.P. & Patronas, N.J. (1999). Incidental findings on brain magnetic resonance imaging from 1000 asymptomatic volunteers. *J. Am. Med. Assoc.*, **282**, 36–9.

Klibanski, A. & Zervas, N.T. (1991). Diagnosis and management of hormone-secreting pituitary adenomas. *N. Engl. J. Med.*, **324**, 822–31.

Knepper, M.A., Vervalis, G. & Nielsen, S. (1997). Role of aquaporins in water balance disorders. *Curr. Opin. Nephrol. Hypertens.*, **6**, 367–71.

Kojima, M., Hosoda, H., Date, Y., Natazato, M., Matsuo, H. & Kangawa, K. (1999). Ghrelin in a growth hormone-releasing acylated peptide from stomach. *Nature*, **402**, 656–60.

Krasner, A.S. (1999). Glucocorticoid-induced adrenal insufficiency. *J. Am. Med. Assoc.*, **282**, 671–6.

Laws, E.R. Jr. & Thapar, K. (1999). Pituitary surgery. *Endocrinol. Metab. Clin. North Am.*, **28**, 119–31.

Lee, P.A. (1999). Central precocious puberty. An overview of diagnosis, treatment, and outcome. *Endocrinol. Metab. Clin. North Am.*, **23**, 901–18.

Mindermann, T. & Wilson, C.B. (1993). Thyrotropin-producing pituitary adenomas. *J. Neurosurg.*, **79**, 521–7.

Molitch, M.E. (1995). Prolactinoma. In *The Pituitary*, ed. S. Melmed, pp. 443–77. Cambridge, MA: Blackwell Science.

Molitch, M.E. (1998). Pituitary diseases in pregnancy. *Semin. Perinatol.*, **22**(6), 457–70.

Naidich, M.J. & Russell, E.J. (1999). Current approaches to imaging of the sellar region and pituitary. *Endocrinol. Metab. Clin. N. Am.*, **28**, 45–79.

Oelkers, W. (1996). Adrenal insufficiency. *N. Engl. J. Med.*, **335**, 1206–12.

Randeva, H.S., Schoebel, J., Byrnet, J. et al. (1999). Classical pituitary apoplexy: clinical features, management and outcome. *Clin. Endocrinol. (Oxf.)*, **51**, 181–8.

Refetoff, S. (1996). Resistance to thyroid hormones. In Werner and Ingbar's *The Thyroid: a Fundamental and Clinical Text*, 7th edn., ed. L.E. Braverman & R.D. Utiger, pp. 1032–48. Philadelphia: JB Lippincott.

Santoro, N., Banwell, T., Tortoriello, D. et al. (1998). Effects of aging and gonadal failure on the hypothalamic-pituitary axis in women. *Am. J. Obstet. Gynecol.*, **178**, 732–41.

Schally, A.V. (1999). LH-RH analogues: Their impact on reproductive medicine. *Gynecol. Endocrinol.*, **13**(6), 401–9.

Schlechte, J., Walkner, L. & Kathol, M. (1992). A longitudinal analysis of premenopausal bone loss in healthy women and women with hyperprolactinemia. *J. Clin. Endocrinol. Met.*, **75**, 698–702.

Shimon, I. & Melmed, S. (1998). Management of pituitary tumours. *Ann. Intern. Med.*, **129**, 472–83.

Snyder, P. (1995). Gonadotroph adenomas. In *The Pituitary*, ed. S. Melmed, pp. 559–75. Cambridge, MA, Blackwell Science.

Tauber, M., Moulin, P., Pienkowski, C. et al. (1997). Growth hormone (GH) retesting and auxological data in 131 GH=deficient patients after completion of treatment. *J. Clin. Endocrinol. Metab.*, **82**, 352–6.

Trainer, P.J., Drake, W.M., Katznelson, L. et al. (2000). Treatment of acromegaly with the growth hormone-receptor antagonist pegvisomant. *N. Engl. J. Med.*, **342**, 1171–7.

Vance, M.L. (1997). The empty sella. *Curr. Ther. Endocrinol. Metab.*, **6**, 38–40.

Vance, M.L. & Mauras, N. (1999). Growth hormone therapy in adults and in children. *N. Engl. J. Med.*, **314**, 1206–16.

Verbalis, J.G. & Martinez, A.J. (1991). Neurological and neuropathological sequelae of correction of chronic hyponatremia. *Kidney Int.*, **39**, 1274–82.

Wand, G.S. (1996). Pituitary disorders. In *The Principles and Practice of Medicine*, ed. J.D. Stobo, D.B. Hellmann, P.W. Ladenson, B.G. Petty & T.A. Traill, pp. 274–81. Stamford: Appleton & Lange.

Webb, S.M., Rigla, M., Wagner, A. et al. (1999). Recovery of hypopituitarism after neurosurgical treatment of pituitary adenomas. *J. Clin. Endocrinol. Metab.*, **84**, 3696–700.

Part VII

Headache and pain

58

Peripheral nociception and genesis of persistent pain

Richard J. Mannion and Clifford J. Woolf

Neural Plasticity Research Group, Department of Anesthesia and Critical Care,
Massachusetts General Hospital and Harvard Medical School, Charlestown, Massachusetts, USA

Pain can be divided into two distinct categories, nociceptive and clinical. The detection of, or reaction to damaging or noxious stimuli, the phenomenon of nociception, is mediated in the periphery by highly specialized primary sensory neurons, the nociceptors. These have peripheral terminals that are activated only by high intensity mechanical, thermal and chemical stimuli. Nociceptive pain, the 'ouch' pain typically experienced on touching a hot object or stubbing a toe, is the readout from a protective system fundamental to maintaining bodily integrity in a potentially lethal environment. The key physiological role of this system is well illustrated by the tissue destruction produced both in the denervated (Charcot) joints and neuropathic ulcers in diabetic patients, or in the mutilating injuries seen in patients with congenital insensitivity to pain due to a loss of nociceptor sensory neurons during development, as a result of a mutation of the TrkA receptor (Indo et al., 1996). Nociceptive pain contributes to the pain associated with the onset of acute trauma and is amenable to a variety of therapies that directly target the nociceptor neuron. These include blocking input to the spinal cord with local anesthetic nerve blockade, epidural or spinal anesthesia or reducing transmission from the nociceptor to the CNS with high dose opioids.

Clinical pain has two general manifestations, that associated with tissue injury and inflammation, inflammatory pain, and that generated as a result of damage to the nervous system, neuropathic pain. Multiple distinct, but commonly coexisting pathophysiological mechanisms are responsible for the generation of clinical pain and these typically involve the recruitment of pain in response to sensory inputs other than just nociceptors (the pain is no longer purely nociceptive). Clinical pain, is moreover, the manifestation of profound alterations in sensory processing within the peripheral and central nervous systems, neuroplasticity. Two key features of clinical pain are that the pain may present in the absence of any obvious peripheral stimulus (spontaneous pain) and that there is typically an abnormal hypersensitivity to applied innocuous and noxious stimuli. Clinical pain can arise from insults to, or changes induced anywhere along, the somatosensory neuraxis from the peripheral innervation targets (as with osteo- or rheumatoid arthritis), in inflammatory pain, along peripheral nerves (postherpetic neuralgia and diabetic neuropathy), in the spinal cord (spinal cord injury) or the brain (stroke), for neuropathic pain. The aim of clinical pain treatment is the elimination of spontaneous pain and the normalization of sensibility, rather than the elimination of pain perception *per se*, but this can be achieved optimally only if the mechanisms responsible can be identified in individual patients and if treatments specific to each mechanism are available. At the moment, however, standard clinical techniques do not enable pain mechanisms to be unambiguously established, nor are there treatments suitable for each mechanism. Accelerating progress in the study of pain makes such a rational approach a realistic possibility for the near future, one that will require, however, considerable effort to translate molecular advances into new clinical diagnostic approaches and therapies. The aim of this chapter is to highlight the advances in our understanding of pain mechanisms and their clinical implications.

Primary sensory neurons and the dorsal horn

Sensory neurons are a heterogeneous group of neurons whose cell bodies are located within the dorsal root and trigeminal ganglia, and which have either myelinated A, or unmyelinated C, axons (Lawson, 1979). Making up approximately two-thirds of the population are the C-fibre neurons, the majority of which are nociceptors (some are

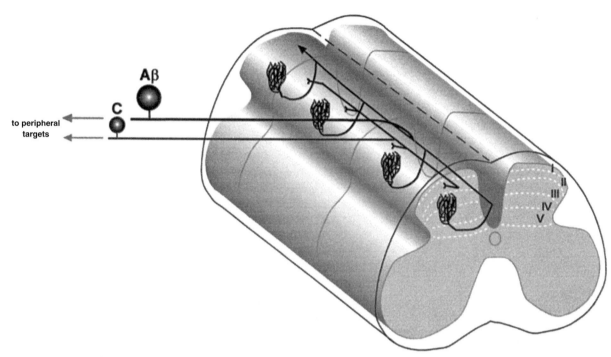

Fig. 58.1. Diagram showing Aβ- and C-fibre central axons entering the spinal cord. C-fibres synapse directly in the superficial dorsal horn. Aβ-fibre central axons enter the ipsilateral dorsal column pathway to travel up to the brain, synapsing in the dorsal column nuclei within the medulla. In addition, they give off multiple collateral axons that synapse within the deep dorsal horn over a few spinal segments.

innocuous warm receptors) (Willis & Coggeshall, 1991). Although some nociceptors are modality-specific, most are polymodal, responding to thermal, mechanical and chemical stimuli (Willis & Coggeshall, 1991). In addition, some are silent, unresponsive to all stimuli even at a very high intensities, but become active under pathological conditions, e.g. during inflammation (McMahon & Koltzenburg, 1990). The remaining sensory neurons (~30–40%) are the A-fibres, which are larger and are classified into three groups: the thinly myelinated Aδ fibres, which are predominantly nociceptive but include cool detectors; the myelinated Aβ fibres, many of which are cutaneous mechanoreceptors responsible for the detection of vibration, pressure and brush; and the large myelinated Aα fibres innervating muscle spindles and golgi-tendon organs, responsible for proprioceptive afferent input (Bonica, 1990).

The central terminal projections of primary sensory neurons in the dorsal horn of the spinal cord are highly ordered rostrocaudally, mediolaterally and dorsoventrally to form a somatotopic map of the body surface with minimal overlap between adjacent nerves (Willis & Coggeshall, 1991). C-fibres synapse directly onto second-order neurons in the ipsilateral dorsal horn either at the

same spinal level that they enter the cord or within a few segments rostrocaudally. A-fibre central axons on entering the spinal cord via a dorsal root give off collateral axons to the dorsal horn before entering the dorsal column pathways and ascending to the brainstem (Fig. 58.1). Dorsoventrally, specific types of afferent innervate cytoarchitectonically distinct laminae in the dorsal horn. Aδ-fibres project to laminae I and V, Aβ-fibre collaterals project to the deeper dorsal horn laminae (III-V, with some input to lamina II inner (II$_i$)), while C-fibres project to lamina II. Lamina II outer (II$_o$), is therefore, innervated almost exclusively by C-fibres (Woolf, 1994) (Fig. 58.2(a), see colour plate section). In addition to producing excitation of pain projection pathways, afferent input also activates segmental inhibitory interneurons which feed back onto the projection neurons in a reciprocal arrangement to dampen down and functionally focus the effect of the input (Woolf, 1994) (Fig. 58.3(a)).

The spinal cord is the site of the first relay along the sensory neuraxis at which the transfer of sensory information can be controlled. The dorsal horn also receives descending innervation from brainstem regions like the periaqueductal grey via the raphe nuclei and locus ceruleus. These tonic and phasic inputs are both excitatory (e.g.

5HT) and inhibitory (e.g. NA and opioids) and act to modulate spinal transmission through the dorsal horn. In this way the amount and nature of sensory input transferred to the brain following a particular stimulus can be either facilitated or inhibited altering the relationship between peripheral stimulus and perceptual response. This form of sensory adaptability was a key feature of Melzack & Wall's gate control theory of pain (1965) and both increased facilitation and reduced inhibition have been implicated in persistent pain states.

Primary sensory neurons can be classified on the basis of their chemical phenotype (i.e. what genes they express). Sensory neuron phenotype is thought to be actively maintained by signalling molecules extrinsic to the neuron, such as growth factors expressed by cells in the peripheral targets and Schwann cells lining the axons (McMahon & Bennett, 1999), and molecules intrinsic to the neurons such as cell specific transcription factors (Wood et al., 1999). For unmyelinated C-fibres, one major phenotypic distinction made is that between peptidergic and non-peptidergic afferents, each forming approximately half of the population. The former express neuropeptide neuromodulators (e.g. SP, CGRP) while the latter do not. The former also express the high affinity NGF receptor TrkA, while the latter express the GDNF receptor binding complex and the $P2X_3$ purinoreceptor (McMahon & Bennett, 1999). The NGF and GDNF sensitive nociceptor populations terminate in laminae I / II_o and II_i respectively (Snider & McMahon, 1998) (Fig. 58.2(b), see colour plate section).

Activation: transduction, transmission and use-dependent augmentation

Primary nociceptor activation

For most of the time the 'protective pain system' lies quiescent, being activated only on exposure to damaging or potentially damaging events. The detection by nociceptors of noxious stimuli is the consequence of their selective expression of specialized transducer molecules, that when activated result in the opening of cation channels and the generation of inward currents at the peripheral terminal. Examples of these molecules are: the VR1 receptor for capsaicin (the active ingredient in chilli peppers), an ion channel that opens in response to heat (>42 °C); VRL1, another vanilloid receptor also activated by heat but at higher temperatures (>50 °C) (Caterina & Julius, 1999); chemosensitive molecules like $P2X_3$ purinoreceptors that detect ATP (released during tissue damage) and proton-

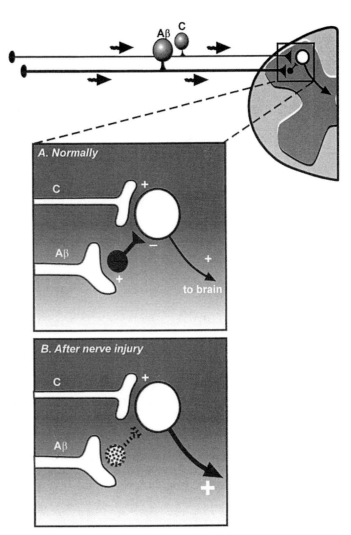

Fig. 58.3. (a) A noxious stimulus leads to the activation of both A- and C-fibres. C-fibres make monosynaptic connections with some spinal neurons that may also receive polysynaptic input from A-fibres that is relayed through an inhibitory interneuron (some $A\beta$ input may also be relayed via excitatory interneurons). Thus, noxious input to spinal projection neurons through C-fibres is controlled to a certain extent by A-fibre activity. The inhibitory input acts to dampen down and functionally focus the effects of the C-fibre input. (b) Following nerve injury, many inhibitory interneurons in lamina II die leading to disinhibition of spinal projection neurons manifesting as increased excitation with a greater level of information being transferred to higher centres.

gated ion channels like ASIC (acid-sensing ion channel) which respond to tissue acidosis (Wood et al., 1999); and molecules that transduce mechanical stimuli, candidates for which are the mDEG ion channels which are homologues of the degenerins, mechanotransducer proteins in the nematode *Caenorhabditis elegans* (Wood et al., 1999).

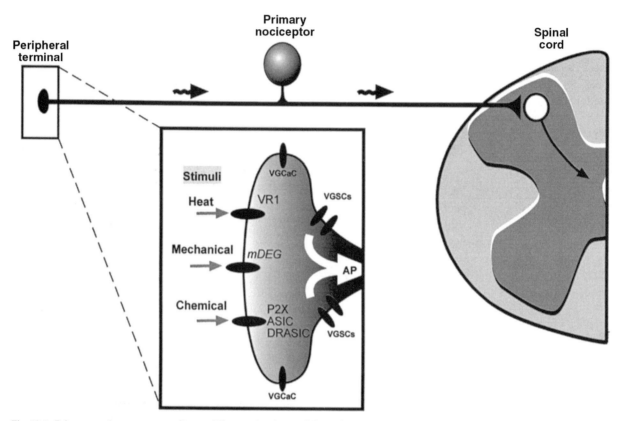

Fig. 58.4. Primary nociceptors responding to different stimulus modalities through the expression of specific transducer proteins on their peripheral terminal membranes. Activation of these proteins leads to the generation of inward currents that further activate voltage gated sodium channels (VGSCs). If stimulus intensity is sufficient to reach activation threshold, action potentials are generated and conducted orthodromically along the axon to the spinal cord. This represents pain normosensitivity.

Once specific transducer receptor/ion channels proteins are activated, depolarization of the nociceptor terminal by cation influx (the generator potential) activates voltage-gated sodium channels (VGSCs) in the terminal axon (Fig. 58.4). VGSCs are responsible for generating the upward phase of the action potential and in sensory neurons can be divided into two types based upon sensitivity to the puffer fish poison tetrodotoxin (TTX), either sensitive (TTXs) or resistant (TTXr) (Gold, 1999). TTXs sodium channels (there are up to six such channels in DRG neurons, most of which are expressed elsewhere in the CNS as well) play a major role in action potential conduction along the axon and are expressed by all sensory neurons. They are inserted into the membrane along unmyelinated axons or selectively at nodes of Ranvier along myelinated axons, mediating fast saltatory conduction (Waxman & Ritchie, 1993) (Fig. 58.5(a), see colour plate section). The TTXr channels, two of which have been cloned (SNS and SNS2) are however, expressed selectively by nociceptors and their electrophysiological properties

are thought to mediate specific functional features of these neurons. For example, TTXr channels have higher activation and inactivation thresholds along with a rapid recovery when compared to TTXs channels, allowing them to remain active during sustained depolarization, a specific feature of nociceptor function (Bevan, 1999). The TTXr channels are likely to contribute both to the generator potential of nociceptors as well as to action potential conduction (Quasthoff et al., 1995).

The threshold of individual transducer proteins in the peripheral nociceptor terminal can be altered by prior activation, as with repetitive peripheral stimuli, an example of activation-dependent plasticity or autosensitization (Woolf & Salter, 2000). Such a lowering of threshold is observed in response to repeated thermal activation of the VR1 receptor producing a drop from 42 °C to about 38 °C and reverses rapidly. Similar thermal threshold changes for the VR1 receptor also occur after capsaicin or proton activation of the receptor. The increased sensitivity may be mediated either by conformational changes or by phos-

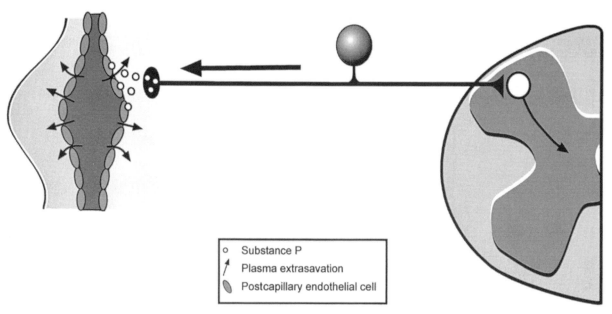

Fig. 58.6. Antidromic conduction of action potentials along nociceptor axons leads to the release of peptides such as CGRP and Substance P into the skin. These molecules bind to receptors on endothelial cells to cause vasodilatation and increase permeability leading to plasma extrasavation. This is known as neurogenic inflammation.

phorylation following calcium entry through the channel, which will activate intracellular kinases.

The selective expression of nociceptor-specific molecules such as VR1 has been exploited by clinicians for treatment targeted at the nociceptor. Topical capsaicin cream has been used to treat postherpetic neuralgia and painful diabetic neuropathy. Initially it results in nociceptor activation (through activation of the VR1 receptor), producing a burning sensation. However, with repeated application over days, the heightened pain is followed by a reduction in sensitivity, a consequence of nociceptor peripheral terminal degeneration that lasts for approximately 4–6 weeks and is thought to be due to prolonged calcium influx (Simone et al., 1998).

Local anesthetic nerve block produces a more rapid and reversible method of blocking primary nociceptor input, but sodium channel blockers such as lignocaine or bupivicaine are both non-selective (motor, sympathetic and proprioceptive sensory axons are also blocked) and limited by their cardiac and central nervous system side effects (they block all sodium channels in a use-dependent fashion). The recent identification of sensory neuron specific sodium channels offers the possibility for the development of highly selective nociceptor blockers/antagonists that will avoid unwanted side effects.

In addition to orthodromic action potentials moving from the peripheral terminal towards the spinal cord, C-

fibres can conduct action potentials antidromically, i.e. from the spinal cord towards the periphery. This is important in producing neurogenic inflammation, where antidromic C-fibre activation causes the release of CGRP and SP from the peripheral terminals, acting on postcapillary venules to produce peripheral vasodilatation and increased capillary permeability respectively (Fig. 58.6). The exact role of neurogenic inflammation is controversial but it has been implicated in pain states, such as migraine, asthma, and arthritis as well as wound healing (Raja et al., 1999). It has also been suggested as a potential mechanism for the trophic skin and nail changes in Reflex Sympathetic Dystrophy (RSD)/Causalgia (Complex Regional Pain Syndrome type II) (Devor & Seltzer, 1999). It is not clear how this antidromic activation occurs; one possibility is that the central terminals of C-afferent fibres are depolarized by presynaptic axo-axonic synapses in the spinal cord, as part of presynaptic inhibition, and this can cause a backfiring of action potentials. Antidromic action potentials also occur as part of the axon reflex producing the flare response (Simone et al., 1998). This process is almost entirely absent in animals with a null mutation in genes for either Substance P or its receptor NK1, suggesting that this is a Substance P mediated phenonemon amenable to treatment with newly developed highly selective tachykinin antagonists (Woolf et al., 1998).

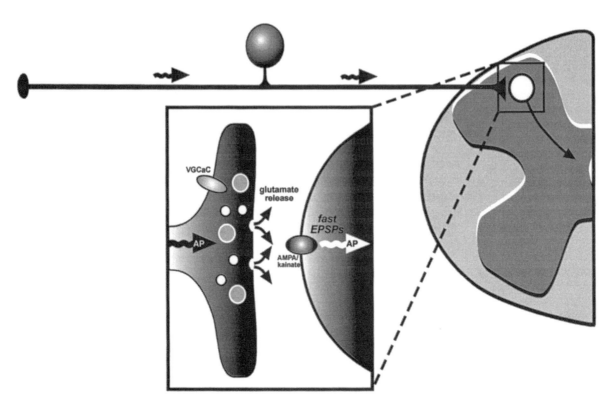

Fig. 58.7. Nociceptor activation leads to the release of glutamate, from primary afferent axon central terminals, that binds postsynaptically to AMPA receptors. If stimulus intensity is sufficient, action potential activation threshold is reached and the spinal projection neuron fires.

Activation of central pain pathways

Primary nociceptor activation leads to the propagation of action potentials to the spinal cord (the frequency of which codes for the intensity of the stimulus (Raja et al., 1999), where they invade central presynaptic terminals to elicit neurotransmitter release. Expressed upon the presynaptic terminal membrane are many different receptors for neurotransmitters/modulators whose activation (both as autoreceptors and from axo-axonic synapses) can alter intracellular calcium levels and the degree of transmitter release from the terminal, e.g. excitatory receptors such as the ionotropic glutamate receptors AMPA, kainate and NMDA, the metabotropic glutamate receptor mGluR, the NK1, P2X3, α_2-adrenoreceptors, 5-HT receptors, ACh_N receptors, EP (prostaglandin) receptors, and receptors which inhibit transmitter release, particularly those for GABA, adenosine and the opioids. A reduction in transmitter release is one of the major mechanisms underlying the analgesic actions of opioids.

Terminals of nociceptor neurons contain two types of synaptic vesicle, small clear glutaminergic vesicles, and large dense-core peptidergic vesicles (containing SP,

BDNF, CGRP, etc). Terminal depolarization, with the influx of calcium through high threshold voltage dependent channels (e.g. N-type) results in the fusion of vesicles with the pre-synaptic membrane and the release of transmitters into the synaptic cleft. N-type calcium channels are inhibited by Ω-conopeptides which reduce inflammatory and neuropathic-related allodynia and hyperalgesia without affecting normal nociceptive responses (Vanegas & Schaible, 2000). The Ω-conopeptides have, however, a narrow therapeutic index and are associated with significant motor and sympatholytic side effects which limit their clinical use.

Following brief, noxious stimulation, spinal nociceptive transmission is mediated mainly, if not exclusively by glutamate released from small clear vesicles acting on AMPA and kainate receptors on postsynaptic dorsal horn neurons to produce fast excitatory post-synaptic potentials (EPSPs) (Yoshimura & Jessell, 1990). Much of this postsynaptic activity is subthreshold, but if stimulus intensity is sufficient, action potentials are generated and the spinal neuron fires at a discharge frequency that is linearly related to stimulus intensity (Fig. 58.7). It is this activity that signals the onset, intensity, and duration of transient

Inputs

Outputs

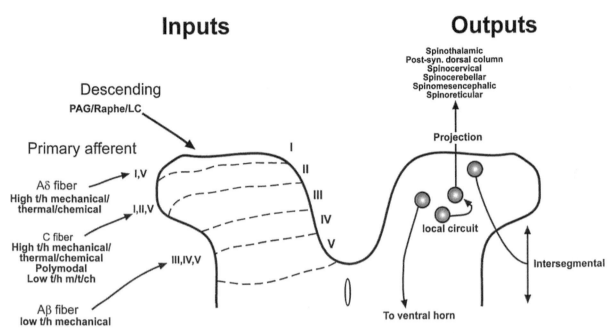

Fig. 58.8. A schematic diagram showing the major sources of inputs into and outputs from the dorsal horn.

noxious stimuli. Spinal neurons are a heterogeneous population often divided into those responding with an action potential output in response only to nociceptor input (nocispecific cells) situated predominantly within superficial regions of the dorsal horn, or those responding to C-, Aδ- and Aβ-fibre inputs, the non-nocispecific (also known as wide dynamic range) cells typically situated in deeper dorsal horn laminae. The electrophysiological properties of dorsal horn neurons are not fixed, however, and change dramatically under different situations such as after a sustained noxious stimulus, after nerve injury or in response to altered descending modulatory inputs. A nocispecific cell may, following a prolonged C-fibre input that induces increased membrane excitability and the recruitment of previously sub-threshold (e.g. Aβ) inputs, become a non-nociceptive specific cell. Similarly, a non-nociceptive cell may become unresponsive to Aβ input if descending modulatory inhibitory inputs increase following electrical stimulation of brain stem nuclei or pharmacologically with morphine (Fields & Basbaum, 1999).

Most neurons in the superficial dorsal horn that project to the thalamus via the spinothalamic tract express the NK1 (Substance P) receptor (Nichols et al., 1999). Neurons that project axons to the brain through the dorsal columns are implicated in visceral pain transmission. Some propriospinal neurons project a few segments along the spinal cord, allowing for the polysynaptic transfer of sensory input to the brain, a pathway implicated in somatosympa-

thetic reflexes, and others project locally/segmentally, forming local excitatory and inhibitory networks (Fig. 58.8). Thus, although the anterolateral spinothalamic tract is sometimes referred to as the 'pain pathway', there actually exist multiple pathways by which primary nociceptor inputs are transferred to the brain. This is seen in patients suffering from chronic pain who, having been rendered 'analgesic' by an anterolateral cordotomy, commonly have their pain return after a period of months (Tasker, 1990). A 'twenty-first century' update of surgical anterolateral cordotomy, recently tested in animals, uses intrathecal infusion of a toxin conjugated to substance P. The substance P toxin conjugate, on binding to NK1 receptors on lamina I spinothalamic tract neurons, and following internalization, selectively kills only these cells (Nichols et al., 1999).

High frequency nociceptor activation following intense or prolonged noxious stimuli leads to the co-release, with glutamate, of neuromodulators such as SP, CGRP and BDNF, possibly controlled by intracellular calcium concentrations (Cao et al., 1998). The corelease of peptides/proteins results in the production of slow synaptic potentials due to activation of ionotropic (AMPA/kainate) and metabotropic (e.g. mGluR, NK1) receptors as well as the NMDA receptor (which at resting membrane potential is blocked by magnesium but opens during depolarization). These slow potentials last for seconds to minutes and have the potential to summate temporally, such that a repetitive noxious stimulation at >0.5 Hz produces a progressively greater postsynaptic response (a cumulative depolarization), which is further augmented by the activation of postsynaptic voltage dependent calcium-activated cation channels. The increased action potential discharge that results is known as wind-up and is an example of spinal autosensitization and represents a short-lasting mechanism for boosting pain transmission. Psychophysical correlates of wind-up can be shown in humans both after repeated heat stimuli and in patients suffering from neuropathic pain (Arendt-Neilsen et al., 1995).

Modulation: reversible alterations in pain processing

The hypersensitivity that accompanies peripheral inflammatory disease or nervous system lesions arises as a consequence of alterations in sensory processing. These alterations can be divided into two mechanistic categories: modulation, a reversible alteration in primary and secondary nociceptor function, brought about by post-translational changes in specific signalling molecules (e.g. through phosphorylation) and modification, longer-term potentially irreversible changes in signalling within the sensory system, involving altered gene expression, neuronal and non-neuronal cell death and the structural reorganization of peripheral terminals and of interneuronal connectivity in the spinal cord (Woolf & Salter, 2000).

Modulating the sensitivity of primary nociceptors

The threshold at which nociceptors are activated determines basal pain sensitivity, the point at which neural activation may lead to the sensation of pain. Inflammatory pain is associated with an increase in nociceptor terminal membrane excitability, increasing basal sensitivity by reducing the activation threshold (enabling normally innocuous inputs to activate the terminal) and increasing suprathreshold responses of the nociceptor terminal to noxious stimuli (peripheral sensitization). This phenomenon accounts for the hypersensitivity to chemical and thermal stimuli at the site of tissue damage in inflammatory pain, but less so for mechanical hypersensitivity, which is largely a central phenomenon.

Peripheral sensitization occurs as a consequence of the local action of inflammatory mediators on the nociceptor terminal. Tissue injury results in the release of ATP and protons from damaged cells, 5-HT and histamine from mast cells, cytokines like TNF and IL-1 from macrophages, prostaglandins, bradykinin and growth factors

like NGF and LIF (Woolf & Costigan, 1999) (Fig. 58.9). Some of these mediators (ATP, bradykinin) can directly activate the terminal eliciting pain, others (NGF, PGE_2) do not activate the terminal but sensitize it. The low levels of NGF produced normally in the target tissue maintain normal basal sensitivity to thermal stimuli (Bennett et al., 1998), but increased NGF increases pain sensitivity (Lewin & Mendell, 1993), which has limited its use as replacement therapy for neuropathies in humans. NGF does not directly depolarize the terminal but sensitizes it, on activation of its tyrosine kinase TrkA receptor, to subsequent thermal and chemical input, both through a short latency (seconds) effect on the VR1 receptor (Shu & Mendell, 1999) as well as slower onset changes (>6 hours) in the level of gene expression in the DRG following retrograde transport of the internalized NGF-TrkA complex to the cell body.

Other peripheral sensitizing agents include prostaglandins particularly PGE_2, 5-HT and adenosine, which activate protein kinase A (PKA), and noradrenaline and bradykinin, which activate PKC (Woolf & Costigan, 1999). The predominant mechanism responsible for peripheral sensitization is phosphorylation of membrane bound receptors and ion channels in the peripheral terminal by the kinases PKC and PKA. Activation of PKC results, for example, in phosphorylation of the TTXr sodium channel SNS/PN3, enhancing nociceptor excitability by increasing the inward current produced by any depolarizing stimulus (Gold, 1999). A similar phosphorylation of the VR1 receptor is likely. Although many PKC isoforms are expressed by primary nociceptors, the PKC' isoform plays a pivotal role in bradykinin (BK), noradrenaline and heat-induced hypersensitivity without involvement in normal nociceptor activation (Cesare et al., 1999).

The molecules that contribute to the generation of this modulation of nociceptor terminal excitability represent potential targets for the development of antihypersensitivity/analgesic treatments for inflammatory pain which could be aimed at reducing the build up or action of inflammatory mediators (IL-1 / $TNF\alpha$ neutralizing antibodies or fusion proteins, NSAIDs, bradykinin antagonists, NGF antibodies/fusion proteins) or kinase inhibitors that block the phosphorylation of nociceptor signalling molecules. The use of cyclo-oxygenase (COX) inhibitors to treat inflammation by reducing prostaglandin synthesis is central to the current management of conditions like rheumatoid arthritis and the introduction of highly selective COX-2 inhibitors (the inducible cyclo-oxygenase isoform) designed to avoid the gastrointestinal and other side effects of COX-1 inhibitors (the constitutive isoform) has been a major advance.

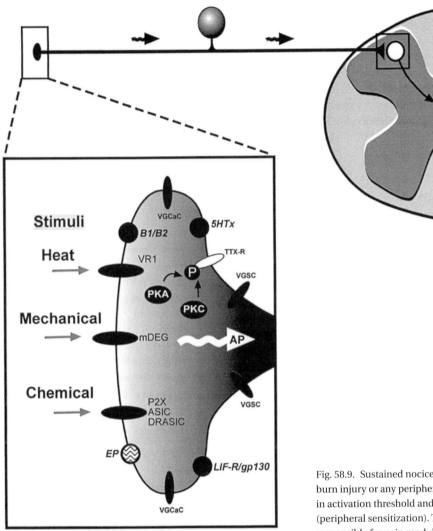

Peripheral sensitization: reduced nociceptor activation threshold

Fig. 58.9. Sustained nociceptor activation such as following a burn injury or any peripheral inflammation leads to a reduction in activation threshold and thereby to pain hypersensitivity (peripheral sensitization). The predominant mechanism responsible for pain modulation in primary nociceptors is activation of kinases in the terminal by sensitizing agents such as PGE2, leading to phosphorylation of ion channels, altering their functional properties.

Peripheral sensitization predominantly contributes to local hypersensitivity where there is local inflammation. In some patients with nerve lesions, however, an increased nociceptor terminal excitability has been detected clinically, particularly in a subgroup of patients with postherpetic neuralgia who can be identified by a reduction in thermal pain threshold at the site of their lesions (Fields et al., 1998). This has led to the recent development of lignocaine patches that can be applied directly to painful areas, limiting systemic action, and these have been used to treat that subtype of postherpetic neuralgia where 'irritable (overactive) nociceptors' are implicated (Fields et al., 1999).

Modulating central pain pathways:

If the intensity/duration of nociceptor input to the spinal cord increases beyond a critical threshold, in addition to the direct fast activation of the dorsal horn neurons during the input, a long-lasting facilitation of sensory transmission occurs in the spinal cord, which is known as central sensitization (Woolf, 1983). Central sensitization manifests as a reduction in the threshold of activation of the dorsal horn neurons, an increase in their receptive field size and an increased response to suprathreshold inputs and is due to a maintained increase in synaptic efficacy. This contributes, with peripheral sensitization, to primary hyperalgesia but is exclusively responsible for the abnormal sensitivity to noxious and innocuous inputs to uninjured tissue adjacent to the site of injury, such as the production of pain on activation of low threshold Aβ fibres (tactile allodynia) and Aδ fibre mediated pin-prick hyperalgesia. In common with peripheral sensitization, this form of central modulation occurs as a consequence of the activation of specific intracellular signal transduction molecules that post-translationally modify receptors and ion channels, but in this case, on the postsynaptic membrane of dorsal horn neurons. This post-translational processing increases membrane excitability such that the stimulus–response relationship of the neuron is augmented, increasing the spinal response to both innocuous and noxious inputs.

The AMPA and NMDA glutamate receptors expressed on dorsal horn neurons are crucial to this functional synaptic plasticity, which may occur either at the activated synapse (homosynaptic facilitation) or spread to neighbouring synapses (heterosynaptic facilitation). Homosynaptic facilitation of spinal AMPA receptor-mediated responses to nociceptor inputs is thought to occur via a mechanism similar to long-term potentiation in CA1 hippocampal neurons. Brief high frequency (100 Hz) inputs lead to the summation of fast AMPA-mediated EPSPs that release the NMDA receptor magnesium block, increasing channel opening and intracellular calcium levels postsynaptically. Calcium-activated kinases, e.g. calcium/calmodulin dependent kinase II (CaMKII) or PKC can then phosphorylate the AMPA receptor on serine or threonine residues increasing AMPA mediated postsynaptic activity for a long period. These changes contribute to the facilitation of responses to subsequent inputs in the same nociceptors that initiated this form of synaptic plasticity. Heterosynaptic facilitation, in contrast, is initiated by much lower stimulation frequencies (1 Hz) in nociceptors and causes a spatially dispersed synaptic enhancement in dorsal horn neurons. This NMDA receptor-mediated increase in membrane excitability leads to the augmentation of the response to subsequent Aβ, Aδ and C-fibre inputs, the first of which leads to tactile allodynia, a major feature of inflammatory and neuropathic pain. This form of NMDA-mediated functional enhancement is the consequence of NK1, mGluR and TrkB receptor activation, secondary to the release from C-fibre terminals of substance P, glutamate and BDNF, followed by convergent activation of second messenger kinases (such as PKCγ) that in turn phosphorylate an intracellular tyrosine kinase src. Src when activated phosphorylates the NMDA receptor on tyrosine residues modifying its channel kinetics and

voltage-dependent characteristics, increasing membrane excitability. Other postsynaptic kinase signalling cascades have also been implicated in central sensitization such as the mitogen-activated protein kinase (MAPK), whose activity is induced in the superficial dorsal horn by nociceptor activity and whose pharmacological inhibition reduces central sensitization experimentally (Ji et al., 1999). Not all the substrates of these kinases have been identified, nor have all the phosphatases involved in regulating their activity. Nitric oxide (NO) generated in dorsal horn neurons following calcium entry is also believed to facilitate NMDA-mediated central sensitization through a positive feedback onto the presynaptic membrane enhancing further transmitter release (Fig. 58.10).

Central sensitization represents a major area for potential new analgesics, ones that could be targeted presynaptically to block neuromodulator release, or postsynaptically to block receptor activation or inhibit intracellular kinases. Since the NMDA receptor is downstream of most of the signalling activity that leads to central sensitization, NMDA receptor antagonists may also have a major role as antihypersensitivity agents. NMDA receptor antagonists, such as ketamine or dextromethorphan, have been found to reduce hypersensitivity in patients with inflammatory and neuropathic pain, but their use is limited by psychotropic side effects due to the widespread distribution of these receptors. Antagonists for the glycine site on the NMDA receptor or those directed at the NR2a NMDA receptor subunit may have a greater therapeutic index and could make a major contribution to normalizing centrally generated pain hypersensitivity.

Central sensitization has been shown to contribute to the generation of both postsurgical and neuropathic pain hypersensitivity (Dahl et al., 1992; Stubhaug et al., 1997; Koltzenburg, 1998). Recently, both peripheral and central sensitization have also been implicated in the pathogenesis of migraine. Early on, pain and associated hypersensitivity in migraine is lateralized on the head, often around or above the orbit, a feature thought to be mediated by peripherally sensitized primary nociceptors (Strassmann et al., 1996). Within hours, hypersensitivity spreads over a much wider area and this has been correlated with the induction of central sensitization within brainstem (Burstein et al., 2000). Treatment early in attack should be targeted, therefore, at preventing/reducing peripheral sensitization, which will then prevent the establishment of central sensitization. If an attack is not aborted early, treatment will have to be targeted at the established central sensitization.

An area where targeting central sensitization contributes to clinical management is use of pre-emptive anal-

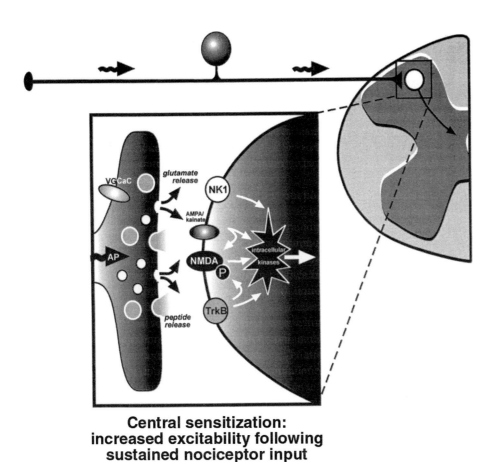

**Central sensitization:
increased excitability following
sustained nociceptor input**

Fig. 58.10. Prolonged nociceptor input to the spinal cord leads to a use-dependent increase in neuronal membrane excitability that long outlasts the duration of the stimulus. A key molecule in this process, known as central sensitization, is the NMDA glutamate receptor. Other receptors such as the substance P receptor NK1 and the BDNF receptor TrkB are involved by means of activating many postsynaptic kinases, which then act to phosphorylate the NMDA and other receptor/ion channels.

gesia to reduce postoperative pain. The rationale is that by blocking C-fibre input to, or action on, the spinal cord before a surgical incision is made, the dorsal horn will remain in a state of normosensitivity and the patient will require less postoperative analgesia. Although this has been borne out in many carefully designed placebo controlled clinical trials using ketamine, opioids and regional anesthesia, this approach has not yet been fully optimized. One problem is that a sensory input sufficient to drive central sensitization will be generated both intraoperatively by surgically induced activation of nociceptors, and postoperatively by input arising from the injured and inflamed tissue. For this reason pre-emptive treatment administered preoperatively alone is insufficient, it needs to continue into the immediate postoperative period.

Modification: long-lasting alterations in pain processing

In addition to the reversible changes in nociceptor and dorsal horn neurons during peripheral and central sensitization, long-term and potentially irreversible changes can occur in these cells, which can be divided into two types: phenotypic and structural, including degeneration, cell death and sprouting and contribute to altered synaptic input, changes in synaptic connectivity as well as disinhibition.

Phenotypic modifications in the sensory system

Both peripheral inflammation and nerve injury can change the phenotype of primary sensory and dorsal horn neurons. The raised levels of NGF at the site of the inflammation results in an increase in NGF-regulated peptide transmitters expressed by sensory neurons (substance P, CGRP and BDNF). This involves both an increase in those cells which normally express these synaptic neuromodulators, as well as novel expression in sensory neurons which normally do not contain them, such as neurons with myelinated axons, a switch from an A-fibre phenotype to a C-fibre phenotype (see Fig. 58.10). In addition to the retrograde transport of NGF, increased activity in sensory neurons appears to be sufficient to alter transcription (Mannion et al., 1999).

For nerve lesions, the disconnection of the neuronal body from its target cuts off the cell body from target-derived peripheral growth factor signals and introduces the neuron to novel signals (such as local inflammation at the site of injury, molecules produced by denervated Schwann cells and altered activity patterns) all of which can lead to a change in sensory neuron phenotype. Nerve injury results in increased excitability in the injured neurons as a consequence of transcriptionally and post-translationally mediated alterations in voltage gated sodium channel function as well as a reduction in potassium channel expression which may be sufficient to generate ectopic activity leading both to spontaneous burning pain and paresthesias (Waxman & Ritchie, 1993). Injured C-fibre afferents dramatically up-regulate a TTXs sodium channel, Brain III, normally only expressed by sensory neurons at high levels during development. This switch to a phenotype resembling developmental (embryonic) neurons is seen for many molecules including structural growth related proteins like growth associated protein-43 (GAP-43). A-fibre neurons distribute sodium channels differently following nerve injury and no longer are they found solely at Nodes of Ranvier (Waxman & Ritchie, 1993) (Fig. 58.5(b), (c), see colour plate section). In particular, sodium channels accumulate at the site of the neuroma and this alters the activation properties of cells and becomes a site for ectopic discharge, as can be demonstrated by tapping the neuroma site as in the Tinel sign in carpal tunnel syndrome. Peripheral nerve injury also results in the development of increased adrenoreceptivity, either due to increased local catecholamine levels following sympathetic axon sprouting into injured tissue and the DRG or following the up-regulation of α_2-adrenoreceptors by sensory neurons which may contribute to the development of sympathetically maintained pain (Devor & Seltzer, 1999).

Although the phenotypic changes in C-fibres after inflammation and nerve injury tend to be in opposite directions, remarkably, both nerve injury and inflammation induce substance P and BDNF expression *de novo* in those large A-fibre neurons normally involved in signalling low threshold innocuous stimuli (Fig. 58.11). A novel feature of both these clinical pain states is that contrary to the normal situation, where only C-fibre input can induce central sensitization, low threshold fibre stimulation can lead to central sensitization and in consequence a build up of pain hypersensitivity known as progressive tactile hypersensitivity (PTH) (Ma & Woolf, 1996). Apart from an increased synaptic drive by virtue of such phenotypic shifts, peripheral nerve injury also results in reduced inhibition as a result of the down-regulation of opioid receptors on injured primary afferents and this may contribute to the relative decrease in morphine sensitivity frequently found in patients with neuropathic pain.

Dorsal horn neurons also show phenotypic changes including up- and down- regulation of receptors such as NK1, TrkB and GABA-R. Alterations in dorsal horn transmitters also occur including increases in dynorphin, GABA and COX-2. These changes may be the result both of alterations in synaptic input as well as systemic signals from cytokines and they may contribute both to an alteration in responsiveness to primary afferent input as well as modifying intrinsic dorsal horn neuronal function.

Postinjury sensory neuron cell death and central sprouting

During development, primary sensory neurons are dependent for survival upon a limited supply of trophic factors expressed in peripheral targets, with around 50% of neurons undergoing apoptosis, known as programmed cell death. After experimental nerve injury in adult animals, although there are small increases in the number of cells undergoing apoptosis (Groves et al., 1998), there are no significant changes in DRG cell or axon number for up to 4 months (Coggeshall et al., 1996), suggesting that adult sensory neurons are independent of target-derived growth factors for survival. The cell death that does occur is predominantly in C-fibres leaving most A-fibre neurons intact. The degree and timing of cell death associated with other insults such as herpes zoster infection remains controversial (Oaklander, 1999) but there is a marked reduced innervation of the epidermis in many of these patients (Oaklander et al., 1998), which contributes to decreased thermal sensitivity and a loss of histamine-induced flare in such patients, while leaving A-fibre terminals in the dermis intact to signal tactile allodynia.

Although nerve injury does not at early time points result in neuronal cell death, it induces the transganglionic degeneration of C-fibre central terminals within the superficial dorsal horn (Doubell et al., 1999). Shortly after, Aβ-

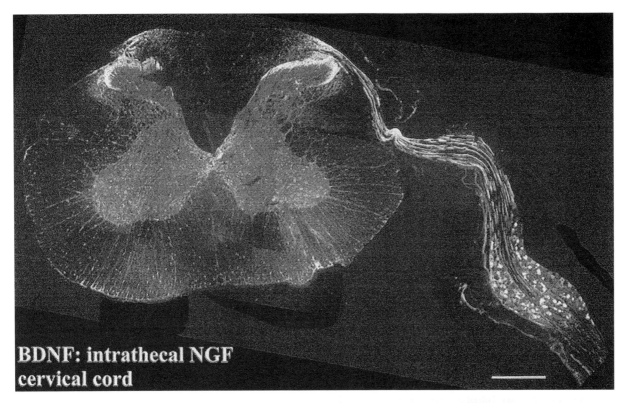

BDNF: intrathecal NGF cervical cord

Fig. 58.11. BDNF is expressed by a subpopulation of sensory neurons in the DRG, predominantly those that express the NGF receptor TrkA. BDNF is synthesized in the cell body and transported centrally into the spinal cord where immunoreactivity can be seen in the superficial laminae of the dorsal horn. Following nerve injury and inflammation and intrathecal NGF administration, BDNF expression is increased and some A-fibres begin to express BDNF. (Printed with permission from Michael et al., 1997.)

fibre collateral central terminals sprout dorsally into superficial regions that normally are innervated specifically by C-fibre neurons (Woolf et al., 1992) (Fig. 58.12, see colour plate section). These sprouted collateral axons make novel synapses with dorsal horn neurons (Woolf et al., 1992; Kohama et al., 2000). Direct monosynaptic input to lamina II may result in the misinterpretation of A-fibre input as C-fibre input, an anatomical substrate for tactile allodynia (Koerber et al., 1999). The spinal A-fibre sprouting in animals is considered a consequence of C-fibre injury (Mannion et al., 1996) possibly as a consequence of peripherally derived growth factor deprivation as suggested by the prevention of the sprouting with intrathecal NGF or BDNF administration (McMahon & Bennett, 1999).

Tonic and phasic central inhibition of sensory transmission, a major part of normal sensory processing, is reduced in superficial laminae following nerve injury as a result of the decreased expression of inhibitory transmitters and receptors and direct cell death of local inhibitory interneurons in this region (Coggeshall et al., 1998; Fig. 58.3(b)). The novel presence of A-fibre terminals in lamina II after nerve

injury may contribute to excitotoxic interneuron death in the superficial dorsal horn, manifesting as progressive disinhibition and worsening neuropathic pain. Such a disinhibition is functionally equivalent to an increase in excitation. In animal models, blocking glycine or GABA receptors locally in the spinal cord produces tactile allodynia. If similar changes occur in patients the issue then is how to prevent/treat this disinhibition. The former may be possible by blocking excitotoxic inhibitory interneuron loss soon after injury with NMDA receptor antagonists, the latter may require administration of GABAergic compounds.

In conclusion, the three functional states of the sensory system: activation, modulation and modification, are distinct but overlapping and will manifest in most patients with chronic pain, to a greater or lesser degree. Thus, successful treatment will never be achieved with single agents which act only on one state. Persistent pain is, therefore, a family of syndromes initiated by diverse etiological factors, the expression of which is a reflection of the activation of diverse neurobiological mechanisms. These syndromes demand a multilayered management strategy targeting not just the mechanisms but also their evolution within the individual. The breakdown of complex symptoms into their cellular and molecular components is expanding our understanding of individual features of pain syndromes as well as identifying new targets to develop rational treatment plans. The key challenges for a rational mechanistically orientated treatment are to be able to identify individual mechanisms within patients using simple, reliable and reproducible clinical tests and to identify specific treatments that have the potential to treat individual mechanisms responsible for hypersensitivity, without the abolition or even reduction of pain normosensitivity. The challenge of conquering pain is enormous and will be difficult but the need is great, as are the opportunities.

References

Arendt-Nielsen, L., Petersen-Felix, S., Fisher, M., Bak, P., Bjerring, P., & Zbinden, A.M. (1995). The effect of NMDA antagonist (ketamine) on single and repeated nociceptive stimuli: a placebo controlled experimental human study. *Anesth. Analg.*, **81**, 63–8.

Bennett, D.L., Koltzenburg, M., Priestley, J.V., Shelton, D.L. & McMahon, S.B. (1998). Endogenous nerve growth factor regulates the sensitivity of nociceptors in the adult rat. *Eur. J. Neurosci.*, **10**(4), 1282–91.

Bevan, S. (1999). Nociceptive peripheral neurons: cellular properties. In *Textbook of Pain*, 4th edn, ed. R. Melzack & P.D. Wall, Edinburgh, UK: Churchill Livingstone.

Bonica, J.J. (1990). Anatomic and physiologic basis of nociception and pain. In *The Management of Pain*, 2nd edn, ed. J.J. Bonica, J.D. Loeser, R. Chapman & R.E. Fordyce, Lea & Febiger.

Cao, Y.Q., Mantyh, P.W., Carlson, E.J., Gillespie, A.M., Epstein, C.J. & Basbaum, A.I. (1998). Primary afferent tachykinins are required to experience moderate to intense pain. *Nature*, **392**, 390–4.

Caterina & Julius, D. (1999). Sense and specificity: a molecular identity for nociceptors. *Curr. Opin. Neurobiol.*, **9**(5), 525–30.

Cesare, P., Dekker, L.V., Sardini, A., Parker, P.J. & McNaughton, P.A. (1999). Specific involvement of PKC-epsilon in sensitization of the neuronal response to painful heat. *Neuron*, **23**(3), 617–24.

Coggeshall, R.E., Jennings, E.A. & Fitzgerald, M. (1996). Evidence that large myelinated primary afferent fibres make synaptic contacts in lamina II of neonatal rats. *Dev. Brain Res.*, **92**, 81–90.

Coggeshall, R.E., Woolf, C.J., White, F.A. & Lekan, H.A. (1998). Further studies on dorsal horn neuron loss following large sensory (A) fibre stimulation of transected rat sciatic nerve *Soc. Neurosci. Abstr.*, **25**, 1680.

Dahl, J.B., Erichsen, C.J., Fuglsang-Frederiksen, A. & Kehlet, H.

(1992). Pain sensation and nociceptive reflex excitability in surgical patients and human volunteers. *Br. J. Anaesth.*, **69**(2), 117–21.

Devor, M. & Seltzer, Z. (1999). Pathophysiology of damaged nerves in relation to chronic pain. *The Textbook of Pain*, 4th edn, ed. R. Melzack & P.D. Wall, London: Churchill Livingstone.

Doubell, P., Mannion, R.J. & Woolf, C.J. (1999). The dorsal horn: state dependent sensory processing, plasticity and the generation of pain. In *The Textbook of Pain*, 4th edn, ed. R. Melzack & P.D. Wall. London: Churchill Livingstone.

Fields, H.L. & Basbaum, A.I. (1999). Central nervous system mechanisms of pain modulation. In *Textbook of Pain*, 4th edn, ed. R. Melzack & P.D. Wall. Edinburgh, UK: Churchill Livingstone.

Fields, H.L., Rowbotham, M. & Baron, R. (1998). Postherpetic neuralgia: irritable nociceptors and deafferentation. *Neurobiol. Dis.*, **5**(4), 209–27.

Fields, H.L., Baron, R. & Rowbotham, M.C. (1999). Peripheral neuropathic pain: an approach to management. In *Textbook of Pain*, 4th edn, ed. R. Melzack & P.D. Wall. Edinburgh, UK: Churchill Livingstone.

Gold, M.S. (1999). Tetrodotoxin-resistant Na^+ currents and inflammatory hyperalgesia. *Proc. Natl. Acad. Sci., USA*, **96**, 7645–9.

Groves, M.J., Christopherson, T., Giometto, B. & Scaravilli, F. (1997). Axotomy-induced apoptosis in adult rat primary sensory neurons. *J. Neurocytol.*, **26**(9), 615–24.

Indo, Y., Tsuruta, M. & Hayashida, Y. (1996). Mutations in the TrkA/NGF receptor gene in patients with congenital insensitivity to pain with anhydrosis. *Nat. Genet*, 13, 485–8.

Ji, R.R., Brenner, G., Schmoll, R., Baba, H. & Woolf, C.J. (1999). Phosphorylation of ERK and CREB in nociceptive neurons after noxious stimulation. In *Proceedings of the 9th World Congress on Pain*, ed. M. Devor, M.C. Rowbotham & Z. Wiesenfeld-Hallin Seattle: IASP Press.

Koerber, H.R., Mirnics, K. & Kavookjian, A.M. & Light, A.R. (1999). Ultrastructural analysis of ectopic synaptic boutons arising from peripherally regenerated primary afferent fibres. *J. Neurophysiol.*, **81**(4), 1636–44.

Kohama, I., Ishikawa, K., Kocsis, J.D. (2000). Synaptic reorganization in the substantia gelatinosa after peripheral nerve neuroma formation: aberrant innervation of lamina II neurons by A-beta afferents. *J. Neurosci.*, **20**(4), 1538–49.

Koltzenburg, M. (1998). Painful neuropathies. *Curr. Opin. Neurol.*, **11**(5), 515–21.

Lawson, S.N. (1979). The postnatal development of large light and small dark neurons in mouse dorsal root ganglia: a statistical analysis of cell numbers and size. *J. Neurocytol.*, **8**(3), 275–94.

Lewin, G.R. & Mendell, L.M. (1993). Nerve growth factor and nociception. *Trends Neurosci.*, **16**(9), 353–9.

Lewin, G.R. & Stucky, C. (2000). Sensory neuron mechanotransduction: regulation and underlying molecular mechanisms. In *Molecular Basis of Pain Induction*, ed. J.N. Wood. New York: Wiley Liss.

McMahon, S.B. & Bennett, D.L.H. (1999). Trophic factors and pain. In *Textbook of Pain*, 4th edn, ed. R. Melzack & P.D. Wall. Edinburgh, UK: Churchill Livingstone.

McMahon, S.B. & Koltzenburg, M. (1990). Novel classes of nociceptors: beyond Sherrington. *Trends Neurosci.*, **13**(6), 199–201.

Ma, Q.P. & Woolf, C.J. (1996). Progressive tactile hypersensitivity: an inflammation-induced incremental increase in the excitability of the spinal cord. *Pain*, **67**(1), 97–106.

Mannion, R.J., Doubell, T.P., Coggeshall, R.E. & Woolf, C.J. (1996). Collateral sprouting of uninjured primary afferent A-fibers into the superficial dorsal horn of the adult rat spinal cord after topical capsaicin treatment to the sciatic nerve. *J. Neurosci.*, **15**, 16(16), 5189–95.

Mannion, R.J., Costigan, M., Decosterd, I. et al. (1999). Neurotrophins: peripherally and centrally acting modulators of tactile stimulus-induced inflammatory pain hypersensitivity. *Proc. Natl. Acad. Sci. USA*, **96**, 9385–90.

Melzack, R. & Wall, P.D. (1965). Pain mechanisms: a new theory. *Science*, **286**, 1558–61.

Michael, G.J., Averill, S., Nitkunan, A. et al. (1997). Nerve growth factor treatment increases brain-derived neurotrophic factor selectively in TrkA-expressing dorsal root ganglion cells and in their central terminations within the spinal cord. *J. Neurosci.*, **17**(21), 8476–90.

Miura, Y., Mardy, S., Awaya, Y. et al. (2000). Mutation and polymorphism analysis of the TRKA (NTRK1) gene encoding a high-affinity receptor for nerve growth factor in congenital insensitivity to pain with anhidrosis (CIPA) families. *Hum. Genet.*, **106**(1), 116–24.

Nichols, M.L., Allen, B.J., Rogers, S.D. et al. (1999). Transmission of chronic nociception by spinal neurons expressing the substance P receptor. *Science*, **286**(5444), 1558–61.

Oaklander, A.L., Romans, K., Horasek, S., Stocks, A., Hauer, P. & Meyer, R.A. (1998). Unilateral postherpetic neuralgia is associated with bilateral sensory neuron damage. *Ann. Neurol.*, **44**(5), 789–95.

Oaklander, A.L. (1999). The pathology of shingles: Head and Campbell's 1900 monograph. *Arch. Neurol.*, **56**(10), 1292–4.

Quasthoff, S., Grosskreutz, J., Schroder, J.M., Schneider, U. & Grafe, P. (1995). Calcium potentials and tetrodotoxin-resistant sodium potentials in unmyelinated C fibres of biopsied human sural nerve. *Neuroscience*, **69**(3), 955–65.

Raja, S.N., Meyer, R.A., Ringkamp, M. & Campbell, J.N. (1999). Peripheral neural mechanisms of nociception. In *Textbook of Pain*, 4th edn, ed. R. Melzack & P.D. Wall. Edinburgh: Churchill Livingstone.

Shu, X.Q. & Mendell, L.M. (1999). Neurotrophins and hyperalgesia. *Proc. Natl. Acad. Sci.*, **96**(14), 7693–6.

Simone, D.A., Nolano, M., Johnson, T., Wendelschafer-Crabb, G. & Kennedy, W.R. (1998). Intradermal injection of capsaicin in humans produces degeneration and subsequent reinnervation of epidermal nerve fibres: correlation with sensory function. *J. Neurosci.*, **18**(21), 8947–59.

Snider, W.D. & McMahon, S.B. (1998). Tackling pain at the source: new ideas about nociceptors. *Neuron*, **20**(4), 629–32.

Strassman, A.M., Raymond, S.A. & Burstein, R. (1996). Sensitization of meningeal sensory neurons and the origin of headaches. *Nature*, **384**(6609), 560–4.

Stubhaug, A., Breivik, H., Eide, P.K., Kreunen, M. & Foss, A. (1997). Mapping of punctuate hyperalgesia around a surgical incision demonstrates that ketamine is a powerful suppresser of central sensitization to pain following surgery. *Acta Anaesthesiol. Scand.*, **41**(9), 1124–32.

Tasker, R.R. (1990). Pain resulting from central nervous system pathology (central pain). In *The Management of Pain*, 2nd edn, Eds J.J. Bonica, J.D. Loeser, R. Chapman & R.E. Fordyce. New York: Lea & Febiger.

Vanegas, H. & Schaible, H. (2000). Effects of antagonists to high-threshold calcium channels upon spinal mechanisms of pain, hyperalgesia and allodynia. *Pain*, **85**(1–2), 9–18.

Waxman, S.G. & Ritchie, J.M. (1993). Molecular dissection of the myelinated axon. *Ann. Neurol.*, **33**(2), 121–36.

Willis, W.D. & Coggeshall, R.E. (1991). *Sensory Mechanisms of the Spinal Cord*. New York: Plenum press.

Wood, J.N., Akopian, A., Cesare, P., Din, Y. et al. (1999). The primary nociceptor: special functions, special receptors. In *Proceedings of the 9th World Congress on Pain*, ed. M. Devor, M.C. Rowbotham & Z. Wiesenfeld-Hallin. Seattle: IASP Press.

Woolf, C.J. (1983). Evidence for a central component of post-injury pain hypersensitivity. *Nature*, **306**(5944), 686–8.

Woolf, C.J. (1994). The dorsal horn. *The Textbook of Pain*, 3rd edn, ed. R. Melzack & P.D. Wall. London: Churchill Livingstone.

Woolf, C.J. & Costigan, M. (1999). Transcriptional and posttranslational plasticity and the generation of inflammatory pain. *Proc. Natl. Acad. Sci., USA*, **96**(14), 7723–30.

Woolf, C.J. & Salter, M. (2000). Neuronal plasticity: increasing the gain in pain. *Science*, **288**(5472), 1765–9.

Woolf, C.J., Shortland, P. & Coggeshall, R.E. (1992). Peripheral nerve injury triggers central sprouting of myelinated afferents. *Nature*, **355**(6355), 75–8.

Woolf, C.J., Mannion, R.J. & Neumann, S. (1998). Null mutations lacking substance: elucidating pain mechanisms by genetic pharmacology. *Neuron*, **20**(6), 1063–6.

Yoshimura, M. & Jessell, T. (1990). Amino acid-mediated EPSPs at primary afferent synapses with substantia gelatinosa neurones in the rat spinal cord. *J. Physiol.*, **430**, 315–35.

59

Central nervous system mechanisms of pain

Frederick A. Lenz[1], Patrick M. Dougherty[2] and Joel D. Greenspan[3]

[1]Department of Neurosurgery, Johns Hopkins University, Baltimore, MD, USA
[2]Department of Anesthesiology, M.D. Anderson Hospital, Houston TX, USA, and
[3]Department of OCBS, Dental School, University of Maryland, Baltimore, MD, USA

Chronic pain is an immense unsolved clinical problem. Current approaches to this condition are limited by uncertainty about mechanisms of acute and chronic pain in man. Although much progress has been made toward understanding peripheral neural mechanisms of human nociception (Willis, 1985; Price & Dubner, 1977), we have a poor understanding of CNS pain mechanisms. Spinal mechanisms of pain processing are the subject of the previous chapter. The purpose of the present chapter is to review the anatomy and physiology of the ascending spinal pathways and supraspinal centres with pain-related activity. This chapter will focus on the primate nervous systems since there are significant differences between pain transmission in primates and other species such as cats and rats.

It is widely recognized that there are different components to the pain sensation (Melzack & Casey, 1968; Casey, 1978). The sensory–discriminative aspect of pain refers to the intensity of the sensory experience of pain. The motivational–affective aspect of pain refers to the unpleasantness of the pain and how likely it is that the pain will motivate the organism to escape the pain. Throughout this chapter we will refer to these different components of the pain sensation.

Ascending spinal pathways

The two main output somatosensory tracts from the spinal cord are the anterior–lateral and the dorsal column spinal systems. The anterior–lateral system terminates in the brainstem and thalamus while the dorsal column system terminates in the dorsal column nuclei (Willis, 1985).

The anterior–lateral spinal column

Anatomy

The cell bodies of origin for the anterior–lateral system are found in the spinal dorsal horn, particularly in lamina I, outer layers of lamina II and in laminae III to V; though some cells are also found in laminae VI to IX (Willis, 1985; Willis & Coggeshall, 1991). The spinal pathway from the spinal cord to the thalamus, the spinothalamic tract (STT) is partly located in the anterior lateral column. The STT system consists of two tracts, one positioned in the ventral lateral and the other in the dorsal lateral spinal funiculus (Cusick et al., 1989; Apkarian & Hodge, 1989b; Craig, 1997; Ralston & Ralston, 1992) and most commonly referred to as the 'ventral' and 'dorsal' STTs, respectively (Ralston & Ralston, 1992; Zhang et al., 2000). The axons of cells in the deeper spinal laminae project via the ventral tract while those from more superficial laminae project in the dorsal STT (Apkarian & Hodge, 1989a,b).

Axons and axon collaterals of the spinal projection neurons that ascend in the ventro-lateral spinal quadrant terminate in a number of nuclei of the medulla, midbrain and diencephalon (Mehler, 1962; Mehler et al., 1960). These include in ascending order, the medullary reticular formation (via the spino-reticular tract) (Kevetter et al., 1982; Menetrey et al., 1982), the mesencephalic periaqueductal grey and neighbouring area (spino-mesencephalic tract) (Bjorkeland & Boivie, 1984; Mehler et al., 1960; Menetrey et al., 1982), the parabrachial nucleus (spino-parabrachial tract) (Saper, 1995; Saper & Loewy, 1980; Slugg & Light, 1994), and the hypothalamus (spino-hypothalamic tract) (Burstein et al., 1987, 1990).

Anterior–lateral spinal columns

Physiology

Neuronal responses

Both non-nociceptive and nociceptive spinoreticular (Blair et al., 1984; Fields et al., 1977; Haber et al., 1982), spinome-sencephalic (Hylden et al., 1986; Yezierski & Schwartz, 1986; Yezierski et al., 1987), spinohypothalamic (Burstein et al., 1991; Katter et al., 1996), spino-parabrachial (Bernard & Besson, 1990), and spinothalamic (Craig & Hunsley, 1991; Palecek et al., 1992a, b; Surmeier et al., 1988), neurons have been demonstrated in many animal species. The non-nociceptive projection cells are termed low-threshold or LT neurons. These are an infrequently observed cell group, usually comprising no more than about 10% of dorsal horn neurons (Dougherty et al., 1993, 1998, 1999). The two types of nociceptive spinal projection neurons identified in the spinal cord include wide dynamic range (WDR) and nociceptive specific (NS) neurons. WDR cells are the most frequently encountered cell group, comprising about 70% of the cells sampled in the dorsal horn. WDR cells are especially concentrated in the deeper laminae of the dorsal horn (III to V) where they receive input from both low-threshold and nociceptive afferent fibres and hence are activated by both innocuous and noxious stimuli. However, the responses of WDR cells to these stimuli are graded so that the noxious stimuli evoke a greater response than non-noxious stimuli. It has been suggested that these properties of WDR neurons account for the discrimination of noxious from non-noxious stimuli (Bushnell et al., 1984; Dubner et al., 1989; Maixner et al., 1989) (the sensory-discriminative aspect of pain). In contrast to WDR cells, NS projection cells respond only to noxious stimuli under physiological conditions. The majority of NS cells are found in the superficial laminae of the dorsal horn (I and outer II).

The dorsal spinal column system

Anatomy

The second set of somatosensory inputs to the brainstem include those primary afferent fibres which ascend in the dorsal (posterior) columns of the spinal cord to form their first synapse at the dorsal column nuclei. In addition, there is input to the dorsal column nuclei from at least two groups of dorsal horn projection neurons, the postsynaptic dorsal column pathway and the spino-cervical tract (Wall & Melzack, 1984; Willis, 1985; Willis & Coggeshall, 1991). Both groups of inputs are organized so that the fibres from the lower extremities are most medial in the nucleus gracilis, and inputs from the upper extremities are most lateral in the nucleus cuneatus. The trunk is represented in a region between these nuclei. Inputs from the most distal body regions are dorsal and the more proximal body regions are ventral. The axons of the second-order cells in the dorsal column nuclei cross the midline and gather into the medial lemniscus on the contralateral side of the brainstem. These fibres then ascend through the brainstem and midbrain toward their site of termination in the ventral posterior lateral (VPL) nucleus of the thalamus.

The dorsal spinal column system

Physiology

The cells of the dorsal column nuclei largely respond to innocuous stimuli alone. The lemniscal system in primates does not appear to encode painful stimuli. The information carried in this path is primarily from hair follicle receptors, pacinian corpuscles, and types I and II slowly adapting receptors (Willis, 1985; Willis & Coggeshall, 1991). In addition, the nucleus cuneatus (but not gracilis) shows responses to muscle afferents (spindles and Golgi tendon organs). However, there are several lines of evidence which suggest a role of the dorsal column nuclei in nociceptive transmission. For example, the dorsal columns might account for the recurrence of pain sensitivity and reference of pain to other regions of the body after lesion of the anterolateral spinal quadrant (Vierck et al., 1990; Vierch, Jr. & Luck, 1979; Nagaro et al., 1993). Neuropathic pains are largely conveyed by myelinated fibre inputs (Campbell et al., 1988), which are the majority of fibres afferent to the dorsal column pathway. In addition, non-myelinated afferents have been shown to project to the dorsal column nuclei (Conti et al., 1990; Fabri & Conti, 1990; Garrett et al., 1992; Patterson et al., 1989, 1990). A small number of nociceptive dorsal column neurons have been reported (Cliffer et al., 1992; Ferrington et al., 1988). Finally, the postsynaptic dorsal column pathway and the spino-cervical tract ascend to the dorsal column nuclei and are often nociceptive (Brown et al., 1983; Brown & Franz, 1969).

Supraspinal nociceptive centres

Brainstem centres

Nociceptive neurons have been shown within the reticular formation (Barbaro et al., 1989; Guilbaud et al., 1973; Haws et al., 1989; Nyquist & Greenhoot, 1974; Villanueva et al., 1990), and the periaqueductal grey (PAG) (Casey, 1971b; Eickhoff et al., 1978). Microstimulation in these nuclei produces a wide spectrum of pain-related responses (Bowsher, 1976; Carstens et al., 1980; Casey, 1971a; Gerhart et al., 1984; Janss et al., 1987; Bandler & Depaulis, 1988; Bandler & Carrive, 1988; Delgado, 1955; Fardin et al., 1984; Lovick, 1993; Nashold, Jr. et al., 1969; Spiegel et al., 1954; Walker, 1938; Wolfle et al., 1971). Electrical or chemical stimulation of the PAG or hypothalamus in animals and humans produces a spectrum of responses from overt nocifensive behaviour and associated cardiopulmonary changes to analgesia. This spectrum of effects in PAG is due to the activation of one of two subdivisions of the PAG, the dorsolateral and ventrolateral columns. Activation of the dorsolateral column of the PAG produces a behavioural response of vocalization, grimacing, attack or escape and a parallel tachycardia and pressor response (Bandler & Shipley, 1994; Lovick, 1993), while activation of the ventrolateral column produces behavioural quiescence, bradycardia and hypotension (Depaulis et al., 1994; Keay et al., 1994). Both of these response profiles have been observed by stimulation within the PAG of humans (Nashold, Jr. et al., 1969; Young, 1989; Young et al., 1985).

Lateral thalamic nuclei

Nociceptive neurons in humans have been observed in the mesencephalon (Amano et al., 1978), hypothalamus (Sano, 1977b; Sano, 1979) and thalamus (Lenz et al., 1993b; Lee et al., 1999). The region of Vc where the majority of cells respond to innocuous cutaneous stimulation is termed the core. Below and behind the core is a less cellular region arbitrarily termed the posterior inferior region in our studies. Receptive field locations for the cells in Vc remain unchanged over distances of several millimetres in the anterior–posterior and dorsoventral directions, but change markedly over similar distances in the mediolateral direction (Lenz et al., 1988). From medial to lateral the sequence of neuronal cutaneous receptive fields progresses from intraoral through face, thumb, fingers (radial to ulnar), and arm to leg. Cells with deep receptive fields are usually located anterior and dorsal in the core but sometime posterior to those with cutaneous receptive fields.

Several lines of evidence demonstrate that the region of Vc is important in human pain-signalling pathways. Studies of patients at autopsy following lesions of the STT show the most dense STT termination in Vc (Mehler, 1962; Mehler, 1966; Bowsher, 1957; Walker, 1943). Additionally,

terminations are observed posterior to Vc in the magnocellular medial geniculate (Mehler, 1962; Mehler, 1969), limitans, and Vc portae nuclei (Mehler, 1966) and inferior to Vc in Vcpc (Mehler, 1966). STT terminations are found in monkey VMpo, posterior to medial Vc, which appears, by immunohistochemistry, to have a human analogue (Craig et al., 1994). It has been suggested that VMpo and the posterior nuclear group are specifically innervated by the dorsal STT (Craig, 1997; Craig et al., 1994), though not all studies have been in agreement (Apkarian & Hodge, 1989a,b; Ralston & Ralston, 1992; Zhang et al., 2000).

The cortical projections of these nuclei in monkeys are as follows: VP (corresponding to human Vc (Hirai & Jones, 1989a)) to primary (S1) and secondary (S2) somatosensory cortices (Jones, 1985; Burton, 1986; Kenshalo, Jr. & Willis, 1991), VPI (corresponding to human Vcpc) to S2 and granular and dysgranular insular cortex (Friedman & Murray, 1986), medial and oral pulvinar (corresponding to human Vcpor) to inferior parietal lobule and outer parietal operculum (7b) plus granular and dysgranular insular cortex (Burton & Jones, 1976; Burton, 1986; Friedman & Murray, 1986), posterior nucleus (as in humans) to retro-, granular and dysgranular insular cortex and S2 (Burton & Jones, 1976; Burton, 1986; Friedman & Murray, 1986), suprageniculate and limitans (as in humans) to granular insular cortex (Burton & Jones, 1976; Burton, 1986) and magnocellular medial geniculate to granular and dysgranular insular cortex (Friedman & Murray, 1986).

Fig. 59.1 shows an example of a cell in Vc with a differential response to painful thermal and mechanical stimuli and with a response to innocuous cool and mechanical stimuli (Lee et al., 1999). Cells in the posterior inferior region have been identified with a significant selective response to noxious heat stimuli (Lenz et al., 1993b) and to cold stimuli (Davis et al., 1999). These reports extend to humans the results of numerous monkey studies in which cells within VP (Casey & Morrow, 1983; Chung et al., 1986; Gautron & Guilbaud, 1982; Apkarian et al., 1991; Casey, 1966; Bushnell et al., 1993; Apkarian & Shi, 1994; Kenshalo et al., 1980; Bushnell & Duncan, 1987) and posterior and inferior to VP respond to noxious stimuli (Apkarian et al., 1991; Casey, 1966; Apkarian & Shi, 1994; Craig et al., 1994).

Cells in the region of Vc that respond to noxious stimuli probably signal pain based on temporary lesioning and stimulation studies. Blockade of the activity in this region by injection of local anesthetic into monkey VP, corresponding to human Vc (Hirai & Jones, 1989a), significantly interferes with the monkey's ability to discriminate temperature in both the innocuous and noxious range (Duncan et al., 1993). Stimulation within Vc and posterior-inferior to it can evoke the sensation of pain (Dostrovsky et al., 1991; Halliday & Logue, 1972; Hassler & Reichert, 1959; Lenz et al., 1993a) and thermal sensations (Lenz et al., 1993a; Davis et al., 1999). Thus, there is strong evidence that the region of Vc is involved in pain signalling pathways: i. it receives input from pain signalling pathways, ii. it contains cells that respond to noxious stimuli, iii. stimulation can evoke pain, and iv. temporary lesioning of monkey VP disables the discrimination of pain and temperature.

Medial and intralaminar thalamic nuclei

In the medial tier of human thalamic nuclei the most dense STT terminal pattern is found in intralaminar nucleus centralis lateralis (Bowsher, 1957; Mehler, 1962; Mehler, 1969) while a much less dense termination is found in other interlaminar nuclei central medial and parafascicularis (Mehler, 1962). These nuclei project to cortex diffusely (Le Gros Clark & Russell, 1940) and to striatum (Oppenheimer, 1967; Vogt & Vogt, 1941). STT terminations are also found in the medial dorsal nucleus (Mehler, 1969) which project to lateral prefrontal cortex (Meyer, 1947; Van Buren & Borke, 1972). An STT projection to human submedius has not been identified although regions of dense neurokinin staining in medial Vcpc (Hirai & Jones, 1989b) may correspond to monkey nucleus submedius (Burton & Craig, Jr., 1983). The nuclear pattern of STT terminations and projection patterns of these nuclei in humans is similar to that demonstrated in more precise anatomic studies in monkeys.

In monkeys, dense STT terminations are observed in central lateral (Mehler et al., 1960; Boivie, 1979; Mantyh, 1983; Berkley, 1980), while a light projection is found in central medial and parafascicularis (Mehler et al., 1960; Burton & Craig, Jr., 1983; Berkley, 1980; Apkarian & Hodge, 1989c; Kerr, 1975). These intralaminar nuclei project to caudate and putamen (Sadikot et al., 1990; Smith & Parent, 1986; Nakano et al., 1990; Kalil, 1978; Sadikot et al., 1992a,b) and diffusely to cortex (Macchi & Bentivoglio, 1986; Strick, 1975; Powell & Cowan, 1967). STT terminations are also found in monkey submedius (Apkarian & Hodge, 1989c), particularly the dorsal (Craig & Burton, 1981) and rostral (Mantyh, 1983; Craig, 1990) portion. The cortical projections of submedius have not been reported in monkey although projections to deep presylvian sulcus have been reported in cats (Craig et al., 1982). The medial dorsal nucleus receives STT input (Apkarian & Hodge, 1989c; Rothwell et al., 1983; Kerr, 1975) and projects to dorsolateral prefrontal cortex (Kievit & Kuypers, 1975; Tobias,

1975; Goldman-Rakic & Porrino, 1985). Therefore, the pattern of STT terminations in monkeys largely confirms that described in humans.

Nociceptive neurons have been identified in the human central medial nucleus (Ishijima et al., 1975; Jeanmonod et al., 1993, 1994; Rinaldi et al., 1991; Tsubokawa & Moriyasu, 1975). Ishijima et al. found that one-quarter (20/80) of the cells they recorded from the central medial/parafascicularis complex of man responded to noxious pinprick and two of these responded to application of noxious heat to the skin (Ishijima et al., 1975). None of these cells responded to non-noxious cutaneous stimuli. They identified nociceptive cells which responded at short latency to the application of stimuli, and terminated discharges shortly after discontinuation of the stimulus. A second group of cells responded with a long latency and showed prolonged after-discharges. Both types of cells had receptive fields that were large and often bilateral. The two types of cells were distributed in different areas of the central medial/parafascicularis, with the first type of cells in the medial basal parts of the nucleus, while the second type were scattered throughout the central medial and in the dorsal parts of parafascicularis. Tsubokawa and Moriyasu (Tsubokawa & Moriyasu, 1975) also found a relatively large number of nociceptive neurons which they localized to the central medial nucleus.

Studies by Rinaldi and coworkers ($n = 81$ cells (Rinaldi et al., 1991)) and Jeanmonod and coworkers ($n = 972$, (Jeanmonod et al., 1993, 1994)) in patients with deafferentation pain rarely found cells with receptive fields, in contrast to previous reports (Ishijima et al., 1975; Tsubokawa & Moriyasu, 1975). Instead cells with very high rates of spontaneous bursting discharge activity were reported ((Rinaldi et al., 1991; Jeanmonod et al., 1993, 1994), see below). The cells with receptive fields to tapping were found in two patients in whom bursting activity was absent (Rinaldi et al., 1991). The receptive fields were very large and often bilateral. Jeanmonod et al. (1993, 1994) found two cells with large, bilateral cutaneous receptive fields to innocuous and noxious stimuli. These cells were found in the medial dorsal nucleus.

Electrical stimulation of the medial regions of thalamus for localization prior to thalamotomy for pain (Amano et al., 1976; Choi & Umbach, 1977; Hithcock & Teixeria, 1981; Laitinen, 1988; Richardson, 1967; Rinaldi et al., 1991; Urabe & Tsubokawa, 1965; Voris & Whisler, 1975) evoked painful sensations (Sano, 1977a; Fairman & Llavallol, 1973; Fairman, 1966). Sano's group (Sano, 1977a, 1979) described two types of sensation evoked by stimulation in medial thalamus. The first type was a diffuse, burning pain

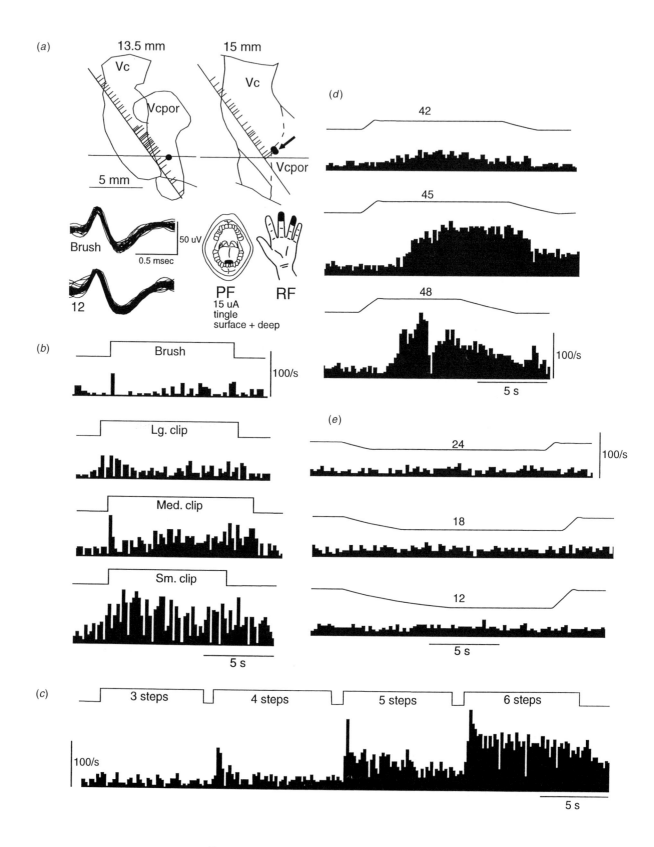

referred to the contralateral half of the body or on occasion the whole body. The sites at which these sensations were produced were usually concentrated near the posterior half of the internal medullary lamina, corresponding to the parvocellular regions of central medial, plus parafascicularis and limitans. The spontaneous pain of the patient was frequently exacerbated by macrostimulation at these sites. The other type of sensation produced by Sano and coworkers was a generalized 'unpleasant' sensation, not localized to a particular body part. The sites at which these sensations were produced were concentrated in the very medial and anterior regions, possibly the medial dorsal and periventricular nuclei. Rinaldi and coworkers have also produced sensations by microstimulation in the medial thalamus, but these were not considered painful (Rinaldi et al., 1991). Instead a sensation of 'pulling' was produced by stimulation in parafascicularis while throbbing was produced by stimulation in the central medial nucleus.

The medial or intralaminar thalamus has often been lesioned for treatment of chronic pain. A decrease in the level of pain was found in 73% of patients on average for these studies (Lenz & Dougherty, 1997). The sensation of pain evoked by an acute experimental paradigm was not altered. Therefore, it is assumed that the medial nuclei subserve the affective–motivational component of pain.

Cortex

Our understanding of cortical areas involved in pain perception has been dramatically altered by the results of functional imaging studies carried out during the application of painful stimuli (Jones et al., 1991; Talbot et al.,

1991a; Casey, 1999; Casey & Bushnell, 2000). These studies have identified four areas metabolically activated by the application of painful stimuli. This section will review anatomy and physiology of each of these areas: primary somatosensory cortex (S1), secondary somatic sensory cortex (S2), insula, and cingulate cortex.

The primary somatosensory cortex (S1)

The S1 cortex located in post-central gyrus is the first cortical target of somesthetic information from the monkey VPL and VPM nuclei of the thalamus. Most of the thalamo-cortical neurons of VPL and VPM project to S1 cortex, including the fraction that receives input from the STT. Human studies suggest a similar picture, such that the ventral caudal nucleus (Vc; corresponding to monkey VP) projects to S1 (Van Buren & Borke, 1972). Multiple case reports describe lesions involving parietal cerebral cortex and underlying white matter, that are associated with hypalgesia (Marshall, 1951; Boivie et al., 1989). Lesions of S1 cortex in old world primates are reported to interfere with discrimination of stimuli into the noxious range (Kenshalo et al., 1991). These results suggest that S1 has a pain-related function.

Neurophysiological studies in primates have demonstrated the existence of nociresponsive neurons in the S1 cortex, although they appear to be a small fraction ($\geqslant 1\%$) of all somatosensory neurons in this area (Kenshalo, Jr. et al., 1988). Nociresponsive neurons in S1 demonstrate response magnitudes that are proportional to the intensity of noxious heat. Thus, these neurons have the capacity to encode the intensity of painful stimuli. This intensity encoding capacity is consistent with S1 being involved in the discriminative aspect of pain.

Fig. 59.1 *(Opposite).* Activity of cell (061093) in Vc responding to painful mechanical and thermal stimuli. (*a*) location of the cell (arrow) relative to the positions of trajectories, nuclear boundaries, and other recorded cells. The ACPC line is indicated by the horizontal line and the trajectories are shown by the oblique lines (left-anterior, up-dorsal). Nuclear location was approximated from the position of the ACPC line. Lateral location of the cell (in millimeters) is indicated above each map. Trajectories have been shifted along the ACPC line until the most posterior cell with a cutaneous RF is aligned with the posterior border of Vc. Since cells responding to innocuous sensory stimuli may be located posterior to Vc (Apkarian & Shi, 1994), this map represents a first approximation of nuclear location and dimensions. The locations of cells are indicated by ticks to the right of each trajectory. Cells with cutaneous RFs are indicated by long ticks, those without definable RFs by short ticks. Filled circles attached to the long ticks indicate that somatic sensory testing was carried out. The scale is as indicated. The shape of action potentials recorded at the beginning of the recording on this cell during application of the brush (upper) and at the end of the recording, during a 12 °C stimulus (lower). Data were collected from upgoing stroke of the action potential by using voltage threshold of 0.15 μV. The RF and PF for the natural, surface and deep, non-painful, tingling sensation evoked by TMIS at the recording site (threshold – 15 μA) are also shown.

(*b*) response to the brush, LC, MC, and SC. (*c*) the response of the neuron to progressive increase in pressure applied with the non-penetrating towel clip, indicated by the number of steps. (*d*) responses to heat stimuli at 42 °C, 45 °C, and 48 °C. (*e*) responses to cold stimuli at 12 °C, 18 °C, and 24 °C. The upper trace in each panel is a footswitch signal indicating the onset and duration of the stimulus in panels (*b*) and (*c*) and the thermode signal in panels (*d*) and (*e*). The scales for the axes for all histograms (binwidth 100 milliseconds) are indicated in each panel. (From Lee et al., 1999 with permission.)

S1 cortex is activated by either innocuous or noxious stimulation in humans, based on magnetoencephalography (MEG), evoked potentials, positron emission tomography (PET), and most recently, functional magnetic resonance imaging (fMRI; see review by Bushnell et al., 1999). Several laser evoked potential (LEP) studies have proposed that LEPs arise in part from generators localized to the contralateral S1 cortex (Tarkka & Treede, 1993). Recent studies have demonstrated that metabolic activation in S1 is significantly related to the magnitude of perceived pain evoked by stimuli of varying intensity (Coghill et al., 1999). Thus, there is clear evidence that S1 is involved in the discriminative dimension of pain.

The secondary somatosensory cortex (S2)

There are several regions in the posterior parietal operculum and posterior insula that show somesthetic responsive neurons in the non-human primate. A part of that area has been identified as S2 cortex, by nature of its connectivity to ventrobasal thalamus and the S1 cortex (Burton, 1986). It is located in the parietal operculum, immediately posterior to the most lateral aspect of S1 cortex. Surrounding S2 cortex are several other electophysiologically defined somatotopic maps, which have been identified as PV (parietal ventral – just anterior to S2 in the parietal operculum; (Krubitzer et al., 1995)), area 7b (lateral to S2), posterior insula (medial to S2), and retroinsula (in the lateral fissure posterior to the insula proper) (Burton, 1986). Together, these areas are referred to as parasylvian cortical areas. Neurophysiological studies in primates have identified cells responsive to painful stimuli in S2 and area 7b (Dong et al., 1989, 1994).

Human studies suggest that the subnuclei in and around Vc project to the posterior parietal operculum (including S2; (Van Buren & Borke, 1972)). Human LEP studies provide evidence of nociceptive inputs to this area. LEPs are the potentials evoked by cutaneous application of a laser which is a pure pain stimulus. Subdural studies demonstrate that LEPs arise from a generator between the sylvian and the central fissures anterior to auditory cortex and discrete from the generator for the P3 event-related potentials (Lenz et al., 1998b). This suggests that the positive component of the LEP is not a potential related to the P3, a potential related to the attention evoked by infrequent events (cf Zaslansky et al., 1996).

The maximum of the LEP is identified just above the sylvian fissure and just anterior to a generator of the AEP – the primary auditory cortex located in Heschl's transverse gyrus on the temporal operculum (Celesia & Puletti, 1969). The polarity of the AEP is opposite at recording sites on opposite sides of the sylvian fissure (Fig. 59.2), consistent with the known location of the AEP generator. If we assume a generator in S2 on the parietal operculum (Burton et al., 1993), facing the temporal operculum, the polarity of the LEP should be opposite on opposite sides of the sylvian fissure, by analogy to the AEP. However, LEPs recorded on opposite sides of the sylvian fissure have the same polarity (Fig. 59.2), suggesting that this generator of the LEP is not located in S2 (Kakigi et al., 1995; Tarkka & Treede, 1993). Comparisons of LEPs with auditory evoked potentials recorded through the same electrodes suggest that the LEP generator is not in S2 but in the dorsal insula at the level of the central sulcus (Lenz et al., 2000).

It has not been possible for PET studies to resolve those regions around the lateral sulcus which are activated by this painful stimulus. Recent fMRI studies have demonstrated multiple loci of activation on the parietal operculum–posterior insula region with both innocuous (Disbrow et al., 2000) and noxious stimuli (Moulton et al., 1999). Hypalgesia has been reported in patients with cerebral lesions involving the parietal operculum, posterior insula, and/or underlying white matter (thereby involving the S2 region), while apparently sparing S1 (Biemond, 1956; Greenspan & Winfield, 1992; Greenspan et al., 1999).

One major issue to be addressed is whether these somatosensory regions demonstrate intensity encoding capacity within the noxious range. Single-unit neurophysiological studies in primates show that some neurons in 7b (adjacent to S2) show responses that can encode for the intensity of noxious heat stimuli (Dong et al., 1994). One PET study reported that responses in the S2 regions (among other areas) were graded in relation to noxious heat intensity (Coghill et al., 1999). Thus there is strong evidence that nociceptive information reaches S2 cortex, and that the activity in this area is related to pain intensity.

The insular cortex

In monkey, portions of the insular cortex have neuroanatomical connectivity suggestive of a role in somatosensory information processing, including inputs from S1 and S2 (Mufson & Mesulam, 1982; Friedman et al., 1986). Additionally, the insula receives input from several thalamic nuclei, including VPI, the oral and medial pulvinar nuclei, the centromedian-parafasicular nuclei, the medial dorsal nucleus, and the VMpo portion of thalamus, which receive nociceptive input from the spinal cord (Burton & Jones, 1976; Jones & Burton, 1976; Friedman et al., 1980; Mesulam & Mufson, 1985; Friedman & Murray, 1986). Stimulation in human Vcpc can evoke previously experienced pain, and the emotional tone associated with that previously experi-

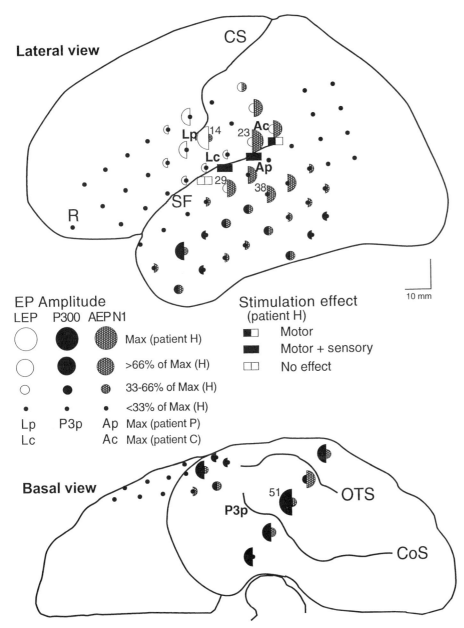

Fig. 59.2. Amplitude distribution of facial LEP P2, AEP, and P3 potentials in patient H and location of maximums for patients C and P. For patient H the LEP P2 amplitude was expressed as a percentage of the maximum (electrode 14) as indicated by the size of the circle. The same conventions were applied to circles for AEPs and P3s so that the location indicates electrode position, the size indicates amplitude as a percentage of the maximum, and the shading indicates the potential (LEP P2, AEP or P3) represented by the circle (Fig. 59.1, left inset). Amplitudes of greater than 33% of maximum were never found at the same electrode for both the LEP P2 and the auditory P3 so that the potentials not represented at any site were less than 33% of maximum.

In patient H, large LEP P2 potentials (>66% maximum) were seen over a restricted area adjacent to the inferior central sulcus, which was confirmed as facial sensorimotor area by stimulation mapping (right inset). LEP P2 maximums in patients C and P (Lc and Lp) were located close to that for patient H. AEPs were maximal posterior and superior to the maximum for LEPs. In patient H, large P3 potentials (>66% maximum) were widespread over basal, anterior, and lateral temporal areas with a maximum over the fusiform gyrus of the temporal base. CS, central sulcus; SF, sylvian fissure; OTS, occipital temporal sulcus; CoS, collateral sulcus. (From Lenz et al., 2000, with permission.)

enced pain. This finding suggests that nuclei in the posterior group may be connected to limbic structures (Lenz et al., 1994b, 1995), through insular connections to the medial temporal lobe (Mishkin, 1979). This suggestion is consistent with anatomic studies demonstrating that the granular portion of insula projects to limbic structures, including the amygdala and perirhinal cortex (Friedman et al., 1986).

There is also evidence that the insula plays a role in human somesthetic perception. Penfield and Faulk (Penfield & Faulk, Jr., 1955) documented somesthetic experiences evoked in patients by direct electrical stimulation of insular cortex. Berthier et al. (1987) described six patients with insular lesions who had reduced motivational–affective responses to pain, but normal sensory--discriminative capacity. A recent report described the perceptual alterations in a group of people with lesions involving portions of the insula and the parietal operculum (Greenspan et al., 1999). Those individuals with lesions encompassing the posterior parietal operculum showed elevated pain thresholds contralaterally, regardless of whether the lesion involved the neighbouring insula. Those individuals with lesions involving the insula, but sparing the parietal operculum showed normal pain thresholds, but demonstrated greater pain tolerance contralaterally. This was interpreted to show that the parietal operculum (containing S2) has a role in the sensory–discriminative aspect of pain (evidenced by elevation of the pain threshold), while the insula has a role in the motivational–affective aspect of pain (evidenced by elevation of pain tolerance).

The insula's significance to thermal and nociceptive information processing has been highlighted by PET studies (Casey et al., 1994, 1996; Coghill et al., 1994; Craig et al., 1996). These reports describe significant activation of a mid/anterior region of insula, and a separate posterior region of insula, associated with noxious thermal stimuli. Both of these insular areas have been described as showing response levels proportional to stimulus and/or pain intensity (Coghill et al., 1999). It has been suggested that the more posterior region of insula, receiving thalamic input similar to S2 cortex, is more related to sensory discriminative functions.

The cingulate cortex

The anterior cingulate cortex (ACC) also appears to have a role in processing nociceptive input. Brodmann's area 24 in particular receives thalamic input from some of the noci-responsive medial thalamic nuclei and VPI (Craig, Jr. et al., 1982; Vogt et al., 1987; Musil & Olson, 1988; Yasui et al., 1988). Nociresponsive neurons have been recorded (Hutchison et al., 1999) in human ACC and LEPS have a maximum over this area (Lenz et al., 1998c). Surgical lesions

have been made near the genu of the ACC in order to relieve chronic pain, and the effects are described as blunting the affective–motivational aspect of pain (Folz & White, 1962; Gybels & Sweet, 1989). Recently, two detailed psychophysical investigations reported sensory changes following cingulotomy or capsulotomy. In the first case pain intensity and unpleasantness was decreased postoperatively (Talbot et al., 1995); a more complex alteration in pain sensibility was observed in the second case who underwent both a capsulotomy and a cingulotomy (Davis et al., 1994).

Perhaps most compelling is the fact that the ACC is the region most consistently activated by noxious stimuli across all PET and fMRI studies (Casey, 1999; Casey & Bushnell, 2000), while innocuous tactile or thermal stimuli consistently fail to activate this region. It has been argued that the ACC activity associated with painful stimulation is not related to the pain experience *per se*, but rather is related to the attentional shift that occurs with an acute painful stimulus. However, the region of the ACC that is activated by painful stimulation is different from the region that is activated by directing attention to non-painful events (Davis et al., 1997). One PET study showed that hypnotic alteration of perceived unpleasantness of painful stimulation produced correlated changes in the ACC response, while producing no significant change in other cortical regions (Rainville et al., 1997). The part of ACC related to pain may be particularly involved in pain unpleasantness.

Central pain syndrome (CPS)

Although little is known of the fundamental pathophysiology of central pain (Boivie & Leijon, 1991), the condition is considered to involve a primary dysfunction of the somatosensory thalamus (Head & Holmes, 1912) that in turn involves cortical structures. The well-described relay of somatosensory information in the ventral posterior medial and lateral nuclei (VPM and VPL) (Guilbaud et al., 1980; Harris, 1980; Jasper & Bertrand, 1966; Jones, 1985; Mountcastle & Henneman, 1949) has historically been cited as evidence to implicate the thalamus in the paroxysmal pain evoked by acute peripheral stimuli in CPS patients (Head & Holmes, 1912). Consistent with this view, intraoperative studies have shown somatotopic rearrangement, abnormal responsiveness to peripheral stimuli, and abnormal spontaneous discharge patterns in thalamic neurons of CPS patients (Lenz et al., 1989, 1993a, 1998d; Radhakrishnan et al., 1999). Electrical stimulation in these zones of altered cellular activity, in lateral thalamus, provoked the sensation of pain at a higher frequency than would be normally expected (Lenz et al., 1998a), and lesion in areas of altered activity in the medial thalamus successfully relieved CPS (Ishijima et al., 1975; Jeanmonod et al., 1993).

Psychophysical studies uniformly demonstrate that CPS is found in patients with impaired STT function (Boivie & Leijon, 1991; Vestergaard et al., 1997; Boivie et al., 1989; Beric et al., 1988) due to injuries to the STT and it's projections (Cassinari & Pagni, 1969). Acute lesion of the STT in humans produces insensitivity to pain but rarely produces pain (Boivie & Leijon, 1991; Bowsher, 1997; Casey, 1991; Cassinari & Pagni, 1969). However, chronic pain develops in an increasing percentage of patients with increasing length of survival following anterior lateral spinal lesion, so that the risk of CPS becomes a major limiting factor in use of cordotomy for pain relief with prolonged life expectancy (Beric et al., 1988; Casey, 1991). Unfortunately, the extent of spinal lesions was variable in the human neurophysiological studies and so, the specific contribution of STT damage to the observed changes in neurons of CPS patients could not be assessed. In monkeys, acute lesion of the STT reduced sensitivity to pain (Vierck, Jr. et al., 1971, 1983; Vierck, Jr., 1998; Vierck, Jr. & Luck, 1979; Willis, 1985). Over the next 6 months pain sensitivity returned for most in monkeys with STT lesions. In addition, one-third to one-half of all animals developed exaggerated responsiveness to nociceptive stimuli (Vierck et al., 1990). Therefore there is strong evidence that lesions of the STT can evoke features of the CPS.

Anatomic plasticity following peripheral neurological injury has been shown in the thalamus of several species (Albe-Fessard et al., 1983; Albe-Fessard & Rampin, 1991; Lombard & Larabi, 1983; Pollin & Albe-Fessard, 1979; Wall & Egger, 1971) (or for review, see Dougherty & Lenz, 1994). Anatomic rearrangements observed after cervical dorsal rhizotomy in non-human primates included loss of afferent terminals and decreased density of neurons (Rausell et al., 1992). Zones of parvalbumin and cytochrome oxidase staining, characteristic of lemniscal terminals, decreased in size while the calbindin positive zones, characteristic of the spinothalamic terminals, increased (Rausell et al., 1992). The affected areas also demonstrated a decrease in GABA-A receptors (GABA-B and -C receptors were not examined) without a decrease in the number of GABA positive interneurons. Marked changes in GABA synaptic morphology have also been shown following chronic dorsal column lesion (Ralston et al., 1996; Ralston & Ralston, 1994).

Thalamic neurons also show functional signs of plasticity after peripheral or central nervous system injury. Among these changes, receptive field reorganization (Kaas, 1991) and changes in the responses to mechanical and thermal stimuli are common (Koyama et al., 1993). Also, pain is evoked more commonly by stimulation in the region of Vc in patients with chronic pain than in patients with movement disorders (Lenz et al., 1998a). These changes may account for perceptual alterations which occur in patients with chronic pain secondary to peripheral deafferentation. For instance, changes in receptive and projected field organization could explain the telescoping of the limbs experienced by patients with amputations (Jensen & Rasmussen, 1994). Pain and hyperalgesia in patients with chronic pain could be explained by the increased likelihood of provoking pain by stimulation of the region of Vc.

An increase in the rate of action potential bursts has been widely reported in both the thalamus of humans (Jeanmonod et al., 1993; Lenz et al., 1989, 1994a) and in animals following lesion of the nervous system (Albe-Fessard et al., 1983, 1985; Lombard & Larabi, 1983; Rodin & Kruger, 1984). Particular significance has been assigned to the changes in spike train properties of thalamic neurons following deafferentation because the rate of neuronal spike bursts in pain patients is significantly higher in regions of the lateral thalamus (VPL/VPM) representing the painful part of the body (Lenz et al., 1994a). Microstimulation in areas of increased rates of neuronal bursting is more likely to produce pain in both post-amputation and post-stroke CPS patients than in other areas of VPL (Davis et al., 1996; Lenz, 1992; Lenz et al., 1998a). Lesions directed at medial thalamic regions of abnormal bursting have been used as a guide to relieve chronic pain surgically (Ishijima et al., 1975; Jeanmonod et al., 1993). The significance of these findings has been challenged by a study suggesting that the number of bursting cells is equal in patients with pain and in patients with movement disorders (Radhakrishnan et al., 1999). It is unclear how the two patient groups in that study would have compared if the rate of bursting in all cells (Lenz et al., 1994) rather than number of bursting cells were studied (Radhakrishnan et al., 1999).

A recently proposed mechanism of central pain proposes that central pain is the result of an imbalance between two ascending pathways. This hypothesis attempts to explain the burning pain and cold allodynia that can be observed in central pain syndromes. It is proposed that the burning pain of intense cold is mediated by the medial pathway from polymodal nociceptive lamina I spinothalamic neurons (HPC) in monkey lamina I to the cingulate gyrus via the ventral caudal portion of the medial dorsal nucleus (MDvc). It is further proposed that the medial pathway is inhibited by the lateral pathway from cold specific lamina I spinothalamic neurons (COLD) to insula via the posterior portion of the ventral medial nucleus (VMpo) (Craig et al., 1996). Lesions of the lateral pathway are proposed to release inhibition of the medial pathway and so cause a burning pain similar to that evoked by intense cold. The site at which the lateral pathway may inhibit the medial pathway is unclear at present.

The idea that the ongoing pain of central pain syndromes resembles the burn of cold pain is the most basic tenet of this hypothesis. However, many patients with central poststroke pain (CPSP: 40–50%) do not experience a burning pain (Leijon et al., 1989; Bowsher, 1997). The cold allodynia which is predicted by this hypothesis is found in a minority of patients with CPSP (23% – 5/22) (Boivie et al., 1989). Thus, it is not clear that clinical features found in central pain syndromes are explained by this hypothesis done. Nevertheless, it is a useful construct for guiding research into central pain mechanisms.

In conclusion, studies in humans have demonstrated involvement of both lateral and medial thalamus in pain processing. In lateral thalamus, cells responsive to painful stimuli are located in the core area and in the postero-inferior area. Stimulation in the postero-inferior area or at the posterior aspect of the core can evoke pain or visceral pain suggesting involvement of this area in the mechanisms of somatic and visceral pain. Injections of local anesthetic into monkey VP blocks the ability of monkeys to discriminate temperature differences in the noxious and non-noxious ranges. These findings and particularly the presence of sensory loss following lesions of lateral thalamus suggest that the region of Vc signals the sensory discriminative aspect of acute pain in humans. Anatomic studies are consistent with this area projecting to parietal and parasylvian cortex.

In medial and intralaminar thalamus, some cells responsive to noxious stimuli have been recorded. Pain has been reported by macrostimulation at some sites. STT terminates in the nuclei where these recording and stimulation results are reported. These results provide support for the involvement of medial thalamic nuclei in pain signalling pathways in man. These structures project to cingulate cortex and diffusely to a wide area of cortex.

Abnormalities in lateral thalamus in patients with chronic pain point to involvement of this area in chronic pain in humans. Somatotopic reorganization of Vc occurs in patients who have chronic pain secondary to deafferentation or spinal cord injury. A reorganization of modalities occurs in patients with chronic pain so that the number of sites where thermal sensations are normally evoked by thalamic stimulation is decreased by an amount equal to the increase in the number of sites where pain is evoked.

Increased rate of bursting is observed in the deafferented areas of thalamus and is probably related to loss of STT inputs. This abnormal burst firing is most pronounced in the posterior–inferior area of the thalamus involved in signalling pain, suggesting that this firing is involved in the sensation of chronic pain.

Acknowledgements

Supported by grants to FAL from the Eli Lilly Corporation and the National Institutes of Health (P01 NS32386-Project 1, NS38493, NS40059), to JDG from the National Institutes of Health (39337) and to PMD from the National Institutes of Health (P01 NS32386-Project 2, NS39933).

References

Albe-Fessard, D. & Rampin, O. (1991). Neurophysiological studies in rats deafferented by dorsal root section. In *Deafferentation Pain Syndromes: Pathophysiology and Treatment*, ed. B.S. Nashold & J. Ovelmen-Levitt, pp. 125–39. New York: Raven Press.

Albe-Fessard, D. & Lombard, M.C. (1983). Use of an animal model to evaluate the origin of and protection against deafferentation pain. *Adv. Pain Res. Ther.*, **5**, 691–700.

Albe-Fessard, D., Berkley, K.J., Kruger, L., Ralston, H. & Willis, W.D. (1985). Diencephalic mechanisms of pain sensation. *Brain Res. Rev.*, **9**, 217–96.

Amano, K., Kitamura, K., Sano, K. & Sekino, H. (1976). Relief of intractable pain from neurosurgical point of view with reference to present limits and clinical indications – a review of 100 consecutive cases. *Neurol. Medico-chir.*, **16**, 141–53.

Amano, K., Tanikawa, T., Iseki, H., Kawabatke, H., Notani, M., Kawamura, H. & Kitamura, K. (1978). Single neuron analysis of the human midbrain tegmentum. *Appl. Neurophysiol.*, **41**, 66–78.

Apkarian, A.V. & Hodge, C.J. (1989a). A dorsolateral spinothalamic tract in macaque monkey. *Pain*, **37**, 323–33.

Apkarian, A.V. & Hodge, C.J. (1989b). Primate spinothalamic pathways: II. The cells of origin of the dorsolateral and ventral spinothalamic pathways. *J. Comp. Neurol.*, **288**, 474–92.

Apkarian, A.V. & Hodge, C.J. (1989c). Primate spinothalamic pathways: III. Thalamic terminations of the dorsolateral and ventral spinothalamic pathways. *J. Comp. Neurol.*, **288**, 493–511.

Apkarian, A.V. & Shi, T. (1994). Squirrel monkey lateral thalamus. I. somatic nociresponsive neurons and their relation to spinothalamic terminals. *J. Neurosci.*, **14**, 6779–95.

Apkarian, A.V., Shi, T., Stevens, R.T., Kniffki, K-D. & Hodge, C.J. (1991). Properties of nociceptive neurons in the lateral thalamus of the squirrel monkey. *Soc. Neurosci. Abstr.*, **17**, 838.

Bandler, R. & Carrive, P. (1988). Integrated defence reaction elicited by excitatory amino acid microinjection in the midbrain periaqueductal grey region of the unrestrained cat. *Brain Res.*, **439**, 95–106.

Bandler, R. & Depaulis, A. (1988). Elicitation of intraspecific defence reactions in the rat from midbrain periaqueductal gray by microinjection of kainic acid, without neurotoxic effects. *Neurosci. Lett.*, **88**, 291–6.

Bandler, R. & Shipley, M.T. (1994). Columnar organization in the midbrain periaqueductal grey: modules for emotional expression? [published erratum appears in *Trends Neurosci.*, **17**(11), 445] [see comments]. *Trends Neurosci.*, **17**, 379–89.

Barbaro, N.M., Heinricher, M.M. & Fields, H.L. (1989). Putative nociceptive modulatory neurons in the rostral ventromedial medulla of the rat display highly correlated firing patterns. *Somatosens. Motor Res.*, **6**, 413–25.

Beric, A., Dimitrijevic, M.R. & Lindblom, U. (1988). Central dysesthesia syndrome in spinal cord injury patients. *Pain*, **34**, 109–16.

Berkley, K.J. (1980) Spatial relationships between the terminations of somatic sensory and motor pathways in the rostral brainstem of cats and monkeys. I. Ascending somatic sensory inputs to lateral diencephalon. *J. Comp. Neurol.*, **193**, 283–317.

Bernard, J.F. & Besson, J.M. (1990). The spino(trigemino)pontoamygdaloid pathway: electrophysiological evidence for an involvement in pain processes. *J. Neurophysiol.*, **63**, 473–90.

Berthier, M., Starkstein, S. & Leiguarda, R. (1987). Behavioral effects of damage to the right insula and surrounding regions. *Cortex*, **23**, 673–8.

Biemond, A. (1956). The conduction of pain above the level of the thalamus opticus. *Arch. Neurol. Psychiatry*, **75**, 231–44.

Bjorkeland, M. & Boivie, J. (1984). The termination of spinomesencephalic fibers in cat. An experimental anatomical study. *Anat. Embryol.(Berl).*, **170**, 265–77.

Blair, R.W., Ammons, W.S. & Foreman, R.D. (1984). Responses of thoracic spinothalamic and spinoreticular cells to coronary artery occlusion. *J. Neurophysiol.*, **51**, 636–48.

Boivie, J. (1979). An anatomic reinvestigation of the termination of the spinothalamic tract in the monkey. *J. Comp. Neurol.*, **186**, 343–69.

Boivie, J. & Leijon, G. (1991). Clinical findings in patients with central poststroke pain. In *Pain and Central Nervous System Disease*, ed. K.L. Casey, pp. 65–75. New York: Raven Press.

Boivie, J., Leijon, G. & Johansson, I. (1989). Central post-stroke pain – a study of the mechanisms through analyses of the sensory abnormalities. *Pain*, **37**, 173–85.

Bowsher, D. (1957). Termination of the central pain pathway in man: the conscious appreciation of pain. *Brain*, **80**, 606–20.

Bowsher, D. (1976). Role of the reticular formation in responses to noxious stimulation. *Pain*, **2**, 361–78.

Bowsher, D. (1997). Central pain: clinical and physiological characteristics. *J. Neurol. Neurosurg., Psychiatry*, **61**, 62–9.

Brown, A.G. & Franz, D.N. (1969). Responses of spinocervical tract neurons to natural stimulation of identified cutaneous receptors. *Exp. Brain Res.*, **7**, 231–49.

Brown, A.G., Brown, P.B., Fyffe, R.E.W. & Pubols, L.M. (1983). Receptive field organization and response properties of spinal

neurones with axons ascending the dorsal columns in the cat. *J. Physiol., (Lond.)*, **337**, 575–88.

Burstein, R., Cliffer, K.D. & Giesler, G.J., Jr. (1987). Direct somatosensory projections from the spinal cord to the hypothalamus and telencephalon. *J. Neurosci.*, **7**, 4159–64.

Burstein, R., Cliffer, K.D. & Giesler, G.J., Jr. (1990). Cells of origin of the spinohypothalamic tract in the rat. *J. Comp. Neurol.*, **291**, 329–44.

Burstein, R., Dado, R.J., Cliffer, K.D. & Giesler, G.J., Jr. (1991). Physiological characterization of spinohypothalamic tract neurons in the lumbar enlargement of rats. *J. Neurophysiol.*, **66**, 261–84.

Burton, H. (1986). Second somatosensory cortex and related areas. In *Cerebral Cortex*, Vol. 5, *Sensory–Motor Areas and Aspects of Cortical Connectivity*, ed. E.G. Jones & A. Peters, pp. 31–98. New York and London: Plenum Press.

Burton, H. & Craig, A.D., Jr. (1983). Spinothalamic projections in cat, raccoon and monkey: a study based on anterograde transport of horseradish peroxidase. In *Somatosensory Integration in the Thalamus*, ed. G.R.A. Macchi, pp. 17–41. Amsterdam: Elsevier.

Burton, H. & Jones, E.G. (1976). The posterior thalamic region and its cortical projection in new world and old world monkeys. *J. Comp. Neurol.*, **168**, 249–302.

Burton, H., Videen, T.O. & Raichle, M.E. (1993). Tactile-vibration-activated foci in insular and parietal-opercular cortex studied with positron emission tomography: mapping the second somatosensory area in humans. *Somatosens. Motor Res.*, **10**, 297–308.

Bushnell, M.C. & Duncan, G.H. (1987). Mechanical response properties of ventroposterior medial thalamic neurons in the alert monkey. *Exp. Brain Res.*, **67**, 603–14.

Bushnell, M.C., Duncan, G.H., Dubner, R. & He, L.F. (1984). Activity of trigeminothalamic neurons in medullary dorsal horn of awake monkeys trained in a thermal discrimination task. *J. Neurophysiol.*, **52**, 170–87.

Bushnell, M.C., Duncan, G.H. & Tremblay, N. (1993). Thalamic VPM nucleus in the behaving monkey. I. Multimodal and discriminative properties of thermosensitive neurons. *J. Neurophysiol.*, **69**, 739–52.

Bushnell, M.C., Duncan, G.H., Hofbauer, R.K., Ha, B., Chen, J.I. & Carrier, B. (1999). Pain perception: is there a role for primary somatosensory cortex? *Proc. Natl. Acad. Sci. USA*, **96**, 7705–9.

Campbell, J. N., Raja, S.N., Meyer, R.A. & Mackinnon, S.E. (1988). Myelinated afferents signal the hyperalgesia associated with nerve injury. *Pain*, **32**, 89–94.

Carstens, E., Klumpp, D. & Zimmermann, M. (1980). Differential inhibitory effects of medial and lateral midbrain stimulation on spinal neuronal discharges to noxious skin heating in the cat. *J. Neurophysiol.*, **43**, 332–42.

Casey, K.L. (1966). Unit analysis of nociceptive mechanisms in the thalamus of the awake squirrel monkey. *J. Neurophysiol.*, **29**, 727–50.

Casey, K.L. (1971a). Escape elicited by bulboreticular stimulation in the cat. *Int. J. Neurosci.*, **2**, 29–34.

Casey, K.L. (1971b). Responses of bulboreticular units to somatic stimuli eliciting escape behavior in the cat. *Int. J. Neurosci.*, **2**, 15–28.

Casey, K.L. (1978). The problem of defining pain. *Neurosci. Res. Prog. Bull.*, **16**, 9–13.

Casey, K.L. (1991). Pain and central nervous system disease: a summary and overview. In *Pain and Central Nervous System Disease: The Central Pain Syndromes*, ed. K.L. Casey, pp. 1–11. New York: Raven Press.

Casey, K.L. (1999). Forebrain mechanisms of nociception and pain: analysis through imaging. *Proc. Natl Acad. Sci., USA*, **96**, 7668–74.

Casey, K.L. & Bushnell, M.C. (2000). *Pain Imaging*. Seattle: IASP Press.

Casey, K.L. & Morrow, T.J. (1983). Ventral posterior thalamic neurons differentially responsive to noxious stimulation of the awake monkey. *Science*, **221**, 675–7.

Casey, K.L., Minoshima, S., Berger, K.L., Koeppe, R.A., Morrow, T.J. & Frey, K.A. (1994). Positron emission tomographic analysis of cerebral structures activated specifically by repetitive noxious heat stimuli. *J. Neurophysiol.*, **71**, 802–7.

Casey, K.L., Minoshima, S., Morrow, T.J. & Koeppe, R.A. (1996). Comparison of human cerebral activation patterns during cutaneous warmth, heat and deep cold pain. *J. Neurophysiol.*, **76**, 571–81.

Cassinari, V. & Pagni, C.A. (1969). *Central Pain. A Neurosurgical Survey*. Cambridge, Massachusetts: Harvard University Press.

Celesia, G.G. & Puletti, F. (1969). Auditory cortical areas in man. *Neurology*, **19**, 211–20.

Choi, C.R. & Umbach, W. (1977). Combined stereotaxic surgery for relief of intractable pain. *Neurochirurgia*, **20**, 84–7.

Chung, J.M., Lee, K.H., Surmeier, D.J., Sorkin, L.S., Kim, I. & Willis, W.D. (1986). Response characteristics of neurons in the ventral posterior lateral nucleus of the monkey thalamus. *J. Neurophysiol.*, **56**, 370–90.

Cliffer, K.D., Hasegawa, T. & Willis, W.D. (1992). Responses of neurons in the gracile nucleus of cats to innocuous and noxious stimuli: basic characterization and antidromic activation from the thalamus. *J. Neurophysiol.*, **68**, 818–32.

Coghill, R.C., Talbot, J.D., Evans, A.C. et al. (1994). Distributed processing of pain and vibration by the human brain. *J. Neurosci.*, **14**, 4095–108.

Coghill, R.C., Sang, C.N., Maisog, J.M. & Iadarola, M.J. (1999). Pain intensity processing within the human brain: a bilateral, distributed mechanism. *J. Neurophysiol.*, **82**, 1934–43.

Conti, F., De Biasi, S., Giuffrida, R. & Rustioni, A. (1990). Substance P-containing projections in the dorsal columns of rats and cats. *Neuroscience*, **34**, 607–21.

Craig, A.D. (1990). Trigeminothalamic projections in the monkey. *Soc. Neurosci. Abst.*, **16**, 1144.

Craig, A.D. (1998). A new version of the thalamic disinhibition hypothesis of central pain. *Pain*.

Craig, A.D. & Burton, H. (1981). Spinal and medullary lamina I projection to nucleus submedius in medial thalamus: a possible pain center. *J. Neurophysiol.*, **45**, 443–66.

Craig, A.D. & Hunsley, S.J. (1991). Morphine enhances the activity of thermoreceptive cold-specific lamina I spinothalamic neurons in the cat. *Brain Res.*, **558**, 93–7.

Craig, A.D., Weigand, S.J. & Price, J.L. (1982). The thalamo-cortical projection of the nucleus submedius in the cat. *J. Comp. Neurol.*, **206**, 28–48.

Craig, A.D., Bushnell, M.C., Zhang, E-T. & Blomqvist, A. (1994). A thalamic nucleus specific for pain and temperature sensation. *Nature*, **372**, 770–3.

Craig, A.D., Reiman, E.M., Evans, A. & Bushnell, M.C. (1996). Functional imaging of an illusion of pain. *Nature*, **384**, 258–60.

Cusick, C.G., Wall, J.T., Felleman, D.J. & Kaas, J.H. (1989). Somatotopic organization of the lateral sulcus of owl monkeys: Area 3b, S-II, and a ventral somatosensory area. *J. Comp. Neurol.*, **282**, 169–90.

Davis, K.D., Hutchinson, W.D., Lozano, A.M. & Dostrovsky, J.O. (1994). Altered pain and temperature perception following cingulotomy and capsulotomy in a patient with schizoaffective disorder. *Pain*, **59**, 189–199.

Davis, K.D., Kiss, Z.H.T., Tasker, R.R. & Dostrovsky, J.O. (1996). Thalamic stimulation-evoked sensations in chronic pain patients and nonpain (movement disorder) patients. *J. Neurophysiol.*, **75**, 1026–37.

Davis, K.D., Taylor, S.J., Crawley, A.P., Wood, M.L. & Mikulis, D.J. (1997). Functional MRI of pain- and attention related activation in the human cingulate cortex. *J. Neurophysiol.*, **77**, 3370–80.

Davis, K.D., Lozano, A.M., Manduch, M., Tasker, R.R., Kiss, Z.H.T. & Dostovsky, J.O. (1999). Thalamic relay site for cold perception in humans. *J. Neurophysiol.*, **81**, 1970–3.

Delgado, J.M.R. (1955). Cerebral structures involved in transmission and elaboration of noxious stimulation. *J. Neurophysiol.*, **18**, 261–75.

Depaulis, A., Keay, K.A. & Bandler, R. (1994). Quiescence and hyporeactivity evoked by activation of cell bodies in the ventrolateral midbrain periaqueductal gray of the rat. *Exp. Brain Res.*, **99**, 75–83.

Disbrow, E., Roberts, T. & Krubitzer, L. (2000). Somatotopic organization of cortical fields in the lateral sulcus of Homo sapiens: evidence for SII and PV. *J. Comp. Neurol.*, **418**, 1–21.

Dong, W.K., Salonen, L.D., Kawakami, Y., Shiwaku, T., Kaukoranta, E.M. & Martin, R.F. (1989). Nociceptive responses of trigeminal neurons in SII-7b cortex of awake monkeys. *Brain Res.*, **484**, 314–24.

Dong, W.K., Chudler, E.H., Sugiyama, K., Roberts, V.J. & Hayashi, T. (1994). Somatosensory, multisensory, and task-related neurons in cortical area 7b (PF) of unanesthetized monkeys. *J. Neurophysiol.*, **72**, 542–64.

Dostrovsky, J.O., Wells, F.E.B. & Tasker, R.R. (1991). Pain evoked by stimulation in human thalamus. In *International Symposium on Processing Nociceptive Information.*, ed. Y. Sjigenaga, pp. 115–20. Amsterdam: Elsevier.

Dougherty, P.M. & Lenz, F.A. (1994). Plasticity of the somatosensory system following neural injury. *Prog. Pain Res. Managem.*, **3**, 439–60.

Dougherty, P.M., Palecek, J., Zorn, S. & Willis, W.D. (1993). Combined application of excitatory amino acids and substance P produces long-lasting changes in responses of primate spinothalamic tract neurons. *Brain Res. Brain Res. Rev.*, **18**, 227–46.

Dougherty, P.M., Willis, W.D. & Lenz, F.A. (1998). Transient inhibition of responses to thermal stimuli of spinal sensory tract neurons in monkeys during sensitization by intradermal capsaicin. *Pain*, **77**, 129–36.

Dougherty, P.M., Schwartz, A. & Lenz, F.A. (1999). Responses of primate spinomesencephalic tract cells to intradermal capsaicin. *Neuroscience*, **90**, 1377–92.

Dubner, R., Kenshalo, D.R., Jr., Maixner, W., Bushnell, M.C. & Oliveras, J.L. (1989). The correlation of monkey medullary dorsal horn neural activity and the perceived intensity of noxious heat stimuli. *J. Neurophysiol.*, **62**, 450–7.

Duncan, G.H., Bushnell, M.C., Oliveras, J.L., Bastrash, N. & Tremblay, N. (1993). Thalamic VPM nucleus in the behaving monkey. III. effects of reversible inactivation by lidocaine on thermal and mechanical discrimination. *J. Neurophysiol.*, **70**, 2086–96.

Eickhoff, R., Handwerker, H.O., McQueen, D.S. & Schick, E. (1978). Noxious and tactile input to medial structures of midbrain and pons in the rat. *Pain*, **5**, 99–113.

Fabri, M. & Conti, F. (1990). Calcitonin gene-related peptide-positive neurons and fibers in the cat dorsal column nuclei. *Neuroscience*, **35**, 167–74.

Fairman, D. (1966). Evaluation of results in stereotactic thalamotomy for the treatment of intractable pain. *Confinia Neurol.*, **27**, 67–70.

Fairman, D. & Llavallol, M.A. (1973). Thalamic tractotomy for the alleviation of intractable pain in cancer. *Cancer*, **31**, 700–7.

Fardin, V., Oliveras, J.L. & Besson, J.M. (1984). A reinvestigation of the analgesic effects induced by stimulation of the periaqueductal gray matter in the rat. I. The production of behavioral side effects together with analgesia. *Brain Res.*, **306**, 105–23.

Ferrington, D.G., Downie, J.W. & Willis, W.D. Jr. (1988). Primate nucleus gracilis neurons: responses to innocuous and noxious stimuli. *J. Neurophysiol.*, **59**, 886–907.

Fields, H.L., Clanton, C.H. & Anderson, S.D. (1977). Somatosensory properties of spinoreticular neurons in the cat. *Brain Res.*, **120**, 49–66.

Folz, E.L. & White, L.E. (1962). Pain 'relief' by frontal cingulotomy. *J. Neurosurg.*, **19**, 89–100.

Friedman, D.P. & Murray, E.A. (1986). Thalamic connectivity of the second somatosensory area and neighbouring somatosensory fields of the lateral sulcus of the macaque. *J. Comp. Neurol.*, **252**, 348–73.

Friedman, D.P., Jones, E.G. & Burton, H. (1980). Representation pattern in the second somatic sensory area of monkey cerebral cortex. *J. Comp. Neurol.*, **192**, 21–41.

Friedman, D.P., Murray, E.A., O'Neill, J.B. & Mishkin, M. (1986). Cortical connections of the somatosensory fields of the lateral sulcus of macaques: evidence for a corticolimbic pathway for touch. *J. Comp. Neurol.*, **252**, 323–47.

Garrett, L., Coggeshall, R.E., Patterson, J.T. & Chung, K. (1992). Numbers and proportions of unmyelinated axons at cervical levels in the fasciculus gracilis of monkey and cat. *Anat. Rec.*, **232**, 301–4.

Gautron, M. & Guilbaud, G. (1982). Somatic responses of ventrobasal thalamic neurones in polyarthritic rats. *Brain Res.*, **237**, 459–71.

Gerhart, K.D., Yezierski, R.P., Wilcox, T.K. & Willis, W.D. (1984). Inhibition of primate spinothalamic tract neurons by stimulation in periaqueductal gray or adjacent midbrain reticular formation. *J. Neurophysiol.*, **51**, 450–66.

Goldman-Rakic, P. & Porrino, L.J. (1985). The primate mediodorsal nucleus and its projection to the frontal lobe. *J. Comp. Neurol.*, **242**, 535–60.

Greenspan, J.D. & Winfield, J.A. (1992). Reversible pain and tactile deficits associated with a cerebral tumor compressing the posterior insula and parietal operculum. *Pain*, **50**, 29–39.

Greenspan, J.D., Lee, R.R. & Lenz, F.A. (1999). Pain sensitivity alterations as a function of lesion location in the parasylvian cortex. *Pain*, **81**, 273–82.

Guilbaud, G., Besson, J.M., Oliveras, J.L. & Wyon-Maillard, M.C. (1973). Modifications of the firing rate of bulbar reticular units (nucleus gigantocellularis) after intra-arterial injection of bradykinin into the limbs. *Brain Res.*, **63**, 131–40.

Guilbaud, G., Peschanski, M., Gautron, M. & Binder, D. (1980). Neurones responding to noxious stimulation in VB complex and caudal adjacent regions in the thalamus of the rat. *Pain*, **8**, 303–18.

Gybels, J.M. & Sweet, W.H. (1989). *Neurosurgical Treatment of Persistent Pain*, pp. 1–442. Basel: Karger.

Haber, L.H., Moore, B.D. & Willis, W.D. (1982). Electrophysiological response properties of spinoreticular neurons in the monkey. *J. Comp. Neurol.*, **207**, 75–84.

Halliday, A.M. & Logue, V. (1972). Painful sensations evoked by electrical stimulation in the thalamus. In *Neurophysiology Studied in Man*, ed. G.G. Somjen, pp. 221–30. Amsterdam: Excerpta Medica.

Harris, F.A. (1980). Wide-field neurons in somatosensory thalamus of domestic cats under barbiturate anesthesia. *Exp. Neurol.*, **68**, 27–49.

Hassler, R. & Reichert, T. (1959). Klinische und anatomische Befunde bei stereotaktischen Schmerzoperationen im Thalamus. *Arch. Psychiat. Nerverkr.*, **200**, 93–122.

Haws, C.M., Williamson, A.M. & Fields, H.L. (1989). Putative nociceptive modulatory neurons in the dorsolateral pontomesencephalic reticular formation. *Brain Res.*, **483**, 272–82.

Head, H. & Holmes, G. (1912). Sensory disturbances from cerebral lesions. *Brain*, **34**, 102–254.

Hirai, T. & Jones, E.G. (1989a). A new parcellation of the human thalamus on the basis of histochemical staining. *Brain Res. Rev.*, **14**, 1–34.

Hirai, T. & Jones, E.G. (1989b). Distribution of tachykinin-and enkephalin-immunoreactive fibers in the human thalamus. *Brain Res. Rev.*, **14**, 35–52.

Hithcock, E.R. & Teixeira, M.J. (1981). A comparison of results from center-median and basal thalamotomies for pain. *Surg. Neurol.*, **15**, 341–51.

Hutchison, W.D., Davis, K.D., Lozano, A.M., Tasker, R.R. & Dostrovsky, J.O. (1999). Pain-related neurons in the human cingulate cortex. *Nature Neurosci.*, **2**, 403–5.

Hylden, J.L., Hayashi, H., Dubner, R. & Bennett, G.J. (1986). Physiology and morphology of the lamina I spinomesencephalic projection. *J. Comp. Neurol.*, **247**, 505–15.

Ishijima, B., Yoshimasu, N., Fukushima, T., Hori, T., Sekino, H. & Sano, K. (1975). Nociceptive neurons in the human thalamus. *Confinia Neurol.*, **37**, 99–106.

Janss, A.J., Cox, B.F., Brody, M.J. & Gebhart, G.F. (1987). Dissociation of antinociceptive from cardiovascular effects of stimulation in the lateral reticular nucleus in the rat. *Brain Res.*, **405**, 140–9.

Jasper, H.H. & Bertrand, G. (1966). Thalamic units involved in somatic sensation and voluntary and involuntary movements in man. In *The Thalamus*, ed. D.P. Purpura, & M.D. Yahr, pp. 365–90. New York: Columbia University Press.

Jeanmonod, D., Magnin, M. & Morel, A. (1993). Thalamus and neurogenic pain: physiological, anatomical and clinical data. *Neuroreport*, **4**, 475–8.

Jeanmonod, D., Magnin, M. & Morel, A. (1994). A thalamic concept of neurogenic pain. In *Proceedings of the 7th World Congress on Pain. Progress in Pain Research and Management*. Volume 2, ed. G.F. Gebhart, D.L. Hammond & T.S. Jensen, pp. 767–87. Seattle: IASP Press.

Jensen, T.S. & Rasmussen, P. (1994). Phantom pain and related phenomena after amputation. In *Textbook of Pain*, ed. P.D. Wall, & R. Melzack, pp. 651–65. New York: Churchill Livingstone.

Jones, A.K.P., Brown, W.D., Friston, K.J., Qi, L.Y. & Frackowiak, R.S.J. (1991). Cortical and subcortical localization of response to pain in man using positron emission tomography. *Proc. Roy. Soc. Lond. B: Biol. Sci.*, **244**, 39–44.

Jones, E.G. (1985). *The Thalamus*. New York: Plenum.

Jones, E.G. & Burton, H. (1976). Real differences in the laminar distribution of thalamic afferents in cortical fields of the insular, parietal and temporal regions of primates. *J. Comp. Neurol.*, **168**, 197–248.

Kaas, J.H. (1991). Plasticity of sensory and motor maps in adult mammals. *Ann. Rev. Neurosci.*, **14**, 137–67.

Kakigi, R., Koyama, S., Hoshiyama, M., Kitamura, Y., Shimojo, M. & Watanabe, S. (1995). Pain-related magnetic fields following painful CO_2 laser stimulation in man. *Neurosci. Lett.*, **192**, 45–8.

Kalil, K. (1978). Patch-like termination of thalamic fibers in the putamen of the rhesus monkey: an autoradiographic study. *Brain Res.*, **140**, 333–9.

Katter, J.T., Dado, R.J., Kostarczyk, E. & Giesler, G.J., Jr. (1996). Spinothalamic and spinohypothalamic tract neurons in the sacral spinal cord of rats. II. Responses to cutaneous and visceral stimuli. *J. Neurophysiol.*, **75**, 2606–28.

Keay, K.A., Clement, C.I., Owler, B., Depaulis, A. & Bandler, R. (1994). Convergence of deep somatic and visceral nociceptive information onto a discrete ventrolateral midbrain periaqueductal gray region. *Neuroscience*, **61**, 727–32.

Kenshalo, D.R., Jr. & Willis, W.D. Jr. (1991). The role of the cerebral cortex in pain sensation. In *Cerebral Cortex*, Vol. 9 *Normal and Altered States of Function*, ed. A. Peters & E.G. Jones, pp. 153–212. New York and London: Plenum Press.

Kenshalo, D.R., Giesler, G.J., Leonard, R.B. & Willis, W.D. (1980). Responses of neurons in primate ventral posterior lateral nucleus to noxious stimuli. *J. Neurophysiol.*, **43**, 1594–614.

Kenshalo, D.R., Jr., Chudler, E.H., Anton, F. & Dubner, R. (1988). SI nociceptive neurons participate in the encoding process by which monkeys perceive the intensity of noxious thermal stimulation. *Brain Res.*, **454**, 378–82.

Kenshalo, D.R, Thomas, D.A. & Dubner, R. (1991). Primary somatosensory cortical lesions reduce the monkeys' ability to discriminate and detect noxious thermal stimulation. *Soc. Neurosci. Abst.*, **17**, 1206.

Kerr, F.W.L. (1975). The ventral spinothalamic tract and other ascending systems of the ventral funiculus of the spinal cord. *J. Comp. Neurol.*, **159**, 335–56.

Kevetter, G.A., Haber, L.H., Yezierski, R.P., Chung, J.M., Martin, R.F. & Willis, W.D. (1982). Cells of origin of the spinoreticular tract in the monkey. *J. Comp. Neurol.*, **207**, 61–74.

Kievit, J. & Kuypers, H.G.J.M. (1975). Subcortical afferents to the frontal lobe in the rhesus monkey studied by means of retrograde horseradish peroxidase. *Brain Res.*, **85**, 261–6.

Koyama, S., Katayama, Y., Maejima, S., Hirayama, T., Fujii, M. & Tsubokawa, T. (1993). Thalamic neuronal hyperactivity following transection of the spinothalamic tract in the cat: involvement of *N*-methyl-D-aspartate receptor. *Brain Res.*, **612**, 345–50.

Krubitzer, L., Clarey, J., Tweedale, R., Elston, G. & Calford, M. (1995). A redefinition of somatosensory areas in the lateral sulcus of macaque monkeys. *J. Neurosci.*, **15**, 3821–39.

Laitinen, L.V. (1988). Mesencephalotomy and thalamotomy for chronic pain. In *Modern Stereotactic Neurosurgery*, ed. L.D. Lunsford, pp. 269–77. Boston: Martinus Nijhoff Publishers.

Le Gros Clark, W.E. & Russell, W.R. (1940). Atrophy of the thalamus in a case of acquired hemiplegia associated with diffuse porencephaly and sclerosis of the left cerebral hemisphere. *J. Neurol., Neurosurg., Psychiatry*, **3**, 123–40.

Lee, J-L., Antezanna, D., Dougherty, P.M. & Lenz, F.A. (1999). Responses of neurons in the region of the thalamic somatosensory nucleus to mechanical and thermal stimuli graded into the painful range. *J. Comp. Neurol.*, **410**, 541–55.

Leijon, G., Boivie, J. & Johansson, I. (1989). Central post-stroke pain-neurological symptoms and pain characteristics. *Pain*, **36**, 13–25.

Lenz, F.A. (1992). The ventral posterior nucleus of thalamus is involved in the generation of central pain syndromes. *Am. Pain Soc. J.*, **1**, 42–60.

Lenz, F.A. & Dougherty, P.M. (1997). Pain processing in the human thalamus. In *Thalamus*: Volume II., ed. M. Steriade, E.G. Jones & D.A. McCormick, pp. 617–51. Oxford: Elsevier.

Lenz, F.A., Dostrovsky, J.O., Tasker, R.R., Yamashiro, K., Kwan, H.C. & Murphy, J.T. (1988). Single-unit analysis of the human ventral thalamic nuclear group: somatosensory responses. *J. Neurophysiol.*, **59**, 299–316.

Lenz, F.A., Kwan, H.C., Dostrovsky, J.O. & Tasker, R.R. (1989). Characteristics of the bursting pattern of action potentials that occur in the thalamus of patients with central pain. *Brain Res.*, **496**, 357–60.

Lenz, F.A., Seike, M., Lin, Y.C., Baker, F.H., Richardson, R.T. & Gracely, R.H. (1993a). Thermal and pain sensations evoked by microstimulation in the area of the human ventrocaudal nucleus (Vc). *J. Neurophysiol.*, **70**, 200–12.

Lenz, F.A., Seike, M., Lin, Y.C. et al., (1993b). Neurons in the area of human thalamic nucleus ventralis caudalis respond to painful heat stimuli. *Brain Res.*, **623**, 235–40.

Lenz, F.A., Kwan, H.C., Martin, R., Tasker, R., Richardson, R.T. & Dostrovsky, J.O. (1994a). Characteristics of somatotopic organization and spontaneous neuronal activity in the region of the thalamic principal sensory nucleus in patients with spinal cord transection. *J. Neurophysiol.*, **72**, 1570–87.

Lenz, F.A., Kwan, H.C., Martin, R.L., Tasker, R.R., Dostrovsky, J.O. & Lenz, Y.E. (1994b). Single neuron analysis of the human ventral thalamic nuclear group: tremor-related activity in functionally identified cells. *Brain*, **117**, 531–43.

Lenz, F.A., Gracely, R.H., Romanoski, A.J., Hope, E.J., Rowland, L.H. & Dougherty, P.M. (1995). Pain with a strong affective dimension reproduced by stimulation of the human somatosensory thalamus. *Soc. Neurosci. Abstr.*

Lenz, F.A., Gracely, R.H., Baker, F.H., Richardson, R.T. & Dougherty, P.M. (1998a). Reorganization of sensory modalities evoked by stimulation in the region of the principal sensory nucleus (ventral caudal – Vc) in patients with pain secondary to neural injury. *J. Comp. Neurol.*, **399**, 125–38.

Lenz, F.A., Rios, M.R., Chau, D., Krauss, G., Zirh, T.A. & Lesser, R.P. (1998b). Painful stimuli evoke potentials recorded over the parasylvian cortex in humans. *J. Neurophysiol.*, **80**, 2077–88.

Lenz, F.A., Rios, M.R., Zirh, T.A., Krauss, G. & Lesser, R.P. (1998c). Painful stimuli evoke potentials recorded over the human anterior cingulate gyrus. *J. Neurophysiol.*, **79**, 2231–4.

Lenz, F.A., Zirh, A.T., Garonzik, I.M. & Dougherty, P.M. (1998d). Neuronal activity in the region of the principal sensory nucleus of human thalamus (ventralis caudalis) in patients with pain following amputations. *Neuroscience*, **86**, 1065–81.

Lenz, F.A., Krauss, G., Treede, R.D. et al. (2000). Different generators in human temporal–parasylvian cortex account for subdural laser-evoked potentials, auditory-evoked potentials, and event-related potentials. *Neurosci. Lett.*, **279**, 153–6.

Lombard, M.C. & Larabi, Y. (1983). Electrophysiological study of cervical dorsal horn cells in partially deafferented rats. In *Advances in Pain Research and Therapy*, vol 5, ed. J.J. Bonica, U. Lindblom & A. Iggo, pp. 147–54. New York: Raven Press.

Lovick, T.A. (1993). Integrated activity of cardiovascular and pain regulatory systems: role in adaptive behavioural responses. *Prog. Neurobiol.*, **40**, 631–44.

Macchi, G. & Bentivoglio, M. (1986). The thalamic intralaminar nuclei and the cerebral cortex. In *Cerebral Cortex*, Vol. 5 *Sensory–Motor Areas and Aspects of Cortical Connectivity*, ed. E.G. Jones & A. Peters, pp. 355–401. New York and London: Plenum Press.

Maixner, W., Dubner, R., Kenshalo, D.R., Jr., Bushnell, M.C. & Oliveras, J.L. (1989). Responses of monkey medullary dorsal horn neurons during the detection of noxious heat stimuli. *J. Neurophysiol.*, **62**, 437–9.

Mantyh, P.W. (1983). The spinothalamic tract in primate: a re-examination using wheatgerm agglutinin conjugated with horseradish peroxidase. *Neuroscience*, **9**, 847–62.

Marshall, J. (1951). Sensory disturbances in cortical wounds with special reference to pain. *J. Neurol. Neurosurg. Psychiatry*, **14**, 187–204.

Mehler, W.R. (1962). The anatomy of the so-called 'pain tract' in man: an analysis of the course and distribution of the ascending fibers of the fasciculus anterolateralis. In *Basic Research in Paraplegia*, ed. J.D. French & R.W. Porter, pp. 26–55. Springfield, IL: Charles C. Thomas.

Mehler, W.R. (1966). The posterior thalamic region in man. *Confinia Neurol.*, **27**, 18–29.

Mehler, W.R. (1969). Some neurological species differences – a posteriori. *Ann. NY Acad. Sci.*, **167**, 424–68.

Mehler, W.R., Feferman, M.E. & Nauta, W.H.J. (1960). Ascending axon degeneration following anterolateral cordotomy. An experimental study in the monkey. *Brain*, **83**, 718–50.

Melzack, R. & Casey, K.L. (1968). Sensory, motivational, and central control determinants of pain. In *The Skin Senses*, ed. D.R. Kenshalo, pp. 423–43. Springfield, IL: Charles C. Thomas.

Menetrey, D., Chaouch, A., Binder, D. & Besson, J.M. (1982). The origin of the spinomesencephalic tract in the rat: an anatomical study using the retrograde transport of horseradish peroxidase. *J. Comp. Neurol.*, **206**, 193–207.

Mesulam, M-M. & Mufson, E.J. (1985). The insula of Reil in man and monkey. In *Cerebral Cortex*, Vol. 4, ed. A. Peters & E.G. Jones, pp. 179–226. New York: Plenum.

Meyer, M. (1947). Study of efferent connections of frontal lobe in human brain after leucotomy. *Brain*, **72**, 265–96.

Mishkin, M. (1979). Analogous neural models for tactual and visual learning. *Neuropsychology*, **17**, 139–51.

Moulton, E.A., Gullapalli, R.P., Small, S.L., Emge, D.K. & Greenspan, J.D. (1999). Intensity coding of mechanical pain in human S2 cortex. *Soc. Neurosci. Abst.*, **25**(140).

Mountcastle, V.B. & Henneman, E. (1949). Pattern of tactile representation in thalamus of cat. *J. Neurophysiol.*, **12**, 88–100.

Mufson, E.J. & Mesulam, M-M. (1982). Insula of the old world monkey. II: Afferent cortical input and comments on the claustrum. *J. Comp. Neurol.*, **212**, 23–37.

Musil, S.Y. & Olson, C.R. (1988). Organization of cortical and subcortical projections to anterior cingulate cortex in the cat. *J. Comp. Neurol.*, **272**, 203–18.

Nagaro, T., Amakawa, K., Kimura, S. & Arai, T. (1993). Reference of pain following percutaneous cervical cordotomy. *Pain*, **53**, 205–11.

Nakano, K., Hasegawa, Y., Tokushige, A., Nakagawa, S., Kayahara, T. & Mizuno, N. (1990). Topographical projections from the thalamus, subthalamic nucleus and pedunculopontine tegmental nucleus to the striatum of the japanese monkey, macaca fuscata. *Brain Res.*, **517**, 54–68.

Nashold, B.S., Jr., Wilson, W.P. & Slaughter, D.G. (1969). Sensations evoked by stimulation in the midbrain of man. *J. Neurosurg.*, **30**, 14–24.

Nyquist, J.K. & Greenhoot, J.H. (1974). A single neuron analysis of mesencenphalic reticular formation responses to high intensity cutaneous input in cat. *Brain Res.*, **70**, 157–64.

Oppenheimer, D.R. (1967). A case of stiatal hemiplegia. *J. Neurol., Neursurg., Psychiatry*, **30**, 134–9.

Palecek, J., Dougherty, P.M., Kim, S.H. et al. (1992a). Responses of spinothalamic tract neurons to mechanical and thermal stimuli in an experimental model of peripheral neuropathy in primates. *J. Neurophysiol.*, **68**, 1951–66.

Palecek, J., Paleckova, V., Dougherty, P.M., Carlton, S.M. & Willis, W.D. (1992b). Responses of spinothalamic tract cells to mechanical and thermal stimulation of skin in rats with experimental peripheral neuropathy. *J. Neurophysiol.*, **67**, 1562–73.

Patterson, J.T., Head, P.A., McNeill, D.L., Chung, K. & Coggeshall, R.E. (1989). Ascending unmyelinated primary afferent fibers in the dorsal funiculus. *J. Comp. Neurol.*, **290**, 384–90.

Patterson, J.T., Coggeshall, R.E., Lee, W.T. & Chung, K. (1990). Long ascending unmyelinated primary afferent axons in the rat dorsal column: immunohistochemical localizations. *Neurosci. Lett.*, **108**, 6–10.

Penfield, W. & Faulk, M.E., Jr. (1955). The insula: Further observations on its function. *Brain*, **78**, 445–70.

Pollin, B. & Albe-Fessard, D.G. (1979). Organization of somatic thalamus in monkeys with and without section of dorsal spinal tracts. *Brain Res.*, **173**, 431–49.

Powell, T.P.S. & Cowan, W.M. (1967). The interpretation of the degenerative changes in the intralaminar nuclei of the thalamus. *J. Neurol., Neurosurg., Psychiatry*, **30**, 140–53.

Price, D.D. & Dubner, R. (1977). Neurons that subserve the sensory-discriminative aspects of pain. *Pain*, **3**, 307–38.

Radhakrishnan, V., Tsoukatos, J., Davis, K.D., Tasker, R.R. Lozano, A.M. & Dostrovsky, J.O. (1999). A comparison of the burst activity of lateral thalamic neurons in chronic pain and non-pain patients. *Pain*, **80**, 567–75.

Rainville, P., Duncan, G.H., Price, D.D., Carrier, B. & Bushnell, M.C. (1997). Pain affect encoded in human anterior cingulate but not somatosensory cortex. *Science*, **277**, 968–71.

Ralston, H.J. & Ralston, D.D. (1992). The primate dorsal spinothalamic tract: evidence for a specific termination in the posterior nuclei [Po/SG] of the thalamus. *Pain*, **48**, 107–18.

Ralston, H.J. & Ralston, D.D. (1994). Medial lemniscal and spinal projections to the macaque thalamus: an electron microscopic study of differing GABAergic circuitry serving thalamic somatosensory mechanisms. *J. Neurosci.*, **14**, 2485–502.

Ralston, H.J., Ohara, P.T., Meng, X.W., Wells, J. & Ralston, D.D. (1996). Transneuronal changes in the inhibitory circuitry of the macaque somatosensory thalamus following lesions of the dorsal column nuclei. *J. Comp. Neurol.*, **371**, 325–35.

Rausell, E., Bae, C.S., Vineula, A., Huntley, G.W. & Jones, E.G. (1992). Calbindin and parvalbumin cells in monkey VPL thalamic nucleus: distribution, laminar cortical projections, and relations to spinothalamic terminations. *J. Neurosci.*, **12**, 4088–111.

Richardson, D.E. (1967). Thalamotomy for intractable pain. *Confinia Neurol.*, **29**, 139–45.

Rinaldi, P.C., Young, R.F., Albe-Fessard, D.G. & Chodakiewitz, J. (1991). Spontaneous neuronal hyperactivity in the medial and intralaminar thalamic nuclei in patients with deafferentation pain. *J. Neurosurg.*, **74**, 415–21.

Rodin, B.E. & Kruger, L. (1984). Deafferentation in animals as a model for the study of pain: an alternative hypothesis. *Brain Res. Rev.*, **7**, 213–28.

Rothwell, J.C., Obeso, J.A., Traub, M.M. & Marsden, C.D. (1983). The behaviour of long-latency stretch reflex in patients with Parkinson's disease. *J. Neurol., Neurosurg., Psychiatry*, **46**, 35–44.

Sadikot, A.F., Parent, A. & Francois, C. (1990). The centre median and parafascicular thalamic nuclei project respectively to the sensorimotor and associative-limbic territories in the squirrel monkey. *Brain Res.*, **510**, 161–5.

Sadikot, A.F., Parent, A. & Francois, C. (1992a). Efferent connections of the centromedian and parafascicular thalamic nuclei in the squirrel monkey: a PHA-L study of subcortical projections. *J. Comp. Neurol.*, **315**, 137–59.

Sadikot, A.F., Parent, W., Smith, Y. & Bolam, J.P. (1992b). Efferent connections of the centromedian and parafascicular thalamic nuclei in the squirrel monkey: a light and electron microscopic study of the thalamostriatal projection in relation to striatal homogeneity. *J. Comp. Neurol.*, **320**, 228–42.

Sano, K. (1977a). Intralaminar thalamotomy (thalamolaminotomy) and postero-medial hypothalamotomy in the treatment of intractable pain. *Prog. Neurol. Surg.*, **8**, 50–103.

Sano, K. (1977b). Intralaminar thalamotomy (thalamolaminotomy) and posteromedial hypothalamotomy in the treatment of intractable pain. In *Prog. Neurol. Surg.*, ed. H. Krayenbuhl, P.E. Maspes & W.H. Sweet, pp. 50–103. Basel: Karger.

Sano, K. (1979). Stereotaxic thalamolaminotomy and posteromedial hypothalamotomy for the relief of intractable pain. In *Advances in Pain Research and Therapy*. Vol. 2, ed. J.J. Bonica & V. Ventrafridda, pp. 475–85. New York: Raven Press.

Saper, C.B. (1995). The spinoparabrachial pathway: shedding new light on an old path. *J. Comp. Neurol.*, **353**, 477–9.

Saper, C.B. & Loewy, A.D. (1980). Efferent connections of the parabrachial nucleus in the rat. *Brain Res.*, **197**, 291–317.

Slugg, R.M. & Light, A.R. (1994). Spinal cord and trigeminal projections to the pontine parabrachial region in the rat as demonstrated with *Phaseolus vulgaris* leucoagglutinin. *J. Comp. Neurol.*, **339**, 49–61.

Smith, Y. & Parent, A. (1986). Differential connections of the caudate nucleus and putamen in the squirrel monkey (*Saimiri sciureus*). *Neuroscience*, **18**, 347–71.

Spiegel, E.A., Kletzkin, M. & Szekely, E.G. (1954). Pain reactions upon stimulation of the tectum mesencephali. *J. Neuropath. Exp. Neurol.*, **13**, 212–20.

Strick, P.L. (1975). Multiple sources of thalamic input to the primate motor cortex. *J. Neurophysiol.*, **88**, 372–7.

Surmeier, D.J., Honda, C.N. & Willis, W.D., Jr. (1988). Natural groupings of primate spinothalamic neurons based on cutaneous stimulation. Physiological and anatomical features. *J. Neurophysiol.*, **59**, 833–60.

Talbot, J.D., Marrett, S., Evans, A.C., Meyer, E., Bushnell, M.C. & Duncan, G.H. (1991). Multiple representations of pain in human cerebral cortex [see comments]. *Science*, **251**, 1355–8.

Talbot, J.D., Villemure, J.G., Bushnell, M.C. & Duncan. G.H. (1995). Evaluation of pain perception after anterior capsulotomy: a case report. *Somatosens. Motor Res.*, **12**, 115–26.

Tarkka, I.M. & Treede, R.D. (1993). Equivalent electrical source analysis of pain-related somatosensory evoked potentials elicited by a CO_2 laser. *J. Clin. Neurophysiol.*, **10**, 513–19.

Tobias, T. (1975). Afferents to prefrontal cortex from the thalamic mediodorsal nucleus in the rhesus monkey. *Brain Res.*, **83**, 191–212.

Tsubokawa, T. & Moriyasu, N. (1975). Follow-up results of centre median thalamotomy for relief of intractable pain. *Confinia Neurol.*, **37**, 280–4.

Urabe, M. & Tsubokawa, T. (1965). Stereotaxic thalamotomy for the relief of intractable pain. *Tohoku J. Exp. Med.*, **85**, 286–300.

Van Buren, J.M. & Borke, R.C. (1972). *Variations and Connections of the Human Thalamus*. Berlin: Springer Verlag.

Vestergaard, K., Nielsen, J., Andersen, G., Ingeman-Nielsen, M., Arendt-Nielsen, L. & Jensen, T.S. (1997). Sensory abnormalities in consecutive unselected patients with central post-stroke pain. *Pain*, **61**, 177–86.

Vierck, C.J., Jr. (1998). Impaired detection of repetitive stimulation following interruption of the dorsal spinal column in primates. *Somatosens. Motor Res.*, **15**, 157–63.

Vierck, C.J., Jr. & Luck, M.M. (1979). Loss and recovery of reactivity to noxious stimuli in monkeys with primary spinothalamic cordotomies, followed by secondary and tertiary lesions of other cord sectors. *Brain*, **102**, 233–48.

Vierck, C.J., Jr., Hamilton, D.M. & Thornby, J.I. (1971). Pain reactivity of monkeys after lesions to the dorsal and lateral columns of the spinal cord. *Exp. Brain Res.*, **13**, 140–58.

Vierck, C.J., Jr., Cohen, R.H. & Cooper, B.Y. (1983). Effects of spinal tractotomy on spatial sequence recognition in macaques. *J. Neurosci.*, **3**, 280–90.

Vierck, C.J., Greenspan, J.D. & Ritz, L.A. (1990). Long-term changes in purposive and reflexive responses to nociceptive stimulation following anterolateral chordotomy. *J. Neurosci.*, **10**, 2077–95.

Villanueva, L., Cliffer, K.D., Sorkin, L.S., Le Bars, D. & Willis, W.D., Jr. (1990). Convergence of heterotopic nociceptive information onto neurons of caudal medullary reticular formation in monkey (*Macaca fascicularis*). *J. Neurophysiol.*, **63**, 1118–27.

Vogt, C. & Vogt, O. (1941). Thalamusstudien I–III. *J. Psychol. Neurol. (Leipzig).*, **50**, 32–152.

Vogt, B.A., Pandya, D.N. & Rosene, D.L. (1987). Cingulate cortex of the rhesus monkey: I cytoarchitecture and thalamic afferents. *J. Comp. Neurol.*, **262**, 256–70.

Voris, H.C. & Whisler, W.W. (1975). Results of stereotaxic surgery for intractable pain. *Confinia Neurol.*, **37**, 86–96.

Walker, A.E. (1938). The Thalamus of the Chimpanzee. I. Terminations of the somatic afferent systems. *Confinia Neurol.*, **1**, 99–127.

Walker, A.E. (1943). Central representation of pain. *Res. Publi. Assoc. Res. Nerv. Ment. Dis.*, **23**, 63–85.

Wall, P.D. & Egger, M.D. (1971). Formation of new connections in adult rat brains after partial deafferentation. *Nature*, **232**, 542–5.

Wall, P.D. & Melzack, R. (1984). *Textbook of Pain*. Edinburgh: Churchill Livingstone.

Willis, W.D. (1985). *The Pain System*. Basel: Karger.

Willis, W.D. & Coggeshall, R.E. (1991). *Sensory Mechanisms of the Spinal Cord*. New York: Plenum Press.

Wolfle, T.L., Mayer, D.J., Carder, B. & Liebeskind, J.C. (1971). Motivational effects of electrical stimulation in dorsal tegmentum of the rat. *Physiol. Behav.*, **7**, 569–74.

Yasui, Y., Itoh, K., Kamiya, H., Ino, T. & Mizuno, N. (1988). Cingulate gyrus of the cat receives projection fibers from the thalamic region ventral border of the ventrobasal complex. *J. Comp. Neurol.*, **274**, 91–100.

Yezierski, R.P. & Schwartz, R.H. (1986). Response and receptive-field properties of spinomesencephalic tract cells in the cat. *J. Neurophysiol.*, **55**, 76–96.

Yezierski, R.P., Sorkin, L.S. & Willis, W.D. (1987). Response properties of spinal neurons projecting to midbrain or midbrain-thalamus in the monkey. *Brain Res.*, **437**, 165–70.

Young, R.F. (1989). Brain and spinal stimulation: how and to whom! *Clin. Neurosurg.*, **35**, 429–47.

Young, R.F., Kroening, R., Fulton, W., Feldman, R.A. & Chambi, I. (1985). Electrical stimulation of the brain in treatment of chronic pain. *J. Neurosurg.*, **62**, 389–96.

Zaslansky, R., Sprecher, E., Katz, Y., Rozenberg, B., Hemli, J.A. & Yarnitsky, D. (1996). Pain-evoked potentials: what do they really measure? *EEG Clin. Neurophysiol.*, **100**, 384–92.

Zhang, X., Wenk, H.N., Honda, C.N. & Giesler, G.J., Jr. (2000). Locations of spinothalamic tract axons in cervical and thoracic spinal cord white matter in monkeys. *J. Neurophysiol.*, **83**, 2869–80.

60

Management of chronic pain

Russell K. Portenoy

Department of Pain Medicine and Palliative Care, Beth Israel Medical Center, New York, NY, USA

Pain is the most common reason that patients seek medical attention. Most community-based surveys indicate that at least 15% of the population have chronic pain associated with adverse consequences in varied domains of functioning (Smith et al., 2001). The aggregate cost of unrelieved pain for health care systems and national economies is staggering.

All clinicians encounter patients with chronic pain. An understanding of the nature of pain provides a foundation for comprehensive assessment. Assessment, in turn, guides the long-term therapeutic strategy for enhancing the comfort of these patients and addressing their pain-related disability.

Definition of pain

Pain has been defined by the International Association for the Study of Pain (IASP) as 'an unpleasant sensory and emotional experience which we primarily associate with tissue damage or describe in terms of such damage, or both (Mersky & Bogduk, 1994)'. This definition underscores the potential contribution of sensory, emotional, and cognitive processes in the experience of pain, and the complex relationship between tissue injury and pain perception. Although pain is typically perceived to be a primary indicator of tissue injury, the relationship between pain and tissue damage is neither uniform nor constant. Pain may occur in association with progressive or stable chronic disease, or may occur in the complete absence of an identifiable lesion.

This complexity highlights the need to distinguish the neural processes initiated by tissue injury from pain. The mechanisms induced in neural pathways by potentially tissue-damaging stimuli are termed 'nociception', and are neither necessary nor sufficient for the experience of pain.

Pain is the perception of nociception, and like other perceptions, is inherently subjective and can be influenced by a variety of non-nociceptive factors. These factors may be organic, e.g. the aberrant processes in the nervous system that result in neuropathic pain, or psychologic.

Given the subjective nature of pain, pain specialists generally believe that the clinician is best served by assuming that the patient is reporting a true experience, even when a causative lesion cannot be demonstrated. Clinical discussion focused on whether or not a pain is 'real' usually obscures the important issues and is unhelpful. Malingering or factitious pain is rare in clinical practice and, in almost all cases, the clinician is better served by assuming that the pain is truly experienced and then thoughtfully inferring the range of factors – ongoing tissue injury, neuropathic processes and psychologic processes – that may be sustaining the pain.

Early definitions of chronic pain used only a temporal measure, specifically pain persisting longer than 3 months or 6 months. More recently, a broader definition has been preferred. Pain is chronic if it persists for a month beyond the usual course of an acute illness or a reasonable duration for an injury to heal, if it is associated with a chronic pathologic process, or if it recurs at intervals for months or years (Bonica, 1990).

Pain assessment

The complexity of chronic pain underscores the critical importance of a comprehensive assessment as a first step in successful management. This assessment includes characterization of the pain, clarification of the relationship between the symptom and underlying diseases, and evaluation of the various comorbidities that may become important ancillary targets of therapy.

Table 60.1. Pain characteristics

Characteristic	Elements
Temporal	Acute, recurrent or chronic Onset and duration Course Daily variation (including breakthrough pain)
Intensity	Pain 'on average,' Pain 'at its worst,' Pain 'right now' Pain 'at its least'
Location	Focal or multifocal Referred Superficial or deep
Quality	Varied descriptors e.g., aching, stabbing, or 　burning Familiar or unfamiliar
Exacerbating/ relieving factors	Volitional ('incident pain') vs. non-volitional

Source: Adapted from Portenoy & Kanner (1996).

Evaluation of pain characteristics

Like all symptoms, pain is evaluated by the verbal reports used by patients to describe the experience (Portenoy & Kanner, 1996) (Table 60.1). Temporal descriptors are essential and include the onset and duration of the pain, the occurrences of episodic pain, and the fluctuation during the day.

Measurement of pain severity can be performed using simple unidimensional scales or multidimensional questionnaires. The choice of one or another method in clinical practice is probably less important than its systematic application repeatedly over time (Au et al., 1994). Because measuring pain enhances its visibility to clinicians, measurement and documentation are major elements in the new standards of institutional pain care adopted by the United States Joint Commission on the Accreditation of Healthcare Organizations. In clinical practice, the clinician is usually best served by selecting a simple approach, e.g. a four-point verbal rating scale such as 'none', 'mild', 'moderate', or 'severe', or an eleven-point, '0–10' numeric scale, and incorporating it into the routine. The time frame, e.g. 'pain right now' or 'pain during the past day', and the clinical context, e.g. after a dose of pain medication, must be defined to adequately measure pain.

Other important characteristics include pain location, quality, and factors that exacerbate or relieve the pain

(Table 60.1). The medical record of patients with chronic pain should document these characteristics so that they can be tracked over time.

Etiology, inferred pathophysiology, and syndromes

The pain assessment, combined with information from the physical examination and radiographic or laboratory evaluations, may identify a pain syndrome or an etiology for the pain, and allow inferences about the broad set of mechanisms that might be sustaining it. These understandings may suggest additional investigations and guide therapeutic decision making.

If a discrete etiology can be reasonably identified as a cause for the pain, this information may be helpful in clarifying the nature of an underlying disease, indicating prognosis (for the pain or the disease itself), or suggesting the use of specific primary therapies. For example, the identification of a neoplasm impinging on a nerve plexus may allow use of an antineoplastic treatment, such as radiotherapy.

Although the classification of pain according to inferences about the underlying mechanisms oversimplifies complex pathophysiological processes, the approach has utility in clinical practice. Based on the characteristics of the pain and its etiologies, pathophysiology can be labeled 'nociceptive', neuropathic', psychogenic', or 'mixed' (Table 60.2). If pain persists in the absence of an identifiable organic substrate (nociceptive or neuropathic) and there is no evidence of a substantial psychologic contribution, it is best to label the pain 'idiopathic' and reassess in the future.

These pathophysiologic constructs have important therapeutic implications. For example, the response to opioids appears to be relatively better during treatment of nociceptive pains than neuropathic pains (Portenoy et al., 1990). Numerous drugs are now targeted specifically to the treatment of neuropathic pain (see below).

The pain assessment also may identify a discrete pain syndrome, identification of which can guide additional evaluation, indicate the likely etiology, or suggest a therapeutic approach. A very large number of disease-related pain syndromes have been defined and varied systems of classification have been proposed. For example, neuropathic pain may be classified by the presumed site of the sustaining pathophysiology – peripheral vs. central (Table 60.3) (Caraceni & Portenoy, 1998) – or by some combination or neurologic findings and etiology (Table 60.4) (Portenoy, 1996a,b).

In some cases, syndromic labels are imprecise and must be applied cautiously. For example, the generic terms 'chronic pain syndrome', 'chronic non-malignant

Table 60.2. Inferred pathophysiologies

Descriptor	Presumed mechanism	Characteristics
Nociceptive pain	Ongoing activation of somatic or visceral nociceptors as a result of persistent tissue injury; nervous system is presumed to be intact	Quality usually aching, sharp, throbbing; described as 'familiar' pain; evaluation typically reveals a source of tissue injury perceived to be commensurate with the pain
Neuropathic pain	Related to aberrant somato-sensory processing in the peripheral or central nervous systems; presumed to be sustained by neural processes that become independent, in part, from areas of tissue injury	Quality may be like nociceptive pain, e.g. aching from radiculopathy, or may be dysesthetic (abnormal, unfamiliar) and described as burning, shooting, electrical; evaluation may or may not reveal neurologic findings
Psychogenic pain	Predominantly determined by psychologic factors	Quality and characteristics variable; psychiatric assessment allows classification by specific diagnoses, e.g. pain disorder, somatization disorder, etc.
Mixed syndromes	Multiple mechanisms	Varied
Idiopathic pain	Unable to infer	Varied

Table 60.3. Pathophysiologic classification of neuropathic pains

Presumed to be primarily sustained by central mechanisms
Complex regional pain syndrome Type I (reflex sympathetic dystrophy) and type II (causalgia)

Deafferentation pain syndromes
  Central pain
  Postherpetic neuralgia
  Root avulsion pain
  Phantom pain
  Miscellaneous syndromes (anesthesia dolorosa)

Presumed to be primarily sustained by peripheral mechanisms
Painful polyneuropathies

Compressive mononeuropathies, e.g. discogenic radiculopathy

Infiltrative or ischemic mononeuropathies, e.g. malignant plexopathies

Traumatic mononeuropathies, e.g. postamputation neuroma

Presumed to be sustained by both peripheral and central mechanisms
Lancinating neuralgias, e.g. trigeminal neuralgia

Source: Adapted from Caraceni & Portenoy (1998).

Table 60.4. Etiologic classification in two types of neuropathic pain

	Possible etiologies
Central pain (lesion in cord, brainstem, or cerebrum)	Trauma
	Ischemia
	Neoplasm
	Syrinx formation
	Focal demyelination
	Infection
	Other
Painful polyneuropathy	Metabolic disorders
	Diabetes
	Hypovitaminosis
	Hypothyroidism
	Uremia
	Amyloid
	Drugs or toxins
	Neoplasm
	Hereditary painful polyneuropathy
	Others

pain syndrome' and 'chronic intractable pain syndrome' are often used but not well defined in the literature. Typically, these terms refer to patients who have pain that is perceived to be excessive for the identifiable organic substrate and is associated with a high level of disability and psychiatric comorbidity. Although the challenge that such patients pose – to enhance analgesia while address-ing serious functional disturbances – is very real, these labels can be stigmatizing and divert attention from potentially treatable nociceptive or neuropathic pro-cesses. The same risk applies to some site-specific terms, such as atypical facial pain, failed low back surgery syn-drome, chronic tension headache, and chronic pelvic pain of unknown etiology.

Evaluation of associated phenomena

The assessment of the medical condition, physical impairments, psychological and social functioning, and prior therapies is an integral part of the pain evaluation, and is essential in developing the therapeutic strategy. The evaluation of pain-related disability as part of this process is particularly important. In a broad sense, the goal is to first clarify the degree to which pain is accompanied by disability, and then to deconstruct the latter phenomenon and understand the various physical and psychosocial factors that may be sustaining it. This assessment will identify patients whose pain syndromes would be most appropriately managed using a multimodality approach that includes interventions that specifically address functional disturbances or impaired quality of life. Some patients will be identified whose disability is sufficient to justify referral to a multidisciplinary pain management program.

The psychological assessment should address the interaction among pain and a spectrum of psychological concerns, including coping and distress, personality, and both present and past psychiatric disorders. When a significant psychiatric disorder (i.e. major depression, anxiety disorder, panic disorder, somatization, or severe personality disorder) is suspected, referral for psychiatric evaluation and specialized treatment is warranted.

The psychologic assessment also should attempt to identify behavioural contingencies and secondary gains that may be sustaining the pain and disability. Although families can be a source of great support for patients who are attempting to cope with pain, the dynamics in some homes have maladaptive consequences. Behavioural contingencies may be identified that reinforce pain, or pain-related behaviours (such as strong encouragement to stay in bed), and could be directly addressed as part of the treatment plan developed by the physician.

The history of prior drug use is an essential part of the assessment. This history should address all types of drug use, including prescription drugs, over-the-counter remedies, and both licit and illicit recreational drugs. A history of substance abuse is extremely important and deliberate questioning may be required to obtain sufficient detail (Passik and Portenoy, 1998). The history should clarify the use of specific drugs (including alcohol) and determine whether this use is remote, recent or ongoing.

Pain management

A comprehensive assessment allows the development of a therapeutic strategy that combines appropriate interven-

Table 60.5. Interventions for pain and pain-related disability

Category	Examples
Pharmacotherapy	
Non-opioid	numerous NSAIDs,
Opioid	various opioids,
Adjuvant analgesic	antidepressants, anticonvulsants, and many other classes
Rehabilitative	physical/occupational therapy, orthoses
Neurostimulatory	transcutaneous electrical nerve stimulation
Psychologic	cognitive/behavioural therapy
Anesthesiologic	neural blockade, neuraxial infusion
Neurosurgical	neuroma resection, CNS lesions, deep brain stimulation
Complementary and alternative	acupuncture, massage, chiropractic, mind-body approaches, herbal therapies
Lifestyle changes	weight loss, exercise

tions from a very large number of potential candidates (Table 60.5). In some cases, the therapeutic strategy can include a primary treatment directed against an etiology of the pain. In others, the strategy can attempt to address disability and various medical and psychosocial comorbidities, the overall goal of which is to improve function and quality of life in tandem with enhanced comfort. There are many interventions that could be offered in a multimodality approach to the pain itself, and the decision to emphasize one type, e.g. pharmacotherapy, over another, e.g. rehabilitative, or to combine them from the start, must be individualized based on the priorities identified by the assessment.

Pharmacologic therapies

Analgesic drugs can be divided into the non-opioid analgesics, the so-called adjuvant analgesics, and the opioid analgesics. The non-opioid analgesics refer to acetaminophen, dipyrone, and all the non-steroidal anti-inflammatory drugs (NSAIDs). The term 'adjuvant analgesic' can be applied to any drug that has a primary indication other than pain but is known to be analgesic in specific circumstances.

Non-opioid analgesics: NSAIDs

The NSAIDs comprise an extremely diverse group of drugs (Table 60.6). They all inhibit the enzyme cyclo-oxygenase

Table 60.6. Non-steroidal anti-inflammatory drugs

Chemical class	Drug	Recommended starting dose (mg/d)	Recommended maximum dose (mg/d)
Non-selective COX inhibitors			
Salicylates	aspirin	2600	6000
	diflunisal	1000×1	1500
	choline magnesium trisalicylate	1500×1 then 1000	4000
	salsalate	1500×1 then 1000	4000
Propionic acids	ibuprofen	1600	4200
	naproxen	500	1500
	naproxen sodium	550	1375
	fenoprofen	800	3200
	ketoprofen	100	300
	flurbiprofen	100	300
	oxaprozin	600	1800
Acetic acids	indomethacin	75	200
	tolmetin	600	2000
	sulindac	300	400
	diclofenac	75	200
	ketorolac (IM)	30 (loading)	60
	ketorolac (PO)	40	40
	etodolac	600	1200
Oxicams	piroxicam	20	40
	meloxicam	7.5	15
Naphthyl-alkanones	nabumetone	1000	2000
Fenamates	mefenamic acid	500×1	1000
	meclofenamic acid	150	400
Pyrazoles	phenylbutazone	300	400
Selective COX-2 inhibitors			
	celecoxib	200	400
	rofecoxib	12.5–25	25

(COX) and reduce the synthesis of prostaglandins. Prostaglandins are key inflammatory mediators and sensitize primary afferent nerves that respond to noxious stimuli in the periphery. Although inhibition of these peripheral processes can explain both the analgesic and anti-inflammatory effects of the NSAIDs, prostaglandin inhibition in the central nervous system probably also contributes to the analgesia produced by these drugs (Willer et al., 1989). A central mechanism predominates in the analgesia produced by acetaminophen and dipyrone, which have minimal to no peripheral anti-inflammatory effects, and also presumably accounts for he observed disparity between the anti-inflammatory and analgesic potencies of some NSAIDs (McCormack & Brune, 1999).

Cyclo-oxygenase is produced in two isoforms, COX-1 and COX-2. COX-1 is relatively more constitutive and is involved in physiologic processes, whereas COX-2 is gen-erally more inducible and involved in the inflammatory cascade. Although the commercially available NSAIDs vary in the extent which they affect COX-1 and COX-2 (some, such as meloxicam and nambumetone are relatively COX-2 selective), all are considered to be non-selective COX-1 and COX-2 inhibitors. The inhibition of the constitutive isoform produced by these drugs is associated with their gastrointestinal toxicities.

COX-2 selective inhibitors are now commercially available and substantially reduce the gastrointestinal risks associated with NSAID therapy (Simon et al., 1999; Langman et al., 1999). These drugs do not have demonstrably lesser renal toxicity than the non-selective COX-1 and COX-2 inhibitors.

Although the maximal efficacy of the NSAIDs varies with the type of pain, these drugs are generally considered to be non-specific analgesics. Nonetheless, clinical observation suggests that they have relatively better efficacy in pain related to a grossly inflammatory process and bone pain, and relatively poorer efficacy in neuropathic pains. Their dose–response relationships are characterized by a minimal effective dose, dose-dependent analgesic effects, and a ceiling dose for analgesia. The existence of a ceiling dose implies that these drugs have limited maximal efficacy and are usually considered first-line for pains that are mild to moderate in severity.

There is large individual variation in the effective dose range and the dose associated with toxicity. Moreover, the maximal efficacy of the NSAIDs varies across drugs in any individual patient. Although an explanation for this phenomenon is lacking, it has important clinical implications. Sequential trials may demonstrate striking differences in effectiveness.

The potential for toxicity during NSAID therapy influences the decision to initiate therapy, the selection of drugs, and the approach to dosing and monitoring. Clinically important adverse gastrointestinal (GI) symptoms occur in about 10% of patients treated with the non-selective COX-1 and COX-2 NSAIDS, and ulcers occur in about 2% (Loeb et al., 1992). Although some surveys suggest that the risk is limited to gastric ulceration, other data implicate both gastric and duodenal lesions. Nausea and abdominal pain are poor predictors of serious GI toxicity; as many as two-thirds of NSAID users have no symptoms before bleeding or perforation.

The factors that have been associated with an increased risk of ulceration include advanced age, higher NSAID dose, concomitant administration of a corticosteroid, and a history of either ulcer disease or previous GI complications from NSAIDs (Loeb et al., 1992). Heavy alcohol or cigarette consumption may also increase the risk. A role for infection with the bacterium, *Helicobacter pylori*, in NSAID-related gastropathy has been suggested but never proved.

There are differences in the potential for GI toxicity among the various NSAIDs. As noted, the COX-2 selective drugs significantly reduce the risk of both GI symptoms and ulcer formation (Simon et al., 1999; Langman et al., 1999). However, comparative epidemiologic data, for these drugs and others, are limited. It is generally accepted that some NSAIDs have a relatively lesser risk of serious GI toxicity (such as the non-acetylated salicylates, choline magnesium trisalicylate and salsalate; ibuprofen and several other proprionic acids; diclofenac, and nabumetone), whereas others have a relatively greater risk (such as ketorolac, piroxicam and the fenamates).

The risk of ulcer can be reduced by concurrent administration of gastroprotective therapy (La Corte et al., 1999). Misoprostol, a prostaglandin analogue, reduces the incidence of NSAID-induced ulcers without reversing anti-inflammatory and analgesic effects. Proton pump inhibitors, such as omeprazole and lansoprazole, also have established efficacy. Studies of H2 blockers have been mixed, but a trial of higher dose famotidine was positive (Taha et al., 1996). Other interventions, such as antacids and sulcrafate, may reduce symptoms but do not decrease ulcer risk.

At the present time, it is reasonable to consider first-line use of the COX-2 selective drugs for patients at relatively high risk for GI toxicity, such as the elderly. Alternatively, co-administration of a gastroprotective therapy could be considered. There are no data presently by which to judge the relative cost-effectiveness of these approaches. Although changing practice patterns suggest that many clinicians are positioning the COX-2 selective drugs ahead of others in all types of patients, studies that confirm the advantages of doing so are still lacking.

All NSAIDs can cause serious renal toxicity (Murray and Brater, 1993). They must be used cautiously in patients who have nephropathies or are likely to have subclinical disease as a result of advanced age, prior treatment with nephrotoxic therapy (such as platinum-based chemotherapy), or an underlying disease.

Although there are large drug-to-drug differences in the degree to which various NSAIDs affect platelet function, the safety of these drugs in patients predisposed to bleeding has not been established in the clinical setting. All these drugs should be used cautiously in patients with a bleeding diathesis. The COX-2 inhibitors do not affect platelets.

Long-term NSAID therapy should be monitored for adverse effects. This monitoring might include periodic testing for occult fecal blood and an evaluation of hemoglobin, renal function and hepatic function. Patients who are predisposed to adverse effects and those who are receiving relatively high doses should be monitored relatively more frequently.

Although studies of dosing protocols in different patient populations are limited, it is prudent to initiate NSAID therapy with gradual dose escalation from a relatively low starting dose when patients have mild to moderate pain or a relatively increased risk of NSAID toxicity. During therapy, dose escalation can be considered if pain is uncontrolled, side effects are not intolerable, and the conventional maximal dose has not yet been reached. Dose escalation will not yield increased effects if the patient is at the ceiling dose. If a ceiling dose or conventional maximal dose is reached without achieving satisfactory analgesia, an alternative NSAID trial should be considered.

Adjuvant analgesics

The adjuvant analgesics include numerous drugs in diverse classes (Table 60.7) (Portenoy, 1998). The term

Table 60.7. Adjuvant analgesics

Multipurpose analgesics	Examples
Antidepressants	
Tricyclic antidepressants	amitriptyline
	desipramine
SSRIs/SNRIs[a]	paroxetine
	venlafaxine
Others	maprotiline
	buproprion
Alpha-2 adrenergic	clonidine
agonists	tizanidine
Corticosteroids	dexamethasone
	prednisone
For neuropathic pain	
Anticonvulsants	gabapentin
	carbamazepine
	phenytoin
	valproate
	clonazepam
	lamotrigine
	topiramate
	tiagabine
	oxcarbazepine
	zonisamide
	levetiracetam
Oral local anesthetics	mexiletine
	tocainide
NMDA receptor antagonists	ketamine
	dextromethorphan
	amantadine
Miscellaneous	baclofen
	calcitonin
Drugs used for CRPS or	calcitonin
suspected SMP[b]	corticosteroids
	clonidine
	prazosin
	phenoxybenzamine
	nifedipine
Topical agents	capsaicin
	local anesthetics
	NSAIDs
For headache	calcium channel blockers
	beta blockers
	antidepressants
	anticonvulsants
	ergot derivatives
	triptans
	ACE inhibitors
For cancer-related bone pain	bisphosphonates, e.g.
	pamidronate
	calcitonin
	radiopharmaceuticals, e.g.
	strontium-89 and
	samarium-153

Table 60.7 (*cont.*)

Multipurpose analgesics	Examples
For painful bowel obstruction	scopolamine
	glycopyrrolate
	octreotide

Notes:
[a] SSRI = serotonin-selective reuptake inhibitor; SNRI = serotonin- and norepineprine-selective reuptake inhibitors.
[b] CRPS = complex regional pain syndrome; SMP = sympathetically maintained pain.

'adjuvant', which was coined in the context of cancer pain management, has become a misnomer as the role of these drugs has been expanded to the primary treatment of many pain syndromes.

Multipurpose adjuvant analgesics
With clinical trials demonstrating efficacy in diverse types of chronic pain, some drug classes are best considered multipurpose analgesics. In this sense, they are similar to the opioids and the NSAIDs.

Antidepressants
The analgesic efficacy of the tricyclic antidepressants (TCAs) has been established in many painful disorders, including headache, arthritis, low back pain, postherpetic neuralgia, painful polyneuropathy, and fibromyalgia (Monks & Merskey, 1999). Both the tertiary amine TCAs (such as amitriptyline, imipramine and doxepin) and the secondary amine compounds (such as desipramine and nortriptyline) have analgesic effects. The supporting evidence is best for amitriptyline and desipramine (Max et al., 1992). Controlled trials also have established the efficacy of some of the serotonin-selective reuptake inhibitors (such as paroxetine), the serotonin- and norepinephrine-selective reuptake inhibitors (such as venlafaxine), and other antidepressant classes. Together, the extant data suggest that all antidepressants have the potential to be analgesic, and that the TCAs are likely to have higher analgesic efficacy overall than the newer drugs.

The analgesia produced by antidepressant drugs is believed to be due to their actions on endogenous monoaminergic pain modulating systems, particularly those that use norepinephrine or serotonin. Although positive mood effects may be beneficial, they are not required for analgesic efficacy.

It is reasonable to consider a TCA as the first-line drug if pain is a primary indication and the patient is likely to tolerate the drug. A tertiary amine, such as amitriptyline, might be considered first, but avoided if the patient is likely to experience troublesome sedative, anticholinergic, or cardiovascular toxicity. The secondary amine TCAs have fewer side effects and are often used instead. The newer antidepressants usually are better tolerated than the TCAs overall, and should be considered for those who cannot tolerate TCAs or are substantially predisposed to side effects.

Variability in the analgesic responses to antidepressant drugs is common and sequential trials are appropriate in an effort to identify an effective and well tolerated drug. When a TCA is used, the analgesic effect is typically obtained at doses lower than the antidepressant dose and the onset of analgesia is more rapid (within a week) than effects on mood.

Alpha-2 adrenergic agonists

Clonidine and tizanidine are alpha-2 adrenergic agonists with established analgesic effects in a variety of pain syndromes (headache, diabetic neuropathy pain, postoperative pain, postherpetic neuralgia, and cancer pain). A study of systemic clonidine in patients with postherpetic neuralgia supported the potential for analgesia, but suggested that a relatively small proportion of patients respond (Byas-Smith et al., 1995). Tizanidine appears to be better tolerated than clonidine. Somnolence is the most difficult side effect associated with both of these drugs. As a result, it is prudent to initiate a trial with a low dose, then gradually increase the dose if tolerated.

Corticosteroids

The corticosteroids have been shown to improve pain, appetite, nausea, malaise, and overall quality of life in populations with advanced medical illness (Tannock et al., 1989). Non-malignant pain syndromes, including neuropathic pains and pains associated with inflammatory diseases, also may respond. Because the risks associated with this therapy increase with both the dose and duration of use, long-term administration is usually considered only for patients with advanced medical illnesses, such as cancer, and those with chronic inflammatory disorders who are administered the drug as a primary, rather than symptomatic, treatment. Current data are inadequate to evaluate drug-selective differences, dose-response relationships for the various effects, predictors of efficacy, or the durability of effects.

Adjuvant analgesics for neuropathic pain

The advent of a more sophisticated pharmacotherapy for chronic neuropathic pain has been one of the major recent advances in pain management (Sindrup and Jensen, 2000). Although the empirical use of many drugs is occurring before confirmatory trials are done, the clinical experience has been positive and the options for patients with challenging neuropathic pain have never been greater.

Chronic neuropathic pain of any type may be a target of one of the multipurpose adjuvant analgesics. Traditionally, the antidepressants and alpha-2 adrenergic agonists are considered to be among the first drugs considered for neuropathic pain characterized by continuous dysesthesias. Although these drugs also may benefit syndromes characterized by lancinating paroxysmal pains (such as trigeminal neuralgia), they usually are considered after the anticonvulsants or baclofen in this circumstance.

Anticonvulsants

There is extensive experience in the use of anticonvulsant drugs in the treatment of neuropathic pains (Ross, 2000). Concurrent with this role, these drugs also have found an expanding utility in the management of headache and varied psychiatric syndromes.

Older anticonvulsant drugs that have been used for neuropathic pain include carbamazepine, phenytoin, valproate, and clonazepam. These drugs have established analgesic effects in many syndromes characterized by lancinating or paroxysmal neuropathic pains, most notably in trigeminal neuralgia. In recent years, however, they have been administered conventionally for all types of neuropathic pain.

There is now a large and favourable experience with gabapentin, and data from experimental and clinical studies support potential efficacy in any type of neuropathic pain (Sindrup and Jensen, 2000; Ross, 2000). A favourable clinical profile has encouraged its use and, at the present time, it is generally considered a first- or second-line drug for all types of neuropathic pain. The effective dose range for pain appears to be very large. Although some patients respond at a total daily dose of 600 mg, many do not benefit until the daily dose is increased to 3600 mg, and some patients appear to benefit at doses substantially higher.

Other anticonvulsants, including lamotrigine, topiramate, oxcarbazepine, zonisamide, tiagabine, and levetiracetam, have more limited support from clinical trials but are nonetheless used in the management of neuropathic pain. At the present time, the best supporting evidence has been obtained for lamotrigine, which has established efficacy in both trigeminal neuralgia and central pain (Zakrewska et al., 1997; Vestergaard et al., 2001).

In the absence of any contrary data, the administration of the anticonvulsants for pain mirrors the approaches used to manage seizures. To use these drugs optimally, the clinician must appreciate their risks and side effect profiles, and understand appropriate dosing methods and monitoring techniques.

Oral local anesthetics

Systemic administration of local anesthetic drugs may produce analgesia in diverse pain syndromes, including neuropathic pains (Deigard et al., 1988). The availability of oral local anesthetic drugs offers an acceptable approach for long-term therapy. In controlled clinical trials, these drugs have been effective in relieving both continuous and paroxysmal pains. Given the relatively limited experience with these drugs as analgesics, and their side effect profiles, they should be considered second-line approaches. In the United States, mexiletine has been the preferred oral local anesthetic for the treatment of pain, based on a relatively better therapeutic index for serious cardiac and neurological toxicity. Alternative drugs, such as tocainide and flecainide, are also used.

Brief intravenous local anesthetic infusions also are analgesic. This approach, which usually involves the administration of lidocaine in doses of 2–4 mg/kg over 20–30 minutes, may be used in an effort to relieve very severe or rapidly progressive pain, or provide a local anesthetic trial in those patients unable to tolerate the oral drugs. It may be possible to predict the effect of oral therapy with a brief infusion, but the validity of this technique has not yet been sufficiently established to apply it routinely.

Given the side effect and toxicity profiles, oral local anesthetic therapy is best initiated at a low starting dose. Gradual dose escalation should proceed until favourable effects occur, side effects become problematic, or the usual maximal daily dose is reached. The electrocardiogram should be monitored at higher doses and measurement of plasma drug concentrations may be informative.

NMDA receptor antagonists

Recent preclinical studies have established that binding of the excitatory amino acid glutamate at the N-methyl-D-aspartate (NMDA) receptor is involved in the mechanisms that may underlie some neuropathic pains. On the basis of these findings, NMDA receptor antagonists are undergoing intensive investigation as potential analgesics.

Three drugs commercially available in the United States, the antitussive dextromethorphan, the dissociative anesthetic ketamine, and the antiviral amantadine, act at this receptor and may be potentially useful in neuropathic pain (Persson et al., 1995; Nelson et al., 1997). A trial of dextromethorphan may be initiated using a commercially available product that contains neither alcohol nor guaifenasin. It is likely that the analgesic dose will be at least 250 mg per day. Ketamine has been used both via brief infusion and orally. The side effect profile of this drug, which includes nightmares, hallucinations and delirium, is problematic and its use is likely to be limited to patients with severe and refractory neuropathic pain. Experience with amantadine is yet very limited.

Other drugs for neuropathic pain

The GABA agonist baclofen has been shown to be effective in the treatment of trigeminal neuralgia and is now often administered for diverse types of neuropathic pain (Fromm et al., 1984). Similar to its use for spasticity, the usual effective dose range is very broad. Although most patients appear to respond at doses lower than 100 mg per day, some require more than twice this dose to achieve a favourable effect. A serious abstinence syndrome, which includes status epilepticus, can occur with abrupt discontinuation of this drug and the dose always should be tapered before treatment is stopped.

Calcitonin may be effective as a treatment for complex regional pain syndrome (reflex sympathetic dystrophy and causalgia) (Gobelet et al., 1992). Its mode of action in this disorder is unknown. Given the favourable safety profile of this drug, it is empirically considered for a trial in other types of neuropathic pain as well. There are no data by which to judge a dose-response or long-term efficacy.

Other drugs are sometimes used in the treatment of complex regional pain syndrome. Prednisone or some other corticosteroid may be administered on the basis of limited data from clinical trials. Other drugs, such as prazocin and phenoxybenzamine, have been tried based on the observation that sympathetic blockade can help a subset of these patients. Still other drugs, such as nifedipine, are used based on anecdotal observation only.

Topical therapies

The role of topical therapy for pain is enlarging. A lidocaine impregnated patch has now been approved by the U.S. Food and Drug Administration for the treatment of post-herpetic neuralgia (Galer et al., 1999). It is being tried more generally for all types of neuropathic pain and other pain syndromes related to injury to skin. Patients with neuropathic pain due to peripheral nerve injury can also be considered for trials of topical local anesthetic creams and gels, which may begin with lidocaine in varied concentrations and extend to a trial of a commercially available eutectic mixture of lidocaine and prilocaine. The latter cream has the ability to produce cutaneous anesthesia with sufficient contact time (Ehrenstrom-Reiz & Reiz, 1982).

Despite equivocal findings in some studies, capsaicin, which depletes peptides in nociceptors and other small primary afferent neurons, continues to be used for both neuropathic and arthritic pain (McCleane, 2000). An adequate trial is generally believed to require three to four applications daily for one month. Musculoskeletal pains of

Table 60.8. Opioid analgesics used during long-term treatment of chronic pain

Drug	Equianalgesic dose (mg)		Half-Life		Duration comment
	P.O.	I.M./I.V	(Hrs)	(Hrs)	
Morphine	20–30[a]	10	2–3	2–4	Standard for comparison; although a single-dose study showed a P.O.: I.M. ratio of 6: 1, the ratio of 2–3: 1 is appropriate for chronic dosing
Morphine CR	20–30	10	2–3	8–12	Various formulations are not bioequivalent
Morphine SR	20–30	10	2–3	24	—
Oxycodone	20	—	2–3	3–4	
Oxycodone CR	20	—	2–3	8–12	
Hydromorphone	7.5	1.5	2–3	2–4	Potency may be greater, i.e. IV hydromorphone: IV Morphine = 3: 1 rather than 6.7: 1, during prolonged use.
Methadone	20	10	12–190	4–12	Although 1: 1 IV ratio with morphine was in single dose study, there is a change with chronic dosing and large dose reduction (75–90%) is needed when switching to methadone.
Fentanyl	—	—	7–12	—	Can be administered as a continuous IV or SQ infusion; based on clinical experience, 100 μg/hr is roughly equianalgesic to IV morphine 4 mg/h.
Fentanyl TTS	—	—	16–24	48–72	Based on clinical experience, 100μg/hr is roughly equianalgesic to IV morphine 4 mg/h. A ratio of oral morphine: transdermal fentanyl of 70: 1 may also be used clinically.

Notes:

[a] Although the PO: IM morphine ratio was 6: 1 in a single dose study, other observations indicate a ratio of 2–3: 1 with repeated administration.

Source: Adapted from Derby et al. (1998).

all types also are candidates for trials of topical NSAIDs, which can be commercially compounded in various formulations (Galer et al., 2000).

Topical opioids, antidepressants (McCleane, 2000), sodium channel blockers such as mexiletine, ketamine, and other drugs are being tried in challenging cases. The relatively low risk of side effects associated with topical therapy ensures that further efforts will be made to identify drugs that may be effective by this route. Studies are needed to establish the benefits and define appropriate therapeutic candidates.

Opioid analgesics

Opioids are mainstay analgesics for acute pain and chronic pain related to cancer, and the role of these drugs in the management of chronic non-malignant pain is rapidly evolving (Portenoy, 1996). Numerous pure mu agonists are available and are the preferred agents for the treatment of acute and chronic pain (Table 60.8).

Opioid drugs have no long-term major organ toxicity and no ceiling effect to analgesia. During dose titration, analgesia increases until unconsciousness or some other intolerable side effect imposes a practical limit. The goal of therapy is to identify a favourable balance between analgesia and side effects. Responsiveness varies with characteristics of the patient and pain syndrome, but there is no characteristic that imparts opioid resistance. Accordingly, any severe chronic pain is potentially a candidate for an opioid trial. Selection of a patient for a trial must be based on a careful assessment and is influenced by the pain syndrome and conventional practice (first-line therapy for moderate or severe cancer pain, but generally not first-line for non-malignant pains), availability of safe alternative therapies, the risk of side effects, and the likelihood that the patient is able to use the drug responsibly.

The most important opioid side effects are constipation, nausea, vomiting, sedation and mental clouding. Tolerance develops to many side effects, usually in the first

Table 60.9. Common strategies to manage opioid side effects

Constipation
– best managed with combination of cathartic and stool softener
– osmotic or lavage agents can be useful
– refractory constipation can be treated with a trial of oral
  naloxone

Nausea, Vomiting
– metoclopramide or other dopamine antagonists
– scopolamine or other anticholinergic drugs
– ondansetron or other 5-HT antagonists
– change route of administration
– switch opioid

Sedation
– methylphenidate or other psychostimulant
– switch opioid

Source: Adapted from Caraceni & Portenoy (1998).

weeks of therapy. There are numerous strategies for the treatment of common opioid side effects (Table 60.9) (Caraceni and Portenoy, 1998). Long-term opioid therapy is fully consistent with functional restoration. Cognitive impairment can usually be avoided and successful therapy is marked by the capacity to drive, work, enjoy social activities and avocations, and otherwise capitalize on analgesia to improve quality of life.

Opioid therapy may be compromised by confusion concerning the phenomena of tolerance, physical dependence and addiction (Portenoy & Payne, 1997). Tolerance refers to a process by which exposure to a drug at a constant dose results in a decreasing effect, or the need for a higher dose to maintain an effect. It is entirely distinct from addiction. In humans, tolerance to non-analgesic opioid effects, such as somnolence, is favourable and allows safe escalation of the opioid dose. Tolerance to analgesic effects is a concern, but large surveys have established that loss of analgesia rarely occurs in opioid-treated patients with stable pain syndromes.

Physical dependence is a physiological phenomenon characterized by the development of an abstinence syndrome following abrupt discontinuation of therapy, substantial dose reduction, or administration of an antagonist drug. It is distinct from addiction and the term 'addicted' should never be used to refer to the capacity for abstinence. If abstinence is avoided, physical dependence is clinically irrelevant.

A task force of the American Medical Association defined addiction as 'a chronic disorder characterized by the com-

pulsive use of a substance resulting in physical, psychological or social harm to the user and continued use despite that harm' (Rinaldi et al., 1988). This statement emphasizes that addiction is a psychological and behavioural syndrome with several fundamental features: (i) loss of control over drug use, (ii) compulsive drug use, and (iii) continued use despite harm. The syndrome is characterized by a genetic predisposition, which interacts in complex ways with psychosocial factors, situational factors and access to abusable drugs. In treating pain patients, addiction is suggested by the development of aberrant drug-related behaviours consistent with these features (Portenoy & Payne, 1997).

Information about addiction liability derives from limited published surveys that report clinical experience in selected populations. In populations with acute pain and those with chronic cancer pain, iatrogenic addiction is rare. In populations with non-malignant pain, the likelihood of iatrogenic addiction is unknown and presumably relates to various risk factors, such as a prior history of drug abuse, a family history of drug abuse, major psychiatric pathology, and social disruption (Compton et al., 1998). Clinicians who are considering the use of an opioid must assess for these factors and monitor patients for the development of aberrant drug-related behaviours over time. Monitoring is particularly important if treatment is offered to patients with a prior or current history of substance abuse (Portenoy & Payne, 1997).

Guidelines for the long-term administration of opioid drugs are well accepted for populations with cancer pain (Jacox et al., 1994). Although additional guidelines should be considered when treating patients with non-malignant pain (Table 60.10) (Portenoy, 1994), the approach to optimizing pharmacologic outcomes is the same irrespective of the clinical population. The most important principle is individualization of therapy, which is accomplished through gradual dose titration. Doses should be increased until a favourable outcome is achieved or treatment-limiting side effects occur. The absolute dose is immaterial as long as there is a favourable balance between analgesia and side effects. The use of extended-release opioids or opioids of long half-life (particularly methadone) is preferred during chronic therapy.

Other analgesic therapies

Patients with chronic pain may be appropriate for any of a very large number of alternative analgesic therapies (Loeser, 2001). Many patients benefit from a multimodality strategy that combines systemic pharmacotherapy with other approaches (Table 60.5).

Psychological interventions and rehabilitative therapies may improve comfort and are essential elements in a

Table 60.10. Guidelines for opioid therapy in populations with non-malignant pain

1. Therapy is based on a comprehensive assessment, which should judge the nature and consequences of the pain, the availability of alternative therapeutic strategies, and the likelihood of opioid responsiveness and responsible drug use.
2. A history of substance abuse or other factors that may predispose to abuse or addiction suggest the need for a more detailed evaluation and the use of strategies during therapy to improve monitoring of drug-taking behaviour.
3. A single practitioner should take primary responsibility for treatment.
4. Patients should give informed consent before starting therapy; accurate information about addiction liability and the occurrence of physical dependence should be provided and the potential for cognitive impairment and constipation should be discussed.
5. After drug selection, doses should be given around-the-clock; several weeks should be agreed upon as the period of initial dose titration, and although improvement in function should be continually stressed, all should agree to at least partial analgesia as the appropriate goal of therapy.
6. Failure to achieve at least partial analgesia at relatively low initial doses in the non-tolerant patient raises questions about the potential treatability of the pain syndrome with opioids.
7. Emphasis should be given to capitalizing on improved analgesia by gains in physical and social function; opioid therapy should be considered complementary to other analgesic and rehabilitative approaches.
8. In addition to the daily dose determined initially, patients should be permitted to escalate dose transiently on days of increased pain; two methods are acceptable: a) prescription of additional 'rescue doses' of the same drug or an alternative short-acting opioid; b) instruction that one or two extra doses may be taken on any day, but must be followed by an equal reduction of dose on subsequent days.
9. Initially, patients must be seen and drugs prescribed at least monthly. When stable, less frequent visits may be acceptable.
10. Evidence of drug hoarding, acquisition of drugs from other physicians, uncontrolled dose escalation, or other aberrant behaviours must be carefully assessed. In some cases, tapering and discontinuation of opioid therapy will be necessary. Other patients may appropriately continue therapy within rigid guidelines. Consideration should be given to consultation with an addiction medicine specialist.
11. At each visit, assessment should specifically address (a) comfort (degree of analgesia), (b) opioid-related side effects, (c) functional status (physical and psychosocial), and (d) occurrence of aberrant drug-related behaviours; these four outcomes should be documented repeatedly in the medical record.

Source: Adapted from Portenoy (1994).

broader approach that addresses pain-related disability. There is strong evidence that the psychological approaches benefit patients with pain. Support for the various rehabilitative therapies derives from an extensive clinical experience. The psychological approaches usually include cognitive, e.g. relaxation training, biofeedback, hypnosis, and varied other techniques, and behavioural therapies. The rehabilitative interventions include therapeutic exercise, the use of orthoses, and various modalities such as heat and cold. Transcutaneous electrical nerve stimulation also is widely used and supported by abundant clinical experience.

Invasive therapies for pain are typically performed by anesthesiologists (sometimes others) with advanced training in pain management. These techniques include injection therapy, neural blockade, neuraxial analgesia techniques, and central nervous system stimulation approaches. Despite very limited data from controlled clinical trials, local anesthetic and corticosteroid injections are widely used to manage neuropathic pain, myofascial and joint pain, and spinal pain syndromes. There is an extensive experience with long-term intraspinal therapy and dorsal column stimulation, and the utility of both these approaches is expanding with improved technology and new drug development. The availability of these techniques to manage pain that has not responded to conservative therapies has relegated the use of chemical and surgical neuroablative interventions to rare patients.

Many patients with chronic pain seek complementary and alternative medicine approaches. Pain specialists, whose practice includes many conventional interventions supported only by clinical experience, are usually open to those modalities for which there is some limited evidence and a high likelihood of safety. Acupuncture, lumbar chiropractic manipulation, and therapeutic massage are widely used.

Conclusion

The past three decades have witnessed an extraordinary increase in knowledge concerning the neurobiology of pain and the potential of diverse types of analgesic interventions. All clinicians should be able to perform a comprehensive pain assessment that clarifies the nature of the pain and pain-related comorbidities, and facilitates a therapeutic strategy that may enhance comfort and function. The non-specialist can implement and monitor many components of this strategy. Patients with refractory pain, and those with pain associated with severe disability, should be considered for referral to specialists in pain management.

References

Au, E., Loprinzi, C.L., Dhodapkar, M. et al. (1994). Regular use of verbal pain scale improve the understanding of oncology inpatient pain intensity. *J. Clin. Oncol.*, **12**, 2751–55.

Bonica, J.J. (ed.) (1990). Definitions and taxonomy of pain. In *The Management of Pain*, pp. 18–27. Philadelphia: Lea & Febiger.

Byas-Smith, M.G., Max, M.B., Muir, H. & Kingman, A. (1995). Transdermal clonidine compared to placebo in painful diabetic neuropathy using a two-staged 'enriched enrolment' design. *Pain*, **60**, 267–74.

Caraceni, A. & Portenoy, R.K. (1998). Pain. In *Baker's Clinical Neurology on CD-Rom*, ed. R.J. Joynt & R.C. Griggs. Philadelphia: Lippincott Williams & Wilkins.

Compton, P., Darakjian, J. & Miotto, K. (1998). Screening for addiction in patients with chronic pain and 'problematic' substance use: evaluation of a pilot assessment tool. *J. Pain Symptom Managem.*, **16**, 355–63.

Dejgard, A., Petersen, P. & Kastrup, J. (1988). Mexiletine for treatment of chronic painful diabetic neuropathy. *Lancet*, **1**, 9–11.

Derby, S., Chin, J. & Portenoy, R.K. (1998). Systemic opioid therapy for chronic cancer pain. Practical guidelines for converting drugs and routes of administation. CNS Drugs, 9(2), 99–109.

Ehrenstrom, Reiz, G.M. & Reiz, S.L. (1982). EMLA-a eutectic mixture of local anesthetics for topical anesthesia. *Acta Anaesthesiol. Scand*, **26**, 596–8.

Fromm, G.H., Terence, C.F. & Chatta, A.S. (1984). Baclofen in the treatment of trigeminal neuralgia. *Ann. Neurol.*, **15**, 240–7.

Galer, B.S., Miller, K.V. & Rowbotham, M.C. (1993). Response to intravenous lidocaine differs based on clinical diagnosis and site of nervous system injury. *Neurology*, **43**, 123–4.

Galer, B.S., Rowbotham, M.C., Perander, J. & Friedman, E. (1999). Topical lidocaine patch relieves postherpetic neuralgia more effectively than a vehicle topical patch: results of an enriched enrollment study. *Pain*, **80**, 533–8.

Galer, B.S., Rowbotham, M., Perander, J., Devers, A. & Friedman, E. (2000). Topical diclofenac patch relieves minor sports injury pain: results of a multicenter controlled clinical trial. *J. Pain Symptom Managem.*, **19**, 287–94.

Gobelet, C., Waldburger, M. & Meier, G.A.L. (1992). The effect of adding calcitonin to physical treatment of reflex sympathetic dystrophy. *Pain*, **48**, 171–5.

Jacox, A., Carr, D.B., Payne, R. et al. (1994). *Management of Cancer Pain. Clinical Practice Guideline* No. 9. Agency for Health Care Policy and Research, HCPR Publication No. 94–0592. Rockville, MD, US Department of Health and Human Services, Public Health Service.

La Corte, R., Caselli, M., Castellino, G., Bajocchi, G. & Trotta, F. (1999). Prophylaxis and treatment of NSAID-induced gastroduodenal disorders. *Drug Saf.*, **20**, 527–43.

Langman, M.J., Jensen, D.M. & Watson, D.J. et al. (1999). Adverse upper gastrointestinal effects of rofecoxib compared with NSAIDs. *J. Am. Med. Assoc.*, **282**, 1929–33.

Loeb, D.S., Ahlquist, D.A. & Talley, N.J. (1992). Management of gastroduodenopathy associated with use of nonsteroidal anti-inflammatory drugs. *Mayo Clin. Proc.*, **67**, 354–64.

Loeser, J.D. (ed.) (2001). *Bonica's Management of Pain*, pp. 1743–2066. Philadelphia: Lippincott.

McCleane, G. (2000). Topical application of doxepin hydrochloride, capsaicin and a combination of both produces analgesia in chronic human neuropathic pain: a randomized, double-blind, placebo-controlled study. *Br. J. Clin. Pharmacol.*, **49**, 574–9.

McCormack, K. & Brune, K. (1999). Dissociation between the antinociceptive and anti-inflammatory effects of the non-steroidal anti-inflammatory drugs. *Drugs*, **41**, 533–47.

Max, M.B., Lynch, S.A., Muir, J., Shoaf, S.E., Smoller, B. & Dubner, R. (1992). Effects of desipramine, amitriptyline, and fluoxetine on pain in diabetic neuropathy. *N. Engl. J. Med.*, **326**, 1250–6.

Mersky, H. & Bogduk, N. eds. (1994). *Classification of Chronic Pain*, 2nd edn. Seattle: IASP Press.

Monks, R. & Merskey, H. (1999). Psychotropic drugs. In *Textbook of Pain*, 4th edn., ed. P.D. Wall & R. Melzack, pp. 1155–86. Edinburgh: Churchill Livingstone.

Murray, M.D. & Brater, D.C. (1993). Renal toxicity of the nonsteroidal anti-inflammatory drugs. *Annu. Rev. Pharmacol. Toxicol.*, **33**, 435–65.

Nelson, K.A., Park, K.M., Robinovitz, E., Tsigos, C. & Max, M.B. (1997). High-dose oral dextromethorphan versus placebo in painful diabetic neuropathy and post-herpetic neuralgia. *Neurology*, **48**, 1212–18.

Passik, S.D. & Portenoy, R.K. (1998). Substance abuse issues. In *The Management of Pain*, ed. M. Ashburn & L.J. Rice, pp. 51–61. New York: Churchill Livingstone.

Persson, J. & Axelsson, G, Hallin, R.G. & Gustafsson, L.L. (1995). Beneficial effects of ketamine in a chronic pain state with allodynia, possibly due to central sensitization. *Pain*, **60**, 217–22.

Portenoy, R.K. (1994). Opioid therapy for chronic nonmalignant pain: current status. In *Progress in Pain Research and Management*, vol 1., *Pharmacological Approaches to the Treatment of Chronic Pain: New Concepts and Critical Issues*, ed. H.L. Fields and J.C. Liebeskind, p. 274. Seattle: IASP Press.

Portenoy, R.K. (1996a). Neuropathic pain. In *Pain Management: Theory and Practice*, ed. R.K. Portenoy & R.M. Kanner, pp. 83–125. Philadelphia: FA Davis.

Portenoy, R.K. (1996b). Opioid therapy for chronic nonmalignant pain: clinicians' perspective. *J. Law Med. Ethics*, **24**, 296–309.

Portenoy, R.K. (1998). Adjuvant analgesics in pain management. In *Oxford Textbook of Palliative Medicine*, 2nd edn., ed. D. Doyle, G.W. Hanks & N. MacDonald, pp. 361–90. Oxford: Oxford University Press.

Portenoy, R.K. & Kanner, R.M. (1996). Definition and assessment of pain. In *Pain Management: Theory and Practice*, ed. R.K. Portenoy & R.M. Kanner, p. 6. Philadelphia: FA Davis.

Portenoy, R.K. & Payne R. (1997). Acute and chronic pain. In *Comprehensive Textbook of Substance Abuse*, 3rd edn, ed. J.H. Lowinson, P. Ruiz, R.B. Millman, pp. 563–90. Baltimore: Williams and Wilkins.

Portenoy, R.K., Foley, K.M. & Inturrisi, C.E. (1990). The nature of opioid responsiveness and its implications for neuropathic pain: new hypotheses derived from studies of opioid infusions. *Pain*, **43**, 2733–86.

Rinaldi, R.C., Steindler, E.M., Wilford, B.B. & Goodwin, D. (1998).

Clarification and standardization of substance abuse terminology. *J. Am. Med. Assoc.*, **259**, 555–7.

Ross, E.L. (2000). The evolving role of antiepileptic drugs in treating neuropathic pain. *Neurology*, **55**(5 Suppl 1), S41–6.

Simon, L.S., Weaver, A.L., Graham, D.Y. et al. (1999). Anti-inflammatory and upper gastrointestinal effects of celecoxib in rheumatoid arthritis: a randomized controlled trial. *J. Am. Med. Assoc.*, **282**, 1921–8.

Sindrup, S.H. & Jensen, T.S. (2000). Pharmacologic treatment of pain in polyneuropathy. *Neurology*, **55**, 915–20.

Smith, B.H., Elliott, A.M., Chambers, W.A., Smith, W.C., Hannaford, P.C. & Penny, K. (2001). The impact of chronic pain in the community. *Fam. Pract.* **18**, 292–9.

Taha, A.S., Hudson, N., Hawkey, C.J. et al. (1996). Famotidine for the prevention of gastric and duodenal ulcers caused by non-steroidal anti-inflammatory drugs. *N. Engl. J. Med.*, **334**, 1435–9.

Tannock, I., Gospodarowicz, M., Meakin, W., Panzarella, T., Stewart, L. & Rider, W. (1989). Treatment of metastatic prostatic cancer with low-dose prednisone: evaluation of pain and quality of life as pragmatic indices of response. *J. Clin. Oncol.*, **7**, 590–5.

Vestergaard, K., Andersen, G., Gottrup, H., Kristensen, B.T. & Jensen, T.S. (2001). Lamotrigine for central poststroke pain: a randomized controlled trial. *Neurology*, **56**, 184–90.

Willer, J.C., De Brouckner, T., Bussel, B., Roby-Brami, A. & Harrewyn, J.M. (1989). Central analgesic effect of ketoprofen in humans – electrophysiological evidence for a supraspinal mechanism in a double-blind and cross-over study. *Pain*, **38**, 1–7.

Zakrewska, J.M., Chaudhry, Z., Nurmikko, T.J., Patton, D.W. & Mullens, E.L. (1997). Lamotrigine (Lamictal) in refractory trigeminal neuralgia: results from a double-blind placebo-controlled trial. *Pain*, **73**, 223–31.

61

Migraine

Michael D. Ferrari[1] and Joost Haan[1,2]

[1] Department of Neurology, Leiden University Medical Centre, Leiden, The Netherlands
[2] Department of Neurology, Rijnland Hospital, Leiderdorp, The Netherlands

Migraine is a common, chronic, multifactorial, neurovascular disorder, typically characterized by attacks of severe headache, associated autonomic and neurological symptoms, and general malaise (Ferrari, 1998). The disease is beset by myths, including that it is mainly 'a psychological response to stress'. Despite that migraine is among the chronic diseases with the highest disability and socioeconomic impact (Menken et al., 2000), it also is among the most undertreated neurological conditions. More than two-thirds of patients either have never consulted a physician for their migraine, or have stopped doing so. Recent progress in the scientific basis of the diagnosis, epidemiology, pathophysiology, and pharmacology of migraine has, however, significantly improved the diagnostic and therapeutic options for this enigmatic brain disorder.

Clinical features and diagnosis

The International Headache Society (IHS, 1988) has considerably improved the diagnosis of migraine and other headache syndromes. Different types of headache, rather than patients, are diagnosed. Patients may have concurrent types of headache (e.g. migraine and tension-type headache), which should be treated separately. The two main types of migraine are migraine without aura (previously known as common migraine), occurring in 75% of migraineurs, and migraine with aura (previously classic migraine), occurring in one-third of patients (Table 61.1). Up to 33% of migraineurs experience both types of attacks during their lifetime (Russell et al., 1995).

Aura symptoms nearly always include visual (99% of patients), together with sensory (31%) or aphasic (18%) symptoms and, rarely, motor ones (6%) (Russel & Olesen, 1996). Aura symptoms typically progress over minutes, or different symptoms succeed one another. They usually

Table 61.1. Simplified diagnostic criteria for migraine with and without aura

Migraine without aura
- Attacks lasting 4–72 hours[a]
- At least two of the following four headache characteristics:
  - unilateral
  - pulsating
  - moderate to severe[b]
  - aggravated by movement
- At least one associated symptom:
  - nausea or vomiting
  - photophobia
  - phonophobia

Migraine with aura[c]
- One or more transient focal neurological aura symptoms[d]
- Gradual development of aura symptom over >4 minutes, or several symptoms in succession
- The aura symptoms last 4–60 minutes
- Headache follows or accompanies aura within 60 minutes

Notes:
[a] duration applies to untreated or unsuccessfully treated attacks
[b] disturbing or precluding daily activities
[c] criteria for typical aura only; for atypical aura see IHS (1988)
[d] referring to focal cortical or brainstem dysfunction
Source: Adapted from IHS (1998).

occur at alternating body sides in different attacks, nearly always precede the headache and usually last between 5 and 60 minutes; motor symptoms may last longer. Up to 42% of patients may have attacks of migraine aura without headache. In patients with a typical history of migraine and an uneventful standard neurological examination, ancilliary investigations are redundant. The following 'alarm symptoms' may warrant a CT- or MRI-scan: aura symptoms always at the same body side or with acute onset without spread or either very brief (<5 min) or unusually long (> 60 min) duration; sudden change in migraine characteristics or a sudden, substantial increase in attack frequency; onset above age 50; aura without headache; or abnormal neurological examination. EEG is seldomly useful, except in the rare cases when epilepsy is suspected.

Differential diagnosis

Migraine may be difficult to differentiate from tension-type headache (previously known as stress-, tension-, or muscle contraction headache), and many patients have both headache types. The diagnostic criteria are opposite to those for migraine (IHS, 1988). Thus, tension-type headache has at least two of four characteristics: bilateral, non-pulsating, mild to moderate, and no aggravation by movement; there is no or only mild nausea or photophobia and phonophobia.

Overuse of antimigraine or analgesic drugs, especially those which also contain caffeine, frequently complicates migraine. The overuse syndrome is characterized by gradual increase of headache frequency and drug consumption, and a change of the headache characteristics. Ultimately, patients use 'painkillers' or other headache medication daily, to treat daily occurring atypical headaches, alternating with migraine-like aggravations. Anyone who has frequent headaches, should be specifically asked about their consumption of caffeine and analgesics, particularly those obtained without prescription (as these are usually not considered a medication by patients). The number of doses used, rather than the total weekly amount of drug, is important. Thus, daily use of a low dose is much riskier than a very large amount on one day a week. Frequent headache sufferers who regularly use headache drugs more often than 1 or 2 days per week should withdraw abruptly from all these drugs (and caffeine) (Hering & Steiner, 1991). After a few weeks of withdrawal symptoms, the severity and frequency of the headaches usually decrease and after 2 to 3 months the original headache characteristics return, enabling a correct diagnosis and treatment (see Chapter 64).

Epidemiology

Migraine patients are defined as individuals who have had at least two attacks with aura or at least five attacks without aura (IHS, 1988). One-year prevalence figures, i.e. migraine patients who have had at least one attack in the previous year, are remarkably similar across western countries and are primarily dependent on sex and age. Between age 10 and 19 there is a sharp but transient rise of the 1-year prevalence of migraine, with a peak around age 14–16 (Stewart et al., 1994); for women this is followed by a less abrupt second rise until age 40 (Stewart et al., 1994). Thus, overall 10–12% of the general population are active migraineurs. From age 16, migraine is 2–3 times more frequent in females than in males; females around age 40 have the highest prevalence (24%). The lifetime prevalence of migraine is at least 18% of the general population, but these figures are deflated by recall bias at older age (Russell et al., 1995). Onset of migraine may be at all ages, but is nearly always (90%) below age 50; the peak incidence is around puberty. The median attack frequency is 1.5 attacks per month; at least 10% of patients have weekly attacks (Stewart et al., 1994). The median attack duration is just under 1 day; one fifth of the patients have attacks lasting 2–3 days. Thus, more than 5% of the general population have at least 18 migraine days per year and more than 1% at least 54 days.

Pathophysiology

Anyone can have a migraine attack occasionally without necessarily being a migraine patient. It is not the attack but the repeated occurrence that is abnormal. Attacks seem to involve physiological mechanisms, initiated by migraine- and patient-specific triggers. Attacks recur only when the threshold for triggers is reduced or when the triggers are particularly strong and frequent. Genetic factors, most likely involving ion channel and receptor function, appear to set the individual threshold; internal and environmental factors such as hormonal fluctuations, fatigue, relaxation following stress, and substance misuse may modulate this set-point (Haan et al., 1996; Ferrari, 1998; Montagna, 2000).

Complex genetic factors are involved in migraine (Russell & Olesen, 1995; Haan et al., 1996; Montagna, 2000). The study of genetic factors in migraine has mainly focused on familial hemiplegic migraine (FHM), a rare, autosomal dominant subtype of migraine with aura, often misdiagnosed as epilepsy. Attacks are characterized by hemiparesis during the aura (IHS, 1988; Haan et al., 1996; Montagna, 2000). FHM is part of the migraine spectrum and can thus be used to identify candidate genes for migraine. In the majority of patients, FHM is caused by missense mutations in the so-called CACNA1A gene on chromosome 19p13, encoding the α_{1A} subunit of a P/Q type voltage-dependent calcium channel (Ophoff et al., 1996). These neuronal calcium channels are involved in cortical spreading depression (see below) and release of neurotransmitters, including acetylcholine, neuroexcitatory aminoacids such as glutamate and aspartate, monoamines such as 5-HT, and calcitonin-gene-related-peptide (CGRP). Both clinical, genetic, and neurophsyiological evidence is accumulating that dysfunction of ion channels is involved in the pathophysiology of migraine (Ferrari, 1998).

Neurophysiological, magnetic resonance spectroscopy, biochemical, and epidemiological data suggest that migraineurs have an interictal state of cortical hyperexcitability, characterized by a reduced threshold and increased responses (Welch & Ramadan, 1995; Ferrari, 1998; Schoenen & Thomsen, 1999). The excitability level is proportional to the attack frequency. Its physiological basis may be defective mitochondrial oxidative phosphorylation, low intracellular magnesium, increased levels of neuroexcitatory amino acids, inherited dysfunction of calcium or other ionchannels, or a combination of these factors (Ferrari, 1998).

During attacks, PET studies have identified an area of increased cerebral blood flow in the upper brain stem (Weiler et al., 1995). This brainstem area may represent the 'migraine generator' involved in the initiation and maintenance of migraine attacks (Fig. 61.1, see colour plate section).

The migraine aura is most likely caused by 'cortical spreading depression' (CSD) (Lauritzen, 1994), a depolarization wave that propagates across the brain (mainly occipital) cortex at 2–3 mm/min and is associated with transient depression of spontaneous and evoked neuronal activity. The depression wave lasts several minutes and is preceded by a front of brief neuronal excitation and intense spike activity. During CSD there is dramatic failure of brain ion homeostasis and efflux of excitatory amino acids from nerve cells.

Activation of the trigeminovascular system (TVS; Fig. 61.1, see colour plate section) is pivotal to the pathogenesis of the migraine headache and associated symptoms. Afferent fibres, arising from the ophthalmic division of the trigeminal nerve and the upper cervical spinal cord segments, innervate the proximal parts of the large cerebral vessels, the pial vessels, large venous sinuses, and dura mater. These sensory fibres carry nociceptive information and project centrally, terminating within the trigeminal nucleus caudalis in the lower brain stem and upper cervical cord. The information is relayed further via the quintothalamic tract to the thalamus and cortical pain (perception) areas.

Depolarization of the trigeminal ganglion or its perivascular nerve terminals activates the TVS. This gives rise to central transmission of nociceptive information and retrograde release of powerful vasoactive neuropeptides from the perivascular nerve terminals. In animal experiments, these neuropeptides promote a sterile neurogenic inflammation response, consisting of two components: (i) dural vasodilation, mediated via release of CGRP from trigeminal A-delta-fibres; and (ii) dural plasma extravasation, mediated via release of neurokinin A and substance P from trigeminal C-fibres. Neurogenic inflammation has yet to be demonstrated in migraine.

Non-pharmacological treatment

Non-pharmacological treatments for migraine, including avoidance of putative migraine triggers, have no demonstrated efficacy, and are usually disappointing. Migraineurs have an inherited tendency to attacks, which may be triggered by a wide variety of factors. Complete avoidance seems impossible. There is no good evidence that specific diets ameliorate migraine. When overuse of analgesics and caffeine is present, stopping can reduce migraine attack frequency and severity.

Prophylactic drug-treatment

Preventive efficacy has been demonstrated for the β adrenoceptor-blockers propranolol and metoprolol (and probably also atenolol, timolol and nadolol), and the antiepileptic drug valproate (which has GABA-ergic and ion channel activity). Other β-blockers or antiepileptic drugs have no demonstrated efficacy. The 5-HT receptor antagonists pizotifen and methysergide, and the non-selective calcium-channel blocker flunarizine, are probably also effective, but formal evidence is limited (Goadsby, 1997a). The widespread use of amitriptyline is largely based on its efficacy in concurrent tension-type headaches, rather than on preventing migraine attacks. In North America such headaches are often referred to as 'minor migraines', which may explain the confusion. The calcium channel blockers nifedipine, nimodipine and verapamil, the $\alpha2$-adrenoceptor agonist clonidine, some NSAIDs, the herbal drug feverfew, riboflavin, and hormonal manipulation, are often recommended, but evidence for preventive efficacy is lacking or unconvincing. Verapamil, however, is highly effective in preventing cluster headache attacks, and NSAIDs are effective symptomatic treatments of migraine.

The efficacy of the current migraine prophylactics is limited: at most 55% of patients will have a 50% or more reduction of the attack frequency (Ramadan et al., 1997; Goadsby, 1997b). The individual reponse is unpredictable and must be determined by 'trial and error', taking into account individual (contra-)indications. Due to the non-specific pharmacology, there is a high risk of adverse events. Therefore, only patients with two attacks or more per month, which respond unsatisfactory to symptomatic treatment, should be considered for preventive treatment. There is a great need for better prophylactic agents.

Attack treatment

Specific and non-specific symptomatic antimigraine drugs treat the headache and associated symptoms only, not the aura. Non-specific drugs include analgesics such as aspirin and paracetamol, rapidly absorbable NSAIDs, prokinetic and antiemetic compounds such as metoclopramide and domperidone, and narcotics such as codeine, pethidine and morphine (Welch, 1993; Ferrari & Haan, 1997). The use of narcotics and barbiturates is highly controversial, not supported by scientific evidence, and is associated with prominent side effects and a high risk of abuse and dependency. Most patients who require narcotics are in fact over-using headache or migraine agents. After withdrawal, they rarely require narcotics anymore.

In migraine attacks, oral resorption is impaired because of vomiting or gastrointestinal stasis and dilatation, even in not nauseated patients. Thus, to optimize drug administration the parenteral route is usually preferred. However, most patients prefer tablets. Use of metoclopramide or domperidone 30 minutes prior to analgesics, improves their oral resorption and combats the nausea, but there is no evidence that analgesic efficacy is improved. The choice of drug, dose, and route of administration, depends on the characteristics and frequency of the attacks, and on the preferences of and contraindications for the patient. Not all attacks in a given patient are necessarily treated with the same drug or dose. Mild attacks may be treated with analgesics or NSAIDs, while severe, disabling ones usually respond better to specific antimigraine drugs. The Migraine Disability Assessment Scale (MIDAS) has proven to be a useful and easy to use clinical instrument to predict acute treatment needs (Lipton et al., 2000).

Ergot alkaloids

For decades ergots were the only drugs specifically for migraine. Most of our so-called knowledge is, however, based on 'authoritative reviews' and textbooks, largely summarizing uncontrolled studies and personal experiences. This surprising lack of scientific evidence contributes to the

Table 61.2. The triptans (5-HT$_{1B/1D}$ receptor agonists)

Triptan	Recommended oral doses (mg)	Company
In clinical use (year)		
Sumatriptan (1991)	25; 50; 100	GlaxoSK**
Zolmitriptan (1997)	2.5; 5	AstraZeneca
Naratriptan (1997)	2.5	GlaxoSK**
Rizatriptan (1998)	5; 10	Merck
Almotriptan (2001)	12.5	Almirall-Prodesfarma
Approved for registration		
Eletriptan (2001)	20; 40; 80	Pfizer
Frovatriptan (2001)	unknown	Vernalis

striking differences between countries in frequency of use, recommended dosing, formulations, and combinations with other compounds. Recent reviews conclude that ergot derivatives display a complex pharmacology and erratic pharmacokinetics, have poorly justified dose recommendations and only limited evidence for efficacy, and show potent and sustained generalized vasoconstrictor effects (Dahlöf, 1993; Tfelt-Hansen et al., 2000). As a result, their clinical use is complicated, results are unpredictable, and complications (including ischemia of organs and limbs, overuse syndromes, and rebound headaches) are frequent; ergot derivatives are strictly contraindicated in the presence of cardiovascular disease. The major reasons for prescribing ergots today seem to be that they have been around for a long time and are much cheaper than the newer drugs. The European Consensus Committee concluded that generally triptans (see below) are to be preferred but when patients have a satisfactory response to ergots it is not necessary to switch as long as there is no escalation of the use of ergots beyond 1–2 days per week.

Triptans

Advances in the understanding of the neurobiology of migraine have resulted in the development of the novel class of selective 5-HT$_{1B/1D}$ (serotonin; 5-hydroxytryptamine$_{1B/1D}$) receptor agonists, known as the triptans (Table 61.2). It is likely that the 5-HT$_{1B/1D}$ agonist activity is the major basis for their therapeutic effects, although 5-HT$_{1F}$ action may be involved as well. Triptans have three potential mechanisms of action, cranial vasoconstriction, peripheral neuronal inhibition, and inhibition of transmission through second order neurons of the trigeminocervical complex (Ferrari 1998; Goadsby et al., 2002). The relative importance of each of these mechanisms remains uncertain (Fig. 61.1, see colour plate section).

In comparison to ergot derivatives, triptans have a number of distinct advantages. These include selective pharmacology, simple and consistent pharmacokinetics, evidence-based prescribing instructions, established efficacy based on an enormous body of well-designed placebo-controlled and direct comparative clinical trials, modest side effects, and a well-established safety record; their most important disadvantage is the higher price (Goadsby et al., 2002; Ferrari et al., 2001). The triptans are now the leading class of acute migraine medications in many western countries. They have proven to be very effective and generally well-tolerated acute migraine treatments, which have made an enormous difference for many patients. However, although the triptans currently are the most effective antimigraine drugs available, they certainly are no wonder drugs.

Sumatriptan was the first triptan available and undoubtedly is the most extensively investigated antimigraine drug (Plosker & McTavish, 1994; Visser et al., 1996a,b,c; Goadsby et al., 2002; Ferrari et al., 2001). Since its launch, first as a 6 mg subcutaneous auto-injector and 100 and 50 mg oral formulations, and later as 20 mg nasal and 25 mg rectal formulations, six other triptans have been marketed all in oral formulations (Table 61.2). For the oral triptans, the following effects can be expected (Goadsby et al., 2002; Ferrari et al., 2001). Approximately 60% of migraine patients improve by 2 hours postdose and up to 40% are pain free at that time. Up to one-third of the responders may experience recurrence of the headache (relapse) within 24–48 hours; repeated drug administration is then usually effective. Prescribing physicians should explain this to their patients. The mechanism of headache relapse is unknown, but seems, contrary to earlier belief, unrelated to the drug plasma half-life. Adverse events (AEs) are frequent, but in the great majority very mild and of short duration. The most frequent AEs include tingling, paresthesias, and warm and hot sensations in head, neck, chest, and extremities; less frequent AEs are dizziness, flushing, and neck pain or stiffness. Of more relevance are the so-called 'chest symptoms' which mainly consist of short-lived heaviness or pressure in the arms and chest, shortness of breath, anxiety, palpitations, and, very rarely, chest pain (Visser et al., 1998a,b,c; Ferrari et al., 2001). When patients are warned about these events, they rarely cause problems. However, they sometimes closely mimic angina and cause alarm. Severe and sustaining sumatriptan-associated chest symptoms should be taken seriously and should prompt cardiovascular investigation.

The mechanism of triptan-induced chest symptoms is unknown. Triptans may cause constriction of the coronary arteries, which is usually short-lived and mild. In atherosclerotic arteries, however, the constrictor effect of triptans may clinically be more important. Furthermore, use of triptans has been associated with myocardial or cerebral ischemia in some individuals, although very few given the very substantial total human exposure to triptans and mainly with pre-existing coronary or cerebral artery disease (Wilkinson et al., 1995; Welch et al., 2000). Myocardial ischemia can thus not be excluded in some patients with chest symptoms, though it seems an unlikely mechanism in most. Other mechanisms such as esophageal spasms, pulmonary vasoconstriction, intercostal muscle spasm, or bronchospasm, seem more likely (Ferrari, 1998). Thus, when prescribed prudently, i.e. not in patients with cardio- or cerebrovascular disease or risk factors, the triptans are safe. The risk of triptan-induced myocardial ischemia in migraineurs without clinical evidence of cardiovascular disease appears no greater than the risk is of exercise-induced myocardial ischemia in sportsmen (Ferrari, 1998).

A large meta-analysis investigated the relative efficacy and tolerability of the oral triptans (Ferrari et al., 2001; Goadsby et al., 2002). Rizatriptan 10 mg (especially to rapidly and consistently achieve freedom of pain), eletriptan 80 mg (especially when high efficacy and low recurrence are favoured over tolerability) and almotriptan 12.5 mg (especially when very good tolerability in combination with good efficacy are favoured) offer the highest likelihood of success. The lower doses of rizatriptan (5 mg) and eletriptan (40 mg) may be good starting doses in many patients. Sumatriptan 100 mg and 50 mg provide good efficacy and tolerability and by far the longest clinical experience; the 50 mg dose has a slightly better efficacy/tolerability ratio but also a slightly lower consistency. In addition, sumatriptan offers the widest range of formulation options (oral, suppositories, nasal, and subcutaneous), allowing tailor-made treatments for individual patients. Naratriptan 2.5 mg offers very good tolerability coupled to a slower onset of improvement; this can be useful in patients with mild or moderate migraine. Zolmitriptan 2.5 mg and 5 mg are good alternatives in many patients; they offer no specific advantages but there are also no specific flaws. Frovatriptan cannot be fully judged in view of the lack of data but doesn't seem to offer any particular advantage; available efficacy data suggest inferior results compared to most of the other oral triptans.

Sumatriptan is also available in parenteral formulations (for review, see Goadsby et al., 2002). Of all triptans, subcutaneous sumatriptan has the best pharmacokinetic profile (Tmax = 10 min; bioavailability = 96%). It is unaffected by gastro-intestinal disturbances during migraine attacks and has excellent clinical efficacy (response of 76% and pain free of 48% already at 1 hour post dose) and within-patient consistency over multiple attacks (up to 90% for headache response in two out of three treated attacks. The main disadvantages are that patients need to inject themselves, and that the incidence of AEs is higher and the intensity is generally greater than for oral triptans, although still usually acceptable and short-lived. This may be related, among other factors, to the fixed 6mg dose; a 3–4mg dose may suffice in many patients. Subcutaneous sumatriptan is also highly effective in the acute treatment of cluster headache attacks. The efficacy and tolerability profiles of rectal and intranasal sumatriptan are very similar to those of the oral formulation, although many users of the nasal formulation complain about the bitter taste. Both formulations may be useful in nauseated and vomiting patients. Intranasal sumatriptan 20 mg is so far the only triptan with at least some demonstrated efficacy in adolescents. A number of studies of oral triptans in adolescent migraine have failed, most likely because adolescent attacks usually are short lasting and associated with prominent gastrointestinal symptoms; spontaneous early remissions generate high placebo responses.

When selecting a triptan, it is important to realize that patients' characteristics and preferences vary and that response to and tolerability for a triptan cannot be predicted in individual patients. As a consequence, optimizing therapy involves trial-and-error: if the first triptan is not successful one may successfully switch to another. Physicians thus need more than one triptan in their repertoire to optimally treat migraine patients. Differences in efficacy and tolerability among the oral triptans at optimal doses are relatively small, but clinically relevant for individual patients.

In conclusion, migraine is a common, very disabling, multifactorial, neurovascular disorder. Prophylactic treatment to prevent attacks may prove highly effective in individual patients, but often provides rather disappointing results, associated with prominent adverse events. There is a great need for specific and better migraine prophylactic drugs. In contrast, acute attack treatment with the novel class of triptans has greatly improved the life of many patients. They often provide very good efficacy and tolerability. Highest likelihood of consistent success is offered by 6mg subcutaneous sumatriptan (highest efficacy with reasonable tolerability); 10 mg oral rizatriptan (very good efficacy and very good tolerability), 80 mg eletriptan (very good efficacy and good tolerability), and 12.5 mg almotriptan (good efficacy and excellent tolerability). Sumatriptan provides the longest clinical experience and widest range of formulations allowing tailor-made treatments for individual patients. Other triptans and dosages are also good alternatives in many patients. When prescribed prudently (i.e. not in patients with cardio- or cerebrovascular disease or major risk factors), triptans are safe.

References   * denotes key references

Bates, D., Ashford, E., Dawson, R. et al. (1994). For the sumatriptan aura study group. Subcutaneous sumatriptan during the migraine aura. *Neurology*, **44**, 1587–92.

Dahlöf, C. (1993). Placebo-controlled clinical trials with ergotamine in the acute treatment of migraine. *Cephalalgia*, **13**, 166–71.

*Ferrari, M.D. (1998). Migraine. *Lancet*, **351**, 1043–51.

Ferrari, M.D. & Haan, J. (1997). Drug treatment of migraine attacks. In *Headache*, ed. P.J. Goadsby & S.D. Silberstein, pp. 117–31. Boston: Butterworth-Heineman.

Ferrari, M.D. & Saxena, P.R. (1993). Clinical and experimental effects of sumatriptan in humans. *Trends Pharmacol Sci.*, **14**, 129–34.

*Ferrari, M.D., Roon, K.I., Lipton, R.B. & Goadsby, P.J. (2001). Triptans (serotonin, 5-HT$_{1B/1D}$ agonists) in migraine: a meta-analysis of 53 trials. *Lancet*, **358**, 1668–75.

Galer, B.S., Lipton, R.B., Solomon, S., Newman, L.C. & Spierings, E.L.H. (1991). Myocardial ischemia related to ergot alkaloids: a case report and literature review. *Headache*, **31**, 446–51.

Goadsby, P.J. (1997a). A triptan too far? *J. Neurol. Neurosurg. Psychiatry*, **64**, 143–7.

*Goadsby, P.J., Lipton, R.B. & Ferrari, M.D. (2002). Migraine, current understanding and treatment. *N. Engl. J. Med.*, **346**, 257–70.

*Goadsby, P.J. (1997b). How do the currently used prophylactic agents work in migraine? *Cephalalgia*, **17**, 85–92.

Gunasekara, N.S. & Wiseman, L.R. (1997). Naratriptan. *CNS Drugs*, **8**, 402–8.

Haan, J., Terwindt, G.M. & Ferrari, M.D. (1996). Genetics of migraine. In *Neurologic Clinics* (*Advances in Headache*), ed. N.T. Mathew. Philadelphia: WB Saunders Co.

Headache Classification Committee of the International Headache Society (Olesen J. et al.). (1988). Classification and diagnostic criteria for headache disorders, cranial neuralgias and facial pain. *Cephalalgia*, **8**(Suppl. 7), 1–96.

Hering, R. & Steiner, T.J. (1991). Abrupt outpatient withdrawal of medication in analgesic-abusing migraineurs. *Lancet*, **337**, 1442–3.

Lauritzen, M. (1994). Pathophysiology of the migraine aura. The spreading depression theory. *Brain*, **117**, 199–210.

Lipton, R.B., Stewart, W.F., Stone, A.M., Lainez, M.J.A & Sawyer, J.P.C. (2000). Stratified care vs step care strategies for migraine. The Disability in Strategies of Care (DISC) Study: a randomized trial. *J. Am. Med. Assoc.*, **284**, 2599–605.

Meijler, W.J. (1996). Side effects of ergotamine. *Cephalalgia*, **16**, 5–10.

Menken, M., Munsat, T.L. & Toole, J.F. (2000). The global burden of disease study – implications for neurology. *Arch. Neurol.*, **57**, 418–20.

*Montagna, P. (2000). Molecular genetics of migraine headaches: a review. *Cephalalgia*, **20**, 3–14.

Moskowitz, M.A. (1992). Neurogenic versus vascular mechanisms of sumatriptan and ergot alkaloids in migraine. *Trends Pharmacol Sci.*, **13**, 307–12.

Ophoff, R.A., Terwindt, G.M., Vergouwe, M.N. et al. (1996). Familial hemiplegic migraine and episodic ataxia type-2 are caused by mutations in the Ca²⁺ channel gene CACNL1A4. *Cell*, **87**, 543–52.

Palmer, K.J. & Spencer, C.M. (1997). Zolmitriptan. *CNS Drugs*, **7**, 468–78.

Plosker, G.L. & McTavish, D. (1994). Sumatriptan. A reappraisal of its pharmacology and therapeutic efficacy in the acute treatment of migraine and cluster headache. *Drugs*, **47**, 622–51.

Ramadan, N.M., Schultz, L.L. & Gilkey, S.J. (1997). Migraine prophylactic drugs: proof of efficacy, utilization and cost. *Cephalalgia*, **17**, 73–80.

Russell, M.B. & Olesen, J. (1995). Increased familial risk and evidence of genetic factor in migraine. *Br. Med. J.*, **311**, 541–4.

Russell, M.B. & Olesen, J. (1996). A nosographic analysis of the migraine aura in a general population. *Brain*, **119**, 355–61.

Russel, M.B., Rasmussen, B.K., Thorvaldsen, P. & Olesen, J. (1995). Prevalence and sex ratio of the subtypes of migraine. *Intern. J. Epidemiol.*, **24**, 612–18.

Schoenen, J. & Thomsen, L.L. (1999). Neurophysiology and autonomic dysfunction in migraine. In *The Headaches*, 2nd edn, ed. J. Olesen, P., Tfelt-Hansen & K.M.A. Welch, pp. 301–312. Philadelphia: Lippincott Williams & Wilkins.

Stewart, W.F., Schechter, A. & Rasmussen, B.K. (1994). Migraine prevalence. A review of population-based studies. *Neurology*, **44**(Suppl. 4), S17–23.

*Tfelt-Hansen, P., Saxena, P.R. & Dahlof, C. et al. (2000). Ergotamine in the acute treatment of migraine – a review and European consensus. *Brain*, **123**, 9–18.

Visser, W.H., de Vriend, R.H.M, Jaspers, N.M.W.H & Ferrari, M.D. (1996a). Sumatriptan in clinical practice; a two year review of 453 migraine patients. *Neurology*, **47**, 46–51.

Visser, W.H., Jaspers, N.M.W.H., de Vriend, R.H.M. & Ferrari, MD. (1996b). Chest symptoms after sumatriptan: a two-year clinical practice review in 735 consecutive migraine patients. *Cephalalgia*, **16**, 554–9.

Visser, W.H., Terwindt, G.M., Reines, S.A., Jiang, K., Lines, C.R. & Ferrari, M.D. (1996c). For the Dutch/US Rizatriptan Study Group. Rizatriptan vs sumatriptan in the acute treatment of migraine. *Arch. Neurol.*, **53**, 1132–7.

Weiller, C., May, A., Limmroth, V. et al. (1995). Brain stem activation in spontaneous human migraine attacks. *Nat. Med.*, **1**, 658–60.

Welch, K.M.A. (1993). Drug therapy of migraine. *N. Eng. J. Med.*, **329**, 1476–84.

Welch, K.M.A. & Ramadan, N.M. (1995). Mitochondria, magnesium and migraine. *J. Neurol. Sci.*, **134**, 9–14.

*Welch, K.M.A., Mathew, N.T., Stone, P., Rosamund, W., Saiers, J. & Gutterman, D. (2000). Tolerability of sumatriptan and post-marketing experience. *Cephalalgia*, **20**, 687–95.

Wilkinson, M., Pfaffenrath, V., Schoenen, J., Diener, H.C. & Steiner, T.J. (1995). Migraine and cluster headache – their management with sumatriptan: a critical review of the current clinical experience. *Cephalalgia*, **15**, 337–57.

62

Cluster headache, other trigeminal autonomic syndromes and the short-lived headaches

Peter J. Goadsby

Institute of Neurology, The National Hospital for Neurology and Neurosurgery, Queen Square, London UK

Of the primary headache syndromes, cluster headache and the related trigeminal autonomic cephalgias, as well as some of the short-lived headache syndromes (Table 62.1), stand out for their very well-defined phenotypes and considerable associated disability. The trigeminal autonomic cephalgias (Goadsby & Lipton, 1997) offer some exceptional physiological insights (see also Chapter 79 (Volume 2)) (May & Goadsby, 1999) and are very rewarding to treat. Books have been written on cluster headache (Kudrow, 1980; Olesen & Goadsby, 1999; Sjaastad, 1992), and readers are referred to these for greater detail. A further issue arises as to what is short-lived; in this context attacks that commonly are measured in minutes (Table 62.2) will fulfil that definition.

Cluster headache

Cluster headache is a relatively rare very severe episodic primary headache with a population prevalence at about 0.1%. It has been recognized for many years with among the earliest known description appearing in Gerhard van Swieten's medical textbook (Isler, 1993):

A healthy robust man of middle age [was suffering from] troublesome pain which came on every day at the same hour at the same spot above the orbit of the left eye, where the nerve emerges from the opening of the frontal bone: after a short time the left eye began to redden, and to overflow with tears; then he felt as if his eye was slowly forced out of its orbit with so much pain, that he nearly went mad. After a few hours all these evils ceased, and nothing in the eye appeared at all changed.

This description fulfils the International Headache Society diagnostic criteria (Table 62.3) for cluster headache (Headache Classification Committee of The International Headache Society, 1988). Before the term

Table 62.1. Primary headache – cluster headache, other TACs and short-lasting headaches

Trigeminal autonomic cephalgias (TACS)	Other short-lasting headaches
Cluster headache	Primary stabbing headache[b]
Paroxysmal hemicrania	Benign cough headache
SUNCT[a] syndrome	Hypnic headache
Hemicrania continua	

Notes:

[a] Shortlasting unilateral neuralgiform headache with conjunctival injection and tearing.

[b] Currently known as idiopathic stabbing headache but due for change in the second edition of the International Headache Society classification.

cluster headache was widely used, the disease was known by a large number of names (Table 62.4), with perhaps the most remarkable understatement being that of Sir Charles Symons (1956b), who called it a particular variety of headache. It has been suggested for many years that cluster headache was a disorder of the carotid artery at the base of the skull (Moskowitz, 1988) on the basis of inflammation (Hardebo, 1994) and vascular change (Ekbom & Greitz, 1970; Waldenlind et al., 1993). However, neuroendocrine studies (Leone & Bussone, 1993) suggest hypothalamic dysfunction in pacemaker regions of the brain, the suprachiasmatic nucleus (Hofman et al., 1996). Recently, activation on functional imaging with positron emission tomography (PET) in the region of the posterior hypothalamic grey (May et al., 1998), as well as a structural difference in the brain of cluster headache patients when compared with controls (May et al.,1999a), confirms this region of the brain to be pivotal to the syndrome (Fig. 62.1,

Table 62.2. Differential diagnosis for short-lasting primary headaches

With autonomic features	Without autonomic features
Cluster headache	Idiopathic stabbing headache
Paroxysmal hemicrania	Trigeminal neuralgia
SUNCT[a] syndrome	Migraine
	Benign cough headache
	Hypnic headache

Notes:

[a] Short-lasting unilateral neuralgiform headache attacks with conjunctival injection and tearing.

Table 62.3. Diagnostic features of cluster headache modified from the International Headache Society

Headaches must have each of:

Severe unilateral orbital, supraorbital, temporal pain lasting 15 minutes to 3 hours;

Frequency: 1 every second day to 8 per day;

Associated with 1 of:
- lacrimation
- nasal congestion
- rhinorrhea
- forehead/facial sweating
- miosis
- ptosis
- eyelid edema
- conjunctival injection

Source: From Headache Classification Committee of The International Headache Society (1988).

see colour plate section). The physiology of the pain and cranial autonomic activation has been reviewed recently (May & Goadsby, 1999).

Clinical features and differential diagnosis (Table 62.5)

Cluster headache is characterized by intermittent, repeated, brief attacks of very severe unilateral pain that is most usually reported to occur over or behind one eye. There are usually associated autonomic features such as lacrimation, nasal congestion, conjunctival injection and a partial Horner's syndrome (Headache Classification Committee of The International Headache Society, 1988). By these criteria each attack may last from 15 minutes to 3 hours and the fre-

Table 62.4. Older terms for cluster headache

Histaminic cephalagia
Sphenopalatine neuralgia
Petrosal neuralgia
Migrainous neuralgia
Hemicrania periodic neuralgiformis
Erythroprosopalgia of Bing
Horton's headache

quency of attacks varies from one every other day to eight per day. Clearly, these are arbitrary rules that human biology breaks from time to time and when broken may be a sign that a more refractory clinical problem is emerging. Most patients with cluster headache have them in a bout or cluster that may last from 6 weeks to several months and are thus designated episodic cluster headache. Some 10–15 of patients have no substantial breaks and are classified as chronic cluster headache. These can be the most challenging of cases being frequently resistant to simpler treatments.

Emerging clinical features

Two recent large cohorts of cluster headache (Bahra et al., 2002; Silberstein et al., 2000) have revealed clinical aspects of cluster headache that are noteworthy. The reported ratio of males to females has dropped over the last 15 years from 9:1 to 3.5:1, due probably to better case ascertainment with studies from non-clinic populations. While clearly a predominately male disorder, female cases are readily seen. A key feature of acute cluster headache that occurs in more than 90% of patients is restlessness or agitation, which contrasts with acute migraine where slightly more than 90% of patients report aggravation of pain with movement. While not perfect, this completely opposite behaviour is an extremely helpful differentiating factor in clinical practice. It has also become clear that migrainous symptoms, such as nausea, photophobia and phonophobia, which occur in 70–80% of migraineurs, can occur in about 50% of cluster headache sufferers. Lastly, typical migrainous aura can be seen in about 15% of patients with cluster headache and should not preclude the diagnosis of cluster headache.

It is important to differentiate cluster headache from similar conditions, which most often consist of shorter more frequent attacks (Goadsby & Lipton, 1997), and to be aware of the rare but recognized causes of secondary cluster headache (Table 62.5) as they guide logical investigation. It can be both diagnostically profitable and clinically reassuring to the patient to investigate or even

Table 62.5. Differential diagnosis of secondary cluster-like headache

Similar secondary headaches	Secondary cluster headaches
	Lesion involving vessels
Tolosa–Hunt syndrome	vertebral artery dissection (Cremer et al., 1995) or aneurysm (West & Todman, 1991)
Maxillary sinusitis	pseudoaneurysm of intracavernous carotid[a] (Koenigsberg et al., 1994)
Temporal arteritis	aneurysm anterior communicating artery (Greve & Mai, 1988)
Raeder's paratrigeminal neuralgia	carotid aneursym (Greve & Mai, 1988)
	occipital lobe AVM (Mani & Deeter, 1982)
	AVM middle cerebral territory (Muoz et al., 1996)
	Lesions involving the caudal medulla or cervical spinal cord
	high cervical meningioma (Kuritzky, 1984)
	unilateral cervical cord infarction (de la Sayette et al., 1999)
	lateral medullary infarction (Cid et al., 2000)
	Intracranial lesions
	pituitary adenoma (Tfelt-Hansen et al., 1982)
	prolactinoma (Greve & Mai, 1988)
	meningioma of the lesser wing of sphenoid (Hannerz, 1989)
	Facial lesions
	facial trauma (Lance, 1993)
	orbito-sphenoidal aspergillosis (Heidegger et al., 1997)
	Other
	head or neck injury (Hunter & Mayfield, 1949)

Note:
[a] SUNCT, Short-lasting unilateral neuralgiform headache attacks with conjunctival injection and tearing

reinvestigate the most refractory patients. It is certainly conceivable that they may harbour a secondary headache, since secondary cluster can respond to routine treatments (Cremer et al., 1995), and it certainly can be difficult to differentiate on clinical grounds.

Management of cluster headache
Many medical treatments in cluster headache can be used in both episodic and chronic cluster headache patients. In general, the acute medications may be used in both settings, although in chronic cluster headache long-term safety issues make the use of the medicines sometimes problematic. Key issues in difficult cluster headache include providing acute treatment when there are several attacks a day, particularly because of the limits on the use of injectable sumatriptan; finding a drug, or combinations of drugs, that are useful in preventing attacks and making decisions about the place and timing of surgery.

Preventative treatment
Preventative treatments in cluster headache can be used to either arrest a bout of episodic cluster headache or to ameli-

orate symptoms in patients with chronic cluster headache. Although each of the preventatives would probably be useful in either situation, certain practical limitations favour the clinical use of each drug. It is useful to think of preventatives as either being short term, limited usually by side effects and useful in episodic and less so in chronic cluster headache; and long term, usually used for longer bouts of episodic cluster headache or chronic cluster headache.

Short-term prevention: Oral ergotamine may be useful as a regular night-time dose to avoid nocturnal attacks (Ekbom, 1947) and at a dose of 1–2 mg nightly can be very useful. Ergotamine is at its best when given well before the attacks and is ideal for the patient with predictable nocturnal attacks and a short bout. It is problematic in patients with vascular disease although, in contrast to migraine sufferers, ergotamine-induced headache seems relatively uncommon in patients with cluster headache. Another useful strategy can be daily or even twice dihydroergotamine (1 mg) which can suppress attacks very effectively. The author has found both injectable dihydroergotamine and the dihydroergotamine nasal spray useful.

A short burst of oral corticosteroids has been recommended for some years (Jammes, 1975) and is certainly effective. The problem of aspectic necrosis of the hip must be clearly explained to the patient. In this regard bony problems with steroid use have been reviewed by Mirzai and colleagues (Mirzai et al., 1999). The shortest course of prednisolone reported to be associated with osteonecrosis of the femoral head is a 30-day course of 16 mg/day (Fischer & Bickel, 1971). Furthermore, courses of adrenocorticotropic hormone (Good, 1974) have produced osteonecrosis after 16 days and dexamethasone at 16 mg per day after 7 days (Anderton & Helm, 1982). Thus a tapering course of prednisolone for 21 days is effective and seems prudent.

Methysergide can be an extremely effective anticluster agent and, because the bouts are usually short, the exposure can be limited. Patients may require up to 12 mg daily but usually respond reasonably quickly and in up to 70% of cases (Curran et al., 1967).

Longer-term prevention: The first-line treatment for longer-term prevention in cluster headache is verapamil. In an open trial employing large doses of 240–720 mg daily in episodic cluster and 120–1200 mg daily in chronic cluster headache, an improvement of more than 75% was noted in 69% of 48 patients treated with verapamil (Gabai & Spierings, 1989). Since this early report, verapamil has been established as among the most effective preventative agents in cluster headache. It is superior to placebo (Leone et al., 2000), and at least equal to lithium (Bussone et al., 1990). It is generally true that the regular verapamil preparation is more useful than the slow-release preparations and that the upper limit of dosing relates to side effects, particularly cardiac conduction problems. Although most patients will start on doses as low as 40 mg twice daily, doses up to 960 mg daily are now employed (Olesen & Goadsby, 1999). Side effects, such as constipation and leg swelling, can be a problem (Silberstein, 1994), but more difficult is the issue of cardiovascular safety.

Verapamil can cause heart block by slowing conduction in the atrioventricular node (Singh & Nademanee, 1987) as demonstrated by prolongation of the A–H interval (Naylor, 1988). Given that the PR interval on the ECG is made up of atrial conduction, A–H and His bundle conduction, it may be difficult to monitor subtle early effects as verapamil dose is increased. This question needs study in this group of patients but for the moment it seems appropriate to do a baseline ECG and then repeat the ECG at least 10 days after a dose change, usually 80 mg increments, when doses exceed 240 mg daily.

Lithium carbonate has been reported to be useful in up to 40% of patients (Carolis et al., 1988; Kudrow, 1977) and its use requires careful monitoring. Unfortunately, its most recent study was limited by practical problems and came to no clear conclusions on the drug's efficacy (Steiner et al., 1997). More recently, each of valproate (Hering & Kuritzky, 1989), gabapentin and topiramate (Wheeler & Carrazana, 1999) have been suggested to be useful. Blinded studies are required before these can be widely recommended.

Acute attacks of cluster headache

Perhaps the over-riding problem in acute cluster headache is that the attacks come on rapidly and reach a peak very quickly so that therapy to be of any value must be rapid in onset and thus oral preparations used in migraine may not be effective. Parenteral dihydroergotamine (1 mg intramuscularly) (Horton, 1952) and intranasal dihydroergotamine (Andersson & Jespersen, 1986) are effective for some but not all patients. Inhalation of 100% oxygen (10–12 l/min) for 15 minutes has been clearly shown to be of benefit in arresting attacks (Fogan, 1985; Kudrow, 1981). Other options include instillation of lidocaine nasal drops (4–6%) ipsilateral to the side of pain (Kitrelle et al., 1985; Robbins, 1995) or injection of the ipsilateral greater occipital nerve (Anthony, 1987). Sumatriptan, a 5-HT$_{1B/1D}$ receptor agonist developed for the treatment of migraine (Humphrey et al., 1991), has proved highly efficacious and rapid in onset of action (Hardebo, 1993) in the treatment of acute attacks of cluster headache (Ekbom & The Sumatriptan Cluster Headache Study Group, 1991). It has been shown that increasing the dose from 6 mg to 12 mg does not result in either more responders or a quicker effect (Ekbom et al., 1993). It is important clinically that the response is not diminished with time (Ekbom et al., 1992) and the side effect profile is modest as it is for migraine (Goadsby, 1994).

Pre-emptive treatment with sumatriptan in a regimen of 100 mg three times daily does not alter either the timing or frequency of headaches (Monstad et al., 1995). These data are in accordance with published data for migraine with aura that has shown pretreatment of patients prior to headache does not prevent headache (Bates et al., 1994). Rather, sumatriptan is only effective when headache has commenced even if the headache is mild (Aube, 1995; Lipton et al., 2000). Sumatriptan nasal spray has been studied in an open-label fashion and had modest effects (Hardebo & Dahlof, 1998). Recently, it was shown that zolmitriptan 5 mg and 10 mg were effective treatments of acute cluster headache but only in patients with the episodic form (Bahra et al., 2000).

Paroxysmal hemicrania (PH)

Sjaastad et al. first reported cases (Sjaastad & Dale, 1974), 7 of whom were female, of a frequent unilateral severe but short-lasting headache without remission coining the term chronic paroxysmal hemicrania (CPH) (Sjaastad & Dale, 1976). The mean daily frequency of attacks varied from 7 to 22 with the pain persisting from 5 to 45 minutes on each occasion. The site and associated autonomic phenomena were similar to cluster headache, but the attacks of CPH were suppressed completely by indomethacin. A subsequent review of 84 cases showed a history of remission in 35 cases whereas 49 were chronic (Antonaci & Sjaastad, 1989). CPH usually begins in adulthood at the mean age of 34 years with a range of 6 to 81 years. Children with CPH have been reported (Broeske et al., 1993; Gladstein et al., 1994; Kudrow & Kudrow, 1989), although at least one case has been considered to be cluster headache (Solomon & Newman, 1995). The author has seen a 4-year child with an otherwise typical indomethacin-sensitive case. A typical case responding to acetazolamide has been reported (Warner et al., 1994).

By analogy with cluster headache the patients with remission have been referred to as episodic paroxysmal hemicrania (Kudrow et al., 1987). Pareja (1995) has recorded attacks which swap sides, just as is known for cluster headache, and attacks of autonomic features without pain. This has been observed in cluster headache after trigeminal nerve section, by this author and others, and is excellent evidence for a primarily CNS disorder. Event-related potentials which have been reported to be abnormal in migraine (Wang & Schoenen, 1998) are normal in CPH (Evers et al., 1997) as is cognitive processing (Evers et al., 1999).

Some recent cases have broadened our understanding of paroxysmal hemicrania. Boes and colleagues reported otalgia and an interesting sensation of fullness of the external auditory meatus responding to indomethacin (Boes et al., 1998). There has been some interesting speculation from Dodick about extra-trigeminal pain in episodic paroxysmal hemicrania (Dodick, 1998), and I doubt that the full clinical dimensions of these syndromes have been defined.

The essential features of paroxysmal hemicrania as it is now understood are:
- female preponderance;
- unilateral, usually fronto-temporal, very severe pain;
- short-lasting attacks (2–45 mins);
- very frequent attacks (usually more than 5 a day);
- marked autonomic features ipsilateral to the pain;
- robust, quick (less than 72 hours), excellent response to indomethacin, generally.

Other issues

The therapy of CPH has been discussed in relation to its responses to triptans. The issue is not clearly settled and may be both variable and dependent on the length of the attacks (Antonaci et al., 1998b; Dahlof, 1993; Pascual & Quijano, 1998). Greater occipital nerve injection is not useful in CPH (Antonaci et al., 1997). Piroxicam has been suggested to be helpful (Sjaastad & Antonaci, 1995), although again not as effective as indomethacin. By analogy with cluster headache verapamil has been used in CPH (Shabbir & McAbee, 1994), although the response is not spectacular and higher doses require exploration. An important and as yet unresolved issue is whether COX (cycloxygenase) II-selective blockers, such as celecoxib (Mathew et al., 2000) or rofecoxib, would be useful in CPH. An early impression is that some patients will benefit from these compounds.

CPH can coexist with trigeminal neuralgia (Caminero et al., 1998; Hannerz, 1993, 1998), just as does cluster headache (Pascual & Berciano, 1993; Watson & Evans, 1985). Both conditions must be treated to control the entire phenotype of the disorder. Similarly, secondary CPH has also been reported with a syndrome like Tolosa–Hunt (Foerderreuther et al., 1997) and in patients with a pituitary microadenoma and a maxillary cyst (Gatzonis et al., 1996), as well as as a first manifestation of cerebral metastasis of parotid epidermoid carcinoma (Mariano et al., 1998). Although extremely rare, a patient with CPH and typical migraine aura is reported.

Short-lasting unilateral neuralgiform headache attacks with conjunctival injection and tearing (SUNCT) (Fig. 62.6)

This condition was first described by Sjaastad et al. (1989) and its basis has been the subject of speculation, although recently posterior hypothalamic activation with BOLD contrast fMRI has been observed (May et al., 1999b), suggesting a disorder of the central nervous system. The patients are mostly males (Pareja & Sjaastad, 1994) with a gender ratio of approximately 4 to 1 (Pareja & Sjaastad, 1997). The paroxysms of pain usually last between 5 and 250 seconds (Pareja et al., 1996b) although longer duller interictal pains have been recognized, as have attacks up to 2 hours in two patients (Pareja et al., 1996a). Patients may have up to 30 episodes an hour although more usually would have 5–6 per hour. The frequency may also vary in bouts. A systematic study of attack frequency demonstrated a mean of 28 attacks per day with a range of 6 to 77 (Pareja et al., 1996a). The conjunctival injection seen with SUNCT is often the most prominent autonomic feature and tearing may also be very obvious. Other less prominent autonomic symptoms include sweating of the forehead or

Table 62.6. Differential diagnosis of short-lasting headaches

Feature	Cluster headache	Chronic paroxsymal hemicrania	Episodic paroxsymal hemicrania	SUNCT[a]	Idiopathic stabbing headache	Trigeminal neuralgia	Hypnic headache
Gender (M:F)	5:1	1:2	1:1	2:1	F>M	F>M	5:3
Pain							
– type	boring	boring	boring	stabbing	stabbing	stabbing	throbbing
– severity	very severe	very severe	very	severe	severe	very	moderate
– location	orbital	orbital	orbital	orbital	any	V2/V3>V1	generalized
Duration	15–180 min	2–45 min	1–30 min	15–120 s	<5 s	<1 s	15–30 min
Frequency	1–8/d	1–40/d	3–30/d	1/d–30/h	any	any	1–3/night
Autonomic	+	+	+	+	–	–[b]	–
Trigger	Alcohol nitrates	Alcohol	Alcohol nitrates	Cutaneous	none	Cutaneous	sleep
Indomethacin	?	+	+	–	+	–	+

Notes:

[a] Short-lasting unilateral neuralgiform headache with conjunctival injection and tearing.

[b] Cranial autonomic activation may be seen in first division trigeminal neuralgia.

rhinorrhoea. The attacks may become bilateral but the most severe pain remains unilateral.

Secondary SUNCT and associations

There have been several reported patients with SUNCT syndromes secondary to homolateral cerebellopontine angle and brainstem arteriovenous malformations diagnosed on MRI (Bussone et al., 1991; De Benedittis, 1996). One patient had a cavernous hemangioma of the cerebellopontine angle seen only on MRI (Morales et al., 1994), so that MRI of the brain should be part of the investigation of this syndrome when it is recognized. Extratrigeminal pain typical of SUNCT is reported (Wingerchuk et al., 2000) and is a syndrome which bears some consideration.

Management

Unlike some of the other short-lasting headache syndromes, such as the paroxsymal hemicranias that are highly responsive to indomethacin, SUNCT is remarkably refractory to treatment, including indomethacin (Pareja et al., 1995). The relationship between trigeminal neuralgia and SUNCT remains unclear (Sjaastad et al., 1997). There is a single report of a patient with trigeminal neuralgia who developed a SUNCT syndrome (Bouhassira et al., 1994). SUNCT patients may respond to carbamazepine in a partial sense. Case reports of responses with gabapentin, lamotrigine and topiramate can be found; of these topiramate and lamotrigine seem most promising.

Hemicrania continua

Sjaastad and Spierings (1984) reported two patients, a woman aged 63 years and a man of 53, who developed unilateral headache without obvious cause. One of these patients noticed redness, lacrimation and sensitivity to light in the eye on the affected side and the other described superadded 'jabs and jolts'. Both patients were relieved completely by indomethacin while other NSAIDs were of little or no benefit. Newman and colleagues (1994) reviewed the 24 previously reported cases and added 10 of their own, some with pronounced autonomic features resembling cluster headache. They divided their case histories into remitting and unremitting forms. Of the 34 patients reviewed, 22 were women and 12 men with the age of onset ranging from 11 to 58 years. The symptoms were controlled by indomethacin 75–150 mg daily.

Goadsby and Lipton (1997) compared the clinical presentation of hemicrania continua with that of chronic and episodic paroxysmal hemicrania, cluster headache and the SUNCT syndrome, concluding that it is likely to best fit under the general heading of 'trigeminal-autonomic cephalgias' to respect some of the likely shared pathophysiology. Silberstein et al. (1996) proposed that patients with hemicrania continua be subdivided into those with and without medication overuse. Apart from this secondary cause, analgesic overuse (Warner, 1997), and a report in an HIV-infected patient (Brilla et al., 1998), the status of secondary hemicrania continua is unclear.

Treatment

Sjaastad and Antonaci (1995) regard responsiveness to indomethacin as being essential for the diagnosis. Antonaci et al. (1998a) proposed the 'indotest' by which the intramuscular injection of 50 mg of indomethacin could be used as a diagnostic tool. In hemicrania continua, pain was relieved in 73 ± 66 minutes and the pain-free period was 13 ± 8 hours. The time elapsed between the oral administration of 25–50 mg t.i.d. and relief varied from 30 minutes to 48 hours (Pareja & Staastad, 1996). In practice, intramuscular indomethacin can be easily done as a single-blind placebo-controlled crossover *n-of*-1 study to clarify the best clinical management. Some patients may also respond to piroxicam and other NSAIDs (Sjaastad & Antonaci, 1995). Acute treatment with sumatriptan has been employed and reported to be of no benefit (Antonaci et al., 1998b). A useful effect from the COX (cycloxygenase) II-selective blocker, rofecoxib, is reported (Peres & Zukerman, 2000).

Primary (idiopathic) stabbing headache

Short-lived jabs of pain, defined by the International Headache Society as idiopathic jabbing headache (Headache Classification Committee of The International Headache Society, 1988) to be known as primary stabbing headache after the next revision, are well documented in association with most types of primary headache. The essential clinical features are:

- pain confined to the head, although rarely is it facial;
- stabbing pain lasting for a fraction of a second and occurring as a single stab or a series of stabs;
- recurring at irregular intervals (hours to days).

Raskin and Schwartz (1980) first described sharp, jabbing pains about the head resembling a stab from an ice-pick, nail, or needle. They compared the prevalence of such pains in 100 migrainous patients and 100 headache-free controls and only three of the control subjects had experienced ice-pick pains compared with 42 of the migraine patients, of whom 60% had more than one attack per month. The pains affected the temple or orbit more often than the parietal and occipital areas and often occurred before or during migraine headaches. Drummond and Lance (1984) obtained a history of ice-pick pains in 200 of 530 patients with recurrent primary headache. The sites of the ice-pick pains were recorded for 92 patients and coincided with the site of the patients' habitual headache in 37.

Retroauricular and occipital region pains are well described and these respond promptly to indomethacin (Martins et al., 1995). Ice-pick pains have been described in conjunction with cluster headaches (Lance & Anthony, 1971), and generally are experienced in the same area as the cluster pain. Ekbom (1975) noted that ice-pick pains may become more frequent as the attack abates. Sjaastad described what he called 'jabs and jolts' lasting less than a minute in patients with chronic paroxysmal hemicrania (Sjaastad et al., 1979). These seem more the exception, since idiopathic stabbing headache is generally truly stabbing: it is likely that longer lasting pains are a part of this overall spectrum. It is of interest that jabbing pains generally are not accompanied by cranial autonomic symptoms and can be seen with each of the trigeminal-autonomic cephalgias described in this chapter. The response of idiopathic jabbing headache to indomethacin (25–50 mg twice to three times daily) is generally excellent (Matthew, 1981; Medina & Diamond, 1981). As a general rule the symptoms wax and wane, and after a period of control on indomethacin it is appropriate to withdraw treatment and observe the outcome.

Benign cough headache

The clinical features of benign cough headache as defined by the IHS are (Headache Classification Committee of The International Headache Society, 1988):

- bilateral headache of sudden onset, short-lasting (usually < 1 min, but may last 30 min) and precipitated by coughing;
- may be prevented by avoiding coughing;
- may be diagnosed only after structural lesions such as posterior fossa tumour have been excluded by neuroimaging.

The presence of an Arnold–Chiari malformation or any lesion causing obstruction of CSF pathways or displacing cerebral structures must be excluded before cough headache is assumed to be benign. Cerebral aneurysm (Smith & Messing, 1993), carotid stenosis (Britton & Guiloff, 1988; Rivera et al., 1991) and vertebrobasilar disease (Staikov & Mattle, 1994) may also present with cough or exertional headache as the initial symptom.

Sharp pain in the head on coughing, sneezing, straining, laughing, or stooping has long been regarded as a symptom of organic intracranial disease, commonly associated with obstruction of the CSF pathways. Symonds (1956a) presented the case histories of six patients in whom cough headache was a symptom of a space-occupying lesion in the posterior fossa or of basilar impression from Paget's disease. He then described 21 patients with the same symptom in whom no intracranial disease became apparent. Cough headache disappeared in nine patients and improved spontaneously in another six patients. Two patients died of heart disease, and four were lost to follow-up. Symonds (1956a) concluded that there was a syndrome of benign cough headache, which he attributed to the stretching of a pain-producing structure in the posterior fossa, possibly the result of an adhesive arachnoiditis. Of Symonds' 21 patients, 18 were males, and ages ranged from 37 to 77 years, with an average age of 55 years (Symonds, 1956a).

Rooke (1968) considered cough headache as a variety of exertional headache and recorded his experienced with 103 patients who experienced transient headaches on running, bending, coughing, sneezing, lifting, or straining at stool in whom no intracranial disease could be detected and who were followed for 3 years or more. During the follow-up period, reinvestigation discovered structural lesions such as Arnold–Chiari malformations, platybasia, subdural hematoma, and cerebral or cerebellar tumour in 10 patients. Of the remaining 93, 30 were free of headache within 5 years, and 73 were improved or free of headache after 10 years. This type of headache was found in men more often than in women at a ratio of 4:1. Rooke observed that this form of headache may appear for the first time after a respiratory infection with cough and that some patients reported an abrupt recovery after the extraction of abscessed teeth, which had also been noted by Symonds (1956a).

Pathophysiology

Williams (1976) recorded cerebrospinal fluid (CSF) pressures from the cisterna magna and lumbar region during coughing. He found that there was a phase in which lumbar pressure exceeded cisternal pressure, followed by a phase in which the pressure gradient was reversed. He postulated that cough headache may be caused by a valve-like blockage at the foramen magnum, which interferes with the downward or rebound pulsation. Williams (1980) followed up this observation by studying two patients with cough headache whose cerebellar tonsils descended below the foramen magnum without any obvious obstruction and confirmed a severe craniospinal pressure dissociation during the rebound after a Valsalva manoeuvre. Decompression of the cerebellar tonsils relieved the headache and eliminated the steep pressure gradient on coughing. Williams (1980) commented that coughing increased intrathoracic and intra-abdominal pressure, which was transmitted to the epidural veins, causing a pressure wave and CSF to move rostrally. The headache was presumably caused by temporary impaction of the cerebellar tonsils when the subject relaxed and the pressure gradient then reversed. Whether this explanation applies to those patients without an Arnold–Chiari type I malformation remains uncertain.

The possibility of a sudden increase in venous pressure being sufficient by itself to cause headache must be considered. Lance (1991) reported the case of a man with a goitre sufficiently large to cause sudden headache when his arms were elevated and the jugular veins distended. Calendre et al. (1996) suggested the term 'Benign Valsalva's manoeuvre-related headache' to cover headaches provoked by coughing, straining or stooping but *cough headache* is more succinct and unlikely to be displaced.

Management

Mathew (1981) reported two patients with benign cough headache (one of whom had proved unresponsive to ergotamine, propranolol, and methysergide) who improved with indomethacin 50 mg three times daily. When this therapy was compared with placebo, the reduction in cough headache with the active drug was 95% in one case and 85% in the other, while the reductions on placebo medication were 0% and 18%, respectively. One patient who had particularly severe cough headaches unresponsive to indomethacin responded completely to the i.v. injection of dihydroergotamine (Hazelrigg, 1986). Raskin (1995) has reported that some patients with cough headache are relieved by lumbar puncture which is a simple option when compared to prolonged use of indomethacin. The mechanism of this response remains unclear.

Hypnic headache

This syndrome was first described by Raskin (1988) in patients aged from 67–84 who had headache of a moderately severe nature that typically came on a few hours after going to sleep. These headaches last from 15 to 30 minutes, are typically generalized, although may be unilateral (Gould & Silberstein, 1997; Morales-Asin et al., 1998), and can be throbbing (Newman et al., 1990). Patients may report falling back to sleep only to be awoken by a further attack a few hours later with up to three repetitions of this pattern over the night. In a large and very carefully presented series of Dodick's (1998) 19 patients, 16 (84%) were female and the mean age at onset was 61 ± 9 years. Headaches were bilateral in two-thirds and unilateral in one-third and in 80% of cases mild or moderate. Three patients reported similar headaches when falling asleep during the day. None had photophobia or phonophobia (Dodick et al., 1998).

Management

Patients with this form of headache generally respond to a bedtime dose of lithium carbonate (200–600 mg) (Newman et al., 1990; Raskin, 1988) and in those that do not tolerate this verapamil or methysergide at bedtime may be alternative strategies. Two patients who responded to flunarizine 5 mg at night have now been reported (Morales-Asin et al., 1998). Dodick and colleagues (1998) reported that one to two cups of coffee or caffeine 60 mg orally at bedtime was helpful. This author has recently successfully controlled a patient poorly tolerant of lithium using verapamil at night (160 mg) and others have reported a case controlled by indomethacin (Ivanez et al., 1998). This is an important observation in the context of trigeminal autonomic cephalgias (Goadsby & Lipton, 1997). Other strategies are important since, in the age group affected by the condition, lithium may have significant side effects.

Acknowledgements

The work of the author described herein has been supported by the Wellcome Trust and the Migraine Trust.

References

Andersson, P.G. & Jespersen, L.T. (1986). Dihydroergotamine nasal spray in the treatment of attacks of cluster headache. *Cephalalgia*, **6**, 51–4.

Anderton, J.M. & Helm, R. (1982). Multiple joint osteonecrosis following short-term steroid therapy. *J. Bone Joint Surg.*, **64A**, 139–42.

Anthony, M. (1987). The role of the occipital nerve in unilateral headache. In *Current Problems in Neurology*: 4 *Advances in Headache Research*, ed. F.C. Rose, pp. 257–62. London: John Libbey.

Antonaci, F. & Sjaastad, O. (1989). Chronic paroxysmal hemicrania (CPH): a review of the clinical manifestations. *Headache*, **29**, 648–56.

Antonaci, F., Pareja, J.A., Caminero, A.B. & Sjaastad, O. (1997). Chronic paroxysmal hemicrania and hemicrania continua: anaesthetic blockades of pericranial nerves. *Funct. Neurol.* **12**, 11–15.

Antonaci, F., Pareja, J.A., Caminero, A.B. & Sjaastad, O. (1998a). Chronic paroxysmal hemicrania and hemicrania continua. Parenteral indomethacin: the 'Indotest'. *Headache*, **38**, 122–8.

Antonaci, F., Pareja, J.A., Caminero, A.B. & Sjaastad, O. (1998b). Chronic paroxysmal hemicrania and hemicrania continua: lack of efficacy of sumatriptan. *Headache*, **38**, 197–200.

Aube, M. (1995). Treatment of slow-developing migraine with subcutaneous sumatriptan. *Cephalalgia*, **15**(Suppl. 14), 231.

Bahra, A. Gawel, M.J., Hardebo, J.-E. Millson, D., Brean, S.A. & Goadsby, P.J. (2000). Oral zolmitriptan is effective in the acute treatment of cluster headache. *Neurology*, **54**, 1832–9.

Bahra, A., May, A. & Goadsby, P.J. (2002). Cluster headache: a prospective clinical study in 230 patients with diagnostic implications. *Neurology*, **58**, 354–61.

Bates, D., Ashford, E., Dawson, R. et al. (1994). Subcutaneous sumatriptan during the migraine aura. *Neurology*, **44**, 1587–92.

Boes, C.J., Swanson, J.W. & Dodick, D.W. (1998). Chronic paroxysmal hemicrania presenting as otalgia with a sensation of external acoustic meatus obstruction: two cases and a pathophysiologic hypothesis. *Headache*, **38**, 787–91.

Bouhassira, D., Attal, N., Esteve, M. & Chauvin, M. (1994). SUNCT syndrome. A case of transformation from trigeminal neuralgia. *Cephalalgia*, **14**, 168–70.

Brilla, R., Evers, S., Soros, P. & Husstedt, I.W. (1998). Hemicrania continua in an HIV-infected outpatient. *Cephalalgia*, **18**, 287–8.

Britton, T.C. & Guiloff, R.J. (1988). Carotid artery disease presenting as cough headache. *Lancet*, **1**(8599), 1406–7.

Broeske, D., Lenn, N.J. & Cantos, E. (1993). Chronic paroxysmal hemicrania in a young child: possible relation to ipsilateral occipital infarction. *J. Child Neurol.*, **8**, 235–6.

Bussone, G., Leone, M., Peccarisi, C. et al. (1990). Double blind comparison of lithium and verapamil in cluster headache prophylaxis. *Headache*, **30**, 411–17.

Bussone, G., Leone, M., Volta, G.D., Strada, L. & Gasparotti, R. (1991). Short-lasting unilateral neuralgiform headache attacks with tearing and conjunctival injection: the first symptomatic case. *Cephalalgia*, **11**, 123–7.

Calendre, L., Hernandez, L-A. & Lopez-Valdez, E. (1996). Benign Valsalva's maneuver-related headache: an MRI study of six cases. *Headache*, **36**, 251–3.

Caminero, A.B., Pareja, J.A. & Dobato, J.L. (1998). Chronic paroxysmal hemicrania-tic syndrome. *Cephalalgia*, **18**, 159–61.

Carolis, P.D., Capoa, D.D., Agati, R., Baldratti, A. & Sacqnegna, T. (1988). Episodic cluster headache: short and long term results of prophylactic treatment. *Headache*, **28**, 475–6.

Cid, C., Berciano, J. & Pascual, J. (2000). Retro-ocular headache with autonomic features resembling 'continuous' cluster headache in a lateral medullary infarction. *J. Neurol. Neurosurg. Psychiatry*, **69**, 134–41.

Cremer, P., Halmagyi, G.M. & Goadsby, P.J. (1995). Secondary cluster headache responsive to sumatriptan. *J. Neurol. Neurosurg. Psychiatry*, **59**, 633–4.

Curran, D.A. Hinterberger, H. & Lance, J.W. (1967). Methysergide. *Res. Clin. Stud. Headache*, **1**, 74–122.

Dahlof, C. (1993). Subcutaneous sumatriptan does not abort attacks of chronic paroxysmal hemicrania (CPH). *Headache*, **33**, 201–2.

De Benedittis, G. (1996). SUNCT syndrome associated with cavernous angioma of the brain stem. *Cephalalgia*, **16**, 503–6.

de la Sayette, V., Schaeffer, S., Coskun, O., Leproux, F. & Defer, G. (1999). Cluster headache-like attack as an opening symptom of a unilateral infarction of the cervical cord: persistent anaesthesia and dysaesthesia to cold stimuli. *J. Neurol., Neurosurg., Psychiatry*, **66**, 397–400.

Dodick, D.W. (1998). Extratrigeminal episodic paroxysmal hemicrania. Further clinical evidence of functionally relevant brain stem connections. *Headache*, **38**, 794–8.

Dodick, D.W., Mosek, A.C. & Campbell, J.K. (1998). The hypnic ('alarm clock') headache syndrome. *Cephalalgia*, **18**, 152–6.

Drummond, P.D. & Lance, J.W. (1984). Neurovascular disturbances in headache patients. *Clin. Exp. Neurol.*, **20**, 93–9.

Ekbom, K. (1947). Ergotamine tartrate orally in Horton's 'histaminic cephalalgia' (also called Harris's cilary neuralgia). *Acta Psychiat. Scand.*, **46**, 106.

Ekbom, K. (1975). Some observations on pain in cluster headache. *Headache*, **14**, 219–25.

Ekbom, K. & Greitz, T. (1970). Carotid angiography in cluster headache. *Acta Radiol.*, **10**, 177–86.

Ekbom, K. & The Sumatriptan Cluster Headache Study Group. (1991). Treatment of acute cluster headache with sumatriptan. *N. Engl. J. Med.*, **325**, 322–6.

Ekbom, K., Waldenlind, E., Cole, J.A., Pilgrim, A.J. & Kirkham, A. (1992). Sumatriptan in chronic cluster headache: results of continuous treatment for eleven months. *Cephalalgia*, **12**, 254–6.

Ekbom, K., Monstad, I., Prusinski, A., Cole, J.A., Pilgrim, A.J. & Noronha, D. (1993). Subcutaneous sumatriptan in the acute treatment of cluster headache: a dose comparison study. *Acta Neurol. Scand.*, **88**, 63–9.

Evers, S., Bauer, B., Suhr, B., Husstedt, J.W. & Grotemeyr, K.H. (1997). Cognitive processing in primary headache: a study of event-related potentials. *Neurology*, **48**, 108–13.

Evers, S., Bauer, B., Suhr, B., Voss, H., Frese, A. & Husstedt, I.W. (1999). Cognitive processing is involved in cluster headache but not in chronic paroxysmal hemicrania. *Neurology*, **53**, 357–63.

Fischer, D.E. & Bickel, W.H. (1971). Corticosteroid-induced avascular necrosis. A clinical study of 77 patients. *J. Bone Joint Surg.*, **53A**, 859–64.

Foerderreuther, S., Maydell, R.V. & Straube, A. (1997). A CPH-like picture in two patients with an orbitocavernous sinus syndrome. *Cephalalgia*, **17**, 608–11.

Fogan, L. (1985). Treatment of cluster headache: a double blind comparison of oxygen vs air inhalation. *Arch. Neurol.*, **42**, 362–3.

Gabai, I.J. & Spierings, E.L.H. (1989). Prophylactic treatment of cluster headache with verapamil. *Headache*, **29**, 167–8.

Gatzonis, S., Mitsikostas, D.D., Ilias, A., Zournas, C.H. & Papageorgiou, C. (1996). Two more secondary headaches mimicking chronic paroxysmal hemicrania. Is this the exception or the rule? *Headache*, **36**, 511–13.

Gladstein, J., Holden, E.W. & Peralta, L. (1994). Chronic paroxysmal hemicrania in a child. *Headache*, **34**, 519–20.

Goadsby, P.J. (1994). Cluster headache and the clinical profile of sumatriptan. *Eur. Neurol.*, **34**(Suppl), 35–9.

Goadsby, P.J. & Lipton, R.B. (1997). A review of paroxysmal hemicranias, SUNCT syndrome and other short-lasting headaches with autonomic features, including new cases. *Brain*, **120**, 193–209.

Good, A.E. (1974). Bilateral aseptic necrosis of the femur following a sixteen day course of corticotropin. *J. Am. Med. Assoc.*, **228**, 497–9.

Gould, J.D. & Silberstein, S.D. (1997). Unilateral hypnic headache: a case study. *Neurology*, **49**, 1749–51.

Greve, E. & Mai, J. (1988). Cluster headache-like headaches: a symptomatic feature? *Cephalalgia*, **8**, 79–82.

Hannerz, J. (1989). A case of parasellar maningioma mimicking cluster headache. *Cephalalgia*, **9**, 265–9.

Hannerz, J. (1993). Trigeminal neuralgia with chronic paroxysmal hemicrania: the CPH-tic syndrome. *Cephalalgia*, **13**, 361–4.

Hannerz, J. (1998). The second case of chronic paroxysmal hemicrania-tic syndrome. *Cephalalgia*, **18**, 124.

Hardebo, J.E. (1993). Subcutaneous sumatriptan in cluster headache: a time study in the effect of pain and autonomic symptoms. *Headache*, **33**, 18–21.

Hardebo, J.E. (1994). How cluster headache is explained as an intracavernous inflammatory process lesioning sympathetic fibres. *Headache*, **34**, 125–31.

Hardebo, J.E. & Dahlof, C. (1998). Sumatriptan nasal spray (20 mg/dose) in the acute treatment of cluster headache. *Cephalalgia*, **18**, 487–9.

Hazelrigg, R.L. (1986). IV DHE-45 relieves exertional cephalgia. *Headache*, **26**(1), 52.

Headache Classification Committee of The International Headache Society (1988). Classification and diagnostic criteria for headache disorders, cranial neuralgias and facial pain. *Cephalalgia*, **8**(Suppl. 7), 1–96.

Heidegger, S., Mattfeldt, T., Rieber, A. et al. (1997). Orbito-sphenoidal aspergillus infection mimicking cluster headache: a case report. *Cephalalgia*, **17**, 676–9.

Hering, R. & Kuritzky, A. (1989). Sodium valproate in the treatment of cluster headache: an open clinical trial. *Cephalalgia*, **9**, 195–8.

Hofman, M.A., Zhou, J.N. & Swaab, D.F. (1996). Suprachiasmatic nucleus of the human brain: an immunocytochemical and morphometric analysis. *J. Comp. Neurol.*, **305**, 552–6.

Horton, B.T. (1952). Histaminic cephalalgia. *Lancet*, **72**, 92–8.

Humphrey, P.P.A., Feniuk, W., Marriott, A.S., Tanner, R.J.N., Jackson, M.R. & Tucker, M.L. (1991). Preclinical studies on the anti-migraine drug, sumatriptan. *Eur. Neurol.*, **31**, 282–90.

Hunter, C.R. & Mayfield, F.H. (1949). Role of the upper cervical roots in the production of pain in the head. *Am. J. Surg.*, **78**, 743–9.

Isler, H. (1993). Episodic cluster headache from a textbook of 1745: Van Swieten's classic description. *Cephalalgia*, **13**, 172–4.

Ivanez, V., Soler, R. & Barreiro, P. (1998). Hypnic headache syndrome: a case with good response to indomethacin. *Cephalalgia*, **18**(4), 225–6.

Jammes, J.L. (1975). The treatment of cluster headaches with prednisone. *Dis. Nerv. Syst.*, **36**, 375–6.

Kitrelle, J.P., Grouse, D.S. & Seybold, M.E. (1985). Cluster headache: local anesthetic abortive agents. *Arch. Neurol.*, **42**, 496–8.

Koenigsberg, A.D., Solomon, G.D. & Kosmorsky, D.O. (1994). Pseudoaneurysm within the cavernous sinus presenting as cluster headache. *Headache*, **34**, 111–13.

Kudrow, L. (1977). Lithium prophylaxis for chronic cluster headache. *Headache*, **17**, 15–18.

Kudrow, L. (1980). *Cluster Headache: Mechanisms and Management.* Oxford: Oxford University Press.

Kudrow, L. (1981). Response of cluster headache attacks to oxygen inhalation. *Headache*, **21**, 1–4.

Kudrow, D.B. & Kudrow, L. (1989). Successful aspirin prophylaxis in a child with chronic paroxysmal hemicrania. *Headache*, **29**, 280–1.

Kudrow, L., Esperanca, P. & Vijayan, N. (1987). Episodic paroxysmal hemicrania? *Cephalalgia*, **7**, 197–201.

Kuritzky, A. (1984). Cluster headache-like pain caused by an upper cervical meningioma. *Cephalalgia*, **4**, 185–6.

Lance, J.W. (1991). Solved and unsolved headache problems. *Headache*, **31**, 439–45.

Lance, J.W. (1993). *Mechanism and Management of Headache*, 5th edn. London: Butterworth Scientific.

Lance, J.W. & Anthony, M. (1971). Migrainous neuralgia or cluster headache? *J. Neurol. Sci.*, **13**, 401–14.

Leone, M. & Bussone, G. (1993). A review of hormonal findings in cluster headache. Evidence for hypothalamic involvement. *Cephalalgia*, **13**(5), 309–17.

Leone, M., D'Amico, D., Frediani, F. et al. (2000). Verapamil in the prophylaxis of episodic cluster headache: a double-blind study versus placebo. *Neurology*, **54**(6), 1382–5.

Lipton, R.B., Stewart, W.F., Cady, R. et al. (2000). Sumatriptan for the range of headaches in migraine sufferers: results of the Spectrum Study. *Headache*, **40**, 783–91.

Mani, S. & Deeter, J. (1982). Arteriovenous malformation of the brain presenting as a cluster headache – a case report. *Headache*, **22**, 184–5.

Mariano, H.S., Bigal, M.E., Bordini, C.A. & Speciali, J.G. (1998). Chronic paroxysmal hemicrania (CPH)-like syndrome as a first manifestation of cerebral metastasis of parotid epidermoid carcinoma: a case report. *Cephalalgia*, **19**(4), 442.

Martins, J.P., Parreira, E. & Costa, I. (1995). Extratrigeminal ice-pick status. *Headache*, **35**, 107–10.

Mathew, N.T. (1981). Indomethacin-responsive headache syndromes. *Headache*, **21**, 147–50.

Mathew, N.T., Kailasam, J. & Fischer, A. (2000). Responsiveness to celecoxib in chronic paroxysmal hemicrania. *Neurology*, **55**, 316.

May, A. & Goadsby, P.J. (1999). The trigeminovascular system in humans: pathophysiological implications for primary headache syndromes of the neural influences on the cerebral circulation. *J. Cereb. Blood Flow Metab.*, **19**, 115–27.

May, A., Bahra, A., Buchel, C., Frackowiak, R.S.J. & Goadsby, P.J. (1998). Hypothalamic activation in cluster headache attacks. *Lancet*, **351**, 275–8.

May, A., Ashburner, J., Buchel, C. et al. (1999a). Correlation between structural and functional changes in brain in an idiopathic headache syndrome. *Nat. Med.*, **5**, 836–8.

May, A., Bahra, A., Buchel, C., Turner, R. & Goadsby, P.J. (1999b). Functional MRI in spontaneous attacks of SUNCT: short-lasting neuralgiform headache with conjunctival injection and tearing. *Ann. Neurol.*, **46**, 791–3.

Medina, J.L. & Diamond, S. (1981). Cluster headache variant: spectrum of a new headache syndrome. *Arch. Neurol.*, **38**, 705–9.

Mirzai, R., Chang, C., Greenspan, A. & Gershwin, M.E. (1999). The pathogenesis of osteonecrosis and the relationships to corticosteroids. *J. Asthma*, **36**, 77–95.

Monstad, I., Krabbe, A., Micieli, G. et al. (1995). Preemptive oral treatment with sumatriptan during a cluster period. *Headache*, **35**, 607–13.

Morales, F., Mostacero, E., Marta, J. & Sanchez, S. (1994). Vascular malformation of the cerebellopontine angle associated with SUNCT syndrome. *Cephalalgia*, **14**, 301–2.

Morales-Asin, F., Mauri, J.A., Iniguez, C., Espada, F. & Mostacero, E. (1998). The hypnic headache syndrome: report of three new cases. *Cephalalgia*, **18**, 157–8.

Moskowitz, M.A. (1988). Cluster Headache – evidence for a pathophysiologic focus in the superior pericarotid cavernous sinus plexus. *Headache*, **28**, 584–6.

Muoz, C., Diez-Tejedor, E., Frank, A. & Barreiro, P. (1996). Cluster headache syndrome associated with middle cerebral artery arteriovenous malformation. *Cephalalgia*, **16**, 202–5.

Naylor, W.G. (1988). *Calcium Antagonists*. London: Academic Press.

Newman, L.C. Lipton, R.B. & Solomon, S. (1990). The hypnic headache syndrome: a benign headache disorder of the elderly. *Neurology*, **40**, 1904–5.

Newman, L.C., Lipton, R.B. & Solomon, S. (1994). Hemicrania continua: ten new cases and a review of the liturature. *Neurology*, **44**, 2111–14.

Olesen, J. & Goadsby, P.J. (1999). *Cluster Headache and Related Conditions*, ed. J. Olesen. *Frontiers in Headache Research*, vol 9. Oxford: Oxford University Press.

Pareja, J.A. (1995). Chronic paroxysmal hemicrania: dissociation of the pain and autonomic features. *Headache*, **35**, 111–13.

Pareja, J.A. & Sjaastad, O. (1994). SUNCT syndrome in the female. *Headache*, **34**, 217–20.

Pareja, J. & Sjaastad, O. (1996). Chronic paroxysmal hemicrania and hemicrania continua. Interval between indomethacin administration and response. *Headache*, **36**, 20–3.

Pareja, J.A. & Sjaastad, O. (1997). SUNCT syndrome. A clinical review. *Headache*, **37**, 195–202.

Pareja, J.A., Kruszewski, P. & Sjaastad, O. (1995). SUNCT syndrome: trials of drugs and anesthetic blockades. *Headache*, **35**, 138–42.

Pareja, J.A., Joubert, J. & Sjaastad, O. (1996a). SUNCT syndrome. Atypical temporal patterns. *Headache*, **36**, 108–10.

Pareja, J.A., Ming, J.M., Kruszewski, P., Caballero, V., Pamo, M. & Sjaastad, O. (1996b). SUNCT syndrome: duration, frequency and temporal distribution of attacks. *Headache*, **36**, 161–5.

Pascual, J. & Berciano, J. (1993). Relief of cluster-tic syndrome by the combination of lithium and carbamazepine. *Cephalalgia*, **13**, 205–6.

Pascual, J. & Quijano, J. (1998). A case of chronic paroxysmal hemicrania responding to subcutaneous sumatriptan. *J. Neurol., Neurosurg., Psychiatry*, **65**(3), 407.

Peres, M.F.P. & Zukerman, E. (2000). Hemicrania continua responsive to rofecoxib. *Cephalalgia*, **20**, 130–1.

Raskin, N.H. (1988). The hypnic headache syndrome. *Headache*, **28**, 534–6.

Raskin, N.H. (1995). The cough headache syndrome: treatment. *Neurology*, **45**(9), 1784.

Raskin, N.H. & Schwartz, R.K. (1980). Icepick-like pain. *Neurology*, **30**, 203–5.

Rivera, M., del Real, M.A., Teruel, J.L., Gobernado, J.M. & Ortuno, J. (1991). Carotid artery disease presenting as cough headache in a patient on haemodialysis. *Postgrad. Med. J.*, **67**(789), 702.

Robbins, L. (1995). Intranasal lidocaine for cluster headache. *Headache*, **35**, 83–4.

Rooke, E. (1968). Benign exertional headache. *Med. Clin. N. Am.*, **52**, 801–8.

Shabbir, N. & McAbee, G. (1994). Adolescent chronic paroxysmal hemicrania responsive to verapamil monotherapy. *Headache*, **34**, 209–10.

Silberstein, S.D. (1994). Pharmacological management of cluster headache. *CNS Drugs*, **2**, 199–207.

Silberstein, S.D., Lipton, R.B. & Sliwinski, M. (1996). Classification of daily and near-daily headaches: a field study of revised IHS criteria. *Neurology*, **47**, 871–5.

Silberstein, S.D., Niknam, R., Rozen, T.D. & Young, W.B. (2000). Cluster headache with aura. *Neurology*, **54**, 219–21.

Singh, B.N. & Nademanee, K. (1987). Use of calcium antagonists for cardiac arrhythmias. *Am. J. Cardiol.*, **59**, 153B–62B.

Sjaastad, O. (1992). *Cluster Headache Syndrome*. London: W.B. Saunders.

Sjaastad, O. & Antonaci, F. (1995). A piroxicam derivative partly effective in chronic paroxysmal hemicrania and hemicrania continua. *Headache*, **35**(9), 549–50.

Sjaastad, O. & Dale, I. (1974). Evidence for a new (?) treatable headache entity. *Headache*, **14**, 105–8.

Sjaastad, O. & Dale, I. (1976). A new (?) clinical headache entity 'chronic paroxysmal hemicrania'. *Acta Neurol. Scand.*, **54**, 140–59.

Sjaastad, O. & Spierings, E.L. (1984). Hemicrania continua: another headache absolutely responsive to indomethacin. *Cephalalgia*, **4**, 65–70.

Sjaastad, O., Egge, K., Horven, I. et al. (1979). Chronic paroxysmal hemicrania V. Mechanical precipitation of attacks. *Headache*, **19**, 31–6.

Sjaastad, O., Saunte, C., Salvesen, R. et al. (1989). Shortlasting unilateral neuralgiform headache attacks with conjunctival injection, tearing, sweating, and rhinorrhea. *Cephalalgia*, **9**, 147–56.

Sjaastad, O., Pareja, J.A., Zukerman, E., Jansen, J. & Kruszewski, P. (1997). Trigeminal neuralgia. Clinical manifestations of first division involvement. *Headache*, **37**, 346–57.

Smith, W.S. & Messing, R.O. (1993). Cerebral aneurysm presenting as cough headache. *Headache*, **33**(4), 203–4.

Solomon, S. & Newman, L.C. (1995). Chronic paroxysmal hemicrania in a child? *Headache*, **35**, 234.

Staikov, I.N. & Mattle, H.P. (1994). Vertebrobasilar dolicoectasia and exertional headache. *J. Neurol. Neurosurg. Psychiatry*, **57**, 1544.

Steiner, T.J. Hering, R., Couturier, E.G.M., Davies, P.T.G. & Whitmarsh, T.E. (1997). Double-blind placebo controlled trial of lithium in episodic cluster headache. *Cephalalgia*, **17**, 673–5.

Symonds, C. (1956a) Cough headache. *Brain*, **79**, 557–68.

Symonds, C.P. (1956b). A particular variety of headache. *Brain*, **79**, 217–32.

Tfelt-Hansen, P., Paulson, O.B. & Krabbe, A.E. (1982). Invasive adenoma of the pituitary gland and chronic migrainous neuralgia. A rare coincidence or a causal relationship? *Cephalalgia*, **2**, 25–8.

Waldenlind, E., Ekbom, K. & Torhall, J. (1993). MR-Angiography during spontaneous attacks of cluster headache: a case report. *Headache*, **33**, 291–5.

Wang, W. & Schoenen, J. (1998). Interictal potentiation of passive 'oddball' auditory event-related potentials in migraine. *Cephalalgia*, **18**, 261–5.

Warner, J.S. (1997). Analgesic rebound as a cause of hemicrania continua. *Neurology*, **48**, 1540–1.

Warner, J.S., Wamil, A.W. & McLean, M.J. (1994). Acetazolamide for the treatment of chronic paroxysmal hemicrania. *Headache*, **34**, 597–9.

Watson, P. & Evans, R. (1985). Cluster-tic syndrome. *Headache*, **25**, 123–6.

West, P. & Todman, D. (1991). Chronic cluster headache associated with a vertebral artery aneurysm. *Headache*, **31**, 210–12.

Wheeler, S.D. & Carrazana, E.J. (1999). Topiramate-treated cluster headache. *Neurology*, **53**, 234–6.

Williams, B. (1976). Cerebrospinal fluid pressure changes in response to coughing. *Brain*, **99**, 331–46.

Williams, B. (1980). Cough headache due to craniospinal pressure dissociation. *Arch. Neurol.*, **37**, 226–30.

Wingerchuk, D.M., Nyquist, P.A., Rodriguez, M. & Dodick, D.W. (2000). Extratrigeminal short-lasting unilateral neuralgiform headache with conjunctival injection and tearing (SUNCT): new pathophysiologic entity or variation on a theme? *Cephalalgia*, **20**, 127–9.

63

Orofacial pain

Steven B. Graff-Radford

Cedars–Sinai Medical Center, 444 South San Vicente # 1101, Los Angeles CA, USA

Orofacial pain presents clinicians with a daunting task. The most critical task in treating patients is to establish the correct diagnosis. Often with chronic pain, we are faced with limited understanding, resulting too often in patients being labelled psychogenic. Pain as defined by The International Association for the Study of Pain is 'an unpleasant sensory and emotional experience associated with actual or potential tissue damage, or described in terms of such damage' (Mersky, 1986). This definition allows for the pain to be present without nociception (the recordable neural activity in Aδ and C-fibres). Thus the clinician is encouraged to consider assessing the associated suffering and pain behaviour in understanding and treating pain. Pain in the face is often referred, owing to the trigeminal nerves' complex distribution. It is suggested therefore, that an organ system classification may simplify the problem enabling a quick and accurate diagnosis.

Classification

The International Headache Society published a classification system that can be used to describe many orofacial pains (Olesen, 1988). This classification separates many conditions that may produce facial pain and classifies them independently. For this discussion Table 63.1 provides an organ-based classification system that simplifies differential diagnosis. The orofacial pains are divided into six categories and will be reviewed separately.

Extracranial

The eyes, ears, nose, throat, sinuses, teeth, lymph glands, salivary glands may produce pain when infectious, degenerative, edematous, neoplastic or destructive processes

Table 63.1. Organ system classification for orofacial pain

Organ	Presence	Quality	
A	Extracranial	Continuous	Dull
B	Intracranial	Continuous	Variable
C	Psychogenic	Variable	Variable
D	Neurovascular	Intermittent	Throbbing
E	Neuropathic	Intermittent	Sharp, shooting, electric
		Continuous	Burning
F	Musculoskeletal	Continuous	Dull, aching

trigger noxious stimulation. While the musculoskeletal system is an extracranial structure, they are separated in the classification as they are considered as a very common pain condition worthy of special attention.

Eye

Pain in and around the eye usually is caused by local disease but may also be referred from the teeth, jaw or sinuses. In addition migraine and other neurovascular pains are often perceived in the eye. An inflammatory pseudotumour in the orbit associated with Tolosa–Hunt syndrome may produce eye pain. Pseudotumour cerebri, also called benign intracranial hypertension, or idiopathic intracranial hypertension, classically presents with headache, associated with papilledema and sometimes 6th nerve palsy. These patients are best followed by neurophthalmologists to ensure vision is not lost due to persistent papilledema. Eye pain may be differentiated into superficial or corneal pain, deep or inflammatory pains. Eye disease includes iritis, acute angle glaucoma. Other eye disease may involve optic neuritis, eye strain and enucleation. Pain quality is variable depending on the cause or pathology location. It is suggested that localized eye pain be evaluated by an ophthalmologist.

Ear

Pain in the ear is often referred from musculoskeletal structures such as the temporomandibular joint or mastication muscles. Additionally, the teeth or temporomandibular joint may refer pain to the ear. In these cases the pain is described as a dull, achy, or stopped-up sensation. Because the ear is complexly innervated by cranial nerves V, VII, IX, X, and cervical roots C2–3, referred pain to the ear needs to be carefully considered. Ear pain may arise from the external ear canal as an acute inflammatory process, or due to an accumulation of wax producing pressure. Middle ear or mastoid problems are often due to infection of the mucous membranes causing otitis media. If inflammation spreads to the petrous bones, a petrositis may develop or meningitis. Acoustic neuroma, a benign tumour involving the neural sheath of cranial nerve VIII, is associated with hearing loss, a tingling sensation deep in the ear and, if there is trigeminal nerve involvement, pain in the ear or face.

Nose

Pain in the nose may also be refereed from the teeth, sinuses or other structures, but is more likely caused by inflammation or local tumour. When there is inflammation present, it is useful to differentiate inflammatory, allergic, vasomotor or atrophic rhinitis. Referral to an ear nose and throat specialist is recommended if dental etiology is ruled out.

Throat

Throat pain is most often a local inflammatory reaction secondary to infection. Certainly, other local problems such as tumor need be considered. Some neurological problems like glossopharyngeal neuralgia, stomatodynia (burning mouth syndrome) and Eagles syndrome will be discussed under neurogenous pains. Throat tumours may invade various structures and produce pain, often associated with neurological or functional change. Diagnosis requires imaging and careful tissue exploration.

Sinus and paranasal pain

It has been established that pain can emanate from nasal and paranasal structures. Wolff, using mechanical stimuli

Table 63.2. Pain referral from nasal and paranasal mucosa

Site stimulated	Site pain reported
Nasal floor and septum	Local, zygoma, towards ear, outer and inner eye canthus, eye
Nasal turbinates	Lateral wall inside nose, upper teeth, below eye
Maxillary sinus	Local, nasopharynx, posterior teeth, zygoma, temple
Frontal sinus	Local
Ethmoid sinus	Eye, deep in the inner eye canthus
Sphenoid sinus	Pharynx, deep in the head, maxillary teeth, vertex

and faradic current at various sites, elicited an aching or sharp, burning sensation from nose and sinus mucosal linings. The referred pain, following stimulation, occurred in specific patterns. The referral patterns are summarized in Table 63.2.

Sinus inflammation may be acute or chronic. Acute sinusitis is characterized by symptoms indicating active nasal membrane and sinus inflammation. Symptoms including dull persistent pain, associated with a purulent discharge, usually into the nose or pharynx. Malaise and fever are also usually present. Inflammatory sinus disease commonly produces toothache. Usually the maxillary sinus is implicated and pain is felt in the maxillary teeth on the involved side. The pain presents as a continuous dull toothache, accompanied by a feeling that the tooth is extruded.

Chronic sinusitis is characterized by persistent sinus mucous membrane inflammation. Hypertrophy, may induce permanent changes to the nasal ciliary action and mucous glands. There is no evidence that these changes produce headache. Chronic sinusitis may relapse into acute inflammation and then may present with pain.

Sinus evaluation may include sinus transillumination, which often reveals pus in acute sinusitis. Plain radiographs may show fluid levels. Specific radiographic techniques may be needed to clearly identify each sinus, e.g. a Waters view is used for the maxillary sinus. A computerized tomogram (CT) scan or MRI may be helpful in differentiating cystic from solid lesions, but differentiating acute from chronic sinusitis requires the presence of clinical features. Treating acute sinusitis and the presenting orofacial pain is best accomplished with antibiotics and systemic or topical decongestants. Surgical drainage may be required.

Teeth

The most common orofacial pain involves the teeth and their supporting structures. Most frequently the pain is related to dental caries, presenting as a reversible pulpitis. The reversible pulpitis is characterized by poorly localized pain, often sensitive to hot or cold stimuli. The reaction to the noxious stimulus (hot or cold) disappears soon after its removal. Eventually when the carious lesion invades the pulp an irreversible pulpitis begins. This is characterized by a lingering reaction to noxious stimuli such as hot or cold. If the microorganisms and inflammatory products invade the area around the root apex (periapical) this is called a periodontitis and may present with toothache associated with chewing, touch and percussion sensitivity. Periapical pathology may be observed as an area of increased radiolucency on radiograms. The tooth may have an abnormal response to pulp testing where applying heat, cold or electrical stimulus is not perceived. In clinical practice differentiating reversible and irreversible pulpitis is difficult. In situations where the diagnosis is not obvious, careful observation over days or weeks is recommended. Too often endodontic therapy is performed when not indicated.

An intermittent pain that is triggered by biting on an offending tooth characterizes cracked tooth syndrome. Unfortunately the cracks are often difficult to find and don't show on all X-ray images. This pain is often confused with pulpitis or trigeminal neuralgia resulting in frustration and unnecessary treatment. Tomographic imaging 1 mm apart through the tooth's long axis may be beneficial in defining the crack. Further careful clinical examination including meticulous bite tests on each tooth cusp or staining may be useful. Graff-Radford and Gratt have studied cracked teeth with thermography and it appears there is a difference in the patients with cracked teeth and neuropathic facial pain. The cracked tooth patients have normal thermograms and the neuropathic pain patients display asymmetrical thermograms (Graff-Radford et al., 1995). Chronic toothache may be a referred phenomenon. Where no obvious local etiology is evident, neuropathic, muscular or vascular etiologies should be considered (Graff-Radford et al., 1995).

Burning mouth syndrome

Burning mouth syndrome (BMS) is characterized by a burning sensation in one or several oral structures (Tourne & Fricton, 1992). Although no obvious cause has been established, numerous possibilities exist. The pathogenesis may be summarized into local, systemic and psychological etiologies. Local factors include contact allergy, denture irritation, oral habits, infection, and possible reflux esophagitis. The systemic factors include menopause, vitamin and mineral deficiency, diabetes, oral infection and chemotherapy. Psychogenic factors have often been cited but are mostly anecdotal. An essential component to rule out is candida infection. Although this may not be obvious to the eye, swabbing the oral mucosa and culture for fungus often reveals an incipient infection. Patients with fungal infection respond quickly to antifungal preparations such as clotrimazole or fluconazole. The author's experience indicates approximately half the patients with BMS have a candida infection. This often follows steroid, antibiotic or chemotherapy. For those patients where no systemic or local pathology is identified, it is postulated that the cause is neuropathic. Topical clonazepam (0.5–1.0 mg three times per day) has been effective in reducing a burning oral pain (Woda et al., 1998). Patients are instructed to suck a tablet for three minutes (and then spit out) 3 times per day for at least 10 days. Serum concentrations are minimal (3.3 ng/ml) 1 and 3 hours after application. Woda hypothesized clonazepam produced a peripheral not central action disrupting the neuropathologic mechanism. Additional treatments for BMS include medications ranging from tricyclic antidepressants, antiepileptic drugs, benzodiazepines, folic acid and oral rinses. Treatment outcome is varied.

Intracranial

Intracranial pathology presenting as orofacial pain is exceedingly rare. The pain is usually associated with additional neurological signs and symptoms. The meninges, cranial nerves and blood vessels are the pain sensitive structures intracranially. Traction, inflammation, distention or pressure on these structures produces pain referral to distant sites.

Thalamic pain is described as 'unilateral facial pain and dysesthesia attributed to a lesion of the quintothalamic pathway or thalamus. Symptoms may also involve the trunk and limbs of the affected side' (Mersky, 1986). Infarcts in the thalamus involving the primary sensory nuclei, or damage in other sensory pathways, may lead to thalamic pain syndrome. The pain quality is moderate to severe, burning or aching, and localized to the face contralateral to the infarct. The clinical presentation may include a hemiplegia and associated allodynia, hyperesthesia and hyperpathia. MRI or CT scans are used to confirm the diagnosis. Treatment is difficult, but patients respond best to the tricyclic antidepressants or membrane stabilizing medications such as listed in Table 63.5. Stimulation produced analgesia such as acupuncture or TENS or even deep brain stimulation may be treatment considerations.

Intracranial neoplasms produce pain in approximately 60% of cases. This is typically a dull, non-pulsatile, persistent pain aggravated by exertion or postural changes (Bulitt & Tew, 1986). In the patient who presents with non-odontogenic face pain where other cranial nerve abnormalities are present, intracranial pathology must be considered. While certain intracranial tumours are more likely to produce neurological problems, all do not present with the same neurological signs (Rushton & Rooke, 1962). Tumours producing facial pain include meningiomas, schwannomas, neurofibromas, acoustic neuromas and cholesteatomas. Pituitary tumours may result in pain when they erode the sella or place pressure on the gasserian ganglion due to invasion of the cavernous sinus (Cueneo & Rand, 1952). It is suggested that tumours arising from the trigeminal ganglion produce pain, and those arising from the root do not (Schisano & Olivercrona, 1960).

Psychogenic

Labelling a disease process psychogenic without clear documented objective criteria is grossly unfair to the patient. Fordyce has pointed out that too often a patient's pain experiences are labelled 'psychogenic pain' when repeated failures using the biomedical model result in a lengthy medical history (Fordyce & Steger, 1978). Fordyce suggests it is the system that has not provided adequate diagnosis. Psychogenic pain may be interpreted in many ways. Some consider psychogenic pain when the pain behaviour is in excess or is discrepant from the physiological sensation or apparent nociceptive cause. A more useful manner in which the psychogenic pain label may be employed, is when the emotional and psychological factors are the pain's primary. The latter alternative requires positive inclusion criteria and Fordyce suggests these may be divided into four groups (i) somatic delusions, (ii) somatization disorder, (iii) conversion, (iv) depression. Fordyce points out that psychogenic diagnosis is a philosophical one. The fact that the International Association for the Study of Pain's (Mersky, 1986) definition of pain provides an emotional component, should not allow us to confuse the emotional overlay with a psychogenic etiology.

It would be better to label pain problems in which no obvious pathology can be determined as idiopathic rather than psychogenic or atypical. Further in-depth, systematic and objective study of these disorders needs to be carried out so as to understand their etiology. It has been reported

Table 63.3. Orofacial pains of neuro-vascular origin

Migraine
  Migraine with aura
  Migraine without aura
  Exertional migraine
Cluster headache
Chronic paroxysmal hemicrania
Hemicrania continua
Severe unilateral neuralgiform headache with conjunctival injection and tearing, rhinorrhea and subclinical sweating (SUNCT)

that patients described as 'atypical' or 'idiopathic' all have an ascribable diagnosis if evaluated by someone with more experience (Fricton, 1999).

Neurovascular

The problems discussed under the neurovascular organ system may not originate in this system but have the trigemino-vascular pathway as the nociceptive mediator (Moskowitz et al., 1988). Neurovascular pains are largely intermittent and involve a complex mechanism, which is still not fully understood. Table 63.3 lists the neurovascular pains that may present in the orofacial region.

Migraine

Although migraine is traditionally considered to present above the oculo-tragus line, facial migraine is documented well (Lovshin, 1960; Raskin & Prusiner, 1977). Migraine is discussed elsewhere in this text. Exertional migraine is described as 'migraine symptoms lasting minutes and presenting with the other associated symptoms attributed to migraine' (Rooke, 1968). The exertional migraine may also be subclassified into benign cough headache (BCH) and benign exertional headache. BCH is defined as an intermittent pain, usually bilateral, with severe bursting explosive pain brought on by coughing. The pain location is usually in the vertex, occipital, frontal or temporal regions, but has been described as presenting in the tooth (Symonds, 1956; Moncada & Graff-Radford, 1993). This pain is responsive to 25–225 mg / day indomethacin doses. Patients are required to maintain the treatment indefinitely. If decreased, the symptoms usually reoccur. When evaluating BCH, Symonds emphasizes the need to rule out intracranial pathology (Symonds, 1956).

Lovshin (Lovshin, 1960) was the first to describe migraine as a facial pain problem that could occur without headache. This has been further described by Raskin (1988). The pain is described as dull pain with superimposed throbbing occurring once to several times per week. Each attack lasting minutes to hours. In the facial migraine, Raskin describes ipsilatertal carotid tenderness, a finding also present when migraine presents in the head. This condition has also been refereed to as carotidynia (Raskin & Prusiner, 1977). Raskin feels that dental trauma may be a precipitant.

Cluster headache

Cluster headache is described as 'attacks of severe strictly unilateral pain orbitally, supraorbitally and/or temporally, lasting 15–180 minutes and occurring from once every other day to 8 times per day. The pains are associated with one or more of the following autonomic signs: conjunctival injection, lacrimation, nasal congestion, rhinorrhea, forehead and facial sweating, meiosis, ptosis, eyelid edema. Attacks occur in series lasting for weeks or months (so-called cluster periods) separated by remission periods usually lasting months or years. About 10% of the patients have chronic symptoms' (Olesen, 1988).

Cluster headache has been described by Brooks as 'periodic migrainous neuralgia' when it presents as orofacial (Brooke, 1978). Brooke's facial cluster included 53% with toothache and 47% with jaw pain. Bittar and Graff-Radford described 42 cases of cluster headache where 42% received unnecessary dental procedures, provided as therapy (Bittar & Graff-Radford, 1992).

Cluster often presents in the orofacial region especially in the maxilla. Using sphenopalatine ganglion block with local anesthetic is useful as a temporary abortive therapy.

Chronic paroxysmal hemicrania (CPH) is described as 'attacks with largely the same characteristics of pain and associated symptoms and signs as cluster headache, but they are shorter lasting, more frequent, occur mostly in females, and there is absolute effectiveness of indomethacin' (Olesen, 1988). CPH may also present as face pain or involve the teeth. The clinical presentation is unchanged, as is the response to indomethacin (Delcanho & Graff-Radford, 1993).

SUNCT syndrome is described as a pain that is associated with short lasting unilateral neuralgiform headache attacks with conjunctival injection, tearing, rhinorrhea and subclinical sweating. Sjaastad and co-workers in 1978 first described SUNCT (Sjaastad et al., 1978). Most attacks are reported as moderate to severe, 30 to 120 second pain paroxysms. Pain is usually localized to the eye and may

Table 63.4. Neuropathic orofacial pain

Intermittent
  Trigeminal neuralgia
  Glossopharyngeal neuralgia
  Nervous intermedius neuralgia
  Occipital neuralgia
Continuous
  Trigeminal dysesthesia
  Trigeminal dysesthesia – sympathetically maintained

occur in a cluster fashion with some quiet periods. Attack frequency may be up to 30 per day or many per hour (Sjaastad et al., 1989; Sjaastad et al., 1991). Although SUNCT is clinically well identified it is poorly treated. Carbamazepine may be effective in controlling some symptomatology, but not consistently (Sjaastad et al., 1991). Gabapentin may also offer relief in some patients (Graff-Radford, 2000a).

Neuropathic

Neuropathic pain suggests there has been some tissue or nerve injury. With injury there is a permanent peripheral nerve and or central nervous system change. It is surprising that with all that the human endures; falls, scrapes, fractures, surgery, etc., that so few chronic pain patients develop. This is likely due to the brain's ability to inhibit or control the permanent changes seen following tissue injury.

We should start out by differentiating 'transient pain' from 'chronic pain'. Short-lived pain following a stimulus that is potentially tissue damaging, also referred to as acute pain is a protective mechanism. Acute pain resolves in an appropriate time period and then normal function is restored. What happens when the stimulus results in a chronic pain? Once the injury appears to have healed there is pain that is non-protective. It is postulated that this may be due to central and peripheral nervous system change (Ren & Dubner, 1999). These changes may include the presence of ongoing peripheral nociception, CNS sensitization or down-regulation of CNS inhibition.

Clinically neuropathic pain can be divided into continuous and intermittent and may present simultaneously or independently. Table 63.4 is a clinical classification for neuropathic facial pain.

Neuropathic pain presents clinically as an intermittent bright, stimulating, electric sharp or burning pain. This is typically seen in trigeminal neuralgia, glossopharyngeal neuralgia, nervous intermedius neuralgia and occipital neuralgia. These intermittent neuralgias are triggerable, usually by non-noxious stimuli. Vascular nerve compression is the proposed etiology (Fromm & Sessel, 1991). Compression may also be secondary to other structures, including tumours and bony growths (e.g. Eagles syndrome) (Janetta, 1977; Massey & Massey, 1979).

Trigeminal neuralgia

Trigeminal neuralgia (TIC) is described as 'a painful unilateral affliction of the face, characterized by brief electric shock-like (lancinating) pain limited to the distribution of one or more divisions of the trigeminal nerve. Pain is commonly evoked by trivial stimuli including washing, shaving, smoking, talking and brushing the teeth, but may also occur spontaneously. The pain is abrupt in onset and termination may remit for varying periods' (Olesen, 1988). Symptomatic trigeminal neuralgia is described as 'pain indistinguishable from trigeminal neuralgia, caused by a demonstrable structural lesion'. This lesion is usually a tumour such as an acoustic neuroma, or may be due to demyelination as seen in multiple sclerosis. If there is tissue or nerve injury there may be an ensuing continuous trigeminal neuralgia, which is usually referred to as traumatic trigeminal neuralgia or trigeminal dysesthesia (TD) (Graff-Radford, 2000b).

TIC is usually unilateral and only occurs bilaterally in 4% of subjects. There is no genetic link to the disorder. The average age at onset is between the sixth and seventh decades, with women slightly more affected than men in a 3 : 2 ratio. The bright stimulating pain perceived is short-lived lasting seconds to minutes. If not questioned carefully the patient may report the pain lasts all day as there is often a dull pain associated with TIC, or the sharp volleys come and go continuously. The author believes the persistent aching pain may be secondary to a reflex muscle splinting and can be controlled with stretching exercise and a vapocoolant spray. Mechanical manoeuvring the trigeminal sensory system usually triggers TIC pain. The area from which the pain is activated has been described as a trigger zone. Characteristically, trigger zones occur around the supraorbital, infraorbital foramina, the inner canthus of the eye, lateral to the ala and over the mental foramen. Trigger zones are also common intraorally. Pain is not elicited from the trigger zone if deep pressure is used or during a latency period between paroxysms. The second and third trigeminal nerve divisions are most commonly affected. The first division cases occur less frequently than 5% (Fromm & Sessel, 1991). Often there is ipsilateral reflex facial spasm hence the term 'tic

douloureux' which has been used synonymously with TIC (Andre'N, 1756).

It is postulated that TIC may be due to a trigeminal nerve focal demyelination at any point along its course. Exploring the posterior cranial fossa reveals between 60 and 88% of cases have trigeminal nerve root vascular compression. The compression is present in the posterior cranial fossa as it exits the pons (Gardner, 1962). This has been postulated to set up a centrally mediated disinhibition of pain modulation and/or peripheral repetitive ectopic action potentials. Once there is sensitization there may be increased afferent fibre activity and enhanced tactile stimulation resulting in trigeminal nucleus interneuron discharge and trigeminothalamic neuron producing pain. Taarnhoj (1982) have described tumours as a possible cause in up to 6% of cases. These include acoustic neurinomas, cholesteatomas, meningiomas, osteomas and angiomas. Aneurysms and adhesions have also been implicated. Although the pain may be typical of TIC usually there are additional symptoms or cranial deficits present. When patients are in the 20–40-year age range and present with trigeminal neuralgia multiple sclerosis should be ruled out. Fromm suggests that all patients with trigeminal neuralgia obtain a brain MRI or CT scan, with particular attention paid to the posterior cranial fossa (Fromm & Sessel, 1991).

Ratner and Roberts have proposed that bony cavities found in the alveolar bone may be the cause of trigeminal neuralgia and that repetitive curettage of these cavities is curative (Ratner et al., 1976, 1979; Roberts et al., 1984) Graff-Radford et al., have demonstrated, using 15-half-maxillae and 12 half-mandibles from cadavers, that cavities in bone larger than 2 mm in diameter occur throughout normal bone (Graff-Radford et al., 1988b). The cavities do not appear to be unique to trigeminal neuralgia patients. This sheds doubt on the bony cavity theory. Rather, it may be postulated that the curettage may be effective through central mechanisms or peripheral denervation.

TIC treatment may be divided into pharmacological and surgical. Table 63.5 outlines the drugs that may be used in TIC therapy.

The anticonvulsant action in pain management is not well understood. Some like carbamazepine block use dependent sodium channels, inhibiting sustained repetitive firing. There is also an effect in the spinal cord reducing post-tetanic synaptic transmission potentiation. There is also decreased synaptic transmission in the trigeminal nucleus, which may explain anticonvulsants effectiveness in facial pain. Valproic acid increases brain concentrations of gamma-aminobutyric acid (GABA), an inhibitory neurotransmitter in the central nervous system as well as affecting sodium channels. The action of phenobarbital is not at

Table 63.5. Common membrane stabilizing drugs used in neuralgia therapy

Generic	Trade name	Dosage (mg/day)	Blood level (ug/ml)	Serum half-life (h)
Lioresal	Baclofen	10–80	–	
Carbamazepine	Tegretol (XR) Carbitrol	100–2000	4–12	12–17
Phenytoin	Dilantin	200–600	10–20	18–24
Valproic acid	Depakote	125–2500	50–100	6–16
Gabapentin	Neurontin	100–5000	–	
Lamotragine	Lamictal	50–500	2–5	14–59
Klonopin	Clonazepam	0.5–8	–	22–33
Orap	Pimozide	2–12	–	55–154
Depakote	Valproic acid	125–2000	50–100	6–16
Topiramate	Topamax	50–400	–	21
Oxcarbazepine	Trileptal	200–2400	–	9

the trigeminal nucleus but rather in the brain. It is therefore not effective for TIC. Gabapentin may increase GABA by preventing its breakdown or may affect the NMDA receptor.

All drugs used in TIC have side effects and great care must be used in their administration. Baclofen perhaps has the least side effects, but also may be less effective than carbamazepine. Fromm has also described the baclofen L isomer are the effective component (Fromm et al., 1984). Therefore, non-response may be secondary to metabolizing the D isomer only. Baclofen is initiated at 10 mg per day and increased every 2 days to a maximum of 80 mg per day usually in four doses. Drowsiness and confusion are the major side effects and many patients will not tolerate it for this reason. Carbamazepine is without doubt the most effective drug. It is suggested that one begins at 100 mg per day and increases by 100 mg every two days to a maximum of 1200 mg. The side effect of aplastic anemia, although rare, needs to be monitored carefully with routine blood tests. Should there be no relief a carbamazepine blood level should be obtained to ensure a therapeutic blood concentration. A rough level should be obtained and is usually in the range of 5–10 μg/ml. The sustained preparations (Tegretol XR, Carbitrol) have improved compliance and reduced the sedating side effects. Gabapentin, although not formally studied has been useful in doses from 300 mg per day to 3000 mg per day. Phenytoin is a good alternative in doses ranging from 100 – 400 mg per day. Fromm (Fromm & Sessel, 1991) has suggested using some of these drugs in combination to either maximize effect or minimize side effects. Pimozide has been described as more effective than carbamazepine in a double blind cross over design

using 48 subjects with trigeminal neuralgia refractory to medical treatment. Side effects were reported in 83% of subjects who received pimozide and included physical and mental retardation, hand tremors, memory impairment, involuntary movements during sleep and slight Parkinson's disease manifestations. None of the patients stopped treatment because of side effects. It is felt therefore by Lechin et al. (1989) that it is effective but because of the adverse effects it should be reserved for severe and intractable trigeminal neuralgia. A new preparation oxcarbazepine (Trileptal) has proven effective and has fewer side effects than carbamazepine.

The surgical treatments for TIC are summarized in Table 63.6. Less traditional treatments reported for trigeminal neuralgia include the curettage of the bony cavities described above. Ratner and Roberts report a long-term success of 80% (Ratner et al., 1976, 1979; Roberts et al., 1984). Sokolovic et al., have described the using peripheral streptomycin and lidocaine injections (Sokolovic et al., 1986). They studied 20 patients in whom five injections of 2% lidocaine and 1 g of streptomycin sulfate were deposited adjacent to peripheral nerves at one month intervals; 16 of the 20 patients remained pain free after 30 months. No side effects were reported and the authors report there was no loss of sensation after the local anesthetic wore off. Bittar and Graff-Radford completed a double-blind placebo-controlled cross-over study using streptomycin, and the results were not favourable. They also reported significant swelling associated with the injections (Bittar & Graff-Radford, 1993).

Although not suggested as a therapeutic modality for trigeminal dysesthesia, surgery is an excellent alternative for trigeminal neuralgia. The most effective surgical approach

Table 63.6. Surgical management of trigeminal neuralgia

Procedure	Effectiveness	Comment
Alcohol block	Excellent	relief is typically 8–16 months
		paresthesia or dysesthesia occur in 48%
Alcohol gangliolysis	88% at 4 years	corneal anesthesia occurs in 15%
		neuroparalitic keratitis in 4–7%
		postoperative paresthesia in 55%
		paresthesia in 38%
		herpetic outbreak in 26%
		transient masticatory muscle weakness in 45%
Neurectomy	Excellent	relief is typically 26–38 months
		anesthesia dolorosa and corneal anesthesia are rare
Glycerol gangliolysis	89–96%	7–10% have early recurrence
		7–21% develop recurrence over extended follow-up
		facial hyperesthesia occurs in 24–80%
		corneal anesthesia occurs in 9%
		facial dysesthesia occurs in 8–29%
Radiofrequency gangliolysis	78–100%	1–17% early recurrence
		4–32% develop recurrence over extended follow-up
		masseter weakness occurs in 7–23%
		trigeminal dysesthesia in 11–42%
		corneal hyperesthesia in 3–27%
		neuroparalytic keratitis in 1–5%
		anesthesia dolorosa in 1–4%
Microvascular compression	96–97%	16–29% develop recurrence over extended follow-compression
		mortality occurs in 1%
		morbidity occurs in 10–23%
Rhizotomy	85%	15% develop recurrence over extended follow-up
		mortality occurs in 0.5–1.6%
		facial weakness occurs in 7–8%
		paresthesia occurs as a minor complaint in 56%
		paresthesia occurs as a major complaint in 5%
		neuroparalytic keratitis occurs in 15%
Trigeminal		ipsilateral limb ataxia occurs in 10%
Tractotomy		contralateral limb sensory loss occurs in 14%
Gamma knife	80–95%	onset may be 6 weeks or longer
		facial numbness
		trigeminal dysesthesia rare

remains microvascular decompression (Janetta, 1996). Advances in microvascular decompression include the use of an endoscopic approach. This allows clearer observation and is less traumatic (Jarrahy & Shahinian, 2000). Gamma knife radiosurgery is a recent advance for trigeminal neuralgia (Young et al., 1997). This technique offers a relatively non-invasive means for lesioning the trigeminal nerve adjacent to the pons using a 4 mm collimator helmet. Complications are rare and to date the author has seen one case of trigeminal dysesthesia attributed to the procedure.

Pretrigeminal neuralgia

Sir Charles Symonds first described pretrigeminal neuralgia (PRE TIC)(Symonds, 1949). Mitchell later reviewed it (Mitchell, 1980). Fromm et al. (1990) have described a further 16 cases in which patients initially present with a dull continuous aching toothache in the upper or lower jaw and in whom the pain changed to classic trigeminal neuralgia. Further, they describe seven cases in which the continuous pain was successfully treated with traditional trigeminal neuralgia therapies. The diagnosis of pretrigeminal neuralgia is based on the following criteria: (i) description of pain as dull toothache; (ii) normal neurological and dental examination; (iii) normal CT or MRI scan of the head. Of note is that the pain of pretrigeminal neuralgia can be interrupted with somatic anesthetic blockade. Merrill and Graff-Radford have described 61 patients treated for pretrigeminal or trigeminal neuralgia. Of these 61% were incorrectly diagnosed and treated with traditional dental therapies (Merrill & Graff-Radford, 1992). The clinician should be aware of PRETIC prior to surgical intervention in orofacial pain where the etiology is unclear.

Glossopharyngeal neuralgia

This pain presents with similar quality and characteristics to trigeminal neuralgia, but in the distribution of the glossopharyngeal nerve. It may be confused with Eagles syndrome (Massey & Massey, 1979). This syndrome presents as described in glossopharyngeal neuralgia but is associated with an elongated stylohyoid process that irritates or compresses the glossopharyngeal nerve. Rotation of the head, swallowing, chewing are all triggering factors. Patients may complain of persistent sore throats. This pain can be decreased with neural blockade and confirmation of the diagnosis requires demonstration of the calcified stylohyoid ligament on radiogram. Treatment is best achieved with surgical resection of the ligament.

Nervous intermedius neuralgia

This pain is described as similar to trigeminal neuralgia but localized to the middle ear. Patients often complain of 'hot poker' in the ear (Walker, 1966). Treatment is usually similar to that for trigeminal neuralgia.

Occipital neuralgia

Occipital neuralgia is pain located in the distribution of the greater and lesser occipital nerves. Pain is described as paroxysmal, sharp electric-like. There is usually an associated trauma at the onset of pain. Graff-Radford et al., have described myofascial trigger points in the splenius cervicus and capitis muscles that may mimic occipital neuralgia and it is suggested that trigger point injections be used to help rule out this possibility (Graff-Radford et al., 1988a,b). Surgical neurectomy has been described for occipital neuralgia, but the results are often short lived.

The neuropathic pain following tissue or nerve injury in the trigeminal nerve distribution may be called a trigeminal dysesthesia (TD). TD is defined as a continuous pain following complete or partial damage to a peripheral nerve. The pain is described as a continuous, burning numbness and often pulling pain (see Table 63.7).

Table 63.7. Criteria for trigeminal dysesthesia

History of trauma
Continuous pain
Associated hyperalgesia and allodynia
Temperature change
Block effect (sympathetic vs. somatic)

In TD the initiating trauma is usually quite obvious, e.g. postwisdom tooth removal or postimplant placement, but may occur with minor traumas such as crown preparation or following viral infection such as herpes zoster. The discomfort can be self-limiting, depending on nerve regeneration. Campbell has described approximately 5% of patients undergoing root canal therapy have persistent pain (Campbell et al., 1990) which may be attributed to the nerve damage. Elies described 17% of patients with mandibular implants as developing persistent sensory change or pain (Ellies & Hawker, 1993; Ellies, 1992). Thermographic studies of TD reveal all patients have abnormal thermograms with some being hot in the pain distribution and some cold. None are normal. Graff-Radford et al. (1995) have described a hypothesis for these temperature changes that may be helpful in selecting a treatment.

There are three peripheral mechanism, which may be involved in chronic trigeminal neuropathic pain development. These are (i) nerve compression, (ii) nerve regeneration and (iii) sympathetically maintained pain.

Nerve compression

When a peripheral nerve is compressed or injured there is a sustained firing that may be persistent. The closer the damage is to the central nervous system, the longer is the spontaneous neural discharge. The pain following nerve compression can be temporarily relieved with local anesthetic blockade. Following neural trauma receptor sprouting occurs on the damaged nociceptor, on dorsal horn cells and peripheral blood vessels. These receptors may include alpha-receptors, NPY receptors and possibly others. There is also an increased release in trigeminal nucleus substance P, CGRP and other neurotransmitters, resulting in further neurogenic inflammation and chronic pain (Bennett & Xie, 1988). When neural inflammation occurs, a neuritis ensues. The pain presentation is a continuous dull, burning pain with associated allodynia and hyperalgesia. A neuritis involving the facial nerve (cranial nerve VII) may present as a Bell's palsy. There is no pain in Bell's palsy unless the herpes zoster involves the geniculate ganglion. Ramsy Hunt Syndrome requires a facial palsy associated with herpes zoster eruption around the ear (Karnes, 1984).

Nerve regeneration

Neuroma formation is essentially created by nerve regeneration where the path for regrowth is obstructed. The nerve resprouting and the continuous nerve irritation may result in pain. As in nerve compression, receptor sprouting, and neurotransmitter presence will increase the pain. Injecting the neuroma with local anesthetic will temporarily block the pain. The sprouting axons fire spontaneously, develop abnormal sensitization to norepinepherine, cold and mechanical stimulation. This occurs in dorsal root ganglion cells as well as peripheral terminals. Clinically, the neuroma may only produce pain following mechanical stimulation. The pain is an aching, burning pain with associated sharp pain volleys.

Sympathetically maintained pain (SMP)

Campbell best summarizes this phenomenon (Campbell et al., 1992). He reports that the initial trauma to the peripheral nervous system activates nociceptors and produces a sprouting of alpha-adrenergic receptors on the nociceptors. Additionally, the initial sensory barrage sensitizes the CNS causing sympathetic afferent activation, and increased response to non-noxious stimulus. This causes peripheral norepinepherine release, which activates the peripheral nociceptors and keeps the cycle active. There is evidence that following neural injury the sympathetic innervation in the dorsal root ganglia increases with age (Roberts & Foglesong, 1988). It is not surprising that there is a higher incidence of neuropathic pain as we age. SMP is aggravated by non-noxious stimuli and interrupted temporarily by sympathetic block or alpha-adrenergic block with phentolamine.

Most orofacial trigeminal dysesthesia occurs in females usually in their 4th decade (Vickers et al., 1998; Solberg & Graff-Radford, 1988). There must be a lesion in the trigeminal nervous system, peripherally or centrally to cause the continuous dysesthesia (Vickers et al., 1998). Sex-based differences have been seen in many pain disorders. The relationship and role of sex hormones in the generation and perpetuation of central sensitization is not fully understood but is obviously important (Ren & Dubner, 1999). In a neuropathic pain model using partial sciatic nerve legation, female rats were more likely to develop allodynia (Coyle et al., 1995). In studies comparing female rats that have been ovariectomized, there is a greater chance that those with estrogen were more likely to develop allodynia after injury than those without estrogen (Coyle et al., 1996).

The therapy for trigeminal dysesthesia is aimed at reducing peripheral nociceptive inputs and simultaneously enhancing central nervous system pain inhibitory systems (Graff-Radford, 1995).

Topical applications

The use of topical therapies has not been well studied. There is some evidence that capsaicin (Zostrix) applied regularly will result in desensitization and pain relief (Scrivani et al., 1999). The recommended dose is five times per day for 5 days then three times per day for 3 weeks. If the patient cannot withstand the burning produced by the application, the addition of topical local anesthetic, either 4% lidocaine or EMLA is useful. A Lidoderm patch has been useful in postherpetic neuralgia and other neuralgias where it is convenient to apply the material to the skin. Clonadine can be applied to the hyperalgesic region by placing the proprietary subcutaneous delivery patch where it is most tender. Alternatively, a 4% gel can be compounded and delivered over a larger area. For local intra-oral application a neurosensory stent has been conceived. After an oral impression, an acrylic stent is manufactured to cover the painful site (Graff-Radford, 1995). The topical agent is applied to the gingival surface and placed intra-orally 24 hours per day.

Topical clonazepam (0.5–1.0 mg three times per day) has been effective at reducing a burning oral pain (Woda et al., 1998). Patients were instructed to suck a tablet for three minutes (and then spit out) three times per day for at least 10 days. Serum concentrations were minimal (3.3 ng/ml) one and three hours after application. Woda hypothesized there was a peripheral not central action at disrupting the neuropathologic mechanism.

Procedures

Neural blockade is very effective in differentiating SMP from sympathetically independent pain. It may also be effective in controlling SMP if used repetitively. Stellate ganglion blocks, phentolamine infusion and sphenopalatine blocks have been described as useful in obtaining a chemical sympathetic block. The author has not had significant benefit using phentolamine infusion in facial pain. Scrivani who used 30 mg infusion without benefit (Scrivani et al., 1999) supports this.

Lidocaine infusion (200 mg over 1 hour) may be used therapeutically in various forms of neuropathic pain (Boas et al., 1982; Rowbotham et al., 1991). It is suggested that response to intravenous lidocaine may predict who responds to the lidocaine analogue mexilatine. Sinnott et

Table 63.8. Common antidepressants used in trigeminal dysesthesia

Medication trade name	Route	Dosage per day
Amitriptyline	PO	10–150
Desipramine	PO	10–150
Doxepin	PO	10–150
Imipramine	PO	10–150
Nortriptyline	PO	10–150
Trazedone	PO	50–300

al., used an animal model to demonstrate that there is a minimal lidocaine concentration (2.1μg/ml) to abolish allodynia (Sinnott et al., 1999). They also describe a ceiling effect. Many animals with experimentally induced allodynia did not obtain persistent relief. They suggest separate physiological mechanisms, with differing pharmacologies, may account for variability and postulate there are different aspects of neuropathic pain.

Pharmacology

Tricyclic antidepressants

It is well documented that tricyclic antidepressants are effective in many pain problems. Solberg and Graff-Radford have studied the response to amitriptyline in traumatic neuralgia. It is noted that the effective range is 10–150 mg per day usually taken in a single dose at bedtime (Solberg & Graff-Radford, 1988). Many antidepressants may be used, see Table 63.8.

Membrane stabilizers

These medications include the anticonvulsants, lidocaine derivatives and some muscle relaxants. They have been classically used in intermittent sharp electric pains (see Table 63.5).

Behavioural strategies

Prior to beginning therapy, it is common to perform a behavioural assessment with appropriate testing. Following the behavioural evaluation, management is directed at the factors which may impact treatment and determining the most appropriate interventions. Consideration should be given to the following factors: (i) behavioural or operant; (ii) emotional; (iii) characterlogical; (iv) cognitive; (v) side effects; (vi) medication use and (vii) compliance. Therapy such as cognitive and behavioural management techniques, relaxation, biofeedback and psychotherapeutic and psychopharmacological interventions may be useful.

Surgery

Although not suggested as a therapeutic modality for trigeminal dysesthesia, surgery is an excellent alternative for trigeminal neuralgia.

Postherpetic neuralgia

Postherpetic neuralgia (PHN) is a complex problem whose treatment has frustrated clinicians and patients (Loeser, 1986; Watson & Evans, 1986). Herpes zoster (HZ) is primarily a disease affecting older people with some predilection for males (67% males: 33% females to 53% males: 47% females) (Molin, 1969). The localization of HZ in the face is between 15% and 30% of reported cases, this includes involvement of the facial nerve (Molin, 1969). The duration of pain after outbreak of the vesicles varies, but with an increase in age of the subject the pain appears to last longer. The number of subjects who go on to having postherpetic neuralgia (PHN), defined as pain after the vesicles are healed, ranges from 14% of males to 25% of females but almost all are older than 60 years (Molin, 1969). No studies to date have suggested that the subset of HZ patients who go on to have PHN is predictable. The mechanism whereby the herpetic virus produces the neuralgia condition has not yet been determined, reports by Head (Head & Campbell, 1900), and Denny-Brown (Denny-Brown & Adams, 1944), reveal that changes occur in the skin and peripheral nerve endings producing anesthesia or dysesthesia in the dorsal root ganglion characteristic of hemorrhage and lymphocytic infiltration. The adjacent proximal nerves and sensory nerve roots show demyelination and rarely in the spinal cord is cell death evident. There are few controlled studies assessing treatment outcome in this relentless disease. Watson has described the use of amitriptyline, which has by and large been the treatment of choice (Watson & Evans, 1986). This was confirmed by Max who showed amitriptyline but not lorazepam was effective in treatment of PHN (Max et al., 1988). Phenothiazines have been suggested as helpful in the treatment of chronic pain, and in five case studies Taub reported the combination of amitriptyline and fluphenazine to be effective (Taub, 1973). In this report there was a mix of acute (active lesions) and chronic cases (pain lasting longer than 6 months). Graff-Radford has studied the effects of amitriptyline and fluphenazine using a double-blind protocol and found no significant benefit in combining amitriptyline with fluphenazine (Graff-Radford et al., 1986). Sympathetic nerve block is considered by many to be effective in preventing PHN, when used in the first 3–6 months following the outbreak of zoster. It is suggested between 1 and 6 blocks be performed, depending on the effects. There is little purpose in doing more than 3 blocks if the pain relief is not outlasting the anesthetic effects. It may be more appropriate for this category to be in the autonomic nervous system category, but in some situations sympathetic block does not reduce the pain and this may suggest a sympathetically independent pain.

Musculoskeletal system

Musculoskeletal pain is the most common cause for chronic orofacial pain. Broadly speaking the disorders may be divided into arthrogenous and muscular referred to as temporomandibular disorders (TMD). The temporomandibular joint (TMJ) is different from other body joints. The most recognizable difference between the TMJ and other synovial joints is the non-innervated avascular fibrous connective tissue articular covering. This is not hyaline in nature, possibly to aid withstand twisting, turning and compressive forces. The fibroconnective tissue covering may also allow for significant remodelling to occur in the TMJ. Other significant differences include the diarthroidal structure. There is an intracapsular disc dividing the joint into upper and lower compartments providing for the complex hinge and gliding action. The mandible produces a reciprocal effect of one articulation on the other by joining the TMJ's. Also interacting in this system is the dental occlusion, which will result in altered forces on the system if not in equilibrium. The teeth provide a solid end point to joint movement unlike any other joint in which end range of motion is somewhat elastic. Due to the structure's nature, the intracapsular anatomy can remodel when subjected to extraneous forces. Such remodelling can be brought about through tooth loss, poor dental restoration, macro trauma and parafunctional habits such as tooth clenching and grinding. The remodelling may lead to dysfunction if the tissues are unable to compensate for the abnormal load. In addition, muscular hyperactivity may be initiated also as a compensation for the lack of equilibrium.

The joints hinge action allows for about a 25 mm interincisal opening, which occurs primarily in the lower joint space (condylar rotation). The next 20–25 mm requires the disc condyle complex to slide down the temporal eminence, with the disc moving posterior relative to the condyle (translation). Remodelling resulting in a deviation in articular form may interrupt this rhythmic function. The

articular tissues are usually characterized by smooth rounded surfaces until subject to extraneous forces, which produce remodelling (Solberg et al., 1985). The mechanical interferences that are produced by the remodelling may cause noise as they move over each other. Remodelling is an ongoing process and results in a disease process continuum beginning with soft tissue change and progressing to involve the bony structures. One might view the process as a failure for the adaptive process to compensate for the extraneous forces exerted on the joint. If there is sufficient change the articular disc may become displaced. The usual direction for displacement is in an anteromedial direction (Ireland, 1953; Farrar, 1972) although displacement has been reported in a posterior direction (Blankestijn & Boering, 1985). The disc displacement may reduce if the individual can manipulate the condyle onto the disc, producing joint noise. This noise is usually heard after the initial 25 mm rotation in the opening movement and again just before the teeth occlude in the closing path. The closing noise is usually much quieter and may be produced by the relocation of the disc in the anterior position. Joint noise occurs in 20–30% of individuals over the age of 15 years (Egermark-Eriksson et al., 1981; Solberg et al., 1979). Pain associated with joint pathology is usually intermittent and associated with function. In order to confirm an articular TMD, patients should display at least three of the following four criteria: (i) limited range of motion <40 mm); (ii) joint noise (clicking, popping or crepitus); (iii) tenderness to palpation; (iv) functional pain. Continuous pain associated with an articular TMD is unusual and usually is produced by associated inflammation or secondary muscle pain. Pain emanating from the ligamentous attachments, the synovium and fibrous capsules is usually secondary to infection or trauma to these structures. The differences between synovitis and capsulitis is almost impossible to determine clinically (Bell, 1995).

Articular remodelling is a direct result of adaptive changes that help to establish a status quo between joint form and function (Moffett et al., 1964). Osteoarthrosis results when there is destruction of articular tissues secondary to excessive strain on the remodelling mechanism. The problem is therefore non-painful and usually only produces mechanical interference's. De Bont has suggested that the degenerative process is due to disruption of the collagen fibre network and fatty degeneration (De Bont et al., 1985). Inflammation of the articular tissue does not occur due to the unvascularized surface. For inflammation to occur a fundamental arthropathic change must occur such as the proliferation of inflamed synovial membrane into the articular tissue, or the exposure of innervated and vascularized osseous tissue (De Bont et al., 1985).

Osteoarthrosis is a common condition that seems to progress with age. It also appears to affect females more than males (Davis, 1981). Osteoarthrosis is insidious in onset, usually not associated with systemic disease, but perhaps initiated through repetitive loading or a variety of factors that occur over a lifetime. The inflammation that occurs in osteoarthritis requires an innervated and vascular surface. This suggests that the adaptive remodelling that continues has been overwhelmed and the tissues below the fibroconnective tissue surface are exposed allowing the inflammatory process to begin.

Muscle disorders

The disorders involving muscle may be independent of the articular problems but more often than not are involved when joint dysfunction exists. Their involvement may be mild and produce minimal dysfunction or severe and markedly disabling. When muscle pain problems occur, the treatment may differ depending on the subgroup defined below.

Myofascial pain syndromes, as classified by the International Association for the Study of Pain Subcommittee on Taxonomy (Mersky, 1986), may be found in any voluntary muscle, and are characterized by trigger points (TPs) which may cause referred pain and local and referred tenderness (Clark et al., 1981; Moller, 1981). When 'active', TPs are painful to palpation and spontaneously refer pain and autonomic symptoms to remote structures in reproducible patterns characteristic for each muscle (Travell & Simons, 1984). It is this referred pain that is usually the presenting complaint. When 'latent', TPs are still locally tender but do not produce referred phenomena. The pain quality is pressing, tightening, deep, aching, and often poorly circumscribed (Travell & Simons, 1984). It may be associated with sensations of swelling, numbness and stiffness. Pain, although usually constant, may fluctuate in intensity and shift anatomical site (Travell & Simons, 1984). Associated symptoms may include autonomic phenomena, most commonly reactive hyperemia or erythema, although photophobia and phonophobia are described (Butler et al., 1975).

The primary basis for myofascial pain is the referred pain. The referral patterns often do not make neurological sense. As an example, pain from a trigger point in the trapezius, innervated by cranial nerve 11, may refer to the forehead, innervated by cranial nerve 5. Despite the poor mechanistic understanding, clinically myofascial pain is widely accepted. It is imperative that we understand how this referral may take place.

Men described a hypothesis for muscle pain referral to other deep somatic tissues remote from the site of the original muscle stimulation or lesion (Mens, 1994). He criticizes the convergence: projection pain referral theory, by pointing out there is little convergence in the dorsal horns associated with deep tissues. Mens' hypothesis adds two new components to the convergence: projection theory. First, the convergent connections from deep tissues to dorsal horn neurons are opened only after nociceptive inputs from muscle are activated. The connections opened after muscle stimulus are called silent connections. Secondly, the referral to muscle outside the initially activated site is due to spread of central sensitization to adjacent spinal segment (Mens, 1994). The initiating stimulus requires a peripheral inflammatory stimulus. In the animal model described by Mens the noxious stimulus was bradykinin injected into the muscle. It is unclear what triggers the muscle referral in the clinical setting where there is usually no obvious inflammation-producing incident.

This Mens theory has been used by Simons to discuss a neurophysiological basis for trigger point pain (Simons, 1994). Simons hypothesizes that when the tender area in the muscle is palpated there are neurotransmitters released in the dorsal horn (trigeminal nucleus) resulting in nociceptive inputs, openings that were previously silent. This causes distant neurons to produce a retrograde referred pain (Simons, 1994). This model accounts for most of the clinical presentation and therapeutic options seen in myofascial pain, but does not account for what initiates the peripheral tenderness, that must be present to activate the silent connections.

Fields has described a means whereby the central nervous system may switch on nociception (Fields & Heinricher, 1989). He describes the presence of 'on' cells which when stimulated may produce activation of trigeminal nucleus nociceptors. Olesen has used Fields' model to describe a hypothesis for tension-type headache (Olesen, 1991). This model describes the interaction of three systems, the vascular, supraspinal and myogenic. The proposed hypothesis suggests that perceived headache pain is facilitated by the central nervous system depending on inputs from either muscle or blood vessel. In migraine the inputs are proposed as primarily vascular whereas in tension-type headache there are primarily muscular inputs. This model helps explain why the clinical presentation and therapeutic options in migraine and tension-type headache are often similar, as well as why there is temporary relief seen with peripheral treatments such as trigger point injections.

The resultant hyperalgesia or trigger point sensitivity may represent a peripheral sensitization related to serum levels on serotonin (5H-T). Ernberg et al. (1999) showed a significant correlation with serum 5H-T and allodynia associated with muscular face pain (Alstergen et al., 1999). In rheumatoid temporomandibuar pain serum 5H-T concentrations correlated with pain. There was no correlation with circulating serum levels of neuropeptide Y (NPY) or interleukin–1B (Alstergen et al., 1999).

It is therefore proposed that patients presenting with facial pain where the etiology is not obvious may have myofascial pain. In these patients careful physical examination will allow the clinician to reproduce the pain by digitally palpating the muscles. Confirmation with trigger point injections is also helpful. It is suggested that the trigger point be injected with 1–2 cc of 1% procaine for best results.

The therapy for myofascial pain requires enhancing central inhibition through pharmacology or behavioural techniques and simultaneously reducing peripheral inputs through physical therapies including exercises and trigger point specific therapy (Travell & Simons, 1986; Graff-Radford et al., 1987; Davidoff, 1998). It is essential that patients are aware that the goals in therapy are to manage the pain and not to cure. It is important to stress the role patients' play in managing the perpetuating factors (Graff-Radford et al., 1987; Davidoff, 1998).

Discussion

Prior to making the diagnosis of orofacial pain, the evaluation must begin with an in-depth medical history which should include the chief complaint and a narrative history of the complaint, its progression and prior treatment. Not all chronic pain conditions require a psychological evaluation, but it should be kept in mind that all pain, no matter what the etiology, is subject to behavioural and emotional factors. These behavioural issues should be considered and, where there is any doubt as to their contribution, a psychological evaluation is suggested. The psychological evaluation is not done to determine weather the pain is psychogenic, rather, for the purpose of selecting specific cognitive and behavioural strategies useful in pain management. Once these data are gathered, a neurological screening examination, temporomandibular joint examination and myofascial palpation should be carried out. At this time, a differential diagnosis can be established and specific tests outlined above may be required to provide a definitive diagnosis. This process permits effective treatment, for an appropriate diagnosis.

References

Alstergen, P., Ernberg, M., Kopp, S. & Lundeberg, T. (1999). TMJ pain in relation to circulating neuropeptide Y, Serotonin, and interleukin – 1B in rheumatoid arthritis. *Orofacial Pain*, **13**, 49–55.

Andre' N. (1756). *Traite' sur les Maladies de l'Urethre*, pp. 323–43. Paris: Delaguette.

Bell, W.E. (1995). *Orofacial Pains: Classification, Diagnosis, Management*. 3rd edn, Year Book Medical Publishers.

Bennett, G.J. & Xie, Y.K. (1988). A peripheral mononeuropathy in rat that produces disorders of pain sensation like those seen in man. *Pain*, **33**, 87–107.

Bittar, G. & Graff-Radford, S.B. (1992). A retrospective study of patients with cluster headache. *Oral Med., Oral Pathol., Oral Surg.*, **73**, 519–25.

Bittar, G. & Graff-Radford, S.B. (1993). The effect of streptomycin/lidocaine block on trigeminal and traumatic neuralgia. *Headache*, **33**(3),155–60.

Blankestijn, J. & Boering, G. (1985). Posterior dislocation of the temporomandibular disk. *Int. J. Oral Surg.*, **14**, 437–43.

Boas, R.A., Covino, B.G. & Shahnarian, A. (1982). Analgesic responses to i.v. lignocaine. *Br. J. Anesth.*, **54**, 501–4.

Brooke, R.I. (1978). Periodic migrainous neuralgia: a cause of dental pain. *Oral Med.*, **46**, 511–16.

Bulitt, E., Tew, J.M. & Boyd, J. (1986). Intracranial tumours with facial pain. *J. Neurosurg.*, **64**, 865–71.

Burchiel, K.J. (1987). Surgical treatment of trigeminal neuralgia: minor and major operative procedures. In *The Medical and Surgical Management of Trigeminal Neuralgia*, ed. G.H. Fromm, pp. 71–101. New York: Futura Publishing Co.

Butler, J.H., Golke, L.E.A. & Bandt, C.L. (1995). A descriptive survey of signs and symptoms associated with the myofascial pain dysfunction syndrome. *J. Am. Dent. A*, **90**(3), 635–9.

Campbell, R.l., Parks, K.W. & Dodds, R.N. (1990). Chronic facial pain associated with endodontic neuropathy. *Oral Surg. Oral Med. Oral Pathol.*, **69**, 287–90.

Campbell, J.N., Meyer, R.A., Davis, K.D. & Raja, S.N. (1992). Sympathetically mediated pain a unifying hypothesis. In *Hyperalgesia and Allodynia*, ed. W.D. Willis, pp. 141–9. New York: Raven Press.

Clark, G.T., Beemsterboer, P.L. & Rugh, J.D. (1981). Nocternal Masseter muscle activity and the symptoms of masticatory dysfunction. *J. Oral Rehabil.*, **8**, 279.

Coyle, D.E., Sehlorst, C.S. & Mascari, C. (1995). Female rats are more susceptible to the development of neuropathic pain using the partial sciatic nerve ligation (PSNL) model. *Neurosci. Lett.*, **186**, 135–8.

Coyle, D.E., Selhorst, C.S. & Behbehani, M.M. (1996). Intact female rats are more susceptive to the development of tactile allodynia than ovariectomized female rats following partial sciatic nerve ligation (PSNL). *Neurosci. Lett.*, **203**, 37–40.

Cueneo, H.M. & Rand, C.W. (1952). Tumours of the gasserian ganglion. Tumor of the left Gasserian ganglion associated with enlargement of the mandibular nerve. A review of the literature and case report. *J. Neurosurg.*, **9**, 423–32.

Davidoff, R.A. (1998). Trigger points and myofascial pain: toward understanding how they affect headaches. *Cephalalgia*, **18**(7), 436–8.

Davis, M.A. (1981). Sex differences in reporting osteoarthritic symptoms: a sociomedical approach. *J. Health Soc. Behav.*, **22**, 293.

De Bont, L.G.M., Boering, G., Liem, R.S.B. & Havinga, P. (1985). Osteoarthritis of the temporomandibular joint: a light microscopic and scanning electron microscopic study of the articular cartilage of the mandibular condyle. *J. Oral Maxillofac. Surg.*, **43**, 481–8.

Delcanho, R.E. & Graff-Radford, S.B. (1993). Chronic paroxysmal hemicrania presenting as toothache. *J. Orofacial Pain*, **7**, 300–6.

Denny-Brown, D. & Adams, R. (1944). *Arch. Neurol., Psychiatry*, **51**, 216–21.

Egermark-Eriksson, I., Carlsson, G.E. & Ingervall, B. (1981). Prevalence of mandibular dysfunction and orofacial parafunction in 7-, 11, and 15 year old Swedish children. *Eur. J. Orthod.*, **3**, 163–72.

Ellies, L.G. (1992). Altered sensation following mandibular implant surgery: a retrospective study. *J. Prosthet. Dent.*, **68**, 664–7.

Ellies, L.G. & Hawker, P.B. (1993). The prevalance of altered sensation associated with implant surgery. *Int. J. Oral Maxillofac. Implants*, **8**, 674–9.

Ernberg, M., Hadenberg-Magnusson, B., Alstergren, P., Lundberg, T. & Kopp, S. (1999). Pain, Allodynia, and serum serotonin level in orofacial pain of muscular origin. *J. Orofacial Pain*, **13**, 56–62.

Farrar, W.B. (1972). Differentiation of temporomandibular joint dysfunction to simplify treatment. *J. Prosthet Dent.*, **28**, 629–36.

Fields, H.L. & Heinricher, M. (1989). Brainstem modulation of nociceptor-driven withdrawal reflexes. *Ann. NY Acad. Sci.*, **563**, 34–44.

Fordyce, W.E. & Steger, J.C. (1978). Chronic pain. In *Behavior Medicine Theory and Practice*, ed. D.F. Pomerteau & J.P. Brady, p. 125. Baltimore: Williams and Wilkins, 1978.

Fricton, J.R. (1999). Critical Commentary. A unified concept of idiopathic orofacial pain: clinical features. *J. Orofacial Pain*, **13**(3), 185–9.

Fromm, G.H. & Sessel, B.J. (1991). Trigeminal neuralgia. Current Concepts regarding Pathogenesis and Treatment. Boston: Butterworth-Heinemann.

Fromm, G.H, Terrence, C.F. & Chattha, A.S. (1984). Baclofen in the treatment of trigeminal neuralgia: double blind study and long term follow up. *Ann Neurol.*, **15**, 240–4.

Fromm, G.H., Graff-Radford, S.B., Terrence, C.F. & Sweet, W.H. (1990). Can trigeminal neuralgia have a prodrome? *Neurology*, **40**, 1493–5.

Gardner, W.J. (1962). Concerning mechanisms of trigeminal neuralgia and hemifacial spasm. *J. Neurosurg.*, **19**, 947–57.

Graff-Radford, S.B. Orofacial Pain. In *Orofacial Pain and Temporomandibular Disorders*, ed. J. Fricton & R. Dubner, pp. 215–41. New York: Raven Press.

Graff-Radford, S.B. (1995). Orofacial pain of neurogenous origin. In *Temporomandibular disorders and Orofacial Pain*, ed. R.A. Pertes & S.G. Gross, pp. 329–41. Chicago: Quintessence.

Graff-Radford, S.B. (2000a). SUNCT syndrome responsive to Gabapentin. (Neurontin). *Cephalagia*, **20**, pp. 515–17.

Graff-Radford, S.B. (2000b). Facial pain. *Curr. Opin. Neurol.*, **13**, 291–6.

Graff-Radford, S.B., Reeves, J.L. & Jaeger, B. (1987). Management of headache: the effectiveness of altering factors perpetuating myofascial pain. *Headache*, **27**, 186–90.

Graff-Radford, S.B., Brechner, T. & Audell, L. (1988a). McGill Pain Questionnaire changes in postherpetic neuralgia patients undergoing a drug trail (abstr.). *Proc. Am. Pain Soc.*, p69.

Graff-Radford, S.B., Simmons, M., Fox, L., White, S. & Solberg, W.K. (1988b). Are bony cavities exclusively associated with atypical facial pain or trigeminal neuralgia? (Abstr.). *Proc. Western USA Pain Soc.*

Graff-Radford, S.B., Ketelaer, M-C., Gratt, B.M. & Solberg, W.K. (1995). Thermographic assessment of neuropathic facial pain. *J. Orofacial Pain*, **9**, 138–46.

Graff-Radford, S.B., Jaeger, B. & Reeves, J.L. (2000). Myofascial pain may present clinically as occipital neuralgia. *Neurosurgery*, **19**(4), 610–13.

Head, H. & Campbell, A.W. (1900). The pathology of herpes zoster. *Brain*, **23**, 353–523.

Headache Classification Committee of the International Headache Society. (1988). Classification and diagnostic criteria for headache disorders, cranial neuralgias, and facial pain. *Cephalalgia*, **8**, 1–96.

Ireland, V.E. (1953). The problem of the clicking jaw. *J. Prosthet. Dent.*, **3**, 200–12

Janetta, P.J. (1977). Observation on the etiology of trigeminal neuralgia, hemifacial spasm, acoustic nerve dysfunction and glossopharyngeal neuralgia. Definitive microsurgical treatment and results in 117 patients. *Neurochirurgia*, **20**, 145–54.

Janetta, P.J. (1996). Trigeminal neuralgia: treatment by microvascular decompression. In *Neurosurgery*, ed. R.H. Wilkins & S.S. Ragachary, pp. 3961–8. New York: Mc Graw Hill.

Jarrahy, R., Berci, G. & Shahinian, H.K. (2000). Endoscopic-assisted microvascular decompression of the trigeminal nerve. *Otolaryngol. Head, Neck Surg.*, in Press.

Karnes, W.E. (1984). Diseases of the seventh cranial nerve. In *Peripheral Neuropathy*, 2nd edn, ed. P.J. Dyke et al., Chap. 55, pp. 1266–99. Philadelphia: Saunders.

Lechin, F., Van der Dijs, B., Lechin, M.E. et al. (1989). Pimozide therapy for trigeminal neuralgia. *Arch. Neurol.*, **46**, 960–3.

Loeser, J.D. (1986). Herpes zoster and postherpetic neuralgia. *Pain*, **25**, 149–64.

Lovshin, L.L. (1960). Vascular neck pain – a common syndrome seldom recognized: analysis of 100 consecutive cases. *Cleve Clin. Q.*, **27**, 5–13.

Massey, E.W. & Massey, J. (1979). Elongated styloid process (Eagles syndrome) causing hemicrania. *Headache*, **19**, 339–41.

Max, M.B., Schafer, S.C., Culnane, M., Smoller, B., Dubner, R., (1988). Amitriptyline, but not lorazepam, relieves post herpetic neuralgia. *Neurology*, **38**, 1427–32.

Mens, S. (1994). Referral of muscle pain new aspects. *Pain Forum*, **3**(1), 1–9.

Merrill, R.L. & Graff-Radford S.B. (1992). Trigeminal neuralgia: how to rule out the wrong treatment. *JADA*, **123**, 63–8.

Mersky, H. (ed.) (1986). Classification of chronic pain: description of chronic pain syndromes and definition of terms. *Pain*, Suppl. 3, S1.

Mitchell, R.G. (1980). Pre-trigeminal neuralgia. *Br. Dent. J.*, **149**, 167–70.

Moffett, B.C., Johnson, L.C., McCabe, J.B. & Askew, H.C. (1964). Articular remodeling in the adult human temporomandibular joint. *Am. J. Anat.*, **115**, 119–30.

Molin, L. (1969). Aspects of the natural history of herpes zoster. *ActDerm. Venereol.*, **49**, 569–83.

Moller, E. (1981). The myogenic factor in headache and facial pain. In *Oral-facial Sensory and Motor Function*, ed. Y. Kawamura & R. Dubner, p. 225. Tokyo: Quintessence.

Moncada, E. & Graff-Radford, S.B. (1993). Cough headache presenting as toothache. *Headache*, **33**, 240–3.

Moskowitz, M.A., Henrikson, B.M., Markowitz, S. & Saito, K. (1988). Intra- and extravascular nociceptive mechanisms and the pathogenesis of head pain. In *Basic Mechanisms of Headache*, ed. J. Olsen & L. Edvinsson, p. 429. Amsterdam: Elsevier.

Olesen, J. (1991). Clinical and pathophysiological observations in migraine and tension type headache explained by integration of vascular, suprapinal and myofascial inputs. *Pain*, **46**, 125–32.

Raskin, N.H. (1988). *Headache*. 2nd edn. New York: Churchill Livingstone.

Raskin, N.H. & Prusiner, S. (1977). Carotidynia. *Neurology*, **27**, 43–6.

Ratner, E.J., Person, P. & Kleinman, D.J. (1976). Oral pathology and trigeminal neuralgia, I Clinical experiences (abstr). *J. Dent. Res.*, **55**, b299.

Ratner, E.J., Person, P., Kleinman, D.J., Shklar, G. & Socransky, S.S. (1979). Jawbone cavities and trigeminal and atypical facial neuralgias. *Oral Surg.*, **48**, 3–20.

Ren, K. & Dubner, R. (1999). Central nervous system plasticity and persistent pain. *J. Orofacial Pain*, **13**, 155–63.

Roberts, A.M., Person, P., Chandran, N.B., Hori, J.M. & Elkins, W. (1984). Further observations on dental parameters of trigeminal and atypical facial neuralgias. *Oral Surg.*, **58**, 121–9.

Roberts, W.J. & Foglesong, M.E. (1988). Identification of afferents contributing to sympathetically evoked activity in wide-dynamic-range neurons. *Pain*, **34**, 305–14.

Rooke, E. (1968). Benign exertional headache. *Med. Clin. N. Amer.*, **52**(4), 801–8.

Rowbotham, M.C., Reisner-Keller, L.A. & Fields, H.L. (1991). Both intravenous lidocaine and morphine reduce the pain of postherpetic neuralgia. *Neurology*, **41**, 1024–8.

Rushton, J.G. & Rooke, E.D. (1962). Brain tumor headache. *Headache*, **2**, 147–52.

Schisano, G. & Olivercrona, H. (1960). Neuromas of the Gasserian ganglion and trigeminal root. *J. Neurosurg.*, **17**, 306.

Scrivani, S.J., Chaudry, A., Maciewicz, R.J. & Keith, D.A. (1999). Chronic neurogenic facial pain: Lack of response to intravenous phentolamine. *J. Orofacial Pain*, **13**, 89–96.

Simons, D.G. (1994). Neurophysiological basis of pain caused by trigger points. *APS J.*, **3**(1); 17–19.

Sinnott, C.J., Garfield, J.M. & Strichartz, G.R. (1999). Differential efficacy of intravenous lidocaine in alleviating ipsilateral versus contralateral neuropathic pain in the rat. *Pain*, **80**, 521–31.

Sjaastad, O., Russell D., Horven, I. & Bunaes, U. (1978). Multiple neuralgia-form unilateral headache attacks associated with conjunctival injection and tearing and clusters. Noso-logic problem. *Proc. Scand. Migraine Soc.*, 31.

Sjaastad, O., Saunte C., Salvesen R. et al. (1989). Short lasting, unilateral neuralagia-form headache attacks with conjunctival injection, tearing, sweating and rhinorrhea. *Cephalalgia*, 9, 147–56.

Sjaastad, O., Vhaoj, M., Krusvewski, P. & Stoverner, L.J. (1991). Short lasting unilateral neuralgia-form headache attacks with conjunctival injection, tearing, etc. (SUNCT): 3. Another Norwegian case. *Headache*, **31**, 175–7.

Sokolovic, M., Todorovic, L., Stajcic, Z. & Petrovic, V. (1986). Peripheral streptomycin/ lidocaine injections in the treatment of idiopathic trigeminal neuralgia. *J. Max. Fac. Surg.*, **14**, 8–9.

Solberg, W.K. (1986). Masticatory myalgia and its management. *Br. Dent. J.*, **160**, 351.

Solberg, W.K. & Graff-Radford, S.B. (1988). Orodental considerations of facial pain. *Semin. Neurol.*, **8** (4), 318–23.

Solberg, W.K., Woo, M.S. & Huston, J.B. (1979). Prevalence of mandibular dysfunction in young adults. *J. Am. Dent. Assoc.*, **98**, 25–34.

Solberg, W.K., Hansson, T.L. & Nordstrom, B.N. (1985). The temporomandibular joint in young adults at autopsy: a morphologic classification and evaluation. *J. Oral Rehab.*, **12**, 303–21.

Symonds, C. (1949). Facial pain: *Ann. Roy. Coll. Surg. Engl.*, 4, 206–12.

Symonds, C. (1956). Cough headache. *Brain*, 79, 557–68.

Taarnhoj, P. (1982). Decompression of the posterior trigeminal root in trigeminal neuralgia: a 30 year follow up review. *J. Neurosurg.*, **57**, 14–17.

Taub, A. (1973). Relief of post herpetic neuralgia with psychotropic drugs. *J. Neurosurg.*, **39**, 235–9.

Tourne, L.P.M. & Fricton, J.R. (1992). Burning mouth syndrome: critical review and proposed clinical management. *Oral Surg. Oral Med. Oral Pathol.*, **74**, 158–67.

Travell, J. & Simons, D.G. (1986). Myofascial pain and dysfunction. The Trigger Point Manual. Baltimore, Williams and Wilkins, 1984.

Vickers, R.E., Cousins, M.J., Walker, S. & Chisholm, K. (1998). Analysis of 50 patients with atypical odontalgia. A preliminary report on pharmacologic procedures for diagnosis and treatment. *Oral Surg. Oral Med. Oral Pathol. Oral Radiol. Endod.*, **85**, 24–32.

Walker, A.E. (1966). Neuralgias of the glossopharangeal, vagus and nervous intermedius nerves. In *Pain*, ed. P.R. Knighton & P.R. Dumke, pp. 421–9. Boston: Little Brown.

Watson, P.N. & Evans, R.J. (1986). Postherpetic neuralgia: a review. *Arch. Neurol.*, **43**, 836–40.

Woda, A., Navez, M-L., Picard, P., Gremeau, C. & Pichard-Leandri, E. (1998). A possible therapeutic solution for stomatodynia (burning mouth syndrome). *J. Orofacial Pain*, **12**, 272–8.

Young, R.F., Vermeulen, S., Grimm P., Blasko, J. & Posewitz, A. (1997). Gamma knife radiosurgery for treatment of trigeminal neuralgia. Idiopathic and tumor related. *Neurology*, **48**, 608–14.

64

Chronic daily headache

Stephen D. Silberstein[1] and Richard B. Lipton[2]

[1] Jefferson Headache Center, and Department of Neurology, Thomas Jefferson University Hospital, Philadelphia, Pennsylvania
[2] Department of Neurology, Epidemiology, and Social Medicine, Albert Einstein College of Medicine, New York, NY, USA

There is no consensus on the classification of chronic daily headache (CDH). Some authors use the term CDH to refer to chronic or transformed migraine; others use it for any headache disorder that occurs on a daily or near-daily basis, regardless of cause. We use CDH to refer to the broad group of very frequent headaches (15 or more days a month) not related to a structural or systemic illness, but we include those headaches that are associated with medication overuse. Population-based studies in the United States, Europe, and Asia suggest that 4 to 5% of the general population has headache 15 or more days per month (Scher et al., 1998; Castillo et al., 1999; Wang et al., 2000) and that chronic tension-type headache (CTTH) is the leading cause (Rasmussen, 1992). CDH patients account for most consultations in headache subspecialty practices (Silberstein et al., 1994).

An approach to thinking about CDH is presented in Table 64.1. Once secondary headache has been excluded, we subdivide frequent headache sufferers into two groups, based on headache duration. When headache duration is less than 4 hours, the differential diagnosis includes cluster headache, chronic paroxysmal hemicrania, idiopathic stabbing headache, hypnic headache, and other miscellaneous headache disorders. When the headache duration is greater than 4 hours, the major primary disorders to consider are transformed migraine (TM), hemicrania continua (HC), CTTH, and new daily persistent headache (NDPH) (Silberstein et al., 1994).

In this chapter, we discuss the classification and treatment of primary CDH of long duration, highlighting the four categories outlined above. We propose revisions to the International Headache Society (IHS) system and offer criteria for TM, CTTH, NDPH, and HC (Silberstein et al., 1994). We also discuss the role of medication overuse in the development and treatment of these disorders, as well as their mechanisms and treatment.

Table 64.1. Chronic daily headache

Primary chronic daily headache
Headache duration >4 hours
    Chronic migraine (transformed migraine)
    Chronic tension-type headache
    New daily persistent headache
    Hemicrania continua
Headache duration <4 hours
    Cluster headache
    Paroxysmal hemicranias
    Hypnic headache
    Idiopathic stabbing headache

Secondary chronic daily headache
– Post-traumatic headache
– Cervical spine disorders
– Headache associated with vascular disorders (arteriovenous malformation, arteritis (including giant cell arteritis), dissection, and subdural hematoma)
– Headache associated with non-vascular intracranial disorders (intracranial hypertension, infection (EBV, HIV), neoplasm)
– Other (temporomandibular joint disorder; sinus infection)

Transformed (chronic) migraine

Transformed migraine has been variously called transformed or evolutive migraine, chronic migraine or mixed headache (Silberstein et al., 1995; Mathew, 1982; Mathew et al., 1982, 1987; Olesen et al., 1993; Saper, 1983). Patients with TM often have a history of episodic migraine that began in their teens or twenties (Silberstein et al., 1995). Most patients with this disorder are women, 90% of whom have a history of migraine without aura. Patients often report a process of transformation characterized by headaches that have grown more frequent over months to years

Table 64.2. Revised criteria for transformed migraine

1.8 Chronic migraine

A. Daily or almost daily (>15 days/month) head pain for >1 month

B. Average headache duration of >4 hours/day (if untreated)

C. At least one of the following:
    1) History of episodic migraine meeting any IHS criteria 1.1 to 1.6
    2) History of increasing headache frequency with decreasing average severity of migrainous features over at least 3 months.
    3) Headache at some time meets IHS criteria for migraine 1.1 to 1.6 other than duration

D. Does not meet criteria for new daily persistent headache (4.7) or hemicrania continua (4.8)

E. No evidence of organic disease.

Note:

The clinician should attempt to distinguish the coincidental occurrence of migraine and CTTH based on the pattern of headache evolution. If the patient cannot recall the pattern of evolution differentiating the coincidental occurrence of two disorders may be difficult.

Source: Modified from Silberstein et al. (1996).

Table 64.3. Proposed criteria for chronic tension-type headache

2.2 Chronic tension-type headache

Diagnostic criteria

A. Average headache frequency >15 days/month (180 days/year) with average duration of >4 hours/day (if untreated) for 6 months fulfilling criteria B-D listed below.

B. At least 2 of the following pain characteristics:
    1. Pressing/tightening quality
    2. Mild or moderate severity (may inhibit, but does not prohibit activities)
    3. Bilateral location
    4. No aggravation by walking upstairs or similar routine physical activity

C. History of episodic tension-type headache in the past (needs to be tested).

D. History of evolutive headaches which gradually increased in frequency over at least a 3 month period (needs to be tested).

E. Both of the following:
    1. No vomiting
    2. No more than one of nausea, photophobia, or phonophobia (needs to be tested).

F. Does not meet criteria for hemicrania continua (4.8), new daily persistent headache (4.7), or chronic migraine (1.8).

G. No evidence of organic disease.

Source: Modified from Silberstein et al. (1996).

while the associated symptoms of photophobia, phonophobia, and nausea have, on average, become less severe and less frequent (Mathew, 1982; Mathew et al., 1982; Mathew, 1987; Saper, 1983). Patients often develop (transform into) a pattern of daily or nearly daily headaches that resemble CTTH. That is, the pain is mild to moderate and not associated with photophobia, phonophobia, or gastrointestinal features. Other features of migraine, including aggravation by menstruation and other trigger factors, as well as unilaterality and gastrointestinal symptoms, may persist. Many patients have attacks of full-blown migraine superimposed on a background of less severe headaches. Migraine transformation most often develops when there is medication overuse, but transformation may occur without overuse (Mathew et al., 1982, 1990).

Eighty per cent of patients with TM have depression (Mathew, 1993; Saper, 1983) which often lifts when the pattern of medication overuse and daily headache is interrupted. We proposed criteria for TM (Table 64.2). We believe that TM is a form of migraine and that the diagnosis is best made in patients who have a past history of IHS migraine and a process of transformation (Silberstein et al., 1995). Our criteria provide three alternative diagnostic links to migraine: (i) a prior history of IHS migraine; (ii) a clear period of escalating headache frequency with decreasing severity of migrainous features (which were both required in the 1994 criteria); or (iii) current superimposed attacks of headaches that meet all the IHS criteria for migraine except duration. Pascual et al. pointed out that individuals with coincidental migraine and CTTH could meet criteria for TM. If a patient has episodic migraine and independent, coincidental CTTH, there is a risk that the headache may be misclassified as TM.

Chronic tension-type headache (Table 64.3)

Daily headaches may also develop in patients with a history of episodic tension-type headache (ETTH). These headaches are more often diffuse or bilateral, frequently involving the posterior aspect of the head and neck. Prior or coexistent episodic migraine is absent in patients with CTTH, as are most features of migraine. We proposed several modifications to the current classification of CTTH. CTTH (2.2) requires head pain on at least 15 days a month for at least 6 months. Although the pain criteria are identical to ETTH, the IHS classification allows nausea, but not vomiting. The need to include any of these migrainous features in the IHS definition of CTTH may be a result of the practice of including TM under the rubric of CTTH. Coexistent migraine and CTTH might exist with the caveat that the non-migrainous headaches have no migrainous features. Guitera et al. (1999) have suggested, based on population-based epidemiologic data, that CTTH and migraine can coexist if, and only if, the current headache has no migrainous features and there is a remote history of migraine.

Calcitonin gene-related peptide (CGRP) is involved in the pathophysiology of migraine and cluster headache. Its role in CTTH is unknown. Ashina et al. (2000) found that plasma levels of CGRP are normal and unrelated to headache state in patients with CTTH. CGRP levels measured in the peripheral circulation of patients on days without headache, 63±5 pmol/l, tended to be higher than CGRP levels of controls, 53±3 pmol/l, but the difference was not statistically significant ($P=0.06$). No differences were found between CGRP levels assessed ictally and interictally in either the cranial ($P=0.91$) or the peripheral ($P=0.62$) circulation. Plasma CGRP was higher in the external jugular vein than in the antecubital vein on days without headache ($P=0.03$), but not on days with headache ($P=0.82$). Interictal plasma CGRP was increased in patients whose pain quality was pulsating. This study suggests that TTHs that fulfill IHS criteria may be related to migraine, if the headache has a pulsating quality.

Russell et al. (1999) evaluated CTTH in a family study of 122 probands and 377 first-degree relatives. Sensitivity, specificity, predictive values, and chance-corrected agreement rate for the diagnosis of CTTH were 68%, 86%, 53% (PVpos), 92% (PVneg), and 0.48, respectively. The low sensitivity for CTTH in a family member, assessed by a proband report, indicates that 32% of CTTH cases are missed using this method. They concluded that direct interviews of family members are necessary to determine case status, as was previously shown for migraine (Ottman & Lipton, 1994). Clinically interviewed parents, siblings, and children had a 2.1- to 3.9-fold increased risk of CTTH compared with the general population. The proband's gender did not influence the risk of CTTH among first-degree relatives. The significantly increased familial risk, with no increased risk found in spouses, suggests that genetic factors are involved in CTTH, although familial environmental factors are also possible.

New daily persistent headache (Table 64.4)

NDPH is characterized by the relatively abrupt onset of an unremitting CDH (Vanast, 1986); that is, a patient develops

Table 64.4. Proposed criteria for new daily persistent headache

4.7 New daily persistent headache
A. Average headache frequency >15 days/month for >1 month
B. Average headache duration >4 hours/day (if untreated). Frequently constant without medication but may fluctuate.
C. No history of tension-type headache or migraine which increases in frequency and decreases in severity in association with the onset of NDPH (over 3 months).
D. Acute onset (developing over <3 days) of constant unremitting headache
E. Headache is constant in location? (Needs to be tested)
F. Does not meet criteria for hemicrania continua 4.8
G. No evidence of organic disease.

Source: Modified from Silberstein et al. (1994).

a headache that does not remit. NDPH is likely to be a heterogeneous disorder. Castillo et al. (1999) conducted a population study of over 2000 patients; they identified only two cases of this disorder, indicating that it is rare. Some cases may reflect a postviral syndrome (Vanast, 1986). The daily headache develops abruptly, over less than 3 days. Patients with NDPH are generally younger than those with TM (Vanast, 1986).

Since NDPH is not defined by the characteristics of the headache, this disorder overlaps with CTTH. The presence or absence of a past history of headache distinguishes the disorders. NDPH requires the relatively abrupt onset of near daily headache in the absence of a history of evolution from migraine or ETTH. Excluding all patients with a history of ETTH is problematic, as almost 70% of men and 90% of women have had a TTH in the past. We allow a diagnosis of NDPH in patients with migraine or ETTH if these disorders do not increase in frequency to give rise to NDPH. The constancy of location is uncertain and needs to be field-tested. NDPH may or may not be associated with medication overuse (4.7.1., 4.7.2.). A diagnosis of NDPH takes precedence over TM and CTTH.

Hemicrania continua (Table 64.5)

HC is a rare, indomethacin-responsive headache disorder characterized by a continuous, moderately severe, unilateral headache that varies in intensity, waxing and waning without disappearing completely (Newman et al., 1993). It rarely alternates sides (Bordini et al., 1991). HC is frequently associated with jabs and jolts (idiopathic stabbing headache). Exacerbations of pain are often associated with

Table 64.5. Proposed criteria for hemicrania continua

4.8 Hemicrania continua[a]

A. Headache present for at least 1 month
B. Strictly unilateral headache
C. Pain has all 3 of the following present:
    1. Continuous but fluctuating
    2. Moderate severity, at least some of the time
    3. Lack of precipitating mechanisms
D. 1) Absolute response to indomethacin or
    2) One of the following autonomic features with severe pain exacerbation
        (a) Conjunctival infection
        (b) Lacrimation
        (c) Nasal congestion
        (d) Rhinorrhea
        (e) Ptosis
        (f) Eyelid edema
E. May have associated stabbing headaches
F. No evidence of organic disease.

Notes:

[a] HC is usually non-remitting, but rare cases of remission have been reported.

Source: Modified from Goadsby and Lipton (1997).

autonomic disturbances, such as ptosis, miosis, tearing, and sweating. HC is not triggered by neck movements, but tender spots in the neck may be present (Table 64.5). Some patients have photophobia, phonophobia, and nausea.

Although HC almost invariably has a prompt and enduring response to indomethacin, the requirement of a therapeutic response as a diagnostic criterion is problematic. It effectively excludes the diagnosis of HC in patients who were never treated with indomethacin (perhaps because another agent helped) and in patients who failed to respond to indomethacin. Cases have been described that did not respond to indomethacin but meet the phenotype; for this reason a characteristic pattern or a response to indomethacin (Table 64.5) provides an alternative means of diagnosis.

HC exists in continuous and remitting forms. In the remitting variety, distinct headache phases last weeks to months, with prolonged pain-free remissions (Newman et al., 1993; Iordanidis & Sjaastad, 1989; Pareja et al., 1990). In the continuous variety, headaches occur on a daily, continuous basis, sometimes for years. A bilateral case and a patient whose attacks alternated sides (Newman et al., 1993) have been described. HC takes precedence over the diagnosis of other types of primary CDH. Many patients with this disorder overuse acute medication; it must be differentiated from TM.

The relative rarity of HC has made it difficult to study its pathophysiology. In a population study of nearly 2000 patients, no cases were identified (Castillo et al., 1999). Pain pressure thresholds are reduced in patients who have HC, as they are in those who have chronic paroxysmal hemicrania (Antonaci et al., 1994). In contrast, orbital phlebography is relatively normal compared with patients who have chronic paroxysmal hemicrania (Antonaci, 1994), although it should be observed that this area is controversial (Bovim et al., 1992). Pupillometric studies have shown no clear abnormality in HC (Antonaci et al., 1992), and studies of facial sweating have shown modest changes, similar to those seen in chronic paroxysmal hemicrania (Antonaci, 1991).

Espada et al.(1999) reported five men and four women who had HC (eight continuous, one remitting) that was diagnosed using proposed diagnostic criteria (Goadsby & Lipton, 1997). The mean age of onset was 53.3 years (range 29 to 69). All nine patients had initial relief with indomethacin (mean daily dose 94.4 mg, range 50 to 150). Follow-up was possible in eight patients. Indomethacin could be discontinued after 3, 7, and 15 months respectively, and patients remained pain free. Three patients discontinued treatment because of side effects and had headache recurrence; two had relief with aspirin. Two other patients continue to take indomethacin with partial relief.

Drug overuse and rebound headache

Patients with frequent headaches often overuse analgesics, opioids, ergotamine, and triptans (Katsarava et al., 1999). Medication overuse may be both a response to chronic pain and a cause of chronic pain. In headache-prone patients, medication overuse may produce drug-induced 'rebound headache' that is accompanied by dependence on symptomatic medication. In addition, medication overuse can make headaches refractory to prophylactic medication (Mathew et al., 1990; Mathew, 1990; Diamond & Dalessio, 1982; Wilkinson, 1988; Saper, 1987a, 1989). Although stopping the acute medication may result in the development of withdrawal symptoms and a period of increased headache, there is generally subsequent headache improvement (Saper, 1989; Andersson, 1988; Baumgartner et al., 1989; Rapoport et al., 1986; Saper & Jones, 1986).

In subspecialty centres, most patients with drug-induced headache have a history of episodic migraine that has been converted into TM as a result of medication overuse (Mathew et al., 1987, 1990; Mathew, 1990; Rapoport, 1988; Kudrow, 1982; Diener et al., 1984; Rasmussen et al., 1989).

Patients with TTH, HC, and NDPH may also overuse symptomatic medications.

In European headache centres, 5 to 10% of the patients have drug-induced headache. One series of 3000 consecutive headache patients reported that 4.3% had drug-induced headaches (Micieli et al., 1988). Experiences in the United Kingdom (Goadsby, P. personal communication) suggest that drug-associated headache is more common than the literature suggests. In American specialty headache clinics, as many as 80% of patients who presented with primary CDH used analgesics on a daily or near-daily basis (Rapoport, 1988; Solomon et al., 1992). In India, in contrast, medication overuse is less common (Ravishankar, 1997). Diener and Tfelt-Hansen (1993) summarized 29 studies, which included 2612 patients with chronic drug-induced headache. Migraine was the primary headache in 65%, TTH in 27%, and mixed or other headaches in 8% (for example, cluster headache). Women had more drug-induced headache than men (3.5 : 1; 1533 women, 442 men). The number of tablets or suppositories taken daily averaged 4.9 (range 0.25 to 25). Patients averaged 2.5 to 5.8 different pharmacologic components simultaneously (range 1 to 14) (Diener & Tfelt-Hansen, 1993).

Clinical features of rebound headache

Rebound headache has not been demonstrated in placebo-controlled trials. However, stopping daily low-dose caffeine frequently results in withdrawal headache (Silverman et al., 1992). In a controlled study of caffeine withdrawal, 64 normal adults (71% women) with low-to-moderate caffeine intake (the equivalent of about 2.5 cups of coffee a day) were given a two-day caffeine-free diet and either placebo or replacement caffeine. Under double-blind conditions, 50% of the patients who were given placebo had a headache by day two, compared to 6% of those given caffeine. Nausea, depression, and flu-like symptoms were common in the placebo group. This study is relevant since caffeine is frequently used by headache sufferers for pain relief, often in combination with analgesics or ergotamine. The study is a model for short-term caffeine withdrawal but does not demonstrate the long-term consequences of detoxification. In a community-based telephone survey of 11 112 subjects in Lincoln and Omaha, Nebraska, 61% reported daily caffeine consumption, and 11% of the caffeine consumers reported symptoms upon stopping coffee (Potter et al., 2000). A group of those who reported withdrawal were assigned to one of three regimes: abrupt caffeine withdrawal; gradual withdrawal; and no change. One-third of the abrupt-withdrawal group and an occasional member of the gradual-withdrawal group had symptoms that included headache and tiredness.

The actual dose limits and the time needed to develop rebound headaches have not been defined in rigorous studies, nor is the relationship of drug half-life to rebound development known. It is believed that overuse occurs when patients take three or more simple analgesics a day more often than 5 days a week, triptans or combination analgesics containing barbiturates, sedatives, or caffeine more often than 3 days a week, or opioids or ergotamine tartrate more often than 2 days a week (Mathew et al., 1990; Diamond & Dalessio, 1982; Mathew, 1990; Saper, 1987a; Wilkinson, 1988). Rebound headache can develop in patients taking as little as 0.5 to 1mg of ergotamine three times a week (Silberstein, 1993; Wilkinson, 1988; Saper, 1983, 1987b; Saper & Jones, 1986; Baumgartner et al., 1989).

The triptans are selective 5-HT$_1$ agonists that are effective in acute migraine treatment and all of them (sumatriptan, rizatriptan, naratriptan, and zolmitriptan) have been reported to induce rebound headache (Catarci et al., 1994; Diener et al., 1991; Gaist et al., 1996; Katsarava et al., 1999). The weekly dosages necessary to initiate drug-induced headache with the centrally penetrant triptans may be lower than with ergotamines or sumatriptan and the time of onset might be shorter. Increasing attack frequency can be the first sign that drug-induced headache is developing. We recommend limiting triptan use to 3 days a week.

Medication overuse may be responsible, in part, for the transformation of episodic migraine or ETTH into daily headache and for the perpetuation of the syndrome. However, medication overuse is not the sine qua non of TM or CTTH. Some patients develop TM or CTTH without overusing medication, and others continue to have daily headaches long after the overused medication has been discontinued. Medication overuse is usually motivated by a patient's desire to treat the headaches (Kaiser, 1999). However, some headache patients overuse combination analgesics to treat a mood disturbance. Medication overuse rarely represents a form of primary substance abuse.

In addition to exacerbating the headache disorder, drug overuse has other serious effects. The overuse of acute drugs may interfere with the effectiveness of preventive headache medications. Prolonged use of large amounts of medication may cause renal or hepatic toxicity in addition to tolerance, habituation, or dependence.

Psychiatric comorbidity

Anxiety, depression, panic disorder and bipolar disease are more frequent in migraineurs than in non-migraine control subjects (Merikangas et al., 1990; Breslau & Davis, 1993). Since TM evolves from migraine, one would expect to find a similar profile of psychiatric comorbidity in TM. In clinic-based samples, depression occurs in 80% of TM patients. The Minnesota Multiphasic Personality Inventory was abnormal in 61% of primary CDH patients, compared with 12.2% of patients with episodic migraine. Zung and Beck Depression Scale scores were significantly higher in primary CDH patients than in migraine controls (Mathew, 1990, 1991; Mathew et al., 1990; Saper, 1987b). Comorbid depression often improves when the cycle of daily head pain is broken.

Mitsikostas and Thomas (1999) found that the average Hamilton rating scores for anxiety and depression were significantly higher in headache patients. Patients with CTTH, mixed headache, or drug abuse headache had the highest Hamilton rating scores for depression and anxiety. Verri et al. (1998) found current psychiatric comorbidity in 90% of primary CDH patients. Generalized anxiety occurred in 69.3% of patients and major depression in 25%.

Psychiatric comorbidity is a predictor of intractability. The Minnesota Multiphasic Personality Inventory was abnormal in 100% of CDH patients who failed to respond to aggressive management (31% of the primary CDH group), compared to 48% of the responders. Physical, emotional, or sexual abuse, parental alcohol abuse, and a positive dexamethasone suppression test also correlated highly with a poor response to aggressive management. Curioso et al. (1999) found that 31 of 69 (45%) CDH patients had an adjustment disorder, 16 (23%) had major depression, 12 (17%) were dysthymic, 6 (9%) had generalized anxiety disorder, 1 (2%) was bipolar, and 3 (4%) were normal. The risk of a bad outcome after treatment was significantly greater for patients with major depression than those without. CDH patients who have major depression or abnormal Beck Depression Inventory scores have worse outcomes at 3 to 6 months compared with patients who are not depressed.

Epidemiology

In population-based surveys, primary CDH occurs in 4.1% of Americans, 4.35% of Greeks, 3.9% of elderly Chinese, and 4.7% of Spaniards. Population-based estimates for the one-year period prevalence of CTTH are 1.7% in Ethiopia (Tekle Haimanot et al., 1995), 3% in Denmark (Rasmussen, 1995), 2.2% in Spain (Castillo et al., 1999), 2.7% in China (Wang et al., 2000), and 2.2% in the United States (Scher et al., 1998).

Scher et al. (1998) ascertained the prevalence of primary CDH in 13,343 individuals aged 18 to 65 years in Baltimore

County, Maryland. The overall prevalence of primary CDH was 4.1% (5.0% women, 2.8% men; 1.8: 1 women to men ratio). In both men and women, prevalence was highest in the lowest educational category. More than half (52% women, 56% men) met criteria for CTTH (2.2%), almost one-third (33% women, 25% men) met criteria for TM (1.3%), and the remainder (15% women, 19% men) were unclassified (0.6%). Overall, 30% of women and 25% of men who were frequent headache sufferers met IHS criteria for migraine (with or without aura). On the basis of chance, migraine and CTTH would co-occur in 0.22% of the population; the fact that TM occurred in 1.3% of this population would suggest that their co-occurrence is more than random.

Castillo et al. (1999) sampled 2252 subjects over 14 years of age in Cantabria, Spain. Overall 4.7% had CDH. Using the criteria of Silberstein et al. (1994), none had HC, 0.1% had NDPH, 2.2% had CTTH, and 2.4% had TM. Overuse of symptomatic medication occurred in 19% of CTTH and 31.1% of TM patients. Eight patients had a previous history of migraine without aura and now had primary CDH with only the characteristics of TTH. These headaches met the criteria of TM but could have been migraine and coincidental CTTH.

Wang et al. (2000) looked at the characteristics of primary CDH in a population of elderly Chinese (over 65 years of age) in two townships on Kinmen Island in August 1993. Person-to-person biannual follow-up of the primary CDH patients was done in June 1995 and August 1997. Sixty patients (3.9%) had CDH. Significantly more women than men had primary CDH (5.6% and 1.8%, $P<0.001$). Of the primary CDH patients, 42 (70%) had CTTH (2.7%), 15 (25%) had TM (1%), and 3 (5%) had other CDH. By multivariate logistic regression, the significant risk factors of primary CDH included analgesic overuse (OR=79), a history of migraine (OR=6.6), and a Geriatric Depression Scale-Short Form score of 8 or above (OR=2.6). At follow-up in 1995 and 1997, approximately two-thirds of patients still had CDH. Compared with the patients in remission, the patients with persistent primary CDH in 1997 had a significantly higher frequency of analgesic overuse (33% vs. 0%, $P=0.03$) and major depression (38% vs. 0%, $P=0.04$).

Pathophysiology of chronic daily headache

The nucleus caudalis (NC) of the trigeminal complex, the major relay nucleus for head and face pain, receives nociceptive input from cephalic blood vessels and pericranial muscles, as well as inhibitory and facilitatory suprasegmental input. Recent evidence suggests that central pain facilitatory neurons (on-cells) are present in the ventrome-dial medulla. In addition, neurons in the trigeminal NC can be sensitized as a result of intense neuronal stimulation. Chronic pain may be due to ongoing peripheral activation of nociceptors (for example, chronic inflammation), although it may occur in the absence of painful stimuli. Although the source of pain in primary CDH is unknown and may be dependent on the subtype of CDH, recent work suggests several mechanisms that could contribute to the process: (i) abnormal excitation of peripheral nociceptive afferent fibres (perhaps due to chronic neurogenic inflam-mation); (ii) enhanced responsiveness of the NC neurons (central sensitization); (iii) decreased pain modulation; (iv) spontaneous central pain; or (v) a combination of these.

Peripheral mechanisms

In migraine, trigeminal nerve activation is accompanied by the release of vasoactive neuropeptides, including calcito-nin gene-related peptides, substance P (SP), and neuroki-nin A from the nerve terminals. These mediators produce mast cell activation, sensitization of the nerve terminals, and extravasation of fluid into the perivascular space around the dural blood vessels. Intense neuronal stimula-tion causes induction of c-fos (an immediate early gene product) in the trigeminal NC of the brainstem. Neurotropins such as nerve growth factor are synthesized locally and can also activate mast cells and sensitive nerve terminals. Prostaglandins and nitric oxide (a diffusible gas that acts as a neurotransmitter) (Edelman & Gally, 1992) are both endogenous mediators that can be produced locally and can sensitize nociceptors. Repeated episodes of neurogenic inflammation may chronically sensitize noci-ceptors and thus contribute to the development of daily headache.

Central sensitization is manifested by increased sponta-neous impulse discharges, increased responsiveness to noxious and non-noxious peripheral stimuli, and ex-panded receptive fields of nociceptive neurons. Does central sensitization play a role in headache? Brief chemi-cal irritation of the dura with a cocktail of four inflamma-tory mediators (histamine, serotonin, bradykinin, and prostaglandin E2) made meningeal perivascular neurons pain-sensitive for a period of one to two hours, becoming more sensitive to mechanical forces (>2 g) (Strassman et al., 1996). This can explain the intracranial hypersensitivity (i.e. the worsening pain during coughing, bending over, or any head movement) and the throbbing pain of migraine (Anthony & Rasmussen, 1993).

Brief dural chemical irritation may also result in tempo-rary changes in the central trigeminal neurons that receive convergent input from the dura and the skin. Their thresh-old decreased and their excitability increased in response to brushing and heating (<42 °C) of the periorbital skin – stimuli to which they showed only minimal or no response prior to chemical stimulation (Burstein et al., 1998). Sensitization may be the basis of the extracranial tender-ness that accompanies migraine. In addition, the threshold of cardiovascular responses to facial and intracranial stimuli is reduced (Yamamura et al., 1999). The enhanced neuronal responses represent a state of central sensitiza-tion and the enhanced cardiovascular responses represent a state of intracranial hypersensitivity and cutaneous allo-dynia.

Burstein et al. (1998) predicted that cutaneous allodynia is present in migraine patients during attacks. They exam-ined the pain thresholds of patients during and between migraine attacks. Many patients had periorbital cutaneous allodynia ipsilateral to the headache. Patients with allody-nia were significantly older than those without cutaneous allodynia, hinting at a possible correlation between age and sensitization. These findings provide a neural basis for the pathophysiology of migraine pain and suggest a basis for continued head pain.

Bendtsen et al. (1996b) found evidence for sensitization in CTTH patients. Pericranial myofascial tenderness, eval-uated by manual palpation, was considerably higher in patients than in controls ($P < 0.00001$). The stimu-lus–response function from highly tender muscle was qualitatively different than from normal muscle, suggest-ing that myofascial pain may be mediated by low-thresh-old mechanosensitive afferents projecting to sensitized dorsal horn neurons.

Lassen et al. (1997) discovered that nitroglycerin, a nitric oxide (NO) donor, can induce more headache in CTTH patients than in healthy volunteers. Ashina et al. (1999) found that a NO synthesis inhibitor (L-NMMA) reduced headache and muscle hardness in CTTH. CTTH patients may have sensitization of second-order neurons due to prolonged nociceptive input from myofascial tissues. The decrease in muscle hardness following treatment with L-NMMA may be caused by decreased central sensitiza-tion.

Pain modulation

The mammalian nervous system contains networks that modulate nociceptive transmission. In the rostroventro-medial medulla are so-called off-cells that inhibit, and on-cells that facilitate nociception (Fields et al., 1991). Increased on-cell activity could enhance the response to both painful and non-painful stimuli. Opiate withdrawal results in increased firing of the on-cells, decreased firing of the off-cells, and enhanced nociception (Fields et al., 1991). A similar mechanism may occur during drug-induced headaches. Primary CDH may result, in part, from enhanced neuronal activity in the NC as a result of enhanced on-cell or decreased off-cell activity.

Jensen and Olesen (1996) used sustained teeth-clenching to trigger TTH in 58 patients with frequent CTTH or ETTH and 58 matched controls. Within 24 hours, 69% of patients (more than would be expected) and 17% of controls developed TTH. Shortly after clenching, electromyography (EMG) amplitude was significantly increased in the trapezius but not in the temporal muscle, and tenderness (which was increased at baseline in the headache patients) was further increased only in the patients who subsequently developed headache. Mechanical pain thresholds remained unchanged in the group that developed headache but increased in the group that did not develop headache. Pain tolerance decreased in the patients who developed headache, was unchanged in the remaining patients, and increased in controls, suggesting that headache patients do not effectively activate their antinociceptive system. This study clearly shows that peripheral mechanisms alone cannot explain TTH, but they could act as a trigger for a central process. Tenderness, not muscle contraction, correlates to headache development.

Exteroceptive suppression (ES) is the inhibition of voluntary EMG activity of the temporalis muscle induced by trigeminal nerve stimulation (Schoenen et al., 1987). There are two successive periods of ES (ES1 and ES2) (silent periods). ES2, a multisynaptic reflex subject to limbic and other modulation, was originally reported to be absent in 40% of patients with CTTH and reduced in duration in 87%, whereas ES1, an oligosynaptic reflex, was normal (Paulus et al., 1992; Makashima & Takahashi, 1991; Pritchard, 1989). More recent studies have not confirmed these findings. Zwart and Sand found normal ES2 values in a small blinded study of 11 patients with CTTH (Zwart & Sand, 1995). Bendtsen et al. (1996a) and Lipchick et al. (1996, 1997) did not find abnormalities in ES2 in blinded studies of patients with CTTH. Measures of ES2 duration depend on tricky methodologic variables. ES2 may be absent in headache-prone patients (Paulus et al., 1992; Nakashima & Takahashi, 1991).

Schoenen et al. (1987) measured the ES2, pain threshold, EMG activity, anxiety scores, and response to biofeedback in 32 women with CTTH, and found an abnormal EMG in 62.5% of the patients if three different muscles and three states were tested. The EMG was abnormal in only 40% if only one muscle and one state were tested. A decreased pain threshold was found in half the patients tested in one

of three muscles but in only 34% if only one muscle was tested. ES2 duration was reduced in 87% of patients

Schepelmann et al. (1998) found that the duration of ES2 (+SD) in fibromyalgia syndrome patients was $30.6+7.5$ ms and was not significantly different from the control group ($33.1+7.8$ ms), whereas it was significantly shortened in CTTH patients ($22.9+11.5$ ms). Lipchik et al. (1996) evaluated masseter ES2 suppression and tenderness in the pericranial muscles of young adults with CTTH, ETTH, migraine without aura, migraine with aura, and controls. Pericranial muscle tenderness better distinguished diagnostic subgroups and better distinguished recurrent headache sufferers from controls than did masseter ES2. CTTH sufferers had the highest pericranial muscle tenderness and controls exhibited the lowest tenderness ($P<0.01$). The association between pericranial muscle tenderness and CTTH was independent of the intensity, frequency, or chronicity of headaches. Pericranial muscle tenderness may be present early in the development of tension headache, while ES2 suppression may only emerge later.

Reduced Achilles tendon pain thresholds were found in half of CTTH patients when compared with headache-free controls (Schoenen et al., 1991). Biofeedback moderately but significantly increased the pain threshold, perhaps by normalizing limbic input to the brainstem pain modulating system. Increased EMG activity or decreased pain thresholds were found in 72% of the patients (Schoenen et al., 1991), consistent with a diagnosis of 'CTTH associated with disorder of pericranial muscles', but these findings were not present in the remaining 28% of patients, consistent with a diagnosis of 'CTTH unassociated with such disorder'. Headache severity, anxiety, ES2, and response to biofeedback did not differ between these two groups, suggesting that their separation may be artificial or a consequence of the headache.

Spontaneous central pain activation

Post and Silberstein (1994) suggested the kindling model for epilepsy as a model for non-epileptic, progressive disorders such as mania. Post and Silberstein (1994) suggested that spontaneous recurrent migraine headaches might be analogous to the low levels of electrical stimulation in the kindling model in the process of headache transformation. Preventive migraine treatment could provide a dual benefit by preventing the occurrence of episodes and blocking the sensitization process that could lead to syndrome progression.

In primary CDH, hypersensitivity of neurons in the trigeminal NC may exist as a result of supraspinal facilitation. The vascular nociceptor may be hypersensitive in TM; in

CTTH associated with a disorder of the pericranial muscles, the myofascial nociceptor may be hypersensitive. In CTTH not associated with a disorder of the pericranial muscles, there may be less myofascial nociceptor hypersensitivity and a general increase in nociception. CTTH and TM may result from a defective interaction between endogenous nociceptive brainstem activity and peripheral input. Physical or psychologic stress or non-physiologic working positions can increase nociception from strained muscles that could trigger or sustain an attack and produce CTTH in an individual with altered pain modulation. Emotional mechanisms may also reduce endogenous antinociception. Long-term potentiation of nociceptive neurons and decreased activity in the antinociceptive system could cause primary CDH. Sensitization of the trigeminal NC neurons can result in normally non-painful stimuli becoming painful, production spots, an overlap in the symptoms of migraine and TTH, and activation of the trigeminal vascular system.

Drug-induced headache mechanisms

Overuse of analgesics, opioids, barbiturates, ergotamine-containing compounds, or triptans may contribute to the transformation of episodic into transformed migraine. Formulations of drugs that maintain sustained, non-fluctuating levels might avoid the development of drug-induced headache (Post & Silberstein, 1994). Continued high fluctuating doses of ergots, analgesics, opioids, or triptans could result in resetting the pain control mechanisms in susceptible individuals, perhaps by enhancing on-cell activity, enhancing central sensitization through NMDA receptors, or blocking adaptive antinociceptive changes.

Cerebral blood flow increases in the brainstem and cortex of patients with migraine without aura. During the headache, the increased cerebral blood flow in the cortex (but not the brainstem) is reversed by sumatriptan, as is the headache. This area of the brainstem is rich in opioids and includes the pain control centres. Dihydroergotamine (DHE) and centrally penetrant triptans selectively bind to this area of the brainstem, while sumatriptan may not. Perhaps this area of the brainstem integrates the phenomenon we call migraine, or it could be activated as a result of the migraine attack. If the first explanation is correct, ongoing activity in this area of the brainstem could produce recurrent or daily headache. If this area is responsible for controlling pain, then its failure to activate could explain ongoing headache activity. Acute migraine medications may induce daily headache by preventing the development of adaptive changes and perhaps by maintaining brainstem activation (Weiller et al., 1995).

Treatment

Overview

Patients suffering from CDH can be difficult to treat, especially when the disorder is complicated by medication overuse, comorbid psychiatric disease, low frustration tolerance, and physical and emotional dependency (Mathew et al., 1987; Saper, 1987b). The following steps should be taken. First, exclude secondary headache disorders; secondly, diagnose the specific primary headache disorder (i.e. TM, HC); and thirdly, identify comorbid medical and psychiatric conditions, as well as exacerbating factors, especially medication overuse. Limit all symptomatic medications (with the possible exception of the long-acting non-steroidal anti-inflammatory drugs (NSAIDs)). Start the patient on a programme of preventive medication (to decrease reliance on symptomatic medication), with the explicit understanding that the drugs may not become fully effective until medication overuse has been eliminated and detoxification completed (Silberstein & Saper, 1993). Outpatient detoxification options, including outpatient infusion in an ambulatory infusion unit, are available. If outpatient detoxification proves difficult or is dangerous, hospitalization may be required. We have proposed guidelines for hospitalization (Table 64.6). Patients need education and continuous support during this process.

Patients who overuse acute medication may not become fully responsive to acute and preventive treatment for 3 to 8 weeks after overuse is eliminated. Withdrawal symptoms include severely exacerbated headaches accompanied by nausea, vomiting, agitation, restlessness, sleep disorder, and (rarely) seizures. Barbiturates and benzodiazepines must be tapered gradually to avoid a serious withdrawal syndrome (Silberstein et al., 1990; Mathew et al., 1990; Baumgartner et al., 1989; Raskin, 1986).

Psychophysiologic therapy involves reassurance, counselling, stress management, relaxation therapy, and biofeedback. Physical therapy consists of modality treatments (heat, cold packs, ultrasound, and electrical stimulation), improvement of posture through stretching, exercise, and traction, trigger point injections, occipital nerve blocks, and a programme of regular exercise, stretching, balanced meals, and adequate sleep (Silberstein, 1984). It has been our experience that treating painful trigger areas in the neck can result in improvement of intractable primary CDH.

Acute pharmacotherapy

Choice of acute pharmacotherapy depends upon the diagnosis. Transformed migraine patients who do not overuse

Table 64.6. Criteria for hospitalization

I. Emergency or urgent admission
A. Certain migraine variants (e.g. hemiplegic migraine, suspected migrainous infarction, basilar migraine with serious neurologic symptoms such as syncope, confusional migraine, etc.)
    1. When a diagnosis has not been established during a previous similar occurrence
    2. When a patient's established outpatient treatment plan has failed.
B. Diagnostic suspicion of infectious disorder involving CNS (e.g. brain abscess, meningitis) with initiation of appropriate diagnostic testing.
C. Diagnostic suspicion of acute vascular compromise (e.g. aneurysm, subarachnoid hemorrhage, carotid dissection) with initiation of appropriate diagnostic testing.
D. Diagnostic suspicion of a structural disorder causing symptoms requiring an acute setting (e.g. brain tumour, increased intracranial pressure) with initiation of appropriate diagnostic testing.
E. Low cerebrospinal fluid headache when an outpatient blood patch has failed and an outpatient treatment plan has failed or there is no obvious cause.
F. Medical emergency presenting with a severe headache.
G. Severe headache associated with intractable nausea and vomiting producing dehydration or postural hypotension, or unable to retain oral medication, and unable to be controlled in an outpatient setting or with admission to observation status.
H. Failed outpatient treatment of an exacerbation of episodic headache disorder with:
    1. Failure to respond to 'rescue' or backup medications or
    2. Failure to respond to outpatient treatment with IV DHE on a schedule of a minimum of twice daily.

II. Non-emergent admission:
A. Coexistent psychiatric disease documented by psychologic or psychiatric evaluation with sufficient severity of illness such that failure to admit could pose a health risk to the patient or impair the implementation of outpatient treatment.
B. Coexistent or risk of disease (e.g. unstable angina, unstable diabetes, recent transient ischemic attack, myocardial infarction in the past 6 months, renal failure, hypertension, age >65) necessitating monitoring for treatment of headache significant enough to warrant admission.
C. Severe chronic daily headaches involving chronic medication overuse when there is:
    1. Daily use of potent opioids and/or barbiturates
    2. Daily use of triptans, simple analgesics, or ergotamine in a patient with a documented failed trial of withdrawal of these medications.
D. Impaired daily functioning (e.g. threatened relationships, many lost days at work or school due to headache), with a failure to respond to 2 days of outpatient treatment with i.v./DHE, i.v. neuroleptics, or i.v. corticosteroids on a schedule of a minimum of twice daily or equivalent treatment.

Source: S.D., Silberstein, W.B., Young, T.D., Rozen & J. Lenow, Personal communication.

symptomatic medication can treat acute migrainous headache exacerbations with triptans, DHE, and NSAIDs. These drugs must be strictly limited to prevent superimposed rebound headache that will complicate treatment and require detoxification. The risk of rebound is much lower for DHE and triptans than for analgesics, opioids, and ergotamine. CTTH and NPDH can be treated with non-specific headache medications, and HC can be treated with supplemental doses of indomethacin.

Preventive pharmacotherapy

Patients with very frequent headaches should be treated primarily with preventive medications, with the explicit understanding that their medications may not become fully effective until the overused medication has been eliminated. It may take 3 to 6 weeks for treatment effects to develop. The following principles guide the use of preventive treatment: (i) from among the first-line drugs, choose preventive agents based on their side effect profiles, comorbid conditions, and specific indications (for example, indomethacin for HC); (ii) start at a low dose; (iii) gradually increase the dose until you achieve efficacy, until the patient develops side effects, or until the ceiling dose for the drug in question is reached; (iv) treatment effects develop over weeks and treatment may not become fully effective until rebound is eliminated; (v) if one agent fails, choose an agent from another therapeutic class; (vi) prefer monotherapy, but be willing to use combination therapy; (vii) communicate realistic expectations (Silberstein & Lipton, 1994).

Table 64.7. Summary of preventive drugs for use in transformed migraine

Drug	Clinical efficacy	Side effects	Clinical evidence[a]
Antidepressants			
Amitriptyline	+++	++	+++
Doxepin	+++	++	++
Fluoxetine	++	+	+++
Anticonvulsants			
Divalproex	+++	++	++
Topiramate	+++	++	++
Beta-blockers			
Propranolol, Nadolol, etc.	++	+	+
Calcium channel blockers			
Verapamil	++	+	+
Miscellaneous			
Methysergide	+++	+++	+

Notes:

All categories are rated from + to ++++ based on a combination of published literature and clinical experience.

[a] Ratings of +++ for clinical evidence indicate at least one double-blind, placebo-controlled study. A rating of ++ indicates open well-designed studies and + indicates ratings based on clinical experience. A rating of ++++ requires at least two double-blind placebo-controlled trials.

Source: Modified from Tfelt-Hansen and Welch (2000).

Most preventive agents used for primary CDH have not been examined in well-designed double-blind studies. Table 64.7 summarizes an assessment of the efficacy, safety, and evidence for a number of agents (Silberstein & Saper, 1993).

Antidepressants are attractive agents for use in TM, CTTH, and NDPH, since many patients have comorbid depression and anxiety. The most widely used tricyclic antidepressants are nortriptyline (Aventyl, Pamelor), doxepin (Sinequan) (Morland et al., 1979), and amitriptyline (Elavil), which has been effective in many but not all studies (Bussone et al., 1991; Couch et al., 1976; Diamond & Baltes, 1971; Holland et al., 1983; Lance & Curran, 1964; Pluvinage, 1994; Pfaffenrath et al., 1986, 1994; Holroyd et al., 1991; Gobel et al., 1994; Cerbo et al., 1998; Mitsikostas et al., 1997; Bonuccelli et al., 1996). In an open-label study in 82 non-depressed patients with either ETTH or CTTH, Cerbo et al. (1998) found that amitriptyline (25mg a day) significantly reduced ($P<0.05$) analgesic consumption and the frequency and duration of headache in CTTH but not in ETTH.

Fluoxetine (Prozac), a selective serotonin reuptake inhibitor, is coming into wider use for daily headaches; evidence from a double-blind study demonstrates its efficacy in primary CDH (Bussone et al., 1991; Saper et al., 1994). Fluvoxamine appears to be effective (Manna et al., 1994) and may have analgesic properties (Palmer & Benfield, 1994). Other selective serotonin reuptake inhibitors including paroxetine (Foster & Bafaloukos, 1994) and monoamine oxidase inhibitors may have a therapeutic role, but this has not been proven to date (Langemark & Olesen, 1994).

Beta-blockers (propranolol, nadolol) remain a mainstay of therapy for migraine (Silberstein & Saper, 1993) and are used for primary CDH (Pfaffenrath et al., 1986; Mathew, 1981). Clinicians fear that beta-blockers may exacerbate depression; however, this issue is controversial (Bright & Everitt, 1992). Beta-blockers are relatively contraindicated in patients who have asthma and Raynaud's disease.

Calcium channel blockers are very well tolerated (Silberstein & Saper, 1993); anecdotal evidence supports their use for TM. Verapamil (Calan) is the most widely prescribed agent in this family. Diltiazem (Cardizem) and nifedipine (Procardia) may also be considered. Flunarizine (Silberstein & Saper, 1993; Lake et al., 1993) is widely used in Canada and Europe but is not available in the United States.

The anticonvulsant divalproex sodium (Depakote) (Jensen et al., 1994) is an important drug in migraine prophylaxis, even for patients who have failed other agents. Four double-blind placebo-controlled studies have demonstrated its efficacy in migraine (Jensen et al., 1994; Mathew et al., 1995; Hering & Kuritzky, 1998; Klapper, 1995). Smaller open studies support its utility in TM (Mathew & Ali, 1991). Doses lower than those used for epilepsy (250 mg twice a day) may be sufficient. In an open-label study, Edwards et al. (1999) assessed the possible benefit of sodium valproate in 20 consecutive CDH patients who were refractory to multiple standard treatments. Eleven (55%) had a response (mild or no headaches within one to four weeks). The doses ranged from 375 mgs to 1500 mg a day. Two patients (10%) discontinued medication due to side effects (nausea and difficulty thinking).

Topiramate is a new antiepileptic agent that has GABA-agonist properties and few side effects when used in low doses. Its chronic use has been associated with weight loss, not weight gain. In an open-label study, Shuaib et al. (1999) used topiramate (25 to 100 mg per day) to treat 37 patients who had more than ten migraine headaches a month. Most patients had CDH in addition to migraine; all had failed previous preventive treatment. Over a 3- to 9-month follow-up, 11 patients had an excellent result (headache frequency decreased by over 60%); 11 patients had a good result (headaches frequency decreased 40% to 60%); three patients discontinued therapy due to side effects; and eight patients had no improvement. This uncontrolled study suggests that topiramate may be useful for TM.

The NSAIDs can be used for both symptomatic and preventive headache treatment. Naproxen sodium is effective for prevention at a dose of one or two 275 mg tablets twice a day (Miller et al., 1987). Other NSAIDs found to be effective include tolfenamic acid, ketoprofen, mefenamic acid, fenoprofen, and ibuprofen (Johnson & Tfelt-Hansen, 1993; Mylecharane & Tfelt-Hansen, 1993). Aspirin was found to be effective in one study (Kangasniemi et al., 1983) and equal to placebo in another (Scholz et al., 1987). We believe that the short-acting NSAIDs such as ibuprofen and aspirin cause rebound and their use should be limited. The rebound potential of the other NSAIDs is uncertain. Indomethacin is the drug of choice for HC, and the response to this medication defines the disorder. We give indomethacin a therapeutic trial to rule out HC, but otherwise limit the use of NSAIDs.

Although monotherapy is preferred, it is sometimes necessary to combine preventive medications. Antidepressants are often used with beta-blockers or calcium channel blockers and divalproex sodium may be used in combination with any of these medications.

Other treatments

Open and small placebo-controlled trials have suggested that CTTH may improve following injection with botulinum toxin A (Botox® (BTX-A)); whether this is due to paralysis of muscles or to unknown mechanisms is uncertain. Botulinum toxin has been shown to be effective in decreasing the frequency of migraine attacks (Gobel et al., 1999).

Porta et al. (1999), in a randomized, single-blind trial, compared BTX-A to methylprednisolone. Injections were given in the tender points of cranial muscles, which were determined using pressure pain threshold measurements with an electronic algometer. Inclusion criteria included a diagnosis of IHS ETTH or CTTH, age between 18 and 70 years, and no preventive treatment. At 30 and 60 days postinjection, both treatment groups had a significant reduction in pain scores (using a visual analogue scale) compared with baseline. At 60 days postinjection, the reduction in pain scores was statistically significantly greater in BTX-A-treated patients compared with those who received steroid.

Smuts et al. (1999) conducted a double-blind, placebo-controlled, randomized study of 40 CTTH patients (29 women, 11 men) who had previously been unsuccessfully treated with either amitriptyline or sodium valproate. Patients received intramuscular injections of either BTX-A (100U in 2 ml saline) or placebo (2 ml saline) at predefined areas in the neck and temporal muscles. The number of headache-free days was significantly increased in the BTX-A group 3 months following treatment compared with controls. A clear shift toward the lower headache score counts for the BTX-A group was retained throughout the study period. A statistically significant reduction in the average pain score was achieved for the BTX-A group compared with the placebo group over the 3-month period. No serious adverse events were reported.

In a double-blind trial, Gobel et al. (1999) treated ten CTTH patients with either 10 i.u. Botox® injected into the frontal muscle and the auricular muscle on each side and 20 i.u. injected into the splenius capitis muscle on each side, or the corresponding quantity of NaCl as placebo. No significant change in headache intensity, headache hours per day, or frequency of analgesic intake was observed between the treatment groups. Relja and Korsic (1999) reported a significant and rather long-lasting decrease in headache intensity in 16 CTTH patients in a double-blind, placebo-controlled study. Botox® and/or placebo (saline) were injected into the most tender pericranial muscle. Botulinum toxin A treatment resulted in a significant decrease of the total tenderness score, obtained by the palpation method, two weeks, four weeks, and eight weeks after injections. Placebo had no effect. According to patients' diaries, the severity and the duration of the attacks decreased significantly during the BTX-A treatment period (Relja & Korsic, 1999).

Outpatient treatment of medication overuse

Two general outpatient strategies are employed. One approach is to taper the overused medication, gradually substituting a long-acting NSAID as effective preventive therapy is established. The alternative strategy is to abruptly discontinue the overused drug, substitute a transitional medication to replace the overused drug, and subsequently taper the transitional drug. Drugs used for this purpose include NSAIDs, DHE, corticosteroids and triptans (Diener et al., 1991; Bonuccelli et al., 1996; Drucker & Tepper, 1998). Serious withdrawal syndromes that can be produced by the overused drug must be prevented. For example, if high doses of a butalbital-containing analgesic combination are abruptly discontinued, phenobarbital should be used to prevent barbiturate withdrawal syndrome. Similarly, benzodiazepines must be gradually tapered. Outpatient treatment is preferred for motivated patients, but is not always safe or effective.

Patients who do not need hospital-level care but cannot be safely or adequately treated as outpatients can be considered for ambulatory infusion treatment. Outpatient ambulatory infusion must be done in a hospital or a supervised medical setting where the patient can be monitored frequently (as often as every 15 minutes). Under these circumstances, repetitive i.v. treatment can be given twice a day for several days in a row. Although ambulatory infusion is better for many patients than outpatient treatment, major concerns still exist. Contraindications to outpatient ambulatory infusion include the likelihood of withdrawal symptoms at night when patients are withdrawn from long-acting or potent drugs; psychiatric disorders that interfere with treatment (these patients cannot be treated aggressively as outpatients); and comorbid medical illness that requires prolonged monitoring. No long-term observation is available, and many problems manifest themselves in an intensely monitored interactive environment.

Inpatient treatment of medication overuse

If outpatient treatment fails or is not safe, or if there is significant medical or psychiatric comorbidity present, inpatient treatment may be needed (Silberstein & Saper, 1993). The goals of inpatient headache treatment include: (i) medication withdrawal and rehydration; (ii) pain control with parenteral therapy; (iii) establishment of effective preventive treatment; (iv) interruption of the pain cycle; (v) patient education; and (vi) establishment of outpatient methods of pain control. The detoxification process can be enhanced and shortened and the patient's symptoms made more tolerable by the use of repetitive i.v. DHE coadministered with metoclopramide (Raskin, 1986), which helps control nausea and is an effective antimigraine drug in its own right. Following 10 mg of IV metoclopramide, 0.5 mg of DEH is administered i.v. Subsequent doses are adjusted based on pain relief and side effects. Patients who are not candidates for DHE or do not respond to this medication can be given repetitive i.v. neuroleptics, such as chlorpromazine, droperidol, and prochlorperazine, and/or corticosteroids. These agents may also supplement repetitive i.v. DHE in refractory patients (Silberstein et al., 1990). Hospitalization is also used as a time for patient education, for introducing behavioural methods of pain control, and for adjusting an outpatient programme of preventive and acute therapy.

Silberstein et al. (1990) showed that repetitive i.v. DHE is a safe and effective means of rapidly controlling intractable headache. Of 214 patients suffering from daily headache with rebound, 92% became headache free, usually within 2 to 3 days, with an average hospital stay of 7.3 days. With more aggressive treatment, the average length of stay is now 3 days. Pringsheim and Howse (1998) reported similar but less robust results.

Prognosis

The 'natural history' of primary CDH, and rebound headache in particular, has never been studied and probably never will be for ethical and technical reasons. Recognition of the rebound process probably is itself therapeutic and could affect the patient's behaviour or the physician's approach. Retrospective analysis suggests that there may be periods of stable drug consumption and periods of accelerated medication use. Patients who are treated aggressively generally improve. There are no literature reports of spontaneous improvement of rebound headache, although this may happen. Silberstein and Silberstein (1992) performed follow-up evaluations on 50 hospitalized primary CDH drug overuse patients who were treated with repetitive i.v. DHE and became headache free. Once detoxified, treated and discharged, most patients did not resume daily analgesic or ergotamine use. Seventy-two per cent continued to show significant improvement at 3 months, and 87% continued to show significant improvement after 2 years. This would suggest at least a 70% improvement at 2 years in the initial group (35/50), allowing for patients lost to follow-up.

Silberstein and Silberstein (1992) reported a 2-year success rate of 87%, consistent with other reports. In a series of 22 papers (Hering & Steiner, 1991; Andersson, 1975, 1988; Tfelt-Hansen & Krabbe, 1981; Schoenen et al., 1989; Isler, 1982; Dichgans et al., 1984; Granella et al., 1998; Baumgartner et al., 1989; Mathew, 1990; Mathew et al., 1990; Rapoport et al., 1986; Lake et al., 1990; Henry et al., 1984; Diener et al., 1988, 1989, 1992; Silberstein & Silberstein, 1992; Pini et al., 1996; Schnider et al., 1996; Pringsheim & Howse, 1998; Monzon & Lainez, 1998; Suhr et al., 1999) published between 1975 and 1991, the success rate of withdrawal therapy (often accompanied by pharmacologic and/or behavioural intervention) in patients overusing analgesics, ergotamine, or both, ranged from 48% to 91%; success rates of 77% or higher were reported in ten papers (45%).

Why treatment fails (Table 64.8)

When patients fail to respond to therapy or announce at the first consultation that they have already tried everything and nothing will work, it is important to try to identify the reason or reasons that treatment has failed. The

Table 64.8. Why treatment fails

The diagnosis is incomplete or incorrect
An undiagnosed secondary headache disorder is present
A primary headache disorder is misdiagnosed
Two or more different headache disorders are present

Important exacerbating factors may have been missed
Medication overuse (including over-the-counter)
Caffeine overuse
Dietary or lifestyle triggers
Hormonal triggers
Psychosocial factors
Other medications that trigger headaches

Pharmacotherapy has been inadequate
Ineffective drug
Excessive initial doses
Inadequate final doses
Inadequate duration of treatment

Other factors
Unrealistic expectations
Comorbid conditions complicate therapy
Inpatient treatment required

Source: Modified from Lipton et al. (2000).

cause of treatment failure may be an incomplete or incorrect diagnosis (Lipton et al., 2000). For example: (i) an undiagnosed secondary headache disorder is the major source of the head pain; (ii) a primary headache disorder has been misdiagnosed (i.e. HC is mistaken for TM, episodic paroxysmal hemicrania or hypnic headache is mistaken for cluster); or (iii) two or more different headache disorders are present. In addition, pharmacotherapy may have been inadequate or important exacerbating factors such as medication overuse may have been missed.

References

Andersson, P.G. (1975). Ergotamine headache. *Headache*, **15**, 118–21.

Andersson, P.G. (1988). Ergotism: the clinical picture. In *Drug Induced Headache*, ed. H.C. Diener & M.S. Wilkinson, pp. 16–19. Berlin: Springer.

Anthony, M. & Rasmussen, B.K. (1993). Migraine without aura. In *The Headaches*, ed. J. Olesen, P. Tfelt-Hansen, & M.A. Welch, pp. 255–61. New York: Raven Press.

Antonaci, F. (1991). The sweating pattern in hemicrania continua. A comparison with chronic paroxysmal hemicrania. *Funct. Neurol.*, **6**, 371–5.

Antonaci, F. (1994). Chronic paroxysmal hemicrania and hemicrania continua: orbital phlebography and MRI studies. *Headache*, **34**, 32–4.

Antonaci, F., Sand, T. & Sjaastad, O. (1992). Hemicrania continua and chronic paroxysmal hemicrania: a comparison of pupillometric findings. *Funct. Neurol.*, **7**, 385–9.

Antonaci, F., Sandrini, G., Danilov, A. & Sand, T. (1994). Neurophysiological studies in chronic paroxysmal hemicrania and hemicrania continua. *Headache*, **34**, 479–83.

Ashina, M., Bendtsen, L., Jensen, R., Lassen, L.H., Sakai, F., Sakai & Olesen, J. (1999). Possible mechanisms of action of nitric oxide synthase inhibitors in chronic tension-type headache. *Brain*, **122**, 1629–35.

Ashina, M., Bendtsen, L., Jense, R., Schifter, S., Jansen-Olesen, I. & Olesen, J. (2000). Plasma levels of calcitonin gene-related peptide in chronic tension-type headache. *Cephalalgia*, **20**, 92 (Abstract).

Baumgartner, C., Wessly, P., Bingol, C. et al. (1989). Long-term prognosis of analgesic withdrawal in patients with drug-induced headaches. *Headache*, **29**, 510–14.

Bendtsen, L., Jensen, R., Brennum, J., Arendt-Nielsen, L. & Olesen, J. (1996a). Exteroceptive suppression of temporal muscle activity is normal in patients with chronic tension-type headache and not related to actual headache state. *Cephalalgia*, **16**, 251–6.

Bendtsen, L., Jensen, R. & Olesen, J. (1996b). Qualitatively altered nociception in chronic myofascial pain. *Pain*, **65**, 259–64.

Bonuccelli, U., Nuti, A., Lucetti, C., Pavese, N., Dellagnello, G. & Muratorio, A. (1996). Amitriptyline and dexamethasone combined treatment in drug-induced headache. *Cephalalgia*, **16**, 197–200.

Bordini, C., Antonaci, F., Stovner, L.J., Schrader, H. & Sjaastad, O. (1991). 'Hemicrania Continua' – a clinical review. *Headache*, **31**, 20–6.

Bovim, G., Jenssen, G. & Ericson, K. (1992). Orbital phlebography: a comparison between cluster headache and other headaches. *Headache*, **32**, 408–12.

Breslau, N. & Davis, G.C. (1993). Migraine, physical health and psychiatric disorders: a prospective epidemiologic study of young adults. *J. Psychiat. Res.* **27**, 211–21.

Bright, R.A. & Everitt, D.E. (1992). Beta-blockers and depression: evidence against association. *J. Am. Med. Assoc.*, **267**, 1783.

Burstein, R., Yamamura, H., Malick, A. & Strassman, A.M. (1998). Chemical stimulation of the intracranial dura induces enhanced responses to facial stimulation in brainstem trigeminal neurons. *J. Neurophysiol.*, **79**, 964–82.

Bussone, G., Sandrini, G., Patruno, G., Ruiz, L., Tasorelli, C. & Nappi, G. (1991). Effectiveness of fluoxetine on pain and depression in chronic headache disorders. In *Headache and Depression: Serotonin Pathways as a Common Clue*, ed. G. Nappi, G. Bono, G. Sandrini, E. Martignoni, & G. Micieli, pp. 265–72. New York: Raven Press.

Castillo, J., Munoz, P., Guitera, V. & Pascual, J. (1999). Epidemiology of chronic daily headache in the general population. *Headache*, **39**, 190–6.

Catarci, T., Fiacco, F. & Argentino, C. (1994). Ergotamine-induced headache can be sustained by sumatriptan daily intake. *Cephalalgia*, **14**, 374–5.

Cerbo, R., Barbanti, P., Fabbrini, G., Pascali, M.P. & Catarci, T. (1998). Amitriptyline is effective in chronic but not in episodic tension-type headache: pathogenic implications. *Headache*, **38**, 453–57.

Couch, J.R., Ziegler, D.K. & Hassainein, R. (1976). Amitriptyline in the prophylaxis of migraine. *Arch. Neurol.,* **26**, 121–7.

Curioso, E.P., Young, W.B., Shechter, A.L. & Kaiser, R.S. (1999). Psychiatric comorbidity predicts outcome in chronic daily headache patients. *Neurology*, **52**, A471 (Abstract).

Diamond, S. & Baltes, B. (1971). Chronic tension headache treated with amitriptyline: a double blind study. *Headache*, **11**, 110–16.

Diamond, S. & Dalessio, D.J. (1982). Drug abuse in headache. In *The Practicing Physician's Approach to Headache*, ed. S. Diamond & D.J. Dalessio, pp. 114–21. Baltimore: Williams & Wilkins.

Dichgans, J., Diener, H.D., Gerber, W.D. et al. (1984). Analgetika-induzierter dauerkopfschmerz. *Dtsch. Med. Wschr.,* **109**, 369.

Diener, H.C., Dichgans, J., Scholz, E., Geiselhart, S., Gerber, W.D. & Billie, A. (1984). Analgesic-induced chronic headache: long-term results of withdrawal therapy. *J. Neurol.,* **236**, 9–14.

Diener, H.C., Gerber, W.D. & Geiselhart, S. (1988). Short and long-term effects of withdrawal therapy in drug-induced headache. In *Drug-induced Headache*, ed. H.C. Diener & M. Wilkinson, pp. 133–142. Berlin: Springer-Verlag.

Diener, H.C., Dichgans, J., Scholz, E., Geiselhart, S., Gerber, W.D. & Billie, A. (1989). Analgesic-induced chronic headache: long-term results of withdrawal therapy. *J. Neurol.,* **236**, 9–14.

Diener, H.C., Haab, J. Peters, C., Ried, S., Dichgans, J. & Pilgrim, A. (1991). Subcutaneous sumatriptan in the treatment of headache during withdrawal from drug-induced headache. *Headache*, **31**, 205–9.

Diener, H.C., Pfaffenrath, V., Soyka, D. & Gerber, W.D. (1992). Therapie des medikamenten-induzierten dauerkopfschmerzes. *Münch Med. Wschr.,* **134**, 159–62.

Diener, H.C. & Tfelt-Hansen, P. (1993). Headache associated with chronic use of substances. In *The Headaches*, ed. J. Olesen, P. Tfelt-Hansen & K.M.A. Welch, pp. 721–7. New York: Raven press Ltd.

Drucker, P. & Tepper, S. (1998). Daily sumatriptan for detoxification from rebound. *Headache*, **38**, 687–90.

Edelman, G.M. & Gally, J.A. (1992). Nitric oxide: linking space and time in the brain. *Proc. Natl Acad. Sci. USA,* **89**, 11651–2.

Edwards, K., Santarcangelo, V., Shea, P. & Edwards, J. (1999). Intravenous valproate for acute treatment of migraine headaches. *Cephalalgia*, **19**, 356 (Abstract).

Espada, F., Morales-Asín, F., Escalza, I., Navas, I., Iñiguez, C. & Mauri, J.A. (1999). Hemicrania continua: nine new cases. *Cephalalgia*, **19**, 442 (Abstract).

Fields, H.L., Heinricher, M.M. & Mason, P. (1991). Neurotransmitters as nociceptive modulatory circuits. *Ann. Rev. Neurosci.,* **219**–45.

Foster, C.A. & Bafaloukos, J. (1994). Paroxetine in the treatment of chronic daily headache. *Headache*, **34**, 587–9.

Gaist, D., Hallas, J. Sindrup, S.H. & Gram, L.F. (1996). Is overuse of

sumatriptan a problem? A population-based study. *Eur. J. Clin. Pharmacol.,* **50**, 161–5.

Goadsby, P.J. & Lipton, R.B. (1997). A review of paroxysmal hemicranias, SUNCT syndrome and other short-lasting headaches with autonomic features, including new cases. *Brain*, **120**, 193–209.

Gobel, H., Hamouz, V., Hansen, C. et al. (1994). Chronic tension-type headache: amitriptyline reduces clinical headache-duration and experimental pain sensitivity but does not alter pericranial muscle activity readings. *Pain*, **59**, 241–9.

Gobel, H., Lindner, V., Krack, P., Heinze, A., Gaartz, N. & Deuschl, G. (1999). Treatment of chronic tension-type headache with botulinum toxin. *Cephalalgia*, **19**, 455 (Abstract).

Granella, F., Cavallini, A., Sandrini, G., Manzoni, G.C. & Nappi, G. (1998). Long-term outcome of migraine. *Cephalalgia*, **18**, 30–3.

Guitera, V., Munoz, P., Castillo, J. & Pascual, J. (1999). Transformed migraine: a proposal for the modification of its diagnostic criteria based on recent epidemiological data. *Cephalalgia*, **19**, 847–50.

Henry, P., Dartigues, J.F., Benetier, M.P. et al. (1984). Ergotamine- and analgesic-induced headache. 197.

Hering, R. & Kuritzky, A. (1998). Sodium valproate in the prophylactic treatment of migraine: a double-blind study versus placebo. *Cephalalgia*, **12**, 81–4.

Hering, R. & Steiner, T.J. (1991). Abrupt outpatient withdrawal from medication in analgesic-abusing migraineurs. *Lancet*, **337**, 1442–3.

Holland, J., Holland, C. & Kudrow, L. (1983). Proceedings of the first international headache congress.

Holroyd, K.A., Nash, J.M. & Pingel, J.D. (1991). A comparison of pharmacologic (amitriptyline HCl) and nonpharmacologic (cognitive-behavioral) therapies for chronic tension headaches. *J. Cons. Clin. Psychol.,* **59**, 387–93.

Iordanidis, T. & Sjaastad, O. (1989). Hemicrania continua: a case report. *Cephalalgia*, **9**, 301–3.

Isler, H. (1982). Migraine treatment as a cause of chronic migraine. In *Advances in Migraine Research and Therapy*, ed. F.C. Rose, pp. 159–64. New York: Raven Press.

Jensen, R. & Olesen, J. (1996). Initiating mechanisms of experimentally induced tension-type headache. *Cephalalgia*, **16**, 175–82.

Jensen, R., Brinck, T. & Olesen, J. (1994). Sodium valproate has a prophylactic effect in migraine without aura. *Neurology*, **44**, 647–51.

Johnson, E.S. & Tfelt-Hansen, P. (1993). Nonsteroidal antiinflammatory drugs. In *The Headaches*, ed. J. Olesen, P. Tfelt-Hansen & K.M.A. Welch, pp. 391–5. New York: Raven Press.

Kaiser, R.S. (1999). Substance abuse and headache. 41st Annual Scientific Meeting, Boston, MA.

Kangasniemi, P.J., Nyrke, T., Lang, A.H. & Petersen, E. (1983). Femoxetine – a new 5HT uptake inhibitor – and propranolol in the prophylactic treatment of migraine. *Acta Neurol. Scand.,* **68**, 262–7.

Katsarava, Z., Limmroth, V., Fritsche, G. & Diener, H.C. (1999). Drug-induced headache following the use of zolmitriptan or naratriptan. *Cephalalgia*, **19**, 414 (Abstract).

Klapper, J. (1995). Divalproex sodium in the prophylactic treatment of migraine. *Headache*, **35**, 290 (Abstract).

Kudrow, L. (1982). Paradoxical effects of frequent analgesic use. *Adv. Neurol.*, **33**, 335–41.

Lake, A., Saper, J., Madden, S. & Kreeger, C. (1990). Inpatient treatment for chronic daily headache: a prospective long-term outcome. *Headache*, **30**, 299–300. (Abstract).

Lake, A.E., Saper, J.R., Madden, S.F. & Kreeger, C. (1993). Comprehensive inpatient treatment for intractable migraine: a prospective long-term outcome study. *Headache*, 55–62.

Lance, J.W. & Curran, D.A. (1964). Treatment of chronic tension headache. *Lancet*, **i**, 1236–9.

Langemark, M. & Olesen, J. (1994). Sulpiride and paroxetine in the treatment of chronic tension-type headache. *Headache*, **34**, 20–4.

Lassen, L.H., Ashina, M., Christiansen, I., Ulrich, V. & Olesen, J. (1997). Nitric oxide synthase inhibition in migraine. *Lancet*, **349**, 401–2.

Lipchik, G.L., Holroyd, K.A., France, C.R. et al. (1996). Central and peripheral mechanisms in chronic tension-type headache. *Pain*, **64**, 475

Lipchik, G.L., Holroyd, K.A., Talbot, F. & Greer, M. (1997). Pericranial muscle tenderness and exteroceptive suppression of temporalis muscle activity: a blind study of chronic tension-type headache. *Headache*, **37**, 368–76.

Lipton, R.B., Silberstein, S.D., Saper, J. & Goadsby, P.J. (2000). Why headache treatment fails. in press.

Makashima, K. & Takahashi, K. (1991). Exteroceptive suppression of the masseter, temporalis and trapezius muscles produced by mental nerve stimulation in patients with chronic headaches. *Cephalalgia*, **11**, 23–8.

Manna, V., Bolino, F. & DiCicco, L. (1994). Chronic tension-type headache, mood depression and serotonin. *Headache*, **34**, 44–9.

Mathew, N.T. (1981). Prophylaxis of migraine and mixed headache. A randomized controlled study. *Headache*, **21**, 105–9.

Mathew, N.T. (1982). Transformed migraine. *Cephalalgia*, **13**, 78–83.

Mathew, N.T. (1987). Transformed or evolutional migraine. *Headache*, **27**, 305–6.

Mathew, N.T. (1990). Drug induced headache. *Neurol. Clin.*, **8**, 903–12.

Mathew, N.T. (1991). Chronic daily headache: clinical features and natural history. In *Headache and Depression: Serotonin Pathways as a Common Clue*, ed. G. Nappi, G. Bono, G. Sandrini, E. Martignoni & G. Micieli, pp. 49–58. New York: Raven Press.

Mathew, N.T. (1993). Transformed migraine. *Cephalalgia*, **13**, 78–83.

Mathew, N.T. & Ali, S. (1991). Valproate in the treatment of persistent chronic daily headache. An open label study. *Headache*, **31**, 71–4.

Mathew, N.T., Stubits, E. & Nigam, M.R. (1982). Transformation of migraine into daily headache: analysis of factors. *Headache*, **22**, 66–8.

Mathew, N.T., Reuveni, U. & Perez, F. (1987). Transformed or evolutive migraine. *Headache*, **27**, 102–6.

Mathew, N.T., Kurman, R. & Perez, F. (1990). Drug induced refractory headache – clinical features and management. *Headache*, **30**, 634–8.

Mathew, N.T., Saper, J.R. Silberstein, S.D. et al. (1995). Migraine prophylaxis with divalproex. *Arch. Neurol.*, **52**, 281–6.

Merikangas, K.R., Angst, J. & Isler, H. (1990). Migraine and psychopathology: results of the Zurich cohort study of young adults. *Arch. Gen. Psychiatry*, **47**, 849–53.

Micieli, G., Manzoni, G.C., Granella, F., Martignoni, E., Malferrari, G. & Nappi, G. (1988). Clinical and epidemiological observations on drug abuse in headache patients. In *Drug-Induced Headache*, ed. H.C. Diener & M. Wilkinson, pp. 20–8. Berlin: Springer-Verlag.

Miller, D.S., Talbot, C.A., Simpson, W. & Korey, A. (1987). A comparison of naproxen sodium, acetaminophen and placebo in the treatment of muscle contraction headache. *Headache*, **27**, 392–6.

Mitsikostas, D.D. & Thomas, A.M. (1999). Comorbidity of headache and depressive disorders. *Cephalalgia*, **19**, 211–17.

Mitsikostas, D.D., Gatzonis, S., Thomas, A. & Ilias, A. (1997). Buspirone vs amitriptyline in the treatment of chronic tension-type headache. *J. Neurol. Scand.*, **96**, 247–51.

Monzon, M.J. & Lainez, M.J. (1998). Quality of life in migraine and chronic daily headache patients. *Cephalalgia*, **18**, 638–43.

Morland, T.J., Storli, O.V. & Mogstad, T.E. (1979). Doxepin in the prophylactic treatment of mixed 'vascular' and tension headache. *Headache*, **19**, 382–3.

Mylecharane, E.J. & Tfelt-Hansen, P. (1993). Miscellaneous drugs. In *The Headaches*, ed. J. Olesen, P. Tfelt-Hansen & K.M.A. Welch, pp. 397–402. New York: Raven Press.

Nakashima, K. & Takahashi, K. (1991). Exteroceptive suppression of the masseter, temporalis and trapezius muscles produced by mental nerve stimulation in patients with chronic headaches. *Cephalalgia*, **11**, 23–8.

Newman, L.C., Lipton, R.B. & Solomon, S. (1993). Hemicrania continua: 7 new cases and a literature review. *Headache*, **32**, 267

Olesen, J., Tfelt-Hansen, P. & Welch, K.M.A. (1993). *The Headaches*, New York: Raven Press.

Ottman, R. & Lipton, R.B. (1994). Comorbidity of migraine and epilepsy. *Neurology*, **44**, 2105–10.

Palmer, K.J. & Benfield, P. (1994). Fluvoxamine: an overview of its pharmacologic properties and a review of its use in nondepressive disorders. *CNS Drugs*, 1, 57–87.

Pareja, J.A., Palomo, T., Gorriti, M.A., Pareja, J. & Espejo, J. (1990). Hemicrania episodica – a new type of headache or pre-chronic stage of hemicrania continua. *Headache*, **30**, 344–6.

Paulus, W., Raubuchl, O., Schoenen, J. & Straube, A. (1992). Exteroceptive suppression of temporalis muscle activity in various types of headache. *Headache*, **32**, 41–4.

Pfaffenrath, V., Kellhammer, U. & Pollmann, W. (1986). Combination headache: practical experience with a combination of beta-blocker and an antidepressive. *Cephalalgia*, **6**, 25–32.

Pfaffenrath, V., Diener, H.C., Isler, H. et al. (1994). Efficacy and tolerability of amitriptylinoxide in the treatment of chronic tension-type headache: a multicentre controlled study. *Cephalalgia*, **14**, 149–55.

Pini, L.A., Bigarelli, M., Vitale, G. & Sternieri, E. (1996). Headaches associated with chronic use of analgesics: a therapeutic approach. *Headache*, **36**, 433–9.

Pluvinage, R. (1994). Le traitement des migraines et des cephalees psychogenes par l'amitriptyline. *Sem. Hop. Paris*, **54**, 713–16.

Porta, M., Loiero, M. & Gamba, M. (1999). Treatment of tension-type headache by botulinum toxin in pericranial muscles. *Cephalalgia*, 19, 453–4. (Abstract).

Post, R.M. & Silberstein, S.D. (1994). Shared mechanisms in affective illness, epilepsy, and migraine. *Neurology*, **44**, s37–47.

Potter, D.L., Hart, D.E., Calder, C.S. & Storey, J.R. (2000). A double-blind, randomized, placebo-controlled, parallel study to determine the efficacy of Topamax® (topiramate) in the prophylactic treatment of migraine. *Neurology* (in press).

Pringsheim, T. & Howse, D. (1998). Inpatient treatment of chronic daily headache using dihydroergotamine: a long-term followup study. *Can. J. Neurol. Sci.*, **25**, 146–50.

Pritchard, D.W. (1989). EWG cranial muscle levels in headache sufferers before and during headache. *Headache*, **29**, 103–8.

Rapoport, A.M. (1988). Analgesic rebound headache. *Headache*, **28**, 662–5.

Rapoport, A.M., Weeks, R.E., Sheftell, F.D. Baskin, S.M. & Verdi, J. (1986). The 'analgesic washout period': a critical variable evaluation in the evaluation of headache treatment efficacy. *Neurology*, **36**, 100–1.

Raskin, N.H. (1986). Repetitive intravenous dihydroergotamine as therapy for intractable migraine. *Neurology*, **36**, 995–7.

Rasmussen, B.K. (1992). Migraine and tension-type headache in a general population: psychosocial factors. *Int. J. Epidemiol.*, **21**, 1138–43.

Rasmussen, B.K. (1995). Epidemiology of headache. *Cephalalgia*, **15**, 45–68.

Rasmussen, B.K., Jensen, R. & Olesen, J. (1989). Impact of headache on sickness absence and utilization of medical services. *J. Epidemiol. Commun. Health*, **46**, 443–6.

Ravishankar, K. (1997). Headache pattern in India: a headache clinic analysis of 1000 patients. *Cephalalgia*, **17**, 143–4.

Relja, M.A. & Korsic, M. (1999). Treatment of tension-type headache by injections of botulinum toxin type A: double-blind placebo-controlled study. *Neurology*, **52**, a203 (Abstract).

Russell, M.B., Stergaard, S., Endtsen, L. & Olesen, J. (1999). Familial occurrence of chronic tension-type headache. *Cephalalgia*, **19**, 207–10.

Saper, J.R. (1983). *Headache Disorders: Current Concepts in Treatment Strategies*, Littleton: Wright-PSG.

Saper, J.R. (1987a). Ergotamine dependence. *Headache*, **27**, 435–8.

Saper, J.R. (1987b). Ergotamine dependency – a review. *Headache*, **27**, 435–8.

Saper, J.R. (1989). Chronic headache syndromes. *Neurol. Clin.*, **7**, 387–412.

Saper, J.R. & Jones, J.M. (1986). Ergotamine tartrate dependency: features and possible mechanisms. *Clin. Neuropharmacol.*, **9**, 244–56.

Saper, J.R., Silberstein, S.D. Lake, A.E. & Winters, M.E. (1994).

Double-blind trial of fluoxetine: Chronic daily headache and migraine. *Headache*, **34**, 497–502.

Schepelmann, K., Dannhausen, M., Kotter, I., Schabet, M. & Dichgans, J. (1998). Exteroceptive suppression of temporalis muscle activity in patients with fibromyalgia, tension-type headache, and normal controls. *Electroencephalog. Clin. Neurophysiol.*, **107**, 196–9.

Scher, A.I., Stewart, W.F., Liberman, J. & Lipton, R.B. (1998). Prevalence of frequent headache in a population sample. *Headache*, **38**, 497–506.

Schnider, P., Aull, S., Baumgartner, C. et al. (1996). Long-term outcome of patients with headache and drug abuse after inpatient withdrawal: five-year followup. *Cephalalgia*, **16**, 481–5.

Schoenen, J., Jamart, B., Gerard, P., Lenarduzzi, P. & Delwaide, P.J. (1987). Exteroceptive suppression of temporalis muscle activity in chronic headache. *Neurology*, **37**, 1834–6.

Schoenen, J., Lenarduzzi, P. & Sianard-Gainko, J. (1989). Chronic headaches associated with analgesics and/or ergotamine abuse: a clinical survey of 434 consecutive outpatients. In *New advances in headache research*, ed. F.D. Rose, pp. 29–43. London: Smith-Gordon.

Schoenen, J., Bottin, D., Hardy, F. & Gerard, P. (1991). Cephalic and extracephalic pressure pain threshold in chronic tension-type headache. *Pain*, **47**, 145–9.

Scholz, E., Gerber, W.D., Diener, H.C. & Langohr, H.D. (1987). Dihydroergotamine vs. flunarizine vs. nifedipine vs. metoprolol vs. propranolol in migraine prophylaxis: a comparative study based on time series analysis. In *Advances in Headache Research*, ed. E. Scholz, W.D. Gerber, H.C. Diener & H.D. Langohr, pp. 139–45. London: John Libbey & Co.

Shuaib, A., Ahmed, F., Muratoglu, M. & Kochanski, P. (1999). Topiramate in migraine prophylaxis: a pilot study. *Cephalalgia*, **19**, 379–80. (Abstract).

Silberstein, S.D. (1984). Treatment of headache in primary care practice. *Am. J. Med.*, **77**, 65–72.

Silberstein, S.D. (1993). Chronic daily headache and tension-type headache. *Neurology*, **43**, 1644–9.

Silberstein, S.D. & Lipton, R.B. (1994). Overview of diagnosis and treatment of migraine. *Neurology*, **44**, 6–16.

Silberstein, S.D. & Saper, J.R. (1993). Migraine: diagnosis and treatment. In *Wolff's Headache and Other Head Pain*, ed. D.J. Dalessio & S.D. Silberstein, pp. 96–170. New York: Oxford University Press.

Silberstein, S.D. & Silberstein, J.R. (1992). Chronic daily headache: prognosis following inpatient treatment with repetitive IV DHE. *Headache*, **32**, 439–45.

Silberstein, S.D., Schulman, E.A. & Hopkins, M.M. (1990). Repetitive intravenous DHE in the treatment of refractory headache. *Headache*, **30**, 334–9.

Silberstein, S.D., Lipton, R.B., Solomon, S. & Mathew, N.T. (1994). Classification of daily and near daily headaches: proposed revisions to the IHS classification. *Headache*, **34**, 1–7.

Silberstein, S.D., Lipton R.B., & Sliwinski, M. (1995). Assessment for revised criteria of chronic daily headache. *Neurology*, **45**, A394.

Silberstein, S.D., Lipton R.B. & Sliwinski, M. (1996). Classification of daily and near-daily headaches: field trial of revised IHS criteria. *Neurology*, **47**, 871–5.

Silverman, K., Evans, S.M., Strain, E.C. & Griffiths, R.R. (1992). Withdrawal syndrome after the double-blind cessation of caffeine consumption. *N. Engl.. J. Med.*, **327**, 1109–14.

Smuts, J.A., Baker, M.K., Smuts, H.M. Tassen, J.M., Ossouw, E. & Barnard, P.W. (1999). Botulinum toxin type A as prophylactic treatment in chronic tension-type headache. *Cephalalgia*, **19**, 454 (Abstract).

Solomon, S., Lipton, R.B. & Newman, L.C. (1992). Clinical features of chronic daily headache. *Headache*, **32**, 325–9.

Strassman, A.M., Raymond, S.A. & Burstein, R. (1996). Sensitization of meningeal sensory neurons and the origin of headaches. *Nature*, **384**, 560–4.

Suhr, B., Evers, S., Bauer, B., Gralow, I., Grotemeyer, K.H. & Husstedt, I.W. (1999). Drug-induced headache: long-term results of stationary versus ambulatory withdrawal therapy. *Cephalalgia*, **19**, 44–9.

Tekle Haimanot, R., Seraw, B., Forsgren, L., Ekbom, K. & Ekstedt, J. (1995). Migraine, chronic tension-type headache, and cluster headache in an Ethiopian rural community. *Cephalalgia*, **15**, 482–8.

Tfelt-Hansen, P. & Krabbe, A.A. (1981). Ergotamine. Do patients benefit from withdrawal? *Cephalalgia*, **1**, 29–32.

Tfelt-Hansen, P. & Welch, K.M.A. (2000). Prioritizing prophylactic treatment of migraine. In *The Headaches*, ed. J. Olesen, P. Tfelt-Hansen, & K.M.A. Welch, pp. 499–500. Philadelphia: Lippincott Williams & Wilkins.

Vanast, W.J. (1986). New daily persistent headaches: definition of a benign syndrome. *Headache*, **26**, 317.

Verri, A.P., Cecchini, P., Galli, C., Granella, F,. Sandrini, G. & Nappi, G. (1998). Psychiatric comorbidity in chronic daily headache. *Cephalalgia*, **18**, 45–9.

Wang, S.J., Fuh, J.L., Lu, S.R. et al. (2000). Chronic daily headache in Chinese elderly: prevalence, risk factors and biannual follow-up. *Neurology*, **54**, 314–19.

Weiller, C., May, A., Limmroth, V. et al. (1995). Brainstem activation in spontaneous human migraine attacks. *Nat. Med.*, **1**, 658–60.

Wilkinson, M. (1988). Introduction. In *Drug Induced Headache*, ed. H.C. Diener & M. Wilkinson, pp. 1–2. Berlin: Springer-Verlag.

Yamamura, H., Malick, A. et al. (1999). Cardiovascular and neuronal responses to head stimulation reflect central sensitization and cutaneous allodynia in a rat model of migraine. *J. Neurophysiol.*, **81**, 479–93.

Zwart, J.A. & Sand, T. (1995). Exteroceptive suppression of temporalis muscle activity: a blind study of tension-type headache, migraine, and cervicogenic headache. *Headache*, **35**, 338–43.

Index

Note: this is a complete two-volume index

Note: page numbers in *italics* refer to figures and tables; 'Fig.' refers to illustrations in the plates section

Abbreviations of conditions used in subheadings (without explanation):
AD Alzheimer's disease
AIDS Acquired immune deficiency syndrome
ALS Amyotrophic lateral sclerosis
CJD Creutzfeldt–Jakob disease
FTD Frontotemporal dementia
HIV Human immunodeficiency virus
HD Huntington's disease
PD Parkinson's disease
SIADH syndrome of inappropriate secretion of antidiuretic hormone